Brief Contents

P9-DDK-090

CANADIAN CLINICAL NURSING SKILLS + TECHNIQUES

FIRST EDITION

Shelley L. Cobbett, RN, GnT, MN, EdD
Assistant Professor
Dalhousie University School of Nursing
Halifax, Nova Scotia

U.S. Authors

Anne Griffin Perry, RN, MSN, EdD, FAAN
Professor Emerita
School of Nursing
Southern Illinois University—Edwardsville
Edwardsville, Illinois

Patricia A. Potter, RN, MSN, PhD, FAAN
Director of Research
Patient Care Services
Barnes-Jewish Hospital
St. Louis, Missouri

Wendy R. Ostendorf, RN, MS, EdD, CNE
Professor of Nursing
Neumann University
Aston, Pennsylvania

Section Editor for the U.S. 9th Edition

Nancy Laplante, PhD, RN, AHN-BC
Associate Professor of Nursing
School of Nursing
Widener University
Chester, Pennsylvania

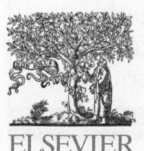

ELSEVIER

CANADIAN CLINICAL NURSING SKILLS & TECHNIQUES, FIRST EDITION   ISBN: 978-1-77172-209-4
Copyright © 2020 Elsevier Inc. All rights reserved.

Adapted from *Clinical Nursing Skills & Techniques*, 9th edition, by Anne Griffin Perry, Patricia A. Potter, and Wendy R. Ostendorf. Copyright © 2018 by Elsevier Inc. Copyright © 2014, 2010, 2006, 2004, 2002, 1998, 1994, 1990, 1986 by Elsevier Inc.

978-0-323-40069-5
(softcover)

Notices

Practitioners and researchers must always rely on their own experience and knowledge in evaluating and using any information, methods, compounds or experiments described herein. Because of rapid advances in the medical sciences, in particular, independent verification of diagnoses and drug dosages should be made. To the fullest extent of the law, no responsibility is assumed by Elsevier, authors, editors or contributors for any injury and/or damage to persons or property as a matter of products liability, negligence or otherwise, or from any use or operation of any methods, products, instructions, or ideas contained in the material herein.

Library of Congress Control Number: 2019941625

VP Education Content: Kevonne Holloway
Content Strategist (Acquisitions): Roberta A. Spinosa-Millman
Director, Content Development Manager: Laurie Gower
Content Development Specialist: Martina van de Velde
Publishing Services Manager: Julie Eddy
Project Manager: Abigail Bradberry
Design Direction: Brian Salisbury

Printed in Canada

Last digit is the print number: 9 8 7 6 5 4 3 2

Working together
to grow libraries in
developing countries

www.elsevier.com • www.bookaid.org

It has been both a pleasure and a privilege to be the editor of the First Canadian Edition of this text, working with expert professional nurses across our country to ensure that the revisions are grounded in our health care system and our Canadian context while balancing jurisdictional differences. I continue to learn from them, as well as the many students who enter my life daily, and I am thankful to be part of such a wonderful profession.

I would like to dedicate this text to my family: my parents, Pat and Bev Gallagher; my husband, Michael, who continues to tell me anything is possible; our sons and their partners, Travis and Megan, Joshua and Annessa; and the youngest members in our family, our grandsons, Jace Michael and Quinn Patrick. Much love to you all!

Shelley L. Cobbett

As always, this book is dedicated to my children. To be their mother brings more joy, honor, and sense of pride than I could have ever imagined. They and their loved ones are truly my shining stars. As they grow, things change, and I now dedicate this book to:

My daughter, Rebecca Lacey Perry Bryan; her husband, Robert Donald Bryan; their three daughters, Cora Elizabeth Bryan, Amalie Mary Bryan, and Noelle Anne Bryan; and their son, Shepherd Charles Bryan; And to my son, Mitch Perry-Cox; and his husband, Samuel Perry-Cox.

Anne Griffin Perry

I wish to dedicate this new edition of our textbook to the exceptional professional nurses at Barnes-Jewish Hospital. It has been my privilege to have worked with so many talented people. They continue to inspire me each day.

Patricia A. Potter

For Toba and Harris, who never saw this achievement but would be proud of its influence on today's and tomorrow's nurses. And, as always, for my always supportive and patient husband.

Wendy R. Ostendorf

About the Authors

SHELLEY L. COBBETT, RN, GNT, MN, EdD

Dr. Shelley Cobbett received her Post-RN BN and her MN from Dalhousie University and her EdD from Charles Sturt University. Her clinical practice background is maternal-child nursing and she has been a nurse educator for over 30 years. Her main research area during the last 15 years has focused on the Scholarship of Learning and Teaching, with over 50 peer-reviewed publications, invited speaker engagements, and oral conference presentations. Dr. Cobbett is the President-Elect for the Atlantic Region Canadian Association of Schools of Nursing and is on the Education Advisory Committee for the College of Registered Nurses of Nova Scotia.

Her commitment to the implementation and evaluation of best pedagogical practices within nursing education was recently recognized, as she was the recipient of a Dalhousie University Teaching Award in 2014, and the Canadian Association of Schools of Nursing Excellence in Teaching Award in 2017. She is currently an Assistant Professor at Dalhousie University School of Nursing, Arctic College BScN Coordinator, and Curriculum Implementation and Evaluation Lead for a new, innovative BScN degree that was initiated in 2016.

ANNE GRIFFIN PERRY, RN, MSN, EdD, FAAN

Dr. Anne G. Perry, Professor Emerita at Southern Illinois University—Edwardsville, is a Fellow in the American Academy of Nursing. She received her BSN from the University of Michigan, her MSN from Saint Louis University, and her EdD from Southern Illinois University—Edwardsville. Dr. Perry is a prolific and influential author and speaker. An author for more than 35 years, her work includes four major textbooks (*Essentials for Nursing Practice*, *Fundamentals of Nursing*, *Nursing Interventions & Clinical Skills*, and *Clinical Nursing Skills & Techniques*) and numerous journal articles, abstracts, and nursing research and education grants. She has presented numerous papers at conferences across the United States and internationally. She was one of a few key consultants on *Mosby's Nursing Video Skills* and *Mosby's Nursing Skills Online*.

Dr. Perry is passionate about nursing education and has been involved in education since 1973, first as an instructor and then achieving the rank of Professor and assuming various leadership roles at Saint Louis University School of Nursing. She was a Professor and Associate Dean and Interim Dean at Southern Illinois University—Edwardsville. As a clinician and researcher, Dr. Perry's contributions to pulmonary nursing and nursing language development involve both research and policy making. She has investigated and published findings regarding topics that include weaning from mechanical ventilation, use of the therapeutic intervention scoring system, critical care, and validation of nursing diagnoses.

PATRICIA A. POTTER, RN, MSN, PhD, FAAN

Dr. Patricia Potter received her BSN at the University of Washington in Seattle and her MSN and PhD at Saint Louis University in St. Louis, Missouri. A groundbreaking author for more than 30 years, her work includes four major textbooks (*Essentials for Nursing Practice*, *Fundamentals of Nursing*, *Nursing Interventions & Clinical Skills*, and *Clinical Nursing Skills & Techniques*) and publications in numerous professional journals. She has been an unceasing advocate of evidence-based practice and quality improvement in her roles as administrator, educator and, more recently, director of research.

Dr. Potter has devoted a lifetime to nursing education, practice, and research. She spent a decade teaching at Barnes Hospital School of Nursing and Saint Louis University. She entered into a variety of managerial and administrative roles, ultimately becoming the director of nursing practice at Barnes-Jewish Hospital. In that capacity she sharpened her interest in the development of nursing practice standards and the measurement of patient outcomes in defining nursing practice. Her most recent passion has been in the area of nursing research, specifically cancer family caregiving, the cancer patient symptom experience, fall prevention, and the effects of compassion fatigue on nurses. Recently Dr. Potter has worked with colleagues to develop an inpatient Innovation Unit, which is designed to incorporate current evidence into the selection and development of a unique work team and the creation of a care delivery model and innovative care practices. Dr. Potter is currently a director of research for patient care services at Barnes-Jewish Hospital.

WENDY R. OSTENDORF, RN, MS, EdD, CNE

Dr. Wendy R. Ostendorf received her BSN from Villanova University, her MS from the University of Delaware, and her EdD from the University of Sarasota. She currently serves as a professor of nursing in the Division of Nursing and Health Sciences at Neumann University in Aston, Pennsylvania. She has contributed more than 30 chapters to multiple nursing textbooks and has served as author for two major textbooks: *Nursing Interventions & Clinical Skills* and *Clinical Nursing Skills & Techniques*. She has presented more than 25 papers at conferences at the local, national, and international levels.

Professionally, Dr. Ostendorf has a diverse background in pediatric and adult critical care. She has taught at the undergraduate and graduate levels for 35 years. With decades of practice as a clinician, her educational experiences have influenced her teaching philosophy and perceptions of the nursing profession. Dr. Ostendorf's current interests include the history and image of nursing as it has been represented in film. Most recently she was a co-primary research investigator on this topic.

Contributors

April Ambalina, RN
Instructor
College of Nursing
University of Manitoba
Winnipeg, MB

Chantal Backman, RN, MHA, PhD
Assistant Professor
School of Nursing
University of Ottawa
Ottawa, ON

Danielle Byrne, RN, MN
Adjunct Lecturer and Clinical Instructor
School of Nursing
Dalhousie University
Yarmouth, NS

Ashley Crane, RN, MN
Instructor
School of Nursing
Memorial University
St. John's, NL

Paula D'Eon, RN, MN-NP
Adjunct Assistant Professor
School of Nursing
Dalhousie University
Yarmouth, NS

Adele deRosenroll, RN
Clinical Resource Nurse, Vascular Access
Island Health
Vancouver, BC

Leslie Graham, RN, MN, CHSE, CNCC
Professor, Nursing
School of Health and Community Studies
Durham College
and
Adjunct Professor
Faculty of Health Sciences
University of Ontario Institute of Technology
Oshawa, ON

Jackie Hartigan-Rogers, RN, MN
Adjunct Assistant Professor
School of Nursing
Dalhousie University
Yarmouth, NS

Giuliana Harvey, RN, MN
Assistant Professor
School of Nursing & Midwifery
Mount Royal University
Calgary, AB

Selena Hebig, BSN, BScKin
Coordinator, Nursing Lab
Department of Health and Human Services
Camosun College (Lansdowne)
Victoria, BC

Christina Hurlock-Chorostecki, NP, MScN, PhD
Professor
Arthur Labatt Family School of Nursing
Western University
London, ON
and
Nurse Practitioner
St. Joseph's Health Care
London, ON

Damilola Funke Iduye, RN, MN
Instructor and Mrs. E.B. Eddy (Bennett) Professor
School of Nursing
Dalhousie University
Halifax, NS

Steve Michael Iduye, RN, MHI
System Analyst
Nova Scotia Health Authority
Halifax, NS

Darlaine Jantzen, RN, RD, MA, PhD
Chair, Baccalaureate of Science Nursing Program
Camosun College (Lansdowne)
Victoria, BC

Rosemary Kohr, RN, MScN, PhD
Corporate Program Lead, Wound/Ostomy/Continence
Saint Elizabeth Health Care
and
Assistant Professor (Clinical Adjunct)
Faculty of Health Sciences
University of Western Ontario
London, ON

Alia Lagace, RN
Instructor
College of Nursing
University of Manitoba
Winnipeg, MB

Nicole Lewis-Power, RN, MN, PhD(c)
Lecturer
School of Nursing
Memorial University
St. John's, NL

Maureen Loft, NP-Adult, MScN, PhD
Nurse Practitioner, CNS
Middlesex Hospital Alliance
Strathroy, ON
and
Adjunct Assistant Professor
School of Nursing
Western University
London, ON

Nancy Logue, RN, MN, PhD
Senior Teaching Associate
Department of Nursing & Health Sciences
University of New Brunswick—Saint John
Saint John, NB

Marian Luctkar-Flude, RN, MScN, PhD
Assistant Professor
School of Nursing
Queen's University
Kingston, ON

Maureen MacInnis-Wheatley, RN, MN
Faculty of Nursing
University of Prince Edward Island
Charlottetown, PEI

Heather MacLean, RN, MN
Assistant Professor
School of Nursing & Midwifery
Mount Royal University
Calgary, AB

Lisa MacNaughton-Doucet, RN, BTHM, MN
Adjunct Assistant Professor
School of Nursing
Dalhousie University
Yarmouth, NS

Joanne Newell, RN, MN
Adjunct Assistant Professor
School of Nursing
Dalhousie University
Yarmouth, NS

Rachel Ollivier, RN, PhD(c)
School of Nursing
Dalhousie University
Halifax, NS

Noelle Ozog, RN, MScN(c)
School of Nursing
Dalhousie University
Halifax, NS

Amanda Parrott, RN, CMSN(c), OHN, CCNE
Instructor
Nursing and Health Science Programs
Nunavut Arctic College (Nunatta Campus)
Iqaluit, NU

Dana Penfound, RN, MACP
Instructor
Nursing and Health Sciences Programs
Nunavut Arctic College (Nunatta Campus)
Iqaluit, NT

Sandra Redmond, RN, MN
Adjunct Assistant Professor
School of Nursing
Dalhousie University
Yarmouth, NS

Holly Richardson, RN, MA, PhD
Assistant Professor
School of Nursing
Dalhousie University
Halifax, NS

Shawna Ryan, RN, COHN, MN
BSN Program Coordinator/BSN Expansion Coordinator
Health, Human and Family Programs
College of the Rockies
Cranbrook, BC

Monakshi Sawhney, RN(EC), NP(Adult), MN, PhD
Assistant Professor
School of Nursing
Queen's University
Kingston, ON
and
Nurse Practitioner, Surgery, Anaesthesia
North York General Hospital
Toronto, ON

Tracy Stephen, RN, MN
Assistant Professor
School of Nursing
Trinity Western University
Langley, BC

Jane Tyerman, RN, MScN, PhD
Professor
Trent/Fleming School of Nursing
Peterborough, ON

Kathryn Weaver, RN, MN, PhD
Professor
Faculty of Nursing
University of New Brunswick
Fredericton, NB

CONTRIBUTORS TO THE U.S. 9ᵀᴴ EDITION

Michelle Aebersold, PhD, RN, CHSE, FAAN
Clinical Associate Professor
Director, Simulation and Educational Innovations
University of Michigan School of Nursing
Ann Arbor, Michigan

Marianne Banas, MSN, RN, CCTN, CWCN
Staff Nurse
University of Chicago Hospitals
Chicago, Illinois

Hope V. Bussenius, DNP, APRN, FNP-BC
Assistant Professor
Nell Hodgson Woodruff School of Nursing
Emory University
Atlanta, Georgia

Janice C. Colwell, RN, MS, CWOCN, FAAN
Advanced Practice Nurse, Ostomy and Wound Care
Department of Surgery
The University of Chicago Medicine
Chicago, Illinois

Jane Fellows, MSN, CWOCN
Wound/Ostomy CNS
Advanced Clinical Practice
Duke University Health System
Durham, North Carolina

Susan Jane Fetzer, BA, BSN, MSN, MBA, PhD
Professor
Department of Nursing
College of Health and Human Services
University of New Hampshire
Durham, New Hampshire

Paula Gray, DNP, CRNP, NP-C
Director, Family (Individual Across the Lifespan) CRNP
    Program
Clinical Assistant Professor of Nursing
Widener University School of Nursing
Chester, Pennsylvania

Stephanie Jeffers, PhD, RN
Assistant Professor
Widener University School of Nursing
Chester, Pennsylvania

Alaine Kamm, BSN, MSN
Nurse Practitioner
General Surgery
The University of Chicago Medicine
Chicago, Illinois

Lori Klingman, MSN, RN
Nurse Educator/Faculty Advisor
Ohio Valley Hospital
McKees Rocks, Pennsylvania

Stephen D. Krau, PhD, CNE
Associate Professor
School of Nursing
Vanderbilt University Medical Center
Nashville, Tennessee

Carol Ann Liebold, RN, BSN, CRNI
President/Owner
CarolAnn Liebold, Inc.
Earlton, New York

Nelda K. Martin, RN, ANP-BC, CCNS
Adult Nurse Practitioner/Clinical Nurse Specialist
Heart and Vascular Center
Barnes-Jewish Hospital at Washington University Medical
    Center
St. Louis, Missouri

**Kristen L. Mauk, PhD, DNP, RN, CRRN, GCNS-BC,
    GNP-BC, ACHPN, FAAN**
Professor of Nursing
Director, RN-BSN and MSN programs
Colorado Christian University;
President, International Rehabilitation Consultants/Senior Care
    Central
Ridgway, Colorado

Angela McConachie, FNP, DNP
Assistant Professor
Faculty
Goldfarb School of Nursing at Barnes-Jewish College
St. Louis, Missouri

**Jennifer Painter, MSN, APRN, CNS, RN-BC, OCN,
    AOCNS**
Staff Education Specialist
Nursing School/Faculty Affiliations Coordinator
Student Nurse Extern Program Coordinator
Nursing Development and Education
Institute for Learning, Leadership, & Development (iLead)
John H. Ammon Education Center
Newark, Delaware

**Ann Petlin, RN, MSN, CCNS, CCRN-CSC,
    ACNS-BC, PCCN**
Clinical Nurse Specialist
Cardiothoracic Surgery
Barnes-Jewish Hospital
St. Louis, Missouri

Theresa Pietsch, PhD, RN, CRRN, CNE
Associate Professor
Neumann University
Aston, Pennsylvania

Diane Rudolphi, MS, RN
Master Instructor
University of Delaware School of Nursing
Newark, Delaware

Jacqueline Raybuck Saleeby, PhD, RN, BCCS
Associate Professor
Catherine McAuley School of Nursing
Maryville University
St. Louis, Missouri

**Felicia Schaps, MSN-Ed, BSN, RN, CRNI, OCN,
    CNSC, IgCN**
Director of Nursing Operations
BioScrip, Inc.
Washington, D.C.

Amy Spencer, MSN, RN-BC
Staff Development Specialist
Christiana Care Health Systems
Newark, Delaware

C.J. Wright-Boon, RN, MSN
Assistant Professor
Saint Francis Medical Center College of Nursing
Peoria, Illinois

Rita Wunderlich, RN, PhD, CNE
Associate Professor
Catherine McAuley School of Nursing
Maryville University
St. Louis, Missouri

Reviewers

Michelle Bayard RN, BscN, MEd(c)
Instructor
Department of Nursing
Vanier College
Montreal, QC

Janine Brown, RN, MSN, PhD(c)
Instructor
Faculty of Nursing
University of Regina
Regina, SK

Alison Cousineau, RN, MN
Professor
School of Nursing
Niagara College
Welland, ON

Joanne Gullison, RN BScN
Instructor
Practical Nurse and Personal Support Worker
New Brunswick Community College—Fredericton
Fredericton, NB

Alexandra Hodson, RN, BSN, MN
Instructor
Faculty of Nursing
University of Regina
Saskatoon, SK

Paula Lynne Littlejohn, CBE, ID, GNC(C), RN, BSN, MA
Instructor
Nursing Department
Camosun College
Victoria, BC

Gail Orr, RN, MA
Instructor
School of Health, Human and Justice Studies
Loyalist College
Belleville, ON

Angela L. Rintoul NP, BScN, MN-ANP
Professor, Coordinator BScN Collaborative Program
Health and Community Studies
Algonquin College/Ottawa University
Pembroke, ON

Monakshi Sawhney, RN(EC), NP(Adult), MN, PhD
Assistant Professor
School of Nursing
Queen's University
Kingston, ON

Laralea Stalkie RN, BNSC, MSN
Professor and Coordinator
School of Baccalaureate Nursing
St. Lawrence College
Kingston, ON

Mary Switzer, BScN
Academic Program Technologist
Health, Wellness and Sciences
Georgian College
Barrie, ON

Elizabeth Ubaldi, RN, BA, MN, CCNE
Professor
Health Sciences
Sault College
Sault Ste. Marie, ON

Jess White, RN, ENC(C)
Instructor
Practical Nursing
Assiniboine Community College
Winnipeg, MB

Cynthia Wilmore, MSN, RN
Instructor
Nursing Education in Southwestern Alberta (NESA) BN
Lethbridge College
Lethbridge, AB

Dawn Winterhalt, RN, MS
Instructor
School of Nursing
Saskatchewan Polytechnic
Saskatoon, SK

Preface to the Student

Numerous features are built into this text to help you identify key pieces of information and study more efficiently. Additional study tools and review questions may be found on the companion Evolve site: http://evolve.elsevier.com/Canada/Perry/clinicalskills/

Objectives highlight the primary aims of chapter content.

Evolve media resources are available for every chapter.

Standards of Care sections summarize the most recent evidence-informed practice standards or professional clinical standards recommended for skills within each chapter

Principles for Practice sections highlight key nursing principles that apply to all skills within a chapter.

---

2 | Transitions in Care

Written by **Michelle Aebersold, PhD, RN, CHSE, FAAN**, and **Paula D'Eon, RN, MN-NP**

SKILLS AND PROCEDURES
Skill 2.1 **Admitting Patients, p. 13**
Skill 2.2 **Transitioning Patients, p. 21**
Skill 2.3 **Discharging Patients, p. 24**

OBJECTIVES
Mastery of content in this chapter will enable the nurse to:
- Describe the role communication plays in maintaining continuity of care through a patient's admission, transition, and discharge from an acute care facility.
- Explain the purpose and importance of discharge planning.
- Identify the ongoing needs of patients in the discharge planning process.
- Explain the role of a patient's caregiver in the admission, transition, or discharge process.

MEDIA RESOURCES
- evolve http://evolve.elsevier.com/Canada/Perry/clinicalskills/
- Review Questions
- Audio Glossary
- Clinical Debrief and Review Questions Answers

PURPOSE
The coordination of resources and planning a patient's care from admission to discharge or transition from one level of care to the next is a key role of a nurse. Nurses identify patients' ongoing health care needs and anticipate physical, psychological, and social deficits that have implications for patients in resuming normal activities. A nurse involves appropriate caregivers, family members, or both in a plan of care; provides interventions, including health education; and assists in making health care resources available to patients.

- Patient care must be integrated across a variety of settings, services, health care practitioners, and care levels to maintain a continuum of care.
- Transitional care involves nursing actions implemented to ensure coordination and continuity of care for patients who transition between different settings or levels of care.
- Transitions of care require careful attention to communication to ensure patient safety.
- Discharge planning begins at the time of admission to a facility, or even earlier when a patient uses an outpatient clinic or testing centre to begin their care journey.

STANDARDS OF CARE
- Accreditation Canada, 2019—Required Organizational Practices Handbook-Version 14 (http://www.wrha.mb.ca/quality/files/2019 ROPHandbook.pdf)
- Accreditation Canada, 2017a—Client- and Family-Centred Care: Its History in Qmentum and a Supporting Literature Review (https://store.accreditation.ca/products/client-and-family-centred-care-its-history-in-qmentum-and-a-supporting-literature-review)
- Accreditation Canada, 2017b—Emergency Department (https://store.accreditation.ca/products/emergency-department)

PRINCIPLES FOR PRACTICE
- Patients and families should be partners in care, sharing in the process of decision making.

PERSON-CENTRED CARE
- Social determinants of health (SDOH) impart an array of cultural, political, economic, social, and environmental conditions that shape the circumstances in which individuals are born, grow up, live, work, and age. In Canada, many individuals face greater obstacles to good health on the basis of one or more of the following factors: age; gender; race; ethnicity; culture; religion; sexual orientation and gender identity; income and social status; education; social support networks; employment or working conditions; social and physical environments; mental health; cognitive, sensory, or physical disability; or other characteristics historically linked to discrimination or exclusion (Mantoura & Morrison, 2016; Mikkonen & Raphael, 2010). As a nurse, your admission assessment should identify relevant SDOH and must

12

STEP	RATIONALE

IMPLEMENTATION

c. Remove sterile seal and cap from bottle in upward motion.

Upward movement prevents contamination of bottle lip.

d. With solution bottle held away from field and bottle lip 2.5 to 5 cm (1 to 2 inches) above inside of sterile receiving container, slowly pour needed amount of solution into container. Hold bottle with label facing palm of hand (see illustration).

Edge and outside of bottle are considered contaminated. Slow pouring prevents splashing. Sterility of contents cannot be ensured if cap is replaced.
Prevents label from becoming wet and illegible.

Clinical Decision Point When liquids permeate sterile field or barrier, it is called strike through, resulting in contamination of the sterile field.

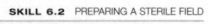

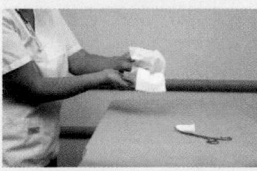
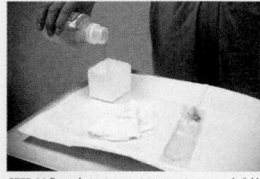

STEP 5c Add items to sterile field.   STEP 6d Pour solution into receiving container on sterile field.

EVALUATION
1. Observe for breaks in sterile technique.

A break in sterile field requires you to set up a new sterile field.

Unexpected Outcomes
1. Sterile field comes in contact with contaminated object or liquid splatters onto drape, causing strike through.
2. Sterile field falls off sterile field.

Related Interventions
- Discontinue field preparation and start over with new equipment.
- Open another package containing new sterile item and add to field unless field becomes contaminated, in which case a new sterile field would need to be established.

Communication and Documentation
- No communication or documentation is required for this set of skills. Document sterile procedure performed and patient status on flow sheet or in nurses' notes in electronic health record (EHR) or chart.

Special Considerations
Care in the Community
- Most care procedures in the home setting involve clean technique. In the event that a sterile environment is required,

the patient and caregiver need to be aware of the principles that apply to the sterile environment. For example, teach patient and caregiver how to correctly use package wrapper as a sterile drape or barrier when applying a sterile dressing or the correct procedure for removing sterile item from the package.
- Assess patient's and caregiver's understanding and ability to provide a sterile environment when needed to perform a specific procedure.

Clinical Decision Points highlight points to consider when performing skills, to ensure effective outcomes and promote safety.

Extensive illustrations demonstrate step-by-step procedures for more thorough understanding.

Quick Response codes may be scanned to link to video clips directly from the text page

Rationales for steps within skills help you learn the why as well as the how of each skill.

+ SKILL 6.3   Sterile Gloving

▶ Video Clip   **NSO** Nursing Skills Online Infection Control Module 2 / Lesson 4

Sterile gloves help prevent the transmission of pathogens by direct and indirect contact. Nurses apply sterile gloves before performing sterile procedures such as inserting urinary catheters or applying sterile dressings. Sterile gloves do not replace hand hygiene.

It is important to verify if the patient or health care providers have a latex allergy. When allergies are present, select latex-free gloves. In an effort to reduce the allergy risk, most health care facilities have a standard practice to use powder-free and latex-free products. Repeated exposure to latex can lead to a latex allergy, in which case latex-free gloves would need to be used. Box 6.2 lists risk factors for a latex allergy. Latex proteins enter the body through skin or mucous membranes, intravascularly, or via inhalation. Reactions to latex range from mild to severe (Box 6.3).

Gloves must be the proper size. The gloves should not stretch so tightly over the fingers that they can tear easily, yet they need to be tight enough that objects can be picked up easily. Sterile gloves are available in various sizes (e.g., 6, 6½, 7). They are also available in "one size fits all" or "small," "medium," and "large."

Delegation and Collaboration

Assisting with skills that include the application and removal of sterile gloves may be delegated to an unregulated care provider (UCP). However, most procedures that require the use of sterile gloves cannot be delegated to a UCP. The nurse instructs the UCP about:

* The reason for using sterile gloves for a specific procedure.

Equipment

* Package of proper-size sterile gloves, latex or synthetic nonlatex. If patient has a latex allergy, ensure that gloves are latex-free and powder-free.

STEP	RATIONALE
ASSESSMENT	
1. Consider the type of procedure to be performed and consult employer policy on use of sterile gloves. In some facilities, double gloving has been recommended for the operating room (Johnson & Osborne, 2016).	Ensures proper use of sterile gloves when needed. Evidence supports the use of double gloving and double gloving with an indicator glove system to decrease the risk of percutaneous injury; such use is an effective barrier to bloodborne pathogen exposure (AORN, 2016).
2. Consider patient's risk for infection (e.g., pre-existing condition and site or extent of area being treated).	Knowledge of risk directs you to follow added precautions (e.g., use of additional protective barriers) if necessary.
3. Select correct size and type of gloves and examine glove package to determine if it is dry and intact with no water stains.	Torn or wet package is considered contaminated. Signs of water stains on package indicate previous contamination by water.

BOX 6.2
Individuals at Risk for Latex Allergy

* Individuals who have had multiple surgeries (e.g., spina bifida surgeries) or medical procedures
* Workers with high latex exposure (e.g., health care employees, greenhouse workers, hair salon workers, estheticians, workers in industries that use gloves routinely)
* Rubber industry workers
* Individuals with a personal or family history
* There is evidence that some people who are allergic to some foods (e.g., avocado, banana, chestnut, kiwi, passion fruit) may also have an allergic reaction to latex.

Canadian Centre for Occupational Health and Safety (CCOHS). (2016). Latex allergy. Retrieved from http://www.ccohs.ca/oshanswers

BOX 6.3
Levels of Latex Reactions

The three types of common latex reactions (in order of severity) are as follows:
1. Irritant dermatitis: Skin reaction isolated to the area of contact
   a. Acute reaction: Red, dry, itchy, and irritated
   b. Chronic reaction: Dry, thick skin, crusting, and possibly cracking or peeling, resulting in open sores
2. Type IV delayed hypersensitivity: Allergic reaction to chemicals used in latex processing

a. Acute reaction: Dry, red, rash, itchy, hives
b. Chronic reaction: Dry, thickened skin, vesicles, peeling (appears 4–96 hours)
3. Type I immediate hypersensitivity: Could be life-threatening, can start as soon as 2–3 minutes after contact
   a. Acute reaction: Hives, swelling, runny nose, cramps, dizziness, low blood pressure, breathing difficulties (shock)

Centers for Disease Control and Prevention. (2013). Frequently asked questions: Contact dermatitis and latex allergy. Retrieved from http://www.cdc.gov/niosh/topics/latex

---

STEP	RATIONALE
EVALUATION	
1. If you are assessing temperature for the first time, establish it as baseline if it is within acceptable range.	Used to compare future temperature measurements.
2. Compare temperature reading with patient's previous baseline and acceptable temperature range for patient's age group.	Body temperature fluctuates within narrow range; comparison reveals presence of abnormality. Improper placement or movement of thermometer can cause inaccuracies. Second measurement confirms initial findings of abnormal body temperature.
3. If patient has fever, take temperature approximately 30 minutes after administering antipyretics and every 4 hours until temperature stabilizes.	Determines if temperature begins to fall in response to therapy.
4. **Use Teach-Back:** "I want to be sure I explained how to check your child's temperature at home. Show me how to swipe his forehead using the thermometer." Develop a revised teaching plan if caregiver is not able to teach back correctly.	Determines caregiver's level of understanding of instructional topic.

Unexpected Outcomes

1. Patient has temperature 1°C (1.8°F) or more above usual range.

Related Interventions

* Initiate measures to lower body temperature:
  * Cool room environment.
  * Reduce external covering on patient's body to promote heat loss but do not induce shivering.
  * Keep clothing and bed linen dry.
  * Apply hypothermia blanket as prescribed.
  * Limit physical activity and sources of emotional stress.
  * Administer antipyretics as prescribed.
  * Increase fluid intake to at least 3 L daily (unless contraindicated).
  * Initiate measures to stimulate appetite and provide nutrients to meet increased energy needs.
  * Prevent or control spread of infection.

2. Patient has temperature 1°C (1.8°F) or more below usual range.

* Initiate measures to raise body temperature:
  * Apply warm blankets and, unless contraindicated, offer warm liquids.
  * Apply hyperthermia blankets if prescribed.
  * Remove wet clothing or linen.

3. Unable to obtain temperature.

* Reassess correct placement of temperature probe or sensor.
* Choose alternative temperature measurement site.
* Obtain alternative temperature measurement device.

Communication and Documentation

* Document temperature and route on vital sign flow sheet or in nurses' notes in EHR or chart.
* Report abnormal findings to nurse in charge or health care provider.
* Document your evaluation of patient and caregiver learning.

Special Considerations
Teaching

* Identify patient's ability to initiate preventive health measures and recognize alteration in body temperature. Educate patient and caregiver about measures to prevent body temperature alterations.
* Educate patients about risk factors for hypothermia and frostbite: fatigue; malnutrition; hypoxemia; cold, wet clothing; alcohol intoxication.
* Educate patients about risk factors for heatstroke: strenuous exercise in hot, humid weather; tight-fitting clothing in hot environments; exercising in poorly ventilated areas; sudden exposures to hot climates; poor fluid intake before, during, and after exercise.

* Educate patients regarding importance of taking and continuing antibiotics as directed until course of treatment for infection is completed.

Pediatric

* Infants and young children may lose more heat to the environment because of their increased body surface area/volume ratios.
* Critically ill children sometimes have cool skin but a high core temperature because of poor perfusion to the skin.
* Use axillary temperatures for screening purposes only; axillary temperature should not be relied on to detect a fever in children.
* Children may assume prone position for rectal temperature measurement.
* With children who cry or become restless, it is best to take temperature as the last vital sign.

Gerontological

* The temperature of older persons is at the lower end of the acceptable temperature range: 36°C (96.8°F).
* Temperatures considered within normal range often reflect a fever in an older person.

Annotations:

NSO icon links to online course lessons

Delegation and Collaboration sections define communication within the patient care team and your responsibility when delegating to unregulated care providers.

Unexpected Outcomes/Related Interventions help you anticipate problems and respond appropriately.

Communication and Documentation guidelines for each skill detail what to document and report.

Special Considerations indicate special teaching considerations, as well as procedure modifications needed for pediatric, gerontological, and self-care teaching in community populations.

Preface to the Instructor

The evolution of technology and knowledge influences the way we teach clinical skills to nursing students, improves the quality of care, and enhances safety for every patient. However, the foundation for success in performing nursing skills remains a competent, evidence-informed nurse who thinks critically, asks the right questions at the right time, and makes timely clinical judgements.

In this First Edition of *Canadian Clinical Nursing Skills & Techniques*, we have consulted with nurses across Canada, including contributors from almost every province and territory. Each chapter opens by introducing students to key concepts: Standards of Practice, Principles for Practice, Person-Centred Care, Evidence-Informed Practice, and Safety Guidelines. We have streamlined these sections into a quick, easy-to-read bulleted format to emphasize, yet simplify, these important concepts.

The importance of interprofessional collaboration has been highlighted and threaded throughout the key concepts. Chapter 1, Evidence-Informed Nursing, prepares students to understand and use evidence-informed practice information that is included in every chapter.

All topics and skills, including sample documentation, have been updated to the most recent Canadian standards in nursing practice.

Your students will find that the First Edition of *Canadian Clinical Nursing Skills & Techniques* provides a comprehensive resource that will serve them well through their nursing education and right into their clinical practice careers.

CLASSIC FEATURES

- **Over 200 basic, intermediate, and advanced nursing skills and procedures** are covered.
- **Five-step nursing process format** provides a consistent presentation that helps students apply the process while learning each skill.
- **Skills and Procedures** list and **Objectives** open each chapter.
- **Over 1200 full-colour photos and drawings** help students master the material covered.
- **Standards of Care** sections summarize the most recent evidence-informed standards, and the professional clinical standards recommended for the skills within each chapter.
- **Principles for Practice** sections highlight the key nursing principles that apply to skills within a chapter.
- **Evidence-Informed Practice** sections present students with the most recent evidence for the procedures presented. Recent research findings are discussed, and their implications for patient care are explored.
- **Person-Centred Care** sections prepare students to recognize the importance of collaborating with patients when performing skills in a compassionate and coordinated way that is based on respect for a patient's cultural preferences, values, beliefs and needs. "Person" in this context means the patient, their family, their caregivers (both formal and informal), and their identified support person(s).
- **Safety Guidelines** sections cover global and Canadian Patient Safety Institute recommendations on the safe execution of the particular skill set covered in each chapter.

- **NSO icon** links text content with the new edition of *Nursing Skills Online*, which has been simultaneously revised with the textbook to provide completely coordinated information.
- **Rationales** are given for steps within skills, so students learn the *why* as well as the *how* of each skill. Rationales include citations from the current literature.
- **Collaboration and Delegation** sections define communication within interprofessional teams and the nurse's responsibility when delegating to unregulated care providers.
- **Clinical Decision Points** alert students to key steps that affect patient outcomes and help them modify care as needed to implement person-centred care.
- **Evaluation** sections highlight steps students must take to evaluate the outcomes of the skills performed.
- **Teach-Back** is included in each evaluation section, where we demonstrate to students how to phrase a Teach-Back question appropriately.
- **Communication and Documentation** sections follow the evaluation discussion and alert students to what information should be documented in each situation.
- **Unexpected Outcomes and Related Interventions** sections inform students to be alert for potential problems and help them determine appropriate nursing interventions.
- **Special Considerations** sections include additional considerations when performing the skill for specific populations of patients or in specific settings and may include:
  - **Teaching Considerations**
  - **Pediatric Considerations**
  - **Gerontological Considerations**
  - **Care in the Community Considerations**
- **Quick Response codes** (scan with smartphone or tablet with camera to view video clips) on the text pages link video clips to the appropriate skill or procedure, allowing students to view the video immediately after reading the implementation section of the skill.
- **End-of-chapter exercises** include a Clinical Debrief case study, examples of SBAR communication, and review questions.
- **Glossary** (on Evolve) defines all key terms.
- **Additional review questions** (on Evolve) include a new set of unique questions for every chapter.
- **TEACH for RN and TEACH for PN instructor manuals** helps you capitalize on the new clinical material in the text, skills video series, and online course. Additional case studies and discussion questions unique to the TEACH manual expand the in-class material available to you.
- An **Image Collection** is available with *Clinical Nursing Skills & Techniques*.

FEATURES OF THE FIRST CANADIAN EDITION

This First Canadian Edition highlights the importance of interprofessional collaboration and patient safety, referencing standards and recommendations from the Canadian Patient Safety Institute.

The most current best practice standards were used, noting that some standards are older than 5 years but are still current in practice. When referencing best practices, we have weighed the strength of the evidence as well as its' currency to choose the most pertinent reference citation. Also, there are some best practice standards in use in Canada that refer to American standards or practices, and this is noted, when applicable.

With continued changes in medication preparation and unit supply, for example, unit-dose systems, the third check for accuracy in medication preparation—which historically is when the nurse returns the stock medication to the cabinet/drawer—may not be possible at all times, because in some instances there is no medication container to return to. In these circumstances, the third check for accuracy is done with the patients MAR at the bedside, prior to administration as part of following the 10 rights of medication administration. Throughout the text we have maintained that the three medication preparation checks for accuracy include: 1) Before removing the medication vial/container from the drawer; 2) When the prescribed amount of the medication is prepared (e.g., poured, drawn up); and, 3) Before returning the medication container to storage or disposing of the single-use vial or ampoule.

Within the Canadian health care context, Registered nurses may "assign" skills to Licensed (Registered) Practical Nurses, but there are very few skills that can be delegated. For a skill to be delegated from a RN to RPN/LPN, the skill must fall outside of the RPN/LPN's scope of practice. Throughout this textbook, when a skill is specific to the role of the RN, we have used "Registered nurse" or "RN"; in all other instances we use the term nurse to refer to a RN and/or RPN/LPN, depending upon jurisdictional regulations. Our rationale for this decision was to align the text with the changing landscape of the Canadian Nurses Association who, in June of 2018, passed a motion that its' membership would include all RNs and RPN/LPNs, and that the membership would be termed "nurses".

As health care continues to change at a fast pace, many employers are developing policies to enable delegation of tasks to unregulated care providers, provided that specific criteria are met relating to knowledge, skills and abilities. It is important for the nurse to be informed of their employer policy in relation to the delegation of tasks. For example, historically, the skill of catheterization could not be delegated to an unregulated care provider; however, currently, in some jurisdictions (e.g., Ontario), this skill can be delegated provided that certain guidelines have been met. Throughout the text the student/reader is always cautioned to check employer policy relating to delegation of skills to an unregulated care provider.

Specific terminology used within this text is grounded in the Canadian health care context to ensure consistency from one chapter to another:

- "Health care provider" can include a physician, nurse practitioner, or an RN who has prescribing of medications and/or treatments within their scope of practice.
- Family member was changed to "caregiver" to be more inclusive; caregivers can be family or friend caregivers, as well as formal or informal caregivers.
- Gender pronouns were removed whenever possible using the terms "they" and "them" as acceptable singular references to achieve gender neutrality (see https://en.oxforddictionaries.com/usage/he-or-she-versus-they).
- "Prescriptions" was used to replace order/medication order, and "prescribing" replaces "ordering".
- "Interprofessional collaboration" is used to refer to any collaboration among health care team members, and others, for example, spiritual care givers.

LEARNING SUPPLEMENTS FOR STUDENTS

- The **Evolve Student Resources** are available online at http://evolve.elsevier.com/Canada/Perry/clinicalskills/ and include the following valuable learning aids, organized by asset:
  - Animations
  - Audio Glossary
  - Calculation Tutorial
  - Examination Review Questions
  - Fluids and Electrolytes Tutorial
  - Printable versions of Chapter Key Points
  - Skills Performance Checklists for each skill in the text
  - Video Clips highlighting common skills
- *Virtual Clinical Excursions Online and Print Workbook for Fundamentals of Nursing* is an exciting package that brings learning to life in a virtual hospital setting. The workbook guides students as they care for patients, providing ongoing challenges and learning opportunities. Each lesson in *Virtual Clinical Excursions* complements the textbook content and provides an environment for students to practice what they are learning. *Virtual Clinical Excursions Online and Print Workbook* are available separately or packaged at a special price with the textbook.

TEACHING SUPPLEMENTS FOR INSTRUCTORS

- The **Evolve Instructor Resources** (available online at http://evolve.elsevier.com/Canada/Perry/clinicalskills/) are a comprehensive collection of the most important tools instructors need, including the following:
  - **TEACH for Nurses** ties together every chapter resource you need for the most effective class presentations, with sections dedicated to objectives, teaching focus, instructor chapter resources, answers to chapter questions, and an in-class case study discussion. Teaching strategies include content highlights, student activities, online activities, and large group activities.
  - The **Test Bank** contains more than 1100 multiple-choice questions with textbook references and answers coded for NCLEX competencies and cognitive level. The ExamView software allows instructors to create new tests; edit, add, and delete test questions; sort questions by category, cognitive level, and question type; and administer and grade online tests.
  - **PowerPoint Presentations** include over 1500 slides for use in lectures.
  - The **Image Collection** contains more than 1200 illustrations from the text for use in lectures.
  - **Simulation Learning System** is an online toolkit that helps instructors and facilitators effectively incorporate medium- to high-fidelity simulation into their nursing curriculum. Detailed patient scenarios promote and enhance the clinical decision-making skills of students at all levels. The system provides detailed instructions for preparation and implementation of the simulation experience, debriefing questions that encourage critical thinking, and learning resources to reinforce student comprehension. Each scenario in the Simulation Learning System complements the textbook content and helps bridge the gap between lectures and clinicals. This system provides the perfect environment for students to practise what they are learning in the text for a true-to-life, hands-on learning experience.

MULTIMEDIA SUPPLEMENTS FOR INSTRUCTORS AND STUDENTS

- **Nursing Skills Online 4.0** contains 19 modules rich with animations, videos, interactive activities, and exercises to help students prepare for their clinical lab experience. The instructionally designed lessons focus on topics that are difficult to master and pose a high risk to the patient if done incorrectly. Lesson quizzes allow students to check their learning curve and review as needed, and the module exams feed out to an instructor grade book. Modules cover Airway Management, Blood Therapy, Bowel Elimination/Ostomy Care, Cardiac Care, Closed Chest Drainage Systems, Enteral Nutrition, Infection Control, Injections, IV Fluid Administration, IV Fluid Therapy Maintenance, IV Medication Administration, Nonparenteral Medication Administration, Safe Medication Preparation, Safety, Specimen Collection, Urinary Catheterization, Vascular Access, Vital Signs, and Wound Care. It is available alone or packaged with the text.

- **Clinical Skills: Essentials Collection** provides videos covering 150-plus essential nursing skills. Each skill in the collection uses a seven-part framework to walk you through every aspect of the skill, including interactive learning tools, including overview information covering skill purpose; safety alerts; patient and family education; delegation guides; equipment lists; preparation procedures; documentation guidelines; demonstration videos and animations; images and illustrations; additional reading suggestions; printable evaluation checklists; and interactive review questions and competency tests, with rationales. It is available online.

Contents

1 | Evidence-Informed Nursing Practice

Written by **Patricia A. Potter, RN, MSN, PhD, FAAN, and Shelley L. Cobbett, RN, GnT, MN, EdD**

OUTLINE

OBJECTIVES

Mastery of content in this chapter will enable the nurse to:

- Discuss how scientific evidence improves the relevance and efficacy of nursing skills.
- Explain the differences between research- and non–research-based evidence.
- Differentiate between evidence-based and evidence-informed practice.
- Discuss critical thinking, clinical reasoning, and clinical judgement.

- Explain the components of a PICO(TS) question.
- Discuss the process for critiquing evidence in the literature.
- Identify the elements to review when critiquing a scientific article.
- Describe the seven steps of the action cycle of the Knowledge-to-Action Framework.
- Discuss ways to apply evidence in nursing practice.
- Explain the importance of identifying outcomes in the evaluation of an evidence-informed practice change.

MEDIA RESOURCES

- evolve http://evolve.elsevier.com/Canada/Perry/clinicalskills/
- Review Questions

- Audio Glossary
- Clinical Debrief and Review Questions Answers
- Case Studies

PURPOSE

The Canadian Nurses Association (CNA) calls for a commitment to innovation, collaboration, and partnerships to achieve an efficient and effective health care system (CNA, 2017a). Knowledge use and translating best evidence into practice result in a more transparent and sustainable health care system (Curtis, Fry, Shaban, et al., 2016). As part of professional nursing practice, nurses advocate for evidence-informed decision-making in their nursing practice (CNA, 2017b). The terms *evidence-informed practice (EIP)* and *evidence-based practice (EBP)* are often used interchangeably, but the definitions provided of each tend to be conflicting in the literature (Kumah et al., 2018). EIP provides more flexibility regarding the nature of the evidence and encompasses a process that is person centred rather than focusing solely on quantitative evidence (Woodbury & Kuhnke, 2014). The CNA's most recent position statement (2010) indicates that in evidence-informed decision-making the many factors that influence decision-making—for example, cultural norms, religious beliefs, and patient values—are taken into account. The process of searching, selecting, appraising, and summarizing evidence is used in partnership with clinical expertise, patient preferences, and values, while grounded in the local context, to implement person-centred, evidence-informed nursing practice. This ongoing process that incorporates evidence and other available resources to make nursing decisions with clients is referred to as *evidence-informed nursing practice* (CNA, 2010).

Nursing is positioned to lead change and advance health through the use of EIP. Using many different levels and types of evidence, nurses ensure that the skills and procedures performed on patients incorporate best practices for efficiency, patient safety, and clinical effectiveness.

STANDARDS OF CARE

There are three recognized nursing professions in Canada: registered nurses (RNs) (including nurse practitioners [NPs]), registered psychiatric nurses, and licensed (registered) practical nurses, with a membership of approximately 365,000 nurses in total (Canadian Council for Practical Nurse Regulators [CCPNR], 2018). At the June 2018 Annual General Meeting of CNA members, a resolution was passed to change their bylaws related to membership—historically, CNA membership had been limited to RNs and NPs. The amended membership bylaw includes the *family of nursing*, that is, the recognized nursing professions noted above.

Nursing registration and licensure is a provincial/territorial responsibility, and each has unique legislation that governs the practice of nursing. Individual provincial and territorial entry-level competencies can be found on the website of each

professional nursing association, for RNs and licensed (registered) practical nurses:

- Canadian Council of Practical Nurse Regulators (CCPNR), 2013a—*Code of Ethics for Licensed Practical Nurses in Canada* (http://www.ccpnr.ca/wp-content/uploads/2013/09/IJLPN-CE-Final.pdf)
- Canadian Council of Practical Nurse Regulators (CCPNR), 2013b—*Entry-to-Practice Competencies for Licensed Practical Nurses* (http://www.ccpnr.ca/wp-content/uploads/2013/09/IJLPN-ETPC-Final.pdf)
- Canadian Council of Registered Nurse Regulators (CCRNR), 2012—*Competencies in the Context of Entry-Level Registered Nurse Practice.* (http://www.ccrnr.ca/assets/jcp_rn_competencies_2012_edition)
- Canadian Nurses Association (CNA), 2015—*Framework for the Practice of Registered Nurses in Canada* (https://www.cna-aiic.ca/~/media/cna/page-content/pdf-en/framework-for-the-pracice-of-registered-nurses-in-canada.pdf)
- Canadian Nurses Association (CNA), 2017b—*Code of Ethics for Registered Nurses* (https://cna-aiic.ca/~/media/cna/page-content/pdf-en/code-of-ethics-2017-edition-secure-interactive.pdf?la=en)

PRINCIPLES FOR PRACTICE

Samantha works on a medical oncology unit where patients undergo chemotherapy and radiation for leukemia, lymphoma, and other forms of cancer. Because of their chemotherapy, many patients experience a drop in their platelet count and clotting factors, increasing their risk for bleeding. Samantha recently cared for an adult male patient who fell while trying to get to the bathroom and hit his head against the bed frame, resulting in a serious intracranial bleed. Samantha discusses the situation with two nurse colleagues and asks, "How can we reduce the number of falls and injuries to our patients on the oncology unit?" The nurse specialist for the unit tells Samantha, "I heard about an approach to fall prevention on one of the surgical floors; it involves hourly rounding. Let's ask this question, "In adult oncology patients, will the use of hourly rounding compared with the current fall prevention protocol affect the incidence of falls during hospitalization?" Feeling frustrated that their existing fall prevention protocol was not effective in reducing falls, the group agrees that the question is the right one to search in the literature.

This clinical case study highlights how professional nurses address problems in their practice.

EIP is a process of making informed decisions about the way nurses care for patients. It begins with asking clinical questions to acquire an evidence base of knowledge. Clinical questions lead nurses such as Samantha and her colleagues to find evidence from the research literature, clinical papers, quality improvement data, risk management trends, and the opinions of nurse experts. In addition to this evidence base, the nurse considers the context of the patient or population, along with their preferences and values, to implement EIP. This process guides the nurse in knowledge translation to make relevant and informed changes in practice, such as fall prevention in the case study.

There are elements of all nursing procedures within this textbook that are evidence based to assist nurses in implementing EIP. For example, the length of time necessary to wash hands, the technique for determining the position of a feeding tube in the stomach, and the technique for giving an intramuscular injection are based on evidence. Clinical research led to the answers for how these nursing procedures should be performed. The use of such evidence in practice enables clinicians to provide the highest quality of care to their patients and families.

Quality Health Care and Patient Safety

According to the CNA (2017b), integrated care is based on six key principles: person-centred care, quality services, health promotion and illness prevention, equitable access to quality care, sustainability, and accountability. The CNA expanded the Institute for Health Care Improvement (IHI) Triple Aim framework (Whittington, Nolan, Lewis, et al., 2015) to a Quadruple Aim concept to include better care, better health, better value, and better engagement for efficient and effective health care. Implementing health care processes or practices that are evidence informed in a reliable and consistent manner is a feature of quality care that maximizes patient safety. Globally, patient harm is thought to be the 14th leading cause of morbidity and mortality (Slawomirski, Auraaen, & Klazinga, 2017), with 1 in 18 patients in Canadian hospitals experiencing a preventable incident of patient harm (CIHI & CPSI, 2016). About 25% of patients receive care that is not needed or is potentially harmful (CIHR, 2015). Implementing new knowledge into practice requires a systematic approach that applies the best available evidence to clinical, educational, and administrative practices. Clinical practice guidelines rely on the best evidence to decide which interventions produce the best outcomes, enhancing patient safety. Nurses play a key role in all areas of health care in questioning outdated, illogical, or unsafe practices and then adopting evidence-informed practices that will alter patients' health status, maximize safety, and achieve desired outcomes.

Critical Thinking, Clinical Reasoning, and Clinical Judgement

The terms *critical thinking, clinical reasoning,* and *clinical judgement* are often used interchangeably, but within nursing, these terms have slightly different meanings. Critical thinking is complex and based on context and has no one "right" definition. Critical thinking is a broad term that refers to purposeful, focused, deliberate, informed, results-oriented thinking and includes both clinical reasoning and clinical judgement (Alfaro-LeFevre, 2016). Critical thinking is essential for sound clinical judgement, identifying nursing diagnoses, planning patient care, and to safely and effectively practise person-centred care. Clinical reasoning is a more specific term that refers to ways of thinking about patient care issues, whereas clinical judgement refers to the outcome of critical thinking and clinical reasoning. It is helpful to think about critical thinking and clinical reasoning as the processes that lead to clinical judgement, the outcome or result (e.g., conclusion, decision, or opinion) (Alfaro-LeFevre, 2016). Critical thinking occurs in clinical settings (e.g., identifying person-centred diagnoses) and nonclinical settings (e.g., test-taking), whereas clinical reasoning and judgement usually occur in the clinical setting. As critical thinkers you will use many skills, knowledge sources, and attitudes; as you progress in your nursing career, your critical thinking skills will continue to improve.

A Case for Evidence

EIP helps the nurse make accurate, timely, and appropriate clinical decisions. It is an interprofessional process for applying the newest knowledge available in health care sciences to the patient's bedside. For example, using a sliding board to transfer a patient from bed to stretcher instead of lifting and using the research-based Braden Scale to routinely assess a patient's risk for skin breakdown are examples of using evidence at the bedside. This textbook demonstrates how to use evidence in nursing procedures or skills and provides the scientific guidelines to perform skills more effectively, improve patient outcomes, and maximize patient safety.

As a professional nurse, you need to stay informed and be aware of the most current evidence. Typically, new students diligently read their textbooks and assigned scientific articles. A good textbook incorporates current evidence into the practice guidelines and nursing skills at the time it is published. However, because a textbook relies on the scientific literature, some information can become outdated by the time the book is published. Articles from nursing and the health care literature are available on almost any topic involving nursing practice. New research is reported every day. Although the scientific basis of nursing practice has grown, there are practices that are still not "research based" (based on findings from well-designed research studies) because findings are inconclusive or researchers have not yet studied the practices. For example, in the past, nurses changed intravenous (IV) site dressings daily and applied antibiotic ointment to reduce the incidence of infection at a site. However, there was no evidence at the time to support this practice. IV care was based on tradition. Subsequent research demonstrated that topical antibiotics offer no benefit, and daily dressing changes are not beneficial unless a dressing becomes soiled or compromised. Today the standard of care is to cleanse an adult's IV site with chlorhexidine antiseptic solution and not use antibiotic ointment on the IV site (Infusion Nurses Society [INS], 2016). A transparent semipermeable membrane (TSM) dressing change should be performed every 5 to 7 days, and gauze dressings every 2 days or when loose, wet, or visibly soiled or when integrity is compromised (INS, 2016). The challenge is to obtain the very best, most current information at the right time, when you need it for patient care.

The best evidence comes from well-designed, systematically conducted research studies that are reported in peer-reviewed scientific journals. The widespread access of online research reports has enhanced the availability of best-practice information in the health care setting, empowering nurses to move away from practices based on tradition, preference, or convenience. It is important for nursing leaders to provide a supportive environment and adequate facilitation of required changes. The leader of today needs to be an agent of change (Porter-O'Grady & Malloch, 2015) to enable nurses to fully engage in critiquing practice and in the translation of knowledge for ongoing efficiency and effectiveness. Information is widely portable, and as such, current practice is continuously evolving and changing, based on the best available evidence. The acceptability of up-to-date information at point-of-care is quickly becoming the norm.

EIP requires nurses to consider many different types and levels of evidence to become informed about practice issues (e.g., fall or infection rates). But remember, as a nurse it is important that you *not* rely on one type of evidence alone. When you face a clinical issue or problem, seek out all sources of evidence, including research, patient preferences, and values, to find the best solution in caring for patients in an evidence-informed, person-centred manner.

Even when you use the best evidence available, application and outcomes will differ based on patients' values, preferences, concerns, and expectations and the local context. It is important to apply critical thinking and clinical reasoning competencies to determine whether evidence is relevant and appropriate to your patients, to aid you in making sound clinical judgements. For example, some evidence suggests that mindfulness has the potential to improve health and well-being (Lomas, Etcoff, Van Gordon, et al., 2017). However, if a patient is reluctant to discuss mindfulness practices, and you are unsure of their beliefs, an attempt to use mindfulness interventions is inappropriate. Using your clinical expertise and considering patients' cultures, values, and preferences ensure that you apply new evidence in practice both ethically and appropriately. EIP requires good nursing judgement; it is not finding research evidence and applying it blindly but, rather, applying the best evidence from a variety of sources from a person-centred perspective.

Ask a Clinical Question

Asking a clinical question is the initial important step of the process, as the question will direct the search for the most relevant and best evidence. Every day, nurses perform interventions (e.g., providing comfort measures, caring for patients with wounds, and offering grief support to a family) that stimulate questions such as "Why do we use this approach?" and "Is there a better way?" or "This step causes patients distress. What other options are available?" Always think about your practice when caring for patients. Question what does not make sense to you and what you think needs clarification. Interprofessional collaboration involves various perspectives and might help to clarify or examine the clinical problem or issue. As practised in the previous case study, think about a patient care problem or an area of interest that is time consuming, costly, or not logical.

Clinical questions often arise because of either a problem- or knowledge-focused trigger. A problem-focused trigger occurs as the nurse cares for a patient or notices a trend on a nursing unit. For example, a problem-focused trigger might arise while caring for an unconscious patient: "Which is the best anti-infective solution to use when giving oral care to unconscious patients?" Examples of problem-focused trends include the increase in the number of pressure injuries to patients' skin or tissues or the incidence of urinary tract infections on a nursing unit. A knowledge-focused trigger arises when the nurse asks a question regarding new information about a topic. For example, "What is the current evidence to reduce bloodstream infection in central venous catheters?" Important knowledge sources often include standards and practice guidelines available from national and provincial/territorial agencies, for example, the Registered Nurses Association of Ontario (http://rnao.ca/bpg), Canadian Stroke Best Practices (http://rnao.ca/bpg), and the Canadian Clinical Practice Guidelines InfoBase (https://www.cma.ca/).

There are two basic types of questions: background and foreground (Thompson, 2017). Think of a forest and the trees. A *background question* gives us a view of a forest. It is broad and general about a condition or idea—for example, "Which interventions reduce falls in oncology patients?" The answer to the question provides general knowledge about the problem, concepts, or topic of interest (e.g., falls, fall occurrence among oncology patients, reasons oncology patients fall). In contrast, a *foreground question* gives us a closer look at the trees in a forest. It is used to find out specific information for making clinical decisions (Thompson, 2017). A foreground question asks which of two interventions is likely to be more effective in addressing a practice issue. For example, "Does hourly rounding compared with a standard fall prevention protocol affect the incidence of falls?" A background question allows you to explore a vast array of options in the literature, whereas a foreground question produces a refined and limited body of evidence specific to your area of interest. In day-to-day clinical practice, it helps to be able to identify foreground questions so that the extent of literature to review is limited.

A well-stated foreground question is clearly worded when you use a PICO(TS) format. Box 1.1 summarizes the elements of a PICO(TS) question. Using key words in a PICO(TS) strategy makes it easier to search for evidence in the scientific literature because it restricts a search to only articles pertinent to the PICO(TS) terms (Brown, 2018). The use of (TS) denotes that T (time) and S (search strategy) are not required elements of every PICO(TS)

Developing a PICO(TS) Question

P	**Patient, population,** or **problem**
	Be as specific as possible to identify the patient, population, or problem
I	**Intervention** or **issue of interest**
	Can be an assessment, intervention, therapy, or evaluation
C	**Comparison** or **context**
	Standard care versus the intervention of interest; context of the question
O	**Outcomes**
	Which result do you wish to achieve or observe as a result of an intervention or issue of interest? Qualitative questions identify this variable as "findings."
T	**Time** (optional component for a clinical question)
S	**Search strategy** (optional component using search limiters)

Adapted from Davies, B., & Logan, J. (2018). *Reading research: A user-friendly guide for health professionals* (6th ed., p. 33). Toronto, ON: Elsevier/Mosby; and Brown, S. (2018). *Evidence-based nursing* (4th ed., p. 253). Burlington, MA: Jones & Bartlett Learning.

question. The words used in the PICO(T) question are the key terms for a literature search, and the (S) limits the search strategy, for example, limiting a search to only randomized control trials (RCTs). Examples of PICO(TS) questions follow: *In abdominal surgery patients (P), does epidural analgesia (I) compared with patient-controlled analgesia (C) affect pain severity (O) the first 24 hours postoperative (T)? In medical patients (P) does the use of a case-management model (I) compared with a telephone call-back system (C) improve patient medication adherence (O) over a 12-month period (T)?*

Well-designed PICO(TS) questions do not have to include all six elements. For example, a comparison intervention is not pertinent when a PICO(TS) question is about meaning, such as *Do family caregivers (P) of hospice patients feel anxiety (O) when providing hands-on care (I)?* Also, if there is no comparison intervention, only the standard of care, a (C) is not required, nor does the time (T) or the search strategy (S) need to be included. The elements of Population, an Intervention or issue of interest, and Outcome are essential for a well-designed PICO(TS) question involving an intervention.

A clearly stated PICO(TS) question helps to identify knowledge gaps for a specific clinical, educational, or managerial problem or situation. When you form well–thought-out questions, the type of evidence you lack for clinical practice becomes clearer when you search the literature. Examples of different knowledge gaps include the following:

- *Diagnosis:* Questions about the selection and interpretation of diagnostic tests. *Example:* Does the use of a disposable oral thermometer compared with an electronic oral thermometer measure body temperature accurately in a patient with an endotracheal tube?
- *Prognosis:* Questions about a patient's likely clinical outcome. *Example:* Is there a difference in the incidence of deep vein thrombosis in surgical patients wearing sequential compression stockings compared to those who wear elastic stockings?
- *Therapy:* Questions about the selection of the most beneficial treatments. *Example:* Which bowel regimen is most effective in relieving constipation caused by the administration of opioid therapy in oncology patients with chronic pain?
- *Prevention:* Questions about screening and prevention methods to reduce the risk of disease. *Example:* Does the use of social

media with education messages compared with informational brochures improve male adolescents' adherence to the human papillomavirus vaccine series?

- *Education:* Questions about best teaching strategies for colleagues, patients, or family members. *Example:* Is the use of motivational interviewing compared with low-literacy teaching booklets more effective to educate low-literacy adults about therapeutic diets?
- *Meaning:* Questions that seek understanding of a phenomenon. *Example:* How do patients with cervical cancer perceive their quality of life?

Search for the Best Evidence

Once you have a clear and concise PICO(TS) question, you are ready to search for evidence. Numerous research and non-research resources are available to aid in your search, including government and professional websites, agency procedure manuals, performance improvement reports, and computerized bibliographical databases. Do not hesitate to ask for help to find appropriate evidence. A reference librarian is an excellent resource with whom to collaborate to conduct a literature search. If one is not available, go to your faculty member or an advanced practice nurse within the health care institution.

A reference librarian knows the relevant databases available to you for a literature search about your PICO(TS) question (Box 1.2). The databases are repositories of published scientific studies, including peer-reviewed research. A peer-reviewed article is preferable for retrieval because it has been evaluated by a panel of experts who are familiar with the topic or subject matter of the article. Working with the librarian, translate the elements of your PICO(TS) question into the language or key words that will yield the best articles for your evidence search. For example, consider this PICO(TS) question: *Does motivational interviewing (I) compared with media instruction (C) improve oncology patients' (P) adherence to chemotherapy medications (O)?* The key words include *oncology patient, motivational interviewing, media instruction, chemotherapy,* and *adherence.* A good librarian will recommend using the indexing language or controlled vocabulary of the database that you are searching. The controlled vocabulary known as Medical Subject Headings (MeSH®) is used in Canada and is updated annually from the U.S. National Library of Medicine (U.S. National Library of Medicine, 2015). Proper use of MeSH® terms facilitates a more thorough and focused literature search than one you might get from simply trying to search combinations of key words on Google or Yahoo. In the previous example the word *oncology* might be entered instead of *cancer* to fit the database language, whereas *adherence* might be also entered as *compliance.*

When working within a database, you need to enter key words to search for articles. Because the vocabulary within published articles is often vague, the words you select sometimes have one meaning to one author and a very different meaning to another. Each key word generates a set of articles. Using Boolean operators or the function of Search Limits enables you to narrow the results of the search by combining key terms from your PICO(TS) question using the Boolean connector *and.* For example, by entering the combination of "oncology patient *and* chemotherapy *and* adherence" into the literature database, you will only obtain a listing of the articles that contain all three terms. A librarian can show you how to use the Search Limits function if needed. Your search can be further narrowed by limiting it by certain categories such as the time frame during which the article was written, types of studies, English-language publications, or age of patients. Use of Boolean connectors and Search Limits reduces the number of articles to a manageable number to review for a PICO(TS) question.

BOX 1.2

Searchable Scientific Literature Databases and Sources

CINAHL	Cumulative Index of Nursing and Allied Health Literature; database for EBSCO nursing resources; includes studies in nursing, allied health, and biomedicine https://www.ebscohost.com/nursing/products/cinahl-databases/cinahl-complete
MEDLINE	U.S. National Library of Medicine®; bibliographical database that contains more than 22 million references to journal articles in life sciences with a concentration on biomedicine https://www.nlm.nih.gov/bsd/pmresources.html
EMBASE	Biomedical and pharmaceutical studies and abstracts and articles from biomedical, drug, and medical device conferences https://www.elsevier.com/solutions/embase-biomedical-research
PsycINFO	Interprofessional bibliographical resources in psychology and the behavioural and social sciences https://www.apa.org/pubs/databases/psycinfo/index.aspx
Cochrane Community—Database of Systematic Reviews	Full text of regularly updated systematic reviews prepared by the Cochrane Collaboration; includes completed reviews and protocols https://www.cochranelibrary.com/
National Guidelines Clearinghouse	Public resource for evidence-informed clinical practice guidelines. Available through the Agency for Healthcare Research and Quality; contains structured abstracts (summaries) about clinical guidelines and their development; also includes condensed version of guidelines for viewing https://www.ahrq.gov/gam/index.html
PubMed	Health science library at the U.S. National Library of Medicine; free access to more than 24 million citations for biomedical literature from MEDLINE, life science journals, and online books https://www.nlm.nih.gov
ERIC (Educational Resources Information Centre)	Consists of resources in education and covers published literature from over 775 periodicals in the discipline of education https://eric.ed.gov/
Joanna Briggs Institute EBP Database	Includes full systematic reviews, protocols, evidence summaries, best practice recommendations, and consumer information http://joannabriggs.org/
RxTx (formerly called eCPS)	Compendium of pharmaceuticals and specialties, drug information, patient information https://www.e-therapeutics.ca/
TRIP (Translating Research into Practice) Database	A clinical search engine that allows hundreds of evidence-informed resources to be search simultaneously. https://www.tripdatabase.com/

The pyramid in Fig. 1.1 represents a hierarchy for rating available scientific evidence obtained in your search. It is important to learn about the types of studies to help you know which ones provide the best scientific evidence to guide you in choosing which articles to review. The strongest level of evidence is at the top of the pyramid; the weakest is at the bottom. You can use the rating scale of I to VIII when you later critique each article that you obtain in your search of the literature. Table 1.1 describes types of studies with examples in the evidence hierarchy, beginning with the study at the top of the hierarchy, a systematic review.

If your PICO(TS) question leads you to an article that is a systematic review, celebrate! A systematic review is the perfect answer to a PICO(TS) question. Basically, a researcher has asked the same PICO(TS) question you have asked and then examined all the well-designed relevant research studies that ask the same question. The researcher creates a detailed and comprehensive plan and uses explicit methods to locate, appraise, and synthesize research on the topic (Davies & Logan, 2018). The researcher sets criteria for the type of studies to review in the search. A systematic review explains if the evidence for which you are searching about a specific question exists and whether it supports a change in practice. A systematic review of well-designed research studies provides the best evidence of the effectiveness of different interventions. A

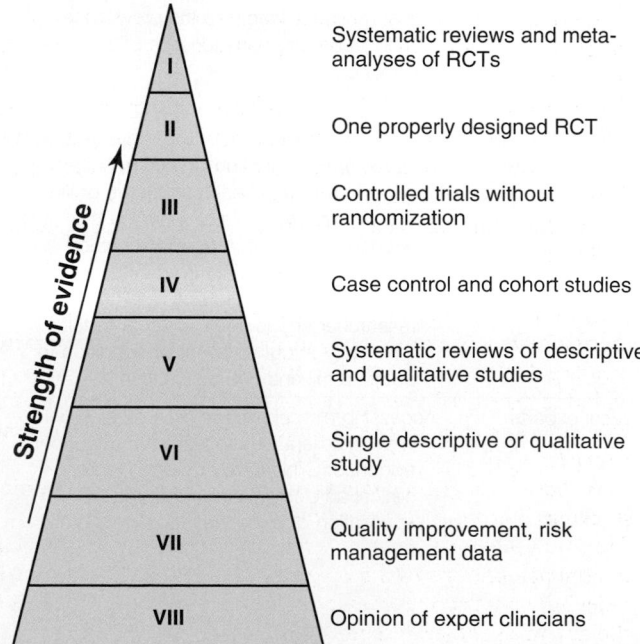

FIG 1.1 The evidence pyramid. *RCT,* Randomized controlled trial.

Strength of evidence

I — Systematic reviews and meta-analyses of RCTs

II — One properly designed RCT

III — Controlled trials without randomization

IV — Case control and cohort studies

V — Systematic reviews of descriptive and qualitative studies

VI — Single descriptive or qualitative study

VII — Quality improvement, risk management data

VIII — Opinion of expert clinicians

TABLE 1.1

Types of Studies in the Evidence Hierarchy

Study Type	Description	Example
Systematic review or meta-analysis	An author or panel of experts reviews the evidence from randomized controlled trials (RCTs) (and other defined types of research studies) about a specific clinical question and summarizes the state of the science. In a meta-analysis, there is the addition of a statistical analysis that combines data from all studies.	This study aimed to examine the validity of using the Braden Scale in long-term care (LTC) settings. Eleven data sets from nine published studies describing 40,361 residents were analyzed. The appropriateness of the Braden Scale in LTC is questionable given its low specificity and positive predictive value. This means that the scale has high probability that subjects with a positive screening test truly have a risk for a pressure injury; however, if the result on the Braden Scale is positive, the certainty of the person actually having a pressure injury is low (Wilchesky & Lungu, 2015).
RCT	A researcher tests an intervention against the usual standard of care. Participants are randomly assigned to either a control group (receives standard care) or a treatment group (receives the experimental intervention), with both measured on the same outcomes to see if there is a difference.	This study, focusing on patient satisfaction, evaluated the impact of providing clinician photographs on inpatients' recall. The RCT involved three groups. A control group received the current standard of care; the second group received handouts with the names and roles of their clinical care team; and the third group received handouts with the names, roles, and photographs of their clinical care team. Patients completed a survey before discharge on their ability to recall their clinicians and rated the quality of communication with the care team. Those who received photos in the handout correctly identified significantly more clinicians by photograph and identified more clinician names. There was no difference in quality of communication (Appel et al., 2015).
Quasi-experimental study	This research approach tries to show that an intervention causes a particular outcome. This type of study is done when one of the three elements of a RCT is not feasible, most commonly randomization (Davies & Logan, 2018).	This one-group pretest–posttest design examined the efficacy of experiential training for improving the empathy of nursing students in terms of capacity building, empathic performance, and increased learning perception and retention of materials. The educational intervention was shown to be effective for improving empathy of the university nursing students in the study. The authors recommend this type of experiential training for students in the health care professions (Bas-Sarmiento, Fernández-Gutiérrez, Baena-Baños, et al., 2017).
Case–control or cohort study	Researchers study one group of subjects with a certain condition (e.g., obesity) at the same time as another group of subjects who do not have the condition to determine if there is an association between the condition and predictor variables (e.g., exercise pattern, family history, history of depression).	The objective of this descriptive cohort design was to validate the Cultural Capability Measurement Tool with a cohort of health professional students to better provide care to Indigenous peoples. The tool was tested for reliability, content, and construct validity using confirmatory factor analysis, and concurrent validity using the Cultural Understanding Self-Assessment Tool. Cronbach's alpha coefficient of 0.86 was obtained and a five-factor solution was confirmed. Measuring nursing students' cultural capabilities can inform their development of a culturally safe nursing workforce (West, Mills, Rowland, et al., 2018).
Descriptive study	Study describes the concepts under study. It sometimes examines the prevalence, magnitude, or characteristics of a concept.	This descriptive study describes nursing activities in primary care settings with patients experiencing chronic illness. The study provides a broad description of nursing activities in five domains: global assessment, care and case management, health promotion, nurse–physician collaboration, and planning services for patients with chronic disease (Poitras, Chouinard, Gallagher, et al., 2018).
Qualitative study	Study examines individuals' perceptions of experiences with health problems or life events and the contexts in which the experiences occur. A qualitative study provides narrative data from extensive interviews with subjects. A qualitative researcher encourages subjects to tell their story about an event or condition to obtain a full and rich description.	Researchers analyzed interviews from patients and their health care providers following abdominal surgery, to develop a conceptual framework for recovery after abdominal surgery. The most important concepts identified were "energy level," "sensation of pain," "general physical endurance," and "carrying out daily routine." Researchers found that no current instruments for measuring recovery include all of these concepts (Lee, Dumitra, Fiore, et al., 2015).
Clinical experts	Accessing clinical experts on a nursing unit is an excellent way to learn about current evidence. Clinical experts often write clinical articles on topics that require application of evidence in the literature.	This article describes how using research and personal experience led to development of an approach to help a preceptor and new nurse make the most of the preceptor experience (Nooe & Kautz, 2015).

meta-analysis involves using statistical techniques to analyze the data from the studies in the systematic review to determine statistically the strength of the evidence.

An RCT is a formal experiment for testing therapies and establishing cause and effect. A researcher tests an intervention (e.g., a mobility program or new type of wound covering) against the usual standard of care. Researchers randomly assign subjects in an RCT to either a control or a treatment group. In other words, all of the subjects in the study have an equal chance of being assigned to either group. In that way, it is not likely for the two groups to be highly different. The treatment group receives the experimental intervention at the same time the control group receives the usual standard of care. Both groups are measured for the same outcomes to determine if the experimental intervention made a difference. Following completion of an RCT, the researcher knows if the intervention leads to better outcomes than the standard of care.

More often you will find articles in the nursing literature that involve controlled trials without randomization (i.e., quasi-experimental studies) or descriptive studies. Regardless of the level of evidence, a study with relevant results helps you decide if your PICO(TS) question can be answered. For example, if a quasi-experimental study resulted in a positive clinical improvement, even though it was not a statistically significant change, the clinical change might be worth strong consideration based on its clinical significance.

The use of clinical experts is at the bottom of the evidence pyramid, but do not consider clinical experts a poor source of evidence. Expert clinicians frequently use evidence as they build their own practice, and they are rich sources of information for clinical problems.

Critique the Evidence

Continuing with the case study presented earlier, the nurses on the oncology unit conduct their unit practice committee (UPC) meeting. During the meeting Samantha and her colleagues decide that it is important to include key members of their interprofessional team (pharmacy and physiotherapy). The UPC then reviews the articles carefully, using a rapid-appraisal checklist. After the group evaluates the articles for the strength of evidence and synthesizes the findings, they decide that there is evidence for implementing hourly rounding with focused patient assessment to prevent falls. The staff notes that one of the articles recommends hourly rounding during daytime hours and rounding every 2 hours during evening and night hours. Another article summarizes fall risks for patients in an acute care hospital and highlights factors to include in a nursing assessment such as medications (e.g., antihistamines, sedatives, analgesics, and antiemetics).

Critically reviewing and analyzing the available evidence requires a systematic approach. Each source of evidence (e.g., journal article, clinical guideline, expert summary) must be reviewed to determine its value, feasibility, and utility of evidence for making a practice change. When you conduct a review, it should enable you to determine if there is evidence that answers your question. It is important to use an approach that does not bog you down by reviewing every single element of each article. The Critical Appraisal Skills Program (CASP), an international collaboration that supports the education of critical appraisal skills and provides several free appraisal tools, advocates answering three important questions when critically appraising evidence (CASP, 2017):

1. Is the study valid? You need to evaluate its methodological quality.
2. What are the results? Consider whether the study is statistically or clinically significant, or both.

3. Are the results useful? Consider how the information applies to your question.

Many organizations use appraisal checklists for recording article reviews; these can be helpful in your own article appraisal. Once you have decided that the article is relevant to your PICO(TS) question, you need to assess the validity of the study. This requires knowing the type of study, using the evidence pyramid. For example, if you have an article on an RCT to review, were subjects randomized in the study? Was the sample of subjects large enough to test the intervention effectively? What approach was used in delivering the intervention and measuring the effects? Were all subjects measured for the same outcomes? In contrast, if you read a qualitative study, did the researcher study a sufficient number and representation of subjects, and did the approach allow for a thorough and objective review of findings? Studies that are not designed well cannot provide definitive support for the evidence they aim to produce.

As you read each article, ask the next question: What are the results? Do the findings apply to your patients and practice setting? If you have an RCT, you will want to know if an intervention worked or not to help decide if it potentially makes sense to use it in your practice. Your analysis of statistics will help. For example, if an intervention was shown to be "statistically significant," the intervention shows benefit. If instead there was no statistically significant difference, you may reject the value of the intervention. However, if the intervention led to improvement even though not statistically significant, you might still consider it to have clinical value. If you have a descriptive study, you will need to decide if the information is relevant to your PICO(TS) question. For example, were characteristics of the patients in the study similar to those of your own patients?

You might also choose to review a clinical article that explains a clinical practice topic relevant to your PICO(TS) question. A clinical article is not rated for its level of evidence, but it can offer useful information, especially if you decide to implement a change related to the practice topic. To learn how to read research and clinical articles, know each of the common elements. This will help you decide if an article is complete and well explained. Articles should include the following elements:

- *Abstract*: A brief summary of the article that tells you if the article is research or clinically based. An abstract summarizes the purpose of the study or clinical topic, the major themes or findings, and the implications for practice.
- *Introduction*: Contains information about the purpose of the article and the importance of the topic for the audience who reads it. There is usually a brief discussion of supporting evidence about why the topic is important from the author's point of view.

After reading the abstract and introduction, decide if you want to continue to read the entire article. You will know if the topic of the article is similar to your PICO(TS) question or related closely enough to provide you useful information. Remember that the research question does not need to be the same as yours but close enough to offer useful information. If this is the case, continue to read the next elements of the article:

- *Literature review or background*: A good author offers a detailed background of the level of scientific or clinical information that exists about the topic of the article. The review explains what led the author to conduct a study or report on a clinical topic. Perhaps the article itself does not address your PICO(TS) question the way you desire but possibly leads you to other more useful articles. The literature review gives you a good idea of how past research led to the researcher's question.
- *Article narrative*: The "middle section" or narrative of an article differs, depending on whether it is an empirical (research) or conceptual article. A conceptual article describes something,

Common Statistical Terms

Sample Size: Number (n) of individuals in a study.

Significance: A measure that gives the likelihood that a finding or a result of a study is caused by the intervention being tested and not simply by chance. Most researchers set the level of significance at a p value of 0.05 or 0.01. For example, if the effects of an intervention (e.g., hourly rounds) are significant at $p < 0.05$, it means that the likelihood of the effect (fewer falls) occurring by chance is less than 5%; thus, it is 95% more likely that the intervention truly had an effect in reducing falls. When a study result has a p value (0.61) greater than that set (e.g., p value 0.05), the researcher has to conclude that the results were possibly by chance and the intervention had no effect.

Confidence interval (CI): The CI tells you the precision of the study with the range (e.g., range of a mean score) in which clinicians judge the confidence of the findings. A 95% CI means that clinicians can be 95% confident that their findings will be within the range given in the study.

Effect size: When the effect of an intervention is statistically significant, it does not necessarily mean that it is big, important, or helpful in decision-making. It simply means that you can be confident that there is a difference.

for example, a clinical topic, which often includes a description of a patient population, the nature of a certain disease or health problem, how it affects patients, and implications for nursing care or how to use a therapy or new technology. A research article describes the conduct of a research study, including its purpose, how the study was designed, and the results. A narrative of a research article contains several standard subsections:

- *Purpose statement:* Explains the focus or intent of a study. It identifies which concepts or variables will be researched.
- *Methods or design:* Explains how a research study is organized and was conducted to answer the research question(s). This is where you learn the type of study (i.e., RCT, case control, or qualitative). You will also learn how many subjects or people are in a study. In health care studies subjects sometimes include patients, family members, or health care staff. The language in the methods section is sometimes confusing if it explains details about how the researcher designs the study to minimize bias so as to obtain the most accurate results possible. Use your faculty member as a resource to help interpret this section.
- *Results or findings:* Conceptual and research articles have a summary section. In a conceptual article the author explains the clinical implications for the topic. In a research article the author explains the results and how the research question was answered. For example, in a qualitative study there is a thorough summary of subject narratives, which provide a description of themes and ideas that arise from the researcher's analysis of data. There is no statistical analysis of the data collected. A quantitative study includes a full description of the study subjects and a statistical analysis of findings. It is important to learn some of the common statistical terms (Box 1.3). A good author discusses limitations to a study in the Results section. The information on limitations will help you decide if you want to use the evidence from the article with your patients.
- *Clinical implications:* A research article includes a section that explains if the findings from the study have clinical implications. The researcher explains how to apply findings in a practice setting for the type of subjects studied.

As you critique each article, complete your critical appraisal checklist. You may choose to rate each article by its level and strength of evidence, using the scale of I to VIII from the evidence pyramid (see Fig. 1.1). It also helps to review multiple articles with a group of colleagues involved in the EIP process. Each person can review a single article; then you can come together as a group to review your total findings. Once all evidence has been reviewed, it is time to discuss the third important question: Are the results useful?

Use critical thinking to consider the scientific rigour of the evidence and how well it answers your area of interest. Scientific rigour is the extent to which the findings of a study are valid, reliable, and relevant to a patient population of interest. Consider the evidence in light of your patients' concerns, preferences, and values. Your review of articles offers a snapshot conclusion based on combined evidence about one focused topical area. Ethically, always consider evidence that will benefit patients and do no harm. Decide if the evidence is relevant, is easily applicable in your setting of practice, and has the potential for improving patient outcomes.

There will be times when you find that there is insufficient or no evidence to answer a PICO(TS) question. This finding warrants no change in practice because the evidence is weak and inconsistent or absent.

KNOWLEDGE-TO-ACTION FRAMEWORK

If a literature review and critique yield evidence that answers your PICO(TS) question and offer evidence that can be applied to practice, the next step is to translate that knowledge to practice. A common conceptual framework, the Knowledge-to-Action (KTA) Framework, includes two components, knowledge creation and an action cycle (Graham et al., 2006), and has been adopted by the Canadian Institutes of Health Research (CIHR) to guide the process of knowledge translation. The framework utilizes a systems perspective that is responsive and adaptive and acknowledges the unpredictability of the environment when moving evidence to action (Crockett, 2017). The action cycle provides a useful framework for knowledge translation and includes seven steps:

1. *Identifying the knowledge-to-action gaps:* Identify a situation or problem that needs to be addressed; compare the evidence and current practice—is there a gap? Involve multiple sources of evidence and engage relevant partners. Critique the evidence that you collected when doing your PICO(TS) search.
2. *Adapting knowledge to local context:* It is critical that the evidence be adapted to fit local circumstances to make it relevant and promote successful implementation of person-centred care. The assimilation of the collected evidence with professional judgement within the local context provides a comprehensive and rational basis for decision-making in patient care.
3. *Assessing barriers/facilitators to knowledge use:* Assess issues related to who will be using the evidence and in what context, as well as the evidence in and of itself, for factors that could potentially enhance or hinder knowledge use. If the barriers to practice change are excessive, adopting a practice change can be difficult, if not impossible. For example, if the oncology unit's fall program is too difficult for staff to complete, if there is inadequate staffing, or if all staff are not able to attend orientation sessions, the practice change may not be successful.
4. *Selecting, tailoring, and implementing interventions:* It is important to select and tailor the interventions to address the identified barriers to knowledge use and to enhance implementation, being mindful of the stakeholders involved, for example, health care

providers, patients, and community groups. A practice change should involve applying evidence in a manner that integrates well with existing practice for all members of the health care team. It is important to understand change theory and lobby for early adopters of the practice change to act as champions while maintaining a focus on communicating the rationale for the change and the anticipated positive outcomes. When practice changes involve other health care team members, interprofessional collaboration related to planning, implementing, and evaluating the change is crucial for optimal success.

Returning to the case study, the oncology UPC has identified evidence from multiple sources and has assessed the barriers and facilitators to knowledge use. The evidence is considered in the context of the committee members' experiences, a review of the unit fall rate reports, and knowledge of their patients' risk factors, to enable the UPC to base the knowledge in the local context of the unit and the patients. The UPC recommends a pilot fall prevention program for a 3-month period. The evidence-informed program includes several features. The patients on the unit fall during all hours of the day and night; therefore, hourly rounding will be implemented around the clock. The evidence revealed information enabling the team to develop a focused fall screening tool and nursing assessments for key fall risk factors. Registered nurses (RNs) and patients are the stakeholders; the UPC will provide professional development sessions for the RNs during scheduled work time related to fall risk factors and the new screening tool. Patients will be informed of the new program, along with the rationale for implementation. The RNs will do rounds on patients on all even hours and conduct the focused assessments of oncology patients' fall risk factors that are identified from the literature, such as lower-extremity weakness, impaired gait, general fatigue, and use of antihistamines. The nurses will inform each patient of their personal fall risks.

The UPC works with the manager to create a staff orientation schedule and sets a date for the start of the hourly rounding program pilot. Before the start date, fall rate data and number of falls with injuries from the last 3 months are collected for baseline measures.

5. *Monitoring knowledge use:* Whether the knowledge use is conceptual, instrumental, or persuasive (CIHR, 2015), once identified it needs to be monitored. There are several ways to monitor knowledge use, for example, recording the frequency of behaviour, observing for a change in attitude, or completing a care pathway.

6. *Evaluating outcomes:* Evaluative measures are to be rigorous, valid, and reliable and should consider both quantitative and qualitative information. Evaluations can be structural, process, or outcome measures (CIHR, 2015). It is important to plan how to collect baseline data on the outcomes that will evaluate the effect of practice change (e.g., the UPC will be able to use the unit's monthly quality performance report that includes fall rate and number of falls with injuries. The UPC collects values for 3 months before implementation of the program and will continue to collect the fall rate and the fall-related injury rate each month, once the new program pilot begins). Collection of outcome measures is critical:

1. Know which outcomes to measure and how to collect the measures consistently (e.g., to measure pain acuity use a self-report pain scale; to measure ambulation determine the distance a patient walks each time).

2. Be sure that the outcomes are measurable (Box 1.4). Use scales (e.g., pain and Braden Scales), physiological measures (e.g., temperature, blood pressure, pulse oximetry), survey tools, and performance improvement reports.

3. Choose outcomes that are not costly to collect. Use existing equipment if possible.

4. Educate team members on the approach to use to collect and record outcomes.

5. Limit the number of staff who collect data to ensure better accuracy and consistency in measurement. Be sure that each person collects data the same way, at the same time or frequency, and accurately.

6. Establish a way to record all data.

Evaluation of outcomes tells you if the practice change has improved conditions, created no change, or worsened conditions. It is important to include all members of the health care team and stakeholders that are involved or affected by the practice change, including patients and their families when applicable.

In the case study, the RNs record the results of the patient-focused assessment every even hour on the patient flow chart and the unregulated care provider (UCP) records during odd hours. Interprofessional collaboration occurs; the nurse consults the physiotherapist if an oncology patient is found to be at high risk for falls, to assess the patient's lower-extremity strength and overall balance and make therapy recommendations; is aware that the pharmacy will place alerts on medication administration records so nurses can monitor patients receiving antihistamines before blood transfusions; and knows that the UCP will do rounds on odd hours and make follow-up observations to be sure that patients have their toileting needs met, are comfortable, and have no further needs, and will document on the patient flow chart. Patients will be told that every hour someone will return to their room for another check. Evaluative measures include comparing fall rates and falls with injuries rates before implementation of the program to the rates 3-months post-implementation. To evaluate the process from the stakeholder's perspective, the UPC will collect short surveys from all members of the interprofessional team to determine their reactions to and acceptance of the program. Patient visits will be completed to ask them to share their experiences regarding the hourly visits by the RNs and the UCPs.

7. *Sustaining knowledge use:* Sustainability needs to be considered in relation to financial and human resources within the health care system or community, to maximize continued knowledge translation. Consider not only if the outcomes were met but also whether or not patients, families, or health care team members were affected in other ways by the change.

In the case study, 3 months after implementing the program, the oncology unit was cautiously optimistic. The average fall rate for the unit dropped from 5.1 to 3.9, and the injury rate also dropped, from 2 during the first 3 months to only 1 after the pilot began. Although it was not an outcome measure, the nurses observed a decline in patients' use of call lights, which was attributed to their knowing that nurses and UCPs would visit frequently. The nursing and physiotherapist surveys revealed that the majority of staff were enthused and agreed that hourly rounding needed to be a routine part of their unit practice. The nursing staff was able to see that the fall prevention program improved patient outcomes and gave them more time to coordinate care because of fewer distractions from patient calls.

Six months after starting the new fall prevention protocol, the fall index of the oncology unit continued to remain low. An added outcome was an improvement in patient satisfaction scores. Cathy submits the protocol for an abstract in the hospital publication, *Nursing Practice.* The outcomes of the oncology UPC

Patient Outcome Measurements

Patient Outcome	Outcome Measure
Fall occurrence	Fall index, falls with injuries
Medication adherence	Pill counts, patient self-report, number of filled prescriptions
Learning discharge instructions (topic specific)	Patient surveys, including questions on topic; nurse observations of patients performing skills (using a rating scale)
Infection occurrence	Monthly infection control reports of laboratory tests on infection incidence

knowledge-to-action project result in the development of hospital-wide hourly rounding protocols. Other units review the literature to customize the nursing assessment to their particular patient needs. The methodical and well-designed knowledge translation project led by the oncology UPC results in establishment of an evidence-informed standard for other nursing units in the hospital.

After applying evidence, it is important to engage in interprofessional collaboration to communicate the change in practice and the results. As a professional, you are responsible for communicating important information about nursing practice. Sharing evidence and the effects of any practice change motivates others within a health care setting and makes them excited about potential practice improvements on their work units. When you successfully adopt an EIP way of thinking, it becomes very natural to talk about available evidence and continue seeking solutions for problems in patient care.

Implementing EIP changes in a health care setting takes time and the commitment to do it well. Competency in EIP requires a commitment to learning new knowledge, adapting it to fit the local context, interprofessional collaboration to appropriately apply and evaluate new interventions in practice, and then finding ways to maintain and continue interventions that are consistently effective. Patients expect nursing professionals to be informed and to use the safest and most appropriate interventions. Use of the action cycle to translate evidence can enhance nursing practice and improve patients' outcomes.

CLINICAL DEBRIEF

An orthopaedic interprofessional team composed of staff nurses, a physiotherapist, and an orthopaedic surgeon has been discussing the care of patients undergoing total hip replacements. The surgeon believes that the patients should be reaching a higher level of mobility before being discharged. The physiotherapist shares concerns about not being able to see all patients in a timely manner since the number of surgeries performed has increased. The staff nurses have noted that patients' family members always seem interested in their loved one's progress. One registered nurse shares a story about a daughter of a patient who spent time coaching her father to walk a bit further, and it seemed to help. The team wonders if the family could be a more involved resource. They want to use an evidence-informed approach to improve patient care over a 6-month period.

1. Write a PICO(TS) question for the orthopaedic team's area of clinical interest.
2. The staff nurse who chairs the unit practice committee contacts the hospital librarian to collaborate on a literature search to find articles pertinent to the PICO(TS) question. The nurse tells the librarian that the team wants to see if there is evidence for their approach to improving patient mobility. The librarian helps the nurse select indexing language from the database that will be searched. Which alternative MeSH® terms might you give the librarian for the term *mobility*?
3. The staff meets to review the articles obtained from the literature review. Each member selects an article to review. The physiotherapist reviews and presents a study involving testing of an educational approach for patients who underwent knee-replacement surgery. Patients were randomly assigned to one of two groups: one group received standard patient education brochures about their surgery, and the other group attended a preoperative teaching class in which their family caregivers participated. The researcher compared the two groups for the discharge outcomes of length of stay and postoperative ambulation.
   a. Which type of study was reviewed by the physiotherapist?
   b. List two reasons why this study might be useful to the interprofessional team in planning their evidence-informed practice (EIP) project.
   c. List two reasons why this study might not be useful to the team in planning their EIP project.
4. Identify two ways members of the interprofessional team might decide to measure mobility and how might they reach that decision in the context of who is on the team.

✦ REVIEW QUESTIONS

1. Place the steps of the action cycle of the Knowledge-to-Action Framework in the correct order:
   1 _____ Select, tailor, and implement intervention(s).
   2 _____ Evaluate outcomes of the practice change.
   3 _____ Adapt the findings to the local context.
   4 _____ Monitor knowledge use.
   5 _____ Assess the barriers and facilitators to knowledge use.
   6 _____ Sustain knowledge use.
   7 _____ Identify the knowledge-to-practice gap or issue.

2. A nurse specialist is reviewing the outcome measures collected during an evidence-informed practice (EIP) project on a surgical unit. The EIP team applied evidence about giving around-the-clock (ATC) analgesics to postoperative patients instead of traditional prn (as needed) medications. The use of ATC analgesics started in September.
   1. Review the graph and describe the change in analgesic doses and pain scores.
   2. Explain if the changes were to be expected as a result of the EIP change.

	June	July	Aug	Sept	Oct	Nov
Average number of analgesic doses per patient/day in first 48 hr	8.5	9.0	8.1	10.1	11.4	12.0
Average pain scores						
24 hr postop		5.4	5.1	4.8	4.1	3.7	3.5
48 hr postop		4.9	4.2	4.6	3.9	4.1	3.3

3. An evidence-informed practice (EIP) committee on a medicine unit has selected a PICO(TS) question and reviewed and critiqued the literature and is now ready to proceed with an EIP project. Which of the following factors are essential for successful EIP project management? *(Select all that apply.)*
   1. A sufficient number of articles providing evidence for the PICO(TS) question
   2. A sponsor who has the commitment and expertise to make the project succeed
   3. Resources to accomplish the project
   4. Time schedule for a pilot project
   5. Adequate number of outcomes to be measured to determine that the EIP practice change is a success.

(e) *Visit the Evolve site for a complete list of Clinical Debrief and Review Questions answers.*

REFERENCES

Alfaro-LeFevre, R. (2016). *Critical thinking, clinical reasoning, and clinical judgment: A practical approach* (6th ed.). Philadelphia, PA: Elsevier.

Appel, L., Abrams, H., Morra, D., & Wu, R. C. (2015). Put a face to a name: A randomized controlled trial evaluating the impact of providing clinician photographs on inpatients' recall. *American Journal of Medicine, 128*(1), 82. doi:10.1016/j.amjmed.2014.08.035

Bas-Sarmiento, P., Fernández-Gutiérrez, M., Baena-Baños, M., & Romero-Sánchez, J. M. (2017). Efficacy of empathy training in nursing students: A quasi-experimental study. *Nurse Education Today, 59,* 59–65. doi:10.1016/j.nedt.2017.08.012

Brown, S. (2018). *Evidence-based nursing* (4th ed.). Burlington, MA: Jones & Bartlett Learning.

Canadian Council of Registered Nurse Regulators (CCRNR). (2012). *Competencies in the context of entry-level registered nurse practice. A report of the 2011–12 jurisdictional competency process: Entry-level registered nurses. JCP entry-level registered nurse competencies.* Ottawa, ON: Author. Retrieved from http://www.ccrnr.ca/assets/jcp_rn_competencies_2012_edition.pdf

Canadian Council of Practical Nurse Regulators (CCPNR). (2013a). *Code of ethics for licensed practical nurses Canada.* Retrieved from http://www.ccpnr.ca/wp-content/uploads/2013/09/IJLPN-CE-Final.pdf

Canadian Council of Practical Nurse Regulators (CCPNR). (2013b). *Entry-to-practice competencies for licensed practical nurses.* Retrieved from http://www.ccpnr.ca/wp-content/uploads/2013/09/IJLPN-ETPC-Final.pdf

Canadian Council of Practical Nurse Regulators (CCPNR). (2018). *Become an LPN/RPN.* Retrieved from http://www.ccpnr.ca/become-an-lpnrpn/

Canadian Institutes of Health Research (CIHR). (2015). *Knowledge translation in health care: Moving evidence to practice.* Ottawa, ON: Author. Retrieved from http://www.cihr-irsc.gc.ca/e/40618.html

Canadian Institutes for Health Information (CIHI) & Canadian Patient Safety Institute (CSPI). (2016). *Measuring patient harm in Canada. What can be done to improve patient safety?* Ottawa, ON: Author.

Canadian Nurses Association (CNA). (2010). *Position statement: Evidence informed decision making and nursing practice.* Ottawa, ON: Author.

Canadian Nurses Association (CNA). (2015). *Framework for the practice of registered nurses in Canada.* Ottawa, ON: Author. Retrieved from https://www.cna-aiic.ca/~/media/cna/page-content/pdf-en/framework-for-the-pracice-of-registered-nurses-in-canada.pdf

Canadian Nurses Association (CNA). (2017a). *Integrating health across the continuum of care.* Ottawa, ON: Author.

Canadian Nurses Association (CNA). (2017b). *Code of ethics for registered nurses.* Ottawa, ON: Author. Retrieved from https://cna-aiic.ca/~/media/cna/page-content/pdf-en/code-of-ethics-2017-edition-secure-interactive.pdf?la=en

Critical Appraisal Skills Program (CASP). (2017). *Critical appraisal skills programme.* Retrieved from https://casp-uk.net/

Crockett, L. (2017). *The knowledge-to-action framework.* Retrieved from https://medium.com/knowledgenudge/kt-101-the-knowledge-to-action-framework-7fbe399723e8

Curtis, K., Fry, M., Shaban, R. Z., & Considine, J. (2016). Translating research findings to clinical nursing practice. *Journal of Clinical Nursing, 26*(5–6), 862–872. doi:10.1111/jocn.13586

Davies, B., & Logan, J. (2018). *Reading research: A user-friendly guide for health professionals* (6th ed.). Toronto, ON: Elsevier Mosby.

Graham, I. D., Logan, J., Harrison, M. B., et al. (2006). Lost in knowledge translation: Time for a map? *Journal of Continuing Education in the Health Professions, 26*(1), 13–24. doi:10.1002/chp.47

Infusion Nurses Society (INS). (2016). Infusion therapy standards of practice. *Journal of Infusion Nursing, 39*(1S).

Kumah, E., McCherry, R., Bettany-Saltikov, J., Hamilton, S., Hogg, J., & Whittaker, V. (2018). *Evidence-informed practice versus evidence-based practice educational interventions for improving knowledge, attitudes, understanding and behavior towards the application of evidence into practice: A comprehensive systematic review of undergraduate health and social care students. The Campbell Collaboration.* Oslo, Norway: Author. Retrieved from https://www.campbellcollaboration.org/library/application-of-evidence-in-practice-health-social-care-undergradates.html

Lee, L., Dumitra, T., Fiore, J., Mayo, N., & Feldman, L. (2015). How well are we measuring postoperative "recovery" after abdominal surgery? *Quality of Life Research, 24*(11), 2583–2590. doi:10.1007/s11136-015-1008-5

Lomas, T., Etcoff, N., Van Gordon, W., & Shonin, E. (2017). Zen and the art of living mindfully: The health enhancing potential of Zen aesthetics. *Journal of Religion and Health, 56*(5), 1720–1739. doi:10.1007/s10943-017-0446-5

Nooe, A., & Kautz, D. D. (2015). Preceptorship: Combining experience with research. *Dimensions of Critical Care Nursing, 34*(2), 81–83. doi:10.1097/DCC.0000000000000100

Poitras, M., Chouinard, M., Gallagher, F., & Fortin, M. (2018). Nursing activities for patients with chronic disease in primary care settings: A practice analysis. *Nursing Research, 67*(1), 35–42. doi:10.1097/NNR.0000000000000253

Porter-O'Grady, T., & Malloch, K. (2015). *Quantum leadership* (4th ed.). Boston, MA: Jones & Bartlett Learning LLC.

Slawomirski, L., Auraaen, A., & Klazinga, N. (2017). *The economics of patient safety: Strengthening a value-based approach to reducing patient harm at the national level.* Paris, France: Organisation for Economic Co-operation and Development. Retrieved from https://psnet.ahrq.gov/resources/resource/30815/the-economics-of-patient-safety-strengthening-a-value-based-approach-to-reducing-patient-harm-at-national-level

Thompson, C. (2017). *Use the 6A's to remember the evidence-based practice process. Nursing Education Expert.* Retrieved from https://nursingeducationexpert.com/evidence-based-practice-process/

U.S. National Library of Medicine. (2015). *Fact Sheet: Medical Subject Headings (MeSH®).* Retrieved from http://wayback.archive-it.org/org-350/20180312141553/https://www.nlm.nih.gov/pubs/factsheets/mesh.html

West, R., Mills, K., Rowland, D., & Creedy, D. (2018). Validation of the First Peoples' cultural capability measurement tool with undergraduate health students: A descriptive cohort study. *Nurse Education Today, 64,* 166–171. doi:10.1016/j.nedt.2018.02.022

Whittington, J. W., Nolan, K., Lewis, N., & Torres, T. (2015). Pursuing the triple aim: The first even years. *Milbank Quarterly, 93*(2), 263–300. doi:10.1111/1468-0009.12122

Wilchesky, M., & Lungu, O. (2015). Predictive and concurrent validity of the Braden Scale in long-term care: A meta-analysis. *Wound Repair and Regeneration, 23*(1), 44–56. doi:10.1111/wrr.12261

Woodbury, M. G., & Kuhnke, J. L. (2014). Evidence-based practice vs. evidence-informed practice. What's the difference? *Wound Care Canada, 12*(1), 26–29.

2 | Transitions in Care

Written by **Michelle Aebersold, PhD, RN, CHSE, FAAN, and Paula D'Eon, RN, MN-NP**

SKILLS AND PROCEDURES

OBJECTIVES

Mastery of content in this chapter will enable the nurse to:
- Describe the role communication plays in maintaining continuity of care through a patient's admission, transition, and discharge from an acute care facility.
- Explain the purpose and importance of discharge planning.
- Identify the ongoing needs of patients in the discharge planning process.
- Explain the role of a patient's caregiver in the admission, transition, or discharge process.

MEDIA RESOURCES

- evolve http://evolve.elsevier.com/Canada/Perry/clinicalskills/
- Review Questions
- Audio Glossary
- Clinical Debrief and Review Questions Answers

PURPOSE

The coordination of resources and planning a patient's care from admission to discharge or transition from one level of care to the next is a key role of a nurse. Nurses identify patients' ongoing health care needs and anticipate physical, psychological, and social deficits that have implications for patients in resuming normal activities. A nurse involves appropriate caregivers, family members, or both in a plan of care; provides interventions, including health education; and assists in making health care resources available to patients.

STANDARDS OF CARE

- Accreditation Canada, 2019—*Required Organizational Practices Handbook–Version 14* (http://www.wrha.mb.ca/quality/files/2019ROPHandbook.pdf)
- Accreditation Canada, 2017a—*Client- and Family-Centred Care: Its History in Qmentum and a Supporting Literature Review* (https://store.accreditation.ca/products/client-and-family-centred-care-its-history-in-qmentum-and-a-supporting-literature-review)
- Accreditation Canada, 2017b—*Emergency Department* (https://store.accreditation.ca/products/emergency-department)

PRINCIPLES FOR PRACTICE

- Patients and families should be partners in care, sharing in the process of decision making.

- Patient care must be integrated across a variety of settings, services, health care practitioners, and care levels to maintain a continuum of care.
- Transitional care involves nursing actions implemented to ensure coordination and continuity of care for patients who transition between different settings or levels of care.
- Transitions of care require careful attention to communication to ensure patient safety.
- Discharge planning begins at the time of admission to a facility, or even earlier when a patient uses an outpatient clinic or testing centre to begin their care journey.

PERSON-CENTRED CARE

- Social determinants of health (SDOH) impart an array of cultural, political, economic, social, and environmental conditions that shape the circumstances in which individuals are born, grow up, live, work, and age. In Canada, many individuals face greater obstacles to good health on the basis of one or more of the following factors: age; gender; race; ethnicity; culture; religion; sexual orientation and gender identity; income and social status; education; social support networks; employment or working conditions; social and physical environments; mental health; cognitive, sensory, or physical disability; or other characteristics historically linked to discrimination or exclusion (Mantoura & Morrison, 2016; Mikkonen & Raphael, 2010). As a nurse, your admission assessment should identify relevant SDOH and must

incorporate patients' cultural beliefs and practices so you can provide a person-centred approach to care.

- Be aware of how SDOH and cultural variables will affect your patient and family assessment, approach to nursing care, and teaching during admission or discharge. It is essential to involve the patient and caregiver(s) in making decisions about care activities.
- Assess the patient's preferences for language, communication and learning styles and modify your approach to meet their needs as appropriate. Inadequate access to language services can compromise patient outcomes (Registered Nurses Association of Ontario [RNAO], 2015).

EVIDENCE-INFORMED PRACTICE

Many of today's patients have complex health needs that often call for more than one discipline to address their health status (Karam, Brault, Van Durme, et al., 2018). Interprofessional collaboration for patients experiencing transitions in care can take on many forms, such as scheduled caregiver meetings to discuss discharge arrangements; formal patient rounds to further explore the effectiveness of interventions; and frequent brief team huddles for providing team members with patient progress updates, to name just a few (McBeth, Durbin-Johnson, & Siegel, 2017).

Regardless of the form it takes, interprofessional collaboration involves the formation of a team or partnership between the patient, caregiver, or both and at least two or more health care providers whose aim is to collaboratively address common goals, such as patient safety, patient satisfaction, provider satisfaction, and improved care outcomes (Karam et al., 2018; McBeth et al., 2017). Nurses have several opportunities to engage in interprofessional collaboration; because of their close relationships with their patients, they are ideally positioned to be advocates for their patients and can offer valuable insights related to their patients' health circumstances and their individual and caregiver strengths and challenges (Karam et al., 2018). The nurse works as part of the interprofessional team to ultimately enhance quality patient care. Through their leadership and communication skills, nurses play a key role in cultivating an environment in which the skills, abilities, and knowledge of all members of the care team are respected and recognized in the shared decision-making process (Karam et al., 2018).

Nurse-to-nurse hand-offs performed effectively during care transitions (e.g., from shift to shift or transitions to different levels of care settings or different facilities) can enhance patient safety by reducing risk of injury in multiple aspects of patient care, including falls (RNAO, 2015) and medication errors (Kear, 2016).

- The use of standardized hand-off tools (e.g., checklists, Situation, Background, Assessment, Recommendation [SBAR]) (see Chapter 3) can reduce hand-off–related errors and helps to ensure patient safety and that critical information is communicated (Accreditation Canada, 2017c; Usher, Nones Cronin, & York, 2018; Zou & Zhang, 2016).
- Verbal hand-offs at the bedside serve important functions beyond information exchanges. They have been shown to improve nurse-to-nurse communication and satisfaction and should be retained in practice. Greater consideration is needed in analyzing hand-offs from a patient-centred perspective (Kear, 2016; Taylor, 2015). Nurse satisfaction with the use of information technology may enhance the effectiveness and standardization of communication processes, benefiting nurse–patient and nurse-to-nurse communications (Chapman, Schweickert, Swango-Wilson, et al., 2016).
- Medication reconciliation involves the process of creating the best possible medication history (BPMH) of the medications a patient is taking, including medication name, dosage, frequency, and route, and comparing that list with the health care provider's prescriptions, with the goal of providing correct medications to the patient at all care transition points (Accreditation Canada, 2019; Canadian Patient Safety Institute [CPSI], 2017; RNAO, 2014).
- Medication reconciliation prevents medication errors such as omissions, duplications, drug errors, or medication interactions (Accreditation Canada, 2017d; RNAO, 2014).
- Protocols and processes for medication reconciliation must be in place. Medications need to be reviewed by either the nursing staff or pharmacy with the patient at the following transition points: on admission, during transitions between levels of care, creating new medication administration records (MARs), and at discharge (Accreditation Canada, 2017d; Buck & Picinbono-Larose, 2018; RNAO, 2014). Medications should be reviewed at discharge, and it should be emphasized to the patient the importance of keeping an updated list of medications and taking it along for future visits to hospital or their health care provider (Accreditation Canada, 2017d; Buck & Picinbono-Larose, 2018; RNAO, 2014).

SAFETY GUIDELINES

- Identify whether a patient has a sensory or communication need (e.g., hearing aid, glasses, need for an interpreter).
- Identify if a patient uses any assistive devices and be sure that each is provided and deemed safe to use.
- Screen all patients on admission to a health care setting for possible discharge needs to ensure that appropriate teaching is completed to ensure a safe discharge.
- Include the patient, caregiver, and relevant health care providers early in planning care to promote successful transition through the health care system.
- Consider a patient's educational background, health literacy level, and ability to understand instructions.
- Use interprofessional collaboration (e.g., dietitian, social worker, pharmacist, physiotherapist) to assess appropriate resources needed as patients transition through the health care system.
- Use interprofessional collaboration to develop a plan of care for discharge to ensure a safe transition to home or an alternate care facility.

◆ SKILL 2.1   Admitting Patients

Patients enter health care systems in a variety of ways (e.g., hospital, clinic, presurgical screening visits, or health care provider's offices). The admission process is typically the first experience a patient has with a health care facility. There are common procedures for admitting patients to these settings (Box 2.1). Most patients enter the health care system through a standardized admission process that often requires an extensive registration. However, some patients require emergency admission. A patient admitted through the emergency department (ED) is often not able to undergo the same registration process that takes place in a hospital admission office. Level of consciousness, pain, or other symptoms may prevent the patient from being a reliable resource. Caregivers or family members

BOX 2.1

Common Procedures for Admission to a Health Care System

- Placement of patient in appropriate receiving area
- Explanation of patient's rights (Accreditation Canada, 2017d; RNAO, 2014) and elements of advance directives
- Orientation to relevant health care employer policies and procedures and room environment
- Assessment of patient's health care problems and needs (e.g., risk for falls, pressure injuries, and allergies)
- Preliminary testing and screening (specific for each facility and patient's condition)
- Development of a person-centred plan of care
- Determination of patient's payment source for facility fees (e.g., ward, semi-private or private room) or health care for non-residents of Canada.

BOX 2.2

The Five Pillars of the *Canada Health Act*

Standard 1: Public Administration
- The provincial and territorial plans must be administered and operated on a nonprofit basis by a public authority.

Standard 2: Comprehensiveness
- The provincial and territorial plans must insure all medically necessary services provided by acute care facilities, physicians, and dentists (when the service must be performed in an acute care facility).
- Medically necessary services are not defined by the *Canada Health Act*. The provincial and territorial health care insurance plans consult with their respective physician colleges or groups. Together, they decide which services are medically necessary for health care insurance purposes.
- If a service is considered medically necessary, the full cost must be covered by the public health care insurance plan.

Standard 3: Universality
- The provincial and territorial plans must cover all residents.

Standard 4: Portability
- The provincial and territorial plans must cover all residents when they travel within Canada. Limited coverage is also required for travel outside the country.
- When a person relocates to another province, they can continue to use their original health care insurance card for 3 months, giving them time to register for the new plan and receive their new health insurance card.

Standard 5: Accessibility
- The provincial and territorial plans must provide all residents reasonable access to medically necessary services. Access must be based on medical need and not the ability to pay.

Adapted from Anthony S. E., & Krahn M. (2015). Healthcare in Canada and issues of health-care reform. In D. Gregory, C. Raymond-Seniuk, L. Patrick, & T. Stephen (Eds.), *Fundamental: Perspectives on the art and science of Canadian nursing* (pp. 28–31). Philadelphia: Wolters Kluwer Health.

usually provide pertinent information for the facility records while the health care team cares for the patient. In contrast, an older person with self-care limitations undergoes extensive screening before being admitted into a long-term care facility.

Hospital registration staff and technicians are often the personnel involved in the preliminary admission process, such as interviewing patients and reviewing information related to provincial/territorial health insurance coverage (e.g., health care card number), demographic data, and facility regulations. A nurse performs the nursing admission assessment (see Chapter 8).

Admission Process

When admitted to hospital, patients should receive information about their safety, patient rights and responsibilities; and privacy (Accreditation Canada, 2017b; RNAO, 2014). A private interview area should be used to provide patients and caregivers a place to reveal important identifying information, including a patient's full legal name, age, date of birth, address, next of kin, health care provider, religious preference, occupation, provincial/territorial health card coverage, and any private insurance coverage. When a patient has severe hearing impairment, the caregiver or a speech and language pathologist may assist. If a patient does not speak English, a professional interpreter may be available, depending on the facility resources, to help during the admission procedure.

An identification (ID) bracelet that legibly states a patient's full legal name, address, acute care facility or provincial/territorial health card number, health care provider, and date of birth is secured to the patient's wrist. Health care providers use information from the ID band to identify a patient when administering medications and performing treatments or procedures. In many health care settings, an ID band contains a patient's unique bar code that then makes it easy to identify a patient for all prescribed procedures. Bar-code wristbands are typically created at the point of admission, and specific patient information is continually updated on the basis of patients' needs (Accreditation Canada, 2017b). If a patient is unconscious, the nurse cannot perform ID until a caregiver or family member arrives. When there is no family available, hospital staff provide an individualized ID band for the patient until the person can be identified. A patient who has been a victim of crime is given an anonymous name on their ID band under the facility's "blackout" or "do not publish" procedure.

Canada's Health Care System

Medicare is a term that refers to Canada's publicly funded national health care system. Instead of having a single national plan, Canada

has 13 provincial and territorial health care insurance plans (Anthony & Krahn, 2015). This system ensures all Canadian residents have reasonable access to medically necessary acute care facility and health care provider services without paying out of pocket (Government of Canada, 2016a). The provincial and territorial governments are responsible for the management, organization, and delivery of health care services for their residents. The federal government is responsible for:

- Setting and administering national standards for the health care system through the *Canada Health Act* (Box 2.2)
- Providing funding support for provincial and territorial health care services
- Supporting the delivery for health care services to specific groups (Indigenous people living on reserves, Inuit, serving members of the Canadian Forces, eligible veterans, inmates in federal penitentiaries, some groups of refugee claimants)
- Providing other health-related functions, such as the regulation of consumer products (e.g., food, pharmaceuticals, cosmetics, chemical, pesticides, medical and medical devices)
- Supporting health research, health promotion and protection, and disease monitoring and prevention
- Providing tax support for health-related costs, such as tax credits and rebates and deductions for those with a disability, caregivers, and dependents living with a disability (Anthony & Krahn, 2015)

Adopted in 1984, the *Canada Health Act* is Canadian government legislation that defines the conditions and criteria to which the

provincial and territorial health insurance programs must conform in order to receive federal transfer payments under the Canada Health Transfer. This financial funding to the provinces and territories assists them with the sustainability of programs and services. There are four main transfers of funds: the Canada Health Transfer (CHT), the Canada Social Transfer (CST), Equalization, and Territorial Formula Financing (TFF). The CHT and CST are transfers that support specific policy areas such as health care, post-secondary education, social assistance and social services, early childhood development, and child care. The equalization and TFF programs provide unconditional transfer funds to the provinces and territories. Equalization enables less prosperous provincial governments to provide their residents with public services that are reasonably comparable to those of other provinces; TFF provides territorial governments with funding to support public services, in recognition of the higher cost of providing programs and services in the North (Anthony & Krahn, 2015; Government of Canada, 2017). In 2018–19, it is estimated that provinces and territories will receive $75.4 billion through major transfers (Government of Canada, 2017).

Patients and families also have responsibilities, including provision of truthful information, observing the rules and regulations of the facility, reporting any safety concerns, and treating others with respect (Accreditation Canada, 2017c; RNAO, 2014). During admission to a facility, a resuscitation care plan should be established outlining what measures the patient would like the health care team to take in the event they stop breathing or their heart stops (e.g., do not resuscitate [DNR], allow natural death [AND]). Patients should also receive information about advance directives and be referred to appropriate resources if they want to discuss or receive help in completing an advance directive document (Box 2.3).

Privacy is a core value deeply rooted in the nursing profession and is a fundamental right of all individuals (CNA, 2017). Privacy has become a matter of increasing concern in health care. With the growing adoption of electronic medical records, there are increasing demands for the use of electronic health care data in health research (CNA, 2018). Federal privacy laws include the *Privacy Act of Canada*, which came into force on July 1, 1983, and the *Personal Information Protection and Electronic Documents Act (PIPEDA)*, effective January 1, 2004. The *Privacy Act* governs the personal-information handling practices of federal government departments and agencies. PIPEDA governs the collection, use, and disclosure of personal information in connection with commercial activities, including personal health information. Under PIPEDA, organizations need to obtain consent from individuals before collecting, using, or disclosing their personal information. They must also have appropriate security safeguards in place to protect personal information. In instances where there may be privacy breach or complaint, PIPEDA outlines an ombudsman model in which complaints are directed to the Office of the Privacy Commissioner of Canada (Office of the Privacy Commissioner of Canada, 2015). Individuals have the right to withhold consent, to access personal information about themselves held by an organization, to have it corrected if necessary, and to have recourse for a suspected information breach (Box 2.4). Several provinces and territories have their own privacy legislation. The Government of Canada requires all provinces and territories to comply with PIPEDA. Provinces whose legislation is deemed "substantially similar" to PIPEDA are exempt, whereas provinces whose legislation is not deemed similar to PIPEDA are not exempt (Office of the Privacy Commissioner of Canada, 2015). The CNA's *Code of Ethics for Registered Nurses* (2017) helps to guide nurses through the decision-making process for ethical dilemmas involving privacy issues.

Role of the Nurse

On admission to a patient care area, nurses complete a thorough nursing assessment, review any advance directives, and ensure that necessary diagnostic testing is completed. If patients were receiving health care before admission (e.g., home health care, long-term care), a nurse from the sending area provides appropriate information to the receiving nurse for continuity of care. In this situation, the nurse from the sending care area or facility should explain to the nurse receiving the hand-off report information about the patient's condition and why the patient is being admitted or transitioned to the particular health care setting (Camicia & Lutz, 2016; RNAO, 2014).

BOX 2.3

Advance Directives

- An advance directive is a document that describes which medical treatment or nonmedical treatment a patient chooses for future medical care or designates another person(s) to make medical decisions if the individual loses decision-making capacity (Dalhousie University Health Law Institute n.d.; Government of Canada, 2016b).
- An advance directive conveys the patient's choices for medical care when the patient is unable to speak or make decisions.
- Advance directives may include a living will, power of attorney for health care, or notarized handwritten document.
- A copy of the document should be available in the patient's medical record. If not available, the details of the advance directive should be documented in the medical record, and a family member should be asked to bring the advance directive to the facility (Accreditation Canada, 2017b).
- The attending health care provider is notified of the patient's advance directive.
- Witnesses for an advance directive document should not be medical personnel, nor should they be related to the patient or heirs to the patient's estate.
- Each province/territory has differing requirements related to advance directives; ensure that you verify your province's/territory's requirements (Walton, 2016).

BOX 2.4

Patients' Rights

Health care laws and regulations vary slightly by province or territory, but generally Canadians share the following rights:
- The right to informed consent
- The right to recognition of a substitute decision-maker
- The right to recognition of an advance care plan
- The right to a second opinion
- The right to confidentiality and privacy of personal health information
- The right to pain and symptom management
- The right to refuse treatment
- The right to request an assisted death
- The right to end-of-life care
- The right to advance directives
- The right to organ procurement

Based on Accreditation Canada. (2017). *Standards: Long-term care services (ver. 11)*. Retrieved from http://intra.nshealth.ca/accreditation/SitePages/Standards.aspx; Dying With Dignity Canada. (2016). *Patient rights booklet*. Retrieved from http://www.dyingwithdignity.ca/patient_rights_booklet; Registered Nurses' Association of Ontario. (2014). *Clinical best practice guidelines care transitions*. Toronto, ON: Author. Retrieved from http://rnao.ca/sites/rnao-ca/files/Care_Transitions_BPG.

Nursing staff should ensure that a patient's room assignment is based on the patient's condition, health care needs, developmental level, activity level, expected length of stay, and personal preferences. For example, the best room for an older person who is acutely ill, at risk for falls, and receiving multiple treatments is one close to the nurses' station. The nurse identifies if a patient has any known allergies and, if any exist, places an allergy band on the patient and properly documents the known allergies in the medical record.

When a patient is admitted through the ED, the ED nurse provides a verbal report over the phone to a unit nurse receiving the patient. The ED nurse provides details on the patient's admission information, including their name; admitting health care provider; chief complaint; and any treatments or testing completed and the outcome, diagnosis, and pertinent information related to the patient's condition (e.g., initial vital signs, allergies, level of consciousness, and intravenous [IV] therapy). A physical hand-off report is seldom given, as most often the patient is brought to the care area by an escort (usually a facility porter or unregulated health care worker), who takes the patient and caregiver to the nursing unit and introduces them to the nurse assuming the patient's care. The ED nurse shares pertinent observations about the patient's behaviour (e.g., anxiety, fear, or level of knowledge regarding need for health care) with the nursing staff to foster continuity of care and help the patient and caregiver adjust to a new health care environment.

Many patients go to an acute care facility in advance for necessary preoperative diagnostic testing. In some cases, these patients and their caregivers also attend preoperative education classes. Other patients have contact with health care providers for the first time when they arrive at an acute care facility. Patients admitted on the morning of a surgical procedure or treatment are "same-day" admissions. A nurse provides basic instructions about the purpose of the surgery or treatment, preparatory procedures, and postsurgical or posttreatment care. Admission and consent forms, diagnostic tests, preoperative patient teaching (see Chapter 37), and instructions are usually completed before the actual day of surgery. When nurses are able to see patients several days in advance, they use a variety of resources, such as Internet sites, classes, videos, information booklets, and telephone calls, for patient teaching.

Nurses actively coordinate the initial admission process for all patients. A patient's condition influences the extent and type of admission activities. The nurse must always note the patient's level of fatigue and comfort. For example, when a critically ill patient reaches a critical care nursing unit, they undergo extensive examination and treatment procedures immediately. There may be little time available for the nurse to orient the patient and caregiver to the unit or learn of the patient's fears or concerns. When a patient enters an acute care facility for elective treatment, the nurse has more time to prepare the person psychologically for the stay and optimize patient outcomes with preadmission planning.

Delegation and Collaboration

The skill of completing the nursing assessment during admission to a health care facility cannot be delegated to an unregulated care provider (UCP). The nurse directs the UCP to:
- Prepare the patient's room with equipment needed before admission.
- Gather and secure the patient's personal care items.
- Escort and orient the patient and caregiver to the nursing unit.

Equipment

- Hospital gown
- Bedpan and urinal (if needed)
- Washbasin, bath towel, and washcloth
- Toiletry items (e.g., soap, toothpaste, hand lotion; *optional* in some facilities)
- Facial tissues
- Water pitcher and drinking cup
- Kidney or emesis basin
- Disposable thermometer (see employer policy)
- Sphygmomanometer
- Stethoscope
- Clean gloves
- Pulse oximeter (*optional*)
- Computer and documentation forms (see employer policy)

STEP	RATIONALE

ROOM PREPARATION

STEP	RATIONALE
1. Perform hand hygiene and prepare room equipment and furniture. Prepare bed by adjusting it to the lowest horizontal position if patient is ambulatory. Place bed in high position if patient is arriving by stretcher. Turn down top sheet and bedspread. Arrange room furniture for easy access to bed. Adjust lights, temperature, and ventilation.	Promotes patient's comfort by preventing delays during admission. Proper position of bed lessens likelihood of patient fall during transfer and also reduces risk of back injuries to staff helping patient into bed.
2. Be sure that equipment is in working order. Assemble any special equipment (e.g., suction, oxygen supplies, or IV pole) in patient's room.	Prevents delays in delivering immediate treatment and provides for smooth transition between caregivers.

ASSESSMENT

STEP	RATIONALE
1. Identify patient using at least two person-specific identifiers (e.g., name and date of birth or name and medical record number) according to employer policy.	Ensures correct patient. Complies with Accreditation Canada's standards and improves patient safety (Accreditation Canada, 2019).
2. Greet patient and caregiver cordially by name. Introduce yourself by full name (unless directed by employer policy to use first name only) and job title; explain your responsibilities in patient's care.	Providing personalized care reduces anxiety about admission, clarifies staff roles, and expedites patient requests.

STEP	RATIONALE

ASSESSMENT

3. If patient does not speak, read, or understand English, arrange for a professional translator to help with the nursing assessment. Use telephone interpreter services as a supplemental system when an interpreter is needed instantly or when services are needed in an unusual or infrequently encountered language (Accreditation Canada, 2017c).

Translation services are preferable to using caregiver or family members to promote effective communication.

4. Use interprofessional collaboration (e.g., speech and language pathologist) when a patient has a severe hearing impairment.

A speech and language pathologist may have augmented hearing devices or resources to facilitate communication of assessment data.

5. Assess patient's general appearance. Note signs or symptoms of physical distress (see Chapter 8).

Provides baseline assessment.

Clinical Decision Point *If patient is having acute physical problems, postpone routine admission procedures and nursing history until their needs are met. Complete a focused assessment at this point.*

6. Assess patient's ability to understand and implement health information by asking a health literacy question, such as "How comfortable are you filling out medical forms by yourself?" The Rapid Estimate of Adult Literacy in Medicine–Short Form (REALM-SF) is a reliable and valid tool with a list of seven words you ask a patient to read to determine their level of health literacy on grade scale. For every correct word, the patient receives 1 point. Patients who score 7 points are considered high school completion level and will be able to read most patient education materials. The tool is available online at https://medicine.osu.edu/sitetool/sites/pdfs/ahecpublic/REALM_SF.pdf.

This helps you determine at what reading level a patient can read, allowing you to select the appropriate level of educational material and teaching methods, such as Teach-Back (CPSI, 2017).

7. Assess patient's and caregiver's psychological status by noting verbal and nonverbal behaviours and responses to greetings and explanations.

Anxiety influences how well a patient adapts to a health care environment and retains instruction.

8. Assess vital signs (see Chapter 7), height and weight (see Chapter 8), and patient's level of discomfort (using an appropriate pain rating scale (see Chapter 16).

Provides baseline measurement to compare future findings. Determines alterations from normal range.

9. Assess for fall risk using an appropriate assessment tool (see employer policy). Ask patient to walk at end of bed and note gait and movement. Consider patient's risk factors (e.g., individual intrinsic factors: comorbidities (neurological disorders), muscle weakness, unsteady gait, and urinary incontinence (Buck, 2018); transient factors: postural hypotension, polypharmacy, and use of high-risk medications (e.g., analgesics, antihypertensives) (Buck, 2018).

Having a patient walk allows you to more objectively assess the patient's gait and level of strength rather than asking the patient if they have walking limitations.

Provides data to determine patient's risk for injury and whether they need to be placed on fall precautions. For acute care facility inpatients, the maximum time frame for completing fall risk admission assessments is 24 hours (Accreditation Canada, 2017b; RNAO, 2014).

10. Have caregivers leave room unless patient wishes to have them help with changing into a hospital gown or pajamas. Close door and curtains. Help patient undress and into comfortable position.

Demonstrates person-centred care because it provides for privacy and prepares patient for examination.

11. Obtain nursing history as soon as possible after patient's arrival to the nursing unit. Apply standards of nursing care adopted by facility (e.g., functional health patterns). Data include the following:

Each patient is to have an admission assessment prepared by a registered nurse (RN) (Accreditation Canada, 2017d). Each facility sets a time frame for completion of admission assessment (maximum time 24 hours).

a. Patient's perception of illness and health care needs

Establishes a baseline of patient's clinical status and enhances the nurse's understanding of the patient's perspective.

b. Past medical history

c. Presenting signs and symptoms and reason for admission or transition in care

Identifies signs and symptoms in case patient's condition deteriorates.

d. Completion of a review of health status based on standards such as elimination, respiration, nutrition and metabolism, activity and exercise, self-concept, values and beliefs, cultural factors, social support, and cognitive function

Provides a holistic view of patient's health issues and response to those issues.

STEP	RATIONALE

ASSESSMENT

e. Risk factors for illness

Allows you to institute preventive care measures and educate patient about health promotion behaviours.

f. History of allergies, including type of substance and a description of the reaction that patient has previously experienced

Patients often have sensitivity to a medication or substance rather than a true allergy; this needs to be clarified. Specify all allergens to prevent accidental exposure.

Clinical Decision Point *Provide patient with allergy arm band listing allergies to foods, medications, latex, or other substances; document allergies according to employer policy.*

g. Detailed medication history, including prescribed, over-the-counter (OTC), and alternative therapies such as herbs, hormones, and natural health products

Assesses potential for medication interactions; information often explains patient's presenting signs and symptoms.

h. Patient's knowledge of health problems and expectations of care

Enables the nurse to recognize and meet patient expectations when possible.

12. Apply clean gloves as appropriate. Conduct physical assessment of appropriate body systems (see Chapter 8). Inform patient of any necessary or additional specimens that need to be collected.

Provides objective data for identifying health problems. Unannounced procedures can make patients anxious. Preparation of patient relieves anxiety.

a. A priority is to assess a patient's skin integrity and any current skin breakdown at admission. Use a risk for pressure injury development scale (e.g., Braden Scale, Norton Scale [see Chapter 39]) to assess risk for potential skin breakdown. After assessment is complete, remove and dispose of gloves and perform hand hygiene.

Provides baseline data for pressure injury prevention and identifies the presence of any previously acquired pressure injuries when patient is admitted. Existing pressure injuries must be documented within 24 hours of admission (Accreditation Canada, 2017c; RNAO, 2014). Pressure injuries that develop while a patient is in an acute care facility are considered an adverse event or incident and become the financial responsibility of the facility responsible for their care.

b. Some facilities are now requiring assessment of risk for obstructive sleep apnea (OSA) in surgical patients (see Chapter 37). See employer policy. The STOP-Bang questionnaire has been specifically developed to meet the need for a reliable, concise, and easy-to-use screening tool. It consists of eight (yes/no) items related to the clinical features of sleep apnea (Snoring, Tiredness, Observed apnea, high blood Pressure, body mass index [BMI], Age, Neck circumference, and male Gender). The total score ranges from 0 to 8. Patients can be classified for their OSA risk based on their respective scores (http://stopbang.ca/translation/pdf/caeng.pdf).

STOP-Bang score was validated in obese and morbidly obese surgical patients. For identifying severe OSA, a STOP-Bang score of 4 has high sensitivity of 88%. For confirming severe OSA, a score of 6 is more specific (Nagappa, Wong, Singh, et al., 2017). Allows you to institute appropriate postoperative observations. OSA is a potentially serious sleep disorder in which breathing repeatedly stops and starts during sleep. Surgical patients with OSA are considered at risk for relaxation of their throat muscles and blockage of the airway during recovery from anaesthesia and sedation (Ross, 2016).

13. Check health care providers' prescriptions for treatment measures to initiate immediately.

Delay can cause deterioration of patient's condition.

14. Ask patient to identify their values regarding health care and needs or expectations of care: "To what extent do you believe being in the hospital will help you? Tell me what you hope will happen during your hospital stay? Tell me what is important to you for your care here to be satisfactory." **NOTE:** Incorporate these questions during the physical examination.

Patient-centred care requires incorporation of patient needs, preferences, and values (Accreditation Canada, 2017b; RNAO, 2014).

15. Orient patient to patient care unit.

a. Introduce staff members who enter room. Always introduce patient by last name unless patient indicates otherwise.

Helps patient recognize caregivers. Demonstrates person-centred care by showing respect for patient.

b. Tell patient and caregiver the name of the nurse in charge of the unit/division and explain that person's role and responsibilities.

Provides means for patient and caregiver to understand unit/division communication structure.

c. Explain visiting hours and their purpose (i.e., to provide time to administer needed procedures and give patient time to rest).

Provides knowledge and increases willingness to observe policy for visiting hours.

STEP	RATIONALE

ASSESSMENT

d. Discuss smoking policy and identify smoking areas for patient and caregiver, if available.

A facility-wide smoking policy that prohibits the use of smoking materials throughout the facility is required. Some facilities may have a designated smoking area.

e. Demonstrate use of equipment (e.g., bed, over-bed table, lighting).

Patient's safety depends on patient understanding correct use of equipment.

f. Show patient how to use nurse call light and position it in a convenient place. Have patient demonstrate use of light. Discuss with patient their specific fall risks and encourage the patient to ask for help when getting out of bed.

Ensures that patient knows why and how to call for assistance.

g. Escort patient to bathroom (if able to ambulate).

Patient's safety depends in part on understanding how to use toilet facilities.

Clinical Decision Point *Ensure that patient knows how to call for help while in bathroom. (An emergency call light is usually in bathrooms.)*

h. Explain hours for mealtime and nourishments to patient and caregiver.

Caregiver often wishes to visit during evening to help with meals.

i. Describe services available (e.g., chaplain, beauty shop, activity therapy).

Offers patient options for making decisions.

NURSING DIAGNOSES

- Acute pain
- Chronic pain
- Anxiety
- Fear

- Insufficient knowledge regarding hospital procedures and planned therapies
- Inadequate coping, individual or caregiver

- Powerlessness
- Potential for injury
- Potential for falls

Related factors/Risk factors are individualized based on patient's condition or needs.

PLANNING

1. Expected outcomes following completion of procedure:

- Patient is able to explain purpose and schedule of planned treatments and procedures.

Understanding treatment plan gives patient a better sense of control and reduces anxiety about the unknown.

- Patient demonstrates how to call for nurse when help is needed.

Falls commonly occur when patients attempt to get out of bed without help.

- Patient is able to ambulate (if condition permits) in room free of obstacles.

Ensures patient safety and mobility in room.

- Patient can safely and efficiently use equipment in the room.

Equipment used in care of patient frequently poses hazards; helps to reduce some anxiety.

- Patient verbalizes understanding of smoking policy, visiting hours, mealtimes, and services available.

Knowledge of facility policies helps patient adapt to the health care environment.

- Patient self-reports improved comfort.

Basic pain and comfort measures are effective.

IMPLEMENTATION

1. Perform hand hygiene. Complete patient medication reconciliation by checking home medication list for duplication, omission, or potential medication interactions with newly prescribed medications. Update medication list based on health care provider's prescriptions for treatment. Follow employer policy.

Medication reconciliation on admission helps to make sure that the patient is taking the correct medications and avoids medication errors (Accreditation Canada, 2017b; RNAO, 2014).

2. Inform patient about procedures or treatments scheduled for the next shift or day (e.g., visits by health care provider or dietitian). These vary based on nature of patient's condition.

Patient has right to be informed of any scheduled procedures or treatments. Being able to anticipate planned therapies minimizes anxiety.

3. Perform basic comfort measures (positioning, temperature of room) and administer analgesic (if prescribed). Remove and dispose of gloves.

Enables patient to participate in planned therapies and education.

STEP	RATIONALE

IMPLEMENTATION

4. Complete learning readiness and learning needs assessment for patient and caregiver.

5. Give patient and caregiver a chance to ask questions about procedures or therapies and to share their personal goals of care. (If patient is unresponsive or unable to understand, review with caregiver.)

6. Collect valuables that patient chooses to keep at bedside. Complete clothing and valuables listing sheet (see employer policy); have patient sign. Place valuables in facility safe or send home with caregiver.

7. Ensure that patient and caregiver have time together alone if desired.

8. Be sure that call light is within easy reach and bed is in low position.

9. Perform hand hygiene.

Rationale column:

Identifies patient's and caregiver's educational needs and learning preferences.

Provides opportunity to clarify expectations and misconceptions. Provides for shared decision making.

Accounts for placement of valuables and prevents loss.

Admission is often stressful and fatiguing. Allows time for decision making.

Provides for patient safety.

Reduces spread of microorganisms.

EVALUATION

1. Have patient explain own fall risks, facility policies, tests, and procedures through discussion and questions.

2. Ask patient to describe characteristics and severity of pain using an appropriate pain rating scale.

3. Have patient demonstrate use of call light.

4. Monitor patient's ability to ambulate independently.

5. Check patient's room setup regularly.

6. **Use Teach-Back:** After providing the patient with education on how to activate the call light system and discussing the importance of preventing falls by calling for assistance before getting out of bed, the nurse uses teach-back to ensure the patient has understood the instructions: "I want to be sure you understand how to use your call bell when you need help from the nurses. Can you show me how to use it and tell me when you should use it?" Develop a revised teaching plan if the patient or caregiver is not able to teach back correctly.

Rationale column:

Patient demonstrates learning and understanding through feedback.

Determines if pain severity has decreased.

Return demonstration confirms learning.

Provides data to assess patient's safety in ambulating without injury.

Determines if care area is free of obstacles.

Determines patient's and caregiver's level of understanding of instructional topic.

Unexpected Outcomes

1. Patient is unable to explain facility policies (e.g., visitation, smoking) or does not know purpose or schedule for tests and procedures.

2. Patient becomes restless, expresses concerns, or displays tension in body movements.

3. Patient falls or is injured.

Related Interventions

- Schedule follow-up session with patient.
- Keep information focused and specific to patient's situation. Include caregiver if appropriate.
- Give patient time to discuss fears and concerns.
- Reassess comfort level or change in health status.
- Demonstrate person-centred care with active listening skills and compassion, to enhance open and honest communication.
- Attend to patient's immediate physical needs.
- Inform health care provider of fall and any injuries.
- Follow the facility falls protocol (e.g., patient must have nursing assessment completed before moving and should have ongoing neurological vital signs monitored as appropriate).
- Reassess patient's environment, alter care plan as needed, ensure that the environment is free of safety hazards.
- Complete adverse event/incident report.

Communication and Documentation

- Document history and assessment findings in appropriate forms or screens of electronic health record (EHR) or chart. Begin to develop nursing plan of care.
- Document your evaluation of patient and caregiver learning.

- If patient has an advance directive, place copy in the medical record. In the absence of an actual advance directive, document the essence of the directive in the medical record (Accreditation Canada, 2017c; RNAO, 2014).

- Notify health care provider of patient's arrival; report any unusual findings. Secure admission prescriptions if not previously provided.

Special Considerations
Teaching
- Explain to patient that a different nurse provides care on each shift. Explain time frame for how assignments are made.
- Teaching occurs throughout the admission process. Provide information regarding physical assessment findings, risks for falling, nature of patient's illness, planned diagnostic and treatment procedures, medications, goals of care, and acute care facility routines.
- In an emergency or if patient is unable to perform aspects of own care, teach caregivers about the rationale for any procedures and routines to be used in patient's care.

Pediatric
- Hospitalization is a major crisis for children who feel stress from separation, loss of control, bodily injury, and pain. Separation anxiety is most common from middle infancy throughout the toddler years, especially ages 16 to 30 months. Preschoolers are better able to tolerate brief periods of separation, but their protest behaviours are more subtle than those in younger children (e.g., refusal to eat, difficulty sleeping, withdrawing from others).

School-age children can cope with separation but have an increased need for parental security and guidance (Perry et al., 2017).
- Explain the rooming-in and visiting policies of the facility. Allow and encourage parental involvement in the child's care. Allow parents to help with routine care activities (e.g., bathing, eating) and, when possible, to remain with the child during procedures.
- Parental input during admission assessment is essential because they can provide information on the child's normal behaviour and deviations caused by illness.

Gerontological
- Hospitalized older persons experience functional declines such as new-onset incontinence, malnutrition, deconditioning, pressure injuries, and falls. Use interprofessional collaboration (e.g., physiotherapy, dietitian) to plan interventions that retain functional status (Buck, 2018).
- Patients who typically fall in the acute care facility are those who have been admitted recently and are unfamiliar with surroundings, have acute illness, take four or more medications, or have been relocated recently. Visual changes that occur with aging often lead to falls in hospitalized older persons (Buck, 2018).

✦ SKILL 2.2   Transitioning Patients

Patients transition to different points of care to receive alternate forms and levels of treatment and services, and to have essential care continued closer to home. Evidence suggests that the use of interprofessional collaboration and standardized tools has a greater influence on positive patient outcomes than without using this approach (Chard & Makary, 2015). When a patient transitions to a different care level, the nurse often assumes the leadership role in ensuring the continuity of care. Nurses interact with patients and caregivers at their most vulnerable times and are often the ones who acquire information critical to successful transition planning. They play a key role in promoting successful transitions by developing, implementing, and evaluating the transition plan and identifying barriers to the plan (Camicia & Lutz, 2016).

When patients move between different points of care or health care facilities for diagnosis, treatment, and ongoing care, there is a safety risk at each interval. The hand-over (or hand-off) communication that occurs between staff on different units and between and among interprofessional teams might not include all the essential information, or information may be misunderstood. Hand-offs serve many functions, from coaching and teaching to team building, but their most important function is information processing—making sure that essential data are transferred for patient safety (Chard & Makary, 2015). Substandard or variable hand-offs have contributed to errors, care omissions, treatment delays, inefficiencies from repeated work, inappropriate treatment, adverse events with minor or major harm, increased length of stay, avoidable readmissions, and increased costs (Camicia & Lutz, 2016).

When providing a hand-off of a patient to another unit, it is essential to clearly communicate information about the patient's care, treatment, services, and current condition and any recent or anticipated changes in prescriptions in order to meet patient safety goals (Accreditation Canada, 2017c). Policies and procedures are usually similar throughout a facility.

Mnemonics such as SBAR (Situation, Background, Assessment, Recommendation) or "I PASS the BATON" (Introduction, Patient, Assessment, Situation, Safety concerns, Background, Actions, Timing, Ownership, Next) are examples of formats to use during communication of patient transitions in care that can be tailored for different clinical areas or purposes. These tools have demonstrated increased confidence for both the speaker and receiver during a hand-off report (Stewart & Hand, 2017).

In the emergency department (ED), when a patient is transferred from one facility to another, a nurse establishes the pertinent information to be included in the hand-off report. Patient circumstances will carry the most significance; however, at a minimum, details typically include the patient's full name and other person-specific identifiers, diagnoses, test results, procedures, contact information for the responsible providers, reason for the transition, and information about allergies, medications, and any advance directives (Accreditation Canada, 2017b; RNAO, 2014). Patient transitions at different points of care must be person centred (i.e., the patient agrees to the transition) and should also take into consideration the following principles:
- Responsibility for the patient's care continues until service has ended or the patient has been transitioned to another care team, service, or facility or organization.
- Use interprofessional collaboration for shared decision making and include the patient and caregiver or substitute decision maker.
- The patient's capacity and ability to make decisions needs to be considered.
- There is open and honest discussion of any risks associated with the transition.

Risk of readmission is assessed, and if applicable, appropriate follow-up is arranged. Follow-up appointment and/or community referrals are made (Accreditation Canada, 2017b; RNAO, 2014).

Delegation and Collaboration

The skill of assessment and decision making conducted during transitions cannot be delegated to an unregulated care provider (UCP). The nurse directs the UCP to:
- Help the patient with dressing.
- Gather and secure the patient's personal belongings and any equipment that goes with the patient.
- Escort the patient to the nursing unit or transport area.

Equipment

- Transfer forms
- Copies of documents such as medical records, radiology films, laboratory test results (as appropriate)

- Special equipment as needed: wheelchair or stretcher, emesis basin, bedpan and urinal, oxygen tank and tubing, intravenous (IV) pole, cardiac monitor, and emergency medications

STEP	RATIONALE

ASSESSMENT

STEP	RATIONALE
1. Identify patient using at least two person-specific identifiers (e.g., name and date of birth or name and medical record number) according to employer policy.	Ensures correct patient. Complies with Accreditation Canada's standards and improves patient safety (Accreditation Canada, 2019).
2. Obtain and review transfer prescription from sending health care provider. Prescription includes name of the receiving facility (when applicable), receiving health care provider's name, and statement of patient's stability for transfer.	Health care provider is legally responsible for releasing patient from medical care and arranging for receiving health care provider. Patient has legal right to refuse transfer against medical advice.
3. In collaboration with health care provider and members of the interdisciplinary team, assess reason for patient's transfer (e.g., change in condition, services available at the facility, patient or caregiver preferences regarding patient's location).	Patient needs to have access to facility with best resources to meet health care needs. Health care provider determines patient's physical stability for transfer.
4. Assess individuals at high risk for transitional care problems (e.g., older persons with multiple health issues, depression, non-English speakers, patients with sensory impairments, and low-income patients).	Identifying patients at risk for transitional care problems enables better continuity of care and improved patient outcomes Stewart & Hand, 2017). Patients may require consultation with needed resources (e.g., care manager, psychologist) when arriving at destination.
5. Explain purpose of transfer at care transitions thoroughly and provide time to discuss patient's and caregiver's feelings about the change in care setting. As necessary, obtain patient's written consent to transfer. If patient is unable to consent, caregiver or substitute decision-maker provides this consent.	Patients need to be informed of transfer plans in a timely manner (Accreditation Canada, 2019; RNAO, 2014). A patient requires adequate psychological preparation. In the event of a clinical emergency in which patient and caregiver are unable to consent, this consent is waived, and patient is transferred to a higher level of care on the basis of the clinical judgement of the health care provider requesting the transfer.
6. Assess patient's current physical condition and determine method for transport. When transferring to a new facility, assess method of transport to transferring vehicle (e.g., wheelchair or stretcher) (consult employer policy).	Determines level of patient stability. Patient's condition often changes quickly and influences stability for transfer and type of support needed during transport.

Clinical Decision Point *Determine if patient's status and safety require life-support equipment. Staff assisting with transfer need training in life-support measures. When transporting to new facility, a vehicle equipped with life-support equipment is necessary.*

STEP	RATIONALE
7. Assess if patient requires pain relief or other medications for symptom management.	Ensures patient's comfort during transfer.
8. Ensure that staff have notified patient's caregiver or significant others of transfer as desired by patient.	Provides adequate communication with caregiver or significant others to help with patient's emotional and psychological adjustment to the transfer (Accreditation Canada, 2019; RNAO, 2014).

NURSING DIAGNOSES

- Anxiety
- Insufficient knowledge regarding transfer procedure
- Fear
- Powerlessness
- Relocation stress syndrome

Related factors are individualized on the basis of patient's condition or needs.

PLANNING

STEP	RATIONALE
1. Expected outcomes following completion of procedure: • Patient's vital signs and physiological status remain the same following transfer. • Patient incurs no injury during transport procedures.	Treatments are planned so as not to interrupt physical support of patient during transfer. Safety measures are successful in transferring patient from wheelchair or stretcher to transport vehicle.

STEP	RATIONALE

PLANNING

- Patient or caregiver explains purpose of transfer and procedure for transport.

  Understanding provides patient with sense of control.

- Receiving nursing staff acquire and confirm written plan of care.

  Ensures continuity of care.

2. Use interprofessional collaboration (e.g., social worker) to arrange for patient's transfer to the facility.

   Transfer needs to occur without delays so that patient has access to all needed resources at all times.

3. When transfer is to a new facility, contact the facility and arrange for bed in appropriate setting. Confirm willingness of the facility to accept patient (usually social worker or discharge coordinator completes confirmation).

   Prevents delays when patient arrives at destination. Receiving facility ensures that space and qualified personnel are available to treat patients and provides confirmation in advance to accept the transferred patient.

IMPLEMENTATION

1. Make sure that documentation in patient's record is complete, with care plan that has individualized nursing care measures.

   Accurate information is necessary for receiving facility to assume patient's care.

2. Complete nursing care transfer form according to employer policy. (When transfer is to a different nursing unit, entire medical record accompanies patient.)

   Form summarizes patient's pertinent nursing care needs to ensure continuity of care and prevent unnecessary duplication of services.

3. Complete medication reconciliation per employer policy. Check patient's current prescriptions for transfer against the most recent medication administration record and the original home medication list. Communicate updated medication list to next provider of care, including last medications given, with times and doses for ongoing consistency in care (e.g., last pain medication, antipyretics, insulin).

   The new medication regimen prescribed at the time of transfer may omit needed medications, unnecessarily duplicate existing therapies, or contain incorrect dosages. Ensures that patient receives correct medications at new facility and decreases medication errors (Accreditation Canada, 2019).

4. Have UCPs gather patient's personal care items, clothing, and valuables. Check the entire room and all storage areas. Secure in suitcase or container.

   Prevents loss of articles during transfer.

5. Anticipate problems that patient frequently develops just before or during transfer. Perform necessary nursing therapies such as suctioning or changing a dressing.

   Ensures patient's comfort and safety during transport.

6. Help to transfer patient to stretcher or wheelchair using safe patient-handling techniques (see Chapter 11).

   It is easier to move a patient being transported to outside facility by stretcher into transport vehicle.

7. Perform and document final assessment of patient's physical stability.

   Minimizes risk of patient developing complications during transfer.

Clinical Decision Point *Priority assessment includes vital signs, clear airway, patency of IV tubing and accuracy of infusion rate, and patient's level of consciousness.*

8. When a patient is physically transferred to an outside facility, accompany patient to transport vehicle.

   Ensures that medically qualified personnel are in attendance until patient leaves facility/unit.

9. Call receiving facility/unit and notify of impending transfer and patient's status (check employer policy).

   Notification of nurse in charge or nurse assuming care of patient ensures better continuity of care at time of patient's arrival.

EVALUATION

1. During the final assessment compare data with the previous findings.

   Determines if patient's condition is changing.

2. Inspect patient's alignment and positioning on stretcher or in wheelchair.

   Proper alignment and positioning reduce risk of an injury occurring during transport.

3. Ensure that equipment needed for transfer is functioning.

   Equipment such as oxygen must last through transport for patient safety.

4. Confirm that patient understands transfer and procedures through discussion and questions.

   Feedback helps to ensure learning.

STEP	RATIONALE

EVALUATION

5. Determine if receiving facility/nurse has questions about patient's care.

6. **Use Teach-Back:** "I want to be sure you understand why you are being transferred to your new unit. Can you tell me why you are being transferred and what the name of your new unit is?" Develop a revised teaching plan if patient or caregiver is not able to teach back correctly.

Provides for clear communication during hand-off and continuity of care.

Determines patient's and caregiver's level of understanding of instructional topic.

Unexpected Outcomes

1. Patient's physical status deteriorates during preparation.

2. Patient is confused or uncertain about transfer.
3. Receiving staff misinterpret directions for patient's care.

Related Interventions

- Call health care provider immediately.
- Initiate interventions to stabilize patient's condition.
- Provide clarification or additional explanation.
- Sending facility has nurse or health care provider call to confirm that there are no questions regarding patient's care.

Communication and Documentation

- The nurse sending the patient documents patient's status, including vital signs and other assessment findings regarding patient's condition, nursing plan of care, date and time of transfer, and method of transport on appropriate transfer form.
- Document your evaluation of patient and caregiver learning.
- The nurse receiving the patient documents patient's arrival at facility by documenting date and time of arrival, reason for transfer, method of transport, patient's condition, and care provided at time of arrival.

Special Considerations
Teaching

- A transfer frequently creates anxiety for a patient and caregivers. Carefully repeat instructions about the transfer when patient and caregiver are better able to understand your explanation. In this situation, be sure to have patient or caregiver restate any critical information.

Pediatric

- Children need their parents' comfort and security; thus, make sure that parents are well informed. Involve older children in

any discussion regarding transfers. Allow a parent to accompany the child in the transfer.

Gerontological

- When transferring an older person to a new facility, relocation can be a stressful time. Ensure that significant support people are still accessible and that patient and caregivers are thoroughly oriented to new surroundings. Practice person-centred care—ensure that the patient's and caregiver's opinions and sensitivities are included when establishing care needs (Accreditation Canada, 2017d; RNAO, 2014).

Long-Term Care

- It is important that patients receive the level of services appropriate to their physical and mental health needs. Use interprofessional collaboration (e.g., continuing care coordinator, social worker, discharge planner) in the transition process to ensure that the placement to a long-term care facility is appropriate.
- Essential components of successful transfer to a long-term care facility are accurate communication of medication lists and advance directives (Accreditation Canada, 2017c; RNAO, 2014).

◆ SKILL 2.3 **Discharging Patients**

Early and comprehensive discharge planning facilitates the transition of a patient or resident from a health care facility to the most independent level of care, whether that is home or another facility. The overall goal of discharge planning is to provide the most appropriate level and quality of care throughout all stages of a patient's illness. Rates of hospital readmission and or return visits to the emergency department are common outcome measures for effective discharge planning (Mabire, Dwyer, Garnier, et al., 2016). Evidence suggests that patients who receive an interprofessional collaborative approach to discharge planning are less likely to experience a readmission or visit to the ED (Mabire et al., 2016). Accreditation Canada (2017d) acknowledges that preparation for discharge begins at the time of admission, and that the patient and caregiver perceptions of the physical and psychosocial readiness for the transition to discharge are incorporated throughout the process. Favourable interventions must include an interprofessional approach that employs good communication between clinicians, patients,

and care settings; areas of education and resources to support patient and caregiver knowledge of self-care management; and medication reconciliation and seamless transition to community resources including primary care follow-up (Accreditation Canada, 2019; Mabire et al., 2016).

The discharge planning process must be comprehensive and interdisciplinary, including all caregivers who are involved in the care of the patient. Every hospitalized patient requires patient-centred discharge planning, and it is equally essential for any patient permanently moving to a different health care facility. The trend toward shorter lengths of stay in acute care settings makes discharge planning increasingly difficult but all the more essential (Mabire et al., 2016).

Development of a discharge plan with outcomes mutually accepted by a patient and health care providers is essential (Accreditation Canada, 2017d; Mabire et al., 2016). Effective discharge planning prepares patients to assume self-care or prepares caregivers to provide needed support and thus can decrease hospital readmission and

promote optimal patient outcomes (Mabire et al., 2016). The discharge process is simple or complex and occurs in three phases: acute, transitional, and continuing care. In the acute phase, medical attention dominates discharge planning efforts. During the transitional phase, the need for acute care is still present; but its urgency declines, and patients begin to address and plan for their future health care needs. In the continuing-care phase, patients are able to participate in planning and implementing continuing-care activities needed after discharge. In acute care facilities, these phases can occur very quickly, even within hours.

The greatest challenge in effective discharge planning is communication. Patients and families should be full partners in the discharge planning process and thus should be engaged in discussing what will be needed to make the transition in care safe and effective (Accreditation Canada, 2017d; Mabire et al., 2016). When team members communicate during end-of-shift hand-offs, consultations, or huddle sessions, a patient's discharge readiness should be a central topic. Communication is enhanced if a facility has a discharge coordinator or case manager. Staff members in these roles thoroughly assess what each patient's needs will be at discharge, identify available and needed resources, and link patients and caregivers to these resources (e.g., community supports, Meals on Wheels, rehabilitation services). The coordination of necessary services (e.g., home health care) and appropriate follow-up on patients' progress after discharge should also occur.

Discharge from a facility can be stressful for a patient and caregiver. Before a patient is discharged, the patient and caregiver need to be prepared with the knowledge and skills to manage care in the home. They also need to know what to expect in regard to any continuing physical problems. Without the necessary equipment and professional resources, a patient risks loss of rehabilitation gains made before discharge. Failure to understand restrictions or implications of health problems often causes a patient to develop complications. Poor discharge planning ignores a patient's needs within the home and increases the chance of the patient needing to re-enter the health care system prematurely.

Delegation and Collaboration

The skills of assessment, care planning, and instruction included in discharging patients cannot be delegated to an unregulated care providers (UCP). The nurse directs the UCP to:

- Gather and secure personal items and any supplies that the patient will take home or to new setting.
- Transport the patient to the discharge transport vehicle.

Equipment

- Wheelchair or stretcher
- Discharge documentation forms (see employer policy)
- Patient instruction sheets
- Plastic bag for personal belongings

STEP	RATIONALE

ASSESSMENT

1. Identify patient using at least two person-specific identifiers (e.g., name and date of birth or name and medical record number) according to employer policy.

   Ensures correct patient. Complies with Accreditation Canada's standards and improves patient safety (Accreditation Canada, 2019).

2. From time of admission, assess patient's discharge needs using nursing history data, including assessments of patient's physical health, functional status, psychosocial support system, financial resources, health values, cultural and ethnic background, level of education, and barriers to care that is needed. Also review ongoing assessment data during your shift of care (e.g., physical examinations and discussions with patient and health care provider). Be sure that the discharge plan is person centred, making the plan culturally appropriate (e.g., learn the patient's preferences and values about continuing health care after discharge).

   Planning for discharge begins at admission and continues throughout patient's stay in a facility to help patient achieve maximum functioning. The discharge planning assessment determines patient's continuing care needs after they leave the acute care setting (Accreditation Canada, 2017d; RNAO, 2014).

3. Identify risk factors that may increase the chance of patient being readmitted after discharge (Accreditation Canada, 2017d; Mabire et al., 2016; RNAO, 2014): diagnoses associated with high readmissions (e.g., heart failure, chronic lung disease); comorbidities; the need for numerous medications; a history of readmissions; psychosocial and emotional factors such as issues relating to mental health, interpersonal relationships, or family matters; the lack of a caregiver who could provide support or help with care; older age; financial distress; deficient living environment (e.g., water supply, heating)

   Allows you to better prioritize care interventions that manage these risk factors during patient stay in facility. Conditions affect either patient's ability to become physically or psychologically ready for discharge or ability and readiness of a caregiver to assume patient's care in the home.

4. If patient's destination at discharge will be the home, assess patient's and caregiver's learning needs as soon as possible (e.g., psychomotor skills, medication management, symptom recognition). Engage patient and caregiver as partners in the discharge teaching plan by having them identify their concerns about discharge.

   Improves understanding of health care needs and ability to achieve self-care at home. Inclusion of caregiver in teaching sessions provides patient with available resource. Engaging patient and caregiver in the assessment supports person-centred nursing care (Accreditation Canada, 2019; Mabire et al., 2016; RNAO, 2014).

STEP	RATIONALE

ASSESSMENT

5. Assess for current barriers to learning (e.g., age, fatigue, pain, lack of motivation). Assess patient's health literacy (see Skill 2.1, Assessment, Step 6).

Determines timing and approach to instruction. Different types of educational materials are effective with different individual learning styles. If printed material is to be used, be sure that material is written at proper reading level.

6. Ask patient, caregiver, or both to describe the home environment and assess for environmental factors that may interfere with self-care (e.g., size of rooms, doorway clearances for wheelchair, steps, lighting, bathroom facilities). (A community-based nurse is usually available on referral to help with assessment.)

Environmental factors within patient's home pose safety risks or problems for self-care (see Chapter 42). Early identification of these factors allows you to arrange for home health referral.

7. Use interprofessional collaboration to assess patient's anticipated needs after discharge and their eligibility for services for care in the community. Ask these questions: "Does patient have an injury or illness that makes it difficult to leave home (e.g., requires the aid of supportive devices such as a wheelchair or walker; requires the use of special transportation; needs the assistance of a caregiver)?" "Does the patient have a 'skilled need' that requires skills from a specific health care provider?"

These conditions are needed for several provinces'/territories' reimbursement of home health care services, and eligibility criteria may differ somewhat. Generally, the patient must have a "skilled need" that requires the skills of a nurse, speech therapist, or physical therapist in order for the patient to perform the task. A health care provider's prescription is needed for nursing services.

8. Assess patient's and caregiver's perceptions of continued health care needs outside the facility. Assess caregivers' perceived ability to provide care to patient, including their level of social and community support and their ability to manage multiple medications with which the patient is discharged.

Caregiving can be a highly stressful experience. Caregivers may or may not be family members, and they may not be properly prepared for caregiving, as many are frequently overwhelmed by patient's needs, which can lead to unnecessary facility readmissions.

9. Provide patient's copy of any written discharge instructions. Return original copy of any advanced directives provided by the patient, provincial/territorial health card, and personal belongings, including home medications.

Evidence confirms that discharge instructions can
- Reduce readmission rates for the same condition.
- Improve quality of patient care.
- Improve patient satisfaction.
- Support patient adherence to patient care plan.

Clinical Decision Point *It is often necessary to talk with the patient and caregiver separately to learn about true concerns or doubts.*

10. Assess patient's acceptance of health problems and related restrictions.

Affects willingness to follow therapies and restrictions.

NURSING DIAGNOSES

- Anxiety
- Caregiver role strain
- Insufficient knowledge regarding home care restrictions

- Inadequate health management
- Interrupted family processes
- Openness to improve health management

- Relocation stress syndrome
- Reduced self-care: feeding, toileting, dressing/grooming, bathing/hygiene

Related factors are individualized on the basis of patient's condition or needs.

PLANNING

1. Expected outcomes following completion of procedure:
- Patient or caregiver explains how health care is to continue in home (or other facility), for which problems to observe and what to do, which treatments or medications patient needs, and when to go to next medical appointment.

Increases likelihood of care not being interrupted in home (or other facility) and reduces chances of unplanned readmission to the acute care facility.

- Patient can demonstrate self-care activities (or caregiver is able to administer care measures).

Feedback ensures learning.

- Obstacles to patient's mobility and hazards to ambulation in home setting are removed.

Patient is often physically weakened or has physical changes resulting from illness that predispose to injury.

STEP	RATIONALE

IMPLEMENTATION

1. Preparation before day of discharge:

   a. Partner with patient and caregiver in identifying ways to change physical arrangement of home that will be required to meet patient's needs (see Chapter 42).

      Maintains patient's level of independence and ability to retain function within safe environment.

   b. Provide patient and caregiver with information about community health care resources (e.g., health link, medical equipment companies, Meals on Wheels, adult day care). Referrals are usually made while patient is in the facility.

      Community resources offer services that patient or caregiver cannot provide.

   c. Conduct teaching sessions with patient and caregiver as soon as possible during hospitalization. Cover these topics: description of what life at home will be like, review of medications and dosing schedules; warning signs of possible health problems; explanation of test results; explanation of how to provide therapies or use home medical equipment; assess knowledge and understanding of applicable community resources; review of restrictions resulting from health alterations; and when to make follow-up appointment. Use appropriate materials such as pamphlets, books, or multimedia resources. Refer patient to reliable and current resources on the Internet.

      Gives patient opportunities to practice new skills, ask questions, and obtain necessary feedback to ensure learning. A combination of written and verbal information is effective in improving patient satisfaction and knowledge (Accreditation Canada, 2017d; RNAO, 2014). In some settings, electronic programs are available that allow you to tailor patient-specific media instructions.

   d. Communicate patient's and caregiver's response to teaching and proposed discharge plan to other health care team members.

      Facilitates continuity and achievement of a person-centred individualized discharge plan.

2. Procedure on day of discharge:

   a. Encourage patient and caregiver to ask questions or discuss issues related to home care. A final opportunity to demonstrate learned skills is helpful.

      Allows for final clarification of information previously discussed. Helps relieve anxiety.

   b. Check health care provider's discharge prescriptions, change in treatments, or need for special medical equipment. (Make sure that prescriptions are written as early as possible.) Arrange for delivery and setup of equipment (e.g., hospital bed, oxygen) before patient arrives home.

      Only a health care provider is able to authorize a discharge. Early check of prescriptions permits you to attend to any last-minute treatments or procedures well before discharge.

   c. Determine whether patient or caregiver has arranged for transportation.

      Patient's condition at discharge determines method of transport.

   d. Provide privacy and assistance as patient dresses and packs all personal belongings. Check closets and drawers for belongings. Obtain copy of list of valuables signed by patient and have security or appropriate administrator deliver valuables to patient.

      Prevents loss of personal items. Patient's signature verifies receipt of items and relieves nursing department of liability for losses.

   e. Complete medication reconciliation per employer policy. Check discharge medication prescriptions against the medication administration record and home medication list. Provide patient with prescriptions or pharmacy-dispensed medications prescribed by health care provider. Offer a final review of information needed to facilitate safe medication self-administration.

      Decreases risk of medication errors and ensures that patient is receiving correct medication at home (Accreditation Canada, 2019, RNAO 2014). The new medication regimen prescribed at the time of discharge may inadvertently omit needed medications, unnecessarily duplicate existing therapies, or contain incorrect dosages (Institute for Safe Medication Practices Canada, 2017). Review provides feedback to determine patient's success in learning about medications.

   f. Provide information on follow-up appointments to health care provider's office.

      Provides patient with contact for questions that arise after discharge. Ensures continuity of care to prevent rehospitalization.

   g. Acquire utility cart to move patient's belongings. Obtain wheelchair for patient. Transport patient leaving by ambulance on ambulance stretcher.

      Provides for safe transport.

STEP	RATIONALE

IMPLEMENTATION

h. Help patient to wheelchair or stretcher using safe patient handling and transfer techniques (see Chapter 11). Escort patient to entrance of facility where source of transportation is waiting (see employer policy) (see illustrations). Lock wheelchair wheels. Help patient transfer into transport vehicle. Help place personal belongings in vehicle.

Prevents injury to nurse and patient. Employer policy requires escort to ensure patient's safe exit. Facility's liability ends once patient is safely in vehicle.

i. Return to unit/division. Notify admitting or appropriate department of time of discharge. Notify housekeeping of need to clean patient's room.

Allows facility to prepare for admission of next patient.

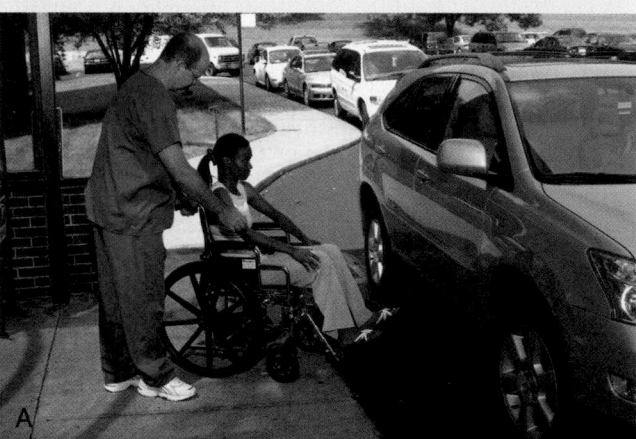 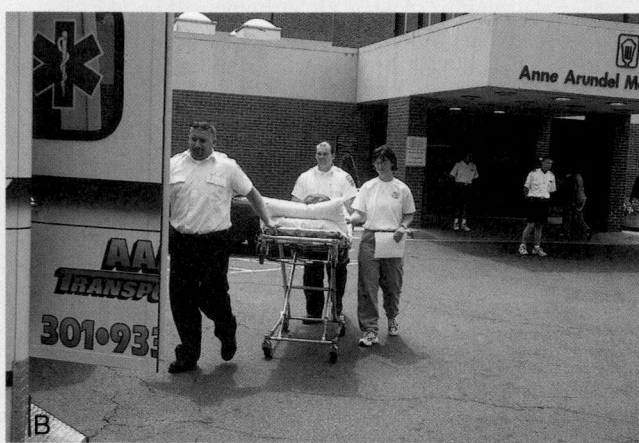

STEP 2h A, Nurse escorts patient to transport vehicle at time of discharge via a wheelchair. **B,** Many patients are discharged via stretcher.

EVALUATION

1. Ask patient or caregiver to describe nature of illness, treatment and medication regimens, and physical signs or symptoms to be reported to a health care provider.

Measures patient's or caregiver's learning.

2. Have patient or caregiver perform any treatments that will continue in the home.

Return demonstrations allow you to evaluate level of learning.

3. Community-based nurse inspects home, identifies obstacles that pose risks for patient, and recommends revisions.

Provides continuity of care.

4. Use Teach-Back: "I want to be sure you understand when your follow-up appointment is. Can you tell me when you require a check-up?" Develop a revised teaching plan if patient or caregiver is not able to teach back correctly.

Determines patient's and caregiver's level of understanding of instructional topic.

Unexpected Outcomes	Related Interventions
1. Patient or caregiver is unable to explain or demonstrate self-care measures.	• Provide immediate clarification or additional instruction. • Plan additional time to demonstrate treatment measures. • Ask patient to explain which aspect of procedure is difficult to perform and why. • If patient or caregiver continues to be unable to correctly demonstrate treatment measures, request referral for home care services.
2. Environmental risks are still present in home.	• Reassess reason for changes not being implemented. • Community-based nurse will problem solve and seek appropriate solution.
3. Patient or caregiver resists discharge plans and refuses assimilation of new roles needed for home care.	• Use interprofessional collaboration (e.g., social work, home care, pastoral care) to provide additional resources.

Communication and Documentation

- Complete documentation of patient's discharge on discharge summary form (Box 2.5). Give patient a signed copy of form.
- Document unresolved problems and description of arrangements made for resolution in nurses' notes in electronic health record (EHR) or chart.
- Document patient's vital signs and status of health problems at time of discharge in nurses' notes in EHR or chart.
- Document your evaluation of patient and caregiver learning.

Special Considerations
Teaching

- Assess patient's fatigue and pain levels before beginning any instruction. Keep focused on the important teaching topics to cover.

Pediatric

- Once caregivers have learned how to perform any necessary caregiver skills, have them assume care before child returns home. Many facilities incorporate a trial period requiring caregivers to manage care before child's discharge home (Perry et al., 2017).
- The nurse is a leader in the interprofessional process of discharge planning in partnership with other health care providers, children, and their parents. Throughout hospitalization, the nurse assesses factors that will affect the caregiver's ability to manage care at home (Perry et al., 2017).

Gerontological

- Older persons and their caregivers often overestimate their ability to manage care after discharge. They may also disagree about what postdischarge care includes. Make referrals to home care to address needs associated with functional decline and help prevent readmission to the acute care facility.

Care in the Community

- Assess availability and skill of primary caregiver (e.g., family member or friend): assess time availability, ability and willingness to give care, emotional and physical stamina, knowledge of caregiving requirements, and type of relationship held with patient. Assess additional resources, including friends or neighbours who are available to help. Ensure that patient and caregiver are aware of how to access additional home care support if needs arise.
- Inform community care services and the patient's health care provider about whether the patient or caregiver will receive home support upon discharge.

BOX 2.5

Nursing Discharge and Referral Summaries

- Description of the patient's status at discharge (e.g., physical, mental, emotional)
- Discharge destination and mode of discharge (e.g., ambulatory, wheelchair, stretcher)
- Identify issues that have been resolved and those that still remain
- Functional and self-care abilities in terms of vision, hearing speech, mobility with or without aids, meal preparation and eating, and medication preparation and administration
- Instructions for continuing self-care needs: activity, diet, medications, special treatments such as wound care, insulin injections, self-catheterization, tracheostomy care
- Reconciled list of current medications with dose, frequency, and route
- Identified restrictions that relate to activity, diet, or personal care
- Patient's and caregiver's comfort level with discharge

- Signs and symptoms of complications or medication reactions for which to be observant
- Signs and symptoms that patient should consider normal
- Referral services (e.g., home health care, occupational therapy, social work)
- Patient support networks, including caregivers, significant other or family members, community self-help groups, home care, and spiritual advisor or other community agencies
- Scheduled follow-up appointment at health care provider's office, clinic
- Name and contact information of health care provider, nursing unit, or both
- Explanation of pertinent emergency procedures
- Patient's signature, showing understanding of instructions

Modified from Foley, V. (2018). Documenting and reporting. In B. Kozier, G. Erb, A. Berman, S. Snyder, G., Frandsen, M. Buck, L. Ferguson, L. Yiu, & L. Leeseberg Stamler (Eds.), *Fundamentals of Canadian nursing: Concepts, process, and practice* (4th ed., p. 471). Don Mills, ON: Pearson Canada Inc.

◆ CLINICAL DEBRIEF

A 69-year-old widow was admitted to the acute care unit with a left-sided stroke. The patient has a history of diabetes mellitus and arthritis. She is able to help with many care activities but requires help with eating. She has a sister who will be her caregiver. On admission, her assessment showed an area of skin breakdown on her left hip, assessed as a stage 1 pressure injury. Her medications on admission were metformin, lisinopril, and St. John's wort. After 3 days she was transferred to the rehabilitation unit. Her medications on transfer were metformin, lisinopril, and warfarin. She has left-sided weakness from her stroke and will likely require a walker.

1. During the patient's admission assessment, which physical assessment findings are a priority to document and why?

2. During her care transition, which key piece of information, reflecting a potential risk, should be shared during the hand-off with the nurse on the rehabilitation unit?

3. At the time the patient is admitted to rehabilitation, the nurse conducts an assessment in an effort to plan for discharge in 2 weeks. The patient will be going home and staying with her sister for at least a month. During the assessment, the nurse learns that the sister is concerned about being able to manage the patient. The sister has heart failure and limited exercise tolerance. Assessment also reveals that her skin has cleared over the left hip. The patient will be trained to use the walker safely in rehabilitation. Write an SBAR to communicate this situation.

✦ REVIEW QUESTIONS

1. The nurse is admitting a patient from the emergency department. Which steps should the nurse take to ensure that the patient is safely admitted? *(Select all that apply.)*
   1. Obtain a list of the patient's medication from the patient
   2. Ask the family to provide interpreter services
   3. Determine patient's level of health literacy
   4. Obtain the patient's history as soon as possible
   5. Wait 24 hours before assessing skin integrity

2. The nurse is orienting a student nurse who asks when medication reconciliation is done. The nurse tells her that it is done: *(Select all that apply.)*
   1. On admission.
   2. On transition to another level of care.
   3. At the change of every shift.
   4. On discharge.
   5. Once every 24 hours.

3. The nurse is preparing the patient on the day of discharge. Which of the following elements are important to address? *(Select all that apply.)*
   1. Reviewing health care providers' prescriptions
   2. Arranging for transportation
   3. Completing medication reconciliation
   4. Reviewing discharge instructions
   5. Beginning discharge planning

ⓔ *Visit the Evolve site for a complete list of Clinical Debrief and Review Questions answers.*

REFERENCES

Accreditation Canada. (2019). *Required organizational practices handbook—Version 14*. Retrieved from http://www.wrha.mb.ca/quality/files/2019ROPHandbook.pdf

Accreditation Canada. (2017a). *Client- and family-centred care: Its history in Qmentum and a supporting literature review*. Retrieved from https://store.accreditation.ca/products/client-and-family-centred-care-its-history-in-qmentum-and-a-supporting-literature-review

Accreditation Canada. (2017b). *Standards: Emergency department (ver. 12)*. Retrieved from http://www.wrh.on.ca/Site_Published/wrh_internet/DocumentRender.aspx?Body.IdType=5&Body.Id=76906&Body.GenericField=

Accreditation Canada. (2017c). *Standards: Long-term care services (ver. 11)*. Retrieved from https://store.accreditation.ca/products/long-term-care-services

Accreditation Canada. (2017d). *Standards: Medication management standards*. Retrieved from http://www.wrh.on.ca/Site_Published/wrh_internet/DocumentRender.aspx?Body.IdType=5&Body.Id=76914&Body.GenericField=

Anthony, S. E., & Krahn, M. (2015). Healthcare in Canada and issues of health-care reform. In D. Gregory, C. Raymond-Seniuk, L. Patrick, & T. Stephen (Eds.), *Fundamentals: Perspectives on the art and science of Canadian nursing* (pp. 28–31). Philadelphia: Wolters Kluwer Health.

Buck, M. (2018). Safety. In B. Kozier, G. Erb, A. Berman, et al. (Eds.), *Fundamentals of Canadian nursing: Concepts, process, and practice* (4th ed., pp. 761–792). Don Mills, ON: Pearson Canada.

Buck, M., & Picinbono-Larose, G. (2018). Medications. In B. Kozier, G. Erb, A. Berman, et al. (Eds.), *Fundamentals of Canadian nursing: Concepts, process, and practice* (4th ed., pp. 792–874). Don Mills, ON: Pearson Canada.

Camicia, M., & Lutz, B. J. (2016). Nursing's role in successful transitions across settings. *Stroke; a Journal of Cerebral Circulation, 47*(11), 246–249. doi:10.1161/STROKEAHA.116.012095

Canadian Nurses Association (CNA). (2017). *Code of ethics for registered nurses*. Ottawa, ON: Author. Retrieved from https://www.cna-aiic.ca/~/media/cna/page-content/pdf-en/code-of-ethics-2017-edition-secure-interactive.pdf?la=en

Canadian Nurses Association (CNA). (2018). *Protection of personal information*. Ottawa, ON: Author. Retrieved from https://www.cna-aiic.ca/en/protection-of-personal-information

Canadian Patient Safety Institute (CPSI). (2017). *Engaging patients in patient safety: A Canadian guide*. Retrieved from http://www.patientsafetyinstitute.ca/en/toolsResources/Patient-Engagement-in-Patient-Safety-Guide/Documents/Engaging%20Patients%20in%20Patient%20Safety.pdf

Chapman, Y. L., Schweickert, P., Swango-Wilson, A., Aboul-Enein, F. H., & Heyman, A. (2016). Nurse satisfaction with information technology enhanced bedside handoff. *Medsurg Nursing, 25*(5), 313–318.

Chard, R., & Makary, M. A. (2015). Transfer-of-care communication: Nursing best practices. *AORN Journal, 102*(4), 329–342. doi:10.1016/j.aorn.2015.07.009

Dalhousie University Health Law Institute. (n.d.). *End of life law and policy in Canada: Advance directives*. Retrieved from http://eol.law.dal.ca/?page_id=231

Government of Canada. (2016a). *Canada's healthcare system*. Retrieved from https://www.canada.ca/en/health-canada/services/canada-health-care-system.html

Government of Canada. (2016b). *End of life care*. Retrieved from https://www.canada.ca/en/health-canada/topics/end-life-care.html

Government of Canada. (2017). *Federal support to provinces and territories*. Retrieved from https://www.fin.gc.ca/fedprov/mtp-eng.asp

Institute for Safe Medication Practices Canada. (2017). *Errors associated with hospital discharge prescriptions: A multi-incident analysis*. Retrieved from https://www.ismp-canada.org/download/safetyBulletins/2017/ISMPCSB2017-01-HospitalDischargePrescriptions.pdf

Karam, M., Brault, I., Van Durme, T., & Macq, J. (2018). Comparing interprofessional and interorganizational collaboration in healthcare: A systematic review of the qualitative research. *International Journal of Nursing Studies, 79*, 70–83. doi:10.1016/j.ijnurstu.2017.11.002

Kear, T. M. (2016). Patient handoffs: What they are and how they contribute to patient safety. *Nephrology Nursing Journal, 43*(4), 339–342.

Mabire, C., Dwyer, A., Garnier, A., & Pellet, J. (2016). Effectiveness of nursing discharge planning interventions on health-related outcomes in discharged elderly inpatients: A systematic review. *Joanna Briggs Institute EBP Database of Systematic Reviews and Implementation Reports*, doi:10.11124/JBISRIR-2016-003085

Mantoura, P., & Morrison, V. (2016). *Policy approaches to reducing health inequalities*. National Collaborating Centre for Healthy Public Policy. Retrieved from http://www.ncchpp.ca/docs/2016_Ineg_Ineq_ApprochesPPInegalites_En.pdf

McBeth, C. L., Durbin-Johnson, B., & Siegel, E. O. (2017). Interprofessional huddle: One children's hospital's approach to improving patient flow. *Journal of Pediatric Nursing, 43*(2), 71–76.

Mikkonen, J., & Raphael, D. (2010). *Social determinants of health: The Canadian facts*. Toronto, ON: York University School of Health Policy and Management. Retrieved from http://thecanadianfacts.org/The_Canadian_Facts.pdf

Nagappa, M., Wong, J., Singh, M., Wong, D. T., & Chung, F. (2017). An update on the various practical applications of the STOP-Bang questionnaire in anesthesia, surgery, and perioperative medicine. *Current Opinion in Anaesthesiology, 30*(1), 118–125. doi:10.1097/ACO.0000000000000426

Office of the Privacy Commissioner of Canada. (2015). *The application of PIPEDA to municipalities, universities, schools, and hospitals*. Retrieved from https://www.priv.gc.ca/en/privacy-topics/privacy-laws-in-canada/the-personal-information-protection-and-electronic-documents-act-pipeda/r_o_p/02_05_d_25/

Perry, S., Hockenberry, M., Lowdermilk, D., Wilson, D., Keenan-Lindsay, L., & Sams, C. (2017). *Maternal child nursing care in Canada* (2nd ed.). Toronto, ON: Elsevier.

Registered Nurses' Association of Ontario (RNAO). (2014). *Clinical best practice guidelines: Care transitions*. Toronto, ON, Canada: Registered Nurses' Association of Ontario. Retrieved from http://rnao.ca/sites/rnao-ca/files/Care_Transitions_BPG.pdf

Registered Nurses' Association of Ontario (RNAO). (2015). *Clinical best practice guidelines: Person- and family-centered care*. Retrieved from http://rnao.ca/sites/rnao-ca/files/FINAL_Web_Version_0.pdf

Ross, C. J. M. (2016). Management of patients with upper respiratory tract disorders. In P. Paul, R. Day, & B. Williams (Eds.), *Brunner & Suddarth's Canadian textbook of medical-surgical nursing* (3rd ed., pp. 539–573). Philadelphia, PA: Wolters Kluwer.

Stewart, K. R., & Hand, K. A. (2017). SBAR, communication, and patient safety: An integrated literature review. *Medsurg Nursing, 26*(5), 297–305.

Taylor, J. (2015). Improving patient safety and satisfaction with standardized bedside handoff and walking rounds. *Clinical Journal of Oncology Nursing, 19*(4), 414–416. doi:10.1188/15.CJON.414-416

Usher, R., Nones Cronin, S., & York, N. L. (2018). Evaluating the influence of a standardized bedside handoff process in a medical-surgical unit. *Journal of Continuing Education in Nursing, 49*(4), 157–163. doi:10.3928/00220124-20180320-05

Walton, N. (2016). Ethics and integrity in practice: Moral dilemmas and moral issues. In D. Gregory, C. Raymond-Seniuk, L. Patrick, & T. Stephen (Eds.), *Fundamentals: Perspectives on the art and science of Canadian nursing* (pp. 146–163). Philadelphia: Wolters Kluwer.

Zou, X. J., & Zhang, Y. P. (2016). Rates of nursing errors and handoff-related errors in a medical unit following implementation of a standardized nursing handoff form. *Journal of Nursing Care Quality, 31*(1), 61–67. doi:10.1097/NCQ.0000000000000133

3 | Communication and Collaboration

Written by **Jacqueline Raybuck Saleeby, PhD, RN, BCCS, and Jackie Hartigan-Rogers, RN, MN**

SKILLS AND PROCEDURES

OBJECTIVES

Mastery of content in this chapter will enable the nurse to:
- Identify guidelines to use in therapeutic communication.
- Explain the communication process.
- Identify the purposes of therapeutic communication and communication in various phases of the nurse–patient relationship.
- Develop skills for therapeutic communication in various phases of the nurse–patient relationship.

- Develop therapeutic communication skills for communicating with patients who have difficulty coping because of feelings such as anxiety, anger, and depression.
- Develop therapeutic communication skills for communication with cognitively impaired patients.
- Develop skills for effective communication with colleagues.

MEDIA RESOURCES

- e∨olve http://evolve.elsevier.com/Canada/Perry/clinicalskills/
- Review Questions
- Audio Glossary

- Clinical Debrief and Review Questions Answers
- Case Studies

PURPOSE

Communication is the interaction between two or more people. Effective communication positively influences how nursing care is delivered and patient satisfaction with that care. A nurse's responsibility to effectively communicate extends beyond the patient to include family members and significant others and interprofessional collaboration with all members of the health care team. The purpose of this chapter is to provide you with a framework to develop effective communication skills that are essential to the delivery of person-centred care.

STANDARDS OF CARE

- Canadian Nurses Association, 2017—*Code of Ethics for Registered Nurses: Part 1. Nursing Values and Ethical Responsibilities A. Providing Safe, Compassionate, Competent and Ethical Care.* Ethical Responsibilities 1, 2, 3 (p. 8) (https://www.cna-aiic.ca/html/en/Code-of-Ethics-2017-Edition/index.html#14)
- Registered Nurses' Association of Ontario, 2015—*Clinical Best Practice Guideline: Person-and Family-Centred Care.* Person- and Family-Centred Care and Its Components (pp. 7–8) (http://rnao.ca/sites/rnao-ca/files/FINAL_Web_Version_0.pdf)

- Registered Nurses' Association of Ontario, 2016—*Clinical Best Practice Guideline: Intra-professional Collaborative Practice among Nurses.* Guiding Principles and Assumptions (p. 8) (http://rnao.ca/sites/rnao-ca/files/bpg/Intra-professional_Collaborative_Practice_042017.pdf)

PRINCIPLES FOR PRACTICE

- Nurses must have knowledge of the principles of therapeutic communication, implement the skills of communicating effectively, and possess the attitude of wanting to improve communication skills (Balzer-Riley, 2017, p. 3).
- Communication is an interaction between two or more people that involves the exchange of information between a sender and a receiver, involving the expression of emotions, ideas, and thoughts through verbal (words or written language) and nonverbal (behaviours) exchanges (Fig. 3.1).
- It is important to establish and understand the purpose of a patient interaction. This is an essential quality of effective communication.
- Communication skills provide information and comfort, promote understanding, clarify misinformation, help to develop plans of care, promote interprofessional collaboration, and facilitate wellness through patient teaching.

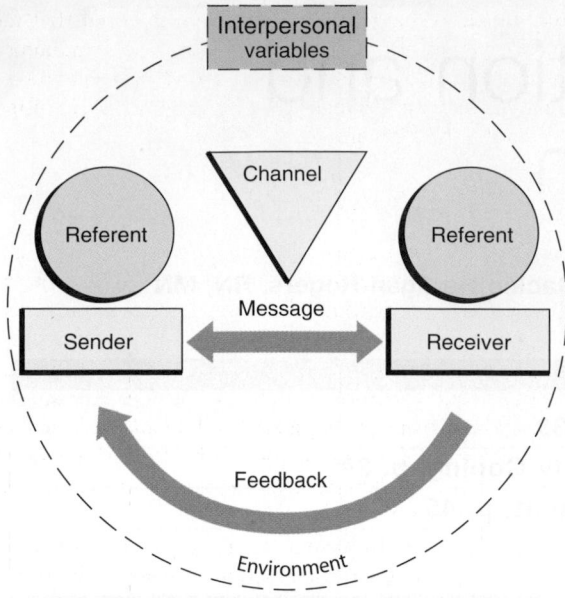

FIG 3.1 Communication is a two-way process.

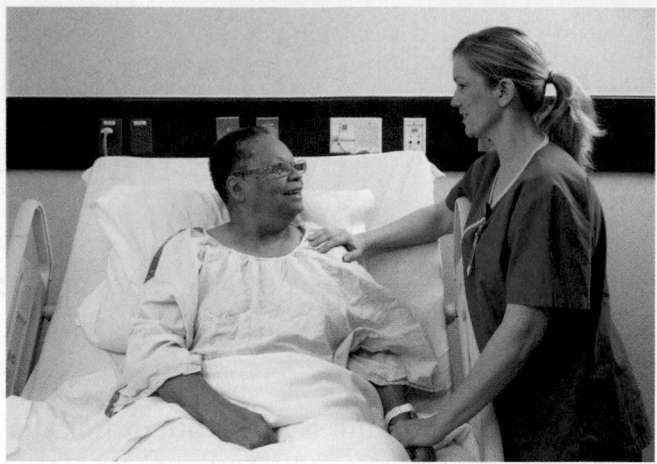

FIG 3.2 An open, relaxed posture conveys interest.

- Communication includes both spoken and written words. To send an accurate message the sender of verbal communication needs to be aware of the tone, volume, and cadence (pace or rate) of voice.
- Nonverbal communication describes all behaviours that convey messages without the use of words. This type of communication includes body movement, physical appearance, personal space, and touch. Be aware of body language, which includes posture, body position, gestures, eye contact, facial expression, and movement. For clarity make sure that nonverbal communication is consistent with the spoken word.
- As a nurse you need to know your attitudes toward a patient or situation. Be aware of your personal feelings to control how you communicate issues. Nurse–patient relationships require special consideration in the use of self-disclosure (Balzer-Riley, 2017, p. 113). Nurses need to identify and recognize actions or behaviours that have the potential for crossing or violating professional boundaries (providing personal information such as address, phone number, sharing social media usernames, participating in social networking, or sharing information about past or current relationships) (College of Registered Nurses of Nova Scotia [CRNNS], 2017, p. 3). You need to use clinical judgement related to the amount of personal information revealed to patients, keeping in mind that anything that is communicated about yourself should be disclosed for the benefit of the patient as the focus of the relationship.

PERSON-CENTRED CARE

- Therapeutic communication enables nurses to deliver person-centred care—care that is respectful of and responsive to individual patient preferences, needs, and values and that ensures patient values guide clinical decisions (Registered Nurses Association of Ontario [RNAO], 2015; Strachan, Kryworuchko, Nouvet, et al., 2017). It also creates a positive relationship with health care providers, promoting interprofessional collaboration, and improves patient adherence to treatment regimens.
- Include patients and significant others in collaboration with health care providers to make decisions related to wellness and

illness care. Benefits include improved satisfaction with care, self-efficacy, quality of life, and empowerment to manage care (Griffiths, 2017; RNAO, 2015, p. 31; Walczak, Butow, Bu, et al., 2016).
- Value the importance of assessing patient and family preferences, values, and beliefs when establishing a therapeutic nurse–patient relationship and planning care for a patient (RNAO, 2015, p. 28).
- Understand how culture affects patients and their knowledge and values about health. Nurses need to recognize their own attitudes about working with patients from different backgrounds.
- It is essential to understand the impact that the residential school system and colonization has had on the overall wellness of Indigenous peoples in Canada (Bourque Bearskin, 2016). Through knowledge and understanding, nurses can work toward eliminating the significant power imbalance that still exists between non-Indigenous health care providers and Indigenous peoples and that continues to create adverse experiences within the health care system (Boyer, 2017).
- Be mindful of cultural differences, such as in the use of touch, and of religious and ethnic practices because these influence methods of communication (Fig. 3.2).
- To avoid misinterpretation of nonverbal cues, be aware of any cultural norms or values (e.g., eye contact) that patients may have (see Skill 3.1).
- Adopt a flexible, respectful attitude that also communicates interest in a patient to bridge any communication barriers that exist because of cultural differences between patient and caregiver.
- When using language assistance:
  - Provide easy-to-understand print and multimedia materials and signage in languages commonly used by populations in the health care employer service area (Deerfield, Barnum, & Pugh-Yi, 2017).
  - Address the patient and family directly when using an interpreter; do not direct questions or comments to the interpreter. Take care to determine if the patient understood (Box 3.1).

EVIDENCE-INFORMED PRACTICE

Recent studies have examined specific interventions used to effectively communicate with people of varying developmental levels and people who may have difficulty communicating with others

BOX 3.1

Suggested Approaches for Patients Who Speak Different Languages

- Use a caring tone of voice and facial expressions to help alleviate patients' fears and anxieties.
- Speak slowly and distinctly, but not loudly.
- Use gestures, pictures, and role playing to help patients understand.
- Repeat a message in different ways if necessary.
- Be alert to and use words that a patient seems to understand and use them frequently.
- Keep messages simple and repeat them frequently.
- Avoid using medical terms that a patient may not understand.
- Use an appropriate language dictionary or have an interpreter or family member make flash cards to communicate key phrases.

From Balzer-Riley, J. (2017). *Communication in nursing* (8th ed., pp. 54–57). St. Louis, MO: Elsevier.

because of a physical or mental illness (Bingham & O'Brien, 2018; Lewis, Gaffney, & Wilson, 2017).

- Speech and language therapy intervention programs have been implemented to help people with brain damage to maximize their communication skills (Byram et al., 2016).
- Information and communication technology, including the use of telephones, television, radio, computers, and handheld devices, to deliver information promotes treatment adherence among people with severe mental illness. These strategies help those with mental illness who have difficulty remembering to take medication or appointment times (Sheehan & Hassiotis, 2017).
- Effective communication and support from health care providers often reduces psychological distress in patients in a variety of settings—for example, those undergoing cancer treatment. Health care providers benefit from communication skills training to interact more therapeutically with their patients who have cancer (Lin et al., 2017).
- Health care providers need to consider the needs of older persons in order for person-centred communication to occur. Specific strategies include use of hearing support, nonverbal communication matching verbal communication, and cultural competence as tools to prompt participation and improve functional independence (Daly, 2017).

- Communicate using printed educational material that focuses on message readability and plain language. Clear communication sends messages that can influence a patient's understanding, with resulting behaviour changes (Deerfield et al., 2017; Grabeel, Russomanno, Oelschlegel, et al., 2018).

SAFETY GUIDELINES

- Listen to what and how a patient communicates, including content and verbal and nonverbal messages. Some patients express themselves clearly without difficulty. However, indirect and nonverbal cues can also communicate a patient's needs (e.g., pain, perceived stress).
- Control external factors in both the environmental setting (temperature of room, privacy issues) and the psychological setting (emotional state of the nurse and patient) that influence communication. When talking with a patient about personal concerns, privacy is important.
- When teaching, try to have a caregiver present with whom to reinforce the content of the instruction. Use language-appropriate print and multimedia materials. This is necessary for caregivers to provide needed support when patients return home.
- Controlling noise level and interruptions is also important to maintain privacy boundaries when communicating with patients (Lee, Park, Kim, et al., 2016).
- Establish and understand the purpose of interaction. This is an essential quality of effective communication.
- Guide an interaction according to the patient's condition and response. For example, the purpose of an interaction may be patient teaching; however, the patient has just learned about the death of a loved one and expresses the need to talk about the death. Help the patient grieve first, and remain flexible in the interaction. Or, if the patient indicates increased pain, provide relief measures.
- When communicating with colleagues, it is important to communicate clearly and to recognize and report errors and near misses that may compromise patient safety (Omura, Maguire, Levitt-Jones, et al., 2016).
- Effective communication is the groundwork for efficient inter-professional collaboration.

◆ SKILL 3.1 **Establishing the Nurse–Patient Relationship**

A therapeutic nurse–patient relationship is the foundation of nursing care and involves using a variety of person-centred therapeutic communication skills (Box 3.2). Communication is essential in nursing as effective communication among patients, families, and health care providers is an essential part of quality care (Hull, 2017; Sanders, Curtis, & Tulsky, 2018). The primary goal of therapeutic communication for a nurse is to promote patients' wellness and personal growth. Therapeutic communication empowers patients to make decisions but differs from social communication in that it is person centred and goal directed with limited disclosure from the professional.

Social communication involves equal opportunity for personal disclosure, and both participants seek to have personal needs met (Balzer-Riley, 2017, p. 112). Nurses do not routinely share intimate details of their personal lives with patients. However, they use personal self-disclosure (e.g., outside interests, thoughts about local news, experience as a nurse) cautiously in selected situations. Personal self-disclosure is useful for the following goals: (1) to educate patients, (2) to build therapeutic alliances with patients, and (3) to encourage patients' independence (Balzer-Riley, 2017, p. 113). There are times when empathy is essential to establishing and maintaining the nurse–patient relationship. *Empathy* is being warm and genuine; it conveys an understanding of a patient's or family's feelings and communicating this understanding to them. Empathetic communication requires an accurate verbal reflection of what the patient said, accompanied by genuine caring (e.g., "You seem to be very upset" expressed with a concerned facial expression or gentle touch on the shoulder, if appropriate). Empathy differs from sympathy, because sympathy often shifts the emphasis to the nurse's feelings, which may prevent the patient from expressing feelings and inhibit the nurse's ability to view the patient's needs objectively. Barriers to therapeutic communication include giving an opinion, offering false reassurance, making insincere comments, being defensive, showing approval or disapproval, stereotyping, and asking, "Why?"

BOX 3.2

Therapeutic Communication Techniques

Technique: Listening

Definition: An active process of receiving information and examining one's reaction to messages received

Example: Consider the cultural practices of your patient, maintain appropriate eye contact, and be receptive to nonverbal communications.

Therapeutic Value: Nonverbally communicates your interest and acceptance to a patient

Technique: Broad Openings

Definition: Encouraging patient to select topics for discussion

Example: "Can you tell me what you are thinking about?"

Therapeutic Value: Indicates your acceptance and valuing of patient's initiative

Technique: Restating

Definition: Repeating main thought that patient has expressed

Example: "You say that your mother left you when you were 5 years old."

Therapeutic Value: Indicates that you are listening and validates, reinforces, or calls attention to something important that has been said

Technique: Clarification

Definition: Attempting to improve your understanding of words, vague ideas, or patient's unclear thoughts or asking patient to explain what they mean

Example: "I'm not sure what you mean. Could you tell me again?"

Therapeutic Value: Helps to clarify patient's feelings, ideas, and perceptions and provide an explicit correlation between them and patient's actions

Technique: Reflection

Definition: Directing back to patient ideas, feelings, questions, or content

Example: "You're feeling tense and anxious, and it's related to a conversation you had with your sister last night?"

Therapeutic Value: Validates your understanding of what patient is saying and signifies empathy, interest, and respect for patient

Technique: Informing

Definition: Demonstrating skills or giving information

Example: "I think it would be helpful for you to know more about how your medication works."

Therapeutic Value: Helpful for patient education about relevant aspects of patient's well-being and self-care

Technique: Focusing

Definition: Asking questions or making statements that help patient expand on a topic of importance

Example: "I think it would be helpful if we talk more about your relationship with your father."

Therapeutic Value: Allows patient to discuss central issues related to problem and keeps communication process goal directed

Technique: Silence

Definition: Using silence or nonverbal communication for a therapeutic reason

Example: Sitting with patient and nonverbally communicating interest and involvement

Therapeutic Value: Allows patient time to think and gain insights, slows the pace of the interaction, and encourages patient to initiate conversation while you convey support, understanding, and acceptance

Modified from Townsend, M. C., & Morgan, K. I. (2018). *Psychiatric mental health nursing: Concepts of care in evidence-based practice* (9th ed., pp. 152–154). Philadelphia: F.A. Davis Company.

The use of "why" questions causes increased defensiveness in patients and hinders communication. The therapeutic nurse–patient relationship is goal directed, with a patient moving toward productive modes of interpersonal functioning.

The therapeutic relationship between nurse and patient is supported through the interrelated phases of pre-interaction, orientation, working, and termination. The pre-interaction phase occurs prior to meeting the patient. The nurse uses self-reflection to become aware of personal feelings, values, and beliefs. This self-awareness allows a nurse to practise using a person-centred approach to develop the relationship and meet the patient's needs. The orientation phase is important in developing a foundation for the therapeutic relationship. The working phase of the helping relationship has two main components: exploring thoughts and feelings and facilitating and taking action (Kennedy, 2018, p. 397). The final phase is the termination phase, which may occur at the end of shift, patient transfer, discharge, or death. Skills such as summarizing or reviewing what has been accomplished can assist in the termination process.

Delegation and Collaboration

All health care providers must practise effective communication. The skill of establishing therapeutic communication cannot be delegated to an unregulated care provider (UCP). The nurse instructs the UCP about:

- The proper way to interact verbally and nonverbally with select patients.
- The need to keep all patient communication confidential.
- Ways to arrange the environment to ensure privacy and confidentiality.
- Special considerations pertaining to communication with patients who are cognitively or sensorially impaired, older, children, or anxious and with potentially violent patients.

STEP	RATIONALE

ASSESSMENT

1. Prepare for orientation phase of therapeutic communication. Formulate individualized patient goals, consider time allocation (e.g., patient acuity and medical priorities), formulate initial questions, and mentally prepare to keep your mind clear of other concerns or distractions. Select the assessment questions most relevant to the clinical situation.

Preparation is part of a planned communication process that facilitates interaction. Planning for the orientation phase helps in identifying actual or potential problems, current health status, and experience. Without preparation, a risk exists for casual, non–goal-oriented communication.

STEP	RATIONALE

ASSESSMENT

2. Address patient by preferred name and introduce yourself and role on health care team ("Hello, my name is Jane Smith, and I am the registered nurse assigned to take care of you today. …") Use clear, specific communication, including verbal and nonverbal techniques (e.g., good eye contact, relaxed, comfortable position) to provide information and clarify concerns (see Fig. 3.2). Create a climate of warmth and acceptance.

Refer to provincial/territorial standards of nursing practice and employer policy related to relaying your full name. Professional presence "includes a registered nurse's verbal and nonverbal communications and the ability to articulate a positive role and professional image, including the use of full name and title" (CRNNS, 2017, p. 22). However, some employers recommend the use of first name only, for personal safety and security reasons. Ensure that when you are introducing yourself to a member or members of the interprofessional team that you include your full name and title.

Congruent verbal and nonverbal communication expresses warmth and respect and helps to establish rapport. The quality of communication in interactions between nurse and patient has important influences on patient outcomes (Griffiths, 2017).

3. Assess the following during initial interaction: patient's needs, coping strategies, defenses, and adaptation styles.

Recognizing recurrent themes in patient's responses helps in identifying problem areas related to health status (e.g., avoidance of questions, request for information, expression of a loss).

4. Determine patient's need to communicate (e.g., constant use of call light, crying, patient who does not understand an illness or who has just been admitted).

Patients in need of support, comfort, knowledge, or encouragement benefit from individualized meaningful communication.

5. Assess reason patient needs health care. Ask patient about health status, lifestyle, support systems, patterns of health and illness, and strengths and limitations.

Nature of illness affects patient's coping ability and effectiveness in communicating needs and concerns. For example, patients who are fearful of a cancer diagnosis and patients who are having joint replacement surgeries probably have differing needs and concerns.

6. Assess for factors about yourself and patient that normally influence communication. Examples of factors include perceptions, values, and beliefs; emotions; sociocultural background; severity of illness; knowledge; age; verbal ability; roles and relationships; environmental setting; physical comfort or discomfort (see illustration).

Communication is a dynamic process influenced by interpersonal and intrapersonal processes. By assessing factors that influence communication, you can more accurately assess a patient's perception of health status (Sim, Crookes, Walsh, et al., 2017).

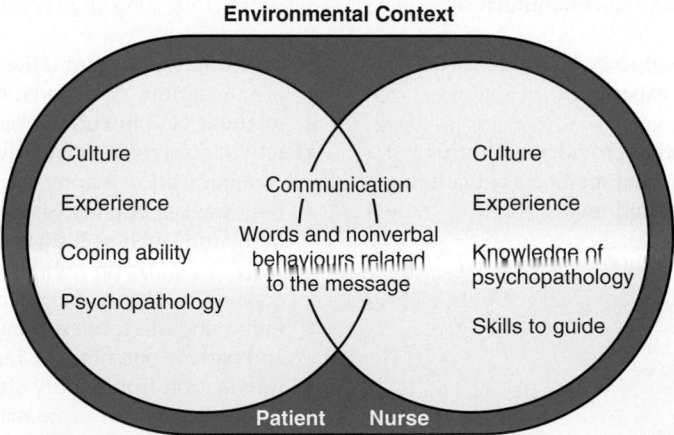

STEP 6 Essential and influencing variables of the therapeutic communication environment. (*Modified from Keltner, N., & Steele, D. [2019]. Psychiatric nursing [8th ed.]. St. Louis: Mosby.*)

7. Assess personal barriers to communicating with patient (e.g., bias toward patient's condition, anxiety from inexperience).

Barriers prevent you from conveying empathy and caring and from obtaining relevant assessment information.

STEP	RATIONALE

ASSESSMENT

8. Assess patient's language and ability to speak. Does patient have difficulty finding words or associating ideas with accurate word symbols? Does patient have difficulty with expression of language, reception of messages, or both? What is patient's primary language?

Assessment determines need for special techniques to address the communication needs of patients with limited English proficiency, hearing impairments, or literacy levels (Balzer-Riley, 2017, p. 55). Examples include picture boards, computers, sign language, or an interpreter (see illustration).

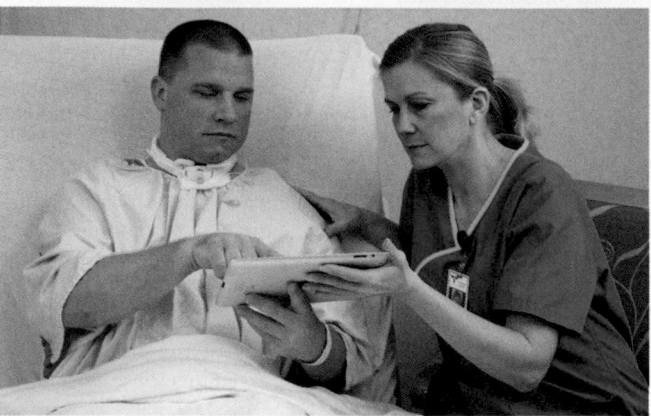

STEP 8 Communication tools for patient who cannot speak.

9. Assess patient's literacy level. Does the patient skip over uncommon or hard words, avoid asking questions, or have difficulty discussing concepts about illness?
Option: Use health literacy resources such as the Rapid Estimate of Adult Literacy in Medicine (REALM), Newest Vital Sign (NVS), or Health Literacy Universal Precautions Toolkit (Health Quality Ontario, 2016).

Health literacy has a direct effect on health outcomes. Assessing patient's level of health literacy allows you to design more effective communication and patient teaching approaches (Deerfield et al., 2017). Assess for patients who avoid questions, show signs of nervousness, or make excuses, which can be indicators of limited health literacy (Wittenberg, Ferrell, Kanter, et al., 2018).

10. Assess patient's ability to hear. Be sure that hearing aid is functional if worn. Be sure that patient hears and understands words (see Chapter 19).

Patients with hearing deficits require techniques to enhance hearing reception (e.g., speaking in normal tone, speaking so patient can see face).

11. Observe patient's pattern of communication and verbal or nonverbal behaviour (e.g., gestures, tone of voice, eye contact).

Observation determines type and manner of communication that you will use.

12. Assess resources available in selecting communication methods:

a. Review information in medical record and reflect on your past patient communication experiences.

Relying totally on information from patient restricts the quality of interaction. Additional resources provide insight into best methods of communicating.

b. Consult with family, health care provider, and other interprofessional health care team members concerning patient's condition, problems, and impressions.

Effective interprofessional collaboration centres on effective communication among team members and facilitates your response to patients, based on integration of knowledge. A framework such as Situation-Background-Assessment-Recommendation (SBAR) requires that communication be concise in relaying pertinent patient information, thus improving interprofessional collaboration, communication, and patient outcomes (Chute, 2015, p. 625). Seek information from family after receiving patient approval. Patient privacy must be maintained (Bell, 2016).

13. Before initiating the working phase of nurse–patient relationship, assess patient's readiness to work toward goal attainment: "We want to work together with you to improve your health. Tell me your goals or what it is that you feel is important for you to recover."

Patient's goals are identified and agreed on by effective communication skills such as restating and clarifying.

14. Consider when patient is due to be discharged or transferred from health care facility. Share that information with patient and caregiver.

This allows you to anticipate the amount of time available to work with the patient and when termination of relationship is to occur.

STEP	RATIONALE

NURSING DIAGNOSES

- Anxiety
- Fear
- Inadequate coping
- Altered verbal communication

- Deficient knowledge regarding communication skills
- Altered social interaction
- Deficient knowledge regarding communication skills

- Nonadherence
- Readiness for enhanced decision making

Related factors are individualized on the basis of patient's condition or needs.

PLANNING

1. Expected outcomes following completion of procedure:
   - Patient expresses ideas, fears, and concerns clearly, asks questions, and openly expresses relief of anxiety.

   - Patient health care goals are identified and achieved.
   - Patient verbalizes understanding of information communicated by nurse.
2. Before engaging in the working phase, prepare patient physically (e.g., deliver pain relief measures, provide for hygiene or elimination), provide a quiet environment, maintain privacy, and reduce distractions or interruptions before beginning discussion.
3. Working phase
   a. Use appropriate communication tools such as iPads or other electronic devices for patients whose initial language is not English.
   b. Prepare open-ended questions to identify strategies for developing a realistic plan to meet identified health goals of patients (e.g., "Let's talk more about the goals you shared earlier for this hospitalization/visit").

Once patients can talk directly about emotions, the focus is on coping more effectively with them (Balzer-Riley, 2017, p. 28). Asking questions shows an openness to communication.
Interaction remains patient focused.
This provides a means to build trust and develop a knowledge base for patient to make decisions.
Taking care of basic needs promotes an environment for interaction and decreases patient distractions and interruptions.

Electronic devices help with communication and provide translation resources.

Open-ended questions promote goal attainment and avoid risk of misinterpretation.

IMPLEMENTATION

1. Working phase: Observe patient's nonverbal behaviours, including body language. If verbal behaviours do not match nonverbal behaviours, seek clarification from patient.
2. Explain purpose of interaction when information is to be shared.
3. Continue to use therapeutic communication skills (see Box 3.2).
4. Identify patient's expectations in seeking health care.

5. Encourage patient to ask for clarification at any time during the communication.
6. Set mutual goals.
   a. Use therapeutic communication skills such as restating, reflecting, and paraphrasing to identify and clarify strategies for attainment of mutually agreed-on goals.
   b. Discuss and prioritize problem areas.

   c. Provide information to patient and help to express needs and feelings.

   d. Use questions carefully and appropriately. Ask one question at a time and allow sufficient time to answer. Use direct questions. Use open-ended statements as much as possible, such as "Tell me about how you're feeling today."

Congruence between patient's verbal and nonverbal behaviours ensures that you receive the correct message.

Information and explanation can decrease anxiety about the unknown.
Fosters open, interactive communication with patient as a participant and the focus of the discussion.
Identifying expectations conveys a level of interest in patient's needs.
This gives patient a sense of control and keeps channels of communication open.

For communication between nurse and patient to be effective, both need to possess the skills and knowledge required for participation within the communicative interaction.
A patient, nonjudgemental, supportive approach minimizes patient anxiety.
Patient can respond to help, develop workable solutions based on goals, and fully participate in a realistic plan for their well-being.
This strategy helps patient express self and allows for thorough collection of information about needs and concerns.

STEP	RATIONALE

IMPLEMENTATION

Clinical Decision Point *Avoid asking questions about information that may not yet have been disclosed to the patient (e.g., human immunodeficiency virus [HIV] status, diagnostic test results). Avoid asking "why" questions; this can cause increased defensiveness in the patient and prevents communication.*

e. Avoid communication barriers (see Box 3.2).	Barriers result in a message not being received, being distorted, or not being understood.
7. Termination phase: Communicate with the patient.	
a. Prepare by identifying methods of summarizing and synthesizing information pertinent to patient's aftercare (e.g., "What are your plans for follow-up once you return home to maintain your health status?").	Effective communication by summarizing and synthesizing information reinforces behaviour change.
b. Use therapeutic communication skills to discuss discharge or termination issues and guide discussion related to specific patient changes in thoughts and behaviours.	Reinforces behaviours and skills learned during working phase of relationship.
c. Summarize with patient what you discussed during interaction, including goal achievement.	The termination phase consists of evaluation and summary of progress toward prescribed goals. Provides a sense of closure and mutual understanding.

EVALUATION

1. Observe patient's verbal and nonverbal responses to your communication, noting their willingness to share information and concerns during orientation phase.	Verbal and nonverbal feedback reveals patient's interest and willingness to communicate and reflects ability to form a therapeutic relationship.
2. Note your response to patient and patient's response to you. Reflect on effectiveness of therapeutic techniques used in establishing rapport with patient.	Sensitivity to one's ability in using therapeutic communication skills helps improve ability to adjust techniques when necessary.
3. During working phase evaluate patient's ability to work toward identified goals. Elicit feedback (verbal and nonverbal) to determine success of goal attainment. Evaluate patient's health status in relation to identified goals. Re-evaluate and identify barriers if patient goals are not met.	Feedback is an essential step in evaluating new behaviours. Modifications are necessary if goals cannot be met.
4. During termination phase summarize and restate. Reinforce patient's strengths, outline issues still requiring work, and develop an action plan.	Evaluates patient progress in terms of attainment of mutually agreed-on goals.
5. Use Teach-Back: "I want to make sure that I explained things clearly. Show me how you would take your blood pressure." Revise the teaching plan if patient or caregiver is not able to teach back correctly.	Determines patient's and caregiver's level of understanding of teaching.

Unexpected Outcomes	**Related Interventions**
1. Patient continues to verbally and nonverbally express feelings of anxiety, fear, anger, confusion, distrust, and helplessness. Patient often responds to internal and external factors and cues.	• Reassess patient's level of anxiety, fear, and distrust. Attempt to determine the cause of anxiety or fear. • Repeat message to patient at a later time. • Determine influence affecting clear communication (e.g., cultural, language, literacy issues, physical limitations).
2. Feedback between you and the patient reveals a lack of understanding and ineffective communication.	• Assess for and remove barriers to communication such as literacy level, language issues (Wittenberg et al., 2018). • Repeat message using another approach, if possible. • Consider cultural norms associated with eye contact, use of touch, personal space, and nonverbal behaviours (Gasiorek & van de Poel, 2018). • Avoid using medical terms that patient does not understand.
3. You are unable to acquire information about patient's ideas, fears, and concerns. Communication techniques do not promote patient's willingness to communicate openly. Trust is not established. Goals are not identified and therefore cannot be achieved.	• Use alternative communication techniques to promote patient's willingness to communicate openly. • Offer another professional with whom patient can talk to obtain necessary information.

STEP	RATIONALE

EVALUATION

4. Caregiver answers for patient even when patient can answer.	• Direct question to patient, using patient's name. • Acknowledge answer given by caregiver; then state that you are interested in patient's response. • Resume interaction after caregiver has left or encourage caregiver to take a break for coffee or a meal.

Communication and Documentation

- Document in nurses' notes in electronic health record (EHR) or chart the communication pertinent to patient's health, response to illness or therapies, and responses that demonstrate understanding or lack of understanding (include verbal and nonverbal cues).
- Document teach-back and any changes to teaching plan.
- Report any relevant information obtained through patient's verbal and nonverbal behaviours to members of interprofessional team.

Special Considerations
Teaching

- Use gestures, pictures, and role playing to help patient understand. Be alert to literacy status; determine if patient can access health information adequately. Be alert to words that patient seems to understand and use them frequently.
- Individualize patient teaching to meet patient needs. Always conduct teaching with the purpose of meeting patient's learning needs with consideration for preferred methods for learning.

Mental Health

- Communicating with patients who are experiencing anxiety, sadness, fear, and worry requires clear communication in order to ensure high quality of care.
- Focus on developing a level of trust with the patient by providing support and empathy to encourage the patient to feel safe in expressing anxieties and symptoms.
- Use simple words in a calm and clear manner in order to understand the reason for the patient's distress.
- Teach the patient signs and symptoms of increasing anxiety and ways to control its progression (calming/relaxation skills) and how to apply these skills during periods of distress (Townsend & Morgan, 2018, p. 575).

Pediatric

- Communicating with children requires an understanding of feelings and thought processes from the child's perspective (McKinney, James, Murray, et al., 2018, p. 48).
- Use vocabulary that is familiar to the child, based on their level of understanding (age and developmental level). Try to be on same eye level as the patient.
- Understand the child's cognitive, developmental, and functional level to select the most appropriate communication techniques. Some age-appropriate communication techniques include story-telling and drawing (McKinney et al., 2018, p. 54).
- Nurses need to utilize effective communication skills to ensure that parents have received education for the child's acute or preventive care and have been provided rationales to facilitate transition from the hospital to home setting (McKinney et al., 2018, p. 48).

Gerontological

- Be aware of any cognitive or sensory impairment. Assess each patient individually and avoid stereotyping older persons who have cognitive or sensory impairments (Ondrejka, 2018, p. 8).
- It is important to understand the value of effective communication skills, history, and personality among older persons in terms of providing both human and therapeutic responses.
- Ensure that older persons with visual or hearing impairment use assistive devices such as eyeglasses, large-print reading material, or hearing aids to assist in communication (Ondrejka, 2018, p. 58).

Care in the Community

- Identify primary caregiver for patient and adapt techniques to assess level of understanding regarding patient's condition.
- Incorporate communication into patient's daily activities (e.g., bathing and dressing).

✦ SKILL 3.2   Communicating With Patients Who Have Difficulty Coping

Patients in the health care setting may have difficulty coping for a variety of reasons and thus experience anxiety, anger, depression, or a combination of these feelings. The nurse can help the patient decrease or manage ineffective coping symptoms and behaviours through effective communication. Examples of factors that cause anxiety are newly diagnosed illness, separation from loved ones, threat associated with diagnostic tests or surgical procedures, and expectations of life changes. How successfully a patient copes with anxiety depends in part on previous experiences, the presence of other stressors, the significance of the event causing anxiety, and the availability of supportive resources. There are four stages of anxiety with corresponding behavioural manifestations: mild, moderate, severe, and panic (Box 3.3).

Anger is a common underlying factor associated with potential for violence. Patients become angry for a variety of reasons. Anger is often directly related to a patient's experience with illness, or it is associated with previous problems. In the health care setting the nurse has frequent contact with a patient and thus often becomes the target of this anger. Understanding how to use de-escalation skills is a useful technique to manage an angry or violent patient and help ensure a safe health care environment for other patients and health care personnel.

BOX 3.3

Behavioural Manifestations of Anxiety: *Stages of Anxiety*

Mild Anxiety
- Increased auditory and visual perception
- Increased awareness of relationships
- Increased alertness
- Able to problem solve

Moderate Anxiety
- Selective inattention
- Decreased perceptual field
- Focus only on relevant information
- Muscle tension; diaphoresis

Severe Anxiety
- Focus on fragmented details
- Headache, nausea, dizziness
- Unable to see connections between details
- Poor recall

Panic State of Anxiety
- Does not notice surroundings
- Feeling of terror
- Unable to cope with any problem

BOX 3.4

Symptoms of Depression

Common Symptoms
- Apathy
- Decreased socialization
- Sadness
- Sleep disturbances
- Hopelessness
- Helplessness
- Powerlessness
- Low self-esteem
- Difficulty experiencing pleasure in activities

Other Symptoms
- Fatigue
- Decrease in performance of activities of daily living
- Thoughts of death
- Decreased libido
- Anorexia or overeating

Data from Townsend, M. C., & Morgan, K. I. (2018). *Psychiatric mental health nursing: Concepts of care in evidence-based practice* (9th ed., pp. 511–512). Philadelphia: F.A. Davis Company.

Depression is a state of feelings that is more than just sadness. It is a common psychiatric condition that affects a person's ability to function in day-to-day activities. Major depression is the fourth leading cause of years lived with disability (YLD) (Hancock, 2018). Approximately one in four Canadians experience depression that requires treatment (Ontario Ministry of Health and Long-Term Care, 2015). There are many symptoms of depression, the most common being apathy, feelings of sadness, fatigue, guilt, poor concentration, sleep disturbances, and suicidal thoughts. Depression results in both subjective and objective behaviours and patient reports of increased physical complaints (Box 3.4). Some patients report feeling anxious when depressed.

Delegation and Collaboration

The skill of communicating with a patient with difficulty coping cannot be delegated to an unregulated care provider (UCP). The nurse instructs the UCP about:
- Basic communication skills needed to interact verbally and nonverbally with anxious, angry, or depressed patients.
- Their support role as the nurse uses de-escalation techniques.
- Appropriate safety measures for themselves and other patients.

STEP	RATIONALE

ASSESSMENT

1. Provide a brief, simple introduction; introduce yourself and explain purpose of interaction.

Ineffective coping behaviours may limit amount of information patient can understand.

2. Assess factors influencing communication with patient (e.g., environment, timing, presence of others, values, experiences, need for personal space because of heightened anxiety).

Identifies effective communication strategies.

3. Assess for possible factors causing patient anxiety (e.g., hospitalization, unknown diagnosis, fatigue).

Understanding the source of anxiety helps in patient support and communication.

4. Discuss possible causes of patient's anxiety, anger, or depression with family members, including past history of the illness, if necessary.

Gathering information about patient from a family perspective is useful because family provides new information or understanding of the situation (Ondrejka, 2018, p. 57).

5. Observe for physical, behavioural, and verbal cues that indicate that patient is anxious, such as dry mouth, sweaty palms, tone of voice, frequent use of call light, difficulty concentrating, wringing of hands, and statements such as "I'm scared."

Anxiety interferes with the usual manner of communication and thus interferes with patient's care and treatment. Extreme anxiety interferes with comprehension, attention, and problem-solving abilities.

6. Assess for physical, behavioural, and verbal cues that indicate patient is depressed, such as feelings of sadness, tearfulness, difficulty concentrating, increase in reports of physical complaints, and statements such as "I'm sad/depressed."

Depression interferes with the usual manner of communication and thus with patient's care and treatment. If depression is severe, it interferes with comprehension, attention, and problem-solving abilities.

STEP	RATIONALE

ASSESSMENT

7. Assess for possible factors causing patient's depression (e.g., acute or persistent illness, personal vulnerability, recent loss).

Patient's depressive state is sometimes unknown. Understanding the possible cause of depression helps in patient support and communication.

8. Observe for behaviours that indicate the patient is angry (e.g., pacing, clenched fist, loud voice, throwing objects) and expressions that indicate anger (e.g., repeated questioning of nurse, not following requests, aggressive outbursts, threats).

Anger is a normal expression of frustration or response to feeling threatened. However, its expression often interferes with or blocks communication and interactions.

9. Assess factors that influence the angry patient's communication, such as refusal to adhere to treatment goals, use of sarcasm or hostile behaviour, having a low frustration level, or being emotionally immature.

Allows you to accurately evaluate the situation or patient experiences that block or facilitate communication.

10. Assess for resources (e.g., social worker, pastoral care, or family) available to help in communicating with a potentially violent patient.

This helps to clarify cause and intervention required to deal with patient's anger.

11. Assess for underlying medical conditions that may potentially lead to violent behaviour.

Patients with medical conditions such as traumatic brain injury, dementia, or substance or alcohol withdrawal may exhibit hostile, aggressive behaviours.

Clinical Decision Point *With some violent behaviours (e.g., physical aggression) you may not be able to de-escalate the situation. When this potential situation exists, know whom to call for assistance (e.g., Code White). Personal safety is essential.*

NURSING DIAGNOSES

- Anxiety
- Hopelessness
- Decisional conflict

- Defensive coping
- Inadequate coping
- Altered verbal communication

- Altered role performance
- Potential for other-directed violence
- Potential for self-directed violence

Related factors/Risk factors are individualized on the basis of patient's condition or needs.

PLANNING

1. Expected outcomes following completion of procedure:
   - Patient discusses factors causing anxiety, anger, or depression.

   Reflects success in ability to communicate openly and building trust.

   - Patient can discuss methods to cope with anxiety, anger, or depression.

   Gains resources (e.g., use of breathing exercises, guided imagery) to cope with situations that cause anxiety, anger, or depression.

   - Patient states that sensations of anxiety or depression are reduced.

   Eases symptoms associated with anxiety and depression and allows patient to focus on problem.

Clinical Decision Point *First acknowledge and address the anxious patient's physical and emotional discomfort. Focus on understanding the patient, providing feedback and helping to problem solve, and providing atmosphere of warmth and acceptance.*

   - Patient no longer exhibits verbal and nonverbal expressions of anger.

   De-escalation techniques successfully allow patient to express anger in a constructive way.

2. Prepare for therapeutic intervention by considering patient goals, time allocation, and resources.

   Allows patient to establish rapport, achieve a sense of calm, and begin to analyze source of anxiety.

3. Recognize personal level of anxiety and consciously try to remain calm (breathe slowly and deeply) when communicating with an anxious, angry, or depressed patient. Be aware of nonverbal cues that indicate your own anxiety (e.g., body language, posture, cadence of speech). Remain nonjudgemental.

   Your anxiety increases patient's anxiety. Your personal feelings and values may negatively affect interaction with patient.

4. Prepare a quiet, calm area, allowing personal space.

   Decreasing stimuli has a calming effect. Invasion of personal space increases anxiety, anger, or depression.

STEP	RATIONALE

PLANNING

Clinical Decision Point *First acknowledge and address the depressed patient's physical and emotional discomfort. Focus on understanding patient, providing feedback, and helping to problem solve.*

5. Prepare for de-escalation for an angry patient.
   a. Pause to collect own thoughts, feelings, and reactions.

   b. Determine what patient is saying.

   c. Prepare the environment to de-escalate a potentially violent patient.

   (1) Encourage other people, particularly those who provoke anger, to leave room or area.
   (2) Maintain an adequate distance and open exit. Position yourself closest to door to facilitate escape from a potentially violent situation. Do not block exit so patient feels that escape is unattainable.
   (3) When anger begins to disturb others, close door. This is particularly important when patient becomes agitated.

	Awareness and control of your reaction and responses facilitate more constructive interaction.
	Clarification of patient need or concern may help to de-escalate situation.
	Potentially violent patient needs to be in an environment with decreased stimuli and have protection from injury to self or against others.
	Encourages patient's expression of anger rather than provoking it.
	Avoids pressuring patient; helps to prevent injury if anger becomes out of control.
	Prevents feeling of being trapped for both you and patient. Feeling trapped may cause a violent outburst. Safety of both parties is essential.
	Agitation and anxiety can spread to others. Some hospital rooms are equipped with security windows and cameras to allow for observation of patients.

Clinical Decision Point *Some patients are disruptive to one another, especially those who are hyperactive, intrusive, or threatening or exhibit bizarre behaviours. For these patients, first try the least restrictive measures before using more restrictive measures such as seclusion.*

   (4) Reduce disturbing factors in room (e.g., noise, drafts, inadequate lighting). | Reduces irritants that may heighten anger. |

IMPLEMENTATION

1. Use appropriate nonverbal behaviours and active listening skills such as staying with patient at bedside and having a relaxed posture. Focus on understanding the patient's issues.	Patients experiencing emotionally charged situation may not comprehend a verbally delivered message. Nonverbal messages to patient express interest and help alleviate anxiety.
2. Use appropriate verbal techniques that are clear and concise to respond to anxious patient. Use brief statements that acknowledge current state of feelings and provide direction to patient, such as "It seems to me that you're anxious" or "I notice that you seem to want to be alone. Would you like to go to your room to rest?"	Promotes effective communication so patient can explore reasons for anxiety, anger, or depression. Appropriate techniques and statements provide reassurance.
3. Help patient acquire alternative coping strategies such as progressive relaxation, breathing exercises, and visual imagery (see Chapter 16).	Coping strategies help patient reduce anxiety and depression and, in some cases, reduce anger.
4. Provide necessary comfort measures such as analgesics, positioning, or hygiene.	Pain heightens patient's anxiety or depression and can contribute to their anger.
5. Use open-ended questions, such as "Tell me about how you're feeling" or "You seem sad. Tell me about your sadness."	Encourages patient to continue talking, facilitating an in-depth discussion of symptoms.
6. Encourage and reward small decisions and independent actions. When necessary, make decisions that patients are not ready to make. Present situations that require no decision making.	Depressed patients are often overly dependent and indecisive.
7. Accept patient and focus on positive aspects. Provide positive feedback.	Depressed patients often have low self-esteem. This approach helps to focus on their strengths.
8. Be honest and empathic.	Honesty and empathy facilitate the development of trust.

STEP	RATIONALE

IMPLEMENTATION

Clinical Decision Point *If your patient seems depressed, ask the person about suicidal ideation. Ask, "Have you thought about hurting yourself? Tell me how you would do it. Do you have the means to carry out your plan?" The risk of suicide is greatly increased if the patient has developed a plan, has strong intentions, and has the means to complete the plan. Listen actively and encourage expression of feelings, including anger, in a nonjudgemental way. It is critical that the nurse be direct with the patient and communicate openly and matter-of-factly about suicide. Refer to an appropriate mental health care provider (if available) (Townsend & Morgan, 2018, pp. 304–306).*

9. De-escalation for an angry patient

a. Maintain personal space. It may be necessary to have someone with you and to keep the room door open. Position yourself between patient and the exit.

> Use of personal space may help to de-escalate patient's anger. Positioning promotes health care provider's safety if patient's anger continues to escalate and patient becomes violent.

b. Maintain nonthreatening verbal and nonverbal approach using a calm, reassuring tone of voice. Use open body language with a concerned, nonthreatening facial expression, open, unfolded arms, relaxed posture, and a safe distance. Use gestures that are slow and deliberate rather than sudden and abrupt.

> Decreases chance of misinterpretation of message and is less threatening.
> A relaxed atmosphere prevents further escalation. Creates climate of acceptance for patient.

c. Use therapeutic silence and allow patient to vent feelings. Use active listening for understanding. Do not argue with patient.

> Often de-escalates anger. Anger expends emotional and physical energy; patient runs out of momentum and energy to maintain anger at high level. Arguing escalates anger.

d. Respond to anger therapeutically; avoid becoming defensive or angry and encourage verbal expression of anger.

> Some depressed patients are angry; understand that anger is a symptom of their depression. Verbal expression often reduces tension.

e. Answer questions calmly and honestly as appropriate. If patient asks power-struggle type of question (challenging or confrontational type) (e.g., "Who said you were in charge?"), redirect and set limits by giving clear, concise expectations. Inform patient of potential consequences without sounding threatening and follow through with consequences if patient does not change behaviours.

> A calm, clear communication style helps to set limits on power-struggle types of questions, provides structure for the interaction, and helps diffuse anger (Balzer-Riley, 2017, p. 272).

f. If patient is making verbal threats to harm others, remain calm yet professional and continue to set limits on inappropriate behaviour.

> Angry patient loses ability to process information rationally and therefore may impulsively express anger through intimidation.

Clinical Decision Point *If imminent harm to another is present on discharge, notify proper authorities (e.g., nurse manager, security). A potentially violent patient can be impulsive and explosive; therefore, you need to keep personal safety skills in mind. In this case, avoid touch.*

g. If patient appears to be calm and anger is defused, explore alternatives to situation or feelings of anger.

> Processing with patient can prevent future explosive outbursts and teach patient effective ways of dealing with anger.

EVALUATION

1. Observe for continuing presence of physical signs and symptoms or behaviours reflecting anxiety, anger, or depression.

> Observation determines extent to which planned interaction relieved patient's emotions.

2. Ask patient to describe ways to cope with anxiety, depression, or anger in the future and make decisions about own care.

> This measures patient's ability to assume more health-promoting behaviour.

3. Evaluate patient's ability to discuss factors causing anxiety, depression, or anger.

> This measures patient's ability to attend to or focus on area of concern.

4. Note patient's ability to answer questions and problem solve.

> Determines whether anger has lessened so patient is able to focus on alternative coping skills.

5. Have patient discuss ways to cope in the future and make decisions about own care.

> Discussion measures patient's ability to assume more health-promoting behaviour.

6. **Use Teach-Back:** "I want to be sure you understand what we went over today. We talked about different ways to help you manage your anxiety along with taking your medication. Tell me about the other methods you are going to use." Develop a revised teaching plan if patient or caregiver is not able to teach back correctly.

> Determines patient's and caregiver's level of understanding of teaching.

STEP	RATIONALE
Unexpected Outcomes	**Related Interventions**
1. Physical signs and symptoms of anxiety/anger continue. Your interaction has increased patient's anxiety/anger; source of anxiety/anger is not resolved.	• Use refocusing or distraction skills such as relaxation or guided imagery to reduce anxiety (Townsend & Morgan, 2018, p. 575). • Reassess factors and remove or alter factors contributing to anxiety/anger. • Take charge with calm, firm directions. Give as-needed (prn) medications as prescribed for anxiety/agitation/escalating behaviours. • Ensure that health care team members are available to help if necessary.
2. Patient displays difficulty making decisions by avoiding your efforts at focusing discussion or is unable to discuss real concerns. Anxiety/anger/depression continues to prevent problem solving. 3. Depressive behaviours continue; interaction has been ineffective at relieving depressive symptoms or patient reports suicidal ideation with or without plan.	• Be clear and direct when communicating with patient to avoid misunderstanding. • When used appropriately, touch helps control feelings of panic. • Continue to use therapeutic communication skills but try different techniques. • Refer patient to mental health provider for consultation regarding use of pharmacological medications, formal psychotherapy to treat depression, or both. • Refer patient to mental health provider for evaluation and possible admission to an inpatient psychiatric treatment facility.

Communication and Documentation

- Document cause of patient's anxiety/anger/depression and any exhibited signs and symptoms of behaviours on flow sheet or in nurses' notes in electronic health record (EHR) or chart.
- Document de-escalation technique used and patient's response to de-escalation efforts on flow sheet or in nurses' notes in EHR or chart.
- Report methods used to relieve anxiety/anger/depression and patient's response to ensure continuity of care between nurses.
- Report technique used to de-escalate and patient's response to nurse in charge.
- Document your evaluation of patient and caregiver learning.

Special Considerations
Teaching

- Teaching patient and caregiver to identify possible sources of anxiety such as illness, hospitalization, knowledge deficits, or other known stressors gives patient knowledge of anxiety and increases sense of control.
- Patients experiencing emotionally charged situations do not always comprehend instruction. Focus on understanding patient; provide feedback and help to problem solve, and provide an atmosphere of safety, warmth, and acceptance.
- Teaching patient and caregiver to identify possible factors that contribute to angry outbursts, such as inadequate coping skills, low frustration levels, illness, hospitalization, knowledge deficits, or other known stressors, may give patient a sense of control.
- Once anger has been de-escalated, teach patient new adaptive methods of coping with anger.
- Teach patient and caregiver to identify possible sources of depression. Knowledge of depression increases patient's sense of control over feelings of depression.

Pediatric

- Children often demonstrate anxiety through physical and behavioural signs but are unable to express anxiety verbally. Some children express anxiety through restless behaviour, physical complaints, or behavioural regression. Note any changes in child's behaviour that occur during illness or hospitalization (McKinney et al., 2018, p. 1314).
- Set limits for inappropriate behaviours exhibited by child such as using a time-out. Apply such limits immediately because children tend to have less internal control over their own behaviours (McKinney et al., 2018, p. 44).
- Children often demonstrate symptoms of depression that differ from those of adults. They manifest depression through physical (increased somatic complaints) and behavioural (poor school performance, social isolation) signs and are often unable to express it verbally. Some children express depression through restless behaviour or behavioural regression. It is important to note any changes in child's behaviour that occur during illness or hospitalization (McKinney et al., 2018, p. 1313).

Gerontological

- Anxiety is one of the most common symptoms seen in older persons. Anxiety develops because of a specific event or a general pattern of change (e.g., decline in health) (Byrd & Luther, 2018, p. 1367).
- Psychosocial factors such as anxiety and confusion, lack of mobility, and spatial organization of a long-term or complex care facility are factors that decrease social contacts, thus hindering communication with peers and health care providers. This leads to further feelings of isolation, boredom, and increased anxiety.
- Older persons who are socially isolated often have multiple health problems and are more likely to have anxious or depressive symptoms. In addition, they are less likely to seek care for these symptoms.
- Depression among older persons is a major health concern. It is important to differentiate between depression and any underlying medical illness, such as cognitive impairment (Byrd & Luther, 2018, p. 1392).
- Suicide risk is increased in older persons because of loss of life partner, health status, independence, and social support system or financial losses (Byrd & Luther, 2018, p. 1411).

Care in the Community

- Anticipation of a home care visit may increase a patient's anxiety (Yamamoto-Mitani, Noguchi-Watanabe, & Fukahori, 2016).
- Personal safety for the nurse against a potentially violent patient or caregiver extends to all health care settings, including the patient's home. Assess patient's home and physical surroundings, including possible exits. You may be in a potentially dangerous situation while giving care to patient at home because you are without support from other team members. Do not enter the home if you feel unsafe; call for help.
- Depression is often present in home care settings. Educate caregivers about how to identify symptoms. Manage depression based on patient's presenting behaviours with a consideration of any cognitive or physical impairment.

✦ SKILL 3.3   Communicating With a Cognitively Impaired Patient

The act of communicating and expressing oneself is affected by a person's ability. Patients with cognitive impairments pose a challenge for nurses because these patients may have disabilities that negatively affect communication (Judd, 2017; Mendes & Palmer, 2018). Acute cognitive impairment or delirium is largely reversible and may be caused by conditions such as infection, polypharmacy, and metabolic changes. Once the cause is identified and treated, the patient's mental status returns to a baseline condition. Persistent types of cognitive impairments are irreversible and progressive. These include dementia (Alzheimer's disease, vascular dementia, frontal-temporal dementia), traumatic brain injury (TBI), and human immunodeficiency virus (HIV)–related cognitive dysfunction.

Cognitive impairments accompanied by communication deficits hinder a patient's ability to initiate conversation and participate in self-care. Since it is time-consuming to interact with these patients, they may be deprived of human contact, which leads to depression, detachment, and isolation. Patients with cognitive impairments may also be at risk for physical status changes such as infection, falls and injury, and poor nutrition.

There is a potential for a lack of quality nurse–patient interaction and communication, which negatively affects patient outcomes. A person-centred approach stresses the individuality of each patient when assessing the patient's ability to communicate.

Delegation and Collaboration

The skill of communicating effectively with a cognitively impaired patient cannot be delegated to unregulated care providers (UCPs). The nurse instructs the UCP about:

- The proper communication skills needed to interact verbally and nonverbally with the cognitively impaired patient.
- The possible causes and signs and symptoms of the patient's cognitive impairment.

STEP	RATIONALE

ASSESSMENT

1. When you first meet a patient, approach from the front. Assess for the physical, behavioural, and verbal cues that indicate a patient is cognitively impaired. Assess orientation status of patient (person, place, time). A mental health examination (see Chapter 8) may be used to assess for the presence of cognitive impairment in a person with suspected dementia or following a head injury.	You may startle and upset a patient if you touch the person unexpectedly or approach from behind. If the patient is unable to think, speak, or understand, you need to adjust communication strategies to communicate effectively.
2. Assess for possible factors causing patient's cognitive impairment (e.g., acute or persistent illness, fever, medications, fluid and electrolyte imbalance).	Understanding the possible cause of mental decline helps in conferring with the health care team on appropriate therapy and has implications for short-term and long-term communication strategies.
3. Assess factors influencing communication with patient (e.g., environment, timing, presence of others, values, experiences, prior sensory loss, poor concentration).	Understanding factors that influence communication helps you to identify effective communication strategies (Sanders et al., 2018).
4. Discuss possible causes of patient's cognitive impairment with family members or caregivers, including current illness, duration, treatment regimen, and past medical history.	Gathering information about the patient from a family perspective is useful because family provides new information or understanding of the situation. It is important to establish patient's baseline mental status.
5. Discuss with family or caregivers how patient typically communicates with them. Consider these questions: Does the patient lose their train of thought, struggle to organize words logically, need more time to understand what you're saying, or curse or use offensive language? (Mayo Clinic, 2016).	Allows you to anticipate pattern of patient's communication so you can use effective communication strategies.
6. Ascertain the most effective means of communication with patient (e.g., verbal or written communication, picture board). Ensure this information is communicated and shared with all members of the interprofessional team.	Knowing how best to communicate and using alternative communication methods can help identify a patient's needs. It is essential that all team members are aware of the strategies that work best for the patient to enhance interprofessional collaboration and improve patient health outcomes.

STEP	RATIONALE

NURSING DIAGNOSES

- Acute confusion
- Hopelessness
- Inadequate coping

- Decisional conflict
- Altered social interaction

- Altered verbal communication
- Altered role performance

Related factors are individualized on the basis of patient's condition or needs.

PLANNING

1. Expected outcomes following completion of procedure:
   - Patient can communicate physical and emotional discomfort needs to nurse.

   Use of relevant communication techniques enables patient to express needs (e.g., physical and emotional discomfort) effectively given the limitations related to cognitive impairment.

2. Prepare for communication by considering type of cognitive and communication impairments, time allocation, and resources.

   Effective communication allows you to establish rapport with patient and have a quality nurse–patient interaction.

3. Be aware of your nonverbal cues that affect communication with the cognitively impaired patient (e.g., body language, posture, cadence of speech). Remain nonjudgemental.

   Frustration in communication with patients with cognitive impairment may negatively affect interaction with patient.

4. Prepare environment physically by providing a quiet, calm area. Reduce distractions such as external noises.

   Decreasing stimuli has a calming effect. Ensuring that the environment is quiet and free from distractions enhances the communication experience.

IMPLEMENTATION

1. Approach patient from the front and face them when speaking.

   This strategy avoids startling the patient and helps to ensure that patient both sees and hears you.

2. Provide brief, simple introduction. Introduce yourself, show respect, and explain purpose of interaction.

   Symptoms associated with cognitive impairment limit amount of information that patient can understand.

3. Use appropriate nonverbal behaviours and active listening skills such as staying with patient at bedside or using touch appropriately.

   Nonverbal messages to patient express your interest and convey empathy. Use of touch may help with concentration and reassurance.

4. Use clear and concise verbal techniques to respond to patient (Mayo Clinic, 2016). Use simple language and speak slowly; use short and simple sentences. Ask yes-or-no questions.

   Appropriate techniques and statements provide reassurance to cognitively impaired patient.

5. Ask one question at a time and allow time for response. Avoid rushing patient. Do not interrupt patient.

   This gives patient time to process the information and respond.

6. Repeat sentences using a steady voice and avoid raising your voice or being too quick to guess what patient is trying to express.

   Repetition allows time for patient to respond; it can be frustrating for patient if you misinterpret their message or pressure them to respond.

7. Use augmentative and assistive communication (AAC) devices such as pictogram grid, talking mats, objects, and iPads to facilitate communication.

   Talking mats are communication aids that use picture symbols, so the patient can place relevant images below a visual scale to indicate feelings (Bunning, Adler, Proudman, et al., 2016).

8. Make sure that patient is wearing eyeglasses or hearing aids to help with communication.

   Some patients with cognitive impairments forget about eyeglasses or hearing aids and need to be reminded to use these to improve clarity of communication.

9. Do not argue with patient or correct if mistakes are made.

   Arguing can lead to increased frustration and agitation.

10. Maintain meaningful interactions with patients and use creative modes of communication based on patient's comfort level and abilities.

    Meaningful interactions help patient engage with family or community and surroundings and help reduce a sense of isolation and detachment.

11. Use individualized coping strategies such as progressive relaxation, breathing exercises, or guided imagery.

    Helps to reduce some anxiety associated with confusion and difficulties in communication.

STEP	RATIONALE

EVALUATION

1. Observe patient's response for clarity and understanding of messages sent and received.
2. Observe verbal and nonverbal behaviours.

3. **Use Teach-Back:** "I want to be sure I explained how this picture board will help you communicate with your family. Tell me how to use the picture board to show your spouse that you want to take a shower or take a walk together." Develop a revised teaching plan if patient or caregiver is not able to teach back correctly.

Observation determines extent to which cognitively impaired patient is able to express self.

Observation reveals if patient is comfortable and needs have been met.

Determines patient's and caregiver's level of understanding of teaching.

Unexpected Outcomes

1. Messages that are sent and received are not understood.

2. Patient becomes frustrated, and communication with nurse becomes more challenging.

Related Interventions

- Continue to use therapeutic communication skills when interacting with cognitively impaired patient. Be creative in using alternative strategies (e.g., involving family members).
- Remain patient and calm and speak in a soft voice (Twigg & Schwartzkopf, 2018, p. 404).
- Allow time for patient to respond and distract if possible.
- Avoid touching, waiting until patient is calmer.
- Identify and address unmet needs (hunger, pain, toileting).
- Allow for periods of adequate rest; make frequent attempts to interact to minimize social isolation.

Communication and Documentation

- Document both objective and subjective behaviours (associated with cognitive impairment) that patient is displaying on flow sheet or in nurses' notes in electronic health record (EHR) or chart.
- Document and report the methods used to communicate and patient's response.
- Document your evaluation of patient and caregiver learning.

Special Considerations
Teaching

- Teach patient and caregiver how to use various methods to communicate, such as pictorial board or communication aids.
- Make teaching modifications with consideration of impaired concentration and memory related to patient's cognitive status (e.g., present a small amount of material at a time; use simple and short phrases; repeat information as needed).

Pediatric

- Children may exhibit cognitive impairments because of acute or persistent metabolic or neurological conditions. Communication

strategies with children should take into consideration their developmental level. Use pictures and drawings for patients who are unable to read.

Gerontological

- Many older persons have cognitive impairments that pose serious barriers to the reliability of your assessment; therefore, it is important to use effective verbal and nonverbal communication strategies. Poor communication can compromise care, leading to increased anxiety and frustration.
- Patients who have cognitive impairments may exhibit tantrum-like behaviours in response to real or perceived frustration. Use distraction techniques to remove a cognitively impaired older person from disturbing stimuli or redirect patient to activity that is pleasurable (Twigg & Schwartzkopf, 2018, p. 1137).

Care in the Community

- Manage care based on patient's presenting behaviours with consideration of any cognitive or physical impairment. Include the caregiver, family, and friends in using effective communication strategies.

✦ SKILL 3.4   Communicating With Colleagues

In health care settings communicating is a key part of everyday practice. As a nurse, you communicate with patients, members of the interprofessional health care team, and external colleagues. This communication occurs face to face, over the phone, and in writing. The quality of these interactions is a key component of error prevention; clarity and comprehension of treatment plans and adherence to them; and patient outcomes. Nevertheless, communication problems are common in health care settings, and failures in communication can have serious consequences (Stewart & Hand, 2017). The Canadian Patient Safety Institute (CPSI) implements programs and publishes guides to improve patient safety and quality in the Canadian health care system. Patient engagement improves communication between patients and health care providers (CPSI, 2017, p. 11). Interprofessional collaboration increases team members' awareness of each other's type of knowledge and skills, leading to continued improvement in decision making and patient outcomes. Moreover, teamwork and interprofessional collaboration are essential to quality patient care. Be aware of the differences in communication styles among members of the interprofessional team and adapt your style of communicating to effectively interact with team members (McKibben, 2017).

Conflicts among colleagues can indirectly influence the therapeutic nurse–patient relationship and negatively affect the delivery of care and patient and health care provider satisfaction (Balzer-Riley, 2017, p. 330; McKibben, 2017). Effective communication is necessary to resolve conflict among members of the health care team. Good communication in the form of conflict resolution skills can decrease the risk of conflict and its negative effects.

Standardized communication with SBAR is structured to optimize effective communication among members of the health care team. Using SBAR, nurses are better prepared before calling a health care provider and when formulating a recommendation based on solid assessment. Nurses are more confident in their clinical judgement, resulting in better patient outcomes (Stewart & Hand, 2017). Improved communication using structured communication techniques, including bedside reporting with the SBAR framework, streamlines information exchanges and promotes patient safety (e.g.,

communicating accurate information about test results or medications) (Stewart & Hand, 2017). The evidence suggests that bedside reporting gives the oncoming nurse a chance for direct observation of a patient and a chance to ask questions related to the patient's status. This type of interaction promotes accountability between shifts. Bedside reporting and effective communication with the use of SBAR help to decrease adverse events and increase patient and family satisfaction (Stewart & Hand, 2017).

Delegation and Collaboration

The skill of communicating effectively with colleagues can be delegated to an unregulated care provider (UCP). The nurse instructs the UCP about:

- The proper communication skills needed to effectively interact verbally and nonverbally with colleagues.

STEP	RATIONALE
ASSESSMENT	
1. Identify purpose of interaction with colleague.	This sets the stage for the interaction; all members of the communication exchange are aware of purpose of the conversation.
2. Assess factors influencing communication with others (e.g., environment, timing, presence of others' cultural beliefs and values, prior experiences).	Assessment allows you to accurately evaluate any barriers to communication or issues that may need to be considered to maintain open, clear channels of communication.
3. Consider level of stress in the situation; do you feel threatened?	Feeling threatened results in a sympathetic stress response that can impair judgement, emotional control, and ability to communicate clearly.

NURSING DIAGNOSES

- Decisional conflict
- Fear
- Altered coping

- Deficient knowledge regarding communication skills
- Inadequate role performance

- Reduced social interaction
- Altered verbal communication

Related factors are individualized on the basis of patient's condition or needs.

STEP	RATIONALE
PLANNING	
1. Prepare for communication with members of the health care team who may have differing needs or concerns. Example: If you feel stressed, try to relax and use breathing exercises.	Effective communication allows members of the health care team to establish rapport and have a quality interaction. Adapt own style of communicating (e.g., relaxation) to meet the needs of the health care team.
2. Be aware of your nonverbal cues that affect communication with others. Remain nonjudgemental.	Frustration in communication may negatively affect interaction with others.
3. Prepare environment physically; go to a quiet, calm area. Reduce distractions such as external noises.	Factors to consider include privacy, noise control, seating space, and convenience to help to ensure the space needed for effective teamwork.
4. Be aware of hierarchical differences among members of the health care team as a common barrier to effective communication and collaboration.	Intimidating behaviour by individuals at the top of a hierarchy can hinder open communication.
IMPLEMENTATION	
1. Approach colleague from the front and face directly when speaking. Maintain appropriate eye contact.	This strategy ensures that the colleague both sees and hears you and conveys an attitude of respect.
2. Provide a brief, simple introduction; introduce yourself and explain purpose of interaction.	This strategy ensures that the colleague understands purpose of interaction.
3. Be aware of your own body language and tone. Assume an open stance; do not fold arms across your chest.	Nonverbal messages convey empathy. Be aware of how your nonverbal communication style may impact others.

STEP	RATIONALE

IMPLEMENTATION

4. Acknowledge and respond to a range of views. Allow equal time for all members to participate in expressing opinions.

Understand the perspectives of others and support the value of collaboration and teamwork.

5. Use oral communication skills such as ask open-ended questions, do not assume, do not interrupt, and do not blame others. Provide feedback. Use active listening and recognize nonverbal triggers. Ask for clarification when necessary.

Effective communication skills should be used for communicating and for resolving conflict.

6. Use a range of workplace written communication methods (e.g., oral, written notes, memos, letters, charts, diagrams).

Standardized communication such as the SBAR method of communication can help streamline information exchanges and promote patient safety.

7. Encourage discussion of both positive and negative feelings to increase opportunities for members to express all their concerns.

Discussion fosters active listening and understanding. All members of the exchange are valued, and their contributions are recognized.

8. Summarize key themes in the discussion and help to develop alternative solutions to the issue.

Conflict resolution involves examining alternative solutions to an issue. It values the influence of system solutions in achieving effective functioning among colleagues (McKibben, 2017).

EVALUATION

1. Confirm clarity and understanding of messages sent and received.

Determines extent to which members of the exchange understand.

2. Observe verbal and nonverbal behaviours.

Observation reveals if there are any negative emotions or further concerns that contradict a message.

Unexpected Outcomes

1. Messages that are sent and received are not understood.

2. Frustration among colleagues persists, and communication becomes more challenging.

Related Interventions

- Continue to use therapeutic communication skills when interacting with others. Be creative in using alternative strategies.
- Conflict among colleagues can have a direct impact on the nurse–patient relationship, affecting delivery of care (College of Nurses of Ontario [CNO], 2017, p. 5).
- Nurses should address conflict directly (CNO, 2017, p. 7). Talk to the colleague first and if that is not effective, consult your manager/director as appropriate for resolution. Follow your employer policy related to whom to contact, and when, following the chain of command as outlined by your employer. Continue to have empathy and use active listening to better understand colleagues.

Communication and Documentation

- As needed, document and report successful communication strategies and pertinent changes to patient's plan of care on flow sheet or in nurses' notes in electronic health record (EHR) or chart.

◆ CLINICAL DEBRIEF

You are assigned to care for Mrs. Adams, an older patient who was admitted to the hospital 2 days ago after falling at her son's home. She recently moved in with her son, her only child, following the sudden death of her husband. Her husband had been her primary caregiver since she was diagnosed with Alzheimer's disease 3 years ago. Neither her husband nor her son wanted to put her into a long-term or complex care facility. She had emergency surgery to repair a fractured wrist. During shift report on a medical-surgical unit, the nurse tells you that the patient is withdrawn and confused. In addition, she has difficulty understanding verbal direction from the interprofessional team members.

When you approach the patient to perform an initial assessment, she is looking out the window and seems disoriented. She appears dishevelled, and her lunch tray is untouched. You ask her if she needs help with bathing, dressing, and feeding; but you get a response that you cannot understand. Her impaired communication is causing her increased anxiety, which is further hindering her communication with others and her ability to follow directions.

1. Which steps are necessary to effectively communicate with a cognitively impaired patient?
2. Which strategies would you use to manage or decrease Mrs. Adams' anxiety level? Explain your choice or choices.
3. Using the SBAR format, describe strategies to communicate with the interprofessional team regarding the treatment plan for Mrs. Adams.

◆ REVIEW QUESTIONS

1. The nurse is learning about barriers to effective nurse–patient communication. Which of the following approaches would be considered a barrier? *(Select all that apply.)*
   1. Discussing fears about a patient with members of the health care team
   2. Interrupting patient when the patient does not answer the question posed
   3. Obtaining information about a critically ill patient from their family
   4. Admitting a mistake to a patient's family
   5. Giving advice to the patient's health care provider
   6. Minimizing concerns and issues of a patient
2. The nurse is caring for a patient recovering from a bilateral mastectomy for breast cancer who tearfully states that she is feeling depressed and worthless as a woman. Which of the following responses are therapeutic statements for the nurse to make? *(Select all that apply.)*
   1. "Many women have body image concerns after undergoing this surgery."
   2. "You will feel better soon."
   3. "Tell me more about how you feel."
   4. "Why do you feel depressed and worthless?"
   5. "How long have you been feeling this way?"
   6. "I am sure your husband will still love you no matter what you look like."
3. The nurse is caring for a patient with a cognitive impairment who is upset about not being able to describe what he wants to eat. The patient is talking loudly, which is annoying other patients. Which of the following actions would be **most** appropriate for the nurse to take? *(Select all that apply.)*
   1. Approach the patient from the front and make eye contact.
   2. Explain to the patient that he will benefit by acting calmer and not talking loudly.
   3. Ask the patient one question at a time about what he would like to eat.
   4. Use nonverbal communication methods.
   5. Ask family members which communication measures are successful at home.

ⓔ *Visit the Evolve site for a complete list of Clinical Debrief and Review Questions answers.*

REFERENCES

Balzer-Riley, J. (2017). *Communication in nursing*. St. Louis, MO: Elsevier.
Bell, L. (2016). Communicating to help patients and families. *American Journal of Critical Care*, 25(6), 508. doi:10.4037/ajcc2016589
Bingham, H., & O'Brien, A. J. (2018). Educational intervention to decrease stigmatizing attitudes of undergraduate nurses towards people with mental illness. *International Journal of Mental Health Nursing*, 27(1), 311–319. doi:10.1111/inm.12322
Bourque Bearskin, R. L. (2016). Through the lens of truth and reconciliation: Next steps. *Canadian Nurse*, 112(2), 36.
Boyer, Y. (2017). Healing racism in Canadian healthcare. *Canadian Medical Association Journal*, 189(46), E1408–E1409. doi:10.1503/cmaj.171234
Bunning, K., Adler, R., Proudman, L., & Wyborn, H. (2016). Co-production and pilot of a structured interview using Talking Mats® to survey the television viewing habits and preferences of adults and young people with learning dis-
abilities. *British Journal of Learning Disabilities*, 45(1), 1–11. doi:10.1111/bld.12167
Byram, A., Lee, G., Owen, A., et al. (2016). Ethical and clinical considerations at the intersection of functional neuroimaging and disorders of consciousness: The experts weigh in. *Cambridge Quarterly of Healthcare Ethics*, 25(4), 613–622. doi:10.1017/S0963180116000347
Byrd, L., & Luther, C. (2018). Anxiety and depression in the older adult. In K. Mauk (Ed.), *Gerontological nursing: Competencies for care* (4th ed., pp. 1362–1430). Burlington, MA: Jones & Bartlett Learning.
Canadian Nurses Association (CNA). (2017). *Code of Ethics for Registered Nurses*. Ottawa, ON: Author. Retrieved from https://www.cna-aiic.ca/~/media/cna/page-content/pdf-en/code-of-ethics-2017-edition-secure-interactive.pdf?la=en
Canadian Patient Safety Institute (CPSI). (2017). *Engaging patients in patient safety: A Canadian guide*. Retrieved from http://www.patientsafetyinstitute.ca/en/toolsResources/Patient-Engagement-in-Patient-Safety-Guide/Documents/Engaging%20Patients%20in%20Patient%20Safety.pdf
Chute, A. (2015). Communication: At the heart of nursing practice. In D. Gregory, C. Raymond-Seniuk, L. Patrick, & T. Stephen (Eds.), *Fundamentals: Perspectives on the art and science of Canadian nursing* (pp. 599–636). Philadelphia: Wolters Kluwer Health/Lippincott Williams & Wilkens.
College of Nurses of Ontario (CNO). (2017). *Practice guideline: Conflict prevention and management*. Toronto: ON: Author. Retrieved from https://www.cno.org/globalassets/docs/prac/47004_conflict_prev.pdf
College of Registered Nurses of Nova Scotia (CRNNS). (2017). *Professional boundaries and the nurse-client relationship: Keeping it safe and therapeutic*. Halifax, NS: Author. Retrieved from https://crnns.ca/wp-content/uploads/2015/02/ProfessionalBoundaries2012.pdf
Daly, L. (2017). Effective communication with older adults. *Nursing Standard*, 31(41), 55–62. doi:10.7748/ns.2017.e10832
Deerfield, C. T., Barnum, A. J., & Pugh-Yi, R. H. (2017). Adapting Paulo Friere's pedagogy for health literacy intervention. *Humanity & Society*, 4(12), 182–208. doi:10.1177/0160597616633253
Gasiorek, J., & van de Poel, K. (2018). Language-specific skills in intercultural healthcare communication: Comparing perceived preparedness and skills in nurses' first and second languages. *Nurse Education Today*, 61, 54–59. doi:10.1016/j.nedt.2017.11.008
Grabeel, K. L., Russomanno, J., Oelschlegel, S., Tester, E., & Heidel, R. E. (2018). Computerized versus hand-scored health literacy tools: A comparison of Simple Measure of Gobbledygook (SMOG) and Flesch-Kincaid in printed patient education materials. *Journal of the Medical Library Association*, 106(1), 38–45. doi:10.5195/jmla.2018.262
Griffiths, J. (2017). Person-centred communication for emotional support in district nursing: SAGE and THYME model. *British Journal of Community Nursing*, 22(12), 593–597. doi:10.12968/bjcn.2017.22.12.593
Hancock, T. (2018). Mental health promotion must be a priority. *Canadian Medical Association Journal*, 190(16), ES22. doi:10.1503/cmaj.180464
Health Quality Ontario. (2016). *Transitions between hospital and home*. Retrieved from http://www.hqontario.ca/Portals/0/documents/qi/health-links/transition-asses s-health-literacy-en.pdf
Hull, R. H. (2017). Communication strategies for a successful practice. *The Hearing Journal*, 70(5), 22–23. doi:10.1097/01.HJ.0000516778.69034.05
Judd, M. (2017). Communication strategies for patients with dementia. *Nursing*, 47(12), 58–61. doi:10.1097/01.NURSE.0000524758.05259.f7
Kennedy, E. (2018). Caring and communicating. In B. Kozier, G. Erb, A. Berman, et al. (Eds.), *Fundamentals of Canadian nursing: Concepts, process and practice* (4th ed., pp. 381–410). Don Mills, ON: Pearson.
Lee, S. J., Park, K. W., Kim, L.-S., & Kim, H. H. (2016). Effects of noise level and cognitive function on speech perception in normal elderly and elderly with amnestic mild cognitive impairment. *Cognitive & Behavioral Neurology*, 29(2), 68–77. doi:10.1097/WNN.0000000000000092
Lewis, P., Gaffney, R. J., & Wilson, N. J. (2017). A narrative review of acute care nurses' experiences nursing patients with intellectual disability: Underprepared, communication barriers and ambiguity about the role of caregivers. *Journal of Clinical Nursing*, 26(11–12), 1473–1484. doi:10.1111/jocn.13512
Lin, M., Hsu, W., Huang, M., Su, Y., Crawford, P., & Tang, C. (2017). "I couldn't even talk to the patient": Barriers to communicating with cancer patients as perceived by nursing students. *European Journal of Cancer Care*, 26(4), 1–9. doi:10.1111/ecc.12648
Mayo Clinic. (2016). *Alzheimer's: Tips for effective communication*. Retrieved from http://www.mayoclinic.org/healthy-lifestyle/caregivers/in-depth/alzheimers/art-20047540
McKibben, L. (2017). Conflict management: Importance and implications. *British Journal of Nursing*, 26(2), 100–103. doi:10.12968/bjon.2017.26.2.100

McKinney, E. S., James, S. R., Murray, S. S., Nelson, K. A., & Ashwill, J. W. (2018). *Maternal-child nursing* (5th ed.). St. Louis: Elsevier.

Mendes, A., & Palmer, S. (2018). Communicating effectively with a person living with dementia. *British Journal of Nursing*, 27(2), 101. doi:10.12968/bjon.2018.27.2.101

Omura, M., Maguire, J., Levitt-Jones, T., & Stone, T. E. (2016). Effectiveness of assertive communication training programs for health professionals and students. *JBI Database of Systematic Reviews and Implementation Reports*, 2016, 64–71. doi:10.1124/JBISRIR-2016-003158

Ondrejka, O. (2018). Teaching and communication with older adults and their families. In K. Mauk (Ed.), *Gerontological nursing: Competencies for care* (4th ed., pp. 524–619). Burlington, MA: Jones & Bartlett Learning.

Ontario Ministry of Health and Long-Term Care. (2015). *Mental health: Depression.* Retrieved from http://www.health.gov.on.ca/en/public/publications/mental/depression.aspx

Registered Nurses' Association of Ontario (RNAO). (2015). *Person- and family-centred care.* Toronto, ON: Author. Retrieved from http://rnao.ca/sites/rnao-ca/files/FINAL_Web_Version 0.pdf

Registered Nurses' Association of Ontario (RNAO). (2016). *Intra-professional collaborative practice among nurses* (2nd ed.). Toronto, ON: Author. Retrieved from http://rnao.ca/sites/rnao-ca/files/bpg/Intra-professional_Collaborative_Practice_042017.pdf

Sanders, J. J., Curtis, J. R., & Tulsky, J. A. (2018). Achieving goal-concordant care: A conceptual model and approach to measuring serious illness communication and its impact. *Journal of Palliative Medicine*, 21(S2), S17–S27. doi:10.1089/jpm.2017.0459

Sheehan, R., & Hassiotis, A. (2017). Digital mental health and intellectual disabilities: State of the evidence and future directions. *Evidence-Based Mental Health*, 20(4), 107–111. doi:10.1136/eb-2017-102759

Sim, J., Crookes, P., Walsh, K., & Halcomb, E. (2017). Measuring the outcomes of nursing practice: A Delphi study. *Journal of Clinical Nursing*, 27(1–2), e368–e378. doi:10.1111/jocn.13971

Stewart, K. R., & Hand, K. A. (2017). SBAR, communication and patient safety: An integrated literature review. *Medsurg Nursing*, 26(5), 297–305.

Strachan, P. H., Kryworuchko, J., Nouvet, E., Downar, J., & You, J. J. (2017). Canadian hospital nurses' roles in communication and decision-making about goals of care: An interpretive description of critical incidents. *Applied Nursing Research*, 40, 26–33. doi:10.1016/j.apnr.2017.12.014

Townsend, M. C., & Morgan, K. I. (2018). *Psychiatric mental health nursing: Concepts of care in evidence-based practice* (9th ed.). Philadelphia: F.A. Davis Company.

Twigg, P., & Schwartzkopf, C. E. (2018). Nursing management of dementia. In K. Mauk (Ed.), *Gerontological nursing: Competencies for care* (4th ed., pp. 1091–1180). Burlington, MA: Jones & Bartlett Learning.

Walczak, A., Butow, P., Bu, S., & Clayton, J. M. (2016). A systematic review of evidence for end-of-life communication interventions: Who do they target, how are they structured and do they work? *Patient Education and Counseling*, 99(1), 3–16. doi:10.1016/j.pec.2015.08.017

Wittenberg, E., Ferrell, B., Kanter, E., & Buller, H. (2018). Health literacy: Exploring nursing challenges to provide support and understanding. *Clinical Journal of Oncology Nursing*, 22(1), 53–61. doi:10.1188/18.CJON

Yamamoto-Mitani, N., Noguchi-Watanabe, M., & Fukahori, H. (2016). Caring for clients and families with anxiety: Home care nurses' practice narratives. *Global Qualitative Nursing Research*, 3, 1–11. doi:10.1177/2333393616665503

4 | Documentation and Informatics

Written by **Theresa Pietsch, PhD, RN, CRRN CNE, and Joanne Newell, RN, MN**

SKILLS AND PROCEDURES

Procedural Guideline 4.1 **Giving a Hand-Off Report, p. 59**

Procedural Guideline 4.2 **Documenting Nurses' Progress Notes, p. 63**

Procedural Guideline 4.3 **Adverse Event/Incident Reporting, p. 64**

Procedural Guideline 4.4 **Guidelines for Meaningful Use of an Interoperable Electronic Health Record (iEHR), p. 66**

OBJECTIVES

Mastery of content in this chapter will enable the nurse to:
- List guidelines for effective communication and reporting.
- Describe measures to maintain confidentiality of patient information.
- Identify the purpose of the patient record.
- Describe the elements of a hand-off report and when it would be used.
- Discuss the role of computerization in documentation.
- Write a nurse's progress note using SBAR, SOAP, SOAPIE, PIE, and focus (DAR) charting formats.

- Describe information found in a patient care profile and nursing Kardex.
- Accurately complete a nursing flow sheet.
- Explain guidelines used in documentation of long-term care and care in the community.
- Describe the role of critical pathways in multidisciplinary documentation.
- Complete an adverse event/incident report accurately.
- Describe the importance of medication reconciliation.

MEDIA RESOURCES

- evolve http://evolve.elsevier.com/Canada/Perry/clinicalskills/
- Review Questions
- Audio Glossary
- Clinical Debrief and Review Questions Answers
- Case Studies

PURPOSE

Documentation is anything entered into a patient's electronic health record (EHR) or written in a patient record. The EHR (Fig. 4.1) is a longitudinal electronic record of patient health information generated by one or more encounters in a care delivery setting (Canada Health Infoway [CHI], 2018b). Nursing documentation ensures continuity of care, provides legal evidence, and evaluates patient outcomes. The nurse's documentation provides a detailed account of a patient's plan of care, assessment, and treatment, which must be an accurate and timely evaluation of information. Electronic tools such as computers support documentation and patient care. Nursing informatics focuses on best practices with information and communication technology (Chauvette, 2016).

STANDARDS OF CARE

- Accreditation Canada, 2019—*Required Organizational Practices Handbook—Version 14* (http://www.wrha.mb.ca/quality/files/2019ROPHandbook.pdf)
- Canadian Health Infoway (CHI), 2018c—*Nursing Data Standards* (https://infocentral.infoway-inforoute.ca/en/standards/other-canadian/nursing-data-standards)

- Canadian Nurses Association (CNA), 2017a—*Code of Ethics for Registered Nurses* (https://www.cna-aiic.ca/~/media/cna/page-content/pdf-en/code-of-ethics-2017-edition-secure-interactive)
- Canadian Nurses Association (CNA), 2017b—*Nursing Informatics: Joint Position Statement* (https://www.cna-aiic.ca/en/~/media/cna/page-content/pdf-fr/nursing-informatics-joint-position-statement)
- College of Licensed Practical Nurses Association of Nova Scotia (CLPNNS) & College of Registered Nurses Association of Nova Scotia (CRNNS), 2017—*Documentation Guidelines for Nurses* (https://crnns.ca/wp-content/uploads/2017/12/Documentation-Guidelines-for-Nurses-Final.pdf)
- College of Registered Nurses of British Columbia (CRNBC), 2018—*Documentation: Practice Standards* (https://crnbc.ca/Standards/PracticeStandards/Lists/GeneralResources/334DocumentationPracStd.pdf)
- College of Registered Nurses of Manitoba (CRNM), n.d. —*Documentation Guidelines for Registered Nurses* (https://www.crnm.mb.ca/support/practice-and-standards-consultation/documentation)
- Ordre des infimieres et infirmiers du Quebec (OIIQ), 2015—*Code of Ethics of Nurses* (https://www.oiiq.org/documents/20147/237836/8450_doc.pdf)

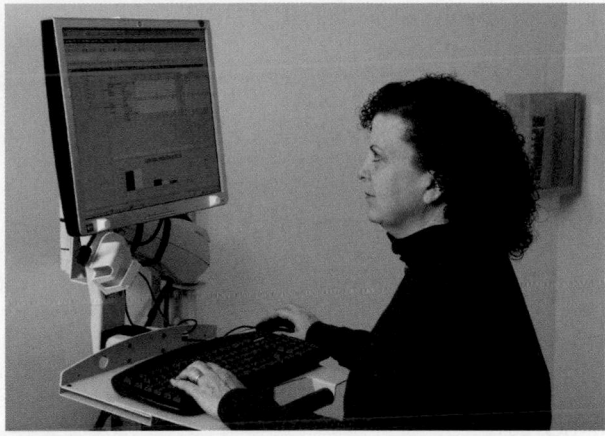

FIG 4.1 Computerized documentation provides many benefits.

PRINCIPLES FOR PRACTICE

- All members of the health care team are legally and ethically obligated to keep patient information confidential and to adhere to documentation standards (CNA, 2017a; Canadian Nurses Protective Society [CNPS], 2007).
- Documentation occurs within the context of the nursing process, including evidence of patient and family teaching and discharge planning (CLPNNS & CRNNS, 2017). Employer standards or policies often state the frequency of assessment; thus, it is essential to know the standards of your health care employer.
- Nursing diagnoses (clinical judgement about potential and actual issues) should be included in a nursing care plan (CRNNS, 2017b). They can be standardized (e.g., International Classification for Nursing Practice [ICNP]; North American Nursing Diagnosis Association International [NANDA-I], 2018; White, 2017) or employer or unit specific.
- Nursing Interventions Classification (NIC) provides a list of nursing actions that are recognized internationally (Butcher, Bulechek, Dochterman, et al., 2018).
- Nursing Order Sets (NOS) provide a standardized list of evidence-informed interventions to address clinical conditions (Registered Nurses Association of Ontario [RNAO], n.d.).
- The Canadian Health Outcomes for Better Information and Care (C-HOBIC, 2015) data set includes a list of measurable standardized clinical outcomes as a result of nursing care that can be retrieved from EHRs and fosters interprofessional collaboration with improved information exchange among the health care team. The use of outcomes is essential when evaluating the achievement of patient care goals and the appropriateness of patient interventions.
- The Canadian Personal Information Protection and Electronic Documents Act [PIPEDA] (Government of Canada, 2018) and individual provincial/territorial-specific acts (e.g., the Personal Health Information Act [PHIA] of Nova Scotia) (Province of Nova Scotia, 2018) govern all areas of health information management (collection, use, disclosure, retention, disposal, and destruction) of personal health information, including safeguards for electronic systems.
- Numerous nursing and medical professional organizations have developed guidelines and strategies for safe computer charting (Box 4.1).
- Although incentives exist to transition from paper health records to EHRs, paper records are still in use in some health care facilities

BOX 4.1

Use of the Electronic Health Record

- Sign on to the electronic health record (EHR) using only your password.
- Never share passwords and keep your password private.
- Only open EHRs for patients for whom you are caring.
- Review assessment data, problems or issues identified (nursing diagnoses), goals and expected outcomes, and interventions and patient responses during contact with each patient before data entry.
- Follow procedures for entering information in all appropriate program functions.
- Review previously documented entries with those that you enter, noting if there is significant change in patient's status. Report changes to patient's health care provider.
- The copy-and-paste features in EHRs should be used sparingly because of the potential for error (Healthcare Insurance Reciprocal of Canada [HIROC], 2017).
- Do not leave information about a patient displayed on a monitor where others can see it. Keep a log that accounts for every copy of a computerized file that you have generated from the system.
- Follow employer confidentiality procedures for documenting sensitive material (e.g., diagnosis of human immunodeficiency virus [HIV] infection).
- Know and implement employer protocol to correct documentation errors.
- Never create, change, or delete records unless your employer provides you with this authority.
- Software programs have a system for backup files. If you inadvertently delete part of the permanent record, follow employer policy. It is necessary to type an explanation into the computer file with the date, time, and your initials and submit an explanation in writing to your supervisor.
- Save information as documentation is completed.
- Protect printouts from computerized records. Shredding printouts and logging in the number of copies generated by each caregiver minimize duplicate records and protect the confidentiality of patient information. Workarounds can occur when EHRs are poorly designed; health care providers may fall back on paper charting (Gephart, Bristol, Dye, et al., 2016). Medication errors may increase when nurses are working in a hybrid system. This system uses two formats—a paper and an electronic medical record for the same patient (Aziz & Alsharabasi, 2015).
- Sign off when you leave the computer.

(CHI, CNA, & Canadian Nurses Informatics Association [CNIA], 2017).

- Comprehensive computer systems in health care delivery have unlimited potential for improving the accuracy, efficiency, and quality of documentation. *Meaningful use* refers to the use of certified EHRs to improve outcomes, increase patient engagement, and reduce health disparities (see Procedural Guideline 4.4) (CHI, 2010b, CHI, CNA, & CNIA, 2017).
- Examples of core objectives for meaningful use include clinical-decision support rules, computerized prescriptions, and real-time drug interaction checks. The EHR can support the nurse's decision making by verifying safety steps in procedures such as medication administration. In addition, clinical data from an EHR can be exchanged more efficiently among the interprofessional team and at transition points in care (RNAO, 2017).
- Accreditation Canada (2019) specifies guidelines for documentation and requires health care facilities to monitor and evaluate patient outcomes and appropriateness of care.
- Primary health care principles encourage person-centred care with patients as active participants in their health care. The use

of patient portals enables patients to have access to their personal health information (Zychla, 2017).

- Working in a digital world requires nurses to be competent with the appropriate use of information and communication technologies. Nurses have the responsibility to acquire nursing informatics knowledge (CNA, 2017b). The NurseOne portal provides Canadian nurses access to an online Health Informatics Training System (HITS). CNIA also offers webinars to members on nursing and health care informatics initiatives (see https://cnia.ca/).
- Student nurses are also expected to be able to use digital technology in practice settings. Nursing faculty have a responsibility to design and implement curricula to foster the development of entry-level informatics competencies for newly graduated nurses (White, 2017).

PERSON-CENTRED CARE

- A patient's record or chart is a confidential, permanent legal document containing information relevant to a patient's health care. Nurses and other health care providers record information about a patient's health care after each patient contact. The record is a continuing account of the patient's health status and needs, treatments delivered, results of diagnostic tests, and response to therapy.
- Documents within the patient's record communicate specific information about a patient's health status and the interventions that all health care team members contribute toward improving patient health and outcomes. Interprofessional collaboration is facilitated and enhanced with quality documentation. For example, a nurse may seek clarification on a patient's ability to participate in their morning care from the occupational therapist and share that information in a patient's record to improve care delivery and patient outcomes.
- Reports are oral or written exchanges of information among caregivers (Fig. 4.2). Reports include information about a patient's clinical status, observations made about their behaviour, data pertaining to diagnostic tests, and directions for changes in therapy. Common reports given by nurses include telephone reports, transfer reports, and adverse event/incident reports (see Procedural Guideline 4.3).
- When a nurse receives a verbal prescription or critical test result, the nurse writes down the prescription or critical test result as it is given and then reads it back to the individual who has given the prescription. By stating the information back (called

the *read-back*) to the individual giving the prescription or test result, the nurse verifies that the complete prescription or test result has been received and understood (CRNNS, 2017a).
- Patient hand-off reports (see Procedural Guideline 4.1), a standardized approach to communication of patient information among caregivers, are being used by many health care facilities.

EVIDENCE-INFORMED PRACTICE

Computer-based health care records, informatics, and implementation of the electronic patient record all have major implications for person-centred care, patient engagement, and evidence-informed practice (RNAO, 2017). Basic nursing care interventions can be documented to provide meaningful data to the health care team (CRNBC, 2018).

- Use of EHRs demonstrates improvement in patient outcomes for trauma patients (Stimson & Botruff, 2017) and those diagnosed with diabetes mellitus (Graetz et al., 2015).
- Quality EHRs allow retrieval of data to improve patient outcomes. For example, data are retrieved from EHRs when patients are identified to their active medication lists. The bar coding of medications can reduce errors because the data retrieved match the right patients to the right medications (Strudwick et al., 2018).
- Recent studies have examined benefits of EHRs and opportunities for further research about EHRs.
  - Nursing outcomes can be measured efficiently with EHRs. Incorporating an EHR promoted decision making and was connected with positive outcomes in the practice setting in relation to catheter-associated urinary tract infection, central-line infections, and patient falls (Walker-Czyz, 2016).
  - Nursing management of chronic diseases such as chronic obstructive pulmonary disease (COPD) can be done more effectively with EHRs. Evidence suggests that the use of EHRs supporting the implementation of complex interventions is effective in managing exacerbations of COPD. Data can be shared in a more timely manner across the health care continuum as patients move among the levels of care. Extraction of data is more efficient because of the standardization of language found in EHRs (Liu, Zou, Huang, et al., 2015).
  - After 5 years of using an EHR system in an acute care hospital, nurses identified opportunities to improve interprofessional communication and clinical decision making by strengthening the system. Researchers suggest that nurses conduct time-motion studies to evaluate the nursing resources used to maintain and improve EHRs (Harmon, Fogle, & Roussel, 2015).
  - Patients need education, guidance, and support as the health care system transitions to EHRs. The evidence suggests that medical language used in EHRs can be difficult for patients to understand. Some patients are concerned about the security of their health information in cyberspace (Wallace, 2015). Challenges for health care providers include improving access for patients and conveying the value of the EHR to patients.

SAFETY GUIDELINES

- Quality documentation and reporting must be factual, accurate, complete, current, and organized.
  - Factual data contain descriptive, objective information about what a nurse sees, hears, feels, and smells. The only subjective data included in a record are what the patient verbalizes.

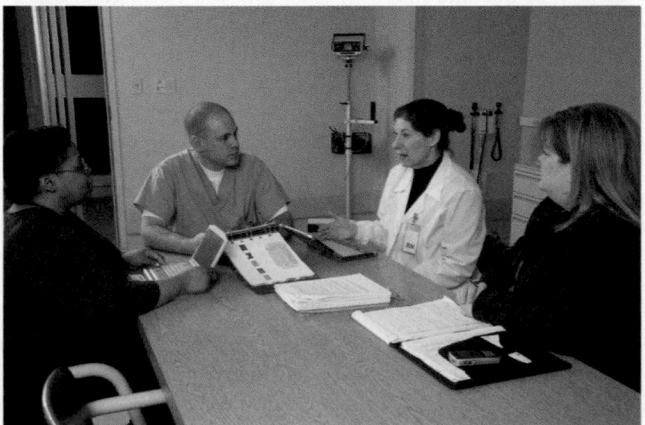

FIG 4.2 Communication among members of the health care team.

Write subjective information with quotation marks, using the patient's exact words whenever possible. For example, record, "Patients states, 'My stomach hurts.'"

- The use of exact measurements in documentation establishes accuracy. For example, charting that an abdominal wound is "5 cm in length without redness, edema, or drainage" is more descriptive than "large wound healing well." It is essential to avoid unnecessary words and irrelevant details. For example, the fact that a patient is watching television is only necessary when this activity is significant to the patient's status and plan of care.
- The information within a recorded entry or a report must be complete, containing appropriate and essential information. Criteria for reporting and documenting information for health problems or nursing activities exist (Table 4.1).
- All entries in medical records must be dated and a method established to identify the authors of entries. Therefore, each

entry in a patient's record ends with the caregiver's full name or initials and status. A nursing student enters full name, student nurse abbreviation (e.g., SN, NS), and educational institution, such as "David Jones, DalSN" (Dalhousie University [Dal] student nurse). An EHR generates the nurse's name and initials when the entry is submitted (CRNBC, 2015).

- Current documentation includes making timely entries in a patient's record, which avoids omissions and delay in patient care (CRNBC, 2018; HIROC, 2017). To increase accuracy and decrease unnecessary duplication, many health care facilities locate medical records near a patient's bedside, which facilitates immediate documentation of care activities. The following activities or findings should be documented at the time of occurrence:
  - Vital signs
  - Pain assessment and evaluation
  - Administration of medications and treatments
  - Preparation for diagnostic tests or surgery
  - Change in patient's status and who was notified
  - Treatment for a sudden change in patient's status
  - Patient response to intervention
  - Admission, transfer, discharge, or death of a patient
- Military time, a 24-hour system that avoids misinterpretation of AM and PM times, is recommended to record the time of events. The military clock ends with midnight at 2400 and begins 1 minute after midnight at 0001. For example, 1:00 PM is 1300 military time; 10:22 AM is 1022 military time. Fig. 4.3 compares military and civilian times. An EHR generates time of entry when the nurse submits the entry.
- The Canadian Patient Safety Institute (CPSI, 2016a) requires health care facilities to standardize abbreviations, symbols, acronyms, and dose designations and establish a list of abbreviations that are in accordance with Institute for Safe Medication Practices (ISMP) Canada's List of Error-Prone Abbreviations, Symbols, and Dose Designations (ISMP, 2015). It is essential to know your employer abbreviation list and to use only the accepted abbreviations, symbols, and measures (e.g., metric) so all documentation is accurate and in compliance with standards. For

TABLE 4.1

Examples of Criteria for Communicating and Documenting

Topic	Criteria to Communicate or Document
Assessment	
Subjective data	Description of episode/event in patient's words in quotation marks. Clarify onset, location, description of condition (severity; duration; frequency; precipitating, aggravating, and relieving factors)
Patient behaviour (e.g., anxiety, confusion, hostility)	Onset, behaviours exhibited, precipitating factors
Objective data (e.g., rash, tenderness, breath sounds)	Onset, location, description of condition (severity; duration; frequency; precipitating, aggravating, and relieving factors)
Nursing Interventions and Evaluation	
Treatments (e.g., enema, bath, dressing change)	Time administered, equipment used (if appropriate), patient's response (objective and subjective changes) compared to previous treatment (e.g., rated pain 2 on a scale of 0–10 during dressing change or "patient reported no abdominal cramping during enema")
Medication administration	Immediately after administration document: time medication given, dose, route, any preliminary assessment (e.g., pain level, vital signs), patient response or effect of medication (e.g., 1200 "Pain reported at 7 [scale 0 being no pain and 10 being worst pain ever])." Acetaminophen 650 mg given PO. 1230: "Patient reports pain level 2 (scale 0–10) at 1330"
Patient teaching	Information presented; method of instruction (e.g., discussion, demonstration, videotape, booklet); patient response, including questions and evidence of understanding such as return demonstration or change in behaviour
Discharge planning	Measurable patient goals or expected outcomes, progress toward goals, need for referrals

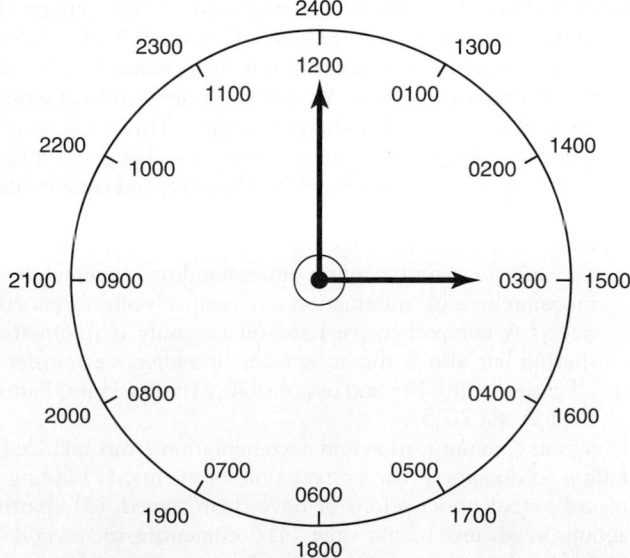

FIG 4.3 Military time clock. Instead of two 12-hour cycles, the military clock is one 24-hour time cycle (e.g., 3 PM is 1500 military time).

BOX 4.2

Official "Do Not Use" Abbreviations

Do Not Use	Potential Problem	Use Instead
U, u (unit)	Mistaken for "0" (zero), the number "4" (four), or "cc"	Use "unit"
IU (International Unit)	Mistaken for "IV" (intravenous) or the number "10" (ten)	Use "International Unit"
Q.D., QD, q.d., qd (daily)	Mistaken for one another	Use "daily"
Q.O.D., QOD, q.o.d, qod (every other day)	Period after the Q mistaken for "I" and the "O" mistaken for "I"	Use "every other day"
Trailing zero (X.0 mg)	Decimal point is missed	Use X mg
Lack of leading zero (.X mg)		Use 0.X mg
MS	Can mean morphine sulphate or magnesium sulphate	Use "morphine sulphate"
MSO$_4$ and MgSO$_4$	Confused for one another	Use "magnesium sulphate"

The Joint Commission. (2015). Facts about the official "Do Not Use" list. Retrieved from http://www.jointcommission.org/facts_about_do_not_use_list/. Accessed February 4, 2019.

example, the abbreviation for *every day (qd)* **is no longer used** (Box 4.2). If a treatment or medication is needed daily, the written prescription or care plan should write out "daily" or "every day." The abbreviation *qd (every day)* can be misinterpreted to mean *O.D. (right eye)*. Neither abbreviation (i.e., qd, OD) is acceptable for use.

- Hand-off occurs during shift change or any time the patient changes caregivers. During a hand-off communication process the patient and patient information are transferred to the next caregiver. Hand-off is also used across the health care continuum when patients leave one health system for another. Effective hand-off allows for face-to-face communication when available, which allows the person receiving care of the patient the opportunity to ask questions (Usher, Cronin, & York, 2018).
  - During hand-off the sender of the patient information initially presents the patient name, room number, age, gender, diagnosis, medical history, and discharge planning. This is followed by patient vital signs and clinical assessments, changes in clinical condition, medication review, fluid balance, and patient safety risk assessment factors. Once hand-off is completed, the receiver of the information is given an opportunity to ask questions and confirm understanding. Incomplete or incomprehensible information can negatively affect a patient's safety. A comprehensive hand-off not only is information sharing but also is the acceptance and effective transfer of all patient authority and responsibility (Foster-Hunt, Parush, Ellis, et al., 2015).
- Common communication and documentation errors include (1) failing to document the correct time of events, (2) failing to record verbal prescriptions or have them signed, (3) charting actions in advance to save time, (4) documenting incorrect data, and (5) failing to give a report or giving an incomplete report to an oncoming shift. Nurses must be aware of the legal guidelines for documentation and reporting (Table 4.2).

COMMON RECORD-KEEPING FORMS OR SCREENS

The patient chart or medical record contains evidence of a patient's health status. The chart includes a variety of forms or screens (as in the case of EHRs) to facilitate quick and comprehensive documentation. Use of these forms or screens helps avoid duplication of information within the record.

Admission Nursing History Forms or Screens

A nurse completes a comprehensive nursing history form or screen to gather baseline assessment data when a patient is admitted to a nursing care unit. The nurse uses the admission data to form a plan of care and compare it to any changes in a patient's condition. The nursing history guides the admitting nurse through a complete assessment to identify relevant nursing issues or problems for the patient's care plan. Examples of information included in the nursing history are patient allergies, primary spoken/written language, advance directives, disabilities, mobility and fall risk, and medication reconciliation.

Flow Sheets and Graphic Records

Flow sheets and graphic records, used in both EHRs and paper charts, enable concise documentation of nursing information and patient data over time. They are especially useful for the documentation of routine observations or repeated specific measurements for a patient, such as vital signs (see Chapter 7), intake and output, hygiene measures, medication administration (see Chapter 20), and pain assessment. Flow sheets have a format or system for entry of information, usually every 24 hours (Fig. 4.4). When you are documenting a significant change that you recognize on a flow sheet, describe the change in the progress notes, including the patient's response to nursing interventions. For example, if a patient's blood pressure becomes dangerously low, record in the progress notes the blood pressure, relevant assessment such as pallor or dizziness, and any interventions to raise the blood pressure. Also include an evaluation of the interventions, such as repeated blood pressures and relief of dizziness. Other health care providers may have the responsibility to document on nursing flow sheets or screens.

Patient Education Record

Many employers have an education record that identifies a patient's knowledge base about their diagnosis, treatment, and medications. The goal of patient and family education is to promote person-centred care by involving the patient, family, or both in self-care and decisions, which improves health outcomes. Standards for patient education include assessment of needs, functional abilities, learning styles, and readiness to learn (Flanders, 2018). The nurse should base patient education needs on the assessment and then teach patients about topics such as safe and effective use of medications, nutrition and dietary modifications, safe use of medical equipment, pain control, rehabilitative methods to promote and improve functional abilities, and self-care activities. When documenting on a patient teaching record, it is important to be specific about the information and skills taught, the patient's learning response, and information given to the patient.

Patient Care Summary or Kardex

Many health care facilities have computerized systems that provide a concise record of patient information in the form of a patient care summary or computer-generated Kardex. This summary prints out for each patient during each shift. Data are updated automatically as new prescriptions and nursing decisions enter the system.

TABLE 4.2

Legal Guidelines for Documentation and Reporting

Guidelines	Rationale	Correct Action
Use only your unique user identification and password to log onto the EHR.	An electronic signature is associated with each user identification and password log-in.	Protect the security of your user identification and password. Once logged on to the computer, do not leave the computer screen unattended.
Do not erase, apply correction fluid, or scratch out errors made while recording in a paper record.	Charting becomes illegible: it appears as if you were attempting to hide information or deface record.	Draw single line through error, write word *error* above it, and sign your name or initials. Then document note correctly. Check employer policy.
Do not write retaliatory or critical comments about patient or care by other health care providers.	Statements can be used as evidence for nonprofessional behaviour or poor quality of care.	Enter only objective descriptions of patient's behaviour; use quotations for patient's comments.
Need to add patient information.	New information is acquired.	If additional information is to be added to an existing entry, write the date and time of the new entry on the next available space and mark it as an addendum (date and time of prior note).
	Forgot to chart during a shift.	Write the current date and time in the next available space and mark it as a late entry (date and time/shift missed).
Correct all errors promptly.	Errors in recording can lead to errors in treatment.	Avoid rushing to complete charting; be sure that information is accurate.
Document all facts.	Record must be accurate and reliable.	Be certain that entry is factual; do not speculate or guess.
Document all entries legibly and in black ink for paper records (HIROC, 2017)	Illegible entries can be misinterpreted, causing errors and lawsuits; ink cannot be erased; black ink is more legible when records are photocopied or scanned.	**Never** erase entries, use correction fluid/tape or pencil. Use enough pressure so the ink will be dark in colour.
If prescription is questioned, record that you sought clarification.	If you perform an incorrect prescription, you are just as liable for prosecution as the health care provider that prescribed it.	Do not document "physician made error." Instead, chart that "Dr. Smith was called to clarify prescription for analgesic."
Chart only for yourself.	You are accountable for information that you document on the chart.	Never document for someone else. **EXCEPTION:** If caregiver has left unit for day and calls with information that needs to be documented, include the name of the source of information in the entry and that the information was provided via telephone.
Avoid using generalized, empty phrases such as "status unchanged" or "had good day."	Specific information about patient's condition or case can be deleted accidentally if information is too generalized.	Use complete, concise descriptions of care.
Begin each entry with time and end with your signature and title.	This guideline ensures that correct sequence of events is documented; signature indicates who is accountable for care delivered.	Do not wait until end of shift to document important changes that occurred several hours earlier; be sure to sign each entry.

EHR, Electronic health record.

In some health care settings, a written Kardex produced on a "cardboard flip-over" file is kept at the nurses' station. Parts of the Kardex have information recorded in pencil, allowing changes to be made to patient information, which prevents it from being considered a legal document. The updated information in the patient summary or Kardex eliminates the need for repeated referral to the chart for routine information throughout the day. The effectiveness of these forms as a communication tool is contingent on timely updates to patient information and transfer of prescriptions. Failure of the nurse to transfer a prescription to the Kardex could result in an adverse event/incident and the nurse being liable. The patient care summary or Kardex does not always become part of the permanent record (check employer policy). Information commonly found on the patient care summary or Kardex includes the following:

- Basic demographic data (e.g., age, religion)
- Primary medical diagnosis
- Current health care provider's prescriptions (e.g., diet, activity, dressing changes)
- Plan of care
- Nursing orders or interventions (e.g., intake and output, comfort measures, teaching)
- Scheduled tests and procedures
- Safety precautions used in the patient's care

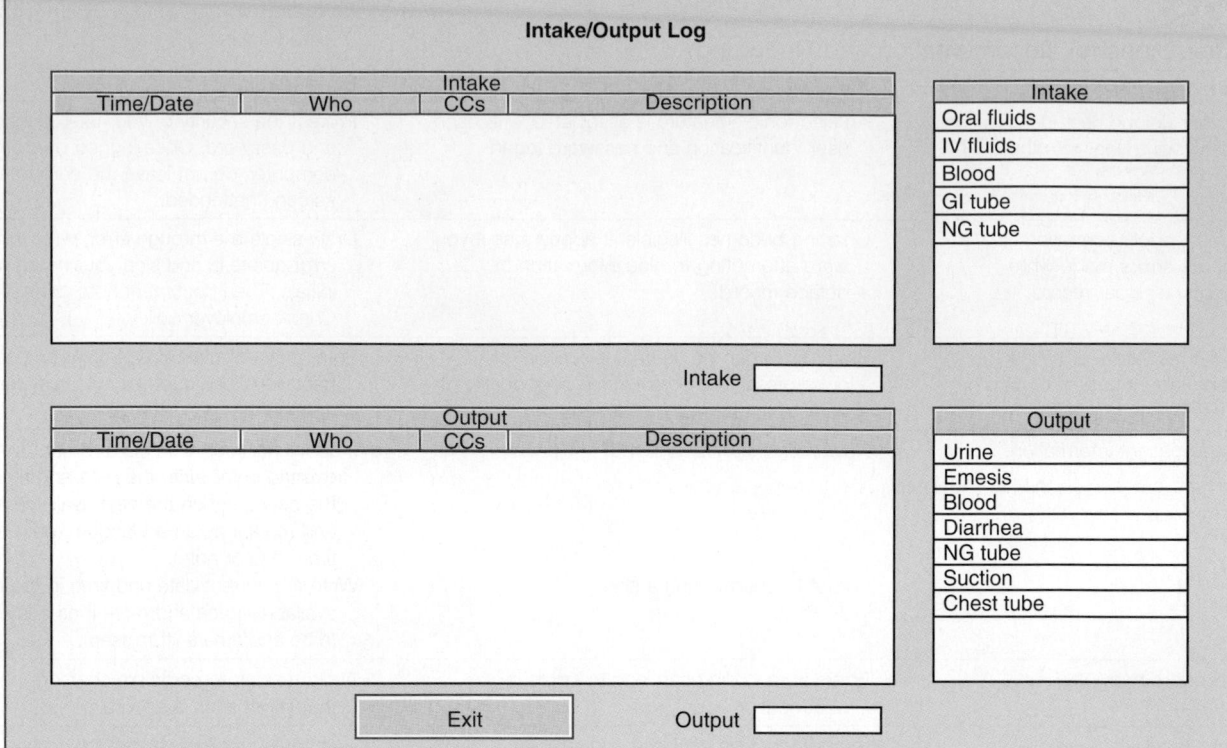

FIG 4.4 Graphic and intake-output record, electronic version. *(Courtesy ER Choice, Irving, TX.)*

- Factors related to activities of daily living
- Nearest relative or guardian or person to contact in an emergency
- Resuscitative care plan information (e.g., do not resuscitate [DNR], allow natural death [AND])
- Allergies

Acuity Records

Many health care facilities use a patient acuity system as a method of determining the intensity of nursing care required for a group of patients. Acuity measurements for patients on a unit serve as a guide for determining staffing needs. An acuity recording system determines the hours of nursing care and number of staff required for a nursing unit.

Typically, nurses enter acuity data into a computerized system in the morning. The administrative staff collects the acuity data electronically and uses them to make appropriate staffing decisions. Acuity levels allow the nursing staff to compare patients with one another. For example, an acuity system might rate bathing patients from 1 to 5 (1 is totally dependent, 5 is independent); a patient returning from surgery who requires frequent monitoring and extensive care has an acuity level of 1. On the same continuum, another patient awaiting discharge after a successful recovery from surgery has an acuity level of 5. Accurate acuity ratings justify the number and qualifications of staff needed to safely care for patients on a particular unit.

Standardized Care Plans

The trend among many health care facilities is to computerize care plans. These systems provide daily computer-generated care plans, which incorporate several nursing diagnoses or problems in a single nursing or interprofessional plan of care. These systems improve documentation and facilitate high-quality care that is based on scientific evidence and past experience (CHI, 2018c). Standardized care plans are based on standards of clinical practice and are established guidelines used to care for patients with similar health problems. Standardized care plans are often used with postoperative patients—for example, a care plan for patient having bowel surgery. As the nurse, after completing a nursing assessment, identify the patient's nursing diagnosis or health problem and select an appropriate standardized care plan for the patient medical record. Always individualize it for each patient. Most standardized care plans allow for the addition of patient-specific outcomes and target dates for achieving these outcomes (Foley, 2018).

One advantage of standardized care plans is the establishment of evidence-informed standards of care. By using standardized plans nurses learn to recognize the accepted requirements of care for patients. Implementation of digital standardized plans improves continuity of care among professional nurses (de Lima Silva, Dora Martinez Évora, & Santana Justo Cintra, 2015; Foley, 2018).

One disadvantage of standardized care plans is an increased risk that the unique, individualized therapies needed by patients will go unrecognized. Standardized care plans do not replace clinical judgement, critical thinking, and clinical reasoning. In addition, care plans need to be updated on a regular basis to ensure that content is current and appropriate.

Discharge Summaries

The discharge summary includes essential information for the patient, caregiver, and health care facility (Box 4.3) and is based on data obtained from the discharge planning process. Discharge planning is a comprehensive process with emphasis placed on preparing a patient for discharge. Nurses enhance discharge planning when they are responsive to changes in a patient's condition and involve the patient and caregiver in the planning process (An, 2015).

There must be evidence of involvement of the patient and caregiver in the discharge planning process so that they have the

Discharge Summary Information

- Use clear, concise descriptions in patient's own language.
- Provide step-by-step description of how to perform a procedure (e.g., home medication administration). Reinforce explanation with printed instructions for the patient to take home.
- Provide a detailed list of all prescribed medications.
- Identify precautions to follow when performing self-care or administering medications.
- Review any restrictions that may relate to activities of daily living (e.g., bathing, ambulating, and driving).
- Review signs and symptoms of complications to report to health care provider.
- List names and phone numbers of health care providers and community resources for the patient to contact.
- Identify any unresolved problems, including plans for follow-up and continuous treatment.
- List actual time of discharge, mode of transportation, and who accompanied patient.

necessary information and resources to return home (Health Quality Ontario [HQO], 2018). Accreditation Canada (2019) has standards for patient education required for effective discharge planning. When a patient is discharged from a health care facility, the members of the health care team prepare a discharge summary. It provides important information relating to the patient's ongoing health problems and need for health care after discharge.

Discharge planning achieves specific outcomes that include identifying patients with ongoing health needs, collaborating with other health care professionals to determine level of care, matching patients with appropriate referrals and resources, and streamlining the transition to the next level of care (Trossman, 2015). Included in the discharge summary are the reason for hospitalization; significant findings; current status of the patient; and the teaching plan that is given to the patient or caregiver, home care, rehabilitation, or long-term care facility (Accreditation Canada, 2019). Discharge summaries make the summary concise and instructive. They emphasize previous learning by the patient and caregiver and care that needs to continue in any restorative care setting.

PROCEDURAL GUIDELINE 4.1 *Giving a Hand-Off Report*

In addition to written documentation, a nurse provides a change-of-shift report to the next nurse assuming responsibility for patient care. The purpose of the report is to provide continuity of care for the patient. An inaccurate or incomplete shift report can contribute to sentinel events (Mardis et al., 2016). Nurses give a hand-off report face to face, through a written report, with the electronic health record (EHR), or during bedside rounds at each patient's bedside. Bedside reporting can increase patient satisfaction and improve outcomes and is becoming increasingly popular (Usher et al., 2018). It is important to have some type of guidelines for reporting to avoid repetitive, irrelevant, and speculative communication (Foster-Hunt et al., 2015). Regardless of the form of the hand-off report, the nurse must maintain confidentiality.

Delegation and Collaboration

The skill of giving a hand-off report cannot be delegated to an unregulated care provider (UCP). The nurse directs the UCP to:
- Report to the nurse (e.g., increased pain, changes in vital signs) so there can be assessment, validation, and reporting of any changes in the hand-off report.

Equipment
- Worksheets, patient care summary or nursing Kardex, plan of care, critical pathway, or interprofessional treatment plan
- EHR (if implemented by employer)

Procedural Steps
1. Use an organized format for delivering report that provides a description of patient needs and problems. SBAR (Situation, Background, Assessment, Recommendation) can be used to organize and streamline report (Usher et al., 2018).
2. Identify the electronic patient record using at least two identifiers (e.g., name and date of birth or name and medical record number) according to employer policy (Accreditation Canada, 2019).

3. Gather information from documentation sources, UCP report, or other relevant documents.

Clinical Decision Point *Report only relevant information to next shift to ensure staff's timely responsiveness.*

4. Prioritize information based on patient's needs and problems.
5. For each patient SBAR include the following:
   S Situation: Patient's name, gender, age, chief concern on admission, and current situation
   B Background information: Allergies, emergency code status (i.e., do not resuscitate [DNR] and allow natural death [AND]), medical and surgical histories, special needs as related to any physical challenges (e.g., visual impairment, hearing deficit, amputee), and immunizations
   A Assessment data: Objective observations and measurements made by the nurse during the shift; emphasis on any recent changes

   Include any relevant information reported by patient, caregiver, or health care team members such as laboratory data and diagnostic test results. Include therapies or treatments administered during shift and expected outcomes (e.g., medication changes, use of oxygen, referral visits). Describe education given in the teaching plan and caregiver's ability to demonstrate learning. Report on evaluation by explaining patient's response and whether outcomes are met.

   Review patient's progress toward discharge during each change-of-shift report.
   R Recommendation: Explanation of the priorities to which oncoming nurse must attend, including referrals, nursing orders, and core measures

Ask staff from oncoming shift if they have any questions regarding information provided.

CHARTING SYSTEMS

A variety of documentation systems (computerized and written) exist for recording patient information and progress (see Box 4.4). The documentation system selected by nursing reflects the philosophy of the health care facility. The same documentation system is used throughout a specific facility, but there are several acceptable methods for recording health care data.

Narrative Documentation

Narrative charting uses a story-like format to document specific information about a patient's conditions and nursing care, usually presented in chronological order. It is useful in emergency situations when the time and order of events are important. A narrative should be organized in a clear, concise way (e.g., by using the nursing process to order the data).

Problem-Oriented Medical Records

A problem-oriented medical record (POMR) is a structured method of documenting narratives that emphasizes a patient's problems. This method organizes data using the nursing process, which facilitates communication about patient needs. Data are organized by problem or diagnosis. Ideally interprofessional collaboration should occur so that all members of the health care team can contribute to the list of identified patient issues. This approach helps to coordinate an individualized plan of care with the following sections: database, problem list, care plan, and progress notes.

Patient Database

A database contains all available information pertaining to a patient. This section is the foundation for identifying patient issues and

---

BOX 4.4

Formats for Recording Progress Notes

Narrative Note
Describes patient data in a narrative paragraph

Example:
Patient states, "I'm dreading this surgery because last time I had a terrible reaction to the anaesthesia and such terrible pain when they made me get out of bed." Noted muscle tension and loud, agitated voice. Notified anaesthesiologist of patient's prior experience. Discussed alternatives for anaesthesia and pain control options. Stressed importance of activity for circulation and healing. Encouraged patient to keep nurses informed of pain level and need for medication and that pain may be present but manageable.

SBAR (Acronym for *S*ituation, *B*ackground, *A*ssessment, and *R*ecommendation)
System of structured communication used to share information about a patient's condition

Example:
S (Situation): Patient verbalized preoperative fears. Nurse noted muscle tension and loud, agitated voice.
B (Background): Patient fearful of surgery because of past experiences with anaesthesia and pain.
A (Assessment): BP: 160/84, T: 37°C (98.6°F); P: 86; R: 18. O₂ Saturation: 96%. Skin warm and dry to touch. Respirations even and nonlaboured.
R (Recommendation): Encourage patient to discuss preoperative fears. Assess pain level at least every 4 hours after surgery. Provide nonpharmacological pain management techniques and administer prescribed medication as needed.

SOAP (Acronym for *S*ubjective Data, *O*bjective Data, *A*ssessment, and *P*lan)
Usually based on a numbered list of problems or nursing diagnoses

Example:
S (Subjective data) (the patient's statements regarding the problem): Patient states, "I'm dreading this surgery because last time I had a terrible reaction to the anaesthesia and such terrible pain when they made me get out of bed."
O (Objective data) (observations that support or are related to subjective data): Noted muscle tension and loud, agitated voice.
A (Assessment/Analysis) (conclusions reached on basis of data): Fear related to pain/anaesthesia.
P (Plan) (plan for dealing with the situation): Notified anaesthesiologist, Dr. Martin, of patient's prior experience. Discussed alternatives for

anaesthesia and pain control options. Stressed importance of activity for circulation and healing. Encouraged patient to keep nurses informed of pain level and need for medication and that pain may be present but manageable.

PIE (Acronym for *P*roblem, *I*ntervention, and *E*valuation)
Problem-oriented system in which progress notes are written on the basis of a list of identified problems; detailed data may be entered by any member of the health care team

Example:
P (Problem): Patient states, "I'm dreading this surgery because last time I had a terrible reaction to the anaesthesia and such terrible pain when they made me get out of bed." Noted muscle tension and loud, agitated voice.
I (Intervention): Notified anaesthesiologist, Dr. Martin, of patient's prior experience. Discussed alternatives for anaesthesia and pain control options. Stressed importance of activity for circulation and healing. Encouraged patient to keep nurses informed of pain level and need for medication and that pain may be present but manageable.
E (Evaluation): Patient stated that she was "very relieved." Stated that she would tell the nurses about pain.

Focus or DAR Charting (Acronym for *D*ata, *A*ction, and *R*esponse)
A way to organize progress notes to make them clearer and organized

Example:
D (Data): Patient states, "I'm dreading this surgery because last time I had a terrible reaction to the anaesthesia and such terrible pain when they made me get out of bed." Noted muscle tension and loud, agitated voice.
A (Nursing Action): Notified anaesthesiologist of patient's prior experience. Discussed alternatives for anaesthesia and pain control options. Stressed importance of activity for circulation and healing. Encouraged patient to keep nurses informed of pain level and need for medication and that pain may be present but manageable.
R (Patient Response): Patient stated that she was "very relieved." Stated understanding of the importance of informing the nurses about pain.
NOTE: Some facilities add **P (Plan)** and refer to this as DARP charting.

Example:
P (Plan): Assess pain level at least every 4 hours after surgery. Provide nonpharmacological pain management techniques and administer medication as needed.

problems and planning care. The database remains active and current for each patient and is revised as new data become available.

Problem List

The problem list includes the patient's physiological, psychological, sociocultural, spiritual, developmental, and environmental needs. Not all facilities refer to this information as a "problem list." For example, in Quebec, the nurse determines a list of priority health problems that require clinical follow-up as part of the therapeutic nursing plan (TNP) (OIIQ, 2006). To develop a patient's problem list, first analyze the assessment data. Identify and list priority problems in chronological order to serve as an organizing guide for the patient's care. Add new problems as they are identified during the ongoing nursing assessment. When a problem is resolved, record the date and draw a line through the problem and its number. In an electronic system, the problem is marked as resolved.

Plan of Care

Interprofessional collaboration is used to ensure that all health team members involved in a patient's care contribute to the development of an interprofessional plan of care. For example, for a patient having a nutritional deficit, a nurse recommends feeding approaches, and a dietitian recommends types of dietary supplements. Care plan standards require that a plan of care be developed for all patients on admission to a health care facility (CRNNS, 2017b; HQO, 2018). Generally, these plans include nursing diagnoses, expected outcomes, interventions, and evaluations.

Progress Notes

Health care team members use progress notes to monitor and record the progress of a patient's problem (Box 4.4). Narrative notes, flow sheets, and discharge summaries are formats used to document patient progress (see Procedural Guideline 4.2).

SBAR Documentation. SBAR (Situation, Background, Assessment, Recommendation) is a concrete approach for framing conversations, especially critical ones that require a nurse's immediate attention and action. It allows for an easy and focused way to set expectations for what the team will communicate. SBAR promotes the provision of safe, efficient, timely, and person-centred communication (Stewart & Hand, 2017). This method is used for written and verbal communication when a patient's condition changes, for a brief targeted report (e.g., a preprocedure or postprocedure report), or as a change-of-shift report (Stewart & Hand, 2017).

SOAP Documentation. One way to structure narrative notes to document patient progress is the SOAP (Subjective data, Objective data, Assessment, and Plan) format. Some facilities add an I and E (i.e., SOAPIE). The *I* stands for intervention, and the *E* represents evaluation. The logic for SOAP(IE) notes is like that of the nursing process: collect data about a patient's problems, draw conclusions, and develop a plan of care. Number each SOAP note, and title it according to the problem on the list.

PIE Documentation. The PIE (Problem, Intervention, Evaluation) note format of documentation is like that of SOAP charting in its problem-oriented nature. However, it differs from the SOAP method in that PIE charting has a nursing origin, whereas SOAP originated from a medical model.

The PIE format simplifies documentation by combining the care plan and progress note into one record. It differs from that of SOAP because there are no assessment data in the narrative note. Assessment data are included in documentation on the flow sheets of each shift. The nurse numbers or labels the PIE notes according to a patient's problems. Resolved problems are dropped from daily documentation after the nurse's review. Continuing problems are documented daily.

Focus Charting. Another narrative format is focus charting or DAR (*D*ata, *A*ction, *R*esponse). One distinction of focus charting is that it places less importance on patient problems and focuses on patient concerns such as a sign or symptom, condition, nursing diagnosis, behaviour, significant event, or change in condition. Each entry includes data (subjective and objective), actions or nursing interventions, and patient response (e.g., evaluation of effectiveness). Focus charting saves time because it is easy for caregivers to understand, is adaptable to most health care settings, and enables all caregivers to track a patient's condition and progress.

Source Records

In a source record a patient's chart is organized so each profession (e.g., nursing, medicine, respiratory therapy) has a separate section in which to record data. The advantage of a source record is that it is easy for each professional to locate the proper section of the record in which to make entries.

A disadvantage of the source record is that information about a specific problem may be distributed throughout the record. For example, the nurse describes the character of a patient's fractured femur pain and use of repositioning and analgesia in the nurses' notes and EHR. The health care provider notes in a separate section of the record the patient's bone healing and the plan for casting or surgery. The results of radiographic examinations that show bone healing are in the radiology section of the record. The method makes it difficult to find chronological information about patient care or how the team is coordinating care to meet all the patient's needs.

Interprofessional Documentation

Interprofessional documentation involves members of the health care team charting in the same record and sharing documentation tools. When interprofessional teams collaborate, they develop and modify the plan of care for the patient together. This method eliminates duplication and improves patient outcomes (CRNM, n.d.).

Charting by Exception

Charting by exception (CBE) is a system of documentation that aims to eliminate redundancy, makes documentation of routine care more concise, emphasizes abnormal findings, and identifies trends in clinical care. CBE is a shorthand method for documenting based on clearly defined standards of practice and predetermined criteria for nursing assessments and interventions (Fig. 4.5). This system involves completing a flow sheet that incorporates standard assessment and intervention criteria by placing a check mark in the appropriate standard box on the flow sheet to indicate normal

2200	Pt states that she feels nauseated. Vomited 100 mL of clear fluid.
	Sally Smith, RN
2205	Gravol 50 mg IV administered.
	Sally Smith, RN
2235	Pt states no longer feels nauseated.
	Sally Smith, RN

FIG 4.5 Charting by exception. Change in patient's condition requiring a narrative note.

findings and routine interventions. The nurse writes a narrative nurse's note *only* when there is an exception to the established standard or abnormal data are present (e.g., presence of pain, change in oral intake and physical activity, emotional distress, and actions the nurse took to address these concerns).

The presumption with CBE is that the nurse assessed the patient and all standards are met unless otherwise documented. Nurses must be careful to not leave fields blank and assume that documentation was not required because a finding was normal. The nurse needs to initial or indicate "not applicable" in charting templates to communicate that the assessment was complete (HIROC, 2017).

Changes in a patient's condition require thorough and precise descriptions of what happened, actions taken, and patient response to treatment. Legal risks in using CBE include difficulty in proving safe care if nurses are not disciplined in documenting exceptions. Nurses need to chart more frequently and thoroughly when patients have complex health needs, are acutely ill, or are deemed high risk (CNPS, 2007; HIROC, 2017).

Critical Pathways

Critical pathways are a system of documentation that states the goals and important treatment interventions on the basis of best practice and patient expectations by documenting, monitoring, and evaluating variances. Key interventions and expected outcomes are established within an expected time frame for specific diseases (Fig. 4.6). Variances are unexpected occurrences, unmet goals, and interventions not specified within the critical pathway time frame and reflect a positive or negative change. A positive variance occurs when a patient progresses more rapidly than the pathway expected

(e.g., use of a Foley catheter is discontinued a day early). A negative variance occurs when the activities on the critical pathway do not happen as predicted or outcomes are unmet (e.g., oxygen therapy is necessary for a new-onset breathing problem). The nurse documents the variance and includes causative factors, actions taken, patient response, and outcomes. Over time, the recurrence of similar variances leads the health care team to revise a critical pathway, particularly if it affects quality of care or length of stay.

Mobile Communication Devices

Use of mobile devices for communication of health care provider prescriptions is discouraged. The risk involved includes disclosure of confidential health information and not delivering complete communication of a patient's health status. Mobile devices can store and retain personal health information (PHI) and given their small size can be easily lost or stolen. Encryption of devices and the use of strong passwords are the only means to reduce risk of PHI from being disclosed (CLPNNS & CRNNS, 2017). Text or email communication should only occur if it is in the best interest of the patient and if employer policies are in place to support this practice. Health care systems should have policies and procedures in place for health care teams to interact with each other and to access patient records (CLPNNS & CRNNS, 2017).

Liability Issues Related to Documentation

Failure to secure patient information that has been documented may result in a breach of information, liability for wrongful act, and professional misconduct. Any changes made to a health record must follow employer policies to protect the integrity of the record.

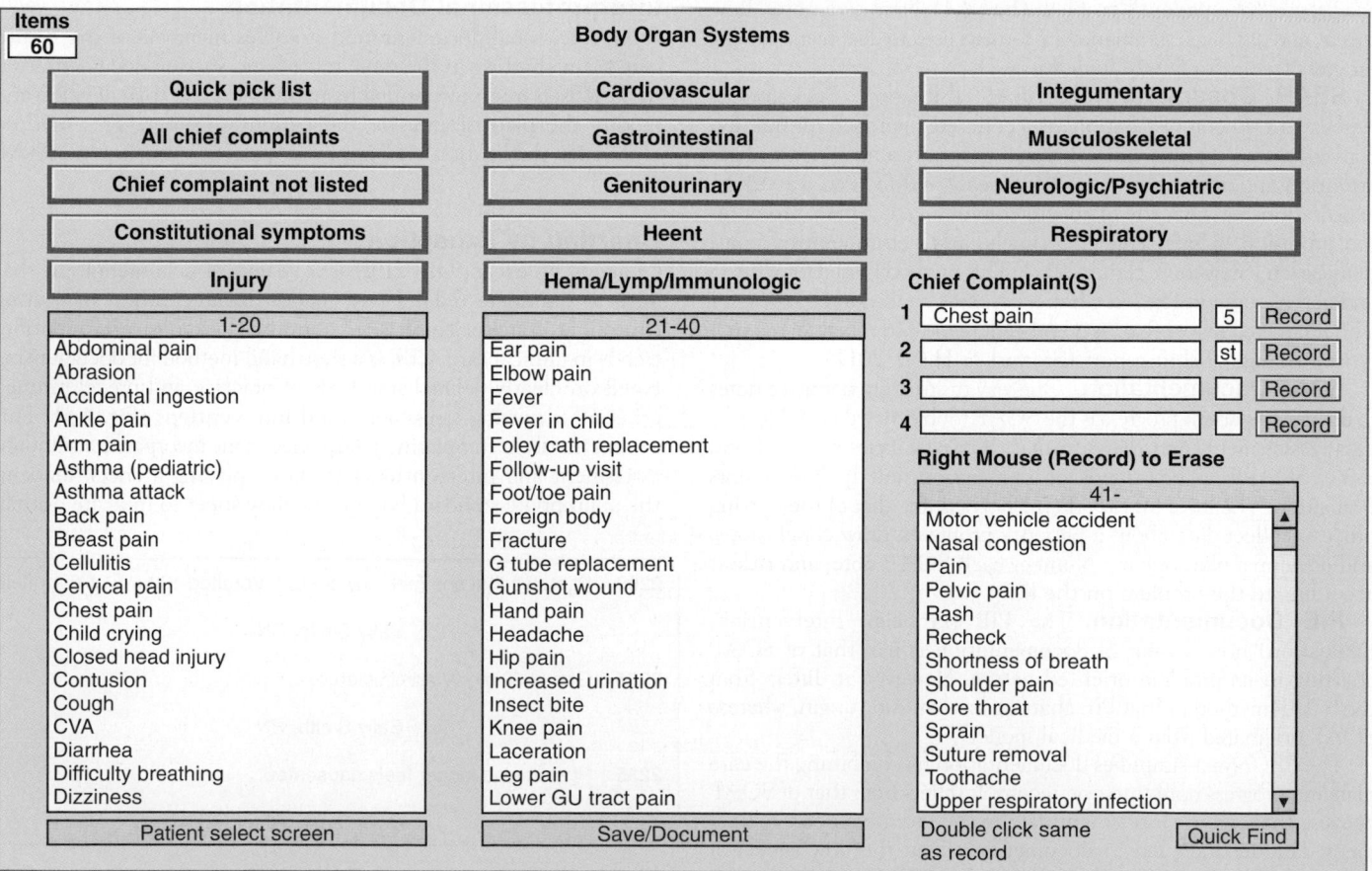

FIG 4.6 Electronic documentation, nursing record. (*Courtesy ER Choice, Irving, TX.*)

PROCEDURAL GUIDELINE 4.2 *Documenting Nurses' Progress Notes*

Accurate documentation reflects the quality of care and provides evidence of each health care team member's accountability in giving care. The purpose of a patient's record is to provide information for communication, education, assessment, research, financial billing, auditing, and legal documentation (Table 4.3).

Because the nursing process directs a nurse's approach to patient care, documentation needs to reflect this process. Nurses record assessment data, changes in a patient's condition, nursing interventions, and an evaluation of the patient's progress toward established outcomes. Prompt documentation of these data increases accuracy and promotes effective communication to all health care team members. The nurse caring for the patient is responsible for writing and signing each progress note, which includes full name and title. All caregivers need to be able to read the progress note and have a clear picture of the problem, level of care required, and results of interventions.

Delegation and Collaboration

The skill of documenting nurse progress notes cannot be delegated to an unregulated care provider (UCP). The nurse instructs the UCP about:

- Which repetitive care activities to document on flow sheets (e.g., vital signs, intake and output [I&O], routine care).
- What to report to the nurse (e.g., increased pain, changes in vital signs) so the nurse can reassess, validate, and document any changes in the progress note.

Equipment

- Progress note form (written or electronic)
- Black pen or electronic health record (EHR)

Procedural Steps

1. Identify the electronic patient record using at least two person-specific identifiers (e.g., name and date of birth or name and medical record number) according to employer policy (Accreditation Canada, 2019).
2. Review assessment data, problems identified, goals and expected outcomes, nursing interventions, and patient response during contact with each patient and before documentation.
3. Document patient information in the format indicated by employer policy for charting to ensure quality documentation.
4. After each patient contact, identify information that needs to be documented. Consider:
   a. Abnormal findings
   b. Changes in status
   c. New problems identified
5. Document in a timely fashion without leaving open spaces between notes and include date and time. In an EHR the date and time are entered automatically by the system.
6. Using employer format, document in chronological order the following:
   a. Pertinent, factual, objective data
   b. Selected subjective data that validate or clarify
   c. Nursing actions taken
   d. Patient responses to actions taken
   e. Additional plans needing to be implemented
   f. To whom information has been reported, including name and status
7. Sign progress note with full name or first initial and last name and status according to employer policy. Do not leave any open space between this note and the previously written note. Students are usually required to indicate their level of education and school affiliation. In an EHR an electronic signature will be generated when the note is submitted electronically.
8. Review previously documented entries with those that you enter, noting if there is significant change in the patient's status. Report any changes to the patient's health care provider.

TABLE 4.3

Purposes of Records

Purpose	Description
Communication	The record is a means for health care team members to communicate a patient's *needs* (e.g., individual therapies, patient education, discharge planning) and *progress* (e.g., response to therapies). Anyone reading the record should have a clear understanding of the plan of care.
Education	The record contains a variety of information, including medical and nursing diagnoses, signs and symptoms of disease, successful and unsuccessful therapies, diagnostic findings, and patient behaviours. Students use records as educational resources.
Assessment	Records provide data that nurses use to identify and support nursing diagnoses and plan proper interventions for care. Information from records adds to the nurse's own observations and assessment. Information in medical progress notes allows a nurse to anticipate the status of a patient and conduct an assessment that augments, validates, or confirms health care provider findings.
Research	Statistical data relating to the frequency of clinical disorders, complications, use of specific medical and nursing therapies, recovery from illness, and death can be gathered from patient records. Records describe characteristics of patient populations in a health care facility.
Financial billing	The record is a document that shows the extent to which hospitals should be reimbursed for services.
Auditing and monitoring	A regular review of information in patient records gives a basis for evaluation of the quality and appropriateness of care provided in a facility. Accreditation Canada (2019) requires health care facilities to establish quality improvement programs to conduct objective, ongoing reviews of patient care. Review of records reveals information about the processes and outcomes of care.

continued

TABLE 4.3
Purposes of Records—cont'd

Purpose	Description
Legal documentation	A medical record must be accurate because it is a legal document. In case of a lawsuit, the medical record, not the nursing care, is on trial. Nursing care may have been excellent; however, care not documented is care not done as far as a court of law is concerned.

PROCEDURAL GUIDELINE 4.3 *Adverse Event/Incident Reporting*

An adverse event/incident is any event not consistent with the routine operation of a health care unit or routine care of a patient. Examples include patient falls, needle-stick injuries, medication errors, or a visitor becoming ill. Patient safety events involve the patient and are events that harm the patient, reach the patient but do not harm the patient, or did not reach the patient (known as a "near miss"), such as a medication error (CPSI, 2011). The CPSI and HQO (2015) identified a standardized list of preventable, never events, a subset of patient safety events, that facilitate reporting of such events (Box 4.5). Completion of a report happens when there is actual or potential patient injury (a "near miss"). The process involves documentation first in the patient health record and in an adverse event/incident report as per employer policy (also referred to as a "serious event report" or an "occurrence report"). Document in the patient's record an objective description of what you observed and follow-up actions taken without reference to the adverse/incident report. The actual report does not become part of the health record. Nurses are accountable to help develop quality practice environments. Reporting helps to identify high-risk trends in nursing care or daily unit operations that warrant correction. You need to complete the report even if an injury does not occur or is not apparent. This information helps nursing staff find solutions to prevent repeated incidents. The reports are an important part of the quality improvement program of a unit.

Adverse event/incident reports are important sources of data for enhancing understanding of underlying causes of events that, when analyzed, can improve patient safety (CPSI, 2016b). Nurses are active participants in examining the cause of errors and redesigning systems to minimize repeat errors. By focusing on systems rather than on individual failures, there is greater opportunity to improve patient safety (CPSI, 2016b). For example, a patient is administered the wrong medication by a nurse. A review of the event focuses primarily on the medication process instead of placing blame.

Nurses are ethically responsible to report near misses and take immediate action to prevent harm to persons receiving care (CNA, 2017a). CPSI (2011; 2016b) disclosure guidelines indicate that communication of near misses takes place immediately following the event, in order to prevent further harm to others. Such disclosure allows patients and families involved to heal and promotes patient safety practices.

Delegation and Collaboration
- Ensure that documentation is completed by the person who performed the action or witnessed the event (CNPS, 2007).

Equipment
- Adverse event/incident report form or screen
- Black pen or digital technology

Procedural Steps
1. Identify the electronic patient record using at least two person-specific identifiers (e.g., name and date of birth or name and medical record number) according to employer policy (Accreditation Canada, 2019).
2. Use clinical reasoning skills to systematically and carefully determine what was involved in the event. The person who witnessed the event is the person who documents the event. Document the exact sequence of events involved, including time and type of event; injury to patient, nurse, visitor, or other staff; and observation of factors that possibly contributed to the event (e.g., wet floor discovered in area of patient fall). Notify risk management per employer policy.

Clinical Decision Point *Prepare the report on any questionable event. Do not avoid reporting because of concerns that punitive actions will occur if reports are filed.*

3. Assess extent of any injury to patient or others, including patient's subjective report and objective physical examination findings.
4. If the adverse event/incident involves an injury, take steps to restore individual's safety, such as stabilizing patient's position after a fall and assessing for further injuries.
5. When patient sustains an injury, notify health care provider immediately.
6. When visitor or staff member sustains an injury, refer to emergency department or appropriate treatment setting.
7. Complete adverse event/incident report form.

Clinical Decision Point *Document on report form as quickly as possible. The closer to the event it is documented, the more accurate the recording.*

    a. Record time of event and describe exactly what occurred or was observed, using objective findings and observations. Use language that does not allow for subjective interpretation. Do not include personal opinions or feelings. Document person's interpretation of event by using quotes.
    b. Objectively describe person's condition when event was discovered or observed.
    c. Describe measures taken by any caregivers at time of event.
    d. Submit report as per employer policy
8. When patient is involved, document events of incident in patient's chart.
    a. Only enter objective description of what happened.
    b. Record any assessment and intervention activities initiated because of event.
    c. Do not duplicate all information from report.
    d. Do not document that report was completed.
9. Submit the report properly with the risk-management department or designated people.

BOX 4.5

15 Never Events for Hospital Care in Canada

- Surgery on the wrong body part or the wrong patient, or conducting the wrong procedure
- Wrong tissue, biological implant, or blood product given to a patient
- Unintended foreign object left in a patient following a procedure
- Patient death or serious harm arising from the use of improperly sterilized instruments or equipment provided by the health care facility
- Patient death or serious harm due to a failure to inquire whether a patient has a known allergy to medication, or due to administration of a medication to a patient whose allergy had been identified
- Patient death or serious harm due to administration of the wrong inhalation or insufflation gas
- Patient death or serious harm as a result of one of five pharmaceutical events (e.g., wrong route used for chemotherapy, IV administration of a concentrated potassium solution)
- Patient death or serious harm as a result of failure to identify and treat metabolic disturbances (e.g., hypoglycoomia or hyperbilirubinemia)
- Patient death or serious harm due to uncontrolled movement of a ferromagnetic object in a magnetic resonance imaging (MRI) area
- Patient death or serious harm due to an accidental burn
- Patient under the highest level of observation leaves a secured facility or ward without the knowledge of staff (e.g., patient with dementia or suicide risk)
- Patient suicide, or attempted suicide that resulted in serious harm, in instances where suicide prevention protocols were to be applied to patients under the highest level of observation
- Infant abducted, or discharged to the wrong person
- Patient death or serious harm as a result of transport of a frail patient, or patient with dementia, when protocols were not followed to ensure the patient was left in a safe environment

Based on Canadian Patient Safety Institute (CPSI) and Health Quality Ontario (HQO). (2015). *Never events for hospital care in Canada: Safer care for patients.* Retrieved from http://www.patientsafetyinstitute.ca/en/toolsResources/Never-Events/Documents/Never%20Events%20for%20Hospital%20Care%20in%20Canada.pdf.

BOX 4.6

Forms for Documentation for Care in the Community

The usual forms used to document care in the community include the following:
- Patient assessment
- Referral source information/intake form
- Discipline-specific care plans
- Health care provider's plan of treatment
- Medication sheet
- Clinical progress notes
- Miscellaneous (conference notes, verbal prescription forms, telephone calls)
- Discharge summary
- Reports to third-party payers

Changing another person's entry in the health record can result in being accused of falsification of a record and professional misconduct (CLPNNS & CRNNS, 2017).

Students are accountable for their actions and are to document the care they provide in the health record. Student documentation notes should not be co-signed (unless required by certain employer policies), as this may result in accountability issues for the co-signer (CLPNNS & CRNNS, 2017). However, students must be aware of practices that require supervision and confirming signature of a witnessed event (e.g., high-alert medications such as insulin, potassium, anticoagulants) (ISMP, 2014). In such events, a third nurse may be involved as a witness and co-signer in addition to the student nurse and instructor/preceptor. Employer policies provide guidance to nurses regarding documentation requirements for student nurses (CLPNNS & CRNNS, 2017).

Poor documentation can affect the integrity of the health record. Lawyers rely on charting to show if a nurse met the standard of care and did not cause harm to the patient that resulted in the legal act of negligence (HIROC, 2017). Working notes should become part of the health record in a timely manner and should be shredded following transcription into the health record. Such notes can be used as evidence in a legal proceeding (HIROC, 2017).

Privacy and Ethics Around Digital Health Information

Patients have the right to confidentiality and security of their health information. Every effort should be made to ensure that those who are not involved in the care of the patient do not have access to patients' digital information. Nurses must follow professional standards, provincial privacy legislation, and employer policies in relation to documentation and protection of personal health information.

Patients have the right to access their health care information and nurses should advocate and assist patients in the retrieval process in accordance with provincial/territorial legislation and employer policies (CNA, 2017a).

DOCUMENTATION OF CARE IN THE COMMUNITY

Care in the community continues to grow with shorter hospitalizations and increasing numbers of persons requiring care in the home. Documentation when caring for a patient at home has different implications than in other areas of nursing. One primary difference is that the patient and family rather than the nurse witness the majority of care. In addition, documentation systems need to provide the entire health care team with the necessary information to maximize the efficiency of interprofessional collaboration (Box 4.6).

Computerized patient records are evolving in the community setting. The EHR facilitates clarity, continuity of care, and comprehensiveness because of increased standardization of language (CNA, 2016; C-HOBIC, 2015). Patient information stored electronically should be encrypted to prevent privacy breaches. Users need to make every effort to keep personal health information secure by avoiding use of public wireless networks and free email services when accessing patient health information from an EHR (Canadian Medical Protective Association [CMPA], 2013).

LONG-TERM HEALTH CARE DOCUMENTATION

Increasing numbers of older persons and people living with disability in Canada require care in long-term health care facilities. Nursing personnel face documentation challenges much different from those in the acute care setting (Michel et al., 2017). EHRs in long-term care facilities improve documentation management, clinical decision-making, and health outcomes (Kruse, Mileski, & Chidambaram, 2017).

A nurse is responsible for coordinating the plan of care. Documentation supports the assessment and planning process for patients using an interprofessional approach. Communication among all health care team members is essential in the documentation process. The overall goal is a system of clinical documentation that identifies potential or actual problems and provides improved actions for each

problem, which results in improved care for residents (Wysocki, Thomas, & Mor, 2015).

CLINICAL DEBRIEF

A 55-year-old retired teacher will be discharged this evening from the ambulatory care unit following his surgical hernia repair. His admission medication list includes hydrochlorothiazide 12.5-mg tablet orally once per day; fluoxetine 40-mg tablet orally once daily in the morning.

Immediately after surgery he rates his pain as 10 on a scale of 0–10 (0 being no pain, 10 being worst pain ever), and he is medicated with hydromorphone 1 mg IV at 0930.

1. Based on his admission medication list, which medications should you expect to find on the discharge medication list?
2. At 1400, he rates his surgical pain as 9 on a scale of 0–10 (0 being no pain, 10 being worst pain ever). He receives two oxycodone 10 mg tablets orally for his pain at 1410. Thirty minutes later, he rates his pain as 2 on a scale of 0–10. At discharge the medication list reads: hydrochlorothiazide 12.5-mg tablet orally once per day and fluoxetine 40-mg tablet orally once daily in the morning. What are your nursing actions?
3. Using SBAR, show how you would communicate with the health care provider about the medication omission.

PROCEDURAL GUIDELINE 4.4 *Guidelines for Meaningful Use of an Interoperable Electronic Health Record (iEHR)*

A Canadian Health Infoway (CHI) (2018a) goal is to improve the health and health care experiences of Canadians by connecting health care information through iEHR. In addition, health care facilities across the country are connecting health care information through technology to facilitate patient transitions across the continuum of care. Meaningful use means that health care providers effectively use iEHRs to improve patient care (CIHI, 2016; C-HOBIC, 2015).

When health care facilities participate in meaningful use initiatives, health care providers use iEHRs to record universal patient data, practise person-centred care, and transmit critical patient data at care transition points (CIHI, 2016; C-HOBIC, 2015). An example of a care transition is a patient discharge from a hospital to a long-term care facility. During transitions, there is a transfer of specific patient data collected from the sending facility to the new provider. Examples of data sent include history of allergies, cognitive status, functional status, immunizations, medications, and smoking history.

An important component of care transitions is the process of medication reconciliation. *Medication reconciliation* is the assessment of the patient's current medications compared to medications actually prescribed at a care transition point. This process minimizes medication errors and adverse events (Jaggi et al., 2018). The EHR provides efficiencies for all health care providers performing medication reconciliation (Electronic Medication Reconciliation Group [EMRG], 2017). Medication reconciliation is one of World Health Organization's top five mandated core objectives for reducing medication errors globally (ISMP Canada, 2018). Medication reconciliation, which is a complex process requiring interprofessional collaboration (ISMP & HQO, 2015), is also a National Patient Safety Goal and a requirement of Accreditation Canada (2019). By using a standardized process to assess a patient's medications at a care transition point, medication discrepancies such as omissions, duplications, contraindications, and vague information can be reduced (EMRG, 2017). Although some facilities may assign other disciplines as the accountable discipline for medication reconciliation, the nurse plays an active collaborative role in the process (College of Nurses of Ontario [CNO], 2017; Jaggi et al., 2018).

Delegation and Collaboration

The skill of using an iEHR for medication reconciliation cannot be delegated to an unregulated care provider (UCP). The nurse instructs the UCP to:

- Report to the nurse any pertinent information the patient or caregiver reports about their medications.

Equipment
- Admission medication list
- Current medication list
- Discharge medication list
- Medication reconciliation work screen or worksheet (follow employer policy)
- iEHR

Procedural Steps
1. Use an organized format for medication reconciliation. Gathering the best possible medication history (BPMH) and using an e-MedRec tool may effectively reduce medication errors for patients transitioning across points of care (EMRG, 2017).
2. Identify the electronic patient record using at least two person-specific identifiers (e.g., name and date of birth or name and medical record number) according to employer policy (Accreditation Canada, 2019).
3. Gather information from electronic documentation sources such as admission medications, active medications, or discharge medications.
4. Include two nurses to complete the medication reconciliation at time of care transition. Assess the current medications prescribed to the medications prescribed for the care transition. If the patient is being discharged from a facility, assess the medications on admission and current medications to the discharge medications (Ruggiero, Smith, Copeland, et al., 2015).
5. Discrepancies are assessed by the two nurses.

Clinical Decision Point *If discrepancies still exist after nurse review, a nurse-to-physician reconciliation occurs.*

6. If the patient is being discharged from a facility, reconcile the medication list before giving information to the patient. Provide the patient with the written reconciled list of medications.
7. Teach the patient how to keep their medication list current.
8. Educate the patient about the medications and importance of sharing the current medication list at every health care visit.
   Use Teach-Back: "It is important to keep your medication list up to date. Tell me how you plan on doing this?" Develop a revised teaching plan if patient or caregiver is not able to teach back correctly.

✦ REVIEW QUESTIONS

1. The patient falls on the unit. Which actions should the nurse perform? *(Select all that apply.)*
   1. Assess extent of any injury to the patient
   2. Document the adverse event report in the electronic health record (EHR)
   3. Identify the patient using at least two person-specific identifiers
   4. Complete an adverse event report on the basis of the nurse's initial reaction
   5. Document the nurse's clinical assessment in the EHR

2. During a hand-off report, the nurse will: *(Select all that apply.)*
   1. Use the patient's first and last name as the two person-specific identifiers.
   2. Provide background information about the patient.
   3. Recommend the priority of care for the next shift.
   4. Include in the assessment the patient's response to pain medications.
   5. Exclude the patient from the hand-off report.

3. The patient is being transitioned from the hospital to a long-term care facility. Place the following criteria in correct order for an SBAR report.
   1. Medical history, allergies, code status, isolation, significant interventions, pain management, responses to interventions, report of abnormal studies, who was notified, any interventions, intravenous [IV] access
   2. Admission date, chief complaint, and diagnosis
   3. Review of systems: neurological, respiratory, cardiac, gastrointestinal, genitourinary, musculoskeletal, peripheral vascular, skin, hematological, endocrine, and psychosocial
   4. Patient's daily goals, consultations, planned treatments, upcoming tests or surgery, discharge planning, and patient education

ⓔ *Visit the Evolve site for a complete list of Clinical Debrief and Review Questions answers.*

REFERENCES

Accreditation Canada. (2019). *Required organizational practices: handbook—Version 14.* Retrieved from http://www.wrha.mb.ca/quality/files/2019ROPHandbook.pdf

An, D. (2015). Cochrane review brief: Discharge planning from hospital to home. *Online J Issues in Nursing,* 20(2), doi:10.3912/OJIN.Vol20No02CRBCol01

Aziz, H. A., & Alsharabasi, O. A. (2015). Electronic health records uses and malpractice risks. *Clinical Laboratory Science,* 28(4), 250–255.

Butcher, H., Bulechek, G., Dochterman, J., & Wagner, C. (2018). *Nursing interventions classification (NIC)* (7th ed.). St. Louis, MO: Elsevier.

Canada Health Infoway (CHI). (2018a). *Connected health information in Canada: A benefits evaluation study.* Retrieved from https://www.infoway-inforoute.ca/en/component/edocman/resources/reports/benefits-evaluation/3510-connected-health-information-in-canada-a-benefits-evaluation-study?Itemid=101

Canada Health Infoway (CHI). (2018b). *Electronic health records.* Retrieved from http://www.infoway-inforoute.ca/en/solutions/electronic-health-records

Canada Health Infoway (CHI). (2018c) *Nursing data standards.* Retrieved from https://infocentral.infoway-inforoute.ca/en/standards/other-canadian/nursing-data-standards

Canada Health Infoway (CHI), Canadian Nurses Association (CNA), & Canadian Nursing Informatics Association (CNIA). (2017, May). *2017 National survey of Canadian nurses. Use of digital health technology in practice, final executive report.* Retrieved from https://www.infoway-inforoute.ca/en/component/edocman/3320-2017-national-survey-of-canadian-nurses-use-of-digital-health-technology-in-practice/view-document?Itemid=0

Canadian Health Outcomes for Better Information and Care (C-HOBIC). (2015). *C-HOBIC Phase 2 final report.* Retrieved from https://c-hobic.cna-aiic.ca/documents/pdf/Canadian-Health-Outcomes-for-Better-Information-and-Care_C-HOBIC-Phase-2_Final-Report_January-2015.pdf

Canadian Institute for Health Information (CIHI). (2016). *CIHI's annual report 2015–2016. Charting a new course.* Retrieved from https://secure.cihi.ca/free_products/2016_AnnualReport_EN-web.pdf

Canadian Medical Protective Association (CMPA). (2013). *Duties and responsibilities: Expectations of physicians in practice. Protecting patient health information in electronic records.* Retrieved from https://www.cmpa-acpm.ca/en/advice-publications/browse-articles/2013/protecting-patient-health-information-in-electronic-records

Canadian Nurses Association (CNA). (2016). *National nursing data standards symposium proceedings.* Retrieved from https://www.cna-aiic.ca/-/media/cna/page-content/pdf-en/national-nursing-data-standards-symposium-proceedings-report.pdf

Canadian Nurses Association (CNA). (2017a). *Code of ethics for registered nurses.* Retrieved from https://www.cna-aiic.ca/html/en/Code-of-Ethics-2017-Edition/index.html

Canadian Nurses Association (CNA). (2017b). *Nursing informatics: Joint position statement.* Retrieved from https://cna-aiic.ca/~/media/cna/page-content/pdf-en/nursing-informatics-joint-position-statement.pdf

Canadian Nurses Protective Society (CNPS). (2007). *Quality documentation: Your best defense.* Retrieved from https://www.cnps.ca/index.php?page=85

Canadian Patient Safety Institute (CPSI). (2011). *Canadian disclosure guidelines: Being open with patients and families.* Retrieved from http://www.patientsafetyinstitute.ca/en/toolsResources/disclosure/Documents/CPSI%20Canadian%20Disclosure%20Guidelines.pdf#search=near%20misses

Canadian Patient Safety Institute (CPSI). (2016a). *Medication incidents: Standards and required organizational practices.* Retrieved from http://www.patientsafetyinstitute.ca/en/toolsResources/Hospital-Harm-Measure/Improvement Resources/Medication-Incidents-Introduction/Pages/Medication-Incidents-Standards-and-Required-Organizational-Practices.aspx

Canadian Patient Safety Institute (CPSI). (2016b). *Patient safety and incident management toolkit.* Retrieved from http://www.patientsafetyinstitute.ca/en/toolsResources/PatientSafetyIncidentManagementToolkit/Pages/default.aspx

Canadian Patient Safety Institute (CPSI) & Health Quality Ontario (HQO). (2015). *Never events for hospital care in Canada: Safer care for patients.* Retrieved from http://www.patientsafetyinstitute.ca/en/toolsResources/NeverEvents/Documents/Never%20Events%20for%20Hospital%20Care%20in%20Canada.pdf

Chauvette, A. (2016). History of nursing informatics in Canada. *Canadian Journal of Nursing Informatics,* 11(4). Retrieved from http://cjni.net/journal/?p=5032

College of Licensed Practical Nurses of Nova Scotia (CLPNNS) & College of Registered Nurses of Nova Scotia (CRNNS). (2017). *Documentation guidelines for nurses.* Retrieved from https://crnns.ca/wp-content/uploads/2017/12/Documentation-Guidelines-for-Nurses-Final.pdf

College of Nurses of Ontario (CNO). (2017). *Practice standard: Medication.* Retrieved from http://www.cno.org/globalassets/docs/prac/41007_medication.pdf

College of Registered Nurses of British Columbia (CRNBC). (2015). *Appropriate use of titles practice standard.* Retrieved from https://www.crnbc.ca/Standards/PracticeStandards/Lists/GeneralResources/343AppropriateUseofTitlesPracStd.pdf

College of Registered Nurses of British Columbia (CRNBC). (2018). *Practice standard for registered nurses and nurse practitioners: Documentation.* Retrieved from https://crnbc.ca/Standards/PracticeStandards/Lists/GeneralResources/334DocumentationPracStd.pdf

College of Registered Nurses of Manitoba (CRNM). (n.d.). *Documentation guidelines for registered nurses.* Retrieved from https://www.crnm.mb.ca/uploads/ck/files/Documentation%20Guidelines%20for%20Nurses%20-%20web%20version.pdf

College of Registered Nurses of Nova Scotia (CRNNS). (2017a). *Medication guidelines for registered nurses.* Retrieved from https://crnns.ca/wp-content/uploads/2015/05/Medication-Guidelines.pdf

College of Registered Nurses of Nova Scotia (CRNNS). (2017b). *Nursing plan of care: Practice guideline.* Retrieved from https://crnns.ca/wp-content/uploads/2015/12/Nursing-Plan-of-Care-Practice-Guideline.pdf

de Lima Silva, K., Dora Martinez Évora, Y., & Santana Justo Cintra, C. (2015). Software development to support decision making in the selection of nursing diagnoses and interventions for children and adolescents. *Revista Latino-Americana de Enfermagem,* 23(5), doi:10.1590/0104-1169.0302.2633

Electronic Medication Reconciliation Group (EMRG). (2017). *Paper to electronic MedRec implementation toolkit* (2nd ed.). Toronto: ISMP Canada & Canadian Patient Safety Institute. Retrieved from http://www.patientsafetyinstitute.ca/en/toolsResources/pages/paper-to-electronic-medrec-implementation-toolkit.aspx

Flanders, S. A. (2018). Nurses as educators. Effective patient education: Evidence and common sense. *Medsurg Nursing,* 27(1), 55–58.

Foley, V. (2018). Documenting & reporting. In B. Kozier, G. Erb, A. Berman, et al. (Eds.), *Fundamentals of Canadian nursing: Concepts, process, & practice* (4th ed., pp. 460–481). Toronto: Pearson Canada.

Foster-Hunt, T., Parush, A., Ellis, J., Thomas, M., & Rashotte, J. (2015). Information structure and organization in change of shift reports: An observational study of nursing hand-offs in a paediatric intensive care unit. *Intensive & Critical Care Nursing,* 31(3), 155–164. doi:10.1016/j.iccn.2014.09.004

Gephart, S. M., Bristol, A. A., Dye, J. L., Finley, B. A., & Carrington, J. M. (2016). Validity and reliability of a new measure of nursing experience with unintended consequences of electronic health records. *Computer, Informatics, Nursing,* 34(10), 436–447. doi:10.1097/CIN.0000000000000285

Government of Canada. (2018). *The Personal Information Protection and Electronic Documents act (PIPEDA).* Ottawa, ON: Author. Retrieved from https://www.priv.gc.ca/en/privacy-topics/privacy-laws-in-canada/the-personal-information-protection-and-electronic-documents-act-pipeda/

Graetz, I., Jie, H., Brand, R., et al. (2015). The impact of electronic health records and teamwork on diabetes care quality. *American Journal of Managed Care*, 21(12), 878–884.

Harmon, C. S., Fogle, M., & Roussel, L. (2015). Then and now: Nurses' perceptions of the electronic health record. *Online Journal of Nursing Informatics*, 19(1), 5.

Healthcare Insurance Reciprocal of Canada (HIROC). (2017). *Strategies for improving documentation: Lessons from medical legal claims*. Retrieved from https://www.hiroc.com/getmedia/9b3d1ed1-b2e1-45fc-ae18-bfc998177d15/Documentation-Guide-2017.pdf.aspx

Health Quality Ontario (HQO). (2018). *Adopting a common approach to transitional care planning: Helping health links improve transitions and coordination of care*. Ontario: Queen's Printer for Ontario. Retrieved from http://www.hqontario.ca/Portals/0/documents/qi/health-links/bp-improve-package-traditional-care-planning-en.pdf

Institute for Safe Medication Practices (ISMP). (2014). *ISMP list of high-alert medications in acute care settings*. Retrieved from https://www.ismp.org/sites/default/files/attachments/2018-01/highalertmedications%281%29.pdf

Institute for Safe Medication Practices (ISMP). (2015). *ISMP's list of error-prone abbreviations, symbols, and dose designations*. Retrieved from https://www.ismp.org/sites/default/files/attachments/2017-11/Error%20Prone%20Abbreviations%202015.pdf

Institute for Safe Medication Practices (ISMP) Canada. (2018). *Medication reconciliation (MedRec)*. Retrieved from https://www.ismp-canada.org/medrec/

Institute for Safe Medication Practices (ISMP) Canada & Health Quality Ontario (HQO). (2015). *Ontario primary care medication reconciliation guide*. Retrieved from https://www.ismp-canada.org/download/PrimaryCareMedRecGuide_EN.pdf

Jaggi, P., Tomlinson, R., McLelland, K., Ma, W., Manson-McLeod, C., & Bullard, M. J. (2018). Nursing duties and accreditation standards and their impacts: The nursing perspective. *Applied Nursing Research*, 40, 61–67. doi:10.1016/j.apnr.2017.12.009

Kruse, C. S., Mileski, M., & Chidambaram, Y. (2017). Impact of electronic health records on long-term care facilities: Systematic review. *JMIR Medical Informatics*, 5(3), e35. doi:10.2196/medinform.7958

Liu, F., Zou, Y., Huang, Q., Zheng, L., & Wang, W. (2015). Electronic health records and improved nursing management of chronic obstructive pulmonary disease. *Patient Preference and Adherence*, 9, 495–500. doi:10.2147/PPA.S76562

Mardis, T., Mardis, M., Davis, J., et al. (2016). Bedside shift-to-shift handoff. *Journal of Nursing Care Quality*, 31(1), 54–60. doi:10.1097/NCQ.0000000000000142.

Michel, L., Waelli, M., Allen, D., & Minvielle, E. (2017). The content and meaning of administrative work: A qualitative study of nursing practices. *Journal of Advanced Nursing*, 73(9), 2179–2190. doi:10.1111/jan.13294

NANDA-I. (2018). *About us*. Retrieved from http://www.nanda.org/about-us/

Ordre des infimieres et infirmiers du Quebec [OIIQ]. (2006). *The therapeutic nursing plan: The track of clinical nursing decisions*. Montreal: Author. Retrieved from https://www.oiiq.org/documents/20147/237836/222A_doc.pdf

Ordre des infimieres et infirmiers du Quebec [OIIQ]. (2015). *Code of ethics of nurses*. Montreal: Author. Retrieved from https://www.oiiq.org/documents/20147/237836/8450_doc.pdf

Province of Nova Scotia. (2018). *Personal Health Information Act*. Retrieved from https://novascotia.ca/just/regulations/regs/phipershealth.htm

Registered Nurses Association of Ontario. (n.d.). *eHealth & Technology: The Nursing and eHealth Project*. Retrieved from http://rnao.ca/ehealth/nursingordersets

Registered Nurses Association of Ontario. (2017). *Adopting eHealth solutions: Implementation strategies*. Retrieved from http://rnao.ca/sites/rnao-ca/files/bpg/Adopting_eHealth_Solutions_WEB_FINAL.pdf

Ruggiero, J., Smith, J., Copeland, J., & Boxer, B. (2015). Discharge time out: An innovative nurse-driven protocol for medication reconciliation. *Medsurg Nursing*, 24(3), 165–172.

Stewart, K. R., & Hand, K. A. (2017). SBAR, communication, and patient safety: An integrated literature review. *Medsurg Nursing*, 26(5), 297–305.

Stimson, C. E., & Botruff, A. L. (2017). Daily electronic health record reports meet meaningful use requirements, improve care efficiency, and provide a layer of safety for trauma patients. *Journal of Trauma Nursing*, 24(1), 53–56. doi:10.1097/JTN.0000000000000262

Strudwick, G., Reisdorfer, E., Warnock, C., et al. (2018). Factors associated with barcode medication administration technology that contribute to patient safety: An integrative review. *Journal of Nursing Care Quality*, 33(1), 79–85. doi:10.1097/NCQ.0000000000000270.

Trossman, S. (2015). Stopping the revolving door. *Am Nurs*, 47(1), 9.

Usher, R., Cronin, S. N., & York, N. L. (2018). Evaluating the influence of a standardized bedside handoff process in a medical–surgical unit. *Journal of Continuing Education in Nursing*, 49(4), 157–163. doi:10.3928/00220124-20180320-05

Walker-Czyz, A. (2016). The impact of an integrated electronic health record adoption on nursing. *JONA*, 46(7/8), 366–372. doi:10.1097/NNA.0000000000000360

Wallace, I. (2015). Is patient confidentiality compromised with the electronic health record? *Computer, Informatics, Nursing*, 32(2), 58–62. doi:10.1097/CIN.0000000000000126

White, P. (2017). Adopting national nursing data standards in Canada. *Canadian Nurse*, 113(3), 18–22.

Wysocki, A., Thomas, K. S., & Mor, V. (2015). Functional improvement among short-stay nursing home residents in the MDS 3.0. *Journal of the American Medical Directors Association*, 16(6), 470. doi:10.1016/j.jamda.2014.11.018

Zychla, L. (2017). Patient portals in an information demanding society. *Canadian Journal of Medical Laboratory Science*, 79(1), 24–27.

5 | Medical Asepsis

Written by **Angela McConachie, FNP, DNP and Sandra Redmond, RN, MN**

OBJECTIVES

Mastery of content in this chapter will enable the nurse to:
- Discuss how to apply critical thinking in the prevention of the transmission of infection.
- Explain the difference between medical and surgical asepsis.
- Identify nursing care measures intended to break the chain of infection.

- Describe how each element of the infection chain contributes to infection.
- Describe the factors that influence nursing staff adherence to hand hygiene.
- Perform proper procedures for hand hygiene.
- Perform correct routine practices and additional precautions.

MEDIA RESOURCES

- evolve http://evolve.elsevier.com/Canada/Perry/clinicalskills/
- Review Questions
- ▶ Video Clips

- Audio Glossary
- **NSO** Nursing Skills Online
- Clinical Debrief and Review Questions Answers

PURPOSE

Infection prevention and control practices reduce or eliminate sources and transmission of infection. These prevention and control practices are designed to protect patients and health care providers from disease. Medical asepsis, or clean technique, includes procedures used for reducing the number of organisms and preventing their transfer.

STANDARDS OF CARE

- Infection Prevention and Control (IPAC) Canada, 2017—*IPAC Canada Practice Recommendations: Hand Hygiene in Health Care Settings* (https://ipac-canada.org/photos/custom/Members/pdf/17JulHand%20Hygiene%20Practice%20Recommendations_final.pdf)
- Ontario Agency for Health Protection & Promotion (Public Health Ontario [PHO]), Provincial Infectious Diseases Advisory Committee (PIDAC), 2014—*Best Practices for Hand Hygiene in all Health Care Settings*, 4th edition (https://www.publichealthontario.ca/en/eRepository/2010-12%20BP%20Hand%20Hygiene.pdf)
- Public Health Agency of Canada (PHAC), 2017—*Routine Practices and Additional Precautions for Preventing the Transmission of Infection in Healthcare Settings* (https://www.canada.ca/en/public-health/services/infectious-diseases/nosocomial-occupational-infections/routine-practices-additional-precautions-preventing-transmission-infection-healthcare-settings.html)

PRINCIPLES FOR PRACTICE

- Hand hygiene practices are major principles of infection control and are essential to safe patient care (IPAC 2017; World Health Organization [WHO], 2009).
- Patients in all health care settings are at risk of becoming colonized or infected because of an impaired immune response, exposure to an increased number of pathogenic organisms, and performance of invasive procedures (Yallew, Kumie, & Yehuala, 2017).
- Know a patient's susceptibility to infection. Age, nutritional status, stress, disease processes, and forms of medical therapy place patients at risk (Rojas-Garcia et al., 2018).
- Health care–associated infections (HAIs) result from delivery of health services in a health care setting that were not present at the time of admission. A hospital is one of the most likely settings for acquiring an HAI because staff, patients, and environmental factors support a high population of pathogens that are resistant to antibiotics. Health care workers transmit many HAIs through direct contact during the delivery of care (Farhoudi et al., 2016).

- Using interprofessional collaboration optimizes the prevention and control of infection and enhances patient safety.
- Recognize elements of the chain of infection and initiate measures to prevent the onset and spread of infections. The presence of a pathogen does not mean that an infection will occur. Infection occurs in a cycle, often referred to as the *chain of infection*. An infection develops if this chain remains intact (Fig. 5.1). In patient care it is important to use infection control practices to break an element of the chain so as not to transmit infection (Table 5.1). The six elements in the chain are as follows:
  - An infectious agent or pathogen
  - A reservoir or source for pathogen growth
  - A portal of exit from the reservoir
  - A mode of transmission
  - A portal of entry to the host
  - A susceptible host

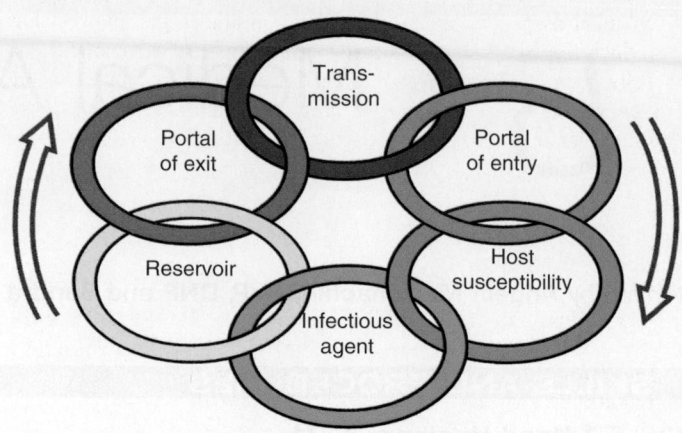

FIG 5.1 Chain of infection.

TABLE 5.1

Breaking the Chain of Infection

Element of Infection Chain	Medical Asepsis Practices
Infectious agent (pathogenic organism capable of causing disease)	Clean contaminated objects. Clean, disinfect, and sterilize.
Reservoir (site or source of microorganism growth)	Perform hand hygiene before and after patient contact with appropriate antiseptic (e.g., alcohol-based hand rub) or soap and water. Control sources of body fluids and drainage. Bathe patient with soap and water, or disposable bath. If a patient is critically ill, chlorhexidine baths are more effective for infection prevention (Raines & Rosen, 2016; Swan et al., 2016). Change soiled dressings. Dispose of soiled tissues, dressings, or linen in moisture-resistant bags. Place syringes, uncapped hypodermic needles, and intravenous needles in designated puncture-proof containers. Keep table surfaces clean and dry. Do not leave bottled solutions open for prolonged periods. Keep solutions tightly capped. Keep surgical wound drainage tubes and collection bags patent. Empty and dispose of drainage suction bottles according to employer policy.
Portal of exit (means by which microorganisms leave a site)	Respiratory • Avoid talking, sneezing, or coughing directly over wound or sterile dressing field. • Cover nose and mouth when sneezing or coughing. • Wear mask if suffering respiratory tract infection. Urine, feces, emesis, and blood • Wear clean gloves when handling blood and body fluids. • Wear gowns and eyewear if there is a chance of splashing fluids. • Handle all laboratory specimens as if infectious.
Transmission (means of spread)	Reduce microorganism spread: • Perform hand hygiene. • Use personal set of care items for each patient. • Avoid shaking bed linen or clothes; dust with damp cloth. • Avoid contact of soiled item with uniform. • Discard any item that touches the floor. • Follow routine practices or additional precautions as indicated (e.g., transmission-based precautions).
Portal of entry (site through which microorganisms enter a host)	Skin and mucosa • Maintain skin and mucous membrane integrity; lubricate skin, offer frequent hygiene, turn and position. • Cover wounds as needed. • Clean wound sites thoroughly. • Dispose of used needles in puncture-proof container. Urinary • Keep all drainage systems closed and intact, maintaining downward flow.
Host (patient)	Reduce susceptibility to infection. Provide adequate nutrition. Ensure adequate rest. Promote body defenses against infection. Provide immunizations.

- Medical asepsis, or clean technique, includes procedures that reduce the number of organisms and prevent their transfer.
- Principles of hand hygiene, barrier techniques, and routine environmental cleaning are examples of medical asepsis. These principles are common in the health care and home environment (e.g., washing hands before preparing food).

PERSON-CENTRED CARE

- Nurses are responsible for educating patients and their families about infection control, including information concerning signs and symptoms of infection, modes of transmission, methods of prevention, knowledge of the infectious process, disease transmission, and critical thinking skills associated with use of aseptic techniques and barrier protection.
- Some infections require transmission-based precautions, leading to isolation of the patient. This may result in loneliness or changes in self-concept or body image (Gammon & Hunt, 2018).
- Know the cultural views and preferences of your patients. Some may choose to rely on alternative health care practices (Abrahamson, Hass, Morgan, et al., 2016)
- When a patient from another culture requires transmission-based precautions that include isolation, use caution to be sure that the patient and caregiver understand the therapeutic purpose (Gammon & Hunt, 2018). For example, the isolation of a loved one may be considered disrespectful and uncaring behaviour in collectivistic cultures.

EVIDENCE-INFORMED PRACTICE

- Bundled interventions such as ongoing education, reminders (e.g., posters), administrative support, wall-mounted alcohol dispensers, and pocket-size bottles improve hand hygiene practices (PHO-PIDAC, 2014).
- Handwashing with plain soap sometimes results in paradoxical increases in bacterial counts on the skin (WHO, 2009, 2016). A systematic review supports the WHO-5 Moments for Hand Hygiene, and compliance with hand hygiene practices among health care providers is increased through goal setting, incentives, and accountability (Farhoudi et al., 2016; PHO-PIDAC, 2014).
- Alcohol-based products are more effective for standard handwashing or hand antisepsis than soap or antiseptic soaps (WHO,

2009). Moreover, brisk alcohol-based rinses or gels containing emollients cause substantially less skin irritation and dryness than plain or antimicrobial soaps (PHO-PIDAC, 2014; Haas, 2015).
- Soap and water are still necessary for hand hygiene if hands are visibly soiled or when caring for patients infected with *Clostridium difficile* (IPAC, 2017).

SAFETY GUIDELINES

- Hand hygiene with an appropriate alcohol-based hand antiseptic or soap and water is an essential part of patient care and infection prevention and is fundamental to patient safety (PHO-PIDAC, 2014).
- Always know a patient's susceptibility to infection. Age, nutritional status, stress, disease processes, and forms of medical therapy can place patients at risk.
- Recognize the elements of the chain of infection and initiate measures to prevent its onset and spread.
- Health care workers should not wear artificial nails or nail enhancements because of bacterial buildup (Alberta Health Services, 2017; IPAC, 2017).
- Fingernails should not be longer than 0.625 cm (1/4 inch) in length, and recent evidence suggests that nail polish should not be worn (Cimon & Featherstone, 2017).
- Consistently incorporate the basic principles of medical asepsis into patient care.
- Ensure that patients, caregivers, and health care workers follow "cough hygiene practices" and cover the mouth and nose with your arm when coughing or sneezing, use tissues to contain respiratory secretions, dispose of tissues in the waste receptacle, and wash their hands (British Columbia Centre for Disease Control, 2018).
- Use clean gloves when you anticipate contact with body fluids, nonintact skin, or mucous membranes when there is a risk of drainage.
- Use barrier protection (e.g., gown, mask, and eye protection) when there is a splash risk.
- Protect other health care workers from exposure to infectious agents through proper use and disposal of equipment.
- Be aware of body sites where HAIs are most likely to develop (e.g., urinary or respiratory tract). This enables you to direct preventive measures.

✦ SKILL 5.1   Hand Hygiene

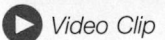 ▶ *Video Clip*   **NSO**   *Nursing Skills Online Infection Control Module 2 / Lessons 1 and 2*

The most important and basic technique in preventing and controlling transmission of infection is hand hygiene. *Hand hygiene* is a general term that applies to handwashing, antiseptic hand wash, antiseptic hand rub, or surgical hand antisepsis. *Handwashing* refers to washing hands with plain soap and water. An *antiseptic hand wash* is defined as washing hands with water and soap or other detergents containing an antiseptic agent. An *antiseptic hand rub* means applying an antiseptic hand rub product to all surfaces of the hands to reduce the number of microorganisms present. *Surgical hand antisepsis* is the use of an antiseptic hand wash or antiseptic hand rub before surgery by surgical personnel to eliminate transient and reduce resident hand flora (see Chapter 38, Skill 38.1).

The decision to perform hand hygiene depends on four factors: (1) the intensity or degree of contact with patients or contaminated

objects, (2) the amount of contamination that may occur with the contact, (3) the patient or health care worker's susceptibility to infection, and (4) the procedure or activity to be performed (Haas, 2015). It is a critical responsibility for all health care workers to follow these guidelines for hand hygiene (IPAC, 2017):

- Wash hands with either plain soap and water or an antibacterial soap and water when they are visibly dirty or soiled with blood or other body fluids, before eating, and after using the toilet.
- Wash hands if exposed to spore-forming organisms such as *Clostridium difficile* (IPAC, 2017).
- If hands are not visibly soiled, use an alcohol-based hand rub for routinely decontaminating hands in the following clinical situations:

- Before and after having direct contact with patients
- Before applying sterile gloves and inserting an invasive device such as in-dwelling urinary catheters and intravenous peripheral vascular catheters
- After contact with body fluids or excretions, mucous membranes, and nonintact skin
- After contact with wound dressings (if hands are not visibly soiled)
- When moving from a contaminated body site to a clean body site during patient care
- After contact with inanimate objects (e.g., medical equipment) in the immediate vicinity of a patient
- After removing gloves

Delegation and Collaboration

The skill of hand hygiene is performed by all caregivers. Hand hygiene is not optional.

Equipment

- Antiseptic hand rub
  - Alcohol-based waterless antiseptic containing emollients
- Handwashing
  - Easy-to-reach sink with warm running water
  - Antimicrobial or regular soap
  - Paper towels or air dryer
  - Disposable nail cleaner (optional)

STEP	RATIONALE

ASSESSMENT

1. Inspect surface of hands for breaks or cuts in skin or cuticles. Cover any skin lesions with a dressing before providing care. If lesions are too large to cover, you may be restricted from direct patient care.

Open cuts or wounds can harbour high concentrations of microorganisms. Employer policy may prevent nurses from caring for high-risk patients if open lesions are present on hands (WHO, 2009).

2. Inspect hands for visible soiling.

Visible soiling requires handwashing with soap and water.

3. Inspect condition of nails. Natural tips should be no longer than 0.625 cm (¼ inch) long. Be sure that fingernails are short, filed, and smooth.

Subungual areas of hand harbour high concentrations of bacteria. Long nails and chipped or old polish increase the number of bacteria residing on hands (IPAC, 2017). Artificial nail applications increase microbial load on hands (Alberta Health Services, 2017).

NURSING DIAGNOSES

This skill is required for all patients with a variety of nursing diagnoses.
Related factors are individualized on the basis of patient's condition or needs.

PLANNING

1. Expected outcomes following completion of procedure:
   - Hands and areas under fingernails are clean and free of debris.

Transient bacteria have been removed.

IMPLEMENTATION

1. Push wristwatch and long uniform sleeves above wrists. Avoid wearing rings. If worn, remove during hand hygiene.

Provides complete access to fingers, hands, and wrists. The skin underneath rings carries higher bacterial count; bacteria include Gram-negative bacilli, enterobacteria, and *Staphylococcus aureus* (Cimon & Featherstone, 2017).

2. **Antiseptic hand rub**
   a. According to manufacturer directions, dispense ample amount of product into palm of one hand (see illustration).

   Use enough product to cover hands thoroughly.

   b. Rub hands together, covering all surfaces of hands and fingers with antiseptic (see illustration).

   Provides enough time for product to work.

   c. Rub hands together until alcohol is dry. Allow hands to dry completely before applying gloves.

   Ensures complete antimicrobial action.

3. **Handwashing using regular or antimicrobial soap:**
   a. Stand in front of sink, keeping hands and uniform away from sink surface. (If hands touch sink during handwashing, repeat sequence.)

   Inside of sink is contaminated area. Reaching over sink increases risk of touching edge, which is contaminated.

STEP	RATIONALE

IMPLEMENTATION

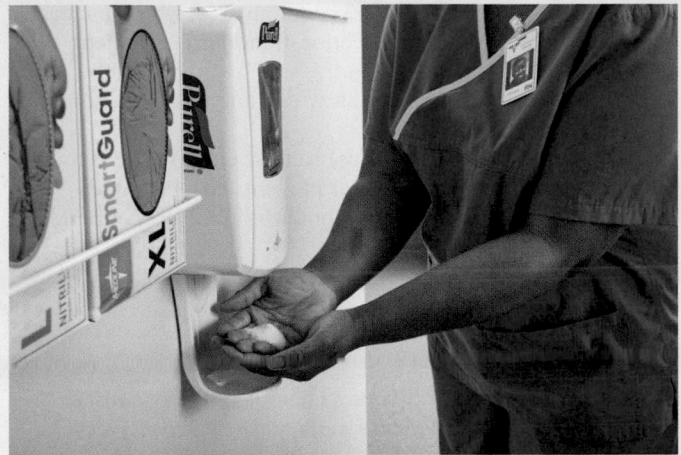

STEP 2a Apply waterless antiseptic to hands.

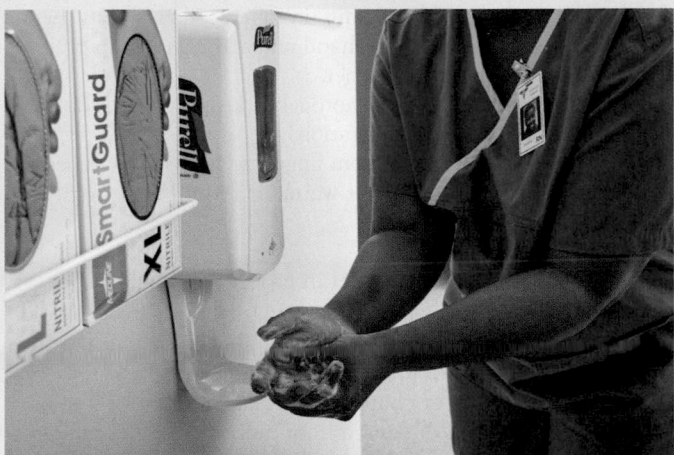

STEP 2b Rub hands thoroughly.

b. Turn on water. Turn on faucet (see illustration) or push knee pedals laterally or press pedals with foot to regulate flow and temperature.

Knee pads within operating room and treatment areas are preferred, to prevent hand contact with faucet. Faucet handles are likely to be contaminated with organic debris and microorganisms and should be manipulated using paper towel (IPAC, 2017).

c. Avoid splashing water against uniform.

Microorganisms travel and grow in moisture.

d. Regulate flow of water so temperature is warm.

Warm water removes less of protective oils on hands than hot water.

e. Wet hands and wrists thoroughly under running water. Keep hands and forearms lower than elbows during washing.

Hands are the most contaminated parts to wash. Water flows from least to most contaminated area, rinsing microorganisms into sink.

f. Apply 3 to 5 mL of antiseptic soap and rub hands together (see illustration).

Ensure that all surfaces of hands and fingers are cleaned.

g. Perform hand hygiene using plenty of lather and friction for at least 15 seconds. Interlace fingers and rub palms and back of hands with circular motion at least 5 times each. Keep fingertips down to facilitate removal of microorganisms.

Soap cleans by emulsifying fat and oil and lowering surface tension. Friction and rubbing mechanically loosen and remove dirt and transient bacteria. Interlacing fingers and thumbs ensures that all surfaces are cleaned. Adequate time is needed to expose skin surfaces to antimicrobial agent.

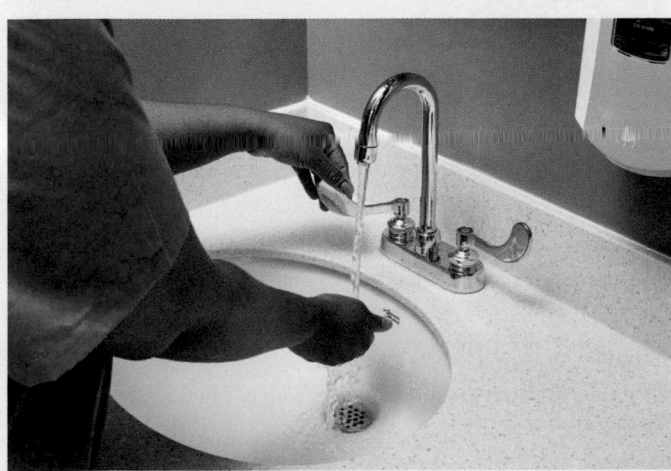

STEP 3b Turn on water.

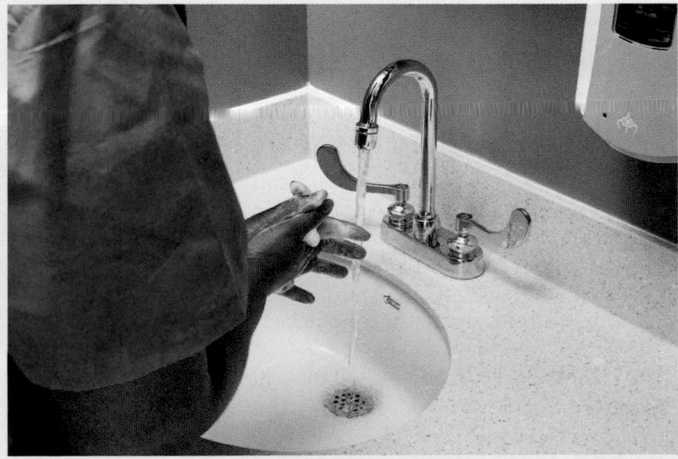

STEP 3f Lather hands thoroughly.

STEP	RATIONALE

IMPLEMENTATION

h. Areas underlying fingernails are often soiled. Clean them with fingernails of other hand and additional soap or with disposable nail cleaner.

i. Rinse hands and wrists thoroughly, keeping hands down and elbows up (see illustration).

j. Dry hands thoroughly from fingers to wrists with paper towel, single-use cloth, or warm air dryer.

k. If used, discard paper towel in proper receptacle.

l. To turn off hand faucet, use clean, dry paper towel; avoid touching handles with hands (see illustration). Turn off water with foot or knee pedals (if applicable).

m. If hands are dry or chapped, use small amount of lotion or barrier cream dispensed from individual-use container.

Area under nails can be highly contaminated, which increases risk for transmission of infection from nurse to patient.

Rinsing mechanically washes away dirt and microorganisms.

Drying from cleanest (fingertips) to least clean (wrist) avoids contamination. Drying hands prevents chapping and roughened skin. Do not tear or cut skin under or around nail.

Prevents transfer of microorganisms.

Wet towel and hands allow transfer of pathogens from faucet by capillary action.

Helps to minimize skin dryness. There is risk of organism growth in lotion; therefore, only apply after patient care activities are complete.

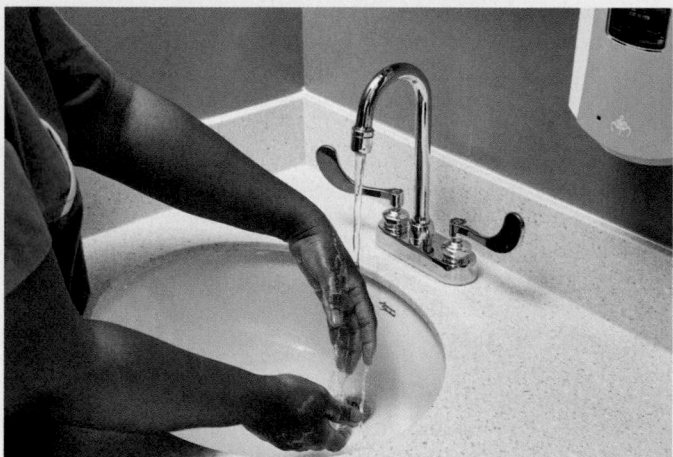

STEP 3i Rinse hands.

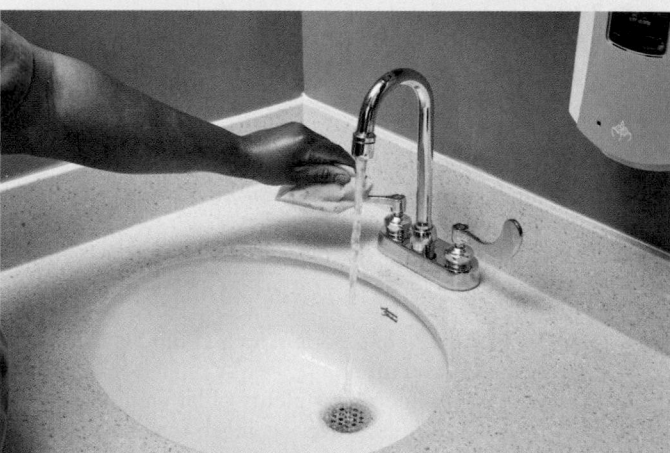

STEP 3l Turn off faucet.

EVALUATION

1. Inspect surface of hands for obvious signs of dirt or other contaminants.

2. Inspect hands for dermatitis or cracked skin.

3. **Use Teach-Back:** "Can you tell me when you or your caregiver would wash your hands, and the different ways you can wash your hands?" Develop a revised teaching plan if patient or caregiver is not able to teach back correctly.

Determines if hand hygiene is adequate.

Breaks in skin integrity increase risk for transmission of microorganisms.

Determines patient's and caregiver's level of understanding of instructional topic.

STEP	RATIONALE

Unexpected Outcomes

1. Hands or areas under fingernails remain soiled.
2. Repeated use of soaps or antiseptics causes dermatitis or cracked skin.

Related Interventions

- Repeat handwashing with soap and water.
- Rinse and dry hands thoroughly after using soap and water; avoid excessive amounts of soap or antiseptic; try various products.
- Use approved hand lotions or barrier creams. Small individual-use containers are preferred because large containers have been found to harbour pathogens.

Special Considerations

Teaching

- Instruct patient and caregiver in proper techniques and situations for hand hygiene.
- When patients are educated about the risks for infections, they can play an important role in improving hand hygiene adherence in health care settings by reminding visitors and health care workers to perform hand hygiene.

Gerontological

- The impact of infections is greater in older persons. Hand hygiene by staff attending older persons is of utmost importance and should be an ongoing continuing-education requirement.

Care in the Community

- Evaluate patient and caregiver to determine their understanding of the transmission of microorganisms and their ability and motivation to perform hand hygiene correctly.
- Evaluate the hand hygiene facilities in the home to determine the possibility of contamination, proximity of the facilities to the patient, and ability to maintain supplies and equipment.

✦ SKILL 5.2 **Caring for Patients Under Transmission-Based Precautions**

 Video Clip

When a patient has a known or suspected source of colonization or infection, health care workers follow specific infection prevention and control practices to reduce the risk of cross-contamination to other patients. Certain procedures performed at a patient's bedside require the application of personal protective equipment (PPE) such as a mask, cap, eyewear, gown, or gloves. Routine practices require the nurse to wear clean gloves before coming in contact with mucous membranes, nonintact skin, blood, body fluids, or other infectious material. Clean gloves are worn routinely when performing a variety of procedures (e.g., nasogastric tube insertion). Masks are worn when there is the risk of splash during a procedure or when certain sterile procedures such as changing a central line dressing are performed. Protective eyewear and masks become important when there is a risk for splash of blood or other body fluids to the eyes or mouth.

Assess the need for PPE for each task you plan and for all patients, regardless of their diagnoses. Because of increased attention to the prevention of bloodborne pathogens and tuberculosis (TB) (Box 5.1), the Public Health Agency of Canada (PHAC, 2017) has stressed the importance of barrier protection. The PHAC (2017) has published guidelines for infection control and prevention, including the use of PPE.

Routine practices are for the care of all patients, regardless of risk or presumed infection status (Box 5.2). Routine practices are the primary strategies for prevention of infection transmission and apply to all patient interaction in all health care and community settings.

Additional precautions (Table 5.2) include precautions designed for care of patients who are known or suspected to be infected, or colonized, with microorganisms transmitted by the contact, droplet, or airborne route (PHO-PIDAC, 2014) or by contact

---

BOX 5.1

Special Tuberculosis Precautions

The Public Health Agency of Canada (PHAC) published guidelines for preventing tuberculosis (TB) transmission in health care facilities. While the overall number of cases of TB continues to decline in Canada, there are notable exceptions where there is a resurgence of TB, including among Indigenous and foreign-born individuals (PHAC, 2012, 2018).

- Current PHAC (2014) guidelines for preventing and controlling TB focus on early detection of infection, preventing close contact with patients with active TB disease, and applying effective infection control measures in health care settings. Suspect TB in any patient with respiratory symptoms lasting longer than 3 weeks accompanied by other suspicious symptoms such as unexplained weight loss, night sweats, fever, and a productive cough often streaked with blood.
- Consider the potential for infectious pulmonary or laryngeal TB from documented positive acid-fast bacilli (AFB) smear or culture, cavitation on chest X-ray film, or history of recent TB exposure.
- Transmission-based precautions for patients with suspected or confirmed TB include placing the patient on airborne precautions in a single-patient negative-pressure room.
- Health care workers who care for patients with suspected or confirmed TB must wear special respirators (e.g., N95 or P100) (British Columbia Centre for Disease Control [BCCDC], 2015). These respirators are high-efficiency particulate masks that have the ability to filter particles at a 95% or better efficiency (BCCDC, 2015; PHAC, 2014).
- The PHAC (2014) recommends that diagnosis of active TB be made with chest radiography and microbiological testing, including sputum smear microscopy, mycobacterial culture, phenotypic drug sensitivity testing, and nucleic acid amplification testing. The use of blood testing may be appropriate in specific circumstances.
- Health Canada (2016) has developed a monitoring and performance framework for TB programs for Indigenous people to guide continuous quality improvement and assist with decreasing the incidence of TB.

BOX 5.2

Provincial Infectious Diseases Advisory Committee (PIDAC) Isolation Guidelines

Routine Practices for Use With All Patients

- Perform hand hygiene using alcohol-based hand rub or soap and water: before and after patient contact; before and after providing direct care; before handling food; before donning gloves and personal protective equipment (PPE) and after removing PPE; when contact with secretions, excretions, blood, or body fluid may occur; after personal body functions; and after contact with items in the patient environment.
- Use a mask and eye protection or face shield based on risk assessment.
- Wear a long-sleeved gown if contamination of skin or clothing is anticipated.
- Wear gloves if there is a risk of contact with blood, body fluids, non-intact skin or mucous membranes, or contaminated surfaces or objects. Glove use is not a substitute for hand hygiene.
- All equipment that is being used by more than one patient must be cleaned between patients.
- Handle soiled linen and waste appropriately to prevent personal contamination and transfer to other patients.
- A private room is unnecessary unless the patient's hygiene is unacceptable (e.g., uncontained secretions, excretions, or wound drainage). Perform hand hygiene on exiting the room.
- Never recap used needles. Discard all contaminated sharp instruments and needles in a puncture-resistant sharps container. Where possible, use safety-engineered medical devices.

Modified from Ontario Agency for Health Protection and Promotion (Public Health Ontario [PHO], Provincial Infectious Diseases Advisory Committee [PIDAC]). (2012). *Routine practices and additional precautions in all health care settings* (3rd ed., p. 63 [Appendix E]). Retrieved from https://www.publichealthontario.ca/en/eRepository/RPAP_All_HealthCare_Settings_Eng2012.pdf.

with contaminated surfaces (see Table 5.2). The three types of transmission-based precautions—airborne, droplet, and contact—may be combined for diseases that have multiple routes of transmission (e.g., chickenpox). Whether used singly or in combination, use these precautions in addition to routine practices.

Delegation and Collaboration

The skill of caring for patients on transmission-based precautions can be delegated to an unregulated care provider (UCP). However, the nurse must assess the patient's status and transmission-based precaution indications. The nurse instructs the UCP about:

- Reason patient is on transmission-based precautions.
- Precautions for bringing equipment into the patient's room.
- Special precautions regarding individual patient needs such as transportation to diagnostic tests.

Equipment

- PPE determined by type of transmission-based precautions required: clean gloves, mask, eyewear or goggles, face shield, and gown (gowns may be disposable or reusable, depending on employer policy)
- Other patient care equipment (as appropriate) (e.g., hygiene items, medications, dressing supplies, sharps container, disposable blood pressure [BP] cuff)
- Soiled linen bag and trash receptacle
- Sign for door indicating type of transmission-based precaution and for visitors to come to the nurses' station before entering room (signs can be text, colour-coded, or both)
- TB transmission-based precautions
  - Room with negative airflow
  - N95 or P100 respirator

TABLE 5.2

Provincial Infectious Diseases Advisory Committee (PIDAC): Routine Practices and Additional Precautions in All Health Care Settings for Use With Specific Types of Patients

Transmission-Based Precaution	Indication for Use	Barrier Protection
Contact Precautions	When contamination of the environment or intact skin is of consideration, such as: • Contamination of the patient environment • Infectious agents of very low infective dose (e.g., norovirus, rotavirus) • Patients who are infected or colonized with epidemiologically important microorganisms that may be transmitted by contact with intact skin or with contaminated environmental surfaces (e.g., MRSA, VRE, *C. difficile*)	Private-room or cohort patients with dedicated sink and toilet (see employer policy), gloves, gowns. Patients may leave their room for procedures or therapy if infectious material is contained or covered and are placed in a clean gown and hands cleaned.
Droplet Precautions (droplet within 1 metre [3 feet] of patient)	When droplets carrying an infectious agent exit the respiratory tract of a person, such as: • Respiratory tract viruses (e.g., adenovirus, influenza and parainfluenza viruses, rhinovirus, human metapneumovirus, respiratory syncytial virus [RSV]) • Rubella, mumps, and Bordetella pertussis	Private room with a dedicated toilet and patient sink, and door may remain open or there may be cohort patients. Mask or respirator (refer to employer policy).
Airborne Precautions	When airborne particles remain suspended in the air, travel on air currents, and are then inhaled by others, such as: • Microorganisms transmitted by the airborne route (e.g., *Mycobacterium tuberculosis* [TB], varicella virus [chickenpox virus], and measles virus)	Private room with own toileting facilities. Room with negative-pressure ventilation, with room air exhausted outside through HEPA filter. Door must remain closed; monitor negative pressure daily while in use. N95 respiratory; patient to wear mask during transport.

Modified from Ontario Agency for Health Protection and Promotion (Public Health Ontario [PHO]), Provincial Infectious Diseases Advisory Committee (PIDAC). (2012). *Routine practices and additional precautions in all health care settings* (3rd ed., pp. 31–38). Retrieved from https://www.publichealthontario.ca/en/eRepository/RPAP_All_HealthCare_Settings_Eng2012.pdf.

STEP	RATIONALE

ASSESSMENT

1. Assess patient's medical history for possible indications for transmission-based precautions (e.g., risk factors for TB, major draining wound, or purulent productive cough). Review specific transmission-based precautions system, including appropriate barriers to apply for each type (e.g., airborne, contact, droplet) (see Table 5.2).

Mode of transmission for infectious microorganism determines type and degree of precautions followed. Ensures adequate protection.

2. Review laboratory test results (e.g., wound culture, acid-fast bacillus [AFB] smears, changes in white blood cell [WBC] count).

Reveals type of microorganism for which patient is being isolated, body fluid in which it was identified, and whether patient is immunosuppressed.

3. Review employer policy for transmission-based precautions necessary for patient circumstance and consider types of care measures that you will perform while in patient's room (e.g., medication administration or dressing change).

Allows you to organize care items for procedures and time spent in patient's room.

4. Review nursing care plan notes or confer with colleagues regarding patient's emotional state and reaction or adjustment to transmission-based precautions. Also assess patient's understanding of purpose of transmission-based precautions.

Provides opportunity to plan for patient's need for emotional support and teaching.

5. Assess whether patient has known latex allergy. If allergy is present, refer to employer policy and resources available to provide full latex-free care.

Protects patient from serious allergic response.

NURSING DIAGNOSES

- Insufficient knowledge regarding purpose of transmission-based precautions
- Reduced social interaction
- Inadequate protection
- Potential for infection

Related factors/Risk factors are individualized on the basis of patient's condition or needs.

PLANNING

1. Expected outcomes following completion of procedure:
- Patient asks for information about disease transmission.

Active interaction reveals patient's willingness and ability to communicate and be taught and understand information.

- Patient explains purpose of transmission-based precautions.

Instruction about precautions improves patient's ability to cooperate in care.

IMPLEMENTATION

1. Perform hand hygiene (see Skill 5.1).

Reduces transmission of microorganisms.

2. Prepare all equipment to be taken into patient's room. In many cases dedicated equipment such as stethoscopes, BP equipment, and thermometers should remain in room until patient is discharged. If patient is infected or colonized with resistant organism (e.g., vancomycin-resistant enterococcus, methicillin-resistant *Staphylococcus aureus* [MRSA]), equipment remains in room and is thoroughly disinfected before removal (see employer policy).

Prevents you from making more than one trip into room. PHO-PIDAC (2012) recommends use of dedicated noncritical patient care equipment.

3. Prepare for entrance into patient room according to appropriate transmission-based precautions. Ideally, before applying PPE, step into patient's room and stay by door. Introduce yourself and explain care that you are providing. If this is not possible, apply PPE outside of the room.

Proper preparation ensures protection from microorganism exposure. Allows patient to see you without PPE and without exposing yourself to risk of infection transmission.

a. Apply gown, being sure that it covers all outer garments. Pull sleeves down to wrist. Tie securely at neck and waist (see illustration).

Prevents transmission of infection; protects you when patient has excessive drainage or discharges.

STEP	RATIONALE

IMPLEMENTATION

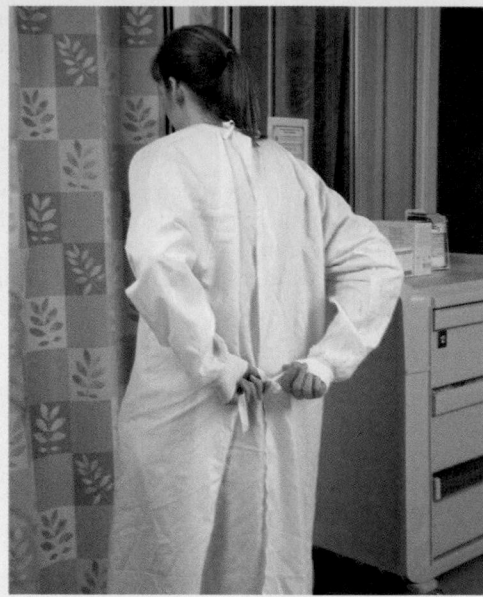

STEP 3a Tie isolation gown at waist.

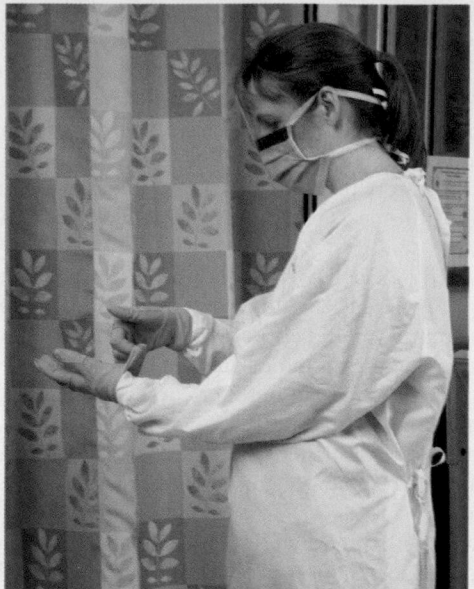

STEP 3d Apply gloves over gown sleeves.

b. Apply either surgical mask or fitted respirator around mouth and nose (type and fit-testing depend on type of transmission-based precaution and employer policy). You must have a medical evaluation and be fit-tested before using a respirator.	Prevents exposure to airborne microorganisms or to microorganisms from splashing of fluids.
c. If needed, apply eyewear or goggles snugly around face and eyes. If you wear prescription glasses, side shields may be used.	Protects you from exposure to microorganisms that may occur during splashing of fluids.
d. Apply clean gloves. (**NOTE:** Wear unpowdered, latex-free gloves if you, patient, or another health care worker has latex allergy.) Bring glove cuffs over edge of gown sleeves (see illustration).	Reduces transmission of microorganisms.
4. Enter patient's room. Arrange supplies and equipment. (**NOTE:** If equipment will be reused, place on clean paper towel.)	Prevents extra trips entering and leaving room. Minimizes contamination of care items.
5. Explain purpose of transmission-based precautions for patient and caregiver to take. Offer opportunity to ask questions. If patient is on TB precautions, instruct to cover mouth with tissue when coughing and to wear disposable surgical mask when leaving room.	Improves patient's and caregiver's ability to participate in care and minimizes anxiety. Identifies opportunity for planning social interaction and diversional activities. Reduces TB microorganism transmission.
6. Assess vital signs (see Chapter 7).	
a. If patient is infected or colonized with resistant organism (e.g., vancomycin-resistant enterococci [VRE], MRSA), equipment remains in room, including stethoscope and BP cuff (PHO-PIDAC, 2012).	Decreases risk of infection being transmitted to another patient.
b. If stethoscope is to be reused, clean earpieces and diaphragm or bell with 70% alcohol or employer-approved germicide. Set aside on clean surface.	Systematic disinfection of stethoscopes with alcohol or approved germicide minimizes chance of spreading infectious agents between patients (Breen, 2017).
c. Use individual or disposable thermometers and BP cuffs when available.	Prevents cross-contamination.

Clinical Decision Point *If disposable thermometer indicates a fever, assess for other signs and symptoms. Confirm fever using an alternative thermometer. Do not use electronic thermometer if patient has suspected or confirmed Clostridium difficile (Balsells et al., 2016).*

STEP	RATIONALE

IMPLEMENTATION

7. Administer medications (see Chapters 20, 21, and 22).

   a. Give oral medication in wrapper or cup.

   b. Dispose of wrapper or cup in plastic-lined receptacle.

   c. Wear gloves when administering an injection.

   d. Discard needleless syringe or safety-sheathed needle into designated sharps container.

8. Administer hygiene, encouraging patient to ask any questions or express concerns about transmission-based precautions. Provide informal teaching at this time.

   a. Avoid allowing isolation gown to become wet; carry washbasin outward away from gown; avoid leaning against wet tabletop.

Handle and discard supplies to minimize transfer of microorganisms.

Reduces risk of exposure to blood.

Needleless devices should be used to reduce risk of needle-sticks and sharps injuries to health care workers.

Hygiene practices further minimize transfer of microorganisms. Quality time should be spent with patient when in room.

Moisture allows organisms to travel through gown to uniform.

Clinical Decision Point *When there is a risk for excess soiling, wear a gown impervious to moisture.*

   b. Help patient remove own gown; discard in leak-proof linen bag.

   c. Remove linen from bed; avoid contact with isolation gown. Place in leak-proof linen bag.

   d. Provide clean bed linen.

   e. Change gloves and perform hand hygiene if gloves become excessively soiled and further care is necessary. Reglove.

9. Collect specimens (see Chapter 9).

   a. Place specimen container on clean paper towel in patient's bathroom and follow procedure for collecting specimen of body fluids.

   b. Follow employer procedure for collecting specimen of body fluids (see Chapter 9).

   c. Transfer specimen to container without soiling outside of container. Place container in plastic bag and place label on outside of bag or per employer policy. Label specimen in front of patient (PHO, 2017). Perform hand hygiene and don gloves if additional procedures are needed.

   d. Check label on specimen for accuracy. Send to laboratory (warning labels are often used, depending on employer policy). Label containers of blood or body fluids with biohazard sticker (see illustration).

Reduces transfer of microorganisms.

Handle linen soiled by patient's body fluids to prevent contact with clean items.

Container will be taken out of patient's room; prevents contamination of outer surface.

Specimens of blood and body fluids are placed in well-constructed containers with secure lids to prevent leaks during transport. Proper labeling prevents diagnostic error.

Ensures that health care providers who transport or handle containers are aware of infectious contents.

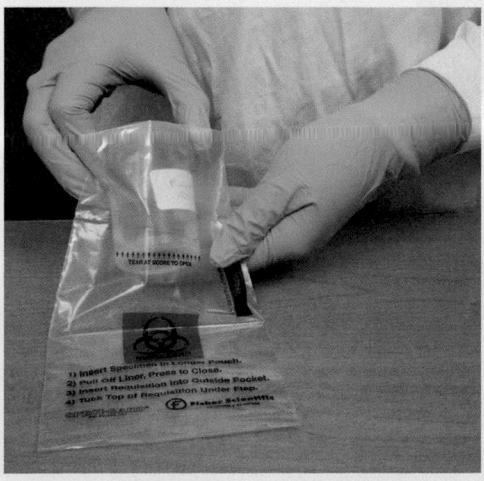

STEP 9d Place specimen container in biohazard bag.

STEP	RATIONALE

IMPLEMENTATION

10. Dispose of linen, trash, and disposable items.
   a. Use sturdy moisture-impervious bags to contain soiled articles. Use double bag if necessary for heavily soiled linen or heavy wet trash.

Linen or refuse should be contained totally to prevent exposure of personnel to infectious material.

   b. Tie bags securely at top in knot (see illustration).

11. Remove all reusable pieces of equipment. Clean and disinfect any contaminated surfaces according to employer policy.

All items must be properly cleaned, disinfected, or sterilized for reuse.

12. Resupply room as needed. Have staff colleague hand new supplies to you.

Limiting trips of personnel into and out of room reduces your and patient's exposure to microorganisms.

13. Leave patient room. Order of removal of PPE depends on what you wear in room. This sequence describes steps to take if all barriers were worn. PPE worn in room must be removed before leaving room.

Order of removal minimizes exposure to any infectious material on barriers.

   a. Remove gloves. Remove one glove by grasping cuff and pulling glove inside out over hand. Hold removed glove in gloved hand (see illustration). Slide fingers of ungloved hand under remaining glove at wrist. Peel glove off over first glove. Discard gloves in proper container.

Technique prevents contact with outer contaminated surface of glove.

Change gloves between exposures to body sites and patient equipment. Inadequate glove changes and hand hygiene can lead to contamination, increasing the risk of health care–associated infections (HAIs) (Haas, 2015).

   b. Remove gown: Untie neck strings and then untie back strings of gown. Allow gown to fall from shoulders (see illustration); touch inside of gown only. Remove hands from sleeves without touching outside of gown. Hold gown inside at shoulder seams and fold inside out into bundle; discard in laundry bag. Perform hand hygiene.

Hands do not come in contact with soiled front of gown.

   c. Remove eyewear, face shield, or goggles. Handle by headband or earpieces. Discard in proper container.

Outside of goggles is contaminated. Hands have not been soiled.

   d. Remove mask. If mask secures over ears, remove elastic from ears and pull mask away from face. For tie-on mask, untie *bottom* mask string and then top strings, pull mask away from face (see illustration A), and drop into trash receptacle (see illustration B). (Do not touch outer surface of mask.)

Ungloved hands are not contaminated by touching only elastic or mask strings. Prevents top part of mask from falling down over uniform.

Clinical Decision Point *If patient is on TB precautions, place reusable mask in labeled paper bag for storage, being careful not to crush mask (check employer policy for number of times reusable masks can be used).*

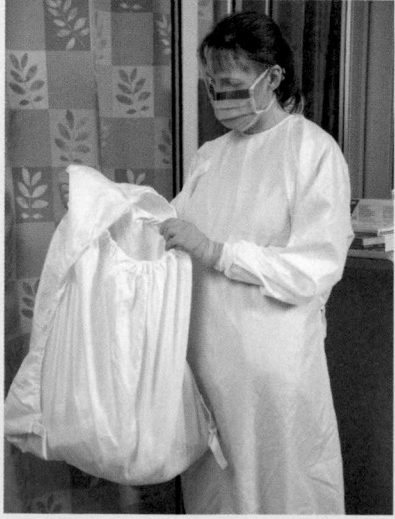

STEP 10b Tie bag securely.

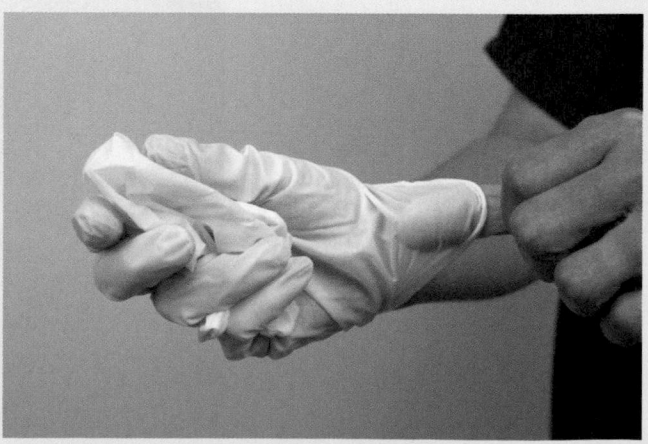

STEP 13a Remove gloves.

STEP	RATIONALE

IMPLEMENTATION

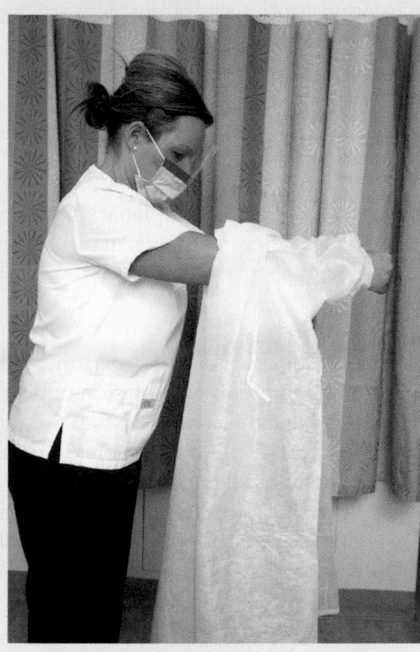

STEP 13b Remove gown by allowing it to fall from shoulders.

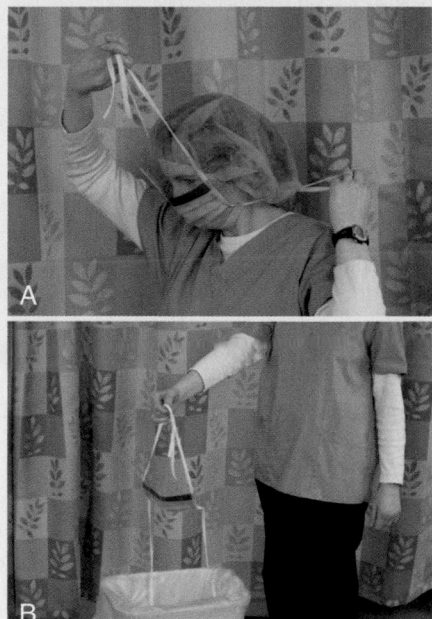

STEP 13d A, Pull mask away from face. **B,** Drop into trash receptacle.

e. Perform hand hygiene.	Reduces transmission of microorganisms.
f. Retrieve wristwatch and stethoscope (unless items must remain in room).	
g. Explain to patient when you plan to return to room. Ask whether patient requires any personal care items. Offer books, magazines, electronic devices.	Diversions can help to minimize boredom and feeling of social isolation.
h. Dispose of all contaminated supplies and equipment in manner that prevents spread of microorganisms to other people (see employer policy). Perform hand hygiene.	
i. Leave room and close door if necessary. Close door if patient is on airborne precautions or in negative-airflow room.	Maintains negative-airflow environment and reduces transmission of microorganisms.

EVALUATION

1. Observe patient's and caregiver's use of transmission-based precautions when visiting.	Promptly identifies any improper use of precaution.
2. While in room, ask if patient has had sufficient chance to discuss health problems, course of treatment, or other topics important to them.	Measures patient's perception of adequacy of discussions with caregivers.
3. **Use Teach-Back:** "I want to be sure I explained when these precautions are needed. Can you tell me when you need to use these precautions?" Develop a revised teaching plan if patient or caregiver is not able to teach back correctly.	Determines patient's and caregiver's level of understanding of instructional topic.

STEP	RATIONALE

Unexpected Outcomes

1. Patient avoids social and therapeutic discussions.

2. Patient or health care worker may have an allergy to latex gloves.

Related Interventions

- Confer with caregiver, significant other, or both and determine best approach to reduce patient's sense of loneliness and depression.
- Notify health care provider or employee health and treat sensitivity or allergic reaction appropriately.
- Use latex-free gloves for future care activities.

Communication and Documentation

- Document procedures performed and patient's response to social isolation. Also document any patient or family education performed and reinforced on flow sheet or in nurses' notes in electronic health record (EHR) or chart.
- Document type of transmission-based precautions in use and the microorganisms (if known).

Special Considerations

Teaching

- Teach visitors and caregivers how to follow the recommended transmission-based precautions when visiting a patient.

Pediatric

- Patient isolation is inherent in many transmission-based precautions, and this creates a sense of separation from family and loss of control. A strange environment adds to the confusion that a child feels when experiencing isolation. Preschoolers are unable to understand the cause–effect relationship for being isolated. Older children may be able to understand the cause but still fantasize.
- Children require simple explanations (e.g., "You need to be in this room to help you get better.") Show all barriers to a child.

Actively involve parents in any explanations. Nurses should let child see their faces before applying masks so child does not become frightened.

Gerontological

- Isolation can be a concern for older persons, especially those who have signs and symptoms of confusion or depression. Many times, patients become more confused when they are confronted with a nurse using barrier precautions or when they are left in a room with the door closed. Nurses must assess need for closing door (negative-airflow room) along with safety of patient and additional safety measures that may need to be taken.
- Assess older persons for signs of depression, such as loss of appetite or decrease in verbal communications. If necessary, report to the health care team for appropriate interventions.

Care in the Community

- Although transmission-based precautions followed in the hospital are not directly applicable to care in the community, caregivers should be aware of potential sources of contamination in the home (see Box 5.2) and practice good hand hygiene at all times.

PROCEDURAL GUIDELINE 5.1 *Caring for Patients With Multidrug-Resistant Organisms (MDROs) and Clostridium Difficile*

Multidrug-resistant organisms (MDROs) such as methicillin-resistant *Staphylococcus aureus* (MRSA) and vancomycin-resistant enterococcus (VRE) have become increasingly common as a cause of colonization and health care–associated infections (HAIs). MRSA is a frequently identified pathogen associated with increased mortality. In recent reports, MRSA caused upward of 19% of health care–associated bloodstream infections (Becker & Kahl, 2015). VRE, another MDRO, poses a greater risk to immune-compromised and debilitated patients (Archibald, 2015). *Clostridium difficile* (*C. difficile*) infection is one of the most common and costly HAIs (Ngam et al., 2017). In most instances patient susceptibility to *C. difficile* infection requires prior treatment with antibiotics. Unlike MRSA and VRE, *C. difficile* is more difficult to eliminate from the environment because it is a spore-forming organism, meaning that it can remain on surfaces in its dormant state for long periods of time. No matter which MDRO is involved, the most common means of transmission is by way of a health care worker's hands. To reduce the risk of cross-contamination among patients, transmission-based precautions (contact) should be used in addition to routine practices when caring for these patients.

Delegation and Collaboration

Assessment of a patient's status and type of care required cannot be delegated to an unregulated care provider (UCP). Basic care procedures performed using transmission-based precautions can be delegated to UCP. The nurse instructs the UCP to:

- Clarify personal precautions used under transmission-based precautions (e.g., contact).
- Explain the type of changes in patient status to report to the nurse.

Equipment

- Clean gloves, gown, protective eyewear, surgical mask (based on patient's clinical condition)
- Basic care items (e.g., medication equipment, hygiene items)

Procedural Steps

1. Perform hand hygiene.
2. Prepare all equipment needed in patient's room.
3. Before entering room apply gown, being sure that it covers all outer garments. Pull sleeves down to wrists. Tie securely at neck and waist.

> **PROCEDURAL GUIDELINE 5.1** *Caring for Patients With Multidrug-Resistant Organisms (MDROs) and Clostridium Difficile—cont'd*

4. Apply clean gloves.
5. Explain purpose of contact precautions to patient and caregivers.
6. Provide personal care and treatments.
7. Leave room after telling patient when you will return and asking if they have questions concerning their care.
8. Remove gloves and discard per employer policy.

9. Untie neck and waist ties on gown. Remove gown, allowing it to fall from shoulders. Discard in appropriate receptacle per employer policy.
10. Perform hand hygiene. If patient is being treated for *C. difficile* infection, clean hands with soap and water. Alcohol-based hand rubs are not effective against the spores of *C. difficile*.

CLINICAL DEBRIEF

A 78-year-old man is admitted from the nursing home to an acute care hospital. He is confused and has a fever, and his urinary output is decreased. After greeting the patient, the nurse begins to conduct a physical assessment.

As the nurse turns the patient to check the condition of his skin, she notices moisture on the skin. As she looks more closely, she realizes that the moisture is from an open, oozing 2 × 2–cm lesion on the patient's sacral area.

1. What should the nurse do next?
2. A few hours later the nurse prepares to enter the patient's room. Wearing gloves, she assesses the wound and quickly checks the position and function of the in-dwelling urinary catheter. She performs hand hygiene before leaving the patient's room. Critique the nurse's approach. Did she use correct technique?
3. Two days later the patient is complaining of increased pain at wound sight. On further assessment, the nurse sees that the wound is now 3 × 3 cm; is red; and has thick, yellow drainage. Use SBAR to communicate this finding to the health care team.

◆ REVIEW QUESTIONS

1. Which of the following are true statements in relation to hand hygiene? *(Select all that apply.)*
   1. The percentage of health care workers using hand hygiene has been decreasing over the last few years.
   2. The incidence of health care–associated infections has decreased because of hand hygiene.
   3. There must be a mode of transmission for an infection to occur.
   4. Soap and water must be used when hands are visibly soiled.
   5. Hand hygiene can be antiseptic hand wash, antiseptic hand rub, or handwashing.
2. A nurse is taking care of a patient on airborne precautions for tuberculosis. Which interventions are appropriate for this patient? *(Select all that apply.)*
   1. Place patient in a private room.
   2. Explain why the patient across the hall is not on precautions.
   3. Wear gloves when giving an intramuscular injection.
   4. Educate patient regarding their specific transmission-based precautions.
   5. Wear a surgical mask into the room to take vital signs.
3. The nurse is having a complication of dermatitis related to repeated handwashing. Which interventions could be used to help the nurse with the situation? *(Select all that apply.)*
   1. Use personal hypoallergenic soap instead of soap provided.
   2. Use only approved hand lotions or barrier creams.
   3. Rinse and dry hands thoroughly after every handwashing.
   4. Quickly wash hands when needed to avoid excess damage to skin.
   5. Wear gloves and change them frequently instead of washing hands.

ⓔ *Visit the Evolve site for a complete list of Clinical Debrief and Review Questions answers.*

REFERENCES

Abrahamson, K., Hass, Z., Morgan, K., Fulton, B., & Ramanujam, R. (2016). The relationship between nurse-reported safety culture and the patient experience. *The Journal of Nursing Administration*, 46(12), 662–668. doi:10.1097/NNA .0000000000000423

Alberta Health Services. (2017). *Artificial nails in the healthcare environment: Why we care.* Retrieved from https://www.albertahealthservices.ca/assets/info/hp/hh/ if-hp-hh-artificial-nails-in-healthcare.pdf

Archibald, L. (2015). Enterococci. In P. Grota (Ed.), *APIC text of infection control and epidemiology* (4th ed.). Washington, DC: Association for Professionals in Infection Control and Epidemiology (APIC). Chapter 76.

Balsells, E., Filipescu, T., Kyaw, M., Wiuff, C., Campbell, H., & Nair, H. (2016). Infection prevention and control of *Clostridium difficile*: A global review of guidelines, strategies, and recommendations. *Journal of Global Health*, 6(2), 020410. doi:10.7189/jogh.06.020410

Becker, K., & Kahl, B. (2015). Staphylococci. In P. Grota (Ed.), *APIC text of infection control and epidemiology* (4th ed.). Washington, DC: Association for Professionals in Infection Control and Epidemiology (APIC). Chapter 93.

Breen, A. E. (2017). Stethoscopes: Friend or fomite? *Nursing Management*, 48(12), 9–11. doi:10.1097/01.NUMA.0000526917.85088.eb

British Columbia Centre for Disease Control (BCCDC). (2015). *Tuberculosis manual.* Vancouver: Provincial Health Services Authority. Retrieved from http:// www.bccdc.ca/health-professionals/clinical-resources/communicable-diseas e-control-manual/tuberculosis

British Columbia Centre for Disease Control (BCCDC). (2018). *Hand hygiene.* Vancouver, BC: Provincial Health Services Authority. Retrieved from http:// www.bccdc.ca/health-info/preventing-infection/hand-hygiene

Cimon, K., & Featherstone, R. (2017). *Jewellery and nail polish worn by health care workers and the risk of infection transmission: A review of clinical evidence and guidelines.* Ottawa, ON: Canadian Agency for Drugs and Technologies in Health. Retrieved from https://www.cadth.ca/sites/default/files/pdf/htis/2017/RC0858%20 Jewellery%20and%20Nail%20Polish%20Risk%20Final.pdf

Farhoudi, F., Sanaei Dashti, A., Hoshangi Davani, M., Ghalebi, N., Sajadi, G., & Taghizadeh, R. (2016). Impact of WHO hand hygiene improvement program implementation: A quasi-experimental trial. *BioMed Research International*, 2016, 1–7. doi:10.1155/2016/7026169

Gammon, J., & Hunt, J. (2018). Source isolation and patient wellbeing in healthcare settings. *British Journal of Nursing*, 27(2), 88–91. doi:10.12968/bjon.2018.27 .2.88

Haas, J. (2015). Hand hygiene. In P. Grota (Ed.), *APIC text of infection control and epidemiology* (4th ed.). Washington, DC: Association for Professionals in Infection Control and Epidemiology (APIC). Chapter 27.

Health Canada. (2016). *Health Canada's monitoring and performance framework for tuberculosis programs for First Nations on-reserve*. Ottawa, ON: Author.

Infection Prevention and Control Canada (IPAC). (2017). *IPAC Canada practice recommendations for hand hygiene in health care settings*. Retrieved from https://ipac-canada.org/photos/custom/Members/pdf/17JulHand%20Hygiene%20Practice%20Recommendations_final.pdf

Ngam, C., Schoofs Hundt, A., Haun, N., Carayon, P., Stevens, L., & Safdar, N. (2017). Barriers and facilitators to *Clostridium difficile* infection prevention: A nursing perspective. *American Journal of Infection Control*, 45(12), 1363–1368. doi:10.1016/j.ajic.2017.07.009

Ontario Agency for Health Protection and Promotion (Public Health Ontario [PHO]), Provincial Infectious Diseases Advisory Committee (PIDAC). (2012). *Routine practices and additional precautions in all health care settings* (3rd. ed.). Retrieved from https://www.publichealthontario.ca/en/eRepository/RPAP_All_HealthCare_Settings_Eng2012.pdf

Ontario Agency for Health Protection and Promotion (Public Health Ontario [PHO]), Provincial Infectious Diseases Advisory Committee (PIDAC). (2014). *Best practices for hand hygiene in all health care settings* (4th ed.). Toronto, ON: Queen's Printer for Ontario. Retrieved from http://www.publichealthontario.ca/en/eRepository/2010-12%20BP%20Hand%20Hygiene.pdf

Public Health Agency of Canada (PHAC). (2012). *Hand hygiene practices in health-care settings*. Ottawa, ON: Centre for Communicable Disease and Infection Control. Retrieved from http://publications.gc.ca/collections/collection_2012/aspc-phac/HP40-74-2012-eng.pdf

Public Health Agency of Canada (PHAC). (2014). *Canadian tuberculosis standards* (7th ed.). Ottawa: Author. Retrieved from http://www.phac-aspc.gc.ca/tbpc-latb/pubs/tb-canada-7/assets/pdf/tb-standards-tb-normes-ch15-eng.pdf

Public Health Agency of Canada (PHAC). (2017). *Routine practices and additional precautions for healthcare settings* (Cat. No. HP40-83/2013E-PDF). Retrieved from https://www.canada.ca/en/public-health/services/publications/diseases-conditions/routine-practices-precautions-healthcare-associated-infections.html

Public Health Agency of Canada (PHAC). (2018). *The time is now: Chief Public Health Officer spotlight on eliminating tuberculosis in Canada*. Retrieved from https://www.canada.ca/en/public-health/corporate/publications/chief-public-health-officer-reports-state-public-health-canada/eliminating-tuberculosis.html

Public Health Ontario (PHO). (2017). *Specimen collection, handling and transportation*. Retrieved from https://www.publichealthontario.ca/en/ServicesAndTools/LaboratoryServices/Pages/Specimen-Collection.aspx

Raines, K., & Rosen, K. (2016). The effect of chlorhexidine bathing on rates of nosocomial infections among the critically ill population: An analysis of current clinical research and recommendations for practice. *Dimensions of Critical Care Nursing*, 35(2), 84–91. doi:10.1097/DCC.0000000000000165

Rojas-García, A., Turner, S., Pizzo, E., Hudson, E., Thomas, J., & Raine, R. (2018). Impact and experiences of delayed discharge: A mixed-studies systematic review. *Health Expectations: An International Journal of Public Participation in Health Care and Health Policy*, 21(1), 41–56. http://doi.org/10.1111/hex.12619

Swan, J. T., Ashton, C. M., Bui, L. N., et al. (2016). Effect of chlorhexidine bathing every other day on prevention of hospital-acquired infections in the surgical ICU: A single-center, randomized controlled trial. *Critical Care Medicine*, 44(10), 1822–1832. doi:10.1097/CCM.0000000000001820

World Health Organization (WHO). (2009). *WHO guidelines on hand hygiene care*. Geneva, Switzerland: World Health Organization (WHO) Press.

World Health Organization (WHO). (2016). *Five moments for hand hygiene*. Geneva, Switzerland: World Health Organization (WHO) Press. Retrieved from http://who.int/gpsc/tools/Five_moments/en/

Yallew, W. W., Kumie, A., & Yehuala, F. M. (2017). Risk factors for hospital-acquired infections in teaching hospitals of amhara regional state, Ethiopia: A matched-case control study. *PLoS ONE*, 12(7), e0181145. doi:10.1371/journal.pone.0181145

6 | Sterile Technique

Written by **Angela McConachie, FNP, DNP, and Sandra Redmond, RN, MN**

SKILLS AND PROCEDURES

Skill 6.1 **Applying and Removing Cap, Mask, and Protective Eyewear, p. 86**
Skill 6.2 **Preparing a Sterile Field, p. 90**
Skill 6.3 **Sterile Gloving, p. 96**

OBJECTIVES

Mastery of content in this chapter will enable the nurse to:
- Discuss settings where surgical aseptic techniques are necessary.
- Describe conditions when surgical asepsis is necessary.
- Identify the principles of surgical asepsis.
- Explain the importance of organization and caution when using surgical aseptic techniques.

- Apply and remove a cap, mask, and protective eyewear correctly.
- Identify individuals at risk for a latex allergy.
- Perform the following skills: preparing a sterile field, applying sterile gloves using open-glove method, and applying a sterile drape correctly.

MEDIA RESOURCES

- **evolve** http://evolve.elsevier.com/Canada/Perry/clinicalskills/
- Review Questions
- ▶ Video Clips

- Audio Glossary
- **NSO** Nursing Skills Online
- Clinical Debrief and Review Questions Answers

PURPOSE

Sterile technique and aseptic practices maintain an area that is free from pathogenic organisms, serve to isolate an operative area from the unsterile environment, and maintain a sterile field for surgery and invasive procedures. Proper sterile asepsis minimizes patient exposure to infection-causing agents, therefore reducing the patient's risk for infection. These techniques are common in the operating room, labour and delivery area, and major diagnostic areas, but they are also used at the bedside (e.g., when inserting an intravenous [IV] or urinary catheter).

STANDARDS OF CARE

- Association of Perioperative Registered Nurses (AORN), 2016—*Guidelines for Perioperative Practice* (https://www.aorn.org/guidelines/about-aorn-guidelines)
- Ontario Agency for Health Protection and Promotion Public Health Ontario (PHO), Provincial Infectious Diseases Advisory Committee (PIDAC), 2012—*Routine Practices and Additional Precautions in All Health Care Settings* (3rd edition) (https://www.publichealthontario.ca/en/eRepository/RPAP_All_HealthCare_Settings_Eng2012.pdf)
- Public Health Agency of Canada (PHAC), 2017—*Routine Practices and Additional Precautions for Preventing the Transmission of Infection*

in Healthcare Settings (https://www.canada.ca/en/public-health/services/publications/diseases-conditions/routine-practices-precautions-healthcare-associated-infections/part-b.html#B.IV)

PRINCIPLES FOR PRACTICE

- The majority of sterile technique practices are used in the operating room (OR) or diagnostic procedure areas, including using personal protective equipment (PPE) (e.g., applying a mask, protective eyewear, a gown, and a cap); performing a surgical hand scrub; applying a sterile gown; and applying sterile gloves.
- As with medical asepsis, proper hand hygiene with an appropriate cleaner or antiseptic is required before initiating any sterile procedure.
- Surgical aseptic technique is also used at the bedside in the following situations: during procedures that require intentional puncture of the skin or insertion of devices into an area of the body that is normally sterile (e.g., sterile dressing change) or in a situation in which skin integrity is compromised because of incision or burn (Box 6.1).
- When sterile procedures are carried out in the OR or procedure area, health care providers must follow a series of steps to maintain sterile asepsis: applying a mask, protective eyewear, and cap; performing a surgical hand scrub; and applying sterile gown and gloves.

BOX 6.1

Principles of Surgical Asepsis

1. All items used within a sterile field must be sterile.
2. A sterile barrier that has been permeated by punctures, tears, or moisture must be considered contaminated.
3. Once a sterile package is opened, a 2.5-cm (1-inch) border around the edges is considered unsterile.
4. Tables draped as part of a sterile field are considered sterile only at table level.
5. If there is any question or doubt about the sterility of an item, the item is considered to be unsterile.
6. Sterile contacting sterile equals sterile; sterile contacting unsterile equals unsterile. Movement around and in the sterile field must not compromise or contaminate the field.
7. A sterile object or field out of the range of vision or an object held below a person's waist is contaminated.
8. A sterile object or field becomes contaminated by prolonged exposure to air; stay organized and complete any procedure as soon as possible.

- When sterile procedures such as a sterile dressing change are carried out at the bedside, the health care provider must perform hand hygiene and apply sterile gloves. When the risk of splash is present, other PPE is required.
- When completing a sterile procedure at the bedside, communicate with the patient about which steps are being taken to prevent infection, including which actions the patient should avoid, to keep the field sterile. These actions include avoiding sudden body movements, refraining from touching sterile supplies, and avoiding coughing or talking over sterile area.

PERSON-CENTRED CARE

- Whether performed in a hospital, ambulatory care setting, the person's home, or health care provider's office, invasive procedures such as starting an IV line or inserting a urinary catheter pose a risk for infection. As a nurse it is your responsibility to protect patients from infection by adhering strictly to the principles of surgical asepsis when performing invasive procedures or when helping with such a procedure and to intervene to stop it when a break in sterile technique occurs. Maintaining surgical asepsis is a shared responsibility for those providing care to the patient (Barnes, 2015).
- Take into consideration the patient's cultural background or beliefs when sterile asepsis is required. Individualized person-centred education for patients and families before any aseptic procedure reduces fears and misconceptions about sterile asepsis attire. This also provides an opportunity for patients,

caregivers, and families to ask questions and express their concerns regarding surgical attire.

EVIDENCE-INFORMED PRACTICE

- Recommendations such as person-centred education, insertion of devices only when necessary, using sterile technique, and removing devices that are no longer needed have decreased the number of health care–associated infections (HAIs). It is estimated that 5 to 10% of all hospitalized patients will develop an HAI (PHAC, 2017).
- Prevention of contamination of a sterile work area is an overall goal to reduce HAIs and is a shared interprofessional responsibility. This can be done by minimizing traffic; comprehensive cleaning and disinfecting; changing skin preparation; administering antibiotics; and removing watches, jewellery, and artificial nails (Cimon & Featherstone, 2017; Infection Prevention and Control Canada [IPAC], 2017).
- Use of additional antiseptics such as chlorhexidine reduces bacterial count on the patient's skin (AORN, 2016; Raines & Rosen, 2016)
- Most health care facilities have policies against artificial nails, including extensions or tips, gels and acrylic overlays, and resin wraps (Wood & VanWicklin, 2015). The subungual area (under a fingernail) of the hand and the 'lifting' of the product from the nail bed contain a high concentration of bacteria, more specifically coagulase-negative staphylococci, Gram-negative rods, and fungal growth (Cimon & Featherstone, 2017). These organisms are not removed effectively after hand hygiene.

SAFETY GUIDELINES

- Follow routine practices with all patients (PHAC, 2017).
- Review employer policies before conducting a sterile procedure.
- Assess the potential for splash, transmission of infection, or both before choosing the PPE to be used, such as masks or protective eyewear.
- Nurses use barrier techniques to decrease the transmission of microorganisms from health care personnel and the environment to a patient.
- Remain organized while performing any sterile procedure; keep bedside surfaces free of clutter.
- Remember that hand hygiene is essential before and after initiating any sterile procedure, to reduce HAIs (PHAC, 2017; PIDAC, 2014).
- Apply the principles of surgical asepsis when conducting any sterile procedure.

✦ SKILL 6.1   **Applying and Removing Cap, Mask, and Protective Eyewear**

NSO *Nursing Skills Online Infection Control Module 2 / Lesson 1*

Although masks and caps are usually worn in surgical procedure areas (e.g., the operating room [OR]), certain aseptic procedures performed at a patient's bedside also require the application of additional PPE, such as eyewear, gown, and gloves. For example, it may be employer policy for a nurse to wear a mask during the changing of a central-line dressing or insertion of a peripherally inserted central catheter (PICC). Other policies might require that a nurse wear a mask and a cap to secure hair during dressing changes on a patient with extensive burns or a central line (Infusion Nurses Society [INS], 2016). When there

is a risk of splattering blood or body fluid, there is also the need to apply protective eyewear (PHAC, 2017). This skill summarizes how to apply a mask, cap, and protective eyewear, which are not considered sterile. The additional application of clean or sterile gloves depends on the type of procedure being performed.

Assess a patient's potential for acquiring an infection and the splash risk before deciding whether to apply a mask (e.g., Does the patient have a large open wound? Is the person immunosuppressed? Is there a splash risk from the wound?). If you wear a mask, change

it when it becomes moist or soiled (e.g., splattered with blood). Wear eyewear when there is a risk of body fluids splashing into your eyes.

Delegation and Collaboration

The skill of applying and removing cap, mask, and protective eyewear is required of all caregivers when working in areas in which sterile procedures are performed. However, the procedures performed at a patient's bedside that require cap, mask, gown, or eyewear generally cannot be delegated to an unregulated care provider (UCP). The skill of applying PPE can be delegated to a UCP. The nurse instructs the UCP to:

- Be available to hand off equipment or help with patient positioning during a sterile procedure.

If the procedure is to use sterile technique, the nurse must educate the UCP regarding the sterile field.

Equipment

- Surgical mask (different types are available for people with different skin sensitivities)
- Surgical cap (**NOTE:** Use in OR, or if employer policy requires. Use to secure hair if there is a possibility of contamination of a sterile field.)
- Hairpins, rubber bands, or both
- Protective eyewear (e.g., goggles or glasses with appropriate side shields). *Option:* Clean or sterile gloves (applied after cap, mask, or eyewear are applied). See Chapter 5 and Skill 6.3.

STEP	RATIONALE

ASSESSMENT

1. Review type of sterile procedure to be performed and consult employer policy for use of mask, caps, gown, or protective eyewear.

2. If you or other health care providers have symptoms of a respiratory infection, either avoid participating in procedure or apply a mask.

3. Assess patient's risk for infection (e.g., older person, neonate, or immunocompromised patient).

Not all sterile procedures require mask, cap, gown, or protective eyewear. Ensures that nurse and patient are properly protected.

A greater number of pathogenic microorganisms reside within the respiratory tract when infection is present.

Some patients are at a greater risk for acquiring an infection; thus, use additional protective barriers.

NURSING DIAGNOSES

- Insufficient protection
- Potential for infection

Related factors/Risk factors are individualized on the basis of patient's condition or needs.

PLANNING

1. Expected outcome following completion of procedure:
   - Patient does not develop signs of localized infection (e.g., redness, tenderness, edema, drainage) or systemic infection (e.g., fever, change in white blood cell [WBC] count) 24 hours after procedure.

2. Prepare equipment and inspect packaging for integrity and exposure to sterilization.

Indicates lack of microorganism transfer to patient and sterile field.

Ensures availability of equipment and sterility of supplies before procedure begins.

IMPLEMENTATION

1. Perform hand hygiene (see Chapter 5).

2. *Option:* In cases in which you are performing or assisting with a procedure at a patient's bedside, apply a clean gown if there is a risk of splatter or soiling. Apply the gown with opening to the back. Be sure that it covers all outer garments. Pull sleeves down to wrist. Tie securely at neck and wrist.

3. Apply a cap.
   a. If hair is long, comb back behind ears and secure.
   b. Secure hair in place with pins.

   c. Apply cap over head as you would apply a hairnet. Be sure that all hair fits under edges of cap (see illustration).

Reduces transient microorganisms on skin.

Proper draping prevents transmission of infections when patient has excessive drainage or discharges.

Cap must cover all hair entirely.

Long hair should not fall down or cause cap to slip and expose hair.

Loose hair hanging over sterile field or falling dander contaminates objects on sterile field.

STEP	RATIONALE

IMPLEMENTATION

4. Apply a mask.

  a. Find top edge of mask, which usually has a thin metal strip along edge.

  b. Hold mask by top two strings or loops, keeping top edge above bridge of nose.

  c. Tie two top strings at top of back of head, over cap (if worn), with strings above ears (see illustration). Alternatively place loops over ears.

  d. Tie two lower ties snugly around neck with mask well under chin (see illustration).

  e. Gently pinch upper metal band around bridge of nose.

5. Apply protective eyewear.

  a. Apply protective glasses, goggles, or face shield comfortably over eyes and check that vision is clear (see illustration).

  b. Be sure that face shield fits snugly around forehead and face.

Pliable metal fits snugly against bridge of nose.

Position prevents contact of hands with clean facial part of mask. Mask covers all of nose.

Position of ties at top of head provides tight fit. Strings over ears may cause irritation.

Tying prevents escape of microorganisms through sides of mask as you talk and breathe.

Pinching prevents microorganisms from escaping around nose and eyeglasses from steaming up.

Positioning affects clarity of vision.

Snug fitting ensures that eyes are fully protected.

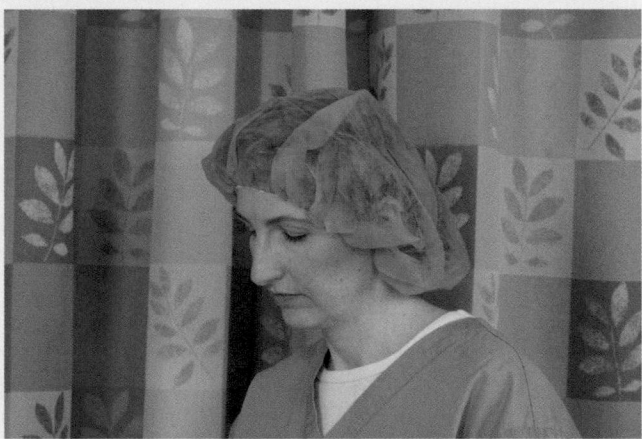

STEP 3c Apply cap over head, covering all hair.

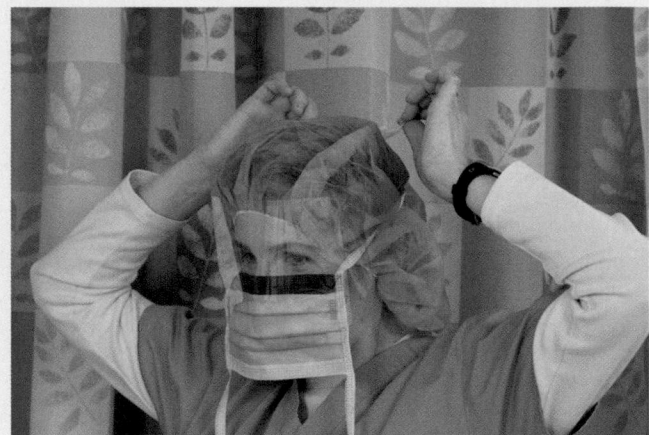

STEP 4c Tie top strings of mask.

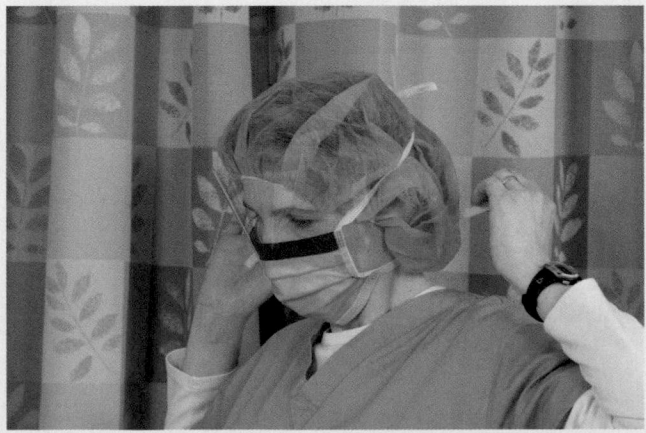

STEP 4d Tie bottom strings of mask.

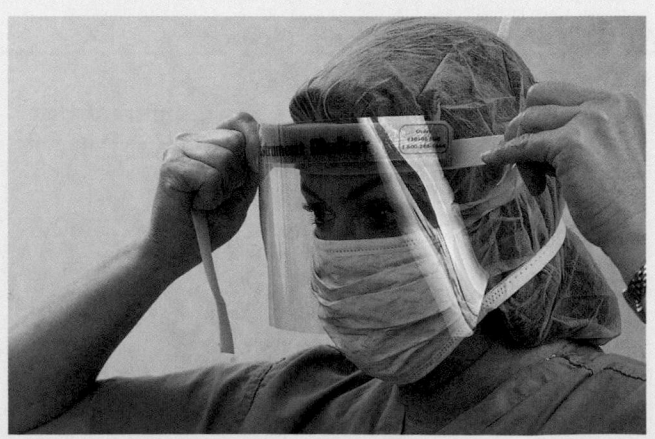

STEP 5a Apply face shield over cap.

STEP	RATIONALE

IMPLEMENTATION

6. If performing a sterile procedure, apply sterile gown (see Skill 6.3) at this time. After applying cap, mask, and eyewear, apply clean gloves for nonsterile procedures and sterile gloves (see Skill 6.3) for sterile procedures. Pull up clean gloves to cover each wrist (see illustration). **NOTE:** Provide a latex-free environment if patient or nurse has a latex allergy.

7. Remove protective barriers.

   a. Remove gloves first if worn (see Chapter 5 or Skill 6.3). Remove gloves by grasping cuff and pulling glove inside out over hand. Hold removed glove in other golved hand. Slide fingers of ungloved hand under remaining glove at wrist (see illustration). Peel glove off over first glove. Discard gloves in proper container.

   b. Remove eyewear. Avoid placing hands over soiled lens. **NOTE:** If wearing a face shield, remove it before removing mask.

   c. Remove gown by unfastening neck ties and pulling away from neck and shoulders. Touching only inside of gown, turn gown inside out, roll, or fold into a bundle and discard.

   d. Untie bottom strings of mask. First hold strings, untie top strings, and pull mask away from face while holding strings. Remove mask from face and discard in proper receptacle (see illustrations).

   e. Grasp outer surface of cap and lift from hair.

Proper removal prevents contamination of hair, neck, and facial area.

Proper removal prevents transmission of microorganisms.

Front and sleeves of gown are contaminated. This method of disposal prevents transmission of infection.

Proper removal prevents top part of mask from falling down over uniform. If mask falls and touches uniform, uniform will be contaminated.

Proper removal minimizes contact of hands with hair.

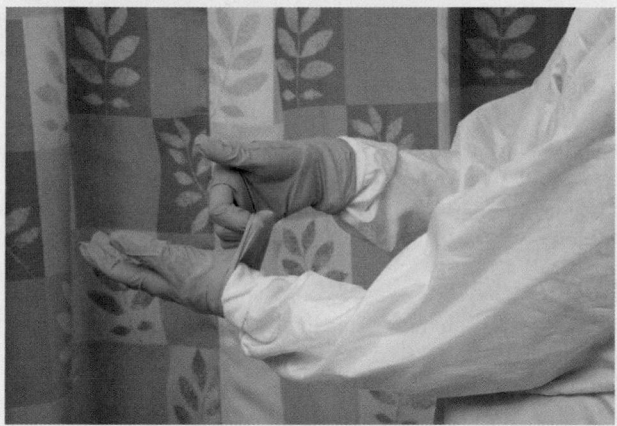

STEP 6 Apply gloves over gown sleeves.

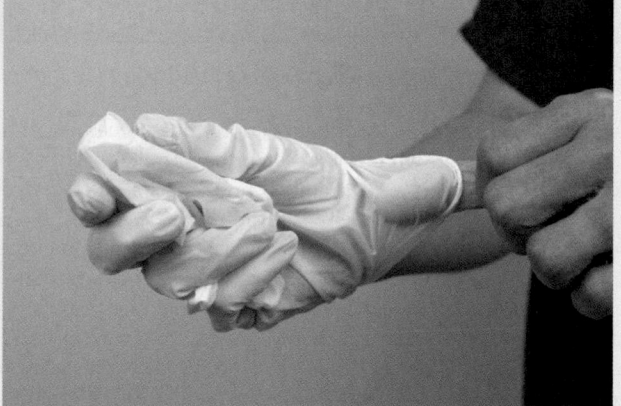

STEP 7a Remove second glove while holding soiled glove.

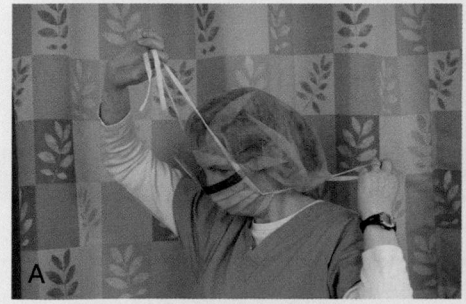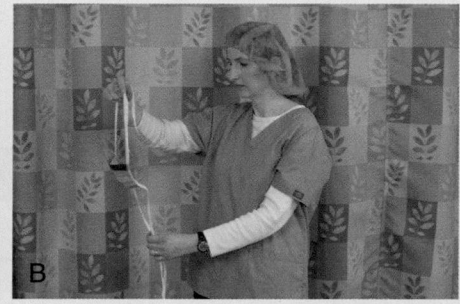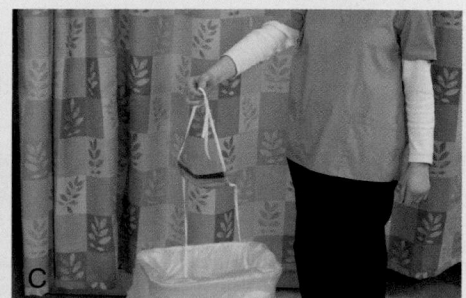

STEP 7d A, Untie top mask strings. **B,** Remove mask from face. **C,** Discard mask.

STEP	RATIONALE

IMPLEMENTATION

STEP	RATIONALE
f. Discard cap in proper receptacle and perform hand hygiene.	Routine reduces transmission of infection.

EVALUATION

STEP	RATIONALE
1. Following the procedure and as part of ongoing assessment, assess patient for signs of systemic infections or local area of body treated for drainage, tenderness, edema, or redness.	Assessment rules out presence of localized infection.

Unexpected Outcomes	Related Interventions
1. Redness, heat, edema, pain, or purulent drainage develops at wound or treatment site, indicating possible infection.	• Notify health care provider of change in condition of affected area and initiate appropriate treatments as prescribed.

Communication and Documentation

- It is unnecessary to document use of PPE.
- Communicate required use of PPE to patients, families, caregivers and all interprofessional team members.

Special Considerations
Care in the Community

- Instruct family, caregiver, or both about specifics of when to use PPE and how to dispose of properly.
- Determine ability of family, caregiver, or both to use equipment safely.
- Observe for the signs and symptoms of infection.

✦ SKILL 6.2   Preparing a Sterile Field

▶ *Video Clip*   **NSO** *Nursing Skills Online Infection Control Module 2 / Lesson 3*

When performing sterile aseptic procedures, it is necessary to have a sterile work area in which objects can be handled with minimal risk for contamination. A sterile field provides a sterile surface for placement of sterile equipment. Sterile drapes establish a sterile field around a treatment site such as a surgical incision, venipuncture site, or site for introduction of an in-dwelling urinary catheter. Sterile drapes also provide a work surface for placing sterile supplies and manipulating items with sterile gloves. After a sterile kit is opened, the inside surface of the cover can be used as a sterile field. Prior to establishing the sterile field, the nurse should gather the equipment and supplies necessary to perform the procedure. Once a sterile field is created, the interprofessional team is responsible for performing the procedure and making sure that the field is not contaminated.

Delegation and Collaboration

Interprofessional collaboration may be a part of sterile field preparation. Surgical technicians may prepare a sterile field (see employer policy); however, an unregulated care provider (UCP) cannot prepare a sterile field. The nurse can direct the UCP to:

- Help with patient positioning and obtain any necessary supplies.

Equipment

- Sterile pack (commercial or institution wrapped)
- Sterile drape or kit that is to be used as a sterile field
- Sterile gloves (*optional*)
- Sterile solution and equipment specific to a procedure
- Waist-high table or countertop surface
- Appropriate personal protective equipment (PPE): gown, mask, cap, protective eyewear (see employer policy)

STEP	RATIONALE

ASSESSMENT

STEP	RATIONALE
1. Identify patient using at least two person-specific identifiers (e.g., name and date of birth or name and medical record number) according to employer policy.	Ensures correct patient. Complies with Accreditation Canada's standards and improves patient safety (Accreditation Canada, 2019).

STEP	RATIONALE

ASSESSMENT

2. Verify with employer policy that procedure requires surgical aseptic technique.

Some procedures require medical rather than surgical aseptic technique.

3. Assess patient's comfort, positioning, oxygen requirements, and elimination needs before preparing for procedure.

Certain procedures that require a sterile field may last a long time. Anticipates patient's needs so patient can relax and avoid any unnecessary movement that might disrupt procedure.

4. Instruct patient (and caregiver if present) not to touch work surface or equipment during procedure.

Instruction prevents contamination of sterile field.

5. Assess for latex allergies.

A review may reveal latex allergies and determine the need to use latex-free supplies.

6. Check sterile package integrity for punctures, tears, discoloration, moisture, or any other signs of contamination. If using commercially packaged supplies or those prepared by employer, check for sterilization indicator (e.g., marker that changes colour when exposed to heat or steam).

Inspection of packaging ensures that only sterile items are presented to sterile field (AORN, 2016).

7. Anticipate number and variety of supplies needed for procedure.

Not all sterile kits contain sufficient amounts or types of supplies. Failure to have necessary supplies can cause you to leave sterile field, increasing risk for contamination.

NURSING DIAGNOSES

- Insufficient protection
- Potential for infection

Related factors/Risk factors are individualized on the basis of patient's condition or needs.

PLANNING

1. Expected outcomes following completion of procedure:
    - Sterile field is not contaminated.
    - Patient is not exposed to microorganisms.

Correct surgical aseptic practice is performed.

Lack of exposure prevents likelihood of infection transmission.

2. Complete all other nursing interventions (e.g., medication administration, suctioning patient) before beginning procedure.

Prepare sterile fields as close as possible to time of use to reduce potential for contamination (AORN, 2016).

3. Ask visitors to step out briefly during procedure. Instruct staff helping with procedure not to move.

Traffic or movement can increase potential for contamination through spread of microorganisms by air currents.

4. Arrange equipment at bedside.

Ensures availability before procedure and prevents break in sterile technique. (**NOTE:** Povidone-iodine and chlorhexidine are not considered sterile solutions and require separate work surfaces for preparation.)

5. Position patient comfortably for specific procedure to be performed. If a body part is to be examined or treated, position patient so area is accessible. Have UCP help with positioning as needed.

Patient should be able to lie still in one position comfortably during procedure. Movement can contaminate sterile field.

6. Explain to patient purpose of procedure and importance of sterile technique.

Explanation ensures patient's ability to cooperate with procedure. Performing patient teaching before procedure reduces need to talk during procedure, which can cause air-droplet contamination of sterile area.

IMPLEMENTATION

1. Apply PPE as needed (see employer policy) (see Skills 6.1 and 6.3).

PPE controls spread of airborne microorganisms.

2. Select a clean, flat, dry work surface above waist level.

A sterile object placed below a person's waist is considered contaminated.

3. Perform hand hygiene (see Chapter 5).

Hand hygiene reduces number of microorganisms on hands, thus reducing transmission to patient. Do not allow rinse water to run down arms onto clean hands (i.e., arms are considered dirty).

STEP	RATIONALE

IMPLEMENTATION

4. Prepare sterile work surface.
   a. **Use sterile commercial kit or pack containing sterile items.**

   (1) Place sterile kit or pack on the prepared work surface.

   (2) Open outside cover (see illustration) and remove package from dust cover. Place on work surface.

   (3) Grasp outer surface of tip of outermost flap.

   (4) Open outermost flap away from body, keeping arm outstretched and away from sterile field (see illustration).

   (5) Grasp outside surface of edge of first side flap.

   (6) Open side flap, pulling to side, allowing it to lie flat on table surface. Keep arm to side and not over sterile surface (see illustration).

   (7) Repeat Step (6) for second side flap (see illustration).

Sterile object placed above waist level is considered sterile.

Inner kit remains sterile.

Outer surface of package is considered unsterile. There is a 2.5-cm (1-inch) border around any sterile drape or wrap that is considered contaminated and can be touched with clean fingers.
Reaching over sterile field contaminates it.

Outer border is considered unsterile.

Drape or wrapper should lie flat so it does not accidentally rise up and contaminate inner surface or sterile contents.

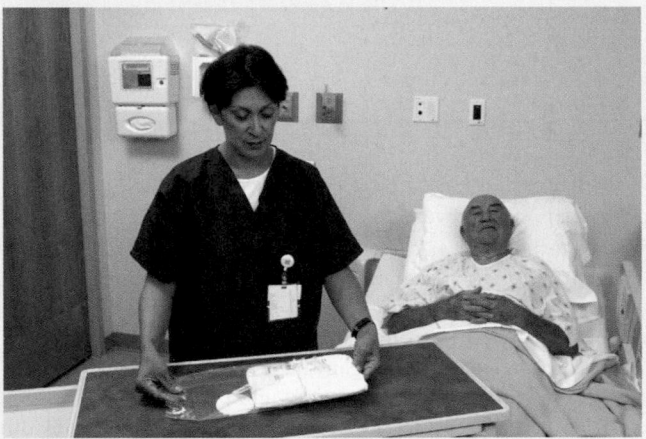

STEP 4a(2) Open outside cover of sterile kit.

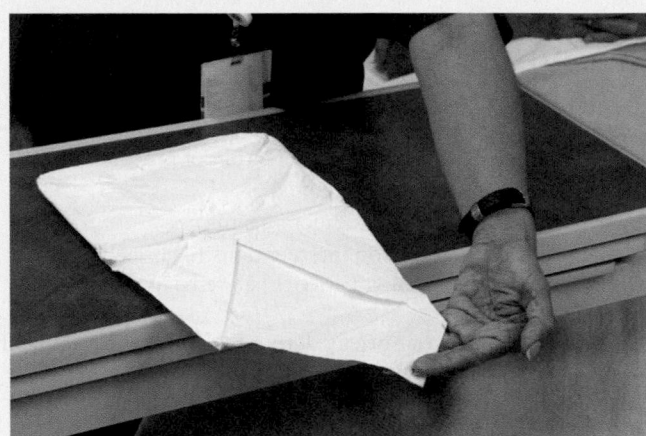

STEP 4a(4) Open outermost flap of sterile kit away from body.

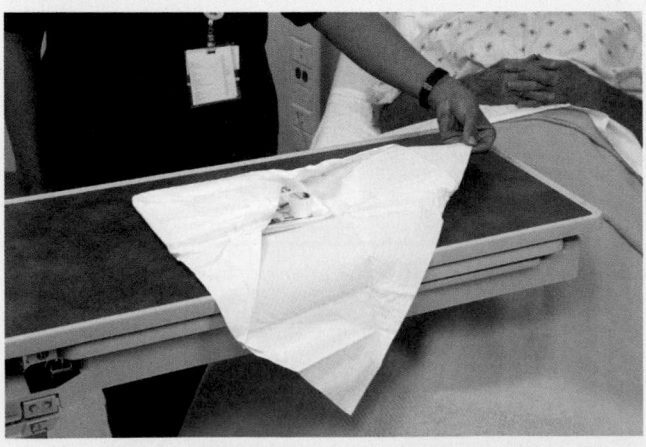

STEP 4a(6) Open first side flap, pulling to side.

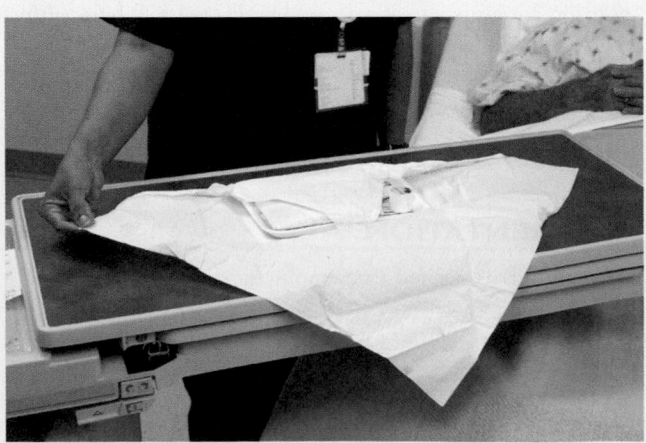

STEP 4a(7) Open second side flap, pulling to side.

STEP	RATIONALE

IMPLEMENTATION

(8) Grasp outside border of last and innermost flap (see illustration). Stand away from sterile package and pull flap back, allowing it to fall flat on table. Kit is ready to be used.

Outer border is considered unsterile.
Never reach over a sterile field.

b. Open sterile linen-wrapped package.

(1) Place package on clean, dry, flat work surface above waist level.

Sterile items placed below waist level are considered contaminated.

(2) Remove sterilization tape seal and unwrap both layers following same steps (see Steps 4a [2] through 4a [8]) as for sterile kit (see illustration).

Linen-wrapped items have two layers. The first is a dust cover. The second layer must be opened to view chemical indicator that verifies the sterility of the item.

(3) Use opened package wrapper as sterile field.

Inner surface of wrapper is considered sterile.

c. Prepare sterile drape.

(1) Place pack containing sterile drape on flat, dry surface and open as described (see Steps 4a [2] through 4a [8]) for sterile package.

Packaged drape remains sterile.

(2) Apply sterile gloves (*optional,* see employer policy). You may touch outer 2.5-cm (1-inch) border of drape without wearing gloves.

Sterile object remains sterile only when touched by another sterile object. Gloves are not necessary as long as fingers grasp the 2.5-cm (1-inch) unsterile border of the drape.

(3) Using fingertips of one hand, pick up folded top edge of drape along 2.5-cm (1-inch) border. Gently lift drape up from its wrapper without touching any object. Discard wrapper with other hand.

If sterile object touches any nonsterile object, it becomes contaminated.

(4) With other hand, grasp an adjacent corner of drape and hold it straight up and away from body. Allow drape to unfold, keeping it above waist and work surface and away from body (see illustration). (Carefully discard wrapper with other hand.)

An object held below a person's waist or above chest is contaminated.
Drape can now be placed properly with two hands.

(5) Holding drape, position bottom half over top half of intended work surface (see illustration).

Proper positioning prevents nurse from reaching over sterile field.

(6) Allow top half of drape to be placed over bottom half of work surface (see illustration).

Proper positioning creates flat, sterile work surface for placement of sterile supplies.

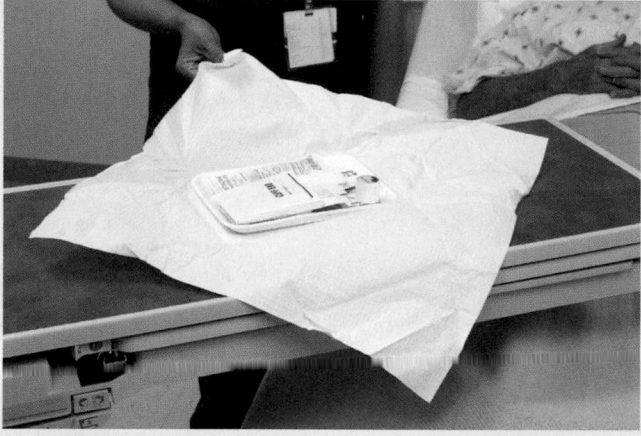

STEP 4a(8) Open last and innermost flap.

STEP	RATIONALE

IMPLEMENTATION

5. **Add sterile items to sterile field.**

   a. Open sterile item (following package directions) while holding outside wrapper in nondominant hand.

   b. With dominant hand, carefully peel wrapper over nondominant hand.

   c. Be sure that the wrapper does not fall down onto the sterile field. Place the item onto the field at an angle (see illustration). **Do not hold arms over sterile field.**

Use of nondominant hand frees dominant hand for unwrapping outer wrapper.

Item remains sterile. Inner surface of wrapper covers hand, making it sterile.

Secured wrapper edges prevent flipping wrapper and contaminating contents of sterile field (AORN, 2016).

Clinical Decision Point *Do not flip or toss objects onto sterile field.*

   d. Dispose of outer wrapper.

6. **Pour sterile solutions.**

   a. Verify contents and expiration date of solution.

   b. Place receptacle for solution near table or work surface edge. Sterile kits have cups or plastic moulded sections into which fluids can be poured.

Disposal prevents accidental contamination of sterile field.

Verification ensures proper solution and sterility of contents.

Proper placement prevents reaching over sterile field during pouring of solution.

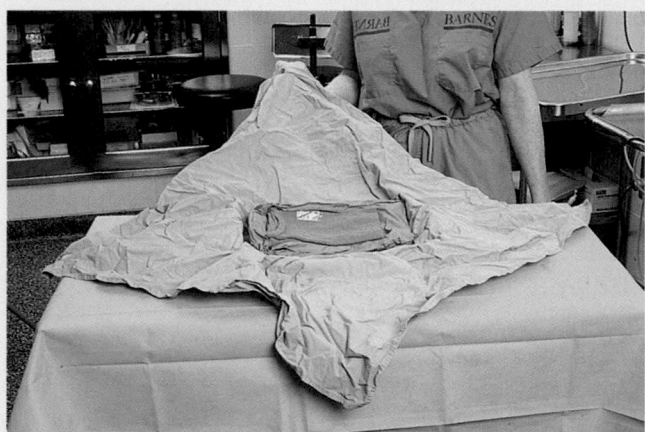

STEP 4c(1) Open sterile linen-wrapped package.

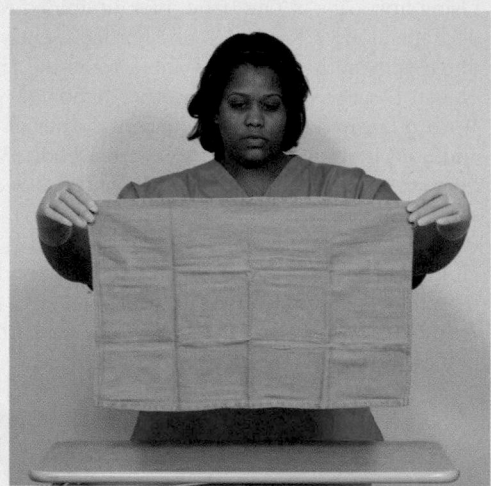

STEP 4c(4) Grasp corners of sterile drape, then hold up and away from body.

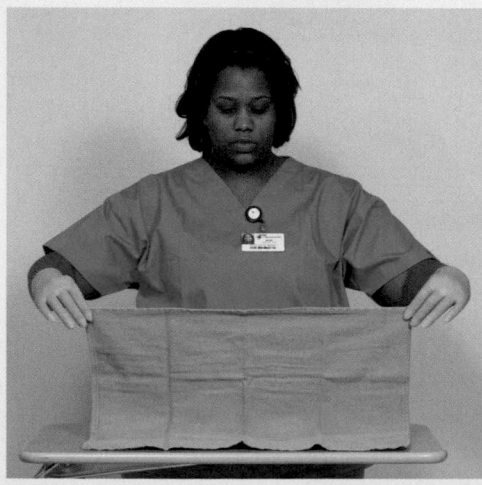

STEP 4c(5) Position bottom half of sterile drape over top half of work space.

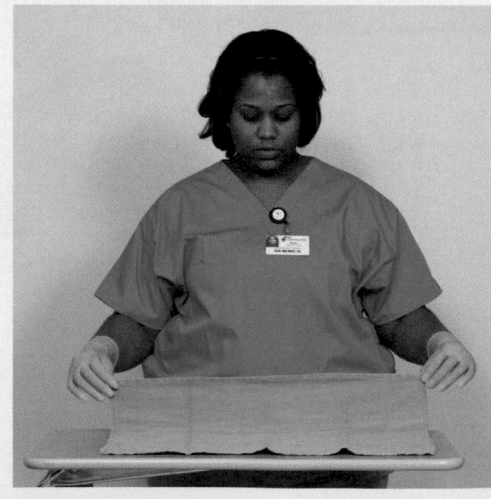

STEP 4c(6) Allow top half of drape to be placed over bottom half of work surface.

STEP	RATIONALE

IMPLEMENTATION

c. Remove sterile seal and cap from bottle in upward motion.

Upward movement prevents contamination of bottle lip.

d. With solution bottle held away from field and bottle lip 2.5 to 5 cm (1 to 2 inches) above inside of sterile receiving container, slowly pour needed amount of solution into container. Hold bottle with label facing palm of hand (see illustration).

Edge and outside of bottle are considered contaminated. Slow pouring prevents splashing. Sterility of contents cannot be ensured if cap is replaced.

Prevents label from becoming wet and illegible.

Clinical Decision Point *When liquids permeate sterile field or barrier, it is called strike through, resulting in contamination of the sterile field.*

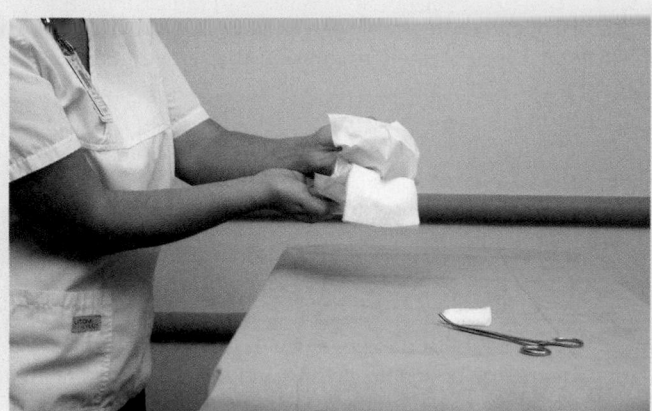

STEP 5c Add items to sterile field.

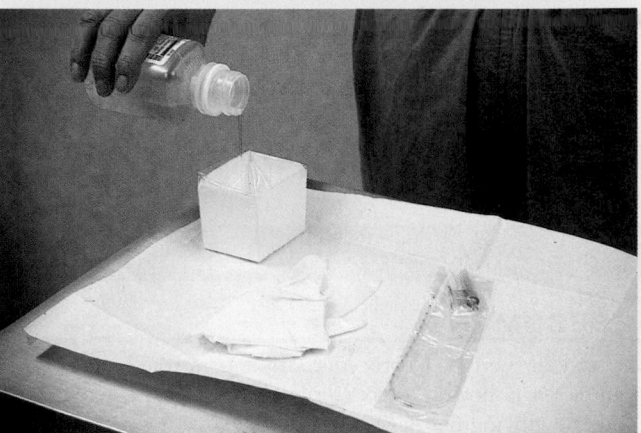

STEP 6d Pour solution into receiving container on sterile field.

EVALUATION

1. Observe for breaks in sterile technique.

A break in sterile field requires you to set up a new sterile field.

Unexpected Outcomes

1. Sterile field comes in contact with contaminated object or liquid splatters onto drape, causing strike through.
2. Sterile item falls off sterile field.

Related Interventions

- Discontinue field preparation and start over with new equipment.

- Open another package containing new sterile item and add to field unless field becomes contaminated, in which case a new sterile field would need to be established.

Communication and Documentation

- No communication or documentation is required for this set of skills. Document sterile procedure performed and patient status on flow sheet or in nurses' notes in electronic health record (EHR) or chart.

Special Considerations
Care in the Community

- Most care procedures in the home setting involve clean technique. In the event that a sterile environment is required,

the patient and caregiver need to be aware of the principles that apply to the sterile environment. For example, teach patient and caregiver how to correctly use package wrapper as a sterile drape or barrier when applying a sterile dressing or the correct procedure for removing sterile item from the package.

- Assess patient's and caregiver's understanding and ability to provide a sterile environment when needed to perform a specific procedure.

✦ SKILL 6.3   Sterile Gloving

▶ *Video Clip* **NSO** *Nursing Skills Online Infection Control Module 2 / Lesson 4*

Sterile gloves help prevent the transmission of pathogens by direct and indirect contact. Nurses apply sterile gloves before performing sterile procedures such as inserting urinary catheters or applying sterile dressings. Sterile gloves do not replace hand hygiene.

It is important to verify if the patient or health care providers have a latex allergy. When allergies are present, select latex-free gloves. In an effort to reduce the allergy risk, most health care facilities have a standard practice to use powder-free and latex-free products. Repeated exposure to latex can lead to a latex allergy, in which case latex-free gloves would need to be used. Box 6.2 lists risk factors for a latex allergy. Latex proteins enter the body through skin or mucous membranes, intravascularly, or via inhalation. Reactions to latex range from mild to severe (Box 6.3).

Gloves must be the proper size. The gloves should not stretch so tightly over the fingers that they can tear easily, yet they need to be tight enough that objects can be picked up easily. Sterile gloves are available in various sizes (e.g., 6, 6½, 7). They are also available in "one size fits all" or "small," "medium," and "large."

Delegation and Collaboration

Assisting with skills that include the application and removal of sterile gloves may be delegated to an unregulated care provider (UCP). However, most procedures that require the use of sterile gloves cannot be delegated to a UCP. The nurse instructs the UCP about:

- The reason for using sterile gloves for a specific procedure.

Equipment

- Package of proper-size sterile gloves, latex or synthetic nonlatex. If patient has a latex allergy, ensure that gloves are latex-free and powder-free.

STEP	RATIONALE

ASSESSMENT

1. Consider the type of procedure to be performed and consult employer policy on use of sterile gloves. In some facilities, double gloving has been recommended for the operating room (Johnson & Osborne, 2016).

Ensures proper use of sterile gloves when needed. Evidence supports the use of double gloving and double gloving with an indicator glove system to decrease the risk of percutaneous injury; such use is an effective barrier to bloodborne pathogen exposure (AORN, 2016).

2. Consider patient's risk for infection (e.g., pre-existing condition and size or extent of area being treated).

Knowledge of risk directs you to follow added precautions (e.g., use of additional protective barriers) if necessary.

3. Select correct size and type of gloves and examine glove package to determine if it is dry and intact with no water stains.

Torn or wet package is considered contaminated. Signs of water stains on package indicate previous contamination by water.

BOX 6.2

Individuals at Risk for Latex Allergy

- Individuals who have had multiple surgeries (e.g., spina bifida surgeries) or medical procedures
- Workers with high latex exposure (e.g., health care employees, greenhouse workers, hair salon workers, estheticians, workers in industries that use gloves routinely)
- Rubber industry workers
- Individuals with a personal or family history of allergies
- There is evidence that some people who are allergic to certain foods (e.g., avocado, banana, chestnut, kiwi, passion fruit) may also develop an allergic reaction to latex.

Canadian Centre for Occupational Health and Safety (CCOHS). (2016). *Latex allergy.* Retrieved from http://www.ccohs.ca/oshanswers/diseases/latex.html

BOX 6.3

Levels of Latex Reactions

The three types of common latex reactions (in order of severity) are as follows:

1. *Irritant dermatitis:* Skin reaction isolated to the area of contact
   a. Acute reaction: Red, dry, itchy, and irritated
   b. Chronic reaction: Dry, thick skin, crusting, and possibly cracking or peeling, resulting in open sores
2. *Type IV delayed hypersensitivity:* Allergic reaction to chemicals used in latex processing

   a. Acute reaction: Dry, red, rash, itchy, hives, small blisters
   b. Chronic reaction: Dry, thickened skin, crusting, scabbing sores, vesicles, peeling (appears 4–96 hours after exposure)
3. *Type I immediate hypersensitivity:* Could be life-threatening, and reactions can start as soon as 2–3 minutes after contact, up to several hours
   a. Acute reaction: Hives, swelling, runny nose, nausea, abdominal cramps, dizziness, low blood pressure, bronchospasm, anaphylaxis (shock)

Centers for Disease Control and Prevention. (2013). *Frequently asked questions: Contact dermatitis and latex allergy.* Retrieved from http://www.cdc.gov/oralhealth/infectioncontrol/faq/latex.htm

STEP	RATIONALE

ASSESSMENT

4. Inspect condition of hands for cuts, hangnails, open lesions, or abrasions. In some settings, you can cover any open lesion with a sterile, impervious transparent dressing (check employer policy). In some cases, presence of such lesions may prevent you from participating in a procedure.

Cuts, abrasions, and hangnails tend to ooze serum, which possibly contains pathogens. Breaks in skin integrity permit microorganisms to enter and increase the risk for infection for both patient and nurse (AORN, 2016).

5. Assess patient for the following risk factors before applying latex gloves:

Risk factors determine level of patient's risk for latex allergy.

   a. Previous reaction to the following items within hours of exposure: adhesive tape, dental or face mask, golf club grip, ostomy bag, rubber band, balloon, bandage, elastic underwear, intravenous (IV) tubing, rubber gloves, condom

Items are known to lead to latex allergy.

   b. Personal history of asthma, contact dermatitis, eczema, urticaria, rhinitis

Patients with a history of these conditions are at higher risk of having a reaction.

   c. History of food allergies, especially avocado, banana, peach, chestnut, passionfruit, raw potato, kiwi, tomato, papaya

Patients with a history of food allergies are at higher risk of developing a reaction.

   d. Previous history of adverse reactions during surgery or dental procedure

Previous history suggests allergic response.

   e. Previous reaction to latex product

Previous reaction suggests allergic response.

NURSING DIAGNOSES

- Insufficient protection
- Potential for infection
- Potential for injury

Related factors/Risk factors are individualized on the basis of patient's condition or needs.

PLANNING

1. Expected outcomes following completion of procedure:
   - Patient does not develop signs or symptoms of infection after procedure.

Lack of signs of infection indicates that microorganisms are not introduced into sterile body cavities or sites (such as skin or urinary tract).

   - Patient does not develop latex sensitivity or latex allergy reaction.

Patient at risk for latex allergy is not exposed to latex proteins.

Clinical Decision Point *Nonlatex gloves (latex-free/powder-free) must be used when patients are at risk or if nurse has sensitivity or allergy to latex.*

IMPLEMENTATION

1. Apply sterile gloves.
   a. Perform thorough hand hygiene. Place glove package near work area.

Hand hygiene reduces number of bacteria on skin surfaces and transmission of infection. Proximity to work area ensures availability before procedure.

   b. Remove outer glove package wrapper by carefully separating and peeling apart sides (see illustration).

Proper removal prevents inner glove package from accidentally opening and touching contaminated objects.

   c. Grasp inner package and lay on clean, dry, flat surface at waist level. Open package, keeping gloves on inside surface of wrapper (see illustration).

Sterile object held below waist is contaminated. Inner surface of glove package is sterile.

   d. Identify right and left glove. Each glove has a cuff approximately 5 cm (2 inches) wide. Glove dominant hand first.

Proper identification of gloves prevents contamination by improper fit. Gloving of dominant hand first improves dexterity.

   e. With thumb and first two fingers of nondominant hand, grasp glove for dominant hand by touching only inside surface of cuff.

Inner edge of cuff will lie against skin and thus is not sterile.

   f. Carefully pull glove over dominant hand, leaving a cuff and being sure that cuff does not roll up wrist. Be sure that thumb and fingers are in proper spaces (see illustration).

If outer surface of glove touches hand or wrist, it is contaminated.

STEP	**RATIONALE**

IMPLEMENTATION

g. With gloved dominant hand, slip fingers underneath cuff of second glove (see illustration).

Cuff protects gloved fingers. Sterile touching prevents glove contamination.

h. Carefully pull second glove over fingers of nondominant hand (see illustration).

Contact of gloved hand with exposed hand results in contamination.

Clinical Decision Point *Do not allow fingers and thumb of gloved dominant hand to touch any part of exposed nondominant hand. Keep thumb of dominant hand abducted back.*

i. After second glove is on, interlock hands together and hold away from body above waist level until beginning procedure (see illustration).

Ensures smooth fit over fingers and prevents contamination.

2. Perform procedure.

3. Remove gloves.

a. Grasp outside of one cuff with other gloved hand; avoid touching wrist.

Procedure minimizes contamination of underlying skin.

b. Pull glove off, turning it inside out, and place it in gloved hand.

Outside of glove does not touch skin surface.

c. Take fingers of bare hand and tuck inside remaining glove cuff (see illustration). Peel glove off inside out and over previously removed glove. Discard both gloves in receptacle.

Fingers do not touch contaminated glove surface.

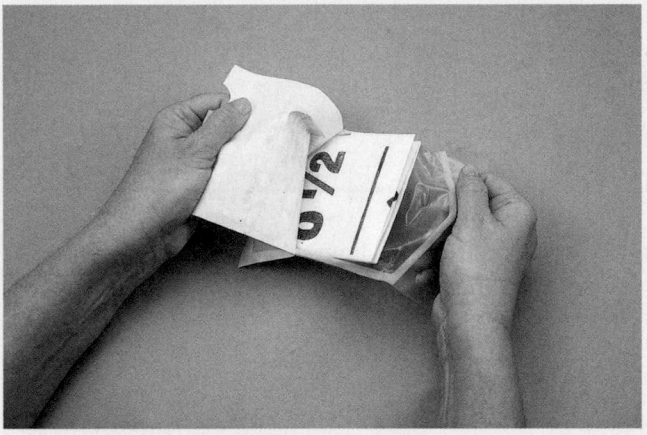

STEP 1b Open outer glove package wrapper.

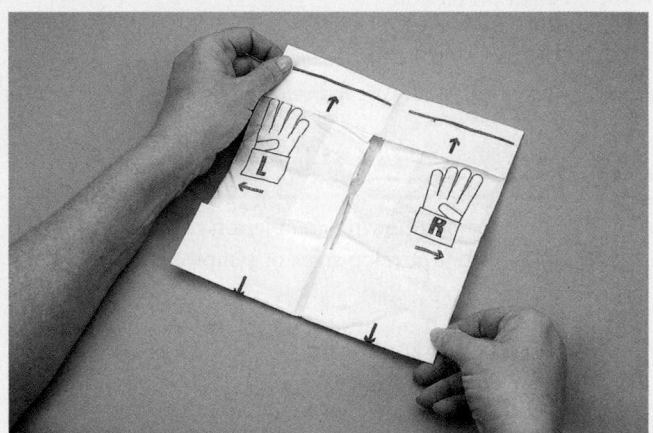

STEP 1c Open inner glove package on work surface.

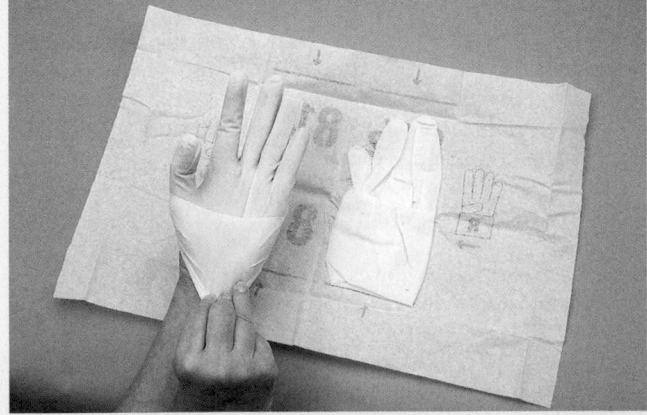

STEP 1f Pick up glove at cuff of dominant hand and insert fingers. Pull glove completely over dominant hand (example is for left-handed person).

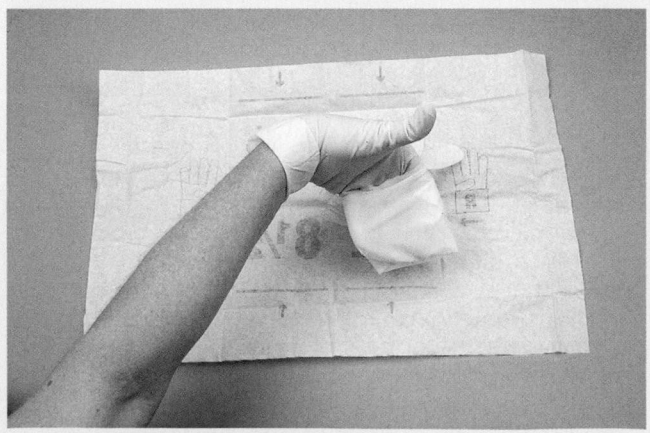

STEP 1g Pick up glove for nondominant hand.

STEP	RATIONALE

IMPLEMENTATION

d. Perform thorough hand hygiene.

Hand hygiene protects health care worker from contamination resulting from any unseen tears or pinholes in gloves; also removes powder from hands to prevent skin irritation.

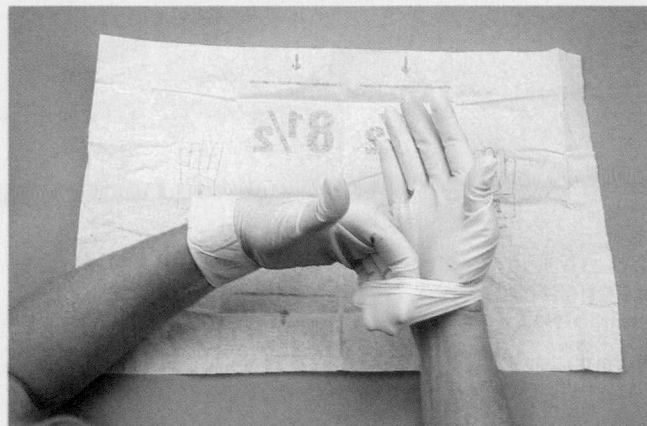

STEP 1h Pull second glove over nondominant hand.

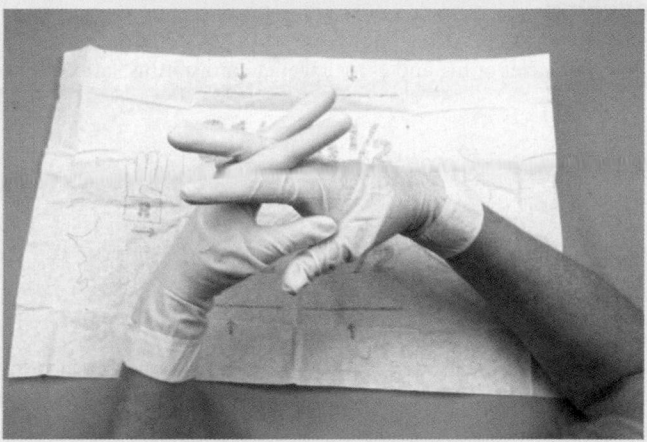

STEP 1i Interlock gloved hands.

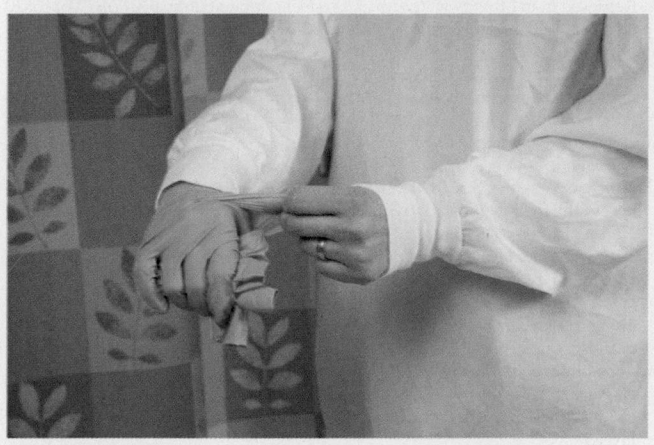

STEP 3c Remove second glove by turning it inside out.

EVALUATION

1 Assess patient for signs of infection, focusing on area treated.

2. Assess patient for signs of latex allergy.

Improper technique contributes to development of an infection. Assessment establishes baseline for patient's reaction to latex.

Unexpected Outcomes

1. Patient develops localized signs of infection (e.g., urine becomes cloudy or odorous; wound becomes painful, edematous, or reddened with purulent drainage).
2. Patient develops systemic signs of infection (e.g., fever, malaise, increased white blood cell count).
3. Patient develops allergic reaction to latex (see Box 6.3).

Related Interventions

- Contact health care provider and implement appropriate treatments as prescribed.

- Contact health care provider and implement appropriate treatments as ordered.
- Immediately remove source of latex.
  Bring emergency equipment to bedside. Have epinephrine injection ready for administration, and be prepared to initiate IV fluids and oxygen.

Communication and Documentation

- It is not necessary to document application of gloves. Document specific procedure performed and patient's response and status.
- In the event of a latex allergy reaction, document patient's response on flow sheet or in nurses' notes in electronic health record (EHR) or chart. Note type of response and patient's reaction to emergency treatment.

Special Considerations
Teaching

- Nurse or patient with a known latex allergy should wear a medical alert bracelet or tag and carry a wallet card stating "latex allergy."

- Individuals with known latex allergies should always carry a quick-acting oral antihistamine and an epinephrine autoinjector.
- Due to risk of severe allergic response, some health care facilities only use powder- and latex-free gloves and products.

◆ CLINICAL DEBRIEF

A 78-year-old woman who is visually impaired is being admitted for a cholecystectomy. You enter her room to begin a series of procedures: inserting an in-dwelling urinary catheter, irrigating a nasogastric tube, suctioning the oral cavity, and measuring her blood pressure.

1. Which procedure requires use of sterile gloves?
2. The health care provider is planning to insert a central venous line. You obtained the necessary equipment, prepared a sterile drape, and opened the sterile pack. You removed the outer wrapper and placed the item on the sterile field. While doing this, you noticed that the item touched the drape 5 cm (2 inches) from the border of the drape. What should you do next?
3. The patient tells you that she develops dermatitis when she uses rubber gloves while doing the dishes and develops a rash when she eats bananas or avocados. How would you use SBAR (Situation-Background-Assessment-Recommendation) to communicate this information to the rest of the health care team?

◆ REVIEW QUESTIONS

1. When opening a sterile pack, which action compromises the sterility of the contents? *(Select all that apply.)*
   1. Positioning the contents of the pack at the very edge of the drape
   2. Holding or moving the object below the waist
   3. Opening the pack just before the procedure
   4. Allowing minimal movement around the sterile field
   5. Obtaining a nonlatex catheter for the procedure
2. When performing a sterile procedure at the bedside, the UCP can assist by helping the nurse _____ the patient.
3. Which of the following procedures requires sterile (aseptic) technique? *(Select all that apply.)*
   1. Urinary catheterization
   2. Insertion of a feeding tube
   3. Tracheal suctioning
   4. Lumbar puncture
   5. Insertion of a rectal suppository
   6. Sitz bath

ⓔ *Visit the Evolve site for a complete list of Clinical Debrief and Review Questions answers.*

REFERENCES

Accreditation Canada. (2019). *Required organizational practices handbook—Version 14*. Retrieved from http://www.wrha.mb.ca/quality/files/2019ROPHandbook.pdf

Association of periOperative Registered Nurses (AORN). (2016). *Guidelines for perioperative practice*. Denver: AORN.

Barnes, S. (2015). Infection prevention: The surgical care continuum. *AORN Journal, 101*(5), 512–518. doi:10.1016/j.aorn.2015.02.006

Cimon, K., & Featherstone, R. (2017). *Jewellery and nail polish worn by health care workers and the risk of infection transmission: A review of clinical evidence and guidelines*. Ottawa, ON: Canadian Agency for Drugs and Technologies in Health. Retrieved from https://www.cadth.ca/sites/default/files/pdf/htis/2017/RC0858%20Jewellery%20and%20Nail%20Polish%20Risk%20Final.pdf

Infection Prevention and Control Canada (IPAC). (2017). *IPAC Canada practice recommendations: Hand hygiene in health care settings*. Retrieved from https://ipac-canada.org/photos/custom/Members/pdf/17JulHand%20Hygiene%20Practice%20Recommendations_final.pdf

Infusion Nurses Society (INS). (2016). Infusion therapy standards of practice. *Journal of Intravenous Nursing, 39*(Suppl. 1), S1–S159.

Johnson, J., & Osborne, S. (2016). Surgical hand antisepsis, gowning and gloving—not necessarily the way it has always been done. *ACORN: The Journal of Perioperative Nursing in Australia, 29*(2), 52–54.

Ontario Agency for Health Protection and Promotion Public Health Ontario (PHO), Provincial Infectious Diseases Advisory Committee (PIDAC). (2012). *Routine practices and additional precautions in all health care settings* (3rd ed.). Retrieved from https://www.publichealthontario.ca/en/eRepository/RPAP_All_HealthCare_Settings_Eng2012.pdf

Provincial Infectious Diseases Advisory Committee (PIDAC). (2014). *Best practices for hand hygiene in all health care settings* (4th ed.). Retrieved from http://www.publichealthontario.ca/en/eRepository/2010-12%20BP%20Hand%20Hygiene.pdf

Public Health Agency of Canada (PHAC). (2017). *Routine practices and additional precautions for preventing the transmission of infection in healthcare settings*. Ottawa, ON: Author. Retrieved from https://www.canada.ca/en/public-health/services/publications/diseases-conditions/routine-practices-precautions-healthcare-associated-infections.html. (Cat. No. HP40-83/2013E-PDF).

Raines, K., & Rosen, K. (2016). The effect of chlorhexidine bathing on rates of nosocomial infections among the critically ill population: An analysis of current clinical research and recommendations for practice. *Dimensions of Critical Care Nursing, 35*(2), 84–91. doi:10.1097/DCC.0000000000000165

Wood, A., & VanWicklin, S. A. (2015). Ultraviolet (UV)-cured nail polish. *AORN Journal, 101*(6), 702–704. doi:10.1016/j.aorn.2016.08.001

7 | Vital Signs

Written by **Susan Jane Fetzer, MSN, MBA, PhD, and Tracy Stephen, RN, MN**

SKILLS AND PROCEDURES

OBJECTIVES

Mastery of content in this chapter will enable the nurse to:
- Identify when it is appropriate to assess each vital sign.
- Accurately assess a patient's oral, rectal, axillary, tympanic membrane, and temporal artery temperatures.
- Describe factors that cause variations in body temperature, pulse, respirations, blood pressure, and oxygen saturation.
- Discuss factors in selecting temperature measurement sites.
- Accurately assess a patient's radial and apical pulses.
- Explain implications of a pulse deficit.
- Accurately assess a patient's respirations.
- Accurately measure a patient's blood pressure using techniques of auscultation and palpation.
- Discuss benefits and disadvantages of using an automatic blood pressure machine.
- Describe factors in selecting an extremity to measure blood pressure.
- Accurately assess a patient's oxygenation status using pulse oximetry.
- Identify ranges of acceptable vital sign values for infant, child, and adult.
- Correctly record vital signs.
- Appropriately delegate vital sign measurements to unregulated care providers (UCP).

MEDIA RESOURCES

- evolve http://evolve.elsevier.com/Canada/Perry/clinicalskills/
- Review Questions
- Audio Glossary
- ▶ Video Clips
- Animations
- Clinical Debrief and Review Questions Answers
- Case Studies

PURPOSE

Vital signs, temperature, pulse, blood pressure, respirations, and oxygen saturation reflect the physiological status of the body and its response to physical, environmental, and psychological stressors. Pain, a subjective symptom, is often referred to as a vital sign. As a nurse, you will frequently perform an assessment of a patient's level of comfort and pain during vital sign measurements (see Chapter 16).

Vital signs reveal both sudden changes in a patient's condition and changes that occur progressively over time. Any difference between a patient's normal baseline measurement and present vital signs may indicate the need for interprofessional collaboration with other health care team members, nursing therapies, and necessary medical interventions.

STANDARDS OF CARE

- Canadian Agency for Drugs and Technologies in Health (CADTH), 2017—*The Assessment of Postoperative Vital Signs: Clinical Effectiveness and Guidelines* (https://www.cadth.ca/sites/default/files/pdf/htis/2017/RA0897%20Assessment%20of%20Postop%20Vital%20Signs%20Final.pdf)
- Canadian Paediatric Society (CPS), 2017—*Position Statement: Temperature Measurement in Paediatrics* (https://www.cps.ca/en/documents/position/temperature-measurement)
- Hypertension Canada, 2018—*Accurate Measurement of Blood Pressure* (http://guidelines.hypertension.ca.chep-resourses/)
- SickKids (The Hospital for Sick Children, Toronto), 2014—*Vital Signs* (http://www.sickkids.ca/Nursing/Education-and-learning/

Nursing-Student-Orientation/module-two-clinical-care/vitals/index.html)

PRINCIPLES FOR PRACTICE

- Vital signs are included in a routine health assessment (see Chapter 8).
- Always obtain a baseline measurement of vital signs on first contact with a patient to provide a means for comparison with later vital sign measurements.
- Frequency of vital sign measurements depends on the specific patient's condition (Box 7.1).
- Use interprofessional collaboration and apply clinical reasoning and judgement to decide which vital sign to measure, when to obtain measurements, and the frequency of assessments.

PERSON-CENTRED CARE

- Interprofessional collaboration and patient involvement regarding vital signs and every other area of the patient's health are important in optimizing patient health and wellness and practising person-centred care. Patients should be actively engaged in the prevention, promotion, and management of their health (Canadian Nurses Association [CNA], 2011).
- Vital sign measurements can require removal of clothing or exposing areas considered inappropriate or offensive to patients from other cultures. Nurses must be sensitive to each patient's need for privacy and observe cultural norms. Provide privacy as part of person-centred care when performing apical pulse assessment.
- Always inform patients about their vital sign measurements. Many patients monitor their own vital signs at home and can be valuable partners in letting the nurse know which values are normal for them.
- Procedures that are normally noninvasive sometimes produce anxiety because of cultural variables of touch, privacy, and gender.
- When reporting findings, patients from some cultures rely on a male elder to receive information on their behalf.

BOX 7.1

When to Take Vital Signs

- On admission to a health care facility
- In a hospital or care facility on a routine schedule according to a health care provider's prescription or employer policy
- When assessing patient during home care visits
- Before, during, and after a surgical or invasive diagnostic procedure
- Before, during, and after the administration of medications or application of therapies that affect cardiovascular, respiratory, or temperature-control functions
- Before, during, and after a transfusion of any type of blood products
- Before, during, and after nursing interventions influencing a vital sign (e.g., before and after patient previously on bed rest ambulates, before and after range-of-motion exercises)
- When patient reports specific symptoms of physical distress (e.g., feeling "funny" or "different")
- When patient's general physical condition changes (e.g., loss of consciousness, increased intensity of pain)
- Before a patient is sent home on a day or weekend pass and upon their return to the facility.

- Provide culturally competent nursing care and assess patient preference related to decision making (e.g., independent or interdependent in health-related issues). Nurses must be aware that patients may make a decision based on what they think is best for their family, not necessarily themselves, and be prepared to advocate for and support the patient (Lewis et al., 2019).

EVIDENCE-INFORMED PRACTICE

Obtaining an accurate and reliable measurement of blood pressure requires consideration of measurement conditions.
- Slow breathing decreases systolic blood pressure measurement about 10 mm Hg (Jones, Sangthong, Pachirat, et al., 2015).
- Talking with a health care provider can increase systolic blood pressure 9.1 mm Hg and diastolic pressure 4.5 mm Hg (Qi et al., 2017).
- The blood pressure cuff should be placed on a bare arm (Hypertension Canada, 2015).

SAFETY GUIDELINES

- A nurse caring for a patient is responsible for measuring vital signs. Nurses analyze vital signs to interpret their significance and make decisions about appropriate interventions.
- Equipment must be clean, functional, properly calibrated, and appropriate for the patient's size, age, condition, and characteristics.
- As the nurse it is your responsibility to know each patient's usual range of vital signs. A patient's usual values may differ from the acceptable range for that age or physical state. They serve as a baseline for comparison with later findings, enabling you to detect changes in condition over time.
- You are also responsible for knowing a patient's medical history, therapies, and prescribed medications. Some illnesses or treatments cause predictable vital sign changes. Most medications affect at least one of the vital signs.
- Control or minimize environmental factors that affect vital signs. For example, assessing a patient's temperature in a warm, humid room may yield a value that is not a true indicator of their condition.
- Use an organized, systematic (step-by-step) approach when taking vital signs to ensure accurate findings.
- Based on a patient's condition, use interprofessional collaboration to decide the minimum frequency of vital sign assessment for each patient. Following surgery or treatment intervention, measure vital signs more frequently to detect complications. In a clinic or outpatient setting take vital signs before the health care provider examines the patient and after any invasive procedures. As a patient's physical condition worsens, it is important to monitor vital signs as often as every 5 to 15 minutes. Use your clinical reasoning and judgement to determine whether more frequent assessments are necessary.
- Analyze the results of vital sign measurements and incorporate all the clinical findings about a patient in determining nursing diagnoses. Do not interpret vital signs in isolation. You need to know related physical signs or symptoms and be aware of the patient's ongoing health status.
- Verify, communicate, and document significant changes in vital signs. Baseline measurements allow you to identify changes in vital signs. When vital signs appear abnormal, it helps to have another nurse repeat the measurement. Inform the health care

provider when vital signs become abnormal and report any changes to the nurse in charge.

- Always practice infection control. Perform hand hygiene before and after care of the patient, use personal protective equipment (PPE) when there is a risk of exposure to or possible transmission of infections, and, if possible, use disposable or dedicated patient-care equipment (e.g., blood pressure cuffs). If disposable or dedicated equipment is not available, clean and disinfect the equipment before use on another patient (Centers for Disease Control and Prevention [CDC], 2017a).

✦ SKILL 7.1   Measuring Body Temperature

▶ *Video Clip* NSO *Nursing Skills Online Vital Signs Module 1, Lessons 1 and 2*

Body temperature is the difference between the amount of heat produced by body processes and the amount lost to the external environment. The core temperature, or temperature of the deep body tissues, is under control of the hypothalamus and remains within a narrow range. The thermostat regulated in the hypothalamus maintains this homeostasis by balancing heat production (from metabolism, exercise, food digestion, external factors) with heat loss (through radiation, evaporation of sweat, convection, conduction) (Jarvis, 2019). Skin or body surface temperature can also fluctuate dramatically as it rises and falls with the changing temperature of the surrounding environment.

The body tissues and cells function best within a relatively narrow temperature range, from 36° to 38°C (96.8° to 100.4°F), but no single temperature is normal for all people. For healthy young adults, the average oral temperature is 37°C (98.6°F). In clinical practice nurses learn the temperature range of individual patients. An acceptable temperature range for adults depends on age, gender, range of physical activity, hydration status, and state of health (Fig. 7.1).

Many factors affect body temperature, but physiological and behavioural control mechanisms act to maintain a constant core temperature. For example, the mechanism of peripheral vasodilation increases blood flow to the skin, which increases the amount of heat radiated to the environment. Control mechanisms have failed when heat produced by the body is not equal to heat lost to the environment. For example, patients without sweat gland function are unable to tolerate warm temperatures because they cannot adequately cool themselves. Fever occurs when heat-loss mechanisms are unable to keep pace with excess heat production, resulting in an abnormal rise in body temperature. When an individual has a febrile condition (i.e., pyrexia), the nurse needs to initiate temperature-control measures, such as administering prescribed antipyretics; providing a tepid sponge bath; applying cool compresses to the patient's forehead, wrists, and other body sites; dressing the patient in lightweight clothing; or in cases of a high fever providing a cooling blanket. It is important to carefully monitor the patient for shivering when using these cooling interventions as shivering increases core body temperature (Smith, 2016).

The purpose of measuring body temperature is to obtain a representative average temperature of core body tissues. Average usual temperature varies, depending on the measurement site used. Research findings from numerous studies are contradictory; however, it is generally accepted that rectal temperatures are usually 0.5°C (0.9°F) higher than oral temperatures. Axillary temperatures are usually 0.5°C (0.9°F) lower than oral temperatures (Potter et al., 2019) (Box 7.2) .

To ensure accurate temperature readings each site needs to be measured correctly. Use the same site when repeated measurements are necessary or when comparing temperature measurements over time. Each site has advantages and disadvantages (Box 7.3). Determine the safest and most accurate site for a patient.

Several types of thermometers are commonly available to measure body temperature (Box 7.4). The mercury-in-glass thermometer, once the standard device found in the clinical setting, is now prohibited because of the potential mercury hazards. However, mercury-in-glass thermometers can still be found in patients' homes.

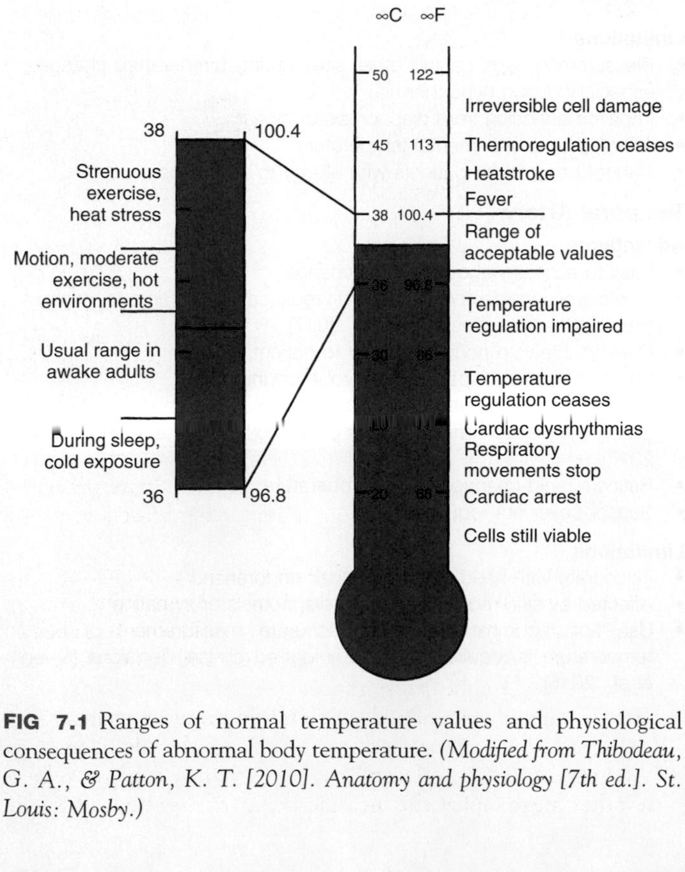

FIG 7.1 Ranges of normal temperature values and physiological consequences of abnormal body temperature. *(Modified from Thibodeau, G. A., & Patton, K. T. [2010]. Anatomy and physiology [7th ed.]. St. Louis: Mosby.)*

BOX 7.2
Core and Surface Temperature Measurement Sites

Core Site
- Rectum
- Tympanic membrane
- Temporal artery
- Esophagus
- Pulmonary artery
- Urinary bladder

Surface Site
- Skin
- Oral cavity
- Axilla

BOX 7.3

Advantages and Limitations of Select Temperature Measurement Sites

Oral

Advantages

- Easily accessible—requires no position change
- Comfortable for patient
- Provides accurate surface temperature reading
- Reflects rapid change in core temperature
- Reliable route to measure temperature for intubated patients

Limitations

- Causes delay in measurement if patient recently ingested hot/cold fluids or foods, chewed gum, or smoked
- Not used with patients who have had oral surgery or facial trauma, are unable to position in mouth, or have shaking chills or history of seizures
- Not used with infants; small children; or confused, unconscious, or uncooperative patients
- Risk for body fluid exposure

Tympanic Membrane

Advantages

- Easily accessible site
- Obtained without disturbing, waking, or repositioning patient
- Used for patients with tachypnea without affecting breathing
- Sensitive to core temperature changes
- Very rapid measurement (2 to 5 seconds)
- Unaffected by oral intake of food or fluids or smoking

Limitations

- More variability of measurement than with other core temperature devices
- Requires removal of hearing aids before measurement
- Requires disposable sensor cover with only one size available
- Readings possibly distorted with otitis media and cerumen impaction
- Not used with patients who have had surgery of the ear or tympanic membrane
- Environmental temperatures can affect the measurement reading, making it invalid
- Does not accurately measure core temperature changes during and after exercise
- Affected by ambient temperature devices such as incubators, radiant warmers, and facial fans
- Recent evidence indicates that tympanic temperature is only a stable measure if the probe is directed at a specific site on the membrane and is influenced by head cooling (Yeoh et al., 2017).
- Anatomy of the ear canal makes it difficult to correctly position in neonates, infants, and children younger than 2 years of age. The thermometer probe is too large in relation to the size of the ear canal, so it will detect infrared emissions from both the tympanic membrane and the proximal meatus wall. The average of these two surface temperatures can produce an erroneously low reading. A slight tug of the pinna to straighten the ear canal can improve accuracy and consistency (Canadian Paediatric Society, 2017).
- Inaccuracies reported because of incorrect positioning of handheld unit

Rectal

Advantages

- Purported to be reliable when oral temperature is difficult or impossible to obtain
- Although controversial, it is still referred to as the gold standard for use in children under 3 years of age (Forrest, Conley, Juliano, et al., 2016); however, emerging research indicates that axillary thermometry is the most accurate for this age group (Otto, 2017).

Limitations

- Lags behind core temperature during rapid temperature changes
- Not used for patients with diarrhea or those who have had rectal surgery, rectal disorders, bleeding tendencies, or neutropenia
- Requires positioning that can be a source of patient embarrassment and anxiety
- Risk for body fluid exposure
- Requires lubrication
- Not used for routine vital signs in newborns because of a risk for possible bowel perforation
- Readings influenced by impacted stool
- Should not be used with patients receiving chemotherapy because it increases the risk for infection

Axilla

Advantages

- Safe and inexpensive
- Reliable in stable neonates and those in the neonatal intensive care unit (NICU) (Joseph, Derstine, & Killian, 2017)

Limitations

- Long measurement time
- Requires continuous positioning to ensure placement over axillary artery
- Poorly reflects core temperature (Niven et al., 2015)
- Not recommended for detecting fever in infants and young children
- Requires exposure of thorax, which can result in temperature loss, especially in newborns
- Affected by exposure to the environment, including time it takes to place thermometer
- Underestimates core temperature

Skin

Advantages

- Inexpensive
- Provides continuous reading
- Safe and noninvasive
- Used for neonates

Limitations

- Measurement lags behind other sites during temperature changes, especially during hyperthermia
- Impaired adhesion from diaphoresis or sweat
- Affected by environmental temperature
- Cannot be used for patients with allergy to adhesives

Temporal Artery

Advantages

- Easy to access without position change
- Provides a considerable reduction in required nursing time to measure (Hayes, Shepard, Cesarec, et al., 2017)
- Comfortable with no risk of injury to patient or nurse
- Eliminates need for patient to disrobe or unbundle
- Can be used for premature infants, newborns, and children; however, axillary temperature measurement is the most accurate method (Otto, 2017)
- Reflects rapid change in core temperature
- Sensor cover not required

Limitations

- Inaccurate with head covering or hair on forehead
- Affected by skin moisture such as diaphoresis or sweating
- Use not recommended when accurate measurement of body temperature is required to make informed clinical decisions (Niven et al., 2015)

BOX 7.4

Types of Thermometers

Electronic Thermometer (Fig. 7.2)

- The thermometer is a rechargeable battery-powered display unit with a thin wire cord and a temperature-processing probe covered by a disposable cover.
- Within 1 minute after placement the thermometer displays a digital temperature reading.
- Separate probes are available for oral and axillary temperature measurement (blue tip) and rectal temperature measurement (red tip).

Tympanic Membrane Thermometer

- The probe consists of an otoscope-like speculum with an infrared sensor tip that detects heat radiated from the tympanic membrane of the ear (Fig. 7.3).
- Within seconds after placing in the ear canal and depressing the scan button, a digital reading appears on the display unit. A sound signals when the peak temperature has been measured.

Temporal Artery Thermometer

- An infrared scanner is swept across the forehead, lifted, and then placed behind the ear. If the patient is diaphoretic, a scan just behind the ear verifies the measurement accuracy (Fig. 7.4).

- Within seconds after scanning, a digital reading appears on the display unit.

Chemical Dot Single-Use or Reusable Thermometer

- The thermometer consists of thin strips of plastic with a temperature sensor at one end and chemically impregnated dots formulated to change colour at different temperatures, usually within 60 seconds (Fig. 7.5).
- It is useful for screening temperatures, especially in infants, during invasive procedures, for a patient on protective isolation, and in orally intubated critical care patients.
- It is not appropriate for monitoring fever in acutely ill patients or for temperature therapies.
- It can be used at axillary or rectal site if covered by a plastic sheath with a placement time of 3 minutes.
- Home disposable thermometers are useful for temperature screening but are not as accurate as nondisposable electronic thermometers (Counts et al., 2014).

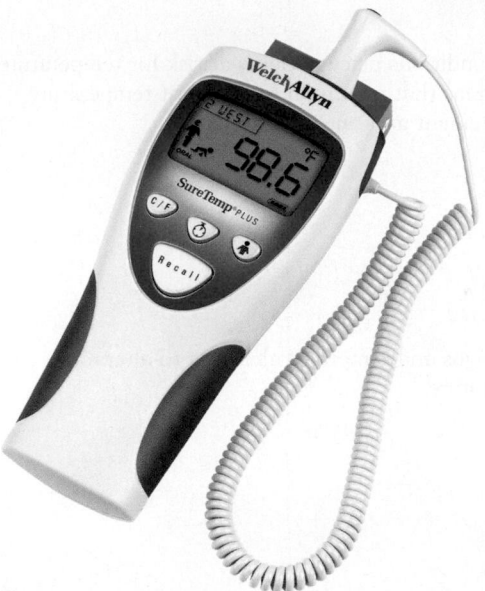

FIG 7.2 Electronic thermometer with disposable plastic probe cover. (*Photo courtesy Welch Allyn.*)

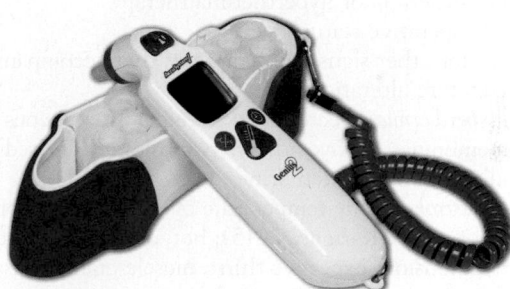

FIG 7.3 Tympanic membrane thermometer with disposable plastic probe cover. (*Copyright © Covidien. All rights reserved.*)

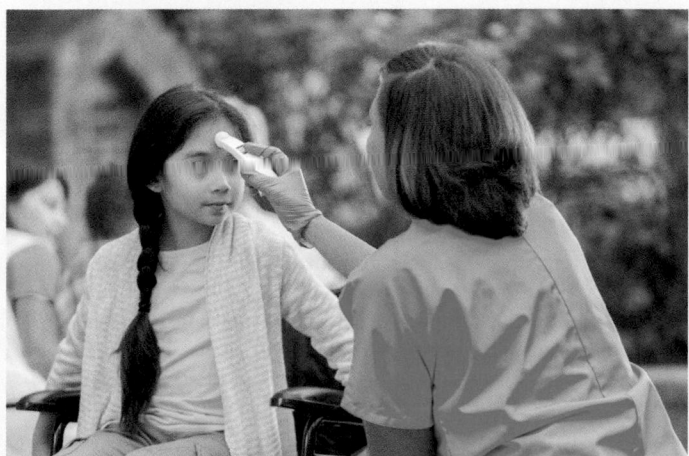

FIG 7.4 A temporal artery thermometer measures the heat from blood flowing through the superficial temporal artery. (*Steve Debenport/ iStockphoto*)

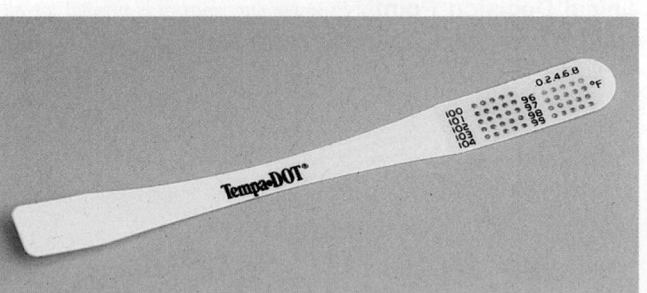

FIG 7.5 Chemical dot, disposable, single-use thermometer.

Delegation and Collaboration

The skill of temperature measurement can be delegated to an unregulated care provider (UCP). The nurse instructs the UCP by:

- Communicating the appropriate route, device, and frequency of temperature measurement.
- Explaining any precautions needed in positioning the patient (e.g., for rectal temperature measurement).
- Reviewing the usual temperature values and significant changes to report to the nurse.

Equipment

- Thermometer (selected based on site used; see Box 7.3)
- Soft tissue or wipe
- Alcohol swab
- Water-soluble lubricant (for rectal measurements only)
- Pen and vital sign flow sheet, record form, or electronic health record (EHR)
- Clean gloves (optional), plastic thermometer sleeve, disposable probe or sensor cover
- Towel

STEP	RATIONALE

ASSESSMENT

STEP	RATIONALE
1. Identify patient using at least two person-specific identifiers (e.g., name and date of birth or name and medical record number) according to employer policy.	Ensures correct patient. Complies with Accreditation Canada's standards and improves patient safety (Accreditation Canada, 2019).
2. Determine need to measure patient's body temperature:	
a. Note patient's risks for temperature alterations: • Expected or diagnosed infection • Open wounds or burns • White blood cell count below $5–10 \times 10^9$/L • Immunosuppressive drug therapy • Injury to hypothalamus • Exposure to temperature extremes • Blood product infusion • Hypothermia or hyperthermia therapy • Postoperative status	Certain conditions place patients at risk for temperature alterations that require more frequent temperature measurement and nursing assessment.
b. Assess for other signs and symptoms that accompany temperature alteration: • *Hyperthermia:* Decreased skin turgor, dry mucous membranes; tachycardia; hypotension; decreased venous filling; concentrated urine • *Heatstroke:* Body temperature of 40°C (104°F) or more (Goforth & Kazman, 2015); hot, dry skin; tachycardia; hypotension; excessive thirst; muscle cramps; visual disturbances; confusion or delirium • *Hypothermia:* Pale skin; skin cool or cold to touch; bradycardia and dysrhythmias; uncontrollable shivering; reduced level of consciousness; shallow respirations	Physical signs and symptoms alert you to alterations in body temperature.
c. Assess for factors that normally influence temperature:	Allows you to accurately assess for presence and significance of temperature alteration.
• Age	Older persons have narrower range of temperature than younger persons.

Clinical Decision Point *No single temperature is normal for all people. A temperature within an acceptable range in an adult may reflect a fever in an older person. Undeveloped temperature-control mechanisms in infants and children cause temperature to rise and fall rapidly.*

STEP	RATIONALE
• Exercise	Muscle activity increases metabolism, which increases heat production and raises temperature.
• Hormones	Females have wider temperature fluctuations than males because of menstrual cycle hormonal changes, because body temperature varies during menopause, and because women have a thicker layer of subcutaneous fat.
• Stress	Stress elevates temperature.
• Medications	Some drugs impair or promote sweating, vasoconstriction, or vasodilation or interfere with ability of hypothalamus to regulate temperature.

STEP	RATIONALE

ASSESSMENT

• Daily fluctuations	Body temperature normally changes 0.5° to 1°C (0.9° to 1.8°F) during a 24-hour period. Temperature is lowest during early morning. Most patients have maximum temperature elevation between 5 PM and 7 PM; temperature falls gradually during night.
• Damage to the hypothalamus	Damage to the hypothalamus caused by nervous system trauma, intracerebral bleeding, and increased intracranial pressure can cause a fever (sometimes called a neurogenic fever). This is a fever of high temperature where the patient does not sweat, and it is resistant antipyretics (Hannon & Porth, 2017).
• Environment	Environment influences body temperature. Infants, older persons, and those with spinal cord injuries are most likely to be affected as their temperature-regulating mechanisms are less efficient. People with spinal cord injuries are often poikilothermic (body temperature adjusts to the temperature in the surrounding environment). The higher the level of injury the greater the degree of poikilothermism, with high cervical injuries having a greater loss of ability to regulate temperature (Lewis et al., 2019).
3. Determine appropriate measurement site and device for patient (see Box 7.3). Use disposable thermometer for patient on isolation precautions.	Determines if patient's status contraindicates selection of a specific method or site.
4. Determine previous baseline temperature and measurement site (if available) from patient's record.	Allows you to assess for change in condition. Provides comparison with future temperature measurements.
5. Assess patient's knowledge of procedure.	Encourages cooperation; minimizes risks and anxiety. Identifies teaching needs.

NURSING DIAGNOSES

• Hyperthermia	• Potential for hyperthermia	• Potential for perioperative hypothermia
• Hypothermia	• Potential for imbalanced body temperature	
• Inadequate thermoregulation		

Related factors/Risk factors are individualized on the basis of patient's condition or needs.

PLANNING

1. Expected outcomes following completion of procedure:	
• Body temperature is within acceptable range for patient's age group.	Thermoregulation is maintained.
• Body temperature returns to baseline range following therapies for abnormal temperature.	Environmental factors that alter temperature are controlled.
2. Explain to patient how you will measure temperature and the importance of maintaining proper position until reading is complete.	Promotes patient cooperation and increases adherence to procedure. Patients are often curious about their temperatures and should be cautioned against prematurely removing thermometer to read results.
3. Collect and bring appropriate supplies to patient's bedside.	Ensures an organized approach for body temperature measurement.
4. Verify that patient has not had anything to eat or drink in the last 20 minutes and has not chewed gum for 5 minutes or smoked within the past 2 minutes (Potter et al., 2019) if having oral temperature measured.	Oral food and fluids, smoking, and gum can alter oral temperature measurement (Potter et al., 2019).

IMPLEMENTATION

1. Perform hand hygiene.	Reduces transmission of microorganisms.
2. Help patient to comfortable position that provides easy access to temperature measurement site.	Ensures patient's comfort and accuracy of temperature reading.

STEP	RATIONALE

IMPLEMENTATION

3. Obtain temperature reading.
   a. **Oral temperature (electronic):**
      (1) *Optional:* Apply clean gloves when there is risk for exposure to respiratory secretions or facial or mouth wound drainage.

      (2) Remove thermometer pack from charging unit. Attach oral thermometer probe stem (blue tip) to thermometer unit. Grasp top of probe stem, being careful not to apply pressure on ejection button.

      (3) Slide disposable plastic probe cover over thermometer probe stem until cover locks in place (see illustration).

      (4) Ask patient to open mouth; gently place thermometer probe under tongue in posterior sublingual pocket lateral to centre of lower jaw (see illustration).

      (5) Ask patient to hold thermometer probe with lips closed.

      (6) Leave thermometer probe in place until audible signal indicates completion and patient's temperature appears on digital display; remove thermometer probe from under patient's tongue.

      (7) Push ejection button on thermometer probe stem to discard plastic probe cover into appropriate receptacle.

      (8) If wearing gloves, remove, dispose in appropriate receptacle, and perform hand hygiene.

      (9) Return thermometer probe stem to storage position of thermometer unit.

      (10) If possible, use a disposable single-use thermometer for patients when there is a risk of exposure or transmission of infection. If disposable or dedicated equipment is not available, clean and disinfect the equipment before use on another patient (CDC, 2017b).

An oral probe cover is removable without physical contact, thus does not require gloves.

Charging provides battery power. Ejection button releases plastic cover from probe stem.

Soft plastic cover will not break in patient's mouth and prevents transmission of microorganisms between patients.

Heat from superficial blood vessels in sublingual pocket produces temperature reading. With electronic thermometer, temperatures in right and left posterior sublingual pocket are significantly higher than in area under front of tongue.

Maintains proper position of thermometer during recording.

Probe must stay in place until signal occurs to ensure accurate reading.

Reduces transmission of microorganisms.

Reduces transmission of microorganisms.

Protects probe stem from damage. Returning thermometer probe stem automatically causes digital reading to disappear.

Reduces transmission of microorganisms.

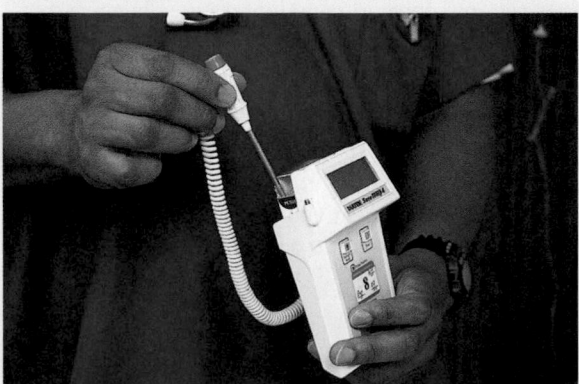

STEP 3a(3) Nurse inserts electronic thermometer probe stem into probe cover. Cover snaps in place.

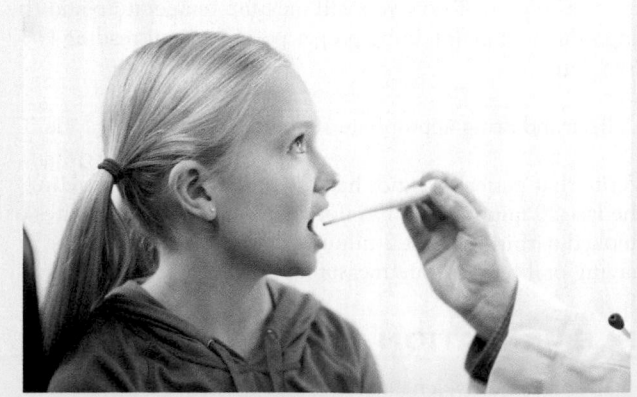

STEP 3a(4) Probe placed under tongue in posterior sublingual pocket. *(YinYang/iStockphoto)*

STEP	RATIONALE

IMPLEMENTATION

b. Rectal temperature (electronic):

(1) Draw curtain around bed and close room door. Help patient to side-lying or Sims' position with upper leg flexed. Move aside bed linen to expose only anal area. Keep patient's upper body and lower extremities covered with sheet or blanket.

Maintains patient's privacy, minimizes embarrassment, and promotes person-centred care and comfort.

(2) Apply clean gloves. Cleanse anal region when feces or secretions are present. Remove soiled gloves and reapply clean gloves.

Maintains standard precautions when exposed to items soiled with body fluids (e.g., feces).

(3) Remove thermometer pack from charging unit. Attach rectal thermometer probe stem (red tip) to thermometer unit. Grasp top of probe stem, being careful not to apply pressure on ejection button.

Ejection button releases plastic cover from probe stem.

(4) Slide disposable plastic probe cover over thermometer probe stem until cover locks in place.

Soft plastic probe cover prevents transmission of microorganisms between patients.

(5) Using a single-use package, squeeze a liberal amount of lubricant on tissue. Dip probe cover of thermometer, blunt end, into lubricant, covering 2.5 to 3.5 cm (1 to 1½ inches) for adult.

Lubrication minimizes trauma to rectal mucosa during insertion. Tissue avoids contamination of remaining lubricant in container.

(6) With nondominant hand separate patient's buttocks to expose anus. Ask patient to breathe slowly and relax.

Fully exposes anus for thermometer insertion. Relaxes anal sphincter for easier thermometer insertion.

(7) Gently insert thermometer into anus in direction of umbilicus 3.5 cm (1½ inches) for adult. Do not force thermometer.

Ensures adequate exposure against blood vessels in rectal wall.

(8) If you feel resistance during insertion, withdraw immediately. Never force thermometer.

Prevents trauma to mucosa.

Clinical Decision Point *If you cannot adequately insert thermometer into rectum or resistance is felt during insertion, remove thermometer and consider alternative method for obtaining temperature.*

(9) Once positioned, hold thermometer probe in place until audible signal indicates completion and patient's temperature appears on digital display; remove thermometer probe from anus (see illustration).

Probe must stay in place until signal occurs to ensure accurate reading.

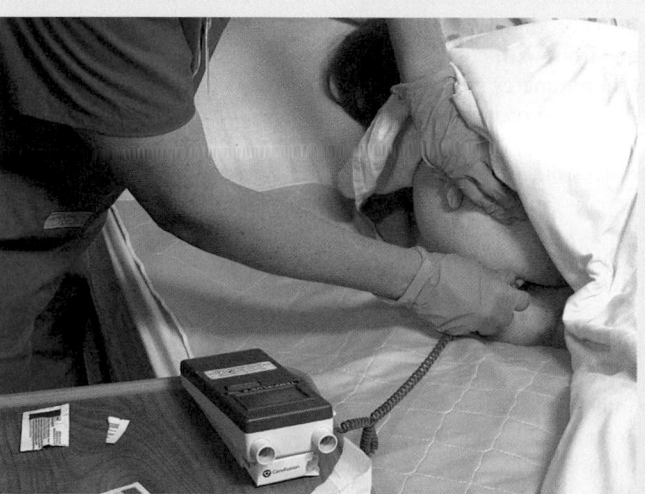

STEP 3b(9) Probe inserted into anus.

STEP	RATIONALE

IMPLEMENTATION

STEP	RATIONALE
(10) Push ejection button on thermometer stem to discard plastic probe cover into appropriate receptacle. Wipe probe stem with alcohol swab, paying particular attention to ridges where probe stem connects to probe, then remove gloves.	Reduces transmission of microorganisms.
(11) Return thermometer stem to storage position of recording unit. Don new gloves.	Protects probe stem from damage. Returning thermometer stem automatically causes digital reading to disappear.
(12) Wipe patient's anal area with soft tissue to remove lubricant or feces and discard tissue. Help patient to assume a comfortable position.	Provides for comfort and hygiene.
(13) Remove and dispose of gloves in appropriate receptacle. Perform hand hygiene.	Reduces transmission of microorganisms.
(14) If possible, use a disposable single-use thermometer for patients when there is a risk of exposure to or possible transmission of infection. If disposable or dedicated equipment is not available, clean and disinfect the equipment before use on another patient (CDC, 2017b).	

c. Axillary temperature (electronic):

STEP	RATIONALE
(1) Draw curtain around bed and close room door. Help patient to supine or sitting position. Move clothing or gown away from shoulder and arm.	Maintains patient's privacy, minimizes embarrassment, and promotes comfort. Exposes axilla for correct thermometer probe placement.
(2) Remove thermometer pack from charging unit. Attach oral thermometer probe stem (blue tip) to thermometer unit. Grasp top of thermometer probe stem, being careful not to apply pressure on ejection button.	Charging provides battery power. Ejection button releases plastic cover from probe stem.
(3) Slide disposable plastic probe cover over thermometer stem until cover locks in place.	Soft plastic probe cover prevents transmission of microorganisms between patients.
(4) Raise patient's arm away from torso. Inspect for skin lesions and excessive perspiration; if needed, dry axilla or select alternative site. Insert thermometer probe into centre of axilla (see illustration), lower arm over probe, and place arm across patient's chest.	Maintains proper position of thermometer against blood vessels in axilla.

Clinical Decision Point *Do not use axilla if skin lesions are present because local temperature is sometimes altered and area may be painful to touch.*

STEP	RATIONALE
(5) Once thermometer probe is positioned, hold it in place until audible signal indicates completion and patient's temperature appears on digital display; remove thermometer probe from axilla.	Thermometer probe must stay in place until signal occurs to ensure accurate reading.
(6) Push ejection button on thermometer stem to discard plastic probe cover into appropriate receptacle.	Reduces transmission of microorganisms.
(7) Return thermometer stem to storage position of recording unit.	Returning thermometer stem to storage position automatically causes digital reading to disappear. Protects stem from damage.
(8) Help patient to assume comfortable position, replacing linen or gown.	Restores comfort and sense of well-being.
(9) Perform hand hygiene.	Reduces transmission of microorganisms.
(10) If possible, use a disposable single-use thermometer for patients when there is a risk of exposure to or possible transmission of infection. If disposable or dedicated equipment is not available, clean and disinfect the equipment before use on another patient (CDC, 2017b).	

STEP	RATIONALE

IMPLEMENTATION

d. Tympanic membrane temperature:

(1) Help patient to assume comfortable position with head turned toward side, away from you. If patient has been lying on one side, use other ear. Obtain temperature from patient's right ear if you are right-handed. Obtain temperature from patient's left ear if you are left-handed.

Ensures comfort and facilitates exposure of auditory canal for accurate temperature measurement.
Heat trapped in ear facing down causes false-high temperature reading.
The less acute the angle of approach, the better the probe seal.

(2) Note if there is an obvious presence of cerumen (earwax) in patient's ear canal.

Cerumen impedes lens cover of speculum. Switch to other ear or select alternative measurement site.

(3) Remove thermometer handheld unit from charging base, being careful not to apply pressure to ejection button.

Charging base provides battery power. Removal of handheld unit from base prepares it to measure temperature. Ejection button releases plastic probe cover from thermometer tip.

(4) Slide disposable speculum cover over otoscope-like lens tip until it locks in place. Be careful not to touch lens cover.

Soft plastic probe cover prevents transmission of microorganisms between patients. Lens cover should not have dust, fingerprints, or cerumen obstructing optical pathway.

(5) Insert speculum into ear canal following manufacturer instructions for tympanic probe positioning (see illustration):

Correct positioning of probe with respect to ear canal allows maximal exposure of tympanic membrane.

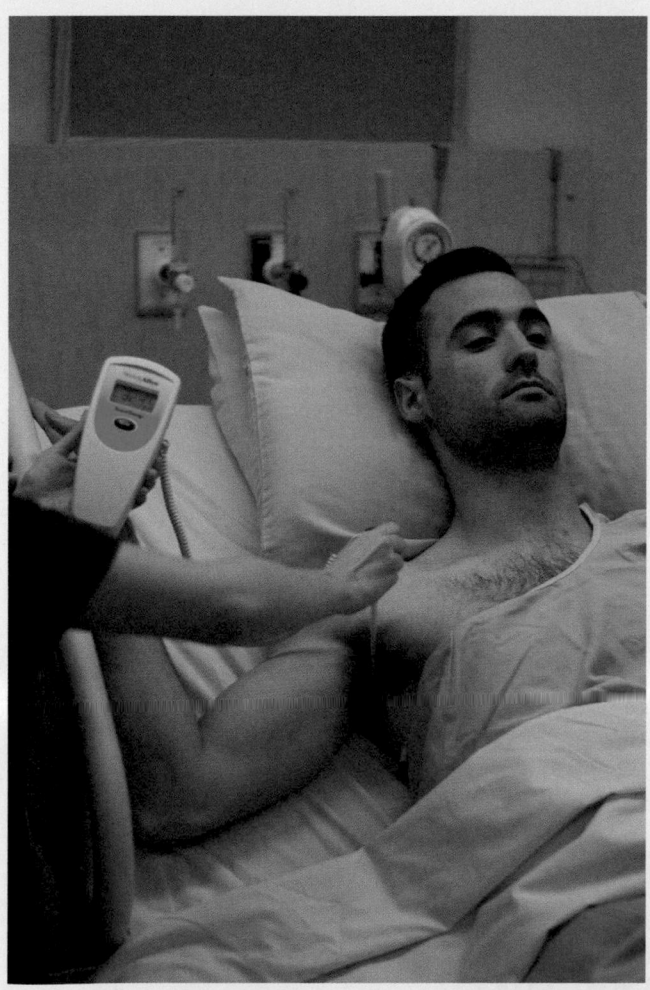

STEP 3c(4) Insert thermometer probe into centre of axilla. (*Courtesy Barbara J. Astle, RN, PhD.*)

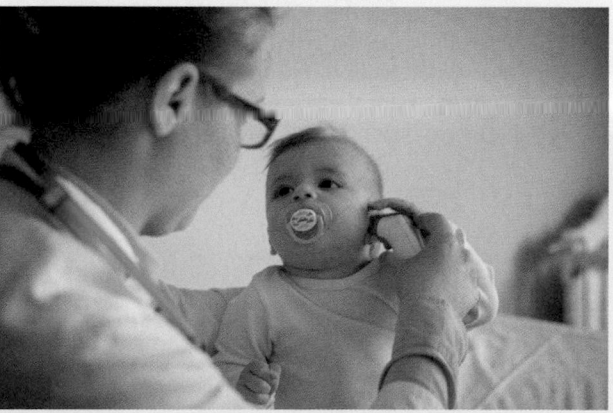

STEP 3d(5) Tympanic membrane thermometer with probe cover placed in patient's ear. (*aywan88/iStockphoto*)

STEP	RATIONALE

IMPLEMENTATION

(a) Pull ear pinna backward, up, and out for an adult. For children less than 3 years of age, pull pinna down and back; point covered probe toward midpoint between eyebrow and sideburns. For children older than 3 years, pull pinna up and back (Hockenberry & Wilson, 2015).

Ear tug straightens external auditory canal, allowing maximum exposure of tympanic membrane and therefore correctly positioning speculum (Hockenberry & Wilson, 2015).

(b) Fit speculum tip snug in canal, pointing toward nose.

Gentle pressure seals ear canal from ambient air temperature, which alters readings as much as 2.8°C (5°F).

(c) Move thermometer in figure-eight pattern.

Some manufacturers recommend movement of speculum tip in figure-eight pattern that allows sensor to detect maximum tympanic membrane heat radiation.

(6) Once positioned, press scan button on handheld unit. Leave speculum in place until audible signal indicates completion and patient's temperature appears on digital display.

Pressing scan button causes detection of infrared energy. Speculum probe tip must stay in place until device has detected infrared energy noted by audible signal.

(7) Carefully remove speculum from auditory meatus. Push ejection button on handheld unit to discard speculum cover into appropriate receptacle.

Reduces transmission of microorganisms. Automatically causes digital reading to disappear.

(8) If temperature is abnormal or second reading is necessary, replace probe cover and wait 2 minutes before repeating in same ear or repeat measurement in other ear. Consider an alternative temperature site or instrument.

Lens cover must be free of cerumen to maintain optical path. Time allows ear canal to regain usual temperature.

(9) Return handheld unit to thermometer base.

Protects sensor tip from damage.

(10) Help patient assume comfortable position.

Restores comfort and sense of well-being.

(11) Perform hand hygiene.

Reduces transmission of microorganisms.

(12) Disinfect thermometer unit regularly when visibly soiled, after every use or once daily (CDC, 2017b).

e. Temporal artery temperature:

(1) Ensure that forehead is dry; dry with towel if needed.

Moisture interferes with thermometer sensor.

(2) Place sensor firmly on patient's forehead.

Flush contact avoids measurement of ambient temperature.

(3) Press red scan button with your thumb. Slowly slide thermometer straight across forehead while keeping sensor flat and firmly on skin (see Fig. 7.4). Keeping scan button depressed, lift sensor after sweeping forehead and touch sensor on neck just behind earlobe. Read temperature when clicking sound during scanning stops. Release scan button.

Thermometer continuously scans for highest temperature when scan button is depressed. Area behind earlobe is less affected by diaphoresis and verifies temperature.

(4) Gently clean sensor with alcohol swab, return to storage unit, and perform hand hygiene.

Prevents transmission of microorganisms.

(5) If possible, use a disposable single-use sensor for patients on isolation precautions or disinfect before using it on another patient (CDC, 2017b).

4. Inform patient of temperature reading and record measurement.

Promotes participation in care and understanding of health status.

5. Return thermometer to charger.

Maintains battery charge of thermometer unit.

STEP	RATIONALE

EVALUATION

1. If you are assessing temperature for the first time, establish it as baseline if it is within acceptable range.

   Used to compare future temperature measurements.

2. Compare temperature reading with patient's previous baseline and acceptable temperature range for patient's age group.

   Body temperature fluctuates within narrow range; comparison reveals presence of abnormality. Improper placement or movement of thermometer can cause inaccuracies. Second measurement confirms initial findings of abnormal body temperature.

3. If patient has fever, take temperature approximately 30 minutes after administering antipyretics and every 4 hours until temperature stabilizes.

   Determines if temperature begins to fall in response to therapy.

4. **Use Teach-Back**: "I want to be sure I explained how to check your child's temperature at home. Show me how to swipe his forehead using the thermometer." Develop a revised teaching plan if caregiver is not able to teach back correctly.

   Determines caregiver's level of understanding of instructional topic.

Unexpected Outcomes

1. Patient has temperature 1°C (1.8°F) or more above usual range.

2. Patient has temperature 1°C (1.8°F) or more below usual range.

3. Unable to obtain temperature.

Related Interventions

- Initiate measures to lower body temperature:
  - Cool room environment.
  - Reduce external covering on patient's body to promote heat loss but do not induce shivering.
  - Keep clothing and bed linen dry.
  - Apply hypothermia blanket as prescribed.
  - Limit physical activity and sources of emotional stress.
  - Administer antipyretics as prescribed.
  - Increase fluid intake to at least 3 L daily (unless contraindicated).
  - Initiate measures to stimulate appetite and provide nutrients to meet increased energy needs.
  - Prevent or control spread of infection.
- Initiate measures to raise body temperature:
  - Apply warm blankets and, unless contraindicated, offer warm liquids.
  - Apply hyperthermia blankets if prescribed.
  - Remove wet clothing or linen.
- Reassess correct placement of temperature probe or sensor.
- Choose alternative temperature measurement site.
- Obtain alternative temperature measurement device.

Communication and Documentation

- Document temperature and route on vital sign flow sheet or in nurses' notes in EHR or chart.
- Report abnormal findings to nurse in charge or health care provider.
- Document your evaluation of patient and caregiver learning.

Special Considerations
Teaching

- Identify patient's ability to initiate preventive health measures and recognize alteration in body temperature. Educate patient and caregiver about measures to prevent body temperature alterations.
- Educate patients about risk factors for hypothermia and frostbite: fatigue; malnutrition; hypoxemia; cold, wet clothing; alcohol intoxication.
- Educate patients about risk factors for heatstroke: strenuous exercise in hot, humid weather; tight-fitting clothing in hot environments; exercising in poorly ventilated areas; sudden exposures to hot climates; poor fluid intake before, during, and after exercise.

- Educate patients regarding importance of taking and continuing antibiotics as directed until course of treatment for infection is completed.

Pediatric

- Infants and young children may lose more heat to the environment because of their increased body surface area/volume ratios.
- Critically ill children sometimes have cool skin but a high core temperature because of poor perfusion to the skin.
- Use axillary temperatures for screening purposes only; axillary temperature should not be relied on to detect a fever in children.
- Children may assume prone position for rectal temperature measurement.
- With children who cry or become restless, it is best to take temperature as the last vital sign.

Gerontological

- The temperature of older persons is at the lower end of the acceptable temperature range: 36°C (96.8°F).
- Temperatures considered within normal range often reflect a fever in an older person.

- Adults without teeth or older persons with poor muscle control may be unable to close their mouth tightly enough to obtain accurate oral temperature readings.
- Older persons are very sensitive to slight changes in environmental temperature because their thermoregulatory systems are not as efficient (Touhy, Jett, Boscart, et al., 2019, pp. 195–96).
- Oral temperature measurement is more reliable in older persons because cerumen tends to be drier and cilia become stiff, contributing to buildup of cerumen impaction, which interferes with accurate tympanic temperature measurement.
- A decrease in sweat gland activity in the older person results in a higher threshold for sweating at high temperatures, which can lead to hyperthermia.
- With aging a loss of subcutaneous fat reduces the insulating capacity of the skin.

- Older persons are at high risk for hypothermia because of diminished sensation to cold, abnormal vasoconstrictor responses, and impaired shivering.

Care in the Community

- Assess temperature and ventilation of patient's environment to determine existence of any environmental conditions that influence patient's temperature.
- In the home, some patients continue to use mercury-in-glass thermometers. Assess safe storage of these thermometers to protect from breakage and mercury spills. Educate patient and caregiver on proper use of the thermometer, mercury hazards, and proper disposal of any mercury-containing devices. Suggest alternative temperature measurement devices for home use.

✦ SKILL 7.2 Assessing Radial Pulse

▶ *Video Clip* **NSO** *Nursing Skills Online Vital Signs Module 1, Lesson 3*

The ejection of blood from the heart distends the walls of the aorta. Because of the force of the blood exiting the heart, aortic distension creates a pulse wave that travels rapidly toward the extremities. When the pulse wave reaches a peripheral artery, you can feel it by palpating the artery lightly against underlying bone or muscle. The pulse is the palpable bounding of the blood flow. The number of pulsing sensations occurring in 1 minute is the pulse rate.

Assessing a patient's peripheral pulses determines the integrity of the cardiovascular system. An abnormally slow, rapid, or irregular pulse indicates the inability of the heart to deliver adequate blood to the body; a pulse deficit may be present. The strength or amplitude of a pulse reflects the volume of blood ejected against the arterial wall with each heart contraction. If the volume decreases, the pulse

often becomes weak and difficult to palpate. In contrast, a full bounding pulse is an indication of increased volume.

The integrity of peripheral pulses indicates the status of blood perfusion to the area distributed by the pulse (Table 7.1). For example, assessment of the right femoral pulse determines whether blood flow to the right leg is adequate. If a peripheral pulse distal to an injured or treated area of an extremity feels weak on palpation, the volume of blood reaching tissues below the affected area may be inadequate, and surgical intervention may be necessary.

While any artery can be used to assess for pulse rate, the radial and carotid arteries are commonly used because they are easy to palpate (Fig. 7.6). When a patient's condition suddenly worsens, the carotid site is recommended for finding a pulse quickly.

TABLE 7.1

Pulse Sites

Site	Location	Rationale for Selection
Temporal	Over temporal bone of head, above and lateral to eyebrow	Easily accessible site to assess pulse in children
Carotid	Along medial edge of sternocleidomastoid muscle in neck	Easily accessible site to assess character of peripheral pulse; used during physiological shock or cardiac arrest when other sites are not palpable
Apical	Fourth to fifth intercostal space at left midclavicular line	Site used to auscultate apical pulse
Brachial	Groove between biceps and triceps muscles at antecubital fossa	Site used to auscultate upper-extremity blood pressure; assesses status of circulation to lower arm
Radial	Radial or thumb side of forearm at wrist	Common site to assess character of peripheral pulse; assesses status of circulation to hand
Ulnar	Ulnar side of forearm at wrist	Site used to assess status of circulation to ulnar side of hand; used to perform Allen's test
Femoral	Below inguinal ligament, midway between symphysis pubis and anterior superior iliac spine	Site used to assess character of pulse during physiological shock or cardiac arrest when other pulses are not palpable; assesses status of circulation to leg
Popliteal	Behind knee in popliteal fossa	Site used to auscultate lower-extremity blood pressure; assesses status of circulation to lower leg
Posterior tibial	Inner side of each ankle, below medial malleolus	Site used to assess status of circulation to foot
Dorsalis pedis	Along top of foot between extension tendons of great and first toe	Site used to assess status of circulation to foot

Assessment of other peripheral pulse sites, such as the brachial or femoral artery, is unnecessary when routinely obtaining vital signs. Other peripheral pulses are assessed when a complete physical examination (see Chapter 8) is conducted or when the radial artery is not available for assessment because of surgery, trauma, or impaired blood flow.

Delegation and Collaboration

The skill of radial pulse measurement can be delegated to an unregulated care provider (UCP) if a patient's condition is stable. The skill cannot be delegated when a patient's condition is unstable (e.g., acute cardiac problem) or when the nurse is evaluating a patient's response to a treatment or medication. The nurse instructs the UCP by:

• Indicating the appropriate site for measuring pulse rate; frequency of measurement; and factors related to the patient history, such as risk for abnormally slow, rapid, or irregular pulse.
• Reviewing patient's usual pulse rate and significant changes to report to the nurse.
• Reviewing the specific changes or abnormalities to report to the nurse for further assessment.

Equipment

• Wristwatch with second hand or digital display
• Pen and vital sign flow sheet in chart or electronic health record (EHR)

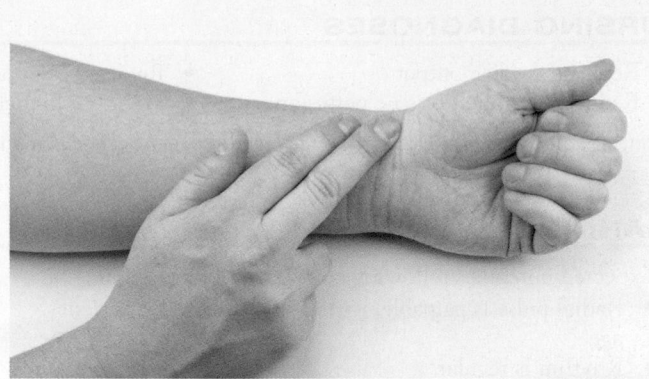

FIG 7.6 Palpating radial pulse. *(Maksim Sheliakin/iStockphoto)*

STEP	RATIONALE

ASSESSMENT

1. Identify patient using at least two person-specific identifiers (e.g., name and date of birth or name and medical record number) according to employer policy.

Ensures correct patient. Complies with Accreditation Canada's standards and improves patient safety (Accreditation Canada, 2019).

2. Determine need to assess radial pulse:
   a. Assess for any risk factors for pulse alterations:
   • History of heart disease
   • Cardiac dysrhythmia
   • Onset of sudden chest pain or acute pain from any site
   • Invasive cardiovascular diagnostic tests
   • Surgery
   • Sudden infusion of large volume of intravenous (IV) fluid
   • Internal or external hemorrhage
   • Administration of medications that alter cardiac function

Certain conditions place patients at risk for pulse alterations. A history of peripheral vascular disease often alters pulse rate and quality.

   b. Assess for signs and symptoms of altered cardiac function such as presence of dyspnea, fatigue, chest pain, orthopnea, syncope, palpitations, edema of dependent body parts, cyanosis or pallor of skin (see Chapter 8).

Physical signs and symptoms often indicate alteration in cardiac function, which affects radial pulse rate and rhythm

   c. Assess for signs and symptoms of peripheral vascular disease such as pale, cool extremities; thin, shiny skin with decreased hair growth; thickened nails.

Physical signs and symptoms indicate alteration in local arterial blood flow.

   d. Assess for factors that influence radial pulse rate and rhythm: age, exercise, position changes, fluid balance, medications, temperature, sympathetic stimulation (e.g., caffeine or nicotine).

Anticipate factors that alter pulse, ensuring accurate interpretation.
Dysrhythmics, cardiotonics, antihypertensives, vasodilators, and vasoconstrictors affect pulse rate and rhythm.

3. Determine patient's previous baseline pulse rate (if available) from patient's record.

Allows you to assess for change in condition. Provides comparison with future pulse measurements.

4. If you anticipate need for patient or caregiver to monitor heart rate at home, assess their knowledge of the procedure and rationale for measurement.

Determines need for patient or caregiver instruction.

STEP	RATIONALE

NURSING DIAGNOSES

- Reduced cardiac output
- Reduced peripheral tissue perfusion
- Reduced stamina
- Potential for dehydration
- Insufficient knowledge regarding pulse assessment

Related factors are individualized on the basis of patient's condition and needs.

PLANNING

1. Expected outcomes following completion of procedure:
   - Radial pulse is palpable, within usual range for patient's age.
   - Rhythm is regular.
   - Radial pulse is strong, firm, and elastic.
2. Explain to patient that you will assess radial pulse rate (heart rate [HR]). Encourage patient to relax as much as possible. If patient has been active, wait 5 to 10 minutes before assessing pulse. If patient has been smoking or ingesting caffeine, wait 15 minutes before assessing pulse.
3. Collect appropriate equipment and bring to patient's bedside

Usual range for adults is 60 to 100 beats/min.

Cardiac status is stable.
Radial artery is patent.
Anxiety, activity, caffeine, and smoking elevate heart rate. Assessing radial pulse rate at rest allows for objective comparison of values.

Ensures an organized approach for assessing a radial pulse.

IMPLEMENTATION

1. Perform hand hygiene.
2. If necessary, draw curtain around bed or close door.

3. Help patient to assume a supine or sitting position.
4. If patient is supine, place their forearm straight alongside or across lower chest or upper abdomen (see illustration A). If sitting, bend patient's elbow 90 degrees and support lower arm on chair or on your arm. Place tips of first two or middle three fingers of hand over groove along radial or thumb side of patient's inner wrist (see illustration B). Slightly extend or flex wrist with palm down until you note strongest pulse.
5. Lightly compress pulse against radius, losing pulse initially; relax pressure so pulse becomes easily palpable.

Reduces transmission of micro-organisms.
Maintains privacy and minimizes embarrassment. Helps patient relax.
Provides easy access to pulse sites.
Fingertips are most sensitive parts of hand to palpate arterial pulsation. Your thumb has pulsation that interferes with accuracy.

Pulse assessment is more accurate when using moderate pressure. Too much pressure occludes pulse and impairs blood flow.

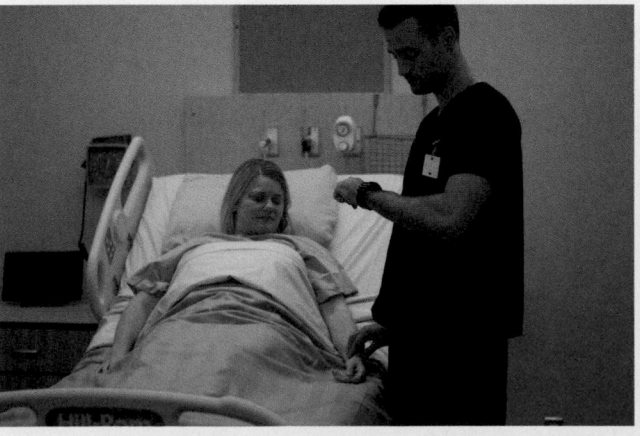
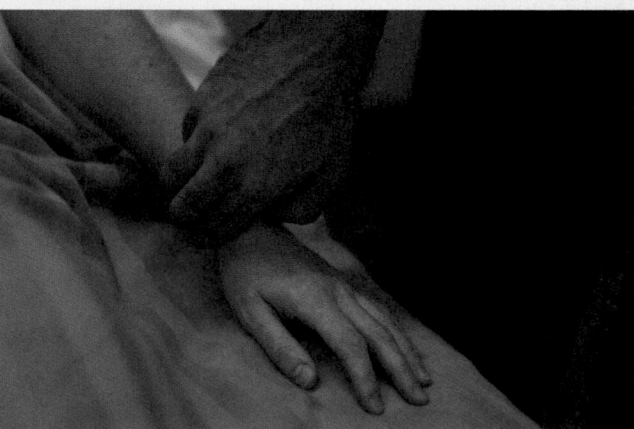

STEP 4 A, Pulse check with patient's forearm at side with wrist extended. **B,** Hand placement for pulse check. (*Courtesy Barbara J. Astle, RN, PhD.*)

STEP	RATIONALE

IMPLEMENTATION

6. Determine strength of pulse. Note whether thrust of vessel against fingertips is bounding (4+); full increased, strong (3+); expected (2+); barely palpable, diminished (1+); or absent, not palpable (0).

Strength reflects volume of blood ejected against arterial wall with each heart contraction. Decreased stroke volume (e.g., shock) is indicated by a "weak thready" pulse, while increased stroke volume (e.g., anxiety, exercise and some abnormal conditions) is indicated by a "full bounding pulse" (Jarvis, 2019). Accurate description of strength improves communication, patient safety, and interprofessional collaboration.

7. After palpating a regular pulse, look at watch second hand and begin to count rate. Count the first beat after the second hand hits the number on the dial; count as one, then two, and so on.

Rate is determined accurately only after pulse has been palpated. Timing begins with zero. Count of one is first beat palpated after timing begins.

8. If pulse is regular, count rate for 30 seconds and multiply total by 2.

A 30-second count is accurate for rapid, slow, or regular pulse rates.

9. If pulse is irregular, count rate for a full 60 seconds. Assess frequency and pattern of irregularity.

Inefficient contraction of heart fails to transmit pulse wave, resulting in irregular pulse. Longer time ensures accurate count.

10. When pulse is irregular, compare radial pulses bilaterally and assess apical pulse for 1 full minute.

A marked difference between pulses indicates that arterial flow is compromised to one extremity, and as a nurse you need to take action.

11. Help patient return to comfortable position.

Promotes comfort and sense of well-being.

12. Discuss findings with patient.

Promotes participation in care and understanding of health status.

13. Perform hand hygiene.

Reduces transmission of microorganisms.

EVALUATION

1. If assessing pulse for first time, establish radial pulse as baseline if it is within acceptable range.

Used to compare future pulse assessments.

2. Compare pulse rate and character with patient's previous baseline and acceptable range for patient's age.

Allows for assessment of change in patient's condition and presence of cardiac alteration.

3. **Use Teach-Back:** "I want to be sure I explained why it is important to check your pulse at home. Tell me why it is important to check your pulse when you have a pacemaker." Develop a revised teaching plan if patient or caregiver is not able to teach back correctly.

Determines patient's and caregiver's level of understanding of instructional topic.

Unexpected Outcomes

1. Patient has weak, thready, or difficult-to-palpate radial pulse.

Related Interventions

- Assess both radial pulses and compare findings.
- Observe for symptoms associated with ineffective tissue perfusion, including pallor and cool skin distal to weak pulse.
- Assess for swelling in surrounding tissues or any encumbrance (e.g., dressing or cast) that may impede blood flow.
- Obtain Doppler or ultrasound stethoscope to detect low-velocity blood flow (see Chapter 8).
- Have another nurse assess pulse.

STEP	RATIONALE

EVALUATION

2. An adult patient's pulse rate is less than 60 beats/min (bradycardia) or more than 100 beats/min (tachycardia).

- Assess the patient's baseline history of pulse rate to determine patient's "normal" and any medications the person is taking (e.g., beta blockers) that can affect pulse rate.
- Identify related data, including fever, pain, fear or anxiety, recent exercise, low blood pressure, blood loss, or inadequate oxygenation.
- Observe for signs and symptoms associated with abnormal cardiac function, including dyspnea, fatigue, chest pain, orthopnea, syncope, palpitations, edema of body parts, cyanosis, or pallor of skin.
- Auscultate apical pulse (see Skill 7.3).
- Use interprofessional collaboration and prepare for possible electrocardiogram.

3. Patient has irregular pulse.

- Auscultate apical pulse (see Skill 7.3).
- Assess for pulse deficit: (a) nurse auscultates apical pulse while second provider palpates radial pulse; (b) nurse begins 60-second pulse count by calling out loud when to begin counting pulses; (c) the two pulse rates are compared. If pulse count differs by more than 2, a deficit exists; assess for other signs and symptoms of decreased cardiac output (see Chapter 8).

Communication and Documentation

- Document pulse rate and assessment site on vital sign flow sheet or in nurses' notes in EHR or chart.
- Document measurement of pulse rate after administration of specific therapies in nurses' notes EHR or chart.
- Document your evaluation of patient and caregiver learning.
- Check patient's baseline pulse and most recent pulse measurement and then report abnormal findings to nurse in charge or health care provider.

Special Considerations
Teaching

- Patients taking certain prescribed cardiotonic or antidysrhythmic medications need to learn to assess their own pulse rates to detect adverse effects of medications.
- Patients undergoing cardiac rehabilitation need to learn to assess their own pulse rates to determine their response to exercise.
- Teach patients taking heart medications or starting a prescribed exercise regimen how to monitor carotid pulse rate.

Pediatric

- The radial artery is difficult to assess in an infant. Apical, femoral, or brachial pulse is the best site for assessing pediatric heart rate and rhythm until 2 years of age.

- Children often have a sinus dysrhythmia, which is an irregular heartbeat that speeds up with inspiration and slows down with expiration.
- Breath holding in a child temporarily lowers pulse rate.

Gerontological

- Older persons have a reduced heart rate with exercise because of a decreased responsiveness to catecholamines.
- It takes longer for the heart rate to rise in the older person to meet sudden increased demands that result from stress, illness, or excitement. Once elevated, the pulse rate of an older person takes longer to return to normal resting rate.
- Peripheral vascular disease is more common among older persons, making radial pulse assessment difficult.

Care in the Community

- Patients taking certain prescribed cardiac medications should learn to assess their own pulse rates to detect adverse effects of medications.

✦ SKILL 7.3   Assessing Apical Pulse

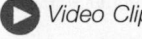 *Video Clip* **NSO** *Nursing Skills Online Vital Signs Module 1, Lesson 3*

The apical pulse is the most reliable noninvasive way to assess cardiac function. The apical pulse rate is the assessment of the number and quality of apical heart sounds in 1 minute. A single apical pulse is the combination of two heart sounds, S_1 and S_2. S_1 is the sound of the tricuspid and mitral valves closing at the end of ventricular filling, just before systolic contraction begins. S_2 is the sound of the pulmonic and aortic valves closing at the end of the systolic contraction. As you listen for sound waves with a stethoscope, you will hear the characteristic "lub-dub" as a single pulsation.

A stethoscope (Fig. 7.7) is a closed cylinder that amplifies sound waves as they reach the surface of the body. The five major parts

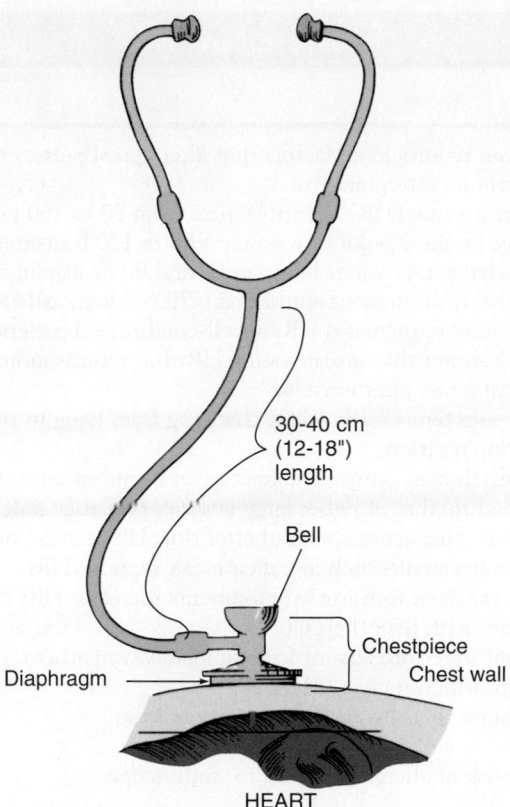

30-40 cm
(12-18")
length

Bell

Chestpiece

Diaphragm

Chest wall

HEART

FIG 7.7 Acoustic stethoscope.

of the stethoscope are the earpieces, binaurals, tubing, bell, and diaphragm. The plastic or rubber earpieces should fit snugly and comfortably in your ears. Binaurals should be angled and strong enough so the earpieces stay firmly in place without causing discomfort. The earpieces follow the contour of the ear canal, pointing toward the face when the stethoscope is in place.

The polyvinyl tubing should be flexible and 30 to 45 cm (12 to 18 inches) in length; longer tubing decreases sound transmission. Stethoscopes can have one or two tubes. At the end of the tubing is the chest piece, consisting of a bell and diaphragm that you rotate into position, depending on which part you choose to use.

The diaphragm is the larger, circular, flat-surfaced part of the chest piece. It transmits high-pitched sounds created by high-velocity movement of air and blood. Position the diaphragm to make a tight seal against a patient's skin. Exert enough pressure to complete the seal, leaving a temporary red ring on the patient's skin after you remove the diaphragm.

The bell is the cone-shaped part of the chest piece, usually surrounded by a rubber ring to avoid chilling the patient during placement. It transmits low-pitched sounds created by the low-velocity movement of blood. Hold the bell lightly against the skin for sound amplification.

Some stethoscopes have one chest piece that combines features of the bell and diaphragm. When you apply light pressure, the chest piece is a bell, whereas exerting more pressure converts the bell into a diaphragm. With the earpieces in your ears tap lightly on the diaphragm and note which side you hear most clearly. This determines which side of the chest piece is functioning.

Delegation and Collaboration

The skill of apical pulse measurement cannot be delegated to an unregulated care provider (UCP). Often the apical pulse is measured when you suspect an irregularity in the radial pulse, before giving some medications, or when a patient's condition requires a more accurate assessment.

Equipment

- Stethoscope
- Wristwatch with second hand or digital display
- Pen and vital sign flow sheet in chart or electronic health record (EHR)
- Alcohol swab

STEP	RATIONALE

ASSESSMENT

1. Identify patient using at least two person-specific identifiers (e.g., name and date of birth or name and medical record number) according to employer policy.

   Ensures correct patient. Complies with Accreditation Canada's standards and improves patient safety (Accreditation Canada, 2019).

2. Determine need to assess apical pulse:

   a. Assess for any risk factors for apical pulse alteration: heart disease, onset of sudden chest pain or acute pain from any site, invasive cardiovascular diagnostic tests, surgery, sudden infusion of large volume of intravenous (IV) fluid, internal or external hemorrhage, administration of medications that alter heart function.

   Certain conditions place patients at risk for pulse alterations.

   b. Assess for signs and symptoms of altered cardiac function such as dyspnea, fatigue, chest pain, orthopnea, syncope, palpitations, edema of dependent body parts, cyanosis, or pallor of skin (see Chapter 8).

   Physical signs and symptoms indicate alteration in cardiac output or stroke volume.

STEP	RATIONALE

ASSESSMENT

c. Assess for factors that normally influence apical pulse rate and rhythm:	Allows you to anticipate factors that alter apical pulse, ensuring an accurate interpretation.
• Age	Infant's heart rate (HR) at birth ranges from 90 to 160 beats/min at rest; by age 2 pulse rate slows to 80 to 120 beats/min; by adolescence rate varies between 50 and 90 beats/min and remains so throughout adulthood (PEDS Cases, 2016).
• Exercise	Physical activity increases HR; a well-conditioned patient may have a slower-than-usual resting HR that returns more quickly to resting rate after exercise.
• Position changes	HR increases temporarily when changing from lying to sitting or standing position.
• Medications	Antidysrhythmics, sympathomimetics, and cardiotonics affect rate and rhythm of pulse; large doses of narcotic analgesics can slow HR; general anaesthetics slow HR; central nervous system stimulants such as caffeine can increase HR.
• Temperature	Fever or exposure to warm environments increases HR; HR declines with hypothermia.
• Sympathetic stimulation	Emotional stress, anxiety, or fear stimulates sympathetic nervous system, which increases HR.
3. Determine previous baseline apical rate (if available) from patient's record.	Allows nurse to assess for change in condition.
4. Determine any report of latex allergy. If patient has latex allergy, ensure that stethoscope is latex free.	Reduces risk of allergic reaction to stethoscope.
5. Determine if patient takes apical heart rate at home. Assess patient's knowledge and skill level.	Determine level and type of instruction required by patient or caregiver.

NURSING DIAGNOSES

- Reduced cardiac output
- Reduced peripheral tissue perfusion
- Reduced stamina

- Insufficient knowledge regarding heart rate monitoring for latex allergy response

- Potential for latex allergy response

Related factors/Risk factors are individualized on the basis of patient's condition or needs.

PLANNING

1. Expected outcomes following completion of procedure:	
• Apical HR is within acceptable range.	Adults average 60 to 100 beats/min.
• Rhythm is regular.	Cardiovascular status is stable.
2. Explain to patient that you will assess apical pulse rate. Encourage patient to relax and not speak. If patient has been active, wait 5 to 10 minutes before assessing pulse. If they have been smoking or ingesting caffeine, wait 15 minutes before assessing pulse.	Anxiety, activity, caffeine, and smoking elevate HR. Patient's voice interferes with nurse's ability to hear sound when measuring apical pulse. Assessing apical pulse rate at rest allows for objective comparison of values.
3. Collect and bring appropriate supplies to patient's bedside.	Ensures an organized approach for assessing radial pulse.

IMPLEMENTATION

1. Perform hand hygiene.	Reduces transmission of microorganisms.
2. If necessary, draw curtain around bed or close door.	Maintains privacy and minimizes embarrassment. Helps patient relax.
3. Help patient to supine or sitting position. Move aside bed linen and gown to expose sternum and left side of chest.	Exposes part of chest wall for selection of auscultatory site. Stethoscope diaphragm must touch skin for best sounds.

STEP	RATIONALE

IMPLEMENTATION

4. Locate anatomical landmarks to identify point of maximal impulse (PMI), also called apical *impulse* (see Chapter 8). The heart is located behind and to left of sternum with base at top and apex at bottom. Find angle of Louis just below suprasternal notch between sternal body and manubrium; it feels like a bony prominence (see illustration A). Slip fingers down each side of angle to find second intercostal space (ICS) (see illustration B). Carefully move fingers down left side of sternum to fifth ICS and laterally to left midclavicular line (MCL) (see illustration C). A light tap felt within area 1 to 2.5 cm ($\frac{1}{2}$ to 1 inch) of PMI is reflected from apex of heart (see illustration D).

Use of anatomical landmarks allows correct placement of stethoscope over apex of heart. This position enhances ability to hear heart sounds clearly. If unable to palpate PMI, reposition patient on left side. In presence of serious heart disease, you may locate PMI to left of MCL or at sixth ICS. PMI may not be palpated in obese adults or patients with severe pulmonary disease that has changed shape of thorax.

5. Place diaphragm of stethoscope in palm of hand for 5 to 10 seconds.

Warming of metal or plastic diaphragm prevents patient from being startled and promotes comfort.

6. Place diaphragm of stethoscope over PMI at fifth ICS, at left MCL, and auscultate for normal S_1 and S_2 heart sounds (heard as "lub-dub") (see illustrations).

Allow stethoscope tubing to extend straight without kinks that would distort sound transmission. Normal sounds S_1 and S_2 are high pitched and best heard with diaphragm.

7. When you hear S_1 and S_2 with regularity, use second hand of watch and begin to count rate: when sweep hand hits number on dial, start counting with zero, then one, two, and so on.

Apical rate is determined accurately only after you are able to auscultate sounds clearly. Timing begins with zero. Count of one is first sound auscultated after timing begins.

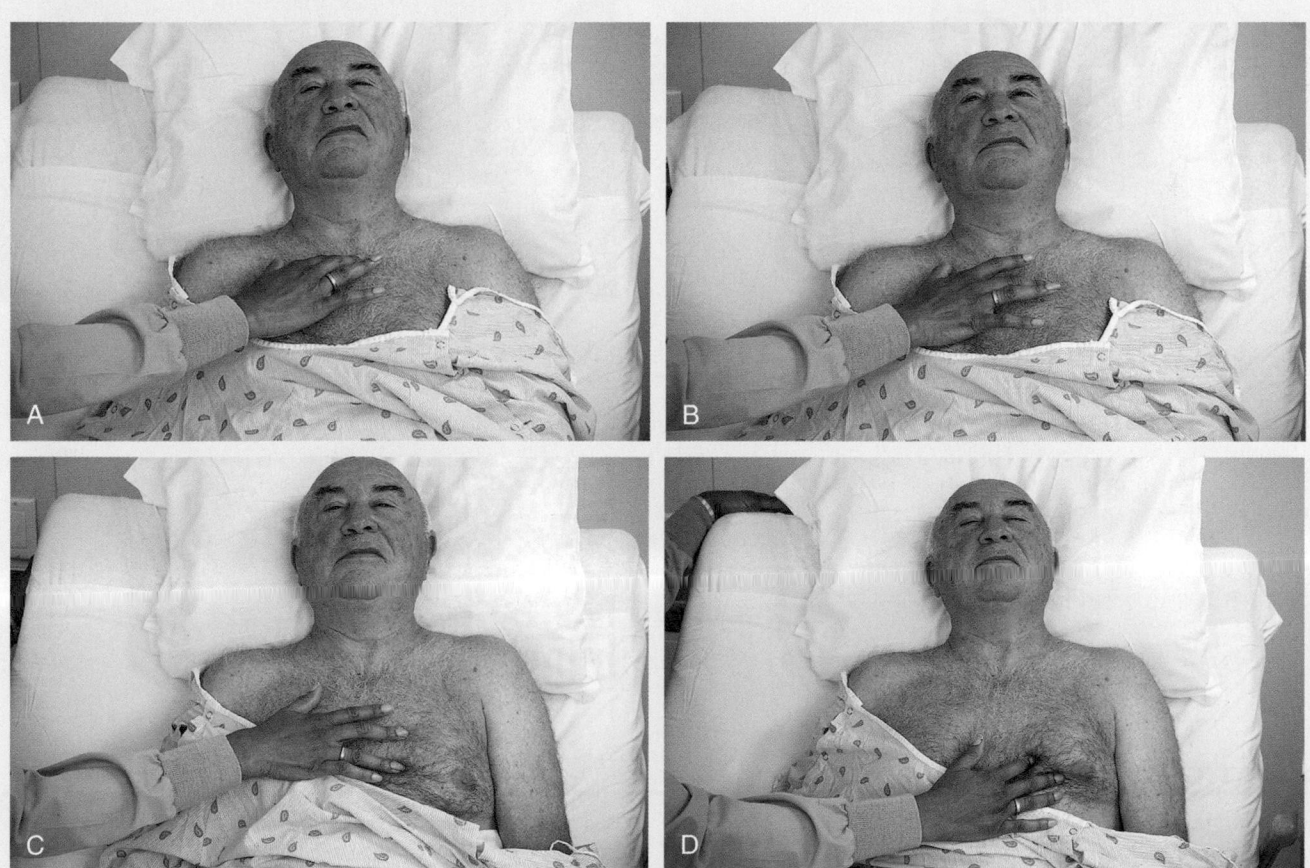

STEP 4 A, Nurse locates sternal notch. **B,** Nurse locates second intercostal space. **C,** Nurse locates fifth intercostal space. **D,** Nurse locates point of maximal impulse at fifth intercostal space at left midclavicular line.

STEP	RATIONALE

IMPLEMENTATION

8. If apical rate is regular, count for 30 seconds and multiply by 2.

   You can assess regular apical rate within 30 seconds.

9. If HR is irregular or patient is receiving cardiovascular medication, count for 1 full minute (60 seconds).

   Irregular rate is more accurately assessed when measured over longer interval.

10. Note regularity of any dysrhythmia (S_1 and S_2 occurring early or late after previous sequence of sounds) (e.g., every third or every fourth beat is skipped).

    Regular occurrence of dysrhythmia within 1 minute indicates inefficient contraction of heart and potential alteration in cardiac output.

11. Replace patient's gown and bed linen; help them return to comfortable position.

    Restores comfort and promotes sense of well-being.

Clinical Decision Point *If apical rate is abnormal or irregular, repeat measurement or have another nurse conduct measurement. Original measurement may be incorrect. Second measurement confirms initial findings of an abnormal HR.*

12. Discuss findings with patient.

    Promotes person-centred care and understanding of health status.

13. Perform hand hygiene.

    Reduces transmission of microorganisms.

14. Clean earpieces and diaphragm of stethoscope with alcohol swab routinely after each use.

    Stethoscopes are frequently contaminated with microorganisms. Regular disinfection can control hospital-acquired infections (Breen & Hessels, 2017).

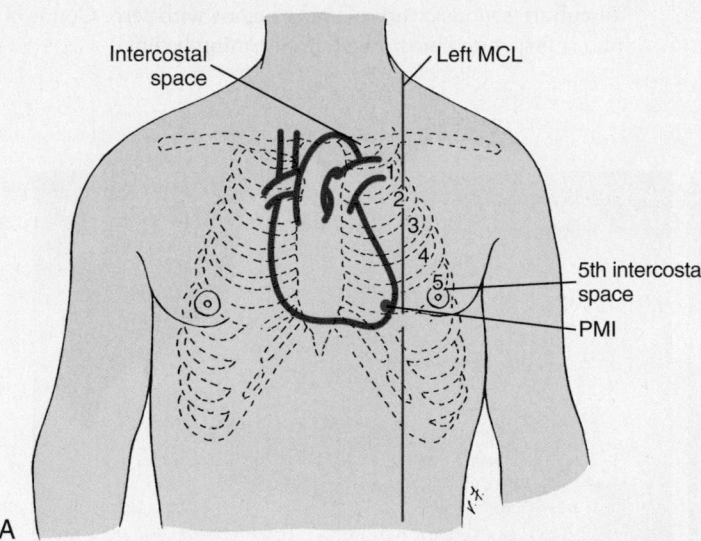

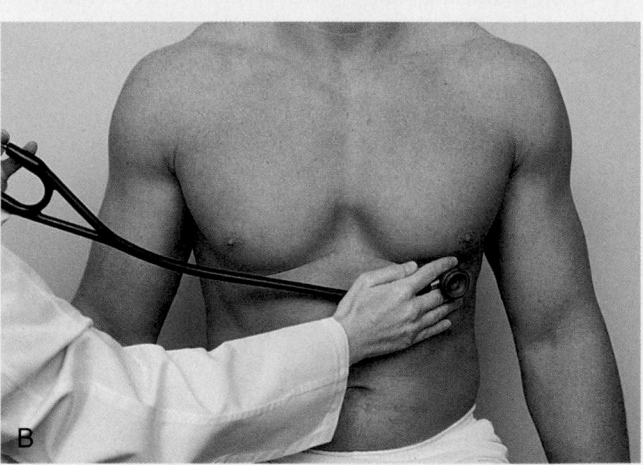

STEP 6 A, Location of point of maximal impulse (PMI) in adult. **B,** Listening to PMI in adult.

EVALUATION

1. If assessing pulse for first time, establish apical rate as baseline if it is within an acceptable range.

   Used to compare future pulse assessments.

2. Compare apical rate and character with patient's previous baseline and acceptable range of HR for patient's age.

   Allows you to assess for change in patient's condition and for presence of cardiac alteration.

STEP	RATIONALE

EVALUATION

3. Use Teach-Back: "I want to be sure I explained why it is important to check your heart rate at home. Tell me which medication you are taking that may decrease your heart rate." Develop a revised teaching if patient or caregiver is not able to teach back correctly.

Determines patient's and caregiver's level of understanding of instructional topic.

Unexpected Outcomes	Related Interventions
1. Adult patient's apical pulse is greater than 100 beats/min (tachycardia).	• Identify related data, including fever, pain, fear or anxiety, recent exercise, low blood pressure, blood loss, or inadequate oxygenation. • Observe for signs and symptoms associated with abnormal cardiac function, including dyspnea, fatigue, chest pain, orthopnea, syncope, palpitations, edema of body parts, cyanosis, or dizziness.
2. Patient's apical pulse is less than 60 beats/min (bradycardia).	• Assess for factors that decrease HR, such as beta blockers and antiarrhythmic drugs. • Observe for signs and symptoms associated with abnormal cardiac function, including dyspnea, fatigue, chest pain, orthopnea, syncope, palpitations, edema of body parts, cyanosis, or dizziness. • Have another nurse assess apical pulse. • Report findings to nurse in charge, health care provider, or both. It may be necessary to withhold prescribed medications that alter HR until health care provider can evaluate need to alter dosage.
3. Patient's apical rhythm is irregular.	• Assess for pulse deficit (see Skill 7.2): (a) nurse auscultates apical pulse while second provider palpates radial pulse; (b) nurse begins 60-second pulse count by calling out loud when to begin counting pulses; (c) if pulse count differs by more than 2, assesses for other signs and symptoms of decreased cardiac output (see Chapter 8). • Report findings to nurse in charge and/or health care provider, who may prescribe an electrocardiogram to detect cardiac conduction alteration.

Communication and Documentation

- Document apical pulse rate and rhythm on vital sign flow sheet or in nurses' notes in EHR or chart. If apical pulse is not found at fifth ICS and left MCL, document location of PMI.
- Document measurement of apical pulse rate after administration of specific therapies in appropriate area in EHR per employer policy.
- Report abnormal findings to nurse in charge or health care provider.
- Document your evaluation of patient and caregiver learning.

Special Considerations
Teaching

- Teach caregivers of patients taking prescribed cardiotonic or antidysrhythmic medications how to assess apical pulse rates to detect adverse effects of medications.

Pediatric

- The PMI of an infant is usually located at the third to fourth ICS near the left sternal border.

- In infants and children younger than 2 years, an apical pulse is more reliable and is counted for 1 full minute because of possible irregularities in rhythm.
- Breath holding in an infant or child temporarily lowers apical pulse rate.

Gerontological

- The PMI can be difficult to palpate in some older persons because the anterior-posterior diameter of the chest increases with age and the heart becomes repositioned because of left ventricular enlargement.
- When assessing older females, you may have to gently lift the breast tissue and place the stethoscope at the fifth ICS or the lower edge of the breast.
- Heart sounds are sometimes muffled or difficult to hear in older persons because of an increase in air space in the lungs.
- The older person normally has a decreased HR at rest.

Care in the Community

- Assess home environment and, if possible, use a room that affords a quiet, private environment for auscultation of apical rate.

◆ SKILL 7.4   Assessing Respirations

▶ *Video Clip* **NSO** *Nursing Skills Online Vital Signs Module 1, Lesson 4*

Respiration is the exchange of oxygen (O_2) and carbon dioxide (CO_2) between cells of the body and the atmosphere. Three processes of respiration are ventilation (i.e., mechanical movement of gases into and out of the lungs), diffusion (i.e., movement of oxygen and carbon dioxide between the alveoli and the red blood cells), and perfusion (i.e., distribution of red blood cells to and from the

pulmonary capillaries). Ventilation is assessed by observing the rate, depth, and rhythm of respiratory movements. Accurate assessment of respirations depends on recognizing normal thoracic and abdominal movements. Normal breathing is both active and passive. On inspiration the diaphragm contracts, and the abdominal organs move down to increase the size of the chest cavity. At the same time, the ribs and sternum lift outward to promote lung expansion. On expiration the diaphragm relaxes upward, and the ribs and sternum return to their relaxed position (Fig. 7.8). During quiet breathing the chest wall gently rises and falls. The body uses more energy during inspiration than during expiration. Expiration is an active process only during exercise, voluntary hyperventilation, and certain disease states.

Delegation and Collaboration

The skill of counting respirations can be delegated to an unregulated care provider (UCP) unless the patient is considered unstable (e.g., evidence of dyspnea). The nurse instructs the UCP by:

- Communicating the frequency of measurement and factors related to patient history or risk for increased or decreased respiratory rate or irregular respirations.
- Reviewing any unusual respiratory values and significant changes to report to the nurse.

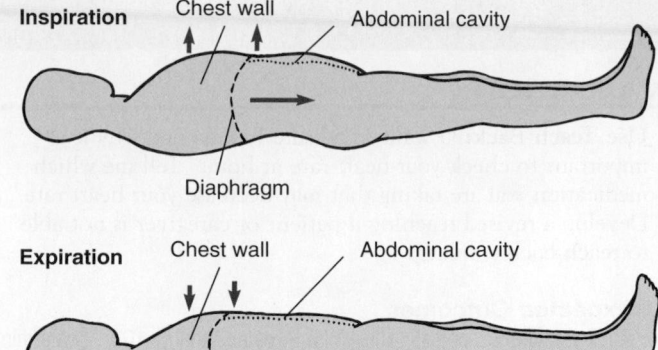

FIG 7.8 Diaphragmatic and chest wall movement during inspiration and expiration.

Equipment

- Wristwatch with second hand or digital display
- Pen and vital sign flow sheet in chart or electronic health record (EHR)

STEP	RATIONALE

ASSESSMENT

1. Identify patient using at least two person-specific identifiers (e.g., name and date of birth or name and medical record number) according to employer policy.

    Ensures correct patient. Complies with Accreditation Canada's standards and improves patient safety (Accreditation Canada, 2019).

2. Determine need to assess patient's respirations:
   a. Assess for risk factors of respiratory alterations:
   - Fever
   - Pain and anxiety
   - Diseases of chest wall or muscles
   - Constrictive chest or abdominal dressings
   - Presence of abdominal incisions
   - Gastric distension
   - Chronic pulmonary disease (emphysema, bronchitis, asthma)
   - Traumatic injury to chest wall with or without collapse of underlying lung tissue
   - Presence of chest tube
   - Respiratory infection (pneumonia, acute bronchitis)
   - Pulmonary edema and emboli
   - Head injury with damage to brainstem
   - Anemia

    Certain conditions place patient at risk for ventilatory alterations detected by changes in respiratory rate, depth, and rhythm.

   b. Assess for signs and symptoms of respiratory alterations, such as:
   - Bluish or cyanotic appearance of nail beds, lips, mucous membranes, and skin
   - Restlessness, irritability, confusion, reduced level of consciousness
   - Pain during inspiration
   - Laboured or difficult breathing
   - Orthopnea
   - Use of accessory muscles
   - Adventitious breath sounds (see Chapter 8)
   - Inability to breathe spontaneously
   - Thick, frothy, blood-tinged, or copious sputum production

    Physical signs and symptoms indicate alterations in respiratory status.

STEP	RATIONALE

ASSESSMENT

c. Assess for factors that influence character of respirations: | Allows you to anticipate factors that influence respirations, ensuring a more accurate interpretation.

- Exercise

Respirations increase in rate and depth to meet need for additional oxygen and rid body of carbon dioxide.

- Anxiety

Anxiety causes increase in respiration rate and depth because of sympathetic nervous system stimulation.

- Acute pain

Pain alters rate and rhythm of respirations; breathing becomes shallow. Patient inhibits or splints chest wall movement when pain is in area of chest or abdomen.

- Smoking

Chronic smoking changes pulmonary airways, resulting in increased respiratory rate at rest when not smoking.

- Medications

Opioids, analgesics, general anaesthetics, and sedative hypnotics depress rate and depth; amphetamines and cocaine increase rate and depth; bronchodilators cause dilation of airways, which ultimately slows respiratory rate.

- Body position

Standing or sitting erect promotes full ventilatory movement and lung expansion; stooped or slumped posture impairs ventilatory movement; lying flat prevents full chest expansion.

- Neurological injury

Damage to brainstem impairs respiratory centre and inhibits rate and rhythm.

- Hemoglobin function

Decreased hemoglobin levels lower amount of oxygen carried in blood, which results in increased respiratory rate to increase oxygen delivery. An increase in altitude lowers amount of saturated hemoglobin, which increases respiratory rate and depth.

3. Assess pertinent laboratory/clinical values:

a. *Arterial blood gases (ABGs)*: Normal ranges (values vary slightly among agencies):
- pH, 7.35–7.45
- $PaCO_2$, 35–45 mm Hg
- HCO_3, 21–28 mmol/L
- PaO_2, 80–100 mm Hg
- SaO_2, 95–100%

ABG values measure arterial blood pH, partial pressure of oxygen and carbon dioxide, and arterial oxygen saturation, which reflect patient's ventilation and oxygenation status.

b. *Pulse oximetry (SpO_2)*: Normal SpO_2 ≥95–100%; less than 90% may be a clinical emergency or may be due to a chronic condition (e.g., chronic obstructive pulmonary disease [COPD]) where a value in the upper 80s would not be considered an emergency (see Procedural Guideline 7.2).

SpO_2 less than 90% is often accompanied by changes in respiratory rate, depth, and rhythm.

- *Complete blood count (CBC)*: Normal CBC for adults (values vary within agencies):
- *Hemoglobin:* 140–180 g/L in male patients; 120–160 g/L in female patients
- *Hematocrit:* 0.42–0.52 in male patients; 0.37–0.47 in female patients
- *Red blood cell count:* 4.6–6.2 × 10^{12}/L in male patients; 4.2–5.4 × 10^{12}/L in female patients

CBC measures red blood cell count; volume of red blood cells; and concentration of hemoglobin, which reflects patient's capacity to carry oxygen.

4. Determine previous baseline respiratory rate (if available) from patient's record.

Assesses for change in condition. Provides comparison with future respiratory measurements.

NURSING DIAGNOSES

- Inadequate airway clearance
- Reduced spontaneous ventilation
- Inadequate breathing pattern
- Reduced gas exchange
- Reduced stamina

Related factors are individualized on the basis of patient's condition or needs.

STEP	RATIONALE

PLANNING

1. Expected outcomes following completion of procedure:
   - Respiratory rate is within acceptable range.
   - Respirations are regular and of normal depth.

Adults average 12 to 20 breaths/min.
Respiratory status is stable.

2. If patient has been active, wait 5 to 10 minutes before assessing respirations.

Exercise increases respiratory rate and depth. Assessing respirations while patient is at rest allows for objective comparison of values.

3. After taking the pulse measurement in an adult, immediately start counting respirations without informing the patient.

Assessing respirations immediately after the pulse without informing the patient prevents the patient from consciously or unintentionally altering rate and depth of breathing and provides a more accurate assessment.

4. Be sure that patient is in comfortable position, preferably sitting or lying with head of bed elevated 45 to 60 degrees.

Sitting erect promotes full ventilatory movement. Position of discomfort causes patient to breathe more rapidly.

Clinical Decision Point *Assess patients with difficulty breathing (dyspnea), such as those with heart failure or abdominal ascites or in late stages of pregnancy, in the position of greatest comfort. Repositioning may increase the work of breathing, which increases respiratory rate.*

IMPLEMENTATION

1. Perform hand hygiene.

Prevents transmission of microorganisms.

2. Draw curtain around bed or close door.

Maintains privacy.

3. Be sure that patient's chest is visible. If necessary, move bed linen or gown.

Ensures clear view of chest wall and abdominal movements.

4. Place patient's arm in relaxed position across abdomen or lower chest or place your hand directly over patient's upper abdomen.

A similar position used during pulse assessment allows respiratory rate assessment to be inconspicuous. Patient's or your hand rises and falls during respiratory cycle.

5. Observe complete respiratory cycle (one inspiration and one expiration).

Rate is accurately determined only after viewing a complete respiratory cycle.

6. After observing a cycle, look at second hand of watch and begin to count rate: when sweep hand hits number on dial, begin time frame, counting one with first full respiratory cycle.

Timing begins with count of one. Respirations occur more slowly than pulse; thus, timing does not begin with zero.

7. If rhythm is regular, count number of respirations in 30 seconds and multiply by 2. If rhythm is irregular, less than 12, or greater than 20, count for 1 full minute.

Respiratory rate is equivalent to number of respirations per minute. Suspected irregularities require assessment for at least 1 minute (Box 7.5).

8. Note depth of respirations by observing degree of chest wall movement while counting rate. In addition, assess depth by palpating chest wall excursion or auscultating posterior thorax after you have counted rate (see Chapter 8). Describe depth as shallow, normal, or deep.

Character of ventilatory movement reveals specific disease states restricting volume of air from moving into and out of lungs.

9. Note rhythm of ventilatory cycle. Normal breathing is regular and uninterrupted. Do not confuse sighing with abnormal rhythm.

Character of ventilations reveals specific types of alterations. Periodically, people unconsciously take single deep breaths or sighs to expand small airways prone to collapse.

Clinical Decision Point *Any irregular respiratory pattern or periods of apnea (cessation of respiration for several seconds) are symptoms of underlying disease in the adult, and you need to report this to the health care provider or nurse in charge. Further assessment and immediate intervention are often necessary.*

10. Replace bed linen and patient's gown.

Restores comfort and promotes sense of well-being.

11. Perform hand hygiene.

Reduces transmission of microorganisms.

12. Discuss findings with patient.

Promotes person-centred care and understanding of health status.

STEP	RATIONALE

EVALUATION

1. If assessing respirations for first time, establish rate, rhythm, and depth as baseline if within acceptable range.

Used to compare future respiratory assessment.

2. Compare respirations with patient's previous baseline and usual rate, rhythm, and depth.

Allows you to assess for changes in patient's condition and presence of respiratory alterations.

3. Correlate respiratory rate, depth, and rhythm with data obtained from pulse oximetry and ABG measurements if available.

Evaluations of ventilation, perfusion, and diffusion are interrelated.

4. Use Teach-Back: "I want to be sure I explained why you will be reminded to take deep breaths after surgery. Tell me why deep breathing is important." Develop a revised teaching plan if patient or caregiver is not able to teach back correctly.

Determines patient's and caregiver's level of understanding of instructional topic.

Unexpected Outcomes

1. Adult patient's respiratory rate is below 12 breaths/min (bradypnea) or above 20 breaths/min (tachypnea). Breathing pattern is sometimes irregular (see Box 7.5). Depth of respirations is increased or decreased. Patient indicates dyspnea.

2. Patient demonstrates Kussmaul's, Cheyne-Stokes, or Biot's respirations (see Box 7.5).

Related Interventions

- Assess for related factors, including obstructed airway, abnormal breath sounds, productive cough, restlessness, anxiety, and confusion (see Chapter 8).
- Help patient to supported sitting position (semi- or high-Fowler's) unless contraindicated.
- Provide oxygen as prescribed (see Chapter 23).
- Assess for environmental factors that influence patient's respiratory rate, such as secondhand smoke, poor ventilation, or gas fumes.
- Notify health care provider or nurse in charge if alteration continues.
- Notify health care provider for additional evaluation and possible medical intervention.

Communication and Documentation

- Document respiratory rate, depth, and rhythm on vital sign flow sheet or in nurses' notes in EHR or chart.
- Document measurement of respiratory rate after administration of specific therapies in nurses' notes in EHR or chart.
- Document your evaluation of patient and caregiver learning.
- Document type and amount of oxygen therapy, if used, in nurses' notes in EHR or chart.
- Review patient's baseline and previous respiratory measurement to report abnormal findings to nurse in charge or health care provider.

Special Considerations
Teaching

- Patients who demonstrate decreased ventilation (e.g., after surgery) often benefit from learning deep-breathing and coughing exercises (see Chapter 37).
- Instruct caregiver to contact community nurse or health care provider if unusual fluctuations in respiratory rate occur.

Pediatric

- Assess respiratory rates before other vital signs or assessments if you are able to view movement of chest wall or abdomen. This

---

BOX 7.5

Alterations in Breathing Pattern

Alteration	Description
Apnea	Respirations cease for several seconds. Persistent cessation results in respiratory arrest.
Biot's respiration	Irregular respirations varying in depth that are followed by periods of apnea associated with central nervous system disorders.
Bradypnea	Rate of breathing is regular but abnormally slow (<12 breaths/min).
Cheyne-Stokes respiration	Respiratory rate and depth are irregular, characterized by alternating periods of apnea and hyperventilation. Respiratory cycle begins with slow, shallow breaths that gradually increase to abnormal rate and depth. The pattern reverses; breathing slows and becomes shallow, climaxing in apnea before respiration resumes.
Hyperpnea	Respirations are increased in depth and increased in rate (>20 breaths/min); occurs normally during exercise.
Hyperventilation	Rate and depth of respirations increase. Hypocarbia, an abnormally low level of carbon dioxide in the blood, may occur.
Hypoventilation	Respiratory rate is abnormally low; depth of ventilation may be depressed. Hypercarbia, an abnormally elevated level of carbon dioxide in the blood, may occur.
Kussmaul's respiration	Respirations are abnormally rapid, deep, and laboured but regular; common with conditions that cause metabolic acidosis (e.g., diabetic ketoacidosis).
Tachypnea	Rate of breathing is regular but abnormally rapid (>20 breaths/min).

allows assessment of rate and rhythm before child becomes anxious because of stranger anxiety or fear of other assessment procedures.

- Average respiratory rate (breaths per minute) for infants is 30 to 53; toddler (1–2 years) is 22 to 37; and school age (6–11 years) is 18 to 25 (PEDS Cases, 2016).
- Children up to age 7 breathe abdominally; thus, respirations are observed by abdominal movement.
- An irregular respiratory rate and short apneic spells are normal for newborns.
- You can simply observe infant or young child while chest and abdomen are exposed.
- Use cardiorespiratory monitors for infants or newborns who are at risk for respiratory compromise or sustained apnea.

Gerontological

- Aging causes ossification of costal cartilage and downward slant of ribs, resulting in a more rigid rib cage, which reduces chest

wall expansion. Kyphosis and scoliosis, frequent in older persons, may also restrict chest expansion.

- Depth of respirations tends to decrease with aging.
- Change in lung function with aging results in respiratory rates generally higher in older persons, with a range of 16 to 24 breaths/min (Hirst, Lane, & Miller, 2015, p. 441).
- Some older persons depend more on accessory abdominal muscles than weakened thoracic muscles during respiration.

Care in the Community

- Assess for environmental factors in the home that influence patient's respiratory rate, such as secondhand smoke, poor ventilation, or gas fumes.

✦ SKILL 7.5   Assessing Arterial Blood Pressure

NSO *Nursing Skills Online Vital Signs Module 1, Lesson 5*

Blood pressure (BP) is the force exerted by blood against the vessel walls. The peak pressure or systolic pressure occurs when the ventricular contraction of the heart forces blood under high pressure into the aorta. When the ventricles relax, the blood remaining in the arteries exerts a minimal or diastolic pressure against the arterial walls at all times.

The standard unit for measuring BP is millimeters of mercury (mm Hg). The most common technique of measuring BP is auscultation with a sphygmomanometer and stethoscope. As the sphygmomanometer cuff is deflated, the five different sounds heard over an artery are called *Korotkoff phases*. The sound in each phase has unique characteristics (Fig. 7.9). BP is recorded with the systolic reading (first sound) before the diastolic (beginning of the fifth sound). The difference between systolic and diastolic pressure is the pulse pressure. For a BP of 120/80, the pulse pressure is 40.

Hypertension

Hypertension is a major factor underlying death from heart attack and stroke in Canada. According to Hypertension Canada, BP recording revealing a high systolic or diastolic BP does not usually qualify as a diagnosis of hypertension unless the non-automated office blood pressure (non-AOBP) mean or automated office blood pressure (AOBP) measurements show a reading of a systolic blood pressure (SPB) ≥180 mm Hg and/or diastolic blood pressure (DBP) ≥110 mm Hg (Leung et al., 2017). The (non-AOBP) mean is calculated by discarding the first BP reading and then averaging the next two readings. If AOBP is used, the mean calculated and displayed by the device is used. If the mean of the AOBP from the first visit is a SBP of 135–179 mm Hg and/or DBP is 85–109 mm Hg or the mean non-AOBP SBP is 140–179 mm Hg and/or DBP is 90–109 mm Hg, out-of-office BP measurements should be performed before the second visit (Leung et al., 2017) (Fig. 7.10). In patients with diabetes mellitus, diagnostic thresholds for AOBP, ambulatory BP monitoring, and home BP have yet to be established (and might be lower than 130/80 mm Hg). If it is thought that a patient has hypertension, a history and physical exam should be performed and diagnostic tests prescribed. Annual BP measurement is recommended for all adults in order to detect progression to hypertension (Leung et al., 2017).

Hypotension

Hypotension occurs when the systolic BP falls to 90 mm Hg or below. Although some adults normally have a low BP, for most people a low BP is an abnormal finding associated with illness (e.g., hemorrhage or myocardial infarction). Orthostatic hypotension is a sustained reduction in systolic pressure by at least 20 mm Hg or a drop in diastolic pressure by at least 10 mm Hg within 3 minutes of standing

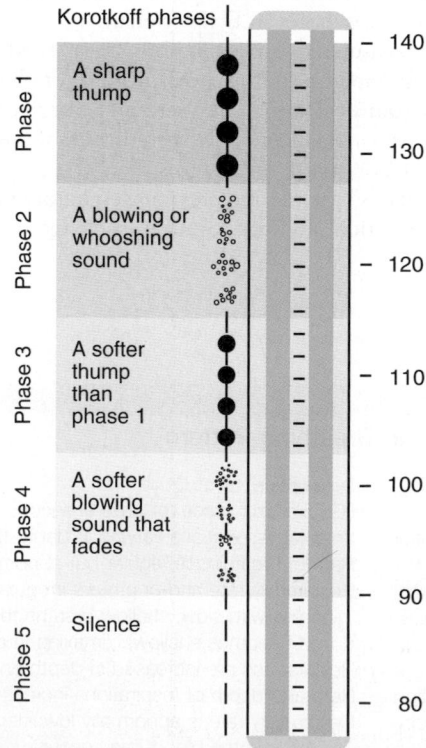

FIG 7.9 The sounds auscultated during blood pressure measurement can be differentiated into five phases. In this example, the blood pressure is 140/90 mm Hg.

or a head-up tilt greater than 60°. The symptoms of cerebral hypoperfusion, including light-headedness, dizziness, blurred vision, fatigue, and headache, often accompany orthostatic hypotension; however, many patients are asymptomatic (Amy, Arnold, & Raj, 2017). Loss of consciousness may occur in severe cases. Orthostatic changes in vital signs are effective indicators of blood volume depletion. Some medications cause orthostatic hypotension, especially in young patients and older persons. Orthostatic hypotension occurs more frequently in older persons and can lead to an increased risk for falls and fall-related injuries (Hirst et al., 2015, p. 413).

Blood Pressure Equipment

Arterial BP is measured either directly (invasively) or indirectly (noninvasively). The direct method requires electronic monitoring equipment and the insertion of a thin catheter into an artery. The risks associated with invasive BP monitoring require a patient to be in a critical care setting.

Electronic or automatic BP machines consist of an electronic sensor positioned inside a BP cuff attached to an electronic processor (see Procedural Guideline 7.1). Cloth or disposable vinyl compression cuffs contain an inflatable bladder and come in several different sizes. The size selected is proportional to the circumference of the limb being assessed. Ideally the bladder width should be close to 40% of arm circumference and bladder length should cover 80–100%

of arm circumference (Hypertension Canada, 2015) (Fig. 7.11). Many adults require a large adult cuff. A regular-size cuff holds a bladder the width of 12 to 13 cm (4.8 to 5.2 inches) and length of 22 to 23 cm (8.5 to 9 inches). An improperly fitting cuff produces inaccurate BP measurements (Box 7.6).

According to Hypertension Canada (2015) measurement using validated electronic devices is preferred over auscultation because they minimize errors (e.g., provider hearing deficits, rounding the reading to a 0 or 5, and rapid deflation) (Leung et al., 2017) (Box 7.7). A recent survey of Canadian family physicians showed, however, that 52% still use aneroid or mercury devices with auscultation to manually measure BP instead of following the current Canadian guidelines (Kaczorowski et al., 2017). It is important that, unless specified otherwise, electronic measurement of BP be used; however, until manual BP is no longer being utilized, it is important for nurses to know proper technique.

Delegation and Collaboration

The skill of BP measurement can be delegated to an unregulated care provider (UCP) unless the patient is considered unstable (e.g., hypotensive or hypertensive). The nurse instructs the UCP by:

- Explaining the appropriate limb to use for measurement, BP cuff size, and equipment (manual or electronic) to be used.
- Communicating the frequency of measurement and factors related to the patient's history, such as risk for orthostatic hypotension.
- Reviewing the patient's usual BP values and significant changes or abnormalities to report to the nurse.

Equipment

- Aneroid sphygmomanometer
- Cloth or disposable vinyl pressure cuff of appropriate size for patient's extremity
- Stethoscope
- Alcohol swab
- Pen and vital sign flow sheet in chart or electronic health record (EHR)

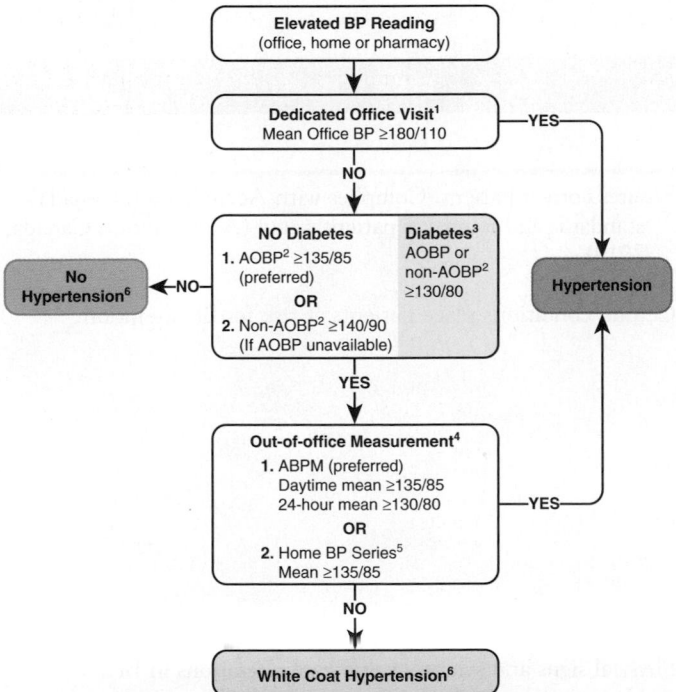

FIG 7.10 Criteria for diagnosis of hypertension and guidelines for follow-up. AOBP is performed with the patient unattended in a private area. Non-AOBP is performed using an electronic upper arm device with the provider in the room. *AOBP,* Automated office blood pressure measurement; *APBM,* ambulatory blood pressure measurement; *BP,* blood pressure; non-AOPB, non-automated office blood pressure measurement. (*From Leung, A. A., Daskalopoulou, S. S., Dasgupta, K., McBrien, K., Butalia, S., Zarnke, K. B., … Rabi, D. M. [2017]. Hypertension Canada's 2017 guidelines for diagnosis, risk assessment, prevention, and treatment of hypertension in adults. Canadian Journal of Cardiology 33[5], 563.*)

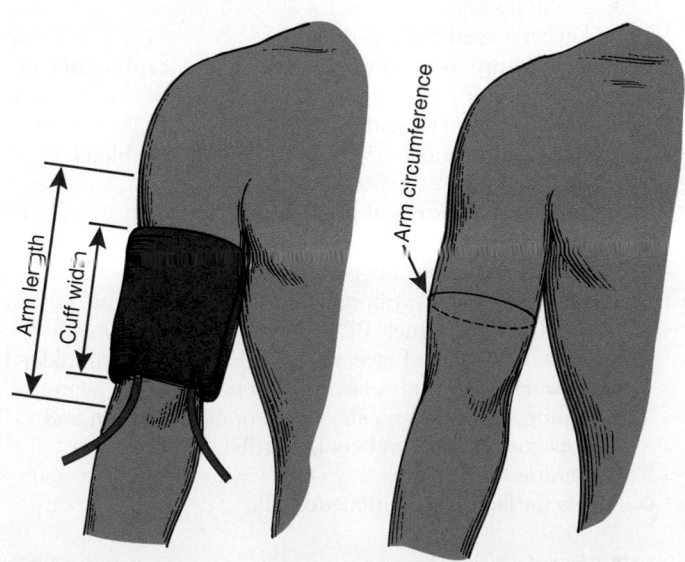

FIG 7.11 Guidelines for proper blood pressure cuff size. Cuff width equals 40% of circumference around bladder, length should cover 80–100% of arm circumference.

BOX 7.6

Common Mistakes in Blood Pressure Assessment

Error	Effect
Bladder or cuff too wide	False-low reading
Bladder or cuff too narrow or too short	False-high reading
Cuff wrapped too loosely or unevenly	False-high reading
Deflating cuff too slowly	False-high diastolic reading
Deflating cuff too quickly	False-low systolic and false-high diastolic reading
Arm below heart level	False-high reading
Arm above heart level	False-low reading
Arm not supported	False-high reading
Stethoscope that fits poorly or impairment of examiner's hearing, causing sounds to be muffled	False-low systolic and false-high diastolic reading
Stethoscope applied too firmly against antecubital fossa	False-low diastolic reading
Inflating too slowly	False-high diastolic reading
Repeating assessments too quickly	False-high systolic reading
Inaccurate inflation level	False-low systolic reading
Multiple examiners using different sounds for diastolic readings	False-high systolic and false-low diastolic reading

---

BOX 7.7

Advantages and Limitations of Assessing Blood Pressure Electronically

Advantages
- Ease of use
- Efficient when frequent repeated measurements are indicated
- Stethoscope not required
- Allows blood pressure to be recorded more frequently, as often as every 15 seconds, with accuracy

Limitations
- Expensive
- Requires source of electricity
- Requires space to position machine
- Pressure from cuff on the arm may cause some patients discomfort and anxiety and lead to bruising of the arm, especially in older persons
- Sensitive to outside motion interference and cannot be used in patients with seizures, tremors, or shivers or in patients unable to cooperate
- May not be accurate for patients with irregular heart rate or hypotension or in conditions with reduced blood flow (e.g., hypothermia)
- Accuracy standards for electronic blood pressure machine manufacturers are voluntary
- Vulnerable to error among older persons and obese patients

STEP	RATIONALE

ASSESSMENT

1. Identify patient using at least two person-specific identifiers (e.g., name and date of birth or name and medical record number) according to employer policy.

   Ensures correct patient. Complies with Accreditation Canada's standards and improves patient safety (Accreditation Canada, 2019).

2. Determine need to assess patient's BP:

   a. Assess risk factors for BP alterations:

   Certain conditions place patients at risk for BP alteration.

   - History of cardiovascular disease
   - Renal disease
   - Diabetes mellitus
   - Circulatory shock (hypovolemic, septic, cardiogenic, or neurogenic)
   - Acute or chronic pain
   - Rapid intravenous (IV) infusion of fluids or blood products
   - Increased intracranial pressure
   - Postoperative status
   - Pregnancy-induced hypertension

   b. Assess for signs and symptoms of BP alterations. In patients at risk for high BP, assess for headache (usually occipital), flushing of face, nosebleed, and fatigue in older persons. Hypotension is associated with dizziness; mental confusion; restlessness; pale, dusky, or cyanotic skin and mucous membranes; and cool, mottled skin over extremities.

   Physical signs and symptoms indicate alterations in BP. Hypertension is often asymptomatic until pressure is very high.

   c. Assess for factors that influence BP:

   Allows you to anticipate factors that influence BP, ensuring a more accurate interpretation.

   - Age

   Acceptable values for BP vary throughout life (see Pediatric and Gerontological Considerations).

   - Gender identity

   During and after menopause women often have higher BP than men of same age.

STEP	RATIONALE

ASSESSMENT

- Daily (diurnal) variation

BP varies throughout day; pressure is highest during the day between 10:00 AM and 6:00 PM and lowest in early morning.

- Position

BP falls as person moves from lying to sitting or standing position; normally postural variations are minimal.

- Exercise

Increases in oxygen demand by body during activity increase BP.

- Weight

Obesity is an independent predictor of hypertension.

- Sympathetic stimulation

Pain, anxiety, or fear stimulates sympathetic nervous system, causing BP to rise.

- Medications

Antihypertensives, diuretics, beta-adrenergic blockers, vasodilators, calcium channel blockers, angiotensin-converting enzyme (ACE) inhibitors, angiotensin receptor blockers (ARBs), and antidysrhythmics lower BP; opioids and general anaesthetics also cause a drop in BP.

- Smoking

Nicotine in cigarette smoke results in vasoconstriction, a narrowing of blood vessels, which raises BP. Smoking also makes BP medications less effective (Diabetes Canada, 2018).

- Ethnicity

Incidence of hypertension is higher among First Nations, Inuit, African, and South Asian people (Heart & Stroke Foundation of Canada, 2018).

3. Determine best site for BP assessment. Avoid applying cuff to extremity when IV fluids are infusing or when breast or axillary surgery has been performed on that side. BP should also not be done on extremities that have dialysis access in the form of an arteriovenous graft (AVG) or arteriovenous fistula (AVF) (Lewis et al., 2019). In addition, avoid applying cuff to traumatized or diseased extremity or one that has a cast or bulky bandage. After a stroke, BP should be measured in the unaffected arm (Maduagwu et al., 2018). Use lower extremities when brachial arteries are inaccessible.

Inappropriate site selection may result in poor amplification of sounds, causing inaccurate readings. Application of pressure from inflated bladder temporarily impairs blood flow and can further compromise circulation in extremity that already has impaired blood flow.

Studies have not directly determined the risk of lymphedema with BP measurement; however, BP cuffs on the affected arm of a person who has had a mastectomy *should be avoided*, as they use high-pressure focal compression that can lead to excessive constriction if not properly used (Lewis et al., 2019).

Avoiding BP on extremities with AVG and AVF helps prevent possible infection and thrombosis in the vascular access (Lewis et al., 2019).

BP measurement in hemiplegic arm is often inaccurate due to changes in muscle tone (Maduagwu et al., 2018).

4. Determine previous baseline BP and site (if available) from patient's record. Determine any report of latex allergy.

Assesses for change in condition. Provides comparison with future BP measurements. If patient has latex allergy, verify that stethoscope and BP cuff are latex free.

5. Assess patient's knowledge of procedure and any BP alteration that exists.

Encourages cooperation; minimizes risks and anxiety. Identifies teaching needs.

NURSING DIAGNOSES

- Reduced cardiac output
- Inadequate tissue perfusion
- Dehydration
- Fluid overload
- Potential for falls

Related factors/Risk factors are individualized on the basis of patient's condition or needs.

PLANNING

1. Expected outcome following completion of procedure:
   - BP is within acceptable range for patient's age.

Cardiovascular status is stable.

2. Explain to patient that you will assess BP. Have patient rest at least 5 minutes before measuring lying or sitting BP and 1 minute before measuring standing BP. Ask patient not to speak while you are measuring BP.

Reduces anxiety that can falsely elevate readings. Exercise causes false elevations in BP. Deep breathing lowers BP. Talking to a patient during assessment increases BP (Qi et al., 2017).

3. Be sure that 1 hour before measurement, patient has had no caffeine or tobacco. Make sure patient has not exercised within past 30 minutes (Hypertension Canada, 2015).

Smoking increases BP immediately and increase lasts up to 15 minutes. The effects of coffee or caffeine increase BP up to 3 hours (Hypertension Canada, 2015).

STEP	RATIONALE

PLANNING

4. Select appropriate cuff size (see Fig. 7.11) and ensure that other equipment is in patient's room.

Use of improper-size cuff causes false-low or false-high reading (see Box 7.6).

IMPLEMENTATION

1. Perform hand hygiene.

Reduces transmission of microorganisms.

2. Have patient assume sitting or lying position. Be sure that room is warm, quiet, and relaxing. Close room curtains.

Maintains patient's comfort during measurement. Patient's perceptions that physical or interpersonal environment is stressful affect BP.

3. Assess BP by auscultation:

a. *Upper extremity:* With patient sitting or lying, position their forearm at heart level with palm turned up (see illustration). If sitting, instruct patient to keep feet flat on floor without legs crossed. If supine, patient should not have legs crossed. If patient cannot be placed in prone position, position them supine with knee slightly bent.

If arm is extended and not supported, patient will perform isometric exercise that can increase diastolic pressure. Placement of arm above level of heart causes false-low reading, 2 mm Hg for each 2.5 cm (1 inch) above heart level.

Lower extremity: With patient prone, position patient so knee is slightly flexed.

Leg crossing can falsely increase BP.

b. Expose extremity (arm or leg) fully by removing constricting clothing.

Ensures proper cuff application.

c. Palpate brachial artery (arm, see illustration A) or popliteal artery (leg). With cuff fully deflated, apply bladder of cuff above artery by centring arrows marked on cuff over artery (see illustration B). If cuff does not have any centre arrows, estimate centre of bladder and place this centre over artery. Position cuff 2.5 cm (1 inch) above site of pulsation (antecubital or popliteal space). With cuff fully deflated, wrap it evenly and snugly around upper arm (see illustration C) or leg (see illustration D).

Brachial artery is along groove between biceps and triceps muscles above elbow at antecubital fossa. Popliteal artery is just below patient's thigh, behind knee.

Placing bladder directly over artery ensures that you apply proper pressure during inflation. A loose-fitting cuff causes false-high readings.

d. Position manometer gauge vertically at eye level. You should be no farther than 1 metre (approximately 1 yard) away.

Looking up or down at scale can result in distorted readings.

e. Measure BP using two-step method:

(1) Relocate brachial or popliteal pulse. Palpate artery distal to cuff with fingertips of nondominant hand while inflating cuff rapidly to pressure 30 mm Hg above point at which pulse disappears. Slowly deflate cuff and note point when pulse reappears. Deflate cuff fully and wait 30 seconds.

Estimating prevents false-low readings. Determine maximal inflation point for accurate reading by palpation. If unable to palpate artery because of weakened pulse, use ultrasonic stethoscope (see Chapter 8). Completely deflating cuff prevents venous congestion and false-high readings.

(2) Place stethoscope earpieces in ears and be sure that sounds are clear, not muffled.

Ensure that each earpiece follows angle of ear canal to facilitate hearing.

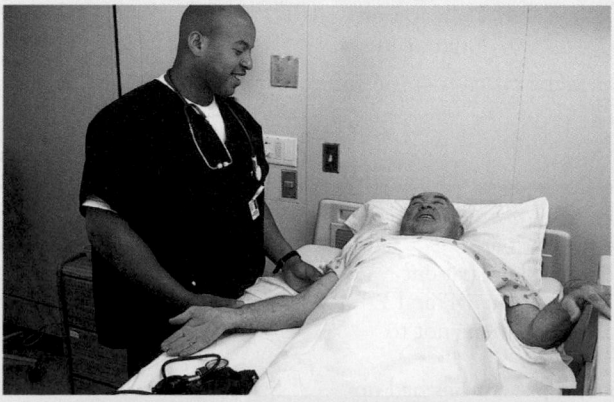

STEP 3a Patient's forearm supported on bed.

STEP	RATIONALE

IMPLEMENTATION

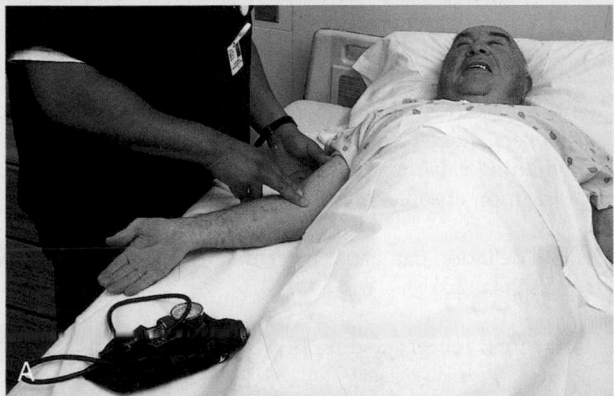

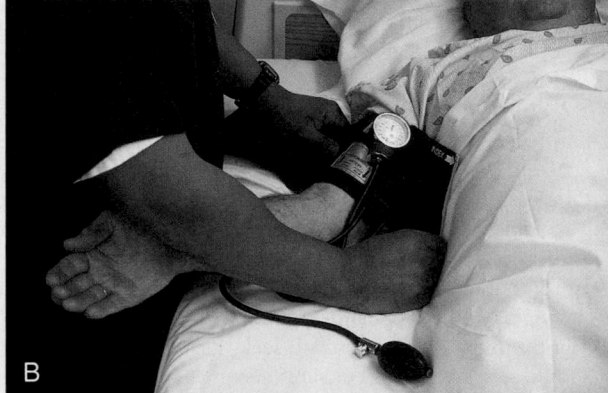

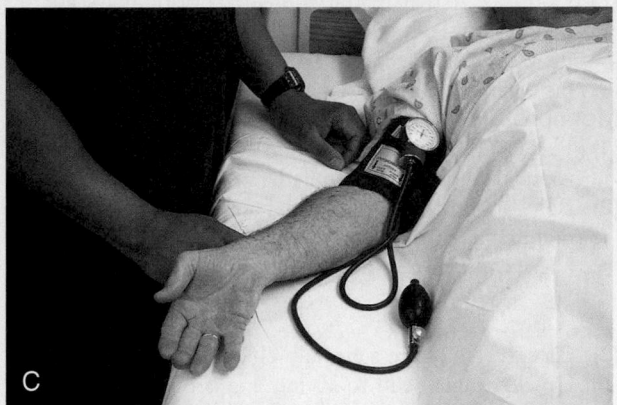

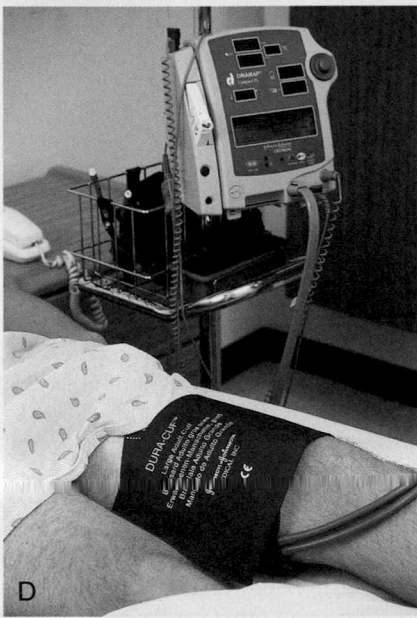

STEP 3c A, Palpating brachial artery. **B,** Aligning blood pressure cuff arrow with brachial artery. **C,** Blood pressure cuff wrapped around upper arm. **D,** Blood pressure cuff applied around thigh. (A–C, *Courtesy Barbara J. Astle, RN, PhD.*)

STEP	RATIONALE

IMPLEMENTATION

(3) Relocate artery and place bell or diaphragm chest piece of stethoscope over it. Do not allow chest piece to touch cuff or clothing.

Proper stethoscope placement ensures best sound reception. Stethoscope improperly positioned causes muffled sounds that often result in false-low systolic and false-high diastolic readings. The bell provides better sound reproduction, whereas the diaphragm is easier to secure with fingers and covers a larger area.

(4) Close valve of pressure bulb clockwise until tight. Quickly inflate cuff to 30 mm Hg above patient's estimated systolic pressure.

Tightening valve prevents air leak during inflation. Rapid inflation ensures accurate measurement of systolic pressure.

(5) Slowly release pressure bulb valve and allow manometer needle to fall at rate of 2 to 3 mm Hg/second.

Rapid deflation can cause inaccurate readings (Hypertension Canada, 2015).

(6) Note point on manometer when you hear first clear sound. Sound will slowly increase in intensity.

First sound reflects systolic BP.

(7) Continue to deflate cuff gradually, noting point at which sound disappears in adults. Note pressure to nearest 2 mm Hg. Listen for 20 to 30 mm Hg after last sound and allow remaining air to escape quickly.

Beginning of last or fifth sound is indication of diastolic pressure in adults whereas in children, the distinct muffling of sounds indicates diastolic pressure (Mattoo, Stapleton, & Fulton, 2018).

f. Measure BP using one-step method:

(1) Place stethoscope earpieces in ears and be sure that sounds are clear, not muffled.

Earpieces should follow angle of ear canal to facilitate hearing.

(2) Relocate brachial or popliteal artery and place bell or diaphragm chest piece of stethoscope over it. Do not allow chest piece to touch cuff or clothing.

Proper stethoscope placement ensures optimal sound reception. Stethoscope improperly positioned causes muffled sounds that often result in false readings. Bell provides better sound reproduction, whereas diaphragm is easier to secure with fingers and covers larger area.

(3) Close valve of pressure bulb clockwise until tight. Quickly inflate cuff to 30 mm Hg above patient's usual systolic pressure.

Tightening valve prevents air leak during inflation. Inflation above systolic level ensures accurate measurement of systolic pressure.

(4) Slowly release pressure bulb valve and allow manometer needle to fall at rate of 2 to 3 mm Hg/second. Note point on manometer when you hear first clear sound. Sound will slowly increase in intensity.

Rapid deflation can cause inaccurate readings (Hypertension Canada, 2015). First sound reflects systolic pressure.

(5) Continue to deflate cuff gradually, noting point at which sound disappears in adults. Note pressure to nearest 2 mm Hg. Listen for 10 to 20 mm Hg after last sound and allow remaining air to escape quickly.

Beginning of last or fifth sound is indication of diastolic pressure in adults, whereas in children the distinct muffling of sounds indicates diastolic pressure (Mattoo et al., 2018).

(6) Leung and colleagues (2017) recommend that if non-AOBP is used to measure BP, the mean of at least three readings is used, discarding the first and calculating the remaining ones.

Three sets of BP measurements help to prevent false-positive readings based on patient's sympathetic response (alert reaction). Averaging minimizes effect of anxiety, which often causes first reading to be higher than subsequent measures (Basilie & Bloch, 2018).

5. Remove cuff from patient's arm or leg unless you need to repeat measurement.

Continuous cuff inflation causes arterial occlusion, resulting in numbness and tingling of patient's arm or leg.

6. If this is first assessment of patient, repeat procedure on other arm or leg.

Different BP readings in the right and left arms that vary by a few mm Hg is not worrisome; however, a significant difference in pressure (greater than 10) in the right and left arms can signal circulatory problems that may lead to stroke, peripheral artery disease, or other cardiovascular problems. Use arm with higher pressure for repeated measurements (Corliss, 2016).

7. Assess systolic BP by palpation:

a. Follow Steps 3a through 3d of auscultation method.

b. Locate and then continually palpate brachial, radial, or popliteal artery with fingertips of one hand. Inflate cuff to pressure 30 mm Hg above point at which you can no longer palpate pulse.

Ensures accurate detection of true systolic pressure once pressure valve is released.

STEP	RATIONALE

IMPLEMENTATION

Clinical Decision Point *If unable to palpate artery because of weakened pulse, use a Doppler ultrasonic stethoscope (Fig. 7.12).*

c. Slowly release valve and deflate cuff, allowing manometer needle to fall at rate of 2 mm Hg/second. Note point on manometer when pulse is again palpable.

Rapid deflation can cause inaccurate readings (Hypertension Canada, 2015). Palpation helps identify systolic pressure only.

d. Deflate cuff rapidly and completely. Remove cuff from patient's extremity unless you need to repeat measurement.

Continuous cuff inflation causes arterial occlusion, resulting in numbness and tingling of extremity.

8. Measure orthostatic hypotension:

a. Have patient lie down for 5 minutes, then measure BP and pulse.

This is to give a baseline BP and pulse.

b. Have patient stand for 1 minute, then retake BP and pulse.

c. Have patient continue to stand, and retake BP and pulse after 3 minutes (CDC, 2017b).

d. Always make sure patient has a safe place to sit or land while standing. If patient is too dizzy or weak to stand, have person sit at edge of the bed and dangle legs (Jarvis, 2019).

Rapid cardiovascular adaptations driven primarily by the autonomic nervous system maintain BP upon assumption of upright posture. A drop in BP upon standing can indicate failure of these compensatory mechanisms and can result in orthostatic hypotension (Amy et al., 2017).

9. Help patient return to comfortable position and cover upper arm or leg if previously clothed.

Restores comfort and provides sense of well-being.

10. Discuss findings with patient.

Promotes participation in care and understanding of health status. Makes patient accountable for follow-up assessment. Systolic BP in leg is 10 to 40 mm Hg higher than arm, but diastolic BP is same.

11. Clean earpieces and diaphragm of stethoscope with alcohol swab as needed. Wipe cuff with employer-approved disinfectant if used between patients. Perform hand hygiene.

Controls transmission of microorganisms when nurses share stethoscope.

Reduces transmission of microorganisms.

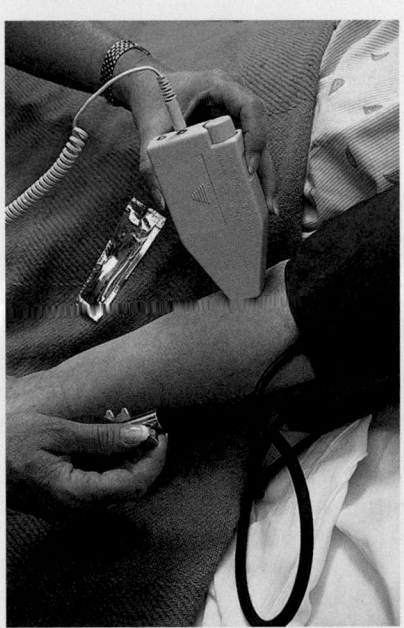

FIG 7.12 Doppler ultrasonic stethoscope over brachial artery to measure blood pressure.

STEP	RATIONALE

EVALUATION

1. If assessing BP for first time, establish baseline BP if it is within acceptable range.

Used to compare future BP measurements.

2. Compare BP reading with patient's previous baseline and usual BP for patient's age.

Allows you to assess for change in condition. Provides comparison with future BP measurements.

3. **Use Teach-Back:** "I want to be sure I explained why it is important to stand up slowly since you have high blood pressure. Tell me which of your medications might make you dizzy if you stand up too fast." Develop a revised teaching plan if patient or caregiver is not able to teach back correctly.

Determines patient's and caregiver's level of understanding of instructional topic.

Unexpected Outcomes	Related Interventions
1. Patient's BP is above acceptable range.	• Repeat measurement in other extremity and compare findings.
	• Verify correct size and placement of BP cuff.
	• If BP was taken manually, have another nurse repeat measurement in 1 to 2 minutes to ensure it is not due to human error.
	• Observe for related symptoms that are not apparent unless BP is extremely high, including headache, facial flushing, nosebleed, and fatigue in older patients.
	• Report BP to nurse in charge or health care provider to initiate appropriate evaluation and treatment.
	• Administer antihypertensive medications as prescribed.
2. Patient's BP is not sufficient for adequate perfusion and oxygenation of tissues.	• Compare BP value to baseline.
	• Position patient in supine position to enhance circulation and restrict activity that decreases BP further.
	• Assess for signs and symptoms associated with hypotension, including tachycardia; weak, thready pulse; weakness; dizziness; confusion; and cool, pale, dusky, or cyanotic skin.
	• Assess for factors that contribute to low BP, including hemorrhage, dilation of blood vessels resulting from hyperthermia, anaesthesia, or medication adverse effects.
	• Report BP to nurse in charge or health care provider to initiate appropriate evaluation and treatment.
	• Increase rate of IV infusion or administer vasoconstriction drugs if prescribed.
3. Unable to obtain BP reading.	• Determine that no immediate crisis is present by obtaining pulse and respiratory rate.
	• Assess for signs and symptoms of decreased cardiac output; if present, notify nurse in charge or health care provider immediately.
	• Use alternative sites or procedures to obtain BP: use Doppler ultrasonic instrument (see Chapter 8); palpate systolic BP.
4. Patient experiences orthostatic hypotension.	• Maintain patient safety.
	• Return patient to safe position in bed or chair.

Communication and Documentation

• Document BP and site assessed on vital sign flow sheet or in nurses' notes in EHR or chart.

• Document measurement of BP and any signs or symptoms of BP alterations after administration of specific therapies in nurses' notes in EHR or chart.

• Document your evaluation of patient and caregiver learning.

• Review baseline and previous BP measurement and report abnormal findings to nurse in charge or health care provider.

Special Considerations
Teaching

• Educate patient about risks for hypertension. People with family history of hypertension, premature heart disease, lipidemia, or

renal disease are at significant risk. Obesity, cigarette smoking, heavy alcohol consumption, high serum lipids, high dietary sodium intake, sedentary lifestyle, and continued exposure to psychosocial stress are factors linked to hypertension (Leung et al., 2017).

• Primary prevention and treatment of hypertension include health behaviour management: smoking cessation, physical exercise, weight reduction, decreased alcohol consumption, decreased sodium intake, stress management, and increased intake of dietary potassium in those who are not at risk for hyperkalemia (Leung et al., 2017).

• Instruct primary caregiver to take BP at same time each day and after patient has had a brief rest. Take BP sitting or lying down; use same position and arm each time pressure is taken.

• Instruct caregiver that if the BP is difficult to hear, it is probably caused by one of the following: cuff too loose, not large enough,

or too narrow; stethoscope not over arterial pulse; cuff deflated too quickly or too slowly; or cuff not pumped high enough for systolic readings.

Pediatric

- BP measurement is not a routine part of assessment in children younger than 3 years.
- BP measurement can frighten children. Prepare child for squeezing feeling of inflated BP cuff by comparing sensation to elastic band on finger or a tight hug on the arm.
- Obtain BP in child before performing anxiety-producing tests or procedures.
- BP sounds are difficult to hear in children because of low frequency and amplitude. Using the bell of a pediatric stethoscope is often helpful.

Gerontological

- Older persons, especially frail older persons, have lost upper-arm mass, requiring special attention to selection of BP cuff size.
- Skin of older persons is more fragile and susceptible to cuff pressure when measurements are frequent. More frequent assessment of skin under cuff or rotation of measurement sites is recommended.
- Older persons commonly have pseudohypertension, which is elevated systolic pressure readings resulting from the inability of the BP cuff to adequately compress the arteries in those with arteriosclerosis (Hirst et al., 2015, p. 415) related to decreased vessel elasticity.
- Older persons often experience a fall in BP after eating.
- Instruct older persons to change position slowly and wait after each change to avoid postural hypotension and prevent injuries.

Care in the Community

- Assess home noise level to determine room that provides the quietest environment for assessing BP.
- Instruct patient in the importance of an appropriate-size BP cuff for home use.

- Assess family's financial ability to afford an electronic BP machine for performing BP evaluations on a regular basis. They should purchase and use only BP monitoring devices that have met the standards of the Association for the Advancement of Medical Instrumentation, the most recent requirements of the British Hypertension Society protocol, or the International Protocol for validation of automated BP-measuring devices. Patients should also be encouraged to use devices that can record date or have automatic data transmission to increase reliability of reported home BP monitoring (Leung et al., 2017).
- Teach patient and caregiver on the correct way to measure BP in the home and if necessary repeat training (Box 7.8). They should be observed to determine that they can measure BP correctly and interpret the readings (Leung et al., 2017).

BOX 7.8

Standardized Protocol for Home Blood Pressure Measurement

- Measurements should be taken using a validated electronic device.
- Choose a cuff with an appropriate bladder size matched to the size of the arm. Bladder width should be close to 40% of arm circumference and bladder length should cover 80–100% of arm circumference. Select the cuff size as recommended by its manufacturer.
- Cuff should be applied to the nondominant arm unless the systolic blood pressure difference between arms is >10 mm Hg, in which case the arm with the highest value obtained should be used.
- The patient should be resting comfortably for 5 minutes in the seated position with back support.
- The arm should be bare and supported with the blood pressure cuff at heart level.
- Measurement should be performed before breakfast and 2 hours after dinner, before taking medication.
- No caffeine or tobacco used in the hour and no exercise done 30 minutes preceding the measurement.
- Duplicate measurement should be taken in the morning and in the evening for 7 days (i.e., 28 measurements in total).
- Average the results excluding the first day's readings.

From Hypertension Canada. (2015). *Home BP measurement* (Table 1). Retrieved from http://guidelines.hypertension.ca/diagnosis-assessment/home-measurement/.

PROCEDURAL GUIDELINE 7.1 *Noninvasive Electronic Blood Pressure Measurement*

NSO *Nursing Skills Online Vital Signs Module 1 / Lesson 5*

Many different styles of electronic blood pressure (BP) machines are available to determine blood pressure automatically (Fig. 7.13). Electronic machines rely on an electronic sensor to detect the vibrations caused by the rush of blood through an artery. They are easy to use and efficient and a stethoscope is not needed. The devices can be preprogrammed to take either single measurements or a series of measurements then average the results. Hypertension Canada strongly encourages the use of these validated electronic digital oscillometric devices as they can minimize or eliminate many auscultation-induced errors (Leung et al., 2017).

Delegation and Collaboration

The skill of BP measurement using an electronic BP machine can be delegated to an unregulated care providers (UCP) unless the patient is considered unstable (e.g., hypotensive). The nurse instructs the UCP by:

- Explaining the frequency and extremity to use for measurement.
- Reviewing how to select an appropriate-size BP cuff for designated extremity and appropriate cuff for the machine.
- Reviewing patient's usual BP and reporting significant changes or abnormalities to the nurse.

Equipment

- Electronic BP machine
- BP cuff of appropriate size as recommended by manufacturer
- Pen and vital sign flow sheet in chart or electronic health record (EHR)

Procedural Steps

1. Identify patient using at least two person-specific identifiers (e.g., name and date of birth or name and medical record number) according to employer policy (Accreditation Canada, 2019).

Continued

PROCEDURAL GUIDELINE 7.1 *Noninvasive Electronic Blood Pressure Measurement*—cont'd

2. Assess need to measure BP (see Skill 7.5, Assessment Step 2) and determine patient's baseline BP.
3. Perform hand hygiene. Determine best site for cuff placement; inspect condition of extremities.
4. Collect and bring appropriate equipment to patient's bedside. Select appropriate cuff size for patient extremity (Table 7.2) and appropriate cuff for machine. Electronic BP cuff and machine must be matched by manufacturer and are not interchangeable.
5. Help patient to comfortable position, either lying or sitting. Plug device into electric outlet and place it near patient, ensuring that connector hose between cuff and machine reaches.
6. Locate on/off switch and turn on machine to enable device to self-test computer systems.

7. Remove constricting clothing to ensure proper cuff application.
8. Prepare BP cuff by manually squeezing all the air out of the cuff and connecting it to connector hose.
9. Wrap flattened cuff snugly around extremity, verifying that only one finger can fit between cuff and patient's skin. Make sure that "artery" arrow marked on outside of cuff is placed correctly (see illustration).

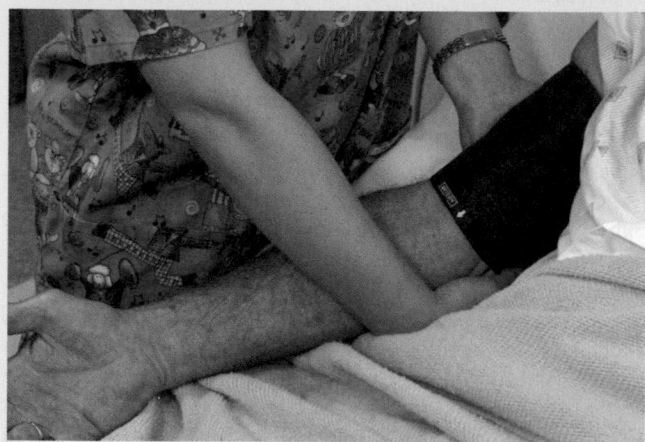

STEP 9 Aligning blood pressure cuff arrow with brachial artery.

10. Verify that connector hose between cuff and machine is not kinked. Kinking prevents proper inflation and deflation of cuff.
11. Following manufacturer directions, set frequency control for automatic or manual and press the start button. The first BP measurement pumps cuff to a peak pressure of approximately 180 mm Hg. After this pressure is reached, the machine begins a deflation sequence that determines the BP. The first reading determines peak pressure inflation for additional measurements.
12. When deflation is complete, digital display provides most recent values and flash time in minutes that have elapsed since the measurement occurred (see illustration).

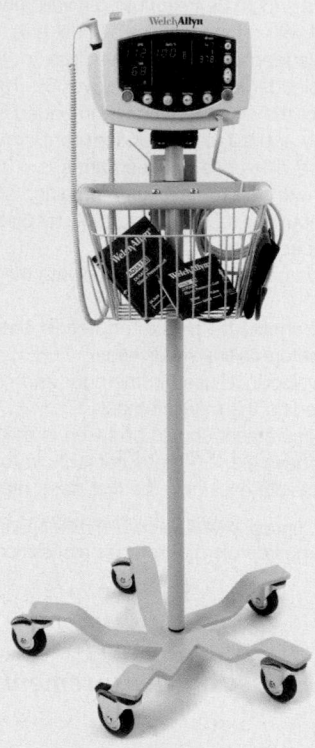

FIG 7.13 Noninvasive electronic blood pressure machine. (*Photo courtesy Welch Allyn.*)

TABLE 7.2	
Correct Blood Pressure Cuff Size for Electronic Monitor*	
Cuff Size	**Limb Circumference (cm)**
Small adult	17–25
Adult	23–33
Large adult	31–40
Thigh	38–50

*A 3.7 to 7.3 metre (12 to 24 foot) cord is usually required for electronic adult BP monitoring.

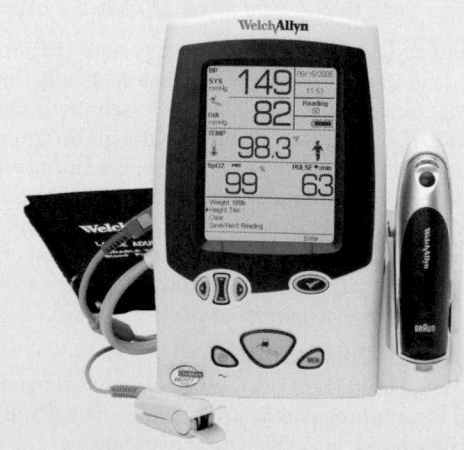

STEP 12 Digital electronic blood pressure display. (*Image courtesy Welch Allyn.*)

PROCEDURAL GUIDELINE 7.1 *Noninvasive Electronic Blood Pressure Measurement—cont'd*

Clinical Decision Point *If unable to obtain blood pressure with electronic device, verify machine connections (e.g., plugged into working electrical outlet, hose-cuff connections tight, machine on, correct cuff). Repeat electronic blood pressure; if unable to obtain, use auscultatory technique (see Skill 7.5).*

13. Set frequency of measurements and upper and lower alarm limits for systolic, diastolic, and mean BP readings. Intervals between measurements can be set from 1 to 90 minutes. A nurse determines frequency and alarm limits on the basis of patient's acceptable range of BP, nursing judgement, and health care provider prescription.

14. Obtain additional readings at any time by pressing the start button. Pressing the cancel button immediately deflates the cuff.

15. If frequent measurements are required, the cuff may be left in place. Remove it at least every 2 hours to assess underlying skin integrity and, if possible, alternate measurement sites. Patients with abnormal bleeding tendencies are at risk for microvascular rupture from repeated inflations. When patient no longer requires frequent BP monitoring, remove and clean cuff according to employer policy to reduce transmission of microorganisms. Disinfect electronic BP unit regularly when visibly soiled, after every use or once daily (CDC, 2017b). If possible, leave the machine in the room for patients on isolation precautions or disinfect before using it on another patient.

16. Perform hand hygiene. Discuss findings with patient.

17. Record BP and site assessed on vital sign flow sheet or in nurses' notes in EHR or chart; record any signs or symptoms of BP alterations in narrative form in nurses' notes; compare patient's baseline and most current previous BP findings to current readings; report abnormal findings to nurse in charge or health care provider.

18. **Use Teach-Back:** "I want to be sure I explained why you need to keep your arm straight while the machine is taking your blood pressure. Tell me why it is important to remain still." Develop a revised teaching plan if patient or caregiver is not able to teach back correctly.

PROCEDURAL GUIDELINE 7.2 *Measuring Oxygen Saturation (Pulse Oximetry)*

NSO *Nursing Skills Online Airway Management Module 1 / Lesson 6* 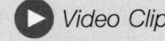 *Video Clip*

Pulse oximetry is the noninvasive measurement of arterial blood oxygen saturation, the percent to which hemoglobin is filled with oxygen. A pulse oximeter is a probe with a light-emitting diode (LED) connected by cable to an oximeter. The LED emits light wavelengths that are absorbed differently by the oxygenated and deoxygenated hemoglobin molecules. The more hemoglobin saturated by oxygen, the higher the oxygen saturation. Normally oxygen saturation (SpO_2) is greater than 95%. A saturation less than 90% is a clinical emergency (World Health Organization [WHO], 2011).

Pulse oximetry measurement of SpO_2 is simple and painless and has few of the risks associated with more invasive measurements of oxygen saturation such as arterial blood gas sampling. A vascular, pulsatile area is needed to detect the change in the transmitted light when making measurements with a finger or earlobe probe. Conditions that decrease arterial blood flow such as peripheral vascular disease, hypothermia, pharmacological vasoconstrictors, hypotension, or peripheral edema affect accurate determination of oxygen saturation in these areas. For patients with decreased peripheral perfusion, you can apply a forehead sensor. Factors that affect light transmission such as outside light sources or patient motion also affect the measurement of oxygen saturation. Carbon monoxide in the blood, jaundice, and intravascular dyes can influence the light reflected from hemoglobin molecules.

In adults, you can apply reusable and disposable oximeter probes to the earlobe, finger, toe, bridge of the nose, or forehead (Box 7.9). Pulse oximetry is indicated in patients who have an unstable oxygen status or are at risk for impaired gas exchange.

Delegation and Collaboration
The skill of SpO_2 measurement can be delegated to an unregulated care provider (UCP). The nurse instructs the UCP by:

BOX 7.9

Characteristics of Pulse Oximeter Sensor Probes and Sites

Finger Probe
- Easy to apply, conforms to various sizes

Earlobe Probe
- Clip-on is smaller and lighter, although more positional than finger probe
- Yields strong correlation with oxygen saturation
- Good when uncontrollable or rhythmic movements (e.g., hand tremors during exercise) are present
- Vascular bed least affected by decreased blood flow

Forehead Sensor
- Greater accuracy during decreased perfusion (Nesseler et al., 2012)
- Reliable for patients on vasoactive medications
- Detects desaturation quicker than other sites (Yont, Korhan, & Khorshid, 2011)
- Does not require a pulsatile vascular bed
- Good when uncontrollable or rhythmic movements (e.g., hand tremors) are present
- Requires headband to secure sensor

Disposable Sensor Pad
- Can be applied to a variety of sites: earlobe of adult, nose bridge, palm or sole of infant
- Less restrictive for continuous oxygen saturation monitoring
- Expensive
- Contains latex
- Skin under adhesive may become moist and harbour pathogens
- Available in variety of sizes; pad can be matched to infant weight

Continued

PROCEDURAL GUIDELINE 7.2 *Measuring Oxygen Saturation (Pulse Oximetry)—cont'd*

- Communicating specific factors related to the patient that can falsely lower SpO_2.
- Informing the UCP about appropriate sensor site and probe.
- Notifying frequency of SpO_2 measurements for a specific patient.
- Instructing to notify nurse immediately of any reading lower than SpO_2 of 95% or value for a specific patient.
- Instructing the UCP to refrain from using pulse oximetry to obtain heart rate because oximeter will not detect an irregular pulse.

Equipment
- Oximeter
- Oximeter probe appropriate for patient and recommended by oximeter manufacturer
- Acetone or nail polish remover if needed
- Pen and vital sign flow sheet in chart or electronic health record (EHR)

Procedural Steps
1. Identify patient using at least two person-specific identifiers (e.g., name and date of birth or name and medical record number) according to employer policy (Accreditation Canada, 2019).
2. Determine need to measure patient's oxygen saturation. Assess risk factors for decreased oxygen saturation (e.g., acute or chronic compromised respiratory problems, change in oxygen therapy, chest wall injury, recovery from anaesthesia).
3. Perform hand hygiene. Assess for signs and symptoms of alterations in oxygen saturation (e.g., altered respiratory rate, depth, or rhythm; adventitious breath sounds [see Chapter 8]; cyanotic nails, lips, mucous membranes, or skin; restlessness; difficulty breathing).
4. Determine if patient has a latex allergy; disposable adhesive sensors are made of latex.
5. Assess for factors that influence measurement of SpO_2 (e.g., oxygen therapy, respiratory therapy such as postural drainage and percussion; hemoglobin level, hypotension, temperature, nail polish [Jubran, 2015]; medications such as bronchodilators).
6. Review patient's medical record for health care provider's prescription and employer policy for standard of care for measurement of SpO_2.
7. Determine previous baseline SpO_2 (if available) from patient's record.
8. Perform hand hygiene. Determine most appropriate patient-specific site (e.g., finger, earlobe, bridge of nose, forehead) for sensor probe placement by measuring capillary refill (see Chapter 8). If capillary refill is greater than 2 seconds, select alternative site.
   - Site must have adequate local circulation and be free of moisture.
   - If patient has tremors or is likely to move, use earlobe or forehead. Motion artifact is the most common cause of inaccurate readings (Jubran, 2015).
   - If patient's finger is too large for the clip-on probe, as may be the case with obesity or edema, the clip-on probe may not fit properly; obtain a disposable (tape-on) probe.
9. Arrange equipment at the bedside.
10. Position patient comfortably. Instruct them to breathe normally.
11. Attach sensor to monitoring site (see illustration). If using finger, remove fingernail polish from digit with acetone or polish remover. Instruct patient that clip-on probe will feel like a clothespin on the finger but will not hurt.

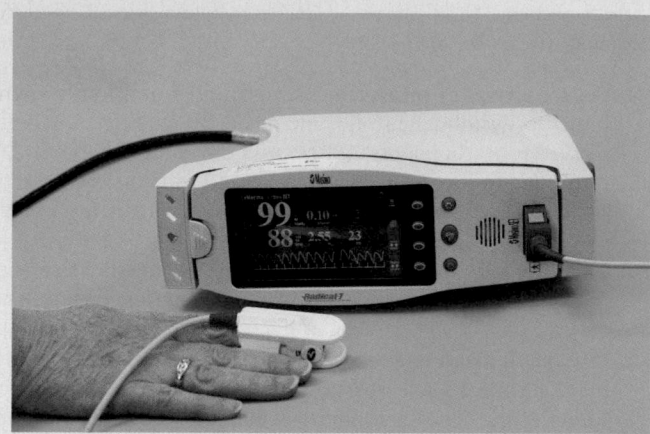

STEP 11 Oximeter sensor attached to finger.

Clinical Decision Point *Do not attach probe to finger, ear, or bridge of nose if area is edematous or skin integrity is compromised. Do not use earlobe and bridge of nose sensors for infants and toddlers because of skin fragility. Do not attach sensor to fingers that are hypothermic. Select ear or bridge of nose if adult patient has a history of peripheral vascular disease. Do not use disposable adhesive sensors if patient has a latex allergy. Do not place sensor on same extremity as electronic blood pressure cuff because blood flow to finger will be interrupted temporarily when cuff inflates and cause inaccurate reading that can trigger alarms (Skirton et al., 2011).*

12. Once sensor is in place, turn on oximeter by activating power. Observe pulse waveform/intensity display and audible beep. Correlate oximeter pulse rate with patient's radial pulse.
13. Leave sensor in place 10 to 30 seconds or until oximeter readout reaches constant value and pulse display reaches full strength during each cardiac cycle. Inform patient that oximeter alarm will sound if sensor falls off or patient moves it. Read SpO_2 on digital display.
14. If you plan to monitor SpO_2 continuously, verify SpO_2 alarm limits preset by manufacturer at a low of 85% and a high of 100%. Determine limits for SpO_2 and pulse rate as indicated by patient's condition. For example, patients receiving oxygen because of an acute exacerbation of chronic obstructive pulmonary disease (COPD) should have their oxygen saturation levels maintained between 88 and 92% (National Institute for Health Care and Excellence [NICE], 2016). Verify that alarms are on. Assess skin integrity under sensor probe every 2 hours; relocate sensor at least every 4 hours and more frequently if skin integrity is altered or tissue perfusion compromised.
15. If you plan intermittent or spot-checking of SpO_2, remove probe and turn oximeter power off. Clean sensor and store sensor in appropriate location.
16. Discuss findings with patient. Perform hand hygiene.
17. Compare SpO_2 with patient's previous baseline and acceptable SpO_2.

PROCEDURAL GUIDELINE 7.2 *Measuring Oxygen Saturation (Pulse Oximetry)—cont'd*

18. Record SpO_2 on vital sign flow sheet in chart or EHR; indicate type and amount of oxygen therapy used by patient during assessment; record any signs or symptoms of alterations in oxygen saturation in narrative form in nurses' notes in EHR or chart.

19. Report abnormal findings to nurse in charge or health care provider.

20. Use Teach-Back: "I want to be sure I explained why you need to keep the probe on your finger. Tell me why this measurement is important and how moving your finger affects the reading." Develop a revised teaching plan if patient or caregiver is not able to teach back correctly.

◆ CLINICAL DEBRIEF

The nurse is caring for a 56-year-old university professor who is admitted from the trauma unit following a motorcycle-automobile accident. The patient has a fractured left humerus and pelvis. Although he was wearing a helmet, he suffered a concussion. When doing your admission assessment, you note a cast on his left arm and an intravenous (IV) line in his right antecubital fossa. His sister is present and tells you that he is on a beta-blocker for mild hypertension. He received IV morphine sulphate 15 mg in the emergency department and is very sleepy. He awakens only to touch.

1. Which admission vital signs can you assign to the unregulated care provider (UCP)? Which directions should the nurse provide the UCP regarding obtaining routine vital signs for this patient?

2. An hour after admission the patient has stabilized. One hour later, the UCP reports the radial pulse rate is 54 beats/min. The nurse notes that the emergency department nurse recorded a heart rate of 108. What might explain the change in heart rate? Which interventions should the nurse consider at this time?

3. Two hours after admission the respiratory rate is 12 breaths/min, oxygen saturation 90%, blood pressure 112/60 mm Hg, pulse 92 beats/min. The nurse repeats and confirms these vital signs and notes that the patient is very difficult to rouse. Using SBAR, show how the nurse should communicate with the health care team about this patient.

◆ REVIEW QUESTIONS

1. Which of the following conditions should the nurse identify as possibly causing a falsely elevated blood pressure measurement? *(Select all that apply.)*
   1. Arm positioned above heart level
   2. Deflating the cuff too slowly
   3. Inflating the cuff too fast
   4. Loose-fitting cuff
   5. Using an adult cuff on a toddler

2. Which site should the nurse use to auscultate the heart rate at the point of maximal impulse (PMI)?
   1. A
   2. B
   3. C
   4. D

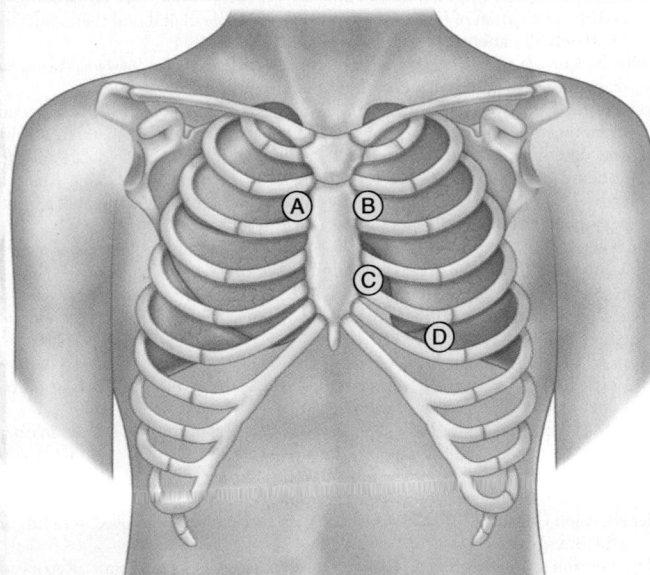

3. Which of the following conditions should the nurse expect to cause an error in SpO_2 measurement? *(Select all that apply.)*
   1. Probe placed on finger with clear pink nail polish
   2. Finger probe on patient with a temperature of 35°C (95°F)
   3. Ear probe on patient with a temperature of 38.5°C (101.3°F)
   4. Foot probe on infant who is actively moving
   5. Forehead probe on patient who is perspiring

ⓔ *Visit the Evolve site for a complete list of Clinical Debrief and Review Questions answers.*

REFERENCES

Accreditation Canada. (2019). *Required organizational practices handbook—Version 14*. Retrieved from http://www.wrha.mb.ca/quality/files/2019ROPHandbook.pdf

Arnold, A. C., & Raj, S. R. (2017). Orthostatic hypotension: A practical approach to investigation and management. *The Canadian Journal of Cardiology, 33*(12), 725–728. doi:10.1016/j.cjca2017.05.007

Basilie, J., & Bloch, M. J. (2018). *Overview of hypertension in adults*. UpToDate, 2018. Retrieved from http://www.uptodate.com/contents/overview-of-hypertension-in-adults

Breen, A., & Hessels, A. (2017). Stethoscopes: Friend or fomite? *Nursing Management, 48*(12), 9–11. doi:10.1097/01.NUMA.0000526917.85088.eb

Canadian Agency for Drugs and Technologies in Health (CADTH). (2017). *The assessment of postoperative vitals: Clinical effectiveness and guidelines*. Retrieved from https://www.cadth.ca/assessment-postoperative-vital-signs-clinical-effectiveness-and-guidelines

Canadian Nurses Association (CNA). (2011). *Position statement: Interprofessional collaboration*. Retrieved from https://www.cna-aiic.ca/-/media/cna/page-content/pdf-en/interproffessional-collaboration_position-statement.pdf?la=en&hash=5695B7264EB8EE6FA1A4B1A73A44A052F0FEA40F

Canadian Paediatric Society. (2017). *Position statement: Temperature measurement in paediatrics*. Retrieved from https://www.cps.ca/en/documents/position/temperature-measurement

Centers for Disease Control and Prevention (CDC). (2017a). *Guideline for disinfection and sterilization in healthcare facilities*. Retrieved from https://www.cdc.gov/infectioncontrol/pdf/guidelines/disinfection-guidelines.pdf

Centers for Disease Control and Prevention (CDC). (2017b). *Infection control: Standard precautions for all patient care*. Retrieved from https://www.cdc.gov/infectioncontrol/basics/standard-precautions.html

Corliss, J. (2016). *Big arm-to-arm difference in blood pressure linked to higher heart attack risk*. Harvard Health Blog. Retrieved from https://www.health.harvard.edu/blog/big-arm-arm-difference-blood-pressure-linked-higher-heart-attack-risk-201403057064

Counts, D., Acosta, M., Holbrook, H., Foos, E., Hays-Ponder, K., & Twiss, E. J. (2014). Evaluation of temporal artery and disposable digital oral thermometers in acutely ill patients. *Medsurg Nursing, 23*(4), 239–244.

Diabetes Canada. (2018). *Hypertension*. Retrieved from https://www.diabetes.ca/diabetes-and-you/complications/high-blood-pressure

Forrest, A., Conley, S., Juliano, M., Nicholson, M., & Auten, J. (2016). Rectal thermometry comparison to temporal artery and axillary thermometry in infants and children. *Annals of Emergency Medicine, 68*(4), S92. doi:10.1016/j.annemergmed.2016.08.249

Goforth, C., & Kazman, J. (2015). Exertional heat stroke in navy and marine personnel: A hot topic. *Critical Care Nurse, 35*(1), 52.

Hannon, R. A., & Porth, C. M. (2017). *Porth pathophysiology: Concepts of altered health states* (2nd Can. ed.). Philadelphia: Wolters Kluwer.

Hayes, K., Shepard, A., Cesarec, A., & Likić, R. (2017). Cost minimisation analysis of thermometry in two different hospital systems. *Postgraduate Medical Journal, 93*, 603–606.

Heart & Stroke Foundation of Canada. (2018). *Risk factors you cannot change*. Retrieved from https://www.heartandstroke.ca/heart/risk-and-prevention/risk-factors-you-cannot-change

Hirst, S. P., Lane, A. M., & Miller, C. A. (2015). *Millers nursing for wellness in older adults* (Cdn. ed.). Philadelphia: Wolters Kluwer.

Hockenberry, M. J., & Wilson, D. (2015). *Wong's nursing care of infants and children* (10th ed.). St. Louis: Mosby.

Hypertension Canada. (2015). *Hypertension Canada guidelines*. Retrieved from http://guidelines.hypertension.ca

Hypertension Canada. (2018). *Accurate measurement of blood pressure*. Retrieved from http://guidelines.hypertension.ca/diagnosis-assessment/measuring-blood-pressure/

Jarvis, C. (2019). *Physical examination and health assessment* (3rd Can. ed.). Toronto: Elsevier.

Jones, C., Sangthong, B., Pachirat, O., & Jones, D. (2015). Slow breathing training reduces resting blood pressure and the pressure responses to exercise. *Physiological Research, 64*(5), 673–682.

Joseph, R., Derstine, S., & Killian, M. (2017). Ideal site for skin temperature probe placement on infants in the NICU: A review of the literature. *Advances in Neonatal Care, 17*(2), 114–122. doi:10.1097/ANC.0000000000000369

Jubran, A. (2015). Pulse oximetry. *Critical Care : The Official Journal of the Critical Care Forum, 19*(1), 272. doi:10.1186/s13054-015-0984-8

Kaczorowski, J., Myers, M. G., Gelfer, M., et al. (2017). How do family physicians measure blood pressure in routine clinical practice? National survey of Canadian family physicians. *Canadian Family Physician, 63*(3), e193–e199.

Leung, A. A., Daskalopoulou, S. S., Dasgupta, K., et al. (2017). Hypertension Canada's 2017 guidelines for diagnosis, risk assessment, prevention, and treatment of hypertension in adults guidelines. *The Canadian Journal of Cardiology, 33*, 557–576. doi:10.1016/j.cjca2017.03.005

Lewis, S. L., Bucher, L., Heitkemper, M., et al. (2019). *Medical-surgical nursing in Canada: Assessment and management of clinical problems* (4th Cdn. ed.). Toronto: Elsevier Canada.

Maduagwu, S., Umeonwuka, C., Mohammad, H., et al. (2018). Reference arm for blood pressure measurement in stroke survivors. *Middle East Journal of Rehabilitation and Health Studies, 5*(1), e62368. doi:10.5812/mejrh.62368

Mattoo, T., Stapleton, F., & Fulton, D. (2018). *Definition and diagnosis of hypertension in children and adolescents*. UpToDate, 2018. Retrieved from https://www.uptodate.com/contents/definition-and-diagnosis-of-hypertension-in-children-and-adolescents?search=children%20blood%20pressure&source=search_result&selectedTitle=1~150&usage_type=default&display_rank=1

National Institute for Health and Care Excellence (NICE). (2016). *Chronic obstructive pulmonary disease in adults*. Retrieved from https://www.nice.org.uk/guidance/qs10/chapter/quality-statement-6-emergency-oxygen-during-an-exacerbation#quality-statement-6-emergency-oxygen-during-an-exacerbation

Nesseler, N., Frenel, J. V., Launey, Y., Morcet, J., Malledant, Y., & Seguin, P. (2012). Pulse oximetry and high-dose vasopressors: A comparison between forehead reflectance and finger transmission sensors. *Intensive Care Medicine, 38*(10), 1718.

Niven, D., Gaudet, J., Laupland, K., Mrklas, K., Roberts, D., & Stelfox, H. (2015). Accuracy of peripheral thermometers for estimating temperature: A systematic review and meta-analysis. *Annals of Internal Medicine, 163*(10), 768–777. doi:10.7326/M15-1150

Otto, M. A. (2017). *Axillary thermometry is the best choice for newborns*. Pediatric News. Retrieved from https://www.mdedge.com/pediatricnews/article/145346/neonatal-medicine/axillary-thermometry-best-choice-newborns

PEDS Cases. (2016). *Pediatric vital signs reference chart*. Retrieved from http://www.pedscases.com/sites/default/files/Vital%20Signs%20Reference%20Chart%201.2_1.pdf

Potter, P. A., Perry, A. G., Ross-Kerr, J. C., et al. (Eds.). (2019). *Canadian fundamentals of nursing* (6th ed.). Toronto, ON: Elsevier Canada.

Qi, W., Wu, Q., Wu, Y., et al. (2017). Talking with a doctor during a visit elicits increases in systolic and diastolic blood pressure. *Blood Pressure Monitoring, 22*(5), 265–267. doi:10.1097/MBP.0000000000000270

SickKids (The Hospital for Sick Children). (2014). *Vital signs*. Toronto: Author. Retrieved from http://www.sickkids.ca/Nursing/Education-and-learning/Nursing-Student-Orientation/module-two-clinical-care/vitals/index.html

Skirton, H., Chamberlain, W., Lawson, C., Ryan, H., & Young, E. (2011). A systematic review of variability and reliability of manual and automated blood pressure readings. *Journal of Clinical Nursing, 20*(5–6), 602–614. doi:10.1111/j.1365-2702.2010.03528.x

Smith, N. (2016). *Nursing practice and skill*. Fever: Managing fever in older adults. Retrieved from https://www.ebscohost.com/assets-sample-content/NRC_Managing_Fever_in_Older_Adults_NSP.pdf

Touhy, T. A., Jett, K., Boscart, V., & McCleary, L. (2019). *Ebersole and Hess' gerontological nursing & healthy aging* (2nd Cdn ed.). Toronto: Elsevier.

World Health Organization (WHO). (2011). *Pulse oximetry training manual*. Geneva: Author. Retrieved from http://www.who.int/patientsafety/safesurgery/pulse_oximetry/who_ps_pulse_oxymetry_training_manual_en.pdf

Yeoh, W., Lee, J., Lim, H., Gan, C., Liang, W., & Tan, K. (2017). Re-visiting the tympanic membrane vicinity as core body temperature as a measurement site. *PLoS ONE, 12*(4), e0174120. doi:10.1371/journal.pone.0174120

Yont, G. H., Korhan, E., & Khorshid, L. (2011). Comparison of oxygen saturation values and measurement times by pulse oximetry in various parts of the body. *Applied Nursing Research, 24*(4), e39. doi:10.1016/j.apnr.2010.03.002

8 | Health Assessment

Written by **Paula Gray, DNP, CRNP, NP-C, and Marian Luctkar-Flude, RN, MScN, PhD**

SKILLS AND PROCEDURES

OBJECTIVES

Mastery of content in this chapter will enable the nurse to:
- Discuss the purposes of health assessment.
- Describe the techniques used with each physical assessment skill.
- Describe proper patient positioning during each phase of the examination.
- Describe how to conduct a physical examination on patients from diverse cultures.
- List techniques to promote a patient's physical and psychological comfort during an examination.
- Make environmental preparations before an assessment.
- Identify data to collect from the nursing history before an examination.

- Discuss normal physical findings for patients across the lifespan.
- Discuss ways to incorporate health promotion and health teaching into an assessment.
- Identify self-screening assessments commonly performed by patients.
- Identify preventive screenings and the appropriate age(s) for each screening.
- Apply physical assessment techniques and skills during routine nursing care.
- Document assessment findings on appropriate forms.
- Use interprofessional collaboration to communicate abnormal findings to appropriate team members.

MEDIA RESOURCES

- evolve http://evolve.elsevier.com/Canada/Perry/clinicalskills/
- Review Questions
- Audio Glossary
- ▶ Video Clips

- Animations
- Case Studies
- Clinical Debrief and Review Questions Answers

PURPOSE

Systematic interviews and physical assessments are regularly performed by nurses to assess the status of a patient's health and their perception of health. The information gathered is documented in the patient's database.

STANDARDS OF CARE

- Canadian Task Force on Preventive Health Care, 2018—*Published Guidelines* (https://canadiantaskforce.ca/guidelines/published-guidelines/)

- College of Family Physicians of Canada, 2013—*Annual Physical Examination Practices by Province/Territory in Canada* (http://www.cfpc.ca/CFPC-PT-Annual-Exam/)
- Health Canada, 2015—*Clinical Practice Guidelines for Nurses in Primary Care* (https://www.canada.ca/en/indigenous-services-canada/services/first-nations-inuit-health/health-care-services/nursing/clinical-practice-guidelines-nurses-primary-care.html)
- Infection Prevention and Control Canada, 2018—*Guidelines and Standards* (https://ipac-canada.org/evidence-based-guidelines.php)

PRINCIPLES FOR PRACTICE

- Use ongoing objective and comprehensive assessment to promote continuity of care.
- An admission assessment involves a detailed review of a patient's condition and includes a health history and physical examination.
- Use open-ended questions and be sure that patients have exhausted their descriptions. For example, as a patient is describing a symptom, you can say "go on" to encourage more information sharing.
- Use critical thinking skills and clinical judgement for evaluation and interpretation of findings.
- Initial assessment and examination provide a baseline for a patient's functional status and serve as a comparison for future assessment findings. In addition, the information is useful in making clinical decisions about the management of a patient's health problems.
- Use diagnostic or clinical reasoning to analyze health data and draw conclusions to identify actual or potential diagnoses and prioritize care.
- Immediately address any *first-level priority problems* encountered, such as life-threatening airway, breathing, or cardiac problems (Jarvis, Browne, MacDonald-Jenkins, et al., 2019).
- Promptly intervene to address *second-level priority problems*, such as acute pain or mental status changes, to prevent further deterioration.
- Address *third-level priority problems*, such as knowledge deficits and health promotion, after more urgent health problems are resolved or stabilized.
- Use interprofessional collaboration to assess, diagnose, and manage patient health problems.
- Practise person-centred nursing care and ensure patient safety and confidentiality.

PERSON-CENTRED CARE

- Conduct a person-centred interview to learn about issues from the patient's perspective.
- Show respect to patients, their families, and caregivers in seeking their involvement in the patient's plan of care.
- Have patients explain their symptoms by allowing them to offer details.
- After gathering data, group significant findings into patterns of data (clusters) that reveal actual or potential nursing diagnoses (Table 8.1).
- Be open to continually informing, communicating with, and educating patients and caregivers regarding patient care.
- Integrate health promotion and education into physical assessment activities. It is an ideal time to offer individualized patient teaching and to encourage promotion of health practices such as breast (Box 8.1) and genital (see Box 8.6) self-examination.
- A patient should understand any symptoms with which they present and symptoms for which to look in detecting problems. For example, educate patients about the Canadian Cancer Society (CCS) guidelines (2018f) for early detection of breast, colorectal, and genital cancers.
- Ensure that the patient is comfortable and free from pain.
- Provide emotional support.
- Respect patients' cultural diversity and beliefs when completing a physical assessment; eye contact or physical touch may be considered inappropriate or offensive in some cultures (Agency for Healthcare Research and Quality [AHRQ], 2015).

TABLE 8.1

Development of Individualized Nursing Diagnoses

Assessment Method	Findings	Patterns	Nursing Diagnosis
Inspection of skin	Skin along sacral area is intact. There is a 3-cm area of redness around coccyx; skin blanches on palpation. No skin lesions are observed.	There is tissue injury area around coccyx.	Potential for impaired skin integrity
Palpation of skin	Skin is moist from diaphoresis. There is tenderness to palpation at sacral area. Skin turgor is elastic.	Skin moisture promotes maceration.	
Historical data	Patient suffered fractured left leg. Patient is immobilized because of left leg traction.	Continued pressure is exerted over sacrum.	

BOX 8.1

Breast Self-Examination (BSE)

The Canadian Task Force on Preventive Healthcare (2011) released updated guidelines for breast cancer screening in average-risk women aged 40–74 years and recommended not advising these women to routinely practise BSE. Neither clinical breast examination nor breast self-examination has been shown to reduce mortality due to breast cancer. Although research does not support a clear benefit of regular BSE, it is important for all women to become aware of their breasts' normal appearance and feel, even if they get regular screening tests. There is not a right or a wrong way for women to examine their breasts, but women need to be familiar with the entire area of breast tissue up to the collarbone and under the armpits and including the nipples (Canadian Cancer Society [CCS], 2018b). Teach women to disrobe to the waist and inspect their breasts in front of a mirror, and palpate their breasts while lying supine, which flattens the breast tissue, or in the shower using soap and water, which assists with palpation (Jarvis et al., 2019). Women should be told about the benefits and limitations of BSE and to report any breast changes to their health care provider right away. Reinforce that the great majority of breast lumps are benign.

- Communicate respect through proper use of distance, attention, eye contact, tone, and loudness of voice.
- Use a professional interpreter familiar with a patient's culture and language if required.
- Obtain information about health risks common to a cultural group. Certain diseases are prevalent in some groups.
- Provide gender-affirming care of people by asking patients if they have preferred pronouns or terms they would like used to address them (Deutsch, 2016).
- Ask permission before you touch a patient.
- Drape the patient thoroughly and use the bedside screen or curtains. This is an important part of person-centred care for patients from all cultures.

EVIDENCE-INFORMED PRACTICE

Agencies such as the CCS support research and develop practice guidelines regarding prevention and management of certain diseases such as skin cancer. The CCS (2018a) recommends that people check their skin regularly and protect themselves from ultraviolet

radiation (UVR). Risk factors for melanoma include exposure to UVR (from the sun or indoor tanning equipment); having many moles or an atypical mole; having congenital melanocytic nevi or familial atypical multiple mole melanoma (FAMMM) syndrome; having light-coloured skin, eyes and hair; having a personal or family history of skin cancer or *CDKN2A* gene mutation; having a weakened immune system or history of blistering sunburn; or having an inherited condition such as xeroderma pigmentosum, Werner syndrome, or retinoblastoma (CCS, 2018i). The CCS recommendations for prevention and early detection of skin cancer include the following:

- People should recognize symptoms of melanoma and non-melanoma skin cancer and report symptoms or skin changes to their health care provider promptly (CCS, 2018j).
- People should inform their health care provider promptly about any of the following: a sore that does not heal; areas of skin that are smooth and pearly, look waxy and sometimes bleed, a firm spot or lump that may have a hard, rough, scaly or crusted surface; a flat reddish patch of skin; any new moles; moles or spots that look different from other spots on the skin, or any change in the colour, size, and shape of existing skin lesions.
- People at higher-than-average risk should talk to their health care provider about a personal plan for testing that may include having regular skin exams by a health care provider.
- People should practise the six principles of sun safety: (1) check the UV index every day; (2) seek shade; (3) cover up; (4) wear sunglasses; (5) use sunscreen properly; and, (6) not use indoor tanning beds.

SAFETY GUIDELINES

- Prioritize an assessment based on a patient's presenting signs and symptoms or health care needs. For example, when a patient develops sudden shortness of breath, first assess the lungs and thorax. If a patient is acutely ill, you may choose to assess only the involved body systems. Use clinical judgement to ensure that an examination is relevant and inclusive.
- Organize an examination. Compare both sides of the body for symmetry. If a patient becomes fatigued, offer rest periods. Perform painful or intrusive procedures near the end of an examination.
- Use a head-to-toe approach following the sequence of inspection, palpation, percussion, and auscultation (except during abdominal assessment). This sequence facilitates an effective assessment.
- Encourage a patient's active participation. Patients usually know about their physical condition. Often a patient can let you know when certain findings are normal or when there have been changes.
- Perform hand hygiene in the patient's presence.
- Follow routine practices for infection control with all patients and additional precautions when warranted. During an assessment, you may have contact with body fluids and discharge. Always wear clean gloves when there are breaks in the skin, lesions, or wounds or when having contact with mucous membranes. In some circumstances, you will need to wear a gown and face or eye protection.
- Consider the possibility of latex allergy. The incidence of serious allergic reaction to latex has increased dramatically (Ball, Dains, Flynn, et al., 2015).
- Record quick notes to facilitate accurate documentation. Inform the patient that you will be recording the data.
- Record a summary of the assessment using appropriate medical terminology and in the sequence that findings are gathered. Use employer-approved medical abbreviations to keep notes concise. Avoid using abbreviations that have more than one meaning. Be thorough and descriptive, especially for abnormal findings.

ASSESSMENT TECHNIQUES

Use assessment techniques during each patient contact, including activities such as bathing, administering medications, other therapies, or while talking with a patient. This practice will help you learn to become more observant and better able to identify changes quickly.

Inspection, palpation, percussion, auscultation, and olfaction are the five basic assessment techniques. Each skill allows you to collect a broad range of physical data about patients. Nurses need experience to recognize normal variations among patients and ranges of normal for an individual. Cultural diversity is one factor that influences both normal variations and potential alterations that you may find during an assessment. It is important to take the time needed to carefully assess each body part. Hurrying can cause you to overlook significant signs and make incorrect conclusions about a patient's condition.

Inspection

Inspection is the visual examination of body parts or areas. An experienced nurse learns to make multiple observations almost simultaneously while becoming very perceptive of any abnormalities. The secret is to always pay attention to patients. Watch all movements and look carefully at the body part you are inspecting. It is important to recognize normal physical characteristics of patients of all ages before trying to distinguish abnormal findings.

Inspection requires good lighting and full exposure of body parts. Inspect each area for size, shape, colour, symmetry, position, and the presence of abnormalities. If possible, inspect each area compared with the same area on the opposite side of the body. When necessary, use additional light such as a penlight to inspect body cavities such as the mouth and throat. *Do not hurry. Pay attention to detail.* Verify and clarify all abnormalities with subjective patient data. In other words, ask the patient for further information about each abnormality or change, such as whether the change is recent.

Palpation

Palpation involves the sense of touch. Through palpation the hands make delicate and sensitive measurements of specific physical signs. It is used to detect resistance, resilience, roughness, texture, temperature, moisture, and mobility. Nurses often use it with or after visual inspection. Use different parts of the hand to detect specific characteristics. For example, the dorsum (back) of the hand is sensitive to temperature variations. The pads of the fingertips detect subtle changes in texture, shape, size, consistency, and pulsation of body parts. The palm of the hand is especially sensitive to vibration. Measure position, consistency, and turgor by lightly grasping a body part with the fingertips.

Help a patient relax and assume a comfortable position because muscle tension during palpation impairs the ability to palpate correctly. Asking the patient to take slow, deep breaths enhances muscle relaxation. Palpate tender areas last because they could cause the patient to become tense and impede the assessment. Ask the patient to point out areas that are more sensitive and note any nonverbal signs of discomfort. Patients appreciate clean, warm hands; short fingernails; and a gentle approach. Palpation is either light or deep and is controlled by the amount of pressure applied with the fingers or hand. Light palpation precedes deep palpation. Consider a patient's condition, the area being palpated, and the reason for using palpation. For example, when a patient is admitted to the

emergency department after an automobile accident, consider the factors surrounding the patient's injury and inspect the chest wall carefully before performing any palpation around the area of the ribs.

For light palpation, apply pressure slowly, gently, and deliberately, depressing approximately 1 cm (Fig. 8.1A). Check tender areas further, using light, intermittent pressure. After light palpation, nurses in advanced practice roles may use deeper palpation to examine the condition of organs (Fig. 8.1B). Depress the area you are examining by approximately 2 cm (0.8 inch). Caution is the rule. Bimanual palpation involves one hand placed over the other while applying pressure. The upper hand exerts downward pressure as the other hand feels the subtle characteristics of underlying organs and masses. Seek the help of a qualified instructor before attempting deep palpation.

Percussion

Percussion involves tapping the body with the fingertips to vibrate underlying tissues and organs. The vibration travels through body tissues, and the character of the resulting sound reflects the density of underlying tissue. The denser the tissue, the quieter the sound. By knowing various densities of organs and body parts, you learn how to locate organs or masses, map their edges, and determine their size. An abnormal sound suggests a mass or substance such as air or fluid in a body cavity. The skill of percussion is used more often by advanced practice nurses (APNs) than by nurses in daily practice at the bedside.

The most commonly used percussion technique is the indirect technique. This is performed by placing the middle finger of the nondominant hand firmly against the body surface. With palm and fingers remaining off the skin, the tip of the middle finger of the dominant hand strikes the base of the distal joint of the finger (Fig. 8.2). Use a quick, sharp stroke, keeping the forearm stationary. Relax the wrist to deliver the proper blow. Once the finger has struck, the wrist snaps back. If the blow is not sharp, if the hand is held loosely, or if the palm rests on the body surface the sound is softened, and you will not detect the presence of underlying structures. A light, quick blow produces the clearest sounds. Table 8.2 describes the five different percussion sounds.

Auscultation

Auscultation is listening with a stethoscope to sounds produced by the body. To auscultate correctly, listen in a quiet environment for both the presence of sound and its characteristics. To be successful in auscultation, you must first recognize normal sounds from each body structure, including the passage of blood through an artery, heart sounds, and movement of air through the lungs. These sounds vary according to the location in which they can be heard most easily. Likewise, you become familiar with areas that normally do

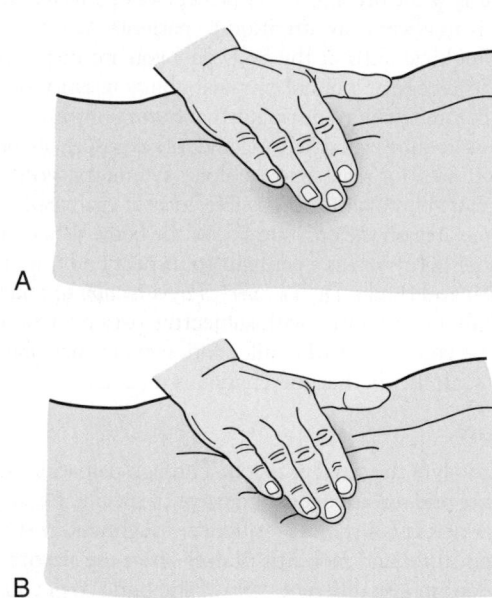

FIG 8.1 A, During light palpation gentle pressure against underlying skin and tissues can be used to detect areas of irregularity and tenderness. **B,** During deep palpation depress tissue to assess condition of underlying organs. (*From Ball, J. W., et al. [2015]. Seidel's guide to physical examination [8th ed.]. St. Louis: Mosby.*)

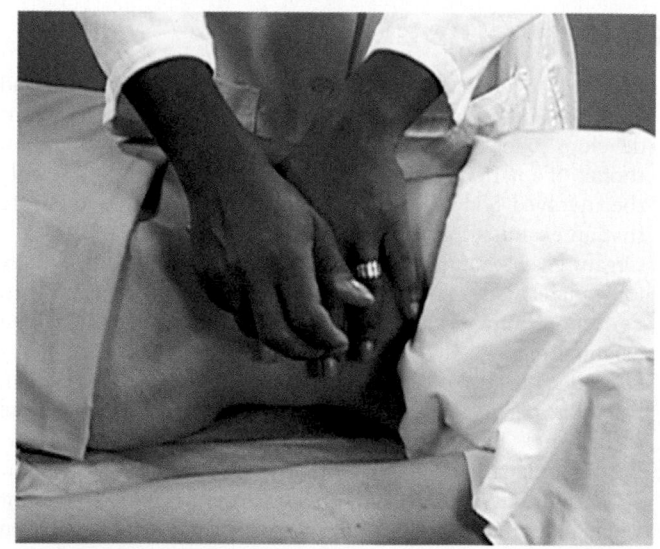

FIG 8.2 Percussion technique: tapping the interphalangeal joint. (*From Ball, J. W., et al. [2015]. Seidel's guide to physical examination [8th ed.]. St. Louis: Mosby.*)

TABLE 8.2					
Sounds Produced by Percussion					
Sound	**Intensity**	**Pitch**	**Duration**	**Quality**	**Common Location**
Tympany	Loud	High	Moderate	Drumlike	Gastric air bubble, puffed-out cheek
Resonant	Loud	Low	Long	Hollow	Healthy lung
Hyperresonant	Very loud	Low	Longer than resonance	Booming	Emphysematous lung
Dull	Soft to moderate	Moderate to high	Moderate	Thudlike	Over liver
Flat	Soft	High	Short	Very dull	Over muscle

Using a Stethoscope

1. Place earpieces in both ears with tips of earpieces turned toward the face. *Lightly* blow against the diaphragm (flat side of chest piece). Now place the earpieces in both ears with the tips turned toward the back of the head and again blow against the diaphragm. Compare comfort in the ears and amplification of sounds with earpieces in both directions. After you have learned the right fit for the loudest amplification, wear the stethoscope the same way each time. Earpieces should fit snugly and comfortably.

2. If the stethoscope has both a diaphragm (flat side) and a bell (bowl-shaped with a rubber ring) (see Fig. 7.7), put earpieces in ears and lightly blow against the diaphragm. The chest piece can be turned to allow sound to be carried through either side (bell or diaphragm). If sound is faint, lightly blow into the bell. Then turn the chest piece and blow again against both the diaphragm and the bell. The diaphragm is used for higher-pitched heart sounds, bowel sounds, and lung sounds. The bell is used for lower-pitched heart sounds and vascular sounds.

3. With earpieces in place and using the diaphragm, move the diaphragm lightly over the hair on your arm. The bristling sound mimics a sound heard in the lungs. When listening for significant sounds, hold the diaphragm still and firmly make a tight seal against the skin to eliminate extraneous sounds.

4. Place the diaphragm over the front of your chest directly on your skin and listen to your own breathing, comparing the bell and the diaphragm. Repeat the process while listening to your own heartbeat. Ask someone to speak in a conversational tone and note how the speech detracts from hearing clearly. When using a stethoscope, both you and the patient should remain quiet.

5. With the earpieces in your ears, gently tap the tubing. Note that it generates extraneous sounds. When listening to a patient, maintain a position that allows the tubing to extend straight and hang free. Movement may allow it to rub or bump objects, creating extraneous sounds. Kinked tubing muffles sounds.

6. *Care of a stethoscope:* Remove earpieces regularly and clean or remove cerumen (earwax). Keep the bell and diaphragm free of dust, lint, and body oils. Keep the tubing away from your body oils. Avoid draping the stethoscope around the neck next to the skin. To clean, wipe the entire stethoscope (e.g., diaphragm, tubing) with alcohol or soapy water. Be sure to dry all parts thoroughly. Follow manufacturer recommendations.

7. *Infection control:* Harmful bacteria, even antibiotic-resistant microorganisms, can be transferred from patient to patient when using portable equipment such as stethoscopes (Breen & Hessels, 2017). Follow employer infection control guidelines, especially contact precautions, to decrease this risk. Clean the stethoscope diaphragm, bell, tubing and earpieces between patients with isopropyl alcohol or ethanol-based cleaning products (Breen & Hessels, 2017).

Assessment of Characteristic Odours

Odour	Site or Source	Potential Causes
Alcohol	Oral cavity	Ingestion of alcohol; diabetes mellitus
Ammonia	Urine	Urinary tract infection, renal failure
Body odour	Skin, particularly in areas where body parts rub together (e.g., under arms, beneath breasts, perineal area)	Poor hygiene, excess perspiration (hyperhidrosis), foul-smelling perspiration (bromhidrosis)
	Wound site	Wound abscess; infection
	Vomitus	Abdominal irritation, contaminated food
Feces	Rectal area	Fecal incontinence; fistula
	Vomitus/oral cavity (fecal odour)	Bowel obstruction
Fetid, sweet odour	Tracheostomy or mucus secretions	Infection of bronchial tree (*Pseudomonas* bacteria)
Foul-smelling stools in infants	Stool	Malabsorption syndrome
Halitosis	Oral cavity	Poor dental or oral hygiene, gum disease; sinus infection
Musty odour	Casted body part	Infection inside cast
Stale urine	Skin	Uremic acidosis
Sweet, fruity ketones	Oral cavity	Diabetic acidosis
Sweet, heavy, thick odour	Draining wound	*Pseudomonas* (bacterial) infection

not emit sounds. Practise listening to many normal sounds so you can recognize abnormal sounds when they arise.

To auscultate the nurse needs good hearing acuity, a good stethoscope, and knowledge of how to use the stethoscope properly (Box 8.2). Nurses with hearing disorders may purchase stethoscopes with greater sound amplification and may need to ask colleagues to verify some findings through auscultation. It is essential to place the stethoscope directly on a patient's skin because clothing obscures and changes sound. Through auscultation the nurse notes that there are four characteristics of sound:

- *Frequency:* Number of sound wave cycles generated per second by a vibrating object. The higher the frequency, the higher the pitch of a sound and vice versa.
- *Loudness:* Amplitude of a sound wave. Auscultated sounds are described as loud or soft.
- *Quality:* Sounds of similar frequency and loudness from different sources. Terms such as *blowing* or *gurgling* describe quality of sound.
- *Duration:* Length of time that sound vibrations last. Duration of sound is short, medium, or long. Layers of soft tissue dampen the duration of sounds from deep internal organs.

A nurse cannot be successful at auscultation without knowing how to use a stethoscope properly. Chapter 7 describes the parts of the acoustic stethoscope and use of the bell and diaphragm.

Olfaction

Olfaction uses the sense of smell to detect abnormalities that go unrecognized by any other means. Some alterations in body function and certain bacteria create characteristic odours (Table 8.3).

PREPARATION FOR ASSESSMENT

Preparation of the environment, equipment, and patient facilitates a smooth assessment. Ensure the environment is warm, quiet, private, and well lit (Jarvis et al., 2019). Practise person-centred care during the physical assessment by providing patient privacy. If possible, place the bed or examination table at waist level so you can assess a patient easily. During an examination, you must protect the patient

from falls and injury and return the bed to a safe height at the completion of the assessment (Jarvis et al., 2019).

Preparing the Patient

Prepare patients both physically and psychologically for accurate assessments. A tense, anxious patient may have difficulty understanding, following directions, or cooperating with your instructions. To prepare a patient:

- Implement comfort measures (e.g., positioning, hygiene) and provide the opportunity to empty the bowel or bladder (a good time to collect needed specimens).

- Minimize the patient's anxiety and fear by conveying an open, receptive, and professional approach. Using simple terms, thoroughly explain what will be done, what the patient should expect to feel, and how they can participate. Even if a patient appears unresponsive, it is still important to explain your actions.
- Provide access to body parts while draping areas that are not being examined.
- Help the patient assume positions during assessment so body parts are accessible and so patient stays comfortable (Table 8.4). Patients' ability to assume positions depends on their physical strength and limitations. Some positions are uncomfortable or

TABLE 8.4

Positions for Physical Assessment

Position		Areas Assessed	Rationale	Limitations
Sitting		Head and neck, back, posterior thorax and lungs, anterior thorax and lungs, breasts, axillae, heart, vital signs, upper extremities	Sitting upright provides full expansion of lungs and better visualization of symmetry of upper body parts.	Physically weakened or developmentally challenged patient is sometimes unable to sit. Use supine position with head of bed elevated instead.
Supine		Head and neck, anterior thorax and lungs, breasts, axillae, heart, abdomen, extremities, pulses	This is normally the most relaxed position. It provides easy access to pulse sites.	If patient becomes short of breath easily, raise head of bed.
Dorsal recumbent		Head and neck, anterior thorax and lungs, breasts, axillae, heart, abdomen	Position is for abdominal assessment because it promotes relaxation of abdominal muscles.	Patients with painful disorders are more comfortable with knees flexed.
Lithotomy		Female genitalia and genital tract	This position provides maximal exposure of genitalia and facilitates insertion of vaginal speculum.	Lithotomy position is embarrassing and uncomfortable; thus, examiner minimizes time that patient spends in it. Keep patient well draped. Patients with arthritis or other joint deformities may be unable to tolerate the position.
Sims'		Rectum and vagina	Flexion of hip and knee improves exposure of rectal and genitourinary areas.	Joint deformities hinder patient's ability to bend hip and knee.
Prone		Musculoskeletal system	This position is for assessing extension of hip joint, skin, and buttocks.	Patients with respiratory difficulties do not tolerate this position well.
Lateral recumbent		Heart	This position aids in detecting murmurs.	Patients with respiratory difficulties do not tolerate this position well.
Knee–chest		Rectum	This position provides maximal exposure of rectal area.	This position is embarrassing and uncomfortable. Patients with arthritis or other joint deformities may be unable to assume it.

embarrassing; keep the patient in position no longer than is necessary.

- Pace assessment according to an individual's physical and emotional tolerance.
- Use a relaxed tone of voice and facial expressions to put the patient at ease.
- Encourage patient to ask questions and report discomfort felt during the examination.
- Given the potential for accusations of inappropriate conduct (e.g., during a genital exam), it is advisable to have a second health care provider assist in the examination room.
- Maintain a dialogue throughout the examination to explain your actions, ask and answer questions, and provide health teaching.
- At conclusion of an assessment, ask the patient if there are any concerns or questions.

PHYSICAL ASSESSMENT OF VARIOUS AGE GROUPS

Children and Adolescents

- Routine assessments of children focus on health promotion and illness prevention, particularly for care of well children with competent parenting and no serious health problems (Hockenberry & Wilson, 2015). Focus on growth and development, sensory screening, dental examination, and behavioural assessment.
- Children who are living with chronic illness, physical or cognitive challenges, in foster care, or foreign-born adopted may require additional assessments because of unique health needs or risks.
- When obtaining histories of infants and children, gather all or part of the information from parents or guardians.
- Parents may think that the examiner is testing or judging them. Offer support during examination and do not pass judgement.

- Call children and their parents by their preferred names.
- Open-ended questions often allow parents to share more information and describe more of the child's problems.
- Older children and adolescents respond best when treated as adults and individuals and often can provide details about their health history and severity of symptoms.
- The adolescent has a right to confidentiality. After talking with parents about historical information, arrange to be alone with the adolescent to speak privately and perform the examination.

Older Persons

- Do not assume that aging is always accompanied by illness or disability. Older persons can adapt to change and maintain functional independence (Touhy, Jett, Boscart, et al., 2019).
- A thorough assessment of an older person provides critical information that can be used to maximize independence.
- Provide adequate space for an examination, particularly if the patient uses a mobility aid.
- Plan the history and examination, considering an older person's energy level, physical limitations, pace, and adaptability. You may need more than one session to complete the assessment (Touhy et al., 2019).
- Measure performance under the most favourable conditions. Take advantage of natural opportunities for assessment (e.g., during bathing, grooming, mealtime) (Touhy et al., 2019).
- Sequence the examination to keep position changes to a minimum. Be efficient throughout the examination to limit patient movement.
- Be sure that examination of an older person includes review of mental status.

✦ SKILL 8.1 **General Survey**

The general survey begins a review of a patient's primary health problems and includes assessment of vital signs, height and weight, general behaviour, and appearance. It provides information about characteristics of an illness, a patient's hygiene, skin condition and body image, emotional state, recent changes in weight, and developmental status. The survey reveals important information about a patient's behaviour that influences how you communicate instructions and continue an assessment.

Equipment

- Stethoscope
- Sphygmomanometer and cuff
- Thermometer
- Digital watch or wristwatch with second hand
- Tape measure
- Clean gloves (use nonlatex if necessary)
- Tongue blade
- Appropriate electronic record or documentation form

STEP	RATIONALE
ASSESSMENT	
1. Identify patient using at least two person-specific identifiers (e.g., name and date of birth or name and account number) according to employer policy.	Ensures correct patient. Complies with Accreditation Canada's standards and improves patient safety (Accreditation Canada, 2019).
2. Note if patient has or has had any acute distress: difficulty breathing, pain, or anxiety. If such signs are present, defer general survey until later and focus immediately on affected body system.	Signs establish priorities regarding which part of examination to conduct first.
3. Review graphic sheet for previous vital signs and consider factors or conditions that may alter values (see Chapter 7).	Provides baseline and historical data about patient's vital signs.

STEP	RATIONALE

ASSESSMENT

4. Determine patient's primary language. If you identify need for an interpreter, determine availability of a professional interpreter. It is best to have an interpreter of the same gender who is older and mature. Have interpreter translate verbatim if possible.

Facilitates patient understanding and promotes accuracy of information provided by patient.

5. After reviewing history, confirm primary reason patient has sought health care.

Keeps assessment focused on patient to ensure their expectations are addressed.

6. Identify patient's normal height, weight, and body mass index. If sudden gain or loss in weight has occurred, determine amount of weight change and period of time in which it occurred. Assess if patient has recently been dieting or following an exercise program. Use growth chart for children under 18 years of age.

Generally, a body mass index of 25 to 29.9 kg/m² for men and women is overweight, whereas 30 kg/m² and over is obese (Ball et al., 2015). Fluid retention is one factor that must be ruled out. A person's weight can fluctuate daily because of fluid loss or retention (1 L of water weighs 1 kg [2.2 lb]).

7. Ask if patient has noticed any changes in condition of skin (e.g., dryness, changes in colour or lack of pigment, changes in moles or new skin lesions).

Skin changes can indicate underlying illnesses (e.g., dry skin may be associated with hypothyroidism, changes in moles may indicate early signs of skin cancers) (Table 8.5).

8. Review patient's past fluid intake and output (I&O) records.

Fluid and electrolyte balance affects health and function in all body systems. Intake includes all liquids taken orally, by feeding tube, and parenterally. Liquid output includes urine, diarrhea stool, vomitus, drainage from fistulas and gastric suction, and drainage from postsurgical tubes such as chest tubes or Jackson-Pratt drains.

9. Identify patient's general perceptions about personal health.

Assessment of patient's general appearance coupled with patient's own perceptions may reveal specific problem areas.

10. Assess for history of latex allergy, which may include contact dermatitis or systemic reactions. Ask if patient has risk factors such as food allergies (papaya, avocado, banana, peach, kiwi, or tomato); has high latex exposure (housekeepers, food handlers, health care worker); or must avoid products containing latex (rubber bands, adhesive tape, certain paints or carpets).

Gloves are worn during certain aspects of the assessment. Repeated exposure to latex may result in more serious reactions, including asthma, itching, and anaphylaxis (Ball et al., 2015).

TABLE 8.5

Skin Colour Variations

Colour	Condition	Cause	Assessment Location
Bluish (cyanosis)	Increased amount of deoxygenated hemoglobin (associated with hypoxia and is a late sign of decreased oxygen levels)	Heart or lung disease, cold environment	Nail beds, lips, base of tongue, skin (severe cases)
Pallor (decrease in colour)	Reduced amount of oxyhemoglobin	Anemia Shock	Face, conjunctivae, nail beds, palms of hands
	Reduced visibility of oxyhemoglobin resulting from decreased blood flow		Skin, nail beds, conjunctivae, lips
Loss of pigmentation	Vitiligo	Congenital autoimmune condition causing lack of pigment	Patchy areas on skin over face, hands, arms
Yellow-orange (jaundice)	Increased deposit of bilirubin in tissues	Liver disease, destruction of red blood cells	Sclerae, mucous membranes, skin
Red (erythema)	Increased visibility of oxyhemoglobin caused by dilation or increased blood flow	Fever, direct trauma, blushing, alcohol intake	Face; area of trauma; and areas at risk for pressure such as sacrum, shoulders, elbows, and heels
Tan-brown	Increased amount of melanin	Suntan, pregnancy	Areas exposed to sun: face, arms; areolae, nipples

STEP	RATIONALE

NURSING DIAGNOSES

- Inadequate breathing pattern
- Inadequate peripheral tissue perfusion
- Pain (acute, chronic)
- Inadequate fluid volume
- Excessive fluid volume

- Inadequate nutrition
- Reduced physical mobility
- Reduced skin integrity
- Anxiety
- Fear

- Decreased self-care: bathing
- Latex allergy response
- Obesity

Related factors are individualized on the basis of patient's condition or needs.

PLANNING

1. Expected outcomes following completion of procedure:
   - Patient demonstrates alert, cooperative behaviour without evidence of physical or emotional distress during assessment.

   - Patient provides appropriate subjective data related to physical condition.
2. *Prepare patient:* Tell patient that you will be using a routine process to check for areas of concern. Ask patient to tell you if any area that you examine hurts when touched.
3. Perform hand hygiene. Assemble necessary equipment. Position patient initially, either sitting or lying supine with head of bed elevated.

Use calm and confident approach during assessment. Patient has no abnormal findings.

Patient is able to cooperate with assessment.

Understanding promotes patient's cooperation. Pain is an important finding during assessment.

Reduces transmission of infection. Promotes efficiency of examination.

IMPLEMENTATION

1. Throughout assessment note patient's verbal and nonverbal behaviours. Determine patient's level of consciousness (LOC) and orientation by observing and talking to patient (Box 8.3).

2. If patient's responses are inappropriate, ask short, to-the-point questions regarding information patient should know (e.g., "Tell me your name." "What is the name of this place?" "Tell me where you live." "What day is this?" "What month is this?" or "What season of the year is this?").
3. If patient is unable to respond to questions of orientation, offer simple commands (e.g., "Squeeze my fingers" or "Move your toes.").
4. Obtain temperature, pulse, respirations, and blood pressure unless taken within last 3 hours or if serious potential change is noted (e.g., change in LOC or difficulty breathing) (see Chapter 7). Inform patient of vital signs.

Behaviours may reflect specific physical abnormalities. Dementia and LOC influence ability to cooperate. Decreased LOC, such as lethargy or confusion, requires further investigation into causes such as fluid and electrolyte imbalance, oxygenation and circulation problems, and metabolic problems.
Measures patient's orientation to person, place, and time. You may note this in documentation as "Oriented × 3." If disoriented in any way, include subjective and objective data rather than just documenting "disoriented."

LOC exists along a continuum ranging from full responsiveness, to inability to consciously initiate meaningful behaviours, to unresponsiveness to stimuli.
Vital signs provide important information regarding physiological changes related to oxygenation and circulation.

BOX 8.3

Characteristics of Dementia

Cognition
- Memory impaired: trouble recalling recent conversations, events, and appointments
- Frequently misplaces objects

Speech/Language
- Struggles to find words
- Conversation possibly incoherent

Activity
- Unchanged from usual behaviour
- Difficulty performing tasks that require many steps

Mood and Affect
- Depressed
- Apathetic
- Uninterested

Delusions/Hallucinations
- Can be some delusions
- No hallucinations

Modified from Ball, J. W., et al. (2015). *Seidel's guide to physical examination* (8th ed.). St. Louis: Mosby.

STEP	RATIONALE

IMPLEMENTATION

5. Ask patients about their preferred names and pronouns (he, she, they) rather than making assumptions based on their physical appearance or gender expression.

A person's gender identity may be the same or different from their assigned sex at birth, and chosen names and pronouns are common ways of expressing gender. As part of person-centred care, use respectful and gender-affirming language that aligns with the patient's self-identification (Bourns, 2015).

6. If uncertain whether patient understands a question, rephrase or ask a similar question.

Inappropriate response from a patient may be caused by language barriers or deterioration of mental status, preoccupation with illness, or decreased hearing acuity.

7. Assess affect and mood: Note if verbal expressions match nonverbal behaviour and if appropriate to situation.

Reflects patient's mental and emotional status, consciousness, and feelings.

8. Watch patient interact with family members or caregiver. Be alert for indications of fear, hesitancy to report health status, or willingness to let caregiver control assessment interview. Does partner or caregiver have a history of violence, alcoholism, or substance misuse? Is person unemployed, ill, or frustrated with caring for a patient? Note if patient has any obvious physical injuries.

Suspect abuse in patients who have suffered obvious physical injury or neglect, show signs of malnutrition, or have ecchymosis (bruises) on extremities or trunk. Health care providers are often the first to identify evidence of abuse because patients may not be able to tell family or friends. Partners or caregivers may have a history of abusive or addictive behaviours.

Clinical Decision Point *Be discreet in how you conduct the interview. Ask direct questions about abuse in private. It is often necessary to delay assessment to a later time when the partner or caregiver is not present. Asking a partner or caregiver to leave during an assessment creates an awkward situation, but inquiring about possible abuse in front of an abuser puts a patient at risk for further abuse. Patients are more likely to reveal any problems when the suspected abuser is absent from the room.*

9. Observe for signs of interpersonal violence (abuse):

    a. *Child:* Blood on underclothing, pain in genital area, difficulty sitting or walking, pain on urination, vaginal or penile discharge, itching or unusual colour in genital area, physical injury inconsistent with parent's or caregiver's account of how injury occurred.

Suggests child sexual abuse (Ball et al., 2015; Hockenberry & Wilson, 2015). Suggests child physical abuse.

    b. *Female patient:* Injury or trauma inconsistent with reported cause or obvious injuries to head, face, neck, breasts, abdomen, and genitalia (e.g., black eyes, abrasions, bruises/welts, broken nose, lacerations, broken teeth, strangulation marks, burns, human bites, orbital fractures, fractured skull).

Suggests intimate partner violence (Ball et al., 2015). These signs also apply to a male patient being abused by his partner.

    c. *Older person:* Injury or trauma inconsistent with reported cause, injuries in unusual locations (e.g., neck or genitalia), pattern injuries (left when an object with which a person is struck leaves an imprint), parallel injuries (e.g., bilateral ecchymosis on upper arms suggesting that patient was held and shaken), burns (shaped like cigarette, iron, rope), fractures, poor hygiene, and poor nutrition.

Suggests elder abuse or neglect (Ball et al., 2015; Touhy et al., 2019). Prolonged interval between injury and time patient sought medical care also indicates elder abuse or neglect.

Clinical Decision Point *Interpersonal violence includes intimate partner abuse, sexual assault, child abuse, and elder abuse or neglect. If abuse is suspected, ask the patient directly and in a nonjudgemental manner about the presence of interpersonal violence. A pattern of findings indicating abuse in children has mandatory reporting requirements in all Canadian provinces and territories, and some have reporting requirements for abuse of older persons or people with developmental challenges. Use immediate interprofessional collaboration to facilitate placement in a safer environment.*

10. Assess posture and position, noting alignment of shoulders and hips while patient stands, sits, or both. Observe whether patient is slumped, erect, or has bent posture (see illustration).

Reveals musculoskeletal problem, mood, or presence of pain.

STEP	RATIONALE

IMPLEMENTATION

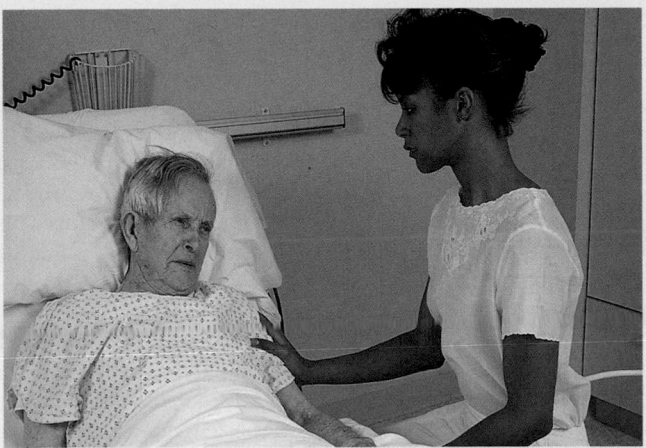

STEP 10 Observe patient's position and posture.

11. Assess body movements. Are they purposeful? Are there tremors of extremities? Are any body parts immobile? Are movements coordinated or uncoordinated?

May indicate neurological or muscular problem or emotional stress (see Skill 8.7).

12. Assess speech. Is it understandable and moderately paced? Is there association with patient's thoughts?

Alterations reflect neurological impairment, injury or impairment of mouth, improperly fitting dentures, differences in dialect or language, and some mental illnesses.

13. Observe hygiene and grooming for presence or absence of makeup, type of clothes (hospital or personal), and cleanliness. Hair, teeth, and nails are good places to assess for hygiene status.

Grooming may reflect activity level before examination, resources available to purchase grooming supplies, patient's mood, and self-care practices. It may also reflect culture, lifestyle, economic status, and personal preferences.

    a. Observe colour, distribution, quantity, thickness, texture, and lubrication of hair.

Changes in hair may reflect hormonal changes, changes from aging, poor nutrition, or use of certain hair-care products.

    b. Inspect condition of nails (hands and feet). Note colour, length, symmetry, cleanliness, and shape. Nails are normally transparent, smooth, and well rounded, with smooth, intact cuticle.

Changes indicate inadequate nutrition or grooming practices, nervous habits, or systemic diseases.

    c. Assess presence or absence of body odour.

Body odour may result from physical exercise, deficient hygiene, or physical or mental abnormalities. Inadequate oral hygiene or unhealthy teeth cause bad breath.

14. Inspect exposed areas of skin and ask if patient has noted any changes, including:

Determines presence of abnormalities and cancerous lesions. Melanoma is an aggressive form of skin cancer; detection and prompt treatment are critical (Box 8.4).

    a. Pruritus, oozing, bleeding

Itching could result from dry skin. Oozing could indicate infection, and bleeding may indicate a blood disorder.

    b. Appearance of mole (nevus), bump, or nodule; change in sensation; itchiness, tenderness, or pain

These are key indicators that a lesion may be cancerous.

    c. Petechiae (pinpoint-size red or purple spots on skin caused by small hemorrhages in skin layers)

Petechiae may indicate serious blood clotting disorder, medication reaction, or liver disease.

15. Inspect skin surfaces. Compare colour of symmetrical body parts, including areas unexposed to sun. Look for any patches or areas of skin colour variation.

Changes in colour can indicate pathological alterations (see Table 8.5).

Clinical Decision Point *Be alert for basal cell carcinomas such as an open sore that does not heal, a shiny nodule, a pink or reddish growth, or scarlike area. These are often seen in sun-exposed areas and frequently occur in sun-damaged skin.*

16. Carefully inspect colour of face, oral mucosa, lips, conjunctiva, sclera, palms of hands, and nail beds.

Abnormalities are easier to identify in areas of body where melanin production is lowest.

STEP	RATIONALE

IMPLEMENTATION

Clinical Decision Point *When assessing the skin of a patient with bandages, cast, restraints, or other restrictive devices, note report of pain or tingling and areas of pallor, decreased temperature, decreased movement, and impaired sensation, which may indicate impaired circulation. Immediate release of pressure from the restrictive device may be necessary.*

17. Use ungloved fingertips to palpate skin surfaces to feel texture and moisture of intact skin.

   a. Stroke skin surfaces lightly with fingertips to detect texture of surface of skin. Note whether skin is smooth or rough, thick or thin, or tight or supple and if localized areas of hardness or lesions are present.

   b. Palpate any areas that appear irregular in texture.

   c. Using dorsum (back) of hand, palpate for temperature of skin surfaces. Compare symmetrical body parts. Compare upper and lower body parts. Note distinct temperature difference and localized areas of warmth.

Changes in texture may be first indication of skin rashes in dark-skinned patients. Hydration, body temperature, and environment may affect skin. Older persons are prone to xerosis, presenting as dry, scaly skin (Touhy et al., 2019). Localized texture changes result from trauma, surgical wounds, or lesions.

Allows detection of localized areas of hardness and/or tenderness within subcutaneous skin layers.

Skin on dorsum of hand is thin, which allows detection of subtle temperature changes. Cool skin temperature often indicates decreased blood flow. A stage 1 pressure injury may cause warmth and erythema (redness) of an area. Environmental temperature and anxiety may also affect skin temperature.

Clinical Decision Point *In patients who receive routine injections (e.g., insulin, heparin), localized areas of hardness (lipodystrophy) may be palpated over injection sites; however, the use of human insulin reduces the risk for lipodystrophy. Rotation of insulin injection sites to different anatomical sites is no longer recommended as this causes variability in insulin absorption. Instead, advise patients to rotate injections within one particular site, such as the abdomen (Lewis, Bucher, Heitkemper, et al., 2019).*

18. Apply clean gloves. Inspect character of any secretions; note colour, odour, amount, and consistency (e.g., thin and watery, thick and oily). Remove gloves. Perform hand hygiene.

19. Assess skin turgor by grasping fold of skin on sternum, forearm, or abdomen with fingertips. Release skinfold and note ease and speed with which skin returns to place (see illustration).

20. Assess condition of skin for pressure areas, paying particular attention to regions at risk for pressure (e.g., sacrum, greater trochanter, heels, occipital area, clavicles). If you see areas of redness, place fingertip over area, apply gentle pressure, and release. Look at skin colour.

Description of secretions helps to indicate type of lesion, presence of infection, or wound healing.

With reduced turgor skin remains suspended or "tented" for a few seconds before slowly returning to place, indicating decreased elasticity and possible dehydration. With altered turgor, provide measures for prevention of pressure injuries (see Chapter 39).

Normal reactive hyperemia (redness) is visible effect of localized vasodilation, the normal response of the body to lack of blood flow to underlying tissue. Affected area of skin normally blanches with fingertip pressure. If area does not blanch, suspect tissue injury.

BOX 8.4

Malignant Melanoma Mnemonics

The ABCDE Rule of Melanoma
Here is a simple way to remember the characteristics that should alert you to the possibility of malignant melanoma.
1. *Asymmetry* of lesion: One side different than the other
2. *Borders*: Irregular (uneven, lumpy edges)
3. *Colour*: Blue/black or variegated; pigmentation not uniform; variations/multiple colours (tan, black) with areas of pink, white, grey, blue, or red
4. *Diameter* greater than 6 mm
5. *Evolving*: Change in size, shape, colour; itching or bleeding

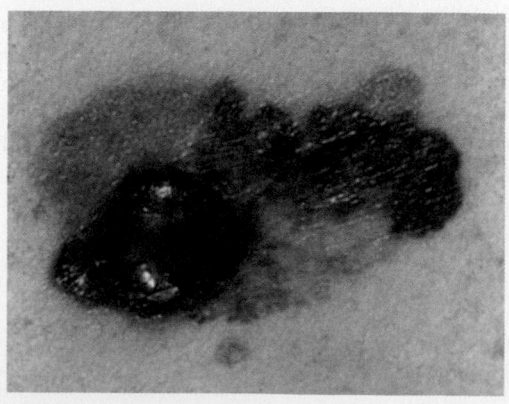

Figure from Ball, J. W., et al. (2015). *Seidel's guide to physical examination* (8th ed.). St. Louis: Mosby.

STEP	RATIONALE

IMPLEMENTATION

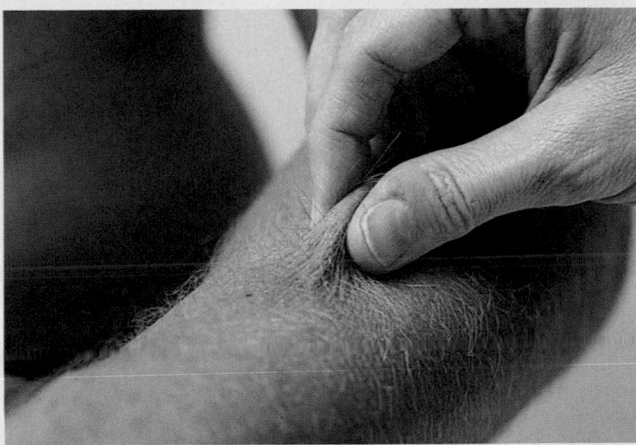

STEP 19 Checking skin turgor.

Clinical Decision Point *When assessing darkly pigmented skin, visual inspection techniques to identify skin problems are ineffective. Skin inspection techniques for individuals with darkly pigmented skin must include assessment of temperature, edema, and changes in tissue consistency as compared with the surrounding skin (Wound Ostomy and Continence Nurses [WOCN] Society, 2016).*

Clinical Decision Point *With evidence of normal reactive hyperemia, reposition patient and develop a turning schedule if the person is dependent.*

21. When you detect a lesion, use adequate lighting to inspect colour, location, texture, size, shape, and type (Box 8.5). Also note grouping (e.g., clustered or linear) and distribution (e.g., localized or generalized).	Observation of skin lesions allows for accurate description and identification.
a. Apply gloves if lesion is moist or draining. Gently palpate any lesion to determine mobility, contour (e.g., flat, raised, or depressed), and consistency (e.g., soft or hard).	Gentle palpation prevents rupture of underlying cysts. Gloves reduce transmission of microorganisms.
b. Note if patient reports tenderness with or without palpation.	Tenderness may indicate inflammation or pressure on body part.
c. Measure size of lesion (height, width, depth) with centimetre ruler.	Provides for baseline to assess changes in lesion over time.
22. Remove gloves. Discard used supplies and gloves in proper receptacle. Help patient to comfortable position. Perform hand hygiene.	Prevents transmission of infections.

EVALUATION

1. Observe throughout assessment for evidence of physical or emotional distress, which may alter assessment data.	Interaction during assessment reveals emotional problems. Manoeuvres used during physical examination reveal presence of physical problems.
2. Compare assessment findings with previous observations	Determines if change has occurred.
3. Ask patient if there is information about physical condition that you have not discussed.	Some patients think that they are bothering you by asking questions unless opportunity for questions is provided.
4. **Use Teach-Back:** "I want to be sure I explained everything about the bleeding mole I found on your back during assessment. Tell me why it is important to see a dermatologist." Develop a revised teaching plan if patient or caregiver is not able to teach back correctly.	Determines patient's and caregiver's level of understanding of instructional topic.

Unexpected Outcomes	Related Interventions
1. Patient demonstrates acute distress (e.g., shortness of breath, acute pain, severe anxiety).	• Respond immediately to identified need (e.g., repositioning, oxygen, or medication as appropriate). • Obtain vital signs. • Notify health care provider.

Types of Skin Lesions

Macule: Flat, nonpalpable change in skin colour; smaller than 1 cm (e.g., freckle, petechia)

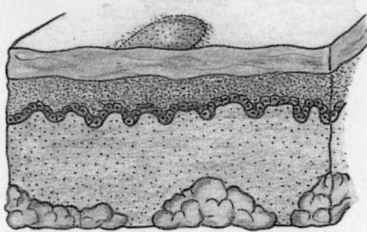

Vesicle: Circumscribed elevation of skin filled with serous fluid; smaller than 0.5 cm (e.g., herpes simplex, chickenpox)

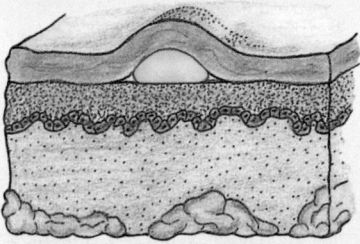

Papule: Palpable, circumscribed, solid elevation in skin; smaller than 0.5 cm (e.g., elevated nevus)

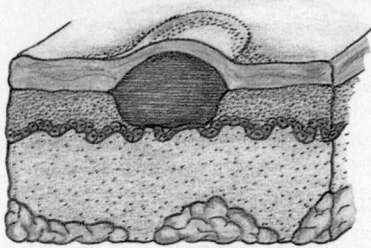

Pustule: Circumscribed elevation of skin similar to vesicle but filled with pus; varies in size (e.g., acne, staphylococcal infection)

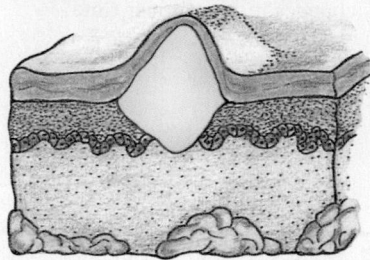

Nodule: Elevated solid mass, deeper and firmer than papule; 0.5 to 2 cm (e.g., wart)

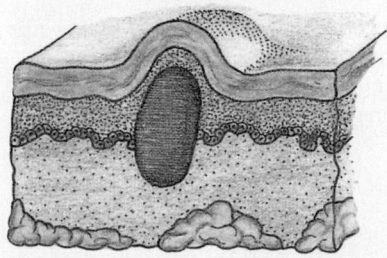

Ulcer: Deep loss of skin surface that may extend to dermis and frequently bleeds and scars; varies in size (e.g., venous stasis ulcer)

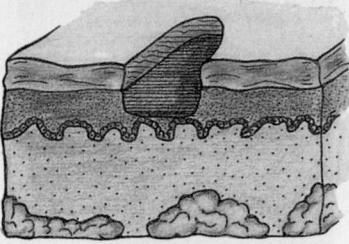

Tumour: Solid mass that may extend deep through subcutaneous tissue; larger than 1 to 2 cm (e.g., epithelioma)

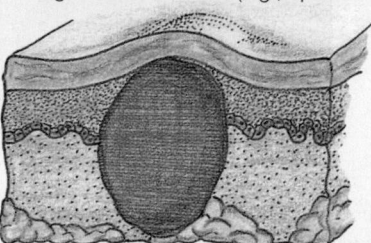

Atrophy: Thinning of skin with loss of normal skin furrow, with skin appearing shiny and translucent; varies in size (e.g., arterial insufficiency)

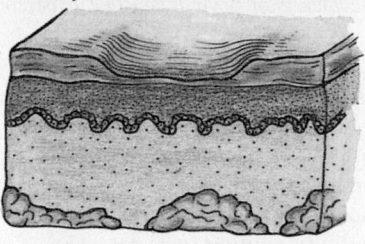

Wheal: Irregularly shaped, elevated area or superficial localized edema; varies in size (e.g., hive, mosquito bite)

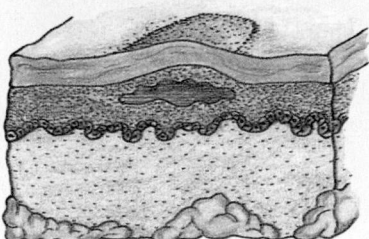

STEP	RATIONALE

EVALUATION

2. Patient has abnormal skin condition (e.g., change in colour of a mole, dry texture, reduced turgor, lesions, or erythema).
3. Patient is unwilling or unable to provide adequate information relating to identified concerns.

- Identify contributing factors and prevent continued irritation or damage as appropriate.
- Seek information from caregiver if present.
- Review patient's record for baseline data.

Communication and Documentation

- Document patient's vital signs on vital sign flow sheet in the electronic health record (EHR) or chart.
- Document description of alterations in patient's general appearance in the EHR or chart.
- Document patient's behaviours using objective terminology. Include patient's self-report of signs and symptoms.
- Document your evaluation of patient and caregiver learning.
- Report abnormalities and acute symptoms to nurse in charge or health care provider.

Special Considerations
Teaching

- During general survey inform patient about normal range of vital signs for age and physical condition and normal weight for height and body frame.
- If patient is on established diet, discuss any problems that they have preparing a diet or selecting food. The best form of weight reduction is to achieve gradual weight loss by increasing exercise and decreasing caloric intake. Use interprofessional collaboration (e.g., dietitian) to obtain specific information.

Pediatric

- Measurement of physical growth is a key element in evaluation of a child's health status. These physical growth parameters include height, length, weight, skinfold thickness, and arm and head circumference (Hockenberry & Wilson, 2015). Use growth charts specific to child's age and condition.
- Weigh infants nude. Weigh children in light underclothes or gown.

- A child's interactions with parents provide valuable information regarding the child's behaviour.

Gerontological

- An older person's presenting signs and symptoms are sometimes deceiving. An older person has a diminished physiological reserve that sometimes masks the usual, or "classic," signs and symptoms of a disease. In older persons, signs and symptoms are often blunted or atypical (Touhy et al., 2019).
- Common skin changes with aging include dryness, thinning, decreased elasticity, and prominent small blood vessels. Common lesions include seborrheic keratosis (pigmented raised, warty lesion); cherry angioma (bright, ruby-red round papules); cutaneous tags (soft pinkish-tan to light-brown pedunculated lesions); and solar lentigines (grey-brown, irregular macular lesions on sun-exposed areas) (Ball et al., 2015).
- Inspection of the feet is critically important in the presence of impaired circulation, impaired vision, and diabetes mellitus. Common foot conditions include ulceration, fungal infection, corns, calluses, bunions, plantar warts, and hammertoe.

Care in the Community

- In the home, the focus may be on the patient's ability to perform basic self-care tasks. Be sure that the home assessment builds on all health concerns identified in other settings.
- The home health nurse takes a small portable scale to monitor weight changes.

✦ SKILL 8.2   Head and Neck Assessment

Examination of the head and neck includes assessment of the head, eyes, ears, nose, mouth, and sinuses. Assessment uses inspection, palpation, and auscultation, with inspection and palpation often used simultaneously.

Delegation and Collaboration

The skill of assessing the head and neck cannot be delegated to an unregulated care provider (UCP). The nurse directs the UCP to:

- Observe for nasal discharge and nasal bleeding.
- Report any findings found during routine care (e.g., oral care, bathing) to the nurse for further assessment.

Equipment

- Stethoscope
- Clean gloves (use nonlatex if necessary)
- Tongue blade
- Pen light

STEP	RATIONALE

ASSESSMENT

1. Assess for history of headache, dizziness, pain, or stiffness.

Headaches and dizziness are signs of stress, a symptom of another underlying problem such as high blood pressure or a result of injury.

STEP	RATIONALE

ASSESSMENT

2. Determine if patient has history of eye disease, diabetes mellitus, or hypertension.

Common conditions predispose patients to visual alterations requiring health care provider referral.

3. Ask if patient has experienced blurred vision, flashing lights, halos around lights, or reduced visual field.

These common symptoms indicate visual problems.

4. Ask if patient has experienced ear pain, itching, discharge, vertigo, tinnitus (ringing in the ears), or change in hearing.

These signs and symptoms indicate infection or hearing loss.

5. Review patient's occupational history.

Patient's occupation can create a risk of injury, potential for eye fatigue, or prolonged noise exposure.

6. Ask if patient has history of allergies, nasal discharge, epistaxis (nosebleeds), or postnasal drip.

History is useful in determining source of nasal and sinus drainage.

7. Determine if patient smokes or chews tobacco.

Tobacco users have greater risk for mouth and throat cancer.

NURSING DIAGNOSES

- Reduced health maintenance
- Insufficient knowledge regarding the need for head and neck assessment
- Inadequate oral mucous membranes
- Potential for injury

Related factors/Risk factors are individualized on the basis of patient's condition or needs.

PLANNING

1. Expected outcomes following completion of procedure:
   - Patient recognizes warning signs and symptoms of eye, ear, sinus, and mouth disease.

   Awareness of warning signs improves adherence to reporting problems to health care provider.

   - Patient takes appropriate safety precautions for occupational injury related to head and neck.

   Awareness of safety precautions improves adherence to healthful behaviours.

   - Patient exhibits good visual acuity, normal hearing, moist and intact oral mucosa, and head and neck without masses or lesions.

   Patient has no abnormal findings.

2. Prepare patient. Tell them that you will be completing routine examination of the head and neck to check for areas of concerns.

Understanding promotes patient's cooperation.

3. Anticipate teaching topics so that during examination you can teach patient about common symptoms of eye, ear, sinus, and mouth problems and occupational health safety.

Enables you to incorporate teaching during examination.

4. Perform hand hygiene. Assemble necessary equipment.

Reduces transmission of infection. Promotes efficiency of examination.

IMPLEMENTATION

1. Position patient sitting upright if possible.

Provides for more thorough examination of head and neck structures.

2. Inspect head. Note head position and facial features. Look for symmetry.

Head tilting to one side may indicate hearing or visual loss. Neurological disorders such as paralysis often affect facial symmetry.

3. Assess eyes (include discussion of signs and symptoms related to eye diseases).
   a. Inspect position of eyes, colour, condition of conjunctiva, and movement.

   Asymmetrical positioning may reflect trauma or tumour growth. Differences in colour are sometimes congenital; changes in colour of conjunctiva may be result of local infection or symptomatic of another abnormality (e.g., pale conjunctiva is associated with anemia).

   b. Assess patient's near vision (ability to read newspaper or magazines) and far vision (ability to follow movement, read clock, watch television, or read signs at a distance).

   Patient with visual acuity or visual field loss indicates need for supporting self-care measures (e.g., feeding, bathing, hygiene, dressing) and teaching.

   c. Inspect pupils for size, shape, and equality (see illustration).

   Normal pupils are round, regular, and equal in size and shape.

STEP	RATIONALE

IMPLEMENTATION

d. Test pupillary reflexes. To test reaction to light, dim room lights. If you cannot dim lights, cup hand over eye to temporarily shield light. As patient looks straight ahead, move penlight from side of patient's face and direct light on pupil. Observe pupillary response of both eyes, noting briskness and equality of reflex (see illustrations A and B).

Darkened room normally ensures brisk response of pupils to light. Pupil that is illuminated constricts. Pupil in other eye should constrict equally (consensual light reflex).

   (1) Test for accommodation by asking patient to focus on distant object, which dilates the pupil. Then have patient shift to near object about 7 to 8 cm (3 to 3.2 inches) from nose and observe for pupil constriction and convergence of eyes. **NOTE:** You can also ask patient to follow an object (e.g., finger, pen) with eyes from far to near point.

Absence of constriction, convergence, or an asymmetrical response requires further ophthalmological assessment (Ball et al., 2015).

4. Assess hearing. Note patient's response to questions and presence or use of hearing aid. If you suspect patient has hearing loss, ask them to repeat random words that you state. Use one- or two-syllable words. Repeat, gradually increasing voice intensity until patient correctly repeats the words.

Patients normally hear three to six sounds clearly when whispered (Ball et al., 2015). For patient with obvious hearing impairment, speak clearly and concisely, stand so patient can see your face, stand toward patient's good ear, use low pitch, and avoid yelling.

Clinical Decision Point *If hearing deficit is present, have a qualified nurse inspect patient's ears because impaired hearing may be the result of impacted cerumen, external otitis, or swelling in ear canal because of allergic reactions to materials in hearing aids.*

5. Inspect nose externally for shape, skin colour, alignment, drainage, and presence of deformity or inflammation. Note colour of mucosa and any lesions, discharge, swelling, or presence of bleeding. If drainage appears infectious, consult with health care provider about obtaining a specimen.

Character of discharge and inflammation indicates allergy or infection. Perforation and erosion of septum and puffiness and/or increased vascularity of mucosa indicate habitual substance use.

6. In patients with nasogastric (NG), nasointestinal (NI), or nasotracheal tube, inspect nares for excoriation, inflammation, or discharge. Using penlight, look up into each naris. Stabilize tube as needed.

Swallowing or coughing reflex causes movement of tubes against nares, and pressure against tissues and mucosa can result in tissue injury.

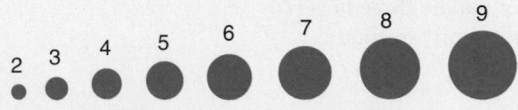

STEP 3c Pupil sizes in millimetres.

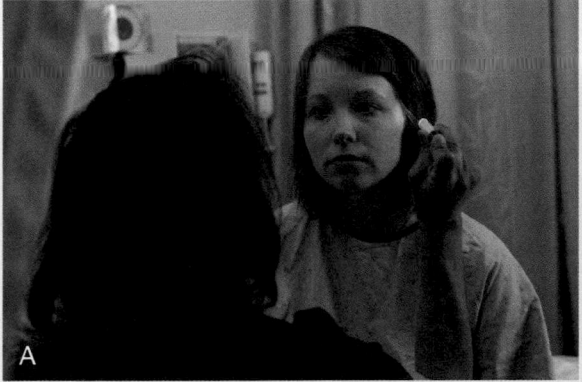
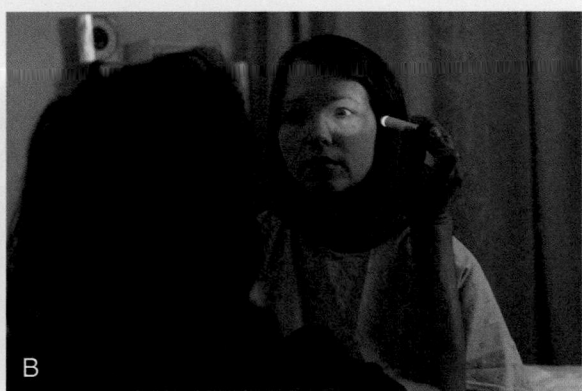

STEP 3d A, Holding penlight to side of patient's face. **B,** Illumination of pupil causes pupillary constriction.

STEP	RATIONALE

IMPLEMENTATION

7. Inspect sinuses by palpating gently over frontal and maxillary areas. Use thumbs to apply pressure up and under eyebrows to assess frontal sinuses. Use thumbs to apply pressure over maxillary sinuses, about 0.4 cm (1 inch) below eyes.

Infection, allergy, or substance use sometimes causes tenderness.

8. Assess mouth (include discussion about signs and symptoms of oral cancer).

   a. Apply clean gloves. Inspect lips for colour, texture, hydration, and lesions. Have females remove lipstick.

   Normal lips are pink, moist, symmetrical, and smooth.

   b. Inspect teeth and note position and alignment. Note colour of teeth and presence of dental caries, tartar, and extraction sites.

   Reveals quality of hygiene and discolouring effects of cola, coffee, and tobacco. Teeth are normally smooth, white, and shiny.

   c. Inspect mucosa and gums. Determine if patient wears dentures or retainers and if they are comfortable. Remove dentures to visualize and palpate gums. Use tongue blade to lightly depress tongue and inspect oral cavity with penlight (see illustration). Inspect oral mucosa, tongue, teeth, and gums for colour, hydration, texture, and obvious lesions.

   Dentures and retainers can cause chronic irritation. Normal mucosa is glistening, pink, smooth, and moist. Precancerous lesions can go unnoticed and progress rapidly.

   d. If oral lesions are present, palpate gently with gloved hand for tenderness, size, and consistency. Remove gloves. Perform hand hygiene.

   Cancerous lesions tend to be hard and nontender.

9. Inspect and palpate the neck:

   Assesses function of all neck structures, including neck muscles, lymph nodes, thyroid glands, and trachea.

   a. Ask patient if there is history of neck pain or difficulty moving neck.

   May indicate muscle strain, head injury, local nerve injury, or swollen lymph nodes.

   b. Neck muscles: Inspect neck for bilateral symmetry of muscles. Ask patient to flex and hyperextend neck and turn head side to side.

   Detects muscle weakness, strain, and range of motion (ROM).

   c. Lymph nodes:

   Lymph nodes are sometimes enlarged from infection or various diseases such as cancer.

   (1) With patient's chin raised and head tilted slightly, inspect area where lymph nodes are distributed and compare both sides (see illustration).

   (2) To examine lymph nodes, have patient relax with neck flexed slightly forward. To palpate, face or stand to side of patient and use pads of middle three fingers of hand (see illustration). Palpate gently in rotary motion for superficial lymph nodes.

   This position relaxes tissues and muscles.

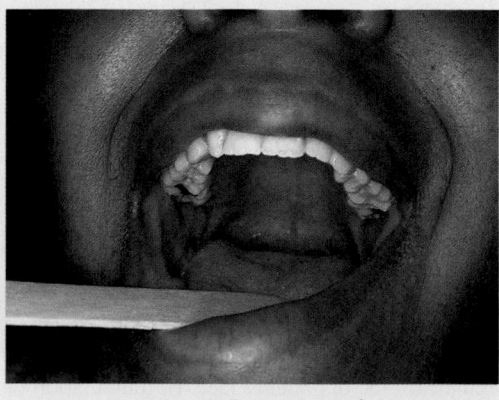

STEP 8c Inspect mouth.

STEP	RATIONALE

IMPLEMENTATION

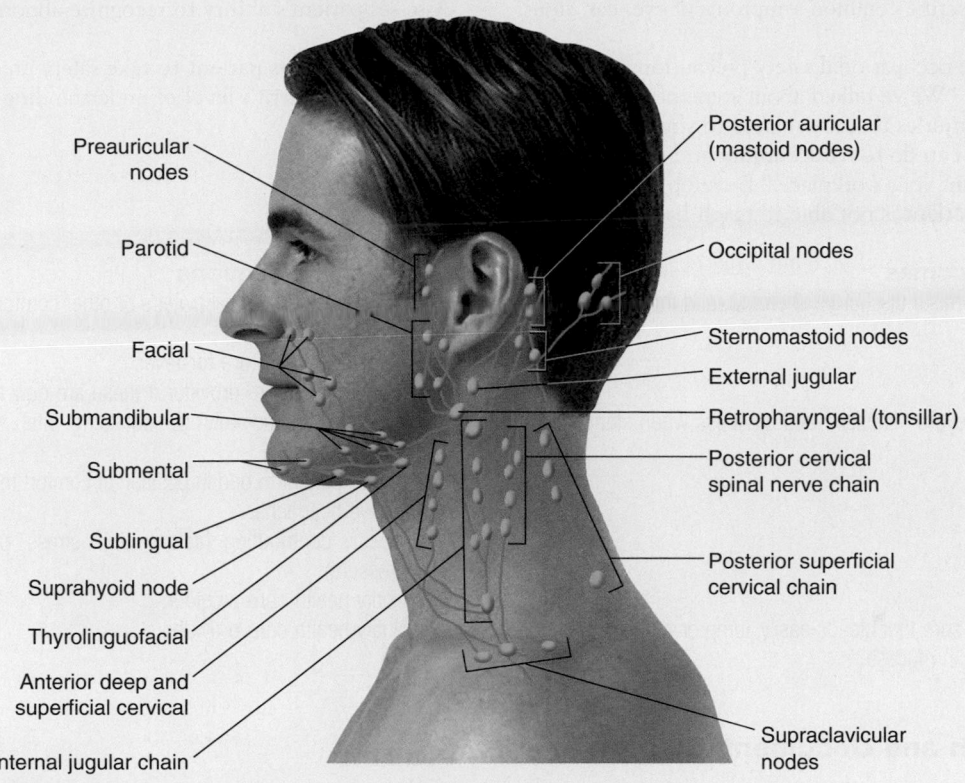

Preauricular nodes

Parotid

Facial

Submandibular

Submental

Sublingual

Suprahyoid node

Thyrolinguofacial

Anterior deep and superficial cervical

Internal jugular chain

Posterior auricular (mastoid nodes)

Occipital nodes

Sternomastoid nodes

External jugular

Retropharyngeal (tonsillar)

Posterior cervical spinal nerve chain

Posterior superficial cervical chain

Supraclavicular nodes

STEP 9c(1) Palpable lymph nodes of head and neck. (*From Ball, J. W., et al. [2015]. Seidel's guide to physical examination [8th ed.]. St. Louis: Mosby.*)

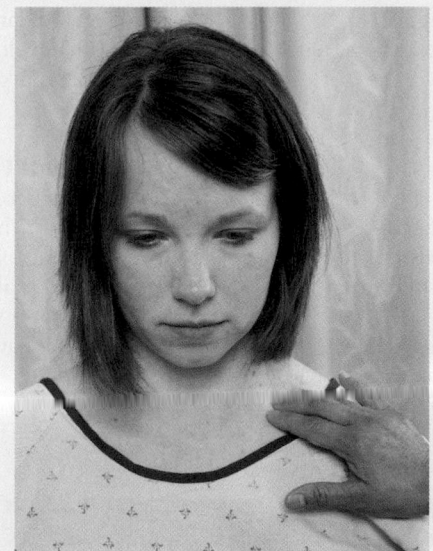

STEP 9c(2) Palpation of cervical lymph nodes.

   (3) Note if lymph nodes are large, fixed, inflamed, or tender.

10. Help patient to comfortable position. Perform hand hygiene.

Large, fixed, inflamed, or tender lymph nodes indicate local infection, systemic disease, or neoplasm.

Reduces transmission of infection.

STEP	RATIONALE

EVALUATION

1. Compare assessment findings with previous observations.	Identifies changes in patient's condition.
2. Ask patient to describe common symptoms of eye, ear, sinus, or mouth disease.	Assesses patient's ability to recognize abnormalities.
3. Ask patient to list occupational safety precautions.	Knowledge allows patient to take safety precautions.
4. **Use Teach-Back:** "We've talked about some of the signs and symptoms of ear injuries that are related to your occupation. Tell me what you can do to reduce injury and potential hearing problems in your workplace." Develop a revised teaching plan if patient is not able to teach back correctly.	Determines patient's level of understanding of instructional topic.

Unexpected Outcomes	Related Interventions
1. Patient has yellow nasal discharge, sneezing, and indicates sinus pain.	• Reposition into semi-Fowler's or other comfortable position to relieve sinus pain. • Monitor temperature for fever. • Notify health care provider if these are new findings.
2. Patient indicates severe headache and dizziness when standing.	• Respond immediately by obtaining vital signs, especially blood pressure. • Return patient to bed in position of comfort to minimize dizziness and relieve headache. • Identify contributing factors (e.g., stress, pain, or elevated blood pressure). • Notify health care provider.
3. Patient has mouth sore that bleeds easily, lump or thickening in cheek, or white or red patch in mucosa.	• Notify health care provider.

Communication and Documentation

• Document all findings, including any abnormal findings such as hearing or visual loss, pain and its location, current infection, and character of drainage in nurses' notes in electronic health record (EHR) or chart.
• Document your evaluation of patient learning.
• Report any unexpected findings or changes to charge nurse or health care provider.

Special Considerations
Teaching

• Explain the common visual changes associated with aging, including reduced acuity (presbyopia), loss of or a reduction in peripheral vision, reduced tearing, and sensitivity to glare or bright lights. Inform patients when to seek help from an eye care professional.
• Teach the visually impaired patient and caregivers how to adjust room arrangements at home to promote safer ambulation. Self-help aids are available to help patient function independently with daily activities.

Pediatric

• Some infants resist eye examination by closing eyes. Using distraction encourages eye opening (Hockenberry & Wilson, 2015).
• Headaches in children are usually caused by loss of sleep, poor nutrition, eye fatigue, and allergies. Children as young as 3 years of age can develop severe migraine headaches, but the symptoms are vague and difficult to diagnose (Hockenberry & Wilson, 2015).

Gerontological

• Older persons commonly have loss of peripheral vision caused by changes in the lens.
• Teach patients older than age 65 to have regular hearing checks.
• Measuring visual acuity helps determine level of assistance that patient requires with daily living activities and ability of patient to safely ambulate and function independently within the home.

◆ Skill 8.3   Thorax and Lung Assessment

Assessment of the thorax and lungs requires review of the ventilatory and respiratory functions of the lungs. It is a critical part of assessment because alterations can be life-threatening. Changes in respiration can occur quickly as a result of immobility, infection, certain analgesic and sedative medications, and fluid overload. Use data from all body systems to determine the nature of pulmonary alterations. You will use inspection, palpation, and auscultation during the examination.

Before assessing the thorax and lungs, know the landmarks of the chest (Fig. 8.3 A–C). These landmarks help you identify findings and use assessment skills correctly. A patient's nipples, angle of Louis at the sternum, suprasternal notch, costal angle, clavicles, and vertebrae are key landmarks. Keep a mental image of the location of the lobes of the lung and the position of each rib (Fig. 8.4 A–C).

Locating the position of each rib is critical to visualizing the lobe of the lung being assessed. To begin, locate the angle of Louis

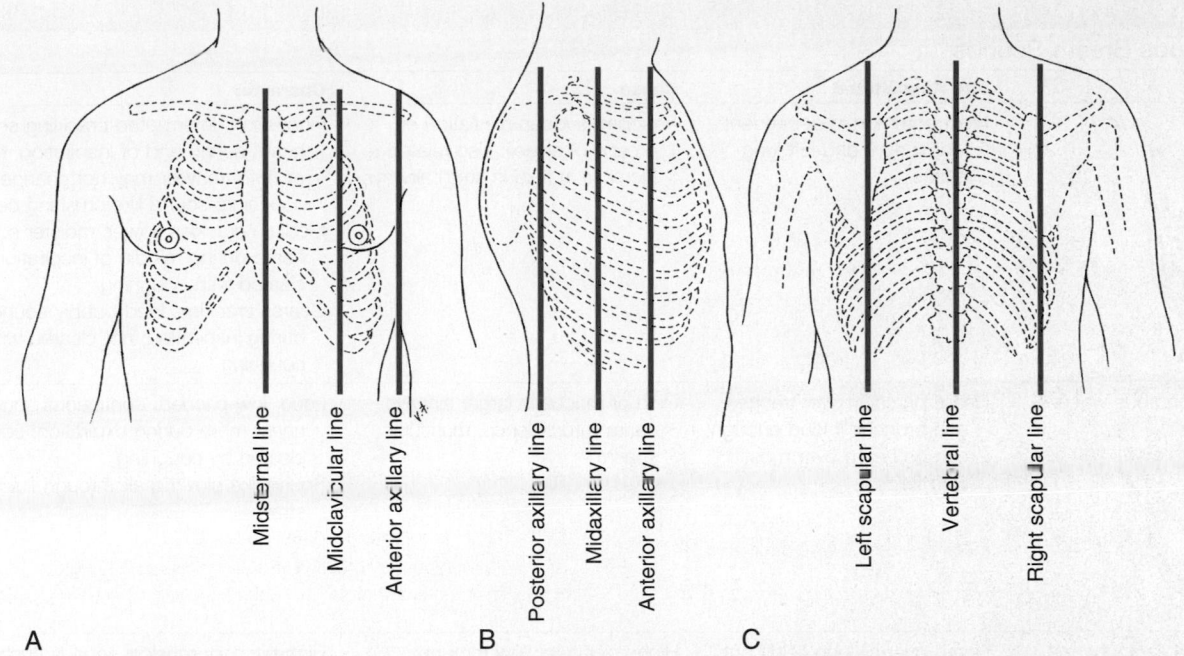

FIG 8.3 Anatomical landmarks and order of progression for examination of thorax. **A,** Anterior thorax. **B,** Lateral thorax. **C,** Posterior thorax.

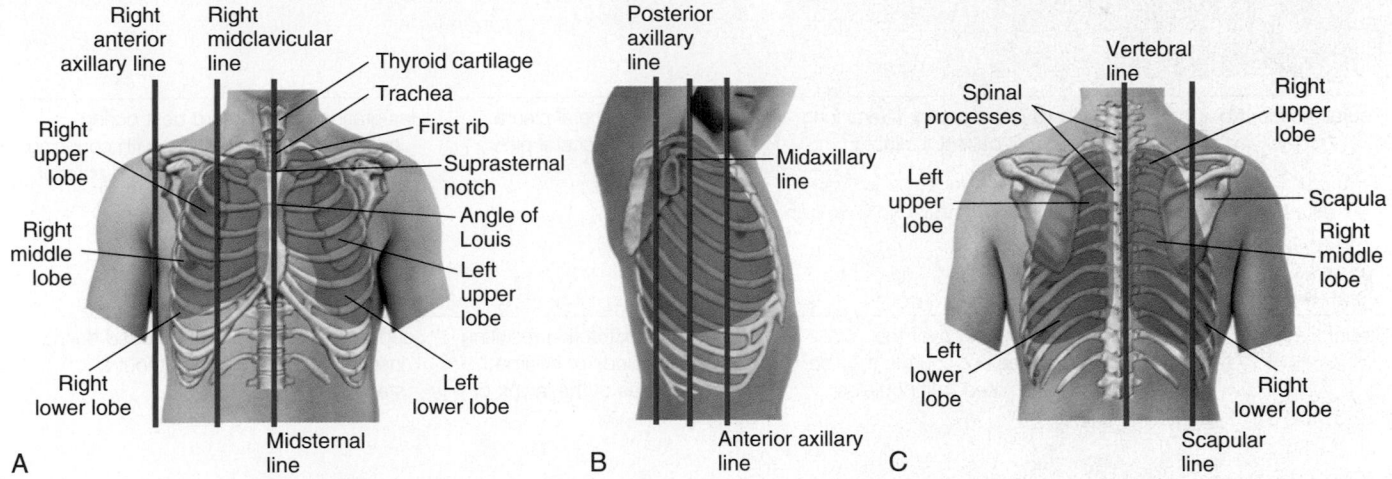

FIG 8.4 Position of lung lobes in relation to anatomical landmarks. **A,** Anterior position. **B,** Lateral position. **C,** Posterior position. *(From Seidel, H. M., et al. [2011]. Mosby's guide to physical examination [7th ed.]. St. Louis: Mosby.)*

on the anterior chest by palpating the "speed bump" at the manubriosternal junction, where the second rib connects with the sternum. The angle is often visible and palpable. Count the ribs and intercostal spaces (between the ribs) from this point. The number of each intercostal space corresponds with that of the rib just above it. The spinous processes of the third thoracic vertebra and the fourth, fifth, and sixth ribs help to locate the lung lobes laterally. The lower lobes project laterally and anteriorly (see Fig. 8.4B). Posteriorly the tip or inferior margin of the scapula lies approximately at the level of the seventh rib (see Fig. 8.4C).

During the examination, use auscultation to listen to breath sounds with a stethoscope. You can hear these sounds best when the person breathes deeply through the mouth. Adventitious sounds (abnormal sounds) result from air passing through fluid, mucus, or narrowed airways or from an inflammation between the pleural linings. The four types of adventitious sounds are crackles, rhonchi, wheezes, and pleural friction rubs (Table 8.6). Additionally, stridor is a high-pitched inspiratory crowing sound originating in the larynx or trachea that is heard louder in the neck than over the chest wall, resulting from an upper airway obstruction from swollen inflamed tissues (e.g., croup or acute epiglottis in children) or foreign body inhalation (Jarvis et al., 2019). Note the location and characteristics of the sounds, diminished breath sounds, or absence of breath sounds. Determine where in the respiratory cycle the abnormal sounds are heard.

Delegation and Collaboration

The skill of assessing the lungs and thorax cannot be delegated to an unregulated care provider (UCP). The nurse directs the UCP to:

TABLE 8.6

Adventitious Breath Sounds

Sound	Site Auscultated	Cause	Character
Crackles	Most common in dependent lobes: right and left lung bases	Random, sudden reinflation of groups of alveoli; also related to increase in fluid in small airways	Fine, short, interrupted crackling sounds heard during end of inspiration, expiration, or both; may or may not change with coughing; sound like crushing cellophane Medium crackles: lower, moister sounds heard during middle of inspiration; not cleared with coughing Coarse crackles: loud bubbly sounds heard during inspiration; not cleared with coughing
Rhonchi (sonorous wheeze)	Heard primarily over trachea and bronchi; if loud enough, can be heard over most lung fields	Fluid or mucus in larger airways causing turbulence; muscular spasm	Loud, low-pitched, continuous sounds heard more during expiration; sometimes cleared by coughing Sound like blowing air through fluid with a straw
Wheezes (sibilant wheeze)	Heard over all lung fields but more distinct over posterior lung fields	High-velocity airflow through severely narrowed or obstructed bronchus	High-pitched, musical sounds such as a squeak heard continuously during inspiration or expiration; usually louder on expiration Not cleared with coughing
Pleural friction rub	Heard over anterior lateral lung field (if patient is sitting upright)	Inflamed pleura, parietal pleura rubbing against visceral pleura	Has grating quality heard best during inspiration; does not clear with coughing; heard loudest over lower lateral anterior surface
Stridor	Heard loudest over the trachea but sounds may be transmitted to lung fields	Upper airway obstruction resulting from foreign body or inflamed, swollen tissues of the larynx or trachea	Loud, high-pitched crowing sound during inspiration, often heard without a stethoscope.

Inspiration — Tonsillar abscess
Epiglottitis — Anaphylaxis
Subglottic stenosis — Laryngomalacia
Vascular ring — Inhaled foreign body

Data from Ball, J. W., et al. (2015). *Seidel's guide to physical examination* (8th ed.). St. Louis: Mosby; Sarkar, M., Madabhavi, I., Niranjan, N., & Dogra, M. (2015). Auscultation of the respiratory system. *Annals of Thoracic Medicine, 10*(3), 158–168.

- Measure the patient's respirations after vital signs confirm that patient is stable.
- Report respiratory distress, difficulty breathing, and changes in rate and depth.

- Keep head of bed elevated for a patient who has respiratory difficulties.

Equipment
- Stethoscope

STEP	RATIONALE

ASSESSMENT

1. Assess history of tobacco or marijuana use, including type of tobacco, duration (number of years), and amount in pack-years. Pack-years equal number of years smoking times number of packs per day (e.g., 4 years × ½ pack per day equals 2 pack-years). If patient has quit, determine length of time since smoking stopped.

Smoking is major cause of lung cancer, heart disease, and chronic lung disease (emphysema and chronic bronchitis). Smoking tobacco is the most important risk factor for lung cancer; other factors include exposure to second-hand smoke, radon, radiation, asbestos, certain chemicals, arsenic in drinking water, pollutants from cooking and heating, and outdoor air pollution (CCS, 2018h). Individuals with weakened immune systems or lupus, or smokers who take beta carotene supplements are also at higher risk for developing lung cancer.

2. Ask if patient experiences any of the following: *persistent cough* (productive or nonproductive), *sputum production*, *blood-streaked sputum*, *chest pain*, shortness of breath, orthopnea, dyspnea during exertion, activity intolerance, or *recurrent attacks of pneumonia or bronchitis*.

Symptoms of respiratory alterations help to localize objective physical findings. (Warning signals for lung cancer are in italics.)

3. Determine if patient works in environment containing pollutants (e.g., asbestos, arsenic, coal dust, or chemical irritants) or requiring exposure to radiation. Does patient have exposure to second-hand cigarette smoke?

Patients with chronic respiratory disease, particularly asthma, have symptoms aggravated by change in temperature and humidity, irritating fumes or smoke, emotional stress, and physical exertion.

4. Review history for known or suspected human immunodeficiency virus (HIV) infection, substance misuse, low income, residence or employment in nursing home or shelter, homelessness, recent imprisonment, being a family member of patient with tuberculosis (TB), and immigration from a country where TB is prevalent.

These are known risk factors for exposure to and development of TB.

5. Ask if patient has history of persistent cough, hemoptysis (bloody sputum), unexplained weight loss, fatigue, night sweats, or fever.

These are signs and symptoms for both TB and HIV infection.

6. Does patient have history of chronic hoarseness?

Hoarseness indicates laryngeal disorder or abuse of cocaine or opioids (sniffing).

7. Assess for history of allergies to pollen, dust, or other airborne irritants and to any foods, medications, or chemical substances.

Allergic response is associated with wheezing on auscultation, dyspnea, cyanosis, and diaphoresis.

8. Review family history for cancer, TB, allergies, or chronic obstructive pulmonary disease (COPD).

Familial history places patient at risk for lung disease.

NURSING DIAGNOSES

- Reduced airway clearance
- Inadequate breathing pattern
- Inadequate gas exchange
- Pain (acute, chronic)
- Fatigue
- Potential for infection

Related factors/Risk factors are individualized on the basis of patient's condition or needs.

PLANNING

1. Expected outcomes following completion of procedure:
   - Respirations are passive, diaphragmatic or costal, and regular (12 to 20 breaths/min in adult) with symmetrical expansion.

   Characteristics of normal respirations.

   - Breath sounds are clear to auscultation and equal bilaterally.

   Air flows without interference or obstruction. Corresponding sides should sound the same.

   - Patient is able to describe factors that predispose to lung disease.

   Awareness of risks can improve patient adherence to healthy behaviour.

   - Patient assumes appropriate posture for optimal breathing.

   Patient can learn about benefits of good posture as examination manoeuvres are performed.

STEP	RATIONALE

ASSESSMENT

2. Anticipate teaching topics so that during the examination you can teach patient about any risk factors for lung disease.

Allows you to incorporate teaching during assessment process.

3. Perform hand hygiene. Assemble necessary equipment.

Reduces transmission of infection. Promotes efficiency of examination.

IMPLEMENTATION

1. Position and prepare patient for examination:
   a. Position patient sitting upright. For bedridden patient elevate head of bed 45 to 90 degrees. If unable to tolerate sitting, use supine and side-lying positions.

   Promotes full lung expansion during examination. Patients with chronic respiratory disease may need to sit up throughout examination because of shortness of breath. Help of another caregiver may be required to position unresponsive patients.

   b. Remove gown or drape first from posterior chest, keeping front of chest and legs covered. As examination progresses, remove gown from area being examined.

   Avoids unnecessary exposure and provides full visibility of thorax. Allows direct placement of diaphragm or bell on patient's skin, which enhances clarity of sounds.

   c. Explain all steps of procedure, encouraging patient to relax and breathe normally through mouth.

   Anxiety alters respiratory function. Breathing through mouth decreases extraneous sounds from air passing through nose.

2. Posterior thorax:
   a. If possible, stand behind patient. Inspect thorax for shape and symmetry. Note any deformities, position of spine, slope of ribs, retraction of intercostal spaces (ICS) during inspiration and bulging of ICS during expiration, and symmetrical expansion during inspiration. Note anteroposterior (AP) diameter.

   Allows for identification of impairment in chest expansion and any symptoms of respiratory distress. Normal chest contour is symmetrical. In a child, the shape of chest is almost circular, with AP diameter in 1:1 ratio. In an adult AP is one-third to one-half of side-to-side diameter. Chronic lung disease causes ribs to be more horizontal and increases AP diameter, resulting in "barrel chest." Patients with breathing problems assume postures that improve ventilation.

Clinical Decision Point *When a patient holds the chest wall during breathing, it indicates localized chest pain. Assess the nature of pain, including onset, severity, precipitating factors, quality, region, and radiation.*

   b. Determine rate and rhythm of breathing (see Chapter 7). Examine thorax as a whole. Have patient relax.

   This is a good time to count respirations, with patient relaxed and unaware of inspection. Awareness could alter respirations.

   c. Systematically palpate posterior chest wall, costal spaces, and ICS, noting any masses, pulsations, unusual movement, or areas of localized tenderness (see illustration). If patient voices pain or tenderness, avoid deep palpation. If there is a suspicious mass, palpate lightly for shape, size, and qualities of lesion (see Skill 8.1). Do not palpate painful areas deeply.

   Palpation is used to assess further characteristics and confirm or supplement findings from inspection. Localized swelling or tenderness indicates trauma to ribs or underlying cartilage. A fractured rib fragment could be displaced.

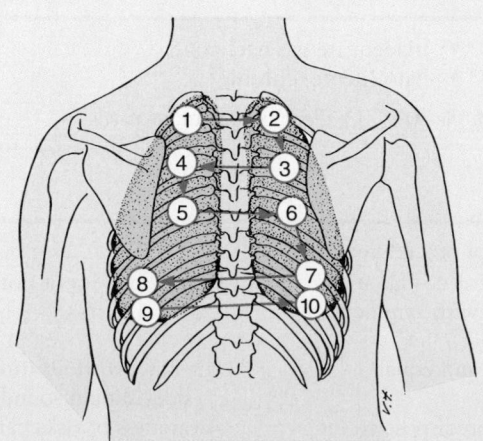

STEP 2c Pattern for assessment of posterior thorax.

STEP	RATIONALE

IMPLEMENTATION

d. Assess chest expansion by standing behind patient and placing thumbs along spinal processes at tenth rib, with palms lightly contacting posterolateral surfaces (see illustration A). Keep thumbs about 5 cm (2 in.) apart, with thumbs pointing toward spine and fingers pointing laterally. Press hands toward patient's spine to form small skinfold between thumbs. After exhalation patient takes deep breath. Note movement of thumbs (see illustration B) and symmetry of chest wall movement. Normally symmetrical separation of thumbs occurs during chest excursion 3 to 5 cm (1.2 to 2 in).

Palpation of chest expansion is used to assess depth of patient's breathing. This technique is a good measure to evaluate patient's ability to perform deep-breathing exercises. Limited movement on one side indicates that patient is voluntarily splinting during ventilation because of pain. Avoid allowing hands to slide over skin, which gives false measure of excursion.

e. Auscultate breath sounds. Instruct patient to take slow, deep breaths with mouth slightly open. For an adult, place diaphragm of stethoscope firmly on chest wall over intercostal spaces (see illustration). Listen to an entire inspiration and expiration at each stethoscope position (see pattern in Step 2c). If sounds are faint, as in obese patients, ask person to breathe harder and faster temporarily. Systematically compare breath sounds over right and left sides, listening for normal and adventitious sounds.

Assesses movement of air through tracheobronchial tree (Table 8.7). Recognition of normal airflow sounds allows detection of sounds caused by mucus or airway obstruction. Characterize sounds by length of inspiratory and expiratory phases.

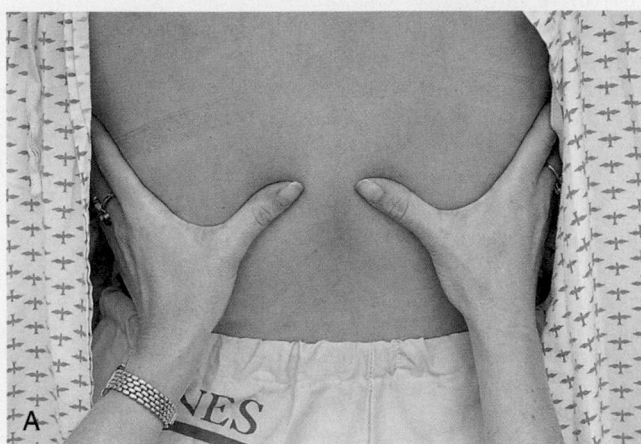
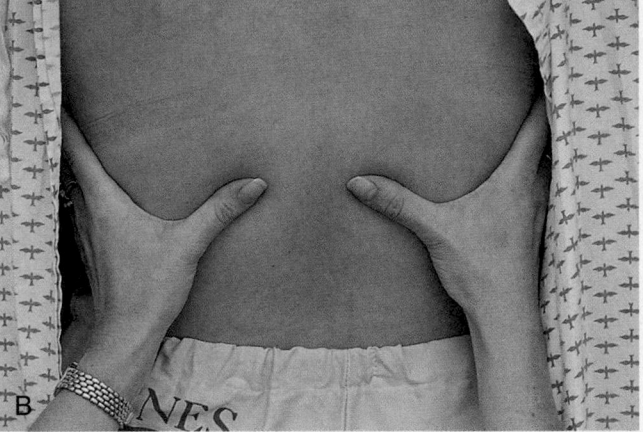

STEP 2d A, Position of hands for palpation of posterior thorax excursion. **B,** As patient inhales, movement of chest excursion separates nurse's thumbs.

TABLE 8.7

Normal Breath Sounds

Type	Description	Location	Origin
Bronchial	Loud and high-pitched sounds with hollow quality Expiration lasts longer than inspiration (3:2 ratio)	Best heard over trachea	Created by air moving through trachea close to chest wall
Bronchovesicular	Medium-pitched and blowing sounds of medium intensity Inspiratory phase equal to expiratory phase	Best heard posteriorly between scapulae and anteriorly over bronchioles lateral to sternum at first and second intercostal spaces	Created by air moving through large airways
Vesicular	Soft, breezy, and low-pitched sounds Inspiratory phase 3 times longer than expiratory phase	Best heard over periphery of lung (except over scapula)	Created by air moving through smaller airways

STEP	RATIONALE

IMPLEMENTATION

f. If you auscultate adventitious sounds, have patient cough. Listen again with stethoscope to determine if sound has cleared with coughing. See Table 8.6 for a description of adventitious breath sounds.

Coughing may clear adventitious sounds. Rhonchi often are eliminated or altered by coughing. Crackles and wheezes are not.

3. Lateral thorax:

a. Instruct patient to raise arms, and inspect chest wall for same characteristics as reviewed for posterior chest.

Improves access to lateral thoracic structures.

b. Extend palpation and auscultation of posterior thorax to lateral sides of chest, except for excursion measurement (see illustration).

Locates abnormalities in lateral lung fields.

4. Anterior thorax:

a. Inspect accessory muscles while patient is breathing: sternocleidomastoid, trapezius, and abdominal muscles; note effort to breathe.

Extent to which accessory muscles are used reveals degree of effort to breathe. Accessory muscles move little with normal passive breathing. Patients who require great effort and rely on these muscles may produce a grunting sound.

b. Inspect width or spread of costal angle made by costal margins and tip of sternum. Angle is usually larger than 90 degrees between margins.

Indicates congenital, acquired, or traumatic alterations that may influence patient's chest expansion.

c. Observe patient's breathing pattern, observing symmetry and degree of chest wall and abdominal movement. Respiratory rate and rhythm are more often assessed on anterior chest wall.

Assesses patient's effort to breathe: symmetrical, passive movement indicates no respiratory distress. Male patient's breathing is diaphragmatic, whereas female's is more costal.

d. Palpate anterior thoracic muscles and ribs for lumps, masses, tenderness, or unusual movement, following a systematic pattern across and down (see illustration).

Localized swelling or tenderness indicates trauma to underlying ribs or cartilage.

e. Palpate anterior chest excursion. Place hands over each lateral rib cage, with thumbs approximately 5 cm apart and angled along each costal margin. As patient inhales deeply, thumbs should symmetrically move apart 3 to 5 cm (1.2 to 2 inches), with each side expanding equally.

Assesses depth of patient's breathing and ability to perform deep-breathing exercises. Certain abnormalities are evident if expansion is not symmetrical.

f. With patient sitting, auscultate anterior thorax following same pattern as in Step 4d. Begin above clavicles; move across and then down as during palpation. Compare right and left sides. Give special attention to lower lobes, where mucus commonly gathers.

A systematic pattern of assessment comparing sides helps to identify abnormal sounds.

5. Clean stethoscope. Perform hand hygiene.

Reduces transmission of infection.

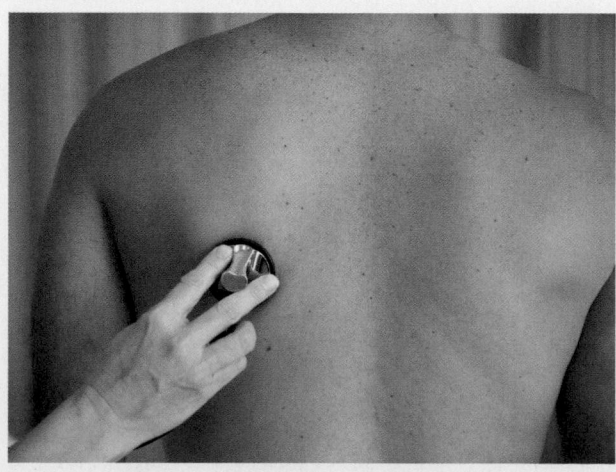

STEP 2e Auscultation with a stethoscope.

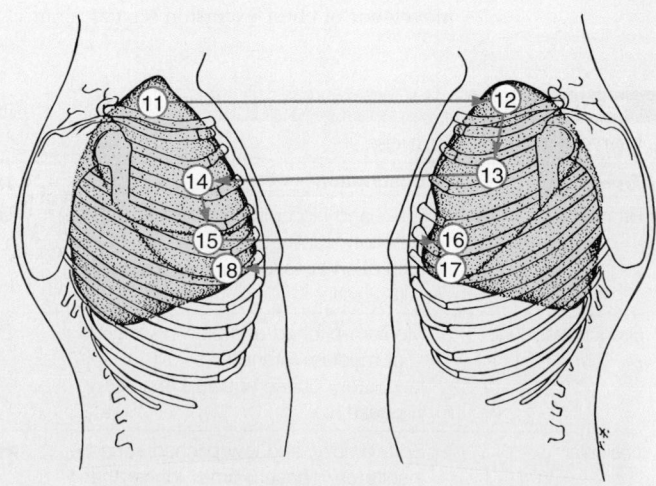

STEP 3b Pattern for assessment of lateral thorax.

STEP	RATIONALE

IMPLEMENTATION

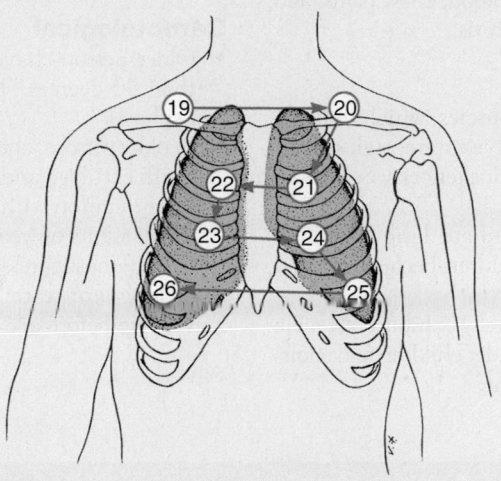

STEP 4d Pattern for assessment of anterior chest.

EVALUATION

1. Compare respiratory findings with assessment characteristics for thorax and lungs.
2. Have patient identify factors leading to lung disease.
3. **Use Teach-Back:** "We've talked about some of the risk factors your occupation poses for lung disease. Tell me what you can to do to reduce exposure in your workplace." Develop a revised teaching plan if patient is not able to teach back correctly.

Determines presence of abnormalities.

Demonstrates learning.

Determines patient's level of understanding of instructional topic.

Unexpected Outcomes	Related Interventions
1. Patient has copious mucus production; audible inspiratory wheezing; or congested cough with thick mucus.	• Help patient cough by splinting chest; teach to inhale slowly through nose, exhale, and cough; encourage expectoration of mucus. • Auscultate breath sounds before and after cough to evaluate cough effectiveness. • Auscultate lungs for adventitious sounds. • Encourage increased oral intake (if permitted). • If unable to clear airway by coughing, suctioning may be indicated. • Monitor vital signs. • Notify health care provider.
2. Respirations are rapid or slow and irregular (see Chapter 7) and bulging of intercostal spaces is present.	• Position patient more upright if appropriate. • Auscultate lungs for adventitious sounds. • Notify health care provider.
3. Chest excursion is reduced. Depth of breathing is reduced by pain, postural deformity, or fatigue.	• Reposition patient more comfortably. • Administer analgesic as prescribed if appropriate.

Communication and Documentation

- Document patient's respiratory rate and character; breath sounds, including type, location, and presence on inspiration, expiration, or both; changes noted after coughing; and other physical assessment findings in nurses' notes in electronic health record (EHR) or chart.
- Report abnormalities immediately to the health care provider.
- Document your evaluation of patient learning.

Special Considerations
Teaching

- Educate patients about risks of cigarette smoking. Smoking accounts for an estimated 30% of all cancer deaths in Canada and 85% of lung cancer cases (CCS, 2018g).
- Individuals who stop smoking have the potential to live longer than those who continue to smoke. The probability of these individuals dying from lung cancer or other related causes continues to decline with further abstinence.

- Explain to patients that exposure to radiation, radon, arsenic, and asbestos from occupational, medical, and environmental sources; air pollution; and second-hand smoke contribute significantly to lung cancer (CCS, 2018h).
- Discuss with patients the warning signs of lung cancer, such as a persistent cough, sputum streaked with blood, chest pains, and recurrent attacks of pneumonia or bronchitis.

Pediatric

- In children observe for use of accessory muscles, which indicate respiratory distress. Retractions may involve intercostal, suprasternal, supraclavicular, or sternal muscles (Hockenberry & Wilson, 2015).
- Use the bell of the stethoscope to auscultate lung sounds in children. Breath sounds are louder in children because of their thin chest walls.
- Children younger than 7 years of age normally exhibit noticeable abdominal or diaphragmatic movement. Older children and adults exhibit more costal or thoracic movement.

- Head bobbing and nasal flaring in infants are signs of significant respiratory distress (Hockenberry & Wilson, 2015).
- Pneumococcal vaccine is recommended for routine immunization of infants and children (Government of Canada, 2016).

Gerontological

- Older persons have a costal angle (anteriorly) of slightly less than 90 degrees. The AP diameter sometimes increases from kyphosis.
- In older persons, chest expansion is reduced because of calcification of rib cartilage and partial contraction of inspiratory muscles.
- Immunization with the pneumococcal vaccine is recommended for all adults 65 years of age and older. Individuals with chronic or immunosuppressed conditions, including asthma, or residents of long-term care facilities should receive the pneumococcal vaccine before age 64 (Government of Canada, 2016).

✦ SKILL 8.4 Cardiovascular Assessment

A patient who presents with signs or symptoms of heart (cardiac) problems such as chest pain may be suffering a life-threatening condition requiring immediate attention. In this situation, you need to act quickly and perform the parts of the examination that are absolutely necessary. This will reveal baseline heart function and any risks for heart disease. The heart, neck vessels, and peripheral circulation are assessed together because the systems work in unison. Then you can conduct a more thorough assessment when the patient is more stable.

Through your assessment you can determine the integrity of the circulatory system. Inadequate tissue perfusion results in an inadequate delivery of oxygen and nutrients to cells, a condition called *ischemia*. This is caused by constriction of vessels or occlusion (blockage) from clot formation. The effects of ischemia depend on the duration of the problem and the metabolic needs of the tissues. Ischemia results in pain. If lack of oxygen to tissues is unrelieved, tissue necrosis (death) occurs. An embolus is a blood clot that breaks loose and travels through the circulation. If the clot obstructs circulation to the lungs or brain, it can be life-threatening.

Assessment of the heart begins after examining the lungs because the patient is already in a suitable position with the chest exposed.

Assessment then proceeds to the neck vessels and ends with evaluating peripheral circulation. The skills of inspection, palpation, auscultation, and percussion are used during the examination.

Delegation and Collaboration

The skill of completing a comprehensive cardiovascular assessment cannot be delegated to an unregulated care provider (UCP). The nurse directs the UCP to:

- Count peripheral pulses after vital signs confirm that patient is stable.
- Recognize skin temperature and colour changes of affected extremities and report any changes to the nurse.
- Recognize changes in peripheral pulses and report any changes to the nurse.

Equipment

- Stethoscope
- Doppler stethoscope (optional)
- Conducting gel (if a Doppler stethoscope is used)
- Clean gloves (use nonlatex if appropriate)

STEP	RATIONALE

ASSESSMENT

STEP	RATIONALE
1. Assess patient for history of smoking, alcohol intake, caffeine intake (e.g., coffee, tea, soft drinks, energy drinks, and chocolate), and recreational substance use or misuse. Determine exercise habits and dietary patterns and intake.	These contribute to risk factors for cardiovascular disease. In addition, caffeine and alcohol cause tachycardia. Insufficient exercise and intake of fatty and salty foods increase risk for cardiovascular disease.
2. Determine if patient is taking medications for cardiovascular function (e.g., antiarrhythmics, antihypertensives, beta-blockers, antianginals) and if they know their purpose, dosage, and adverse effects.	Allows you to assess patient's adherence to and understanding of medications therapies. Medications for cardiovascular function cannot be taken intermittently.
3. Ask if patient has experienced dyspnea, chest pain or discomfort, palpitations, excess fatigue, cough, leg pain or cramps, edema of the feet, cyanosis, fainting, or orthopnea. Ask if symptoms occur at rest or during exercise.	These are the cardinal symptoms of heart disease. Cardiovascular function is sometimes adequate during rest but not during exercise.

STEP	RATIONALE

ASSESSMENT

4. If patient reports chest pain, determine onset (sudden or gradual), precipitating factors, quality, region, and severity and if it radiates. Anginal pain is usually a deep pressure or ache that is substernal and diffuse, radiating to one or both arms, neck, or jaw.

Symptoms reveal acute coronary syndrome or coronary artery disease (CAD).

5. Assess family history for heart disease, diabetes mellitus, high cholesterol or lipid levels, hypertension, stroke, or rheumatic heart disease.

Family history of these conditions increases risk for heart and vascular disease.

6. Ask patient about history of any pre-existing heart conditions (e.g., heart failure, congenital heart disease, CAD, dysrhythmias, or murmurs), heart surgery, or vascular disease (e.g., hypertension, phlebitis, varicose veins).

Knowledge reveals patient's level of understanding of condition. Pre-existing condition influences which examination techniques to use and expected findings.

7. Determine if patient experiences leg cramps; numbness or tingling in extremities; sensation of cold hands or feet; pain in legs; or swelling or cyanosis of feet, ankles, or hand.

These are signs and symptoms of vascular disease.

8. If patient experiences leg pain or cramping in lower extremities, ask if it is relieved by walking or standing for long periods or if it occurs during sleep.

Relationship of symptoms to exercise clarifies if problem is vascular or musculoskeletal. Pain caused by vascular condition tends to increase with activity. Musculoskeletal pain is usually not relieved when exercise ends.

9. Ask women if they wear tight-fitting underwear or hosiery. Ask both men and women if they wear tight-fitting trouser socks and sit or lie in bed with legs crossed.

Tight hosiery around lower extremities and crossing legs can impair venous return, promoting clot formation.

NURSING DIAGNOSES

- Reduced cardiac output
- Inadequate peripheral tissue perfusion
- Pain (acute, chronic)
- Reduced stamina
- Insufficient knowledge regarding the need for a cardiovascular assessment
- Potential for peripheral neurovascular dysfunction

Related factors/Risk factors are individualized on the basis of patient's condition or needs.

PLANNING

1. Expected outcomes following completion of procedure:
   - Heart rate is 60 to 100 beats/min (adolescent through adult), without extra sounds or murmurs.

   Indicates normal rate and sinus rhythm.

   - Point of maximal impulse (PMI) is palpable at fifth intercostal space at left midclavicular line in children older than 7 years of age and in adults.

   Indicates normal heart position.

   - Patient describes changes in own behaviour that could improve cardiovascular function.

   Instruction about cardiovascular disease risks may improve patient's health behaviour habits.

   - Patient describes schedule, dosage, purpose, and benefits of medications being taken for cardiovascular function.

   Information related to health benefits may improve adherence to therapy.

   - Blood pressure is within normal limits for patient (see Chapter 7).

   This is one indicator of normal cardiovascular function.

   - Carotid pulse is localized, strong, elastic, and equal bilaterally. No change occurs during inspiration or expiration; without carotid bruit.

   This indicates a patent vessel.

   - Jugular veins distend when patient lies supine and flatten when patient is in sitting position.

   Venous pressure is normal.

   - Peripheral pulses are equal and strong (2+); extremities are warm and pink, with capillary refill <3 seconds; <1 second for infants.

   Peripheral circulation is intact.

   - There is no clubbing of fingernails.
   - There is no dependent edema.
   - Peripheral hair growth is symmetrical and evenly distributed, and the skin is free of lesions.

STEP	RATIONALE

ASSESSMENT

2. Anticipate teaching topics so that during the examination you can teach patient about risks for heart and vascular disease.

Allows you to incorporate teaching during examination.

3. Perform hand hygiene. Prepare necessary supplies.

Reduces transmission of infection. Promotes efficient examination.

IMPLEMENTATION

1. Help patient be as relaxed and comfortable as possible.

An anxious or uncomfortable patient can have mild tachycardia, which alters findings.

2. Have patient assume semi-Fowler's or supine position.

Provides adequate visibility and access to left thorax and mediastinum. Patient with heart disease often experiences shortness of breath while lying flat.

3. Explain procedure. Avoid facial gestures reflecting concern.

Patients with previously normal cardiac history may become anxious if you show concern.

4. Be sure that room is quiet.

Subtle, low-pitched heart sounds are difficult to hear.

5. Assess the heart:

   a. Form mental image of exact location of the heart (see illustration). Base of heart is the upper part, and apex is the bottom tip. Surface of right ventricle constitutes most of the anterior surface of the heart.

   Visualization improves ability to assess findings accurately and determines possible source of abnormalities.

   b. Find angle of Louis, felt as ridge in sternum approximately 5 cm (2 in.) below suprasternal notch (between sternal body and manubrium). Slip fingers down each side of angle to feel adjacent ribs. Intercostal spaces (ICS) are just below each rib.

   Provides you with landmarks to locate and assess heart sounds.

   c. Find the following anatomical landmarks (see illustration):

   Familiarity with landmarks allows you to describe findings more clearly and ultimately may improve assessment.

   (1) Aortic area is at second ICS, right of patient's sternum, close to sternal border *(1)*.

   Listening to heart sounds from too far away from sternal border decreases ability to hear them clearly.

   (2) Pulmonic area is at second ICS, left of patient's sternum, close to sternal border *(2)*.

   (3) Second pulmonic area is found by moving down left side of sternum to third ICS, close to sternal border *(3)*, also referred to as *Erb's point*.

   (4) Tricuspid area *(4)* is located at fourth left ICS along sternum, close to sternal border.

   (5) Mitral area is found by moving fingers laterally to patient's left to locate fifth ICS at left midclavicular line *(5)*.

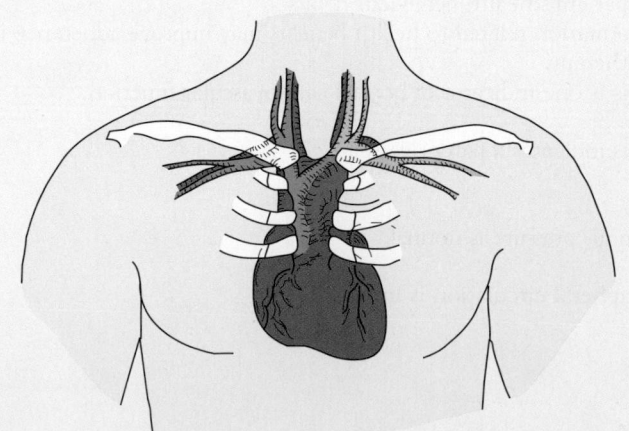

STEP 5a Anatomical position of heart.

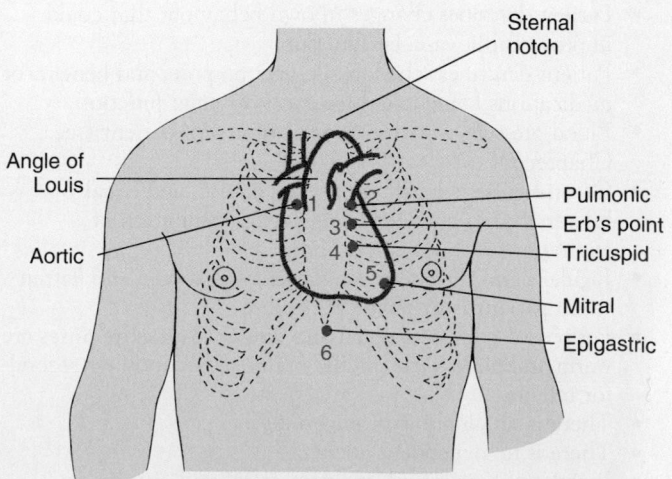

STEP 5c Anatomical sites for assessment of cardiac function.

STEP	RATIONALE

IMPLEMENTATION

(6) Epigastric area *(6)* is at inferior tip of sternum.

d. Stand to patient's right to inspect and palpate precordium with patient supine. Note any visible pulsations and more exaggerated lifts. Closely inspect area of apex. Palpate for pulsations (placing proximal half of four fingers together and then alternating with ball of hand at all anatomical landmarks).

Reveals size and symmetry of heart. Apical impulse may be visible at midclavicular line in fifth intercostal space. Apical impulse (PMI) may become visible only when patient sits up, bringing heart closer to anterior wall. Obesity obscures ability to visualize PMI. There should be no pulsations or vibrations. A thrill is a continuous palpable sensation, like purring of a cat. A thrust is the upward lift felt when palpating the chest wall.

e. Locate PMI by palpating with fingertips along the fifth ICS in midclavicular line (see illustration). Note light, brief pulsation in area 1 to 2 cm (⅓ to ¾ in) in diameter at the apex.

In presence of serious heart disease, PMI is located to left of midclavicular line related to enlarged left ventricle. In chronic lung disease PMI may be to right of midclavicular line as a result of right ventricular enlargement.

Clinical Decision Point *Presence of a palpable thrill is not normal and indicates a disruption of blood flow caused by a defect in closure of a heart valve or atrial septal defect. A stronger-than-expected impulse is a heave or lift, which indicates increased cardiac output or left ventricular hypertrophy. Report to health care provider.*

f. If palpating PMI is difficult, turn patient onto left side.

Manoeuvre moves heart closer to chest wall.

g. Inspect epigastric area and palpate abdominal aorta.
NOTE: You should feel a localized strong beat.

Rules out reduced blood flow or diffuse pulse, which indicates abnormality.

h. Auscultate heart sounds:

(1) Have patient sit up and lean slightly forward; then have the person lie supine; end examination with patient in left lateral recumbent position (see illustration A to C). In female patient, it may be necessary to lift left breast to hear heart sounds more effectively.

Different positions help to clarify type of sounds heard. Sitting position is best to hear high-pitched murmurs (if present). Supine is common position for hearing all sounds. Left lateral recumbent is best position to hear low-pitched sounds.

(2) While auscultating sounds at each anatomical landmark, ask patient not to speak but to breathe comfortably. Begin with diaphragm of stethoscope; alternate with bell. Use very light pressure for bell. Move stethoscope along slowly; avoid jumping from one area to another. Do not try to hear all heart sounds at once.

Auscultation requires you to isolate each heart sound at all auscultation sites, especially in patients with soft heart sounds.

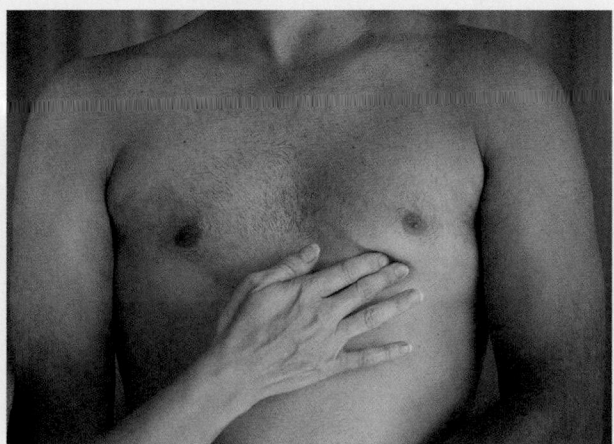

STEP 5e Palpation of point of maximal impulse.

STEP	RATIONALE

IMPLEMENTATION

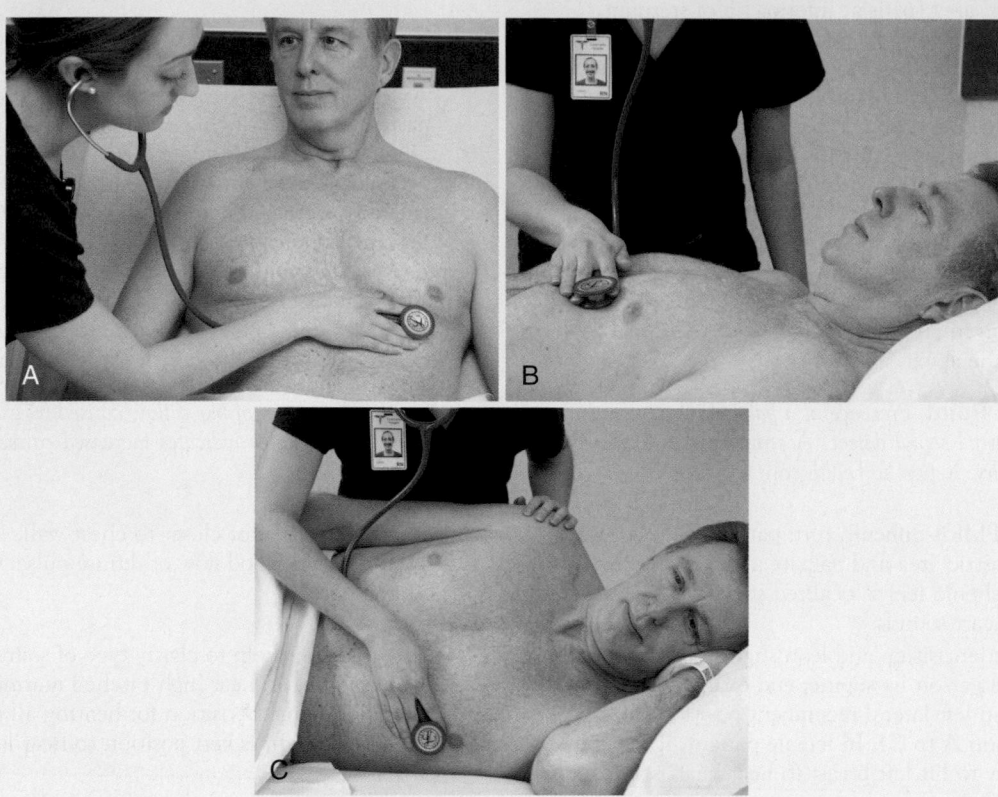

STEP 5h(1) Patient positions for auscultation of heart sounds. **A,** Sitting. **B,** Supine. **C,** Left lateral.

(3) Begin at apex or PMI; move systematically to aortic area, pulmonic area, Erb's point, tricuspid area, and mitral area (see illustration in Step 5c). (**NOTE:** Some examiners use reverse sequence.) S_1 is loudest at apex and is simultaneous with carotid pulse. **NOTE:** Helpful mnemonic for remembering heart sound locations: **A P**ig **E**ats **T**oo **M**uch (**A**ortic, **P**ulmonic, **E**rb's point, **T**ricuspid, **M**itral).

(4) Listen for S_2 at each site. This sound is loudest at the aortic area. Heart sounds vary by pitch, loudness, and duration, depending on auscultatory site (Table 8.8).

(5) After both sounds are heard clearly as "lub-dub," count each combination of S_1 and S_2 as one heartbeat. Count number of beats for 1 minute.

At normal slow rates S_1 is high-pitched and dull in quality and sounds like a "lub." This sound precedes systolic phase of heart contraction.

Normal sounds S_1 and S_2 are high-pitched and best heard with diaphragm. S_2 precedes diastolic phase and sounds like "dub."

Determines apical pulse rate.

TABLE 8.8

Heart Sounds According to Auscultatory Area

	Aortic	**Pulmonic**	**Second Pulmonic**	**Mitral**	**Tricuspid**
Pitch	$S_1 < S_2$	$S_1 < S_2$	$S_1 < S_2$	$S_1 > S_2$	$S_1 = S_2$
Loudness	$S_1 < S_2$	$S_1 < S_2$	$S_1 < S_2$*	$S_1 > S_2$†	$S_1 > S_2$
Duration	$S_1 > S_2$	$S_1 > S_2$	$S_1 > S_2$	$S_1 > S_2$	$S_1 > S_2$

*S_1 is relatively louder in second pulmonic area than in aortic area.
†S_1 may be louder in mitral area than in tricuspid area.
Modified from Ball, J. W., et al. (2015). *Seidel's guide to physical examination* (8th ed.). St. Louis: Mosby.

STEP	RATIONALE

IMPLEMENTATION

(6) Assess heart rhythm by noting time between S_1 and S_2 (systole) and then time between S_2 and the next S_1 (diastole). Listen to full cycle at each auscultation area. Note regular intervals between each sequence of beats. There should be a distinct pause between S_1 and S_2.

Failure of heart to beat at regular intervals is a dysrhythmia, which interferes with ability of heart to pump effectively.

(7) When heart rate is irregular, compare apical and radial pulses (Table 8.9). Auscultate apical pulse and then immediately palpate radial pulse. Also, you can ask a colleague to assess radial pulse while you simultaneously assess apical pulse.

Determines if pulse deficit (radial pulse is slower than apical) exists. Deficit indicates that ineffective contractions of heart fail to send pulse waves to periphery.

i. Auscultate for extra heart sounds at each site. Note pitch, loudness, duration, timing, location on chest wall, and where it is heard in cardiac cycle.

Abnormal sounds include murmurs. Characteristics of murmurs help to identify contributing factors.

(1) Use stethoscope bell and listen for low-pitched extra heart sounds such as S_3 and S_4 gallops, clicks, and rubs. S_3, or a ventricular gallop, occurs just after S_2 at end of ventricular diastole. It sounds like "lub-dub-ee" or "Ken-tuc-ky." S_4, or an atrial gallop, occurs just before S_1 or ventricular systole. It sounds like "dee-lub-dub" or "Ten-nes-see."

Premature rush of blood into a ventricle that is stiff or dilated or an atrial contraction pushing against a ventricle that is not accepting blood causes gallops.

(2) With patient leaning forward or lying on left side, listen for friction rubs as "squeaky" or rubbing sounds.

Rubs result from lungs or inflamed visceral and parietal layers of the pericardium of the heart rubbing against one another.

j. Auscultate for heart murmurs over each auscultation site.

Murmurs are sustained swishing or blowing sounds heard at beginning, middle, or end of systole or diastole. Increased blood flow through a normal valve, forward flow through a stenotic valve or into a dilated vessel or chamber, or backward flow through a valve that fails to close causes murmurs.

(1) When you detect a murmur, listen carefully to note where you hear it best. Note intensity of the murmur.

Intensity is related to rate of blood flow through the heart or amount of blood regurgitated.

(2) Note if murmur is low, medium, or high in pitch, using bell for low-pitched sounds.

Pitch depends on velocity of blood flow through the valves.

6. Assess neck vessels:

a. To assess carotid arteries, have patient remain in sitting position.

Allows easier mobility of neck to expose artery for inspection and palpation.

TABLE 8.9

Abnormalities in Rates and Rhythms

Type	Findings	Description
Atrial fibrillation	Rapid, random contractions of atria cause irregular ventricular beats >100 beats/min and atrial beats at 200–350 beats/min.	Atria discharge very rapidly, with some impulses not reaching ventricles. This condition occurs in rheumatic heart disease and mitral stenosis. It causes reduced cardiac output.
Sinus arrhythmia	Pulse rate changes during respiration, increasing at peak of inspiration and decreasing during expiration.	Blood is momentarily trapped in lungs during inspiration, causing a fall in stroke volume of heart.
Sinus bradycardia	Pulse rhythm is regular, but rate is <60 beats/min.	Sinoatrial node fires less frequently. This is common in well-conditioned athletes and with use of antiarrhythmic medications.
Sinus tachycardia	Pulse rhythm is regular, but rate is accelerated to >100 beats/min.	Exercise, emotional stress, and caffeine or alcohol ingestion are common factors that cause increased firing of sinoatrial node.
Premature ventricular contraction	Premature beat occurs before regularly expected heart contraction. Underlying rhythm can be any rate.	Ventricle contracts prematurely because of electrical impulse bypassing normal conduction pathway. It may occur so early that it is difficult to detect as second beat. It may be followed by a pause.

STEP	RATIONALE

IMPLEMENTATION

b. Inspect neck on both sides for obvious arterial pulsations. Sometimes a pulse wave can be seen.

Carotids are the only sites to assess quality of pulse wave (see illustration). Experience is required to evaluate wave in relation to events of cardiac cycle.

c. Palpate each carotid artery separately with index and middle fingers around medial edge of sternocleidomastoid muscle. Ask patient to raise chin slightly, keeping head straight (see illustration) or slightly away from artery. Note rate and rhythm, strength, and elasticity of artery. Also note if pulse changes as patient inhales and exhales.

If both arteries were occluded simultaneously, patient could lose consciousness from reduced circulation to brain. Turning head improves access to artery. A change indicates a sinus arrhythmia.

Clinical Decision Point *Do not palpate or massage the carotid artery vigorously. Stimulation of carotid sinus causes a reflex drop in heart rate and blood pressure.*

d. Place bell of stethoscope over each carotid artery, auscultating for blowing sound (bruit) (see illustration). Ask patient to exhale and hold breath for a few heartbeats so respiratory sounds do not interfere with auscultation (Ball et al., 2015).

Narrowing of lumen of carotid artery by arteriosclerotic plaques causes disturbance in blood flow. Blood passing through narrowed section creates turbulence and emits blowing or swishing sound. Normally you do not hear a bruit.

e. To estimate the jugular venous pressure (JVP), hold a vertical ruler on the angle of Louis (sternal angle), align a straight edge on the ruler like a T-square, and adjust the level of the horizontal straight edge to the level of pulsation (Jarvis et al., 2019). Read the level of intersection on the vertical ruler and state the patient's position, e.g., "JVP 3 cm above sternal angle when elevated 10 degrees."

7. Peripheral vascular assessment:

a. Inspect lower extremities for changes in colour and condition of skin (Table 8.10). Note skin and nail texture, hair distribution, venous patterns, edema, and scars or impaired skin integrity. Compare skin colour with patient lying and standing.

Changes may reflect impaired peripheral circulation.

b. Palpate edematous areas, noting mobility, consistency, and tenderness.

Helps to determine extent of edema.

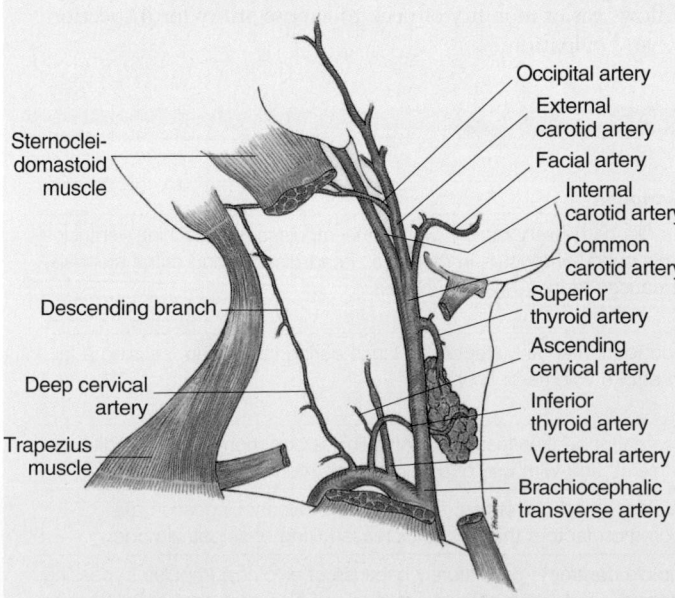

STEP 6b Anatomical position of carotid artery.

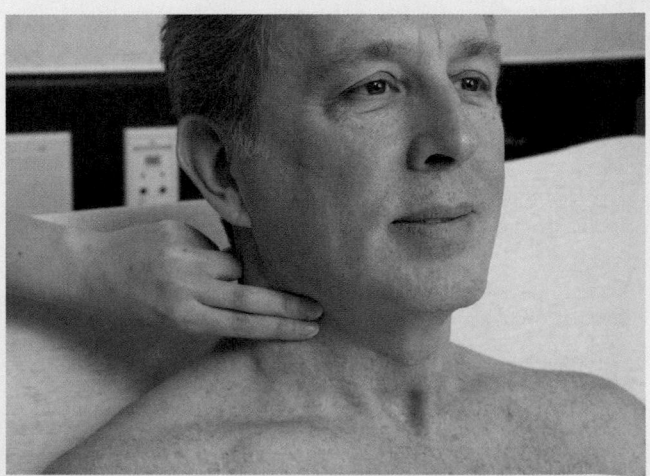

STEP 6c Palpate each carotid artery separately.

STEP	RATIONALE

IMPLEMENTATION

c. Assess for pitting edema by pressing area firmly with one finger for 5 seconds and releasing. Depth of indentation determines severity (see illustration).

    2 mm: 1+ edema
    4 mm: 2+ edema
    6 mm: 3+ edema
    8 mm: 4+ edema

d. Use tape measure to measure circumference of extremity.

e. Check capillary refill by grasping patient's fingernail or toenail and noting colour of nail bed. Apply gentle, firm pressure to nail bed. Release quickly, watching for colour change. Circulation is restored and normally returns to pink colour in less than 2 seconds.

f. Inspect index fingers using the profile sign (viewing the finger from the side); the normal nail bed angle is 160 degrees.

g. Ask if patient experiences pain or tenderness and gently palpate for heat, firmness, or localized swelling of calf muscle, all of which are signs of phlebitis or DVT.

Limb edema is classic sign of deep vein thrombosis (DVT), although this can be seen in other conditions; therefore, if DVT is suspected diagnostic tests must be performed. If DVT is diagnosed, emergency referral is needed due to risk of pulmonary embolism (Jarvis et al., 2019).

Measuring circumference establishes baseline for future comparison.

Capillary refill is measured in seconds; less than 2 seconds is brisk; whereas greater than 4 seconds is sluggish.

Cold environmental temperature with vasoconstriction and vascular disease can delay refill. Local pressure from cast or bandage also slows refill.

Flattening of the nail bed angle suggests early clubbing, which may occur with chronic heart or lung diseases.

A frequent cause of DVT is prolonged immobility, such as in postoperative patients and in individuals after a long trip without adequate movement or exercise. Other factors that contribute to DVT include obesity, trauma, tobacco use, oral contraceptives, advanced age, malignancies, and stroke (Lewis et al., 2019).

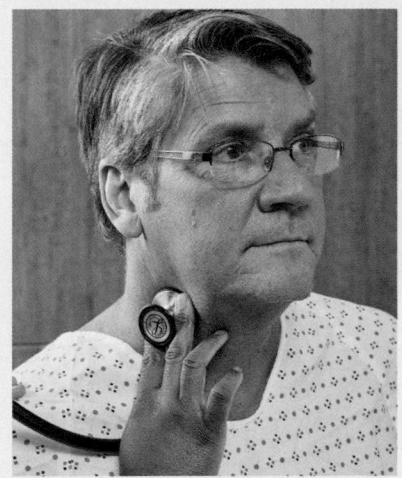

STEP 6d Auscultation for carotid artery bruit.

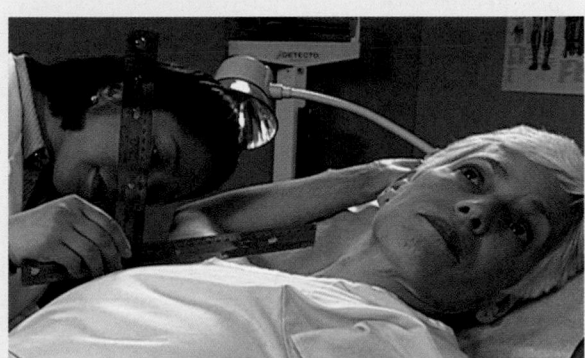

STEP 6e Estimating jugular venous pressure (JVP). *(From Ball, J. W., et al. [2015]. Seidel's Guide to Physical Examination [8th ed., p. 343]. St. Louis: Elsevier.)*

TABLE 8.10

Signs of Venous and Arterial Insufficiency

Assessment Criterion	Venous	Arterial
Pain	Aching; increases in evening and with dependent position	Burning, throbbing, cramping; increases with exercise
Paresthesia	None	Numbness, tingling, decreased sensation
Temperature	Normal to touch	Cool to touch
Colour	Normal or cyanotic	Pale; worsened by elevation of extremity; dusky red when extremity is lowered
Capillary refill	Not applicable	>2 seconds
Pulse	Present	Decreased or absent
Skin changes	Brown pigmentation around ankles	Thin, shiny skin; decreased hair growth; thickened nails
Ulcerations	Shallow ulcers around ankles (chronic venous stasis); edema apparent	Deep, well defined at site of trauma or tips of toes

STEP	RATIONALE

IMPLEMENTATION

Clinical Decision Point *Homans' sign (pain in calf on dorsiflexion of foot) is no longer considered a reliable indicator for the presence or absence of DVT (Ball et al., 2015) and should not be considered a reliable test. Trauma to a vein or muscle, reduced mobility, and increased blood clotting are reliable risk factors. If calf is swollen, tender, or red, notify patient's health care provider for further assessment and evaluation. If there is a strong suspicion of DVT, testing for Homans' sign is contraindicated. If a clot is present, it may become dislodged from its original site during this test. This could result in a pulmonary embolism.*

   h. Palpate peripheral arteries.

     (1) Start at most distal part of each extremity. Palpate each peripheral artery for equality, comparing side to side; elasticity of vessel wall (depress and release artery, noting ease with which it springs back to shape); and strength of pulse (force of blood against arterial wall) using the following rating scale (Ball et al., 2015):

       0   Absent, not palpable

       1+ Diminished, pulse barely palpable, weak and thready, and easy to obliterate

       2+ Normal pulse, easy to palpate

       3+ Full, easy to palpate, increases

       4+ Strong, bounding against fingertips; cannot be obliterated

Comparison of both arteries allows you to determine any localized obstruction or disturbance in blood flow. Pulses should be symmetrical side to side. If asymmetry is noted, look for other factors related to impaired circulation.

     (2) Palpate radial pulse by lightly placing tips of first and second fingers in groove formed along radial side of forearm, lateral to flexor tendon of wrist (see illustration).

Pulse is relatively superficial and should not require deep palpation.

     (3) Palpate ulnar pulse by placing fingertips along ulnar side of forearm (see illustration).

Palpated when arterial insufficiency to hand is expected or when you assess for radial occlusion (e.g., during arterial blood gas sampling), which may affect circulation to hand.

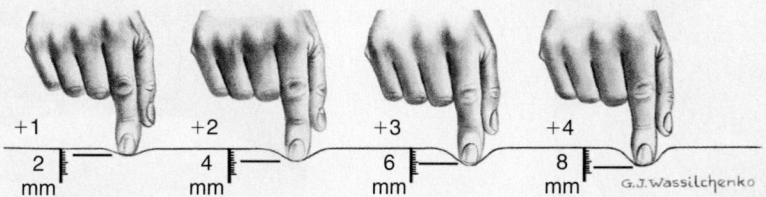

STEP 7c Assessing for pitting edema. *(From Seidel, H. M., et al. [2011]. Mosby's guide to physical examination [7th ed.]. St. Louis: Mosby.)*

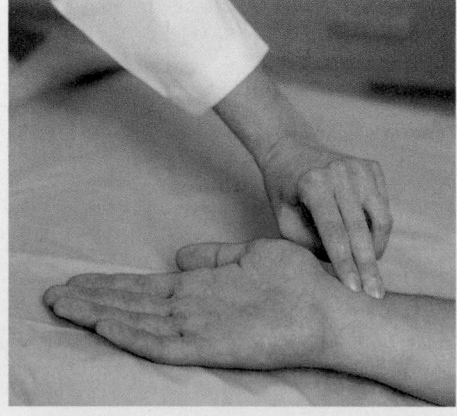

STEP 7h(2) Palpation of radial pulse.

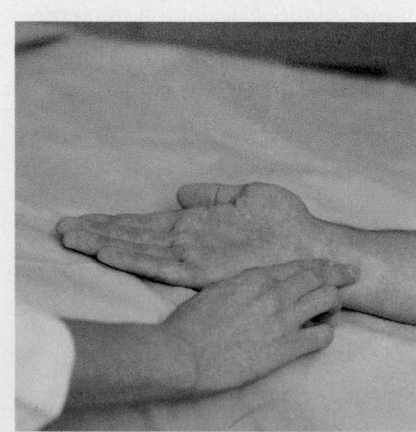

STEP 7h(3) Palpation of ulnar pulse.

STEP	RATIONALE

IMPLEMENTATION

(4) Palpate brachial pulse by locating groove between biceps and triceps muscles above elbow at antecubital fossa (see illustration). Place tips of first two fingers in muscle groove.

Artery runs along medial side of extended arm, requiring moderate palpation. If difficult to palpate, hyperextend arm to bring pulse site closer to the surface.

(5) Have patient lie supine with feet relaxed and palpate dorsalis pedis pulse. Gently place fingertips between great and first toe; slowly move fingers along groove between extensor tendons of great and first toe until pulse is palpable (see illustration).

Artery lies superficially and does not require deep palpation. Pulse may be congenitally absent.

(6) Palpate posterior tibial pulse by having patient relax and extend feet slightly. Place fingertips behind and below medial malleolus (ankle bone) (see illustration).

Artery is easily palpable with foot relaxed.

(7) Palpate popliteal pulse by having patient slightly flex knee with foot resting on table or bed. Instruct patient to keep leg muscles relaxed. Palpate deeply into popliteal fossa with fingers of both hands placed just lateral to midline. Patient may also lie prone to achieve exposure of artery (see illustration).

Flexion of knee and muscle relaxation improve accessibility of artery. Popliteal pulse is one of the more difficult pulses to palpate.

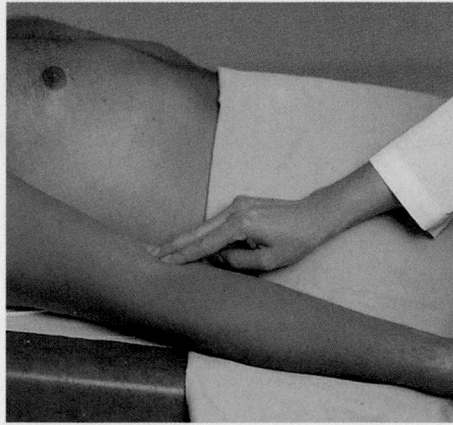

STEP 7h(4) Palpation of brachial pulse.

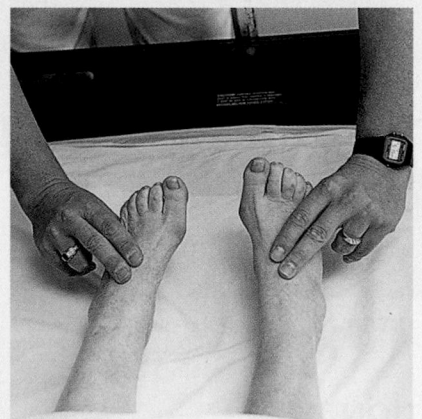

STEP 7h(5) Palpation of dorsalis pedis pulses.

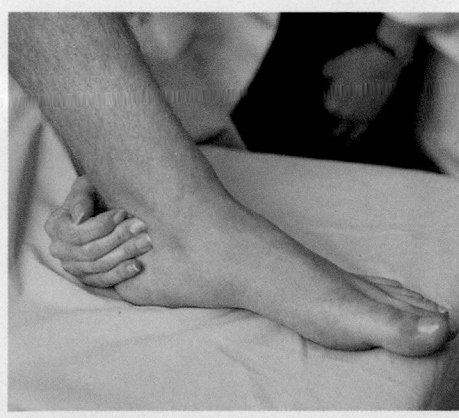

STEP 7h(6) Palpation of posterior tibial pulse.

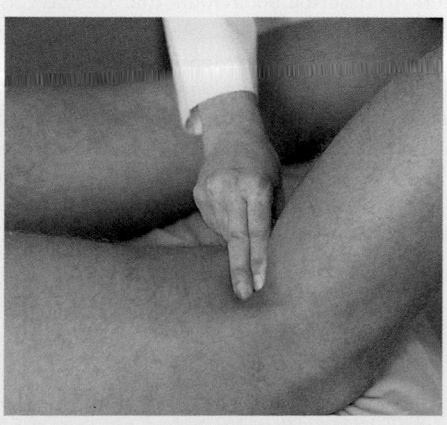

STEP 7h(7) Palpation of popliteal pulse with patient prone.

STEP	RATIONALE

IMPLEMENTATION

(8) Apply clean gloves. With patient supine, palpate femoral pulse by placing first two fingers over inguinal area below inguinal ligament, midway between pubic symphysis and anterosuperior iliac spine (see illustration).

Supine position prevents flexion in groin area, which interferes with artery access.

i. If pulses are difficult to palpate or are not palpable, use a Doppler instrument over pulse site:

(1) Apply conducting gel to patient's skin over pulse site or onto transducer tip of probe. Turn Doppler on.

(2) Gently apply ultrasound probe to skin, changing Doppler angle until pulsation is audible. Adjust volume as needed (see illustration). Wipe off gel from patient and Doppler.

Doppler amplifies sounds, allowing you to hear low-velocity blood flow through peripheral arteries.

8. Remove gloves and discard used supplies and gloves in proper receptacle. Help patient to comfortable position. Perform hand hygiene.

Reduces transmission of infection.

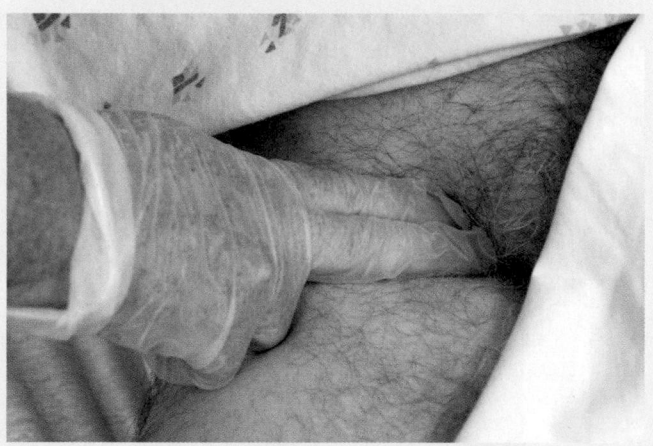

STEP 7h(8) Palpation of femoral pulse.

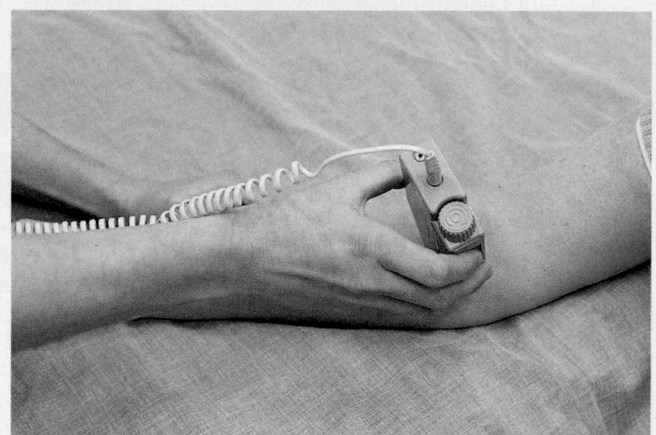

STEP 7i(2) Use of Doppler to assess brachial pulse.

EVALUATION

1. Compare findings with normal assessment characteristics of heart and vascular system.

Determines presence of abnormalities.

2. If heart sounds are not audible or pulses are not palpable, ask another nurse to confirm assessment.

Validates abnormal assessment findings.

3. Ask patient to describe behaviours that increase risk for heart and vascular disease.

Demonstrates learning.

4. Compare pulses and capillary refill bilaterally with previous assessment.

Demonstrates change from baseline measures.

5. **Use Teach-Back:** "I would like to make sure you understand some of the risks and behaviours that can lead to heart disease. Tell me how exercise affects your risk for heart disease." Develop a revised teaching plan if patient or caregiver is not able to teach back correctly.

Determines patient's and caregiver's level of understanding of instructional topic.

STEP	RATIONALE

EVALUATION

Unexpected Outcomes

1. Findings differ from previous assessments, including:
   - Pulsations, vibrations, or both are palpable. These are result of valvular problem, murmur, or both.
   - Extra heart sounds S_3 or S_4 are auscultated. Extra sounds indicate atrial or ventricular gallop.
   - Murmur is auscultated. Impaired blood flow through heart indicates need for immediate medical attention. Some murmurs are benign.
   - JVP is elevated. This is sign of right-sided heart failure or fluid overload.
2. Heart rate is irregular, with rate less than 60 beats/min or more than 100 beats/min.

3. Pulse deficit is noted. There is risk for inadequate cardiac output.

Related Interventions

- Prepare to obtain or help with electrocardiogram (ECG).

- Check blood pressure. If low, dysrhythmia is contributing to inadequate cardiac output.
- Observe for sensations or reports of dizziness or feeling "faint."
- Prepare to obtain ECG.
- Obtain vital signs.

Communication and Documentation

- Document quality (clear or muffled), intensity (weak or pounding), rate, and rhythm (regular, regularly irregular, or irregularly irregular) of heart sounds and peripheral pulses in nurses' notes in electronic health record (EHR) or chart.
- Document additional cardiac findings, JVP, and condition of extremities in nurses' notes in EHR or flow sheet.
- Document activity level and subjective data related to fatigue, shortness of breath, and chest pain.
- Document your evaluation of patient and caregiver learning.
- Report immediately to health care provider any irregularities in heart function and indications of impaired arterial blood flow.
- Report to health care provider changes in peripheral circulation, which may indicate circulatory compromise, which may result in permanent nerve damage or tissue death if untreated.

Special Considerations
Teaching

- Explain risk factors for heart disease: high dietary intake of saturated fat or cholesterol, lack of regular aerobic exercise, smoking, excess weight, stressful lifestyle, hypertension, and family history of heart disease.
- Refer patient (if appropriate) to resources available for controlling or reducing risks (e.g., nutrition counselling, exercise class, and stress-reduction programs).
- Help patient to find resources to help quitting smoking because

this lowers the risk for cardiovascular disease (Anderson, Gregoire, Pearson, et al., 2016). Nicotine in cigarette smoke causes vasoconstriction.
- Patients who are at risk benefit from taking a daily low dose of aspirin. Consult health care provider before starting therapy.

Pediatric

- PMI is at fourth intercostal space at left midclavicular line in children younger than 7 years of age (Hockenberry & Wilson, 2015).
- Capillary refill in infants is usually less than 1 second.
- It is not uncommon for children to have third heart sounds (S_3). Sinus arrhythmia occurs normally in many infants and children (Hockenberry & Wilson, 2015).
- Children have louder, higher-pitched heart sounds because of their thin chest walls.

Gerontological

- PMI may be difficult to find in an older person because anteroposterior diameter of the chest deepens.
- Accidental massage of the carotid sinus during palpation of the carotid artery is a particular problem for older persons, causing a sudden drop in heart rate from vagal nerve stimulation.
- Older persons with hypertension benefit from regular monitoring of blood pressure (daily, weekly, or monthly). Home monitoring kits are available. Teach patient how to use them correctly.

◆ SKILL 8.5   Abdominal Assessment

Abdominal assessment is complex because of the multiple organs located within and near the abdominal cavity. This area of the body is associated with many health complaints; and many people are embarrassed by bowel or bladder dysfunction, reproductive problems, or urinary elimination problems. Abdominal pain is one of the most common symptoms that patients report when seeking medical care. It can be caused by alterations in organs such as the stomach, gallbladder, or intestines; or the pain may be the result of spinal or muscular injury. An accurate assessment requires matching the patient's history with a careful assessment of the location of physical symptoms (Table 8.11).

To perform an effective abdominal assessment, you need to know the location and function of the underlying structures involved, including the lower pelvis, kidneys, rectum, genitalia, liver, gallbladder, stomach, spleen, appendix, pancreas, intestines, and reproductive organs (Fig. 8.5). An abdominal assessment is routine after abdominal surgery, for any patient who has undergone invasive diagnostic tests of the gastrointestinal (GI) tract, and for patients with abnormalities affecting GI function. The order of an abdominal assessment differs from that of other assessments. You begin with inspection and follow with auscultation. It is important to auscultate

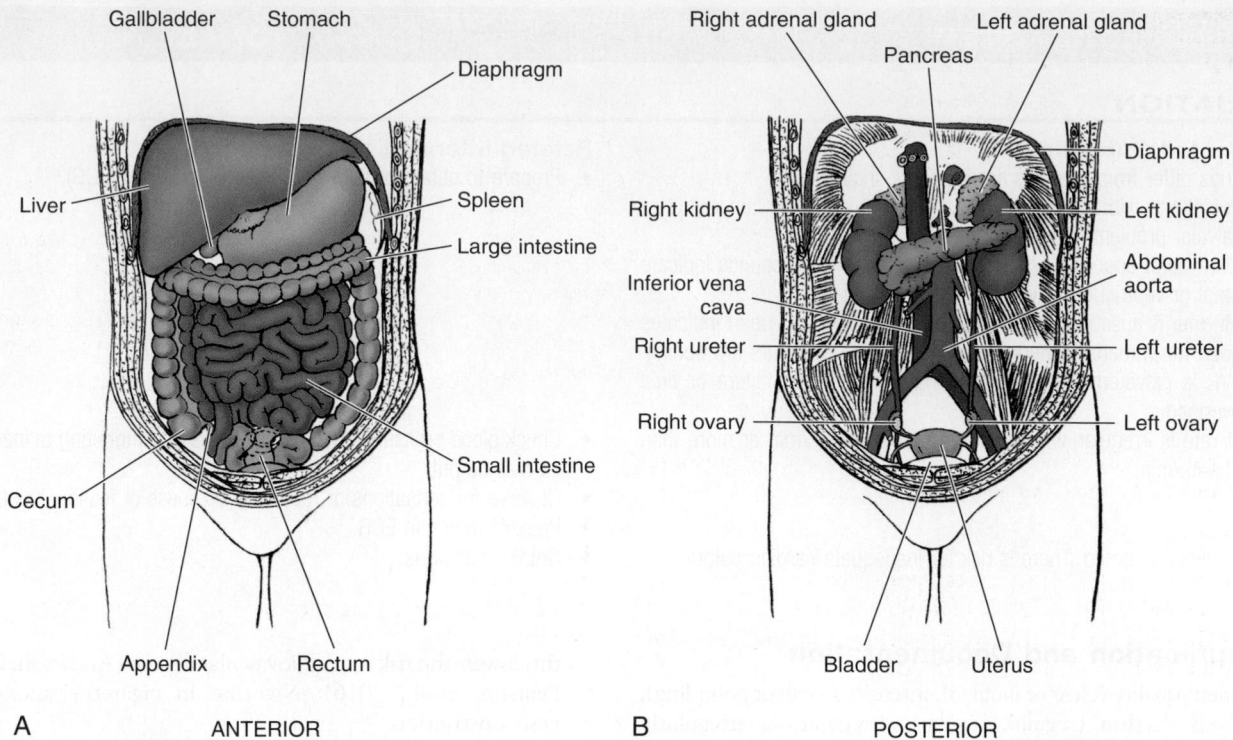

FIG 8.5 Location of organs in abdomen. **A,** Anterior. **B,** Posterior. (*Modified from Mosby's expert 10-minute physical examinations [2nd ed.] [2005]. St. Louis: Mosby.*)

TABLE 8.11

Common Causes of Abdominal Pain

Condition	Physical Alteration	Physical Signs and Symptoms
Appendicitis	Obstruction of appendix associated with inflammation, perforation, and peritonitis. Patient often lies on back or side with knees flexed to decrease pain	Sharp pain directly over the irritated peritoneum 2–12 hours after onset. Often pain localizes in right lower quadrant between anterior iliac crest and umbilicus. Associated with rebound tenderness. Accompanied by anorexia, nausea, and vomiting.
Celiac disease	Damage to small intestine mucosa from ingestion of barley, rye, oats, and wheat	Foul-smelling diarrhea, abdominal distension, and symptoms of malnutrition may be present.
Cholecystitis	Obstruction of cystic duct causing inflammation or distension of gallbladder	*Murphy's sign:* Apply gentle pressure below right subcostal arch and liver margin. Sharp pain and increased respiratory rate occur when patient takes a deep breath (Ball et al., 2015).
Constipation	Disruption in normal bowel pattern, which may occur with opioid use or inadequate fibre and fluid intake	Generalized discomfort accompanied by distension and palpation of a hard mass in the left lower quadrant. Nausea and vomiting may begin after several days.
Crohn's disease	Chronic inflammatory disease of the ileum	Steady colicky pain in the right lower quadrant, with cramping, tenderness, flatulence, nausea, fever, and diarrhea. Often associated with bloody stools, weight loss, weakness, and fatigue. A tender mass of thickened intestine may be palpated in right lower quadrant.
Gastroenteritis	Inflammation of the stomach and intestinal tract	Generalized abdominal discomfort accompanied by anorexia, nausea, vomiting, diarrhea, and abdominal cramping.
Pancreatitis	Inflammation of the pancreas associated with alcoholism, medication reaction, and gallbladder disease	Steady severe epigastric pain close to umbilicus radiates to back. Associated with abdominal rigidity and vomiting. Pain is unrelieved by vomiting, worsens by lying supine.
Paralytic ileus	Obstruction of the small bowel that occurs after abdominal surgery, from abdominal radiation, or from use of anticholinergic medications	Generalized severe abdominal distension, nausea, and vomiting; decreased or absent bowel sounds.

TABLE 8.11

Common Causes of Abdominal Pain—cont'd

Condition	Physical Alteration	Physical Signs and Symptoms
Peptic ulcers (gastric and duodenal)	Damage of gastrointestinal (GI) mucosa at any area of the GI tract May be caused by bacterial infection (Helicobacter pylori) or nonsteroidal anti-inflammatory drugs (NSAIDs) Thought to be unrelated to stress Aggravated by smoking and excessive alcohol use	*Gastric ulcer:* Dull epigastric pain, localized midline. Early satiety; not usually relieved by food or antacids. *Duodenal ulcer:* Pain is episodic, lasting 30 minutes to 2 hours. It is located midline in epigastric region, may radiate around costal border to back; described as aching, burning, or gnawing. Typically occurs 1–3 hours after meals and at night (12 midnight to 3 AM). Often relieved by food or antacid. *Both (dyspepsia syndrome):* symptoms of fullness, epigastric discomfort, vague feeling of nausea, abdominal distension, and bloating; anorexia; weight loss.

before palpation and percussion because these manoeuvres alter the frequency and character of bowel sounds.

Delegation and Collaboration

The skill of abdominal assessment cannot be delegated to an unregulated care provider (UCP). The nurse directs the UCP to:

- Report the development of abdominal pain and changes in the patient's bowel habits or dietary intake to the nurse.

Equipment

- Stethoscope
- Tape measure
- Examination light
- Water-based marking pen
- Drapes

STEP	RATIONALE

ASSESSMENT

1. If patient has abdominal or low back pain, assess the character of pain in detail (location, onset, frequency, precipitating factors, aggravating factors, type of pain, severity, course).

   Knowing pattern of characteristics of pain helps determine its source.

2. Carefully observe patient's movement and position, such as lying still with knees drawn up, moving restlessly to find a comfortable position, or lying on one side or sitting with knees drawn up to chest.

   Positions assumed by patient reveal nature and source of pain (e.g., peritonitis, kidney stone, appendicitis). Patients with peritonitis lie still because movement aggravates pain. Supine position worsens acute pancreatitis pain; flexed knee, curved-back position brings relief. Patients with appendicitis lie on side or back with knees flexed in attempt to decrease muscle strain on abdominal wall.

3. Assess patient's normal bowel habits: frequency of stools; character of stools; recent changes in character of stools; measures used to promote elimination such as laxatives, enemas, and dietary intake; and eating and drinking habits.

   Data compared with information from physical assessment may help identify cause and nature of elimination problems.

4. Determine if patient has had abdominal surgery, trauma, or diagnostic tests of GI tract.

   Surgery or trauma to abdomen may result in altered position of underlying organs. Diagnostic tests may change character of stool.

5. Assess if patient has had recent weight changes or intolerance to diet (nausea, vomiting, cramping, especially in past 24 hours).

   Changes may indicate alterations in upper GI tract (e.g., stomach or gallbladder) or lower colon.

6. Assess for difficulty in swallowing, belching, flatulence, bloody emesis (hematemesis), black or tarry stools (melena), heartburn, diarrhea, or constipation.

   Indicative of GI alterations.

7. Determine if patient takes anti-inflammatory medications (e.g., aspirin, steroids, nonsteroidal anti-inflammatory drugs [NSAIDs]), or antibiotics.

   These medications may cause GI upset or bleeding.

8. Review family history of cancer, kidney disease, alcoholism, hypertension, or heart disease.

   Information may reveal risk for significant abdominal alterations. Chronic alcohol ingestion causes GI and liver problems.

9. Review patient's history for health care occupation, hemodialysis, intravenous medication use, household or sexual contact with hepatitis B virus (HBV) carrier, sexually active heterosexual person (more than one sex partner in previous 6 months), sexually active gay or bisexual man, international traveller in area of high HBV prevalence.

   These are risk factors for HBV exposure. Abdominal findings for hepatitis include jaundice, hepatomegaly, anorexia, abdominal and gastric discomfort, tea-coloured urine, and clay-coloured stools (Lewis et al., 2019).

STEP	RATIONALE

NURSING DIAGNOSES

- Pain (acute, chronic)
- Constipation
- Diarrhea

- Inadequate nutrition
- Excessive nutrition
- Reduced health maintenance

- Nausea
- Insufficient knowledge regarding need for an abdominal assessment

Related factors are individualized on the basis of patient's condition or needs.

PLANNING

1. Expected outcomes following completion of procedure:
   - Abdomen is soft and symmetrical, with smooth and even contour. No mass, distension, or tenderness is palpable. There are no forceful visible pulsations.
   - Bowel sounds are active and audible in all four quadrants.
   - No costovertebral angle (CVA) tenderness is present.
   - Patient denies discomfort or worsening of existing discomfort following examination.
2. Anticipate teaching topics so that during the examination you can teach patient about warning signs of colorectal cancer.
3. Perform hand hygiene. Prepare necessary supplies.

These are normal abdominal assessment findings.

Indicates normal peristaltic activity.
Indicates no inflammation of kidney.
Proper examination procedures have been implemented.

Allows you to incorporate instruction during physical assessment.

Reduces transmission of infection. Ensures efficiency during examination.

IMPLEMENTATION

1. Prepare patient for abdominal assessment:
   a. Ask if patient needs to empty bladder or defecate.

   b. Keep upper chest and legs draped.

   c. Be sure that room is warm.

   d. Have patient lie supine or in dorsal recumbent position with arms down at sides and knees slightly bent. Place small pillow under patient's knees.
   e. Move sheet or blanket to expose area from just above xiphoid process down to symphysis pubis.
   f. Maintain conversation during assessment except during auscultation. Explain steps calmly and slowly.

   g. Ask patient to point to tender areas.

Palpation of full bladder causes discomfort and feeling of urgency and makes it difficult for patient to relax.
Maintains patient's comfort during examination, promoting relaxation.
Promotes patient's comfort. Reduces risk of patient tensing abdominal muscles.
Placing arms under head or keeping knees fully extended causes abdominal muscles to tighten. Tightening of muscles prevents adequate palpation.
Provides full visualization of abdomen.

Patient's ability to relax during assessment improves accuracy of findings. Talking interferes with hearing bowel sounds.
Assess painful areas last. Manipulation of body part increases patient's pain and anxiety and makes remainder of assessment difficult to complete.

2. Abdominal assessment:
   a. Identify landmarks that divide abdominal region into quadrants. Boundary begins at tip of xiphoid process to symphysis pubis with line crossing and intersecting umbilicus, dividing abdomen into four equal sections (see illustration).
   b. Inspect skin of surface of abdomen for colour, scars, venous patterns, rashes, lesions, silvery white striae (stretch marks), and artificial openings (stomas). Observe skin lesions for characteristics described in Skill 8.1.

   c. If you note bruising, ask if patient self-administers injections (e.g., heparin or insulin).

Location of findings by common reference point helps successive examiners confirm findings and locate abnormalities.

Scars reveal evidence that patient has had past trauma or surgery. Striae indicate stretching of tissue from growth, obesity, pregnancy, ascites, or edema. Venous patterns reflect liver disease (portal hypertension). Artificial openings indicate bowel or urinary diversion (see Chapters 34 and 35).
Frequent injections may cause bruising and hardening of underlying tissues.

Clinical Decision Point *Bruising may also indicate physical signs of abuse, accidental injury, or bleeding disorder. When bruising is noted, additional information may be needed from the patient.*

STEP	RATIONALE

IMPLEMENTATION

d. Inspect contour, symmetry, and surface motion of abdomen. Note any masses, bulging, or distension. (Flat abdomen forms a horizontal plane from xiphoid process to symphysis pubis. Round abdomen protrudes in convex sphere from horizontal plane. Concave abdomen sinks into muscular wall. All are normal.)

Changes in symmetry or contour reveal underlying masses, fluid collection, or gaseous distension. Everted umbilicus (protruding outward) indicates distension. Hernia also causes umbilicus to protrude upward.

e. If abdomen appears distended, note if distension is generalized. Look at flanks on each side.

Distension may be caused by the nine F's (*fat, flatus, feces, fluids, fibroid, full bladder, false pregnancy, fatal tumour,* and *fetus*) (Ball et al., 2015). If gas causes distension, flanks do not bulge. If fluid causes distension, flanks bulge. Tumour may cause more unilateral bulging or distension. Pregnancy causes symmetrical bulge in lower abdomen.

f. If you suspect distension, measure size of abdominal girth by placing tape measure under patient and around abdomen at level of umbilicus (see illustration).

Consecutive measurements show any increase or decrease in abdominal distension. Make all subsequent measurements at same level of umbilicus to provide objective means to evaluate changes.

g. If patient has a nasogastric (NG) or nasointestinal (NI) tube connected to suction, turn off momentarily.

Sound of suction obscures bowel sounds.

h. To auscultate bowel sounds, place diaphragm of stethoscope lightly over each of four abdominal quadrants. Ask patient not to talk. Listen until you hear repeated gurgling or bubbling sounds in each quadrant (minimum of once in 5 to 20 seconds). Describe sounds as normal, hyperactive, hypoactive, or absent. If initially there are no bowel sounds, listen 5 minutes over each quadrant before deciding that bowel sounds are absent.

Normal bowel sounds occur irregularly every 5 to 15 seconds. Absence of sounds indicates cessation of gastric motility. Hyperactive bowel sounds not related to hunger or recent meal may indicate diarrhea or early intestinal obstruction. Hypoactive or absent bowel sounds indicate paralytic ileus or peritonitis. It is common for bowel sounds to be hypoactive after surgery for 24 hours or more, especially following abdominal surgery.

Clinical Decision Point *Nausea and vomiting, increasing distension, and inability to pass flatus may accompany severe paralytic ileus.*

i. Place bell of stethoscope over epigastric region of abdomen and each quadrant. Auscultate for vascular (whooshing) sounds.

Determines presence of turbulent blood flow (bruit) through thoracic or abdominal aorta, which may indicate an aneurysm.

Clinical Decision Point *If aortic bruit is auscultated, suggesting presence of an aneurysm, stop assessment and notify health care provider immediately. Percussion or palpation over abdominal bruit could cause rupture of an already weakened vessel wall in the presence of an abdominal aneurysm.*

j. With patient supine, gently percuss each of four abdominal quadrants systematically. Note areas of tympany and dullness.

Reveals presence of air or fluid in stomach and intestines. Normal percussion is tympanic because of swallowed air in GI tract. Presence of fluid or underlying masses is revealed by dull percussion.

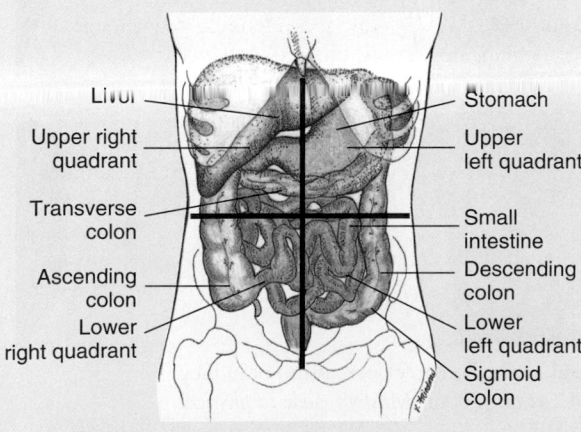

STEP 2a Division of abdomen into quadrants.

Liver
Upper right quadrant
Transverse colon
Ascending colon
Lower right quadrant

Stomach
Upper left quadrant
Small intestine
Descending colon
Lower left quadrant
Sigmoid colon

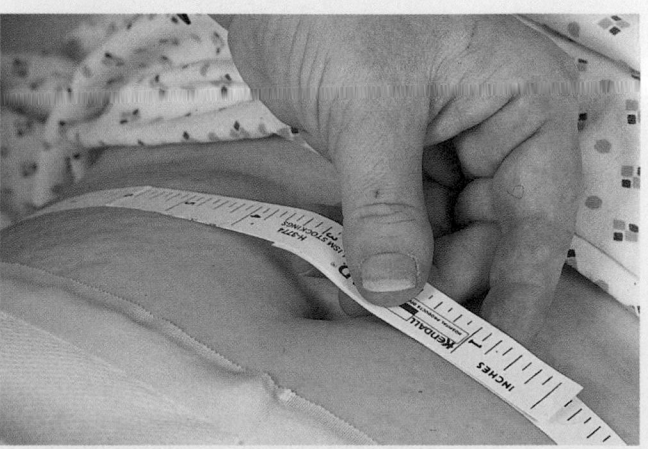

STEP 2f Measuring abdominal girth at level of umbilicus.

STEP	RATIONALE

IMPLEMENTATION

k. Ask patient if abdomen feels unusually tight and determine if this is a recent development.

Continued sensation of fullness helps to detect distension. Feeling of fullness after heavy meal causes only temporary distension. Tightness is not felt with obesity.

l. With patient sitting, gently but firmly percuss over each CVA along scapular lines (see illustration A). Use ulnar surface of fist indirectly by placing nondominant hand flat against CVA and percussing with dominant hand or percuss directly against patient's skin (see illustration B). Note if patient experiences pain.

Determines presence of kidney inflammation.

m. Lightly palpate over each abdominal quadrant, laying palm of hand with fingers extended and approximated lightly on abdomen. Keep palm and forearm horizontal. Pads of fingertips depress skin no more than 1 cm (0.4 inch) in gentle dipping motion (see illustration). Palpate painful areas last.

Detects areas of localized tenderness, degree of tenderness, and presence and character of underlying masses or fluid. Palpation of sensitive area causes guarding (voluntary tightening of underlying abdominal muscles).

   (1) Note muscular resistance, distension, tenderness, and superficial masses or organs while observing patient's face for signs of discomfort.

Patient's verbal and nonverbal cues may indicate discomfort from tenderness. Firm abdomen indicates active obstruction with buildup of fluid or gas.

   (2) Note if abdomen is firm or soft to touch.

Soft abdomen is normal or reveals that obstruction is resolving.

n. Just below umbilicus and above symphysis pubis, palpate for smooth, rounded mass. While applying light pressure, ask if patient has sensation of need to void.

Detects presence of dome of distended bladder.

Clinical Decision Point *Routinely check for distended bladder if patient has been unable to void, patient has been incontinent, or an in-dwelling Foley catheter is not draining well or has been removed recently.*

o. If masses are palpated, note size, location, shape, consistency, tenderness, mobility, and texture.

Descriptive characteristics help to reveal type of mass.

p. When tenderness is present, press one hand slowly and deeply into involved area and let go quickly. Note if pain is aggravated.

Test determines if rebound tenderness is present. Results are positive if pain increases. This indicates peritoneal irritation such as appendicitis (Ball et al., 2015).

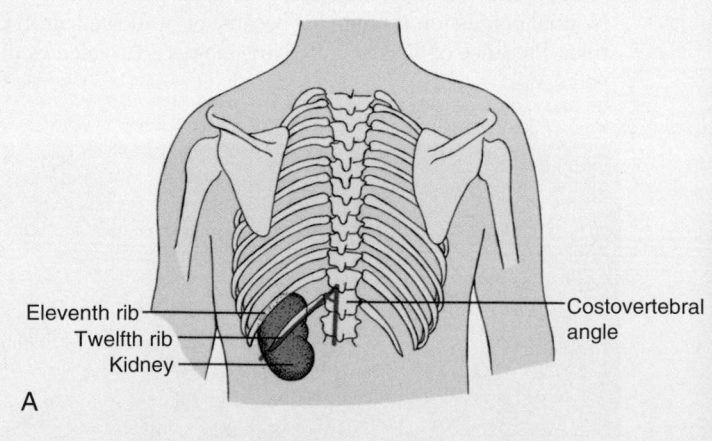

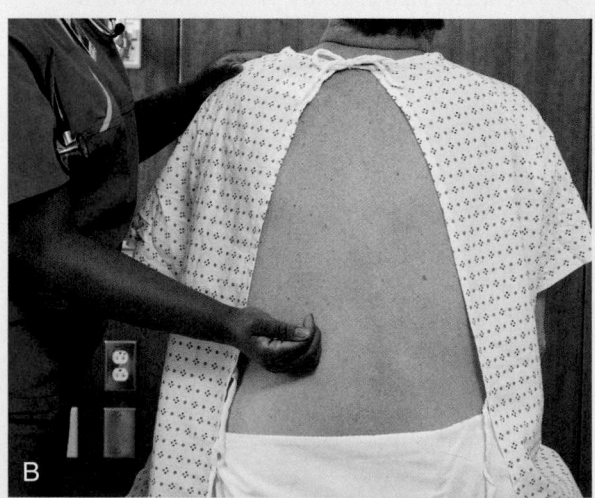

Eleventh rib
Twelfth rib
Kidney
Costovertebral angle

A

B

STEP 2l A, Position of kidney in relation to costovertebral angle. **B,** Direct percussion of kidney for costovertebral angle tenderness. (**A** *From Seidel, H. M., et al. [2006]. Mosby's guide to physical examination [6th ed.]. St. Louis: Mosby.*)

STEP	RATIONALE

IMPLEMENTATION

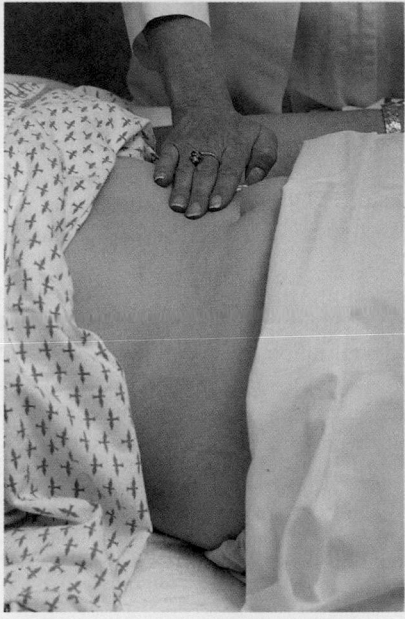

STEP 2m Light palpation of abdomen.

EVALUATION

1. Compare assessment findings with previous assessment characteristics to identify changes.

   Determines presence of abnormalities.

2. **Use Teach-Back:** "I would like to make sure that you understand the signs and symptoms of colorectal cancer. Tell me three changes in your bowel function that might be signs of colorectal cancer." Develop a revised teaching plan if patient or caregiver is not able to teach back correctly.

   Determines patient's and caregiver's level of understanding of instructional topic.

Unexpected Outcomes

1. Abdomen protrudes symmetrically with skin taut; patient complains of tightness, and/or bowel sounds are absent. GI motility has ceased. Patient is vomiting. Signs suggest an obstruction.

2. Hyperactive bowel sounds are evident with GI motility. Commonly they result from anxiety, diarrhea, overuse of laxatives, inflammation of bowel, or reaction of intestines to certain foods.

3. Rebound abdominal tenderness is palpated.

4. Bladder is palpable over symphysis pubis and distended.

Related Interventions

- Keep patient on nothing by mouth (NPO) status and encourage ambulation.
- Notify health care provider.
- Gastric decompression following insertion of NG tube sometimes may be necessary.
- Patient may need to be NPO.
- Contact health care provider to consider prescription for antidiarrheal medication.
- Avoid palpating area a second time.
- Notify health care provider.
- Keep patient NPO.
- Facilitate voiding by placing patient in sitting position or encouraging them to bear down (if not contraindicated); run water within hearing distance or have patient place hand in basin of warm water.
- Use bladder scan to determine extent of bladder fullness (see Chapter 34).
- If unable to void, urinary catheterization is necessary (see Chapter 34).

Communication and Documentation

- Document appearance of abdomen, quality of bowel sounds, presence of distension, abdominal circumference, and presence and location of tenderness in nurses' notes in electronic health record (EHR) or chart.
- Document evaluation of patient and caregiver learning.
- Document patient's ability to void and defecate, including description of output in the EHR or chart.
- Report serious abnormalities such as absent bowel sounds, presence of a mass, or acute pain to nurse in charge and health care provider.

Special Considerations
Teaching

- Explain that factors such as diet, regular exercise, limited use of over-the-counter medications causing constipation, establishment of regular elimination schedule, and adequate fluid intake promote normal bowel elimination.
- If patient is a health care worker or has contact with blood or body fluids of affected people, encourage them to receive series of three HBV vaccine doses.

Pediatric

- The most common palpable abdominal mass in a child is feces, usually palpated in right lower quadrant (Hockenberry & Wilson, 2015).

- Have child stand erect and then lie supine during inspection of abdominal surface. Normal abdomen of infants and young children is cylindrical in erect position and flat in supine position. School-age children may have a rounded abdomen until 13 years of age when standing.
- In infants and children skin of abdomen is usually taut and without wrinkles or creases.
- Infants and children until the age of 7 years are abdominal breathers.
- Some children perceive superficial palpation as tickling. Drawing attention to their laughter only causes it to increase. Have children help by placing their hand on top of yours or have them place their hand on their abdomen with their fingers separated and then palpate between their fingers.

Gerontological

- Older persons often lack abdominal tone; underlying organs are more easily palpable.
- Constipation along with nausea, flatulence, and heartburn is common.
- Stress to older persons the importance of adequate fluid intake; regular exercise; and a diet with at least four servings daily of fresh fruit, vegetables, and high-fibre food to promote normal defecation.

✦ SKILL 8.6   Genitalia and Rectum Assessment

The best time to examine a patient's external genitalia is while performing routine hygiene measures or preparing to insert or care for a urinary catheter. An examination of female and male external genitalia is part of preventive health screenings. Male patients need to learn how to perform self-examinations of the genitalia to detect testicular cancer (Box 8.6). Adolescent and young adults are examined because of the growing incidence of sexually transmitted infections (STIs). The average age of menarche among females has declined, and most teenagers are sexually active by age 19 (Hockenberry & Wilson, 2015). You can easily combine rectal and anal assessments with this examination because the patient assumes a lithotomy or dorsal recumbent position.

Examination of the genitalia of a transgender person must be done with sensitivity and must be relevant to the anatomy present, as sex organs and secondary sex characteristics will vary depending on whether the patient has had gender assignment surgery or hormone therapy (Jarvis et al., 2019).

Delegation and Collaboration

The skill of assessing the genitalia and rectum cannot be delegated to an unregulated care provider (UCP). The nurse directs the UCP to:

- Report changes in patient's genitourinary function and presence of drainage in the perineal area.

Equipment

- Examination light
- Clean gloves (use nonlatex if necessary)
- Drapes

BOX 8.6

Genital Self-Examination

Counselling for routine testicular self-examination in patients with low risk is no longer recommended, as the incidence of testicular cancer is low, and outcomes are favourable (Greig, Constantin, LeBlanc, et al., 2016). However, all males should know what is normal for their testicles. The best time to feel the testicles is during or after a warm bath or shower, which causes the testicles to descend and the scrotal sac to relax. It is normal to feel a soft cord or a small bump at the back of each testicle, which is the epididymis, a tube that collects and carries sperm. It is also normal for one testicle to be larger than the other. The patient should be encouraged to report any changes promptly to a health care provider.

STEPS	RATIONALE

ASSESSMENT

1. Assessment: female genitalia:

    a. Determine if patient has signs and symptoms of vaginal discharge, painful or swollen perianal tissues, or genital lesions.

These signs and symptoms are consistent with an STI or other pathological condition.

    b. Determine if patient has symptoms or history of genitourinary problems, including burning during urination (dysuria), frequency, urgency, nocturia, hematuria, or incontinence.

Urinary problems are associated with gynecological disorders, including STIs.

    c. Ask if the patient has had signs of bleeding outside of normal menstrual cycle or after menopause or unusual vaginal discharge.

These are warning signs for cervical and endometrial cancer or vaginal infection.

    d. Determine if patient has received human papillomavirus (HPV) vaccine.

To protect against cervical cancer, the National Advisory Committee on Immunization (NACI) recommends that healthy females aged 9–14 years receive a 2- or 3-dose schedule of the HPV4 (Gardasil), HPV2 (Cervarix), or HPV9 (Gardasil 9) vaccine, and healthy females age 15 years or older receive a 3-dose schedule of one of the vaccines (Public Health Agency of Canada [PHAC], 2017). The Gardasil vaccine also protects against most genital warts and some cancers of the vulva, vagina, and anus. Gardasil or Gardasil 9 is recommended for males aged 9–14 years (2 or 3 doses) and males aged 15 or older (3 doses) (PHAC, 2017).

    e. Determine if patient has history of HPV infection, smoking, giving birth many times, being sexually active, or weakened immune system, has a low income, is the daughter of a woman who took diethylstilbestrol (DES) during pregnancy, or has taken oral contraceptives for a long period of time.

These are risk factors for cervical cancer (CCS, 2018c).

    f. Determine if patient has a history of breast cancer, *BRCA* gene mutations, Lynch syndrome, hormone replacement therapy, smoking, asbestos exposure, or endometriosis; tall adult height; a family history of ovarian, colorectal, uterine, or pancreatic cancer; Ashkenazi Jewish ancestry; or has never been pregnant or given birth.

These are risk factors for ovarian cancer (CCS, 2018k).

    g. Determine if patient is overweight or obese; had early menarche or late menopause; has never given birth, has history of diabetes mellitus, polycystic ovarian syndrome, Lynch syndrome, or Cowden syndrome; or has a history of estrogen-related exposure (estrogen-only hormone replacement therapy, tamoxifen use), pelvic radiation, or low levels of physical activity.

These are risk factors for endometrial (uterine) cancer (CCS, 2018m).

    h. Determine patient's knowledge of risk factors and signs of cervical and other gynecological cancers.

Provides baseline for patient education.

2. Assessment of male genitalia:

    a. Review normal elimination pattern, including frequency of voiding, history of nocturia; character and volume of urine; daily fluid intake; symptoms of burning, urgency, and frequency; difficulty starting stream; and hematuria.

Urinary problems are directly associated with genitourinary problems because of anatomical structure of men's reproductive and urinary systems.

    b. Ask if patient has noted penile pain or swelling, genital lesions, or urethral discharge.

These are signs and symptoms of STIs.

    c. Determine if patient has noted heaviness, painless enlargement, or irregular lumps of testis.

These signs and symptoms are early warning signs for testicular cancer.

    d. Determine if patient reports any enlargement in inguinal area and assess if intermittent or constant, associated with straining or lifting, and painful. Assess whether coughing, lifting, or straining at stool causes pain.

Signs and symptoms indicate potential inguinal hernia.

STEP	RATIONALE

ASSESSMENT

    e. Ask if patient has experienced urinary frequency or urgency, difficulty starting urine flow, inability to empty the bladder completely, slow or interrupted urine stream, urinary or bowel incontinence, blood in the urine or semen, burning or pain during urination, painful ejaculation, erectile dysfunction, pain or stiffness in the bones of the hips, back, or chest, weakness or numbness in the legs or feet, shortness of breath, or a cough that does not go away.

These are warning signs and symptoms of prostate cancer (CCS, 2018l). Symptoms also may indicate infection or prostate enlargement.

    f. Assess patient's knowledge of risk factors and signs of prostate and testicular cancer.

Provides baseline for patient education.

3. Assessment of all patients:

    a. Determine whether patient has rectal bleeding, black or tarry stools (melena), rectal pain, change in bowel habits (constipation, diarrhea, or stool that looks narrower than usual), or weight loss.

These are warning signs of colorectal cancer (CCS, 2018e) or other gastrointestinal (GI) alterations.

    b. Determine whether patient has personal or family history of colorectal cancer, Ashkenazi Jewish ancestry, polyps, familial adenomatous polyposis, chronic inflammatory bowel disease, or personal history of breast, ovarian, or uterine cancer or Lynch syndrome. Determine if patient is overweight or obese, smokes, drinks alcohol, has sedentary lifestyle, eats a diet high in red and processed meats or low in fibre.

These are risk factors for colorectal cancer (CCS, 2018d).

    c. Assess medication history for use of laxatives or cathartic medications.

Repeated use causes diarrhea and eventual loss of intestinal muscle tone.

    d. Assess for use of opioids or iron preparations.

Opioids cause constipation. Iron turns stool black and tarry.

    e. Assess patient's knowledge of risks and signs of colorectal cancer.

Provides baseline for patient education.

NURSING DIAGNOSES

- Pain (acute, chronic)
- Inadequate health maintenance
- Insufficient knowledge regarding need for a genital and rectal assessment
- Readiness for enhanced immunization status

Related factors are individualized on the basis of patient's condition or needs.

PLANNING

1. Expected outcomes following completion of procedure:

- Patient denies discomfort or worsening of existing discomfort following examination.

Proper examination procedures have been implemented.

- Patient is able to list warning signs of colorectal cancer: female patient (or transgender man): cervical, endometrial, and ovarian cancer; male patient (or transgender woman): testicular and prostate cancer.

Demonstrates learning.

- Patient is able to discuss guidelines for HPV immunization.

Demonstrates learning.

2. Anticipate teaching topics so that during the examination you can teach patient about warning signs of colorectal cancer.

Prepares you for incorporating teaching into assessment activities.

3. Perform hand hygiene. Prepare necessary supplies.

Reduces transmission of infection.

IMPLEMENTATION

1. Prepare patient for assessment:

    a. Ask if patient needs to empty bladder or defecate.

Palpation of full bladder causes discomfort and feeling of urgency and makes it difficult for patient to relax.

    b. Keep upper chest and legs draped and keep room warm.

Maintains patient's comfort during examination, promoting relaxation.

STEP	RATIONALE

IMPLEMENTATION

c. Position patient:

(1) Female should lie in dorsal recumbent position with arms down at sides and knees slightly bent. Place small pillow under the knees.

Placing arms under head or keeping knees fully extended causes tightening of abdominal muscles.

(2) Male should lie supine with chest, abdomen, and lower legs draped; or have him stand during examination.

(3) Transgender patient should be placed in a gender-affirming position. Physical examination should be relevant to the anatomy present.

d. Apply clean gloves.

2. Female genitalia examination. (Use this time to discuss patient's risk for STIs and signs and symptoms of cervical, ovarian, and endometrial cancers.)

a. Expose perineal area, repositioning sheet as needed.

b. Inspect surface characteristics of perineum and retract labia majora; observe for inflammation, edema, lesions, or lacerations. Note if there is any vaginal discharge. Presence of discharge may indicate need for a culture.

Skin of perineum is smooth, clean, and slightly darker than other skin. Mucous membranes are dark pink and moist. Labia majora are symmetrical; may be dry or moist. Normally there is no vaginal discharge.

3. Male genitalia examination. (Use this time to discuss patient's risk for STIs and signs and symptoms of testicular cancer.)

a. Expose perineal area. Observe genitalia for rashes, excoriations, or lesions.

Normally skin is clear without lesions.

b. Inspect and palpate penile surfaces (see also Box 8.6).

(1) Inspect corona, prepuce (foreskin), glans, urethral meatus, and shaft. Retract foreskin in uncircumcised males. Observe for discharge, lesions, edema, and inflammation. Return foreskin to normal position.

Glans should be smooth and pink along all surfaces. Urethral meatus is slitlike and normally positioned at tip of glans. Foreskin should retract easily. Area between foreskin and glans is common site for venereal lesions.

c. Inspect and palpate testicular surfaces.

(1) Inspect size, colour, shape, and symmetry; also gently palpate for lesions and edema.

Left testicle is normally lower than right. Scrotal skin is usually loose, surface is coarse, and skin colour is more deeply pigmented than body skin.

d. Palpate testes (see also Box 8.6).

(1) Note size, shape, and consistency of tissue.

Testes are normally ovoid and approximately 2 to 4 cm (0.8 to 1.6 inches) in size, feel smooth and rubbery, and are free from nodules. Most common symptom of testicular cancer is irregular, nontender fixed mass.

(2) Ask if patient experiences tenderness with palpation.

Testes are normally sensitive but not tender.

4. Assess rectum.

a. Female patient remains in dorsal recumbent position or assumes side-lying (Sims') position.

These positions allow for optimum visualization of the rectum.

b. Male patient stands and bends forward with hips flexed and upper body resting across examination table; examine nonambulatory patient in Sims' position.

c. View perianal and sacrococcygeal areas by gently retracting buttocks with your nondominant hand.

Perianal skin is smooth, more pigmented, and coarser than skin covering buttocks.

d. Inspect anal tissue for skin characteristics, lesions, external hemorrhoids (dilated veins that appear as reddened skin protrusion), inflammation, rashes, and excoriation.

Anal tissues are moist and hairless; voluntary sphincter holds anus closed.

5. Remove and discard gloves. Discard disposable supplies. Help patient to comfortable position. Perform hand hygiene.

Reduces transmission of infection.

EVALUATION

1. Compare assessment findings with previous assessment characteristics to identify changes.

Determines presence of abnormalities.

STEP	RATIONALE

EVALUATION

2. Ask patient to identify guidelines for HPV vaccination.

3. Use Teach-Back:

Male patient: "I would like to make sure that you understand the warning signs of colorectal, testicular, and prostate cancer. Tell me some of the signs and symptoms of testicular cancer." Develop a revised teaching plan if patient is not able to teach back correctly.

Female patient: "I would like to make sure that you understand the warning signs of colorectal, cervical, endometrial, and ovarian cancer. Tell me some of the signs and symptoms of cervical cancer." Develop a revised teaching plan if patient is not able to teach back correctly.

Demonstrates learning.

Determines patient's level of understanding of instructional topic.

Unexpected Outcomes	Related Interventions
1. Patient has vaginal/penile drainage and burning sensation during voiding. Female may have vaginal bleeding between menstrual periods. Symptoms may suggest STI.	• Notify health care provider. • Prepare to collect a culture of the discharge. • Provide additional education.

Communication and Documentation

- Document results of assessment in nurses' notes in electronic health record (EHR) or chart.
- Document patient's ability to void, including description of output, in the EHR or chart.
- Document evaluation of patient learning.
- Report any abnormalities such as presence of a mass or acute pain to nurse in charge and health care provider.

Special Considerations
Teaching

- Discuss the screening guidelines of the Canadian Task Force on Preventive Health (2016) for early detection of colorectal cancer. The guidelines recommend that people aged 60–74 (strong recommendation) and people aged 50–59 (weak recommendation) should be screened every 2 years with guaiac fecal occult blood testing (gFOBT) or fecal immunochemical testing (FIT), or every 10 years by flexible sigmoidoscopy. These recommendations apply to adults aged 50 years and older who are not at high risk for colorectal cancer.
- Discuss warning signs of colorectal cancer, including long-term progressive weight loss, change in bowel habits, and blood in stools.
- Discuss dietary planning and healthy lifestyle choice to maintain or improve colon health.

Female Health Teaching

- Teach patient about purpose and recommended frequency of Papanicolaou (Pap) tests, gynecological examinations, and HPV vaccines.

- Explain warning signs of STIs: pain or burning on urination, pain during sex, pain in pelvic area, bleeding between menstruation, itchy rash around vagina, and abnormal vaginal discharge.
- Teach measures to prevent STIs (e.g., male or female use of condoms, restricting number of sexual partners, avoiding sex with people who have several other partners, and perineal hygiene measures).
- Reinforce the importance of performing perineal hygiene (as appropriate).

Male Health Teaching

- Explain warning signs of STIs: pain on urination and during sex, abnormal penile discharge, swollen lymph nodes, or rash or ulcer on skin or genitalia.
- Teach measures to prevent STIs: use of condoms, HPV vaccines, avoiding sex with infected partner, avoiding sex with people who have multiple partners, and using regular perineal hygiene.
- Tell patients with an STI to inform their sexual partners of the need to have an examination. Instruct patient to seek treatment as soon as possible if partner becomes infected with an STI.

Pediatric

- When examining the testes in a male infant, avoid stimulating the cremasteric reflex, which causes the testes to pull higher into the pelvic cavity.

◆ SKILL 8.7   Musculoskeletal and Neurological Assessment

During the musculoskeletal and neurological assessment you will use the skills of inspection and palpation. During the general survey inspect gait, posture, and body position. A more thorough assessment of major bone, joint, and muscle groups and sensory, motor, and cranial nerve (CN) function is indicated in the presence of abnormalities. The assessment can be performed as you examine other

body systems. For example, while assessing head and neck structures, assess neck range of motion (ROM) and examine select CNs. Integrate assessment into routine activities of care (e.g., while bathing or positioning the patient). Assessment of these systems is important when a patient reports pain, loss of sensation, or impairment of muscle function. Prolonged illness or immobility may result in muscle weakness and atrophy. Neurological assessment is often conducted simultaneously because muscles may be weakened as a result of nerve involvement.

Delegation and Collaboration

The skill of assessing musculoskeletal and neurological function cannot be delegated to an unregulated care provider (UCP). The nurse directs the UCP to:

- Report patients' problems with gait, balance, ROM, and muscle strength.
- Be informed of patients at risk for falls (unsteady gait, foot dragging, weakness of lower extremities).
- Help patients with muscular weakness with transfer and ambulation.

Equipment

- Cotton balls or cotton-tipped applicators
- Penlight
- Tape measure
- Tongue blade
- Tuning fork
- Reflex hammer

STEP	RATIONALE

ASSESSMENT

1. Review patient history for low calcium intake, low physical activity, smoking, consuming large amounts of alcohol, postmenopausal status.

These factors increase risk for osteoporosis (Jarvis et al., 2019).

2. Ask if patient has had a vertebral compression fracture, fragility fracture after age 40, either parent has had a hip fracture, more than 3 months use of a glucocorticoid, or medical conditions or medications that inhibit absorption of nutrients or contribute to bone loss.

These are risk factors for fracture (Osteoporosis Canada, 2018).
Both females and males over the age of 50 should be assessed for risk factors for osteoporosis and fractures (Papaioannou, Morin, Cheung, et al., 2010).

3. Determine if patient has been screened for osteoporosis.

Both females and males aged 65 and older should be screened using bone mineral density (BMD) testing. Menopausal females, and males aged 50 to 64 years with clinical risk factors for fracture should also be tested (Papaioannou et al., 2010).

4. Ask patient to describe history of changes in bone, muscle, or joint function (e.g., recent fall, trauma, lifting heavy objects, bone or joint disease with sudden or gradual onset) and location of alteration.

History helps in assessing nature of musculoskeletal problem. It is estimated that 2 million Canadians are affected by osteoporosis (Osteoporosis Canada, 2018).

5. Assess height and weight (see Skill 8.1). Note if there is a decrease in height among females older than 50 by subtracting current height from recall of maximum adult height.

Body mass index less than 22 kg/m^2 is a risk factor, and loss of height more than 7.5 cm is one of the first clinical signs of osteoporosis (Touhy et al., 2019).

6. Assess nature and extent of patient's musculoskeletal pain: location, duration, severity, predisposing and aggravating factors, relieving factors, and type of pain. If patient reports pain or cramping in lower extremities, ask if walking relieves or aggravates it. Assess distance walked and characteristics of pain before, during, and after activity.

Pain frequently accompanies alterations in bone, joints, or muscle. It has implications for comfort and also ability to perform activities of daily living (ADLs). Pain caused by certain vascular conditions tends to increase with activity.

7. Determine if patient uses analgesics, antipsychotics, antidepressants, nervous system stimulants, or recreational substances.

These medications alter level of consciousness (LOC) or cause behavioural changes. Abuse sometimes causes tremors, ataxia, and changes in peripheral nerve function.

8. Determine if patient has recent history of seizures or convulsions: clarify sequence of events (aura, loss of muscle tone, falling, motor activity, loss of consciousness); character of any symptoms; and relationship to time of day, fatigue, or emotional stress.

Seizure activity often originates from central nervous system (CNS) alteration. Characteristics of seizure help determine its origin.

9. Screen patient for headache, tremors, dizziness, vertigo, numbness or tingling of body part; visual changes; weakness; pain; or changes in speech.

These symptoms commonly result from CNS dysfunction. Identifying patterns aids in diagnosis.

10. Discuss with spouse, family member, or friends any recent changes in patient's behaviour (e.g., increased irritability, mood swings, memory loss, change in energy level).

Behavioural changes may result from intracranial pathology.

11. Determine if patient has noticed change in vision (cranial nerve [CN] II), hearing (CN VIII), smell, (CN I) taste (CN VII), or touch.

Major sensory nerves originate from brainstem. These symptoms help to localize nature of problem during CN examination.

STEP	RATIONALE

ASSESSMENT

12. If patient displays sudden acute confusion (delirium), review history for medication toxicity (e.g., anticholinergics, digoxin, antihistamines, antipsychotics, benzodiazepines, opioid analgesics, sedative/hypnotics, steroids); serious infections; metabolic disturbances (e.g., diabetes mellitus); heart failure; and severe anemia.

Delirium is one of most common mental health disorders in older people (Touhy et al., 2019), but it also occurs in children.

13. Review history for head or spinal cord injury, meningitis, congenital anomalies, neurological disease, or psychiatric counselling.

These neurological symptoms or behavioural changes help to focus assessment on possible cause.

NURSING DIAGNOSES

- Inadequate peripheral tissue perfusion
- Pain (acute, chronic)
- Reduced physical mobility
- Decreased self-care abilities (bathing/ hygiene, dressing/grooming, feeding, or toileting)
- Reduced stamina
- Potential for injury
- Potential for peripheral neurovascular dysfunction
- Potential for trauma

Related factors/Risk factors are individualized on the basis of patient's condition or needs.

PLANNING

1. Expected outcomes following completion of procedure:
  - Patient demonstrates erect posture; strong grasp; steady gait, with arms swinging freely at side.

    Indicates normal alignment, gait, and neuromuscular muscle strength.

  - There is bilateral symmetry of extremities in length, circumference, alignment, position, and skinfolds.
  - Full active ROM is present in all joints, with good muscle tone and absence of contractures, spasticity, or muscular weakness.

    Indicates normal ROM of joints.

  - Patient is alert and oriented to person, place, and time. Behaviour and appearance appropriate for condition and situation.

    Indicates normal cerebral function.

  - Patient demonstrates normal pupil reaction to light and accommodation (see Skill 8.2); external ocular muscles (EOMs) intact; facial sensation intact; symmetrical facial expressions; soft palate and uvula midline and rise on phonation; gag reflex intact; speech clear without hoarseness; no difficulty swallowing.

    Indicates normal functioning of CNs III, IV, V, VI, VII, IX, and X.

  - Patient distinguishes between sharp and dull sensations and light touch on symmetrical areas of extremities. Position sense intact to lower extremities.

    Indicates normal function of sensory nerves.

  - Gait is coordinated, steady with appropriate stance and swing phases. Romberg test negative.

    Indicates normal cerebellar and motor system functioning.

2. Perform hand hygiene. Prepare necessary supplies.

Reduces transmission of infection.

IMPLEMENTATION

1. Prepare patient:
  a. Integrate musculoskeletal and neurological assessments during other parts of physical assessment or during nursing care (e.g., when patient moves in bed, rises from chair, or walks).

  You can conduct assessment as patient performs activities or goes through movements required during complete physical examination. Integration with care conserves patient's energy and allows observation of patient performing more naturally.

  b. Plan time for short rest periods during assessment.

  Movement of body parts and various manoeuvres may tire patient. Always plan rest periods with older person and very ill patients.

2. Assess musculoskeletal system. (Discuss any risks patient may have for falls or other injuries.)
  a. Observe ability to use arms and hands for grasping objects (e.g., pen, utensils).

  Assesses coordination and muscle strength.

STEP	RATIONALE

IMPLEMENTATION

b. To assess hand grasp strength, cross your hands and have patient grasp index and middle fingers of both of your hands and squeeze them as hard as possible (see illustration).

It is common for patient's dominant hand to be slightly stronger than nondominant hand. By crossing your hands, patient's right hand grasps your right hand. This helps with recall of which is patient's right/left hand.

c. To assess strength of lower arms or legs, ask patient first to contract the muscle you indicate by extending or flexing the joint. Then have patient resist as you apply force against that muscle contraction. Have patient maintain pressure until told to stop. Compare symmetrical muscle groups. Note weakness and compare right with left.

Compares strength of symmetrical muscle groups. Upper and lower extremities on dominant side are usually stronger. Rate muscle strength on scale of 0 to 5 as follows:

0   No voluntary contraction
1   Slight contractility, no movement
2   Full ROM, passive
3   Full ROM, active
4   Full ROM against gravity, some resistance
5   Full ROM against gravity, full resistance

Each joint or muscle group requires different position for measurement.

d. Observe body alignment for sitting, supine, prone, or standing positions. Muscles and joints should be exposed and free to move to allow for accurate measurement.

e. Inspect gait as patient walks. Have patient use their assistive device (e.g., cane, walker) if appropriate. Observe for foot dragging, shuffling or limping, balance, presence of obvious deformity in lower extremities, and position of trunk in relation to legs.

Gait is more natural if patient is unaware of your observation. Assesses for neuromusculoskeletal disorder.

f. Perform timed get-up-and-go test: Have adult wear regular footwear, sit back in comfortable chair, and use normal assist devices, if needed. Have watch with a second hand. On the word "Go," begin timing as you have the patient stand from a sitting position without using chair arms for support, stand still momentarily, walk 3 metres (10 feet) in a line, turn around and return to chair; and sit back in chair without using chair arms for support. Observe gait and ability to stand.

The timed get-up-and-go test is an assessment that should be conducted as part of routine evaluation of older persons. The test helps to detect a person's risk for falls. Normally a person completes the task in less than 10 seconds; over 20 seconds is abnormal.

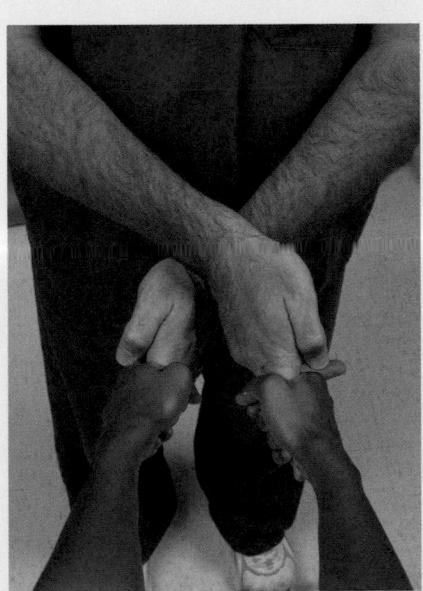

STEP 2b Assessing strength of hand grasps, comparing sides.

STEP	RATIONALE

IMPLEMENTATION

g. Stand behind patient and observe postural alignment (position of hips relative to shoulders). Look sideways at cervical, thoracic, and lumbar curves (see illustration).

Abnormal curves of posture include kyphosis (hunchback, exaggerated posterior curvature of thoracic spine), lordosis (swayback, increased lumbar curvature), and scoliosis (lateral spinal curvature). Postural changes indicate muscular, bone, or joint deformity; pain; or muscular fatigue. Head should be held erect.

h. Make a general observation of extremities. Look at overall size, gross deformity, bony enlargement, alignment, and symmetry.

General review pinpoints areas requiring in-depth assessment.

i. Gently palpate bones, joints, and surrounding tissue in involved areas. Note any heat, tenderness, edema, or resistance to pressure.

Reveals changes resulting from trauma or chronic disease. Do not attempt to move joint when fracture is suspected or joint is apparently "frozen" by lack of movement over a long period of time.

j. Ask patient to put major joint through its full ROM (Table 8.12). Patients with deformities, reduced mobility, joint fixation, or weakness require passive ROM assessment. Observe equality of motion in same body parts:

Assessment of patient's normal ROM provides baseline for assessing later changes after surgery or inactivity.

  (1) *Active motion:* (Patient needs no support or help and is able to move joint independently.) Teach patient to move each joint through its normal range. Sometimes it is necessary to demonstrate and to ask patient to mimic your movements.

Identifies muscle strength and detects limited ROM.

  (2) *Passive motion:* (Joint has full ROM, but patient does not have strength to move it independently.) Have patient relax and move same joints passively until end of range is felt. Support extremity at joint. Do not force joint if there is pain or muscle spasm.

Determines ability to perform joint motion in presence of muscle weakness. Forcing joint causes injury and pain.

k. Palpate joint for swelling, stiffness, tenderness, and heat; note any redness.

Indicates acute or chronic inflammation. ROM causes pain or injury.

l. Assess muscle tone in major muscle groups. Normal tone causes mild, even resistance to movement through entire ROM.

If muscle has increased tone (hypertonicity), any sudden movement of joint is met with considerable resistance. Hypotonic muscle moves without resistance. Muscle feels flabby.

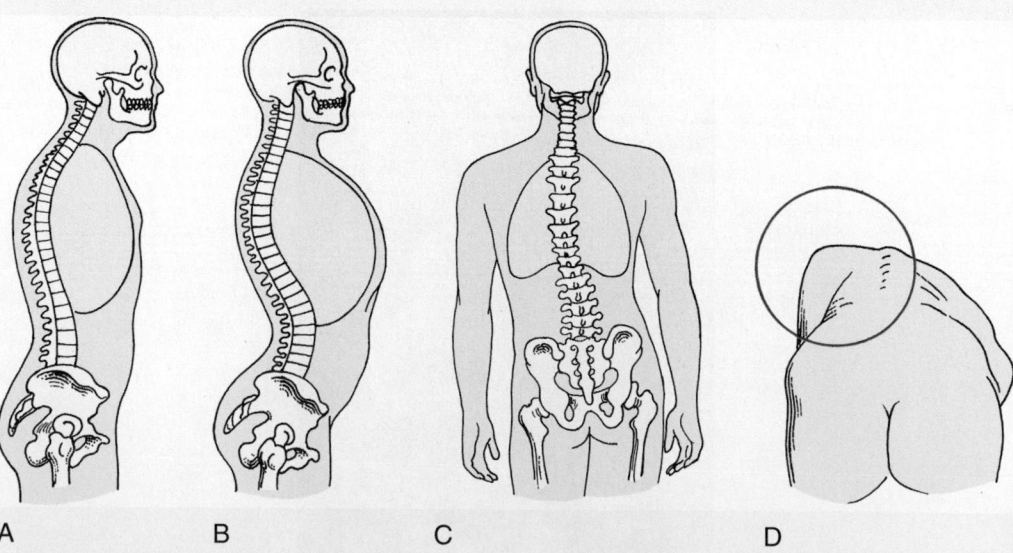

STEP 2g Observe spinal deformities. **A,** Kyphosis. **B,** Lordosis. **C,** Scoliosis. **D,** Scoliosis with patient bending forward.

STEP	RATIONALE

IMPLEMENTATION

3. Neurological assessment

    a. Assess LOC and orientation by asking patient to identify name, location, day of week, and year; note behaviour and appearance. This can be completed during general survey.

A fully conscious patient responds to questions spontaneously. As consciousness declines patient may show irritability, shortened attention span, or unwillingness to cooperate. As consciousness continues to deteriorate patient becomes disoriented to name, time, and place. Behaviour and appearance reveal information about patient's mental status.

TABLE 8.12

Assessing Range of Motion*

Body Part	Assessment Procedure	ROM
Upper Extremities		
Neck	Bend head forward and then backward. Bend neck side to side. Turn head to look over each shoulder.	Flexion, lateral flexion, rotation
Shoulders	Raise both arms to vertical position level at sides of head.	Flexion
	Bring arm across upper chest to touch opposite shoulder.	Adduction
	Place both hands behind neck, with elbows out to sides.	External rotation and abduction
	Place both hands behind small of back.	Internal rotation
	Have patient make small circles with hands, with arms extended at shoulder level.	Circumduction
Elbows	Bend and straighten elbows.	Flexion and extension
	Place hands at waist with elbows flexed.	Internal rotation
Wrists	Flex and extend wrist (bend and straighten).	Flexion and extension
	Bend wrist to radial and then ulnar side.	Radial and ulnar deviation
	Turn palm upward and then downward.	Supination and pronation
Hands	Make a fist with both hands; open hand.	Flexion and extension
	Extend and spread fingers and thumb outward; bring back together.	Adduction and abduction
Lower Extremities		
Hips (with patient supine)	With knees extended, raise one leg upward.	Flexion and extension: Expect 90 degrees flexion
	Cross leg over other leg.	Abduction: Expect 45 degrees
	Swing legs laterally.	Adduction: Expect 30 degrees
	With knee flexed, hold ankle and rotate leg inward and outward.	Internal and external rotation: Expect 40–45 degrees
Knees (with patient sitting)	Raise foot, keeping knee in place.	Extension: Expect full extension and up to 15 degrees hyperextension
Ankles	With foot held off floor, point toes downward and bring them back toward knee.	Plantar flexion: Expect 45 degrees Dorsiflexion: Expect 20 degrees
Toes	Turn foot (sole) inward and sole outward.	Inversion and eversion: Expect to reach 5 degrees
	Bend toes down and back.	Flexion and hyperextension: Expect to reach 40 degrees

AROM, Active range of motion; *PROM*, passive range of motion; *ROM*, range of motion.
*This may be done actively by the patient (AROM) or passively by the nurse (PROM).

STEP	RATIONALE

IMPLEMENTATION

b. Assess cranial nerves (CNs):

(1) For CNs III (oculomotor), IV (trochlear), and VI (abducens), assess EOMs. Ask patient to look straight ahead without moving head and follow movement of your finger through six cardinal positions of gaze; measure pupillary reaction to light reflex and accommodation (see Skill 8.2) using penlight.

These CNs are those most likely to be affected by increasing intracranial pressure (ICP), which causes change in response or size of pupil; pupils may change shape (more oval) or react sluggishly. ICP impairs movements of EOMs. Accommodation is ability of eye to adjust vision from near to far.

(2) For CN V (trigeminal), apply light sensation with cotton ball to symmetrical areas of face.

Sensations should be symmetrical; unilateral decrease or loss of sensation may be caused by CN V lesion.

(3) For CN VII (facial) note facial symmetry. Have patient frown, smile, puff out cheeks, and raise eyebrows.

Expressions should be symmetrical; Bell's palsy causes drooping of upper and lower face; cerebrovascular accident (CVA) causes asymmetry.

(4) For CNs IX (glossopharyngeal) and X (vagus), have patient speak and swallow. Ask them to say "ah" while using tongue blade and penlight. Check for midline uvula and symmetrical rise of uvula and soft palate. Use tongue blade and place on posterior tongue to elicit gag reflex.

Damage to CN IX causes impaired swallowing; damage to CN X causes loss of gag reflex, hoarseness, nasal voice. When palate fails to rise and uvula pulls toward normal side, this indicates a unilateral paralysis.

c. Assess extremities for sensation. Perform all sensory testing with patient's eyes closed so they are unable to see when or where a stimulus strikes skin. Use minimal stimulation initially, increasing gradually until patient is aware of it.

For all sensory stimulus testing, patient should note minimal differences side to side, correctly describe the sensation (sharp or dull, hot or cold), and recognize side of the body tested and location.

(1) *Pain:* Ask patient to indicate when sharp or dull sensation is felt as you alternately apply sharp and dull ends of a broken tongue blade to skin surface. Apply in symmetrical areas of extremities.

Patient should be able to distinguish sharp or dull sensations. Impaired sensations indicate disorders of spinal cord or peripheral nerve roots.

(2) *Light touch:* Apply light wisp of cotton to different points along surface of skin in symmetrical areas of extremities.

Patient should be able to distinguish when touched.

(3) *Position:* Grasp finger or toe, holding it by its sides with your thumb and index finger. Alternate moving patient's finger or toe up and down. Ask patient to state when finger is up or down. Repeat with toes.

Patient should be able to distinguish movements of a few millimetres. Decreased or absent position sense may occur in spinal anaesthesia, paralysis, or other neurological disorders.

d. Assess motor and cerebellar function:

(1) *Gait:* Have patient walk across room, turn, and come back. Similarly note use of assistive devices. This is good time to instruct in proper use of assistive devices.

Neurological and musculoskeletal disorders impair gait and balance.

(2) *Romberg's test:* Have patient stand with feet together, arms at sides, both with eyes open and eyes closed (for 20 to 30 seconds). Protect patient's safety by standing at side; observe for swaying.

Romberg's test should be negative; slight swaying is considered normal.

e. Assess deep tendon reflexes (DTRs):

(1) In patients with back pain or surgery, CVA, or spinal cord compression, it is appropriate to monitor DTRs (Ball et al., 2015). This requires an advanced level of skill. In most settings, this is not part of routine physical assessment.

Muscle spasticity and hyperactive reflexes may result from disorders such as stroke and paralysis. Diminished DTRs and muscle weakness may suggest electrolyte abnormalities or lower motor neuron disorders (e.g., amyotrophic lateral sclerosis [ALS] or Guillain-Barré syndrome).

(2) For each reflex tested, compare sides and assign a grade on the following scale:

0   No response
1+   Sluggish or diminished response
2+   Normal, active or expected response
3+   More brisk than expected; slightly hyperactive
4+   Very brisk; hyperactive, with clonus.

Grade indicates extent of neuron dysfunction. Clonus is described as repeated spasms of muscular contraction and relaxation.

STEP	RATIONALE

IMPLEMENTATION

(3) *Knee reflex:* Palpate patellar tendon just below patella. Tap pointed end of reflex hammer briskly on tendon (see illustration).

Knee reflex is the most common DTR assessment performed. The normal response is knee extension.

(4) *Plantar response (Babinski's reflex):* Using handle end of reflex hammer, stroke lateral aspect of sole from heel to ball of foot.

Toes should flex inward and downward (see illustration).

(5) After stroking soles of feet, if Babinski's reflex is present, great toe dorsiflexes, accompanied by fanning of the other toes.

Indicates CNS dysfunction. Dorsiflexion of great toe and fanning of the others are normal in child younger than age 2 (Hockenberry & Wilson, 2015).

4. Dispose of supplies. Perform hand hygiene.

Reduces transmission of infection.

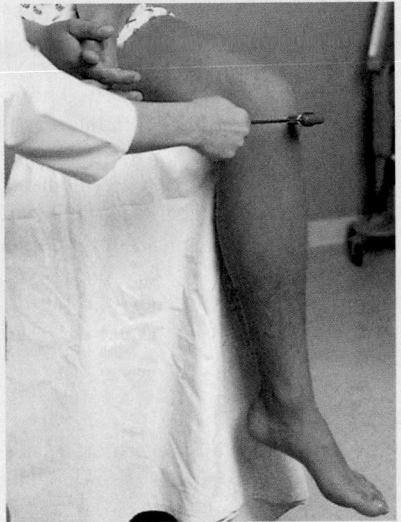

STEP 3e(3) Assessing knee reflex. Knee should extend.

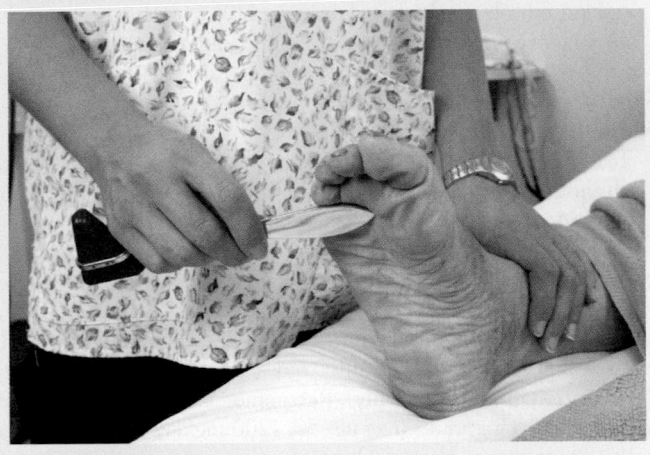

STEP 3e(4) Assessing plantar response. Toes should flex inward and downward.

EVALUATION

1. Compare muscle strength and ROM with previous physical assessment.

Determines presence of abnormalities.

2. Compare neurological status with previous physical assessment.

Determines presence of abnormalities.

3. Evaluate level of patient's discomfort following procedure, using appropriate pain scale.

Determines if manipulation of musculoskeletal structures intensifies patient's discomfort.

4. **Use Teach-Back:** "I want to be sure you understand the reasons why you are at risk for falling that we discussed during your exam. Tell me two reasons why you are at risk for falling." Develop a revised teaching plan if patient or caregiver is not able to teach back correctly.

Determines patients' and caregiver's level of understanding of instructional topic.

Unexpected Outcomes

1. Joints are prominent, swollen, and tender with nodules or overgrowth of bone in distal joints, indicating signs of arthritis.

2. ROM is reduced in one or more major joints: shoulder, elbow, wrist, fingers, knee, hip.

3. Patient demonstrates weakness in one or more major muscle groups or has difficulty with gait or ability to walk and sit during get-up-and-go test, indicating a fall risk.

Related Interventions

- Teach patient proper ROM.
- Determine patient's knowledge regarding use of anti-inflammatory medications and nonpharmacological measures (see Chapter 16).
- Assess further for pain during movement with joint unstable, stiff, painful, or swollen or with obvious deformity.
- Notify health care provider.
- Reduce mobility in extremity until cause of abnormal joint motion is determined.
- Place patient on fall precautions.
- Provide patient safety when ambulating (see Chapter 12).
- Notify health care provider.

STEP	RATIONALE

EVALUATION

4. Patient has changes in mental status and pupillary response or other neurological deficits.

- Notify health care provider immediately.
- Continue to assess patient's vital signs and LOC closely.
- Place on fall precautions.

Communication and Documentation

- Document posture, gait, muscle strength, and ROM in nurses' notes in electronic health record (EHR) or chart.
- Document LOC, orientation, pupillary response, sensation, and reflex responses in nurses' notes in EHR or chart.
- Document evaluation of patient and caregiver learning.
- Report to nurse in charge or health care provider acute pain or sudden muscle weakness, change in LOC, or change in size or pupillary reaction, which require immediate treatment.

Special Considerations
Teaching

- Teach patient about correct postural alignment. Consult with physiotherapist to provide patient with exercises for improving posture.
- To reduce bone demineralization, teach older persons about a proper weight-bearing exercise program (e.g., walking, low-impact aerobics) to be followed three or more times a week.
- Encourage intake of calcium to meet the recommended daily allowance. Increased vitamin D aids calcium absorption (400 to 800 international units daily). Recommendation for daily calcium supplements for adults over age 50: 1200 mg/day. Instruct patient to take no more than 500 mg of calcium supplements at one time (Touhy et al., 2019).
- Explain to patients with low back pain that they can benefit from modification of work-related risk factors (e.g., lifting heavy weights, use of protective equipment), regular aerobic exercise, exercises that strengthen the back and increase trunk flexibility, and learning how to lift properly.
- Explain measures to ensure safety (e.g., use of ambulation aids or safety bars in bathrooms or stairways) for patients with sensory or motor impairments.

Pediatric

- Examine infants carefully for musculoskeletal anomalies resulting from genetic or fetal insults. An examination includes review of posture, generalized movement, symmetry and skin creases of the extremities, muscle strength, and hip alignment.
- Normally the back of a newborn is rounded, or **C** shaped from the thoracic and pelvic curves.
- Scoliosis, or lateral curvature of the spine, is an important childhood problem, especially in females, usually identified at puberty. (For closer examination have child stand erect wearing only underclothes. Observe from behind, looking for asymmetry of shoulders and hips. Then observe from the back as child bends forward.) Uneven dress hems or trouser hems or uneven fit of clothing at the waist is an indication of scoliosis.
- Watching a child during play reveals information about musculoskeletal function.
- Children ages 13 to 19 years need 1300 mg of calcium daily with 400 international units of vitamin D (Hockenberry & Wilson, 2015).

Gerontological

- Teach older persons about fall prevention. Make modifications in the home environment to reduce the risk of falls (see Chapter 42).
- Teach older persons and those with osteoporosis about proper body mechanics, ROM exercises, and moderate weight-bearing exercises (e.g., swimming, walking) to minimize trauma.
- Functional assessment is a measurement of an older person's ability to perform ADLs (Ball et al., 2015). When patient is unable to perform self-care easily, determine need for assistive devices (e.g., zippers on clothing instead of buttons, elevation of chairs to minimize bending of knees and hips).
- Older persons tend to assume a stooped, forward-bent posture with hips and knees somewhat flexed, arms bent at the elbows, and level of arms raised.

PROCEDURAL GUIDELINE 8.1 *Monitoring Intake and Output*

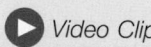 *Video Clip*

Measuring and recording intake and output (I&O) during a 24-hour period is part of the assessment database for fluid and electrolyte balance (Table 8.13). Nurses are responsible for accurate recording of all intake (liquids taken orally, by enteral feedings, and parenterally) and output (urine, diarrhea, vomitus, gastric suction, and drainage from surgical tubes). Monitoring a patient on I&O requires cooperation and help from the patient and caregivers. Accuracy is critical, as physicians will use findings in prescription of medications and intravenous (IV) fluids.

Monitor I&O for patients with a fever or edema or with a urinary catheter; receiving diuretic or intravenous (IV) therapy; or on restricted fluids as per employer policy or health care provider prescription. It is also important when a patient has electrolyte losses associated with vomiting, diarrhea, gastrointestinal drainage, or extensive open wounds such as burns. Total and evaluate I&O at the end of each shift or at specified times such as every 8 hours. Significant alterations are apparent by comparing 24-hour totals over several days. Because fluid imbalance occurs at any time, be aware of I&O for all patients, even when documentation is not required. Certain disease processes (e.g., renal failure) and postoperative patients also require monitoring and documentation of I&O.

Delegation and Collaboration

The skills of assessing I&O totals at the end of each shift; comparing 24-hour totals over several days; and monitoring and recording intravenous (IV) therapy, wound or chest tube drainage, and tube

PROCEDURAL GUIDELINE 8.1 *Monitoring Intake and Output—cont'd*

feedings cannot be delegated to an unregulated care provider (UCP). The nurse needs to emphasize maintaining routine practices and additional precautions (e.g., transmission-based precautions) related to body fluids, accurately measuring and recording I&O, and using the metric system with standard containers. The nurse directs the UCP to:

- Measure and record oral intake, urinary output, liquid diarrheal stools, vomitus, and wound drainage device output.
- Report changes in patient's condition such as alteration in intake or changes in colour, amount, or odour of output.

Equipment

- Sign to alert personnel of I&O measurement
- Daily I&O record form or computer graphic
- Graduated measuring container
- Bedpan, urinal, bedside commode, or urine "hat" (a receptacle that fits under the toilet seat)
- Clean gloves
- Mask, eye protection, and gown (optional)

Procedural Steps

1. Identify patients with conditions that increase fluid loss (e.g., fever, diarrhea, vomiting, surgical wound drainage, chest tube drainage, gastric suction, major burns, or severe trauma).
2. Identify patients with impaired swallowing, unconscious patients, and patients with impaired mobility.
3. Identify patients on medications that influence fluid balance (e.g., diuretics and steroids).
4. Assess signs and symptoms of dehydration and fluid overload (e.g., bradycardia versus tachycardia, hypotension versus hypertension, and reduced skin turgor versus edema).
5. Weigh patients daily using the same scale, the same time of day, and with comparable clothing.
6. Monitor laboratory reports:
   - Urine specific gravity (normal is 1.010 to 1.030)
   - Hematocrit (Hct) (normal range is 37 to 47% for females and 42 to 52% for males).
7. Assess patient's and caregiver's knowledge of purpose and process of I&O measurement.
8. Explain to patient and caregiver the reasons that I&O are important.
9. Perform hand hygiene.
10. Measure and record all fluid intake:
    a. Liquids with meals, gelatin, custards, ice cream, popsicles, sherbets, ice chips (recorded as 50% of measured volume [e.g., 100 mL of ice chips equals 50 mL of water]). Convert household measures to the metric system: 1 oz equals 30 mL; therefore 12 oz (pop can) equals 360 mL.
    b. Count liquid medicines such as antacids and fluids with medications as fluid intake.
    c. Calculate fluid intake from tube feedings (see Chapter 32).
    d. Calculate fluid intake from parenteral fluids, blood components, and total parenteral nutrition solutions (see Chapters 29, 30, and 33).

Clinical Decision Point *Record intake as soon as you measure it to maintain accuracy. If more than one patient is in the same room, each must have urine receptacles labelled with name and bed location.*

11. Instruct patient and caregiver to call you or the UCP to empty contents of urinal, urine hat, or commode each time patient uses it. Have patient and caregiver monitor incontinence, vomiting, and excessive perspiration and report it to the nurse.
12. Inform patient and caregiver that Foley catheter drainage bag and wound, gastric, or chest tube drainage are closely monitored, measured, and recorded and who is responsible for performing these tasks. Each patient must have a graduated container clearly marked with name and bed location and used only for the patient indicated.
13. Apply clean gloves. Measure drainage at the end of the shift or as indicated, using appropriate containers and noting colour and characteristics. If splashing is anticipated, wear mask, eye protection, and/or gown.
    a. Measure urine drainage using a "hat" into which patient voids or a graduated container (see illustration).
    b. Observe colour and characteristics of urine in Foley tubing and drainage bag. Sometimes a measuring device is part of the drainage bag (see illustration). Otherwise measure with a graduated container.
    c. Measure chest tube drainage by marking and recording the time on the collection chamber at specified intervals (see illustration) (see Chapter 27). Chest tube collection devices are changed when they become full.
    d. Measure Jackson-Pratt/Hemovac drainage with a medicine cup (see illustration) (see Chapter 39).
    e. Measure gastric drainage or larger drainage pouches by opening clamp and pouring into graduated cup with a 240-mL capacity (see illustration).

TABLE 8.13

Adult Average Fluid Gains and Losses

Fluid Intake and Output	Volume (mL)	Fluid Intake and Output	Volume (mL)
Fluid Intake		**Fluid Output**	
Oral fluids	1100–1400	Kidneys	1200–1500
Solid foods	800–1000	Skin	500–600
Oxidative metabolism	300	Lungs	400
		Gastrointestinal	100
Total Gains	2200–2700	**Total Losses**	2200–2700

From Hall, J. E. (2016). *Guyton and Hall textbook of medical physiology* (13th ed.). Philadelphia: Saunders.

Continued

PROCEDURAL GUIDELINE 8.1 *Monitoring Intake and Output—cont'd*

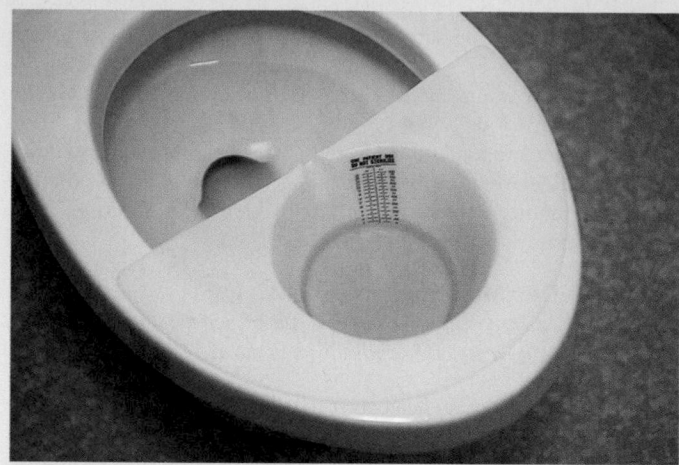

STEP 13a Urine "hat."

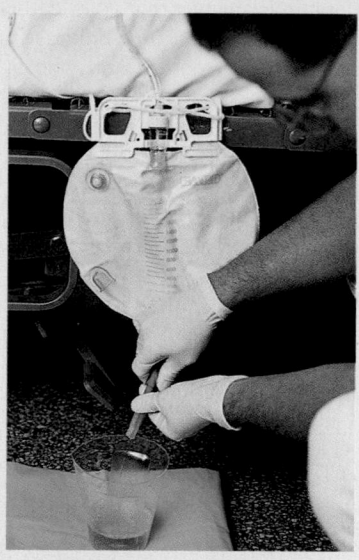

STEP 13b Device for monitoring hourly urine output.

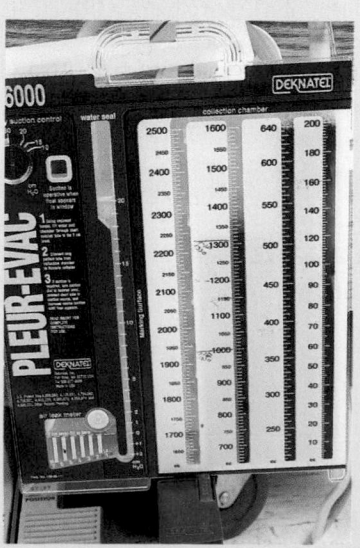

STEP 13c Collection chamber for measuring chest tube drainage.

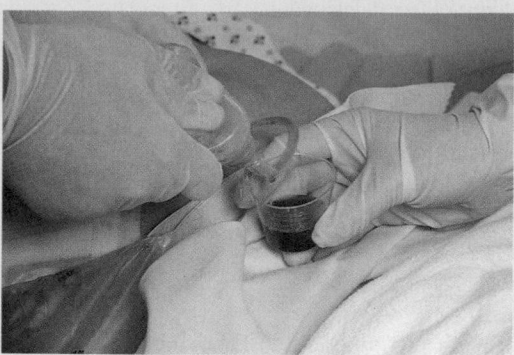

STEP 13d Measuring wound drainage through Jackson-Pratt drain.

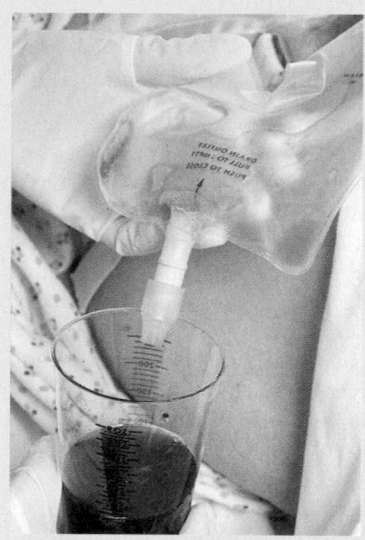

STEP 13e Measuring drainage from large drainage pouch.

14. Remove gloves and dispose of them in appropriate receptacle. Perform hand hygiene.
15. Note I&O balance or imbalance and report to health care provider any urine output less than 30 mL/hr or significant changes in daily weight.
16. Document on I&O forms or electronic record.

◆ CLINICAL DEBRIEF

You are performing your morning assessment on a 69-year-old male patient 3 days post coronary artery bypass surgery (CABG). When asked about pain, the patient states, "My heart hurts. I feel short of breath and very hot."

1. Which body systems should you assess on the patient and why?
2. You check his last recorded temperature, which was 1 hour ago, and it reads 37.7°C (100°F); you check it again and it is now 38.3°C (101°F). What could cause this change in temperature?
3. On auscultation of his heart you hear a "squeaky" or rubbing sound. Which cardiac abnormality should you suspect?
4. Your assessment of vital signs reveals BP 140/86 mm Hg, T 38.3°C (101°F), HR 90 beats/min, RR 22 breaths/min, oxygen saturation 91%. How should you document your assessment findings using SBAR and what should be your next step?

◆ REVIEW QUESTIONS

1. Which of the following are characteristics of malignant melanoma? *(Select all that apply.)*
   1. An irregularly shaped lesion
   2. A lesion with lumpy edges
   3. A small papule with a dry, rough scale
   4. A pearly papule with a central crater and a waxy border
   5. A lesion with blue/black or variegated colour
   6. A lesion of greater than 6 mm in size
2. In conducting a general survey of a patient, the nurse knows that the survey should include which of the following? *(Select all that apply.)*
   1. Appearance
   2. Obtaining peripheral pulses
   3. Measuring chest expansion
   4. Conducting a detailed history
   5. Behaviour
   6. Pupillary response
   7. Posture
3. You are about to begin an abdominal assessment on your patient. Place the following sequence in order.
   1. Auscultation
   2. Inspection
   3. Palpation
   4. Percussion

ⓔ *Visit the Evolve site for a complete list of Clinical Debrief and Review Questions answers.*

REFERENCES

Accreditation Canada. (2019). *Required organizational practices handbook—Version 14.* Retrieved from http://www.wrha.mb.ca/quality/files/2019ROPHandbook.pdf

Agency for Healthcare Research and Quality (AHRQ). (2015). *Consider culture, customs, and beliefs: Tool #10.* Rockville, MD: Author. Retrieved from https://www.ahrq.gov/professionals/quality-patient-safety/quality-resources/tools/literacy-toolkit/healthlittoolkit2-tool10.html

Anderson, T. J., Gregoire, J., Pearson, G. J., et al. (2016). 2016 Canadian Cardiovascular Society guidelines for the management of dyslipidemia for the prevention of cardiovascular disease in the adult. *Canadian Journal of Cardiology, 32,* 1263–1282. doi:10.1016/j.cjca.2016.07.510

Ball, J. W., Dains, J., Flynn, J., Solomon, B., & Stewart, R. (2015). *Seidel's guide to physical examination* (8th ed.). St. Louis: Mosby.

Bourns, A. (2015). *Guidelines and protocols for hormone therapy and primary health care for trans clients.* Toronto: Sherbourne Health Centre. Retrieved from http://sherbourne.on.ca/guidelines-protocols-for-trans-care/

Breen, A. E., & Hessels, A. J. (2017). Stethoscopes: Friend or fomite? *Nursing Management, 48*(12), 9–11. doi:10.1097/01.NUMA.0000526917.85088.eb

Canadian Cancer Society (CCS). (2018a). *Be sun safe.* Retrieved from http://www.cancer.ca/en/prevention-and-screening/reduce-cancer-risk/make-healthy-choices/be-sun-safe/?region=on

Canadian Cancer Society (CCS). (2018b). *Breast cancer: Screening for breast cancer.* Retrieved from http://www.cancer.ca/en/cancer-information/cancer-type/breast/screening/?region=on

Canadian Cancer Society (CCS). (2018c). *Cervical cancer: Risk factors for cervical cancer.* Retrieved from http://www.cancer.ca/en/cancer-information/cancer-type/cervical/risks/?region=on

Canadian Cancer Society (CCS). (2018d). *Colorectal cancer: Risk factors for colorectal cancer.* Retrieved from http://www.cancer.ca/en/cancer-information/cancer-type/colorectal/risks/?region=on

Canadian Cancer Society (CCS). (2018e). *Colorectal cancer: Symptoms of colorectal cancer.* Retrieved from http://www.cancer.ca/en/cancer-information/cancer-type/colorectal/signs-and-symptoms/?region=on

Canadian Cancer Society (CCS). (2018f). *Find cancer early.* Retrieved from http://www.cancer.ca/en/prevention-and-screening/reduce-cancer-risk/find-cancer-early/?region=bc

Canadian Cancer Society (CCS). (2018g). *Live smoke free.* Retrieved from http://www.cancer.ca/en/prevention-and-screening/reduce-cancer-risk/make-healthy-choices/live-smoke-free/?region=on

Canadian Cancer Society (CCS). (2018h). *Lung cancer: Risk factors for lung cancer.* Retrieved from http://www.cancer.ca/en/cancer-information/cancer-type/lung/risks/?region=on

Canadian Cancer Society (CCS). (2018i). *Melanoma.* Retrieved from http://www.cancer.ca/en/cancer-information/cancer-type/skin-melanoma/melanoma/?region=on

Canadian Cancer Society (CCS). (2018j). *Non-melanoma skin cancer.* Retrieved from http://www.cancer.ca/en/cancer-information/cancer-type/skin-non-melanoma/non-melanoma-skin-cancer/?region=on

Canadian Cancer Society (CCS). (2018k) *Ovarian cancer: Risk factors for ovarian cancer.* Retrieved from http://www.cancer.ca/en/cancer-information/cancer-type/ovarian/risks/?region=qc

Canadian Cancer Society (CCS). (2018l). *Prostate cancer: Symptoms of prostate cancer.* Retrieved from http://www.cancer.ca/en/cancer-information/cancer-type/prostate/signs-and-symptoms/?region=on

Canadian Cancer Society (CCS). (2018m). *Uterine cancer: Risk factors for uterine cancer.* Retrieved from http://www.cancer.ca/en/cancer-information/cancer-type/uterine/risks/?region=on

Canadian Task Force on Preventive Health Care. (2011). Recommendations on screening for breast cancer in average-risk women aged 40–74 years. *Canadian Medical Association Journal, 183*(17), 1991–2001. doi:10.1503/cmaj.110334

Canadian Task Force on Preventive Health Care. (2016). Recommendations on screening for colorectal cancer in primary care. *Canadian Medical Association Journal, 188*(5), 340–348. doi:10.1503/cmaj.151125

Canadian Task Force on Preventive Health Care. (2018). *Published guidelines.* Retrieved from https://canadiantaskforce.ca/guidelines/published-guidelines/

College of Family Physicians of Canada. (2013). *Annual physical examination practices by province/territory in Canada.* Retrieved from http://www.cfpc.ca/CFPC-PT-Annual-Exam/

Deutsch, M. B. (2016). *Guidelines for the primary and gender-affirming care of transgender and gender nonbinary people.* Retrieved from http://transhealth.ucsf.edu/protocols

Government of Canada. (2016). *Canadian immunization guide: Part 4—Active vaccines.* Retrieved from https://www.canada.ca/en/public-health/services/publications/healthy-living/canadian-immunization-guide-part-4-active-vaccines/page-16-pneumococcal-vaccine.html

Greig, A. A., Constantin, E., LeBlanc, C. M., Riverin, B., Li, P. T., & Cummings, C. (2016). An update to the Greig Health Record: Preventive health care visits for children and adolescents aged 6 to 17 years—Technical report. *Paediatrics & Child Health, 21*(5), 265–268.

Health Canada. (2015). *Clinical practice guidelines for nurses in primary care.* Retrieved from https://www.canada.ca/en/indigenous-services-canada/services/first-nations-inuit-health/health-care-services/nursing/clinical-practice-guidelines-nurses-primary-care.html

Hockenberry, J. N., & Wilson, D. (2015). *Wong's nursing care of infants and children* (10th ed.). St. Louis: Elsevier.

Infection Prevention and Control Canada. (2018). *Guidelines and standards.* Retrieved from https://ipac-canada.org/evidence-based-guidelines.php

Jarvis, C., Browne, A. J., MacDonald-Jenkins, J., & Luctkar-Flude, M. (2019). *Physical examination & health assessment* (3rd ed.). Toronto: Elsevier Canada.

Lewis, S. L., Bucher, L., Heitkemper, M. M., Harding, M. M., Barry, M. A., & Goldsworthy, S. (2019). *Medical-surgical nursing in Canada: Assessment and management of clinical problems* (4th ed.). Toronto, ON: Elsevier Canada.

Osteoporosis Canada. (2018). *Osteoporosis: Fast facts.* Retrieved from https://osteoporosis.ca/about-the-disease/fast-facts/

Papaioannou, A., Morin, S., Cheung, A. M., et al. (2010). 2010 clinical practice guidelines for the diagnosis and management of osteoporosis in Canada: Summary. *Canadian Medical Association Journal, 182*(17), 1864–1873. doi:10.1503/cmaj.100771

Public Health Agency of Canada (PHAC). (2017). *Updated recommendations on human papillomavirus (HPV) vaccines: 9-valent HPV vaccine 2-dose immunization schedule and the use of HPV vaccines in immunocompromised populations.* Retrieved from https://www.canada.ca/en/public-health/services/publications/healthy-living/updated-recommendations-human-papillomavirus-immunization-schedule-immunocompromised-populations.html

Touhy, T. A., Jett, K. F., Boscart, V., & McCleary, L. (2019). *Ebersole and Hess' gerontological nursing & healthy aging* (2nd ed.). Toronto: Elsevier Canada.

Wound Ostomy and Continence Nurses (WOCN) Society. (2016). *Guideline for prevention and management of pressure ulcers.* WOCN clinical practice guideline series. Mt. Laurel, NJ: Author.

9 | Specimen Collection

Written by **Rita Wunderlich, RN, PhD, CNE, April Ambalina, RN, and Alia Lagace, RN**

OBJECTIVES

Mastery of content in this chapter will enable the nurse to:

- Explain the rationale for the collection of each specimen.
- Identify special conditions necessary for collection of each specimen.
- Provide patient education to promote patient cooperation during specimen collection.
- Identify measures to minimize anxiety and promote safety during specimen collection.
- Discuss nursing responsibilities for processing a specimen after collection.
- Document appropriate information in a patient's electronic health record (EHR) or written record after collection of a specimen.

- Use correct technique for collecting clean-voided, timed, and catheterized urine specimens.
- Use correct technique for collecting specimens and cultures for blood and other body fluids.
- Use correct technique to perform venipuncture.
- Use infection control practices during specimen collection techniques.
- Use correct technique to perform arterial puncture for blood gas measurement.
- Identify nursing responsibility for reporting laboratory results to the health care provider.

MEDIA RESOURCES

- evolve http://evolve.elsevier.com/Canada/Perry/clinicalskills/
- Review Questions
- ▶ Video Clips

- Audio Glossary
- **NSO** Nursing Skills Online
- Clinical Debrief and Review Questions Answers

PURPOSE

Laboratory test results aid in the diagnosis of health care problems, provide information about the stage and activity of a disease process, and measure a patient's response to therapy. Nurses are accountable for correctly collecting specimens, monitoring patient outcomes, and ensuring that these tests are collected and shared with the interprofessional team in a timely manner.

STANDARDS OF CARE

- Accreditation Canada, 2019—*Required Organizational Practices Handbook—Version 14* (http://www.wrha.mb.ca/quality/files/2019 ROPHandbook.pdf)
- Public Health Agency of Canada (PHAC), 2016—*Canadian Biosafety Handbook, Second Edition* (https://www.canada.ca/content/dam/phac-aspc/migration/cbsg-nldcb/cbs-ncb/assets/pdf/cbsg-nldcb-eng.pdf)

PRINCIPLES FOR PRACTICE

- Proficiency and judgement in obtaining specimens minimize patient discomfort, promote patient safety, and ensure accuracy and quality of diagnostic procedures.
- Everyone who handles body fluids is at risk for exposure. The use of hand hygiene and personal protective equipment (PPE) is necessary to protect health care workers and patients. Proper labelling in a container marked as biohazard protects and informs laboratory personnel and others who may come in contact with the specimen (PHAC, 2016).
- Each employer may establish its own values for each test, which are printed on the employer laboratory forms. When questions arise, consult the employer procedure manual or call the laboratory.

PERSON-CENTRED CARE

- Patients often experience embarrassment or discomfort when giving a sample of body excretions or secretions, especially urine, urogenital, or stool samples. It is important to handle excretions or secretions discretely and provide a patient with as much privacy as possible. Given clear instructions, patients can obtain their own specimens of urine, stool, and sputum without unnecessary exposure (Pagana, Pagana, & Pike-MacDonald, 2019).
- Consider both cultural and language barriers when delegating specimen collection to patients and caregivers. Language barriers make it difficult to explain the purpose of tests and collection techniques. Be sure to use strategies such as diagrams or illustrations and repeated return demonstrations (Awua, Wiredu, Afari, et al., 2017).
- Whenever possible, use gender-congruent caregivers when collecting vaginal, rectal, and urinary specimens from patients whose cultural values demand modesty and distinct separation of gender roles.

EVIDENCE-INFORMED PRACTICE

- Hemolysis of blood specimens causes delayed treatment of patients and increases health care costs (McCaughey, Vecellio, Lake, et al., 2017).
- Venipuncture is recommended over the use of obtaining a blood sample from an intravenous (IV) site, to prevent hemolysis when possible (Long & Koyfman, 2016).
- Hemolysis may result from vigorously shaking a blood sample, which invalidates the test. Promptly deliver blood specimens to the laboratory for processing to prevent hemolysis.

SAFETY GUIDELINES

- Verify the type of procedure scheduled and the procedure site with the patient.
- Follow standard precautions (see Chapter 5) when collecting specimens of blood or body fluids.
- Properly label all specimens and confirm requisitions with patient's identification, date and time the specimen is obtained, name of the test, and source of the specimen/culture for each container.
- Deliver specimens to the laboratory within the recommended time, or ensure that they are stored properly for later transport.
- Follow procedures for special conditions (e.g., iced specimens, special containers with preservatives) required for transport of specimens. Specific required prerequisite conditions include fasting and nothing by mouth (NPO) and may need to be completed before the collection of a specimen (Pagana et al., 2019).
- Know employer policy regarding infection control practices for transportation of all specimen containers of body substances.
- Follow procedures for medications or dietary intake that may result in some deviations from normal values.
- Follow precautions for collecting specimens from patients who require transmission-based precautions (e.g., protective isolation).

✦ SKILL 9.1 **Urine Specimen Collection: Midstream (Clean-Voided) and Sterile Urinary Catheter**

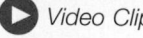 *Video Clip* **NSO** *Nursing Skills Online Specimen Collection Module 3 / Lessons 1 and 2*

A urinalysis provides information about kidney or metabolic function, nutrition, and systemic diseases. Urine collection uses a variety of methods, depending on the purpose of the urinalysis and the presence or absence of a urinary catheter. Guidelines for assessment, planning, and evaluation are similar, regardless of the method of collection. Routine urinalysis includes measurement of nine or more elements, including urine pH, protein and glucose levels, ketones, specific gravity, white blood cell (WBC) count, and presence of bacteria, blood, or both (Pagana et al., 2019).

Types of Urine Tests and Specimens

- A *random urine specimen for routine urinalysis* is collected using a specimen "hat" (Fig. 9.1), which is placed under a toilet seat to collect voided urine. The nurse then places approximately 120 mL of urine in a specimen container, properly labelled, and sends it to the laboratory.
- A *timed urine specimen for quantitative analysis* requires urine to be collected over 2 to 72 hours. The 24-hour timed collection

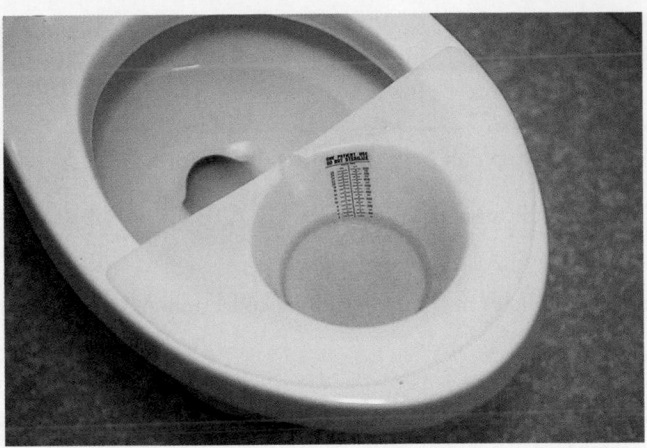

FIG 9.1 Specimen hat.

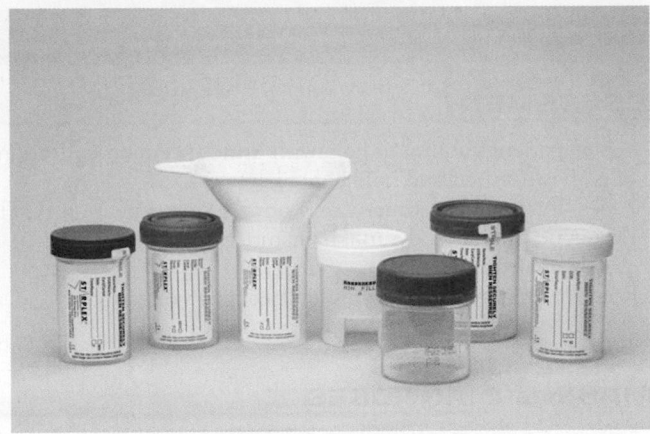

FIG 9.2 Various specimen collection containers. ((*Image courtesy of Starplex Scientific Inc.*)

(see Procedural Guideline 9.1) is most common and allows for measurement and quantitative analysis of elements such as amino acids, creatinine, hormones, glucose, and adrenocorticosteroid excretion.

- *A urine specimen for culture and sensitivity (C&S)* is performed to identify if bacteria are present (culture) and determine the most effective antibiotic for treatment (sensitivity). Specimens for C&S are collected either as a clean-voided midstream specimen or under sterile technique from a urinary catheter. Urine collected by these methods may also be analyzed for the same components as a routine urinalysis.

- *Chemical properties of urine* are tested by immersing a specially prepared test strip of paper (Chemstrip) into a clean urine specimen. The test detects the presence of glucose, ketones, protein, or blood not normally present in the urine (see Procedural Guideline 9.2). When the screening test for the presence of substances in the urine is positive, additional laboratory tests are used to determine a patient's diagnosis or measure the effectiveness of treatment.

Delegation and Collaboration

Interprofessional collaboration often occurs with urine specimen collections. The skill of collecting urine specimens may be delegated to an unregulated care provider (UCP) or collaboration may occur with parts of the skill such as monitoring, skill implementation, teaching, and documentation. The nurse may collaborate with the UCP on the following:

- Obtaining the specimens at a specified time when appropriate.
- Positioning patient as necessary when mobility restrictions are present.

- Communicating if the urine is not clear (e.g., contains blood, cloudiness, or excess sediment).
- Communicating when a patient is unable to initiate a stream or has pain or burning on urination.

Equipment

- Completed identification labels with appropriate patient identifiers
- Completed laboratory requisition
- Small plastic biohazard bag (or container)

Midstream (Clean-Voided) Urine Specimen

- Sterile specimen container (Fig. 9.2)
- Antiseptic towelettes
- Clean gloves
- Soap, water, washcloth, and towel
- Specimen hat (see Fig. 9.1) or bedpan (for nonambulatory patient)

Sterile Urine Specimen From Urinary Catheter

- Specimen container (nonsterile for routine urinalysis, sterile for culture)
- 20-mL Luer-Lok syringe for routine urinalysis or 3-mL Luer-Lok syringe for culture
- Antiseptic swab
- Clean gloves
- Clamp

STEP	RATIONALE

ASSESSMENT

1. Identify patient using at least two person-specific identifiers (e.g., full name, date of birth, personal identification number, etc.) according to employer policy. Compare identifiers with information on patient's medical record and laboratory requisition.

Ensures correct patient. Complies with Accreditation Canada standards and improves patient safety (Accreditation Canada, 2019).

2. Assess patient's or caregiver's understanding of purpose of test and method of collection.

Information allows you to clarify misunderstanding; promotes patient cooperation.

STEP	RATIONALE

ASSESSMENT

3. Assess patient's ability to help with urine specimen collection (e.g., position self and hold container).

Determines degree of help patient requires.

4. Assess for signs and symptoms of urinary tract infection (UTI) (frequency, urgency, dysuria, hematuria, flank pain, fever; cloudy, malodorous urine).

These are indicators of UTI.

5. Refer to employer procedures for specimen collection methods.

Employer policies may vary regarding collection and/or handling of specimens.

NURSING DIAGNOSES

- Potential for infection
- Insufficient knowledge regarding specimen collection

Related factors/Risk factors are individualized on the basis of patient's condition or needs.

PLANNING

1. Expected outcomes following completion of procedure:
- Specimen free of contaminants is collected.

  Proper collection technique prevents substances from changing normal characteristics of urine.

- Patient discusses procedure for specimen collection.

  Procedure is performed safely.

- Patient discusses purpose and benefits of specimen collection.

  Evaluates patient's learning.

IMPLEMENTATION

1. Perform hand hygiene, check labels, and complete laboratory requisition for specimen container.

Reduces transfer of microorganisms. Organizes procedure.

2. Provide privacy for patient; close curtains around bed or close room door. Allow mobile patients to collect specimen in bathroom.

Privacy allows patient to relax and produce specimen more easily.

3. Collect clean-voided, midstream urine specimen.

   a. Apply clean gloves. Give patient cleaning towelette or towel, washcloth, and soap to clean perineum or help with cleaning perineum. Help bedridden patient onto bedpan to facilitate access to perineum. Remove and dispose of gloves.

Patients prefer to wash their own perineal areas when possible. Cleaning prevents contamination of specimen after urine passes from urethra.

   b. Using aseptic technique, open outer package of commercial specimen kit.

Maintains sterility of equipment.

   c. Apply clean gloves.

Prevents contact of microorganisms on your hands.

   d. Pour antiseptic solution over cotton balls (unless kit contains prepared antiseptic towlettes).

Cotton ball or towelette is used to clean perineum.

   e. Open specimen container, maintaining sterility of the inside of the container, and set cap aside with sterile side up. Do not touch inside of cap or container.

Maintains sterility of equipment. Contaminated specimen is most frequent reason for inaccurate reporting of urine C&S.

   f. Use aseptic technique to help patient or allow patient to independently clean perineum and collect specimen. Amount of help needed varies with each patient. Inform patient that antiseptic solution will feel cold.

Maintains patient's dignity and comfort.

     (1) *Male:*

       (a) Hold penis with one hand; using circular motion and antiseptic towelette, clean meatus, moving from centre to outside three times with different towelettes (see illustration). Have uncircumcised male patient retract foreskin for effective cleaning of urinary meatus and keep retracted during voiding. Return foreskin when done.

Reduces number of microorganisms at urethral meatus and moves from areas of least to most contamination. Return of foreskin prevents stricture of penis.

STEP	RATIONALE

IMPLEMENTATION

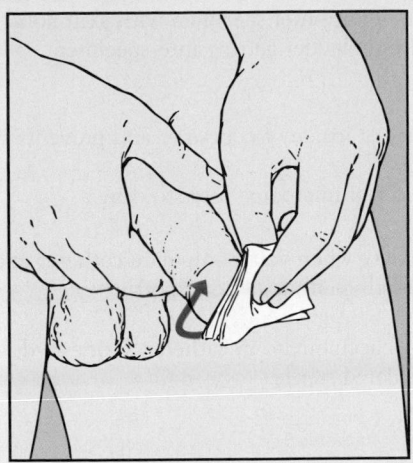

STEP 3f(1)(a) Cleaning technique (male).

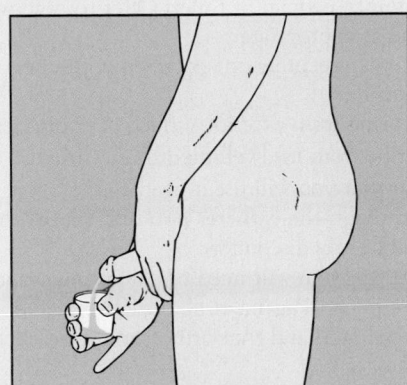

STEP 3f(1)(c) Collecting midstream urine specimen (male).

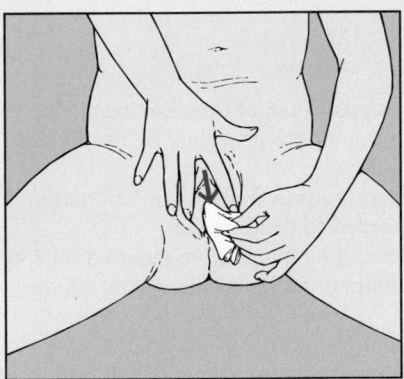

STEP 3f(2)(b) Clean from front to back, holding labia apart.

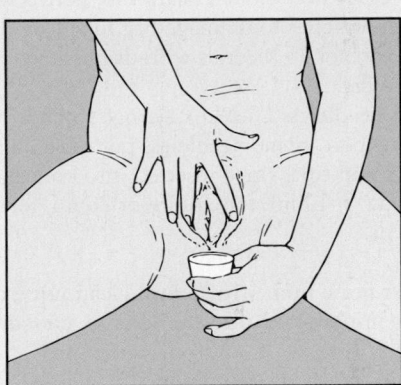

STEP 3f(2)(d) Collecting midstream urine specimen (female).

(b) If employer procedure indicates, rinse area with sterile water and dry with gauze.

Prevents contamination of specimen with antiseptic solution.

(c) After patient initiates urine stream into toilet or bedpan, have him pass urine specimen container into stream and collect 90 to 120 mL of urine (Pagana et al., 2019) (see illustration).

Initial urine flushes out microorganisms that normally accumulate at urinary meatus and prevents transfer into specimen.

(2) *Female:*

(a) Either nurse or patient spreads labia minora with fingers of nondominant hand.

Provides access to urethral meatus.

(b) With dominant hand clean urethral area with antiseptic swab (cotton ball or gauze). Move from front (above urethral orifice) to back (toward anus). Use fresh swab each time; clean three times; begin with labial fold farthest from you, then labial fold closest, and then down centre (see illustration).

Prevents contamination of urinary meatus with fecal material Cleaning down centre last decreases contamination from labia.

(c) If employer procedure indicates, rinse area with sterile water and dry with cotton ball.

Prevents contamination of specimen with antiseptic solution.

(d) While continuing to hold labia apart, patient initiates urine stream into toilet or bedpan; after stream is achieved, pass specimen container into stream and collect 90 to 120 mL of urine (Pagana et al., 2019) (see illustration).

Initial stream flushes out resident microorganisms that accumulate at urethral meatus and prevents transfer into specimen.

STEP	RATIONALE

IMPLEMENTATION

g. Remove specimen container before flow of urine stops and before releasing labia or penis. Patient finishes voiding into bedpan or toilet. Offer to help with personal hygiene as appropriate.

Prevents contamination of specimen with skin flora. Prevents sediment from bladder getting into specimen.

h. Replace cap securely on specimen container, touching only outside.

Retains sterility of inside of container and prevents spillage of urine.

i. Clean urine from exterior surface of container.

Prevents transfer of microorganisms to others.

4. Collect urine from in-dwelling urinary catheter.

a. Explain that you will use a needleless syringe to remove urine through the catheter port and that patient will not experience any discomfort.

Minimizes anxiety when you manipulate catheter and aspirate urine with syringe from catheter port.

b. Explain that you will need to clamp the catheter for 15 to 30 minutes (Pagana et al., 2019) before obtaining a urine specimen and that urine cannot be obtained from the drainage bag.

Allows urine to accumulate in catheter. Urine in drainage bag is not considered sterile.

c. Apply clean gloves. Clamp drainage tubing with clamp or rubber band for as long as 30 minutes below catheter port (see illustration).

Permits collection of fresh sterile urine in catheter tubing rather than draining into bag.

d. After 15 minutes, position patient so catheter sampling port is easily accessible. Location of port is where catheter attaches to drainage bag tube (see illustration). Clean port for 15 seconds with disinfectant swab and allow to dry.

Prevents entry of microorganisms into catheter.

e. Attach needleless Luer-Lok syringe to built-in catheter sampling port. Some needleless ports use blunt plastic valve or slip-tip syringe inserted into port diaphragm.

Guideline recommends use of Luer-Lok needleless system. Needleless system prevents injury by needlestick.

f. Withdraw 5–10 mL for culture or 20 mL for routine urinalysis.

Allows collection of urine without contamination. Proper volume is needed to perform test.
Increased volume of sample may be required for specific tests.

g. Transfer urine from syringe into clean urine container for routine urinalysis or into sterile urine container for culture.

Prevents contamination of urine during transfer procedure.

h. Place lid tightly on container.

Prevents contamination of specimen by air and loss by spillage.

i. Unclamp catheter and allow urine to flow into drainage bag. Ensure that urine flows freely.

Allows urine to drain by gravity and prevents stasis of urine in bladder.

5. Securely attach label to container (not lid). In patient's presence, confirm label information (two person-specific identifiers, specimen source, and collection date and time). If patient is female, indicate if patient is menstruating.

Ensures that specimen is identified correctly for proper diagnosis (Accreditation Canada, 2019).

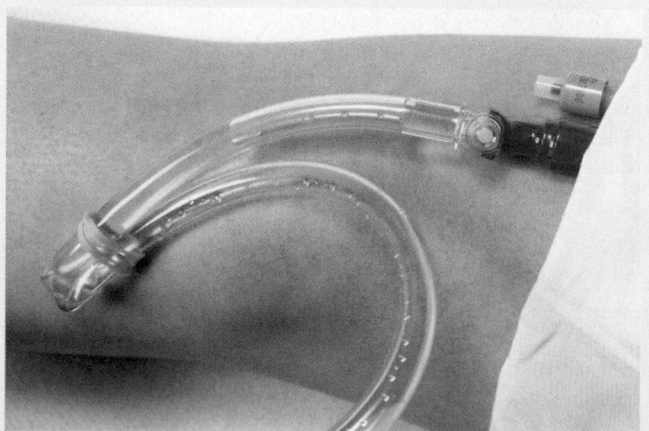

STEP 4c Rubber band used to clamp drainage tube.

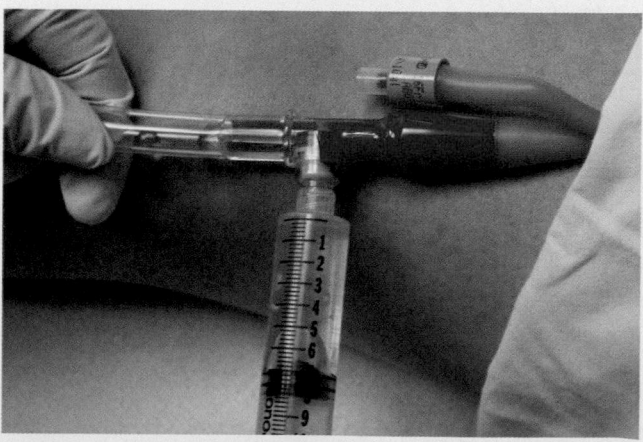

STEP 4d Access urinary catheter port with Luer-Lok syringe or syringe with blunt plastic valve.

STEP	RATIONALE

IMPLEMENTATION

6. Dispose of soiled supplies. Remove and dispose of gloves and perform hand hygiene.	Prevents transmission of microorganisms.
7. Send specimen and completed requisition to laboratory within 20 minutes. Refrigerate specimen if delay cannot be avoided.	Delay of analysis may significantly alter test results (Pagana et al., 2019).

EVALUATION

1. Inspect clean-voided midstream specimen for contamination with toilet paper or stool.	Contaminants prevent specimen from being used.
2. Evaluate patient's urine C&S report for bacterial growth.	Routine cultures identify organism(s), and sensitivity study identifies antimicrobial medications that may be effective against pathogen.
3. Observe urinary drainage system in catheterized patient to ensure that it is intact and patent.	System must remain closed to remain sterile.
4. **Use Teach-Back:** "I want to be sure I explained clearly the way to obtain a urine sample. Can you tell me how you would take the sample?" Develop a revised teaching plan if patient or caregiver is not able to teach back correctly.	Determines level of understanding of instructional topic.

Unexpected Outcomes

1. Urine specimen is contaminated with stool or toilet paper.

2. Patient is unable to void, or urine does not collect in drainage tube.

3. Urine culture reveals bacterial growth (determined by colony count of more than 10 000 organisms per millilitre).

4. Lumen leading to balloon that holds catheter in place is punctured.

Related Interventions

- Repeat patient instruction and specimen collection. If unable to obtain specimen through clean voiding, patient may need catheterization (see Skill 34-1).
- Ensure patency of tube, then offer fluids if permitted to enhance urine production.
- Report findings to health care provider.
- Administer medications as prescribed.
- Monitor patient for fever and dysuria.
- Notify health care provider.
- Prepare for removal of existing catheter and insertion of new catheter.

Communication and Documentation

- Document collection of specimen in nurses' notes in electronic health record (EHR) or chart or per employer policy; note method used to obtain specimen, date and time collected, type of test prescribed, appearance, odour and colour of urine, and time sent to laboratory.
- Document your evaluation of patient and caregiver learning.
- Report any abnormal findings to health care provider.

Special Considerations
Teaching

- Explain significance of cleaning genital area before collecting specimen.
- Discuss signs and symptoms of UTI (e.g., burning or pain with urination, urgency, increased frequency, cloudy urine) with patient

and caregiver if appropriate.
- Self-catheterization may be an alternative for urine collection and taught to patients, if appropriate.

Pediatric

- Urine collection bags may be used with infants and young children who are not toilet trained, for some forms of analysis (such as glucose, ketones, or proteins) (Naimer, 2017; Perry et al., 2017). Ensure that you cut a small slit in the diaper and pull the urine collection bag through the slit so that urine collected is visible outside the diaper (Fig. 9.3). Remove the bag as soon as the urine specimen is visible (Naimer, 2017; Perry et al., 2017).
- For some forms of analysis, urine may also be aspirated with a syringe directly from the diaper (Perry et al., 2017).

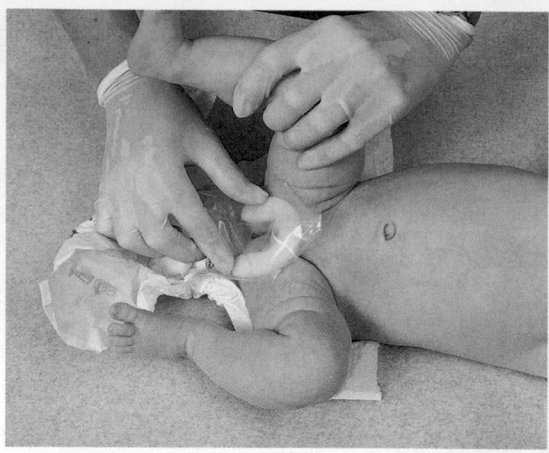

FIG 9.3 Application of urine collection bag. *(From Warekois, R. S., & Robinson, R. [2012]. Phlebotomy worktext and procedures manual [3rd ed.]. St. Louis: Mosby.)*

- To collect a urine specimen for culture, use the clean-voided midstream collection method (Larocco, Franek, Leibach, et al., 2016). Collection using sterile urine-collecting bags or directly from diapers is not recommended as results are often contaminated and, therefore, inaccurate when analyzing for pathogenic microorganisms (Larocco et al., 2016). However, it is challenging to collect a urine specimen via the clean-voided midstream method with infants and younger children; thus, when infection is suspected and an accurate specimen is critical, suprapubic urine aspiration or insertion of a sterile catheter is recommended (Perry et al., 2017).

Gerontological

- Older persons may need help in positioning to obtain a specimen. In confused patients, use interprofessional collaboration to obtain information about how best to help the patient in collecting a specimen (Touhy, Jett, Boscart, et al., 2019).

Care in the Community

- Instruct a patient collecting a sample at home to keep it refrigerated or on ice until it reaches the laboratory to minimize bacterial growth before applying it to a culture medium in the laboratory setting.

PROCEDURAL GUIDELINE 9.1 *Collecting a Timed Urine Specimen*

Some tests of renal function and urine composition require urine to be collected over 2 to 72 hours. The 24-hour timed collection method is used most often and to measure elements such as amino acids, creatinine, hormones, glucose, and adrenocorticosteroids. A timed urine collection provides a means to measure the concentration or dilution of urine.

To ensure the accuracy of a 24-hour timed urine specimen, the patient and staff must work together to collect all voided urine in a 24-hour period. Obtain an appropriate container with or without preservative. The type of analysis for the 24-hour timed specimen determines the need for any preservative. The specimen container can be placed in the patient's bathroom or the "soiled" utility room. Post a sign to remind the patient and staff that a test is in progress. Label the specimen container with all appropriate identification information and the number of containers sequentially if more than one container is needed. Documentation and collection of all urine are necessary for an accurate test result.

Delegation and Collaboration

The skill of collecting a timed urine specimen can be delegated to an unregulated care provider (UCP). The nurse informs the UCP about:

- When timed collection begins, proper method to store the collected urine, where to place signs that a timed urine collection is in progress, and saving all urine.
- Reporting when blood, mucus, or foul odours are present in the urine specimen or if there is a break in the collection procedure.

Equipment

- Large collection bottle with cap that usually contains a chemical preservative
- Bedpan, urinal, specimen hat, bedside commode, or pediatric potty-chair

- Graduated measuring container for intake and output (I&O) measurement
- Large basin to hold collection bottle surrounded by ice if immediate refrigeration is required
- Specimen identification label and completed laboratory requisition
- Instructional signs that remind patient and staff of timed urine collection
- Clean gloves
- Plastic biohazard plastic bag or container

Procedural Steps

1. Identify patient using at least two person-specific identifiers (e.g., full name, date of birth, personal identification number, etc.) according to employer policy. Compare identifiers with information on patient's medical record and laboratory requisition (Accreditation Canada, 2019).
2. Explain the reason for specimen collection, how the patient can help, and that urine must be free of feces and toilet tissue.
3. Place specimen collection container in the bathroom and, if indicated, in a pan of ice. Post signs to remind staff, family and visitors, and patient of timed urine collection on patient's door and toileting area. If patient leaves unit, be sure that personnel in receiving area collect and save all urine.
4. If possible, have patient drink two to four glasses of water about 30 minutes before times of collection to facilitate ability to void at the appropriate time for test to begin.
5. Perform hand hygiene and apply clean gloves. Discard the first voided specimen as the test begins. Indicate time test began on laboratory requisition. For accurate results the patient must begin the test with an empty bladder. Begin collecting all urine for designated time.

PROCEDURAL GUIDELINE 9.1 *Collecting a Timed Urine Specimen—cont'd*

6. Measure volume of each voiding if I&O are to be recorded. Place all voided urine in labelled specimen bottle with appropriate additives.

7. Unless instructed otherwise, keep specimen bottle in specimen refrigerator or container of ice in bathroom to prevent decomposition of urine.

8. Encourage patient to drink two glasses of water 1 hour before timed urine collection ends. Encourage patient to empty bladder during last 15 minutes of urine collection period.

9. Perform hand hygiene and apply clean gloves. Collect final specimen at end of collection period. Label specimen (two person-specific identifiers, specimen source, collection date and time, number of bottle) in patient's presence, attach appropriate requisition, and send to laboratory. Remove gloves and perform hand hygiene.

10. Remove signs. Tell patient that specimen collection period is completed.

PROCEDURAL GUIDELINE 9.2 *Urine Screening for Glucose, Ketones, Protein, Blood, and pH*

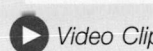 *Video Clip*

Tests for chemical properties of urine are part of the routine urinalysis completed in the laboratory or as a point-of-care test performed at the bedside or in the home. A Multistix reagent test strip may simultaneously be used to assess for up to nine chemical properties: specific gravity, pH, protein, glucose, ketones, blood bilirubin, urobilinogen, leukocytes, and nitrates. The test is easy to perform and causes no pain. This type of screening is used when more detailed laboratory testing is not available (e.g., health care provider's office, clinic, or long-term care setting). The use of urine testing for managing blood glucose is no longer recommended but continues to be useful in detecting presence of ketones in patients with diabetes (Diabetes Canada Clinical Practice Guidelines Expert Committee, 2018). Capillary blood monitoring is an accurate assessment of serum glucose levels (Pagana et al., 2019).

Delegation and Collaboration

The skill of urine screening for chemical properties can be delegated to an unregulated care provider (UCP). The nurse informs the UCP to:

- Obtain the specimen correctly (e.g., before meals, following a "double-voided" specimen).
- Report the results of the test or any odour, blood, or mucus in the urine specimen.

Equipment

- Bedpan, urinal, specimen hat, bedside commode, or pediatric potty-chair
- Container for urine from catheter
- Watch with second hand or digital counter
- Reagent test strip (check expiration date on container)
- Test strip colour chart
- Paper towel
- Clean gloves
- Small biohazard plastic bag for delivery of specimen to laboratory (or container specified by employer)

Procedural Steps

1. Identify patient using at least two person-specific identifiers according to employer policy. Compare identifiers with information on medical record and laboratory requisition (Accreditation Canada, 2019).

2. Determine if double-voided specimen is needed for glucose testing. If required, ask patient to void, discard, and then drink a glass of water.

3. Perform hand hygiene and apply clean gloves. Ask patient to collect a fresh, random urine specimen. If patient is catheterized, remove a 5- to 10-mL specimen from the catheter port (see Skill 9.1).

4. Immerse end of reagent strip into urine container. Remove the strip immediately and tap it gently against the side of the container to remove excess urine.

5. Hold strip in horizontal position to prevent mixing of chemical reagents (see illustration).

6. Precisely time the number of seconds specified on container and compare colour of strip with colour chart on container (Table 9.1).

7. When appropriate, discuss test results with patient. Discard urine. Remove and discard gloves. Perform hand hygiene.

8. Record results immediately on appropriate flow sheet. Report reading to health care provider.

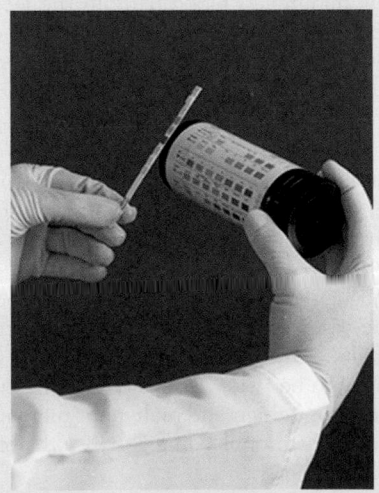

STEP 5 Testing urine using reagent strip.

Continued

PROCEDURAL GUIDELINE 9.2 *Urine Screening for Glucose, Ketones, Protein, Blood, and pH—cont'd*

TABLE 9.1

Example of a Chart for a Reagent Strip*

Test	When to Read	Range of Results
pH	60 seconds	5.0–9.0
Protein	60 seconds	(–) or 3+ (5 g/L)
Glucose	10 seconds (qualitative)	(–) to 4+ (55 mmol/L)
	30 seconds (quantitative)	(–) to 4+ (55 mmol/L)
Ketones	40 seconds	(–) to 3+ (large)
Blood	60 seconds	(–) to 4+ (large)

*Based on Roche Canada's Chemstrip 7 product line.

◆ **SKILL 9.2** **Measuring Occult Blood in Stool**

▶ *Video Clip* **NSO** *Nursing Skills Online Specimen Collection Module 3 / Lesson 4*

Hemoccult testing is useful for screening for the presence of occult (not visible) blood in the stool for conditions such as colon cancer, bleeding gastrointestinal (GI) ulcers, and localized gastric or intestinal irritation. Use caution; a false-positive result may occur if a patient has ingested red meat within 3 days of testing or is taking certain medications (e.g., iron). A false-negative may result if that patient is taking vitamin C (Pagana et al., 2019). The test measures microscopic amounts of blood in the stool. Normally a person loses small amounts of blood daily in the feces as a result of minor abrasions of the nasopharyngeal or oral mucosa. If greater than 50 mL of blood enters the feces from the upper GI tract, the blood causes melena (darkening of feces). When blood is present, further testing is indicated to determine the source of the bleeding.

Patients are often instructed on how to collect stool specimens for the test in the home. Only a small amount of stool is needed to perform the test successfully. The common types of stool tests used are the gFOBT (guaiac-based fecal occult blood test) and the FIT (fecal immunochemical test) (Canadian Cancer Society, 2018). Methods of guaiac-based testing include the Hemoccult slides and the Hematest tablets. A new deoxyribonucleic acid (DNA) stool sample test promises to be twice as sensitive as the current guaiac testing for precancerous benign and malignant tumours. The DNA stool sample test identifies nonbleeding polyps with abnormal DNA (Pagana et al., 2019).

Delegation and Collaboration

The skill of testing stool for occult blood can be delegated to an unregulated care provider (UCP). The nurse informs the UCP to:

• Report immediately if any blood is detected and not to discard stool from a positive test so the nurse may repeat the testing.

Equipment

• Soap, water, washcloth, and towel
• Paper towel
• Clean gloves
• Wooden applicators

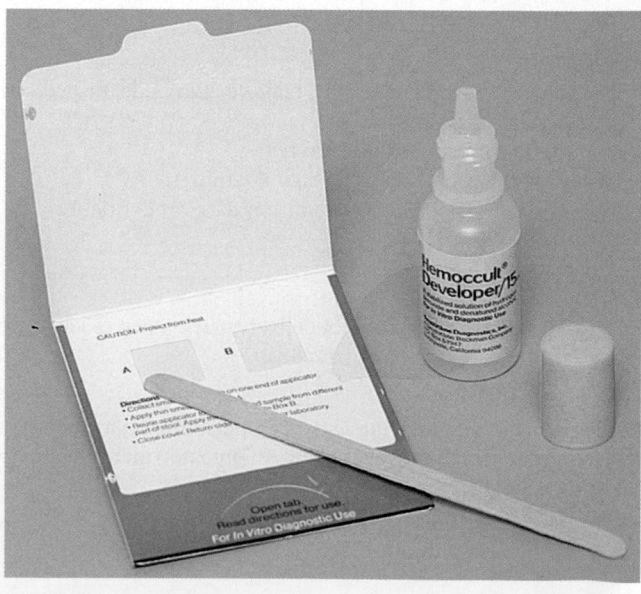

FIG 9.4 Hemoccult testing kit for measuring occult blood.

Hemoccult Test
- Cardboard Hemoccult slide (Fig. 9.4)
- Hemoccult developing solution

Hematest
- Hematest tablets (must be protected from moisture, heat, and light)
- Guaiac paper
- Clean container of tap water

STEP	RATIONALE

ASSESSMENT

1. Identify patient using at least two person-specific identifiers (e.g., full name, date of birth, personal identification number, etc.) according to employer policy. Compare identifiers with information on patient's medical record and laboratory requisition.

Ensures correct patient. Complies with Accreditation Canada standards and improves patient safety (Accreditation Canada, 2019).

2. Assess patient's or caregiver's understanding of need for stool test.

Provides information on which to base necessary health teaching.

3. Assess patient's ability to cooperate with procedure and collect specimen.

To avoid embarrassment, patients often prefer to collect own stool specimen. Some patients require help.

4. Assess patient's medical history for GI disorders (e.g., history of bleeding, colitis, or hemorrhoids).

You can institute routine screening. Hemorrhoids can cause bleeding that may be misinterpreted as upper GI bleeding.

5. Review patient's medications for medications that contribute to GI bleeding.

Anticoagulants increase risk for bleeding in GI tract, even from minor trauma to mucosa. Long-term use of steroids, nonsteroidal anti-inflammatory medications (NSAIDs), and acetylsalicylic acid (aspirin) can irritate mucosa and result in bleeding (Pagana et al., 2019).

6. Refer to health care provider's prescriptions for medication or dietary modifications or restrictions before test.

Specimens will be positive if contaminated by menstrual blood, hemorrhoid blood, or povidone-iodine. Diets rich in meats, green leafy vegetables, poultry, and fish may produce false-positive results.

NURSING DIAGNOSES

- Anxiety
- Bowel incontinence
- Constipation
- Insufficient knowledge regarding collection and testing of stool specimen
- Diarrhea

Related factors are individualized on the basis of patient's condition or needs.

PLANNING

1. Expected outcomes following completion of procedure:
   - Test for occult blood is negative.

Patient has only small amount of blood in feces because of normal nasopharyngeal and oral mucosa abrasions.

   - Patient discusses purpose and benefits of testing stool for blood.

Validates learning

2. Explain procedure to patient and/or caregiver. Discuss reason for specimen collection and how patient can help. Explain that feces must be free of urine and toilet tissue.

Patient who understands procedure is more likely to cooperate and may be able to obtain specimen independently. Also prevents accidental disposal of specimen.

3. Arrange for any needed dietary or medication restrictions.

Ensures accuracy of test results.

IMPLEMENTATION

1. Perform hand hygiene.

Reduces transmission of microorganisms.

2. Apply clean gloves. Obtain uncontaminated stool specimen and place in clean, dry container not contaminated with urine, water, or toilet tissue.

Prevents transmission of microorganisms. Allows for accurate testing when specimen is not contaminated with other products.

3. Use tip of wooden applicator to obtain small part of feces.

Small specimen is sufficient for measuring blood content.

STEP	RATIONALE

IMPLEMENTATION

4. Measure for occult blood.

   a. Perform Hemoccult slide test:

      (1) Open flap of Hemoccult slide. Apply thin smear of stool on paper in first box.

Guaiac paper inside box is sensitive to fecal blood content.

      (2) Using same applicator, obtain second fecal specimen from different part of stool and apply thinly to second box of slide (see illustration).

Occult blood from upper GI tract is not always dispersed equally throughout stool. Findings of occult blood are more conclusive for GI bleeding when entire specimen is found to contain blood.

      (3) Close slide cover and turn slide over to reverse side. Open cardboard flap and apply 2 drops of Hemoccult developing solution on each box of guaiac paper (see illustration).

Developing solution penetrates underlying fecal specimen. Change in colour of guaiac paper indicates blood.

      (4) Read results of test after 30 to 60 seconds. Note colour changes.

Ensures correct results. Bluish discoloration indicates occult blood (guaiac positive). No change in colour of guaiac paper indicates negative results.

      (5) Dispose of test slide in proper receptacle.

Reduces transfer of microorganisms.

   b. Perform test using Hematest tablets:

Tablet contains solid form of developing solution.

      (1) Place stool on guaiac paper. Then place Hematest tablet on top of stool specimen. Apply 2 to 3 drops of tap water to tablet, allowing water to flow onto guaiac paper.

Tap water dissolves Hematest tablet and thus dispenses developing solution over specimen and guaiac paper.

      (2) Observe colour of guaiac paper within 2 minutes.

Bluish discoloration is guaiac positive. Do not read colour after 2 minutes. False findings may occur.

      (3) Dispose of tablet and paper in proper receptacle.

Reduces transfer of microorganisms.

5. Wrap wooden applicator in paper towel, grasp in nondominant hand, remove gloves over wrapped applicator. Discard in proper receptacle. Perform hand hygiene.

Reduces transfer of microorganisms.

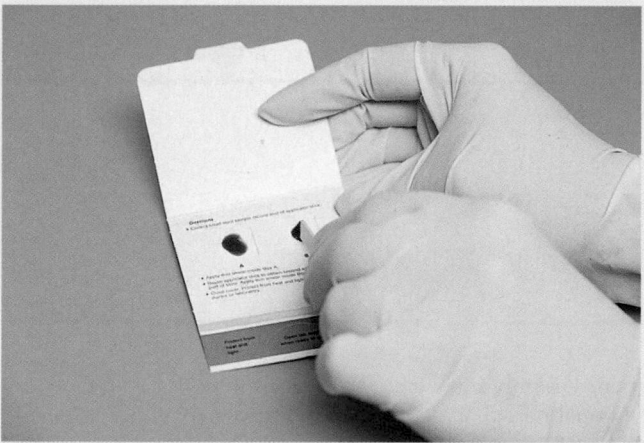

STEP 4a(2) Applying stool specimen to both spots on Hemoccult slide.

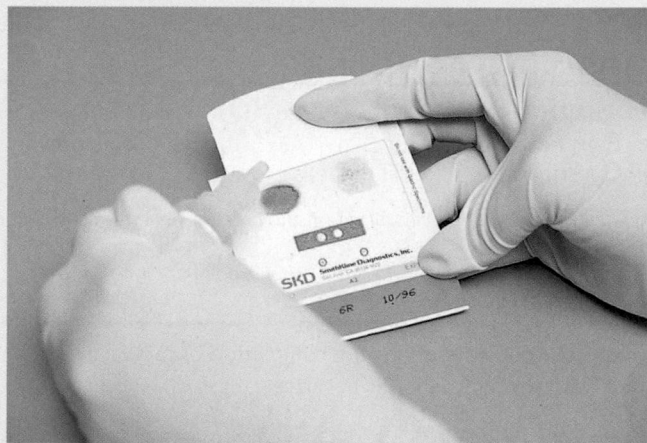

STEP 4a(3) Applying developing solution.

STEP	RATIONALE

EVALUATION

1. Note colour changes in guaiac paper.	Reveals blood in feces.
2. **Use Teach-Back:** "You will need to check your stool two more times for blood when you go home. I want to be sure I explained the procedure correctly. Tell me the steps you will use to collect this specimen." Develop a revised teaching plan if patient or caregiver is not able to teach back correctly.	Determines level of understanding of instructional topic.

Clinical Decision Point *A single positive test result does not confirm bleeding or indicate colorectal cancer. To confirm positive results, the test must be repeated while the patient is on a meat-free, high-residue diet and with more in-depth diagnosis (Van Leeuwen & Bladh, 2015).*

3. Note character of stool specimen.	Certain abnormal constituents of stool may be visible.

Unexpected Outcomes	Related Interventions
1. Test for occult blood is positive.	• Continue to monitor patient. • Notify health care provider.

Communication and Documentation

- Document results of test and include stool characteristics in nurses' notes in electronic health record (EHR) or chart.
- Document your evaluation of patient and caregiver learning.
- Report positive test results to health care provider.

Special Considerations
Pediatric

- Children of school age and older are concrete thinkers, are often very curious, and may ask many questions about the test. Answer questions honestly and at the child's level of understanding.
- Allow child to watch, if desired, while performing test (Hockenberry & Wilson, 2015).
- Testing reagent is often poisonous; thus, keep it out of reach of the small child.

Care in the Community

- Many patients or caregivers are instructed to collect specimens at home and return them to the health care provider's office immediately after collection. Be sure they know infection control principles. Be sure they are aware of diet and medication restrictions before and after the stool collection period.

✦ SKILL 9.3 Measuring Occult Blood in Gastric Secretions (Gastroccult)

NSO *Nursing Skills Online Specimen Collection Module 3 / Lesson 3*

Analysis of gastric secretions or emesis can detect blood that is not always visible. Gastroccult testing helps to reveal bleeding in the esophagus or stomach. The test can verify the presence of blood when red or black coloration of the gastric contents is noted or when the gastric contents or emesis has the appearance of coffee grounds. The test measures microscopic amounts of blood in the gastric secretions. Gastric aspirate obtained by either nasogastric tube, nasoenteral tube, or emesis is an appropriate sample for use with this test. It is a useful diagnostic tool for conditions such as upper gastrointestinal (GI) ulcers or bleeding. Because the test is easy to perform, patients are often taught how to test emesis in the home.

Delegation and Collaboration

The skill of Gastroccult testing can be delegated to an unregulated care provider (UCP) for test on emesis. You cannot delegate the skill of Gastroccult testing to an UCP if the specimen is collected from a nasogastric (NG) or nasoenteral (NE) tube. The nurse informs the UCP to:

- Report immediately if blood or coffee-ground emesis is visible in NG or NE tube secretions.
- Save specimen for repeat testing.

Equipment

- Facial tissues
- Emesis basin
- Wooden applicator or 3-mL syringe
- Catheter tip syringe
- Cardboard Gastroccult test slide
- Gastroccult developing solution
- Clean gloves

STEP	RATIONALE

ASSESSMENT

1. Identify patient using at least two person-specific identifiers (e.g., full name, date of birth, personal identification number, etc.) according to employer policy. Compare identifiers with information on patient's medical record and laboratory requisition.

Ensures correct patient. Complies with Accreditation Canada standards and improves patient safety (Accreditation Canada, 2019).

2. Assess patient's or caregiver's understanding of need for test.

Provides you with information on which to base necessary health teaching.

3. Assess patient's medical history for bleeding or GI disorders.

You can institute routine screening.

4. Assess patient's medical history for GI disorders (e.g., history of bleeding, colitis).

Anticoagulants increase risk for bleeding in GI tract, even from minor trauma to mucosa. Long-term use of steroids, nonsteroidal anti-inflammatory medications (NSAIDs), and acetylsalicylic acid (aspirin) can irritate mucosa.

NURSING DIAGNOSES

- Anxiety
- Insufficient knowledge regarding occult blood testing
- Fear

Related factors are individualized on the basis of patient's condition or needs.

PLANNING

1. Expected outcomes following completion of procedure:
   - Test for occult blood is negative.

Patient has only small or no amount of blood in gastric secretions.

   - Patient discusses purpose and benefits of testing gastric contents for blood.

Validates learning.

2. Explain procedure to patient and/or caregiver. Discuss why specimen collection is necessary.

Patient who understands procedure is more likely to be less anxious and more cooperative.

IMPLEMENTATION

1. Perform hand hygiene.

Reduces transmission of microorganisms.

2. Verify NG tube placement (see Chapter 32).

Ensures aspiration of gastric contents.

3. Obtain specimen by disconnecting suction or gravity drainage tube from NG or NE tube. Using a syringe, aspirate 0.5 to 5 mL of fluid from NG or NE tube.

Only a small amount of specimen is needed. In pediatric settings, even smaller amounts would be required.

Clinical Decision Point *Observe specimen. If you find red blood or coffee-ground material, report these findings immediately to health care provider.*

4. To obtain sample of emesis, use 3-mL syringe or wooden applicator to obtain sample from emesis basin.

A small specimen is sufficient for measuring blood content.

5. *Perform Gastroccult test:*
   a. Using wooden applicator or syringe, apply 1 drop of gastric sample to Gastroccult blood test slide.

Sample must cover test paper for test reaction to occur.

   b. Apply 2 drops of commercial developer solution over sample and 1 drop between positive and negative performance monitors (see illustration).

   c. Verify that performance monitor turns blue in 30 seconds.

Indicates proper function of testing paper.

   d. After 60 seconds compare colour of gastric sample with that of performance monitor.

If sample turns blue, test is positive for occult blood. If sample turns green, it is negative for occult blood.

   e. Dispose of test slide, wooden applicator, and syringe in proper receptacle. If needed, reconnect NG or NE tube to drainage system or suction. Remove gloves. Perform hand hygiene.

Reduces transmission of microorganisms.

STEP	RATIONALE

IMPLEMENTATION

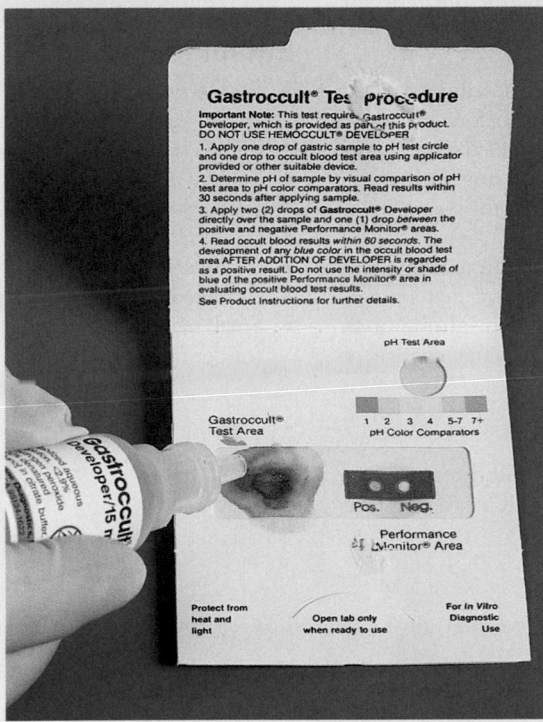

STEP 5b Applying developing solution to Gastroccult test area.

EVALUATION

1. Note character of gastric secretions.

2. Note colour changes on Gastroccult blood test slide.
3. **Use Teach-Back:** "I want make sure you know the purpose of the procedure and understand it. Can you tell me what we will need to do to obtain a gastric specimen from your emesis (or NG/NE tube)?" Develop a revised teaching plan if patient or caregiver is not able to teach back correctly.

Blood may be visible, or coffee-ground material denoting blood may be observed.
Reveals blood in gastric secretions.
Determines level of understanding of instructional topic.
Generally, patients only self-test with emesis in the home environment, and not via NG or NE tube.

Unexpected Outcomes
1. Test for occult blood is positive.

Related Interventions
• Continue to monitor patient.
• Notify health care provider.

Communication and Documentation

• Document results of test and presence of any unusual characteristics of gastric contents in nurses' notes in electronic health record (EHR) or chart.
• Document your evaluation of patient and caregiver learning.
• Report positive test results to health care provider.

Special Considerations
Pediatric

• Children of school age and older are concrete thinkers, often very curious, and may ask many questions about the test. Answer

questions honestly and at the child's level of understanding. Allow the child to watch, if desired, while test is performed (Hockenberry & Wilson, 2015).

Care in the Community

• Many patients or caregivers can perform the Gastroccult test on emesis. Be sure they know infection control principles.

✦ SKILL 9.4   Collecting Nose and Throat Specimens for Culture

When patients have signs and symptoms of an upper respiratory or sinus infection, and for the purposes of screening for methicillin-resistant *Staphylococcus aureus* (MRSA), a nose or throat culture, or both, is a simple diagnostic tool to identify the presence and type of microorganisms. Other sites may be prescribed to be sampled when screening for MRSA. Cultures should be obtained before antibiotic therapy is initiated because antibiotics may interrupt the growth of the organisms in the laboratory. If a patient is receiving antibiotics, notify the laboratory and identify which specific antibiotics they are receiving (Pagana et al., 2019).

Collection of a specimen from the nose and throat can cause discomfort and gagging because of sensitive mucosal membranes. It is important to collect a throat culture before mealtime or at least 1 hour after eating or drinking to decrease the chance of inducing vomiting.

Delegation and Collaboration

The skill of obtaining specimens from the nose and throat cannot be delegated to an unregulated care provider (UCP). The nurse informs the UCP to:

- Report shortness of breath, difficulty breathing, and other signs of respiratory distress.

Equipment

- Sterile swab(s) in culture transport tube(s) (flexible swab with cotton tip may be used for nasopharyngeal cultures)
- Emesis basin or clean container (*optional*)
- Tongue depressor and penlight
- Facial tissues
- Clean gloves
- Completed identification labels with proper patient identifiers
- Completed laboratory requisition
- Small biohazard plastic bag for delivery of specimen to laboratory (or container specified by employer)

STEP	RATIONALE

ASSESSMENT

1. Identify patient using at least two person-specific identifiers (e.g., full name, date of birth, personal identification number, etc.) according to employer policy. Compare identifiers with information on patient's medical record and laboratory requisition.	Ensures correct patient. Complies with Accreditation Canada standards and improves patient safety (Accreditation Canada, 2019).
2. Assess patient's understanding of purpose for procedure and ability to cooperate. You may need help to obtain throat cultures from confused, combative, or unconscious patients.	Provides basis to determine need for health teaching and assistance.
3. Inspect condition of nares and drainage from nasal mucosa and sinuses.	Reveals signs that indicate infection or allergic irritation. Clear drainage usually indicates allergy. Yellow, green, or brown drainage usually indicates infection.
4. Determine if patient experiences postnasal drip, sinus headache or tenderness, nasal congestion, sore throat, or exposure to others with similar symptoms.	Symptoms help reveal nature of problem.
5. Apply clean gloves. Assess condition of posterior pharynx (see Chapter 8).	Reveals local inflammation or lesions of pharynx.
6. Assess patient for signs of infection, including fever, chills, and/or fatigue.	Infection originating within nasopharynx can become systemic, requiring antibiotic therapy.
7. Review health care provider's prescriptions to determine if nose, throat, or both cultures are needed.	Prevents exposing patient to unnecessary discomfort of repeated cultures.

NURSING DIAGNOSES

- Acute pain
- Persistent pain

- Insufficient knowledge regarding specimen collection

- Potential for infection

Related factors/Risk factors are individualized on the basis of patient's condition or needs.

PLANNING

1. Expected outcomes following completion of procedure:	
• There is no bacterial growth in specimens.	Absence of bacterial infection.
• Patient does not experience bleeding of nasal mucosa.	Procedure is atraumatic.

STEP	RATIONALE

PLANNING

• Specimen is not contaminated.	Evidenced by results of laboratory analysis.
• Patient discusses purpose of nose and throat cultures.	Validates learning.
2. Plan to do culture before mealtime or at least 1 hour after eating.	Procedure often induces gagging; timing decreases patient's chances of vomiting.
3. Explain procedure to patient and caregiver. Discuss reason for specimen collection and how patient can help.	Understanding procedure usually decreases anxiety and promotes cooperation.
4. Explain that patient may have tickling sensation or gagging during swabbing of throat. Nasal swab may create urge to sneeze. Each procedure only takes a few seconds to complete.	Helps patient relax.

IMPLEMENTATION

1. Ask patient to sit erect in bed or chair facing you. An acutely ill patient or young child may lie back against bed with head of bed raised to 45-degree angle in semi-Fowler's position.	Provides easy access to nasal or oral structures.
2. Perform hand hygiene. Loosen cap and have swab in tube ready for use.	Reduces transmission of microorganisms. Allows you to grasp swab easily without danger of contamination. Most commercial tubes have tops that fit securely over end of swab. Allows touching outer tops without contaminating swab stick.
3. Collect throat culture	
a. Apply clean gloves.	Reduces transmission of microorganisms.
b. Instruct patient to tilt head backward. For patients in bed, place pillow behind shoulders.	Facilitates visualization of pharynx.
c. Ask patient to open mouth and say "ah." If necessary to visualize pharynx, use penlight and depress tongue with tongue depressor and note inflamed areas of pharynx or tonsils. Depress anterior third of tongue only.	Permits exposure of pharynx, relaxes throat muscles, and minimizes gag reflex. Area to be swabbed should be visualized clearly.

Clinical Decision Point *Do not attempt throat culture in a pediatric patient if you suspect acute epiglottitis because trauma from swab might cause increase in edema, resulting in occlusion of airway (Hockenberry & Wilson, 2015).*

d. Insert swab without touching lips, teeth, tongue, cheeks, or uvula.	Prevents contamination with organisms from oral cavity (Pagana et al., 2019).
e. Gently but quickly swab posterior pharynx, tonsils, and inflamed areas.	These areas contain most microorganisms.
f. Carefully withdraw swab without touching oral structures.	Collects microorganisms from throat tissues without contamination from mouth and tongue.
4. Collect nasal culture	
a. Apply clean gloves.	Reduces transmission of microorganisms.
b. Encourage patient to blow nose and then check nostrils for patency with penlight. Select nostril with greatest patency. For MRSA, ensure both nostrils are clear.	Clears nasal passages of mucus containing resident bacteria.
c. With patient in sitting position have patient tilt head backward. Patients in bed should have a small pillow behind shoulders.	Provides access to nasal passages and facilitates visualization of nasal septum and sinuses.
d. Carefully pass swab approximately 2–2.5 cm (0.8–1 inch) into nostril. Rotate swab against the nasal mucosa (Diagnostic Services Manitoba, 2015). **NOTE:** If you need to obtain **nasopharyngeal culture**, use special swab that can be flexed downward to reach nasopharynx.	Swab should remain sterile until it reaches area to be cultured. Rotating swab covers all surfaces where exudate is present.
e. Remove swab without touching sides of nasal canal. If screening for MRSA, use same swab and repeat procedure with other nostril.	Prevents contamination of swab by resident bacteria.
f. Offer patient facial tissue and/or wash cloth.	Minimizes period of time that patient experiences discomfort.

STEP	RATIONALE

IMPLEMENTATION

5. Carefully insert swab into culture transport tube and recap tube securely. If using specific type of culture kit, crush the culture transport tube with fingers at the appropriate area and make sure the specimen is in contact with the medium (see illustrations).

Placing swab within culture transport tube maintains life of bacteria for testing.
Crushing tube releases culture medium.

6. Attach completed identification label to culture transport tube and confirm identifiers, specimen source, and collection date and time in front of patient (see employer policy). Note on laboratory requisition if patient is taking antibiotic or if specific organism is suspected (e.g., *Bordetella pertussis*).

Incorrect identification of specimen could result in diagnostic or therapeutic errors.

7. Enclose specimen in biohazard bag and send immediately to laboratory.

Specimen not sent to laboratory immediately or refrigerated allows growth of organisms and inaccurate results.

8. Ensure patient is comfortable. Dispose of gloves and perform hand hygiene.

Provides for patient comfort. Reduces transmission of microorganisms.

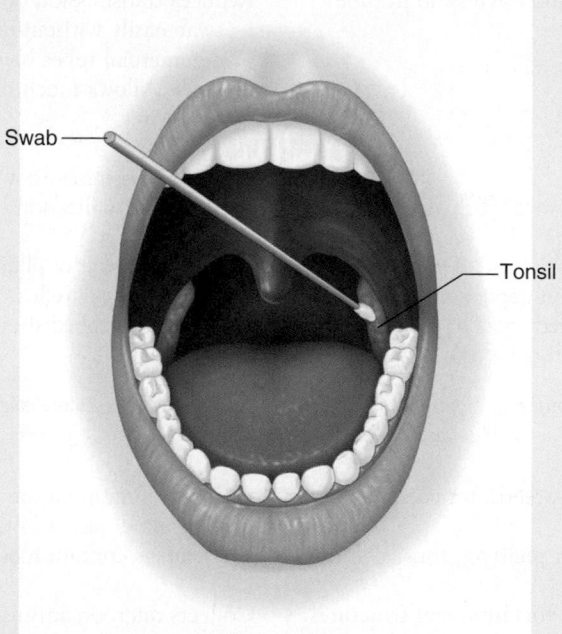

STEP 3e Collecting specimen from posterior pharynx.

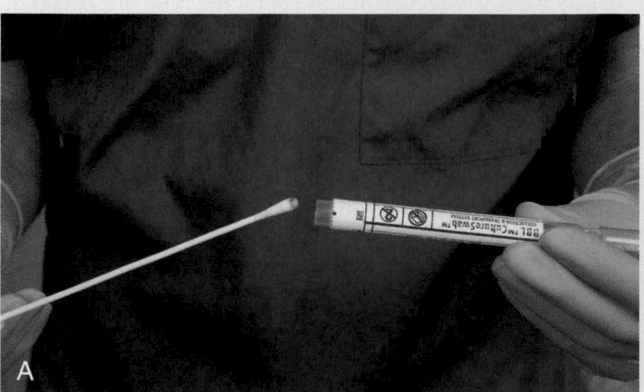
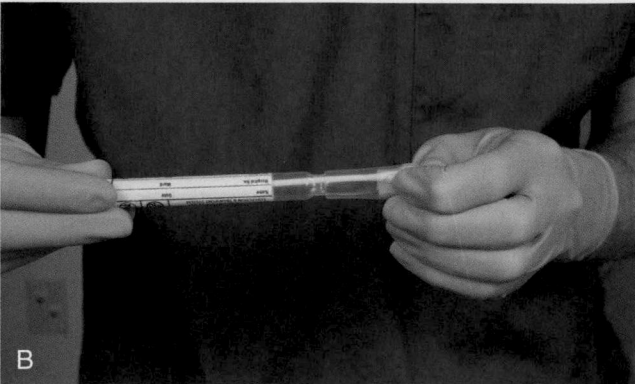

STEP 5 Activating culture tube. **A,** Place swab into tube. **B,** Crush tube to release liquid medium.

STEP	RATIONALE

EVALUATION

1. Check laboratory record for results.

Results reveal type of organisms in nose or pharynx and antibiotics most likely to be effective.

2. Use Teach-Back: "I want to be sure I explained the purpose and procedure for obtaining a throat culture. Please tell me why we are obtaining this culture." Develop a revised teaching plan if patient or caregiver is not able to teach back correctly.

Determines level of understanding of instructional topic.

Unexpected Outcomes	**Related Interventions**
1. Nose and throat cultures reveal bacterial growth.	• Notify health care provider of findings. • Administer medications as prescribed.
2. Patient experiences minor nasal bleeding.	• Apply mild pressure and ice pack over bridge of nose. • Notify health care provider of patient's condition.
3. Specimen is contaminated.	• Repeat specimen collection.

Communication and Documentation

- Document appearance of nasal and oral mucosal structure and specimen collection, date, time, and disposition in nurses' notes in electronic health record (EHR) or chart.
- Document your evaluation of patient and caregiver learning.
- Report unusual test results to health care provider.

Special Considerations
Teaching

- Teach patient that procedure may cause slight discomfort and that gagging is common.
- Discuss reason for time delay in receiving culture results.

Pediatric

- Immobilization of child's head and arms is important when obtaining specimen. You should do this in a firm, gentle, kind manner. Ask another nurse to help if necessary.

- Ask parents to act as coach and suggest that they hold their child on their lap. Do not ask parents to restrain child (Hockenberry & Wilson, 2015).
- Showing tongue depressor and penlight to child and demonstrating how to say "ah" helps to decrease anxiety.
- School-age children will be more cooperative if given opportunity to ask questions about procedure and results.

Gerontological

- Some older persons need help in keeping mouth open to obtain specimen.
- Some older persons have poor dentition. Take care not to break a tooth and consider removal of dentures.

✦ SKILL 9.5   Obtaining Vaginal or Urethral Discharge Specimens

Normally drainage from the vagina or urethra is thin, nonpurulent, whitish or clear, and small in amount. Factors such as poor hygiene practices can cause an accumulation of discharge. If a patient develops an increased amount of discharge or if there is a change in the character of discharge from the vagina or urethra, health care provider follow-up is necessary.

Patients most commonly requiring cultures of vaginal or urethral discharge have signs and symptoms of a sexually transmitted infection (STI) or urinary tract infection (UTI). Patients suspected of having an STI may be embarrassed by their condition. Show respect and understanding toward the patient. When collecting vaginal or urethral specimens, work quickly and calmly, practising person-centred care to maintain the patient's privacy at all times.

Delegation and Collaboration

The skill of obtaining vaginal or urethral discharge specimens cannot be delegated to an unregulated care provider (UCP).

Equipment

- Sterile swab in sterile culture tube (commercially available culture tubes have swab and tube with ampule containing special transport medium)
- Sheet, blanket, or paper drape
- Clean gloves
- Penlight or gooseneck lamp
- Completed identification labels with proper patient identifiers
- Completed laboratory requisition
- Small biohazard plastic bag for delivery of specimen to laboratory (or container specified by employer)

STEP	RATIONALE

ASSESSMENT

1. Identify patient using at least two person-specific identifiers (e.g., full name, date of birth, personal identification number, etc.) according to employer policy. Compare identifiers with information on patient's medical record and laboratory requisition.

Ensures correct patient. Complies with Accreditation Canada standards and improves patient safety (Accreditation Canada, 2019).

2. Assess patient's understanding of need for specimen collection and ability to cooperate with procedure.

Provides you with information on which to base necessary health teaching.

3. Perform hand hygiene and apply clean gloves. Assess condition of external genitalia and urethra, meatus, and vaginal orifice. Observe for redness; swelling; verbalizes of tenderness; and discharge that is whitish, mucoid, or purulent or a whitish discharge such as cottage cheese. Remove and discard gloves and perform hand hygiene. **NOTE:** This step may be done during collection.

Reduces transmission of microorganisms. Assessment findings and specimen test results reveal nature of problem.

4. Ask patient about dysuria, localized pruritus of genitalia, or lower abdominal pain.

Symptoms of urinary tract or vaginal infection.

5. If symptoms suggest STI, gather and record patient's sexual history.

Determines sexual activity and if there has been sexual contact with a person known to have an STI. If culture results are positive, inform patient of need to receive treatment, have sexual partners evaluated if applicable, and refrain from sexual activity during treatment (Pagana et al., 2019).

6. Refer to health care provider's prescription to determine if culture is to be vaginal or urethral.

Patient may require one or both types of cultures.

NURSING DIAGNOSES

- Acute pain
- Anxiety
- Insufficient knowledge regarding specimen collection
- Potential for infection

Related factors/Risk factors are individualized on the basis of patient's condition or needs.

PLANNING

1. Expected outcomes following completion of procedure:
- Specimen is not contaminated.

Results will reveal whether skin cells or mucosal cells have contaminated specimen.

- Vaginal or urethral cultures do not reveal growth of microorganisms.

Evidence of absence of infection.

2. Explain procedure to patient, caregiver, or both. Discuss reason for specimen collection and how patient can help. Instruct female patient not to douche 24 hours before culture is obtained. Male is not to urinate 1 hour before urethral culture is obtained.

Patients who understand procedure are less anxious and more likely to cooperate. Douching of vaginal canal would remove discharge containing pathogens. Urinating by male washes secretions out of urethra (Pagana et al., 2019).

IMPLEMENTATION

1. Perform hand hygiene. Apply clean gloves.

Reduces transmission of microorganisms.

2. Draw bedside curtains or close room door. Place "Do Not Enter" sign on door (if available).

Provides privacy and demonstrates respect as part of person-centred nursing care.

3. Help patient to proper position, raise gown, and drape body parts to be exposed:
a. *Female:* Dorsal recumbent position with sheet draped over each leg and genitalia.
b. *Male:* Sitting on chair or bed or lying supine with sheet draped across lower trunk and genitalia.

Provides easy access to perineal area. Draping minimizes exposure of body parts, minimizing anxiety.

STEP	RATIONALE

IMPLEMENTATION

4. Direct light source onto perineum (may not be needed for male patient). — Allows better visualization of external urethral or vaginal structures.

5. Open culture tube and hold swab in dominant hand. — Provides for easier manipulation of swab during culture collection.

6. Instruct patient to deep breathe slowly. — Helps patient relax. Tensing of muscles around pelvic floor may cause discomfort during swabbing.

7. Obtain specimens.

   a. Female:

   (1) With nondominant hand, fully separate labia to expose vaginal orifice. — Exposes perineum and ensures that specimen is of vaginal discharge.

   (2) Touch tip of swab into discharge pool, being careful not to touch skin or mucosa along perineum or vaginal canal. If no discharge is visible, gently insert swab 1 to 2.5 cm ($\frac{1}{3}$ to 1 inch) into vaginal orifice and rotate before removal. — Discharge contains greatest concentration of microorganisms.

   (3) To expose urethral meatus, use nondominant hand to pull gently on labia minora upward and back to separate. — Allows better visualization of urethral orifice.

   (4) Use swab; gently apply to tip of meatus where discharge is visible. Avoid touching labia. — Discharge contains greatest concentration of microorganisms.

Clinical Decision Point *If discharge near vagina appears different from discharge along perineum, collect separate specimens from each area because, if two organisms are present, they could be cross-contaminated on a single swab. Label specimen with area of patient's body that you swabbed.*

   b. Male:

   (1) Grasp patient's penis proximal to glans with nondominant hand; if male is uncircumcised, gently retract foreskin. — Provides clear exposure of urethral meatus.

   (2) Use dominant hand to hold swab. Apply gently to area of discharge at urinary meatus. — Discharge contains greatest number of microorganisms.

   (3) If no discharge is apparent, health care provider may prescribe swab to be introduced into urinary meatus. Hold male genitalia firmly but gently. — Excess manipulation can cause erection.

   (4) Return foreskin to natural position. — Tightening of foreskin around shaft of penis can cause localized discomfort, edema, and potential necrosis.

8. Return each swab to culture tube and secure top. — Retains microorganisms within tube.

9. If using commercial culture tube, wrap ampule with gauze to prevent injury to your fingers while crushing. Immediately squeeze end of tube to crush ampule (see Skill 9.4). Push tip of swab into fluid medium. — Medium supports life of microorganisms until culture is analyzed.

10. Remove and discard gloves. Perform hand hygiene. — Reduces transmission of microorganisms.

11. Label each culture tube with identification label, affix completed requisition, and confirm identifiers in front of patient (Accreditation Canada, 2019). — Incorrect specimen identification could lead to diagnostic or therapeutic error.

12. Send specimen to laboratory immediately or refrigerate. — Bacteria multiply quickly. Prompt analysis ensures accurate results.

13. Help patient to comfortable position, help with personal hygiene, and remove and discard drape. — Reinforces patient's sense of self-esteem. Reduces transmission of microorganisms.

EVALUATION

1. Review laboratory results for evidence of pathogens. — Results will reveal type of organisms present. Certain organisms are common to vaginal tract. Urethra should be free of microorganisms.

2. Continue to monitor whether discharge is present; if so, observe colour and amount. — Characteristics of discharge indicate specific type of infection.

STEP	RATIONALE

Unexpected Outcomes

1. Vaginal or urethral cultures reveal growth of pathogenic microorganisms.

2. Specimen is contaminated with feces or epidermal cells.

Related Interventions
- Notify health care provider of findings and follow new prescriptions.
- Continue to monitor patient.
- Repeat specimen collection.

Communication and Documentation

- Document types of cultures obtained, and date and time sent to laboratory in nurses' notes in electronic health record (EHR) or chart.
- Document your evaluation of patient and caregiver learning.
- Report laboratory results to health care provider.

Special Considerations
Teaching

- Discuss sexuality and safer sex practices with patient if appropriate.

- Patients with urethral or vaginal discharge often require instruction about perineal hygiene measures.
- Teach patient proper administration route of medication prescribed (e.g., suppositories, topical) (see Chapter 21).

Pediatric

- A second nurse can help with specimen collection from an infant or young child by gently holding child's legs apart in froglike position. Have parent present to encourage cooperation.
- Ensure parents understand that obtaining a vaginal specimen will not affect virginity of the child.

PROCEDURAL GUIDELINE 9.3 *Collecting a Sputum Specimen by Expectoration*

Sputum is mucus produced by cells of the lungs, bronchi, and trachea. A specimen is collected either by having a patient cough and expectorate into a sterile specimen container or by suctioning into a sterile sputum trap (see Skill 9.6). In a healthy patient sputum production is minimal; a disease state can increase the amount and character of sputum. Sputum specimens are collected to identify cancer cells, for culture and sensitivity (C&S), and for acid-fast bacillus to diagnose pulmonary tuberculosis.

Delegation and Collaboration

The skill of collecting a sputum specimen by expectoration can be delegated to an unregulated care provider (UCP). The nurse instructs the UCP to:
- Immediately report the presence of blood in the sputum or changes in patient's vital signs.

Equipment

- Completed identification labels with appropriate patient identifiers
- Completed laboratory requisition
- Small biohazard plastic bag for delivery of specimen to laboratory (or container as specified by employer)
- Sterile specimen container (screw-capped)
- Clean gloves
- Facial tissues
- Emesis basin *(optional)*
- Toothbrush *(optional)*
- Disinfectant swab *(optional)*

Procedural Steps

1. Identify patient using at least two person-specific identifiers according to employer policy. Compare identifiers with information on medical record and laboratory requisition (Accreditation Canada, 2019).
2. Provide opportunity to rinse mouth with water. Patient should not use mouthwash or toothpaste because the products may alter culture results.
3. Perform hand hygiene and apply clean gloves. Provide sputum cup and instruct patient not to touch the inside of the container.
4. Have the patient take three to four deep, slow breaths with full exhalation. Then have patient take full inhalation followed immediately by a forceful cough, expectorating sputum directly into specimen container.
5. Repeat until 5 to 10 mL of sputum (not saliva) has been collected. A minimum of 3 mL must be collected.
6. Secure lid on container tightly. If any sputum is present on outside of container, wipe it off with disinfectant.
7. Offer patient tissues after patient expectorates, dispose of tissues, and offer mouth care.
8. Remove and dispose of gloves. Perform hand hygiene.
9. Securely attach properly completed identification label and laboratory requisition to side of specimen container (not lid). Confirm identifiers in patient's presence.
10. Enclose specimen in a biohazard bag.
11. Send specimen to laboratory immediately.

◆ SKILL 9.6   Collecting a Sputum Specimen by Suction

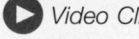 *Video Clip*

Sputum is produced by cells lining the respiratory tract. Although production is minimal in the healthy state, disease states can increase the amount or change the character of sputum. Examination of

sputum aids in the diagnosis and treatment of several conditions, ranging from simple bronchitis to lung cancer.

Suctioning is often indicated to collect sputum from patients unable to spontaneously expectorate a sample for laboratory analysis. Sometimes suctioning provokes violent coughing, which can induce vomiting and constriction of pharyngeal, laryngeal, and bronchial muscles. In addition, it may cause hypoxemia or vagal overload, causing cardiopulmonary compromise and increased intracranial pressure.

Delegation and Collaboration

The skill of collecting sputum specimens by suction cannot be delegated to an unregulated care provider (UCP). The nurse instructs the UCP to:

- Notify the nurse if the patient expectorates bloody sputum.

Equipment

- Completed identification labels with proper patient identifiers
- Completed laboratory requisition
- Suction device (wall or portable)
- Sterile suction catheter (size 14, 16, or 18 Fr or suction catheter with sleeve [see Chapter 25]).
- Sterile gloves and clean gloves
- Sterile water
- In-line specimen container or sputum trap
- Small plastic bag (or a container)
- Oxygen therapy equipment (if indicated)
- Protective eyewear
- Disinfectant wipe

STEP	RATIONALE
ASSESSMENT	
1. Identify patient using at least two person-specific identifiers (e.g., full name, date of birth, personal identification number, etc.) according to employer policy. Compare identifiers with information on patient's medical record and laboratory requisition.	Ensures correct patient. Complies with Accreditation Canada standards and improves patient safety (Accreditation Canada, 2019).
2. Check health care provider's prescriptions for type of sputum analysis and specifications (e.g., amount of sputum, number of specimens, time of collection, method to obtain). Specimens for acid-fast bacillus (AFB) require three consecutive morning samples.	Specific test dictates when or how frequently specimens are collected. The ideal time to collect sputum is early morning because bronchial secretions tend to accumulate during the night. Bacteria also accumulate as secretions pool.
3. Assess patient's level of understanding of procedure and its purpose.	Provides baseline to establish teaching plan.
4. Assess when patient last ate a meal (or had tube feeding).	It is best to obtain specimen 1 to 2 hours after or 1 hour before meal to minimize gagging, which can cause vomiting and aspiration.
5. Determine if help is needed by patient to obtain specimen.	Positioning, postural drainage, and deep-breathing and coughing exercises may improve ability to cough productively. Suctioning is often indicated when patient is unable to cough and expectorate.
6. Assess patient's respiratory status, including respiratory rate, depth, pattern, and colour of mucous membranes.	Active coughing may alter respiratory status. Respiratory status can depend on amount of sputum in tracheobronchial tree.

NURSING DIAGNOSES

- Inadequate airway clearance
- Inadequate breathing pattern
- Insufficient knowledge regarding specimen collection procedures
- Potential for aspiration
- Potential for infection

Related factors/Risk factors are individualized on the basis of patient's condition or needs.

PLANNING

1. Expected outcomes following completion of procedure:	
• Patient's respirations are same rate and character before and after procedure.	Specimen collection did not alter respiratory status.
• Patient maintains comfort level and experiences minimal anxiety.	Suctioning tends to cause anxiety.
• Sputum is not contaminated by saliva or oropharyngeal flora.	Sputum must originate from tracheobronchial tree for accurate results.
• Patient discusses purpose and benefit of sputum collection.	Validates learning.
2. Explain procedure and purpose. Instruct patient to breathe normally during suctioning to prevent hyperventilation.	Promotes understanding and cooperation.

STEP	RATIONALE

IMPLEMENTATION

1. Close curtains or room door.	Provides privacy as part of person-centred care.
2. Position in high- or semi-Fowler's position for suctioning.	Promotes full lung expansion and facilitates ability to cough.

Clinical Decision Point *If patient has surgical incision or localized area of discomfort, have them place pillow or hands firmly over affected area. Splinting of painful area minimizes muscular stretching and discomfort during coughing and thus makes cough more productive.*

3. Perform hand hygiene and apply clean glove to nondominant hand. Prepare suction machine or device and determine if it functions properly.	Adequate amount of suction is necessary to aspirate sputum.
4. Connect suction tube to adapter on sputum trap. Open sterile water (see Chapter 25).	Establishes suction that passes through sputum trap to aspirate specimen.
5. Using sterile technique, apply sterile glove to dominant hand or use clean glove if suction catheter has plastic sleeve.	Tracheobronchial tree is sterile body cavity. Allows you to manipulate suction catheter without contamination.
6. With gloved hand connect sterile suction catheter to rubber tubing on sputum trap.	Aspirated sputum will go directly to trap instead of to suction tubing.
7. Lubricate suction catheter tip with sterile water (*with suction off*).	Lubrication allows for easier insertion of catheter.
8. Gently insert tip of suction catheter through nasopharynx, endotracheal tube, or tracheostomy tube without applying suction (see Chapter 25).	Minimizes trauma to airway as catheter is inserted.
9. Gently and quickly advance catheter into trachea. Warn patient to expect to cough.	Entrance of catheter into larynx and trachea triggers cough reflex.
10. As patient coughs, apply suction for 5 to 10 seconds, collecting 2 to 10 mL of sputum.	Ensures collection of sputum from deep within tracheobronchial tree. Suctioning longer than 10 seconds can cause hypoxia and mucosal damage.
11. Release suction and remove catheter; turn off suction.	Suction can damage mucosa if applied during withdrawal.
12. Detach catheter from specimen trap and dispose of catheter in appropriate receptacle.	Decreases risk for spreading microorganisms.
13. Secure top on specimen container tightly. For sputum trap, detach suction tubing and connect rubber tubing on sputum trap to plastic adapter (see illustration).	Contains microorganisms within container, preventing exposure to personnel handling specimen.
14. If any sputum is present on outside of container, wipe it off with disinfectant.	Prevents spread of infection to people handling specimen.
15. Offer patient tissues after suctioning. Dispose of tissues in emesis basin or appropriate container.	Maintains cleanliness and comfort.
16. Remove and dispose of gloves. Perform hand hygiene.	Reduces transmission of microorganisms.

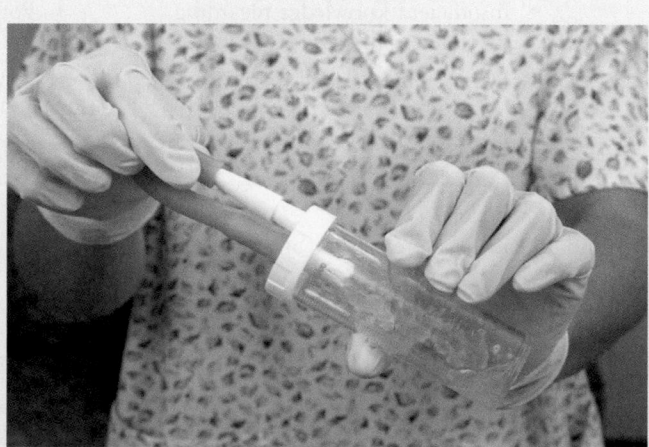

STEP 13 Closing sputum specimen trap.

STEP	RATIONALE

IMPLEMENTATION

17. Label specimen with identification label on side of specimen container (not lid). Confirm person-specific identifiers in front of patient (Accreditation Canada, 2019). Place specimen in small plastic bag (or container specified by employer) and attach requisition.

Incorrect identification could lead to diagnostic or therapeutic error. Plastic bag or container reduces risk of health care worker's exposure to sputum.

18. Send specimen immediately to laboratory or refrigerate.

Bacteria multiply quickly. Prompt analysis ensures accurate results.

19. Offer patient mouth care if desired.

Promotes comfort.

EVALUATION

1. Observe patient's respiratory status throughout procedure, especially during suctioning. If under distress, measure oxygen saturation with pulse oximeter.

Excessive coughing or prolonged suctioning can alter respiratory pattern and cause hypoxia. Determines oxygenation status.

2. Note anxiety or discomfort in patient.

Procedure can be uncomfortable. If patient becomes short of breath, anxiety will develop.

3. Observe character of sputum: colour, consistency, odour, volume, viscosity, and/or presence of blood.

Characteristics may indicate disease entities.

4. Refer to laboratory reports for test results.

Indicates if abnormal cells or microorganisms are present in sputum.

5. Use Teach-Back: "I want to make sure you understand this procedure. Can you repeat back to me the steps we need to do to get this sputum sample?" Develop a plan for revised patient or caregiver teaching if they are not able to repeat back correctly.

Determines level of understanding of instructional topic.

Unexpected Outcomes

1. Patient becomes hypoxic with increased respiratory rate and effort and shortness of breath.

2. Patient remains anxious or reports discomfort from suction catheter.

3. Patient reports pain when coughing to produce sputum.

Related Interventions

- Discontinue suctioning immediately.
- Administer oxygen (if prescribed).
- Notify health care provider of patient's condition.
- Continue to monitor patient's vital signs and pulse oximetry.
- Discontinue procedure until stable.
- Administer oxygen (if prescribed).
- Notify health care provider of patient's change in condition.
- Continue to monitor patient's vital signs and pulse oximetry.
- Encourage patient who is recovering from surgical procedure to splint incision before coughing.
- Obtain prescription for pain medication as needed (prn).
- Inform health care provider of changes in patient's condition.

Communication and Documentation

- Document in nurse's notes in electronic health record (EHR) or chart the method used to obtain specimen, date and time collected, type of test prescribed, and transport to laboratory in nurses' notes. Describe characteristics of sputum specimen. Describe patient's tolerance of procedure.

- Report unusual sputum characteristics to nurse in charge or health care provider.
- Document your evaluation of patient and caregiver learning.
- When laboratory reports are available, report abnormal findings to health care provider. If AFB sputum culture is positive, initiate appropriate isolation techniques.

* Most employer policies require nurses to note on specimen requisition if patient is receiving antibiotics.

Special Considerations
Teaching
* Demonstrate proper splinting technique for postoperative patients.
* If aerosol treatment is indicated, teach patient purpose of procedure, explaining that it will stimulate coughing and sputum expectoration.

Pediatric
* Children need very clear instructions or demonstration for deep breathing. Infants and young children will be unable to cooperate; aerosol treatment may be indicated.
* Use smaller catheter size for young children. It may be possible to elicit a cough by tickling the back of the throat with the suction catheter.

✦ SKILL 9.7 Obtaining Wound Specimens for Culture

NSO *Nursing Skills Online Specimen Collection Module 3 / Lesson 5*

When caring for a patient with a wound, assess the condition of the wound and observe for signs of infection. Localized inflammation, tenderness, warmth, and purulent drainage are signs and symptoms of wound infection. Identification of the causative organism confirms an infection and provides guidelines for accurate treatment. A wound specimen is analyzed to determine the type and number of pathogenic microorganisms. Additionally, a specimen may be collected from a wound site or other sites such as the rectum, groin, or nares for the purpose of screening to identify patients colonized by methicillin-resistant *Staphylococcus aureus* (MRSA), vancomycin-resistant enterococci (VRE), or both. Identification of these patients ensures infection prevention measures are put in place.

Collect a wound specimen from fresh exudate in the centre of a wound, from an area of viable tissue (Copeland-Halperin, Kaminsky, Bluefeld, et al., 2016). Cleansing the wound with sterile normal saline prior to obtaining a sample is necessary to rid the wound of old exudate, and recover specimen at and below the level of the wound bed surface (Spichler, Hurwitz, Armstrong, et al., 2015). This minimizes the risk of contaminating the sample with skin flora, necrotic tissue, or slough (Copeland-Halperin, et al., 2016). Resident colonies of bacteria on the skin grow in wound exudate and may not be the true causative organisms of infection. Deeper wound tissue specimens provide a collection of bacteria that is a more accurate indication of the causative organisms (Haalboom, Blokhuis-Arkes, Beuk, et al., 2018). Use separate techniques to collect specimens for measuring aerobic versus anaerobic microorganisms. Aerobic organisms grow in superficial wounds exposed to the air. Anaerobic organisms grow deep within body cavities, where oxygen is not normally present.

Delegation and Collaboration
The skill of obtaining wound tissue specimens cannot be delegated to an unregulated care provider (UCP). The nurse instructs the UCP to:
* Report foul odour, increase in drainage, and increase in temperature or if patient reports discomfort.

Equipment
* Sterile swab in culture tube for aerobic culture (with transport medium)
* Sterile swab in culture tube for anaerobic culture (contains carbon dioxide or nitrogen gas)
* 30–60 mL irrigation syringe and 19- to 20-gauge cathlon
* 5–10 mL safety syringe and 19-gauge needle (for anaerobic culture) (**NOTE:** *Syringe sampling may not be done in some facilities; check employer policy.*)
* Two pairs of clean gloves
* Protective eyewear (optional)
* Sterile dressing tray and materials (determined by type of dressing, to redress wound)
* Paper or plastic disposable bag
* Completed specimen identification label with proper patient identifiers
* Completed laboratory requisition
* Small plastic biohazard bag (or container)

STEP	RATIONALE

ASSESSMENT

1. Identify patient using at least two person-specific identifiers (e.g., full name, date of birth, personal identification number, etc.) according to employer policy. Compare identifiers with information on patient's medical record and laboratory requisition.

Ensures correct patient. Complies with Accreditation Canada standards and improves patient safety (Accreditation Canada, 2019).

2. Assess patient's understanding of need for wound culture and ability to cooperate with procedure.

Use data to develop teaching plan. A wound is a painful site. Collection of specimen may cause anxiety or fear.

3. Assess patient for signs of fever, chills, or excessive thirst. Note in medical record laboratory results if white blood cell (WBC) count is elevated.

Signs and symptoms indicate systemic infection.

STEP	RATIONALE

ASSESSMENT

4. Assess patient's pain at wound site using an appropriate pain assessment tool. If patient requires analgesic before dressing changes, give medication 30 minutes before beginning procedure to reach peak effect.

Pain at wound site often increases with infection.

5. Determine when dressing change is scheduled (see Chapters 39 and 40). Perform wound assessment as part of actual procedure.

6. Review health care provider's prescriptions for aerobic or anaerobic culture.

Specimens are taken from different sites and placed in different containers, depending on type of culture.

NURSING DIAGNOSES

- Acute pain
- Persistent pain
- Reduced tissue integrity

- Insufficient knowledge regarding wound drainage culture procedure
- Anxiety

- Potential for infection
- Potential for injury

Related factors/Risk factors are individualized on the basis of patient's condition or needs.

PLANNING

1. Expected outcomes following completion of procedure:
   - Wound culture does not reveal bacterial growth.
   - Culture swab is free of contamination from skin bacteria.
   - Patient discusses purpose and procedure for specimen collection.

Wound remains free of pathogenic microorganisms.
Test results indicate type of cells present.
Validates learning.

2. Determine if analgesia is necessary. Administer analgesic 30 minutes before dressing change and/or specimen collection.

Minimizes discomfort during procedure. Provides person-centred care.

3. Explain reason for wound culture and how it will be collected.

Promotes understanding and cooperation and eases anxiety.

4. Explain that patient may feel tickling sensation when wound is swabbed.

Anticipation of expected sensations minimizes anxiety.

IMPLEMENTATION

1. Close bedside curtains or door to room.

Provides privacy.

2. Perform hand hygiene and apply clean gloves.

Gloves minimize exposure to microorganisms.

3. Remove old dressings covering wound. Fold soiled sides of dressing together and dispose. Remove soiled gloves, perform hand hygiene, then apply clean gloves. Observe wound for swelling, separation of wound edges, inflammation, and drainage.

Signs indicate wound infection.
Provides baseline for condition of wound.

4. Thoroughly cleanse wound with sterile normal saline or sterile water as per employer policy. Ensure peri-wound skin is cleansed from edges outward.

Removes old exudate containing skin flora, preventing possible contamination of specimen.
Larger amounts of solution may be required for larger wounds.

5. Use sterile gauze to remove excess normal saline or water from the wound surface. Ensure a 1 cm × 1 cm (0.4 × 0.4 inch) area of viable wound bed tissue is visible.

Ensures that the swab is collected from viable tissue, not necrotic slough, pooled exudates, or eschars (as surface pathogens are often contaminants).

6. Obtain cultures:
   a. **Aerobic culture**
      (1) Carefully open sterile swab in culture tube. Rotate tip of swab over 1 cm × 1 cm (0.4 × 0.4 inch) area of viable tissue in centre of wound for 5 seconds (Levine technique). Use sufficient pressure to extract exudate from wound. Avoid touching wound edge or peri-wound skin with swab. Immediately place swab into culture tube and ensure tip of swab is in contact with medium.

For dry wounds, the swab can be pre-moistened in the transport medium or with sterile normal saline before swabbing wound.
The swab should be coated with fresh exudate from wound.
If there are multiple wounds in the same location, use separate swabs for each.
Medium preserves bacteria until laboratory analysis is complete.

STEP	RATIONALE

IMPLEMENTATION

b. Anaerobic culture

(1) Take swab from special anaerobic culture tube, swab deeply into draining body cavity, and rotate gently. Remove swab and return to culture tube.

Specimen is taken from deep cavity where oxygen is not present. Carbon dioxide or nitrogen gas keeps organisms alive until analysis is complete. Air injected into tube would cause organisms to die.

Or

(2) Insert tip of syringe (without needle) into wound and aspirate 5 to 10 mL of exudate. Attach 19-gauge needle, expel all air, and inject drainage into special culture tube.

Sterile large-bore needle (19-gauge) allows exudate to be transferred from sterile syringe into special culture tube without contamination.

7. Remove and dispose of gloves. Perform hand hygiene.

Reduces transfer of microorganisms.

8. Place correct specimen label on each culture tube. Verify person-specific identifiers in front of patient (Accreditation Canada, 2019). **NOTE:** Indicate on specimen if patient is receiving antibiotics.

Ensures correct results for correct patient.

9. Send specimens to laboratory immediately.

Bacteria multiple rapidly. Prompt analysis ensures accurate results.

10. Perform wound dressing change as per health care provider's prescription and/or employer policy. Apply new sterile dressing (see Chapters 39 and 40) using aseptic technique.

Protects wound from further contamination; aids in absorbing drainage and debridement of wound.

11. Remove and dispose of gloves and soiled supplies in appropriate receptacle according to employer policy. Perform hand hygiene.

Reduces transmission of microorganisms.

12. Help patient to comfortable position.

Promotes patient's ability to relax.

EVALUATION

1. Obtain laboratory report for results of cultures.

Report indicates if pathogenic organisms are identified.

2. Observe character of wound drainage.

Characteristics can reveal abnormal status and infection.

3. Observe edges of wound for redness and bleeding.

Indicates trauma to healing tissue.

4. **Use Teach-Back:** "I want to make sure you understand what needs to be done to get this sample. Can you tell me the steps of the procedure?" Develop a revised teaching plan if patient or caregiver is not able to teach back correctly.

Determines level of understanding of instructional topic.

Unexpected Outcomes	Related Interventions
1. Wound cultures reveal bacterial growth.	• Monitor patient for fever, chills, or excessive thirst, which indicate systemic infection.
	• Inform health care provider of findings.
2. Wound culture is contaminated from superficial skin cells.	• Monitor patient for fever and pain.
	• Inform health care provider of findings.
	• Repeat collection of specimen as prescribed.
3. Patient reports increased pain.	• Provide analgesia.
	• Notify health care provider.

Communication and Documentation

- Document types of specimens obtained, source, and time and date sent to laboratory and describe appearance of wound and characteristics of drainage in nurses' notes in electronic health record (EHR) or chart.
- Report any evidence of infection to the health care provider.
- Document your evaluation of patient and caregiver learning.
- Document patient's reaction to procedure and response to analgesics.

Special Considerations
Teaching

- Instruct patient to inform you if procedure causes pain or if you need to stop because patient is unable to tolerate pain.
- Teach patient to assess status of wound for changes and signs and symptoms of infection.

Pediatric

- If procedure is to be performed on a child and is anticipated to be painful, some agencies prefer performing it in an area other

than child's room to maintain feeling that child's room is a safe place (Hockenberry & Wilson, 2015).

- It is often helpful to have an additional nurse or other adult available to help with specimen collection in a young child or infant.

Care in the Community
- Teach patient antiseptic practices (e.g., handwashing, disposal of dressings, and clean technique for applying dressing).

✦ **SKILL 9.8**	**Collecting Blood Specimens and Culture by Venipuncture (Syringe and Vacutainer Method)**

NSO *Nursing Skills Online Caring for Central Vascular Access Devices (CVAD) Module 14 / Lesson 2*

Blood tests are one of the most common diagnostic aids in the care and evaluation of patients. Tests allow health care providers to screen patients for early signs of physical illness, monitor changes in acute or chronic diseases, and evaluate responses to therapies.

With some employers, the nurse is responsible for collecting blood specimens; however, many employers have specially trained phlebotomists who are responsible for drawing venous blood. Be familiar with your employer policies and procedures for drawing blood samples.

The three methods of obtaining blood specimens are (1) venipuncture, (2) skin puncture, and (3) arterial puncture. All procedures require sterile technique. Venipuncture is the most common method of obtaining blood specimens. This method involves inserting a hollow-bore needle into the lumen of a large vein to obtain a specimen using either a needle and syringe or a Vacutainer device that allows the drawing of multiple samples. Because veins are major sources of blood for laboratory testing and routes for intravenous (IV) fluid or blood replacement, maintaining their integrity is essential. The nurse needs to be skilled in venipuncture to avoid unnecessary injury to veins.

Skin puncture, also called *capillary puncture*, is the least traumatic method of obtaining a blood specimen. A sterile lancet or needle is used to puncture a vascular area on a finger or earlobe in an adult or child. The nurse places a drop of blood on a test slide, wicks a drop of blood to a test slide, or collects it within a thin glass capillary tube for laboratory analysis. Changes in health care economics and delivery have resulted in the increased use of skin puncture. Point-of-care clinical laboratory tests at the bedside most frequently involve skin puncture (Pagana et al., 2019).

Blood cultures aid in detection of bacteria in the blood. It is important that at least two culture specimens be drawn from two different sites. Because bacteremia may be accompanied by fever and chills, blood cultures should be drawn when these symptoms are present (Pagana et al., 2019). Bacteremia exists when both cultures grow the infectious agent. Only one culture growing bacteria is considered contamination. All cultures should be drawn before antibiotic therapy begins because the antibiotic may interrupt the growth of an organism in the laboratory. If the patient is receiving antibiotics, notify the laboratory and inform them of specific antibiotics the patient is receiving (Pagana et al., 2019).

Delegation and Collaboration

The skill of collecting blood specimens by venipuncture can be delegated to a specially trained unregulated care provider (UCP). In some facilities phlebotomists obtain the venipuncture samples. Employer and government regulations and policies differ regarding personnel who may draw blood specimens. The nurse informs the UCP to:

- Report any patient discomfort or signs of excessive bleeding from the puncture site to the nurse.

Equipment
All Procedures
- Clean gloves
- Small pillow or folded towel
- Tourniquet
- Chlorhexidine 2% in 70% alcohol swabs or other antiseptic (check employer policy)
- Sterile 5 × 5–cm (2 × 2–inch) gauze
- Adhesive bandage or adhesive tape
- Completed identification labels with proper patient identifiers
- Completed laboratory requisition
- Small plastic biohazard bag (or container)
- Sharps container

Venipuncture With Syringe
- Sterile safety needles (20- to 21-gauge for adults; 23- to 25-gauge for children)
- Sterile 10- to 20-mL Luer-Lok syringes
- Blood transfer device (needleless)
- Appropriate blood specimen tubes

Venipuncture With Vacutainer
- Vacutainer with Luer-Lok adapter
- Sterile double needles or butterfly needles (20- to 21-gauge for adults; 23- to 25-gauge for children)
- Appropriate blood specimen tubes

Blood Cultures
- Sterile double needles or butterfly needles (20- to 21-gauge for adults; 23- to 25-gauge for children)
- Two or three 20- to 30-mL sterile syringes
- Culture bottle adapters
- Anaerobic and aerobic culture bottles (check employer policy)

Central Venous Catheter Collection
- Two empty 10-mL sterile syringes
- Sterile 10-mL normal saline flushes
- Vacutainer with Luer-Lok adapter
- Culture bottle adapters
- Appropriate blood specimen tubes

STEP	RATIONALE

ASSESSMENT

1. Identify patient using at least two person-specific identifiers (e.g., full name, date of birth, personal identification number, etc.) according to employer policy. Compare identifiers with information on patient's medical record and laboratory requisition.

Ensures correct patient. Complies with Accreditation Canada standards and improves patient safety (Accreditation Canada, 2019).

2. Determine whether patient understands purpose of procedure and ability to cooperate.

Provides data for you to establish teaching plan and provides emotional support. Some patients' past experiences increase anxiety.

3. Determine if special conditions need to be met before specimen collection (e.g., patient allowed nothing by mouth [NPO], specific time for collection in relation to medication given, need to ice specimen).

Some tests require meeting specific conditions to obtain accurate measurement of blood elements (e.g., fasting blood sugar, drug peak and trough level, timed endocrine hormone levels).

4. Assess patient for possible risks associated with venipuncture: anticoagulant therapy, low platelet count, bleeding disorders (history of hemophilia). Review medication history.

Patient history may include abnormal clotting abilities caused by low platelet count, hemophilia, or medications that increase risk for bleeding and hematoma formation.

5. Assess patient for contraindicated sites for venipuncture: presence of IV infusion, hematoma at potential site, arm on side of mastectomy, or hemodialysis shunt.

Drawing specimens from such sites can result in false test results or may injure patient. Samples taken from vein near IV infusion may be diluted or contain concentrations of IV fluids. Postmastectomy patients may have reduced lymphatic drainage in arm on operative side, increasing risk for infection from needle-sticks. Never use arteriovenous shunt to obtain specimens because of risks for clotting and bleeding. Hematoma indicates existing injury to vessel wall.

6. Identify presence of tape sensitivities or latex allergies.

Requires voiding exposure to these items.

7. Before drawing blood cultures, assess for systemic signs and symptoms of bacteremia, including fever and chills.

Three blood culture samples should be drawn at least 1 hour apart, beginning at the earliest signs of sepsis (Pagana et al., 2019).

8. Review health care provider's prescriptions for type of tests.

Multiple samples are often needed. A health care provider's prescription is required.

Clinical Decision Point *Some specimens have special collection requirements before or after specimen collection; examples follow:*
- *Cryoglobulin levels: Place tube in warm water for transport.*
- *Ammonia and ionized calcium levels: Place tube in ice for transport.*
- *Lactic acid levels: Do not use tourniquet.*
- *Vitamin levels: Avoid exposure of test tube to light.*

NURSING DIAGNOSES

- Anxiety
- Fear

- Insufficient knowledge regarding blood specimen collection process

- Potential for injury
- Potential for infection

Related factors/Risk factors are individualized on the basis of patient's condition or needs.

PLANNING

1. Expected outcomes following completion of procedure:
- Venipuncture site shows no evidence of continued bleeding or hematoma at venipuncture site after specimen collection.

Indicates that hemostasis is achieved.

- Patient denies anxiety or discomfort.

Explanation relieves anxiety; procedure is performed quickly. Removal of painful stimulus lessens anxiety.

- An adequate sample is collected for testing (see employer policy or laboratory manual).

Appropriate laboratory analysis can be conducted.

- Patient discusses purpose, procedure, and benefits of venipuncture.

Validates learning.

2. Explain procedure to patient: describe purpose of tests; explain how sensation of tourniquet, alcohol swab, and needle-stick will feel.

Anticipatory guidance helps to reduce anxiety.

STEP	RATIONALE

IMPLEMENTATION

1. Bring equipment to bedside and organize.

   Facilitates procedure.

2. Close bedside curtain or room door. Perform hand hygiene.

   Provides for privacy. Reduces transmission of infection.

3. Raise or lower bed to comfortable working height.

   Reduces strain on your back muscles and improves access to venipuncture site.

4. Help patient to supine or semi-Fowler's position with arms extended to form straight line from shoulders to wrists. Place small pillow or towel under upper arm. (*Option:* Lower arm briefly so it fills veins in hand and lower arm with blood.)

   Helps to stabilize extremity because arms are most common sites of venipuncture. Supported position in bed reduces chance of injury to patient if fainting occurs.

5. Apply tourniquet so it can be removed by pulling an end with single motion.

   Tourniquet blocks venous return to heart from extremity, causing veins to dilate for easier visibility.

   a. Position tourniquet 5 to 10 cm (2 to 4 inches) above venipuncture site selected (antecubital fossa site is most often used).

   b. Cross tourniquet over patient's arm (see illustration). You may place it over gown sleeve to protect skin.

   Older person's skin is very fragile.

   c. Hold tourniquet between your fingers close to arm. Tuck loop between patient's arm and tourniquet so you can grasp free end easily (see illustration).

   Pull free end to release tourniquet after venipuncture.

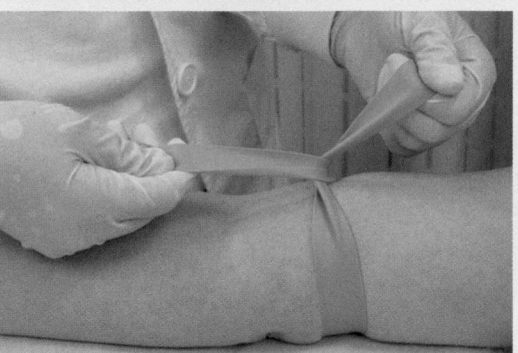

STEP 5b Cross tourniquet over arm.

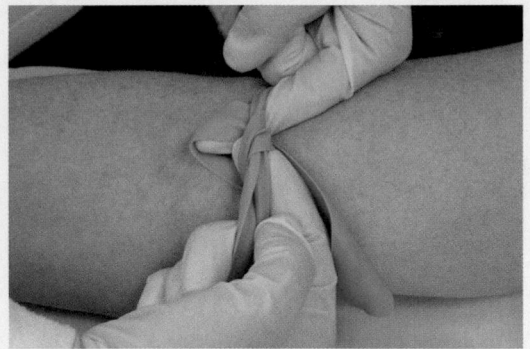

STEP 5c Tuck loop between patient's arm and tourniquet.

Clinical Decision Point *Palpate distal pulse (e.g., radial) below tourniquet. If pulse is not palpable, remove tourniquet, wait 60 seconds, and reapply it more loosely. If tourniquet is too tight, pressure will impede arterial blood flow.*

6. Do not keep tourniquet on patient longer than 1 minute.

   Prolonged tourniquet application causes stasis, localized acidemia, and hemoconcentration (Pagana et al., 2019).

7. Quickly inspect extremity for best venipuncture site, looking for straight, prominent vein without swelling or hematoma. Of three veins located in antecubital area, median cubital vein is preferred (see illustration).

   Straight and intact veins are easiest to puncture.

8. Apply clean gloves. Palpate selected vein with finger (see illustration). Note if vein is firm and rebounds when palpated or if it feels rigid or cordlike and rolls when palpated. Avoid vigorously slapping vein, which can cause vasospasm.

   Patent, healthy vein is elastic and rebounds on palpation. Thrombosed vein is rigid, rolls easily, and is difficult to puncture.

9. Obtain blood specimen.

   a. Syringe method

   (1) Have syringe with appropriate needle securely attached.

   Needle must not dislodge from syringe during venipuncture.

   (2) Clean site with antiseptic, with first swab moving back and forth on horizontal plane, another swab on vertical plane, and last in circular motion from site outward a 5 cm × 5 cm (2 inch × 2 inch) area for 30 seconds. Allow to dry for approximately 30 seconds.

   Antimicrobial agent cleans skin surface of resident bacteria so that organisms do not enter puncture site. Allowing antiseptic to dry completes its antimicrobial task and reduces "sting" of venipuncture. Alcohol left on skin can cause hemolysis of sample and retraction of tissue away from puncture site.

STEP	RATIONALE

IMPLEMENTATION

(a) If drawing sample for blood alcohol level or blood cultures, use only antiseptic swab rather than alcohol swab.

Ensures accurate test results.

(3) Remove needle cover and inform patient that "stick" lasts only a few seconds.

Patient has better control over anxiety when prepared for what to expect.

(4) Place thumb or forefinger of nondominant hand 2.5 cm (1 inch) below site and gently pull skin taut. Stretch skin steadily until vein is stabilized.

Stabilizes vein and prevents rolling during needle insertion.

(5) Hold syringe and needle at 10- to 30-degree angle from patient's arm with bevel up.

Reduces chance of penetrating both sides of vein during insertion. Bevel up decreases chance of contamination by not dragging bevel opening over skin and allows point of needle to first puncture skin, reducing trauma.

(6) Slowly insert needle into vein, stopping when "pop" is felt as needle enters vein (see illustration).

Prevents puncture through vein to opposite side.

(7) Hold syringe securely and pull back gently on plunger.

Syringe held securely prevents needle from advancing. Pulling on plunger creates vacuum needed to draw blood into syringe. If plunger is pulled back too quickly, pressure may collapse vein.

(8) Observe for blood return (see illustration).

If blood flow fails to appear, needle may not be in vein.

(9) Obtain desired amount of blood, keeping needle stabilized.

Test results are more accurate when required amount of blood is obtained. Some tests cannot be performed without minimal blood requirement. Movement of needle increases discomfort.

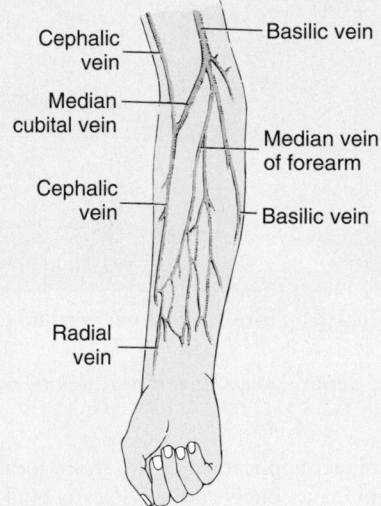

Cephalic vein
Basilic vein
Median cubital vein
Median vein of forearm
Cephalic vein
Basilic vein
Radial vein

STEP 7 Location of antecubital veins.

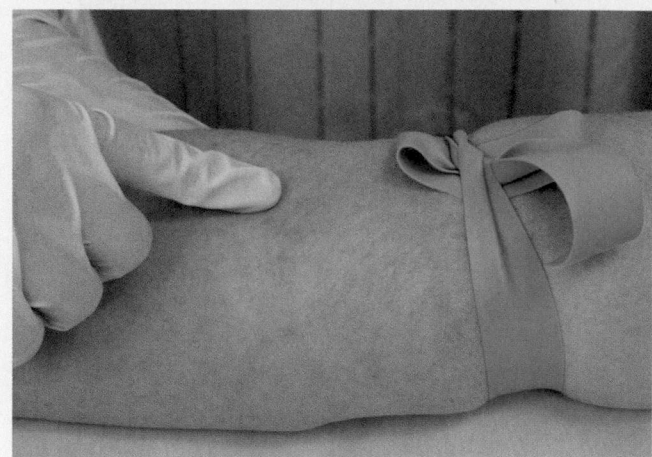

STEP 8 Palpate vein.

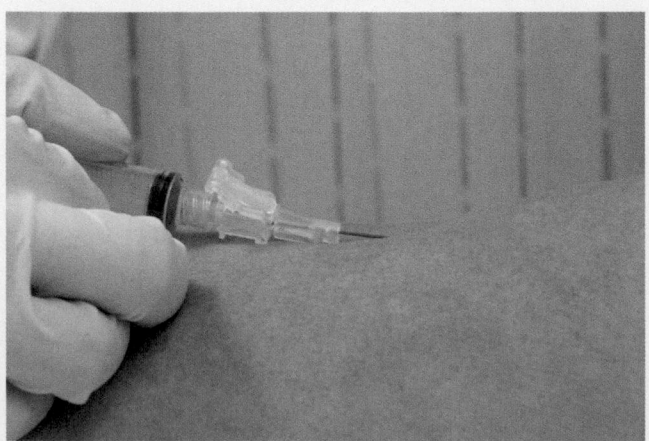

STEP 9a(6) Insert needle into vein.

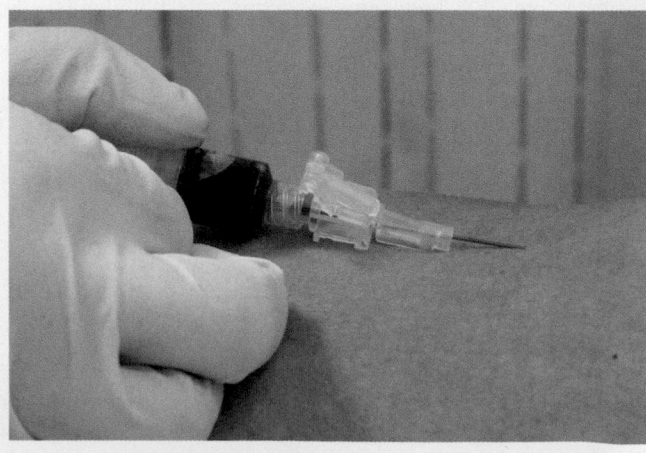

STEP 9a(8) Observe for blood return.

STEP	RATIONALE

IMPLEMENTATION

(10) After obtaining specimen, release tourniquet.

(11) Apply 5 × 5–cm (2 × 2–inch) gauze over site without applying pressure. Quickly but carefully withdraw needle from vein and apply pressure following removal of needle (see illustration) for 2 to 3 minutes or until bleeding stops. Check for hematoma.

(12) Activate safety cover and immediately discard needle in sharps container.

(13) Attach blood-filled syringe to needle-free blood transfer device. Attach tube and allow vacuum to fill tube to specified level. Remove and fill other tubes as appropriate (see illustration). Gently rotate each tube back and forth per specified tube or test requirements.

b. Vacutainer system method

(1) Attach double-ended needle or butterfly needle to Vacutainer tube (see illustration for double-ended needle).

Reduces bleeding at site when needle is withdrawn.

Pressure over needle can cause discomfort. Careful removal of needle minimizes discomfort and vein trauma.

Hematoma may cause compression injury (McCall & Tankersley, 2015).

Prevents needle-stick injury.

Additives prevent clotting. Proper mixing of tubes ensures that culture medium is blended with blood (Alberta Health Services, 2017). Shaking can cause hemolysis of red blood cells (RBCs).

Over-mixing of coagulation tubes may trigger the blood-clotting cascade pathway (Alberta Health Services, 2017).

Long end of needle is used to puncture vein. Short end covered with rubber is inserted into Vacutainer and is used to puncture blood tubes.

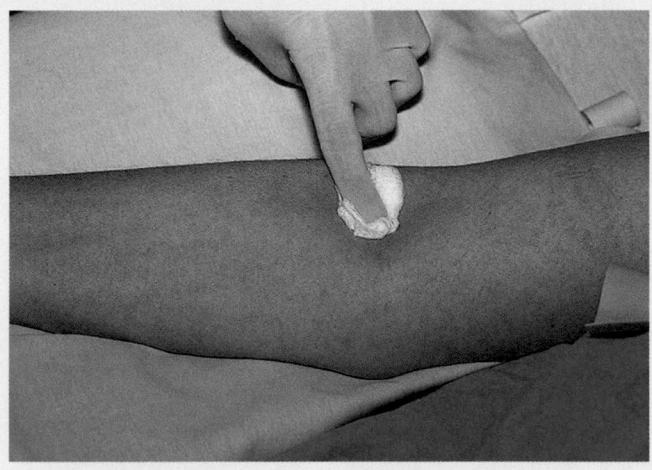

STEP 9a(11) Apply gauze to puncture site.

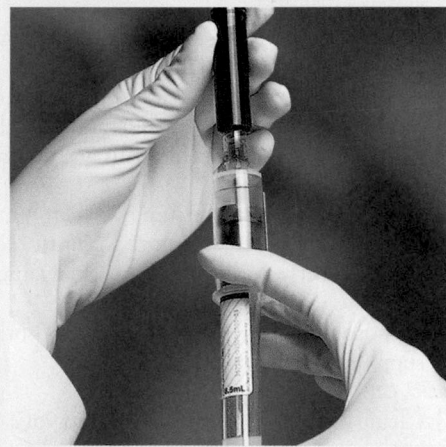

STEP 9a(13) Attach blood-filled syringe to needle-free blood transfer device.

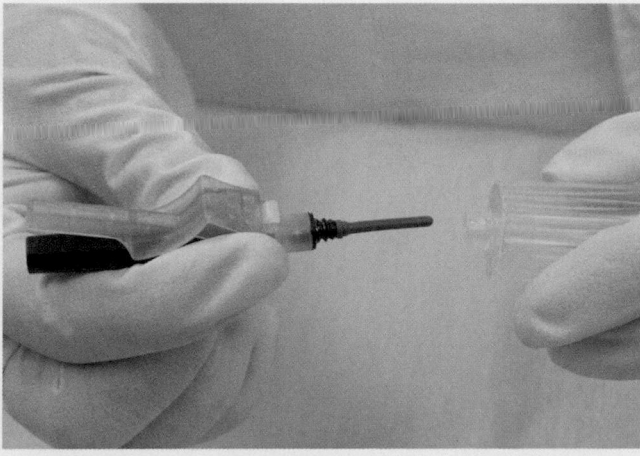

STEP 9b(1) Attach double-ended needle to Vacutainer tube.

STEP	RATIONALE

IMPLEMENTATION

(2) Have proper blood tube resting inside Vacutainer device but do not puncture rubber stopper on tube.

Puncturing causes loss of tube vacuum.

(3) Clean venipuncture site by following Steps 9a(2) and 9a(2)(a) for antiseptic swab. Allow to dry.

Cleans skin surface of resident bacteria so organisms do not enter puncture site. Drying maximizes effect of antiseptic.

(4) Remove needle cover and inform patient that "stick" will occur, lasting only a few seconds.

Patient has better control over anxiety when prepared about what to expect.

(5) Place thumb or forefinger of nondominant hand 2.5 cm (1 inch) *below* site and gently pull skin taut. Stretch skin down until vein stabilizes.

Helps to stabilize vein and prevent rolling during needle insertion.

(6) Hold needle at 10- to 30-degree angle from patient's skin with bevel up.

Smallest and sharpest point of needle will puncture skin first. Reduces chance of penetrating sides of vein during insertion. Keeping bevel up causes less trauma to vein.

(7) Slowly insert needle into vein (see illustration).

Prevents puncture on opposite side.

(8) Grasp Vacutainer securely and advance tube into needle with rubber (do not advance other needle end into vein).

Pushing tube through stopper breaks vacuum and causes flow of blood into tube. If needle in vein advances, vein may become punctured on other side.

(9) Note flow of blood into tube, which should be fairly rapid (see illustration).

Failure of blood to appear indicates that vacuum in tube is lost or needle is not in vein.

(10) After filling specimen tube, firmly grasp Vacutainer firmly and remove tube. Insert additional tubes as needed (and in the correct order). Gently rotate each tube back and forth as per specified tube or test requirements.

Vacuum in tube stops flow at amount to be collected. Grasping prevents needle from advancing or dislodging. Tube should fill completely because additives in certain tubes are measured in proportion to filled tube. Ensures proper mixing with additive to prevent clotting.

(11) After last tube is filled and removed from Vacutainer, release tourniquet.

Reduces bleeding at site when needle is withdrawn.

(12) Apply 5 × 5–cm (2 × 2–inch) gauze over puncture site without applying pressure and quickly but carefully withdraw needle with Vacutainer from vein.

Pressure over needle can cause discomfort. Careful removal of needle minimizes discomfort and vein trauma.

(13) Immediately apply pressure over venipuncture site with gauze for 2 to 3 minutes or until bleeding stops. Observe for hematoma. Tape gauze dressing securely.

Direct pressure minimizes bleeding and prevents hematoma formation. Hematoma may cause compression and nerve injury. Pressure dressing controls bleeding.

(14) Dispose of syringe, needle, gauze, and other supplies in appropriate containers.

Safe disposal of supplies exposed to body fluids prevents transfer of microorganisms.

c. Blood culture

(1) Clean venipuncture site as in Step 9a(2) with antiseptic swab or follow employer policy. Allow to dry.

Antimicrobial agent cleans skin surface so that organisms do not enter puncture site or contaminate culture. Drying ensures complete antimicrobial action and decreases stinging.

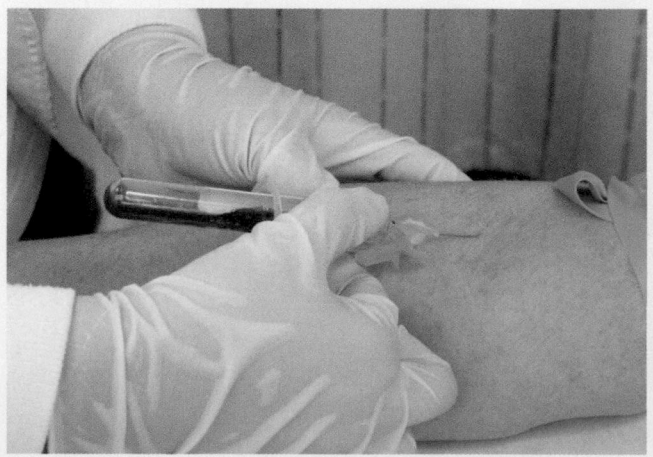

STEP 9b(9) Blood flowing into tube.

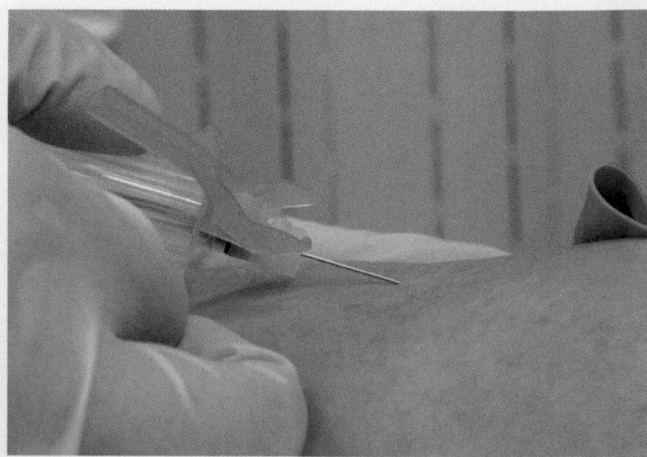

STEP 9b(7) Insert needle into vein.

STEP	RATIONALE

IMPLEMENTATION

(2) Remove caps off culture bottles and cleanse tops for 30 seconds with antiseptic. Allow to dry for 1 minute.

Ensures that bottle top is sterile.

(3) Collect required volumes of blood (as per employer policy), using syringe method (see Step 9a) with two 20- or 30-mL syringes **or** using a double-ended needle or butterfly needle attached directly to culture bottle via bottle adapter. Ensure collection of specimen from two separate venipuncture sites.

The optimum blood volume level for each culture bottle is 20 mL; the minimum required for each culture bottle is 5 mL (Long & Koyfman, 2016, p. 535). Pediatric volumes and collection methods may vary (e.g., less volume required, less number of bottles, etc.).

At least two blood cultures must be collected from two different sites to confirm culture growth (Long & Koyfman, 2016, p. 535).

(4) With each specimen, activate needle safety guard and remove and discard needles. If using **syringe method**, replace with new sterile needles and then inject each blood specimen into culture bottles. If using **double-ended needle** or **butterfly needle**, use bottle adapters to allow direct flow of blood into culture bottles.

Maintains sterile technique and prevents contamination of specimen.

(5) If both aerobic and anaerobic cultures are needed, fill aerobic bottle first.

(6) Gently mix blood in each culture bottle.

Mixes medium and blood.

d. Central venous catheter (CVC) collection

(1) Select appropriate port on catheter (see illustration). Turn off all infusions and clamp lumens.

If more than one lumen, select distal lumen, if possible. Prevents dilution of sample with medication or total parenteral nutrition (TPN).

(2) Cleanse selected port's Luer-Lok access cap with antiseptic and/or remove Luer-Lok disinfecting cap (e.g., DualCap, SwabCap) (see illustrations). Attach 10-mL prefilled normal saline syringe to selected port. Open clamp. Aspirate for blood return. Flush 10 to 20 mL normal saline (NS) using turbulent (push-pause) flow (or as per employer policy). Do not use syringe smaller than 10 mL.

Antiseptic-impregnated caps are recommended for use in conjunction with frictional antiseptic wiping between applications and access (Moureau & Flynn, 2015). The disinfecting cap eliminates issue of disinfecting CVC ports adequately. Aspirating and flushing ensures patency of selected lumen and catheter in vein. Check employer policy for specified flushing volume.

Pressure from small syringe may damage catheter.

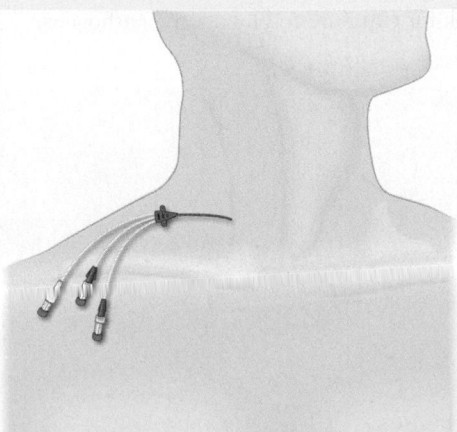

STEP 9d(1) Triple-lumen central venous catheter; select appropriate distal lumen port.

STEP 9d(2a) Disinfecting cap system. Disinfects and protects both IV catheter needleless Luer access and end of IV tubing.

STEP	RATIONALE

IMPLEMENTATION

(3) For **syringe method**, use same syringe and immediately aspirate 5–7 mL of blood for discard, reclamp catheter, then remove and discard syringe. Attach 10- to 20-mL Luer-Lok syringe, unclamp catheter, and aspirate desired amount of blood for sample. Reclamp catheter and remove specimen syringe. To transfer blood from syringe to specimen tube, use blood transfer device with Luer-Lok adapter. Attach specimen syringe to blood transfer device via Luer-Lok, then insert tube into blood transfer device.

Discard ensures that blood sample is not contaminated with IV fluids, medication, or other products.
Check employer policy for specific discard amounts.
Tubes have vacuum and automatically fill to necessary amount.

(4) For **Vacutainer method,** clamp catheter, and remove syringe used for flushing. Attach Vacutainer with Luer-Lok adapter, unclamp catheter, and advance tube into Vacutainer to activate blood flow. Allow blood to fill tube, clamp catheter, and discard first tube. Attach specimen tube to Vacutainer, unclamp catheter, and obtain blood specimen (see illustration). Remove Vacutainer after all specimens collected.

Tubes have vacuum and automatically fill to necessary amount.

(5) After all specimens are collected, clamp catheter.

(6) Attach prefilled NS syringe(s) and flush with 10 to 20 mL NS using push-pause method (volume as per employer policy). To lock lumen, ensure correct solution (heparin or saline) and pressure for cap is instilled. Neutral and positive pressure caps are designed for syringe to be removed, and the lumen will be automatically locked. For caps without automatic neutral or positive pressure, hold syringe plunger steady at completion of flush, lock off lumen with clamp, and remove syringe.

Push-pause creates turbulence that helps to clear lumen. Neutral fluid displacement cap designs (e.g., One-Link [Baxter]) prevent blood from flowing into tip of catheter and forming clot and lower the risk of bloodstream infections.

(7) Blood tubes contain additives; gently rotate back and forth 8 to 10 times (or as per specific test requirements).

Additives mix with blood to prevent clotting. Shaking can cause hemolysis of RBCs, producing inaccurate test results.

10. Check tubes for any sign of external contamination with blood. Decontaminate with antiseptic if necessary.

Prevents cross-contamination. Reduces risk for exposure to pathogens present in blood.

11. Remove gloves and perform hand hygiene after specimen is obtained and any spillage is cleaned.

Reduces risk for exposure to bloodborne pathogens.

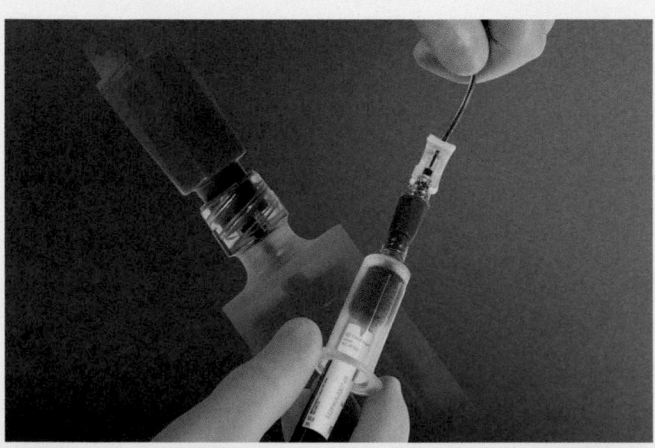

STEP 9d(4) Male Luer-Lok Vacutainer adapter attaches to port; blood draws directly into specimen tubes. (*Courtesy and copyright © Becton Dickinson.*)

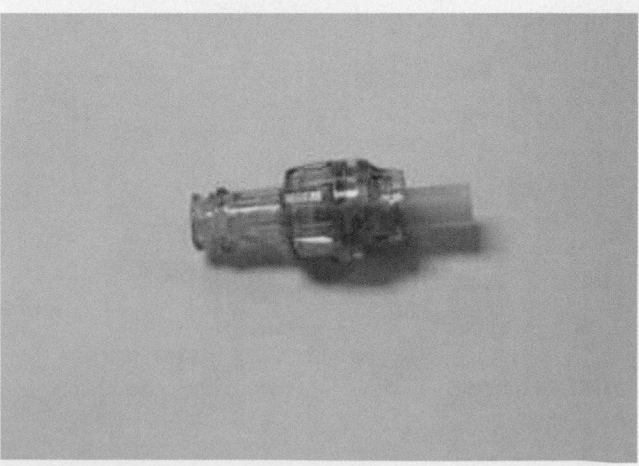

STEP 9d(6) Neutral-pressure cap helps maintain patency of vascular access device. (*Image courtesy of April Ambalina.*)

STEP	RATIONALE

IMPLEMENTATION

12. Help patient to comfortable position, and ensure any infusions are re-established and/or required lumens are locked as prescribed or per employer policy.

13. Attach completed identification label to each tube and affix proper requisition. Verify identifiers in front of patient (Accreditation Canada, 2019). | Incorrect identification of specimen could result in diagnostic or therapeutic errors.

14. Place specimens in biohazard bag and send to laboratory. Cultures must be sent to laboratory within 30 minutes (Pagana et al., 2019). | Minimizes spread of microorganisms.

15. Perform hand hygiene. | Reduces transfer of microorganisms.

EVALUATION

1. Inspect venipuncture site for homeostasis. | Determines if bleeding has stopped or hematoma has formed.

2. Determine if patient remains anxious or fearful. | Some patients require more blood tests in future. Address concerns and let patient express anxiety.

3. Check laboratory report for test results. | Reveals constituents of blood specimen.

4. Use Teach-Back: "I want to be sure you understand the purpose and procedure for obtaining a blood specimen. Tell me why we are collecting this blood specimen." Develop a revised teaching plan if patient or caregiver is not able to teach back correctly. | Determines level of understanding of instructional topic.

Unexpected Outcomes

1. Hematoma forms at venipuncture site.

2. Bleeding at site continues.

3. Signs and symptoms of infection at venipuncture site occur.

Related Interventions

- Apply pressure using 5 × 5–cm (2 × 2–inch) gauze dressing.
- Continue to monitor patient for pain and discomfort.
- Apply pressure to site; patient may also apply pressure.
- Monitor patient.
- Notify health care provider.
- Notify health care provider.

Communication and Documentation

- Document in electronic health record (EHR) or chart the method used to obtain blood specimen, date and time collected, type of test prescribed, disposition of specimen, and description of venipuncture site.
- Document your evaluation of patient and caregiver learning.
- Report any STAT or abnormal test results to health care provider.

Special Considerations

Teaching

- Instruct patient to briefly apply pressure to venipuncture site. Patients with bleeding disorders or those undergoing anticoagulant therapy should apply pressure for at least 5 minutes.
- Instruct patient to notify nurse or health care provider if persistent or recurrent bleeding or expanding hematoma develops at venipuncture site.

Pediatric

- Explain procedure to child at developmentally appropriate age and provide atraumatic care (Hockenberry & Wilson, 2015).
- Because children often fear that loss of their blood is a threat to their lives, explain to them that their blood is continually being produced. An adhesive bandage gives them assurance that their blood will not leak out through puncture site (Hockenberry & Wilson, 2015).
- At times it is advantageous to draw children's blood specimens in a treatment room instead of in their bed or room to maintain feeling that their room is a safe place (Hockenberry & Wilson, 2015).
- When performing venipuncture on children, explore sources for vein access: scalp, antecubital fossa, saphenous, and hand veins.
- Application of eutectic mixture of local anaesthetics (EMLA) cream to the venipuncture site may be prescribed before the stick to reduce pain in infants and young children (Hockenberry & Wilson, 2015).
- Vacutainers are not recommended in children under 2 years of age because of possible vein collapse with their use.

Gerontological

- Older persons have fragile veins that are easily traumatized during venipuncture. Sometimes application of warm compresses may help in obtaining samples. Use of a small-bore catheter may be beneficial.

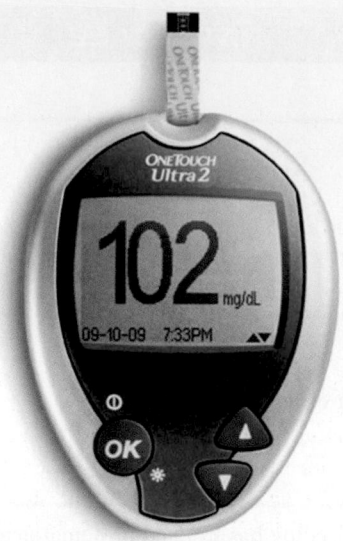

FIG 9.5 Blood glucose monitor. (*Courtesy LifeScan, Milpitas, CA.*)

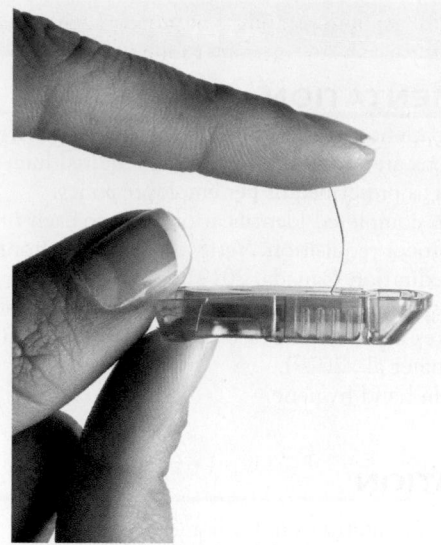

FIG 9.6 Tiny sensor implanted under skin transmits continuous reading to receiver. (*Courtesy DexCom.*)

✦ SKILL 9.9 Blood Glucose Monitoring

Blood glucose monitoring (BMG) is an essential component of any diabetes mellitus self-management program (Lecklider, 2015). The procedure is less painful than venipuncture, and the ease of the skin puncture method makes it possible for patients to perform this procedure at home. The development of reagent strips, home glucose monitors, and the skin puncture method has revolutionized home-management care of patients with diabetes mellitus.

Blood glucose reflectance meters are lightweight and run on batteries (e.g., Accu-Chek III, OneTouch) (Fig. 9.5). After a drop of blood from the skin puncture is dropped or wicked onto a reagent strip, the meter provides an accurate measurement of blood glucose level in 5 to 50 seconds. Point-of-care blood glucose testing meters must be cleaned and disinfected after each patient use (Canadian Agency for Drugs and Technologies in Health [CADTH], 2017).

The meters differ in several ways, including amount of blood needed for each test, testing speed, overall size, ability to store test results in memory, cost of the meter, and cost of test strips. Some larger meters are voice activated, which provides support for the older person or patient with visual impairments. Most meters now allow for the use of an alternative site or forearm capillary testing. Through improved technology a method for glucose measurement is now available on the market. A minimally invasive glucose meter uses a very small, fine plastic sensor inserted through the abdomen and provides continuous readings of blood glucose levels (Fig. 9.6). A disadvantage is that the patient must wear the meter at all times for continuous blood glucose monitoring (CBM). Initiatives and clinical trials are under way to develop noninvasive glucose

testing that evaluates intermittent blood glucose levels (Lecklider, 2015).

Testing of glycosylated hemoglobin (HbA1$_c$) evaluates the amount of glucose available in the bloodstream over the 120-day lifespan of a red blood cell. HbA1$_c$ provides an accurate long-term index of a patient's average blood glucose level drawn by venous puncture (Pagana et al., 2019).

Delegation and Collaboration

Assessment of a patient's condition cannot be delegated to an unregulated care provider (UCP). When the patient's condition is stable, the skill of obtaining and testing a sample of blood for blood glucose level may be delegated to an UCP, depending on employer policy. The nurse informs the UCP by:
- Explaining appropriate sites to use for puncture and when to obtain glucose levels.
- Reviewing expected blood glucose levels and when to report unexpected glucose levels to the nurse.

Equipment

- Antiseptic swab
- Cotton ball
- Lancet device (either self-activating or button activated)
- Blood glucose meter (e.g., Accu-Chek III, OneTouch)
- Blood glucose test strips appropriate for meter brand used
- Clean gloves
- Sterile 5 × 5–cm (2 × 2–inch) gauze

STEP	RATIONALE

ASSESSMENT

1. Identify patient using at least two person-specific identifiers (e.g., full name, date of birth, personal identification number, etc.) according to employer policy. Compare identifiers with information on patient's medical record.

Ensures correct patient. Complies with Accreditation Canada standards and improves patient safety (Accreditation Canada, 2019).

2. Assess patient's understanding of procedure and purpose of blood glucose monitoring. Determine if patient understands how to perform test and its importance in glucose control.	Provides baseline for developing teaching plan.
3. Determine if specific conditions need to be met before or after collection (e.g., fasting, postprandial, after certain medications, before insulin doses).	Dietary intake of carbohydrates and ingestion of concentrated glucose preparations alter blood glucose levels.
4. Determine if risks exist (e.g., low platelet count, anticoagulant therapy, bleeding disorders).	Abnormal clotting mechanisms increase risk for local ecchymosis and bleeding.
5. Assess potential puncture site. Inspect site for edema, inflammation, cuts, or sores. Avoid areas of bruising and open lesions. Avoid using hand on side of mastectomy.	Sides of fingers are commonly selected because they have fewer nerve endings. Measurements from alternative sites are meter specific and may be different from those at traditional sites. Puncture site should not be edematous, inflamed, or recently punctured because these factors cause increased interstitial fluid and blood to mix and also increase risk for infection.
6. Review health care provider's prescription for time or frequency of measurement.	Health care provider determines test schedule on the basis of patient's physiological status and risk for glucose imbalance.
7. For patient with diabetes mellitus who performs test at home, assess ability to handle devices. Patient may choose to continue self-testing while in hospital.	Patient's physical health may change (e.g., vision disturbance, fatigue, pain, disease process), preventing them from performing test.

NURSING DIAGNOSES

- Inadequate health maintenance
- Anxiety
- Insufficient knowledge regarding blood glucose monitoring

Related factors are individualized on the basis of patient's condition or needs.

PLANNING

1. Expected outcomes following completion of procedure:	
• Puncture site shows no evidence of bleeding or tissue damage.	Hemostasis is achieved. Lancet or needle did not puncture skin too deeply.
• Blood glucose measurements are accurate.	Normal fasting glucose is 4.0 to 7.0 mmol/L, indicating good metabolic control (Diabetes Canada Clinical Practice Guidelines Expert Committee, 2018). Values may vary slightly; check employer policy.
• Patient can verbalize procedure for self-monitoring blood glucose.	Demonstrates psychomotor learning.
• Patient explains test results.	Validates knowledge.
2. Explain procedure and purpose. Offer patient and caregiver opportunity to practice testing procedures. Provide resources and teaching aids.	Promotes understanding and cooperation.

IMPLEMENTATION

1. Perform hand hygiene. Instruct patient to perform hand hygiene, including forearm (if applicable), with soap and water. Rinse and dry.	Promotes skin cleansing and vasodilation at selected puncture site. Reduces transmission of microorganisms.
2. Position patient comfortably in chair or in semi-Fowler's position in bed.	Ensures easy access to puncture site. Patient assumes position when self-testing.
3. Remove reagent strip from container and tightly reseal cap. Check code on container. Use only test strips recommended for meter. Some newer meters do not require code and/or have disk or drum with 10 or more test strips.	Protects strips from accidental discoloration caused by exposure to air or light.
4. Insert strip into meter (refer to manufacturer directions [see illustration]). Do not bend strip. Meter turns on automatically.	Some machines must be calibrated; others require zeroing of timer. Each meter is adjusted differently.
5. Meter displays code on screen that must match code from test strip vial. Press proper button on meter to confirm matching codes. Meter is ready for use.	Codes must match for meter to operate. Meters have different messages that confirm that meter is ready for testing and blood can be applied.

STEP	RATIONALE

ASSESSMENT

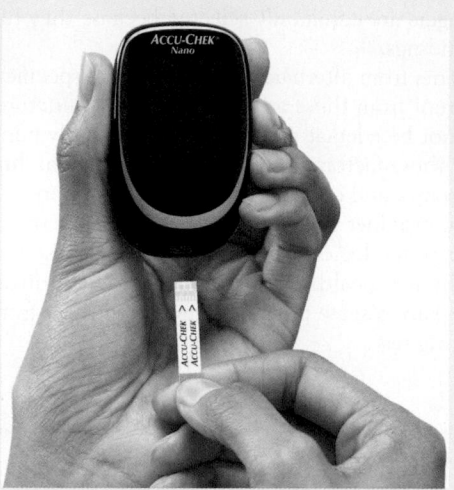

STEP 4 Load test strip into meter. *(Courtesy Accu-Chek Glucometer.)*

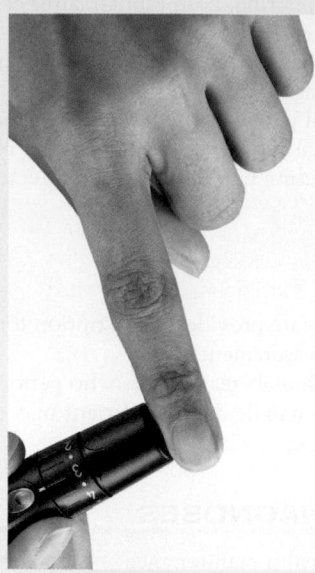

STEP 7c Prick side of finger with lancet. *(Courtesy Accu-Chek Glucometer.)*

6. Perform hand hygiene and apply clean gloves. Prepare single-use lancet or multiple-use lancet device. **NOTE:** Some meters recommend that this step be completed before preparing test strip. Remove cap from lancet device; insert new lancet. Some lancet devices have disk or cylinder that rotates to new lancet.

    a. Twist off protective cover on tip of lancet. Replace cap of lancet device.

    b. Cock lancet device, adjusting for proper puncture depth.

7. Obtain blood sample.

    a. Cleanse patient's finger lightly with antiseptic and allow to dry. Choose vascular area for puncture site. In stable adults, select lateral side of finger. Avoid central tip of finger, which has denser nerve supply (Pagana et al., 2019).

    b. Hold area to be punctured in dependent position. Do not milk or massage finger site.

    c. Hold tip of lancet device against area of skin chosen for test site (see illustration). Press release button on device. Some devices allow you to see blood sample forming. Remove device.

    d. With some devices a blood sample begins to appear. Otherwise, gently squeeze or massage fingertip until round drop of blood forms (see illustration).

8. Obtain test results.

    a. Be sure that meter is still on. Bring test strip in meter to drop of blood. Blood will be wicked onto test strip (see illustration). Follow specific meter instructions to be sure that you obtain adequate sample.

Reduces transmission of microorganisms.
Never reuse a lancet because of risk of infection.

Each patient varies as to depth of insertion needed.

Removes microorganisms. Side of finger is less sensitive to pain.

Increases blood flow to area before puncture. Milking may hemolyze specimen and introduce excess tissue fluid (Pagana et al., 2019).
Placement ensures that lancet enters skin properly.

Adequate-size blood sample is needed to test glucose.

Exposure of blood to test strip for prescribed time ensures proper results.

Clinical Decision Point *Do not scrape blood onto the test strips or apply it to wrong side of test strip. This prevents accurate glucose measurement.*

STEP	RATIONALE

IMPLEMENTATION

b. Blood glucose test result will appear on screen (see illustration). Some devices "beep" when completed.

9. Turn meter off. Some meters turn off automatically. Offer patient cotton ball and hold over puncture site until bleeding stops. Dispose of test strip, lancet, cotton ball, and gloves in proper receptacles.

Meter is battery powered. Proper disposal reduces risk for needle-stick injury and spread of infection.

10. Perform hand hygiene.

11. Discuss test results with patient and encourage questions and eventual participation in care if this is a new diabetes diagnosis.

Reduces transmission of microorganisms.
Promotes participation in and adherence to therapy.

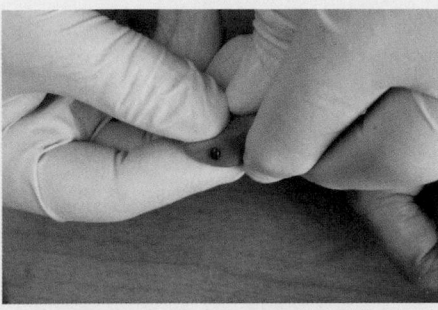

STEP 7d Gently squeeze puncture site until drop of blood forms.

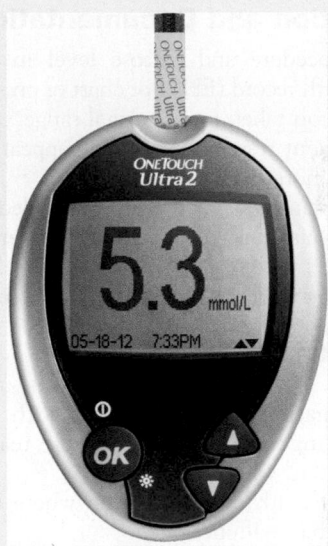

STEP 8b Results appear on meter screen. (*Courtesy Accu-Chek Glucometer.*)

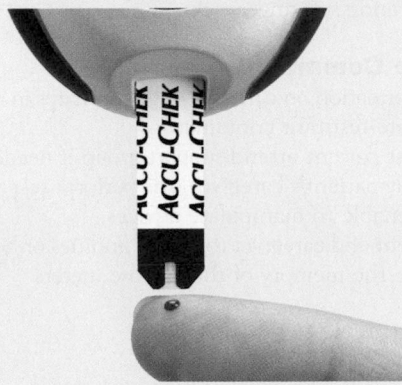

STEP 8a Touch test strip to blood drop. Blood wicks into test strip. (*Courtesy Accu-Chek Glucometer.*)

EVALUATION

1. Inspect puncture site for bleeding or tissue injury.
2. Compare glucose meter reading with normal blood glucose levels and previous test results.
3. **Use Teach-Back:** "I want to be sure I explained clearly the way to obtain a blood glucose reading. Show me the steps you will use to obtain your blood glucose measurement." Develop a revised teaching plan if patient or caregiver is not able to teach back correctly.

Site can be source of discomfort and infection.
Determines if glucose level is normal.

Determines level of understanding of instructional topic.

STEP	RATIONALE

EVALUATION

Unexpected Outcomes	Related Interventions
1. Puncture site is bruised or continues to bleed.	• Apply pressure. • Notify health care provider if bleeding continues. • Continue to monitor patient.
2. Blood glucose level is above or below target range.	• Check for medication prescriptions for deviations in glucose level. • Notify health care provider. • Administer insulin or carbohydrate source as prescribed, depending on glucose level.
3. Glucose meter malfunctions.	• Review instructions for troubleshooting glucose meter. • Repeat test.

Communication and Documentation

• Document procedure and glucose level in nurses' notes in electronic health record (EHR) or chart or on special flow sheet. Document action taken for abnormal range.
• Document patient response, including appearance of puncture site, in nurses' notes in EHR or chart.
• Document explanations or teaching provided in nurses' notes in EHR or chart and evaluation of patient and caregiver learning.
• Document and report abnormal blood glucose levels.

Special Considerations
Teaching

• Provide information on where patient with diabetes mellitus can obtain testing supplies. When possible, teach with the same meter that patient will use at home.
• Provide patient with information on where to obtain help if glucose meter has malfunctioned.
• Stress importance of the timing of blood glucose levels, particularly in patients with diabetes mellitus.

Pediatric

• Allow young children to choose puncture site; outer aspect of heel and great toe are common puncture sites in infants.

• Heel warming helps to obtain specimen from a neonate.
• Infection or abscess of the heel and necrotizing osteochondritis are the most serious complications of heelstick puncture in infants. To avoid osteochondritis, make sure that puncture is not deeper than 2 mm (0.1 inch) and is made at the outer aspect of the heel (Hockenberry & Wilson, 2015).
• Allow young child with parent to demonstrate technique; incorporate a play activity for further understanding.

Gerontological

• Warming fingertips with warm water may facilitate obtaining specimen.
• Some older persons have vision or dexterity problems that interfere with performing self-fingersticks.

Care in the Community

• Provide information on correct disposal of sharps in nonpermeable and puncture-resistant container.
• Suggest that patient attend support group if needed.
• Be sure that patient's caregiver can perform test when patient is ill or is unable to manipulate devices.
• Teach patient and caregiver to record findings or how to retrieve results from the memory of the glucose meters.

◆ SKILL 9.10   Obtaining an Arterial Specimen for Blood Gas Measurement

Effectiveness of oxygenation and ventilation is assessed by measuring arterial blood gases (ABGs). Measurement of ABGs provides valuable information in assessing and managing a patient's respiratory and metabolic disturbances (Pagana et al., 2019). The parameters measured in an ABG include arterial blood pH, partial pressure of oxygen (PaO_2), partial pressure of carbon dioxide ($PaCO_2$), and arterial oxygen saturation (SaO_2).

Each employer has a policy regarding which health care providers can obtain ABG samples. Many employers allow nurses in specialty areas (e.g., critical care) to obtain them; others specify a certified respiratory therapist or a physician, and some require institutional certification of this skill. Always check employer policy.

Delegation and Collaboration

The skill of obtaining an ABG sample cannot be delegated to an unregulated care provider (UCP). The nurse informs the UCP to:
• Report any bleeding from an arterial puncture site.
• Report any changes in patient vital signs, level of consciousness, or restlessness.

Equipment

Commercial blood gas kit or individual supplies, including:
• 3-mL heparinized syringe
• 23- or 25-gauge needle with safety guard
• Filter cap (allows expelling of air and retains blood)

- Alcohol swabs (2)
- 5 × 5–cm (2 × 2–inch) gauze pad
- Tape
- Sodium heparin (1 : 1000 solution)
- Cup or plastic bag with crushed ice

- Clean gloves
- Protective eyewear
- Completed identification labels with proper patient identifiers
- Completed laboratory requisition
- Small plastic biohazard bag (or container)

STEP	RATIONALE

ASSESSMENT

1. Identify patient using at least two person-specific identifiers (e.g., full name, date of birth, personal identification number, etc.) according to employer policy. Compare identifiers with information on patient's medical record.	Ensures correct patient. Complies with Accreditation Canada standards and improves patient safety (Accreditation Canada, 2019).
2. Assess for factors that influence ABG measurements:	Allows you to eliminate factors that interfere with accurate measurement.
a. Hypoventilation or hyperventilation	Hypoventilation can cause retention of CO_2, and hyperventilation can cause decreased CO_2 levels (Hockenberry & Wilson, 2015).
b. Body temperature	Change in body temperature by as little as 0.6°C (1°F) can alter ABG values (Hockenberry & Wilson, 2015).
3. Identify medications or herbal products that may influence ABG measurement (e.g., anticoagulants, diuretics, St. John's wort).	Certain medications increase risk for bleeding at puncture site or may cause hemoconcentration.
4. Assess respiratory status, including rate, depth, rhythm, adventitious sounds, and use of accessory muscles.	Physical signs and symptoms may indicate need for ABG sample.
5. Review criteria for choosing site for ABG sample.	Prevents causing compromised circulation from puncture.

Clinical Decision Point *Factors that contraindicate the use of arterial site include amputation, contractures, localized infection, dressing or cast, mastectomy, or arteriovenous shunts.*

a. Assess collateral blood flow. *Perform Allen test.*	Allen test is used to assess collateral circulation before performing arterial puncture on radial artery. A positive Allen test ensures that there is collateral circulation to the hand in case thrombosis of radial artery occurs following puncture (Pagana et al., 2019).
(1) Have patient make tight fist and raise hand above heart.	Removes as much blood from hand as possible.
(2) Apply direct pressure to both radial and ulnar arteries (see illustration).	Obstructs arterial blood flow to hand.
(3) Have patient lower and open hand (see illustration).	Fingers and hand should be pale and blanched, indicating lack of arterial blood flow.

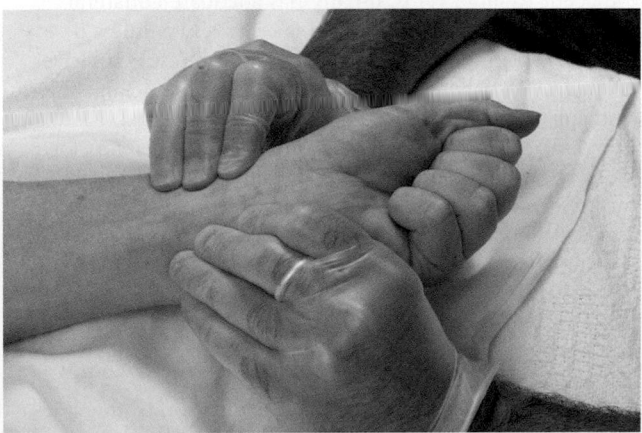

STEP 5a(2) Apply pressure to radial and ulnar arteries.

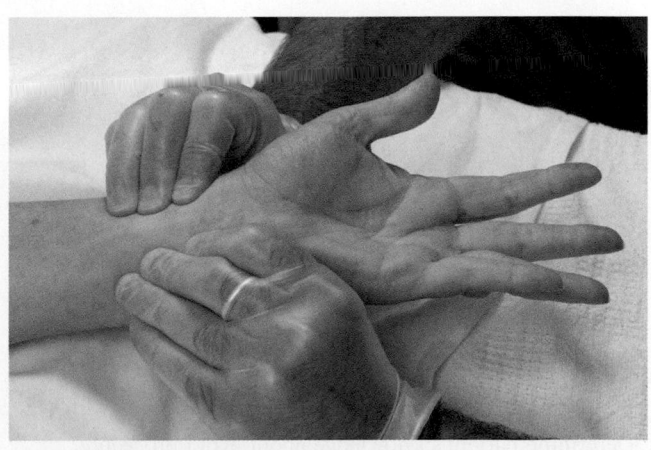

STEP 5a(3) Patient opening hand; note colour.

STEP	RATIONALE

ASSESSMENT

(4) Release pressure over ulnar artery; observe colour of fingers, thumbs, and hand (see illustration).

Flushing identifies that circulation through the ulnar artery is good and that the ulnar artery alone is capable of providing blood supply to the entire hand. Therefore, you can use the radial artery for puncture.

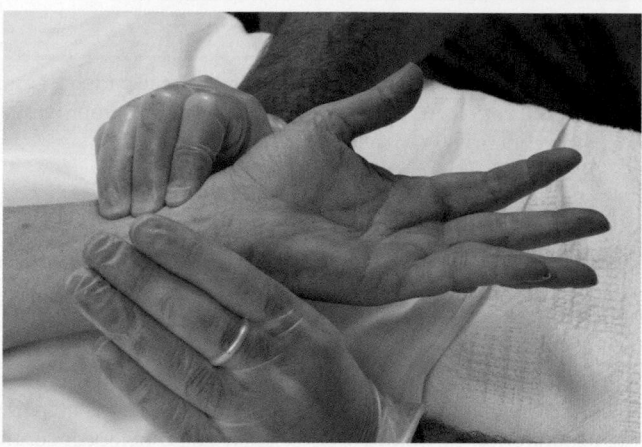

STEP 5a(4) Release pressure over ulnar artery and note colour of hand.

Clinical Decision Point *If there is no flushing in 15 seconds, Allen test is negative and you should repeat it on the other arm or choose another artery for puncture (Pagana et al., 2019).*

b. Assess accessibility of vessel.

Palpating, stabilizing, and performing venipuncture of superficial artery is easier. Superficial arteries are located at distal ends of extremities.

c. Assess tissue surrounding artery.

Muscle, tendon, and fat have decreased sensation to pain. Bony periosteum and nerves are highly sensitive to pain.

d. Assess that arteries are not directly adjacent to veins.

Helps reduce chance of venous puncture and possibility of inaccurate samples.

6. Assess arterial sites for use in obtaining specimen.

Arterial blood may be obtained from areas where strong pulses are palpable (i.e., radial, brachial, or femoral artery) (Pagana et al., 2019).

Clinical Decision Point *Previous puncture sites or pre-existing conditions may eliminate potential sites (see employer policy). Artery should be easily accessible.*

a. Radial artery

Safest, most accessible site for puncture. It is superficial, is not adjacent to large veins, usually has adequate collateral circulation by ulnar artery, and is relatively painless if periosteum is avoided. Used when Allen's test is positive.

b. Brachial artery

Has reasonable collateral blood flow, is less superficial, is more difficult to palpate and stabilize, carries increased risk for venous puncture, and results in increased discomfort for patient if brachial nerve is punctured. It is used when radial artery is inaccessible or Allen's test is negative.

c. Femoral artery

Nurses without specialized training should not use this artery. It has no adequate collateral flow if obstructed below inguinal ligament, is difficult to stabilize, is deep, and is directly adjacent to the femoral vein. It is the best artery to use in emergency (e.g., cardiac arrest or hypovolemic shock when pulses are difficult to palpate).

7. Review baseline ABG values for patient.

Provides baseline for comparison and evaluation of therapies.

8. Determine patient's knowledge about ABG procedure.

Obtaining blood specimen is painful. Patient who is knowledgeable will be more cooperative.

STEP	RATIONALE

NURSING DIAGNOSES

- Reduced gas exchange
- Reduced airway clearance
- Inadequate breathing pattern
- Inadequate peripheral tissue perfusion
- Anxiety
- Insufficient knowledge regarding arterial blood gases
- Potential for injury

Related factors/Risk factors are individualized on the basis of patient's condition or needs.

PLANNING

STEP	RATIONALE
1. Expected outcomes following completion of procedure:	
• Patient's ABG values are within normal range.	Indicates adequate oxygenation.
• Patient's extremity distal to puncture remains warm and pink, has adequate capillary refill, and is free of pain.	Indicates adequate arterial circulation to extremity.
• Patient denies anxiety, and respiratory rate remains within baseline.	Anxiety increase respiratory rate, which can alter ABG results.
• Patient correctly discusses ABG procedure.	Indicates learning.
2. Prepare heparinized syringe (if not in commercial kit).	Heparin mixes with specimen to prevent clotting.
a. Aspirate 0.5 mL sodium heparin (1000 units/mL) into syringe from vial or ampule.	Prevents blood sample from clotting before reaching laboratory. Excessive heparin can affect pH of arterial sample.
b. Withdraw plunger entire length of syringe. Maintain asepsis.	Coats inside of barrel of syringe with heparin.
c. Eject all heparin in barrel out of syringe.	In hub of syringe 0.15 to 0.25 mL of sodium heparin remains; 0.05 mL of sodium heparin adequately anticoagulates 1 mL of blood; 0.15 mL adequately anticoagulates 3 mL without affecting pH level.
3. Explain steps and purpose of procedure to patient.	Reduces anxiety and promotes understanding and cooperation.

IMPLEMENTATION

STEP	RATIONALE
1. Perform hand hygiene.	Reduces transmission of infection.
2. Palpate selected radial, femoral, or brachial site with fingertips.	Determines area of maximal impulse for puncture site.
3. Using radial artery, elevate patient's wrist with small pillow and ask them to extend fingers downward. Stabilize artery through slight hyperextension of wrist.	Flexes wrist and positions radial artery closer to surface. Reduces mobility of artery and makes insertion of needle easier.
4. Apply clean gloves. Clean area of maximal impulse with alcohol swab or antiseptic swab (check employer or manufacturer recommendation). Wipe in circular motion away from site or use back-and-forth strokes. Allow to dry.	Reduces number of resident bacteria on surface of skin. Drying maximizes antibacterial effects.
5. Hold 5 × 5–cm (2 × 2–inch) gauze with same fingers used to palpate artery.	Keeps gauze pad accessible for covering puncture site when necessary.
6. Use corner of sterile gauze pad or alcohol wipe to point to chosen site.	Maintaining location of artery improves likelihood of successful puncture.
7. Hold needle bevel up and insert at 30- to 45-degree angle into artery. Prepare patient for needle-stick because radial sticks are painful.	Angle allows for better arterial flow into needle. Prepared patient will be less likely to withdraw arm.
8. Stop advancing needle when blood is noted returning into hub of needle or syringe.	Quick return of blood indicates that arterial flow is obtained. Prevents puncturing through both sides of artery.
9. Allow arterial pulsations to pump 2 to 3 mL of blood into heparinized syringe slowly (see illustration).	Allowing pulsations to help fill syringe reduces presence of air bubbles in sample. Bubbles alter ABG results.
10. When sampling is complete, hold 5 × 5–cm (2 × 2–inch) gauze over puncture site, withdraw syringe and needle, and activate safety guard over needle.	Pad minimizes pulling of skin as needle is withdrawn. Decreases contamination from blood and accidental needlestick.
11. Apply pressure over and just proximal to puncture site with pad (see illustration).	Insertion of needle into artery is just proximal to insertion site through skin. Gauze absorbs any blood that might ooze from site.

STEP	RATIONALE

IMPLEMENTATION

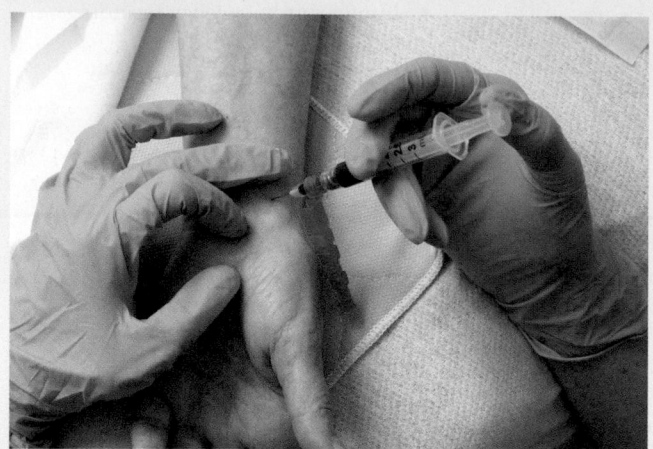

STEP 9 Blood flowing into syringe.

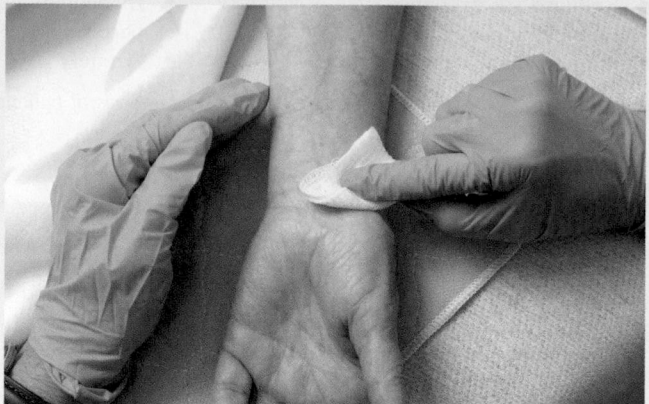

STEP 11 Apply firm pressure to arterial puncture site.

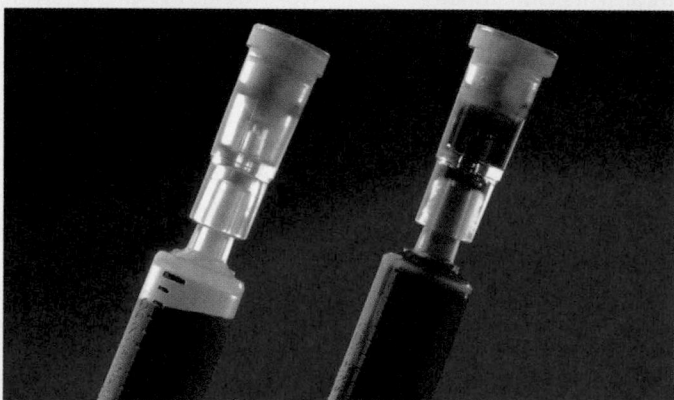

STEP 15 Filter-Pro Air Bubble Removal Device expels air safely from syringe without accidentally expelling blood and aerosolizing sample. *(With permission from Smiths Medical, Carlsbad, CA.)*

12. Maintain continuous pressure on and proximal to site for 3 to 5 minutes (approximately 15 minutes if patient is undergoing anticoagulant therapy or has bleeding disorder) (Pagana et al., 2019). Have another nurse remove safety needle and attach filter cap to syringe (see Step 15 below) if prolonged pressure is needed.

To avoid hematoma formation, apply and hold pressure or apply a pressure dressing to arterial puncture site for 3 to 5 minutes (Pagana et al., 2019). Prevents delay in preparing syringe in ice.

13. Visually inspect site for signs of bleeding or hematoma formation.

Determines if continued need exists to exert pressure. Because artery rather than vein has been accessed, monitor puncture site for bleeding.

14. Palpate artery below or distal to puncture site.

Determines if pulse quality has changed, indicating alteration in arterial flow.

15. Take syringe, remove safety needle, and discard needle in appropriate biohazard container. Attach filter cap to syringe (available in kit) to expel air or cover tip of syringe with 5 × 5–cm (2 × 2–inch) sterile gauze to expel air (see employer procedure). Some kits may have all supplies, including syringe with heparin, needle with safety needle cap, and filter cap that allows air to vent and not blood (see illustration).

Decreases chance of contamination from room air. Air bubbles in specimen can falsely elevate or decrease results, depending on patient's blood gas concentration (Van Leeuwen & Bladh, 2015).

STEP	RATIONALE

IMPLEMENTATION

16. Prepare syringe for laboratory analysis (according to employer policy).

    a. Place patient identification label on syringe in front of patient; confirm person-specific identifiers (Accreditation Canada, 2019). — Ensures proper identification of sample.

    b. Place syringe in cup of crushed ice (check employer policy). — Failure to place ABG sample on ice can affect results of pH, PaO_2, and $PaCO_2$ (Pagana et al., 2019).

    c. Attach properly labelled laboratory requisition to blood gas sample. Add appropriate patient data (e.g., hemoglobin, mode and flow of supplemental oxygen, and patient's body temperature) (check employer policy). — Prevents mislabelled specimens. Hemoglobin level, supplemental oxygen, and hypothermia or hyperthermia affect PaO_2 or $PaCO_2$ values.

17. Place sample in biohazard bag. Send sample to laboratory immediately. — Prevents alteration in gas tensions resulting from metabolic processes that continue after blood is drawn.

18. Remove gloves and perform hand hygiene. — Reduces transmission of microorganisms.

EVALUATION

1. Inspect puncture site and area distal to puncture site for complications. — An artery can be obstructed, or important structures anatomically juxtaposed to an artery can be penetrated (Pagana et al., 2019).

2. Review results of sample as soon as possible. — Identifies any abnormality and expedites initiation of treatment.

3. **Use Teach-Back:** "I want to be sure I explained the way I will obtain your blood sample. Tell me the steps I will use to obtain this specimen." Develop a revised teaching plan if patient or caregiver is not able to teach back correctly. — Determines level of understanding of instructional topic.

Unexpected Outcomes

1. Patient has abnormal ABG values.

2. Patient has hematoma formation at puncture site.

3. Puncture site is bruised or continues to bleed.

Related Interventions

- Continue to monitor patient.
- Notify health care provider of findings and obtain further prescriptions.
- Continue to monitor patient.
- Notify health care provider.
- Apply pressure.
- Notify health care provider if bleeding continues.

Communication and Documentation

- Document results of Allen test, location and condition of puncture site, patient's tolerance of procedure, and disposition of specimen to laboratory in nurses' notes in electronic health record (EHR) or chart.
- Communicate ABG results to health care provider as soon as available.
- Document patient's fraction of inspired oxygen concentration (FiO_2) and any ventilator settings (e.g., tidal volume [V_t], respiratory frequency [RF], mode of ventilation).
- Document your evaluation of patient and caregiver learning.
- Document results of test in nurses' notes in EHR or chart.

Special Considerations
Teaching

- Teach patient to report numbness, burning, and/or tingling during and after in hand that had radial artery puncture.

Pediatric

- In neonatal and pediatric patients, you can use capillary blood gas. Procedures are similar to those for obtaining heelsticks.
- When caring for neonatal patients, especially premature infants, normal values for ABGs often differ from those of adults.
- Arterial blood samples from punctures are painful and cause crying and breath holding that affect the accuracy of ABG values (decreases PaO_2) (Hockenberry & Wilson, 2015).

Gerontological

- Pay special attention during interpretation of ABGs for patients with chronic pulmonary conditions. In these patients, compensatory mechanisms may allow normal pH in face of markedly elevated $PaCO_2$.

◆ CLINICAL DEBRIEF

1. An 88-year-old female is admitted from home to the health care facility. She has an in-dwelling Foley catheter. Her urine is dark and cloudy. She is pulling at her Foley catheter, temperature is 38.4°C (101.2°F), blood pressure 88/50 mm Hg, pulse 128 beats/min, and she is restless and confused. On the basis of these findings, which laboratory specimens would you expect to obtain?

2. A male patient was diagnosed with type 1 diabetes mellitus 2 years ago. He was admitted with diabetes ketoacidosis (DKA) related to an upper respiratory infection associated with his past history of chronic obstructive pulmonary disease (COPD). He states that he quit taking his insulin because he was nauseated and vomiting. You observe that he has multiple puncture sites that are reddened on the central tip of his fingers. He states that his fingertips are sore. He is expected to be discharged home the next day. Which instructions will you provide to the patient to help in his self-management of type 1 diabetes mellitus?

3. This same patient was to be discharged today, but during the night he developed shortness of breath. He has received multiple respiratory treatments over the past 3 hours, yet you observe that his work of breathing has increased dramatically. Using SBAR, show how you would communicate with the health care team.

◆ REVIEW QUESTIONS

1. A urine specimen for culture and sensitivity is being collected from a male patient. Which steps should be used to obtain an accurate specimen? *(Select all that apply.)*
   1. Check two person-specific identifiers.
   2. Help patient to perform pericare before the sterile part of the procedure.
   3. Wipe head of the penis back and forth three times with each swab.
   4. Collect 10 to 20 mL for the sample.
   5. Have patient initially void into a bedpan or clean container.
   6. Have patient hold penis above the sterile specimen cup without touching the container.

2. The nurse is preparing to obtain a throat culture on a 22-year-old female. Which step(s) would facilitate obtaining an accurate specimen? *(Select all that apply.)*
   1. Placing patient in a sitting position or with head elevated at a 45-degree angle
   2. Having patient lean head forward
   3. Inserting swab without touching lips, teeth, tongue, or cheeks
   4. Swabbing the tonsillar area
   5. Swabbing the uvula
   6. Having patient blow her nose

3. Place the following steps for collecting a sterile urine specimen for a culture and sensitivity from a Luer-Lok catheter port in the correct order.
   1. Attach Luer-Lok syringe to Luer-Lok port.
   2. Clamp drainage tube with clamp or rubber band for 15 minutes.
   3. Clean catheter entry port and wait for disinfectant to dry.
   4. Unclamp catheter and allow urine to flow into drainage bag.
   5. Aspirate 3 mL of urine into syringe attached to Luer-Lok.

ⓔ *Visit the Evolve site for a complete list of Clinical Debrief and Review Questions answers.*

REFERENCES

Accreditation Canada. (2019). *Required organizational practices handbook—Version 14*. Retrieved from http://www.wrha.mb.ca/quality/files/2019ROPHandbook.pdf

Alberta Health Services. (2017). *Performing blood culture collections*. Retrieved from https://www.albertahealthservices.ca/assets/wf/lab/wf-lab-prc-performing-bc-collection.pdf

Awua, A. K., Wiredu, E. K., Afari, E. A., Tijani, A. S., Djanmah, G., & Adanu, R. M. K. (2017). A tailored within-community specimen collection strategy increased uptake of cervical cancer screening in a cross-sectional study in Ghana. *BMC Public Health*, 18, doi:10.1186/s12889-017-4631-y

Canadian Agency for Drugs and Technologies in Health (CADTH). (2017). *Point-of-care testing: An environmental scan*. Ottawa: Author. Retrieved from https://www.cadth.ca/sites/default/files/pdf/es0308_point_of_care_testing.pdf

Canadian Cancer Society. (2018). *Screening for colorectal cancer*. Retrieved from http://www.cancer.ca/en/cancer-information/cancer-type/colorectal/screening/?region=on

Copeland-Halperin, L., Kaminsky, A., Bluefeld, N., & Miraliakbari, R. (2016). Sample procurement for cultures of infected wounds: A systematic review. *Journal of Wound Care*, 25(4), S4–S6, S8–10. doi:10.12968/jowc.2016.25.Sup4.S4

Diabetes Canada Clinical Practice Guidelines Expert Committee. (2018). Diabetes Canada 2018 clinical practice guidelines for the prevention and management of diabetes in Canada. *Canadian Journal of Diabetes*, 42(Suppl. 1), S1–S325.

Diagnostic Services Manitoba. (2015). *Clinical microbiology procedure manual: Sample collection–DSM Document # 120-10-05, V05*. Retrieved from http://dsmanitoba.ca/wp-content/uploads/2014/05/1478_120-10-05-V05-Clinical-Microbiology-Sample-Collection-Manual-ALL.pdf

Haalboom, M., Blokhuis-Arkes, M. H. E., Beuk, R. J., Klont, R., Guebitz, G., & Heinzle, A. (2018). Wound swab and wound biopsy yield similar culture results: Culture results of swab versus biopsy. *Wound Repair and Regeneration*, 26(5), 192–199. doi:10.1111/wrr.12629

Hockenberry, M. J., & Wilson, D. (2015). *Wong's nursing care of infants and children* (10th ed.). St. Louis: Mosby.

Larocco, M., Franek, J., Leibach, E., et al. (2016). Effectiveness of preanalytic practices on contamination and diagnostic accuracy of urine cultures: A laboratory medicine best practices systematic review and meta-analysis. *Clinical Microbiology Reviews*, 29(1), 105–147. doi:10.1128/CMR.00030-15

Lecklider, T. (2015). Monitoring blood glucose levels. *Evaluation Engineering*, 54(8), 22.

Long, B., & Koyfman, A. (2016). Best clinical practice: Blood culture utility in the emergency department. *Journal of Emergency Medicine*, 51(5), 529–539. doi:10.1016/j.jemermed.2016.07.003

McCall, R., & Tankersley, C. (2015). *Phlebotomy essentials* (6th ed.). Philadelphia: Lippincott Williams & Wilkins.

McCaughey, E., Vecellio, E., Lake, R., et al. (2017). Key factors influencing the incidence of hemolysis: A critical appraisal of current evidence. *Critical Reviews in Clinical Laboratory Sciences*, 54(1), 59–72.

Moureau, N., & Flynn, J. (2015). Disinfection of needleless connector hubs: Clinical evidence systematic review. *Nursing Research and Practice*, 2015, 1–20.

Naimer, S. A. (2017). Diaper slit perineal bag urine sampling. *Pediatric Emergency Care*, 33(6), 446–448. doi:10.1097/PEC.0000000000001160

Pagana, K., Pagana, T., & Pike-MacDonald, S. A. (2019). *Mosby's Canadian manual of diagnostic and laboratory tests* (2nd Canadian ed.). Toronto, ON: Elsevier Canada.

Perry, S., Hockenberry, M., Lowdermilk, D., Wilson, D., Keenan-Lindsay, L., & Sams, C. (2017). *Maternal child nursing care in Canada* (2nd ed.). Toronto, ON: Elsevier Canada.

Public Health Agency of Canada. (2016). *Canadian biosafety handbook* (2nd ed.). Ottawa: Author. Retrieved from https://www.canada.ca/en/public-health/services/canadian-biosafety-standards-guidelines/handbook-second-edition.html

Spichler, A., Hurwitz, B. L., Armstrong, D. G., & Lipsky, B. A. (2015). Microbiology of diabetic foot infections: From Louis Pasteur to 'crime scene investigation'. *BMC Medicine*, 13(1), 2. doi:10.1186/s12916-014-0232-0

Touhy, T., Jett, K., Boscart, V., & McCleary, L. (2019). *Ebersole and Hess' gerontological nursing and healthy aging* (2nd Canadian ed.). Toronto, ON: Elsevier Canada.

Van Leeuwen, A., & Bladh, M. (2015). *Davis's comprehensive handbook of laboratory and diagnostic tests with nursing implications* (6th ed.). Philadelphia: FA Davis.

10 | Diagnostic Procedures

Written by **Nancy LaPlante, PhD, RN, AHN-BC, Stephen D. Krau, PhD, CNE, and Leslie Graham, RN, MN, CHSE, CNCC**

SKILLS AND PROCEDURES

OBJECTIVES

Mastery of content in this chapter will enable the nurse to:
- Identify the physiological indications for diagnostic procedures.
- Describe the health care team collaboration and teamwork required before, during, and after procedures, including delegation to unregulated care providers (UCPs).
- Perform appropriate physical and psychosocial assessments before, during, and after diagnostic procedures.

- Assist health care providers with arteriogram (angiogram), cardiac catheterization, intravenous pyelogram, bone marrow aspiration/biopsy, lumbar puncture, paracentesis, thoracentesis, bronchoscopy, and endoscopy.
- Explain nursing responsibilities related to the use of intravenous sedation during diagnostic and surgical procedures.

MEDIA RESOURCES

- evolve http://evolve.elsevier.com/Canada/Perry/clinicalskills/
- Review Questions

- Audio Glossary
- Clinical Debrief and Review Questions Answers

PURPOSE

Diagnostic procedures are performed at the patient's bedside or in specially equipped rooms within a hospital or outpatient care setting. Before beginning, check the employer protocol specific to the procedure you will be performing or with which you are assisting. As the nurse, you are responsible for assessing the patient's knowledge of a procedure; preparing the patient; and providing a safe environment and emotional support throughout the procedure. The role of the nurse continues in providing preprocedure and postprocedure assessment, care, and documentation and providing discharge teaching. Before the procedure the health care provider is responsible for providing the patient with an explanation of the test or procedure, the risks, benefits, and treatment options, and expected outcomes, as part of the *informed consent* process.

STANDARDS OF CARE

- Accreditation Canada, 2019—*Required Organizational Practices Handbook—Version 14* (http://www.wrha.mb.ca/quality/files/2019ROPHandbook.pdf)

- Canadian Anesthesiologists' Society (CAS), 2018a—*Guidelines to the Practice of Anesthesia* (http://www.cas.ca/English/Guidelines)
- Canadian Association for Interventional Radiology (CAIR), 2010—*Guidelines and Standards* (https://www.cairweb.ca/en/publications/guidelines-and-standards/)
- Canadian Association of Radiologists (CAR), 2011—*National Practice Guidelines* (https://car.ca/patient-care/practice-guidelines/)
- Canadian Medical Protective Association (CMPA)—*Good Practices Guide: Informed Consent* (https://www.cmpa-acpm.ca/serve/docs/ela/goodpracticesguide/pages/communication/Informed_Consent/informed_consent-e.html)
- Canadian Patient Safety Institute (CPSI), 2014—*A Surgical Care Safety Action Plan* (http://www.patientsafetyinstitute.ca/en/About/PatientSafetyForwardWith4/Documents/Surgical%20Care%20Safety%20Action%20Plan.pdf)
- Hospital for Sick Children (HSC), 2017—*Clinical Practice Guidelines: Pain Management* (http://www.sickkids.ca/clinical-practice-guidelines/clinical-practice-guidelines/export/CLINH142/Main%20Document.pdf)

- Registered Nurses' Association of Ontario (RNAO), 2004/2008—*Best Practice Guideline: Assessment and Device Selection for Vascular Access* (https://rnao.ca/bpg/guidelines/assessment-and-device-selection-vascular-access)

PRINCIPLES FOR PRACTICE

- It is essential for nurses to ensure that patients who require diagnostic testing understand the purpose, preparation, and postprocedural care.
- Some tests require intravenous (IV) sedation to facilitate the diagnostic procedure, such as a gastrointestinal endoscopy.
- Diagnostic procedures pose some risk to the patient. It is important for the nurse to understand the purpose of the diagnostic procedure, the appropriate preprocedural assessments required, the role of the nurse during the procedure, expected outcomes, potential risks, the appropriate actions in event of unexpected outcomes, and appropriate postprocedural nursing care. Patient safety principles guide all aspects of the procedure (National Patient Safety Consortium, 2017).
- IV sedation is used for diagnostic or surgical procedures that do not require complete or general anaesthesia. Sedation classifications include "minimal," "moderate," or "deep" sedation/analgesia, depending on the depth of sedation (CAS, 2018d).
- The Canadian Anesthesiologists' Society (CAS) has adopted the American Society of Anesthesiologists' (ASA) physical status classification (Box 10.1) system to determine if patients are at risk for undesirable outcomes. Use of this objective scale can reduce the risk for complications by determining when it is prudent to use interprofessional collaboration (e.g., anaesthesiologist) to assist in the collaborative management of a complicated patient condition (CAS, 2018c).
- These scales incorporate evidence-informed guidelines to reduce the risk for sedation-induced complications such as cardiac arrhythmias, respiratory failure, renal insufficiency, and neurological sequelae related to the use of paralytic agents.
- Proper sequencing of tests improves efficiency and quality of the outcomes.

BOX 10.1

ASA Physical Status Classification System

P1/ASA I = Normal healthy patient (nonsmoker, minimal or no alcohol use)

P2/ASA II = Patient with mild systemic disease (mild diseases; controlled hypertension or diabetes mellitus, current smoker/social alcohol drinker, obesity, pregnancy)

P3/ASA III = Patient with severe systemic disease (poorly controlled diabetes or hypertension, COPD, morbid obesity, alcohol misuse, stroke, myocardial infarction greater than 3 months)

P4/ASA IV = Patient with severe systemic disease that is a constant threat to life (stroke, myocardial infarction less than 3 months, ongoing cardiac ischemia, sepsis)

P5/ASA V = Moribund patient who is not expected to survive without the operation (ruptured abdominal/thoracic aneurysm, massive trauma, ischemic bowel, multi-organ dysfunction)

P6/ASA VI = Declared brain-dead patient whose organs are being removed for donor purposes

The letter "E" is added if the procedure is performed as an emergency.

COPD, Chronic obstructive pulmonary disease.
From Canadian Anesthesiologists' Society (CAS). (2018). *Appendix 2: American Society of Anesthesiologists' classification of physical status.* Retrieved from https://cas.ca/English/Page/Files/97_Appendix%202.pdf.

- An interprofessional team-based approach to care, where all health care team members work to the full scope of practice with a common vision, is optimal (Coffey & Anyinam, 2015).

PERSON-CENTRED CARE

- Any diagnostic procedure can create a sense of powerlessness for patients. The unknown (i.e., not knowing what a test may reveal or not completely understanding what a test involves) can also create fear and anxiety.
- Involve patients in a discussion of what to expect when a test is performed and provide ample opportunity for questions. Explore with patients their concerns to identify a mutual plan to address their apprehension. For example, if a patient is worried about being physically exposed during a procedure, communicate with procedure staff to minimize exposure through the use of draping.
- When a patient is chronically ill or fatigued with decreased functional status, plan the diagnostic testing schedule to provide rest periods between multiple tests performed on the same day.
- Having a nursing presence and using an empathetic approach throughout the procedure to provide explanations and reassurance will decrease anxiety and expedite the process.

EVIDENCE-INFORMED PRACTICE

- Topical anaesthetics (e.g., eutectic mixture of local anaesthetics [EMLA]) should be used for all skin-breaking procedures in children, unless contraindicated (HSC, 2017).
- Preprocedural fasting should be in accordance to the CAS standards and individualized for each patient according to the level of sedation, patient comorbidities, and procedure. Evidence has not demonstrated an increased aspiration of gastric contents with liberal fasting guidelines (CAS, 2018a).
- The literature demonstrates a wide variation in patient positioning post–cardiac catheterization. However, there is no agreement on the length of bed rest, which ranges from 2 to 24 hours, or head elevation (Suggs, Lewis, Troutman-Jordan, et al., 2017). The literature suggests there is no increase in complications with position change and early mobilization in post–cardiac catheterization (Suggs et al., 2017).
- An updated review of the literature concluded that there was no evidence suggesting that routine bed rest after lumbar puncture (LP) is beneficial for the prevention of postprocedure headache (PPH). The role of fluid supplementation in the prevention of PPH also remains unclear (Arevalo-Rodriguez, Ciapponi, Roqué i Figuls, et al., 2016).

SAFETY GUIDELINES

Before a Procedure

- The use of two person-specific identifiers to ensure positive patient identification is required prior to any procedure. The first includes verbal verification using acceptable identifiers (i.e., patient's name, hospital/encounter number, date of birth, health card number) and the second one involves checking the identification against a source such as a requisition or prescription to confirm the correct procedure for the correct patient (Accreditation Canada, 2019; World Health Organization, 2007).
- Patient requirements prior to a procedure include informed consent, history and physical that includes findings to verify indication of the proposed procedure, past health-identifying comorbidities (e.g., sleep apnea), ASA classification, height, weight, vital signs, evaluation of the airway, auscultation of heart sounds and breath

sounds, allergies, history of tobacco, alcohol or substance use/misuse, electrocardiogram (ECG), laboratory tests, consultations with other health care team members, and medications (prescription, nonprescription, vitamins, and over-the-counter). Review of the discharge process, including adult accompaniment who will be able to report any complications should they occur (Quality Management Partnership [QMP], 2015). Follow the employer policy regarding accompaniment by a responsible person postprocedure. Factors to consider are age, general health status, type of procedure, and procedural medications.

- On the day of the procedure, updates to the documentation include any changes to medical history or medications taken prior to the procedure. Anticoagulant or antiplatelet medications are assessed. Baseline vital signs are documented, along with a blood glucose for patients with diabetes mellitus; as well, time and nature of last oral intake are documented. A two-stage verification process is used: The patient's name and date of birth must be confirmed with the patient or substitute decision maker. The second verification must be completed by a different team member, with the entire care team present. All members of the interprofessional team are to introduce themselves and identify their role (QMP, 2015). A *time-out* may be called as part of the preprocedure safety review, where the team verifies the right procedure, correct patient, that the procedure is being performed on the correct site, allergies, presence of renal failure, and last dose of anticoagulants. If the team agrees, the procedure may commence with the premedication (Kern, Sorajja, & Lim, 2016). Instruct the patient to put on a patient gown, remove undergarments as necessary, and secure jewellery from area to be imaged (Pagana, Pagana, & Pike-MacDonald, 2019).

- Identify any medications for which uninterrupted dosing is required (e.g., anticonvulsants, antibiotics, and certain cardiac medications). If the procedure requires the patient to have nothing by mouth (NPO), discuss medications with the health care provider for further prescriptions. When insulin or oral hypoglycemic medications are given to patients before procedures, arrange to have either the patient's meal or other nutritional support available on completion of the procedure. Verify that informed consent was obtained before administering any sedatives. The health care provider performing the procedure is responsible for obtaining informed consent from the patient. *When there is no evidence of informed consent in the patient medical record, hold any preprocedure medications that may alter the patient's level of consciousness and notify the health care provider performing the procedure and staff in any receiving area.*

- Verify that emergency equipment is readily available and functioning (e.g., oxygen, suction, defibrillator, airway management equipment).

- Confirm presence of medications for routine administration and resuscitation, as required (i.e., reversal agents for opioids and benzodiazepines, anaphylaxis) (CAS, 2018a).

During a Procedure

- When a procedure involves the use of ionizing radiation (radiation with enough energy to alter the molecular components), for example, chest X-ray or computer tomography (CT):
  - Minimize the amount of radiation exposure by using protective shielding devices such as a lead apron and lead eyeglasses, radioprotective gloves, and a thyroid shield.
  - Routinely monitor all personnel's radiation exposure through the use of a dosimeter or radiation badge, as radiation exposure is cumulative (Kern et al., 2016).
  - Personnel should remain positioned as far away from the radiographic equipment as possible while performing required patient care.

- Monitor physiological parameters indicated by the procedure. Position patients carefully to avoid musculoskeletal or neurological injury.

- Label any specimens obtained accurately and transport to lab according to employer policy.

After the Procedure

- Assess for possible procedural complications for early detection and intervention.
- Monitor oxygen saturation and vital signs to detect adverse effects from sedation (i.e., vomiting, hypoxic events) (CAS, 2018d).
- Be familiar with the use, side effects, and complications of sedative and reversal drugs administered.
- Prepare to monitor for cardiac dysrhythmias.
- Institute fall precautions until the patient has recovered from effects of sedatives.
- Conduct neurovascular assessments for early identification of postprocedure limb ischemia or other arterial complications.

✦ SKILL 10.1   Intravenous Moderate (Conscious) Sedation

Certain diagnostic or therapeutic procedures require patients to receive intravenous (IV) moderate sedation. Moderate sedation or analgesia produces a minimally depressed level of consciousness induced by administration of pharmacological agents during which a patient has the ability to maintain protective reflexes and a patent airway. Moderate sedation improves the patient's assistance with the procedure, allowing for a rapid return to their preprocedure status and minimizing risk for injury. It often raises a patient's pain threshold and provides amnesia of the procedural events. Deep sedation is one risk associated with moderate or conscious sedation, which results in significant depression of the patient's level of consciousness. Owing to the patient's decreased level of consciousness, the patient may not have the capacity to protect their own airway, necessitating insertion of an artificial airway and manual ventilation with a bag-valve mask. Because of this risk of respiratory compromise, the use of IV moderate sedation is closely controlled and normally restricted to health care providers who receive specialized training (CAS, 2018d).

The most common types of medications used to achieve moderate sedation include benzodiazepines and opioids. Benzodiazepines reduce anxiety and promote muscle relaxation. Midazolam also produces an amnesic effect. Opioids such as morphine or fentanyl maintain pain control while achieving sedation.

Patient risks during IV moderate sedation include hypoventilation, airway compromise, hemodynamic instability, and deeper level of sedation resulting in a depressed level of consciousness or agitation and combativeness (Metzner & Domino, 2015). Emergency equipment appropriate for the patient's age and size (see Chapter 27) and health team members well trained in airway management, oxygen delivery, and use of resuscitation equipment are essential (CAS, 2018a). During a procedure, continuous monitoring (documented at least every 5 minutes) is required: heart rate and rhythm, respiratory rate, blood pressure, oxygen saturation, and level of consciousness (CAS, 2018a). End-tidal carbon dioxide (CO_2) is also becoming a common parameter for monitoring ventilation status during administration of IV sedation (Metzner & Domino,

2015). An end-tidal CO_2 monitoring device is placed between the endotracheal tube and the bag-valve mask; it detects the level of CO_2, which reflects the effectiveness of ventilation. Monitoring of the parameters just listed continues after the procedure.

Delegation and Collaboration

The skill of assisting with IV moderate sedation, including the preprocedure assessment, cannot be delegated to an unregulated care provider (UCP). In most facilities, a health care provider assesses and monitors a patient's level of sedation, airway patency, and level of consciousness. Roles in monitoring depend on scope-of-practice guidelines as determined by provincial/territorial regulations and employer policy.

Equipment

- Personal protective equipment (PPE): Gloves, mask, head cover, gown, eye protection
- Sedation as prescribed: benzodiazepines, opioids, and short-acting anaesthetic agents
- Emergency equipment: Crash cart, cardiac monitor/defibrillator, and endotracheal intubation/airway management equipment in various sizes and appropriate for patient's age, resuscitation drugs
- Equipment for insertion of a peripheral IV catheter (see Chapter 29)
- Oxygen and airway supplies; bag-valve mask device, oral/nasopharyngeal airways
- Suction equipment (see Chapter 25)
- Sphygmomanometer or noninvasive blood pressure monitor
- Pulse oximeter and/or end-tidal CO_2 monitor
- Electrocardiogram (ECG) monitor
- Appropriate reversal drugs (e.g., flumazenil for reversal of benzodiazepines, naloxone for reversal of opioids)
- Analgesia (opioids) for procedures anticipated to cause discomfort

STEP	RATIONALE

ASSESSMENT

1. Identify patient using at least two person-specific identifiers (i.e., name and date of birth or name and medical record number) according to employer policy. Compare identifiers with information in patient's medication administration record (MAR) or medical record.	Ensures correct patient. Complies with Accreditation Canada's standards and improves patient safety (Accreditation Canada, 2019).
2. Verify type of procedure scheduled and procedure site with patient, and identify interprofessional team.	Ensures correct procedure for correct patient.
3. Verify that a preprocedure medication reconciliation (see employer policy) and history and physical examination were completed.	Accrediting agencies, such as the CAS (2018d), require a documented preprocedure medication history and history and physical examination before administration of procedural IV sedation.
4. Verify that informed consent was obtained before administering any sedatives.	Federal regulations, provincial/territorial laws, and accreditation agencies require informed consent for procedures.
5. Assess patient's past history of adverse reaction to IV sedation (e.g., hemodynamic instability, nausea or vomiting, airway compromise, altered level of consciousness).	Patients with a history of these reactions are at higher risk for procedural complications if IV sedation is used.
6. Verify patient's ASA physical status classification (see Box 10.1).	ASA recommends that patients receiving classification of 3 or higher have anaesthesia consultation before receiving IV sedation (CAS, 2018b).

Clinical Decision Point *Consultation with an anaesthesiologist is often required by the facility if a patient has an ASA classification of 3 to 6 or a history of or evidence for difficult intubation, sleep apnea, or complications related to sedation/anaesthesia.*

7. Assess patient for history of airway abnormalities, liver failure, lung disease, heart failure, hypotonia, morbid obesity, severe gastroesophageal reflux, and history of adverse reaction to sedatives (CAS, 2018a).	These risk factors increase likelihood of adverse event (CAS, 2018a).
8. Assess patient's current status or history regarding substance use/misuse or liver/kidney disease.	A history of substance use or misuse, liver or kidney disease, or both usually requires dose adjustment of sedative agents.
9. Verify that patient has not ingested food or fluids, except for oral medications, for at least 4 hours.	Because risk of moderate sedation is loss of airway protection, an empty stomach reduces risk for aspiration.
10. Determine if patient is allergic to latex, antiseptic, tape, or anaesthetic solutions.	Allergic reactions to latex or tape range from mild skin reaction to anaphylaxis. Common allergic reactions to local anaesthetic agents include central nervous system (CNS) depression, respiratory difficulty, and hypotension.
11. Assess patient's level of understanding of procedure, including any concerns.	Determines extent of instruction or level of support required.
12. Assess baseline heart rate, breath sounds, respiratory rate, blood pressure, level of consciousness, pain level, and pulse oximetry (SpO_2).	Establishes baseline for comparison during and after procedure.

STEP	RATIONALE

ASSESSMENT

13. Determine patient's height and weight.
14. Assess patient's baseline status via designated scoring system of employer. A variety of tools are available for scoring (e.g., Aldrete score; National Association of Perioperative Nurses of Canada [NAPAN], 2018; Table 10.1).

Needed to calculate drug dosages.
Establishes baseline for comparison after procedure.

NURSING DIAGNOSES

- Acute pain
- Anxiety
- Potential for aspiration
- Potential for injury

Related factors/Risk factors are individualized on the basis of patient's condition or needs.

PLANNING

1. Expected outcomes following completion of procedures:
   - Adhere to the Surgical Safety Checklist (CPSI 2009) or employer-specific checklist (Box 10.2).
   - Patient's airway remains patent.

   - Patient's level of comfort is equivalent to score of 4 or less on pain scale of 0 to 10.
2. Explain to patient that IV sedation will cause relaxation and amnesia but that they will be awake during the procedure. If patient will not be able to verbalize because of nature of procedure, teach patient agreed-on nonverbal signals for words such as *yes*, *no*, and *pain*.
3. Reassure patient of nursing presence by explaining that close monitoring of vital signs and frequent assessment to determine if patient is awake are normal procedure.
4. Explain to patient major steps of procedure.
5. Position patient as needed for procedure.

Maintains patient safety (CPSI, 2009, 2014).

Moderate sedation is monitored successfully without progression to deep sedation.
Procedure managed to minimize patient's pain.

Encourages patient participation and minimizes risks and anxiety about procedure.

Reduces patient anxiety during procedure.

Reduces patient anxiety during procedure.

IMPLEMENTATION

1. Establish peripheral IV access (RNAO, 2004/2008) (see also Chapter 29).
2. Complete Surgical Safety Checklist with all health care team members (as applicable) and in accordance with employer policy (see Box 10.2).
3. During diagnostic procedure, monitor heart rate and SpO_2 continuously via pulse oximetry equipment. Some agencies also use end-tidal CO_2 monitoring (capnography) (Metzner & Domino, 2015). Monitor patient's airway patency, respiratory rate and depth, blood pressure, and level of consciousness and responsiveness every 5 to 15 minutes (Lewis, Bucher, Heitkemper, et al., 2019).

Provides access for administration of sedation and any emergency medications (as needed).
Ensures patient safety by correctly identifying correct patient with correct procedure.

Vital signs, oximetry, and capnography provide comparison with patient's baseline status.

BOX 10.2

Surgical Safety Checklist

- Anaesthesia equipment safety check completed.
- Verification of correct person, consent, correct site, and correct procedure occurs.
- Procedure site is marked before moving to procedure area.
- A "time-out" is performed immediately before starting procedures.

- When patient is in preprocedure area (immediately before moving them to procedure room), a checklist (i.e., paper, electronic, or other medium such as a wall-mounted white board) is used to review and verify that required items are available and accurately matched to the patient.

From Canadian Patient Safety Institute (CPSI). (2009). *Surgical safety checklist.* Retrieved from http://www.patientsafetyinstitute.ca/en/toolsResources/pages/surgicalsafety-checklist-resources.aspx.

STEP	RATIONALE

IMPLEMENTATION

4. Assess verbal or nonverbal evidence of pain, such as grimacing, crying, and restlessness (Lewis et al., 2019).

Physical responses augment pain assessment.

5. Assess level of sedation using a sedation scale such as the Motor Assessment Activity Scale (MASS), Sedation Agitation Scale (SAS), or Modified Ramsay Sedation Scale (Table 10.2) or other criteria as per employer policy.

Determines patient's level of sedation. A valid and reliable rating scale offers consistent assessment and accurate judgement of patient's changing status and verbal and physical stimulation.

Clinical Decision Point *Report a Ramsay Sedation score higher than 3 (responsive to commands only) to the health care provider (see Table 10.2).*

6. Reposition patient as needed without interrupting diagnostic procedure.

Prevents pressure- and position-related injuries (Lewis et al., 2019).

EVALUATION

1. Monitor patient throughout procedure using the Modified Ramsay Sedation Scale (or other criteria per employer policy).

Provides data to verify patient's expected return to baseline status.

2. After procedure: Use Aldrete score (see Table 10.1) or similar scale to monitor level of consciousness, respiratory rate, SpO_2, blood pressure, heart rate and rhythm, and pain score according to employer policy (Taslakian & Sridhar, 2017) (e.g., every 5 minutes for at least 30 minutes, then every 15 minutes for an hour, and then every 30 minutes until patient meets discharge criteria).

Enables prompt detection of any airway compromise or protective reflexes caused by delayed action of medications.

3. Ask patient to repeat back what they understand regarding procedure or any postprocedure patient instructions, including medication prescriptions and instructions.

Verifies patient understanding of procedure or discharge education.

TABLE 10.1

Aldrete Scoring System—Modified

		Score
Activity (moving voluntarily on command)	4 extremities	2
	2 extremities	1
	0 extremities	0
Respiration	Able to breathe deeply and cough freely	2
	Dyspnea, shallow or limited breathing	1
	Apneic	0
Circulation	BP ± 20 mm Hg of presedation level	2
	BP ± 20–50 mm Hg of presedation level	1
	BP ± 50 mm Hg of presedation level	0
Consciousness	Fully awake	2
	Arousable on having name called	1
	Not responding	0
Pulse oximetry	92% while breathing room air	2
	Needs supplemental oxygen to maintain saturation >90%	1
	90% even with supplemental oxygen	0

From International Anesthesia Research Society (IARS). (2018). PACU bypass: Stage 1 bypass criteria: Aldrete's original scoring system modified. *Open Anesthesia*. Retrieved from https://www.openanesthesia.org/pacu_bypass_stage_i_bypass_criteria/.

BP, Blood pressure.

TABLE 10.2

Modified Ramsay Sedation Scale

Value	Description	Assessment
1	Awake: Anxious and agitated or restless or both	Observe the patient
2	Awake: Cooperative, oriented, and tranquil	Observe the patient. Does the patient make eye contact and respond to commands?
3	Awake: Patient responds to commands only	Talk to the patient. Does patient make eye contact and respond to commands?
4	Asleep: Brisk response to a light glabellar (forehead) tap or loud auditory stimulus	Physically stimulate the patient by shaking the shoulder while speaking loudly. Does patient respond after 10 seconds?
5	Asleep: Sluggish response to a light forehead tap or loud auditory stimulus	Physically stimulate the patient by shaking the shoulder while speaking loudly. Does patient respond after 10 seconds?
6	Asleep: No response to pain	Use painful stimuli. No response.

Data from Canadian Anesthesiologists' Society (CAS). (2018). *Appendix 6: An official position paper of the CAS.* Retrieved from https://cas.ca/English/Page/Files/97_Appendix%206.pdf.

STEP	RATIONALE

EVALUATION

STEP	RATIONALE
4. Have patient's "designated driver" or responsible person explain any postprocedure education and sign appropriate documents.	Patients who receive conscious sedation are restricted from driving for 24 to 48 hours, depending on procedure, type of sedation, and postprocedure restrictions (CAS, 2018a).
5. **Use Teach-Back:** "I want to be sure I explained everything clearly to you. Please tell in your own words what you heard me say about the medications that you will be taking once you are home." Develop a revised teaching plan if patient or caregiver is not able to teach back correctly.	Determines patient's and caregiver's level of understanding of instructional topic.

Unexpected Outcomes	Related Interventions
1. Oversedation, evidenced by decreasing SpO_2 (cyanosis, slow shallow respirations with periods of apnea), tachycardia, sedation score of 4 (exhibiting brisk response to light glabellar [forehead] tap or loud auditory stimulus) or higher on Modified Ramsay Sedation Scale or less than 8 on Aldrete scale.	• Support ventilation through positioning, insertion of nasal or oral airway, and use of a bag-valve mask • Immediately notify health care provider. • Be prepared to administer reversal agents. Naloxone is for reversal of opioids, and flumazenil is for reversal of benzodiazepines.

Clinical Decision Point *Naloxone or flumazenil can be used as reversal agents for opioids and benzodiazepines. Caution must be used, because the duration of action of the reversal agents is shorter than the duration of the opioids or sedation agents (CAS, 2018d).*

2. Patient develops cardiac instability evidenced by irregular heart rate, change in pulse rate, or change in blood pressure.	• Initiate oxygen therapy, ensure IV access, and obtain ECG as prescribed. • Immediately notify health care provider.

Communication and Documentation

- Document vital signs, SpO_2, end-tidal CO_2, and sedation level at baseline, then every 5 minutes during the procedure, and every 15 minutes for at least 30 minutes after the procedure according to employer policy.
- Document dosage, route, and time of administration for drugs given during and after the procedure, including reversal agents, in the electronic health record (EHR) or chart.
- Document significant patient reactions during the procedure.
- Document intake and output, including IV fluids and blood products if administered.
- Immediately report to patient's health care provider any respiratory distress, cardiac compromise, or unexpected altered mental status, using SBAR format.
- Document discharge teaching, medication reconciliation, discontinuation of IV access, final/discharge assessment, and to whom and how discharged (e.g., designated driver, ambulance or transporter, nursing home).
- Document your evaluation of patient and caregiver learning.

Special Considerations

Teaching

- Explain that it is unlikely for patients to remember the procedure because of the amnesic effect of the sedative(s).
- Before the procedure, instruct patient to arrange for transportation home after the procedure because patient usually will not be permitted to drive for 24 hours after receiving sedation.
- Provide patients and caregivers with discharge instructions that include complications that may occur; how to manage complications; and physical signs and symptoms to report to the health care provider, including contact information and postprocedure medication reconciliation and instructions. Prior to engaging in discharge teaching, perform a needs assessment so that the discharge instructions are tailored to the patient's and caregiver's learning styles and provide information they require to safely transition to their home.

Pediatric

- Often, children undergoing surgery are healthy when compared with adults, but pediatric patients have some unique surgical risks: physiological challenges (e.g., neonatal circulation, high propensity to suffer fluid losses and hypothermia); airway anatomy that is smaller and narrower than an adult's; smaller blood volumes; and immature immune system (Lagoo, Lopushinsky, Haynes, et al., 2017).
- The pediatric patient often has limited understanding of the surgical procedure and the parent or guardian is usually the decision maker and advocate for the child (Lagoo et al., 2017).
- During the preprocedure assessment answer the parent's questions in a relaxed and confident manner. When communicating with children, demonstrate person-centred care and consider the child's developmental stage.

Gerontological

- Closely monitor the effects of analgesia, sedation, and anaesthetic agents on older persons' respiratory and hemodynamic status. These medications may interfere with the respiratory rate or heart rate as a result of reduced drug clearance through the kidneys or liver (Lewis et al., 2019).
- Physical limitations of the patient, including hearing and vision loss, contribute to frustration and confusion, compounding the sense of loss of control.
- In older persons, some medications are not metabolized as rapidly, leading to drug toxicity and overdose (Lewis et al., 2019).

Care in the Community

- Instruct patient to avoid making any legally binding decisions until at least 24 hours after the procedure.

- The patient and caregiver should be instructed in wound care; pain management; resuming medications, activity, driving, or dietary restrictions; follow-up appointment with health care provider; and complications to observe for and report (CAS, 2018d).

- The patient should be alerted to complications that require urgent assessment at the health care provider clinic or emergency department, for example, bleeding.

◆ SKILL 10.2 **Contrast Media Studies: Arteriogram (Angiogram), Cardiac Catheterization, and Intravenous Pyelogram**

Contrast media studies involve visualization of blood vessels and internal organs by intravascular injection of a radiopaque medium. An arteriogram (angiogram) permits visualization of the vasculature and arterial system of an organ (Fig. 10.1). Arteriography is performed by an interventional radiologist to diagnose arterial or venous occlusions such as stenosis, emboli, thromboses, aneurysms, and tumours; congenital malformations; or traumas.

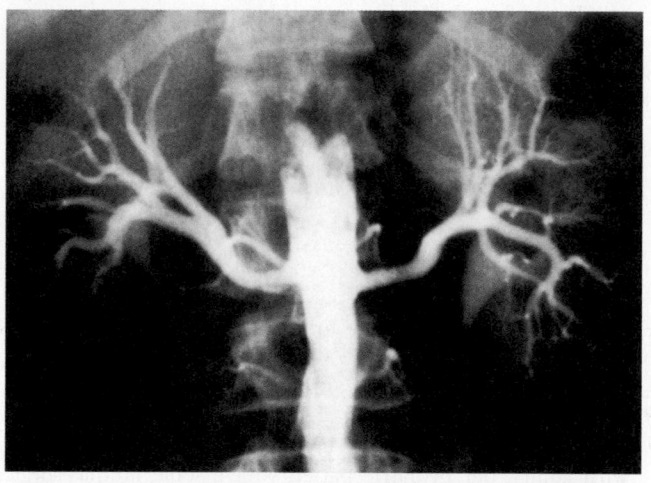

FIG 10.1 Renal arteriogram. *(From Pagana, K., Pagana, T., & Pike-Mac-Donald, S. [2019]. Mosby's Canadian manual of diagnostic and laboratory tests [2nd Cdn ed., p. 1027, Fig. 12-1]. Toronto, ON: Elsevier Inc.)*

Cardiac catheterization is a specialized form of angiography performed by an interventional cardiologist. An intravenous (IV) or intra-arterial catheter introducer is inserted into the left or right side of the heart via a major peripheral vessel, usually the femoral artery or vein. The test studies pressures within the heart, cardiac volumes, valvular function, and patency of coronary arteries. Cardiac catheterizations are performed in specially equipped laboratories (Fig. 10.2). A contrast medium is injected, and the structures and functions of the heart and lungs are assessed.

Cardiac catheterizations are contraindicated in patients who would refuse needed surgery, are allergic to iodine contrast media, are uncooperative or cannot lie still during the entire procedure, or are susceptible to dye-induced renal failure. People at particular risk for renal issues or contrast-induced nephrotoxicity (CIN) are those with pre-existing renal dysfunction, diabetes mellitus, heart failure, hypertension or hypotension, advanced age, anemia, or previous chemotherapy; those taking nephrotoxic medications (e.g., loop diuretics, vancomycin, NSAIDs); and Indigenous people (Kern et al., 2016). Interventions to help prevent dye-induced renal failure are controversial and include prehydrating the patient with bicarbonate solution or sodium chloride with or without prophylactic N-acetylcysteine (Honicker & Holt, 2016).

IV pyelography (IVP) is an examination of the kidneys, ureters, and bladder using contrast medium to investigate an obstruction, hematuria, stones, bladder injury, or renal artery occlusion. Dye is injected intravenously via a peripheral vein, followed by serial radiographs taken over the subsequent 30 minutes (Pagana et al., 2019).

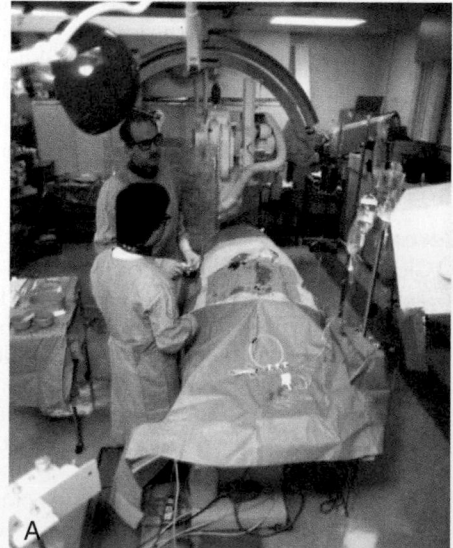
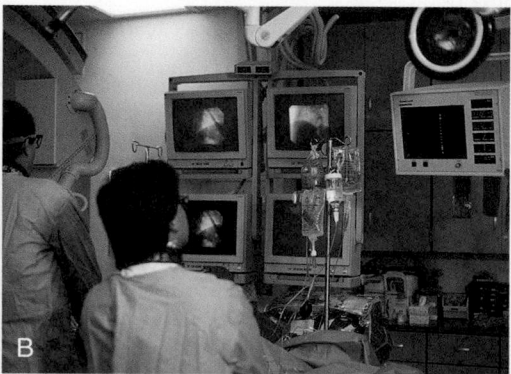

FIG 10.2 A, Clinical setting for cardiac catheterization. **B,** Monitoring of cardiac catheterization procedure. *(From Pagana, K., Pagana, T., & Pike-MacDonald, S. [2015]. Mosby's Canadian manual of diagnostic and laboratory tests [1st Cdn ed., p. 1146, Fig. 12-8]. Toronto, ON: Elsevier Canada.)*

Delegation and Collaboration

Interprofessional collaboration is required when caring for a patient who is having a cardiac catheterization, to maximize patient safety. Each team member is a valued contributor to ensure the patient expediently undergoes the procedure. The team includes the primary health care provider or interventional cardiologist; a circulating nurse or technologist who is capable of assisting in all aspects of the procedure, including emergency cardiovascular care (Kern et al., 2016); a scrub nurse or technician who assists the interventional cardiologist with equipment and supplies during the catheterization; and a radiology technician with the ability to monitor and archive ECG and hemodynamic data. A culture of patient safety is promoted through interprofessional collaboration using effective communication (Kern et al., 2016).

The skill of assisting with an angiography, IVP, and cardiac catheterization can be delegated to an unregulated care provider (UCP) if the patient is stable, no IV sedation is used, the nurse is always present, and employer policy indicates this role for the UCP. The nurse directs the UCP about:

- When to obtain and report vital signs, urinary output, and weight
- Which signs and symptoms to report to the nurse
- Assistance with patient transport, positioning, and obtaining supplies

Equipment

- Personal protective equipment (PPE): Mask, sterile gown, head cover, eye protection, and sterile gloves
- Sterile packs containing catheters and equipment for performing procedures
- Equipment for peripheral IV access
- Medications such as sedatives (e.g., diazepam, midazolam, propofol) for IV sedation, or analgesics for relaxation and pain control
- Emergency equipment: Oxygen, endotracheal intubation and airway management equipment, emergency cart with resuscitation medications, cardiac monitor and defibrillator, sedative reversal agents
- Pulse oximeter, end-tidal carbon dioxide (CO_2) monitor, blood pressure (BP) equipment

STEP	RATIONALE

ASSESSMENT

1. Identify patient using at least two person-specific identifiers (e.g., name and date of birth or name and medical record number) according to employer policy. Compare identifiers with information on patient's medication administration record (MAR) or medical record.

Ensures correct patient. Complies with Accreditation Canada's standards and improves patient safety (Accreditation Canada, 2019).

2. Verify type of procedure scheduled and procedure site with patient.

Ensures correct procedure and patient (CAS, 2018a).

3. Verify that informed consent was obtained before administering any sedatives.

Federal regulations, many provincial/territorial laws, and accreditation agencies require informed consent for procedure.

4. Determine if patient is taking anticoagulants, aspirin, or any nonsteroidal medication.

Some medications increase risk for bleeding and are often stopped before the procedure according to employer policy or health care provider's prescriptions (e.g., 24 hours, 3–4 days prior to procedure, depending on the medication).

5. Assess patient for history of any allergies to iodine dye, shellfish, or latex and whether patient has had previous reaction to contrast agent. If so, notify cardiologist or radiologist (Pagana et al., 2019).

Allergic individuals may be at a mildly increased risk for developing adverse reactions to radiocontrast media (hypoallergenic contrast medium is sometimes used). Whenever a patient is receiving contrast medium, a health care team trained in resuscitation procedures should be available (Kern et al., 2016).

6. Review medical record for contraindications:
   a. *All contrast media:* Pregnancy unless benefits of test outweigh risks to fetus.
   b. *Angiography:* Anticoagulant therapy, bleeding disorders, thrombocytopenia, dehydration, uncontrolled hypertension, renal insufficiency, and pregnancy.

   c. *Cardiac catheterization:* History of severe cardiomyopathy, severe dysrhythmias, uncontrolled heart failure (HF).
   d. *IVP:* History of dehydration, known renal insufficiency (with blood urea nitrogen [BUN] level greater than 35 mmol/L or creatinine greater than 247 mmol/L (Pagana et al., 2019).

Radioactive iodinated contrast medium crosses blood–placental barrier.
Anticoagulants and bleeding disorders interfere with patient's blood-clotting abilities and may cause blood loss.
Dehydration and renal insufficiency are contraindications to use of ionic radiographic contrast medium because patient has impaired ability to excrete contrast medium via kidneys.
Introduction of catheters into the heart increases risk for dysrhythmias (Pagana et al., 2019).
Iodinated dye is nephrotoxic and worsens existing renal disease.

STEP	RATIONALE

ASSESSMENT

e. Determine whether patient took metformin hydrochloride within previous 48 hours. If so, notify health care provider immediately.

Metformin hydrochloride, an oral hypoglycemic prescribed for type 2 diabetes mellitus, may or may not be discontinued 1 day before the procedure and 2 days after catheterization because of the possibility of causing lactic acidosis, leading to acute renal failure (Pagana et al., 2019).

7. Assess patient's bleeding and coagulation status (i.e., complete blood count [CBC], platelets, prothrombin time [PT], activated partial thromboplastin time [aPTT], international normalized ratio [INR]) and patient's renal function (e.g., BUN, creatinine levels) before procedure. Assess electrolytes (sodium and potassium).

The procedure may be cancelled or modified in the presence of abnormal laboratory results. Most significant risks are hemorrhage and/or renal failure. Hypokalemia may precipitate lethal arrhythmias (Pagana et al., 2019).

8. Obtain vital signs and weight and assess peripheral pulses. For arterial procedures, mark patient's peripheral pulses before procedure. For cardiac catheterization, auscultate heart and lungs.

Provides baseline data of location of peripheral pulses for comparison during and after procedure. Many emergency medications are weight based; therefore, having an accurate weight permits accurate dosing. Breath sounds are assessed to detect changes such as mild heart failure for early intervention. Heart sounds are assessed for early detection of complications.

9. Assess patient's hydration status, including condition of mucous membranes, and recent 24-hour intake.

Severe dehydration can lead to renal failure (Pagana et al., 2019).

10. Assess patient's level of procedural understanding, exploring any concerns.

Determines extent of instruction or level of support required.

11. Determine type of arteriogram scheduled (i.e., carotid, femoral, brachial). If cardiac catheterization, verify if test is for right or left heart or both. For IVP, confirm if study is for one or both kidneys.

Enables nurse to anticipate patient teaching needs and postprocedure interventions.

12. Determine and document last time of ingested food, drink, or medications. Patients should be NPO for 2 to 8 hours before procedure (see employer policy).

Prevents possible aspiration due to patient sedation. Excessive hydration causes dilution of contrast medium, making structures more difficult to visualize. (Pagana et al., 2019).

Clinical Decision Point *Exceptions occur for patients at risk for contrast media–induced renal impairment who are specifically instructed to drink increased fluids in the hours before the procedure or those instructed by the health care provider to take medications before the procedure. Preprocedure hydration reduces the risk for renal impairment caused by contrast media (Pagana et al., 2019).*

13. Review health care provider's prescriptions for preprocedure medications, hydration, antihistamines, and IV sedation:

Increased sedation is necessary for anxious or confused patients. Increased hydration is often required for renal insufficiency and antihistamines for possible allergic reaction.

a. Atropine

Decreases salivary secretions and increases heart rate when bradycardia is present.

b. Diphenhydramine

Used prophylactically to block histamine and decrease allergic response.

c. Preprocedural sedation

Decreases anxiety and promotes relaxation.

NURSING DIAGNOSES

- Decreased cardiac output
- Acute pain
- Fear of the unknown
- Anxiety
- Potential for infection
- Potential for injury

Related factors/Risk factors are individualized on the basis of patient's condition or needs.

PLANNING

1. Expected outcomes following completion of procedure:
- Patient does not experience any procedure or postprocedure complications such as significant changes in vital signs, diminished or absent peripheral pulses, allergic response, or decreased or absent urine output.

Procedure performed without complication.

- Patient is assessed using an appropriate pain rating scale. Expected discomfort includes soreness at catheter insertion site and possible backache.

Patient tolerates procedure.

STEP	RATIONALE

PLANNING

- Patient tolerates increased fluid intake and urinates sufficiently (at least 30 mL/hr or 0.5 mL/kg/hr) to excrete radiographic dye. / Adequate renal function.
- Patient recovers from IV sedation without respiratory complications or change in level of consciousness. / Appropriate level of sedation.

2. Explain to patient purpose of procedure and what will happen during it. / Helps to minimize patient's anxiety.

3. Remove all of patient's jewellery, metal objects, and body piercings. / Eliminates objects that interfere with radiography visualization of vessels and could be conductive material during electrocautery.

4. Preprocedure preparation:

   a. *For IVP*: Verify that patient has completed necessary bowel preparation of orally administered evacuation preparation 24 hours before test and evacuation enema 8 hours before test (check employer policy). / An evacuated lower intestine and bowel improve visualization of urinary structures.

   b. *For cardiac catheterization*: Determine whether hair at site of catheter insertion needs clipping or preparation with antiseptic just before procedure. Allow antiseptic to dry. Do not shave site. / Reduces risk for site-related infection. Drying promotes maximal antibacterial activity. Shaving results in increased chance for infection.

5. For cardiac catheterization, it is common to verify availability of emergent cardiac surgery because of risk for complete coronary artery occlusion from dislodged plaque or inadvertent perforation of vasculature. Also verify patient's American Society of Anesthesiologists (ASA) classification before procedure (see Box 10.1). / Prepares backup plan for possible procedural outcomes that would require emergency surgery.

IMPLEMENTATION

1. Have patient empty bladder or bowels before procedure. / Ensures that patient's elimination needs are met prior to the procedure.

2. Prepare cardiac monitor, pulse oximeter, and/or end-tidal CO_2 monitor. / Provides easy access to equipment for monitoring patient status during and after procedure.

3. Perform hand hygiene and apply appropriate protective equipment. / Reduces transmission of microorganisms.

4. Provide IV access using large-bore cannula. Remove gloves. / Provides access for delivery of IV fluids and medications.

5. Help patient assume a comfortable supine position on X-ray table. Immobilize extremity that will be injected. Pad any bony prominences. / For arterial procedures, patient may need to maintain a specific position after the procedure (e.g., with femoral artery use, the extremity is extended for 1 to 3 hours postprocedure). Padding the bony prominences reduces the risk for impaired skin integrity or pressure ulcers.

6. Complete "time-out" to verify patient's name, type of procedure to be performed, and procedure site with patient. / "Time-out" verification just before starting an invasive procedure includes health care provider and all involved personnel and is a safety precaution to prevent wrong-patient, wrong-site, and wrong-procedure errors (CPSI, 2009; Kern et al., 2016).

7. Monitor vital signs, pulse oximetry (SpO_2), and end-tidal CO_2, and, for arterial procedures, palpate peripheral pulses. / Data provide comparison with baseline to determine patient's response to procedure.

8. Inform patient that during injection of dye it is common to experience some chest pain and a severe hot flash that is quite uncomfortable but lasts only a few seconds. / Dye causes feeling of warmth, flushing, or metallic taste shortly after injection.

9. All health care team members apply PPE (mask, goggles, sterile gown, head cover, and sterile gloves). Use sterile drapes to prepare the sterile field, leaving puncture site exposed. / Maintains surgical asepsis.

10. Health care provider cleanses arterial puncture site for catheter insertion (femoral, radial, carotid, or brachial) with antiseptic. / Reduces transmission of microorganisms.

11. Health care provider anaesthetizes skin overlying arterial puncture site. / Provides local anaesthetic to area of incision or puncture to minimize discomfort.

STEP	RATIONALE

IMPLEMENTATION

12. For arterial procedures health care provider does the following:

    a. Punctures artery, inserts introducer into artery, inserts guidewire through introducer and advances, and inserts flexible catheter over guidewire and advances into heart. Introducers allow for use of various procedure catheters, depending on need (e.g., balloon angioplasty, stent placement, ablation).

> Permits access to coronary arteries for diagnosis and intervention.

    b. Advances catheter to desired artery or cardiac chamber, removes guidewire, and injects contrast medium through catheter.

> Permits radiographic visualization of structures, aneurysms, occlusions, or other anomalies.

13. During dye injection, specialized machinery takes rapid sequence of X-ray films.

> Permits radiographic records of visualization of dye through artery and any abnormalities present.

14. If iodinated dye is used, observe patient for signs of anaphylaxis, including respiratory distress, palpitation, itching, and diaphoresis.

> Allergic reactions can be life threatening.

15. During cardiac catheterization the nurse helps with measuring cardiac volumes and pressure.

> Provides data related to cardiac output, central venous pressure (CVP), ventricular pressures, and pulmonary artery pressure.

Clinical Decision Point *Be prepared to end the cardiac catheterization procedure early in the event of severe unrelieved chest pain, neurological symptoms of a cerebrovascular accident, cardiac dysrhythmias, or hemodynamic changes (Pagana et al., 2019).*

16. Health care provider or nurse (see employer policy) administering IV sedation monitors levels of sedation, level of consciousness, and vital signs (see Skill 10.1).

> Achieving the correct level IV sedation does not cause loss of consciousness and the patient is able to maintain the airway.

17. Health care provider withdraws catheter and applies manual pressure to puncture site until homeostasis occurs (5 to 15 minutes or longer).

> Five to fifteen minutes of manual pressure is often enough to stop active site bleeding. However, a certain amount of bed rest is needed to achieve reliable hemostasis. Check employer policy for postprocedure bed rest requirements. This may vary from 2 to 6 hours when no arteriotomy closure device is used.

    a. *Option:* Health care provider may choose to use an arteriotomy closure device (ACD), which can be categorized as either passive- or active-closure devices. Passive-closure devices help with compression such as clamps or tamping devices, assisted or enhanced coagulation, and sealants. Some facilities use an elasticized pressure dressing and sandbag over the site to assist with hemostasis and to immobilize the limb. If the radial site is used, a compression bracelet is used to provide hemostasis. Active-closure devices or devices causing immediate closure using suture devices, clips, and collagen plug devices permit early ambulation.

> Use of ACDs is reasonable after invasive cardiovascular procedures performed via femoral artery to achieve faster hemostasis, shorter duration of bed rest, and improved patient comfort. Use of devices should be weighed against risk of complications (Kern et al., 2016).

Clinical Decision Point *Before removing catheter sheath, check health care provider's prescriptions for instructions for treating a vasovagal reaction. Manual pressure applied to the groin or femoral area can stimulate the baroreceptors and cause a vasovagal reaction in which the patient becomes bradycardic and hypotensive. Vasovagal reactions are usually brief and self-limiting. When applying pressure to the groin after sheath removal, be alert for a vasovagal reaction and be prepared to treat it by lowering the head of the bed to the flat position and giving a bolus of IV fluids.*

18. If a percutaneous coronary intervention (PCI) such as a percutaneous transluminal coronary angioplasty (PTCA) or directional coronary atherectomy (DCA) was performed during cardiac catheterization, a femoral introducer/sheath is often left in place and removed in several hours.

> Postinterventional sheaths provide emergency access to vasculature in the event that the coronary artery becomes occluded.

19. Remove and discard gloves. Perform hand hygiene.

> Reduces transmission of microorganisms.

STEP	RATIONALE

IMPLEMENTATION

20. Postprocedure

    a. For arterial procedures:

        (1) Patient keeps affected extremity extended and immobilized for 2 to 6 hours after removal of sheath (see employer policy). Patient uses bedpan as needed for bowel or bladder evacuation while on bed rest.

        There is evidence of no benefit relating to bleeding and hematoma formation in patients who have more than 3 hours of bed rest following transfemoral diagnostic cardiac catheterization. There is evidence of benefit relating to decreased incidence and severity of back pain after 3 hours of bed rest.

        (2) Emphasize to patient the need to lie flat for 6 to 12 hours (and possibly overnight if sheath is left in groin).

        Helps to prevent disruption of hemostasis.

    b. Encourage patient to drink fluids after procedure.

    Facilitates elimination of contrast material and prevents renal damage (Pagana et al., 2019).

EVALUATION

1. Evaluate patient's body position and comfort during procedure.

Position can cause stress on cannulation site and patient's musculoskeletal structures.

2. Monitor vital signs and SpO$_2$ and assess for signs of cardiac complications every 15 minutes for 1 hour, every 30 minutes for 2 hours, or until vital signs are stable.

Verifies patient's physiological status and evaluates effect of procedure. Signs of cardiac complications include chest pain or pressure, new dysrhythmias, and shortness of breath.

3. Monitor for complications:

    a. Perform neurovascular checks by palpating peripheral pulses on affected extremity and comparing right and left extremities for skin colour, temperature, and sensation. Use Doppler ultrasound to locate pulses that are not palpable (see Chapter 8).

Enables prompt detection of circulatory impairment caused by intravascular clotting or bleeding at procedure site. Signs of reduced circulation include diminishing distal pulses and/or coolness, mottling, pallor, pain, numbness, and tingling in affected extremity.

    b. When performing vital signs, assess vascular access site for bleeding and hematoma formation.

Verifies expected sealing of puncture.

    c. Auscultate heart and breath sounds for preprocedural comparison.

Evaluates patient response to procedure and identifies early deterioration.

    d. Observe patient for possible delayed reaction to iodine dye (if used)—dyspnea, hives, tachycardia, and rash (Pagana et al., 2019).

Reaction may occur up to 6 hours after injection of dye.

4. Evaluate level of sedation, level of consciousness, and SpO$_2$. Use Aldrete scale or a similar scale (see Table 10.1).

Determines patient's response to IV sedation.

5. Assess postprocedure laboratory values—CBC, PT, aPTT, INR, electrolytes, BUN/creatinine.

Detects changes in laboratory values that indicate onset of complications such as bleeding.

6. Have patient rate discomfort on pain scale of 0 to 10.

Pain is early sign of complications.

7. Use Teach-Back: "I want to be sure I have explained signs to be aware of to indicate an allergic reaction from the dye after this procedure. Tell me what you have heard that would make you think you might be having an allergic reaction." Develop a revised teaching plan if patient or caregiver is not able to teach back correctly.

Determines patient's and caregiver's level of understanding of instructional topic.

Unexpected Outcomes

1. Vasovagal response occurs (at time of femoral puncture or after procedure with femoral pressure). Symptoms include feeling faint, dizzy, and light-headed and possible momentary loss of consciousness. Bradycardia is caused by stimulation of vagus nerve via baroreceptors.

2. Evidence of oversedation:
   - Prolonged reduced level of consciousness.

3. Pedal pulses are no longer palpable bilaterally 2 hours after arteriogram with change in skin colour and temperature.

Related Interventions

- Support airway (through positioning).
- Lower table or head of bed to flat position.
- Be prepared to administer bolus of IV fluid (normal saline).

- See Skill 10.1.

- Assess pulse with Doppler ultrasound.
- Immediately notify health care provider.

STEP	RATIONALE
Unexpected Outcomes 4. Hematoma or hemorrhage is present at catheter insertion site.	**Related Interventions** • Apply pressure over insertion site. • Monitor catheter site every 15 to 30 minutes for 2 to 3 hours; follow employer policy. • Notify health care provider if interventions do not stop bleeding or if patient has symptoms of acute blood loss (hypotension, tachycardia, decreased level of consciousness).
5. Patient has allergic reaction to contrast medium with symptoms of flushing, itching, and urticaria.	• Monitor vital signs and observe for symptoms of anaphylaxis. • Notify health care provider. • Follow specific postprocedure prescriptions related to findings. • Prepare to administer antihistamine or epinephrine if prescribed.
6. Renal toxicity from contrast medium occurs: • Urine output less than 30 mL/hr or 0.5 mL/kg/hr.	• Place on strict intake and output monitoring. • Monitor closely for signs of fluid overload. Auscultate breath sounds (e.g., assess for crackles). • Review electrolyte, urea nitrogen, and creatinine levels.
7. Patient experiences retroperitoneal bleeding (when femoral access site is used): • Low back pain radiating to both sides of body (hallmark sign) • Tachycardia	• Prepare patient for emergency surgery. • Monitor vital signs every 5 to 15 minutes. • Monitor distal pulses hourly.

Communication and Documentation

- Document patient's status: vital signs, SpO_2/end-tidal CO_2, status of peripheral pulses for equality and symmetry, blood pressure for hypotension, temperature and colour of catheterized extremity, condition of IV site, and level of patient responsiveness in electronic health record (EHR) or chart. Document any drainage from puncture site, appearance of dressing, and condition of puncture site.
- Report to health care provider any vital sign change, excessive bleeding or increasing hematoma at puncture site, decreased or absent peripheral pulses, persistent pain, altered neurological status, dysrhythmias, decreased SpO_2 or increased end-tidal CO_2, or decreased responsiveness after sedation.
- Document your evaluation of health teaching provided to patient and caregiver.

Special Considerations
Teaching
- See Skill 10.1, Teaching Considerations.
- Prepare patient to stay in the hospital if complications occur or if an intervention necessitates prolonged postprocedure vascular checks.

Pediatric
Infants and children are particularly susceptible to the diuretic effects of radiocontrast dyes because of their small body size and immature renal and hepatic systems. In addition, those with congenital cardiac anomalies develop compensatory erythrocytosis and thus experience complications from dehydration very quickly. Emphasize to the parent(s) or caregiver the importance of fluid intake with the child after the procedure. Urinary output should exceed 1 mL/kg/hr (Perry, Hockenberry, Lowdermilk, et al., 2017).

Gerontological
- Physical exposure and low room temperature contribute to hypothermia in frail older persons who are unable to communicate that they are cold. Use heated blankets or forced-air heat to maintain core temperature at comfortable, safe levels (Lewis et al., 2019).
- In older persons, slight alterations in vital signs or behaviour are signs for impending problems; therefore, close monitoring is important.

Care in the Community
- On discharge provide patient with written instructions to contact the health care provider (or affiliated emergency department) if the following occur after arteriogram or cardiac catheterization:
  - Bleeding from the catheterization puncture site; apply gentle pressure with a clean gauze or cloth
  - Formation of a knot or lump under the skin that increases in size
  - Worsening of a bruise or its movement down the extremity rather than disappearing
  - Pain at puncture site or in the extremity used for the catheterization
  - Extremity is pale and cool to the touch where arterial puncture is made
  - Appearance of redness, swelling, or warmth of the affected extremity
- It is helpful to have patient or caregiver repeat these instructions back to you and to acknowledge clear understanding.
- After arteriogram or cardiac catheterization, instruct patient not to drive or climb stairs for 24 hours; to avoid sports, strenuous activity or housework, and lifting (e.g., groceries, children) for 3 days; and to avoid taking tub baths or swimming until wound is healed.
- On discharge after an IVP, instruct patient to:
  - Drink at least 1 to 2 L (34 to 68 ounces) of water to help flush the contrast medium through the kidneys.
  - Observe for signs of a delayed reaction to the contrast medium up to 24 hours after the procedure. If signs of allergic reactions occur call the health care provider or go to the nearest emergency department.

Assisting With Aspirations: Bone Marrow Aspiration/Biopsy, Lumbar Puncture, Paracentesis, and Thoracentesis

Aspirations are sterile invasive procedures involving the removal of body fluids or tissue for diagnostic procedures (Table 10.3). The nurse helps the health care provider during an aspiration procedure. Informed consent is obtained for invasive procedures.

Marrow aspiration is the removal of a small amount of the liquid organic material in the medullary canals of selected bones. The sternum and the posterior superior iliac crests are the most common in adults. In children, the anterior or posterior iliac crests are used, and in infants the proximal tibia is used (Pagana et al., 2019; Perry et al., 2017). A biopsy is the removal of a core of marrow cells for laboratory analysis. Both aspiration and biopsy are used to diagnose and differentiate leukemia, certain malignancies, anemia, and thrombocytopenia. The marrow is examined in a laboratory to reveal the number, size, shape, and development of red blood cells (RBCs) and megakaryocytes (platelet precursors). Bone marrow cultures help differentiate infectious diseases such as tuberculosis (TB) or histoplasmosis. This procedure takes approximately 20 minutes to perform. Potential complications of bone marrow aspiration or biopsy include bleeding, especially if coagulopathy is present; infection; and, less commonly, organ puncture.

A lumbar puncture (LP), called a *spinal puncture* or *tap*, involves the introduction of a needle into the subarachnoid space of the spinal column. The purpose of the test is to measure pressure in the subarachnoid space; obtain cerebrospinal fluid (CSF) for visualization and laboratory examination; and inject anaesthetic, diagnostic, or therapeutic agents. CSF is examined in a laboratory to help diagnose spinal cord tumours, central nervous system (CNS) infections, hemorrhage, and degenerative brain disease. The procedure takes approximately 30 minutes to perform.

The major contraindication for LP is evidence of increased intracranial pressure (ICP). The LP causes a sudden release of pressure and possible herniation of the brain structures through the foramen magnum. This herniation compresses the brainstem, which contains the vital cardiac, respiratory, and vasomotor centres, and sudden

TABLE 10.3

Summary of Aspiration Procedures

Aspiration Procedure	Preparation/Assessment Specific to Test	Position and Site	Special Considerations
Bone marrow aspiration	Assess complete blood count for abnormalities.	Sternum — Superior iliac crest — Proximal tibia	Patients with arthritis or orthopnea may have difficulty assuming the positions. Pressure is applied to the site following procedure.

"X" marks site of aspiration. (*From Ignatavicius, D. D., & Workman, M. L. [2010]. Medical-surgical nursing: Patient-centered collaborative care [6th ed.]. St. Louis: Saunders.*)

Bone marrow aspiration from the iliac crest. (*From Ignatavicius, D. D., & Workman, M. L. [2013]. Medical-surgical nursing: Patient-centered collaborative care [7th ed.]. St. Louis: Saunders.*)

Continued

TABLE 10.3			

Summary of Aspiration Procedures—cont'd

Aspiration Procedure	Preparation/Assessment Specific to Test	Position and Site	Special Considerations
Lumbar puncture	Assess neurological status, including movement, sensation, and muscle strength of legs to provide a baseline for comparison.	Lateral decubitus position L1 L3 L5 L2 L4 Subarachnoid space (From Ignatavicius, D. D., & Workman, M. L. [2013]. Medical-surgical nursing: Patient-centered collaborative care [7th ed.]. St. Louis: Saunders.)	*Risk for spinal headache*: Instruct patient to remain flat and logroll according to health care provider's prescriptions. Observe for excessive drainage at site. Fluid loss at site can predispose patient to headache and infection.
Paracentesis	Assess bladder for distension and determine last voiding. Weigh patient, inspect and palpate abdomen, and measure abdominal girth at largest point. Mark location for consistent reference point.		After fluid is removed, pressure on diaphragm is released, and breathing becomes much easier. *Risk for trauma:* Prevent inadvertent puncture of bladder by voiding prior to procedure. Monitor for signs of hypovolemia (Pagana et al., 2019)
Thoracentesis	Assess respiratory rate and depth, breath sounds, symmetry of chest on inspiration and expiration, cough, and sputum. Assist patient to remain immobile during procedure to prevent trauma to visceral pleura. Patient will need to hold breath and avoid coughing during procedure.	Area for needle insertion Ribs Parietal pleura Visceral pleura Lung tissue (parenchyma) Pleural effusion Syringe Diaphragm	Monitor blood pressure for hypotension if large quantity of fluid is removed. *Risk for pneumothorax:* Observe for sudden shortness of breath, tracheal deviation, anxiety, altered vital signs, and decreased oxygen saturation.

death results. In elective LP preprocedure computed tomography results are reviewed for evidence of brain shift to rule out ICP. Spinal punctures are contraindicated in patients who are suspected of having it.

Abdominal paracentesis involves aspiration of peritoneal fluid from the abdomen. Cytological analysis of the aspirate determines presence of bacteria, blood, glucose, and protein to help diagnose the causes of an abdominal effusion. Paracentesis may also be a palliative measure to provide temporary relief of abdominal and respiratory discomfort caused by severe ascites. Lavage paracentesis, in which a lavage of solution is instilled and then withdrawn, is done to detect the presence of bleeding, as in cases of blunt abdominal trauma or tumour cells when cancer is suspected. Although not contraindicated, paracentesis is performed with caution in patients with coagulopathies, with portal hypertension accompanied by abdominal collateral circulation, and in those who are pregnant. The procedure takes approximately 30 minutes to perform.

Thoracentesis is performed to analyze or remove pleural fluid or instill medications intrapleurally. Cytological studies of specimens reveal presence of blood, glucose, amylase, lactate dehydrogenase (LD), and cellular composition. Cytological specimens are also examined for malignancy, differentiated between transudative and exudative characteristics, and cultured for pathogens. The following cause transudate in the pleural space: ascites, cirrhosis (hepatic), heart failure, hypertension (pulmonary, systemic), nephritis, and nephrosis. Therapeutic thoracentesis relieves pain, dyspnea, and signs of pleural pressure. The test takes approximately 30 minutes to perform.

Delegation and Collaboration

The skill of helping with aspirations can be delegated to an unregulated care provider (UCP) if the patient is stable (check employer policy). However, assessment of the patient's condition and health teaching must be completed by the nurse and cannot be delegated to a UCP. The nurse directs the UCP about:

- Proper positioning of the patient during the procedure.
- When to take and report vital signs.
- Which signs and symptoms experienced by the patient would be of immediate concern.

Equipment

- PPE: Masks, goggles, gowns, head cover, sterile gloves for all health care members performing the procedure
- Test tubes, sterile specimen containers, laboratory requisitions, and labels
- Analgesia (if prescribed)
- Antiseptic solution

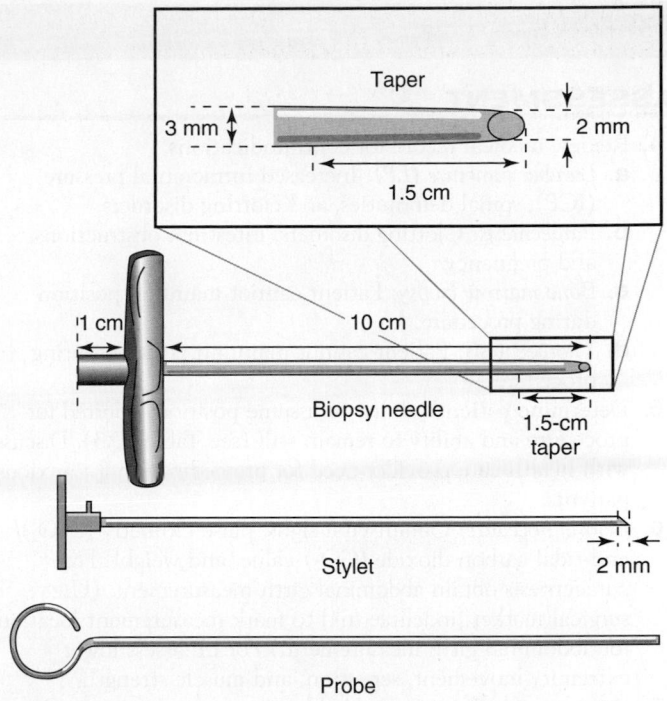

FIG 10.3 Bone marrow biopsy needle showing shape and size. *(From Monahan, F., et al. [2007]. Phipps' medical-surgical nursing: Health and illness perspectives [8th ed.]. St. Louis: Mosby.)*

- 10 × 10–cm (4 × 4–inch) sterile gauze pads, tape, Band-Aid
- Sphygmomanometer, pulse oximeter/end-tidal CO$_2$ monitor
- Aspiration tray: Most facilities provide trays specific to the aspiration procedure. A standard tray includes antiseptic solution (e.g., povidone-iodine, chlorhexidine); gauze sponges (10 × 10 cm [4 × 4 inch]); sterile towels; local anaesthetic solution (e.g., lidocaine); and two 3-mL sterile syringes with 16- to 27-gauge needles.

Additional Equipment for Specific Aspirations

- Bone marrow aspiration: Two bone marrow needles with inner stylet (Fig. 10.3)
- LP: Manometer to measure spinal pressure and at least four test tubes
- Paracentesis: Intravenous (IV) fluids as prescribed, vacuum bottles to collect fluid, stopcock with extension tubing, sterile collection containers, measuring tape
- Thoracentesis: Vacuum bottles to collect fluid, stopcock with extension tubing

STEP	RATIONALE

ASSESSMENT

1. Identify patient using at least two person-specific identifiers (e.g., name and birthday or name and medical record number) according to employer policy. Compare identifiers with information on patient's medication administration record (MAR) or medical record.

Ensures correct patient. Complies with Accreditation Canada's standards and improves patient safety (Accreditation Canada, 2019).

2. Verify type of procedure scheduled, purpose, and procedure site with patient and medical record.

Ensures correct patient and procedure (QMP, 2015).

3. Verify that informed consent was obtained before administering any analgesia or antianxiety drugs.

Federal regulations, many provincial/territorial laws, and accreditation agencies require informed consent for procedures.

STEP	RATIONALE

ASSESSMENT

4. Review medical record for contraindications.
   a. *Lumbar puncture (LP):* Increased intracranial pressure (ICP), spinal deformities, and clotting disorders.
   b. *Paracentesis:* Clotting disorders, intestinal obstructions, and pregnancy.
   c. *Bone marrow biopsy:* Patient cannot maintain position during procedure.
   d. *Thoracentesis:* Patient cannot maintain position during procedure.

   Factors can cause hemorrhage, and ICP may cause brainstem herniation.
   Paracentesis in pregnant woman may injure fetus.

5. Determine patient's ability to assume position required for procedure and ability to remain still (see Table 10.3). Discuss with health care provider need for premedication for anxious patients.

   Movement during procedure can cause complications such as bleeding and injury to nerves or tissue. Required position depends on site used for aspiration.

6. *Before procedure:* Obtain vital signs, pulse oximetry (SpO_2)/end-tidal carbon dioxide (CO_2) value, and weight. For paracentesis obtain abdominal girth measurement. (Use surgical marker [indelible ink] to mark measurement location for abdominal girth measurement.) For LP assess lower extremity movement, sensation, and muscle strength.

   Provides baseline for comparison with vital signs during and after procedure. Patients will have decreased abdominal girth and lose weight after paracentesis.

7. Instruct patient to empty bladder.

   Reduces risk for bladder trauma during paracentesis. Promotes patient comfort.

8. Assess patient's coagulation status: use of anticoagulants, complete blood count (CBC), platelet count, clotting factors, activated partial thromboplastin time (aPTT)/international normalized ratio (INR), and prothrombin time (PT).

   Invasive procedures are contraindicated in patients with coagulation disorders because of risk for bleeding (Pagana et al., 2019).

9. Determine whether patient is allergic to antiseptic, latex, or anaesthetic solutions.

   Precautions can be taken to decrease chance of allergic reactions.

10. Assess patient's level of understanding of procedure, including any concerns.

   Determines extent of instruction and level of support required.

11. Assess baseline pain level, using an appropriate pain scale.

   Determines need for preprocedure analgesia.
   Pain control helps patients maintain proper position and tolerate aspiration procedure.

NURSING DIAGNOSES

- Reduced gas exchange
- Acute pain
- Anxiety
- Fear of the unknown
- Insufficient knowledge
- Reduced mobility
- Potential for infection
- Potential for injury

Related factors/Risk factors are individualized on the basis of patient's condition or needs.

PLANNING

1. Expected outcomes following completion of procedure:
   - Patient describes purpose of procedure.

     Demonstrates understanding and improves likelihood of cooperation.

   - Patient assumes and maintains required position and remains still throughout procedure.

     Correct position facilitates safe and timely completion of procedure.

   - There is scant to no bleeding at needle insertion site.

     Precautions during procedure prevent bleeding.

   - Amount of aspirate is sufficient to perform laboratory testing.

     Usually 0.5 to 2 mL of bone marrow is aspirated, smeared on slides, and allowed to dry (Pagana et al., 2019).

   - Patient's level of comfort is assessed using an appropriate scale.

     Procedure is performed with minimal discomfort to patient.

   - Vital signs, SpO_2, and end-tidal CO_2 remain within normal limits during and after aspiration procedure.

     Removal of abdominal (ascites) or pleural fluid increases lung expansion and improves gas exchange.

   - Patient undergoing paracentesis has reduced abdominal girth and improved respirations.

     Fluid is successfully removed from peritoneal space.

2. Explain steps of skin preparation, anaesthetic injection, needle insertion, and position required.

   Anticipation of expected sensations and procedural activities reduces anxiety.

STEP	RATIONALE

PLANNING

3. If prescribed, premedicate 30 minutes before procedure. *Option:* In some cases, patients will receive antianxiety medications.

Pain and anxiety control helps patient to remain in the required position, minimizes discomfort from needle insertion, and decreases anxiety.

4. Before thoracentesis verify recent chest X-ray film examination.

Provides preprocedure baseline to determine location of pleural fluid.

IMPLEMENTATION

1. Perform hand hygiene.

Reduces transmission of microorganisms.

2. Set up sterile tray or open supplies to make accessible for health care provider.

Maintains integrity of sterile field and promotes prompt completion of procedure.

3. Complete "time-out" to verify patient's name, type of procedure scheduled, and procedure site with patient and health care team.

"Time-out" verification just before starting procedure includes health care provider and all personnel and is a safety precaution to prevent wrong-patient, wrong-site, and wrong-procedure errors (QMP, 2015).

4. Help patient maintain correct position. Reassure patient while explaining procedure.

Decreases chance of complications occurring during procedure. Explanations increase patient comfort and relaxation.

   a. Bone marrow
   - *Adults:* For sternal biopsy place patient in supine position. For iliac crest biopsy place in prone or lateral recumbent position.
   - *Children:* For iliac crest biopsy place patient in prone or lateral recumbent position.

Provides best access to bone containing marrow.

   b. LP
   Position patient in lateral recumbent (fetal) position with head and neck flexed (see Table 10.3).

Provides full curvature and flexion of spinal column to allow maximal space between vertebrae.

   c. Paracentesis
   Position patient in bed in semi-Fowler's position or sitting upright on side of bed or in chair with feet supported (see Table 10.3).

Position uses gravity to cause fluid to accumulate in lower abdominal cavity, where it is drained more easily.

   d. Thoracentesis
   Place patient in orthopneic position (upright position with arms and shoulders raised and supported on padded over-bed table) (see Table 10.3). If patient is unable to tolerate this, help patient to side-lying position with affected lung positioned upward.

Expands intercostal space for needle insertions.

Clinical Decision Point *Emphasize the importance of remaining immobile during the procedure to prevent trauma, especially with the LP. Sudden movement is a risk for spinal cord nerve root damage. Sudden movement during paracentesis or thoracentesis risks damage of the abdominal or pulmonary structures. Also instruct patient not to cough, sneeze, or breathe deeply during the procedures because these actions increase the risk for needle displacement and damage of other structures.*

5. Explain to patient that pain may occur when lidocaine (local anaesthetic) is injected into tissues. Pressure may also occur when tissue or fluid is aspirated.

Aspiration is painful but lasts for only a few moments. If patient is having bone marrow aspirate, deep pressure feeling is frequently experienced as bone marrow is withdrawn (Pagana et al., 2019).

6. Health care provider applies PPE (e.g., sterile gloves, mask, gown, and goggles), cleans patient's skin with antiseptic solution, and drapes site with sterile drape.

Removes surface bacteria from skin at area of puncture site. Creates sterile field.

7. Health care provider injects local anaesthetic and allows time for anaesthesia to occur.

Provides optimal effect of local anaesthesia.

8. Health care provider inserts needle or trocar into spinal space or body cavity involved (see Table 10.3). To aspirate tissue or body fluids for specimen analysis, syringe is attached to trocar or needle, and aspirate is placed into specimen container.

Success depends on positioning, accurate insertion site, and patient remaining still.

9. Nurse assesses patient's condition during procedure, including respiratory status, vital signs if indicated, and any indications of pain.

Identifies any changes that indicate complication.

STEP	RATIONALE

IMPLEMENTATION

Clinical Decision Point *Increased or worsening abdominal or thoracic pain is significant in paracentesis and thoracentesis. Severe abdominal pain indicates a possible bowel perforation following a paracentesis. Following a thoracentesis abdominal pain results from diaphragmatic, liver, or spleen perforation. Inspiratory chest pain results from perforation of the lung.*

10. Note characteristics of aspirate:	
a. *Bone marrow aspirate:* Marrow may appear red or yellow.	Normal marrow.
b. *LP:* Record opening pressure; observe fluid for colour, cloudiness, or blood.	Normal CSF is clear and colourless. Cloudiness is a result of protein, which indicates an infection.
c. *Paracentesis:* Fluid may appear yellow, cloudy, bile-stained green, or blood tinged. Peritoneal lavage fluid may appear bright red.	Blood-tinged fluid is caused by traumatic tap. In patient with abdominal trauma bloody lavage identifies active bleeding.
d. *Thoracentesis:* Pleural fluid may appear clear yellow, puslike, or cloudy.	Clear yellow is normal. Transudate and exudates are typically yellow, straw colour. Blood-tinged fluid indicates malignancy, pulmonary infarction, or severe inflammation. Puslike fluid indicates infection (empyema); milky fluid indicates chylothorax (i.e., leak from thoracic duct resulting in lymphatic drainage in pleural cavity).
11. Properly label specimens in presence of patient and transport to laboratory in proper containers. Label specimens in order of collection.	Ensures that correct laboratory results are assigned to right patient. Test tubes are numbered in sequence of collection (i.e., 1 through 4).
12. Health care provider removes needle/trocar and applies pressure over insertion site until drainage ceases. If necessary, help with direct pressure and application of adhesive pressure dressing.	Helps in homeostasis and secures insertion site.
13. All health care team members in procedure remove PPE, discard in appropriate receptacle, and perform hand hygiene.	Reduces transmission of infection.

EVALUATION

1. Monitor level of consciousness, vital signs, and SpO_2/end-tidal CO_2. Closely monitor vital signs every 15 minutes for 2 hours, according to employer policy.	Verifies patient's physiological status in response to procedure or any potential complications.
2. Inspect dressing over puncture site for bleeding, swelling, tenderness, and erythema. Inspect area under patient for bleeding. Avoid disrupting healing clot at site if pressure dressing is present.	Determines further blood loss from puncture site. Infection is a potential complication, especially if patient is leukopenic (Pagana et al., 2019).
3. Evaluate pain score to determine if patient's level of comfort is equivalent to a score of 4 or less on pain scale of 0 (no pain) to 10 (worst pain ever).	Determines if patient is having increased pain to warrant postprocedure analgesia.
4. Following paracentesis, measure abdominal girth and respirations and compare to preprocedure measurements.	Determines amount of change in abdominal size and ability to ventilate.
5. Use Teach-Back: "I want to be sure I explained everything clearly about this procedure. Please tell me in your own words what you heard me say." Develop a revised teaching plan if patient or caregiver is not able to teach back correctly.	Demonstrates patient's and caregiver's level of understanding of instructional topic.

Unexpected Outcomes	**Related Interventions**
1. Oversedation occurs.	• See Skill 10.1.
2. Site complications occur:	• Notify health care provider and obtain further prescriptions.
a. *Bone marrow:* Tenderness or erythema at site.	• Administer analgesic as prescribed.
	• Continue to monitor site.
b. *LP:*	
(1) Postprocedure headache (PPH) is evidenced by headache, blurred vision, and tinnitus.	• Monitor fluid loss.
	• Health care provider may inject blood patch into epidural space.
	• Medicate for pain as prescribed.

STEP	RATIONALE

Unexpected Outcomes

    (2) Excess loss of CSF is indicated by decreased level of consciousness, hearing loss, dilated pupils, and decreased ICP.

  c. *Paracentesis:* Leakage of fluid from site and acute abdominal pain occur.

  d. *Thoracentesis:* Pneumothorax is evidenced by sudden dyspnea, tachypnea, and asymmetrical chest excursion.

Related Interventions
- Maintain airway.
- Transfer to critical care unit (CCU) per health care provider prescription.
- Reinforce dressing; may also be instructed to place sterile collection bag over site to keep site dry to maintain skin integrity.
- Monitor vital signs and SpO_2.
- Assess abdomen for bowel sounds.
- Administer oxygen.
- Monitor vital signs and SpO_2.
- Anticipate chest X-ray film examination and possible chest tube insertion.

Communication and Documentation

- Document name of procedure; preprocedure preparation; location of puncture site; amount, consistency, and colour of fluid drained or specimen obtained; duration of procedure; patient's tolerance (e.g., vital signs, SpO_2) and comfort level; laboratory tests prescribed and specimen sent; type of dressing; postprocedure activities (e.g., chest X-ray film examination); and other procedure-specific assessments (e.g., extremity assessment, abdominal girth, level of consciousness) in nurses' notes in electronic health record (EHR) or chart.
- Immediately report to health care provider any change in vital signs and SpO_2, unexpected pain or discomfort, and any excessive drainage from dressing over puncture site.
- Document your evaluation of patient and caregiver learning.

Special Considerations
Teaching

- Instruct patient that some people experience tenderness at the puncture site for several days after the procedure and that mild analgesia often helps to relieve some of the discomfort.

Pediatric

- Conscious or unconscious sedation is commonly used. If using unconscious sedation for the procedure, interprofessional collaboration will include an anaesthesiologist or nurse anaesthetist.

- Prepare preschool children before the procedure; make a game out of having child recall the next procedural step, which can serve as a distraction (Perry et al., 2017).

Gerontological

- Older persons with limited mobility (e.g., arthritis) need help to stay in the required position.
- Older persons have reduced elastic lung recoil, weaker cough efficiency, and decreased chest expansion. Restlessness may indicate hypoxia following thoracentesis.
- Be aware that older persons may have specific fears and anxiety related to postprocedure falling and fatigue.

Care in the Community

- Teach patients and caregivers about specific postprocedure complications and when to report them to the health care provider.
- If patient is transferred to a long-term care facility, ensure thorough communication between facilities results of procedure and patient condition.

◆ SKILL 10.4   Care of a Patient Undergoing Bronchoscopy

Bronchoscopy is the examination of the tracheobronchial tree through a lighted tube containing mirrors. A flexible fibreoptic bronchoscope has lumens that allow both visualization and simultaneous administration of oxygen (Fig. 10.4). The fibreoptic bronchoscope is used for obtaining sputum, foreign bodies, and biopsy specimens. Laser ablation of endotracheal lesions may also be performed through the bronchoscope.

Bronchoscopy may be an emergency or elective procedure and may be performed for diagnostic or therapeutic reasons. The main purposes of this procedure include aspirating excessive sputum or mucous plugs that airway suctioning cannot remove; visualizing the tracheobronchial tree for assessment of abnormalities of the mucosa, abscesses, aspiration pneumonia, strictures, and tumours; obtaining deep-tissue biopsy and sputum specimens; and removing foreign bodies. This procedure is contraindicated in patients who cannot tolerate interruption of high-flow oxygen unless intubated. Potential complications of bronchoscopy include fever, infection, hypoxemia, bronchospasm and laryngospasm, pneumothorax, aspiration, dysrhythmias and hypotension, hemorrhage (after biopsy), and

cardiac arrest (Pagana et al., 2019). The procedure is performed at the bedside or in a specially equipped endoscopy room. Usually a pulmonary specialist or surgeon performs it in approximately 30 to 45 minutes.

Delegation and Collaboration

The skill of assisting with a bronchoscopy cannot be delegated to an unregulated care provider (UCP). The nurse assesses the patient postprocedure, monitoring vital signs, pulse oximetry, and respiratory status. The nurse monitors for the presence of a gag reflex prior to offering fluids or food. If there is any respiratory distress or expectoration of blood, the nurse needs to notify the health care provider. If prescribed, the chest radiograph should be completed to assess for a pneumothorax (Pagana et al., 2019).

The nurse directs the UCP to:
- Help position the patient appropriately.
- Immediately report to the nurse if the patient has possible respiratory distress or is coughing up blood after the procedure.

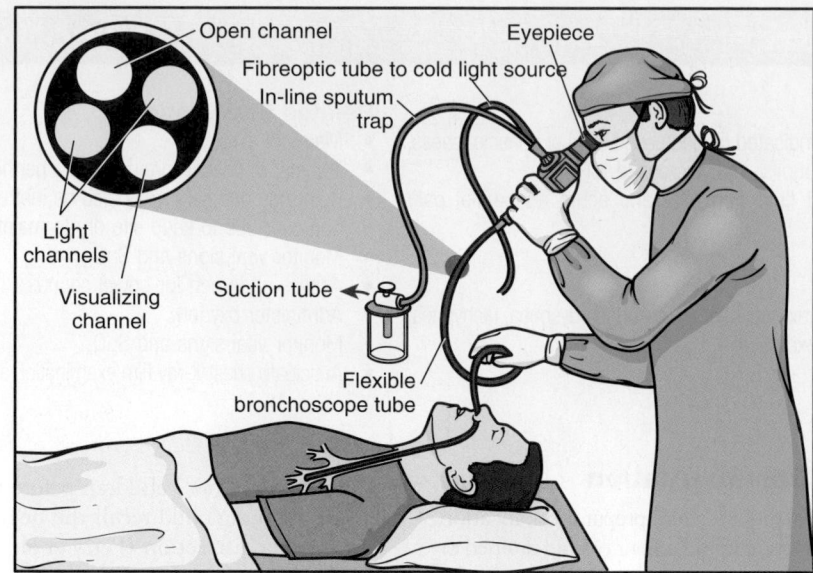

FIG 10.4 Flexible fibreoptic bronchoscopy. *(From Pagana, K., Pagana, T., & Pike-MacDonald, S. [2019]. Mosby's Canadian manual of diagnostic and laboratory tests [2nd Cdn ed., p. 613, Fig. 4-4]. Toronto, ON: Elsevier Canada.)*

Equipment

- PPE: Mask, gown, gloves, head cover, and goggles for all health care providers
- Bronchoscopy tray, includes flexible fibreoptic bronchoscope (see Fig. 10.4); 10 × 10–cm (4 × 4–inch) gauze sponges; local anaesthetic spray (lidocaine); sterile tracheal suction catheters; diazepam, midazolam, or other sedative for intravenous (IV) sedation required for the procedure
- Oxygen, resuscitative equipment, and emergency medications
- Pulse oximeter/end-tidal carbon dioxide (CO_2) monitor, cardiac monitor
- Sterile gloves
- Sterile water-soluble lubricating jelly (**NOTE**: Petroleum-based lubricants are not used because of the hazard of aspiration and subsequent pneumonia.)
- Emesis basin
- Suction machine and connecting tube
- Blood pressure equipment

STEP	RATIONALE

ASSESSMENT

1. Identify patient using at least two person-specific identifiers (i.e., name and birthday or name and medical record number) according to employer policy. Compare identifiers with information on patient's medication administration record (MAR) or medical record.

Ensures correct patient. Complies with Accreditation Canada's standards and improves patient safety (Accreditation Canada, 2019).

2. Verify type of procedure scheduled and procedure site with patient.

Ensures procedure and correct patient. Complies with CPSI (2009) standards and improves patient safety.

3. Verify that informed consent was obtained before administration of any sedatives.

Federal regulations, many provincial/territorial laws, and accreditation agencies such as Accreditation Canada require informed consent for procedure.

4. Assess patient's history for inability to tolerate interruption of high-flow oxygen unless intubated.

Determines need for oxygen administration during procedure.

5. Obtain baseline vital signs and pulse oximetry (SpO_2) and end-tidal CO_2 values.

Baseline data provide for comparison with findings during and after procedure.

6. Assess type of cough, sputum produced, and heart and lung sounds.

Provides for comparison with respiratory status during and after procedure.

7. Determine purpose of procedure: for sputum aspiration, assessment, tissue biopsy, or removal of foreign body.

Anticipates equipment needs of health care provider and type of information to convey to patient during teaching.

8. Determine whether patient is allergic to local anaesthetic used for spraying throat (usually lidocaine).

Allergy causes laryngeal edema or laryngospasm.

9. Assess need for preprocedure medication (e.g., atropine and opioid or sedative).

Atropine decreases secretions and inhibits vagally stimulated bradycardia; opioids or sedatives relieve anxiety and decrease discomfort.

STEP	RATIONALE

ASSESSMENT

10. Assess time patient last ingested food, fluids, or medications. Patient must be NPO for at least 8 hours before a bronchoscopy; however, some medications may be taken before procedure by health care provider prescription.

Reduces risk for aspiration.

11. Assess patient's level of understanding of procedure, including any concerns.

Determines extent of instruction and level of support required.

NURSING DIAGNOSIS

- Inadequate breathing pattern
- Reduced airway clearance
- Reduced gas exchange

- Anxiety
- Insufficient knowledge
- Fear of the unknown

- Potential for aspiration
- Potential for infection

Related factors/Risk factors are individualized on the basis of patient's condition or needs.

PLANNING

1. Expected outcomes following completion of procedure:
- Patient recovers from sedation without respiratory complications or change in level of consciousness.

Sedation adequate, and patient tolerates procedure.

- Patient's level of comfort is equivalent to score of 4 or less on pain scale of 0 to 10.

Minimal trauma caused by bronchoscope.

- Health care provider is able to observe, suction, and obtain specimens from tracheobronchial tree.

Indicates that purpose of procedure was achieved.

- Patient explains procedure and assumes appropriate position.

Demonstrates patient's understanding.

2. Administer atropine, opioid, or antianxiety agent 30 minutes before procedure.

Ensures that medication takes effect before procedure.

3. Explain procedure to patient.

Reduces anxiety and increases cooperation.

4. Remove and safely store patient's dentures and/or eyeglasses.

Minimizes chance of airway obstruction.

IMPLEMENTATION

1. Assess current IV access or establish new IV access with large-bore cannula (see Chapter 29).

Provides immediate access for IV fluids or medications if emergency occurs.

2. Help patient assume position desired by health care provider: usually semi-Fowler's.

Provides maximal visualization of lower airway and adequate lung expansion.

3. Complete "time-out" to verify patient's name, type of procedure scheduled, and procedure site with patient and health care team.

"Time-out" verification just before starting procedure includes entire health care team and is a safety precaution to prevent wrong-patient, wrong-site, and wrong-procedure errors (CPSI, 2009).

4. Perform hand hygiene and apply PPE. Position tip of suction catheter for easy access to patient's mouth.

Reduces transmission of microorganisms. Removes secretions to reduce risk for aspiration.

5. Health care provider usually sprays nasopharynx and oropharynx with topical anaesthetic. Lidocaine is commonly used 10 to 15 minutes before procedure. When a patient is intubated or has tracheostomy, anaesthetic spray is usually not needed.

Provides swift anaesthesia of oropharynx.

6. Instruct patient not to swallow local anaesthetic; provide emesis basin for expectorating it.

Reduces unintended anaesthesia of esophagus.

7. Another health care team member attaches bronchoscope to machine light source.

Enhances visualization during procedure.

8. Health care provider applies PPE, introduces bronchoscope into mouth to pharynx, and passes it through glottis and into trachea and bronchi (see Fig. 10.4). More anaesthetic spray may be used at glottis to prevent cough reflex. For intubated patients, flexible bronchoscope is introduced through their endotracheal tube.

Bronchoscope must be passed through upper airway structures to promote visualization of lower airways. Trachea and bronchi are observed for lesions and obstructions. Adaptor accompanies bronchoscope and is used for bag-valve mask or ventilator use.

STEP	RATIONALE

IMPLEMENTATION

9. Health care provider suctions mucus and performs bronchial washing with cytological specimens taken with wire brush or curette. Biopsy specimens may also be obtained.

Cytological specimens are obtained to diagnose carcinoma.

10. Help patient through procedure by providing explanations, verbal reassurance, and support.

Although patient is premedicated and drowsy, remind patient not to change position and to cooperate. Reinforce that patient will be able to breathe during procedure.

11. Assess patient's pulse, blood pressure, respirations, SpO_2, end-tidal CO_2, and breathing capacity during procedure; observe degree of restlessness, capillary refill, and colour of nail beds.

Bronchoscope can cause feelings of suffocation and vasovagal response and laryngospasm. Because airway is partially occluded, patient can develop hypoxia during procedure.

12. Note characteristics of suctioned material. Expect small amount of blood mixed with aspirate because of tissue trauma.

Information used to document and report and make further patient observations.

13. Using gloved hand, wipe patient's mouth and nose to remove lubricant after bronchoscope is removed.

Promotes hygiene and comfort.

14. Instruct patient not to eat or drink until local anaesthesia has worn off and gag reflex has returned, usually in 2 hours. Use tongue depressor to touch pharynx to test for presence of gag reflex.

Prevents aspiration.

15. Remove PPE, discard, and perform hand hygiene.

Reduces transmission of microorganisms.

EVALUATION

1. Monitor vital signs, SpO_2, and end-tidal CO_2 on a regular basis, according to employer policy.

Verifies physiological response to procedure.

2. Observe character and amount of sputum. Health care provider may prescribe serial sputum collection for 24 hours for cytological examination.

Evaluates for complication of bronchial perforation, indicated by severe hemoptysis.
Slight blood-tinged sputum is normal after this procedure.

3. Observe respiratory status closely; palpate for facial or neck crepitus.

Detects early sign of bronchial or esophageal perforation.

4. Assess for return of gag reflex. It usually returns in approximately 2 hours.

Helps prevent aspiration pneumonia, which is risk until gag reflex returns.

5. **Use Teach-Back:** "I want to be sure I explained what are considered postprocedure normal and abnormal symptoms. Tell me what you heard me say about these symptoms." Develop a revised teaching plan if patient or caregiver is not able to teach back correctly.

Demonstrates patient's and caregiver's level of understanding of instructional topic.

Unexpected Outcomes

1. Vasovagal response caused by stimulation of baroreceptors during bronchoscope insertion, causing symptoms of:
   - Feeling nauseous, faint, dizzy, and/or light-headed.
   - Diaphoresis with slow, steady pulse.
   - Unconsciousness for a few seconds.
2. Laryngospasm and bronchospasm as evidenced by:
   - Sudden, severe shortness of breath.

3. Hypoxemia as evidenced by:
   - Gradual shortness of breath.
   - Decreasing level of consciousness.
4. Hemorrhage as evidenced by:
   - Acute blood loss
   - Hypotension and tachycardia
   - Decreasing level of consciousness
5. Oversedation

Related Interventions

- Lower head of table.
- Continue vital signs monitoring.
- Lower head of table.
- Support airway (positioning/suctioning).

- Call health care provider immediately.
- Support airway (positioning).
- Prepare emergency resuscitation equipment.
- Anticipate possible cricothyrotomy.
- Monitor SpO_2.
- Maintain airway and breathing.
- Notify health care provider immediately.
- Notify health care provider immediately.
- Monitor vital signs.
- Be prepared to administer IV fluids.

- See Skill 10.1.

Communication and Documentation

- Document procedure(s) performed (e.g., biopsy); character of sputum; duration of procedure, patient's tolerance and, if any, complications; and the collection and disposition of specimen(s) in nurses' notes in electronic health record (EHR) or chart. Document time of gag reflex return.
- Report bleeding or respiratory distress following the procedure or any changes in vital signs beyond patient's normal limits to health care provider immediately. Report results of procedure to appropriate health care personnel.
- Document your evaluation of patient and caregiver learning.

Special Considerations
Teaching

- Before the procedure instruct patient to perform good mouth care to decrease risk of introducing bacteria into lungs during the procedure.
- In some cases, patients may receive IV sedation (see Skill 10.1, Teaching Considerations).
- If prescribed, teach patient how to perform controlled coughing techniques for obtaining serial sputum samples (see Chapter 9).

Pediatric

- In children the procedure is most frequently performed under general anaesthesia to remove foreign bodies from the larynx or trachea. Follow-up care after the foreign body is removed includes chest physiotherapy, monitoring for respiratory distress, and education of parent or guardian.
- Children are at higher risk for hypoxemia than adults because their bronchus is smaller and the bronchoscope decreases the available breathing space (Pagana et al., 2019).

Gerontological

- Physical exposure and room temperature contribute to hypothermia in frail older persons who are unable to communicate that they are cold. Use warmed blankets or forced-air heat to maintain core temperature at comfortable, safe levels (Lewis et al., 2019).
- Postprocedure restlessness often indicates hypoxemia or pain. Thoroughly assess pulmonary capacity before administering opioids, which may depress the respiratory control.

Care in the Community

- Instruct ambulatory care patients to notify the health care provider if the following symptoms develop: fever, chest pain or discomfort, dyspnea, wheezing, or hemoptysis.
- Throat discomfort is managed with throat lozenges or warm saline gargles.

♦ SKILL 10.5 | **Care of a Patient Undergoing Endoscopy**

Endoscopy allows direct visualization of an internal organ or structure by means of a long, flexible fibreoptic scope. The tip of the scope has a light source and camera lens that allows visualization of the lining of the gastrointestinal (GI) structures on a large display screen (Fig. 10.5, A–C). For visualization of the upper GI tract, esophagoscopy, gastroscopy, gastroduodenojejunoscopy (GDJ), or duodenoscopy is performed, or, more frequently, esophagogastroduodenoscopy (EGD), which permits visualization of the esophagus, stomach (Fig. 10.6), and duodenum in one examination. Besides direct observation, endoscopy enables biopsy of suspicious tissue, polyp removal, and performance of many other procedures such as direct visual guidance for fine-needle aspiration biopsies and dilation and stenting of strictures. For visualization of the hepatobiliary tree and pancreatic ducts, an endoscopic retrograde cholangiopancreatography (ERCP) is performed. For visual examination of the lower GI tract, proctoscopy, sigmoidoscopy, or colonoscopy is performed. Typically, these patients receive intravenous (IV) moderate sedation.

Risks of endoscopic procedures include intestinal perforation, hemorrhage, peritonitis, aspiration, respiratory depression, and myocardial infarction secondary to vasovagal response. Both upper and lower GI endoscopic examinations may be performed in a specially equipped endoscopic unit or at the patient's bedside.

Delegation and Collaboration

The skill of helping with endoscopy cannot be delegated to an unregulated care provider (UCP). The nurse is responsible for

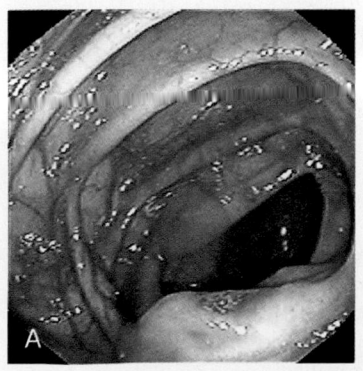
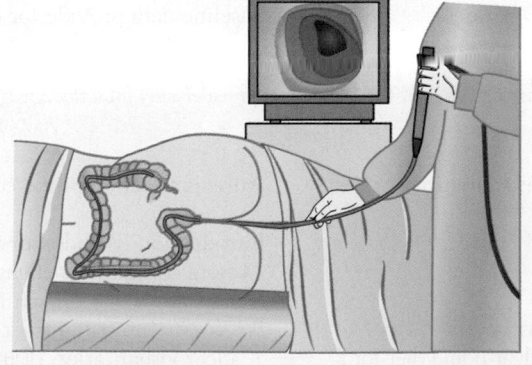
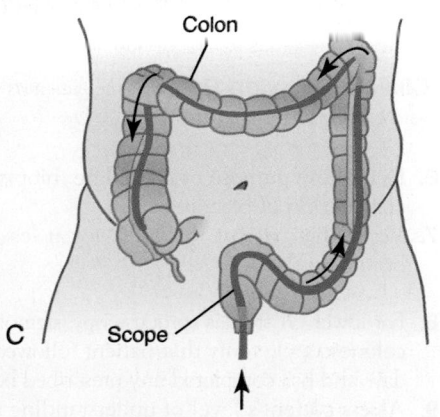

FIG 10.5 A, Scope view of healthy colon. **B,** Overview of colonoscopy process. **C,** Path of scope through colon.

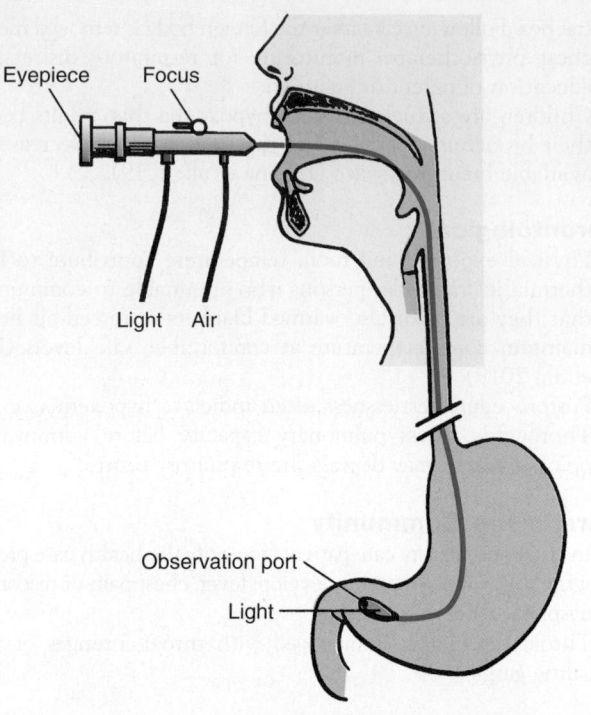

FIG 10.6 Stomach may be visualized by means of a fibrescope. (*From Ignatavicius, D. D., & Workman, M. L. [2010]. Medical-surgical nursing: Patient-centered collaborative care [6th ed.]. St. Louis: Saunders.*)

assessing the patient preprocedure, assisting with the procedure, and providing postprocedure care. The nurse directs the UCP about:

- How to help with patient positioning.

Equipment

- PPE: Mask, gown, gloves, head cover, goggles for all health care personnel
- Endoscopy tray
- Fibreoptic endoscope and camera
- Solutions for biopsy specimens
- Local anaesthetic spray
- Tracheal suction equipment (see Chapter 25)
- Blood pressure equipment
- Sterile water-soluble jelly
- Sterile gloves for health care provider
- Emesis basin
- IV fluid and equipment for IV start (*optional*)
- Diazepam, midazolam, or other sedative for IV sedation (*optional*)
- Sedative reversal agents
- Carbon dioxide (CO_2) source to inflate colon (for lower GI procedures)
- Oxygen, resuscitative equipment, SpO_2/end-tidal CO_2 monitor

STEP	RATIONALE

ASSESSMENT

STEP	RATIONALE
1. Identify patient using at least two person-specific identifiers (i.e., name and date of birth or name and medical record number) according to employer policy. Compare identifiers with information in patient's medication administration record (MAR) or medical record.	Ensures correct patient. Complies with Accreditation Canada's standards and improves patient safety (Accreditation Canada, 2019).
2. Verify type of procedure scheduled and procedure site with patient.	Ensures correct procedure and patient. Complies with the CPSI (2009) standards and improves patient safety.
3. Verify that informed consent was obtained before administering sedation.	Federal regulations, many provincial/territorial laws, and accreditation agencies such as Accreditation Canada require informed consent for procedure.
4. Determine if GI bleeding is present. Observe character of emesis, stool, and nasogastric (NG) tube drainage for frank blood or material that looks like coffee grounds.	Test is completed in patients with upper GI bleeding to identify sources of bleeding, as well as to facilitate passage of instruments used for sclerosing and probes to control or stop bleeding (Lewis et al., 2019).
5. Obtain vital signs and SpO_2/end-tidal CO_2 values.	Baseline data provide for comparison with findings during and after procedure.

Clinical Decision Point *If the patient is bleeding actively, the health care provider may prescribe lavage of the stomach and aspiration to clear clots before the procedure is attempted.*

STEP	RATIONALE
6. Determine purpose of procedure: biopsy, examination, or coagulation of bleeding sites.	Anticipates appropriate equipment needs.
7. Verify that patient was NPO for at least 8 hours for endoscopy of upper GI tract.	Introduction of endoscope increases risk for vomiting resulting from stimulation of gag reflex. Empty stomach reduces risk for aspiration of stomach contents.
8. For lower GI studies (proctoscopy, sigmoidoscopy, or colonoscopy), verify that patient followed clear-liquid diet for 2 days and has completed any prescribed bowel-cleansing regimen.	An empty intestinal tract promotes endoscopic insertion and clear visualization of interior walls.
9. Assess patient's level of understanding and previous experience with procedure, including any concerns.	Determines extent of instruction and level of support required.

STEP	RATIONALE

NURSING DIAGNOSES

- Inadequate breathing pattern
- Reduced gas exchange
- Anxiety

- Insufficient knowledge regarding procedure
- Fear of the unknown

- Potential for aspiration
- Potential for injury
- Potential for infection

Related factors/Risk factors are individualized on the basis of patient's condition or needs.

PLANNING

1. Expected outcomes following completion of procedure:	
• Patient does not aspirate and has no postprocedure bleeding.	Indicates absence of complications and tolerance of procedure.
• Patient's level of comfort is equivalent to score of 4 or less on pain scale of 0 (no pain) to 10 (worst pain ever).	Provides reliable detection of increasing pain so postprocedure analgesia is given.
• Patient is without respiratory complications or change in level of consciousness.	Recovers from sedation.
• Patient describes purposes and steps of procedure.	Documents patient understanding.
2. Prepare patient:	
a. Explain steps of procedure, including sensations to expect.	Relieves anxiety and answers patient's questions.
b. Administer pain medication or preprocedure medication.	Promotes relaxation and reduces anxiety.

IMPLEMENTATION

1. Perform hand hygiene and apply PPE.	Reduces transmission of microorganisms.
2. Remove patient's eyeglasses, dentures, or other dental appliances.	Prevents damage to eyeglasses or damage or dislodgement of dental structures during intubation phase.
3. Complete "time-out" to verify patient's name, type of procedure scheduled, and procedure site with patient and health care team.	"Time-out" verification just before starting procedure includes entire health care team and is a safety precaution to prevent wrong-patient, wrong-site, and wrong-procedure errors (CPSI, 2009; QMP, 2015)
4. Ensure that IV line is patent and administer IV sedation as prescribed (see Skill 10.1).	Provides route for emergency medications and creates immediate conscious sedation.
5. Help patient assume proper position for procedure and apply appropriate drape.	Improves efficiency of procedure and ability of health care provider to visualize site. Drape provides comfort and minimizes exposure.
a. *Upper GI procedures:* Help patient maintain left lateral Sims' position (lying on left side with knees flexed).	Sims' position allows easy passage of upper or lower endoscope. Provides airway clearance if patient gags and vomits gastric contents.
b. *Lower GI procedures:* Help patient maintain left lateral decubitus position. Drape patient for privacy.	Left lateral decubitus position provides access to lower GI tract.
6. Health care provider performs hand hygiene and puts on protective equipment.	Reduces transmission of microorganisms.
7. **Upper GI procedures:**	
a. Help health care provider spray nasopharynx and oropharynx with local anaesthetic.	Topical anaesthetic decreases gag reflex caused by passage of endoscope, thus improving safety and comfort.
b. Administer atropine if prescribed.	Reduces quantity of secretions, therefore reducing risk for aspiration.
c. Position tip of suction cannula for easy access in patient's mouth.	Drains oral secretions to reduce risk for aspiration.
8. **Lower GI procedures:**	
a. Prepare lubricant for fibreoptic endoscope.	Facilitates passage of tubing.
9. Health care provider slowly passes endoscope into mouth or through anus to view esophagus, stomach, colon, or rectum and advances to desired depth while visualizing lining of structures.	Provides visualization of all structures to detect polyps, cancerous lesions, or areas of inflammation and stricture.
10. Health care provider insufflates air through endoscope into upper GI tract or CO_2 into lower GI tract in case of colonoscopy.	Distends GI structures for better visualization. CO_2 insufflation produces less postprocedure abdominal cramping than air insufflation because it is more readily absorbed.

STEP	RATIONALE

IMPLEMENTATION

11. Help patient throughout procedure.

    a. Anticipate needs and promote comfort.

    Demonstrates person-centred care. Patient is unable to speak after tube is passed into throat.

    b. Tell patient what is happening as each part of procedure is carried out (e.g., abdominal cramping).

    Reassures patient about procedure and how long it will last.

    c. For upper GI procedures, suction if there are excessive oral secretions or vomitus.

    Prevents aspiration of oral secretions or gastric contents.

12. Place tissue specimens in proper laboratory containers or on proper slides. Seal as needed. Date, time, and initial all specimen containers before sending to laboratory.

    Ensures proper specimen preservation and labelling and preparation of specimens for microscopic examination.

13. Help patient return to comfortable position.

    Promotes relaxation.

14. Help to dispose of equipment and perform hand hygiene.

    Reduces transmission of infection.

15. In recovery, after sedation resolves, inform patient not to eat or drink until gag reflex returns.

    Reduces risk for aspiration.

EVALUATION

1. Monitor vital signs and SpO$_2$ according to employer policy (e.g., every 15 minutes for 1 hour, every 30 minutes for 1 hour, every hour until stable).

    Change in vital signs may indicate new bleeding in GI tract or oversedation.

2. Assess for levels of sedation and consciousness (see Skill 10.1).

    Determines patient's response to IV sedation.

3. Ask patient to describe level of comfort using an appropriate pain scale.

    Monitors for sudden abdominal pain, which can indicate rupture of abdominal organs.

4. Evaluate emesis or aspirate for frank or occult blood (see Chapter 9).

    Monitors for GI bleeding.

5. Assess for return of gag reflex, usually in 2 to 4 hours. Provide oral hygiene when gag reflex returns.

    Determines when effects of anaesthetic have disappeared. Gag reflex prevents aspiration.

6. **Use Teach-Back:** "I want to be sure I explained the postprocedure diet and activity limitations clearly to you. Tell me what you know about postprocedure dietary and activity limitations." Develop a revised teaching plan if patient or caregiver is not able to teach back correctly.

    Determines patient's and caregiver's level of understanding of instructional topic.

Unexpected Outcomes	Related Interventions
1. Vasovagal response caused by stimulation of baroreceptors during endoscope insertion as evidenced by: • Feeling nauseous, faint, dizzy, and/or light-headed. • Diaphoresis with slow, steady pulse. • Few seconds of unconsciousness.	• Lower head of table. • Support airway.
2. For upper GI procedures: Laryngospasm and bronchospasm as evidenced by: • Sudden, severe shortness of breath.	• Call health care provider immediately. • Support airway (positioning). • Prepare emergency resuscitation equipment. • Anticipate possible cricothyrotomy.
3. For upper GI procedures: Hypoxemia as evidenced by: • Gradual shortness of breath. • Decreasing level of consciousness.	• Monitor SpO$_2$. • Maintain airway and breathing. • Notify health care provider immediately.
4. Pulmonary aspiration as evidenced by: • Dyspnea, tachypnea, decreasing levels of oxygen saturation.	• Support airway. • Follow specific postprocedural prescriptions related to findings. • Monitor oxygen saturation.
5. Abdominal pain, fever, or bleeding, indicating damage to intestinal wall.	• Continue to monitor vital signs. • Notify health care provider of findings.
6. Oversedation with decreasing level of consciousness.	• See Skill 10.1.

Communication and Documentation

- Document the procedure, duration, patient's tolerance, complications and interventions, and collection and disposition of specimen in nurses' notes in electronic health record (EHR) or chart.
- Report onset of bleeding, abdominal pain, dyspnea, and vital sign changes to health care provider.
- Document your evaluation of patient and caregiver learning.

Special Considerations
Teaching
- Upper GI endoscopy:
  - Explain method for endoscope insertion. Prepare patient for a slight feeling of not being able to breathe. Assure them that this feeling is common, but that air is delivered through the endoscope and suffocation will not occur.
  - Teach patient simple hand signals for pain or discomfort because they will not be able to speak after the endoscope is positioned in the esophagus.
- Lower GI procedures (colonoscopy, sigmoidoscopy, proctoscopy):
  - Explain that it is normal to experience increased flatus and abdominal cramping.
  - Small amounts of blood in the stool are common if a biopsy was taken.

Pediatric
- Introduction of the endoscope in infants and small children who have a narrow and collapsible airway may result in respiratory distress.

Gerontological
- Older persons frequently have reduced drug clearance from decreased glomerular filtration rate (GFR) and nephron activity or decreased hepatic function. It is important to monitor the effects of medications given to older persons (Lewis et al., 2019).
- Because of age-related changes in older persons, the gastric mucosa is thinner, which increases the incidence of irritation, ulceration, and perforation.
- Physical exposure and room temperature contribute to hypothermia in frail older persons who are unable to communicate that they are cold. Use warmed blankets or forced-air heat to maintain core temperature at comfortable, safe levels (Lewis et al., 2019).
- Some older persons experience dehydration, electrolyte imbalance, and exhaustion from pretest preparation. If the procedure is done on an ambulatory care basis, it is helpful to have someone stay with the patient for at least 24 hours.

Care in the Community
- Explain that patient might have hoarseness or a sore throat after an upper GI procedure. Patient can have ice chips or anaesthetic lozenges after gag reflex returns.
- Instruct patient or caregiver to notify health care provider if patient has a fever, abdominal pain, rigid abdomen, and rectal bleeding or stool in blood.

✦ CLINICAL DEBRIEF

A 67-year-old male of Métis descent currently living in Toronto with his sister has recently experienced what he describes as "mild discomfort" in his chest when he walks to the park. He also has experienced fatigue with the chest pain. He has been engaging his Indigenous cultural practices of smudging to help with the chest pain. After constant chest pain, he goes to the emergency department to "check it out." His tests are suggestive of coronary artery disease and he is scheduled for an urgent cardiac catheterization under moderate sedation. Currently he is taking warfarin for an irregular heartbeat.

1. Which laboratory data would you review as part of your preparation of for his procedure?
2. He has arrived in the waiting area of the catheterization laboratory; you are the nurse assigned to this case. Describe the steps you would take to perform patient verification safety procedures for the patient.
3. The patient's cardiac catheterization procedure is finished, and he is now in the recovery area. The right femoral site was used for catheter insertion. Using SBAR, show how you would communicate with the health care team about this patient.

✦ REVIEW QUESTIONS

1. Place the steps listed here in the correct order for helping a patient who is undergoing a lumbar puncture.
   1. Help patient maintain lateral recumbent position with head and neck flexed.
   2. Properly label specimen in presence of patient.
   3. Assess patient's condition during procedure.
   4. Take "time-out" to verify patient's name, type of procedure scheduled, and procedure site.
   5. Explain to patient that pain may occur when lidocaine (local anaesthetic) is injected into the site.
   6. Document the opening intracranial pressure; observe fluid for colour.
2. A patient underwent a bronchoscopy and is now entering the recovery area. The patient develops sudden, severe shortness of breath. Which actions should the nurse take? (Select all that apply.)
   1. Support the patient's airway and monitor SpO₂.
   2. Call the health care provider immediately and prepare for possible resuscitation.
   3. Measure vital signs and ensure that the patient has patent intravenous (IV) access.
   4. Observe for blood-tinged mucus and suction airway.
   5. Anticipate the need for a possible cricothyrotomy
3. Which patients would be unable to undergo an angiogram? (Select all that apply.)
   1. 44-year-old female who is taking warfarin
   2. 52-year-old male suspected of having an abdominal aneurysm
   3. 77-year-old female suspected of having an arterial occlusion of the renal artery
   4. 65-year-old female who actually is 30 weeks' pregnant
   5. 36-year-old male who has a history of uncontrolled hypertension

Ⓔ *Visit the Evolve site for a complete list of Clinical Debrief and Review Questions answers.*

REFERENCECS

Accreditation Canada. (2019). *Required organizational practices handbook—Version 14*. Retrieved from http://www.wrha.mb.ca/quality/files/2019ROPHandbook.pdf

Arevalo-Rodriguez, I., Ciapponi, A., Roqué i Figuls, M., Muñoz, L., & Bonfill Cosp, X. (2016). Posture and fluids for preventing post-dural puncture headache. *The Cochrane Database of Systematic Reviews*, (3), CD009199.

Canadian Anesthesiologists' Society (CAS). (2018a). Guidelines to the practice of anesthesia—Revised edition 2018. *Canadian Journal of Anesthesia*, 65(1), 76–104. doi:10.1007/s12630-017-0995-9

Canadian Anesthesiologists' Society (CAS). (2018b). Appendix 2: American Society of Anesthesiologists classification of physical status. *Canadian Journal of Anesthesia*, 65(1), doi:10.1007/s12630-017-0995-9. Retrieved from https://www.cas.ca/English/Page/Files/97_Appendix%202.pdf

Canadian Anesthesiologists' Society (CAS). (2018c). Appendix 3: Pre-anesthetic checklist. *Canadian Journal of Anesthesia*, 65(1), doi:10.1007/s12630-017-0995-9. Retrieved from https://www.cas.ca/English/Page/Files/97_Appendix%203.pdf

Canadian Anesthesiologists' Society (CAS). (2018d). Appendix 6: Position paper on procedural sedation: An official position paper of the Canadian Anesthesiologists' Society. *Canadian Journal of Anesthesia*, 65(1), doi:10.1007/s12630-017-0995-9. Retrieved from http://www.cas.ca/English/Page/Files/97_Appendix%206.pdf

Canadian Association for Interventional Radiology (CAIR). (2010). *Guidelines and standards*. Retrieved from https://www.cairweb.ca/en/publications/guidelines-and-standards/

Canadian Association of Radiologists (CAR). (2011). *National practice guidelines*. Retrieved from https://car.ca/patient-care/practice-guidelines/

Canadian Medical Protective Association. (n.d.). *Good practices guide: Informed consent*. Retrieved from https://www.cmpa-acpm.ca/serve/docs/ela/goodpracticesguide/pages/communication/Informed_Consent/informed_consent-e.html

Canadian Patient Safety Institute (CPSI). (2009). *Surgical safety checklist*. Retrieved from http://www.patientsafetyinstitute.ca/en/toolsResources/Documents/Interventions/Surgical%20Safety%20Checklist/Detailed%20Explanation%20of%20the%20Checklist.pdf

Canadian Patient Safety Institute (CPSI). (2014). *A surgical care safety action plan*. Retrieved from http://www.patientsafetyinstitute.ca/en/About/PatientSafetyForwardWith4/Documents/Surgical%20Care%20Safety%20Action%20Plan.pdf

Coffey, S., & Anyinam, C. (2015). *Interprofessional health care practice*. Toronto, ON: Pearson.

Honicker, T., & Holt, K. (2016). Contrast-induced acute kidney injury: Comparison of preventative therapies. *Nephrology Nursing Journal*, 43(2), 109–116.

Hospital for Sick Children (HSC). (2017). *Clinical practice guidelines: Pain management*. Retrieved from http://www.sickkids.ca/clinical-practice-guidelines/clinical-practice-guidelines/export/CLINH142/Main%20Document.pdf

Kern, M., Sorajja, P., & Lim, M. (2016). *The cardiac catheterization handbook* (6th ed.). Philadelphia, PA: Elsevier.

Lagoo, J., Lopushinsky, S., Haynes, A., et al. (2017). Effectiveness and meaningful use of paediatric surgical safety checklists and their implementation strategies: A systematic review with narrative synthesis. *BMJ Open*, 7, e016298. doi:10.1136/bmjopen-2017-0

Lewis, S., Bucher, L., Heitkemper, M., et al. (2019). *Medical-surgical nursing in Canada* (4th ed.). Toronto, ON: Elsevier Canada.

Metzner, J., & Domino, K. (2015). Moderate sedation: A primer for perioperative nurses. *AORN Journal*, 102(5), 527–537. doi:10.1016/j.aorn.2015.09.001

National Association of Perioperative Nurses of Canada (NAPAN). (2018). *Standards for practice resources*. Retrieved from http://napanc.ca/index.php/159-membership/159-standards-resources-2018

National Patient Safety Consortium. (2017). *Integrated patient safety plan*. Retrieved from http://www.patientsafetyinstitute.ca/en/About/PatientSafetyForwardWith4/Pages/Integrated-Patient-Safety-Action-Plan.aspx

Pagana, K., Pagana, T., & Pike-MacDonald, S. (2019). *Mosby's Canadian manual of diagnostic and laboratory tests* (2nd Canadian ed.). Toronto, ON: Elsevier Canada.

Perry, S. E., Hockenberry, M. J., Lowdermilk, D. L., Wilson, D., Keenan-Lindsey, L., & Sams, C. (2017). *Maternal child nursing care in Canada* (2nd ed.). St. Louis: Mosby.

Quality Management Partnership (QMP). (2015). *Pre- and post-procedure guidelines and checklists for endoscopy facilities*. Retrieved from https://www.qmpontario.ca/common/pages/UserFile.aspx?fileId=364570

Registered Nurses' Association of Ontario (RNAO). (2004/2008). *Nursing best practice guideline: Assessment and device selection for vascular access*. Retrieved from https://rnao.ca/bpg/guidelines/assessment-and-device-selection-vascular-access

Suggs, P., Lewis, R., Troutman-Jordan, M., & Hardin, S. (2017). What's your position? Strategies for safely reaching patient comfort goals after cardiac catheterization via femoral approach. *Dimensions of Critical Care Nursing*, 36(2), 87–93. doi:10.1097/DCC.0000000000000232

Taslakian, B., & Sridhar, D. (2017). Post-procedural care in interventional radiology: What every interventional radiologist should know. *Cardiovascular and Interventional Radiology*, 40, 481–495. doi:10.10007/s00270-017-1564-x

World Health Organization (WHO). (2007). *Patient identification. Patient Safety Solutions, Volume 1, solution 2*. Retrieved from http://www.who.int/patientsafety/solutions/patientsafety/PS-Solution2.pdf

11 | Safe Patient Handling, Transfer, and Positioning

Written by **Rita Wunderlich, RN, PhD, CNE, and Chantal Backman, RN, MHA, PhD**

OBJECTIVES

Mastery of content in this chapter will enable the nurse to:

- Describe principles of safe patient handling, transfer, and positioning.
- Explain the importance of using mechanical lifts and other assist devices when moving, positioning, and transferring patients.
- Perform an assessment for determining the type of approach to use and amount of help needed to transfer and position patients safely.

- Describe transfer and positioning procedures to follow to ensure patient and nurse safety.
- Describe positioning techniques for the supported Fowler's, supine, prone, 30-degree lateral side-lying, and Sims' positions.
- Describe the procedures for helping a patient move up in bed, helping a patient to a sitting position, logrolling a patient, and transferring a patient from a bed to a chair.

MEDIA RESOURCES

- **evolve** http://evolve.elsevier.com/Canada/Perry/clinicalskills/
- Review Questions
- ▶ Video Clips

- Audio Glossary
- **NSO** Nursing Skills Online
- Clinical Debrief and Review Questions Answers

PURPOSE

Health care facilities are required to provide employees with safety information and education to properly transfer, position, and lift patients. Relying on proper body mechanics and manual lifting techniques alone is not effective for reducing health care workers' musculoskeletal injuries. A comprehensive safe patient-handling program that combines management commitment with employee involvement, policies, and proper mechanical equipment availability and education is needed (Canadian Centre for Occupational Health and Safety [CCOHS], 2018a). Workers might need to move, roll, steady, and position patients while using lifting equipment. However, because most musculoskeletal injuries in care facilities are cumulative, any steps taken to minimize the potential for musculoskeletal injuries during patient-handling tasks benefit health care workers. Nurses should always refer to their employer's policies. Many patients have conditions resulting in immobility or require limitations in activity imposed by their treatment plan. It is an important nursing role to safely and correctly position and move patients effectively to reduce the risks related to immobilization, such as skin breakdown, pneumonia, and thromboembolism. When performing the skills in this chapter, it is essential to use safe patient-handling techniques.

STANDARDS OF CARE

- Accreditation Canada, 2019—*Required Organizational Practices Handbook—Version 14* (http://www.wrha.mb.ca/quality/files/2019 ROPHandbook.pdf)
- Canadian Centre for Occupational Health and Safety (CCOHS), 2018a—*Ergonomic Safe Patient Handling Program* (http://www.ccohs.ca/oshanswers/hsprograms/patient_handling.html)
- Canadian Centre for Occupational Health and Safety (CCOHS), 2018b—*Patient Lifts and Worker Risks* (http://www.ccohs.ca/newsletters/hsreport/issues/2012/08/ezine.html)

PRINCIPLES FOR PRACTICE

- Body mechanics are the coordinated effort of the musculoskeletal and nervous systems to maintain balance, posture, and body alignment during lifting, bending, moving, and performing activities of daily living (ADLs).

- The use of safe patient transfer and positioning techniques helps patients achieve an optimal level of independence without resultant injury to health care providers.
- Teaching the use of safe patient-handling equipment in combination with proper body mechanics is more effective than either one in isolation (CCOHS, 2018a).
- Key principles in determining the proper handling techniques to use for patients are knowing if a patient is weight bearing and the patient's weight and height, strength, and ability to cooperate and provide help (CCOHS, 2018a).
- Patients who are at high risk for complications from improper positioning and injury during transfer include those with poor nutrition, poor circulation, loss of sensation, alterations in bone formation or joint mobility, and impaired muscle development.

PERSON-CENTRED CARE

- Ultimately, it is a patient's choice to increase their mobility and activity level. Practise person-centred nursing care by considering a patient's knowledge, cultural beliefs, and attitudes about the loss of independent activity and the person's willingness to participate in activity when developing a plan of care.
- Use simple language when providing patients information about the complications of immobility and their unique risks.
- Consider the circumstances surrounding a patient's loss of independent activity and mobility to ensure that a plan of care is realistic and attainable.
- Understand to what extent the patient chooses to have a caregiver involved to learn transfer and positioning techniques for care at home.

EVIDENCE-INFORMED PRACTICE

There is more available evidence with regard to techniques necessary to reduce workplace injuries within health care facilities.

- Inpatient health care facilities have some of the highest rates of injury and illness among all industries. In 2016, the health and social services industry averaged over 43 836 lost time claims out of the total claims of 241 508 in Canada (Association of Workers' Compensation Boards of Canada, 2016).
- CCOHS (2018a) has provided guidelines for how to complete an ergonomics hazard assessment on the basis of patient population, patient-handling tasks, and physical environment. It is critical to educate health care staff about devices, equipment, and handling policies.
- Most organizations have developed "no-lift" policies that discourage manual lifting and require the use of safe handling of equipment and devices as needed (CCOHS, 2018a; Occupational Health Clinic for Ontario Workers Inc., 2018).
- Knowledge about safe, efficient transfer and positioning techniques (Box 11.1) and proper use of assistive equipment and devices promotes safe patient transfer without injury to a patient or health care worker (CCOHS, 2018a).

SAFETY GUIDELINES

- Know how physiological influences on body alignment and mobility affect patients throughout the lifespan. Inactive older

---

BOX 11.1

Principles of Safe Body Mechanics When Transferring and Positioning Patients

Mechanical lifts and lift teams are essential when a patient is unable to help. When a patient is able to help, remember these principles:

- The lower the centre of gravity, the greater the stability of the nurse.
- The equilibrium of an object is maintained as long as the line of gravity passes through its base of support.
- Facing the direction of movement prevents abnormal twisting of the spine.
- Dividing balanced activity between arms and legs reduces the risk for back injury.
- Leverage, rolling, turning, or pivoting requires less work than lifting.
- When friction is reduced between the object to be moved and the surface on which it is moved, less force is required to move it.

BOX 11.2

Bedrail Safety Tips

A patient can get trapped in the bedrails of a hospital bed.
Before using bedrails:

- Assess whether a patient would benefit from the use of bedrails.
- Know the potential areas of entrapment (within the rail, under the rail, between the rail and the mattress, between split bedrails, between the end of the rail and the side edge of the head- or footboard, and between the head- or footboard and the end of the mattress).
- Make sure the mattress is the right size.
- Use a mattress with raised foam edges.
- Contact the manufacturer for the product safety information, and ensure regular maintenance of the bedrail latching system.
When using bedrails:
- Lower sections of the bedrail (if possible).
- Make sure all latches are securely fastened.
- Monitor patient regularly, and report any bed-related incidents.

---

persons are at risk for muscle atrophy, loss of bone mass, contractures of joints, and pressure injury (Harridge & Lazarus, 2017).

- Control the factors that can indirectly affect body mechanics by making the environment safe. Cluttered hallways and bedside areas increase a patient's risk of falling (see Chapter 42).
- Assess a patient's range of motion. Contractures or spasticity limit joint and muscle mobility; take care not to position a patient's limb in an unnatural position. This could result in injury or dysfunction of the affected limb (see Chapter 12).
- Determine a patient's level of sensory perception (vision and hearing) because this affects the person's ability to cooperate during transfer and lifting procedures (see Chapter 8).
- Loss of sensation increases vulnerability to the hazards of immobility because of the inability to sense pain or the need for repositioning.
- Use assistive equipment and devices to transfer and position patients safely.
- Know the risk factors for bed entrapment in the hospital or nursing home and in home health care, and how to prevent it (Box 11.2) (Government of Canada, 2015).

▶ *Video Clip* **NSO** *Nursing Skills Online Safety Module 4 / Lesson 3*

Safe and effective transfer is a nursing skill for assisting dependent patients or patients with restricted mobility to attain positions to regain or maintain optimal independence. For example, transferring from a bed to a chair promotes physical activity to maintain and improve joint motion, increase strength, promote circulation, relieve pressure on the skin, and improve urinary and respiratory functions (see Chapter 12). It also benefits a patient psychologically by increasing social activity and mental stimulation and providing a change in environment (Huether & McCance, 2016).

Consider an individual patient's clinical problems during a transfer. For example, a patient who has been immobile for several days or longer may be weak or dizzy or may develop orthostatic hypotension (decreased blood pressure) when transferred to a chair. To ensure safe patient transfers, always use a gait or transfer belt or an appropriate lift and get help from a colleague (WorkSafe NB, 2015).

Delegation and Collaboration

The skill of effective transfer techniques can be delegated to an unregulated care provider (UCP). The nurse is responsible for initially assessing patient's readiness and ability to transfer. The nurse directs the UCP by:

- Helping and supervising when moving patients who are transferred for the first time after prolonged bed rest, extensive surgery, critical illness, or spinal cord trauma.
- Explaining the patient's mobility restrictions, changes in blood pressure to monitor for, or sensory alterations that may affect safe transfer.
- Explaining what to observe for and reporting back to the nurse conditions such as dizziness or the patient's inability to help.

Equipment

- Transfer belt
- Sling (as needed)
- Nonskid shoes, bath blankets, pillows
- Slide board (friction-reducing board)
- Bedside chair with arms
- Stretcher: Position next to bed, lock brakes on stretcher, lock brakes on bed
- Mechanical/hydraulic lift: Use frame, canvas strips or chains, and hammock or canvas strips; stand-assist lift device
- Sphygmomanometer and stethoscope
- Clean gloves (if risk of soiling)

STEP	RATIONALE
ASSESSMENT	
1. Identify patient using at least two person-specific identifiers (e.g., name and date of birth or name and medical record number, according to employer policy).	Ensures correct patient. Complies with Accreditation Canada's standards and improves patient safety (Accreditation Canada, 2019).
2. Perform hand hygiene.	Reduces transmission of microorganisms.
3. Review medical record or directly assess physical capacity of a patient to transfer and help with transfer (see Chapter 8). Assess the following:	Determines patient's ability to tolerate and help with transfer and whether special adaptive techniques or safe handling devices are necessary.
a. Muscle strength (legs and upper arms) through active range of motion	Immobile patients have decreased muscle strength, tone, and mass. Affects ability to bear weight, raise body, and thus help with transfer.
b. Joint mobility and contracture formation	Immobility or inflammatory processes (e.g., arthritis) may lead to contracture formation and impaired joint mobility.
c. Paralysis or paresis (spastic or flaccid)	Patient with central nervous system (CNS) damage may have bilateral paralysis (requiring transfer by swivel bar, sliding bar, mechanical lift) or unilateral paralysis, which requires belt transfer to strong side. Weakness (paresis) requires stabilization of knee while transferring. Flaccid arm must be supported with sling during transfer.
d. Bone continuity (trauma, amputation) or calcium loss from long bones	Patients with trauma to one leg or hip may be non–weight bearing when transferred. Amputees may use sliding board to transfer. Osteoporosis increases risk for injury.
4. Refer to medical record for most recent recorded weight and height for patient.	These factors are used to determine if mechanical transfer device or friction-reducing device is needed for transfer.
5. Assess for history of presence of weakness, dizziness, or postural hypotension (when sitting or standing).	Determines risk for fainting or falling during transfer. The move from supine to vertical position with a decrease of 20 mm Hg or more in systolic blood pressure results in orthostatic hypotension (Lewis, Bucher, Heitkemper, et al., 2019).
6. Assess medical record for patient's level of fatigue and activity tolerance during previous transfers. Assess endurance by noting patient's participation in activities of daily living (ADLs).	Estimates ability of patient to participate in transfer. Planned rest periods before transfer may enhance function.

STEP	RATIONALE

ASSESSMENT

7. Assess patient's proprioceptive function (awareness of posture and changes in equilibrium):	Determines stability of patient's balance for transfer.
a. Ability to maintain balance while sitting in bed or on side of bed	Determines risk for fainting or falling during transfer.
b. Tendency to sway or position self to one side	Patients with brain dysfunction may have proprioceptive losses. This may cause them to lean to one side or lose balance during transfer.
8. Assess patient's sensory status, including adequacy of vision and hearing and presence of peripheral sensation loss (see Chapter 8).	Determines influence of sensory loss on ability to make transfer. Visual field loss decreases patient's ability to see in direction of transfer. Peripheral sensation loss decreases proprioception. Patients with visual and hearing losses need transfer techniques adapted to deficits.

Clinical Decision Point *Patients with hemiplegia may "neglect" one side of the body (inattention to or unawareness of one side of body or environment), which distorts perceptions of the visual field.*

9. Assess patient for pain (e.g., joint discomfort, muscle spasm) and measure level of pain using appropriate pain rating scale. Offer prescribed analgesic 30 minutes before transfer.	Pain reduces patient's motivation and ability to be mobile. Pain relief before transfer enhances patient participation (Horgas, 2017).
10. Assess patient's cognitive status:	Determines patient's ability to follow directions and help during transfer.
a. Ability to follow verbal instructions	May indicate that patient is at risk for injury.
b. Short-term memory	Patient with short-term memory deficit may have difficulty with transfer, initial learning, or consistent performance.
c. Recognition of physical deficits and limitations to movement	Patient's knowledge of deficits can help you plan a safe transfer.
11. Assess patient's level of motivation, such as their eagerness versus unwillingness to be mobile.	Altered psychological states often reduce patient's desire to engage in activity.
12. Assess previous mode of transfer (if applicable).	Determines mode of transfer and help required to provide continuity.
13. Just before transfer assess patient's vital signs.	Vital sign changes such as increased pulse and respiration may indicate activity intolerance (see Chapter 7). A patient with low blood pressure may not tolerate sudden position change and is at risk for orthostatic hypotension. Provides baseline to determine tolerance to transfer.
14. Refer to safe-handling algorithm (available in most facilities) to determine if a lift device or mechanical transfer device is needed and the number of people needed to help with transfer. Do not start procedure until all required caregivers are available.	Ensures safe patient handling, reducing risk of injury to patient and caregivers.

NURSING DIAGNOSES

- Acute or persistent pain
- Acute confusion
- Reduced physical mobility

- Reduced stamina
- Reduced skin integrity

- Potential for falls
- Potential for injury

Related factors/Risk factors are individualized on the basis of patient's condition or needs.

PLANNING

1. Expected outcomes following completion of procedure:	
• Patient sits on side of bed without dizziness, weakness, or orthostatic hypotension.	Precautions during transfer prevent vascular compromise.
• Patient tolerates increased activity.	Gradual increase in number of transfers and period of time out of bed increases tolerance and endurance.
• Patient can bear more weight.	Repeated transfers usually result in improved endurance and greater independence of patient.

STEP	RATIONALE

PLANNING

- Patient transfers without injury.

  Use of proper techniques avoids injury.
- Patient transfers with minimal discomfort.

  Transfer procedures are performed correctly.

2. Explain to patient (in simple language) how you are going to prepare for transfer technique and safety precautions to be used. Explain benefits and reasons for getting up in a chair. Do so in a way that matches patient's beliefs and values regarding recovery or maintaining health (Shieh, Weaver, Hanna, et al., 2015).

   Provides for clearer understanding by patient. Motivates patient to be involved in transfer.

3. Close room curtains or door.

   Provides for patient privacy.

4. Get additional caregivers, necessary lift or transfer device, or both, to perform transfer.

   Safe-handling algorithms (see employer policy) determine number of caregivers and type of devices needed to transfer a patient if lifting is required.

IMPLEMENTATION

1. Perform hand hygiene.

   Reduces transmission of microorganisms.

2. Help patient from supine to sitting position on edge of bed with bed positioned so top of mattress is even with your elbows. (See Chapter 12, Procedural Guideline 12.4, Step 14 with illustrations.)

   Reduces strain on your back.

3. Allow patient to sit on side of bed for a few minutes. Have patient alternately flex and extend feet, move lower legs up and down. Ask if patient feels dizzy; if so, check blood pressure. Have patient relax and take a few deep breaths until dizziness subsides and balance is gained. If dizziness lasts more than 60 seconds, return patient to bed (Myszenski, 2017). Recheck blood pressure.

   Allows patient's circulation to equilibrate to reduce chance of orthostatic hypotension.

Clinical Decision Point *Remain in front of patient until the person regains balance and continue to provide physical support to weak or cognitively impaired patient.*

4. **Transfer patient from bed to chair:**
   a. Have chair in position at 45-degree angle with one side against bed, facing foot of bed.

      Positions chair with easy access for transfer.
   b. Place bed in low position or to point where patient's feet are comfortably on the floor.

      Provides patient stability when transferring.
   c. If patient has partial weight bearing with upper body strength or caregiver must lift more than 15.9 kg (35 lb), use mechanical lift or transfer aid with minimum of two or three caregivers (see illustration). Follow manufacturer lift guidelines to apply.

      The use of mechanical lift devices is strongly recommended to transfer a patient to reduce risk for musculoskeletal injury (CCOHS, 2018a).

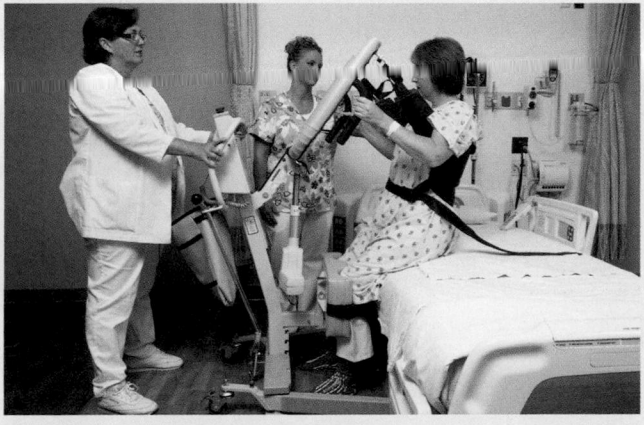

STEP 4c Patient grasps handles as nurse turns on motorized lift.

STEP	RATIONALE

IMPLEMENTATION

Clinical Decision Point *If patient demonstrates weakness or paralysis of one side of the body, place chair on their strong side.*

d. If patient has partial weight bearing, is cooperative and able to stand, and has upper body strength, use stand-and-pivot technique with one caregiver.

(1) Apply transfer belt (see illustration). Be sure that it completely circles waist. Place belt low and be sure that it is snug. Avoid placing belt over any intravenous lines, incisions, or drainage tubes.

Transfer belt allows you to maintain stability of patient during transfer and reduces risk for falling (WorkSafe NB, 2015).

(2) If not already in place, help patient apply stable, nonskid shoes or socks. Place patient's weight-bearing or strong leg forward on floor, with weak foot back.

Nonskid soles decrease risk for slipping during transfer. Always have patient wear shoes during transfer; bare feet increase risk for falls. Patient will stand on stronger, or weight-bearing, leg.

(3) Spread your feet apart. Flex hips and knees, aligning knees with patient's knees.

Ensures balance with wide base of support.

Flexing knees and hips lowers your centre of gravity to object to be raised; aligning knees with those of patient allows for stabilization of knees when patient stands.

(4) Grasp transfer belt, keeping your palms up, along patient's sides (see illustration).

Transfer belt allows you to move patient at centre of gravity. Patients should never be lifted by or under their arms.

(5) Rock patient up to standing position on count of three while straightening hips and legs and keeping knees slightly flexed (see illustration). While rocking patient in back-and-forth motion, make sure that your body weight is moving in the same direction as patient's, to ensure that you and patient are moving in same direction simultaneously. Unless contraindicated, patient may be instructed to use hands to push up, if applicable.

Rocking motion gives patient's body momentum and requires less muscular effort to lift the person.

(6) Maintain stability of patient's weakened leg with your knee.

Ability to stand can often be maintained in weak limb with support of knee to stabilize.

(7) Pivot on foot farthest from chair.

Maintains support of patient while allowing adequate space for patient to move.

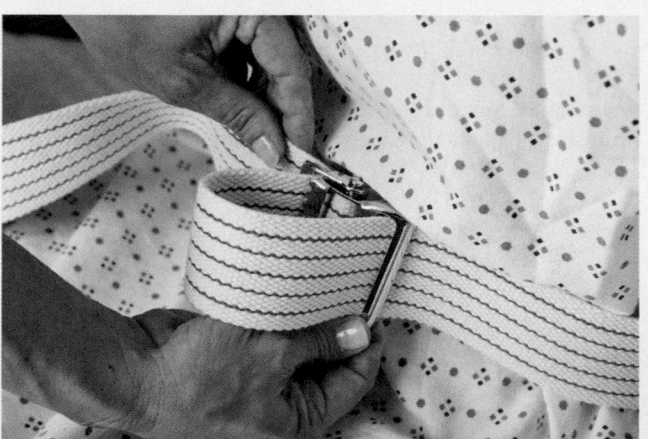

STEP 4d(1) Application of transfer belt.

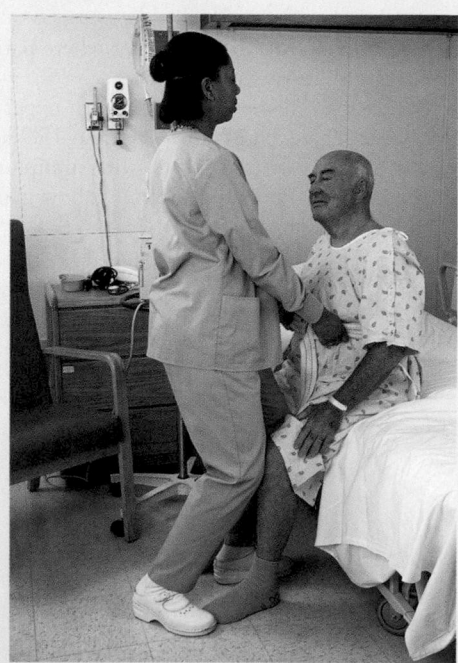

STEP 4d(4) Nurse flexes hips and knees, aligns knees with patient's knee, and grasps transfer belt palms up.

STEP	RATIONALE

IMPLEMENTATION

(8) Instruct patient to use armrests on chair for support and ease into chair (see illustration).

Increases patient stability.

(9) Flex hips and knees while lowering patient into chair.

Prevents injury from poor body mechanics.

(10) Assess patient for proper alignment in sitting position. Provide support for weakened extremity. You can use a sling or lap board to support an injured or flaccid arm. Stabilize leg with bath blanket or pillow.

Prevents injury to patient from poor body alignment.

(11) Proper alignment for sitting position: head is erect, and vertebrae are in straight alignment. Body weight is evenly distributed on buttocks and thighs. Thighs are parallel and in horizontal plane. Both feet are supported on floor, and ankles are comfortably flexed. A 2.5- to 5-cm (1- to 2-inch) space is maintained between edge of seat and popliteal space on posterior surface of knee.

Prevents stress on intravertebral joints. Prevents increased pressure over bony prominences and reduces damage to underlying musculoskeletal system.

e. **If patient is not able to cooperate (regardless of ability to bear weight) or has no upper body strength, use ceiling or floor hydraulic lift to transfer patient from bed to chair.**

Research supports use of mechanical lifts to prevent musculoskeletal injuries (CCOHS, 2018a). Use of ceiling-mounted lifts is a popular choice because of availability of lift in each patient's room (see illustration).

(1) Bring mechanical floor lift to bedside or lower ceiling lift and position properly.

Ensures safe elevation of patient off bed.

(2) Position chair near bed and allow adequate space to manoeuvre the lift.

Prepares environment for safe use of lift and subsequent transfer.

(3) Raise bed to high position with mattress flat. Lower side rail on side near chair.

Allows you to use proper body mechanics.

(4) Have second nurse positioned at opposite side of bed.

Maintains patient safety, preventing fall from bed.

(5) Roll patient on side away from you.

Positions patient for placement of lift sling.

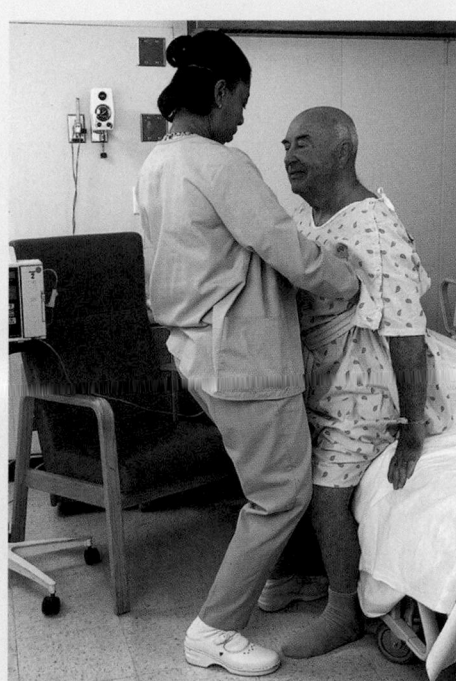

STEP 4d(5) Nurse rocks patient (who is able to help) to standing position.

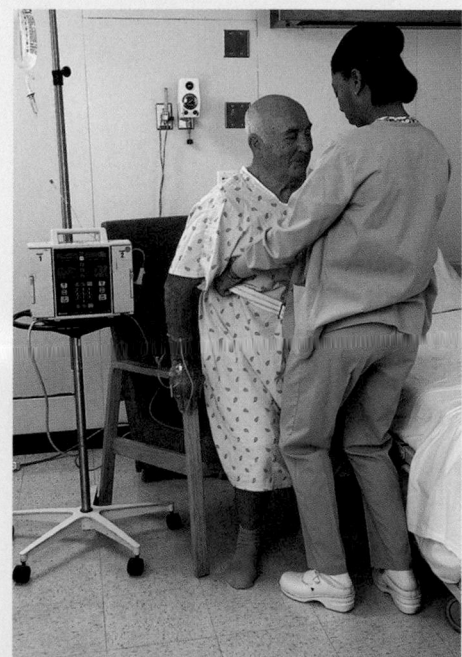

STEP 4d(8) Patient uses armrests and is guided to sit in chair.

STEP	RATIONALE

IMPLEMENTATION

(6) Place hammock or canvas strips under patient to form sling. With two canvas pieces, lower edge fits under patient's knees (wide piece), and upper edge fits under patient's shoulders (narrow piece).

Two types of seats are supplied with a mechanical/hydraulic lift: hammock style is better for patients who are flaccid, weak, and need support; canvas strips can be used for patients with normal muscle tone. Hooks should face away from patient's skin. Place sling under patient's centre of gravity and greatest part of body weight.

(7) Roll patient back toward you as second nurse pulls hammock (straps) through.

Ensures that sling is in proper position before lift.

(8) Return patient to supine position. Be sure that hammock or straps are smooth over bed surface. Sling should extend from shoulders to knees (hammock) to support patient's body weight equally.

Completes positioning of patient on mechanical/hydraulic sling.

(9) Remove patient's glasses if appropriate.

Swivel bar is close to patient's head and could break eyeglasses.

(10) Place horseshoe base of floor lift under patient's bed (on side with chair).

Positions lift efficiently and promotes smooth transfer.

(11) Lower horizontal bar to sling level by following manufacturer directions. Lock valve if required.

Positions hydraulic lift close to patient. Locking valve prevents injury to patient.

(12) Attach hooks on strap (chain) to holes in sling. Short chains or straps hook to top holes of sling; longer chains hook to bottom of sling (see manufacturer directions).

Secures hydraulic lift to sling.

(13) Elevate head of bed to Fowler's position.

Positions patient in sitting position.

(14) Have patient fold arms over chest.

Prevents injury to patient's arms during transfer.

(15) Pump hydraulic handle using long, slow, even strokes until patient is raised off bed (see illustration). For ceiling lift turn on control device to move lift.

Ensures safe support of patient during elevation.

(16) Use lift to raise patient off bed and use steering handle to pull lift from bed as you and another nurse manoeuvre patient to chair. Have second nurse alongside patient.

Lifts patient off the bed safely; nurse's position reduces any risk of patient falling from sling.

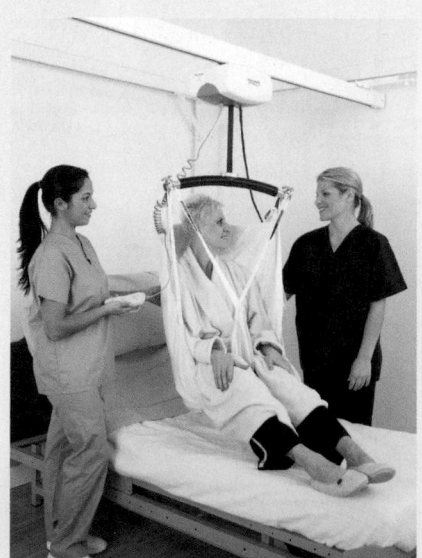

STEP 4e Ceiling lift. (*Courtesy Waverly Glen Systems, a Prism Medical Co.*)

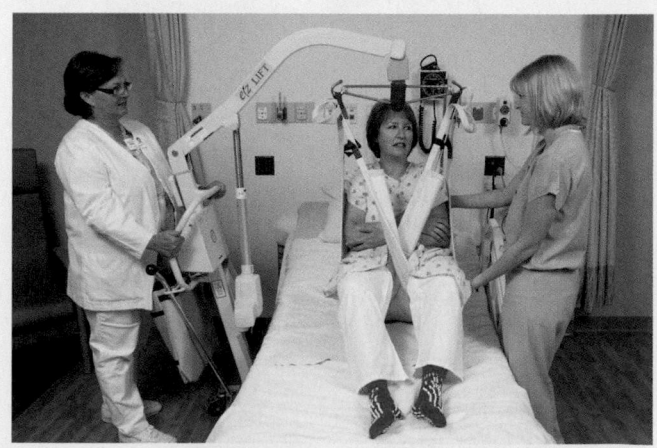

STEP 4e(15) Patient lifted in hydraulic lift above bed.

STEP	RATIONALE

IMPLEMENTATION

(17) Roll base of lift around chair. Release check valve slowly and lower patient into chair (see manufacturer directions) (see illustration).

Positions lift in front of chair into which patient is to be transferred. Safely guides patient into back of chair as seat descends.

(18) Close check valve as soon as patient is down in chair and straps can be released.

If valve is left open, boom may continue to lower and injure patient.

(19) Remove straps and roll mechanical/hydraulic lift out of patient's path.

Prevents damage to skin and underlying tissues.

(20) Check patient's sitting alignment and correct if necessary.

Prevents injury from poor posture.

5. Perform lateral transfer from bed to stretcher:

The three-person lift for horizontal transfer from bed to stretcher is no longer recommended and, in fact, is discouraged (Occupational Safety & Health Association [OSHA], 2014). Physical stress can be decreased significantly by using a slide board or friction-reducing board positioned under drawsheet beneath patient. In addition, patient is more comfortable with this method.

a. Determine if patient can assist.

Patient's level of strength and weight determine level of help required for safe transfer. During any patient-transferring task, if any caregiver is required to lift more than 15.9 kg (35 lb) of patient's weight, patient is considered fully dependent, and an assist device is used (OSHA, 2014).

(1) If patient can assist, caregiver is only needed to stand by for safety, with stretcher and bed locked as patient moves to stretcher.

(2) If patient is partially or not at all able to help and is <90.7 kg (<200 lb), use friction-reducing device or lateral transfer board.

(3) If patient is partially or not at all able to help and is >90.7 kg (>200 lb), use a ceiling lift with supine sling or a mechanical lateral-transfer device with three caregivers.

b. Lateral transfer with friction- reducing device— slide board (see illustration) or air assisted device:

Maintains alignment of spinal column. Ensures that bed does not move inadvertently.

(1) Apply clean gloves if there is risk of soiling. Lower head of bed as much as patient can tolerate. Be sure to lock bed brakes.

Reduces transmission of microorganisms.

(2) Cross patient's arms on chest.

Prevents injury to arms during transfer.

(3) Lower side rails. To place slide board under patient, position two nurses on side of bed toward which patient will be turned. Position third nurse on other side of bed.

Distributes weight equally between nurses.

(4) Fanfold drawsheet on both sides.

Provides strong handles to grip drawsheet without slipping.

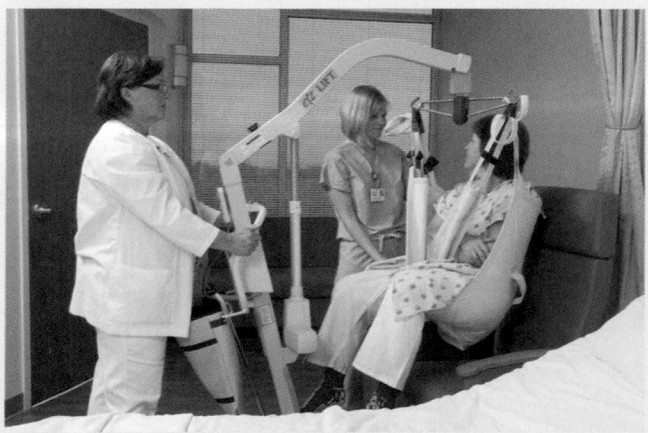

STEP 4e(17) Use of hydraulic lift lowers patient into chair.

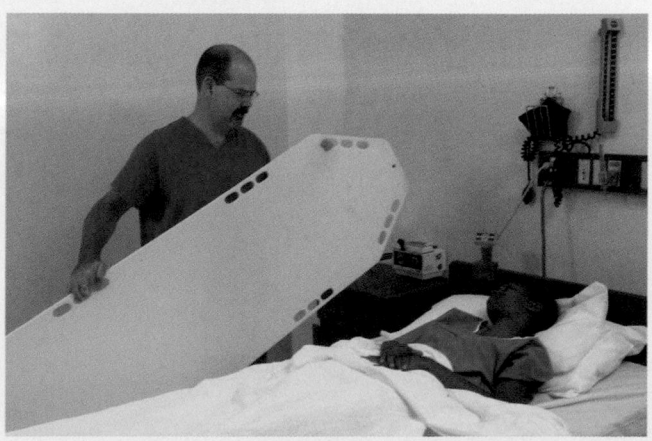

STEP 5b Slide board.

STEP	RATIONALE

IMPLEMENTATION

(5) On count of three logroll patient onto side toward the two nurses. Turn patient as one unit with smooth, continuous motion.

Maintains body in alignment, preventing stress on any part.

(6) Place slide board under drawsheet (see illustration). *Option:* Apply air-assisted device.

Prevents friction from contact of skin with board.

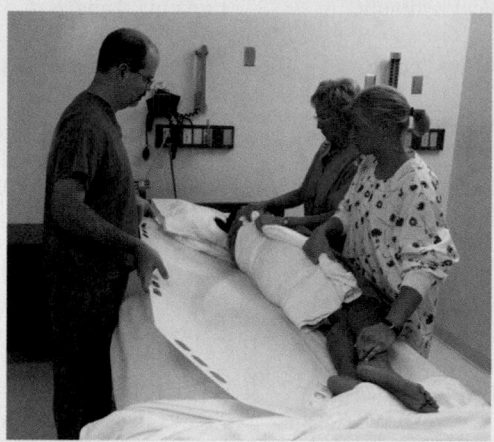

STEP 5b(6) Caregivers placing slide board under drawsheet.

(7) Gently roll patient back onto slide board.

(8) Line up stretcher so surface is 1.3 cm (½ inch) lower than bed. Lock brakes on stretcher. Instruct patient not to move.

Ensures that stretcher does not move inadvertently during transfer.

(9) Two nurses position themselves on side of stretcher while third nurse positions self on side of bed without stretcher. All three nurses place feet widely apart with one foot slightly in front of the other and grasp friction-reducing device.

Clinical Decision Point *A nurse may also be positioned at the head of patient's bed to protect and support the person's head and neck if patient is weak or unable to help.*

(10) Holding fan-folded drawsheet and one nurse counting to three, the two nurses pull drawsheet across slide board, positioning patient onto stretcher (see illustration A). The third nurse holds slide board in place. *Option:* Inflate air-assisted device and slide patient across bed onto stretcher (see illustrations B and C).

Slide board remains stationary, provides slippery surface to reduce friction, and allows patient to transfer easily to stretcher.

STEP	RATIONALE

IMPLEMENTATION

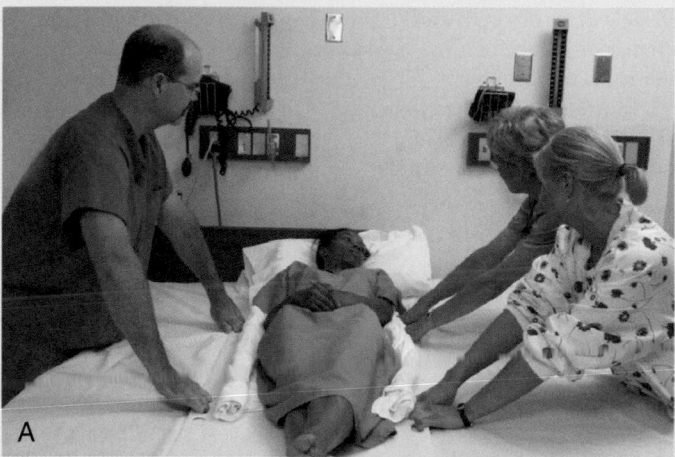

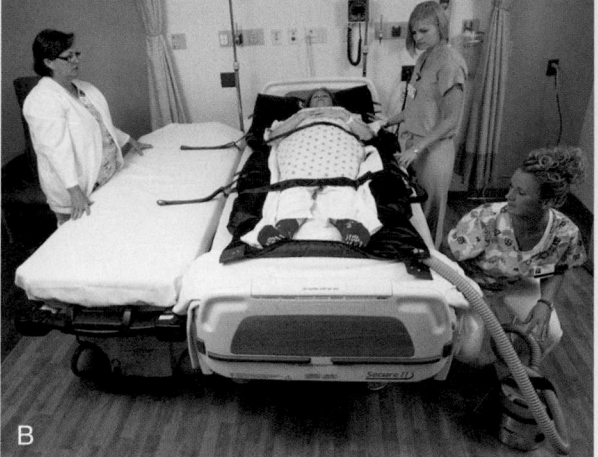
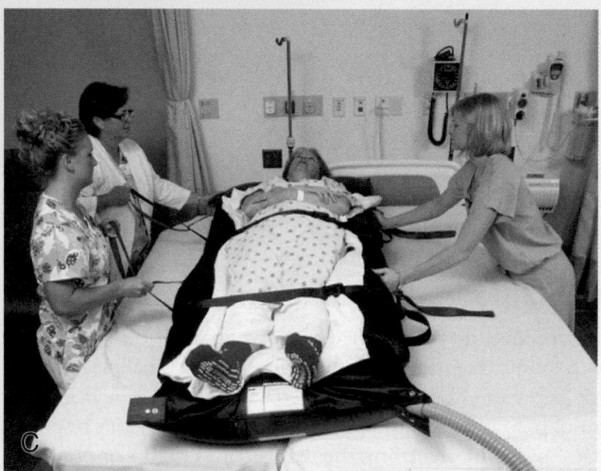

STEP 5b(10) A, Transfer of patient to stretcher using slide board. B, Inflating air-assisted transfer device. C, Transfer of patient using air-assisted transfer device.

STEP	RATIONALE
(11) Position patient in centre of stretcher. Raise head of stretcher if not contraindicated. Raise stretcher side rails. Cover patient with blanket.	Provides for patient comfort.
6. Remove and dispose of gloves (if used) and perform hand hygiene.	Reduces transmission of microorganisms.

STEP	RATIONALE

EVALUATION

1. Monitor vital signs. Ask if patient feels dizzy or tired. Ask patient to rate pain on an appropriate pain scale.

Evaluates patient's response to postural changes and activity.

2. Note patient's behavioural response to transfer.

Reveals level of motivation and self-care potential.

3. **Use Teach-Back:** "We are ready to transfer you to the chair. Do you remember what you can do to help us transfer you safely?" Develop a revised teaching plan if patient is not able to teach back correctly.

Determines patient's level of understanding of instructional topic.

Unexpected Outcomes	Related Interventions
1. Patient is unable to comprehend or is unwilling to follow directions for transfer.	• Reassess continuity and simplicity of your instruction. • If patient is tired or in pain, allow for rest period before transferring. • Consider medicating for pain if indicated. • Consider using hydraulic lift.
2. Patient sustains injury on transfer.	• Evaluate incident that led to injury (e.g., inadequate assessment, change in patient status, improper use of equipment). • Complete adverse event/incident report according to employer policy.
3. Patient is unable to stand for the time required to transfer to chair.	• Consider use of a lateral transfer board (see Procedural Guideline 11.1) or hydraulic lift.

Communication and Documentation

- Document procedure, including pertinent observations: weakness, ability to follow directions, weight-bearing ability, balance, ability to pivot, number of personnel needed to help, assist device used, amount of help (muscle strength) required, and patient's response in nurses' notes in electronic health record (EHR) or chart.
- Document your evaluation of patient and caregiver learning.
- Communicate transfer ability and help needed during hand-off report or to other caregivers.
- Use interprofessional collaboration to discuss patient progress or remission and revise the plan of care as required (e.g., collaborate with physiotherapist, occupational therapist).

Special Considerations

Teaching

- Teach patient and caregiver the importance of increasing activity out of bed.
- Instruct caregiver on how to assess a patient's tolerance to increased activity.

Pediatric

- Whenever possible, it is good to transport a child by stretcher, stroller, or wheelchair outside confines of room to increase environmental stimuli and provide social contact with others (Hockenberry & Wilson, 2015).

- Children confined to bed for any length of time, such as those in traction, need to have dependent skin surfaces assessed at least three times in a 24-hour period.

Gerontological

- A health concern that threatens the function of an older person is the risk for falls (Rasche, Mertens, Bröhl, et al., 2017). Concern increases when an older person enters a health care facility. Assess the patient for the risk for falls on admission and implement a protocol to prevent falls (Lewis et al., 2019) (see Chapter 14).

Care in the Community

- Have caregiver practise and demonstrate transfer skills to achieve success before taking patient home. Alternatively, have patient (if living alone) practise transfer skills in bed that will be used at home. Teach patient to transfer to a chair with arms for ease of rising and sitting. Home should be free of hazards (e.g., throw rugs, electric cords in walkways, slippery floors). If wheelchair is used as chair, access must be possible through all doorways, and space for transfer must be available in bedroom and bathroom (see Chapter 42).
- Aids that enhance transfer ability are shower stools, elevated commodes, handrails on tub, and nonskid shower surface. Medical supply stores provide excellent information and catalogues of such supplies.

PROCEDURAL GUIDELINE 11.1 *Wheelchair Transfer Techniques*

Transferring a patient from a bed to a wheelchair encompasses most of the same principles discussed in Skill 11.1. The following procedural guideline focuses on the safety precautions that need to be considered when a weight-bearing patient is using a wheelchair. This is common when hospitalized patients are taken by wheelchair to procedures. Several additional steps must be taken to maintain safety of a patient and for the nurse to prevent injury when transferring a patient from or to a wheelchair (Fairchild, O'Shea, & Washington, 2018). Check wheelchair locks, wheels, and footplates for proper functioning before use.

Delegation and Collaboration

The skill of transferring a patient to or from a wheelchair can be delegated to an unregulated care provider (UCP). The nurse directs the UCP by:

- Assessing and supervising when moving patients who are transferring for the first time after prolonged bed rest, extensive surgery, critical illness, or spinal cord trauma.
- Explaining the patient's mobility restrictions, changes in blood pressure, or sensory alterations that may affect safe transfer.

Equipment

- Transfer belt, nonskid shoes, wheelchair, transfer board

Procedural Steps

1. Perform hand hygiene.
2. Review medical record to assess patient's weight, height, and strength; cognition; level of pain; and balance during previous transfer. Or complete a full assessment (see Skill 11.1) to determine patient's ability to help with transfer.
3. Explain to patient the steps you will be taking to help in transfer.
4. **Transferring patient from a wheelchair to bed (patient is cooperative and weight bearing) using pivot technique:**
   a. Adjust the height of the bed to the level of the seat of the wheelchair.
   b. Position wheelchair at a 45-degree angle next to the bed midway between the head and foot of the bed, with the wheelchair facing toward the foot of the bed. Remove the armrest nearest the side of the bed.
   c. Lock the wheelchair. Locks are located above the rims of the wheels. Push handle forward to lock.
   d. Raise the footplates.
   e. Place a transfer belt on patient. Be sure that it completely circles patient's waist. Place the belt low and be sure that it is snug. Avoid placing the belt over any intravenous lines, incisions, or drainage tubes.
   f. Have patient place hands on armrests and stand by as you have them move to the front of the wheelchair.
   g. Stand slightly in front of patient to guard and protect the person throughout the transfer.
   h. Instruct patient to stand on a count of three as you place both hands (palms up) under transfer belt while bending your knees.
   i. Allow patient to stand a few seconds to ensure that they are not dizzy and has good balance. Pivot with patient as the person turns to face away from the side of the bed. Then have patient sit on the edge of the mattress.
   j. With patient sitting on the edge of the bed, place your arm nearest the head of the bed under their shoulder while supporting the head and neck. Place your other arm under patient's knees. Bend your knees and keep your back straight.
   k. Tell patient to help lift the legs when you begin to move. On a count of three, standing with a wide base of support, raise patient's legs as you pivot their body and lower the shoulders onto the bed. Remember to keep your back straight.
   l. Help patient return to a comfortable position in bed.
5. **Transferring patient from a wheelchair to bed (patient is non–weight bearing and unable to stand but is cooperative and has upper body strength) using transfer board:**
   a. Position patient in wheelchair at a 45-degree angle next to the bed midway between the head and foot of the bed, with the wheelchair facing toward the foot of the bed.
   b. Remove the armrest nearest the side of the bed.
   c. Lock the wheelchair. Locks are located above the rims of the wheels. Push handle forward to lock.
   d. Raise the footplates.
   e. If not already applied, place a transfer belt on patient. Be sure that it completely circles patient's waist. Place the belt low and be sure that it is snug. Avoid placing the belt over any intravenous lines, incisions, or drainage tubes.
   f. If possible, have the seat of the wheelchair level with the top of the bed mattress. Position a transfer board by placing it across the bed to the chair so the patient can slide across it. Be sure the board overlaps the chair and mattress so that it will not slip out of place.
   g. Stand in front of patient and have the person move to the front of the wheelchair.
   h. Place your legs on the outside of the patient's legs. Be sure that patient's feet are on the floor. Grasp the transfer belt (palms up) along both of patient's sides. Have patient place one hand on the slide board and the other on the mattress surface.
   i. Bend your knees and on a count of three have patient use the arms to slide across the board from the chair to the bed. If patient is struggling to move across the board, try to have them lean the head and shoulders in the opposite way they want the hips to move.
   j. Have patient sit on edge of bed.
   k. Follow Steps 4 j–l when helping patient to comfortable position in bed.
6. Perform hand hygiene.
7. Monitor vital signs after patient has been transferred. Ask if patient feels dizzy or fatigued.
8. Note patient's behavioural response to transfer.
9. **Use Teach-Back:** "I want to be sure I explained what to do as I move you from the chair to the bed. Tell me how you can help move to the bed." Develop a revised teaching plan if patient is not able to teach back correctly.
10. Document patient's ability to tolerate transfer.

✦ SKILL 11.2   Moving and Positioning Patients in Bed

NSO *Nursing Skills Online Safety Module 4 / Lesson 3* ▶ *Video Clip*

Correctly positioning patients in bed is crucial for maintaining their body alignment and comfort; preventing injury to their musculoskeletal and integumentary systems; and providing sensory, motor, and cognitive stimulation. A patient with impaired mobility, decreased sensation, impaired circulation, or lack of voluntary muscle control can suffer damage to the musculoskeletal and integumentary systems while lying down. Proper positioning with correct body alignment minimizes these risks. The term *body alignment* refers to the condition of the joints, tendons, ligaments, and muscles in various body positions. When the body is aligned, whether standing, sitting, or lying, no excessive strain is placed on these structures. Caregivers are at risk for injury during positioning of patients in bed. It is important to follow your employer's safe-handling algorithms and use appropriate repositioning devices.

Delegation and Collaboration

The skills of moving and positioning patients in bed and maintaining correct body alignment can be delegated to an unregulated care provider (UCP). The nurse directs the UCP by:

- Explaining about any moving and positioning restrictions (e.g., avoid prone position, patient has one-sided weakness) and type of safe patient-handling devices needed.
- Designating specific times throughout the shift that the UCP must reposition the patient.
- Providing information regarding patient's individual needs for body alignment (e.g., patient with spinal cord injury), ability to help, and number of other caregivers needed to help.

Equipment

- Pillows, drawsheet
- Appropriate safe patient-handling assistive device (e.g., friction-reducing device, ceiling lift, or mechanical floor lift)
- Therapeutic boots/splints (*optional*)
- Trochanter roll
- Sandbag
- Hand rolls
- Clean gloves

STEP	RATIONALE

ASSESSMENT

1. Identify patient using at least two person-specific identifiers (e.g., name and date of birth or name and medical record number, according to the employer policy).

Ensures correct patient. Complies with Accreditation Canada's standards and improves patient safety (Accreditation Canada, 2019).

2. Perform hand hygiene.

Prevents transmission of microorganisms.

3. Assess patient's range of motion (ROM) (see Chapters 8 and 12) and current body alignment while patient is lying down.

Provides baseline data for later comparisons. Determines ways to improve position and alignment.

4. Assess for risk factors that contribute to complications of immobility:

Increased risk factors require patient to be repositioned more frequently.

   a. *Reduced sensation:* Cerebrovascular accident (CVA), spinal cord injury, or neuropathy

With reduced sensation, patient has difficulty moving and poor awareness of involved body part. Patient is unable to position body part and protect it from pressure.

   b. *Impaired mobility:* Traction, arthritis, CVA, spinal cord injury, hip fracture, joint surgery, or other contributing disease processes

Traction, bone fractures, surgery, or arthritic changes of affected extremity result in decreased ROM. Loss of function caused by CVA or spinal injury can lead to contractures.

   c. *Impaired circulation:* Arterial insufficiency

Decreased circulation predisposes patient to pressure injury.

   d. *Age:* Very young child, older person

Premature and young infants require frequent turning because their skin is fragile. Normal physiological changes associated with aging predispose older persons to greater risks for developing complications of immobility.

5. Assess patient's level of consciousness.

Determines need for special aids or devices. Patients with altered levels of consciousness may not understand instructions and may be unable to help with positioning.

6. Assess patient for presence of pain; rate using appropriate pain rating scale.

Pain reduces patient's motivation and ability to be mobile. Pain relief before transfer enhances patient participation (Horgas, 2017).

7. Assess condition of patient's skin, especially over bony prominences.

Provides baseline to determine effects of positioning.

8. Refer to patient's electronic health record (EHR) or chart for most recent recorded weight and height.

Factors needed to determine if mechanical lift, mechanical transfer device, or friction-reducing device is needed for moving patient up in bed.

9. Assess patient's physical ability to help with moving and positioning, which may be affected by age, level of consciousness, disease process, strength, ROM, and coordination.

Enables you to use patient's mobility, strength, and coordination during positioning. Determines need for additional help. Ensures patient and nurse safety.

STEP	RATIONALE

ASSESSMENT

10. Assess for sensory loss (vision and hearing) (see Chapter 8).

Deficits affect patient's ability to cooperate during repositioning procedures.

11. Apply clean gloves (as needed) to assess for presence of incisions, drainage tubes, and equipment (e.g., traction). Empty drainage bags before positioning. Remove and dispose of gloves. Perform hand hygiene.

Alters positioning procedure and type of position in which to place patient. Eliminates barriers to moving patient.

12. Assess motivation of patient and ability of caregivers to participate in moving and positioning if patient is to be discharged home.

Indicates whether instruction is necessary before discharge.

13. Check health care provider's prescriptions before positioning patient.

Some positions may be contraindicated in certain situations (e.g., spinal cord injury; hip fracture; respiratory difficulties; certain neurological conditions; presence of incisions, drains, or tubing).

NURSING DIAGNOSES

- Acute confusion
- Reduced physical mobility
- Reduced stamina
- Reduced skin integrity
- Potential for impaired skin integrity

Related factors/Risk factors are individualized on the basis of patient's condition or needs.

PLANNING

1. Expected outcomes following completion of procedure:
   - Patient retains ROM.

   Correct positioning allows patient to achieve optimal joint mobility and alignment.

   - Patient's skin shows no evidence of breakdown.

   Frequent position changes decrease occurrence of skin breakdown.

   - Patient's comfort level increases.

   Proper positioning reduces stress on joints.

   - Patient's level of independence in completing activities of daily living (ADLs) increases.

   Maintaining good body alignment and joint mobility increases patient's overall mobility. Patient with inadequate joint mobility may need help to carry out ADLs.

2. If patient perceives level of pain to be enough to avoid movement, offer an analgesic 30 minutes (if prescribed) before repositioning.

Will lessen discomfort when positioning extremities. **NOTE:** The frequency of an analgesic may not be available as frequently as a patient will require turning.

3. Remove all pillows and devices used in previous position.

Reduces interference from bedding during positioning procedure.

4. Get additional caregivers and/or necessary lift or transfer device to perform positioning.

Safe-handling algorithms (see employer policy) determine number of caregivers and type of devices needed to position a patient if lifting is required.

5. Explain positioning procedure to patient using plain language.

Helps to decrease anxiety and increase cooperation.

IMPLEMENTATION

1. Perform hand hygiene.

Reduces transmission of microorganisms.

2. Close door to room or bedside curtains.

Provides for patient privacy.

3. Raise level of bed to comfortable working height, level with your elbows.

Raises level of work toward nurse's centre of gravity and reduces risk for back injuries.

4. **Assist patient to move up in bed:**

This is not a one-person task unless patient can help completely. Pulling patients who have migrated in bed carries an extremely high risk of caregiver injury (OSHA, 2014).

   a. Determine if the patient can assist.

   Determines degree of risk in repositioning patient and technique required to safely help patient.

   (1) Patient is fully able to assist:
       (a) Stand at bedside to help with positioning of tubing and equipment as patient moves.

   Promotes patient independence.

STEP	RATIONALE

IMPLEMENTATION

(b) Have patient place feet flat on mattress, grasp either side rails or overhead trapeze and, on a count of three, lift hips up and push legs so body moves up in bed.

(2) Patient is partially able to assist:

(a) Encourage patient to help using friction-reducing device (e.g., slide board).

Repositioning device reduces friction as patient is moved up in bed.

(b) Patient weighs <90.7 kg (<200 lb): Use friction-reducing sheet or slide board and two or three caregivers.

(c) Patient weighs >90.7 kg (>200 lb): Use friction-reducing device and at least three caregivers.

i. *Using a friction-reducing device (three nurses):* Position patient supine with head of bed flat. A nurse stands on each side of bed.

Prevents friction from contact of skin with board.

ii. Remove pillow from under head and shoulders and place it at head of bed.

iii. Turn patient side to side to place friction-reducing device under drawsheet on bed, with device extending from shoulders to thighs/ankles.

iv. Return patient to supine position.

v. Have two caregivers grasp drawsheet (one on each side of bed) firmly and have third nurse hold onto end of friction-reducing device.

Slide board remains stationary, provides slippery surface to reduce friction, and allows patient to move up in bed easily.

vi. Place feet apart with forward-backward stance. Flex knees and hips. On count of three, shift weight from front to back leg and move patient and drawsheet to desired position up in bed.

Positions patient smoothly without exerting shear against skin and without risk of injury to nurses.

(3) Patient unable to assist:

(a) Use appropriate number of caregivers and appropriate safe-handling devices (e.g., supine sling with ceiling lift or floor-based lift and two or more caregivers).

Repositioning patients manually is associated with high risk of musculoskeletal injury (OSHA, 2014).

Clinical Decision Point *Protect patient's heels from shearing force by having another caregiver lift heels while moving patient up in bed.*

5. Position patient in bed in one of the following positions. Ensure correct body alignment. Protect pressure areas.

Prevents injury to patient's musculoskeletal system and integument.

Even positioning patient side to side requires use of safe-handling techniques.

a. Determine if patient can assist.

Determines degree of risk in repositioning patient and the technique required to safely help patient.

b. Begin with patient lying supine and move up in bed following Steps 4a (1)–(3).

c. Position patient in supported semi-Fowler's (see illustration) or Fowler's position:

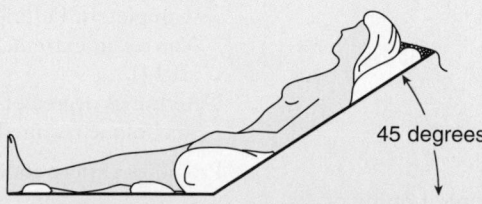

45 degrees

STEP 5c Supported semi-Fowler's position.

STEP	RATIONALE

IMPLEMENTATION

(1) With patient lying supine, elevate head of bed 45 to 60 degrees if not contraindicated.

Increases comfort, improves ventilation, and increases patient's opportunity to socialize or relax.

(2) Rest head against mattress or on small pillow.

Prevents flexion contractures of cervical vertebrae.

(3) Use pillows to support arms and hands if patient does not have voluntary control or use of hands and arms.

Prevents shoulder dislocation from effect of downward pull of unsupported arms, promotes circulation by preventing venous pooling, and prevents flexion contractures of arms and wrists.

(4) Position small pillow at lower back.

Supports lumbar vertebrae and decreases flexion of vertebrae.

(5) Place small pillow or roll under thigh.

Prevents hyperextension of knee and occlusion of popliteal artery from pressure from body weight.

(6) Support calves with pillows.

Heels should not be in contact with bed to prevent prolonged pressure of mattress on heels. This is sometimes referred to as *floating* heels.

d. Position hemiplegic patient in supported semi-Fowler's or Fowler's position:

(1) Elevate head of bed 45 to 60 degrees.

Increases comfort, improves ventilation, and increases patient's opportunity to relax. Adjust head of bed according to patient's condition. For example, those with increased risk for pressure injury remain at 30-degree angle (see Chapter 39).

(2) Position patient in Fowler's position as anatomically straight as possible.

Counteracts tendency to slump toward affected side. Improves ventilation and cardiac output; decreases intracranial pressure. Improves patient's ability to swallow and helps prevent aspiration of food, liquids, and gastric secretions.

(3) Position head on small pillow with chin slightly forward. If patient is totally unable to control head movement, avoid hyperextension of neck.

Prevents hyperextension of neck. Too many pillows under head may cause or worsen neck flexion contracture.

(4) Provide support for involved arm and hand by placing arm away from patient's side and supporting elbow with pillow.

Paralyzed muscles do not automatically resist pull of gravity as they do normally. As a result, shoulder subluxation, pain, and edema may occur.

(5) Place rolled blanket (trochanter roll) firmly alongside patient's legs.

Ensures proper alignment. Prevents external rotation of hips, which contributes to contractures.

(6) Support feet in dorsiflexion with therapeutic boots or splints.

Prevents plantar flexion contractures or footdrop by positioning patient's ankle in neutral dorsiflexion. Positions foot so heel is aligned in opening of splint to prevent pressure. Other therapeutic boots or splints are manufactured with thick padding to cushion heel and prevent pressure injury.

e. Position patient in supported supine position:

(1) Place patient supine with head of bed flat.

Necessary for properly aligning patient.

(2) Place small rolled towel under lumbar area of back.

Provides support for lumbar spine.

(3) Place pillow under upper shoulders, neck, and head.

Maintains correct alignment and prevents flexion contractures of cervical vertebrae.

(4) Place trochanter rolls or sandbags parallel to lateral surface of patient's thighs.

Reduces external rotation of hip.

(5) Place patient's feet in therapeutic boots or splints.

Maintains feet in dorsiflexion. Prevents plantar flexion contractures or footdrop.

(6) Place pillows under pronated forearms, keeping upper arms parallel to patient's body (see illustration).

Reduces internal rotation of shoulder and prevents extension of elbows. Maintains correct body alignment.

STEP	RATIONALE

IMPLEMENTATION

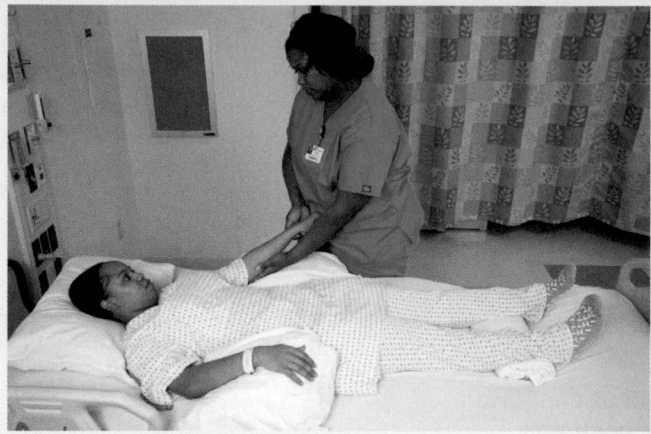

STEP 5e(6) Supported supine position with pillows in place.

(7) Place hand rolls in patient's hands. Consider physiotherapy collaboration for use of hand splints.	Reduces extension of fingers and abduction of thumb. Maintains thumb slightly adducted and in opposition to fingers.
f. Position hemiplegic patient in supine position:	
(1) Place head of bed flat.	Necessary for positioning in supine position.
(2) Place folded towel or small pillow under shoulder of affected side.	Decreases possibility of pain, joint contracture, and subluxation. Maintains mobility in muscles around shoulder to permit normal movement patterns.
(3) Keep affected arm away from body with elbow extended and palm up. Position affected hand in one of recommended positions for flaccid or spastic hand. (Alternative is to place arm out to side, with elbow bent and hand toward head of bed.)	Maintains mobility in arm, joints, and shoulder to permit normal movement patterns. (Alternative position counteracts limitation of ability of arm to rotate outward at shoulder [external rotation]. External rotation must be present to raise arm overhead without pain.)
(4) Place folded towel under hip of involved side.	Diminishes effect of spasticity in entire leg by controlling hip position.
(5) Flex affected knee 30 degrees by supporting it on pillow or folded blanket.	Slight flexion breaks up abnormal extension pattern of leg. Extensor spasticity is most severe when patient is supine.
(6) Support feet with soft pillows at right angle to leg.	Maintains foot in dorsiflexion and prevents footdrop. Pillows prevent stimulation to ball of foot by hard surface, which has tendency to increase muscle tone in patient with extensor spasticity of lower extremity.
g. Position patient in 30-degree lateral (side-lying) position (one nurse):	This position is recommended to prevent development of pressure injury by reducing direct contact of trochanter with support surface (see Chapter 39).
(1) Lower head of bed completely or as low as patient can tolerate.	Provides position of comfort for patient and removes pressure from bony prominences on back.
(2) Lower side rail and position patient on side of bed opposite direction toward which patient is to be turned. Move upper trunk, supporting shoulders first; then move lower trunk, supporting hips.	Provides room for patient to turn to side.
(3) Raise side rail and go to opposite side of bed.	
(4) Flex patient's knee that will not be next to mattress. Keep foot on mattress. Place one hand on patient's upper bent leg near hip and other hand on patient's shoulder.	Use of leverage makes turning to side easy.
(5) Roll patient onto side toward you.	Rolling decreases trauma to tissues. In addition, patient is positioned so leverage on hip makes turning easy.
(6) Place pillow under patient's head and neck.	Maintains alignment. Reduces lateral neck flexion. Decreases strain on sternocleidomastoid muscle.
(7) Place hands under patient's dependent shoulder and bring shoulder blade forward.	Prevents patient's weight from resting directly on shoulder joint.

STEP	RATIONALE

IMPLEMENTATION

(8) Position both arms in slightly flexed position. Support upper arm with pillow level with shoulder; other arm, by mattress.

Decreases internal rotation and adduction of shoulder. Supporting both arms in slightly flexed position protects joint. Ventilation improves because chest is able to expand more easily.

(9) Place hands under dependent hip and bring hip slightly forward so angle from hip to mattress is approximately 30 degrees.

The 30-degree lateral position reduces pressure on trochanter; designed to prevent pressure injury.

(10) Place small tuck-back pillow behind patient's back. (Make by folding pillow lengthwise. Smooth area is slightly tucked under patient's back.)

Provides support to maintain patient on side.

(11) Place pillow under semiflexed upper leg level at hip from groin to foot (see illustration).

Flexion prevents hyperextension of leg. Maintains leg in correct alignment. Prevents pressure on bony prominences.

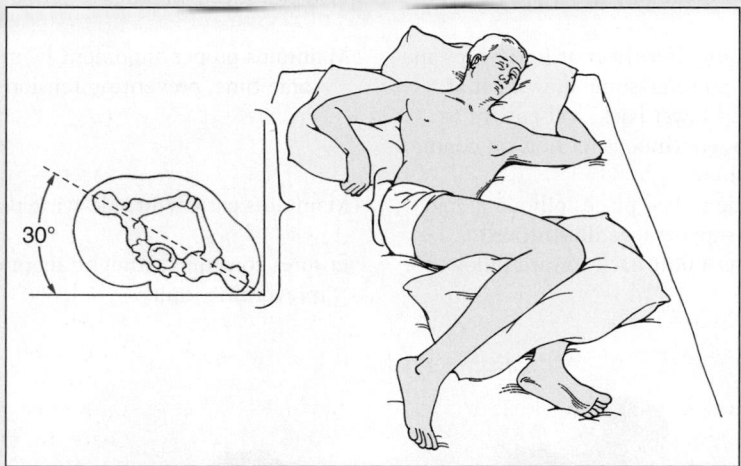

STEP 5g(11) Thirty-degree lateral position with pillows in place.

(12) Place sandbags parallel to plantar surface of dependent foot. May use ankle-foot orthotic on feet if available.

Maintains dorsiflexion of foot.

h. Position patient in Sims' (semiprone) position:

(1) Lower head of bed completely.

Provides for proper body alignment while patient is lying down.

(2) Place patient supine on side of bed opposite direction toward which they are to be turned. Move upper trunk, supporting shoulders first, followed by moving lower trunk, supporting hips.

Prepares patient for position.

(3) Move to other side of bed and turn patient on side. Position in lateral position, lying partially on abdomen, with dependent shoulder lifted out and arm placed at patient's side.

(4) Place small pillow under patient's head.

Maintains proper alignment and prevents lateral neck flexion.

(5) Place pillow under flexed upper arm, supporting arm level with shoulder.

Prevents internal rotation of shoulder. Maintains alignment.

(6) Place pillow under flexed upper legs, supporting leg level with hip.

Prevents internal rotation of hip and adduction of leg. Flexion prevents hyperextension of leg. Reduces mattress pressure on knees and ankles.

(7) Place sandbags parallel to plantar surface of foot (see illustration).

Maintains foot in dorsiflexion. Prevents plantar flexion contractures or footdrop.

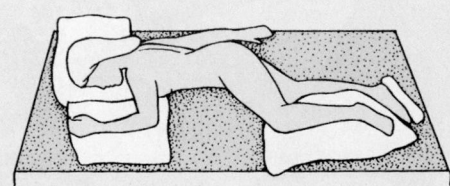

STEP 5h(7) Sandbag supporting right foot in dorsiflexion.

STEP	RATIONALE

IMPLEMENTATION

i. Logroll patient (three nurses):

Clinical Decision Point *A registered nurse can have the UCP assist when there is a health care provider's prescription to logroll a patient. Patients with a spinal cord injury or who are recovering from neck, back, or spinal surgery often need to keep the spinal column in straight alignment to prevent further injury.*

(1) Place small pillow between patient's knees.	Prevents tension on spinal column and adduction of hip.
(2) Cross patient's arms on chest.	Prevents injury to arms.
(3) Position two nurses on side toward which patient is to be turned and one nurse on side where pillows are to be placed (see illustration).	Distributes weight equally between nurses during turning.
(4) Fanfold drawsheet alongside of patient who will be turning.	Provides strong handles to grip drawsheet without slipping.
(5) With one nurse grasping drawsheet at lower hips and thighs and the other nurse grasping drawsheet at patient's shoulders and lower back, roll patient as one unit in a smooth, continuous motion on count of three (see illustration).	Maintains proper alignment by moving all body parts at the same time, preventing tension or twisting of spinal column.
(6) Nurse on opposite side of bed places pillows along length of patient for support (see illustration).	Maintains patient in side-lying position.
(7) Gently lean patient as a unit back toward pillows for support.	Ensures continued straight alignment of spinal column, preventing injury.

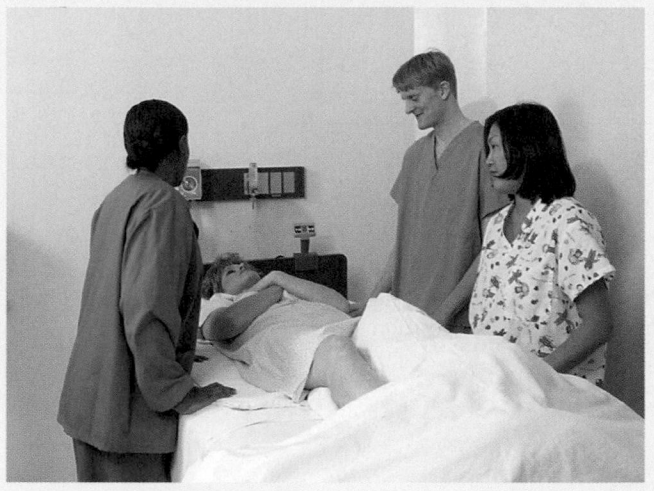

STEP 5i(3) Preparing patient for logrolling.

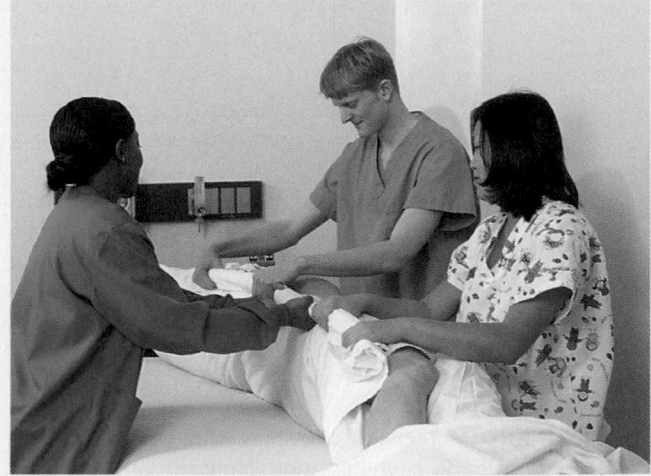

STEP 5i(5) Logrolling patient onto side.

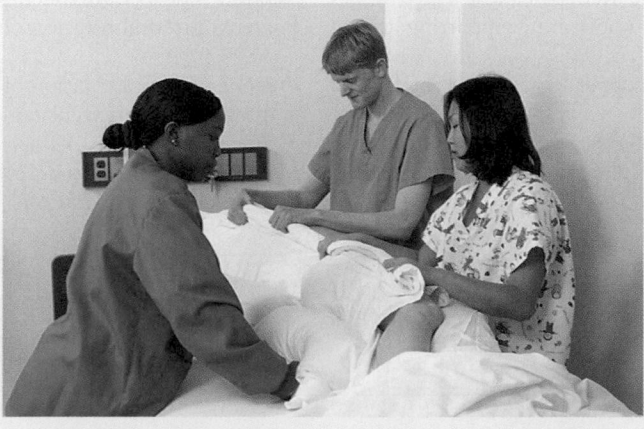

STEP 5i(6) Placing pillows along patient's back for support.

STEP	RATIONALE

IMPLEMENTATION

6. Perform hand hygiene.

Reduces transmission of microorganisms.

EVALUATION

1. Assess patient's body alignment, position, and level of comfort. Patient's body should be supported by adequate mattress, and vertebral column should be without observable curves.

Determines effectiveness of positioning. Additional supports (e.g., pillows, bath blankets) may be added or removed to promote comfort and correct body alignment.

2. Measure ROM.

Determines if joint contracture is developing.

3. Observe for areas of erythema or breakdown involving skin (see Chapter 39).

Provides ongoing observation regarding patient's skin and musculoskeletal systems. Indicates complications of immobility or improper positioning of body part.

4. Use Teach-Back: "I want to be sure I explained the steps we are going to use to move and position you in bed. Can you repeat the steps you can follow to help us move you up in bed?" Develop a revised teaching plan if patient or caregiver is not able to teach back correctly.

Determines patient's and caregiver's level of understanding of instructional topic.

Unexpected Outcomes

1. Joint contractures develop or worsen.

2. Skin shows localized areas of erythema and breakdown.

3. Patient avoids moving.

Related Interventions

- Increase frequency of ROM exercises to affected and immobilized areas (see Chapter 12).
- Consider physiotherapy consultation for different positioning.
- Increase frequency of repositioning.
- Place turning schedule above patient's bed.
- Medicate with analgesia as prescribed by health care provider to ensure patient's comfort before moving.
- Allow pain medication to take effect before repositioning.

Communication and Documentation

- Document time and position change of patient throughout shift, observations (e.g., condition of skin, joint movement, patient's ability to help with positioning), and whether positioning devices are needed, in nurses' notes in electronic health record (EHR) or chart.
- Document your evaluation of patient and caregiver learning.
- Communicate observations at change of shift and document in nurses' notes in EHR or chart.

Special Considerations
Teaching

- Teach caregiver how to position patient, especially when caring for infant, young child, or confused or unconscious patient.

- Teach patient ways to help with positioning and provide opportunity for return demonstration.
- Teach patient and caregiver signs and symptoms of pressure injury and contractures.

Gerontological

- Reposition older persons at least every 1 to 2 hours and maintain a regular program of ROM exercises (Harridge & Lazarus, 2017).

◆ CLINICAL DEBRIEF

A 37-year-old man who may have suffered a spinal cord injury in a motor vehicle accident is admitted to the health care institution. He has sustained multiple deep lacerations on his face and trunk and facial fractures of the maxillary and zygomatic bones. He has a cervical collar in place. He rates his pain at 9 on a scale of 0 to 10 (with 0 = no pain and 10 = worst pain ever). He weighs approximately 88 kg (193.6 lbs). You are preparing to transfer him to a stretcher. The emergency department nurse was extremely busy and was unable to provide a complete report.

1. Which other information would you obtain about this patient before safely transferring him to a stretcher?
2. The unregulated care provider (UCP) states that the patient wants to be turned and that he will be glad to reposition him without help. The health care provider's prescription is for logrolling until the computed tomography (CT) scan is completed and injury to the neck and spine is ruled out. What is the appropriate, safe action in response to turning the patient? Explain your answer.
3. The patient's pain continues to be at a level of 7 after receiving pain medication, his heart rate is 118 beats/min compared to a baseline of 82. The patient states, "I can't take this pain anymore." He refuses to go to radiology for his procedure. Write an SBAR for communicating this situation.

◆ REVIEW QUESTIONS

1. A patient is to sit up in a chair for breakfast 1 day after abdominal surgery per the health care provider's prescriptions. Which of the following would you select to ensure a safe transfer while facilitating cooperation from the patient? *(Select all that apply.)*
   1. Offer pain medication 30 minutes before transferring patient.
   2. Assess presence of weakness, dizziness, and muscle strength.
   3. Determine need for safe patient-handling device.
   4. Tell the unregulated care provider (UCP) to transfer patient to the chair.
   5. Follow prescription to transfer patient even though patient is refusing.
2. Place the following in correct sequence that facilitates safe transfer from a wheelchair to bed.
   1. Position wheelchair at a 45-degree angle next to bed.
   2. Stand by as you have patient move to front of wheelchair.
   3. Raise footplates and apply transfer belt.
   4. Lock wheelchair.
   5. Position self slightly in front of patient.
   6. Have patient stand as you place both hands under transfer belt and pivot to side of bed.
   7. Adjust height of bed to level of wheelchair seat.
3. Place the following in correct sequence that reflects safe use of a mechanical/hydraulic lift to transfer patients from bed to chair.
   1. Release check valve slowly and lower patient into chair.
   2. Roll patient back toward you as second nurse pulls hammock (straps) through holes.
   3. Position chair near bed and allow adequate space to manoeuvre lift.

4. Attach hooks on strap to holes in sling.
5. Roll patient onto side toward second nurse and position sling under patient.
6. Use lift to raise patient off bed and steering handle to pull lift from bed and manoeuvre to chair.
7. Place horseshoe base of floor lift under patient's bed and lower horizontal bar to sling level.
8. Roll patient supine onto canvas seat.

ⓔ *Visit the Evolve site for a complete list of Clinical Debrief and Review Questions answers.*

REFERENCES

Accreditation Canada. (2019). *Required organizational practices handbook—Version 14.* Retrieved from http://www.wrha.mb.ca/quality/files/2019ROPHandbook.pdf

Association of Workers' Compensation Boards of Canada. (2016). *Canadian workers' compensation system—2016 year at a glance.* Retrieved from http://awcbc.org/?page_id=11803

Canadian Centre for Occupational Health and Safety (CCOHS). (2018a). *Ergonomic safe patient handling program.* Retrieved from http://www.ccohs.ca/oshanswers/hsprograms/patient_handling.html

Canadian Centre for Occupational Health and Safety (CCOHS). (2018b). *Patient lifts and worker risks.* Retrieved from http://www.ccohs.ca/newsletters/hsreport/issues/2012/08/ezine.html

Fairchild, S. L., O'Shea, R. K., & Washington, R. (2018). *Pierson and Fairchild's principles & techniques of patient care* (6th ed.). St. Louis: Saunders.

Government of Canada. (2015). *Hospital bed safety.* Ottawa: Author. Retrieved from https://www.canada.ca/en/health-canada/services/drugs-medical-devices/hospital-bed-safety.html

Harridge, S., & Lazarus, N. (2017). Physical activity, aging and physiological function. *Physiology, 32,* 152–161. doi:10.115/physiol.00029.2016

Hockenberry, M. J., & Wilson, D. (2015). *Wong's nursing care of infants and children* (10th ed.). St. Louis: Mosby.

Horgas, A. (2017). Pain management in older adults. *Nursing Clinics, 52*(4), e1–e7. doi:10.1016/j.cnur.2017.08.001

Huether, S. E., & McCance, K. L. (2016). *Understanding pathophysiology* (6th ed.). St. Louis: Mosby.

Lewis, S. L., Bucher, L., Heitkemper, M., et al. (2019). *Medical-surgical nursing in Canada: Assessment and management of clinical problems* (4th Cdn. ed.). Toronto, ON: Elsevier Canada.

Myszenski, A. (2017). The essential role of lab values and vital signs in clinical decision making and patient safety for the acutely ill patient. *PhysicalTherapy.com.* Retrieved from https://www.physicaltherapy.com/articles/essential-role-lab-values-and-3637

Occupational Health Clinic for Ontario Workers Inc. (2018). *Patient handling for healthcare workers.* Retrieved from http://www.ohcow.on.ca/edit/files/general_handouts/Healthcare%20Workers%20Patient%20Handling.pdf

Occupational Safety & Health Association (OSHA). (2014). *Safe patient handling—Preventing musculoskeletal disorders in nursing homes,* OSHA Publication 3108. Retrieved from https://www.osha.gov/Publications/OSHA3708.pdf

Rasche, P., Mertens, A., Bröhl, C., et al. (2017). The "Aachen fall prevention app"—A smartphone application app for the self-assessment of elderly patients at risk for ground level falls. *Patient Safety in Surgery, 11,* 14. doi:10.1186/s13037-017-0130-4

Shieh, C., Weaver, M. T., Hanna, K. M., Newsome, K., & Mogos, M. (2015). Association of self-efficacy and self-regulation with nutrition and exercise behaviors in a community sample of adults. *Journal of Community Health Nursing, 32*(4), 199–211. doi:10.1080/07370016.2015.1087262

WorkSafe NB. (2015). *Transfer belts.* St. John, NB: Author. Retrieved from http://www.worksafenb.ca/docs/Transferdist.pdf

12 | Exercise and Mobility

Written by **Patricia A. Potter, RN, MSN, PhD, FAAN, and Shawna Ryan, RN, COHN, MN**

SKILLS AND PROCEDURES

OBJECTIVES

Mastery of content in this chapter will enable the nurse to:
- Discuss implications for preventing deconditioning and deep vein thrombosis in patient care.
- Describe the evidence that supports early activity and exercise in patient care.
- Explain how to plan a safe exercise program for a patient.
- Discuss indications for performing range-of-motion exercises.
- Discuss risk factors related to the development of deep vein thrombosis.
- Identify complications that may develop in a patient wearing either elastic stockings or a sequential compression device.

- Identify significant assessment data to be noted before assisting with exercise and ambulation.
- Demonstrate assisting with ambulation, assisting with ambulation with the use of an assistive device, assisting with range-of-motion exercises, and applying elastic stockings and a sequential compression device.
- Develop teaching plans for safety in the home while using an ambulation aid, applying and monitoring effects of elastic stockings and sequential compression devices, and performing range-of-motion exercises.

MEDIA RESOURCES

- evolve http://evolve.elsevier.com/Canada/Perry/clinicalskills/
- Review Questions
- Case Studies

- ▶ Video Clips
- Audio Glossary
- Clinical Debrief and Review Questions Answers

PURPOSE

Regular physical activity and exercise contribute to patients' physical and emotional well-being, while positively impacting psychosocial health (Hogana, Catalino, Mata, et al., 2015; Stanhope, Lancaster, Jakubec, et al., 2017). Regular physical activity and exercise should apply in the care of patients in all settings. Functional decline (e.g., the loss of the ability to perform self-care or activities of daily living) may not only result from illness or adverse treatment effects but also can be the result of deconditioning. Deconditioning is associated with inactivity and can lead to generalized weakness and impaired aerobic capacity within a short period of time (Falvey, Mangione, & Stevens-Lapsley, 2015). Deconditioning results in numerous physical changes and is a particular risk for hospitalized patients who spend most of their time in bed, even when they are able to walk. Nurses can play an important role in increasing the overall activity of patients across the continuum of care to minimize the effects of deconditioning (Arnold, 2017). In addition to deconditioning, patients with limited mobility are at risk for developing thromboembolic disease and deep vein thrombosis (Box 12.1). The promotion of early exercise and mobility in health care settings and as a daily therapy for patients is basic to competent nursing practice.

STANDARDS OF CARE

- Accreditation Canada, 2019—*Required Organizational Practices Handbook—Version 14* (http://www.wrha.mb.ca/quality/files/2019ROPHandbook.pdf)
- Canadian Patient Safety Institute, 2017—*Venous Thromboembolism (VTE) Prevention* (http://www.patientsafetyinstitute.ca/en/toolsResources/VTE-Getting-Started-Components/Pages/default.aspx)

BOX 12.1

Risk Factors for Deep Vein Thrombosis

- Injury to a vein, often caused by:
  - Fractures
  - Severe muscle injury
  - Major surgery (e.g., involving the abdomen, pelvis, hip, or legs)
- Decreased blood flow, often caused by:
  - Confinement to bed (e.g., caused by a medical condition or after surgery)
  - Limited movement (e.g., a cast on a leg to help heal an injured bone)
  - Sitting for a long time, especially with crossed legs
  - Paralysis
- Increased estrogen, often caused by:
  - Birth control pills
  - Hormone replacement therapy, sometimes used after menopause
  - Pregnancy, for up to 6 weeks after giving birth
- Certain chronic medical illnesses such as:
  - Heart disease, lung disease, cancer and its treatment, inflammatory bowel disease (Crohn's disease or ulcerative colitis)
- Other factors include:
  - Previous DVT or PE
  - Family history of DVT or PE
  - Age (risk increases as age increases)
  - Obesity
  - A catheter located in a central vein
  - Inherited clotting factors

DVT, Deep vein thrombosis; *PE,* pulmonary embolism. From Canadian Patient Safety Institute (CPSI). (2017). *Venous thromboembolism prevention: Getting started kit.* Retrieved from http://www.patientsafetyinstitute.ca/en/toolsResources/VTE-Getting-Started-Components/Documents/Section%201%20Rationale%20for%20VTE%20Prophylaxis.pdf#search=dvt.

- Registered Nurses Association of Ontario (RNAO)—*Best Practice Guidelines* (http://rnao.ca/bpg):
  - *Person- and Family-Centred Care* (2015) (https://rnao.ca/bpg/guidelines/person-and-family-centred-care)
  - *Preventing Falls and Reducing Injury from Falls,* 4th edition (2017) (https://rnao.ca/bpg/guidelines/prevention-falls-and-fall-injuries)
  - *Strategies to Support Self-Management in Chronic Conditions: Collaboration with Clients* (2010) (https://rnao.ca/bpg/guidelines/strategies-support-selfmanagement-chronic-conditions-collaboration-clients)

PRINCIPLES FOR PRACTICE

- Older persons are at greater risk for a reduction of muscle mass, strength, and power and for developing orthostatic hypotension, decubitus ulcers, syncope, confusion, increased risk for fractures, and functional incontinence because of decreased mobility from bed rest (Arnold, 2017; Liu, Moore, Almaawiy, et al., 2018; Witard, McGlory, Hamilton, et al., 2016).
- Early mobility and activity reduce impairment in cardiovascular and metabolic functioning, risk for pulmonary complications and development of pressure injury, and elimination alterations (Arnold, 2017; Liu, et al., 2018; Saunders, 2015).
- Changes in a patient's mobility and activity can result from a variety of health problems (e.g., musculoskeletal, cardiovascular, and neurological) and therapeutic reasons (e.g., prescribed bed rest or reduced activity from sedation). Direct nursing measures help to maintain or restore optimal mobility and decrease the hazards associated with immobility.
- It is important to act aggressively and to implement early activity and mobility once patients are physiologically stable and able to respond to verbal stimulation (Arnold, 2017).
- When caring for patients with reduced mobility, consider that there may be profound psychosocial and developmental effects (Hogana et al., 2015). Across the lifespan, immobilization often leads to emotional, intellectual, sensory, and sociocultural alterations. For young and older persons, immobility may alter employment, family role functions, and social interactions. Such changes can lead to altered self-concept, lowered self-esteem, and depression.

PERSON-CENTRED CARE

The shift to person-centred care in nursing practice involves integrating the whole person as a partner in care (RNAO, 2015). In exercise and mobility, person-centred care is realized when the nurse:

- Empowers and promotes the patient's proactive and preferred level of engagement in their health (RNAO, 2015). It is important to assess each patient's expectations concerning activity and exercise and determine their perception of what is normal or acceptable.
- Assesses a patient's level of physical and emotional comfort as well as their basic safety needs before implementing activity or exercise therapies (RNAO, 2015, 2017). Patients with pain, nausea, or fatigue have little motivation to engage in physical activity. Patients who are anxious or afraid of injury often resist participation.
- Is sensitive to the nonmedical aspects of care (culture, beliefs, values, and spirituality) (RNAO, 2015). When assisting with exercises or ambulation, the nurse must recognize that these activities may place patients in compromising positions. Provide privacy (e.g., clothing, blanket, close curtains) to preserve the patient's modesty and enhance participation.

EVIDENCE-INFORMED PRACTICE

- It is estimated that more than half of all patients hospitalized are at increased risk for the development of venous thromboembolism (VTE). Current evidence supports early nonpharmacological interventions in addition to pharmacological prophylaxis to prevent VTE (Pai & Douketis, 2016; Zisberg, Shadmi, Gur-Yaish, et al., 2015):
  - Early ambulation
  - Mechanical methods of VTE prevention (e.g., intermittent pneumatic compression, graduated compression stockings, venous foot pump)
  - Continuation of prophylaxis until the patient is ambulatory or discharged
  - Pharmacological prophylaxis for patients at low risk for bleeding who have at least one risk factor for the development of VTE (e.g., prolonged immobility ≥3 days, age ≥60 years of age, previous VTE)
  - A formal program in health care agencies for VTE prevention
- Immobility and the resultant deconditioning of hospitalized patients have led to greater efforts within hospitals to adopt evidence-informed early progressive mobility protocols.
  - Zisberg et al. (2015) studied 684 patients (age 70 and older) admitted to a hospital with a nondisabling condition. Functional decline at discharge was reported by 282 participants (41.2%), and 317 (46.3%) participants reported functional decline at 1 month after discharge. In-hospital low mobility

accounted for immediate and 1-month posthospitalization functional decline (Zisberg et al., 2015). Decreased mobility in hospital is a modifiable risk factor for which exercise programs can be targeted.

- In a systematic review of the literature it was found that safe and effective interventions that support early mobilization and physiotherapy can have a significant impact on functional outcomes in the critical care setting (Cameron, Ball, Cepinskas, at al., 2015; Hashem, Nelliot, & Needham, 2016). In critical care units and immediate post-acute environments, the mobilization of critically ill but stable patients who have required a period of mechanical ventilation can be done safely with minimal risk to patients.

- In a systematic review examining the effects of early mobility protocols on postoperative thoracic and abdominal surgery patients, the researchers concluded that the outcomes achieved are unclear (Castelino, Fiore, Nicolseanu, et al., 2016). Important questions that need to be studied include the following: At what frequency and intensity should patients mobilize after surgery? What mobilization targets should be used? And do patients treated with an early mobilization protocol have better postoperative outcomes than those of patients who mobilize at will? More research is needed in this area, but early mobilization is becoming a more common practice.

- Across the continuum of care, physical activity and exercise are integral aspects for older populations and those with chronic and neuromuscular diseases (i.e., multiple sclerosis [MS], Parkinson's disease, diabetes mellitus) who are negatively affected by immobility. Whether patients are hospitalized or situated in the community, the integration of physical activity and exercise can promote health and prevent risks such as falls.

- Davis, Bryan, Best, et al. (2015) found that mobility is a predictor of health-related quality of life among older adults.

- The benefits of exercise are directly associated with enhanced quality of life, improved cognition, and independence while reducing fatigue, anger, and depression among people with MS (Multiple Sclerosis [MS] of Canada, 2019).

SAFETY GUIDELINES

- Obtain and become familiar with any type of assistive device to be used. Know how to properly prepare and use a device so you can teach patients or caregivers how to use it safely and correctly.

- Prior to any mobilization, prepare yourself, the patient, the environment, and equipment. Ensure that the patient's vital signs are stable, that pain is controlled, and that their energy level supports activity. Obtain assistance from other personnel as needed, ensure the environment is clear from clutter, use safe patient-handling devices, and have the patient wear flat, nonskid shoes or socks.

- Assess the patient's cognitive status for their ability to follow mobility instructions as well as their fear of falling. Ask patients about their fear of falling and whether they have fallen recently and identify ways to reduce falling risks.

- Use appropriate clinical guidelines (see employer protocols) for assessing level of mobility (Chapter 11) and advancing a patient's activity level. Interprofessional collaboration is required to ensure a coordinated, holistic approach to mobility decision making for the patient, with shared, complementary responsibilities among the health care team (MOVE Canada, 2015).

- Know a patient's home care plan. A patient may need to continue the exercise regimen or use an assistive device at home.

✦ **SKILL 12.1** **Promoting Early Activity and Exercise**

In 2017, Canada's Chief Public Health Officer's report highlighted the need to increase the ease with which Canadians access physical activity to improve health, fitness, and quality of life (Tam, 2017). Regular physical activity is strongly linked to improved physical and mental health and healthy development of Canadians of all ages, regardless of whether a chronic disease or disability is present (Statistics Canada, 2016; Tam, 2017). As a nurse, you may work in a variety of settings with the opportunity to engage patients in mobility and plan health promotion activities. It is crucial to educate patients and caregivers about the importance of regular physical activity and exercise and how these activities can be incorporated into daily routines.

In health care settings, health care staff have made a concerted effort to increase patients' activity and mobility levels as soon as possible, to prevent deconditioning and other complications of immobility. Early progressive mobility protocols are the standard of care for critical care patients as well as for those on general nursing units and across the continuum of care (see employer policy for protocols) (Arnold, 2017). However, the success and progression of these protocols require tailoring of early mobility to the individual's condition (Liu et al., 2018). While the positive impact of early mobilization is recognized, nurses often have difficulty routinely helping patients ambulate because of overall patient care demands and heavy workload, have lack of access to equipment, or are unfamiliar with transfer skills and training (see Chapter 11) (Bilodeau, Gallagher, & Tanguay, 2017). Some hospitals have designated special mobility teams or mobility assistants to engage patients in early ambulation and activity. Successful implementation of early progressive mobility protocols and improved patient outcomes are linked to interprofessional collaboration in which all members of the interprofessional team are involved in mobility decisions (Uzdanovich, Regan, & Monagle, 2015). This includes, but is not limited to, the nurse, respiratory therapist, physiotherapist, physician, pharmacist, and patient.

Delegation and Collaboration

The skill of promoting early activity and exercise for patients can be delegated to unregulated care providers (UCPs) trained in transfer and assisted ambulation skills. Across health care settings (e.g., hospitals, long-term care facilities, home and community settings), the nurse directs the UCP by:

- Explaining the level of progressive mobility that a patient has achieved.
- Explaining any restrictions in range-of-motion (ROM) exercises to perform (see Procedural Guideline 12.1).
- Explaining if there are any weight-bearing precautions or if the patient needs to use assist devices.
- Explaining criteria to use to stop assisted ambulation or sitting if the patient cannot tolerate activity.

Equipment

- Inpatient—Pulse oximeter, gait belt, patient-specific mobility tools and assistive devices (see Skill 12.2)
- Outpatient—Patient-specific mobility tools and assistive devices, dependent on type of exercise recommended (e.g., 2.2 kg [5-lb] weights, resistance bands)

STEP	RATIONALE

ASSESSMENT

1. Identify patient using at least two person-specific identifiers (e.g., name and date of birth or name and medical record number) according to employer policy.

Ensures correct patient. Complies with Accreditation Canada's standards and improves patient safety (Accreditation Canada, 2019).

2. Review patient's health record for:
   • Baseline mobility and functional history.
   • Mobility restrictions and weight-bearing status.
   • Medical history conditions that influence or contraindicate mobility/exercise (e.g., dysrhythmias, recent myocardial infarction, stroke, paralyzed extremity, neuromuscular disease, peripheral neuropathy, current pregnancy).
   • Health care provider's prescription for early mobility or exercise program.

Examples of conditions that may contraindicate or require adjustments to activity. Patients should have medical clearance to begin an activity/exercise program.

3. Assess patient's beliefs, values, and perceptions regarding current health status and confidence in being capable of performing exercise.

Perceived self-efficacy is a judgement of capability. The outcomes that people anticipate depend largely on their judgements of how well they will be able to perform in given situations (RNAO, 2010; Selzler, Rodgers, Berry, et al., 2016; Shieh, Weaver, Hanna, et al., 2015).

4. Gather baseline assessment of vital signs and oxygen saturation (if available).

Allows you to assess patient's ability to participate in activity/exercise and evaluate patient's response to activity/exercise.

5. Assess patient's pain level using an appropriate pain rating scale (see Chapter 16 for pain assessment resources).

Determines if there is need for an analgesic before mobilizing or ambulating patient. Allows you to counsel patient as to best time to try more strenuous exercise.

6. Complete a patient mobility assessment (see Chapter 11) within 24 hours from admission (MOVE Canada, 2015).

Allows you to minimize injury to self and patient, determine if it is safe to mobilize a patient independently, and if assistive devices are required.

7. Implement early progressive mobility protocol specific to the acuity of your patient (e.g., critical care).

Mobility protocols are established for acute care patients with specific protocols for critical care. Different mobility protocols and policies exist for various levels of care.

Clinical Decision Point *Terminate physical activity when (Interior Health Authority, 2015; Schmidt et al., 2016):*
• *Heart rate is greater than a 20% increase in resting value or less than 40 beats/min or greater than 130 beats/min.*
• *Oxygen saturation shows greater than 4% drop from baseline or less than 88–90%.*
• *Blood pressure: Systolic pressure is greater than 180 mm Hg or greater than 20% decrease in systolic/diastolic or orthostatic hypotension.*
• *Respirations are less than 5 breaths/min or greater than 40 breaths/min.*
   Terminate exercise if dizziness lasts 60 seconds or fainting or diaphoresis occurs; change in breathing pattern occurs with increase in accessory muscle use, extreme fatigue, or severe dyspnea with respiratory rate greater than baseline by >20/min (Myszenski, 2017; Sommers, Engelbert, Dettling-Ihnenfeldt, et al., 2015).

---

7. **Perform a multisystem assessment** (e.g., cardiac, respiratory, musculoskeletal, and neurological) and safety screening (Arnold, 2017; Delaney, 2017).

If high-risk clinical features are present, then consultation should take place with physician and team prior to mobilization. Allows you to assess patient's ability to participate in activity/exercise.

   Cardiac status: Assess patient's myocardial stability.
   • No evidence of active myocardial ischemia has occurred over last 24 hours.
   • No dysrhythmia requiring new antidysrhythmic drug has occurred over last 24 hours.
   • Heart rate is above 60 and below 120 beats per minute.
   • Stable blood pressure (systolic above 90 mm Hg or no change of >30 mm Hg).
   • No increase of any inotrope/vasopressors agents has occurred for last 2 hours.

Ensures cardiac stability. Exercise can initiate ischemic attack or worsen dysrhythmias (Hopkins, Mitchell, Thomsen, et al., 2016).

Change in inotrope/vasopressor dose could lead to adverse effects such as tachycardia, dysrhythmias, and blood pressure changes such as orthostatic hypotension (Burchum & Rosenthal, 2016).

STEP	RATIONALE

ASSESSMENT

Respiratory status: Assess oxygenation status; must be adequate on:
- FiO_2 ≤60%
- PEEP (on ventilator) <10 cm H_2O
- Respiratory rate <28 (Hopkins et al., 2016)
- Oxygen saturation ≥90% (Schmidt, Knecht, & MacIntyre, 2016)

Musculoskeletal: No unstable major fractures or large open wounds

Neurological status:
- Patient engages to voice of caregiver.
- Patient responds appropriately to verbal stimulation and commands.
- No evidence of spinal precautions, open lumbar drains, or uncontrolled seizures.

8. Assessment to facilitate transition and support of mobility/exercise in community
   a. Identify patient's activity/exercise history:
      - Which type of regular daily exercise do you perform at home?
      - Do you exercise or play a sport at least three times a week? How often in a week do you exercise and how would you describe the intensity of this exercise (i.e., breathless, sweating, increased heart rate)?
      - How long have you been exercising regularly?
   b. Ask patient to what extent they enjoy exercising and what their beliefs are about ability to exercise.
   c. Determine if patient has social support from peers, family, friends, or spouse.
   d. Determine if patient has access to facility or area to exercise. Is neighbourhood considered safe?
   e. Consider these factors in your assessment: patient's age, income level, time available to exercise, rural resident, overweight, being disabled.
   f. Have patient rate level of quality of life based on current activity level.

Rationale column:

Activity assessment criteria allow for early ambulation (Hopkins et al., 2016).

Healing of the unstable fractures and wounds can be compromised if mobilized too early or incorrectly (Lewis, Bucher, Heitkemper, et al., 2019).
Patient must be alert and responsive, able to follow directions.

Provides information on patient's motivation or willingness to exercise regularly.
Allows you to plan exercise that compliments and advances patient's activity level.

Factors positively associated with adult physical activity (Potter, Perry, Ross-Kerr, et al., 2019).
Factors positively associated with adult physical activity (Potter et al., 2019).
Absence of facility or sense of safety discourages activity/exercise.

Factors negatively associated with adult participation in activity (Potter et al., 2019).

Serves as baseline to measure long-term benefits of exercise.

NURSING DIAGNOSIS

- Acute pain
- Persistent pain
- Readiness for enhanced health management
- Reduced physical mobility
- Reduced stamina

Related factors are individualized on the basis of patient's condition or needs.

PLANNING

1. Expected outcomes following completion of procedure:
   - Inpatient: Patient will progress from sitting on edge of bed to sitting in chair 20 minutes three times a day (TID).
   - Inpatient: Patient will gradually increase ambulation distance during hospital stay.
   - Outpatient: Patient will identify and develop an exercise and activity program to perform.
   - Outpatient: Patient will demonstrate adherence to exercise/activity plan at home.
   - Patient will report a perceived improvement in overall mobility and quality of life (**NOTE:** Some employers may use a scale for measurement).

Rationale column:

Early mobility protocol is designed with progressive levels of exercise to promote improved patient function and cognition, reduce length of hospital stay and complications of illness and bed rest, and improve patients' perceived quality of life.
Relevant and appropriate exercise plan increases adherence.

STEP	RATIONALE

PLANNING

2. Inpatient: Consult with physiotherapy regarding role in protocol to provide planned active resistance exercise for patients. Consult physiotherapist on types of exercises suited for patient's mobility restrictions.

Progressive resistance exercise (PRE) is method of increasing ability of muscles to generate force.

3. All patients: Explain benefits and reasons for activity/exercise. Do so in a way that matches patient's beliefs and values regarding recovery or maintaining health.

Exercise self-efficacy is an important predictor of the adoption and maintenance of exercise behaviours. Self-efficacy is the belief and conviction that one can perform a given activity successfully (RNAO, 2010; Selzler et al., 2016; Shieh et al., 2015).

4. Inpatient: Explain precautions that will be taken to prevent falls during ambulation (gait belt, assisted walking, monitoring for dizziness).

Patients may have a fear of falling. Explanation may relieve anxiety.

5. Inpatient: As patient progresses to ambulating, try to schedule ambulation around patient's other activities.

Avoids overexertion of patient. Organizes nursing care activities.

IMPLEMENTATION

1. Early progressive mobility protocol (Interior Health Authority, 2015)

Each patient starts at a different level, depending on their medical status and ability to participate in mobility.

Stage 1: Patient unstable

• Initiate passive ROM exercises TID (see Procedural Guideline 12.1). Turn patient every 2 hours.

• Help patient to sitting position in bed (e.g., stretcher chair or elevating head of bed to 30 degrees) and maintain for 20 minutes TID, or as tolerated.

• Obtain a physiotherapy consultation if patient is alert to determine if strengthening exercises are indicated.

This level is designed for patients who are medically unstable to tolerate activity or have bed rest prescriptions because of a medical condition.

Stage 2: Patient stable

• Continue passive/active ROM exercises TID.

• Turn patient every 2 hours.

• Help patient to sitting position in bed and maintain for 20–30 minutes TID.

• Initiate sitting patient on edge of bed or lift patient to chair.

• Dependent with activities of daily living (ADLs).

• Obtain physiotherapy consultation for mobility/strengthening program (e.g., active resistance exercise).

Patient begins to progress, patient is starting to be able to sit independently on edge of bed or tolerate sitting up in a chair.

Principles of active resistance exercise: (1) to perform small number of repetitions until fatigue, (2) to allow sufficient rest between exercises for recovery, and (3) to increase resistance as ability to generate force increases. There is evidence that PRE improves function and strength and reduces pain, which can improve quality of life and ability to do everyday tasks (Larsson, Palstam, Löfgren, et al., 2015).

Stage 3: Patient stable

• Patient is able to do active ROM exercises TID.

• Patient is able to turn self every 2 hours and assist with ADLs.

• Help patient to sitting position in bed and maintain for 20 minutes TID; sitting on edge of bed unsupported (but supervised).

• Active transfer to chair with the patient sitting up in chair 20–30 minutes TID (use mechanical lift, as needed).

• Physiotherapy to continue with strengthening program as prescribed.

Patient progresses to transfer training, prewalking activities. Patient can still be in CCU during this phase or on nursing unit.

STEP	RATIONALE

IMPLEMENTATION

Stage 4: Patient stable
- Patient is able to do active ROM TID.
- Patient is able to turn self every 2 hours and assist with ADLs.
- Active transfer to chair with patient sitting up in chair 1–2 hours TID sitting on edge of bed unsupported (but supervised).
- Physiotherapy to continue with strengthening program.
- Initiate ambulation. Apply gait belt (if needed). Have patient ambulate (marching in place, walking in halls) (see Procedural Guideline 12.4 and Skill 12.2).

NOTE: Ambulation time and distance should increase daily during hospitalization.

Stage 5: Patient stable
- Patient is able to turn self.
- Patient is able to do active leg and arm exercises.
- Patient is active in ADLs.
- Sitting in chair at bedside minimum of 2 hours, or as tolerated TID.
- Continue to increase ambulation time and distance (5–10 metres) with aides or staff assistance and wheelchair follow as required.

Stage 6: Patient stable
- Same as stage 5 with patient able to progress in distance and frequency of walking with assistance as required.

2. Exercise and activity promotion
   a. Initiate an exercise program that contains any of the following components:
      - Warm-up (5–10 minutes)
      - Strengthening exercises
      - Endurance physiotherapy
      - Balance exercises
      - Flexibility exercises

   Consider consulting physiotherapy to help develop a complete exercise program that would fit the needs of your patient. A good overview of physical activity guidelines across the lifespan can be found at http://www.csep.ca/en/guidelines/links-to-csep-guidelines.

   b. Recommend strength training for adults.

   c. The Heart and Stroke Foundation of Canada (2018) recommends moderate to vigorous aerobic exercise at least 150 minutes per week in bouts of 10 minutes or more. This includes activities (e.g., climbing stairs; playing sports; or aerobic activities such as walking, jogging, swimming, or biking).

   d. Recommend balance exercises for older adults to decrease risk of falls. Have patient be sure to have something sturdy nearby on which to hold (wall or chair) if they become unsteady.
      - Perform exercises: standing on one foot, walking heel to toe, balance walking, back leg raises, side leg raises. Have patient do strength exercises (back leg raises, side leg raises) 2 or more days per week, but not on any 2 days in a row (National Institute on Aging, n.d.; RNAO, 2017).

RATIONALE

Patients can still be in CCU during this phase or out on general nursing unit. Progression of mobility (amount of help required and distance walked) should occur until hospital discharge.

Warm-up directs needed blood flow to muscles and prepares body for exercise. Warming up is important for preventing injury. Flexibility exercises help prevent tightness of muscles and improve joint ROM. Loss of ROM or muscle tightness can impede a person's function.
Cool-downs help body recover from exercises.

Strength training has been shown to improve strength and bone density and can be beneficial for older adults.
Designed to improve overall cardiovascular health.

Helps to improve person's balance while standing or sitting and may decrease risk of falls.

STEP	RATIONALE

IMPLEMENTATION

e. Recommend patient perform cool-down (5 to 10 minutes) after exercising: • Quadriceps stretch • Hamstring/calf stretch • Chest and arm stretch • Neck, upper back, and shoulder stretch	Exercises help muscles relax and become more flexible.

EVALUATION

1. Measure vital signs and oxygen saturation during activity/exercise and compare findings with baseline.	Determines patient's exercise tolerance.

Clinical Decision Point NOTE: *Each employer (or even each critical care unit [CCU]) may have different screening criteria based on the population that it commonly sees.*

2. Evaluate patient's pain severity using appropriate pain rating scale (e.g., on a scale of 0 to 10, 0 being no pain and 10 being worst pain ever) (see Chapter 16 for pain assessment resources).	Exercises can increase muscle discomfort.
3. Monitor number of steps or estimated distance during walking.	Provides objective measure of ambulation progression.
4. After patient has reached each stage of mobility protocol or after patient in the community has been exercising over 2 to 3 months, evaluate level of confidence in performing exercises.	Determines self-efficacy and likelihood of continued participation in exercise.
5. Use Teach-Back: "We've talked about doing a warm-up and cool-down as part of your exercise plan. Tell me why each is important." Develop a revised teaching plan if patient or caregiver is not able to teach back correctly.	Determines patient's and caregiver's level of understanding of instructional topic.

Unexpected Outcomes	Related Interventions
1. Patient has abnormal vital sign response or decrease in oxygen saturation requiring termination of exercise. (In community settings, be sure that patient or caregiver knows patient's normal pulse range and when to terminate exercise.)	• Return patient to chair or bed immediately using safe patient-handling principles. • Notify health care provider. • Continue to monitor vital signs until patient's condition stabilizes.
2. Patient develops chest pain or discomfort during exercise.	• Return patient to chair or bed immediately using safe patient-handling principles. • Notify health care provider. • Use interprofessional collaboration and prepare for possible electrocardiogram. • Continue to monitor vital signs until patient's condition stabilizes. • In community setting have caregiver call 9-1-1.

Communication and Documentation

- Document in the patient medical record or clinic record results of patient screening, type of exercise implemented, pre-exercise and post-exercise assessments, and patient's tolerance in nurses' notes in electronic health record (EHR) or chart.
- Document your evaluation of patient and caregiver learning.
- Report to health care provider any signs or symptoms indicative of exercise intolerance.

Special Considerations
Care in the Community

- Teach patient or caregiver how to measure carotid or radial pulse, what a normal range is for patient, how to monitor exercise tolerance, and when to notify health care provider about problems.
- Have patient or caregiver keep diary to record exercise activities, progression, and patient response.

PROCEDURAL GUIDELINE 12.1 *Performing Range-of-Motion Exercises*

Range of motion (ROM) refers to the distance or amount of freedom a joint can be moved in a certain direction (e.g., rotating, bending, or twisting). ROM exercises may be active, passive, or active assisted. They are active if a patient can move the limb against gravity, active assisted when a caregiver is needed to help the patient move the limb against gravity, and passive when the exercises are performed by a caregiver. Always encourage patients to be as active and independent as possible in every aspect of activities of daily living (ADLs). Incorporate active ROM exercises in a patient's ADLs (Table 12.1) and incorporate passive ROM into bathing and feeding activities. Collaborate with patients to develop schedules for ROM activities.

Delegation and Collaboration

The skill of performing ROM exercises can be delegated to a trained unregulated care provider (UCP). Patients with spinal cord injuries, burns, or orthopaedic trauma usually require ROM exercises by professional nurses or physiotherapists. The nurse directs the UCP to:

- Perform exercises slowly and provide adequate support to each joint being exercised.
- Not exercise joints beyond the point of resistance or to the point of fatigue or pain.
- Be aware of a patient's individual limitations or pre-existing conditions such as arthritis that affect ROM.

Equipment

- No mechanical or physical equipment needed
- Clean gloves (*optional*)

Procedural Steps

1. Identify patient using at least two person-specific identifiers (e.g., name and date of birth or name and medical record number) according to employer policy (Accreditation Canada, 2019).
2. Review patient's chart for physical assessment findings that could affect the performance of ROM exercises (e.g., pain in joint, skin integrity or presence of wound near joint, presence of deformity; level of consciousness and ability to attend); health care provider prescriptions (e.g., any ROM restrictions for medical reasons); medical diagnosis, medical history, and progress.
3. Obtain data on patient's baseline joint function. Observe for obvious limitations in joint mobility, redness, or warmth over joints; joint tenderness; deformities, or edema.
4. Determine patient's or caregiver's readiness to learn (e.g., desire to learn, perceived ability to perform exercise, perceived benefit of exercise). Explain in plain language reason for the ROM exercises and describe and demonstrate exercises to be performed.
5. Assess patient's level of comfort using an appropriate pain rating scale (see Chapter 16) before exercises. Determine if patient would benefit from pain medication before beginning ROM exercises; then administer analgesic 30 minutes before exercise.
6. Perform hand hygiene and apply clean gloves if wound drainage or skin lesions are present.
7. Help patient to a comfortable position, preferably sitting or lying down.

8. When performing passive ROM exercises (Table 12.2), support joint by holding distal part of extremity or using cupped hand to support joint (see illustration).
9. Complete exercises in head-to-toe sequence. Repeat each movement five times during exercise period. Inform patient how these exercises can be incorporated into ADLs (see Table 12.1).

TABLE 12.1

Incorporating Active Range-of-Motion Exercises Into Activities of Daily Living

Joint Exercised	Activity of Daily Living	Movement
Neck	Nodding head "yes"	Flexion
	Shaking head "no"	Rotation
	Moving right ear to right shoulder	Lateral flexion
	Moving left ear to left shoulder	Lateral flexion
Shoulder	Reaching to turn on overhead light	Flexion, extension
	Reaching to bedside stand for book	Hyperextension
	Rotating shoulders toward chest	Internal rotation
	Rotating shoulders toward back	External rotation
Elbow	Eating, bathing, shaving, grooming	Flexion, extension
Wrist	Eating, bathing, shaving, grooming	Flexion, extension, ulnar/radial deviation
Fingers and thumb	All activities requiring fine-motor coordination (e.g., writing, eating, painting)	Flexion, extension, abduction, adduction, opposition
Hip	Walking	Flexion, extension, hyperextension
	Moving to side-lying position	Flexion, extension, abduction
	Moving from side-lying position	Extension, adduction
	Rolling feet inward	Internal rotation
	Rolling feet outward	External rotation
Knee	Walking	Flexion, extension
	Moving to and from side-lying position	Flexion, extension
Ankle	Walking	Dorsiflexion, plantar flexion
	Moving toe toward head of bed	Dorsiflexion
	Moving toe toward foot of bed	Plantar flexion
Toes	Walking	Extension, hyperextension
	Wiggling toes	Abduction, adduction

Continued

PROCEDURAL GUIDELINE 12.1 *Performing Range-of-Motion Exercises—cont'd*

Clinical Decision Point *When resistance is noted within a joint, do not force joint motion. Consult with health care provider or physiotherapist.*

10. Observe patient performing ROM activities.
11. Remove gloves, if worn. Perform hand hygiene.
12. Measure joint motion as needed to determine level of improvement.
13. Evaluate patient during exercise by having them rate the severity of pain on a pain scale.

14. **Use Teach-Back:** "Let's review what I discussed about ways to practice ROM at home. Tell me some exercises you can do at home." Develop a revised teaching plan if patient or caregiver is not able to teach back correctly.
15. Document exercises performed and patient's tolerance in nurses' notes in electronic health record (EHR) or chart.

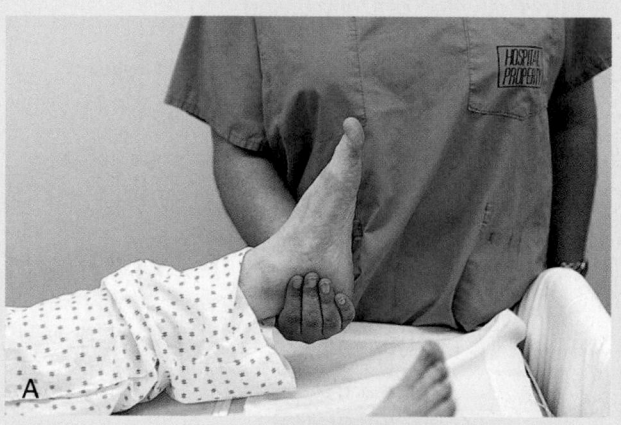
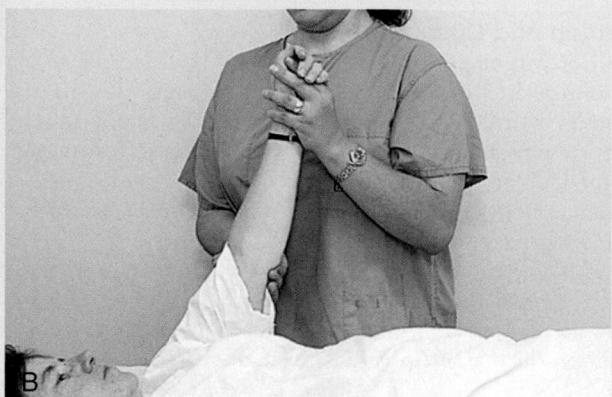
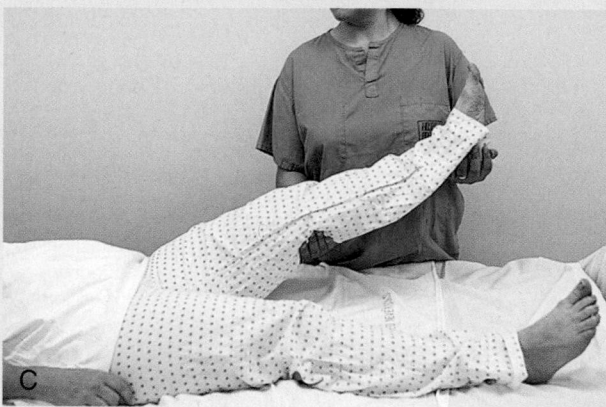

STEP 8 A, Support joint by holding distal and proximal areas adjacent to joint. **B,** Support joint by cradling distal part of extremity. **C,** Use cupped hand to support joint.

PROCEDURAL GUIDELINE 12.1 *Performing Range-of-Motion Exercises—cont'd*

TABLE 12.2

Range-of-Motion Exercises

Body Part	Type of Joint	Type of Movement	Range (Degrees)	Primary Muscles
Neck, cervical spine	Pivotal	Flexion: Bring chin to rest on chest.	45	Sternocleidomastoid
		Extension: Return head to erect position.	45	Trapezius
		Hyperextension: Bend head back as far as possible.	10	Trapezius
		Lateral flexion: Tilt head as far as possible toward each shoulder.	40–45	Scalenus
		Rotation: Turn head as far as possible in circular movement.	180	Sternocleidomastoid, upper trapezius
Shoulder	Ball and socket	Horizontal flexion: Swing arm horizontally forward.	130	Coracobrachialis, deltoid, pectoralis major
		Horizontal extension: Swing arm horizontally backward.	45	Latissimus dorsi, teres major, triceps brachii
		Abduction: Bring arm up sideways.	180	Supraspinatus, deltoid, trapezius, and serratus anterior
		Adduction: Bring arm toward midline of the body.	45	Pectoralis major, triceps, teres major
		Shoulder extension: Move arm behind body, keeping elbow straight.	0–60	Latissimus dorsi, teres major, deltoid
		Circumduction: Move arm in full circle (circumduction is combination of all movements of ball-and-socket joint).	360	Deltoid, coracobrachialis, latissimus dorsi, teres major
Elbow	Hinge	Flexion: Bend elbow so lower arm moves toward its shoulder joint and hand is level with shoulder.	150	Biceps brachii, brachialis, brachioradialis
		Extension: Straighten elbow by lowering hand.	150	Triceps brachii

Continued

PROCEDURAL GUIDELINE 12.1 *Performing Range-of-Motion Exercises—cont'd*

TABLE 12.2

Range-of-Motion Exercises—cont'd

Body Part	Type of Joint		Type of Movement	Range (Degrees)	Primary Muscles
Forearm	Pivotal		Supination: Turn lower arm and hand so palm is up.	70–90	Supinator, biceps brachii
			Pronation: Turn lower arm so palm is down.	70–90	Pronator teres, pronator quadratus
Wrist	Condyloid		Flexion: Move palm toward inner aspect of forearm.	80–90	Flexor carpi ulnaris, flexor carpi radialis
			Extension: Move fingers and hand posterior to midline.	70–80	Extensor carpi radialis brevis, extensor carpi radialis longus, extensor carpi ulnaris
			Hyperextension: Bring dorsal surface of hand back as far as possible.		Extensor carpi radialis brevis, extensor carpi radialis longus, extensor carpi ulnaris
			Radial deviation: Bend wrist medially toward thumb.	Up to 30	Flexor carpi radialis brevis, extensor carpi radialis brevis, extensor carpi radialis longus
			Ulnar deviation: Bend wrist laterally toward fifth finger.	30	Flexor carpi ulnaris, extensor carpi ulnaris
Fingers	Condyloid hinge		Flexion: Make fist.	90	Lumbricales, interosseus volaris, interosseus dorsalis
			Extension: Straighten fingers.	90	Extensor digiti quinti proprius, extensor digitorum communis, extensor indicis proprius
			Hyperextension: Bend fingers back as far as possible.	30–60	Extensor digitorum
			Abduction: Spread fingers apart.	30	Interosseus dorsalis
			Adduction: Bring fingers together.	30	Interosseus volaris

PROCEDURAL GUIDELINE 12.1 *Performing Range-of-Motion Exercises—cont'd*

TABLE 12.2

Range-of-Motion Exercises—cont'd

Body Part	Type of Joint	Type of Movement	Range (Degrees)	Primary Muscles
Thumb	Saddle	Flexion: Move thumb across palmar surface of hand.	90	Flexor pollicis brevis
		Extension: Move thumb straight away from hand.	90	Extensor pollicis longus, extensor pollicis brevis
		Abduction: Extend thumb laterally (usually done when placing fingers in abduction and adduction).	30	Abductor pollicis brevis and longus
		Adduction: Move thumb back toward hand.	30	Adductor pollicis obliquus, adductor pollicis transversus
		Opposition: Touch thumb to each finger of same hand.		Opponens pollicis, opponens digiti minimi
Hip	Ball and socket	Flexion: Move leg forward and up.	110–120	Psoas major, iliacus, sartorius
		Extension: Move leg back beside other leg.	90–120	Gluteus maximus, semitendinosus, semimembranosus
		Abduction: Move leg laterally away from body.	30–50	Gluteus medius, gluteus minimus
		Adduction: Move leg back toward midline position and beyond if possible.	20–30	Adductor longus, adductor brevis, adductor magnus
		Internal rotation: Turn foot and leg toward other leg.	45	Gluteus medius, gluteus minimus, tensor fasciae latae
		External rotation: Turn foot and leg away from other leg.	45	Obturatorius internus, obturatorius externus, quadratus femoris, piriformis, gemellus superior and inferior, gluteus maximus
		Circumduction: Move leg in circle.	120–130	Psoas major, gluteus maximum, gluteus medius, adductor magnus

Continued

PROCEDURAL GUIDELINE 12.1 *Performing Range-of-Motion Exercises—cont'd*

TABLE 12.2

Range-of-Motion Exercises—cont'd

Body Part	Type of Joint	Type of Movement	Range (Degrees)	Primary Muscles
Knee	Hinge	Flexion: Bring heel back toward back of thigh.	120–130	Biceps femoris, semitendinosus, semimembranosus, sartorius
		Extension: Return leg to floor.	120–130	Rectus femoris, vastus lateralis, vastus medialis, vastus intermedius
Ankle	Hinge	Dorsal flexion: Move foot so toes are pointed upward.	20–30	Tibialis anterior
		Plantar flexion: Move foot so toes are pointed downward.	45–50	Gastrocnemius, soleus
Foot	Gliding	Inversion: Turn sole of foot medially.	35 or less	Tibialis anterior, tibialis posterior
		Eversion: Turn sole of foot laterally.	10 or less	Peroneus longus, peroneus brevis
Toes	Condyloid	Flexion: Curl toes downward.	30–60	Flexor digitorum, lumbricalis pedis, flexor hallucis brevis
		Extension: Straighten toes.	30–60	Extensor digitorum longus, extensor digitorum brevis, extensor hallucis longus
		Abduction: Spread toes apart.	15 or less	Abductor hallucis, interosseus dorsalis
		Adduction: Bring toes together.	15 or less	Adductor hallucis, interosseus plantaris

PROCEDURAL GUIDELINE 12.2 *Monitoring a Patient on a Continuous Passive Motion Machine*

The continuous passive motion (CPM) machine is designed to exercise various joints such as the hip, ankle, knee, shoulder, and wrist. It is used most commonly after knee surgery. However, questions have been raised about CPM benefits (Viveen, Doornberg, Kodde, et al., 2017). A recent review of research involving knee arthroplasty surgery showed that CPM probably improves the ability of a patient to bend the knee slightly but may not ease pain or improve function (Gatewood, Tran, & Dragoo, 2017). It is usually prescribed from the first to fourth day following surgery, for 1.5 to 24 hours a day, depending on a surgeon's preference and patient's condition (Lewis et al., 2019). An initial setting is typically 20 to 30 degrees of flexion and full extension at two cycles per minute. The purpose of the CPM machine is to keep a joint mobilized to improve range of motion (ROM), reduce swelling, and ultimately prevent contractures and improve function. Although the value of the therapy is questioned, it continues to be used, and as a nurse you must be able to monitor patients safely on the device.

The electronically controlled CPM machine has Velcro straps to secure an extremity. When the device is turned on, the frame slides slowly back and forth, gently moving the joint through a preset ROM. The CPM machine can weigh up to 11.3 kg (25 lb). Using two caregivers to lift the machine reduces the risk for caregiver back strain and prevents risk of damage to a patient's extremity.

PROCEDURAL GUIDELINE 12.2 *Monitoring a Patient on a Continuous Passive Motion Machine—cont'd*

Delegation and Collaboration

The skill of applying the CPM machine cannot be delegated to an unregulated care provider (UCP). The nurse directs the UCP to:

- Immediately report to the nurse any increase in patient's pain when on CPM.
- To notify nurse of any skin breakdown observed when CPM is off.

Equipment

- CPM machine
- Padding
- Clean gloves

Procedural Steps

1. Review medical record and assess nature of patient's condition and ROM limits prescribed by health care provider. Be sure that prescription designates cycles per minute and time on machine.
2. Assess CPM machine for electrical safety. If you suspect a problem, notify the employer's electrical safety department.
3. Assess setup of machine before placing on bed: Check stability of frame, flexion/extension controls, padding of exposed metal parts or hard surfaces, and on/off switch.
4. Identify patient using at least two person-specific identifiers (e.g., name and date of birth or name and medical record number) according to employer policy (Accreditation Canada, 2019).
5. Perform hand hygiene.
6. Establish a baseline by assessing patient's pain using an appropriate pain rating before and during use.
7. Assess patient's heart rate, blood pressure, and respirations to establish baseline for exercise tolerance.
8. Assess patient's knowledge about CPM and ability and willingness to learn about the CPM machine.
9. Explain procedure and demonstrate CPM machine, turning machine on for patient to observe a cycle before placing on bed.
10. Help patient to comfortable supine position.

> **Clinical Decision Point** *Before placing patient in a CPM device, attend to their elimination needs and, if prescribed, provide an analgesic 30 minutes before a new treatment begins.*

11. Apply clean gloves if wound drainage is present.
12. Place elastic compression stockings on patient (if prescribed) to promote venous return (see Procedural Guideline 12.3).
13. Place CPM machine on bed. Set limits of flexion and extension as prescribed. Set speed control to slow or moderate range as prescribed; turn machine on for it to run one full cycle.
14. Stop CPM machine when in extension. Place padding on CPM machine.
15. Support patient's affected joint while placing extremity in CPM machine frame.
16. Adjust CPM machine to patient's extremity. Lengthen and shorten appropriate sections of frame while centring patient's extremity on it. Align patient's joint with mechanical joint of CPM.

17. Secure patient's extremity on CPM machine with Velcro straps (see illustration). Apply loosely.

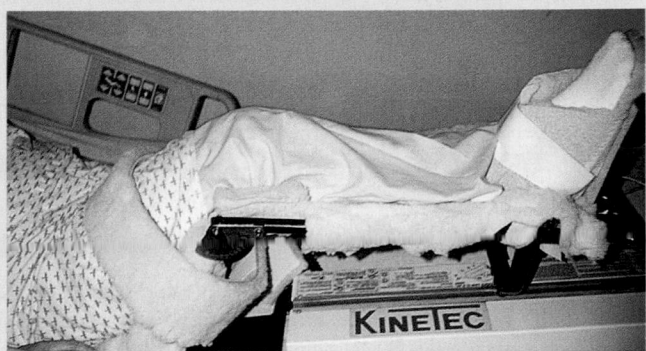

STEP 17 Patient's extremity properly placed and secured on CPM machine.

18. Press power switch to start machine. When it reaches flexed position, stop it and check degree of flexion. Then observe patient and affected extremity for two full cycles.
19. Ask if patient feels comfortable; evaluate pain severity on pain scale.
20. Be sure that CPM on/off power switch is within patient's reach. Instruct patient to turn CPM machine off if malfunctioning, or if patient is experiencing pain, to notify nurse immediately.
21. Discard gloves and perform hand hygiene.
22. **Use Teach-Back:** "I want to be sure you understand what the CPM machine is supposed to do for you. In your own words, tell me the purpose of the CPM machine." Develop a revised teaching plan if patient or caregiver is not able to teach back correctly.
23. Inspect bony prominences and areas of skin in contact with machine at least every 2 hours; look for skin breakdown using an appropriate risk assessment tool (e.g., Braden Scale or Norton Scale—see Chapter 39).
24. Check patient's alignment and positioning at least every 2 hours.
25. Continue to evaluate patient for presence of pain. If patient is on a continuous cycle, provide analgesic at next scheduled dose.
26. Observe patient and CPM machine with each increase in flexion and extension.
27. Record in the nurses' notes in electronic health record (EHR) or chart patient's tolerance for CPM machine, rate of cycles per minute, degree of flexion and extension used, condition of extremity and skin, condition of operative site if present, and length of time CPM machine is in use.
28. Report immediately to nurse in charge or health care provider any resistance to ROM; increased pain; or swelling, heat, or redness in joint.

PROCEDURAL GUIDELINE 12.3 *Applying Graduated Compression (Elastic) Stockings and Sequential Compression Device*

▶ *Video Clip*

The development of deep vein thrombosis (DVT) is a hazard of immobility. Common risk factors include conditions that influence the Virchow's triad: hypercoagulability (e.g., clotting disorders, fever, dehydration); venous wall abnormalities (e.g., orthopaedic surgery, varicose veins); and blood flow stasis (e.g., immobility, obesity, pregnancy) (Dunn & Ramos, 2017; Lewis et al., 2019). Signs of DVT include swelling in the affected leg (rarely swelling in both legs); warm, cyanotic skin; and pain in the leg that often starts in the calf and can feel like cramping or soreness. If a DVT is suspected, keep patient calm and quiet in bed and notify the health care provider.

If patients are at high risk for DVT, mechanical thrombo-prophylaxis (use of elastic stockings or intermittent sequential compression devices [SCDs]) is a recommended form of therapy (CPSI, 2017; Pai & Douketis, 2016), especially in surgical patients after surgery.

Anticoagulant medication is the best approach for preventing DVTs; however, early ambulation, adequate hydration, wearing compression stockings or intermittent SCDs, and using foot pumps are equally important (Gee, 2015; Pai & Douketis, 2016). All intermittent compression systems have a simple objective (i.e., to squeeze blood from the underlying deep veins, which, if the valves are competent, will be displaced proximally). On deflation of the cuff, the veins will refill and, because of the intermittent nature of the system, will ensure periodic flow of blood through the deep veins if there is a supply (Gee, 2015). Compression stockings appear to function more by preventing distension of veins. Reduction of edema and leg pain during the day is accomplished while wearing elastic stockings (Carvalho, Pinto, Godoy, et al., 2015). SCDs pump blood into deep veins, thus removing pooled blood and preventing venous stasis. A venous plexus foot pump promotes venous return by pumping blood through compression, mimicking the natural action of walking (Fig. 12.1). The combination of stockings and foot compression has been shown to be more effective than stockings alone in both DVT and pulmonary embolism incidence (Dunn & Ramos, 2017; Gee, 2015).

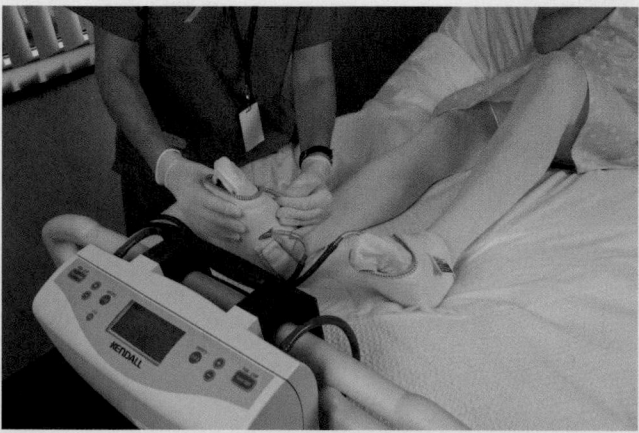

FIG 12.1 Venous plexus foot pump with bedside controls. (*Courtesy Tyco Healthcare Group LP.*)

Delegation and Collaboration

The skill of applying and maintaining graduated compression stockings and intermittent SCDs may be delegated to an unregulated care provider (UCP). The nurse initially determines the size of elastic stockings and assesses the patient's lower extremities for any signs and symptoms of a DVT or impaired circulation. The nurse directs the UCP to:

- Remove the SCD sleeves before allowing a patient to get out of bed.
- Report to the nurse if a patient's calf appears larger than the other or is red or hot, if the patient has calf pain, or if there are signs of skin breakdown or allergic reactions to elastic (redness, itching, or irritation).

Equipment

- Tape measure
- Graduated compression stockings
- SCD insufflator with air hoses attached, adjustable Velcro compression stockings/SCD sleeve
- Hygiene supplies

Procedural Steps

1. Review medical record for prescription for SCDs or graduated compression stocking.
2. Identify patient using at least two person-specific identifiers (e.g., name and date of birth or name and medical record number) according to employer policy (Accreditation Canada, 2019).
3. Assess patient for risk factors for developing DVT (see Box 12.1) (CPSI, 2017).
4. Assess for contraindications for use of elastic stockings or SCDs:
   a. Dermatitis or open skin lesions on area to be covered by stockings/SCD
   b. Recent skin graft to lower leg
   c. Decreased arterial circulation in lower extremities as evidenced by cyanotic, cool extremities or gangrenous conditions affecting the lower limb(s)
   d. If signs or symptoms of a DVT are present, do not manipulate the leg to apply stockings.
5. Assess condition of patient's skin (area to be covered by stockings) and circulation to the legs. Palpate pedal pulses, note any palpable veins, and inspect skin over lower extremities for edema, skin discoloration, warmth, and presence of lesions.
6. Obtain health care provider's prescription.
7. Assess patient's or caregiver's knowledge of previous use of elastic or sequential compression stockings.
8. Explain procedure and reason for applying elastic stockings or SCDs.
9. Position patient in supine position.
10. Perform hand hygiene. Bathe patient's legs as needed. Dry thoroughly. Perform hand hygiene.
11. **Apply graduated compression stocking:**
    a. Use tape measure to measure patient's leg to determine proper elastic stocking size (follow package directions).
    b. *Optional:* Apply a small amount of powder or cornstarch to legs, provided patient does not have sensitivity.

PROCEDURAL GUIDELINE 12.3 *Applying Graduated Compression (Elastic) Stockings and Sequential Compression Device—cont'd*

c. Turn elastic stocking inside out: Place one hand into stocking, holding heel of stocking. Take other hand and pull stocking inside out until reaching the heel (see illustration).

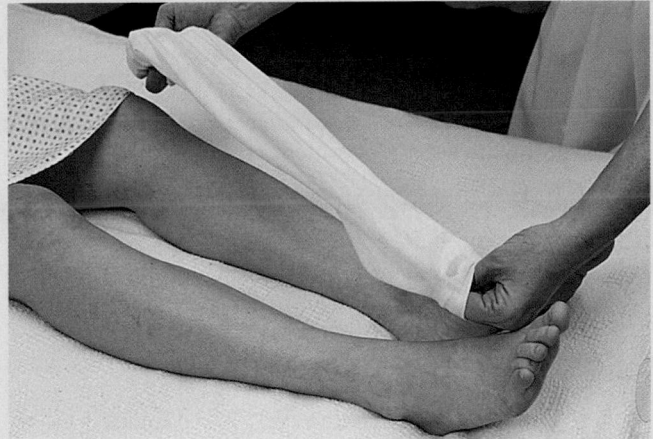

STEP 11c Turn stocking inside out; hold heel and pull through.

d. Place patient's toes into foot of elastic stocking up to the heel, making sure that stocking is smooth (see illustration).

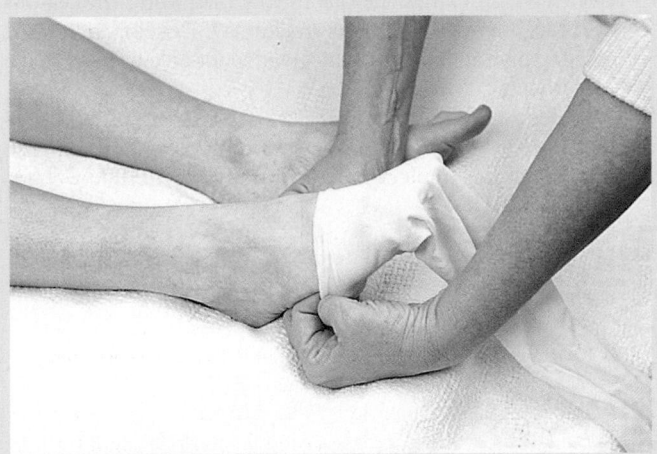

STEP 11d Place toes into foot of stocking.

e. Slide remaining part of stocking over patient's foot, making sure that toes are covered. Make sure that foot fits into toe-and-heel position of stocking. Stocking will now be right side out (see illustration).

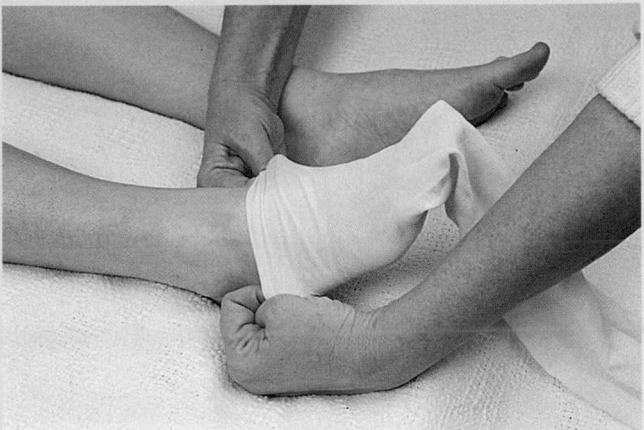

STEP 11e Slide remaining part of stocking over foot.

f. Slide stocking up over patient's calf until sock is completely extended. Be sure that stocking is smooth and that no ridges or wrinkles are present (see illustration).

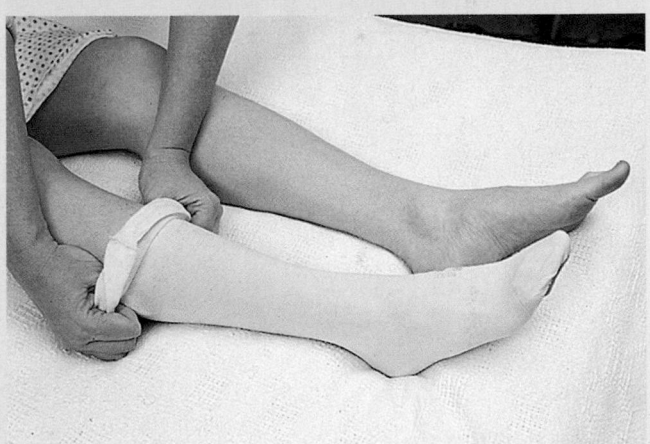

STEP 11f Slide sock up leg until completely extended.

g. Instruct patient not to roll stockings partially down, to avoid wrinkles and crossing legs, and to elevate legs while sitting.

12. **Apply SCD sleeve(s):**
   a. Remove SCD sleeve from plastic cover; unfold and flatten on bed.
   b. Arrange SCD sleeve under patient's leg according to leg position indicated on inner lining of sleeve.
   c. Place patient's leg on SCD sleeve. Back of ankle should line up with ankle marking on inner lining of sleeve.
   d. Position back of knee with popliteal opening on inner sleeve (see illustration).

Continued

PROCEDURAL GUIDELINE 12.3 *Applying Graduated Compression (Elastic) Stockings and Sequential Compression Device—cont'd*

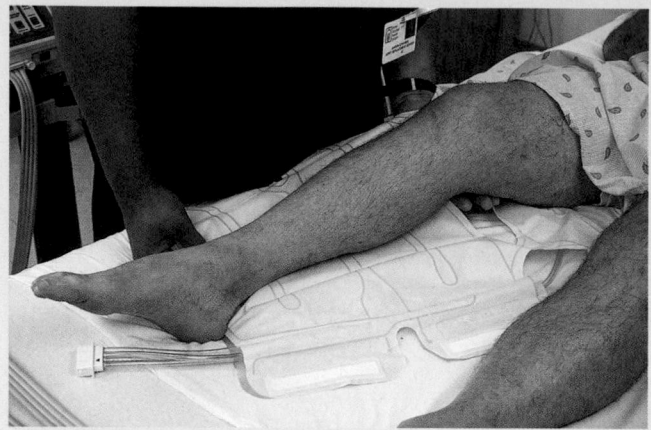

STEP 12d Position back of patient's knee with popliteal opening.

   e. Wrap SCD sleeve securely around patient's leg. Check fit of SCD sleeve by placing two fingers between patient's leg and sleeve (see illustration).

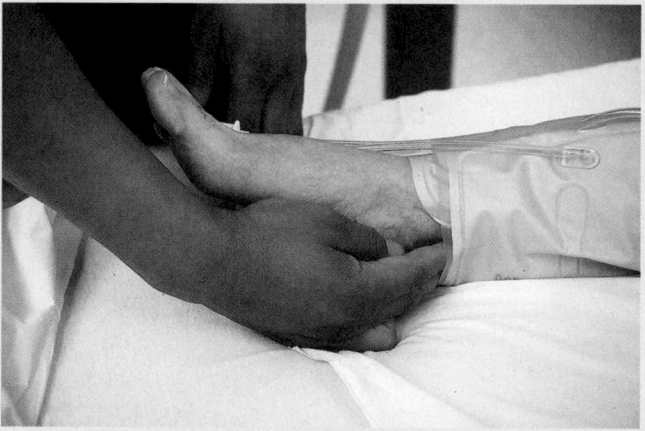

STEP 12e Check fit of SCD sleeve.

   f. Attach SCD sleeve connector to plug on mechanical unit. Arrows on connector line up with arrows on plug from mechanical unit (see illustration).

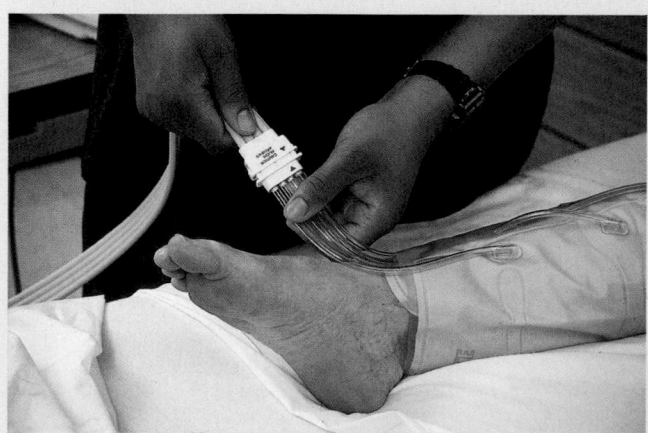

STEP 12f Align arrows when connecting plug to mechanical unit.

   g. Turn on mechanical unit. Green light indicates that unit is functioning. Monitor functioning SCD through one full cycle of inflation and deflation.

13. Position patient comfortably and perform hand hygiene.

Clinical Decision Point *Caution patient not to exit bed and walk with SCDs in place. Have patient call for help.*

14. Remove compression stockings or SCD sleeves at least once per shift (e.g., long enough to inspect skin for irritation or breakdown and determine patient's comfort level).

15. Evaluate skin integrity and circulation to patient's lower extremities as prescribed (see employer policy).

16. Educate patient and caregiver about how to care for elastic stockings (keep two pair and wash one daily) and precautions to take to prevent DVT at home (Alberta Health, 2018):
- Stay active and move around as much as possible.
- When sitting for long periods of time, such as when travelling for more than 4 hours:
  - Get up and walk around every 2 to 3 hours.
  - Drink plenty of water.
  - Exercise legs while sitting by raising and lowering heels while keeping toes on the floor, raising and lowering toes while keeping heels on the floor, tightening and releasing leg muscles.
  - Wear loose-fitting clothes.

17. Use Teach-Back: "I want to be sure you understand why you have elastic stockings. Tell me in your own words the reasons why you are wearing these stockings." Develop a revised teaching plan if patient or caregiver is not able to teach back correctly.

18. Document condition of lower extremities, application of stockings or SCD, patient education, and patient response in nurses' notes in electronic health record (EHR) or chart.

PROCEDURAL GUIDELINE 12.4 *Assisting With Ambulation (Without Assist Devices)*

 Video Clip

Patients who are immobile for even a short time often require help with ambulation. Having patients ambulate early after immobilization is important in preventing deconditioning. The benefits of ambulation include maintenance of muscle tone, strength, and joint flexibility and function of the respiratory, circulatory, and gastrointestinal systems. Although these benefits are well established, patient ambulation requires interprofessional collaboration around decision making related to when and how to ambulate and should always be preceded by assessing the patient's fall risk (see Chapter 13). Using a gait belt to assist a patient in ambulation increases patient safety and decreases a patient's fall risk.

When helping a patient up and out of bed or a chair, there is a risk for orthostatic hypotension. Orthostatic hypotension or postural hypotension is a decrease in blood pressure that occurs when a patient changes from a horizontal to a vertical position. A decrease in blood pressure greater than 20 mm Hg in systolic pressure or 10 mm Hg in diastolic pressure with symptoms of dizziness, light-headedness, nausea, tachycardia, pallor, and fainting indicates orthostatic hypotension (Lewis et al., 2019). Orthostatic hypotension is common among older adults. Although it can be related to the aging process, orthostatic hypotension may also result from a variety of factors, such as anemia, adverse effects of medications, deconditioning, infection, and systemic disease (Arnold & Raj, 2017). When a patient moves from a lying to a sitting position, dangling the legs on the side of the bed (sitting on the edge of the bed with patient moving legs back and forth) and making sure the legs can touch the floor can minimize onset of orthostatic hypotension by allowing the circulatory system to equilibrate. After leg dangling, have patient stand; if they tolerate standing without dizziness, proceed with ambulation. Use safety precautions before and during ambulation to control for orthostatic hypotension and subsequent falling.

Delegation and Collaboration

The skill of assisting patients with ambulation can be delegated to an unregulated care provider (UCP). The nurse directs the UCP to:

- Have a patient dangle following lying in bed and check patient's blood pressure before ambulation.
- Immediately return a patient to the bed or chair if nauseated, dizzy, pale, or diaphoretic and report these signs and symptoms to the nurse immediately.
- Apply safe, nonskid shoes or socks on the patient and ensure that the environment is free of clutter and there is no moisture on the floor before ambulating patient.

Equipment

- Gait belt
- Nonskid shoes or socks

Procedural Steps

1. Review medical record for patient's most recent activity experience, including distance ambulated, use of any assistive device, tolerance to activity, balance, and gait. Note any medications, chronic illnesses, presence of foot or leg deformity, or history of falling, all of which may influence patient's ability to ambulate independently.

2. Review most recently recorded weight for patient; this may indicate need for help from another care provider.

3. Review medical record for any history of or risks for orthostatic hypotension; identify medications or conditions that may place patient at risk.

4. Review health care provider's prescription for activity; note any mobility or weight-bearing restrictions.

5. Determine the best time to ambulate, considering other scheduled activities such as bathing or other medical procedures.

6. Check patient's environment for any barriers or safety risks. When walking, it is helpful within a hospital or rehabilitation centre to walk in an area where handrails are on the walls and chairs are near.

7. Identify patient using at least two person-specific identifiers (e.g., name and date of birth or name and medical record number) according to employer policy (Accreditation Canada, 2019).

8. Perform hand hygiene.

9. Assess patient's physical readiness to ambulate (see employer's protocol for mobility assessment and falls risk assessment [see Chapter 13]):

   a. Assess baseline resting heart rate, blood pressure, oxygen saturation (when available), and respirations.

   b. If patient's strength and endurance have been affected by illness or deconditioning, assess range of motion (ROM) and muscle strength (see Chapter 8) of lower extremities while in bed.

   c. Ask if patient feels excessively tired or is currently experiencing any pain. Determine source and severity of pain using an appropriate pain rating scale (see Chapter 16). This may delay ambulation. Offer an analgesic 30 minutes before ambulation to improve patient's tolerance to exercise.

Clinical Decision Point *Do not administer an analgesic that could make the patient feel dizzy.*

10. Assess patient's level of response to commands. Is the patient able to understand instructions and cooperate during ambulation? Also assess patient's views and perceptions regarding current state of health and willingness to participate in activity.

11. Assess patient for any visual, hearing, or perceptual deficit that may affect their ability to follow instructions.

12. If this is the first time ambulating or if patient has been unsteady in the past, have a chair or wheelchair positioned close to the path you choose for ambulation. You want to be able to move the patient quickly into a safe sitting position if the patient becomes unstable.

13. Explain to patient (in simple language) how you are going to prepare for ambulation (i.e., transfer technique and safety precautions to be used). Explain the benefits and reasons for activity or exercise. Do so in a way that matches patient's beliefs and values regarding recovery or maintaining health (Shieh et al., 2015).

14. Assist patient from a supine position to side of bed:

   a. With patient in supine position in bed, raise head of bed 30 degrees and place bed in low position, ensuring brakes are engaged, level with your hips. Place nonskid shoes or socks on patient.

Continued

PROCEDURAL GUIDELINE 12.4 *Assisting With Ambulation (Without Assist Devices)—cont'd*

b. While standing on side of bed where patient will sit, turn patient onto their side so that they are facing you.

c. Stand opposite patient's hips. Turn diagonally to face patient and far corner of foot of bed.

d. Place your feet apart in wide base of support with foot closer to head of bed in front of other foot.

e. Place your arm nearer to head of bed under patient's lower shoulder, supporting their head and neck. Place your other arm over and around patient's thighs (see illustration).

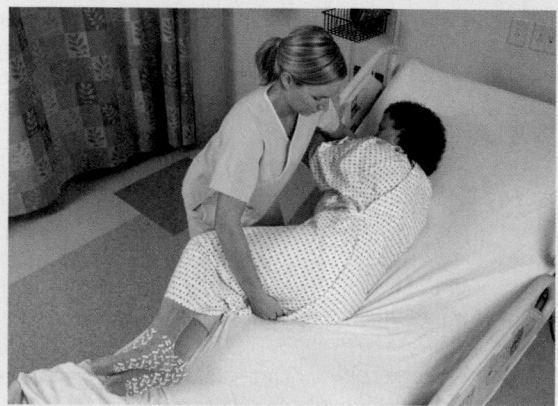

STEP 14e Nurse places arm over patient's thigh, other arm under patient's shoulder.

f. Move patient's lower legs and feet over side of bed. Pivot weight onto your rear leg as you allow patient's upper legs to swing downward (see illustration). At same time, continue to shift weight to your rear leg and elevate patient's trunk to the upright position.

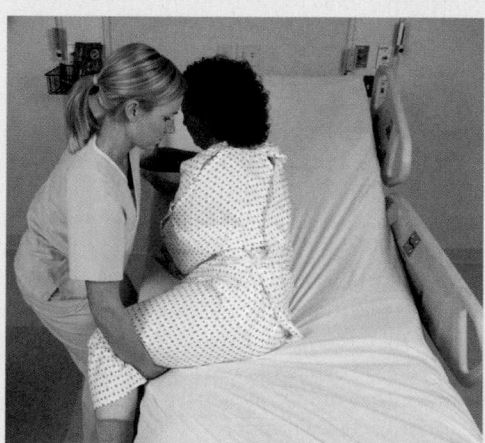

STEP 14f Nurse shifts weight to rear leg and elevates patient to sitting position.

15. Allow patient to sit on side of bed for a few minutes. Have patient alternately flex and extend feet and move lower legs up and down (see illustration). Ask if patient feels dizzy; if so, check the blood pressure. Have patient relax and take a few deep breaths until dizziness subsides and balance is gained. If dizziness lasts more than 60 seconds, return patient to lying position in bed (Myszenski, 2017). Recheck blood pressure.

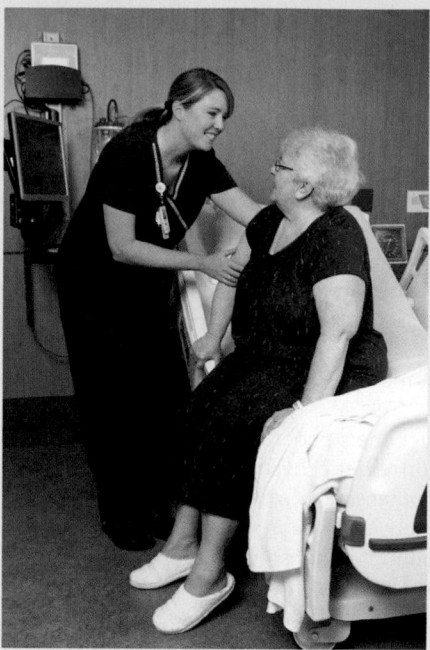

STEP 15 Patient sits on side of bed.

16. Apply gait belt around patient's waist. Be sure that it completely circles the waist. Place belt low and be sure that it is snug. Avoid placing it over any intravenous (IV) lines, incisions, or drainage tubes. You may need to adjust it once patient stands. Hold onto belt along patient's back with your palm facing up. The gait belt controls patient's centre of mass during mobility, controls descent if a fall occurs, and reduces the chance of grabbing patient's upper extremities.

17. Help patient into standing position at bedside. Have patient stand fully erect with shoulders back and looking ahead (not at floor). Next, assess patient's ability to bear weight and balance.

18. If patient is unsteady, place in chair or return to bed immediately and obtain additional help.

19. If patient has an IV line, place IV pole on same side as patient's arm where the infusion is located. Instruct patient where to hold and push the pole while walking.

20. If a Foley catheter is present, empty drainage bag before ambulating patient. You or patient will carry bag below the level of patient's bladder. Sometimes you can pin the bag in the proper position on patient's gown. Be sure that there is no tension on the tubing.

21. Decide with patient how far or how long to ambulate, to set a mutual goal. Walk a distance that patient can tolerate (see employer policy). Plan to increase ambulation time and distance during successive walks, as patient can tolerate.

22. Stand on patient's strong side and slightly behind. If assistive device (e.g., cane, walker) is used (see Skill 12.2), stand on patient's weak side and slightly behind.

23. Grasp gait belt firmly with palm facing up (see illustration). Take a few steps, supporting patient with one hand on the gait belt and the other under the elbow of patient's flexed arm (see illustration). *Optional:* Use ambulation lift or ceiling lift with a gait harness for a more dependent patient who is now walking for first time after being in bed.

PROCEDURAL GUIDELINE 12.4 *Assisting With Ambulation (Without Assist Devices)—cont'd*

24. Have patient take a few steps forward. Then assess their strength and balance before continuing.
25. When ambulating down hallway, position patient between yourself and the wall. Encourage use of handrail (if present).
26. Observe how patient walks (posture, gait, balance, coordination) and evaluate activity tolerance to ambulation (i.e., measure pulse and respirations and compare with baseline).
27. If patient starts to fall (see illustrations):
    a. Grasp patient's gait belt with both hands around their waist with palms up.

    b. Stand with feet apart for a broad base of support (see illustration A).
    c. Extend one leg, pull patient against you, and guide the patient to slide down your leg as you ease them to the floor (see illustration B). *Caution:* If patient is obese, do not risk personal injury.
    d. Bend your knees and lower your body as patient slides to floor (see illustration C).
    e. Stay with patient until help arrives.

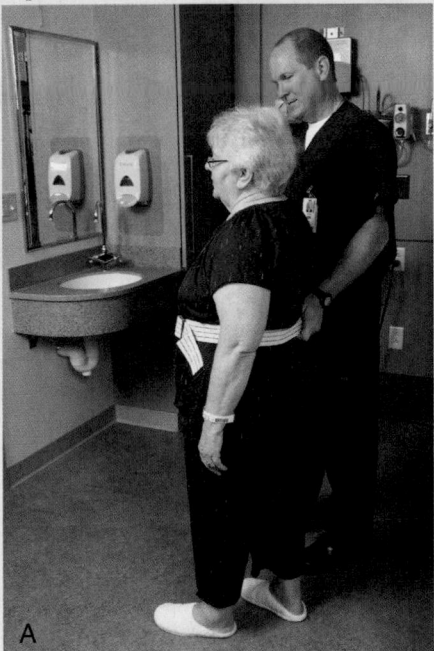
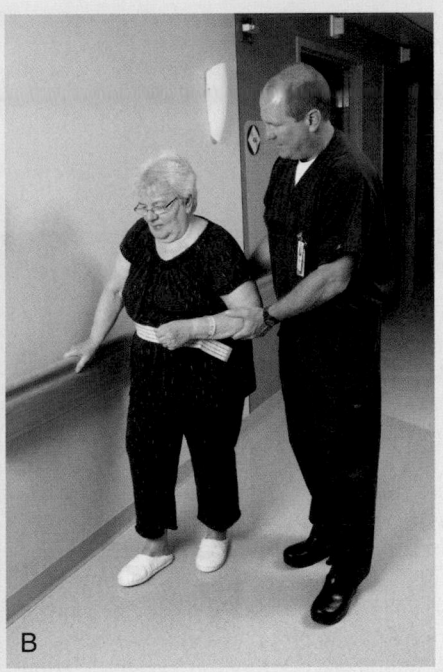

STEP 23 A, Nurse grasps gait belt firmly. **B,** Nurse helps patient by providing support under patient's flexed arm.

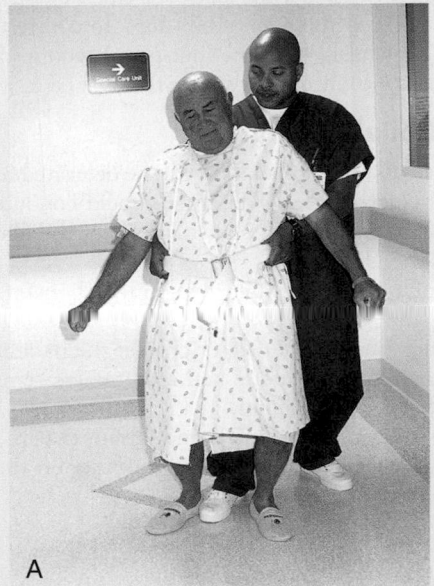
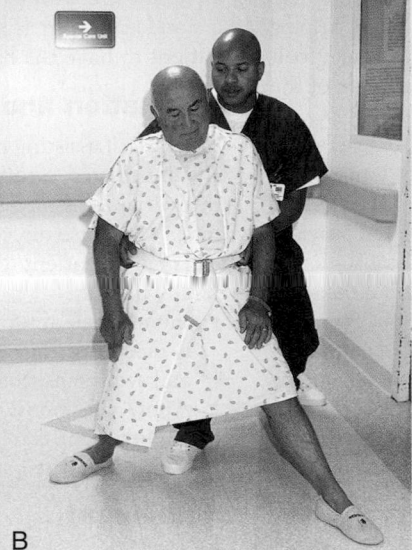
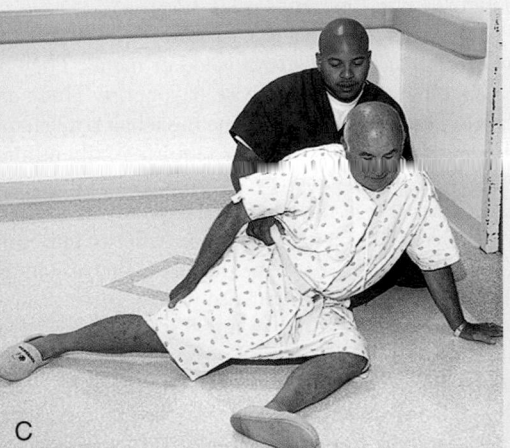

STEP 27 A, Grasp gait belt and stand with feet apart to provide broad base of support. **B,** Extend one leg and let patient slide against it to floor. **C,** Bend knees to lower body as patient slides to floor.

Continued

PROCEDURAL GUIDELINE 12.4 *Assisting With Ambulation (Without Assist Devices)*—cont'd

28. Once patient has completed the walk, return them to a bed or chair and help to assume a comfortable position. Perform hand hygiene.

29. Record time or distance ambulated, any changes in vital signs, and patient's tolerance (symptoms such as pain and fatigue) in nurses' notes in electronic health record (EHR) or chart.

✦ SKILL 12.2 | Assisting With Use of Canes, Walkers, and Crutches

An assistive device is any device that is designed, made, or adapted to help a person perform a particular task or function. For example, canes, crutches, and walkers are assistive devices for walking. An assistive device increases stability during ambulation; supports weak extremities; or reduces the load on weight-bearing structures such as hips, knees, or ankles. These devices range from standard canes, which provide balance and minimal physical support, to crutches and walkers, which are used by patients with weight-bearing limitations on one or more of their legs.

A physiotherapist should be consulted to help choose the proper assistive device, fit the device, and instruct the patient on the correct technique. Selection of an appropriate device depends on a patient's age, diagnosis, muscular coordination, weight-bearing status, and ease of manoeuverability. Use of assistive devices may be temporary (e.g., during recovery from a fractured extremity or orthopaedic surgery) or permanent (e.g., a patient with paralysis or permanent weakness of the lower extremities). As a nurse, you help patients use their devices correctly during ambulation. When helping a patient with an assistive device ambulate, always have a gait belt on the patient and stand slightly behind and off to the side of the patient (on the patient's weak side).

Canes are lightweight, easily movable devices that extend about waist high and are made of wood or metal. They help to maintain balance by widening the base of support. There are three types of canes. The standard crook cane has a half circle handle and provides the least support for patients requiring only minimal assistance to walk. The tripod cane (pyramid cane) has three legs, and the quad cane has four legs; the additional legs provide a wider base of support. These types of canes are useful for patients with unilateral or partial leg paralysis. They also have the advantage of standing alone, freeing the arms to help a patient rise from a chair.

A crutch is a wooden or metal staff that reaches from the ground almost to the axilla. Crutches remove weight from one leg. They are used by patients who must transfer more weight to their arms than is possible with canes. There are two types of crutches: axillary and Lofstrand. Patients of all ages often use axillary crutches short term for various weight-bearing limitations on the lower extremities. A Lofstrand crutch has a handgrip and a metal band that fits around a patient's forearm. Both the metal band and the handgrip are adjusted to fit a patient's height. This type of crutch is useful for patients with a permanent disability such as paraplegia (Lewis et al., 2019; Potter et al., 2019). The metal armband stabilizes and helps to guide the crutch. It also allows patients to use their hands for other activities such as opening doors without dropping the crutches. The anterior opening of the band allows patients to free themselves of the crutches if a fall occurs.

A walker is a lightweight, movable device that stands about waist high, consisting of a metal frame with handgrips, four widely placed sturdy legs, and one open side. It provides a wide base of support and the greatest stability and security during walking. A walker can be used by a patient who is weak, has a weight-bearing limitation on a lower extremity, or has problems with balance. Most of the walkers that are used today are wheeled walkers. These walkers have two wheels on the front posts or four wheels on all posts of the walker, making them easier to use and requiring less energy. This design is safer to use for patients with balance disorders because a patient keeps all four posts on the floor at all times. In contrast, a standard walker (has no wheels, only the four posts) requires a patient to have the balance to lift up the walker to advance it.

Delegation and Collaboration

The skill of assisting patients with ambulation can be delegated to an unregulated care provider (UCP). The nurse should conduct the initial assessment when the patient is ambulating for the first time. The nurse directs the UCP to:

- Have a patient dangle the legs after lying in bed, before ambulation.
- Immediately return a patient to the bed or chair if the patient is nauseated, dizzy, pale, or diaphoretic and report these signs and symptoms to the nurse immediately.
- Apply safe, nonskid shoes on the patient and ensure that the environment is free of clutter and there is no moisture on the floor before the patient ambulates.

Equipment

- Ambulation device (crutch, walker, cane)
- Safety device (gait belt)
- Well-fitting, flat, nonskid shoes for patient
- Goniometer (*optional*)

STEP	RATIONALE

ASSESSMENT

1. Identify patient using at least two person-specific identifiers (e.g., name and date of birth or name and medical record number) according to employer policy.

   Ensures correct patient. Complies with Accreditation Canada's standards and improves patient safety (Accreditation Canada, 2019).

2. Complete assessment steps in Procedural Guideline 12.4, Steps 1–5, 7–11.

   Determines patient's ability to ambulate with a device and readiness for learning necessary gaits and precautions.

3. Determine patient's or caregiver's understanding of type of device to be used in ambulating.

   Allows patient to verbalize concerns. Patients who have been immobile may be hesitant to ambulate. Caregiver may be hesitant to learn how to help with ambulation.

4. Assess degree of assistance that patient needs. Consult with physiotherapy to make this recommendation.

   For safety, another person may be needed initially to help with patient ambulation. Allow patient as much independence as possible.

NURSING DIAGNOSES

- Reduced physical mobility
- Altered health management
- Fatigue
- Potential for falls

- Potential for injury
- Reduced knowledge regarding use of assist device
- Reduced stamina

- Willingness for enhanced health management

Related factors/Risk factors are individualized on the basis of patient's condition or needs.

PLANNING

1. Expected outcomes following completion of procedure:
   - Patient ambulates using assistive device without injury.

     Appropriate level of assistance with device ensures patient's safety.

   - Patient is able to ambulate without excessive fatigue or dizziness and with return of vital signs to baseline 3 to 5 minutes after rest.

     Assistive device chosen requires minimal exertion. Patient tolerates exercise.

   - Patient demonstrates correct use of assist device, gait pattern, and weight-bearing status.

     Demonstrates learning and physical ability to use device.

2. Explain to patient how you are going to prepare for ambulation (e.g., transfer technique out of bed and safety precautions to be used while walking). Explain benefits and reasons for activity/exercise. Do so in a way that matches patient's educational level and beliefs and values regarding recovery or maintaining health.

   Exercise self-efficacy is an important predictor of the adoption and maintenance of exercise behaviours. Self-efficacy is a belief and conviction that one can successfully perform a given activity (RNAO, 2015; Selzler et al., 2016; Shieh et al., 2015).

3. Explain and demonstrate specific gait technique to patient or caregiver.

   Teaching and demonstration enhance learning, reduce anxiety, and encourage cooperation.

4. Check for appropriate height and fit of assist device. If physiotherapist has seen patient, the device should be at appropriate height. **NOTE:** *This is usually done when patient is standing at side of bed and is stable.*

   Ensures that patient is able to ambulate successfully without injury using device.

   a. *Cane measurement:* Cane should extend from greater trochanter of the hip to floor while cane is held 15 cm (6 inches) from foot. Allow 15- to 30-degree elbow flexion. Cane handle should fit comfortably in palm of hand.

      If cane is too short, patient has difficulty supporting weight and is bent over and uncomfortable. As weight is taken on by hands and affected leg is lifted off floor, complete extension of elbow is needed.

   b. *Crutch measurement:* Includes three areas: patient's height, distance between crutch pad and axilla, and angle of elbow flexion. Use one of two methods:

      Promotes optimal support and stability.

      (1) *Standing:* Position crutches with crutch tips at 15 cm (6 inches) to side and 15 cm in front of patient's feet (tripod position). Crutch pads should be 5 to 6.25 cm (2 to 2 ½ inches) or 3–4 finger widths) under axilla (Potter et al., 2019) (see illustration).

          Radial nerve passes under axillary area superficially. If crutch is too long, it places pressure on axilla and radial nerve. Injury to radial nerve causes paralysis of elbow and wrist extensors, commonly called *crutch palsy*. In addition, if crutch is too long, shoulders are forced upward, and patient cannot push body off the ground. If ambulation device is too short, patient is bent over and uncomfortable.

STEP	RATIONALE

PLANNING

    (2) *Supine:* Crutch pad is approximately 5 to 6.25 cm (2 to 2½ inches) or 3 to 4 finger widths under axilla with crutch tips positioned 15 cm (6 inches) lateral to patient's heel (see illustration).

    (3) Height of handgrip must be adjusted so patient's elbow is flexed 15 to 30 degrees or it sits at approximately height of wrist crease. Both height of crutch and handgrip dimensions are adjustable on a well-made crutch. | Low handgrips cause radial nerve damage. High handgrips cause elbow to be sharply flexed, decreasing strength and stability of arms. This allows patient to fully extend the elbow when taking a step.

  c. *Walker measurement:* When patient relaxes arms at side of body and stands up straight, top of walker should line up with crease on inside of wrist (Potter et al., 2019). Elbows should flex about 15 to 30 degrees when standing inside walker, with hands on handgrips. | Walker should be at proper height so that patient does not bend forward. Patient must have sufficient strength to be able to move walker.

5. Make sure that ambulation device has rubber tips. | Prevents device from slipping.

> **Clinical Decision Point** *Remove obstacles from pathways, including throw rugs (in the home), fall pads, and electrical cords, and wipe up any spills immediately. Avoid crowds. Crowds increase the risk of the crutch, cane, or walker being kicked or jarred and patient losing balance.*

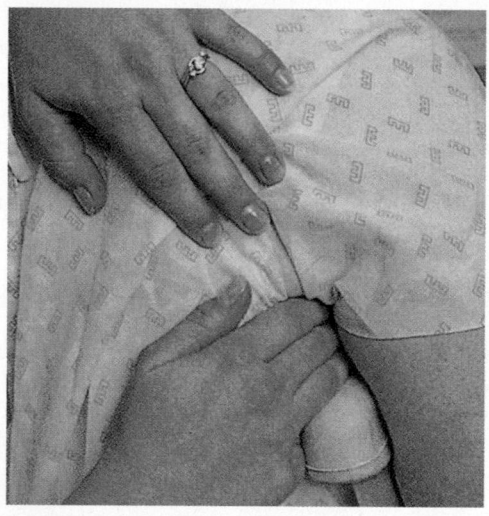

STEP 4b(1) Crutch pad is 3 to 4 finger widths under axilla.

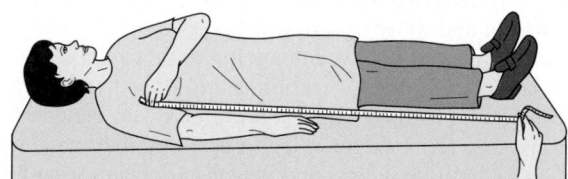

STEP 4b(2) Measuring length of crutch with patient in bed.

IMPLEMENTATION

1. Perform hand hygiene.

2. If using crutches, have patient report any tingling or numbness in upper torso. | Helps to indicate that crutches are being used incorrectly or that they are wrong size.

3. Help patient from lying position to side of bed (see Procedural Guideline 12.4, Step 14) or up from chair. | Ensures that patient is stable and ready to ambulate.

4. Allow patient to sit on edge of bed for a few minutes. Have patient alternately flex and extend feet, move lower legs. Ask if patient feels dizzy. Have patient relax and take a few deep breaths until dizziness subsides and balance is gained. | Determines ability to tolerate standing. If dizziness lasts more than 60 seconds, this may indicate orthostatic hypotension; return patient to bed (Myszenski, 2017). Recheck blood pressure.

5. Apply gait belt around patient's waist. Be sure that it completely circles patient's waist. Place belt low and be sure that it is snug. You may need to adjust belt once patient stands. Hold belt along patient's back with your palms facing up as patient walks. | Belt controls patient's centre of mass during mobility, controls descent if a fall occurs, and reduces chance of grabbing patient's upper extremities.

STEP	RATIONALE

IMPLEMENTATION

6. Help patient stand at bedside. Reassess height of device to make sure that it is correct size. Have patient stand fully erect with shoulders back and looking ahead (not at floor). At this time assess patient's ability to bear weight (e.g., Does patient have discomfort, unsteady stance?) and balance.

7. If patient is unsteady, seat patient in chair or return to bed immediately.

8. Decide with patient how far to ambulate.

9. Implement ambulation around patient's other activities.

10. **Helping patient walk with cane (steps are the same with standard, tripod, or quad cane):**

    a. Have patient hold cane on strong side. Direct patient to place cane forward 10 to 15 cm (4 to 6 inches) and slightly to the side of the foot, keeping body weight on both legs. Allow approximately 15- to 30-degree elbow flexion.

    b. To begin, have patient move cane forward about 15 to 25 cm (6 to 10 inches), keeping body weight on both legs.

    c. Instruct patient to advance involved leg forward, even with the cane. The cane and affected leg swing and strike the ground at the same time.

    d. Have patient advance strong leg 15 to 25 cm (6 to 10 inches) past cane.

    e. Have patient move involved leg forward, even with strong leg, which can go as far forward as bad leg or slightly past it.

    f. Repeat sequences as patient tolerates. Once comfortable, have patient advance cane and weak leg together.

11. **Helping patient crutch walk by using appropriate crutch gait:**

    a. Four-point gait:

    (1) Begin in tripod position (see illustration). Have patient place the crutch tips about 4 to 6 inches (10 to 15 cm) to the side and in front of each foot (Potter et al., 2019). Have patient place weight on handgrips, not under arms.

    (2) Move right crutch forward 10 to 15 cm (4 to 6 inches) (see illustration A).

    (3) Move left foot forward to level of left crutch (see illustration B).

    (4) Move left crutch forward 10 to 15 cm (4 to 6 inches) (see illustration C).

RATIONALE column:

Ensures that patient begins ambulation with correct posture and position.

Patient may require strengthening exercises or evaluation of balance by a physiotherapist.

Determines mutual goal.

Taking scheduled rest periods between activities reduces patient fatigue.

Offers most support when on stronger side of body. Cane and weaker leg work together with each step.

Distributes body weight equally.

Body weight is supported by cane and strong leg.

Aligns patient's centre of gravity. Returns patient body weight to equal distribution.

To use crutches, patient supports self with hands and arms; therefore, ability to balance body in upright position and stamina are necessary. Type of crutch gait depends on patient's weight-bearing status.

This is the most stable crutch gait. It provides at least three points of support at all times. Patient must be able to bear weight on both legs. Patient moves each leg alternately with each opposing crutch so three points of support are on floor all the time. Often used when patient has some form of paralysis, (e.g., children with spastic cerebral palsy) (Hockenberry & Wilson, 2015). May also be used for arthritic patients.

Improves balance by providing wide base of support. Patient should have posture of erect head and neck, straight vertebrae, and extended hips and knees.

Crutch and foot position is similar to arm and foot position during normal walking.

STEP	RATIONALE

IMPLEMENTATION

    (5) Move right foot forward to level of right crutch (see illustration D).

    (6) Repeat above sequence.

  b. Three-point gait (see illustrations):

Requires patient to bear all weight on one foot. Weight is borne on strong leg and then on both crutches. Affected leg does not touch ground during early phase of three-point gait. May be useful for patient with broken leg or sprained ankle.

    (1) Begin in tripod position (see illustration A), with patient standing on weight-bearing foot.

    (2) Advance both crutches and involved leg, keeping foot of involved leg off floor (see illustration B).

    (3) Move weight-bearing leg forward, stepping on floor (see illustration C).

Improves patient's balance by providing wide base of support.

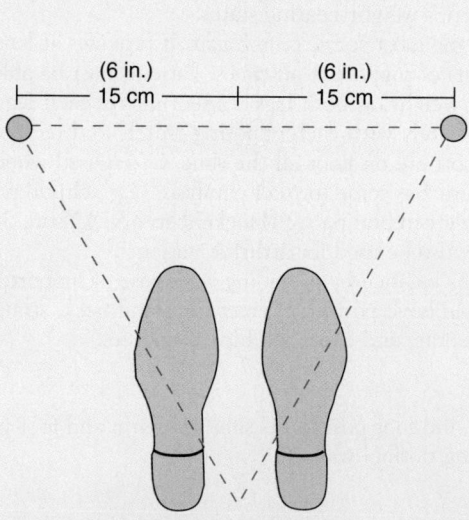

STEP 11a(1) Tripod position.

(6 in.)   (6 in.)
15 cm — 15 cm

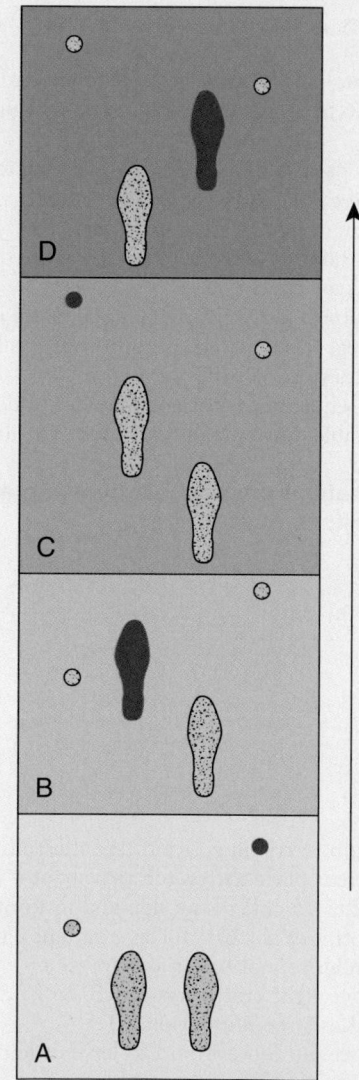

STEP 11a(2) Four-point gait. Solid feet and crutch tips show foot and crutch tip movement in each of four phases. (Read from bottom to top.) **A,** Right tip moves forward. **B,** Left foot moves toward left crutch. **C,** Left crutch tip moves forward. **D,** Right foot moves toward right crutch.

STEP	RATIONALE

IMPLEMENTATION

(4) Repeat sequence.

c. Two-point gait (see illustrations):

Requires at least partial weight bearing on each foot. Is faster than four-point gait. Requires more balance because only two points support body at one time.

(1) Begin in tripod position (see illustration A).

Improves patient's balance by providing wide base of support.

(2) Move left crutch and right foot forward (see illustration B).

Crutch movements are similar to arm movement during normal walking; patient moves crutch at same time as opposing leg.

(3) Move right crutch and left foot forward (see illustration C).

(4) Repeat sequence.

d. Swing-to gait:

Used by patients whose lower extremities are paralyzed or who wear weight-supporting braces on their legs.

(1) Begin in tripod position.

This is the easier of two swinging gaits. It requires ability to partially bear body weight on both legs.

(2) Move both crutches forward.

(3) Lift and swing legs to crutches, letting crutches support body weight.

(4) Repeat two previous steps.

e. Swing-through gait:

Requires that patient have ability to bear partial weight on both feet.

(1) Begin in tripod position.

Improves patient's balance by providing wide base of support.

(2) Move both crutches forward.

Initial placement of crutches increases patient's base of support so, when body swings forward, patient is moving centre of gravity toward additional support provided by crutches.

(3) Lift and swing legs through and beyond crutches.

(4) Repeat previous steps.

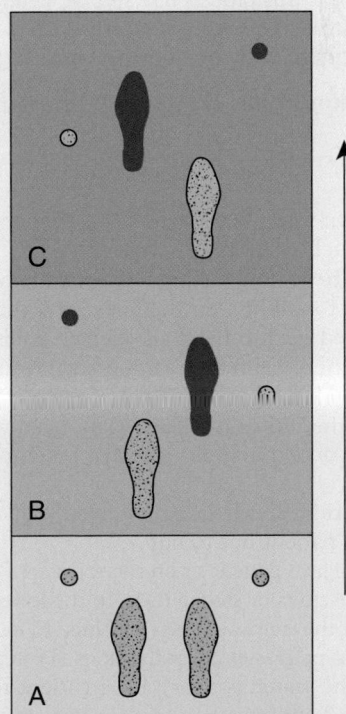

STEP 11b Three-point gait with weight borne on unaffected right leg. Solid foot and crutch tips show weight bearing in each phase **A** to **C**. (Read from bottom to top.)

STEP 11c Two-point gait. Solid areas indicate weight-bearing leg and crutch tips **A** to **C**. (Read from bottom to top.)

STEP	RATIONALE

IMPLEMENTATION

12. Helping patient climb up stairs with a railing with crutches (partial weight bearing, one leg):

Climbing stairs with use of a railing is safest way for patient with crutches to ascend stairs.

Clinical Decision Point *There is a risk for falling using this technique. Monitor patient's balance carefully. See option below.*

  a. Have patient begin in tripod position. Stand on weight-bearing leg.

Improves patient's balance by providing wide base of support.

  b. Patient transfers body weight to crutch.

Prepares patient to transfer weight to strong leg when ascending first stair.

  c. Have patient hold handrail with one hand (strong leg next to railing). As the nurse, you carry crutch positioned next to handrail. Patient holds other crutch.

Ensures patient safety.

  d. Have patient support weight evenly between the handrail and crutch.

Achieves balance.

  e. Patient next places some weight on crutches and then steps up with first step with weight-bearing foot. Have patient get balance.

  f. Patient then straightens uninvolved knee and lifts body weight, bringing crutches and affected leg up the stair.

  g. Repeat sequence of steps until patient reaches top of stairs. Observe patient's balance and level of fatigue.

  h. Option: Have patient sit on the lower stair. If distance and reach allow, place crutches at the top of the staircase. If this isn't possible, have patient place crutches as far up the stairs as they can. Then patient will move them to the top as they progress up the stairs (Potter et al., 2019).

Reaching for inaccessible crutches could lead to a fall.
Moving up by seat avoids risks of losing balance and tripping on stairs.

  (1) In the seated position, have patient reach behind with both arms.

  (2) Then have patient use arms and weight-bearing foot or leg to lift up one step.

  (3) Repeat this process one step at a time.

13. Helping patient descend stairs with a railing with crutch (partial weight bearing, one leg):

Clinical Decision Point *There is a risk for falling using this technique. Monitor patient's balance carefully. See option below.*

  a. Begin in tripod position.

Improves patient's balance by providing wide base of support.

  b. Patient transfers body weight to strong leg and aligns with crutches.

Prepares patient to release support of body weight maintained by crutches.

  c. Have patient hold handrail with one hand (involved leg next to railing). As the nurse, you carry crutch positioned next to handrail. Patient holds other crutch.

  d. Have patient bend their strong knee while moving crutch and involved leg down a step.

  e. Patient then supports their weight evenly between handrail and crutch. Be sure that patient has good balance.

  f. Have patient slowly bring involved leg down step. Caution patient not to hop.

Hopping could injure leg and create risk for fall.

  g. Option: Have patient sit on the top step. Place crutches down the stairs by sliding them to the lowest possible point on the stairway. Then continue to move them down as patient progresses down the stairs (Potter et al., 2019).

Reaching for inaccessible crutches could lead to a fall.
Moving down by seat avoids risk of losing balance and falling down stairs.

  (1) In the seated position, have patient reach behind with both arms.

  (2) Have patient use arms and weight-bearing foot or leg to lift self down one step.

  (3) Repeat this process one step at a time.

STEP	RATIONALE

IMPLEMENTATION

14. Helping patient ambulate with walker:

   a. Have patient stand straight in centre of walker and grasp handgrips on upper bars.

   b. Have patient move walker a comfortable distance forward, about 15 to 20 cm (6 to 8 inches). Patient then takes step forward with involved leg first and follows through with good leg. Instruct patient not to advance leg past the front bar of walker. If patient has equal strength in both legs, it makes no difference which leg advances first.

   c. If patient is unable to bear weight on involved leg, have them slowly hop to centre of walker using strong leg, supporting weight on hands.

   d. Instruct patient not to try to climb stairs with walker unless they have a specific walker for steps.

15. After patient ambulates, help them back to bed or chair and help assume comfortable position.

16. Perform hand hygiene.

Rationale:

Patients who are able to bear partial weight use walkers. Patient balances self before attempting to walk.

Provides broad base of support between walker and patient. Patient then moves centre of gravity toward walker. Keeping all four feet of walker on floor is necessary to prevent tipping walker.

Patient should use handrails as alternative. Using walker could cause a fall.

Prevents transmission of infection.

EVALUATION

1. After ambulation, obtain patient's vital signs, observe skin colour, and ask about comfort and energy levels.

Evaluates how patient tolerated procedure and whether there was progress in ambulation. Assesses stage of patient's illness and degree of convalescence when evaluating process.

2. Evaluate patient's subjective statements regarding experience.

Evaluates activity tolerance.

3. Evaluate patient's gait pattern: Observe body alignment in standing position and balance during gait.

Determines if patient is using supportive aids for ambulation correctly. Keep in mind patient's previous manner of ambulating when assessing gait.

4. Use Teach-Back: "You have done well walking with your walker. We reviewed with your spouse how to place a gait belt. I talked about why it is important for your spouse to use a gait belt to help you at first. Can both of you tell me why a gait belt is important?" Develop a revised teaching plan if patient or caregiver is not able to teach back correctly.

Determines patient's and caregiver's level of understanding of instructional topic.

Unexpected Outcomes

1. Patient is unable to ambulate because of fear of falling, physical discomfort, upper body muscles that are too weak to use ambulation device, or lower extremities that are too weak to support body.

2. Patient sustains an injury.

3. When using cane or walker, patient bends over and does not stand up straight.

Related Interventions

- Consult with physiotherapist about possible exercise program to strengthen muscles or other alternative methods that patient can use for ambulation.
- Provide analgesic for discomfort.
- Discuss with patient fears or concerns about walking using assist device.
- Notify health care provider.
- Return patient to bed if injury is such that it is safe to do so.
- Document per employer policy.
- Reinforce correct posture.

Communication and Documentation

- Document in the medical record assessment findings, type of assist device and gait patient used, amount of help required, distance walked, and activity tolerance in the electronic health record (EHR) or chart.
- Document your evaluation of patient and caregiver learning.
- Immediately report any injury sustained during attempts to ambulate, alteration in vital signs, or inability to ambulate to nurse in charge or health care provider.

Special Considerations
Teaching

- Instruct the patient with exercises such as squeezing a rubber ball, raising and lowering both arms in a slow and rhythmic manner while holding weights, chair push-ups, and pull-ups, which help strengthen the upper extremities.
- Teach patients who use a walker to examine the frame daily. When inspecting a walker, the patient should observe for signs of bending or deformation of the frame, protruding screws that can scratch, and loose or missing screws that weaken the joints

of the frame. Assess handgrips for any cracks or signs of being loose, and ensure proper function of brakes on wheeled walkers.

- Teach patients to use the arms of a chair rather than the assistive device to give them leverage when getting up from a chair; the device is likely to tip if used for this purpose.
- Blistering or soreness of the hands can result from continual pressure between the hand and the handle of a crutch. Advise patient to release pressure intermittently and wear gloves or pad the handle to reduce friction.
- Instruct patient that, if wearing shoes with varying heel sizes, the crutches, canes, and walkers may need to be adjusted to maintain the proper height.
- Caution patients when using an assistive device: **Don't** look down. Look straight ahead as you normally do when you walk. **Don't** walk on slippery surfaces. Avoid snowy, icy, or rainy conditions. **Don't** put *any* weight on the affected foot if your doctor has so advised (Potter et al., 2019).
- For assistive devices such as motorized scooters, clients and caregivers should know how to properly operate the equipment, apply brakes, and adhere to safety standards. Safety information can be accessed through the Canada Safety Council (https://canadasafetycouncil.org/motorized-scooters-and-other-devices/) and Transport Canada (https://www.tc.gc.ca/eng/motorvehiclesafety/tp-tp2436-rs200803-menu-374.htm). Advice on purchasing a device can be accessed through https://www.canada.ca/en/health-canada/services/healthy-living/your-health/lifestyles/seniors-aging-assistive-devices.html.

Pediatric

- For rehabilitation of a small child who has not yet learned to walk or who is unsteady, special crutches with three or four legs provide the needed stability to allow the child to maintain an upright posture and learn to walk (Hockenberry & Wilson, 2015).
- Another option for children who are just learning to walk would be front- or rear-rolling walkers.

Gerontological

- The Public Health Agency of Canada and the Canadian Society for Exercise Physiology (CSEP) have many resources and guidelines about physical activity for older persons. Both agencies offer tips that care providers can use to motivate patients (see https://www.canada.ca/en/public-health/services/health-promotion/healthy-living/physical-activity/physical-activity-tips-older-adults-65-years-older.html; http://www.csep.ca/CMFiles/Guidelines/CSEP_PAGuidelines_older-adults_en.pdf).

Care in the Community

- Teach patient how to use the ambulation aid on various terrains (e.g., carpet, stairs, rough ground, inclines). Teach how to manoeuvre around obstacles such as doors and how to use the aid when transferring to and from a chair, toilet, and tub.
- Teach caregivers how to help and what to observe to ensure that an assistive device is used correctly.

Long-Term Care Facility

- Conduct safety and maintenance checks of ambulation devices on a routine basis.
- Perform periodic assessments to ensure that the patient is using the ambulation device properly.

✦ CLINICAL DEBRIEF

A 72-year-old woman was transferred out of the critical care unit (CCU) following a motor vehicle accident and has progressed through stages 1 and 2 of an early mobility protocol to stage 3, where she will sit in a chair for 20 minutes. She had a fractured right hip that was repaired in surgery and has multiple bruises causing discomfort in her right shoulder and chest area. During surgery, she had significant blood loss. She has been in the CCU for 3 days. Her heart rate per minute since being hospitalized has ranged from 72 to 94, BP 118–146/72–84 mm Hg, and respirations 18 to 26 breaths/minute. The nurse is helping the patient with active range-of-motion (ROM) exercises before getting her to sit on the side of the bed.

1. What should be included in the nurse's assessment before getting the patient up to sit in a chair?
2. The health care provider prescribed graduated compression stockings for the patient to wear. Which risk factors does she have for developing a deep vein thrombosis?
3. The patient is about to move to stage 4 in the mobility protocol. She received an analgesic 30 minutes ago. The nurse completes assessment of vital signs: BP 138/80 mm Hg; R 26 breaths/min, P 88 beats/min, oxygen saturation 96%. The patient has been sitting in a chair for 15 minutes, and her pain score is a 4 before ambulation. The nurse begins to help the woman walk down the hallway for the first time. She walks approximately 7 metres and develops sudden chest pain and dizziness. The nurse returns the patient to a nearby chair immediately. Her vital signs are BP 110/60 mm Hg, P 130 beats/min, R 32 breaths/min. Write an SBAR for this situation.

✦ REVIEW QUESTIONS

1. Place the following steps for a four-point crutch gait in the correct order.

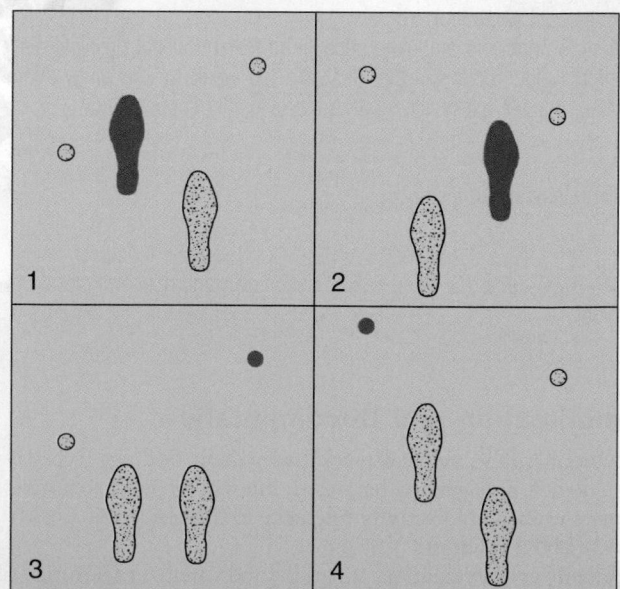

2. Which tips should you recommend to patients for preventing deep vein thrombosis in the home environment? *(Select all that apply.)*
1. Avoid sitting for any period of time over 2 to 3 hours.
2. Limit fluid intake during travelling.
3. Wear loose-fitting clothes if travelling more than 4 hours.
4. When sitting, always keep your legs crossed.
5. Perform foot exercises when flying in a plane for more than 4 hours.

3. A patient is placed on an early progressive mobility protocol. After helping them sit in a chair for 15 minutes, which patient data indicate to the nurse that the patient needs to return to bed immediately? *(Select all that apply.)*
1. Patient is dizzy for 15 seconds.
2. Respiratory rate increases over baseline by 4 breaths per min.
3. Systolic blood pressure (BP) falls 30 mm Hg below baseline systolic level.
4. Patient expresses severe fatigue.
5. Patient becomes diaphoretic.

Ⓔ *Visit the Evolve site for a complete list of Clinical Debrief and Review Questions answers.*

REFERENCES

Accreditation Canada. (2019). *Required organizational practices handbook—Version 14.* Retrieved from http://www.wrha.mb.ca/quality/files/2019ROPHandbook.pdf

Alberta Health. (2018). *AADL compression stockings information.* Retrieved from http://www.health.alberta.ca/services/AADL-compression-stockings.html

Arnold, A. C., & Raj, S. R. (2017). Orthostatic hypotension: A practical approach to investigation and management. *Canadian Journal of Cardiology, 33*(12), 1725–1728. doi:10.1016/j.cjca.2017.05.007

Arnold, M. (2017). Building a foundation of mobility: From the ICU and across the continuum of care. *International Journal of Safe Patient Handling & Mobility (SPHM), 7*(1), 40–44.

Bilodeau, C., Gallagher, F., & Tanguay, A. (2017). Perceived factors influencing early mobilization of mechanically ventilated patients among critical care nurses. *Canadian Journal of Critical Care Nursing, 28*(2), 52–53.

Burchum, J. R., & Rosenthal, L. D. (2016). *Lehne's pharmacology for nursing care* (9th ed.). St. Louis: Elsevier.

Cameron, S., Ball, I., Cepinskas, G., et al. (2015). Early mobilization in the critical care unit: A review of adult and pediatric literature. *Journal of Critical Care, 30*(4), 664–672. doi:10.1016/j.jcrc.2015.03.032

Canadian Patient Safety Institute (CPSI). (2017). *Venous thromboembolism prevention getting started kit, Section 2: Evidence-based appropriate VTE prophylaxis.* Retrieved from http://www.patientsafetyinstitute.ca/en/toolsResources/VTE-Getting-Started-Components/Documents/Section%202%20Evidence%20Based%20Appropriate%20VTE%20Prophylaxis.pdf

Carvalho, C. A., Pinto, R. L., Godoy, M. F. G., & Pereira de Godoy, J. M. (2015). Reduction of pain and edema of the legs by walking wearing elastic stockings. *International Journal of Vascular Medicine, 2015*(2015), doi:10.1155/2015/648074. Retrieved from https://www.hindawi.com/journals/ijvm/2015/648074/

Castelino, T., Fiore, J. F., Niculiseanu, P., Landry, T., Augustin, B., & Feldman, L. S. (2016). The effect of early mobilization protocols on postoperative outcomes following abdominal and thoracic surgery: A systematic review. *Surgery, 159*(4), 991–1003. doi:10.1016/j.surg.2015.11.029

Davis, J. C., Bryan, S., Best, J., et al. (2015). Mobility predicts change in older adults' health-related quality of life: Evidence from a Vancouver falls prevention prospective cohort study. *Health and Quality of Life Outcomes, 13*(101), 1–10. doi:10.1186/s12955-015-0299-0

Delaney, N. (2017). *Early progressive mobility: Adult acute care* [PowerPoint presentation]. British Columbia, Canada: Interior Health Authority.

Dunn, N., & Ramos, R. (2017). Preventing venous thromboembolism: The role of nursing with intermittent pneumatic compression. *American Journal of Critical Care, 26*(2), 164–167. doi:10.4037/ajcc2017504

Falvey, J. R., Mangione, K. K., & Stevens-Lapsley, J. E. (2015). Rethinking hospital-associated deconditioning: Proposed paradigm shift. *Physical Therapy, 95*(9), 1307–1315. doi:10.2522/ptj.20140511

Gatewood, C. T., Tran, A. A., & Dragoo, J. L. (2017). The efficacy of post-operative devices following knee arthroscopic surgery: A systematic review. *Knee Surgery,*

Sports Traumatology, Arthroscopy: Official Journal of The ESSKA, 25(2), 501–516. doi:10.1007/s00167-016-4326-4

Gee, E. (2015). Compression in acute stroke: Nursing considerations. *British Journal of Neuroscience Nursing, 11*(Suppl. 2), 20–22. doi:10.12968/bjnn.2015.11.Sup2.20

Hashem, M. D., Nelliot, A., & Needham, D. M. (2016). Early mobilization and rehabilitation in the ICU: Moving back to the future. *Respiratory Care, 61*(7), 971–979. doi:10.4187/respcare.04741

Heart and Stroke Foundation of Canada. (2018). *How much physical activity do you need?* Retrieved from http://www.heartandstroke.ca/get-healthy/stay-active/how-much-physical-activity-do-you-need

Hockenberry, M. J., & Wilson, D. (2015). *Wong's nursing care of infants and children* (10th ed.). St. Louis: Mosby.

Hogana, C. L., Catalino, L. I., Mata, J., & Fredrickson, B. L. (2015). Beyond emotional benefits: Physical activity and sedentary behaviour affect psychosocial resources through emotions. *Psychology & Health, 30*(3), 354–369. doi:10.1080/08870446.2014.973410

Hopkins, R., Mitchell, L., Thomsen, G. E., Schafer, M., Link, M., & Brown, S. M. (2016). Implementing a mobility program to minimize post-intensive care syndrome. *AACN Advanced Critical Care, 27*(2), 187–203. doi:10.4037/aacnacc2016244

Interior Health Authority. (2015). *Early progressive mobility for critical care patients.* British Columbia: Author.

Larsson, A., Palstam, A., Löfgren, M., et al. (2015). Resistance exercise improves muscle strength, health status and pain intensity in fibromyalgia—A randomized controlled trial. *Arthritis Research & Therapy, 17,* 161. doi:10.1186/s13075-015-0679-1

Lewis, S., Bucher, L., Heitkemper, M. L., Harding, M. M., Barry, M. A., & Goldsworthy, S. (Eds.). (2019). *Medical–surgical nursing in Canada. Assessment and management of clinical problems* (4th ed.). Toronto, ON: Elsevier Canada.

Liu, B., Moore, J. E., Almaawiy, U., et al. (2018). Outcomes of mobilisation of vulnerable elders in Ontario (MOVE ON): A multisite interrupted time series evaluation of an implementation intervention to increase patient mobilization. *Age and Ageing, 47*(1), 112–119. doi:10.1093/ageing/afx128

MOVE Canada. (2015). *Mobilization.* Retrieved from http://movescanada.ca/mobilization

Multiple Sclerosis (MS) Society of Canada. (2019). *Exercise and physical activity.* Retrieved from https://mssociety.ca/hot-topics/exercise-and-physical-activity

Myszenski, A. (2017). The essential role of lab values and vital signs in clinical decision making and patient safety for the acutely ill patient. *Physical Therapy, com.* Retrieved from https://www.physicaltherapy.com/articles/essential-role-lab-values-and-3637

National Institute on Aging (NIA). (n.d.). *Weekly exercise and physical activity plan.* Retrieved from https://go4life.nia.nih.gov/weekly-exercise-and-physical-activity-plan/

Pai, M., & Douketis, J. (2016). Prevention of venous thromboembolic disease in acutely ill hospitalized medical adults. *UpToDate.* Retrieved from http://www.uptodate.com/contents/1346

Potter, P. A., Perry, A. G., Ross-Kerr, J. C., et al. (Eds.). (2019). *Canadian fundamentals of nursing* (6th ed.). Toronto, ON: Elsevier Canada.

Registered Nurses' Association of Ontario (RNAO). (2010). *Strategies to support self-management in chronic conditions: Collaboration with clients.* Toronto, ON: Author. Retrieved from http://rnao.ca/sites/rnao-ca/files/Strategies_to_Support_Self-Management_in_Chronic_Conditions_-_Collaboration_with_Clients.pdf

Registered Nurses' Association of Ontario (RNAO). (2015). *Person- and family-centred care.* Toronto, ON: Author. Retrieved from http://rnao.ca/sites/rnao-ca/files/FINAL_Web_Version_0.pdf

Registered Nurses' Association of Ontario (RNAO). (2017). *Preventing falls and reducing injury from falls* (4th ed.). Toronto, ON: Author. Retrieved from http://rnao.ca/sites/rnao-ca/files/bpg/FALL_PREVENTION_WEB_1207-17.pdf

Saunders, C. B. (2015). Preventing secondary complications in trauma patients with implementation of multidisciplinary mobilization team. *Journal of Trauma Nursing, 22*(3), 170–175. doi:10.1097/JTN.0000000000000127

Schmidt, U. H., Knecht, L., & MacIntyre, N. R. (2016). Should early mobilization be routine in mechanically ventilated patients? *Respiratory Care, 61*(6), 867–875. doi:10.4187/respcare.04566

Selzler, A., Rodgers, W. M., Berry, T. R., & Stickland, M. K. (2016). The importance of exercise self-efficacy for clinical outcomes in pulmonary rehabilitation. *Rehabilitation Psychology, 61*(4), 380–388. doi:10.1037/rep0000106

Shieh, C., Weaver, M. T., Hanna, K. M., Newsome, K., & Mogos, M. (2015). Association of self-efficacy and self- regulation with nutrition and exercise behaviors in a community sample of adults. *Journal of Community Health Nursing, 32*(4), 199–211. doi:10.1080/07370016.2015.1087262

Sommers, J., Engelbert, R., Dettling-Ihnenfeldt, D., et al. (2015). Physiotherapy in the intensive care unit: An evidence-based, expert driven, practical statement

and rehabilitation recommendations. *Clinical Rehabilitation, 29*(11), 1051–1063. doi:10.1177/0269215514567156

Stanhope, M., Lancaster, J., Jakubec, S. L., & Pike-MacDonald, S. A. (2017). *Community health nursing in Canada*. Toronto, ON: Elsevier Canada.

Statistics Canada. (2016). *Healthy people, healthy places (Cat. No. 82-229-X)*. Ottawa: Author. Retrieved from http://www.statcan.gc.ca/pub/82-229-x/82-229-x200900 1-eng.htm

Tam, T. (2017). *The Chief Public Health Officer's report on the state of public health in Canada 2017—designing healthy living*. Retrieved from https://www.canada.ca/ en/public-health/services/publications/chief-public-health-officer-reports-state-pu blic-health-canada/2017-designing-healthy-living.html#a5

Uzdanovich, K., Regan, M., & Monagle, J. (2015). Let's move together: A collaborative approach to implementing early mobility. *Critical Care Nurse, 35*(2), E54.

Viveen, J., Doornberg, J. N., Kodde, I. F., et al. (2017). Continuous passive motion and physical therapy (CPM) versus physical therapy (PT) versus delayed physical therapy (DPT) after surgical release for elbow contractures; a study protocol for a prospective randomized controlled trial. *BMC Musculoskeletal Disorders, 18*, 1–7. doi:10.1186/s12891-017-1854-0

Witard, O., McGlory, C., Hamilton, D., & Phillips, S. (2016). Growing older with health and vitality: A nexus of physical activity, exercise and nutrition. *Biogerontology, 17*(3), 529–546. doi:10.1007/s10522-016-9637-9

Zisberg, A., Shadmi, E., Gur-Yaish, N., Tonkikih, O., & Sinoff, G. (2015). Hospital-associated functional decline: The role of hospitalization processes beyond individual risk factors. *Journal of the American Geriatrics Society, 63*(1), 55–62.

13 | Support Surfaces and Special Beds

Written by **Kristen L. Mauk, PhD, DNP, RN, CRRN, GCNS-BC, GNP-BC, ACHPN, FAAN, and Dana Penfound, RN, MACP**

SKILLS AND PROCEDURES

OBJECTIVES

Mastery of content in this chapter will enable the nurse to:
- Identify the different types of support surfaces and specialty beds used for pressure redistribution.
- Explain why preventive nursing care is still essential when using support surfaces and specialty beds.
- Describe guidelines for placing patients on support surfaces and specialty beds.

- Compare differences between mattress overlays and mattress replacements.
- Describe mechanisms by which skin breakdown can occur on a special bed, a support surface mattress, or wheelchair seat cushion.
- Describe the steps for correct placement of a patient on a special bed or a support surface mattress.

MEDIA RESOURCES

- **evolve** http://evolve.elsevier.com/Canada/Perry/clinicalskills/
- Review Questions

- Audio Glossary
- Clinical Debrief and Review Questions Answers

PURPOSE

Despite increasing technological advances in health care, pressure injuries remain a major problem that affects patient comfort, length of stay in a health care facility, and health care costs. Interprofessional collaboration is key to reducing pressure injuries, with nurses at the forefront of their prevention and treatment in health care settings (Norton, Parslow, Johnston, et al., 2018) and playing an extremely important role in risk assessment and prevention (Registered Nurses' Association of Ontario [RNAO], 2011, p. 15).

STANDARDS OF CARE

- Hanna-Bull, D., 2016—Preventing heel pressure ulcers: Sustained quality improvement initiative in a Canadian acute care facility. *Journal of Wound, Ostomy and Continence Nurses, 43*(2), 129–132 (https://www.ncbi.nlm.nih.gov/pubmed/26473635)
- Registered Nurses Association of Ontario (RNAO), 2005/2011—*Risk Assessment & Prevention of Pressure Ulcers* (https://rnao.ca/sites/rnao-ca/files/Risk_Assessment_and_Prevention_of_Pressure_Ulcers.pdf)
- Wounds Canada, 2018—*Best Practice Recommendations for the Prevention and Management of Pressure Injuries* (https://www.woundscanada.ca/docman/public/health-care-professional/bpr-workshop/165-wc-bpr-prevention-and-management-of-wounds/file)

PRINCIPLES FOR PRACTICE

- Factors contributing to pressure injury formation are both extrinsic (e.g., pressure, moisture, friction, and shear) and intrinsic (e.g., malnutrition, loss of sensation, impaired mobility, aging skin, impaired mental status, infection, incontinence, and low arteriolar pressure) (Norton et al., 2018). Pressure injuries are localized injuries to the skin, underlying tissue, or both, usually over a bony prominence, because of pressure or pressure in combination with shear or friction. Pressure injuries occur in any age group or ethnic population, regardless of socioeconomic status (Norton et al., 2018).
- The major cause of pressure injuries is unrelieved pressure. The greater the pressure and the longer it is applied, the greater the likelihood for pressure injury development. When external pressure on the tissues exceeds 32 mm Hg (the capillary closing pressure), the network of capillaries collapses. This interrupts the supply of oxygen and nutrients to the cells and the removal of metabolic waste products. As a result, there is tissue ischemia and, if unrelieved, tissue death or necrosis.
- The best prevention for pressure injuries is frequent repositioning. Support surfaces are another important aspect of pressure injury prevention; however, their use still requires frequent repositioning for optimal effectiveness. Support surfaces are specialized devices (e.g., mattress overlays, mattress replacements, integrated bed systems, seat cushions, or seat cushion overlays) that redistribute

pressure and are designed for management of tissue loads, microclimate, shear, and other therapeutic functions (Bowman, 2015). Microclimate is the mean skin temperature and skin moisture between the patient's skin and the support surface (Norton et al., 2018; Wound, Ostomy and Continence Nurses Society [WOCN], 2016). Support surfaces are used in acute, rehabilitative, long-term, and home care settings. Support surfaces reduce pressure by redistributing it over a larger surface area. The extent to which a support surface reduces pressure is characterized in two ways. The first is preventive, in which pressure is not consistently reduced below 32 mm Hg (e.g., foam, air, or gel overlay). The second is therapeutic, in which pressure is consistently reduced below 32 mm Hg (e.g., powered overlay air mattress or low-air-loss mattress).

- Preventive surfaces are for patients at risk for skin breakdown and partial-thickness injury.
- Therapeutic surfaces are for patients at high risk for pressure injury development or for those with existing pressure injuries (Norton et al., 2018; WOCN, 2016). Support surfaces are one intervention for redistributing pressure; they are used in conjunction with other pressure injury risk-reduction strategies (see Chapter 39), including frequent repositioning.
- A reliable and valid tool should be used to complete a risk assessment related to pressure injuries (e.g., Braden scale [see Chapter 39] for adults; Braden Q scale [Noonan, Quigley, & Curley, 2011] or Braden DQ scale [Curley, Hasbani, Quigley, et al., 2018] for pediatric patients; the Norton scale [see Chapter 39]).

- Individuals at high risk for pressure injury should be placed on a pressure redistribution support surface (WOCN, 2016). Use specialized support surfaces (e.g., foam, air, or gel mattresses; beds; cushions) to reduce pressure (Qaseem, Mir, Starkey, et al., 2015).
- Pressure-redistribution surfaces are classified as nonpowered (formerly called *static*) support surfaces or powered (formerly called *dynamic*) support surfaces (National Pressure Ulcer Advisory Panel [NPUAP], 2014). Nonpowered support surfaces include mattresses or mattress overlays filled with air, water, gel, foam, or a combination of any of these. Powered support surfaces change the pressure beneath a patient, reducing the duration of any applied pressure. Many studies have reported the benefits demonstrated by pressure-redistribution surfaces in the prevention of pressure injuries (McInnes, Jammali-Blasi, Bell-Syer, et al., 2015).
- Several support surfaces also reduce friction, shear, and moisture. Support surfaces with a slick surface help decrease friction and shear. Surfaces with porous covers allow airflow, which reduces moisture, resulting in decreased risk for skin maceration. Table 13.1 provides a comparison of support surfaces.
- Frequent repositioning, which temporarily relieves pressure, is the backbone of prevention protocols. No bed or mattress eliminates the need for competent, person-centred nursing care and a regular, consistent repositioning regime. As a nurse, it is your responsibility to use appropriate repositioning schedules for patients in bed or in a chair (RNAO, 2005/2011, p. 23). Use lift teams and lifting devices to transfer patients from a regular

TABLE 13.1

Support Surfaces

Category and Mechanism of Action	Indications for Use	Advantages	Disadvantages
Support Surfaces and Overlays			
Foam Overlay (Available as an Overlay or in a Full Mattress)			
Reduces pressure; the cover (top) can reduce friction and shear. Base height of 7.5–10 cm (3–4 inches); see manufacturer guidelines regarding amount of body weight supported	Use for moderate- to high-risk patients	One-time charge No setup fee Cannot be punctured Available in various sizes (e.g., bed, chair, operating room table) Little maintenance Does not need electricity	Elevated body temperature Hot and may trap moisture Limited lifespan Plastic protective sheet needed for incontinent patients or patients with draining wounds Not indicated for those with existing stage 3 or 4 pressure injuries
Water Overlay (Available as an Overlay or in a Full Mattress)			
Reduces pressure and pressure points because surface provides flotation with pressure reduction by redistributing patient's weight evenly over entire support surface	Use for high-risk patients	Readily available Some control over motion sensations Easy to clean	Easily punctured Heavy Fluid motion may make procedures (e.g., dressing changes, CPR) difficult Maintenance needed to prevent microorganism growth Patient transfers out of bed are difficult Difficult to raise and lower head of bed
Gel Overlay			
Reduces pressure and pressure points because surface provides flotation by redistributing patient's weight evenly over entire support surface	Use for moderate- to high-risk patients Use for patients who are wheelchair dependent	Low maintenance Easy to clean Multiple-patient use Impermeable to needle punctures	Heavy Expensive Lacks airflow for moisture control Variable friction control

TABLE 13.1

Support Surfaces—cont'd

Category and Mechanism of Action	Indications for Use	Advantages	Disadvantages
Nonpowered Air-Filled Overlay			
Reduces pressure by lowering mean interface pressure between patient's tissue and mattress	Use for moderate- to high-risk patients Use for patients who can reposition themselves	Easy to clean Multiple-patient use Low maintenance Potential repair of some air-filled products Durable	Damaged by punctures from needles and sharps Requires routine monitoring to determine adequate inflation pressure Patient transfers out of bed are difficult
Low-Air-Loss Overlay (Available as an Overlay or in a Full Mattress)			
Maintains constant and slight air movement against patient's skin; also assists in managing the heat and humidity (microclimate) of the skin	Use for moderate- to high-risk patients	Easy to clean Maintains constant inflation Deflates to facilitate transfer and CPR Moisture control Fabric covering overlay is air permeable, bacteria impermeable, and waterproof Reduces shear and friction Setup provided by manufacturer	Damaged by needles and sharps Noisy Requires electricity, but some are available with short backup battery In home may need to purchase backup generator in case of loss of electrical power
Specialty Beds			
Air-Fluidized Bed			
Bedframe contains silicone-coated beads and provides pressure redistribution by the fluid-like medium that is created by forcing air through beads, resulting in immersion and envelopment of the patient.	Use for high-risk patients Use for patients with stage 3 or 4 pressure injuries or burns	Less frequent turning or repositioning Improved patient comfort Quickly becomes firm for CPR or other treatments when device is turned "off" Reduces shear, friction, and edema to site May facilitate management of copious wound drainage or incontinence Setup provided by manufacturer	Continuous circulation of warm, dry air may increase patient risk for dehydration Possible increase in room temperature Patient may experience disorientation Patient transfer difficult Heavy Expensive May not be wide enough for use with obese patients or patients with contractures Patient cannot lie prone because of risk of suffocation
Low-Air-Loss Bed			
Bedframe with series of connected air-filled pillows. The flow of air controls the amount of pressure in each pillow and assists in managing the heat and humidity (microclimate) of the patient's skin.	Use for patients who need pressure relief, those who cannot be repositioned frequently, or those who have skin breakdown on more than one surface Contraindicated in patients with unstable spinal column	Can raise and lower head and foot of bed Easy transfer in and out of bed Less frequent turning schedule Pillows can be transferred to stretcher with patient Setup provided by manufacturer	Portable motor is noisy Bed surface material is slippery; patients can easily slide down mattress or out of bed when being transferred
Kinetic Therapy			
Provides continuous passive motion to promote mobilization of pulmonary secretions and low air loss, which provides pressure relief	Use primarily for patients needing spinal stabilization Should not be used when the patient is hemodynamically unstable	Reduces pulmonary complications associated with restricted mobility Reduces risk for urinary stasis and urinary tract infections Reduces venous stasis	Does not reduce shear or moisture Cannot be used with cervical or skeletal traction Possible motion sickness initially Possible sensations of claustrophobia

Data from Doughty, D., & McNichol, L. (2016). *Wound, Ostomy and Continence Nurses Society (WOCN): Core curriculum: Wound management.* Philadelphia: Wound, Ostomy, and Continence Society; Wound, Ostomy and Continence Nurses Society (WOCN). (2016). *Guideline for prevention and management of pressure ulcers, WOCN clinical practice guideline series* (2nd ed.). Mt. Laurel, NJ: Author.

CPR, Cardiopulmonary resuscitation.

bed to a special support surface (see Chapter 11). Although useful, turning devices still injure soft tissues, requiring a nurse to be especially observant for signs of pressure formation.

PERSON-CENTRED CARE

- When making decisions about the best support surface for a patient, you must first complete a thorough patient assessment, including individual needs, health care provider needs, and location of the patient.
- Ultimately the features of the support surface must match a patient's unique needs and circumstance, demonstrating person-centred care.
- Always describe to a patient and caregiver which interventions will be instituted and allow time for questions as needed.
- Some cultural groups may hesitate to ask questions or ask for help, especially when they have limited English communication.
- Educate the patient and caregiver on all of the features of the support surface, provide a demonstration, and observe return demonstration of these features.

EVIDENCE-INFORMED PRACTICE

Pressure injuries can be partially controlled by an appropriate support surface. Evidence suggests that pressure redistribution devices can reduce the incidence of pressure injuries by 60% (Doughty & McNichol, 2016).

- Pressure reduction and relief are major nursing interventions for the prevention of pressure injuries (Doughty & McNichol, 2016; McInnes et al., 2015).
- Pressure-redistribution surfaces need to serve as adjuncts and not replacements for repositioning protocols (Doughty & McNichol, 2016).
- There is insufficient evidence to support one specific pressure redistribution surface or design over another for the prevention of pressure injuries (Norton et al., 2018; WOCN, 2016).
- There is emerging evidence that a dressing with a slippery backing placed over areas at risk for pressure injury development reduces friction and shear and may lower the incidence of pressure injuries (Norton et al., 2018).
- High-specification foam mattress compared with a standard hospital mattress with foam overlay is effective in decreasing the incidence of pressure injuries in high-risk patients (WOCN, 2016).
- Encourage patients to be up as soon as medically possible in a specialty chair or wheelchair equipped with a tailored support surface for pressure relief.

- Measure seat cushions so they are properly fitted to the person's body type and chair size to prevent friction and pressure.
- Pressure distribution surfaces should be used in the operating room for individuals assessed to be at high risk for pressure injury development, especially in older adult and bariatric patients. Pressure redistribution has been associated with a decreased incidence of postoperative pressure injuries (Broome, Ayala, Georgeson, et al., 2015; WOCN, 2016).

SAFETY GUIDELINES

- Using a valid and reliable tool, perform a complete assessment to determine patient's risk for pressure injuries. A complete patient assessment includes use of appropriate pressure injury risk scales, which include factors such as presence of shear and friction and a patient's mobility and continence status (RNAO, 2011, p. 9) (see Chapter 39).
- Select a support surface based on the patient's risk for developing pressure injuries, such as impaired mobility, need for microclimate control, reduction of shear, and size and weight of patient.
- Know the reason for and extent of a patient's reduced mobility. A patient who is not easy to reposition or who has pressure injuries involving multiple surfaces benefits from pressure-redistribution support devices.
- Strict monitoring for signs of pressure injury is required with the use of incontinence products or devices, as they may contribute to increased pressure (Norton et al., 2018).
- Continue to provide basic prevention care measures against the hazards of immobility (e.g., regular skin assessment, turning, correct positioning, or range-of-motion exercises).
- Use safe patient-handling techniques and proper body mechanics when positioning or working with patients (see Chapter 11).
- Follow all safety measures to prevent injury to patients from accidental falls or improper positioning when placing them on special beds or mattresses.
- Educate caregivers about the advantages and disadvantages and methods of operation of all support devices to ensure their proper use in all settings.
- Use interprofessional collaboration (e.g., wound care nurse, physiotherapist) to maximize preventative strategies and patient safety.

PROCEDURAL GUIDELINE 13.1 *Selection of a Pressure-Redistribution Support Surface*

Delegation and Collaboration

The selection of a pressure-redistribution support device cannot be delegated to an unregulated care provider (UCP).

Equipment

- Pressure injury risk assessment tool (see employer policy) (see Chapter 39)
- Body chart, tape measure, and/or camera to document existing areas of impaired skin integrity
- Documentation form or electronic health record
- Skin-care products

Procedural Steps

1. Assess patient's risk for skin breakdown using an appropriate risk assessment tool (e.g., Braden Scale score [adult patient]: ≤18 indicates "at risk" or Braden Q score [pediatric patient]: ≤16 indicates "at risk" and ≤9 indicates "very high risk" (see Tables 39.1 and 39.2).
2. Assess patient's existing pressure injuries, including location, stage, areas of blistering, abnormal reactive hyperemia, and abrasion.
3. Consider patient weight and weight distribution and the following risk factors and comorbidities: advanced age, fever,

PROCEDURAL GUIDELINE 13.1 *Selection of a Pressure-Redistribution Support Surface—cont'd*

poor dietary intake of protein, diastolic pressure <60 mm Hg, hemodynamic instability, generalized edema, and anemia (WOCN, 2016).

4. Assess patient's level of comfort using an appropriate pain rating scale (e.g., scale of 0 [no pain] to 10 [worst pain ever]).

5. Determine the need for a pressure-reduction surface from assessment data. Place "at-risk" patients on a pressure-reduction surface, high-specification foam mattress and not on a standard hospital mattress (WOCN, 2016).

6. Identify patient factors when selecting an appropriate surface (Fig. 13.1):

a. Braden Scale score ≤18 and Braden Q scale ≤16.

b. Does the patient need pressure redistribution (e.g., you cannot reposition the patient, or there is an existing pressure injury)?

WOCN Society's Evidence- and Consensus-Based Support Surface Algorithm

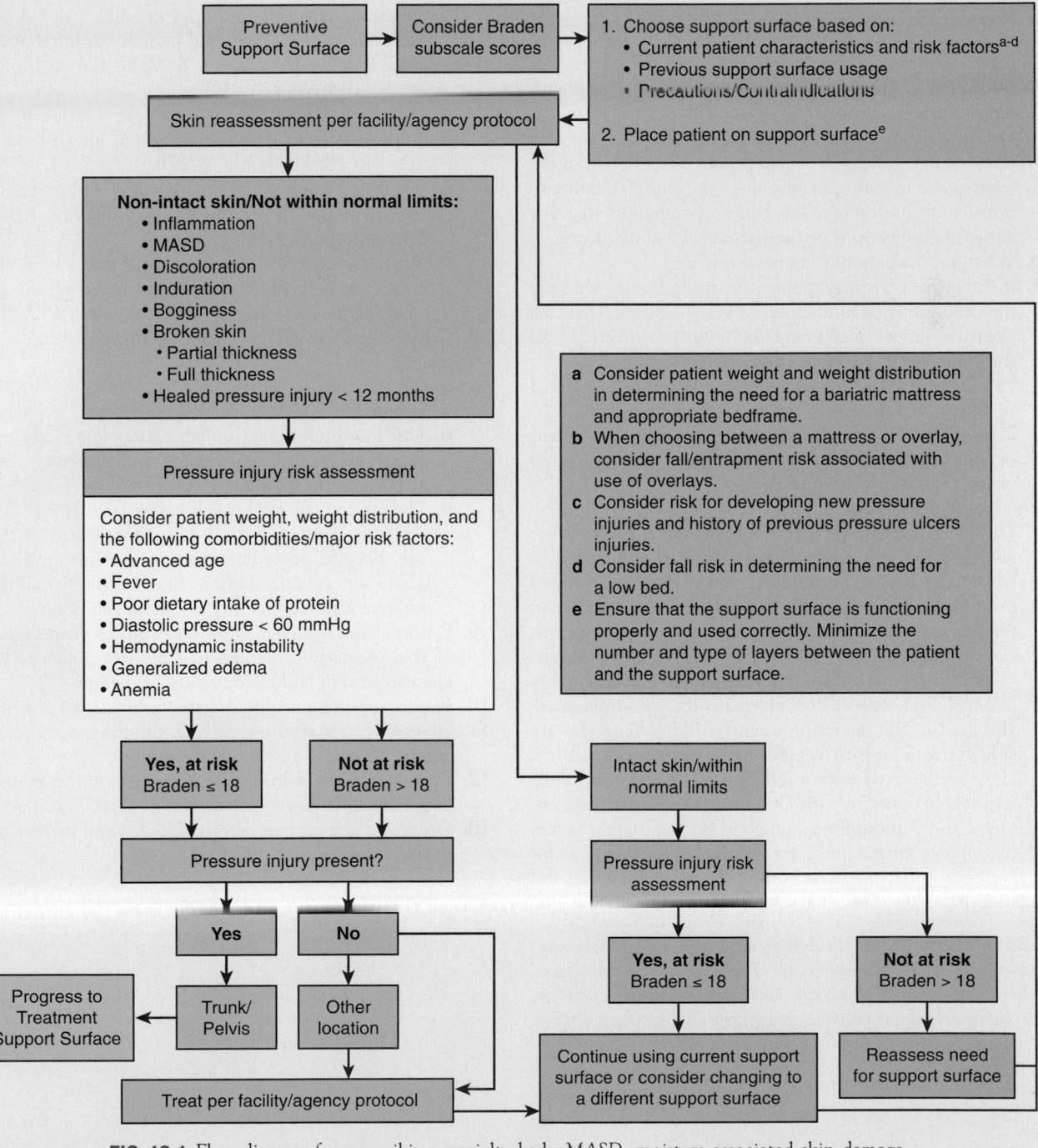

FIG 13.1 Flow diagram for prescribing specialty beds. *MASD,* moisture-associated skin damage. *(Modified from McNichol, L., Watts, C., Mackey, D., Beitz, J. M., & Gray, M. [2015]. Identifying the right surface for the right patient at the right time: Generation and content validation of an algorithm for support surface selection. Journal of Wound, Ostomy and Continence Nursing, 42[1], p. 32 [Fig 1].)*

Continued

PROCEDURAL GUIDELINE 13.1 *Selection of a Pressure-Redistribution Support Surface—cont'd*

c. Is the surface needed for short- or long-term care? A short-term surface is usually needed for an acute illness and hospitalization. A long-term surface is usually needed for extended or home care.

d. What is the potential comfort level achieved by the surface? If the patient is sensitive to noise, a device with a loud motor will increase discomfort.

e. Are the patient and caregiver cooperative and adherent to repositioning? In addition, are they aware that a support surface should never replace repositioning? Is adequate help available for repositioning? In a home setting a support surface is often necessary when the caregiver or patient is unable to reposition independently or help with repositioning.

f. Does the support surface have a potential to interfere with the patient's independent functioning? The height of the overlay and its soft edge may affect the patient's ability to transfer, and a high-air-loss bed is not appropriate for a patient who needs to get in and out of bed frequently.

g. What are the patient's financial resources?

h. If the patient is using the device in the home, what are the environmental limitations? Will the home and existing electrical service accommodate the surface selected? Can the caregiver in the home manage the surface?

i. How durable is the product? Is the surface easily subjected to puncture? How easily can the surface be cleaned?

j. Does the patient need pressure-relief surfaces in a chair or wheelchair? Has the family or caregiver been instructed on appropriate inflation of the device?

7. Choose the appropriate surface (see Table 13.1).

a. Pressure-redistribution devices redistribute the pressure and load over the control area of the patient's body to reduce the overall pressure and avoid areas of localized pressure (WOCN, 2016). Surfaces providing pressure redistribution include therapeutic mattress replacements, nonpowered and powered (e.g., moving) surfaces, low-air-loss beds and mattresses, and air-fluidized beds (Doughty & McNichol, 2016). Pressure-redistribution surfaces are also used in the operating room for individuals who are at high risk or for lengthy procedures (Broome et al., 2015).

b. Use a nonpowered support surface if the patient can assume a variety of positions without bearing weight on a pressure injury and without bottoming out. Bottoming out makes the support surface ineffective because it is inadequate for patient's weight and the body sinks too deeply into the surface.

c. Select a powered support surface when the patient cannot assume a variety of positions without bearing weight on a pressure injury, if patient fully compresses the nonpowered support surface, or if the pressure injury does not show evidence of healing. Alternating or powered mattresses are associated with lower incidence of pressure injuries compared with standard mattresses (Doughty & McNichol, 2016).

d. High-specification foam is effective in decreasing the incidence of pressure injuries in fairly high-risk patients, including older persons and patients with fractures of the neck and femur (Doughty & McNichol, 2016; McInnes et al., 2015; WOCN, 2016).

e. Patients with stage 3 or 4 pressure injuries on multiple turning surfaces often benefit from an air-fluidized bed (Doughty & McNichol, 2016).

f. There is limited evidence that low-air-loss beds reduce the incidence of pressure injuries in critical care units (Doughty & McNichol, 2016).

g. When excess moisture is a potential risk, a support surface that provides airflow is important in drying the skin and reducing the incidence of pressure injuries (WOCN, 2016).

8. Check employer policy regarding implementing a support surface.

a. Obtain a health care provider's prescription. This is usually required for a patient to obtain third-party reimbursement.

b. Use interprofessional collaboration (e.g., case manager, social worker) to help patient and caregiver obtain the required surface product.

c. Use interprofessional collaboration (e.g., home care nurse, discharge planner) if the device is anticipated for long-term use. Specific procedures and evaluations are needed for continuity of surface when patient is transitioning care to an extended care facility or discharged home.

9. Perform hand hygiene. Apply clean gloves. Inspect condition of skin regularly according to employer policy to evaluate changes in skin and effectiveness of therapy.

10. Inspect existing pressure injuries for evidence of healing.

11. Observe for side effects associated with the specific pressure-reducing surface (e.g., nausea, dizziness).

12. Document pressure injury risk assessment and skin assessment in patient's electronic health record (EHR) or chart.

13. Document the support surface selected and patient response to the surface in patient's EHR or chart.

Clinical Decision Point *Hand checks are a satisfactory but subjective method for assessing for "bottoming out" of static air overlay mattresses. According to the NPUAP, the hand check method is inappropriate for replacement mattresses and integrated bed systems (bedframe and support surfaces) (Call, Deppisch, Jordan, et al., 2015; WOCN, 2016).*

◆ SKILL 13.1   Placing a Patient on a Support Surface

There are numerous support surfaces to reduce pressure on tissues overlying bony prominences. These devices are recommended for preventive measures for patients with reduced mobility and risk for developing pressure injuries. Most of the devices are easy to apply and keep clean. The extent to which the devices actually reduce pressure and prevent skin breakdown is highly variable.

Support surfaces are categorized as mattress (or wheelchair) overlays (Fig. 13.2), mattress replacements, or specialty beds. An overlay rests on top of a hospital mattress and uses foam, air, water, gel, or combinations of these products to provide pressure relief. Mattress overlays and mattress replacements are either nonpowered (e.g., foam, gels) or powered (e.g., alternating-pressure surfaces).

A flotation pad is made of a silicone or polyvinyl-chloride gel enclosed in a vinyl-covered square. The pad serves as an artificial layer of fat to protect bony surfaces such as the sacrum and greater trochanters. These flotation pads are available for the bed or wheelchair (Fig. 13.3).

There are two types of foam mattresses. One is the foam mattress overlay, which has a flat smooth surface, foam rubber peaks (egg-crate, Fig. 13.4), or a cut surface. Place one on top of a bed mattress and place a sheet over the foam mattress pad overlay to prevent soiling and provide ease of cleaning. The second type is the high-specification foam specialty mattress, which completely replaces the hospital mattress and is covered by a loose-fitting cover intended to protect the mattress and minimize friction and shear. Some of the newer foam mattresses have memory and an increased lifespan. The memory foam molds to the shape of the body and reduces pressure to the area in contact with the foam.

One type of air mattress is fully integrated into the hospital bed or designed to be placed in a wheelchair (Fig. 13.5). The nurse can adjust this bed surface to a patient's comfort level by adding or removing air through buttons within the patient's reach, or pressures can be automatically adjusted to a patient's position and movement when in the automatic mode. Always use a bedsheet to cover an air mattress to prevent skin from touching the plastic surface. Always be cautious of patient safety: overinflation may cause the patient to fall or "flip" out of the bed; underinflation could result in patient entrapment (i.e., the patient is "trapped" between the mattress and the bed rail). There is inconclusive evidence regarding the effectiveness of the use of constant low-pressure and alternating-pressure air support surfaces in preventing pressure injuries (McInnes et al., 2015).

Air mattress overlays are either nonpowered or powered and consist of interconnected air cells or cushions inflated using a motorized blower (Fig. 13.6). More complex air mattresses contain several layers

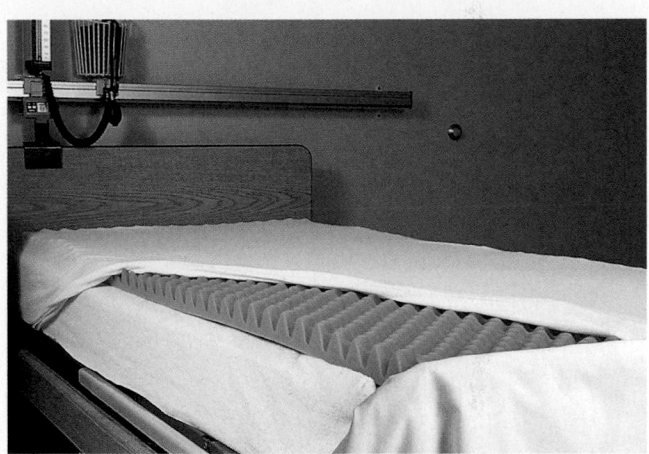

FIG 13.4 Egg-crate foam overlay is primarily for comfort.

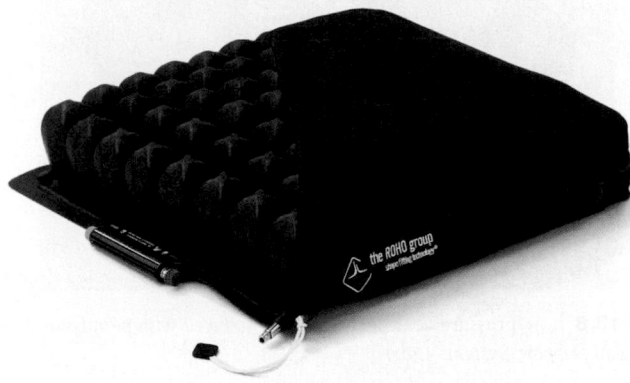

FIG 13.2 ROHO cushion for wheelchair. (© *ROHO Group. Reprinted with permission. All rights reserved.*)

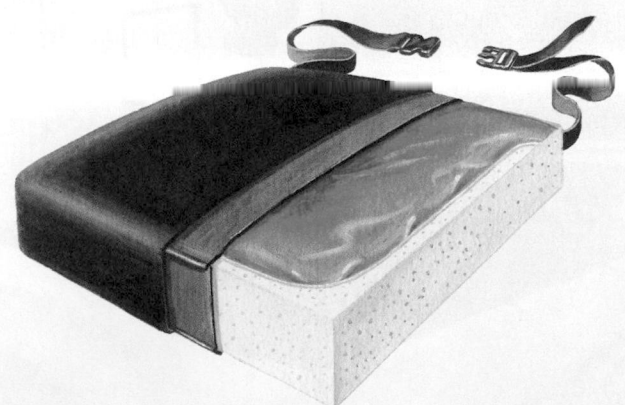

FIG 13.3 Gel cushion for wheelchair. (© *Skil-Care Corp. Reprinted with permission. All rights reserved.*)

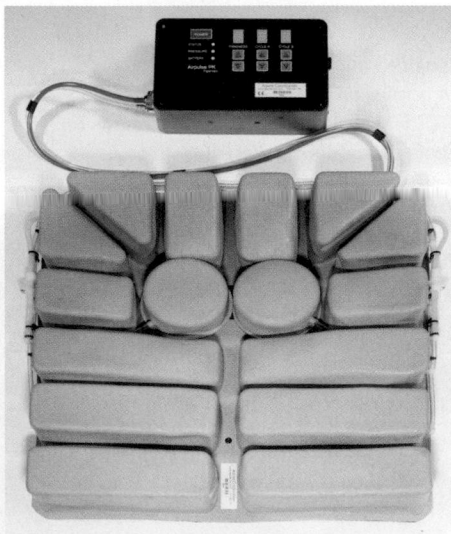

FIG 13.5 Air-filled cushion for wheelchair. (© *Aquila Corporation, Reprinted with permission. All rights reserved.*)

of tubes or support cells. These mattresses use a pressure-cycling device to intermittently inflate and deflate or to maintain a constant inflation and slight air movement in the mattress.

A nonpowered support surface is inflated with a simple air blower after placing the mattress on a bed. An integrated air mattress connects with a pressure-cycling device that intermittently inflates and deflates sections of the mattress, creating a cycling effect that minimizes pressure on bony prominences (Fig. 13.7).

Replacement mattresses have foam, gel, air, or fluid sections that can be customized to the needs of a specific patient with moderate-to-high risk for skin breakdown. Another available option is an air-integrated replacement mattress instead of the conventional mattress. These mattresses may also be fully integrated into the bed. Air mattresses are usually for patients with moderate to high risk for skin breakdown. Air mattresses must be deflated before initiating cardiopulmonary resuscitation (CPR). Many facilities have purchased replacement mattresses to replace their standard hospital mattresses because of improved skin and wound outcomes.

Another preventive intervention is a low-pressure seat cushion (Fig. 13.8) overlaid on a wheelchair, or a dry, nonpowered flotation mattress system (Fig. 13.9) that can be overlaid on a bed. Through a system of controlled dynamics, a cushion maintains low pressures by distributing pressure across a patient's body surface, reducing friction and shear. Although seat cushions may increase patient comfort, their effectiveness in preventing pressure injuries has not yet been determined (McInnes et al., 2015).

Support surfaces aid in reducing pressure on a patient's skin but do not replace regular repositioning, meticulous skin assessment and skin care, or range-of-motion exercises; these interventions are the hallmarks of pressure injury preventative care. Use interprofessional collaboration (e.g., with occupational therapist, physiotherapist) to arrive at evidence-informed decisions to place a patient on a pressure-redistribution surface and to determine which support surface is best for the patient (see Procedural Guideline 13.1).

Delegation and Collaboration

The skill of placing a patient on a support surface can be delegated to an unregulated care provider (UCP). However, the nurse must first complete the assessment, determine the need for a support surface, and select the specific surface. Some types of support surfaces require that a manufacturer representative set up and maintain the support system. The nurse directs the UCP to:

• Notify the nurse of any changes in a patient's skin; the nurse then assesses the condition of the skin.

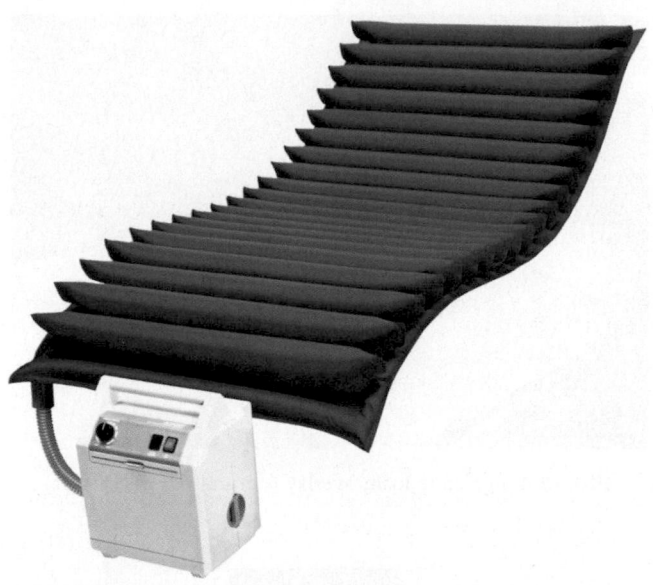

FIG 13.6 Dynamic air mattress overlay. (© 2002 Hill-Rom Services. Reprinted with permission. All rights reserved.)

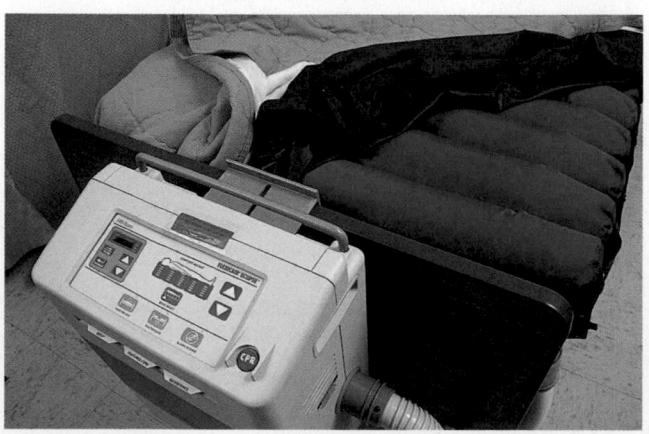

FIG 13.7 Motor for integrated air mattress.

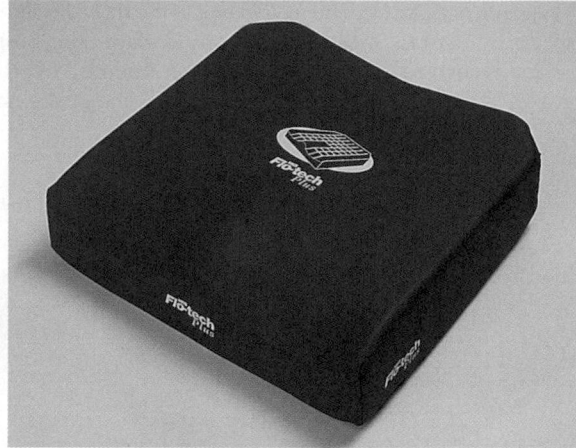

FIG 13.8 Low-pressure seat cushion. (Reproduced with permission from Medical Support Systems Ltd.)

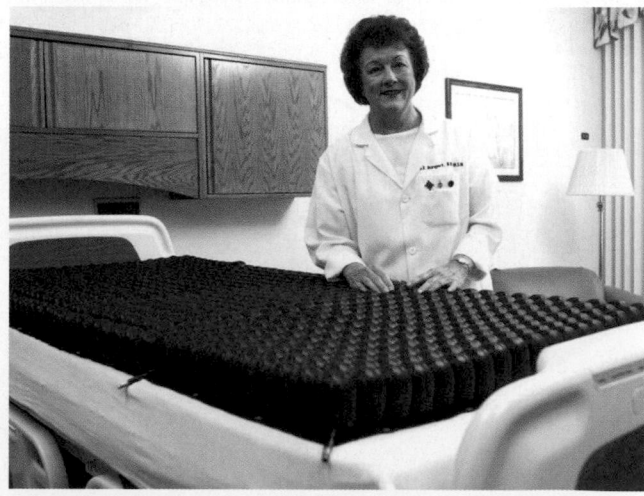

FIG 13.9 ROHO dry flotation mattress for bed. (© The ROHO Group. Reprinted with permission. All rights reserved.)

- Continue to regularly turn and reposition a patient and seek help for patient position changes as necessary in bed or a wheelchair.
- Monitor the normal functioning of the support device, such as inflation and deflation cycles, and report to the nurse any changes in these cycles or leakage of air, water, or gel.

Equipment

- Pressure injury risk-assessment tool (see employer policy) (see Chapter 39)

- Mattress and/or chair overlay support surface of choice: foam overlays, air mattress overlay, bed with integrated surface, air-integrated replacement mattress
- Sheet(s)
- Clean gloves (if soiled linen is being handled)
- Standard bedframe (with mattress) if overlay is to be used (*optional*)

STEP	RATIONALE

ASSESSMENT

STEP	RATIONALE
1. Identify patient using at least two person-specific identifiers (e.g., name and date of birth or name and medical record number) according to employer policy.	Ensures correct patient. Complies with Accreditation Canada's standards and improves patient safety (Accreditation Canada, 2019).
2. Perform hand hygiene.	Reduces transmission of microorganisms.
3. Determine patient's risk for pressure injury formation using a valid assessment tool (e.g., Braden Scale) and assess for risk factors for pressure injuries (e.g., nutritional deficits, shear stress, friction, alterations in mobility and sensory perception, moisture, and abnormal serum albumin and hemoglobin levels) (see Chapter 39).	Risk assessment tools provide an objective, reliable, and valid measure of risk consistent over time (Doughty & McNichol, 2016).

Clinical Decision Point *Patients with unstable conditions do not always tolerate turning or positioning required for thorough assessment or the application of a support surface mattress.*

STEP	RATIONALE
4. Perform skin assessment (see Chapters 8 and 39). Inspect condition of skin, especially over dependent sites and bony prominences.	Provides baseline to determine change in skin integrity or in existing pressure injury.
5. Assess patient's level of comfort using an appropriate pain rating scale.	Provides baseline to determine patient's response to therapy and comfort needs.

Clinical Decision Point *Some patients experiencing pain need pain medication before application of support surface of choice or transfer to another bed (NPUAP, 2014; WOCN, 2016).*

STEP	RATIONALE
6. Assess patient's understanding of purpose of support surface.	Misconceptions affect patient's cooperation in use of mattress.
7. Verify health care provider's prescription for type of support surface.	Health care provider's prescription is usually required to ensure third-party payment of support surface.

NURSING DIAGNOSES

- Insufficient peripheral tissue perfusion
- Reduced physical mobility
- Reduced skin integrity
- Pain (acute, chronic)
- Insufficient knowledge regarding use of support surface mattress
- Potential for impaired skin integrity
- Potential for infection

Related factors/Risk factors are individualized on the basis of patient's condition or needs.

PLANNING

STEP	RATIONALE
1. Expected outcomes following completion of procedure:	
• Patient's skin is without erythema or mottling.	Mottling represents hypoxia, which is an abnormal physiological response in tissues under pressure.
• Existing pressure injury shows signs of healing.	Skin remains free of new pressure injuries. Support surface does not interfere with circulation to dependent areas.
• Patient expresses improved level of comfort.	Equalized pressures have eliminated localized areas of discomfort.
• Patient is removed from therapeutic surface when risk for pressure injuries decreases.	Provides for efficient, cost-effective care while maintaining high-quality outcomes.
2. Explain purpose of mattress and method of application to patient and caregiver.	Reduces anxiety and promotes cooperation.

STEP	RATIONALE

IMPLEMENTATION

1. Close room door or bedside curtain. | Provides patient privacy and demonstrates person-centred care during application of mattress to bed or transfer to alternative bed.

2. Perform hand hygiene. Apply clean gloves (if linens are soiled or wet). Get help to position patient or mattress as needed. | Prevents transmission of microorganisms. Assistance from other caregivers reduces risk for friction and shear in transfer to new surface.

3. Apply support surface to bed or prepare alternative bed (bed may be occupied or unoccupied). Keep sharp objects away from air mattress or air-surface bed.

   a. Replacing mattress:

   (1) Apply mattress to bedframe after removing standard hospital mattress. | Hospital mattress needs to be stored. In some instances, mattress replacements are standard procedure.

   (2) Apply sheet over mattress. Keep linens between surfaces to a minimum. | Sheet reduces soiling. Multiple layers decrease surface effectiveness in reducing pressure (Doughty & McNichol, 2016).

   b. Preparing an air mattress/overlay:

   (1) Apply deflated mattress flat over surface of bed mattress. (There may be directions on pad indicating which side to place up.) | Provides smooth, even surface.

   (2) Bring any plastic strips or flaps around corners of bed mattress. | Secures air mattress in place.

   (3) Attach connector on air mattress to inflation device. Inflate mattress to proper air pressure determined by air pump or blower. | Mattresses vary as to requiring one-time or continuous inflation cycle. Check inflation daily. Manufacturer directions indicate desired air pressure designed to distribute patient's body weight evenly. Directions are included with each mattress.

   (4) Place sheet over air mattress, being sure to eliminate all wrinkles. | Prevents soiling of mattress; reduces direct contact of skin with plastic surface. Wrinkles can cause pressure.

Clinical Decision Point *Avoid placing excessive linens and incontinence pads on top of support surface. This can interfere with functioning of support surface (NPUAP, 2014; WOCN, 2016).*

   (5) Check air pumps to be sure that pressure cycle alternates. | Alternating airflow mattress produces intermittent cycling, inflating only parts of mattress at any one time. Intermittent cycle continually alternates pressure against skin and soft tissue.

   (6) Help patient transfer in and out of bed. | Mattress surface is less firm and slippery. This makes it difficult for some patients to transfer from bed to chair or stretcher.

   c. Using an air-surface bed:

   (1) Obtain and place linen on bed. | In some instances, an air-surface bed is available in patient rooms. If not, an ordering system exists to obtain one as needed (see employer policy).

   (2) Place switch in "prevention" mode. | In "prevention" mode, surface pressures change automatically with patient position to equalize pressure and eliminate points of pressure.

Clinical Decision Point *Most pressure-relieving beds are equipped with a CPR switch to instantly lower head section from an elevated position and deflate the mattress to provide a firm surface for chest compressions (Fig. 13.10). Note this on the patient's record.*

4. Position patient comfortably as desired over support surface. Reposition frequently, according to employer policy. | Location of existing pressure injury might influence type of positioning (Doughty & McNichol, 2016).

5. Remove and dispose of gloves and perform hand hygiene. | Reduces transmission of microorganisms.

STEP	RATIONALE

IMPLEMENTATION

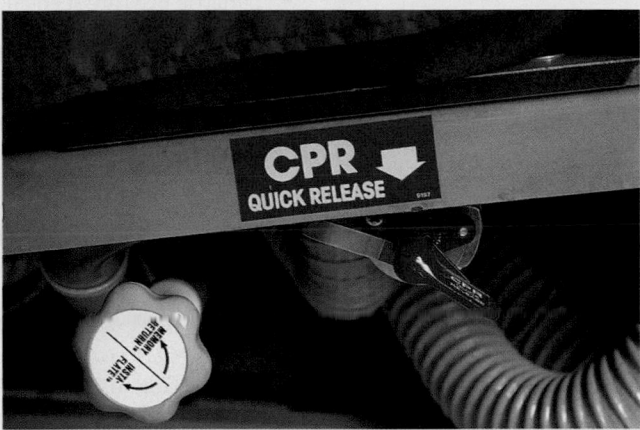

FIG 13.10 Cardiopulmonary resuscitation (CPR) switch deflates low-air-loss bed to provide hard surface.

EVALUATION

1. Reassess patient's risk for pressure injury formation at routine intervals.

Documents change in status, which is critical for evaluating continued need for therapeutic surface.

2. Inspect and compare condition of patient's skin every 8 hours or according to employer policy to determine changes in skin integrity, pressure injury status, and effectiveness of support surface.

Determines if pressure sores develop or if condition of existing sores changes.

3. Ask patient to rate comfort on an appropriate pain rating scale.

If pressure-relief mattress is effective, patient generally experiences less discomfort.

4. Evaluate functioning of support surface periodically.

Regular inspection of mechanical components of mattress ensures proper functioning (WOCN, 2016).

5. **Use Teach-Back:** "I want to be sure I explained why we put your mother on this special bed. Tell me why we placed her on this type of bed." Develop a revised teaching plan if caregiver is not able to teach back correctly.

Determines caregiver's level of understanding of instructional topic.

Unexpected Outcomes

1. Patient develops localized areas of abnormal reactive hyperemia for longer than 30 minutes, mottling, swelling, and tenderness with evidence of skin breakdown.

2. Existing pressure areas fail to heal or increase in size or depth.

3. Patient expresses discomfort while on support surface.

Related Interventions

- Modify skin-care regimen.
- Increase frequency of skin assessment.
- Increase types of pressure-relief interventions.
- Check for proper inflation of support surface.
- Revise turning schedule.
- Consult with skin-care expert.
- Notify health care provider.
- Modify skin-care regimen.
- Revise turning schedule.
- Consult with skin-care expert.
- Notify health care provider.
- Evaluate need for analgesia or mild sedation.
- Evaluate need to modify support surface.
- Reposition patient more frequently.
- Unless contraindicated, provide back massage. Do not massage reddened areas or bony prominences because massage to these areas contributes to skin breakdown (Doughty & McNichol, 2016).

Communication and Documentation

- Document type of support surface applied, extent to which patient tolerated procedure, and condition of patient's skin in nurses' notes in electronic health record (EHR) or chart and/or skin assessment flow sheet.
- Document your evaluation of patient and caregiver learning.
- Report evidence of pressure injury formation to nurse in charge or health care provider.

Special Considerations
Teaching

- Explain risks of immobility and pressure injury formation to patient and caregivers (see Chapter 39).
- Instruct in proper use of body mechanics, positioning, and pressure relief methods.
- Explain purpose and function of the pressure-redistribution surface. Include reminder that the surface augments care and does not replace the need for turning and pressure-relief manouevres.
- Explain precautions regarding sharp objects and fire hazards.

Pediatric

- Use a pressure injury risk assessment tool that has been developed specifically for use in children.
- Parent or guardian can support children in being able to express their pain and treatment preferences related to pressure injuries (Hockenberry & Wilson, 2015).

Gerontological

- Implement preventive measures because an older person's skin is drier, thinner, and less pressure sensitive, increasing the risk for skin breakdown.

- Adding mattress overlays changes the bed height. Use care when transferring and teaching caregiver to transfer a patient from bed to chair.

Patients Living With Obesity

- Bariatric beds are specialized beds designed to support increased weight and provide comfort for patients who are living with obesity.
- Patients living with obesity report a devaluation of self, embarrassment in social situations, embarrassment about appearance, repeated failure of weight loss diets, and frustration arising from activity limitations (Pories & Rose, 2017).
- Evidence suggests that the stigma of obesity and weight bias has increased in recent years. It is important to implement strategies for eliminating negative attitudes toward patients living with obesity on an interpersonal and systemwide basis (Pories & Rose, 2017).
- Practise person-centred care and engage in respectful dialogue when caring for patients living with obesity, recognize societal stigma and biases, and maintain patients' dignity at all times.

Care in the Community

- Most of the devices may be adapted for home use on a standard twin bed or hospital bed.
- Base selection on patient needs and environmental audit as part of person-centred care in the community. For example, a patient on total bed rest who smokes is not an ideal candidate for a foam mattress because of the potential for fire; a patient with pets that sleep in the bed is not suited for an air-filled mattress because of the risk for puncture.
- Address concerns in the home setting related to need for a backup generator or other plan to maintain the support surface during power outages.

✦ SKILL 13.2 **Placing a Patient on a Special Bed**

Air-suspension beds are designed for patients who are immobile or confined to bed. The air-suspension bed supports a patient's weight on air-filled cushions. There are two types of systems: low air loss and high air loss. A low-air-loss system minimizes pressure and reduces shear. In this type of system, air flow is provided to assist in managing the heat and humidity (microclimate) of the patient's skin (WOCN, 2016). If a patient has large stage 3 or 4 pressure injuries on multiple turning surfaces of the skin, a low-air-loss bed or air-fluidized bed may be indicated. If wounds are not healing, a change in support surface is indicated and should be matched to the patient's needs (Doughty & McNichol, 2016).

High-air-loss beds provide for selective drying and do not increase insensible fluid losses. For patients requiring high air loss under a body part (e.g., under the buttocks), high-air-loss cushions can be substituted. It is also possible to adapt the air-suspension beds to individual patient needs with specialty cushions for positioning, foot support, and lateral arm supports.

Another adaptation of the air-suspension bed is the kinetic low-air-loss bed (Fig. 13.11). This bed is used in critical care areas and can provide a pressure-relief surface while rotating approximately 30 to 35 degrees continuously. Do not use this surface with a patient who has an unstable spine or who is in traction.

An air-fluidized or combination bed is a powered device designed to distribute a patient's weight evenly over its support surface (Fig. 13.12). In this type of system, pressure redistribution occurs by a fluid-like medium that is created by forcing air through beads

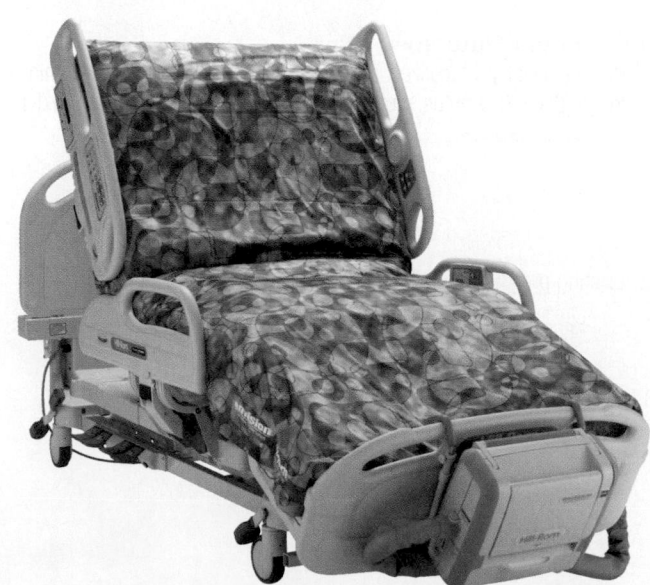

FIG 13.11 Low-air-loss bed. (© 2002 Hill-Rom Services. *Reprinted with permission. All rights reserved.*)

(microspheres). The bed minimizes pressure and reduces shearing force and friction through the principle of fluidization. Fluidization is created by forcing a gentle flow of temperature-controlled air upward through a mass of fine ceramic microspheres (WOCN, 2016). The patient lies directly on a polyester filter sheet that allows air to pass through but does not allow the microspheres to escape. Patients feel as though they are floating on a surface such as a warm waterbed. Air-fluidized beds are effective in promoting positive outcomes (e.g., faster and complete healing, reduced rate of pressure injury–related admissions) for patients with stage 2 or greater pressure injuries compared with other active support surfaces and standard hospital mattresses (Haesler, 2018).

Air-fluidized beds are useful in the care of patients who require minimal movement to prevent skin damage by shearing force and for patients who experience significant pain when being turned or positioned (e.g., burn patients, those who have undergone extensive skin grafts or have existing pressure injuries, and victims of multiple trauma). Patients tend to perspire and lose body fluids while on the bed because the surface of the filter sheet warms. As patients perspire, moisture is quickly absorbed into the circulating microspheres. Diaphoresis often goes undetected; thus, insensible fluid loss is not always evident until a patient develops fluid and electrolyte imbalances. Therefore, the nurse needs to monitor the patient's fluid balance status carefully.

Head-of-bed position changes are not possible with some conventional fluidized beds. Use foam wedges to elevate the head. Combinations of fluidized-low-air-loss beds that allow head-of-bed elevation are also available. These beds use air to lift the upper body while the lower body stays on a fluidized bed surface. The weight of the bed structure makes transport extremely difficult. A pediatric version of this bed is available.

A valuable resource in the care of a morbidly obese patient (a person who weighs more than 45.4 kg [100 lb] above ideal weight) is the bariatric bed (Fig. 13.13). The bariatric bed can allow upright or sitting positions, patient transport, and in-bed scale use. It is equipped with hand controls that allow self-positioning and facilitate independence for an obese patient. The full-function hand controls also allow the nurse to change the bed position and thus facilitate care while reducing risk for staff injury when moving a patient. The in-bed scale provides the nurse with a means of obtaining accurate weights and thus improves health care and patient dignity. The bed is slightly wider than a standard hospital bed; yet it is within the guidelines for standard door width, which allows movement into and out of a room without difficulty. Because the bariatric bed is capable of supporting weights up to 453.6 kg (1000 lb) (Hill-Rom Services, 2018), it provides a stable, balanced surface that limits hospital liability should the standard bedframe collapse or the electric motor burn out.

A limitation of this bed is the lack of pressure reduction or relief in the mattress. An at-risk patient who is obese needs to have some type of pressure-redistribution mattress placed on the bariatric bed. Choices for pressure redistribution include air or gel type of mattresses and low-air-loss replacement systems. These beds also have cardiopulmonary resuscitation (CPR) switches, which permit an immediate hard surface for chest compressions.

The Rotokinetic bed helps maintain skeletal alignment while providing constant rotation (Fig. 13.14). It is used in the care of patients with spinal cord injuries or multiple traumas. The support structure of the bed outlines the body parts and maintains proper alignment when secured properly. This bed improves skeletal alignment with constant side-to-side rotation up to 90 degrees. It rotates from side to side at a 60- to 90-degree angle every 7 minutes. The nurse may adjust turning angles to meet a patient's needs. Constant rotation reduces pressure injury development and stimulates body systems. It is recommended that the bed stay in the rotation mode for at least 20 hours a day. There is an emergency lever that can quickly interrupt rotation when needed. To initiate CPR, return the bed to the horizontal position and lock in place.

The constant motion often leads to sensory distress for patients, especially older persons. This is associated with the constant kinetic stimulation, the limited visual field, and inner ear disequilibrium. Be aware of these complications and provide necessary emotional support.

Delegation and Collaboration

The skill of placing a patient on a specialty bed can be delegated an unregulated care provider (UCP). However, first the nurse completes the assessment, determines the need for a support surface,

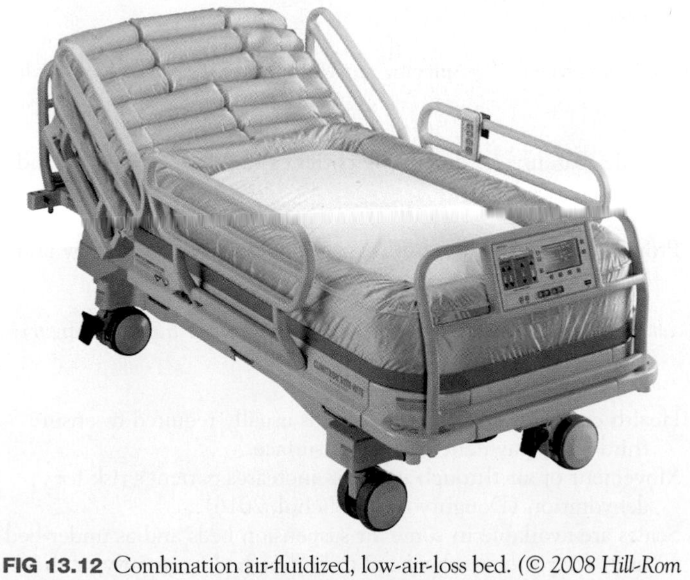

FIG 13.12 Combination air-fluidized, low-air-loss bed. (© 2008 Hill-Rom Services. Reprinted with permission. All rights reserved.)

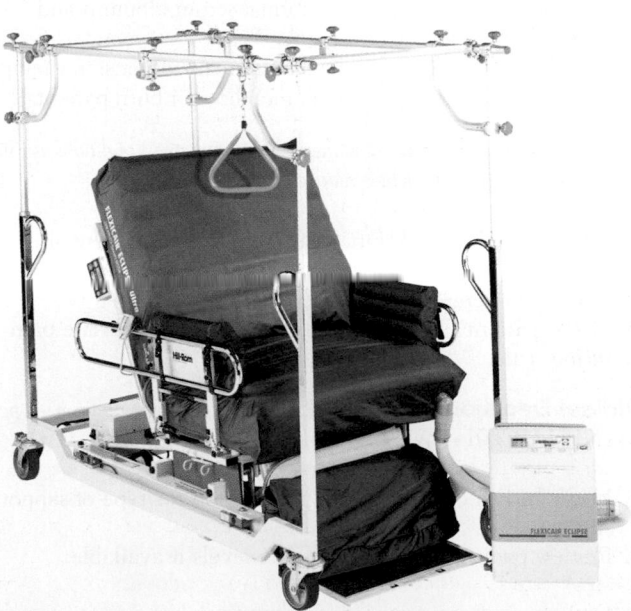

FIG 13.13 Bariatric bed with low-air-loss mattress replacement. (© 2008 Hill-Rom Services. Reprinted with permission. All rights reserved.)

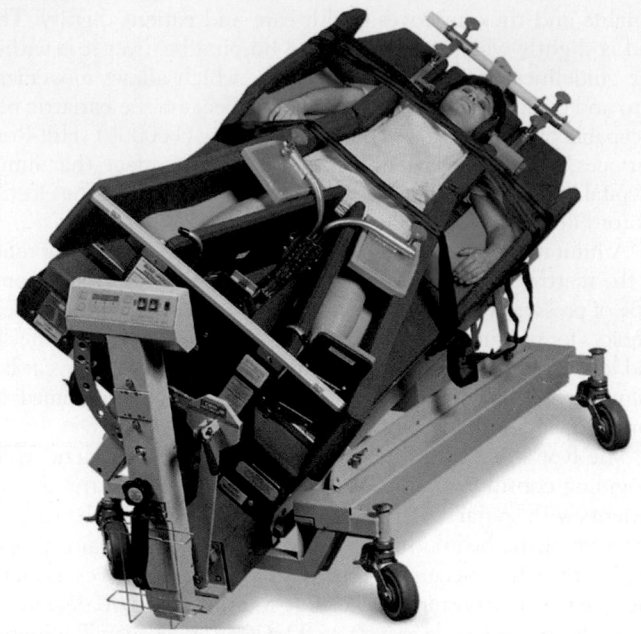

FIG 13.14 Rotokinetic bed. *(RotoRest, Courtesy Kinetic Concepts, San Antonio, TX.)*

and selects the specific surface. Some types of support surfaces require that the manufacturer representative set up and maintain the support system. The nurse directs the UCP to:

- Notify the nurse of any changes in the patient's skin.
- Continue to turn and reposition the patient regularly and seek help for patient position changes as necessary. This is not always necessary for patients who are placed on a lateral-rotation air-suspension bed.
- Monitor the normal functioning of the air-suspension bed, such as inflation and deflation cycles, and report to the nurse any changes in these cycles.
- Notify the nurse if the patient becomes disoriented or restless or complains of nausea.

Equipment

- Disposable bed pads, if indicated
- Clean gloves (*optional*)
- Foam positioning wedges if indicated
- Special sheet (if appropriate, supplied by manufacturer)
- Mechanical lift (if indicated)

STEP	RATIONALE

ASSESSMENT

1. Identify patient using two person-specific identifiers (e.g., name and date of birth or name and medical record number) according to employer policy.	Ensures correct patient. Complies with Accreditation Canada's standards and improves patient safety (Accreditation Canada, 2019).
2. Perform hand hygiene.	Reduces transmission of microorganisms.
3. Determine patient's risk for pressure injury formation using a valid assessment tool (e.g., Braden Scale) and assess for risk factors for pressure injuries (e.g., nutritional deficits, shear stress, friction, alterations in mobility and sensory perception, moisture, and abnormal serum albumin and hemoglobin levels) (see Chapter 39).	Risk assessment tools provide an objective measure of risk consistent over time (Doughty & McNichol, 2016).
4. Identify patients who will benefit from air-suspension therapy or air-fluidized therapy (e.g., immobilized or burn patients).	Determines that patient receives correct type of bed for their needs.

Clinical Decision Point *Patients with unstable conditions do not always tolerate turning or positioning required for thorough assessment or the application of a support surface mattress.*

5. Inspect condition of skin, especially over dependent sites and bony prominences. Note appearance of existing pressure injury and determine stage of injury (see Chapter 39).	Provides baseline to determine patient's response to therapy and comfort needs.
6. Assess patient's level of comfort using an appropriate pain rating scale.	Provides baseline to determine patient's response to therapy and comfort needs.

Clinical Decision Point *Some patients experiencing pain need pain medication before application of support surface of choice or transfer to another bed (NPUAP, 2014; WOCN, 2016).*

7. Verify health care provider's prescription for type of support surface.	Health care provider's prescription is usually required to ensure third-party payment of support surface.
8. Review patient's serum electrolyte levels if available.	Movement of air through mattress increases patient's risk for dehydration (Doughty & McNichol, 2016).
9. Determine if patient needs frequent weights.	Scales are available in some air-suspension beds and as under-bed units for patients who need to be weighed frequently or those who cannot be moved for weighing.

STEP	RATIONALE

ASSESSMENT

10. Assess risk of complications from air-fluidized beds.
   a. Dehydration
       Patients may become dehydrated with use of this bed because of insensible fluid loss.
   b. Aspiration
       Inability to elevate head of bed is limited to placing foam wedges under patient's head and shoulders.
   c. Difficulty with patient positioning
       Repositioning is limited to use of foam wedges.
   d. Level of orientation
       Patients may be at risk for developing delirium from dehydration and floating sensation with air-fluidized bed.

NURSING DIAGNOSES

- Insufficient peripheral tissue perfusion
- Insufficient knowledge regarding use of support surface mattress
- Insufficient fluid volume
- Reduced physical mobility
- Reduced skin integrity
- Pain (acute, chronic)
- Potential for impaired skin integrity

Related factors/Risk factors are individualized on the basis of patient's condition or needs.

PLANNING

1. Expected outcomes following completion of procedure:
   - Patient's skin is without erythema or mottling.
       Mottling represents hypoxia, which is an abnormal physiological response in tissues under pressure.
   - Existing pressure injury shows signs of healing.
       Skin remains free of new pressure injuries. Support surface does not interfere with circulation to dependent areas.
   - Patient expresses improved level of comfort.
       Equalized pressures have eliminated localized areas of discomfort.
   - Patient is removed from therapeutic surface when risk for pressure injuries decreases.
       Provides for efficient, cost-effective care while maintaining high-quality outcomes.
2. Explain purpose of mattress and method of application to patient and caregiver.
       Reduces anxiety and promotes cooperation.
3. Review instructions provided by manufacturer.
       Promotes safe and correct use of bed.
4. Obtain additional personnel needed to transfer patient to bed.
       Ensures safety by having sufficient personnel for transfer.
5. For patients with moderate to severe pain, premedicate approximately 30 minutes before transfer to bed.
       Promotes patient's comfort and ability to cooperate during transfer to bed. Decreases patient's energy expenditure (Doughty & McNichol, 2016).

IMPLEMENTATION

1. Close room door or bedside curtain.
       Provides patient privacy and demonstrates person-centred care during application of mattress to bed or transfer to alternative bed.
2. Perform hand hygiene. Apply clean gloves (if linens are soiled or wet). Get help to position patient or mattress as needed.
       Prevents transmission of microorganisms. Assistance from other caregivers reduces risk for friction and shear in transfer to new surface.
3. Transfer patient to bed using appropriate transfer techniques (see Chapter 11). Bed surface is sometimes slippery; thus, do not attempt transfers without help.
       Appropriate safe patient-handling techniques maintain alignment and reduce risk of injury during procedure. Manufacturer representative adjusts bed to patient's height and weight.
4. Once patient has been transferred, turn bed on by depressing switch; regulate temperature.
       Releasing Instaflate or turning on bed allows pressure cushions to adjust automatically to preset levels to minimize pressure, friction, and shear.
5. Position patient and perform range-of-motion exercises as appropriate.
       Promotes comfort and reduces contracture formation.
6. To turn patient, position bedpans, or perform other therapies, turn on Instaflate or other setting. Once you have completed the procedure, release Instaflate. With air-fluidized bed, use foam wedges to position patient as needed.
       Instaflate firms bed surface to facilitate turning and handling patient. Patient does not receive pressure relief while bed is in this mode.
7. Use special features of bed as needed.

STEP	RATIONALE

IMPLEMENTATION

a. Scales

b. Portable transport units to maintain inflation when primary power is interrupted

c. Specialty cushions for positioning, providing pressure relief, reducing moisture, preventing patient from sliding down in bed, or relieving weight from orthopedic devices

d. Lateral rotation (Fig. 13.15), which allows approximately 30 degrees of turning

Facilitates ability to obtain routine weights.

Provides for continuous pressure reduction.

Reduces pressure, friction, and shearing forces.

Underinflation or improper functioning of certain overlays may result in tissue damage. Likewise, overinflation can result in too firm a surface and create pressure damage.

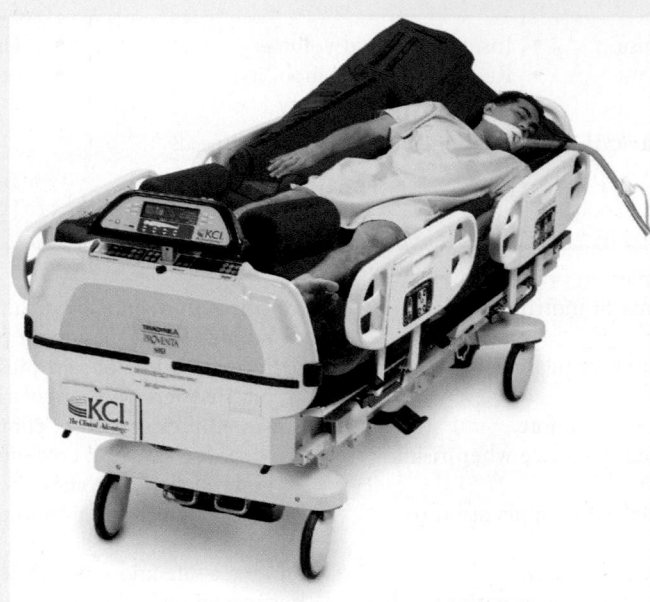

FIG 13.15 Lateral rotation bed. (*Tria Dyne™ Therapy System. Courtesy KCI Licensing, Inc., 2013.*)

Clinical Decision Point *A patient should never be placed in prone position on an air-fluidized bed because of the chance of suffocation.*

8. Assess effectiveness of pressure-relief mattress or seat cushion by placing hand beneath support surface under a bony prominence.

9. Remove and dispose of gloves and perform hand hygiene.

Helps reduce risk and prevent pulmonary and urinary complications of reduced mobility (Doughty & McNichol, 2016).

Reduces transmission of microorganisms.

EVALUATION

1. Reassess patient's risk for pressure injury formation at routine intervals.

2. Inspect and compare condition of patient's skin every 8 hours or according to employer policy to determine changes in skin integrity, pressure injury status, and effectiveness of support surface.

3. Ask patient to rate comfort or pain using an appropriate pain rating scale.

4. Evaluate functioning of support surface periodically, according to employer policy.

5. **Use Teach-Back:** "I want to be sure I explained why your bed is in this position. Tell me why we placed your bed sideways and how you might feel." Develop a revised teaching plan if patient or caregiver is not able to teach back correctly.

Documents change in status, which is critical for evaluating continued need for therapeutic surface.

Determines if pressure sores develop or if condition of existing sores changes.

If pressure-relief mattress is effective, patient generally experiences less discomfort.

Regular inspection of mechanical components of mattress ensures proper functioning.

Determines patient's and caregiver's level of understanding of instructional topic.

STEP	RATIONALE

EVALUATION

Unexpected Outcomes

1. Existing areas of skin breakdown or pressure areas fail to heal or increase in size and depth.

2. Patient becomes nauseated.

Related Interventions

- Modify skin-care regimen.
- Increase frequency of skin assessment.
- Change types of pressure-relief interventions.
- Check for proper inflation of support surface.
- Revise turning schedule.
- Consult with skin-care expert.
- Notify health care provider.
- Provide short-term antiemetic such as prochlorperazine. If using lateral rotation, obtain antiemetic prescription around the clock.
- If using lateral rotation, decrease cycle frequency.
- Notify health care provider.

Communication and Documentation

- Document transfer of patient to bed, amount of help needed for transfer, tolerance of procedure, and condition of skin in nurses' notes in electronic health record (EHR) or chart and/or skin assessment flow sheet.
- Document your evaluation of patient and caregiver learning.
- Report changes in condition of skin, level of orientation, and electrolyte levels to health care provider.

Special Considerations

Teaching

- Explain function and purpose of specialty support surface or bed.
- Explain the need to continue to change position at intervals to diminish the effects of immobility.
- Explain the need for adequate fluid intake because bed surfaces sometimes contribute to dehydration.

Pediatric

- The air-suspension bed is used commonly with older children and for children with significant burns. Make sure that instructions are age-appropriate and include any restrictions, such as raising the head of the bed.
- Parent or guardian needs to know that the child will have some dizziness or nausea when first placed on the air-fluidized or other specialty bed. This is because of the flotation sensation and will disappear as the child becomes adjusted to the bed.

Gerontological

- Some hospitalized older persons experience misperceptions of their environment that are intensified by the constant flotation of these types of beds. Proprioception abnormalities affecting older persons are the result of nervous system and muscle changes (Doughty & McNichol, 2016).

Care in the Community

- The air-fluidized bed is extremely heavy (up to 954 kg [2100 lbs]); therefore, the company leasing the bed needs to inspect the home for accessibility and structural support to ensure safety of use.
- Use interprofessional collaboration (e.g., social worker, home care case manager) to determine third-party reimbursement. Thorough documentation of skin condition is essential in obtaining reimbursement.
- A version of the air-fluidized bed is available for home use for rent or purchase; the bed rental company is responsible for proper cleaning.
- Instruct caregiver in importance of maintaining patient hydration and skin care.
- Instruct caregiver regarding steps to take in the event of a power failure. This may include purchasing a backup generator for the home.

Long-Term Care

- Nurses and UCPs need to be instructed on proper use and inflation of the bed.
- Post signs and have protocols in place for procedures in the event of the need to perform CPR (e.g., how to deflate the bed to provide a flat surface for compressions).

◆ CLINICAL DEBRIEF

The nurse is assigned to admit a 48-year-old male who was involved in a motor vehicle accident that resulted in quadriplegia (causing loss of sensation and movement below the neck). The patient is unable to change positions or transfer without help. He has a language barrier and communicating instructions about his care is difficult. The nurse has arranged for the services of a qualified interpreter to help breach the language barrier.

Following interprofessional collaboration (e.g., physiotherapy, social services) the health care provider prescribes an air-suspension bed with lateral rotation because the patient has some blistering over bony prominences and his impaired mobility and sensation increase his risk for developing pressure injuries. The patient begins experiencing a small amount of nausea and restlessness when placed on the air-suspension bed initially.

1. When this patient indicates sudden dizziness, the nurse checks his blood pressure and notes that on lateral rotation he develops orthostatic hypotension. What should the nurse's initial actions be?
2. While conducting a skin assessment, the nurse notices skin breakdown over the coccyx and left hip, even though this patient has received meticulous skin care and routine repositioning. What is the appropriate nursing action to take first?
3. The patient continues to have nausea and dizziness on the air-suspension bed. Using SBAR, show how you would communicate with the health care team about this patient.

✦ REVIEW QUESTIONS

1. The patient is discharged to home with home health care. He has been prescribed an air-celled cushion that will move with the patient (i.e., a Roho cushion) and is taught to self-adjust the inflation during the day when he is in his wheelchair. The caregiver notes that the patient has small areas of continuing redness on his ischia. Which interventions are indicated? The caregiver should: *(Select all that apply.)*
   1. Report the situation to the nurse or case manager immediately.
   2. Instruct the patient to not change the chair cushion inflation.
   3. Check for proper inflation of the cushion.
   4. Re-inflate the cushion appropriately while the patient is sitting on it and wait to re-evaluate the skin condition later.
   5. Increase frequency of checking the patient's skin.
2. Place the following steps for applying an air mattress overlay in the correct order:
   1. Check air pumps to be sure that pressure cycle alternates.
   2. Bring any plastic strips or flaps around corners of bed mattress.
   3. Apply deflated mattress flat over surface of bed mattress.
   4. Place sheet over air mattress, being sure to eliminate all wrinkles.
   5. Attach connector on air mattress to inflation device and inflate to proper pressure.
3. The nurse is caring for a patient on an air-fluidized bed. Which complications should the nurses assess for in this patient? *(Select all that apply.)*
   1. Back pain from lack of firm support
   2. Dehydration from the amount of warm circulating air
   3. Problems moving the patient out of bed because of the body submersion
   4. Lack of healing of the pressure injury because of high skin and bed pressures
   5. Difficulty moving the bed to another location because of its weight

ⓔ *Visit the Evolve site for a complete list of Clinical Debrief and Review Questions answers.*

REFERENCES

Accreditation Canada. (2019). *Required organizational practices handbook—Version 14.* Retrieved from http://www.wrha.mb.ca/quality/files/2019ROPHandbook.pdf

Bowman, T. (2015). *Preventing and treating pressure sores: A guide for people with spinal cord injuries.* Toronto: Spinal Cord Injury Ontario. Retrieved from www.onf.org/documents/preventing-and-treating-pressure-sores

Broome, C. A., Ayala, E. M., Georgeson, K. A., Heidrich, S. M., Karnes, K., & Wells, J. B. (2015). Nursing care of the super bariatric patient: Challenges and lessons learned. *Rehabilitation Nursing, 40*(2), 92–99. doi:10.1002/rnj.16

Call, E., Deppisch, M., Jordan, R., Sylvia, C., Thurman, K., & Gruccio, P. (2015). *Hand check method: Is it an effective method to monitor support surfaces for bottoming out? A National Pressure Ulcer Advisory position statement.* Retrieved from http://www.npuap.org/wp-content/uploads/2012/01/Hand-Check-Position-Statement-June-2015.pdf

Curley, M., Hasbani, N., Quigley, S., et al. (2018). Predicting pressure injury risk in pediatric patients: The Braden QD scale. *The Journal of Pediatrics, 192,* 189–195. doi:10.1016/j.jpeds.2017.09.045

Doughty, D., & McNichol, L. (2016). *Wound, Ostomy, and Continence Nurses Society (WOCN) core curriculum: Wound management.* Philadelphia: Wound, Ostomy, and Continence Society.

Haesler, E. (2018). Evidence summary: Pressure injuries: Active support surfaces for preventing and treating pressure injuries. *Wound Practice & Research, 26*(1), 50–51.

Hanna-Bull, D. (2016). Preventing heel pressure ulcers: Sustained quality improvement initiative in a Canadian acute care facility. *Journal of Wound, Ostomy and Continence Nurses, 43*(2), 129–132. doi:10.1097/WON.0000000000000181

Hill-Rom Services. (2018). *TriFlex II™ bariatric bed.* Retrieved from https://www.hill-rom.ca/ca/Products/Products-by-Category/Hospital-Beds-and-Long-Term-Care-Beds/TriFlex-II-Bariatric-Beds/

Hockenberry, M. J., & Wilson, J. (2015). *Wong's nursing care of infants and children* (10th ed.). St. Louis: Mosby.

McInnes, E., Jammali-Blasi, A., Bell-Syer, S., Dumville, J., Middleton, V., & Cullum, N. (2015). Support surfaces for pressure ulcer prevention. *Cochrane Database System Review,* (9), CD00173, doi:10.1002/14651858.CD001735.pub5

National Pressure Ulcer Advisory Panel (NPUAP) Support Surfaces Standard Initiative. (2014). *Pressure ulcer treatment recommendations: Clinical practice guidelines.* Washington, DC: National Pressure Ulcer Advisory Panel.

Noonan, C., Quigley, S., & Curley, M. (2011). Using the Braden Q scale to predict pressure ulcer risk in pediatric patients. *Journal of Pediatric Nursing, 26*(6), 566–575. doi:10.1016/j.pedn.2010.07.006

Norton, L., Parslow, N., Johnston, D., et al. (2018). *Best practice recommendations for the prevention and management of pressure injuries.* North York, ON: Wounds Canada. Retrieved from https://www.woundscanada.ca/docman/public/health-care-professional/bpr-workshop/172-bpr-prevention-and-management-of-pressure-injuries-2/file

Pories, M., & Rose, M. (2017). From stigma to empathy: Reframing our view of the bariatric patient. *Bariatric Times, 14*(4), 10–11.

Qaseem, A., Mir, T. P., Starkey, M., Denberg, T. D., & Clinical Guidelines Committee of the American College of Physicians. (2015). Risk assessment and prevention of pressure ulcers: A clinical practice guideline from the American College of physicians. *Annals of Internal Medicine, 162*(5), 359–369. doi:10.7326/M14-1567

Registered Nurses' Association of Ontario (RNAO). (2005/2011). *Risk assessment & prevention of pressure ulcers.* Toronto, ON: Author. Retrieved from http://rnao.ca/sites/rnao-ca/files/Risk_Assessment_and_Prevention_of_Pressure_Ulcers.pdf

Wound, Ostomy and Continence Nurses Society (WOCN). (2016). *Guideline for prevention and management of pressure ulcers* (2nd ed.). (WOCN clinical practice guideline series). Mt. Laurel, NJ: Author.

Wounds Canada. (2018). *Best practice recommendations for the prevention and management of pressure injuries.* Retrieved from https://www.woundscanada.ca/docman/public/health-care-professional/bpr-workshop/165-wc-bpr-prevention-and-management-of-wounds/file

Written by **Patricia A. Potter, RN, MSN, PhD, MAAN, and Shelley L. Cobbett, RN, GnT, MN, EdD**

SKILLS AND PROCEDURES

OBJECTIVES

Mastery of content in this chapter will enable the nurse to:
- Discuss the importance of national standards for patient safety.
- Discuss current evidence in fall prevention.
- Discuss the importance of a fall risk assessment in providing for patient safety.
- Describe nursing interventions specific for reducing patients' risks for falls.
- Describe steps in the design of a restraint-free environment.

- Describe nursing interventions taken in the event of a fire, electrical shock, or chemical spill.
- Discuss precautions used to prevent injury in patients who are restrained.
- Describe nursing interventions for a patient who experiences generalized seizures.
- Describe methods to evaluate safety interventions.

MEDIA RESOURCES

- evolve http://evolve.elsevier.com/Canada/Perry/clinicalskills/
- Review Questions
- ▶ Video Clips
- Audio Glossary
- **NSO** Nursing Skills Online
- Clinical Debrief and Review Questions Answers

PURPOSE

Improving patient safety and the quality of health care delivery is a national priority (Canadian Patient Safety Institute [CPSI], 2016). Health care that is provided in a safe environment, in which nurses practice safety-related skills, reduces the risk for illness and injury and contains the costs of health care by preventing extended lengths of treatment and hospitalization, improving or maintaining a patient's functional status, and increasing the patient's sense of well-being.

STANDARADS OF CARE

- Accreditation Canada, 2019—*Required Organizational Practices Handbook—Version 14* (http://www.wrha.mb.ca/quality/files/2019 ROPHandbook.pdf)
- Canadian Institutes for Health Information (CIHI), 2010–2018—*Patient Safety* (https://www.cihi.ca/en/patient-safety)
- Critical Care Services Ontario (CCSO), 2015—*Provincial Guidelines for Management of Epilepsy in Adults and Children* (https://www.criticalcareontario.ca/EN/Library/Epilepsy%20 Guideline%20Series/Pages/default.aspx)
- Government of Canada, 2012—*Current Patient Safety Organizations in Canada* (https://www.canada.ca/en/health-canada/services/ quality-care/patient-safety/current-patient-safety-organizations -canada.html)
- Registered Nurses' Association of Ontario (RNAO), 2017—*Preventing Falls and Reducing Injuries from Falls*, 4th edition (http://rnao.ca/bpg/guidelines/prevention-falls-and-fall-injuries)
- World Health Organization (WHO), 2017—*Patient Safety: Making Health Care Safer* (http://www.who.int/patientsafety/publications/ patient-safety-making-health-care-safer/en/)

PRINCIPLES FOR PRACTICE

- The integration and implementation of evidence-informed nursing skills and procedures promote a safer health care environment and improves patient outcomes.

- The nurse must be responsible for incorporating critical thinking skills when using the nursing process, assessing each patient and the environment for hazards that threaten safety, and planning and intervening appropriately to maintain a safe environment.
- Safe patient care is a priority, with a focus on reducing the incidence of adverse health care–associated conditions and reducing harm from inappropriate care (CPSI, 2016).
- The CPSI (2016) *SHIFT to Safety* program is designed to assist patients and families in advocating for their health care safety, enable health care providers to prioritize safety when caring for patients, and create a positive patient safety culture.
- As a health care provider, it is essential to share information about any patient injury, learn from errors, and participate in the trending and evaluation of those errors (Health Canada, 2018).

PERSON-CENTRED CARE

- Person-centred care is an approach to health care that involves partnering with patients to enable them to be active participants and have a voice in the design and delivery of the care they receive, to improve their health care experience (Cancer Care Ontario [CCO], 2015).
- Being hospitalized or living in a care facility may place patients at risk for injury in an unfamiliar and confusing environment. Normal life cues such as a bed without side rails and the direction one usually takes to the bathroom are absent. Thought processes and coping mechanisms are affected by physical and psychological illness and the accompanying emotions. Thus, patients are more vulnerable to injury.
- For patients of diverse cultural backgrounds, vulnerability to injury may be intensified. It is a nurse's responsibility to diligently protect all patients, regardless of their cultural background. Most adverse events are related to failures of communication. Health care providers must be particularly attentive to communication during assessment. For example, the nurse must use approaches that recognize a patient's cultural background (e.g., an interpreter or simple language) so appropriate questions can be raised to clearly reveal health behaviours and risks.
- Nurses enhance a patient's safety by considering the whole person and seeing each care situation through "the patient's eyes" and not just a nurse's perspective. The following include some specific person-centred safety guidelines:
    - Nurses should support patients emotionally and empower them to express their values and preferences and ask questions without being inhibited, and be prepared to raise and discuss sensitive issues (CCO, 2015).
    - When restraints are needed, the nurse needs to clarify their meaning to the patient and family. Always use a "least restraints" approach and behaviour management techniques (CPSI, 2017).
    - The nurse collaborates with family members in accommodating a patient's cultural perspectives regarding restraints. Removing restraints when family members are present shows respect and caring for a patient.
    - Nurses should be familiar with employer restraint policies. It is important to identify potential areas for negotiation with a patient's and family's preferences, such as using a mitten instead of arm restraints.
    - Nurses need to inform patients and family members of the reasons a patient is at fall risk. It is important for patients to know their risks, the options that exist to promote safety, and the consequences of not following precautions.

EVIDENCE-INFORMED PRACTICE

Significant research continues in the area of fall prevention, both in community and health care settings.

- Young neurological patients with impaired gait and balance or medium-to-severe motor disability are at increased risk of falling. Patients who are relatively independent and still involved in challenging activities have an increased exposure to fall risk. Improperly fitted canes and walkers, wheelchair characteristics, and environmental hazards are significant environmental risk factors (RNAO, 2017).
- In long-term care settings, multifactorial interventions (using multiple fall prevention strategies) significantly reduce the number of falls and of recurrent fallers (Vlaeyen, Coussement, Leysens, et al., 2015).
- Older persons should be screened routinely for relevant risk factors for falling. These individuals will most likely benefit from a fall prevention program targeted to their risk factors (e.g., frailty, polypharmacy, multimorbidity, vitamin D status, and home hazards). Not all fall prevention strategies are useful for all patients (Tricco, Thomas, Veroniki, et al., 2017).
- Exercise can significantly reduce numbers of falls among older persons with and without cognitive impairment in community and facility-based settings (Tricco et al., 2017).
- Vitamin D and calcium supplementation, home visits, and adjustments within the living environment can reduce the risk of falls among older persons in noninstitutional settings (Tricco et al., 2017). Including an occupational therapist or physiotherapist in a home-hazard assessment may have added benefit.
- An inpatient–nurse ratio of >5 : 1 is associated with a higher incidence of falls (Lee, Jin, Piao, et al., 2016).
- A safety priority for Accreditation Canada (2019) is falls prevention. Fall prevention programs may include team education, risk assessments, balance and strength training, vision care, medication evaluation, physical environment assessments, behavioural assessments, and bed exit alarms. Fall prevention programs need to be interprofessional, collaborative, and person centred to minimize fall injury. Accreditation Canada (2019) identifies three tests for falls prevention compliance:
    - Universal fall precautions are identified and implemented to ensure a safe environment.
    - Team members and volunteers are educated, and clients and caregivers are provided with information to prevent falls and reduce injuries from falling.
    - The effectiveness of fall prevention and injury reduction precautions and education are evaluated to inform improvements when indicated.

SAFETY GUIDELINES

- Accurate patient identification is crucial to their safety before carrying out any procedures. Use at least two person-specific identifiers (Accreditation Canada, 2019).
- Safety begins with a patient's immediate environment (Fig. 14.1). Always keep a bed in the low position and a bed alarm activated and use necessary fall prevention strategies. The call-light/bed-control system allows patients to adjust bed positions and signal caregivers for help. Explain to patients and visitors how to operate a call system correctly and then use teach-back to confirm understanding and have them demonstrate use of device.
- Always be alert to conditions within a patient's environment that pose risks for patient injury (e.g., personal care items out

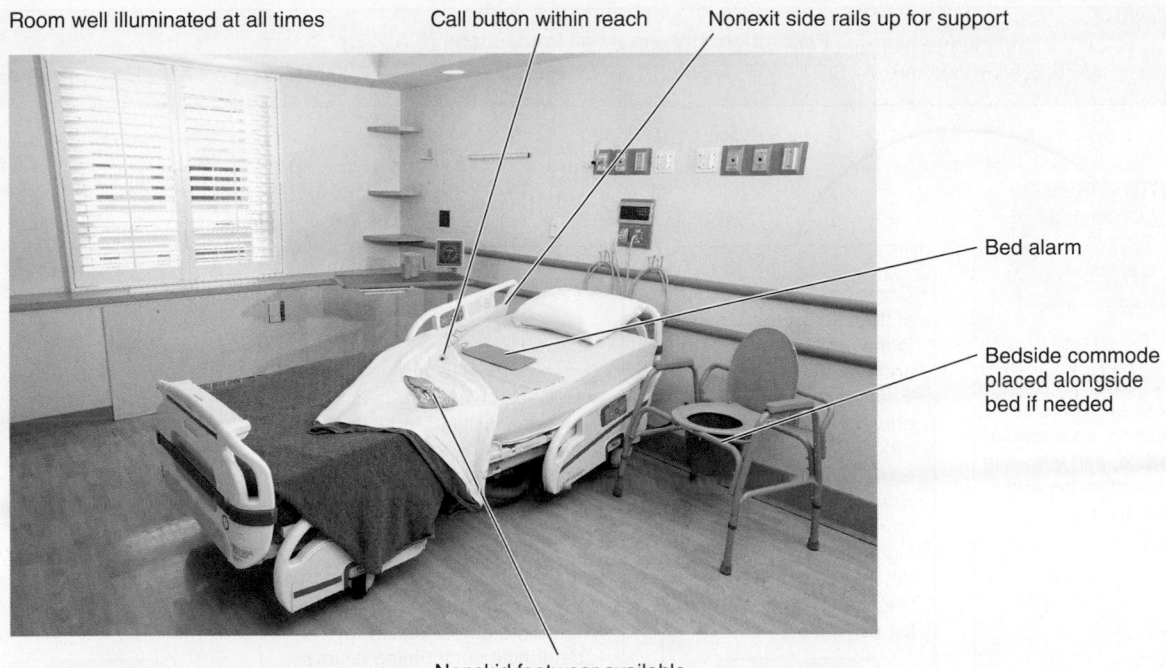

Room well illuminated at all times   Call button within reach   Nonexit side rails up for support

Bed alarm

Bedside commode placed alongside bed if needed

Nonskid footwear available

FIG 14.1 Safe patient room environment with bed in low position, bed alarm activated, nonskid floor mat and call light in place, and bedside commode positioned along bedside.

of reach, hazards along walking paths, liquid spilled on the floor, poorly functioning equipment).
- Do not use work-arounds when performing skills or procedures. A work-around occurs when a person improvises or works around intended work practices.

- Communicate clearly to other health care providers the plan of care, including test results, procedures to be performed, procedures completed, and patient response.

◆ SKILL 14.1   Fall Prevention in Health Care Facilities

NSO *Nursing Skills Online Safety Module 4 / Lesson 1*

Falls are a recurrent problem in health care facilities that affect patients, families, visitors, care providers, and the health care system. A fall may result in fractures, bruises, lacerations, or internal bleeding, leading to increased diagnostic tests and treatments, extended hospital stays, and discharge to rehabilitation or long-term care instead of home. Research shows that approximately one third of falls can be prevented (Public Health Agency of Canada [PHAC], 2014). Fall prevention involves completing a fall risk assessment of the person and the environment to inform safe patient care.

Risk factors for falls are numerous, complex, and interactive. Each person may have a combination of risk factors according to life circumstance, health status, health behaviours, economic status, social supports, and environment. Older persons are at increased risk for falls related to chronic and acute health conditions, balance or gait deficits, sensory factors, inadequate nutrition, and social isolation (PHAC, 2014). As a nurse, your role is to assess these factors in each patient and determine the most suitable preventive interventions that match the patient's risks and behaviour.

The CPSI (2015) defines *never events* as "patient safety incidents that result in serious harm or death, and that can be prevented by using organizational checks and balances" (p. 4). They have identified 15 pan-Canadian "never events," which are incidents that should never occur in a health care setting. One of these "never events" is patient death or serious harm as a result of transport of a frail patient or a patient with dementia, where protocols were

not followed to ensure the patient was left in a safe environment. Organizations are encouraged to report "never events" to share best practices and quality improvement successes to enhance patient safety.

Fall prevention is not simple. The CPSI and the RNAO have updated the evidence relating to reduction of falls and injuries from falls, originally part of the *Safer Healthcare Now Getting Started Kit* (2014). The Fall Prevention/Injury Reduction Intervention Model (Fig. 14.2) focuses on a safe environment, assistance with mobility, fall risk reduction, and engagement with the patient and family (CPSI & RNAO, 2018). The RNAO (2017) has issued a detailed list of the components involved in preventing falls (Box 14.1).

Another area of risk includes wheelchair-related falls involving older persons and those living with disabilities. Patients fall from wheelchairs because of unlocked brakes, overreaching, sliding, tipping the chair, and unassisted transfers. Wheelchair-related injuries from falls include fractures, concussions, dislocations, amputations, and serious head and spinal injuries. An example of a wheelchair characteristic that increases risk for falls is having smaller and harder front wheels that cause a chair to tip when striking uneven terrain. Caregivers are also at risk for injury by not handling patients correctly or not asking for help. Injuries can occur while caregivers transfer patients who are agitated, fearful, unsteady, or too weak to transfer. Tripping over the front foot or leg rest and leaning over the back

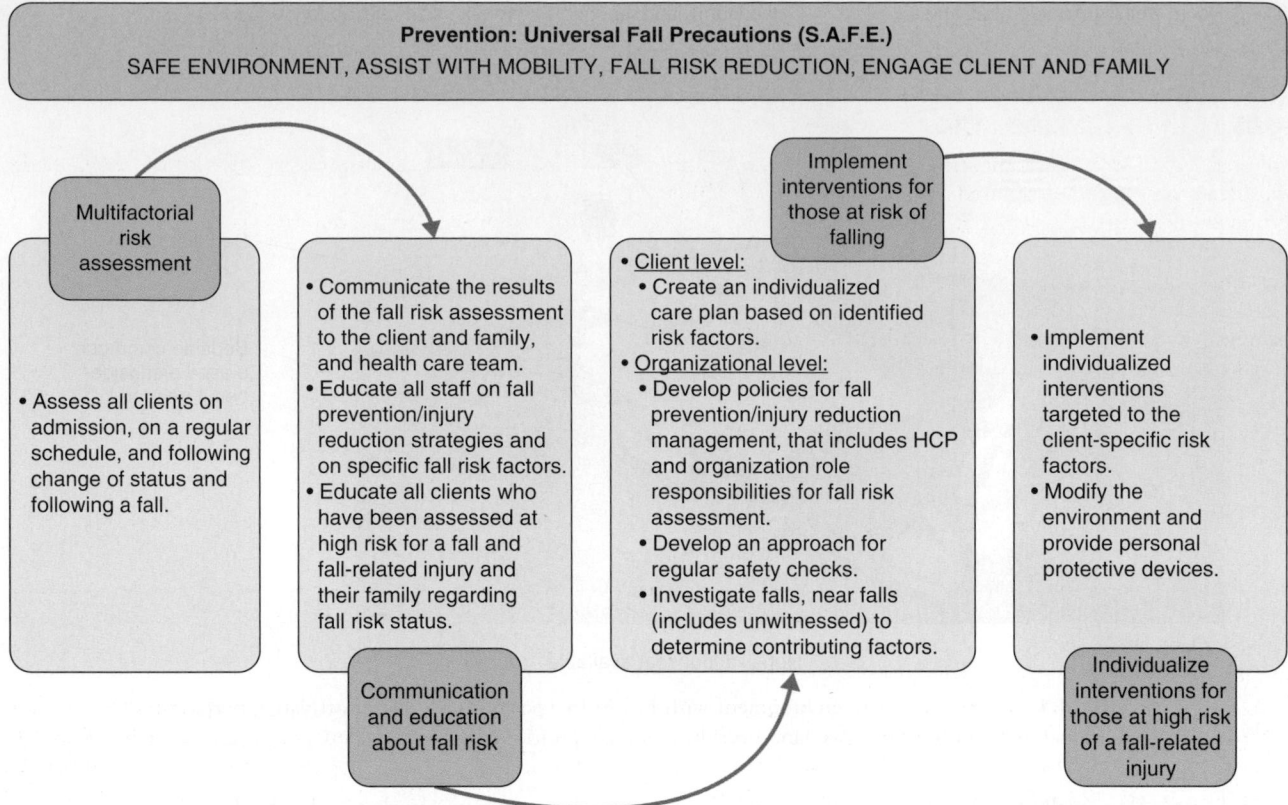

FIG 14.2 CPSI/RNAO Fall Prevention/Injury Reduction Intervention Model (*From Canadian Patient Safety Institute [CPSI] & Registered Nurses Association of Ontario [RNAO]. [2018]. Reducing falls and injuries from falls. A starting kit: Evidence update [p. 5]. Retrieved from http://www.patientsafetyinstitute. ca/en/toolsResources/Documents/Interventions/Reducing%20Falls%20and%20Injury%20from%20Falls/ Falls%20Evidence%20update%202018-01.PDF.*)

BOX 14.1

Components of Evidence-Informed Universal Falls Precautions

- Environmental modifications:
  - Implement universal falls precautions; modify equipment and other factors in the physical and structural environment
  - Bed rails in low position; nurse call bell within reach
- Exercise interventions and physical training:
  - Core strength training, Pilates exercise training, muscle strengthening, stepping training, perturbation-based balance training (lower-limb strengthening exercises)
  - Exergaming (interactive gaming)
  - Fall prevention exercise programs
  - Foot and ankle exercises that strengthen and stretch the foot and ankle
  - Individualized exercise or physiotherapy
  - Interactive cognitive-motor interventions
- Footwear:
  - Antislip shoes; thin, hard-soled footwear with high collars
- Multifaceted podiatry care:
  - Footwear assessment
  - Customized insoles
  - Foot and ankle exercises
- Pacemakers
- Whole-body vibration for postmenopausal women
- Cognitive-motor interference (training for the performance of two simultaneous tasks to prevent falls)
- Continence management (e.g., prompted elimination management schedule)
- Medication management (be aware of medications associated with falling)
- Rounding (e.g., hourly) as a strategy to proactively meet the person's needs and prevent falls
- Vitamin D supplementation

Adapted from Registered Nurses' Association of Ontario (RNAO). (2017). *Preventing falls and reducing injuries from falls* (4th ed.). Toronto, ON: Author.

---

of the wheelchair to engage or disengage the wheel lock are common sources of injury.

It is important for nurses to identify patients' fall risks and communicate these risks to patients, their visitors, and members of the health care team. Person-centred care is important, with nurses making patients their partners in recognizing fall risks and taking preventive action. Fall prevention strategies must be targeted to specific patient risks. For example, if a patient has postural hypotension, a nurse might choose a low bed and have the patient dangle their legs for 5 minutes while sitting on the side of the bed before trying to ambulate. Or a patient with a history of urinary incontinence might be given a bedside commode to use. Remember that patient

situations change. Preventing falls and fall-related injuries requires diligent ongoing nursing assessment and engagement of the entire health care team.

Delegation and Collaboration

The skill of assessing and communicating a patient's risk for falling cannot be delegated to an unregulated care provider (UCP). Skills used to prevent falls can be delegated. The nurse directs the UCP by:

- Explaining a patient's mobility limitations and specific fall prevention measures needed to minimize risks.
- Teaching specific environmental safety precautions to use (e.g., bed locked in low position, call light within reach).

- Explaining patient behaviours (e.g., disorientation, wandering, anxiety) that are precursors to falls and that should be reported immediately.

Equipment

- Validated fall risk assessment tool (Accreditation Canada, 2019; RNAO, 2017)
- Hospital bed with side rails; low bed
- Wedge cushion
- Call-light intercom system
- Gait belt for assisting with ambulation
- Wheelchair and seat belt (as needed)
- Additional safety devices (e.g., bed alarm pad, wedge cushion)

STEP	RATIONALE

ASSESSMENT

1. Identify patient using at least two person-specific identifiers (e.g., name and date of birth or name and medical record number) according to employer policy.

   Ensures correct patient. Complies with Accreditation Canada's standards and improves patient safety (Accreditation Canada, 2019).

2. Complete a person-centred fall risk assessment using critical thinking and clinical judgement. Be sensitive to population being screened: patient's age (over 65), presence of comorbidities, altered memory and cognition, incontinence or urinary frequency and urgency, reduced hearing and vision, orthostatic hypotension, arthritis, impaired gait, weak lower extremities, poor balance, fatigue, need for transfer assistance, and decreased peripheral sensation (CPSI & RNAO, 2018). Also assess for risk for injury during fall (e.g., vitamin D level, osteoporosis, bleeding tendency).

   A variety of physiological factors predispose patients to fall and injury from falling. There are a variety of fall risk assessment tools. Those with a greater number of risk factors are less likely to be sensitive because all patients will be found at risk. Tools based on the risk factors of a population (e.g., older persons, oncology, or neurological patient) are more likely to be sensitive to predicting falls.

Clinical Decision Point *Do not ask patient to provide a self-report of balance, gait, or ability to ambulate. Ask patient to walk a short distance and observe each factor.*

3. Assess level of patient's pain using an appropriate rating scale (e.g., on a scale from 0 to 10, with 0 being no pain, and 10 being worst pain ever).

   Pain has been shown to be a risk factor for falls (PHAC, 2014).

4. Determine if patient has a history of recent falls or other injuries within the home. Use an appropriate risk assessment tool to identify high-risk patients (e.g., St. Thomas Risk Assessment Tool in Falling Elderly In-Patients (STRATIFY), Morse Fall Scale, Hendrich II Fall Risk) (Welch, Ghogomu, & Shea, 2016).

   Symptoms are helpful in identifying a cause for falls. Onset, location, and activity associated with a fall provide further details about causative factors and how to prevent future falls.

5. Review patient's medications (including over-the-counter [OTC] medications and herbal products) for use of antidepressants, sedatives and hypnotics (especially benzodiazepines), anxiolytics, beta-blockers, diuretics, antihypertensives, neuroleptics, anti-Parkinson drugs, hypoglycemics, nonsteroidal anti-inflammatories, opioids, antipsychotics, and laxatives. Assess for polypharmacy (e.g., over four medications, duplicate medications, drugs inappropriate for condition) (CPSI & RNAO, 2018).

   Effects of certain medications and use of multiple medications increase risk for falls and injury (CPSI & RNAO, 2018).

Clinical Decision Point *If patient is on multiple medications, confer with health care provider and pharmacist about possibility of reducing or adjusting doses.*

6. Assess patient for fear of falling: Consider those over 70 years of age, female, lower income, or single and have poor perceived general health (Kiel, 2018).

   Fear of falling is interrelated with incidence of falls, change in way patient walks, curtailment of activities, immobility, functional dependence, falls with serious injury (CPSI & RNAO, 2018).

STEP	RATIONALE

ASSESSMENT

7. Perform the "timed get up and go (TUG)" test if patient is able to ambulate. At a minimum, observe patient walk in room (with or without help). Steps for TUG dual assessment:

- Give patient verbal instructions to stand up from a chair, walk 3 metres (10 feet) as quickly and safely as possible (cross a line marked on the floor), turn around, walk back, and sit down.
- Have patient rise from straight-back chair without using arms for support.
- Begin counting.
- Observe patient's postural stability, gait, stride length, and sway.
- Have patient return to chair and sit down without using arms for support. Check time elapsed.
- For accuracy, a patient should have one practice trial that is not included in the score. The patient must use the same assistive device each time they are tested to be able to compare scores.

The TUG test is a simple and quick clinical, performance-based measure of lower-extremity function, mobility, and fall risk, useful even with healthy adults (Government of British Columbia, 2017). It quantifies a patient's functional mobility. Observing a patient walk allows you to determine if gait and posture are normal. The TUG test is a measure of physical and cognitive performance. Ability to follow simple instructions measures cognitive function. A TUG time of >10 seconds indicates an increased risk for falling for hospitalized patients (Government of British Columbia, 2017) and ≥13.5 seconds for individuals in community settings (Bloch, Jønsson, & Kristensen, 2017). Recent evidence suggests that there should be three trials of the TUG test, and the scores averaged to determine the most accurate result (Bloch et al., 2017).

8. Assess condition of equipment (e.g., legs on bedside commode, tips of walker)

Equipment in poor repair increases risk for fall.

9. Assess patient's medical history for osteoporosis, use of anticoagulants, history of previous fracture, cancer, and recent chest or abdominal surgery.

Factors increase likelihood of injury from fall.

10. Use person-centred approach to determine what patient knows about risks for falling and steps that they can take to prevent falls.

Knowledge of fall risks influences one's ability to take necessary precautions in reducing falling. Matching interventions with factors that patient perceives as relevant may increase success in preventing falls.

11. If patient is assessed to be a fall risk, apply colour-coded wristband (see illustration). Some facilities institute fall risk signs on doors.

Colour-coded bands (e.g., yellow, blue—check employer policy) are easily recognizable.

12. If patient is in a wheelchair, assess their level of comfort, fatigue, boredom, mental status, or level of engagement with others.

These factors can cause patient to make an attempt to exit wheelchair without help.

NURSING DIAGNOSES

- Acute or chronic pain
- Reduced physical mobility
- Inadequate transfer ability

- Reduced urinary elimination
- Reduced stamina
- Reduced memory

- Potential for falls
- Potential for injury
- Potential for trauma

Related factors/Risk factors are individualized on the basis of patient's condition or needs.

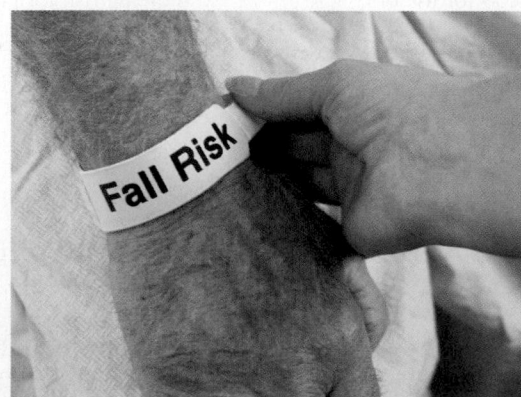

STEP 11 Fall risk armband alerts health care staff to patient's risk of falling.

STEP	RATIONALE

PLANNING

1. Expected outcomes following completion of procedure:
   - Patient's environment is free of hazards
   - Patient and/or caregiver is able to identify fall risks.

   - Patient and/or caregiver verbalizes understanding of fall prevention interventions.
   - Patient does not experience a fall or injury.
2. Gather equipment and perform hand hygiene.
3. Explain what you plan to do. Specifically discuss reasons that patient is at risk for falling. Include caregivers (as appropriate) in discussion. Provide privacy. Be sure that patient is comfortable.

Hazards predispose to tripping and falls.
Patient awareness of risks promotes cooperation and understanding of fall prevention plan.

Demonstrates person-centred care by involving patient and caregiver in decisions about preventive strategies.
Fall precautions show success in preventing falls.
Organizes care. Reduces transmission of microorganisms.
Reduces patient anxiety and promotes cooperation. Results in fall prevention measures that are patient centred and not just routine. Younger patients are very independent and often believe that they are not likely to fall.

IMPLEMENTATION

1. Conduct rounding (hourly) on all patients to determine status of pain, need to toilet, and need to relocate personal items for easy reach; provide pain relief intervention.

2. Adjust bed to low position with wheels locked (see illustration). Place nonslip padded floor mats at exit side of bed.
3. Encourage use of properly fitted skid-proof footwear. *Optional:* Place nonslip padded floor mat on exit side of bed.
4. Orient patient to surroundings, call light, and routines to expect in plan of care.
   a. Provide patient's hearing aid and glasses. Be sure that each is functioning and clean. If patient indicates visual or hearing problems, refer to appropriate health care provider.
   b. Place call-light and bed-control system in an accessible location within patient's reach. Explain and demonstrate how to turn system on and off at bedside and in bathroom (see illustration). Have patient perform return demonstration.

Provides nurses with surveillance mechanism to purposefully keep patients safe and comfortable by proactively meeting their needs. Research that associates rounding with fall reduction needs to be more rigorous (RNAO, 2017).
Height of bed allows ambulatory patient to get in and out of bed easily and safely. Pads provide nonslippery surface on which to stand.
Prevents falls from slipping on floor.

Orientation to room and plan of care provides familiarity with environment and activities to anticipate.
Enables patient to remain alert to conditions in environment.

Knowledge of location and use of call light is essential for patient to be able to call for help quickly. Reaching for an object when in bed can lead to an accidental fall.

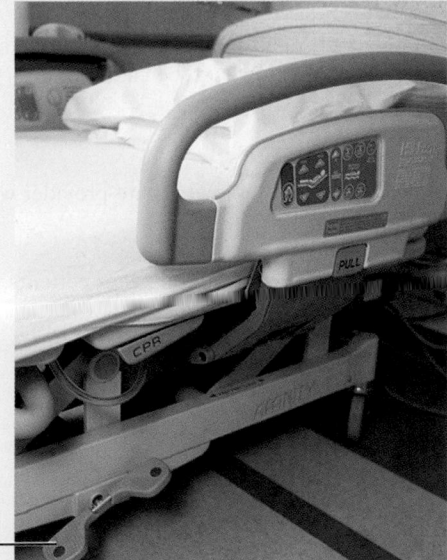

Brake lock

STEP 2 Hospital bed should be kept in lowest position with wheels locked and side rails up (as appropriate).

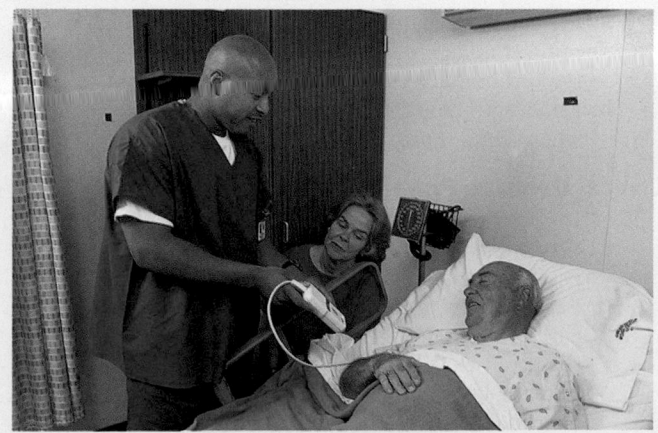

STEP 4b Nurse demonstrates use of call light to patient.

STEP	RATIONALE

IMPLEMENTATION

c. Explain to patient and caregiver when and why to use call system (e.g., report pain, get out of bed, go to bathroom). Provide clear instructions to patient and caregiver regarding mobility restrictions.

Increases likelihood that patient will call for help and of nurse being able to respond to patient's needs in a timely way.

5. Safe use of side rails:

a. Explain to patient and caregiver reason for using side rails: moving and turning self in bed.

Promotes cooperation.

b. Check employer policy regarding side rail use.

(1) Dependent, less mobile patients: In two–side rail bed, keep both rails up. (**NOTE:** Rails on newer hospital beds allow for room at foot of bed for patient to safely exit bed.) In four–side rail bed, leave two upper rails up.

Side rails are restraint devices if they immobilize or reduce ability of a patient to move their arms, legs, body, or head freely.

(2) Patient able to get out of bed independently: In four–side rail bed, leave two upper side rails up. In two–side rail bed, keep only one rail up.

Allows for safe exit from bed.

6. Make patient's environment safe:

a. Remove excess equipment, supplies, and furniture from rooms and halls.

Reduces likelihood of falling or tripping over objects.

b. Keep floors free of clutter and obstacles (e.g., intravenous [IV] pole, electrical cords), particularly path to bathroom.

Reduces likelihood of falling or tripping over objects.

c. Coil and secure excess electrical, telephone, and any other cords or tubing.

Reduces risk of entanglement.

d. Clean all spills promptly. Post sign indicating wet floor. Remove sign when floor is dry (usually done by housekeeping).

Reduces risk of falling on slippery, wet surfaces.

e. Ensure adequate glare-free lighting; use a night-light at night.

Glare may be a problem for older persons because of vision changes.

f. Have assistive devices (e.g., cane, walker, bedside commode) on exit side of bed. Have chair back of commode placed against wall of room if possible.

Provides added support when transferring out of bed. Stabilizes commode.

g. Arrange personal items (e.g., water pitcher, telephone, reading materials, dentures) within patient's easy reach and in logical way.

Facilitates independence and self-care; prevents falls related to reaching for hard-to-reach items.

h. Secure locks on beds, stretchers, and wheelchairs.

Prevents accidental movement of devices during patient transfer.

7. Provide comfort measures, offer ordered analgesics for patients experiencing pain.

Pain can be a factor causing patients to exit bed; thus, pain relief is essential. However, be cautious, as opioids increase fall risk.

8. Interventions for patients at moderate-to-high risk for falling (based on fall risk assessment):

a. Prioritize call-light responses to patients at high risk, using team approach with all staff knowing responsibility to respond.

Ensures rapid response by health care provider when patient calls for help.

b. Establish elimination schedule, using bedside commode when appropriate.

Proactive elimination scheduling keeps patients from being unattended with sudden urge to use toilet.

Clinical Decision Point *The need for elimination is a common event leading to a patient's fall (Berry & Kiel, 2018).*

c. Stay with patient (standing outside bathroom unless patient status indicates you remain in the bathroom).

Patients often try to get up to stand and walk back to their beds from the bathroom without help.

d. Place patient in geri-chair or wheelchair with wedge cushion. Use wheelchair only for transport, not for sitting an extended time.

Maintains alignment and comfort and makes it difficult to exit chair.

e. Use low bed that has low height above floor and apply floor mats.

Reduces fall-related injuries.

f. Activate bed alarm for patient.

Alarm activates when patient rises off sensor. Alarm sounds alert to staff.

STEP	RATIONALE

IMPLEMENTATION

g. Confer with physiotherapy on feasibility of gait training, strength and balance training, and regular weight-bearing activities.

Exercise can reduce falls, fall-related fractures, and several risk factors for falls in individuals with low bone density and in older persons. Strength and balance training has been shown to reduce the rate of injurious falls in older persons (Tricco et al., 2017).

h. Use sitters or restraints only when alternatives are exhausted.

A sitter is a nonprofessional staff member or volunteer who stays in a patient room to closely observe patients who are at risk for falling. Restraints should be used only as final option (see Skill 14.2).

9. When ambulating patient, have patient wear a gait belt or walking sling and walk along their side (see Chapter 12).

Safe patient-handling techniques (e.g., use of walking sling or gait belt) allows for safe patient ambulation and prevention of injury to you and patient.

10. Safe use of wheelchair:

a. Be sure that wheelchair is correct fit for patient: Patient thighs are level while sitting, feet flat on floor; back of chair comes up to mid-shoulder, elbows rest on armrests without leaning over or tucking arms in, and there are two fingers of space between patient and side of chair.

Correctly fitted chair promotes comfort, making it less likely for patient to try to exit it.

b. Transfer patient to wheelchair.

(1) Determine level of help needed to transfer patient to wheelchair. Position wheelchair on same side of bed as patient's strong or unaffected side (see Chapter 11).

Patient's condition may require more than a one-person assist. Positioning of chair facilitates patient's ability to help in transfer.

(2) Place wedge cushion in chair (see illustration).

Prevents patient from slipping out of chair.

(3) Securely lock brakes on both wheels when transferring patient into or out of wheelchair.

Keeps chair steady and secure.

(4) Raise footplates before transfer to chair; then lower footplates, placing patient's feet on them after they are seated.

Prevents tripping over footplate.

(5) Have patient sit with buttocks well back in seat. *Option:* Apply quick-release seat belt.

Prevents patient from sliding out of chair.

(6) Back wheelchair into and out of elevator or door, leading with large rear wheels first (see illustration).

Prevents smaller front wheels from catching in crack between elevator and floor, causing chair to tip.

c. Manage patient's pain and do not allow patient to sit in wheelchair for an extended amount of time; provide alternative sitting option.

Reduces restlessness and discomfort that can lead to wheelchair exit.

11. Remove unnecessary supplies. Perform hand hygiene.

Reduces transmission of microorganisms.

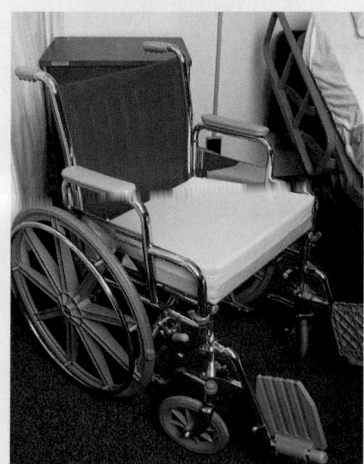

STEP 10b(2) Wheelchair with footplates raised and wedge cushion in place.

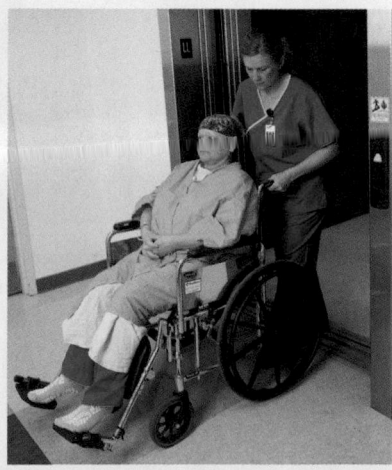

STEP 10b(6) Nurse backing wheelchair into elevator.

STEP	RATIONALE

EVALUATION

1. Ask patient and caregiver to identify patient's fall risks.

   Demonstrates learning.

2. Ask patient and caregiver to describe fall prevention interventions that are implemented.

   Demonstrates learning.

3. Evaluate patient's ability to use assistive devices such as walker or bedside commode.

   Adjustments in devices may become necessary.

4. Evaluate for changes in motor, sensory, and cognitive status and review if any falls or injuries have occurred.

   May require different interventions to be added. Fall outcomes determine success of plan.

5. **Use Teach-Back:** "I want to be sure I explained clearly to you why you are more likely to fall than other patients. Tell me some of those reasons." Develop a revised teaching plan if patient or caregiver is not able to teach back correctly.

   Determines patient's and caregiver's level of understanding of instructional topic.

Unexpected Outcomes	Related Interventions
1. Patient and caregiver are unable to identify fall risks or fall prevention strategies.	• Reinforce identified risks with patient and review safety measures with caregiver.
2. Patient starts to fall while ambulating with nurse or caregiver.	• Put both arms around patient's waist or grasp gait belt. • Stand with feet apart to provide broad base of support (see Chapter 12). • Extend one leg and let patient slide against it to floor (Fig. 14.3 *A*). • Bend knees and lower body as patient slides to floor (see Fig. 14.3 *B*).
3. Patient found after falling.	• Call for assistance. • Assess patient for injury and stay until help arrives. • Notify primary health care provider and caregiver. • Complete report as indicated by employer. • Evaluate patient's environment and risk factors; revise fall prevention plan as needed.

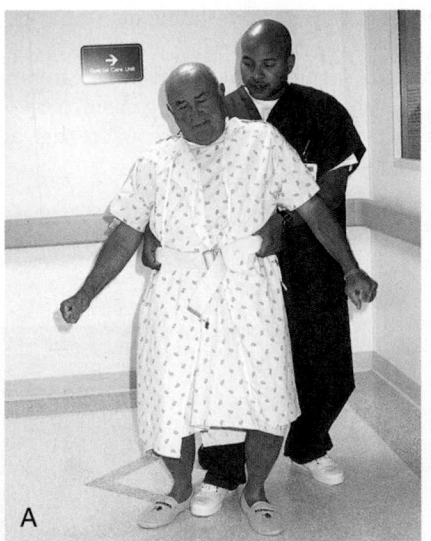
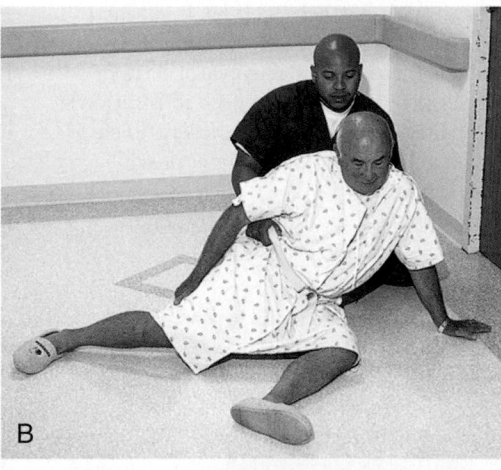

FIG 14.3 A, Stand with feet apart to provide broad base of support; extend one leg against which patient can slide to floor. **B,** Bend knees and lower body as patient slides to floor.

Communication and Documentation

• Document fall risk assessment findings, specific interventions used to prevent falls, and patient's response to teach-back in care plan on flow sheet or in nurses' notes in electronic health record (EHR) or chart.

• Report to health care personnel specific risks to patient's safety and measures taken to minimize risks.

• Document your evaluation of patient and caregiver learning.

• If a fall occurs, document a description of the fall as given by patient or you as witness. Be sure to include baseline assessment,

any injuries noted, tests or treatments given, follow-up care, and additional safety precautions taken after fall. Complete report as per employer policy.

Special Considerations
Teaching
- The website for the Canadian Patient Safety Institute (CPSI) has educational resources on fall prevention for older persons and caregivers at http://www.patientsafetyinstitute.ca/en/Topic/Pages/Falls.aspx.
- Encourage patients to have annual vision and hearing examinations. Adaptive devices such as a hearing aid or glasses are sometimes necessary or need modification.
- Emphasize to patients the need to always look ahead when ambulating and use good posture.
- Teach patients how to use assistive devices and keep them in good repair.

Pediatric
- Encourage parents to follow best practices for falls prevention among children (Children's Health and Safety Association [CHSA], 2015):
  - *Play safely.* Be sure that playground equipment that a child uses is designed and maintained properly and that there is a safe, soft landing surface below; optimal equipment height to reduce risk of head injury is 1.5 m (9–12 inches).
  - *Make the home safer.* Use home safety devices such as guards on windows that are above ground level, stair gates, and guard rails. Canadian legislation prohibits the use of baby walkers.
  - *Keep sports safe.* Be sure that a child wears protective gear such as wrist guards, knee and elbow pads, and a helmet for biking or skating when playing active sports.
  - *Supervision is key.* Supervise young children at all times around fall hazards, whether at home or out to play.
- Keep side rails of hospital beds down to allow toddlers and preschoolers easy exit and decrease the need to crawl over the rails (Hockenberry & Wilson, 2015).
- When caring for infants, keep a hand on the child when you turn away from the bedside.

Gerontological
- Interventions to improve balance confidence has shown benefits, including multicomponent behavioural group interventions and exercise (including Pilates) (Tricco et al., 2017).

Care in the Community
- See Chapter 42.

◆ SKILL 14.2 Designing a Restraint-Free Environment

 Video Clip   **NSO** *Nursing Skills Online Safety Module 4 / Lesson 2*

A physical restraint is any physical, environmental, or chemical (e.g., anxiolytic, sedative) measure that restricts the movement or controls the behaviour of a patient (College of Nurses of Ontario [CNO], 2018). Evidence suggests that the use of restraints increases the severity of falls. Best practice is a least-restraint policy that requires all possible alternative interventions to be exhausted before deciding to use a restraint (CNO, 2018).

Because physical and chemical restraints restrict a patient's physical activity or normal access to the body, serious and often fatal complications can develop, especially when patients try to get out of restraints. As a nurse, always be aware of your employer policy related to the use of restraints. Creating a restraint-free environment allows you to have interventions in place to reduce wandering and risk of patient falls. *A restraint-free environment is the first goal of care for all patients*.

Patients at risk for falls or wandering present special safety challenges. Wandering is a common problem in patients who are confused or disoriented (e.g., patients with dementia). Interrupting a wandering patient can increase their distress. Wandering is a persistent problem in long-term care settings. Common strategies to manage wandering include environmental adaptations, use of signaling tags, distraction, social interaction, regular exercise, and circular design of a patient care unit. More frequent observation of patients, involvement of family during visitation, and frequent reorientation are also helpful measures.

Delegation and Collaboration

The skills of assessing patient behaviours and orientation to the environment and determining the type of restraint-free interventions to use cannot be delegated to an unregulated care provider (UCP). Actions for promoting a safe environment can be delegated to UCPs. The nurse directs the UCP about:
- Using specific diversional or activity measures for making the environment safe.
- Applying appropriate alarm or monitoring devices.
- Reporting patient behaviours and actions (e.g., confusion, getting out of bed unassisted, combativeness) to the nurse.

Equipment
- Visual or auditory stimuli (e.g., calendar, clock, radio, photos, CD or MP3 player, television, smartphone)
- Diversional activities (e.g., puzzle, game, audiobooks, DVD)
- Wedge cushion
- Wrap-around belt
- *Options:* Electronic bracelet or pressure pad alarm sensor; bed enclosure system

---

STEP	RATIONALE

ASSESSMENT

1. Assess patient's medical history for dementia, depression, and the following conditions: is considered dangerous to self or others; lacks cognitive ability (either permanently or temporarily) to make relevant decisions; or has physical limitations that increase their risk.	Wandering is commonly associated with these conditions (Olley & Morales, 2017).

STEP	RATIONALE

IMPLEMENTATION

2. Assess patient's behaviour (e.g., orientation, level of consciousness, ability to understand and follow directions, resistant behaviours, restlessness, agitation), balance, gait, vision, hearing, bowel and bladder routine, level of pain, electrolyte and blood count values, and presence of orthostatic hypotension.

Accurate assessment identifies patients with safety risks and the physiological causes for patient behaviours that prompt caregivers to use restraints. Ensures proper selection of nonrestraint interventions.

3. Review over-the-counter (OTC) and prescribed medications (see Skill 14.1) that pose risk for falling. Assess for interactions and untoward effects.

Medication interactions or adverse effects often contribute to falling or altered mental status.

4. Assess patient's or caregiver's knowledge of condition and prescribed treatments.

Knowledge of treatment protocols and rationales increases patient's cooperation.

5. For patients who wander or have known dementia, assess for cognitive decline using Mini-Mental State Examination (MMSE) (see Chapter 42).

Determines cause and nature of wandering, which leads to effective intervention selection.

6. Assess degree of wandering behaviour using Algase Wandering Scale Version 2 (AWS-V2) (Martin, Biessy-Dalbe, Albaret, et al., 2015) or the Morse Falls Scale Fall Risk Assessment (Nova Scotia Health Authority [NSHA], 2018).

The AWS-V2 is a valid and reliable measure overall and for persistent walking, spatial disorientation, and eloping behaviour subscales.

7. For patients with dementia, ask family or friends about their usual communication style and cues to indicate pain, fatigue, hunger, and need to urinate or defecate.

Enables person-centred care to identify individual patient cues for which patient behaviours often prompt wandering when need is unmet.

8. Inspect condition of any therapeutic medical devices.

Patients who become restless, agitated, or confused will attempt to remove medical devices and then become candidates for physical restraint.

NURSING DIAGNOSES

- Wandering
- Insufficient knowledge regarding need for least-restraint environment
- Potential for falls
- Potential for injury
- Potential for trauma

Related factors/Risk factors are individualized on the basis of patient's condition or needs.

PLANNING

1. Expected outcomes following completion of procedure:
   - Patient is injury free and does not inflict injury on others while in restraint-free environment.
   - Patient does not remove a therapeutic medical device.

Alternative interventions are successful in reducing agitation and preventing injury or least-restraint use.

IMPLEMENTATION

1. Orient patient and caregiver to surroundings, introduce to staff, and explain all treatments and procedures. Be sure that patient is able to read your name badge.

Promotes patient understanding and cooperation.

2. Assign same staff to care for patient as often as possible. Encourage family and friends to stay with patient. In some facilities volunteers are effective companions.

Increases familiarity with individuals in patient's environment, decreasing anxiety and restlessness. Companions are helpful and prevent patient from being alone.

3. Place patient in room that is easily accessible to caregivers, close to nurses' station.

Allows for frequent observation to reduce falls among high-risk patients.

4. Be sure that patient is wearing glasses, hearing aid, or other sensory-aid devices and that all are functioning.

Improves patient's level of orientation to environment.

5. Provide visual and auditory stimuli meaningful to patient (e.g., clock, calendar, radio, CD, or MP3 player [with patient's choice of music], television, and family pictures).

Orients patient to day, time, and physical surroundings. Stimuli must be individualized for this to be effective.

6. Anticipate patient's basic needs (e.g., elimination needs, relief of pain, relief of hunger) as quickly as possible; conduct hourly rounding (RNAO, 2017).

Providing basic needs in timely fashion decreases patient discomfort, anxiety, restlessness, and incidence of falls.

STEP	RATIONALE

IMPLEMENTATION

7. Provide scheduled ambulation, chair activity, and elimination (e.g., during rounding, ask patient about elimination needs). Organize treatments so patient has uninterrupted periods throughout the day.

Regular opportunity to void avoids risk of patient trying to reach bathroom alone. Provides for sleep and rest periods. Constant activity overstimulates patients.

8. Position intravenous (IV) catheters, urinary catheters, and tubes and drains out of patient view. Use camouflage by wrapping IV site with bandage or stockinette. Place undergarments on patient with urinary catheter or cover abdominal feeding tubes and drains with loose abdominal binder.

Maintains medical treatment and reduces patient access to tubes and lines.

9. Decrease wandering: Eliminate stressors from environment such as cold at night, changes in daily routines, and extra visitors.

Reduced stress allows patient's energy to be channelled more appropriately.

10. Use stress-reduction techniques such as back rub, massage, and guided imagery (see Chapter 16).

Reduces level of anxiety and restlessness.

11. Use diversional activities: puzzles, games, music therapy, pet therapy, activity apron, performing purposeful activity (e.g., folding towels, drawing and colouring). Be sure that it is an activity in which patient has interest. Involve caregiver (if appropriate).

Meaningful diversional activities provide distraction, help to reduce boredom, and provide tactile stimulation. Minimize occurrences of wandering.

12. Position patient on wedge cushion and apply wrap-around belt (see illustration).

Cushion prevents slipping in chair and makes it difficult for patient to get out of chair without help. Wrap-around belt allows patient to lift flap for self-release.

13. Use pressure-sensitive bed or chair pad with alarms:

Alarms alert staff to patient who is standing or rising from bed or chair without help.

   a. Explain use of device to patient and caregiver.

   b. When in bed, position device so it is correctly positioned under patient's mid-to-low back or buttocks.

Alarm activates sooner if placed under patient's back. By the time buttocks are off sensor, patient may be almost out of bed.

   c. Test alarm by applying and releasing pressure.

Ensures that alarm is audible through call-light system.

14. Place electronic monitoring bracelet on wrist of patient with dementia.

Tag in bracelet contains radio-frequency circuit that communicates with detection sensor usually installed at an exit door or elevator. Distance between tag and monitor is constantly measured with an alarm, which sounds when predetermined distance is exceeded.

15. Place wandering patient in bed enclosure system (see illustration).

Restraint alternative that allows patient freedom of movement within protected environment.

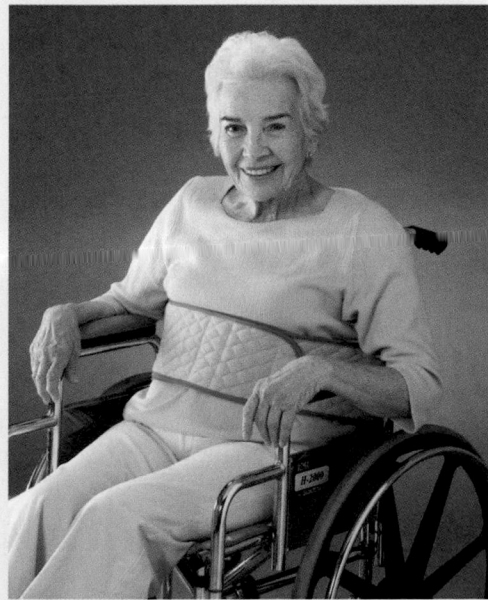

STEP 12 Wrap-around belt. (*Courtesy Posey Company, Arcadia, CA.*)

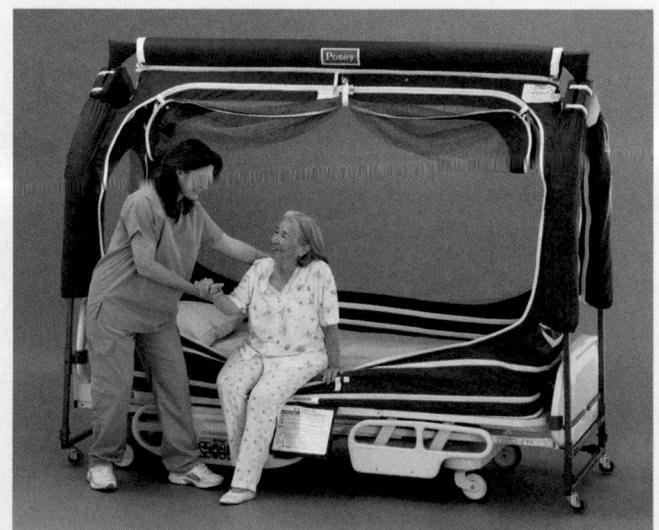

STEP 15 Bed enclosure system. (*Courtesy Posey Company, Arcadia, CA.*)

STEP	RATIONALE

IMPLEMENTATION

16. Consult with physiotherapy, speech, and occupational therapy for activities that provide stimulation and exercise.

17. Minimize invasive treatments (e.g., tube feedings, blood sampling) as much as possible.

Involvement in meaningful and purposeful activities reduces tendency to wander. Exercise improves balance and coordination.
Stimuli increase patients' restlessness.

EVALUATION

1. Monitor patient's behaviour routinely.

2. Observe patient for any injuries.

3. Observe patient's behaviour toward staff, visitors, and other patients.

4. Use Teach-Back: "We've talked about what we are doing to reduce your husband's wandering. Tell me ways you can help. I want to be sure you understand." Develop a revised teaching plan if caregiver is not able to teach back correctly.

Will determine if agitation, wandering, or attempt to remove medical devices has been prevented.
Patient should be injury free.
Ensures that patient's behaviour does not cause injury to others.

Determines caregiver's level of understanding of instructional topic.

Unexpected Outcomes

1. Patient displays behaviours that increase risk for injury to self or others.

2. Patient sustains injury or is agitated and places others at risk for injury.

3. Patient wanders away from facility.

Related Interventions

- Review episodes for pattern (e.g., activity, time of day) that indicates alternatives that would eliminate behaviour.
- Discuss with all caregivers and family alternative interventions.
- Notify health care provider.
- Complete report according to employer policy.
- Identify alternative measures for safety or behavioural control.
- Apply physical restraint (see Skill 14.3) only after all possible alternatives have been exhausted.
- Be prepared to follow employer policy, which should include whom to notify; who will search for patient; which areas will be searched and their priority; who will notify authorities, if necessary; who will notify family members; and who will coordinate search efforts.

Communication and Documentation

- Document restraint alternatives used, patient behaviours that relate to cognitive status, and interventions to mediate these behaviours in nurses' notes in electronic health record (EHR) or chart.
- Document your evaluation of caregiver learning.

Special Considerations
Teaching Considerations

- Teach caregiver ways to involve patient in their visits, keeping patient appropriately stimulated.
- Teach caregiver how to adapt the home environment (see Chapter 42) to minimize wandering.

Gerontological Considerations

- Keep older persons active and ambulatory to increase endurance and function.
- Reminiscence helps older persons remain oriented.

Care in the Community

- Patients with a potential for self-injury or violence to others need intensive supervision. Family members and home health caregivers need to recognize this and take appropriate preventive measures.
- Have caregiver set up an area in the home where it is safe for an older person to wander.

▶ *Video Clip* NSO *Nursing Skills Online Safety Module 4 / Lesson 2*

In health care settings restraints are most commonly used to prevent the disruption of therapy. Restraints are used in critical care settings, where patients who are seriously ill often unknowingly attempt to remove endotracheal tubes, intravenous (IV) catheters, urinary catheters, and feeding tubes (Freeman, Yorke, & Dark, 2018). Unplanned removal of endotracheal tubes has been found to be associated with agitation, inadequate sedation, and reduced patient surveillance by health care staff; however, the effectiveness of the use of physical restraint in adult critical care areas has not been established (Freeman et al., 2018). Nurses often pursue prescriptions for restraints when they are concerned that disruption of therapy can significantly injure patients; however, a least-restraint approach is best practice. Nurses need to implement approaches to appropriately secure medical devices and prevent accidental removal without using restraints (e.g., ensure endotracheal tube is anchored correctly; IV line is secured; long-sleeved robe to IV insertion site). The use of physical and chemical restraints in long-term care has been associated with concerns about patient behaviours (e.g., wandering and aggression) and fall risks and a shortage of nurse staffing (fewer staff to monitor patient safety).

The least-restraint directive is best practice in facilities across Canada. The CPSI (2015) considered adding "patient death or serious harm caused by the use of restraints …" (p. 11) as a "never event" but did not do so because restraints are sometimes needed for both patient and health care provider safety, and they were concerned about balancing benefits with risk of harm (e.g., preventing patient falls). Accreditation Canada (2019) requires health care facilities to have restraint policies and procedures.

The Canadian Medical Protection Agency (CMPA, 2016) has released the following risk management guidelines relating to the use of restraints: (1) attempt other methods prior to using a restraint; (2) obtain an adequate history; (3) conduct a physical exam; (4) explain the restraint plan calmly and clearly to patient and caregiver; (5) document rationale for using restraints and use the least restrictive method; (6) ensure accurate policies for monitoring the patient; and (7) adhere to applicable regulations, laws, and employer policies.

Restraints are a temporary way to keep patients safe. However, there is no evidence that they prevent falls, reduce wandering, or prevent medical devices from being pulled out. Research has shown that patients suffer fewer injuries if left unrestrained (Freeman et al., 2018). The use of mechanical or physical restraints requires a health care provider's prescription and must be based on a face-to-face patient assessment. The nurse must ensure that the patient or caregiver is aware of restraint use and its rationale, because there is a potential liability from restraint use in the absence of informed consent (CPSI, 2017).

The use of physical restraints is never considered to be a part of treatment and they are used only as a last resort (CPSI, 2017). Extreme caution is required in their application when there is no other option to manage the undesired behaviour. Chemical restraint, or *acute control medication* (ACM), refers to "the administration of psychotropic medication in situations where a person may have already lost behavioural control or where there is imminent risk of loss of control in behaviour that will lead to harm to self or others" (CPSI, 2017, p. 4).

Delegation and Collaboration

The skills of assessing a patient's behaviour and level of orientation, the need for restraints, the appropriate restraint type, and the ongoing assessments required while a restraint is in place cannot be delegated to an unregulated care provider (UCP). Applying and routinely checking a restraint can be delegated to a UCP. The nurse directs the UCP by:

- Reviewing correct placement of the restraint and how to routinely check the patient's circulation, skin condition, and breathing.
- Reviewing when and how to change a patient's position and provide range-of-motion (ROM) exercises, elimination assistance, and skin care.
- Instructing the UCP to notify the nurse immediately if there is a change in level of patient agitation, skin integrity, circulation of extremities, or patient's breathing.

Equipment

- Proper restraint (e.g., belt, wrist, mitten)
- Padding (if needed)

STEP	RATIONALE

ASSESSMENT

1. Identify patient using at least two person-specific identifiers (e.g., name and date of birth or name and medical record number) according to employer policy.

Ensures correct patient. Complies with Accreditation Canada's standards and improves patient safety (Accreditation Canada, 2019).

2. Assess for underlying cause(s) of agitation and cognitive impairment leading to patient-initiated medical device removal (Freeman et al., 2018):

   a. Assess for life-threatening physiological impairments.

   Physiological alterations might lead to accidental patient-initiated medical device removal (Freeman et al., 2018). Identification of conditions might lead to more appropriate medical or pharmacological treatment, eliminating need for restraints (see Skill 14.2).

   b. Assess for respiratory and neurological conditions, fever and sepsis, hypoglycemia and hyperglycemia, alcohol or substance withdrawal, and fluid and electrolyte imbalance.

STEP	RATIONALE

ASSESSMENT

c. Notify health care provider of change in mental status and compromised physiological status.

d. Obtain baseline or premorbid cognitive function from caregivers.

Caregivers provide an excellent source of information for patient's behaviour patterns and past history.

e. Establish whether patient has history of dementia or depression.

f. Review medications (including OTC and herbal therapy) that cause risk for falling to identify interactions, adverse effects.

g. Review current laboratory values.

3. Assess patient's current behaviour (e.g., confusion, disorientation, agitation, restlessness, combativeness, inability to follow directions, or repeated removal of tubing, dressing, or other therapeutic devices). Does patient create a risk to other patients?

If patient's behaviour continues despite treatment or restraint alternatives, use of least restrictive restraint is indicated.

4. If restraint alternatives failed earlier, confer with health care provider. Review employer policies and provincial/territorial laws regarding restraints. Obtain current health care provider's prescription, which must include purpose, type, location, and time or duration of restraint. Determine if signed consent for use of restraint is necessary (see employer policy). Some policies require that the prescription be renewed according to time limits for a maximum of 24 consecutive hours (CPSI, 2017).

A health care provider's prescription for least restrictive type of restraint is required (Accreditation Canada, 2019).

Clinical Decision Point *A licensed independent health care provider responsible for the care of the patient evaluates the patient in person within 1 hour of the initiation of restraint used for the management of violent or self-destructive behaviour that jeopardizes the physical safety of the patient, staff, or others. A registered nurse or a physician assistant may conduct the in-person evaluation if they are trained in accordance with the requirements and consult with the above health care provider after the evaluation as determined by facility policy. Always use the least restrictive restraint possible (e.g., mitts, elbow extenders) (CPSI & RNAO, 2018).*

5. Review manufacturer instructions for restraint application before entering patient's room. Determine most appropriate size restraint.

You need to be familiar with all devices used for patient care and protection. Incorrect application of a restraint device can result in patient injury or death.

NURSING DIAGNOSES

- Potential for injury
- Potential for trauma

Risk factors are individualized on the basis of patient's condition or needs.

PLANNING

1. Expected outcomes following completion of procedure:
   - Patient maintains intact skin integrity, pulses, temperature, colour, and sensation of restrained body part.

   Restraints are applied and monitored correctly.

   - Patient is free from injury.

   Restraints are removed in a timely manner.

   - Patient's therapy (e.g., intravenous [IV] tube, catheters) is uninterrupted.

   Disruption of therapy causes patient injury, pain, or discomfort and increases risk of infection.

   - Patient maintains self-esteem and sense of dignity.

   Physical restraints have a detrimental effect on psychosocial well-being of patient.

   - Restraint is discontinued as soon as possible.

   Limits period of time patient is at risk for injury.

2. Gather equipment and perform hand hygiene.

   Promotes organization and reduces transmission of microorganisms.

3. Explain what you plan to do and why. Provide privacy.

   Reduces patient anxiety and promotes cooperation.

STEP	RATIONALE

IMPLEMENTATION

1. Adjust bed to proper height and lower side rail on side of patient contact. Be sure that patient is comfortable and in proper body alignment.

   Allows you to use proper body mechanics and prevents injury during restraint application. Positioning prevents contractures and neurovascular injury while restraint is in place.

2. Inspect area where restraint is to be placed. Note if there is any nearby tubing or device. Assess condition of skin, sensation, adequacy of circulation, and range of joint motion.

   Restraints sometimes compress and interfere with functioning of devices or tubes. Assessment provides baseline to monitor patient's response to restraint.

3. Pad skin and bony prominences (as necessary) that will be under restraint.

   Reduces friction and pressure from restraint to skin and underlying tissue.

4. Apply proper-size restraint. **NOTE:** Refer to manufacturer directions.

   a. *Mitten restraint:* Thumbless mitten device restrains patient's hands. Place hand in mitten, being sure that Velcro strap is around wrist and not forearm (see illustration).

   Prevents patient from dislodging or removing medical device, removing dressings, or scratching but allows greater movement than wrist restraint. It is considered a restraint alternative if untethered and patient is physically and cognitively able to remove it.

   b. *Elbow restraint (freedom splint):* Restraint consists of rigidly padded fabric that wraps around arm and is closed with Velcro. The upper end has a clamp that hooks to sleeve of patient's gown or shirt (see illustration). Insert arm so elbow joint rests against padded area, keeping joint extended.

   Commonly used with infants and children to prevent elbow flexion (e.g., with IV line placed in antecubital fossa). Restraint keeps elbow extended, making it difficult to remove or disrupt a medical device.

   c. *Belt or body restraint:* Have patient in sitting position in bed. Apply belt over clothes, gown, or pajamas. Be sure to place restraint at waist, not chest or abdomen. Slot in belt may be positioned in front for limited movement or rear for increased movement. Remove wrinkles or creases in clothing. Bring ties through slots in belt. Help patient lie down in bed. Have patient roll to side, and avoid applying belt too tightly. Ensure that straps secured to bedframe are snug so belt does not slide to sides of bed (see illustrations). *Option:* Apply restraint net if intent is to limit patient turning.

   Restrains centre of gravity and prevents patient from rolling off stretcher, sitting up while on stretcher, or falling out of bed. Tight application interferes with ventilation if belt moves up over abdomen or chest.

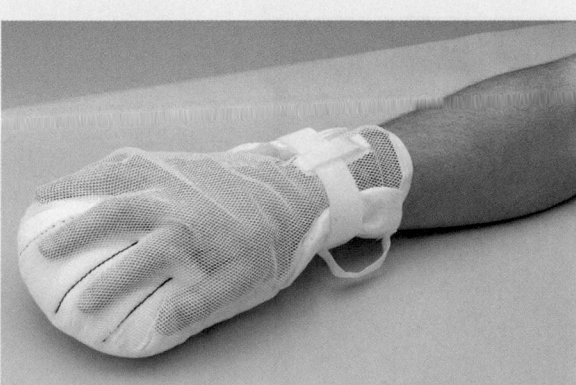

STEP 4a Mitten restraint. (*Courtesy Posey Company, Arcadia, CA.*)

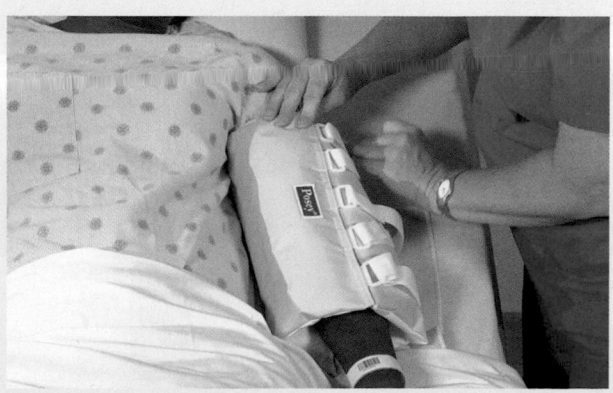

STEP 4b Freedom elbow restraint. (*Courtesy Posey Company, Arcadia, CA.*)

STEP	RATIONALE

IMPLEMENTATION

d. *Extremity (ankle or wrist) restraint:* Restraint made of soft quilted material or sheepskin with foam padding. Wrap limb restraint around wrist or ankle with soft part toward skin and secure snugly (not tightly) in place by Velcro strap (see illustration). Insert two fingers under secured restraint (see illustration).

Restraint is designed to immobilize one or all extremities. Maintains immobilization of extremity to protect patient from fall or accidental removal of therapeutic device (e.g., IV tube, Foley catheter). Tight application interferes with circulation and potentially causes neurovascular injury.

Clinical Decision Point *Patient with wrist and ankle restraints is at risk for aspiration if positioned supine. Place patient in lateral position or with head of bed elevated rather than supine.*

5. Attach restraint straps to part of bedframe that moves when raising or lowering head of bed. Be sure that straps are secure. *Do not attach to side rails.* Attach restraint to chair frame for patient in chair or wheelchair, being sure that buckle is out of patient's reach.

Properly positioned strap does not tighten and restrict circulation when bed is raised or lowered.

6. Secure restraints on bedframe with quick-release buckle (see illustration). *Do not tie strap in a knot.* Be sure that buckle is out of patient reach.

Allows for quick release in emergency.

7. Double-check and insert two fingers under secured restraint one more time. Assess proper placement of restraint, including skin integrity, pulses, skin temperature and colour, and sensation of restrained body part.

Provides baseline to later evaluate if injury develops from restraint.

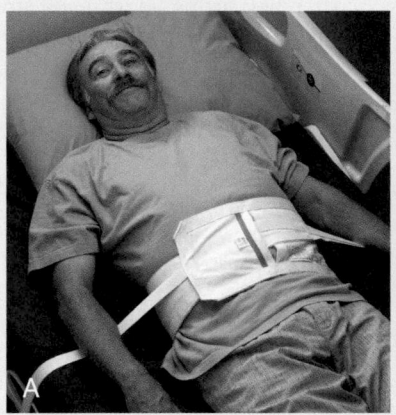 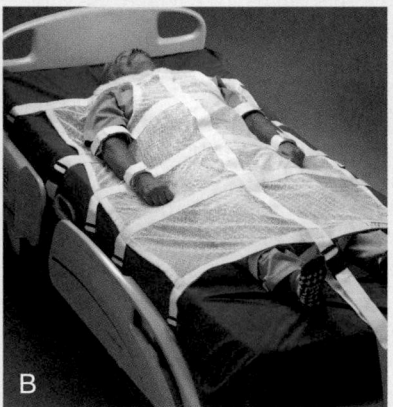

STEP 4c A, Properly applied belt restraint allows patient to turn in bed. **B,** *Option:* Restraint with net limits patient's ability to turn. (A, B, *Courtesy Posey Company, Arcadia, CA.*)

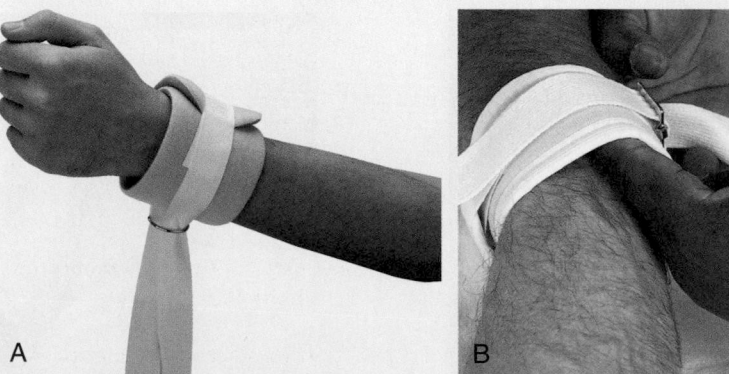

STEP 4d A, Extremity restraint. **B,** Check restraint for constriction by inserting two fingers under restraint.

STEP	RATIONALE

IMPLEMENTATION

8. Remove restraint at least every 2 hours (RNAO, 2012) or more frequently as determined by employer policy. Reposition patient, provide comfort, assess patient need for elimination, and evaluate patient condition each time. If patient is violent or noncompliant, remove one restraint at a time or have staff assistance while removing restraints.

Provides opportunity to attend to patient's basic needs and determine need for continuation.

Clinical Decision Point *Do not leave a patient who is violent or aggressive unattended while restraints are off.*

9. Secure call light or intercom system within patient's reach.

Allows patient, family, or caregiver to get help quickly.

10. Leave bed or chair with wheels locked. Keep bed in lowest position.

Prevents bed or chair from moving if patient tries to get out. If patient falls with bed in lowest position, this reduces chance of injury.

11. Perform hand hygiene.

Reduces transmission of microorganisms.

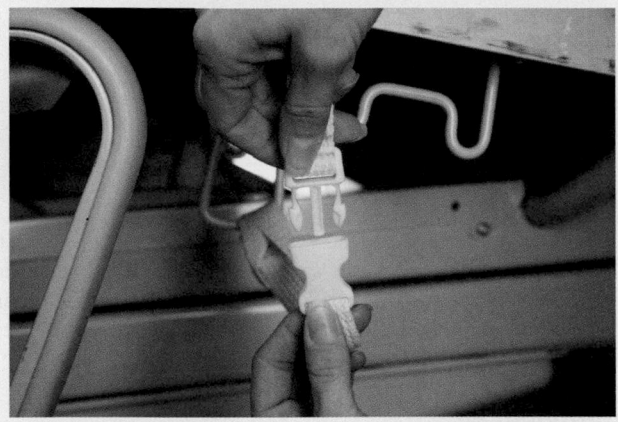

STEP 6 Quick-release buckle makes it easier to disconnect and evacuate patients in an emergency.

EVALUATION

1. After application, evaluate patient for signs of injury every 15–30 minutes (check employer policy) (e.g., circulation, vital signs, ROM, physical and psychological status, and readiness for discontinuation).

Frequent evaluation prevents injury to patient and ensures removal of restraint at earliest possible time. Frequency of monitoring guides staff in determining appropriate intervals for evaluation based on patient's needs and condition, type of restraint used, risk associated with use of chosen intervention, and other relevant factors.

2. Evaluate patient's need for elimination, nutrition and fluids, and hygiene and release restraint at least every 2 hours.

Prevents injury to patient and attends to basic needs.

3. Evaluate patient for any complications of immobility.

Early detection of skin irritation, restricted breathing, or reduction in mobility prevents serious adverse events.

4. Evaluate patient within 1 to 4 hours after initiation of restraints (depending on employer policy).

Determines patient's immediate situation, reaction to restraints, medical and behavioural condition, and need to continue or terminate restraints.

5. After 24 hours, before writing a new prescription, health care provider who is responsible for patient's care must see and reassess patient.

Ensures that restraint application continues to be medically appropriate.

6. Observe IV catheters, urinary catheters, and drainage tubes to determine that they are positioned correctly and that therapy remains uninterrupted.

Reinsertion is uncomfortable and increases risk for infection or interrupts therapy.

7. Observe patient's behaviour and reaction to presence of restraint.

Restraints can increase restlessness and agitation, resulting in harm.

STEP	RATIONALE

EVALUATION

8. Use Teach-Back: "We've talked about the reason we're using restraints on your father. Tell me that reason. I want to be sure you understand." Develop a revised plan if caregiver is not able to teach back correctly.

Determines caregiver's level of understanding of instructional topic.

Unexpected Outcomes	Related Interventions
1. Patient experiences impaired skin integrity.	• Evaluate need for continued use of restraint and if alternatives can be used. • If restraint is still needed, be sure that it is applied correctly and provide adequate padding. • Check skin under restraint for abrasions and remove restraints more often. Provide appropriate skin care and change wet or soiled restraints.
2. Patient becomes more confused or agitated.	• Determine cause of behaviour and eliminate if possible; consult with health care provider. • Determine need for more or less sensory stimulation and make any stimulation meaningful. • Reorient as needed and try restraint-free options.
3. Patient has neurovascular injury (e.g., cyanosis, pallor, and coldness of skin or complains of tingling, pain, or numbness).	• Remove restraint immediately, stay with patient, and have health care provider notified. • Protect extremity from further injury.

Communication and Documentation

- Document nursing interventions and restraint alternatives tried on restraint flow sheet or in nurses' notes in electronic health record (EHR) or chart.
- Document your evaluation of caregiver learning.
- Document purpose for restraint, type and location, time applied, time ending the restraint, and routine observations made every 15 minutes (e.g., skin colour, pulses, sensation, vital signs, behaviour) in flow sheets or nurses' notes.
- Document patient's level of orientation and behaviour after restraint application. Document times patient was evaluated, attempts to use alternatives, and patient's response when restraint was removed.

Special Considerations
Teaching

- Explain thoroughly to patient and caregiver the use of restraints. Caution caregiver against removing, repositioning, or retying restraint.

Pediatric

- Limit the use of restraints to clinically appropriate and adequately justified situations (e.g., examination or treatment that involves the head and neck) after exhausting all appropriate alternatives. Remain with infant while restrained and remove restraint immediately after treatment is completed.

- When a child needs to be restrained for a procedure, it is best if the person applying the restraint is not the child's parent or guardian.
- When an infant or small child requires a restraint, a mummy wrap using a blanket or sheet effectively controls their movements (Hockenberry & Wilson, 2015).

Gerontological

- Restrained older persons often respond with anger, fear, depression, humiliation, demoralization, discomfort, and resignation.
- Consider the risks associated with restraints (e.g., pressure injuries, impaired strength and balance) for older persons (Touhy, Jett, Boscart, et al., 2019). All of the complications of immobility are amplified, leading to greater risk for functional decline.

Care in the Community

- Much of the evidence available relating to the use of restraints has been derived from acute and chronic care facilities, not from the home setting. The family or caregiver has a different role in the home setting and more influence related to care decisions (Scheepmans, Dierckx de Casterlé, Paquay, et al., 2018).
- It is important to educate caregivers about the importance of frequently checking on the patient when restraints are used, in order to ensure safety. In home settings, restraints often involve use of equipment that is already in the person's home instead of professional equipment (e.g., placing a chair close to the table) (Scheepmans et al., 2018).

PROCEDURAL GUIDELINE 14.1 *Fire, Electrical, and Chemical Safety*

There are over 250 health care institution fires annually in Canada (Statistics Canada, 2019). Most are typically electrical or anaesthetic related. Smoking-related fires pose a significant risk because of unauthorized smoking in beds or bathrooms. The CPSI (2015)

"never event" list includes "patient death or serious harm due to an accidental burn" (p. 7) from oxygen fires, unintended burns occurring during surgery, heat or cold burns from assisted bathing, and the use of hot or cold packs and wound care. In the home

PROCEDURAL GUIDELINE 14.1 *Fire, Electrical, and Chemical Safety—cont'd*

setting, oxygen-related fires is a risk for patients requiring oxygen therapy (see Chapter 23). Health care facilities routinely check and maintain all electrical devices. Every biomedical device (e.g., suction machine, infusion pump) must have a safety inspection sticker with an expiration date applied to it. Electrical equipment in good working order requires a three-prong electrical plug for proper grounding. If a patient brings an electrical device to a hospital, an engineer must inspect the device for safe wiring and function before use. Always discourage patients from bringing nonessential electrical devices (e.g., hair dryers or electric tooth-brushes) into a health care facility. Many patients living with disabilities use battery chargers for mobility equipment function. These devices need to be inspected by hospital engineers as well. Prevention is the key to fire safety. Always comply with employer smoking policies, use equipment correctly, and keep combustible materials away from heat sources.

Chemicals in many medications (e.g., chemotherapy drugs), anaesthetic gases, cleaning solutions, and disinfectants are potentially toxic. They injure the body after skin or mucous membrane (e.g., eyes) contact, ingestion, or vapour inhalation. The Workplace Hazardous Materials Information System (WHMIS) (Health Canada, 2015) regulates hazard classification and requirements for labels and safety data sheets (SDS) (previously called *material safety data sheet*) for each hazardous chemical in the workplace. An SDS form contains information about the properties of the particular chemical and handling the substance in a safe manner (Table 14.1).

Delegation and Collaboration

The skill of fire, electrical, and chemical safety can be delegated to an unregulated care provider (UCP). Interprofessional collaboration is a priority in an emergency situation. In the event of fire, collaborate with the fire department; in an electrical or chemical event, collaborate with the safety officer of the facility. The nurse directs the UCP to:

- Identify patients requiring the most help to evacuate or protect.
- Be aware of any risks for chemical exposure.

TABLE 14.1

Safety Data Sheets Requirement Summary

1	Identification	Product identifier, recommended use and restrictions on use, supplier contact information, emergency phone number
2	Hazard Identification	Classification (hazard class and category), label elements (including hazard pictogram, signal word, hazard statement and precautionary statements) and other hazards (e.g., thermal hazards)
3	Composition/Ingredients Information	For a hazardous product that is a substance: the chemical name, synonyms, CAS No. and the chemical name of impurities, stabilizing solvents and stabilizing additives where classified and that contribute to the classification of the product For a hazardous product that is a mixture: for ingredients that present a health hazard, the chemical name, synonyms, CAS No. and concentration **NOTE:** Confidential Business Information Rules may apply.
4	First Aid Measures	First-aid measures by route of exposure as well as most important symptoms or effects
5	Fire Fighting Measures	Suitable (and unsuitable) extinguishing media, specific hazards, special equipment and precautions for fire fighters
6	Accidental Release Measures	Protective equipment, emergency procedures, methods and materials for containment and cleanup
7	Handling and Storage	Precautions for safe handling, conditions for storage, including any incompatibilities
8	Exposure Controls/Personal Protection	Exposure limits, engineering controls, personal protective equipment
9	Physical and Chemical Properties	Appearance, odour, odour threshold, pH, melting/freezing point, boiling point and range, flash point, upper and lower flammable or explosive limits
10	Stability and Reactivity	Reactivity, chemical stability, possible hazardous reactions, conditions to avoid, incompatible materials, hazardous decomposition products
11	Toxicological Information	Description of various toxic effects by route of entry, including effects of acute or chronic exposure, carcinogenicity, reproductive effects, respiratory sensitization
12	Ecological Information	Aquatic and terrestrial toxicity (if available), persistence and degradability, bioaccumulative potential, mobility in soil
13	Disposal Considerations	Safe handling and methods of disposal, including contaminated packaging
14	Transport Information	UN number and proper shipping name, hazard classes, packing group
15	Regulatory Information	Safety, health, and environmental regulations specific to the product
16	Other Information	Other information, including date of the latest revision of the SDS

From Eversafe Media Inc. (2017). *WHMIS 2015 safety data sheets*. Windsor, ON: Author. Retrieved from https://eversafe.ca/whmis-2015-safety-data-sheets/.

Continued

PROCEDURAL GUIDELINE 14.1 *Fire, Electrical, and Chemical Safety—cont'd*

Equipment
Fire
- Appropriate fire extinguisher for fire: type A, B, C, or ABC

Chemical
- Appropriate personal protective equipment (PPE): clean gloves, mask, gown
- SDS form

Procedural Steps
1. Review employer policies for rapid response to fire, electrical, and chemical emergency. Know your responsibilities such as initiating fire alarm and patient evacuation.
2. Know the location of fire alarms, emergency equipment (e.g., fire extinguishers), SDS forms, emergency eyewash stations, and emergency exit routes.
3. Assess patient's mental status and ability to ambulate, transfer, or move to anticipate the procedures that will be needed to evacuate the patient.
4. Be alert to situations that increase the risk of fire (e.g., a patient on oxygen charging a cell phone while in bed). Regularly check a patient room for electrical or fire hazards.
5. Know which patients are on oxygen. Oxygen delivery may be shut off in the event of a severe fire.
6. Inspect equipment for current maintenance sticker. Check electrical equipment for basic safety features (i.e., intact cords and plugs, intact casing). Know employer process for tagging and reporting broken or unsafe equipment.
7. Fire safety:
   a. Follow the acronym *RACE*.
      (1) **R**escue patient from immediate injury by removing from area or shielding from fire to avoid burns.
      (2) **A**ctivate fire alarm immediately. Follow employer policy for alerting staff to respond. (In many situations perform Steps (1) and (2) simultaneously by using call system to alert staff while you help patients at risk.)
      (3) **C**ontain the fire by:
         (a) Closing all doors and windows.
         (b) Turning off oxygen and electrical equipment.
         (c) Placing wet towels along base of doors.

      (4) **E**vacuate patients:
         (a) Direct ambulatory patients to walk by themselves to a safe area. Know the fire exits and emergency evacuation route.
         (b) If patient is on life support, maintain respiratory status manually (Ambu bag) until patient removed from fire area.
         (c) Move bed-bound patients by stretcher, bed, or wheelchair.
         (d) For patients who cannot walk or ambulate use these options:
            (i) Place on blanket and drag patient out of area of danger.
            (ii) *Use two-person swing:* Place patient in sitting position and have two staff members form a seat by clasping forearms together. Lift patient into "seat" and carry out of area of danger (see illustrations A and B).

Clinical Decision Point *Consider the patient's weight and size when choosing an evacuation carry. Use safe patient-handling techniques. Have a staff member help to avoid injury.*

         (e) If fire department personnel are on the scene, they will help with evacuation of patients.
      b. Extinguish fire using appropriate fire extinguisher: type A for ordinary combustibles (e.g., wood, cloth, paper, most plastics); type B for flammable liquids (e.g., gasoline, grease, paint, anaesthetic gas); type C for electrical equipment, type ABC for any type of fire (most common extinguisher in use). To use an extinguisher, follow the acronym *PASS*.
         (1) **P**ull the pin (see illustration A).
         (2) **A**im nozzle at base of fire (see illustration B).
         (3) **S**queeze extinguisher handles (see illustration C).
         (4) **S**weep from side to side to coat area evenly.
      c. Most facilities have fire doors that are held open by magnets and close automatically when a fire alarm sounds. Fire doors should never be blocked.

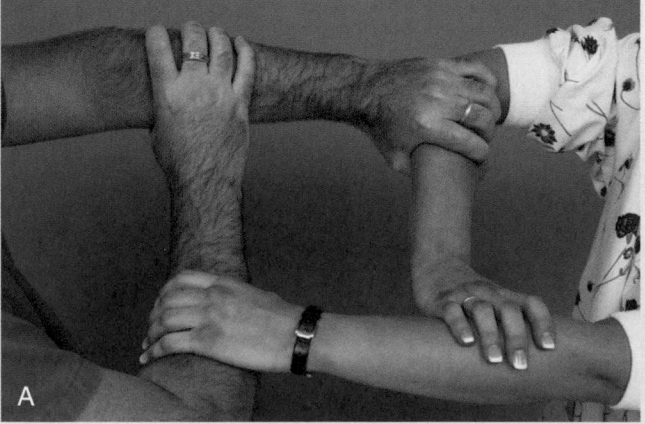
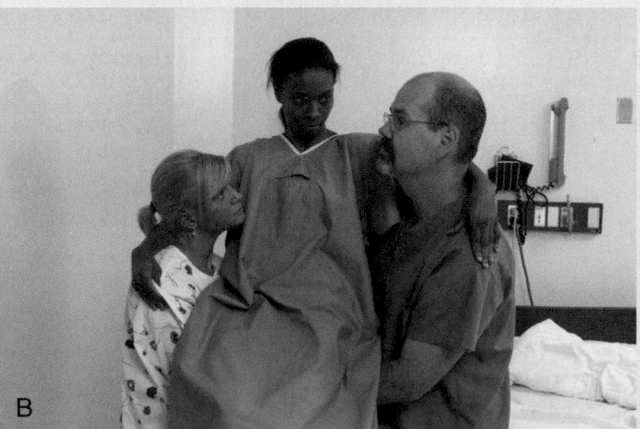

STEP 7a(4)(d)ii A, Hands positioned to form two-person evacuation swing. **B,** Patient seated firmly on swing and holding shoulders of nurses for evacuation.

PROCEDURAL GUIDELINE 14.1 *Fire, Electrical, and Chemical Safety—cont'd*

8. **Electrical safety:**
   a. If patient receives an electrical shock, immediately turn off power to electrical source and assess for presence of a pulse. *Caution:* When disengaging electrical source, check for presence of water on floor.

Clinical Decision Point *Do not touch a person who is being shocked while they are still engaged with the electrical source. If unable to turn off power, call emergency number for help.*

   b. Once the source of electricity is disconnected, provide appropriate assistance. If patient is pulseless, institute emergency resuscitation (see Chapter 28).
   c. Notify emergency personnel and patient's health care provider.
   d. If patient has a pulse and remains alert and oriented, obtain vital signs and assess the skin for signs of thermal injury.

9. **Chemical safety:**
   a. Attend to any person exposed to a chemical. Treat chemical splashes to the eyes immediately; flush eyes with water using clean, lukewarm tap water for 15 to 20 minutes; stand under a shower or place head under running faucet. Remove contact lenses if flushing does not remove them (see Chapter 19).
   b. Notify people in the immediate area of the spill and evacuate all nonessential personnel from area.
   c. Refer to SDS; if spilled material is flammable, turn off electrical and heat sources.
   d. Avoid breathing vapours of spilled material; apply appropriate respirator.
   e. Use appropriate PPE (refer to SDS) to clean up a spill.
   f. Dispose of any materials used in cleanup as hazardous waste.
10. Follow employer policy for reporting any fire and document accordingly.

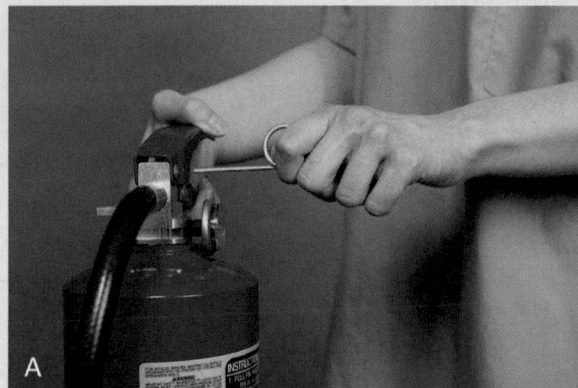
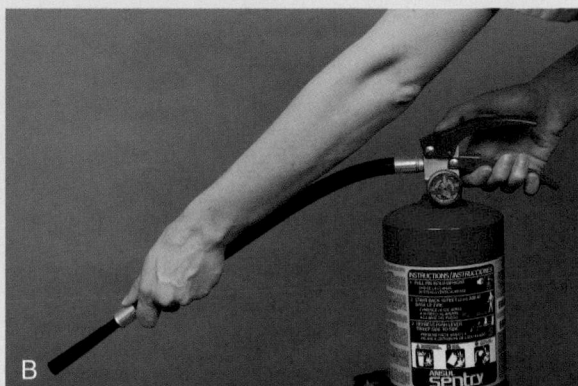
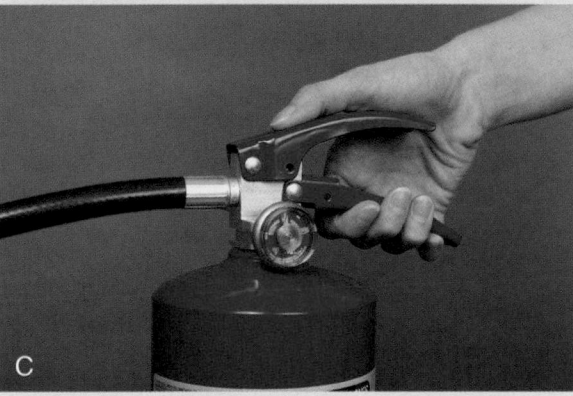

STEP 7b(1) A, Pull safety pin from fire extinguisher. **B,** Aim nozzle of hose at base of fire. **C,** Squeeze handle while sweeping side to side with nozzle.

✦ SKILL 14.4   Seizure Precautions

Approximately 140 000 Canadians have epilepsy (Statistics Canada, 2016), which is a disease in which seizures occur. Seizures are sudden, abnormal, uncontrolled electrical discharge of neurons in the brain that interfere with normal function (Lewis, Bucher, Heitkemper, et al., 2019). Seizures are classified as either focal, generalized, or unknown onset (Fisher, Cross, French, et al., 2017). The International League Against Epilepsy revised the operational classification of seizure types to adopt more transparent names when classifying the type of seizure (Fisher et al., 2017):

- **Focal Onset**—Patient may be aware or have impaired awareness; motor versus nonmotor onset; focal aware seizure (prior term *simple partial seizure*); focal impaired awareness seizure (prior term *complex partial seizure*); focal to bilateral tonic-clonic (prior term *partial onset with secondary generalization*);

hyperkinetic seizure (agitated thrashing or leg pedaling movements); focal seizures can have emotional manifestations (e.g., fear, joy).

- **Generalized Onset**—Can be motor (e.g., tonic-clonic) or nonmotor (absence); myoclonic-tonic-clonic seizure is common in juvenile epilepsy.
- **Unknown Onset**—Can be motor (e.g., tonic-clonic) or nonmotor; referred to as an unclassified seizure and can include additional features (e.g., tonic-clonic, epileptic spasms, behaviour arrest). An unknown onset seizure may later become classified as a focal or generalized seizure.

Prolonged seizures last between 5 and 30 minutes, whereas status epilepticus is more than 30 minutes of continuous clinical or electrographic (shown on an electroencephalogram [EEG]) seizure activity or recurrent seizure activity without recovery between seizures (Glauser, Shinnar, Gloss, et al., 2016). Once a seizure lasts more than 5 minutes it is predicted to be prolonged; thus, treatment protocols use a 5-minute definition to initiate treatment (Glauser et al., 2016). It is a critical care emergency. Status epilepticus can be convulsive (rhythmic jerking of the extremities), nonconvulsive (activity on EEG), and repeated focal motor signs not associated with altered awareness.

Traditionally, patients who have a seizure are immediately placed in the side-lying position to prevent aspiration of oral secretions. This is still a standard of practice. However, the patient should be rolled gently into this position and only if possible without injuring any body part (Smith, Wagner, & Edwards, 2015). Refer to employer policy for positioning guidelines.

The current practice guidelines for patients with status epilepticus include the following (Lewis et al., 2019; Smith et al., 2015):

- Ensure patent airway when patient loses consciousness.
- Provide noninvasive airway protection and gas exchange with head positioning, keeping the airway patent and administering oxygen (see Chapters 23 and 25).
- Monitor vital signs, level of consciousness, oxygen saturation, Glasgow Coma Scale, and pupil size and reactivity, according to employer policy.
- Establish an intravenous (IV) route for emergency medications.
- When seizure begins to subside, intubation (insertion of an artificial airway) should be attempted only if gas exchange is compromised or if patient is believed to have increased intracranial pressure; never force an airway between a patient's clenched teeth.
- Administer IV dextrose if patient is hypoglycemic.

Delegation and Collaboration

The skill of assessing a patient's risk for seizures cannot be delegated to an unregulated care provider (UCP). However, the skills for making a patient's environment safe and the ongoing care of patients on seizure precautions can be delegated. The nurse directs the UCP about:

- The patient's prior seizure history and factors that may trigger a seizure.
- Taking immediate action in the event of a seizure by protecting the patient from falling or injury, not trying to restrain the patient, and not placing anything into the mouth.
- Informing the nurse immediately when seizure activity develops.
- Observing the patient's seizure pattern.

Equipment

- Seizure pads for side rails and headboard
- Suction machine and oral Yankauer suction catheter
- Oral airway
- Oxygen via nasal cannula or face mask
- Equipment for vital signs, pulse oximetry and blood glucose testing (see Chapter 7)
- Equipment for IV insertion (see Chapter 29)
- Emergency antiepileptic medications:
  - For emergent condition, IV lorazepam, midazolam for intramuscular (IM) administration (also nasal or buccal), rectal diazepam; for urgent treatment, oral valproate sodium or phenytoin, IV midazolam (Smith et al., 2015)
  - Clean gloves
  - Equipment for vital signs, pulse oximetry, and blood glucose monitoring

STEP	RATIONALE

ASSESSMENT

1. Assess patient's seizure history (e.g., new diagnosis, seizure within last year), knowledge of precipitating factors (e.g., emotional stress, sleep deprivation), frequency of seizures, presence of aura (e.g., metallic taste, perception of breeze blowing on face, or noxious odour), body parts affected, and sequence of events if known. Use family as resource if necessary.	Knowledge about seizure history and nature of seizures allows you to eliminate triggers that cause seizure, anticipate onset of seizure activity, and take appropriate safety measures.
2. Assess for medical and surgical conditions, including history of head trauma, electrolyte disturbances (e.g., hypoglycemia, hyperkalemia), heart disease, excess fatigue, and alcohol or caffeine consumption. Also assess for any bleeding tendencies.	Common conditions that lead to seizures or worsen existing seizure condition. Bleeding conditions could predispose patient to injury during seizure.
3. Assess medication history (e.g., antidepressants and antipsychotics). Assess for patient's adherence to anticonvulsants and therapeutic drug levels if test results are available.	Certain medications lower seizure threshold. Seizure medications must be taken as prescribed and not stopped suddenly. Stopping or changing dose may precipitate seizure activity.
4. Inspect patient's environment for potential safety hazards (e.g., extra furniture or equipment). Keep bed in low position, side rails up at head of bed.	Protects patient from injury sustained by striking head or body on furniture or equipment.
5. Assess patient's individual and cultural perspective about the meaning of seizures and their treatment.	Demonstrates person-centred care, because some cultures may follow different caring practices for a person with seizures.

STEP	RATIONALE

NURSING DIAGNOSES

- Nonadherence
- Insufficient knowledge regarding seizure precautions
- Potential for aspiration
- Potential for injury
- Potential for inadequate airway clearance
- Reduced self-concept

Related factors/Risk factors are individualized on the basis of patient's condition or needs.

PLANNING

1. Expected outcomes following completion of procedure:

- Patient remains free of traumatic injury while experiencing seizure.

  Seizure precautions prevent patients from incurring injury from a fall or seizure.

- Patient's airway remains patent during seizure activity.

  Airway occlusion and aspiration are potential complications of seizure activity.

- Patient does not experience lowered sense of self-concept following seizure episode.

  Loss of bowel or bladder control is common in generalized seizures, causing patient to feel embarrassment or shame.

2. Inform patient and appropriate caregiver that patient is on seizure precautions.

  May help to relieve patient and caregiver anxiety.

IMPLEMENTATION

1. For patients with history of seizures, keep bed in lowest position with side rails up (see employer policy). Pad rails if patient is at risk for head injury. Have oral suction and oxygen equipment ready for use.

  Modifications to environment minimize risk of injury from seizure activity or related fall. Use padded side rails only when patient is at risk for head injury (see illustration).

2. Place patient with history of seizures in room close to nurse's station or room with video monitor.

  Improves likelihood of quick response with emergency equipment.

3. Focal or generalized seizure response:

    a. Position patient safely.

        (1) If patient is standing or sitting, guide them to floor and protect head by cradling it in your lap or place pillow under head. Position patient to keep head tilted to maximize breathing (if able). Try to position patient on side *but do not force.* Do not lift patient from floor to bed during seizure.

  Position protects patient from aspiration and traumatic injury, especially head injury.

        (2) If patient is in bed, turn them onto side (*do not force*) and raise side rails.

    b. Note time seizure began and call for help immediately to have staff member bring emergency cart to bedside and clear surrounding area of furniture. Provide airway protection and gas exchange by positioning head. Have health care provider notified immediately.

  Timing and description of seizure may help in ultimate identification of type of seizure. Establishing and protecting airway when patient loses consciousness must occur immediately (Fisher et al., 2017).

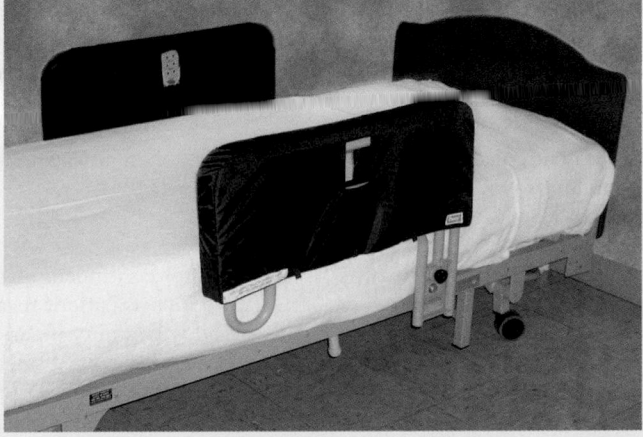

STEP 1 Padded side rails for patients at risk for head injury.

STEP	RATIONALE

IMPLEMENTATION

c. Keep patient in side-lying position (if possible), supporting head and keeping it flexed slightly forward.

Position prevents tongue from blocking airway and promotes drainage of secretions, reducing risk of aspiration.

d. Do not restrain patient; if patient is flailing limbs, hold them loosely. Loosen restrictive clothing or gown to aid breathing.

Prevents musculoskeletal injury. Promotes free ventilatory movement of chest and abdomen.

e. *Never force any object into patient's mouth*, such as fingers, medicine, tongue depressor, or airway, when teeth are clenched.

Prevents injury to mouth and possible aspiration.

Clinical Decision Point *Injury can result from forcible insertion of a hard object into the mouth. Soft objects break and become aspirated. Insert a bite block or oral airway in advance if you recognize the possibility of a generalized seizure.*

f. If possible, provide privacy. Have staff control flow of visitors in area.

Embarrassment is common after a seizure, especially if others witnessed it.

g. Observe sequence and timing of seizure activity. Note type of seizure activity (tonic, clonic, staring, blinking); whether more than one type of seizure occurs; level of consciousness; character of breathing; presence of incontinence; presence of autonomic signs of lip smacking, mastication, or grimacing; rolling of eyes.

Continued observation helps to document, diagnose, and treat seizure disorder.

h. As patient regains consciousness, assess vital signs and reorient and reassure them. Explain what happened and answer patient's questions. Stay with patient until fully awake.

Informing patients of type of seizure activity experienced helps them to participate knowledgeably in their care. Some patients remain confused for a period of time after seizure or become violent.

4. **Status epilepticus is a critical care emergency.**

a. Follow Steps 3a to 3c to stabilize airway and call emergency team.

Ensures rapid response and management of airway and breathing.

b. Assist health care provider with intubation (introduction of endotracheal tube or oral airway) (see Chapter 25) if oxygen saturation is compromised or elevated intracranial pressure is suspected. (**NOTE:** Apply clean gloves if timing allows.) Physician on team will intubate patient when jaw is relaxed (between seizure activity).

Medical emergency requires rapid response. Airway establishes oxygenation (Fisher et al., 2017; Smith et al., 2015).

c. Access and administer oxygen; turn on suction equipment; keep airway patent with oral suctioning (if possible).

Maintains oxygenation.

Clinical Decision Point *Never place hands in patient's mouth during a seizure. The patient may accidentally bite your fingers. Do not force any type of airway into mouth.*

d. Have another nurse on team monitoring vital signs and oxygen saturation according to employer policy, and have team member perform fingerstick to check blood glucose (Smith et al., 2015).

Necessary to monitor and support baseline vital signs and determine if patient is hypoglycemic (common cause of seizure).

e. Member of team will prepare for and insert IV catheter (if one is not in place) with 0.9% sodium chloride infusing and administer IV antiseizure medications (see Chapter 29).

Provides route for IV medication to stop seizure and for fluid resuscitation (Smith et al., 2015).

f. As seizure begins to subside, suction patient's airway if secretions have accumulated. If oral airway was inserted, be sure that it remains in correct position. Continue oxygen administration.

Maintains open airway and oxygenation.

g. Keep patient in side-lying position of comfort in bed with side rails up and bed in lowest position.

Provides for continued safety to reduce risk of aspiration of secretions as patient regains consciousness and lessens risk of fall with injury if patient tries to exit bed.

5. As patient regains consciousness, reorient and reassure them. Explain what happened and provide quiet, nonstimulating environment (e.g., lights low, minimal care interruptions). Place call light or intercom system within reach. Instruct patient not to get out of bed without help.

Provides for continued safety. Patients are often confused and lethargic following seizure. They are at risk for falls if they attempt to get out of bed.

STEP	RATIONALE

IMPLEMENTATION

6. Clean up patient care area; dispose of used supplies. Perform hand hygiene.	Reduces transmission of microorganisms.

EVALUATION

1. Check vital signs and oxygen saturation every 15 minutes postseizure and maintain patent airway.	Determines patient's cardiopulmonary status and response to seizure episode.
2. Recheck blood glucose per health care provider prescription.	Determines if normal blood glucose level has been reached.
3. Examine patient for injury, including oral cavity (broken teeth, laceration of tongue or mucosa) and extremities.	Determines presence of any traumatic injuries resulting from seizure activity.

Clinical Decision Point *If onset of seizure was not witnessed and you suspect that patient fell and struck head, treat as a closed head injury or spinal injury. Place a cervical collar on patient before attempting to turn or reposition.*

4. Evaluate patient's mental status after seizure (level of consciousness, confusion, hallucinations). Encourage them to verbalize feelings.	Temporary mental status changes are common following seizure. Therapeutic interaction enables patient to recognize feelings associated with having a seizure disorder.
5. Help health care provider as needed conduct neurological examination of patient and collect any ordered blood tests (see Chapter 9).	Evaluates for potential life-threatening metabolic alterations (Lewis et al., 2019; Smith et al., 2015).

Unexpected Outcomes	**Related Interventions**
1. Patient suffers traumatic injury.	• Continue to protect patient from further injury. • Notify health care provider immediately. • Administer prescribed treatments. • Reassess patient's environment to ensure that environment is free of safety hazards. • Complete required employer documentation.
2. Patient aspirates oral secretions.	• Turn onto side, insert oral airway (if possible; see Chapter 25), and apply suction to remove material in oral pharynx and maintain patent airway. • Administer oxygen as needed per order.

Communication and Documentation

- Document in nurses' notes in electronic health record (EHR) or chart what you observed before, during, and after seizure. Provide detailed description of the type of seizure activity and sequence of events (e.g., motor activity, level of consciousness, vital signs and oxygen saturation, colour, movement of extremities, incontinence, patient's status immediately following seizure, and time frame of events).
- Document treatments administered: establishment of IV line, fluid infusing, stabilization of airway.
- Alert health care provider immediately as seizure begins. Status epilepticus is a critical care emergency that requires immediate interprofessional collaboration.

Special Considerations
Teaching

- Inform an adult with an unprovoked first seizure that their seizure recurrence risk is greatest early within the first 2 years (21–45%). The patient's health care provider is likely to prescribe immediate antiepileptic drug (AED) therapy to reduce recurrence risk within the first 2 years (Krumholz, Wiebe, Gronseth, et al., 2015).
- Patients need to know that antiseizure medications help control epilepsy. Warn them to take prescribed medications regularly.

They should never stop medications suddenly because this precipitates seizures.
- Advise patient to avoid alcohol, which is often incompatible with anticonvulsive medications and intensifies central nervous system depression.
- Proper oral hygiene and frequent dental care are necessary when patient takes phenytoin long term because gingival hyperplasia is an adverse effect.
- Encourage patient to wear a medical alert bracelet or carry identification card noting presence of seizure disorder and listing medications taken.
- Fatigue, stress, and illness can potentiate seizures. Teach patients to eat a balanced diet regularly, get adequate sleep, and consult their health care provider promptly when ill.
- A seizure disorder usually imposes driving limitations. It is recommended that a waiting period of 6–12 seizure-free months elapse before patient attempts to drive or operate dangerous equipment (refer to specific provincial/territorial law).

Pediatric

- Teach parents what to observe for in their child's seizure.
- Child should wear a medical alert bracelet noting presence of a seizure disorder.

- Encourage children with severe atonic seizures (abrupt loss of muscle tone, often dropping to floor) to wear helmets to protect them when they fall.

Gerontological

- Older persons often have symptoms that make it difficult to recognize a seizure disorder. Confusion lasting several days, receptive and expressive speech problems, and unusual behaviours are often the result of a seizure.
- Older persons metabolize some antiseizure medications more slowly, allowing drugs to accumulate and possibly result in toxicity. Consult a pharmacist for specific information.
- If patient has dentures, do not try to remove them during a seizure. If they loosen, tilt head slightly forward and remove after seizure.

Care in the Community

- Instruct caregiver about steps to take when patient experiences a seizure.
- Complete a fall risk assessment in the patient's home to decrease the potential of injury in the event of a fall.
- Until a seizure condition is well controlled (usually for at least 1 year), make sure that patient does not take a tub bath or engage in activities such as swimming unless another person is present.
- Refer patient to the Epilepsy Canada or a community resource for support groups.

✦ CLINICAL DEBRIEF

A 72-year-old male patient was admitted to an acute medicine division. He has diabetes mellitus, heart disease, and arthritis and has been admitted for acute pneumonia. His home medications include an oral hypoglycemic (glyburide), a nonsteroidal anti-inflammatory drug (NSAID), and a laxative. He has symptoms of fever 39.4°C (103°F), productive cough with dark yellow mucus, and chest pain when breathing and coughing. His appetite has been poor. He has an intravenous (IV) line running with D_5NS at 80 mL/h. He reports feeling very tired. The nurse observes that he is having difficulty standing up from the bed and needs help to walk to the nearby bedside commode. The health care provider orders a colonoscopy to investigate the new development of blood in his stool and abdominal cramping. The patient is placed on nothing by mouth (NPO) status until after the colonoscopy. It has been 7 hours since the test was ordered, and the patient has not eaten.

1. Identify the factors that place the patient at risk for falling and recommend three fall prevention strategies appropriate for this patient.
2. The nurse enters the room to find the patient lying in bed, unresponsive to verbal command with tonic and clonic movement of his extremities. What is the first step the nurse should take and why? What likely caused the seizure?
3. The patient begins to awaken from the seizure. He knows his name but is confused about date and time. He asks, "What happened?" Blood glucose is 3.2 mmol/L. How would the nurse report the patient's clinical situation using SBAR?

✦ REVIEW QUESTIONS

1. A 42-year-old patient is on an orthopaedic floor following a compound fracture of the lower leg. The patient's leg is in a splint enclosed with an Ace bandage. The nurse enters the room and discovers fire in the bedside garbage can. Place in the correct order the actions that should be taken by the nurse.
   1. The nurse turns off the oxygen source at the head of the bed.
   2. The nurse gets help from a staff member, transfers the patient into a wheelchair, and moves him to a different room.
   3. The nurse moves the patient's bed away from the trash can.
   4. The nurse hits the emergency button in the room and instructs the secretary to report a fire emergency.
2. The nurse is caring for an older person with progressive dementia. The nurse is concerned about the patient being at risk for wandering.

Which of the following interventions would be appropriate for this patient? *(Select all that apply.)*
   1. Determine from family the patient's usual communication style and cues to indicate hunger or need to go to bathroom.
   2. Provide a diversional activity that family reports patient enjoys.
   3. Place patient in a bed enclosure.
   4. Use soft wrist restraints for the patient when restlessness increases.
   5. Control room temperature and reduce number of care routines.
3. A nurse is assessing an older patient who reports falling a month ago at home but did not sustain an injury. Which of the following would the nurse assess about the previous fall? *(Select all that apply.)*
   1. The medications the patient is currently taking
   2. The location of the fall in the home
   3. The patient's medical conditions
   4. The activity the patient was engaged in just before the fall
   5. Whether the patient had dizziness or weakness just before falling

ⓔ *Visit the Evolve site for a complete list of Clinical Debrief and Review Questions answers.*

REFERENCES

Accreditation Canada. (2019). *Required organizational practices handbook—Version 14*. Retrieved from http://www.wrha.mb.ca/quality/files/2019ROPHandbook.pdf

Berry, S., & Kiel, D. (2018). Falls: Prevention in nursing care facilities and the hospital setting, *UpToDate 2016*. Retrieved from http://www.uptodate.com/contents/falls-prevention-in-nursing-care-facilities-and-the-hospital-setting

Bloch, M., Jønsson, L., & Kristensen, M. (2017). Introducing a third timed up & go test trial improves performances of hospitalized and community-dwelling older individuals. *Journal of Geriatric Physical Therapy*, 40(3), 121–126. doi:10.1519/JPT.0000000000000080

Canadian Institutes for Health Information (CIHI). (2010–2018). *Patient safety*. Retrieved from https://www.cihi.ca/en/patient-safety

Canadian Medical Protection Agency (CMPA). (2016). *Safety of care. Medical-legal implications when using restraints*. Retrieved from https://www.cmpa-acpm.ca/en/advice-publications/browse-articles/2016/medical-legal-implications-when-using-restraints

Canadian Patient Safety Institute (CPSI). (2015). *Never events for hospital care in Canada. Safer care for patients*. Edmonton, AB: Author. Retrieved from http://www.patientsafetyinstitute.ca/en/toolsResources/NeverEvents/Documents/Never%20Events%20for%20Hospital%20Care%20in%20Canada.pdf

Canadian Patient Safety Institute (CPSI). (2016). *SHIFT to safety*. Edmonton, AB: Author. Retrieved from http://www.patientsafetyinstitute.ca/en/About/Programs/shift-to-safety/Pages/default.aspx

Canadian Patient Safety Institute (CPSI). (2017). *The patient safety education program. Module 13d: Mental health care: Seclusion and restraints: When all else fails.* Edmonton, AB: Author. Retrieved from http://www.patientsafetyinstitute.ca/en/education/PatientSafetyEducationProgram/PatientSafetyEducationCurriculum/Documents/Module%2013d%20Seclusion%20and%20Restraint.pdf

Canadian Patient Safety Institute (CPSI) & Registered Nurses' Association of Ontario (RNAO). (2018). *Reducing falls and injuries from falls. A starting kit: Evidence update.* Retrieved from http://www.patientsafetyinstitute.ca/en/toolsResources/Documents/Interventions/Reducing%20Falls%20and%20Injury%20from%20Falls/Falls%20Evidence%20update%202018-01.PDF

Cancer Care Ontario (CCO). (2015). *Person-centred care guideline.* Retrieved from https://archive.cancercare.on.ca/pcs/person_centred_care/person_centred_care_guideline/

Children's Health and Safety Association (CHSA). (2015). *Home safety checklist.* Etobicoke, ON: Author. Retrieved from https://www.safekid.org/images/SafetyDocuments/HomeSafetyChecklist.pdf

College of Nurses of Ontario (CNO). (2018). *Understanding restraints.* Retrieved from http://www.cno.org/en/learn-about-standards-guidelines/educational tools/restraints/

Critical Care Services Ontario (CCSO). (2015). *Provincial guidelines for management of epilepsy in adults and children.* Retrieved from https://www.criticalcareontario.ca/EN/Library/Epilepsy%20Guideline%20Series/Pages/default.aspx

Fisher, R., Cross, J., French, J., et al. (2017). Operational classification of seizure types by the International League Against Epilepsy: Position paper of the ILAE commission for classification and terminology. *Epilepsia, 58*(4), 522–530. doi:10.1111/epi.13670

Freeman, S., Yorke, J., & Dark, P. (2018). Patient agitation and its management in adult critical care: A systematic review and narrative synthesis. *Journal of Clinical Nursing, 27*(7–8), e1284–e1308. doi:10.1111/jocn.14258

Glauser, T., Shinnar, S., Gloss, D., et al. (2016). Evidence-based guideline: Treatment of convulsive status epilepticus in children and adults. *Epilepsy Currents, 16*(1), 48–61. doi:10.5698/1535-7597-16.1.48

Government of British Columbia. (2017). *Timed up and go (TUG) test.* Retrieved from https://www2.gov.bc.ca/assets/gov/health/practitioner-pro/bc-guidelines/frailty-TUG.pdf

Government of Canada. (2012). *Current patient safety organizations in Canada.* Retrieved from https://www.canada.ca/en/health-canada/services/quality-care/patient-safety/current-patient-safety-organizations-canada.html

Health Canada. (2015). *WHMIS (Workplace Hazardous Materials Information System) 2015.* Retrieved from https://www.canada.ca/en/health-canada/services/environmental-workplace-health/occupational-health-safety/workplace-hazardous-materials-information-system/whmis-2015.html

Health Canada. (2018). *Canada's vigilance program.* Retrieved from https://www.canada.ca/en/health-canada/services/drugs-health-products/medeffect-canada/canada-vigilance-program.html

Hockenberry, M. J., & Wilson, D. (2015). *Wong's nursing care of infants and children* (10th ed.). St. Louis: Mosby.

Kiel, D. (2018). Falls in older persons: Risk factors and patient evaluation, *UpToDate 2016.* Retrieved from http://www.uptodate.com/contents/falls-in-older-persons-risk-factors-and-patient-evaluation

Krumholz, A., Wiebe, A., Gronseth, G., et al. (2015). Evidence-based guideline: Management of an unprovoked first seizure in adults. *Neurology, 84*(16), 1705–1711. doi:10.1212/WNL.0000000000001487

Lee, J., Jin, Y., Piao, J., & Lee, S. (2016). Development and evaluation of an automated fall risk assessment system. *International Journal for Quality in Health Care, 28*(2), 175–182. doi:10.1093/intqhc/mzv122

Lewis, S., Bucher, L., Heitkemper, M., et al. (2019). *Medical-surgical nursing in Canada* (4th ed.). Toronto, ON: Elsevier Canada.

Martin, E., Biessy-Dalbe, N., Albaret, J., & Algase, D. (2015). French validation of the revised Algase Wandering Scale for long-term care. *American Journal of Alzheimer's Disease and Other Dementias, 30*(8), 762–767. doi:10.1177/1533317513494454

Nova Scotia Health Authority (NSHA). (2018). *Morse Falls Scale fall risk assessment.* Retrieved from https://library.nshealth.ca/FallPrevention

Olley, R., & Morales, A. (2017). Systematic review of evidence underpinning non-pharmacological therapies in dementia. *Australian Health Review, 42*(4), 361–369. doi:10.1071/AH16212

Public Health Agency of Canada (PHAC). (2014). *Seniors' falls in Canada. Second report.* Ottawa: Author. Retrieved from http://www.phac-aspc.gc.ca/seniors-aines/publications/public/injury-blessure/seniors_falls-chutes_aines/assets/pdf/seniors_falls-chutes_aines-eng.pdf

Registered Nurses' Association of Ontario (RNAO). (2012). *Promoting safety: Alternative approaches to the use of restraints.* Toronto, ON: Author. Retrieved from http://rnao.ca/sites/rnao-ca/files/Promoting_Safety_-_Alternative_Approaches_to_the_Use_of_Restraints_0.pdf

Registered Nurses' Association of Ontario (RNAO). (2017). *Preventing falls and reducing injuries from falls* (4th ed.). Toronto, ON: Author. Retrieved from https://rnao.ca/sites/rnao-ca/files/bpg/FALL_PREVENTION_WEB_1207-17.pdf

Scheepmans, K., Dierckx de Casterlé, B., Paquay, L., & Milisen, K. (2018). Restraint use in older adults in home care: A systematic review. *International Journal of Nursing Studies, 79*, 122–136. doi:10.1016/j.ijnurstu.2017.11.008

Smith, G., Wagner, J., & Edwards, J. (2015). Epilepsy update: Part 2: Nursing care and evidence-based treatment. *The American Journal of Nursing, 115*(6), 34–44. doi:10.1097/01.NAJ.0000466314.46508.00

Statistics Canada. (2016). *Health reports. Epilepsy in Canada: Prevalence and impact.* Retrieved from https://www.statcan.gc.ca/pub/82-003-x/2016009/article/14654-eng.htm

Statistics Canada. (2019). *Incident-based fire statistics, by type of fire incident and type of structure.* Retrieved from http://www5.statcan.gc.ca/cansim/a26?lang=eng&id=2600001

Touhy, T. A., Jett, K. F., Boscart, V., & McCleary, L. (2019). *Ebersole and Hess' gerontological nursing & healthy aging* (2nd Canadian ed.). Toronto, ON: Elsevier Canada.

Tricco, A., Thomas, A., Veroniki, A., et al. (2017). Comparisons of interventions for preventing falls in older adults: A systematic review and meta-analysis. *JAMA: The Journal of the American Medical Association, 318*(17), 1687–1699. doi:10.1001/jama.2017.15006

Vlaeyen, E., Coussement, J., Leysens, G., et al. (2015). Characteristics and effectiveness of fall prevention programs in nursing homes: A systematic review and meta-analysis of randomized controlled trials. *Journal of the American Geriatrics Society, 63*(2), 211–221. doi:10.1111/jgs.132

Welch, V., Ghogomu, E., & Shea, B. (2016). Evidence-based screening tools and fall risk assessment in continuing care. A bruyère rapid review. *Bruyère Reports, 5.* Retrieved from https://www.bruyere.org/uploads/Falls%20assessment%20in%20continuing%20care.pdf

World Health Organization (WHO). (2017). *Patient safety: Making health care safer.* Retrieved from http://www.who.int/patientsafety/publications/patient-safety-making-health-care-safer/en/

15 | Emergency Preparedness and Disaster Management

Written by **Shelley L. Cobbett, RN, GnT, MN, EdD, and Nancy LaPlante, PhD, RN, AHN-BC**

SKILLS AND PROCEDURES

Skill 15.1 **Care of a Patient After Biological Exposure, p. 391**

Skill 15.2 **Care of a Patient After Chemical Exposure, p. 398**

Skill 15.3 **Care of a Patient After Radiation Exposure, p. 401**

OBJECTIVES

Mastery of content in this chapter will enable the nurse to:
- Describe elements of emergency preparedness and disaster management, including prevention and mitigation, preparedness, response, and recovery.
- Discuss the characteristics of different types of disasters.
- Identify actions to take in the event of biological, chemical, and radiation exposure.

- Discuss guidelines for patient care in the event of a mass casualty incident.
- Identify components of the START and JumpSTART triage systems.
- Describe factors related to the mental health and well-being of patients, nurses, and health care providers postdisaster.

MEDIA RESOURCES

- evolve http://evolve.elsevier.com/Canada/Perry/clinicalskills/
- Review Questions

- Audio Glossary
- Clinical Debrief and Review Questions Answers

PURPOSE

The incidence of natural and human-made disasters and infectious diseases continues to rise throughout the world, increasing the likelihood and frequency of these events happening in Canada. Recent massive wildfires in Fort McMurray, Alberta, were unlike any fire seen before within our borders (Canadian Red Cross, 2019c). In 2017, natural disasters continued to be a cause of concern—the ice storms in New Brunswick, severe flooding in Quebec and Ontario, and the province-wide declaration of a state of emergency in British Columbia in response to wildfires.

Canadian emergency management adopts an all-hazards approach to address natural and human-made disasters. Pandemics and epidemics can also be disasters, for example, the disease outbreak of the Zika virus in 2015. Regardless of the cause of the disaster, the demand for health care providers who are skilled in disaster preparedness and emergency management and able to effectively educate the public and deliver care to diverse populations at times of crisis is of paramount importance. Nurses, as members of the interprofessional health care team, play a key role in the coordination and implementation of emergency preparedness and disaster management. Postdisaster mental health and well-being are important to assess in patients, nurses, and members of the health care team. Many factors may adversely affect mental health status postdisaster—for example, the extent of traumatic exposure, lack of social support, lack of preparedness, and impact of the disaster on one's personal and professional life (Brooks, Dunn, Amlôt, et al., 2016, 2017;

Brooks, Dunn, Sage, 2015). Information gathered from the many postdisaster evaluations that have occurred in recent years has provided a considerable body of knowledge and experience to improve the response of an entire health care team and the many agencies and individuals involved in a disaster response.

STANDARDS OF CARE

- Canadian Nurses Association (CNA), 2012—*Position Statement: Emergency Preparedness and Response* (https://www.cna-aiic.ca/~/media/cna/page-content/pdf-en/ps119_emergency_preparedness_2012_e.pdf?la=en)
- Canadian Red Cross, 2019a—*Emergencies and Disasters in Canada* (http://www.redcross.ca/how-we-help/emergencies-and-disasters-in-canada)
- Public Health Agency of Canada (PHAC), 2005—*Centre for Emergency Preparedness and Response* (https://www.canada.ca/en/public-health/services/emergency-preparedness-response/centre-emergency-preparedness-response.html)
- Public Safety Canada, 2017—*An Emergency Management Framework for Canada*, Third Edition (https://www.publicsafety.gc.ca/cnt/rsrcs/pblctns/2017-mrgnc-mngmnt-frmwrk/index-en.aspx)
- World Health Organization (WHO) and the International Council of Nurses (ICN), 2009—*ICN Framework of Disaster Nursing Competencies* (http://www.wpro.who.int/hrh/documents/icn_framework.pdf)

PRINCIPLES FOR PRACTICE

- A disaster is any unexpected event, the effect of which leads to significant destruction, adverse consequences, or both (Box 15.1).
- Surveillance of the public by the World Health Organization (WHO) focuses on diseases such as the Zika virus for indications of mutations and increased transmission (Box 15.2).
- The most common forms of disaster are natural or human-made. If the public is not adequately protected, the spread of natural-borne disease can create a natural disaster.
- The main purpose of *Canada's Emergency Management Framework, Third Edition* (Public Safety Canada, 2017) is to save lives, preserve the environment, and protect property and the economy. The *Framework* includes information used to assist with collaborative management to enhance the four interdependent emergency management components: prevention and mitigation, preparedness, response, and recovery from potential threats and disaster events.
- *Prevention and mitigation* are focused on eliminating, reducing, or adapting to the risk of disasters; *preparedness* is the state of readiness to respond to a disaster situation and manage its consequences prior to the disaster occurring; *response* is the ability to act during, immediately before, or after a disaster to minimize suffering and losses; and, *recovery* is restoration of conditions to an acceptable level postdisaster (Public Safety Canada, 2017).
- Effective implementation of the four emergency management components is based on an evidence-informed risk assessment, strong public awareness, and community engagement, all of which are key attributes of societal resilience (Public Safety Canada, 2017).
- An all-hazards approach is used to identify, analyze, and prioritize potential natural and human-made threats, considering vulnerabilities, potential consequences, and means to mitigate the risks (Public Safety Canada, 2015a).
- Incident Command System (ICS) Canada (2019) outlines an incident communications plan that addresses preparedness planning related to equipment, systems, and protocols necessary to achieve integrated voice and data communications in the event of a disaster. On an individual level, the 9-1-1 system can be activated.
- The Canadian Red Cross is an invaluable resource in the event of a disaster and provides assistance in disaster situations for people's basic needs, including family reunification, emergency lodging, reception and information, emergency food, emergency clothing, and personal services (Canadian Red Cross, 2019b).
- Most disasters in Canada have been local (community, municipal, provincial) in nature but can be declared federally with Canada's *Emergencies Act* (R.S.C. 1085, c. 22 [4th Supp.]), allowing the implementation of special measures to ensure safety and security and to amend other Acts as required.
- Promoting effective emergency preparedness and response requires collaboration of all levels of government and interprofessional collaboration among nongovernmental agencies such as the health, social services, safety, transportation, meteorology, and voluntary sectors (e.g., Canadian Red Cross, St. John Ambulance)

BOX 15.1

Disaster Definitions and Types

- **Disaster:** A social phenomenon that results when a hazard intersects with a vulnerable community, overwhelming or exceeding the community's ability to cope, and may cause serious harm to the safety, health, welfare, property, or the environment.
- **Mass casualty incident or event (MCI):** Any event or situation (e.g., bombing of a public area) that results in multiple casualties and deaths; exists when health care needs exceed health care resources.
- **All-hazards approach:** This approach addresses vulnerabilities exposed by natural or human-made hazards and disasters; it increases efficiency by integrating common emergency management elements across all hazard types, supplementing with hazard-specific subcomponents as required.
- **Hazard:** A potentially damaging physical event, phenomenon, or human activity that may cause injury or death, property damage, social and economic disruption, or environmental degradation.
- **Hazardscape:** Cumulative emergency management environment, consisting of all hazards, risks, vulnerabilities, and capacities.
- **Casualty:** Any individual who is ill, injured, missing, or killed as a result of an MCI.
- **Emergency:** A present or imminent event that requires immediate coordination of actions concerning persons or property to protect the health, safety, or welfare of people, or to limit damage to property or the environment.
- **Emergency management:** The management of emergencies involving all hazards, including activities and risk-management measures related to prevention and mitigation, preparedness, response, and recovery.
- **Threat:** The presence of a hazard and an exposure pathway to threats that may be natural or human induced, either accidental or intentional.
- **Vulnerability:** Conditions determined by physical, social, economic, and/or environmental factors or processes which increase the susceptibility of a community to the impact of hazards.

Adapted from Public Safety Canada. (2017). *An emergency management framework for Canada* (3rd ed., pp. 20–23). Ottawa, ON: Author.

BOX 15.2

Zika Virus (ZIKV)

- Mainly transmitted to people through the *Aedes* mosquito but can also be transmitted sexually and via blood transfusion.
- ZIKV has been reported in humans since 1952 with mild symptoms (Uganda and Tanzania), but large disease outbreaks in 2007 (Island of Yap), 2013 (Polynesia), and 2015 (Brazil) gained attention because of the associated increase in microcephaly and possible association with Guillain Barré syndrome.
- ZIKV infection in a relatively healthy individual is typically asymptomatic, and for those who do experience symptoms they tend to be mild and include fever, skin rash, conjunctivitis, muscle and joint pain, malaise, and headache.
- The risk of a primary infection in pregnant women is the same as for any other adult, but there is significant risk to the unborn child, who is at risk of congenital Zika virus syndrome (CZVS).
- Diagnosis is based on symptoms and exposure; however, the virus can be confirmed through laboratory tests. ZIKV has been detected in blood, urine, saliva, cerebrospinal fluid, semen, and amniotic fluid.
- Prevention and control focuses on reducing the risk of transmission. The best method for prevention is protecting against mosquito bites—for example, wearing clothes that cover as much of the body as possible; using insect repellent (DEET, IR3535, or icaridin); protecting areas of residence with mosquito nets and window screens; and covering, emptying, or cleaning potential breeding sites for mosquitos.
- The WHO (2017) provides a toolkit for the care and support of people affected by complications associated with ZIKV, with the main goal of enhancing country preparedness for ZIKV outbreaks.

Data from World Health Organization (WHO). (2017). *WHO toolkit: For the care and support of people affected by complications associated with Zika virus.* Retrieved from http://www.who.int/mental_health/neurology/zika_toolkit/en/.

(CNA, 2012). Nurses play a vital role on the interprofessional team related to emergency preparedness and response.

- Some provincial nursing regulatory agencies have regulations that allow a person who is authorized to practice nursing as a registered nurse in another jurisdiction in Canada or the United States to practice nursing in the province during an emergency (e.g., Registered Nurses of Manitoba). A nurse who is eligible for Canadian Nurses Protective Society (CNPS) services and moves to another Canadian jurisdiction to do emergency work remains eligible for CNPS services (CNPS, 2010).

- The National Public Alerting System (NPAS) is a collaborative initiative between federal-provincial-territorial governments and industry partners that provides the capability to rapidly warn the public of imminent or actual hazards, using various communication modalities (Public Safety Canada, 2018a) (Fig. 15.1). A public awareness campaign, Alert Ready, provides information on the types of alerts that can be issued, wireless device compatibility, and what to do if an alert occurs.

- As of April 6, 2018, the NPAS has wireless and smartphone capabilities (for more information see https://www.alertready.ca/).

- The ICS is designed to enable effective, efficient incident management through integration of facilities, equipment, personnel, procedures, and communications within a common organizational structure (ICS Canada, 2018). Refer to Fig. 15.2 for an example of a hospital ICS.

- A mass casualty incident (MCI) occurs when the number of casualties, or the rate of their arrival, overwhelms the local healthcare system, where the needs of people exceed the local resources and capabilities (Ben-Ishay, Mitaritonno, Catena, et al., 2016).

- The Canadian Disaster Database (CDD) describes disasters that have affected Canada since the 1900s (excluding war) (Public Safety Canada, 2018c).

- The Public Health Agency of Canada (PHAC) funds the National Emergency Strategic Stockpile (NESS), which provides health and social service supplies quickly to provinces and territories when their own resources are depleted during an emergency. There is a central depot in Ottawa, with several supply centres located across Canada (PHAC, 2015).

- Support resources required during a disaster include human resources, agencies, facilities, supplies, and vehicles.

- Support is for the victims of disaster and all health care providers involved. Support is holistic, encompassing the body, mind, and spirit. Health care providers (including nurses, first responders, and physicians) are at risk for post-traumatic stress disorder (PTSD).

- Health care providers care for the worried well (those frightened by the events) and sick and injured individuals (including the walking wounded) already admitted to the hospital or emergency department (ED).

- Acute care facility EDs must have an emergency disaster plan and protocols to address high patient volume and surges in the ED (Accreditation Canada, 2019) as well as internal disasters.

- Health care facilities need to be competent in disaster preparedness and management at all levels of the health system—for example, have clear plans related to incident command, triage, mass casualty events or mass gatherings, and hazardous materials (Centre for Excellence in Emergency Preparedness [CEEP], 2011).

- Even with a well-developed acute care facility disaster preparedness and management plan, coping with the consequences of a disaster is a complex challenge. Amid these challenges and demands, interprofessional collaboration in the implementation of priority actions can help facilitate a timely and effective facility-based response (WHO, 2011).

- The WHO (2011) provides a hospital emergency response checklist for an all-hazards approach (refer to http://www.euro.who.int/__data/assets/pdf_file/0008/268766/Hospital-emergency-response-checklist-Eng.pdf).

- Canada has aligned the Workplace Hazardous Materials Information System (WHMIS) with the Globally Harmonized System of Classification and Labelling of Chemicals (Canadian Centre for Occupational Health and Safety [CCOHS], 2015) and developed pictograms for easy identification of potential health hazards (Fig. 15.3).

- Public Safety Canada recommends that communities use the handbook that is part of the United Nations Global Campaign, *Making Cities Resilient: My City Is Getting Ready* (United Nations Office for Disaster Risk Reduction, 2017).

National Public Alerting System (NPAS)

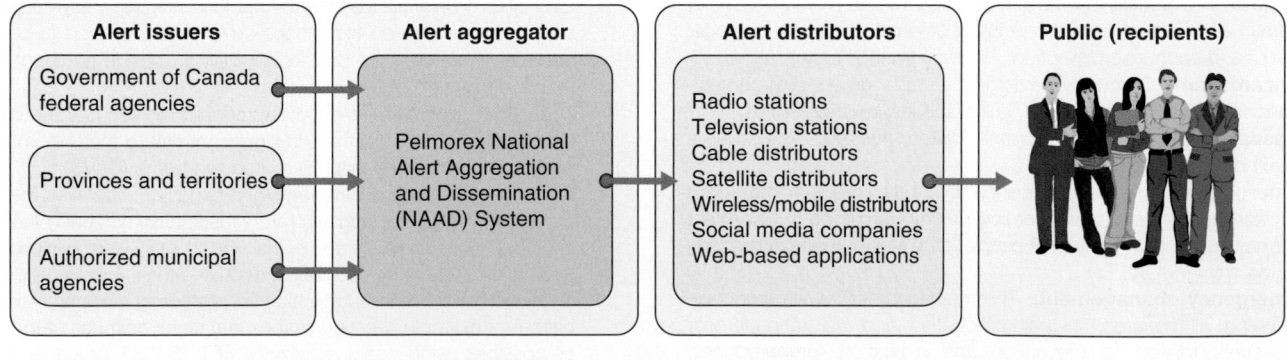

FIG 15.1 National Public Alerting System. (*From Public Safety Canada. [2018]. National public alerting system. Retrieved from https://www.publicsafety.gc.ca/cnt/mrgnc-mngmnt/mrgnc-prprdnss/ntnl-pblc-lrtng-sstm-en.aspx*)

HOSPITAL EMERGENCY INCIDENT COMMAND SYSTEM

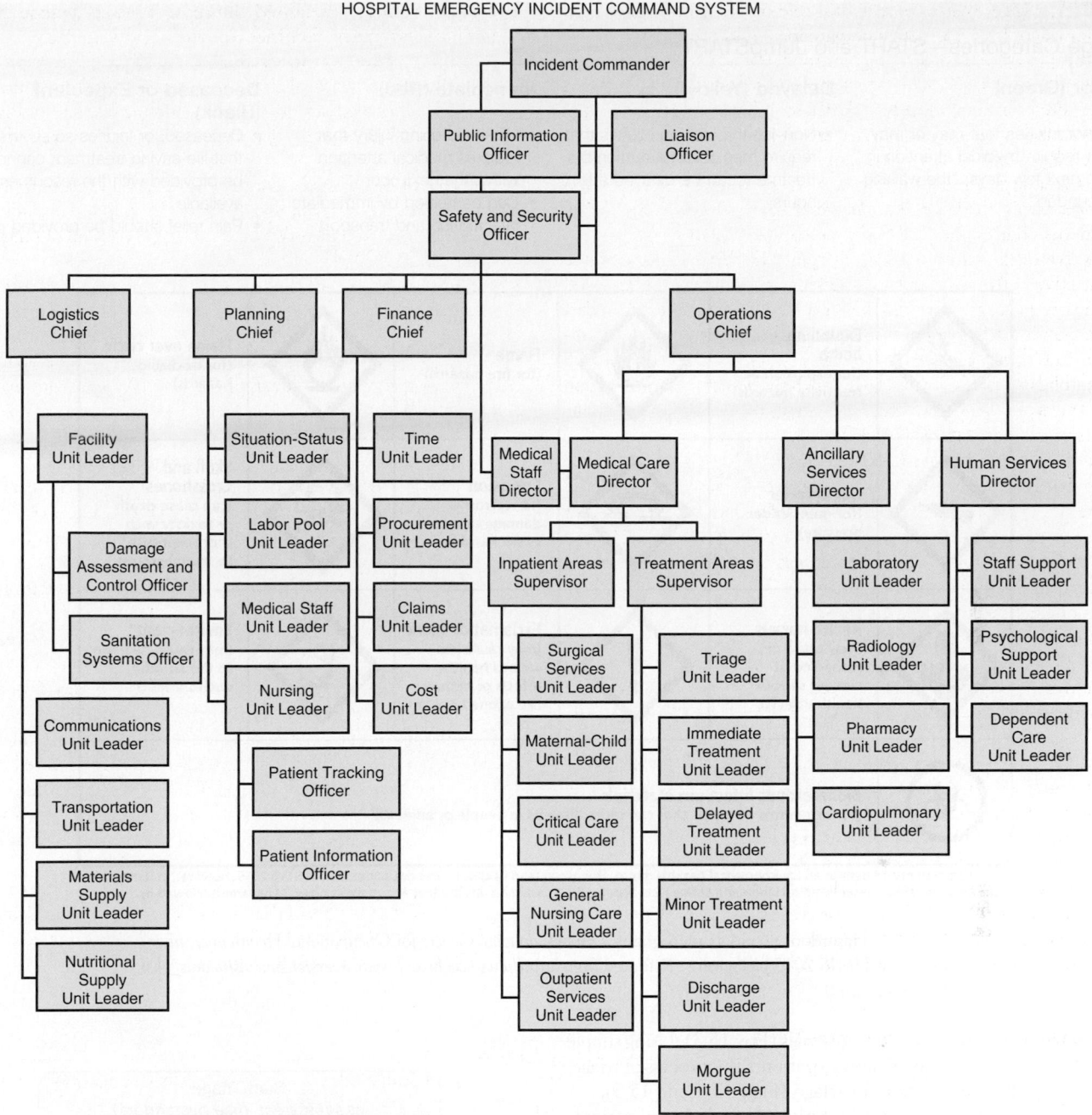

FIG 15.2 The hospital emergency incident command system prepares all response teams to work smoothly in a disaster situation.

- A community disaster resiliency model can help communities be more prepared in the event of a disaster (Cox, 2015) and should include risk reduction and disaster readiness, response, recovery, and rebuild (Community Foundations of Canada, 2017).
- Public Safety Canada (2018d) has announced the Regional Resilience Assessment Program, which is a comprehensive risk assessment program for owners and operators of Critical Infrastructure (CI) facilities within the 10 CI sectors in Canada, which includes health care facilities.
- The Justice Institute of British Columbia and Wilfred Laurier University (2015) have created an online resource, the Aboriginal Disaster Resilience Planning Guide, to help Indigenous communities anticipate and minimize the damage caused by disasters.

- Nurses provide public health education to empower resilience in communities by focusing on individual self-accountability and responsibility and knowing how to access community, municipal, provincial/territorial, and federal resources.

PERSON-CENTRED CARE

- Once a scene is deemed safe for health care providers, triage is initiated to identify the most severely injured patients with the greatest chance of survival. It is important to maintain therapeutic communication while conveying caring and compassion.
- Different models can be used to triage in a mass casualty incident, for example, START (Simple Triage and Rapid Treatment) and JumpSTART (the version of START for pediatric patients). Both

BOX 15.3

Triage Categories—START and JumpSTART

Minor (Green)	Delayed (Yellow)	Immediate (Red)	Deceased or Expectant (Black)
• Minor injuries that may or may not require medical attention in the next few days; "the walking wounded"	• Non–life-threatening injuries that require medication attention but treatment can be delayed a few hours	• Life-threatening injury that requires medical attention within the next hour • Can be helped by immediate intervention and transport	• Deceased, or injuries so severe that life-saving treatment cannot be provided with the resources available • Pain relief should be provided prn

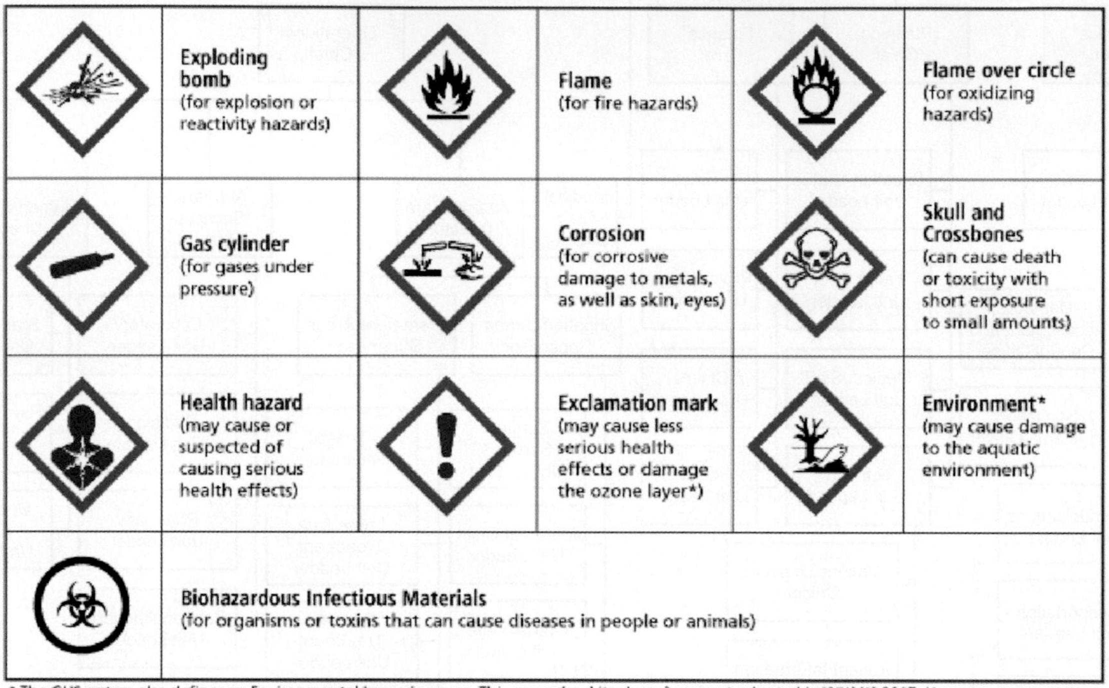

Exploding bomb
(for explosion or reactivity hazards)
Flame
(for fire hazards)
Flame over circle
(for oxidizing hazards)
Gas cylinder
(for gases under pressure)
Corrosion
(for corrosive damage to metals, as well as skin, eyes)
Skull and Crossbones
(can cause death or toxicity with short exposure to small amounts)
Health hazard
(may cause or suspected of causing serious health effects)
Exclamation mark
(may cause less serious health effects or damage the ozone layer*)
Environment*
(may cause damage to the aquatic environment)
Biohazardous Infectious Materials
(for organisms or toxins that can cause diseases in people or animals)

* The GHS system also defines an Environmental hazards group. This group (and its classes) was not adopted in WHMIS 2015. However, you may see the environmental classes listed on labels and Safety Data Sheets (SDSs). Including information about environmental hazards is allowed by WHMIS 2015.

FIG 15.3 Hazardous products pictograms. *(From Canadian Centre for Occupational Health and Safety. [2015]. WHMIS 2015 pictograms. Retrieved from http://www.ccohs.ca/oshanswers/chemicals/whmis_ghs/pictograms.html)*

models sort patients into four categories (Box 15.3). Using simple language, the nurse can explain to patients the process of triage.

- There are three main steps for triage (Figs. 15.4 and 15.5):
  - *Step 1:* Triage begins by instructing all ambulatory patients to move to a designated area, the "green area." Those patients who are able to do this are tagged "green" (minor).
  - *Step 2:* Assess breathing; if the patient is breathing, move to Step 3. If the patient is not breathing, attempt to open the airway.
    - With START, if there are no spontaneous respirations, the patient is triaged black.
    - With JumpSTART, if there are no spontaneous respirations, assess peripheral pulse; if no pulse, the patient is triaged black; if the patient has a palpable pulse, five assisted ventilations (15 sec) are given and if spontaneous respirations, the patient is triaged red; if there is no return of respirations, the patient is triaged black.
  - *Step 3:* Assess respiratory rate, perfusion, and mental status.
- A common mnemonic that can assist with differentiating between the triage categories of yellow and red for START is "RPM-30-2-Can Do." To be triaged yellow, the patient must have a respiratory rate under 30 breaths per minute, capillary

Start Triage
assess, treat, (use bystanders)
when you have a colour
STOP - TAG - MOVE ON
MINOR
-- Move walking wounded
DECEASED
-- No RESPIRATIONS after head tilt
IMMEDIATE
-- Breathing but UNCONSCIOUS
-- Respirations - over 30
-- Perfusion capillary refill > 2 or NO RADIAL PULSE
Control bleeding
-- Mental status unable to follow simple commands
DELAYED
-- Otherwise
Remember:
Respirations - 30
Perfusion - 2
Mental status - can do

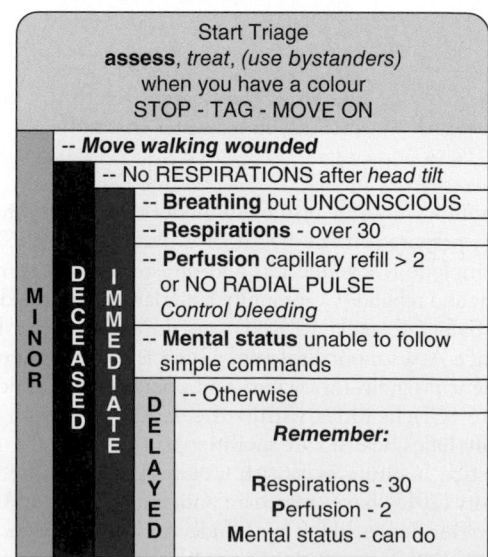

FIG 15.4 START triage. *(From http://www.start-triage.com/)*

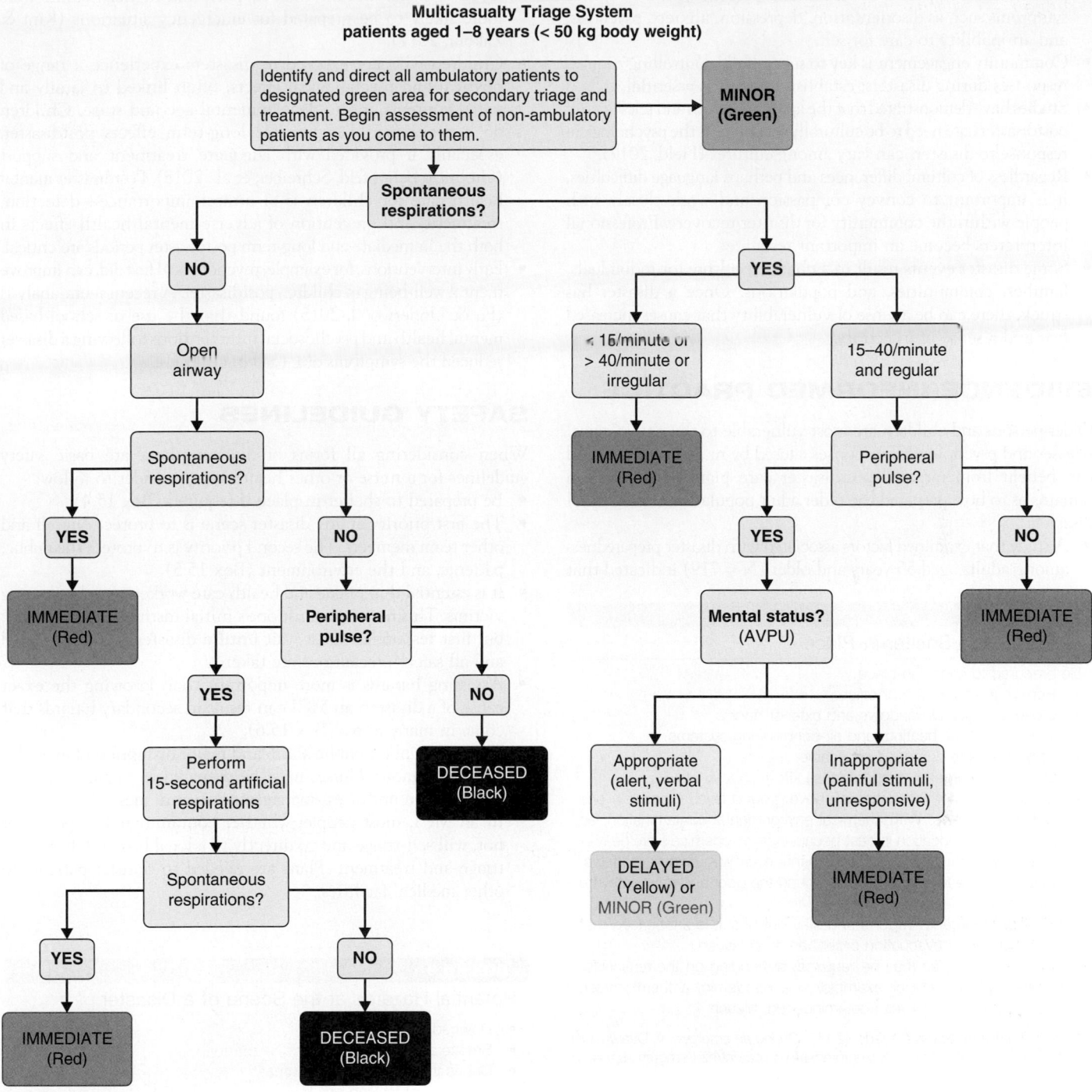

JumpSTART
Field Pediatric
Multicasualty Triage System
patients aged 1–8 years (< 50 kg body weight)

AVPU: alert, voice, pain, unresponsive

FIG 15.5 JumpSTART triage *(From Fire Fighting in Canada. [2007]. EMS focus: Handling the mass casualty incident, creating order out of chaos [Figure 2]. Simcoe, ON: Author. Retrieved from https:// www.firefightingincanada.com/emergency-disaster-management/ems-focus-oct.-06-cff-1448)*

refill must be under 2 seconds, and mental status is adequate; that is, the patient "can do" what they are asked. If any one of these three criteria are not met, the patient is triaged red.

- The mnemonic for JumpSTART is "RPM-30-2-Can Do-15-45," to reflect the differences in the normal respiratory rates between children and adults. In pediatric patients, children who are

breathing under 15 breaths per minute or over 45 breaths per minute are triaged as red.

- In an epidemic situation triage is also used to prevent secondary spread of the disease.
- During triage the nurse provides psychological support to survivors, as well as physical care.

- The nurse must remain calm and assess a patient's immediate psychological response. Some patients present with dissociative symptoms such as disorientation, depression, anxiety, psychosis, and an inability to care for self.
- Community engagement is key to successfully controlling people's responses during disasters; establishing trust is essential.
- Studies have demonstrated that the appropriateness and relevance of postdisaster care need to be culturally sensitive, as the psychological response to disasters can vary among cultures (Field, 2017).
- Regardless of cultural differences and perhaps language difficulties, it is important to convey compassion and work closely with people within the community for disaster recovery. Professional interpreters become an important resource.
- Some disaster events result in a changed culture for individuals, families, communities, and populations. Once a disaster has struck, there can be a sense of vulnerability that causes increased fear and a sense of insecurity.

EVIDENCE-INFORMED PRACTICE

Older persons and children are most vulnerable to the physiological stresses and psychological responses caused by natural disasters and can benefit from targeted postdisaster care plans. The question remains as to how prepared the older adult population is for natural disasters.

- A study that examined factors associated with disaster preparedness among adults aged 55 years and older ($N = 719$) indicated that

BOX 15.4

Guidelines to Shelter-in-Place

Be prepared to shelter-in-place:
- Remain in your home or office.
- Close and lock all windows and exterior doors.
- Turn off all fans, heating, and air-conditioning systems.
- Close fireplace damper if applicable.
- Get your emergency preparedness kit.
- Go to an interior room that is above ground level, if possible one with no windows. With chemical environmental contamination, an above-ground location is best because some chemicals are heavier than air and may seep into basements even with closed windows.
- Use duct tape to seal all cracks around the door and any vents into the room.
- Monitor emergency reports and stay put until it is announced that all is safe or an evacuation order has been issued.
- Additional supplies may be required, depending on the reason for sheltering-in-place—for example, in a pandemic, a thermometer, non-aspirin pain reliever, acetaminophen, bleach.

Adapted from Public Safety Canada. (2017). *During an emergency*. Ottawa, ON: Author. Retrieved from https://www.getprepared.gc.ca/cnt/hzd/drng-en.aspx#a03.

BOX 15.5

Safety and Security

- Trained emergency personnel (e.g., firefighters and police) are responsible for the safety and security of a disaster scene.
- Nurses stay out of a disaster scene unless they are well trained and invited. Call 9-1-1 if emergency personnel have not already been notified.
- Do not disturb the scene; key evidence could be lost or contaminated.
- A health care facility becomes a secondary disaster site when contaminated by the agent from the original disaster scene. For example, a patient exposed to radiation who then enters a health care facility prior to decontamination may inadvertently contaminate health care providers and others.

individuals who had connections to community groups, higher levels of social and informal support, and higher income were more likely to be prepared for emergency situations (Kim & Zakour, 2017).

- Children who are exposed to disasters experience a range of physical and psychological effects, often linked to family and social contexts and to developmental age and stage. Children do not necessarily experience long-term effects postdisaster, especially if provided with adequate treatment and support (Grolnick, Schonfeld, Schreiber, et al., 2018). Postdisaster mental health care for children is of utmost importance—detection, treatment, and prevention of adverse mental health effects in both the immediate and long-term postdisaster periods are critical.
- Early interventions, for example, psychological first aid, can improve mental well-being in children postdisaster. A recent meta-analysis (Fu & Underwood, 2015) found that the use of school-based mental health and psychosocial interventions following a disaster reduced the symptoms of PTSD in children.

SAFETY GUIDELINES

When considering all forms of disaster, there are basic safety guidelines for a nurse or other health care provider to follow:
- Be prepared to shelter-in-place if required (Box 15.4).
- The first priority at any disaster scene is to protect oneself and other team members. The second priority is to protect the public, patients, and the environment (Box 15.5).
- It is essential that rescue and health care workers avoid becoming victims. This may go against one's initial instinct to help others, but first responders must wait until a disaster scene is secured and all safety precautions are taken.
- Assessing hazards is more important than knowing the exact cause of a disaster; an MCI can result in secondary hazards that come in many forms (Box 15.6).
- The potential for public alarm and major disruption of everyday life is enormous. Nurses must be prepared to implement crisis intervention and stress-management techniques.
- In an MCI, most people, whether contaminated, exposed, or not, will self-triage and go directly to a local hospital, bypassing triage and treatment. Plans are needed to transfer patients to other medical facilities.

BOX 15.6

Potential Hazards at the Scene of a Disaster

- Downed power lines
- Smoke and toxic gases
- Debris that can result in trauma
- Fractured or leaking gas lines
- Fire resulting in burns
- Structural collapse
- Blood and other body fluids
- Inclement weather
- Hazardous materials
- Chemical, biological, radiological, or nuclear exposure
- Flooding and the threat of drowning
- Explosion, particularly secondary explosions
- Snipers
- Darkness
- Infection
- High-velocity projectiles and the pressure wave after an explosion
- Becoming incapacitated and being unable to protect yourself or patients

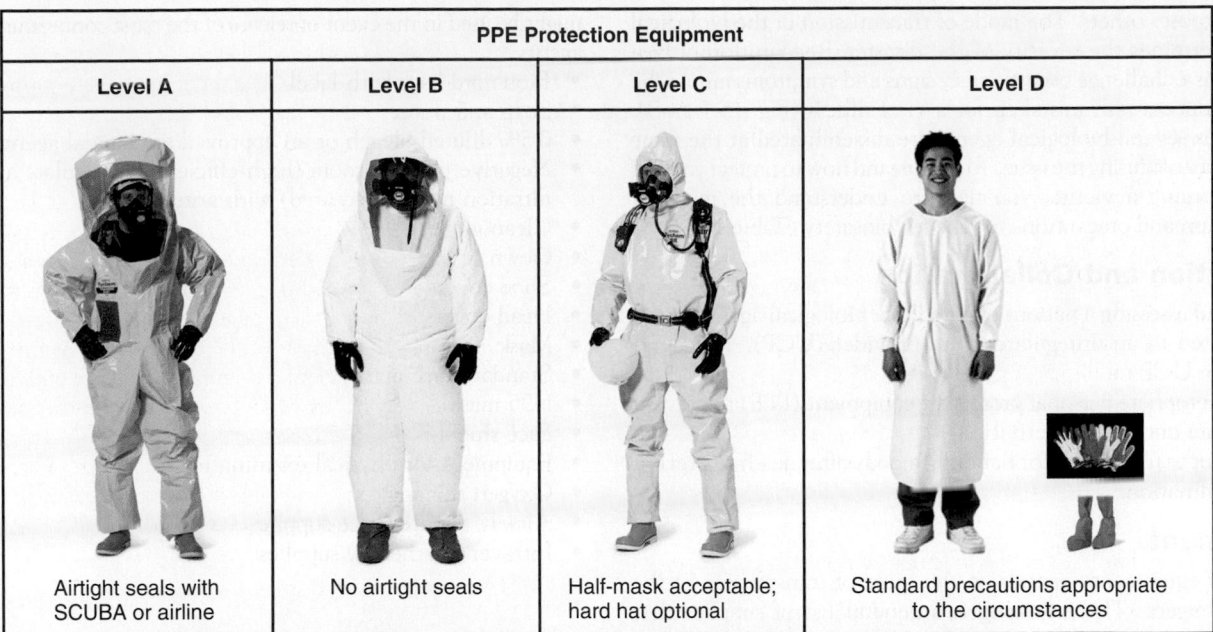

PPE Protection Equipment			
Level A	Level B	Level C	Level D
Airtight seals with SCUBA or airline	No airtight seals	Half-mask acceptable; hard hat optional	Standard precautions appropriate to the circumstances

FIG 15.6 The Occupational Safety and Health Administration (OSHA) defines personal protective equipment for the four levels of hazardous exposure. *PPE*, Personal protective equipment; *SCUBA*, self-contained underwater breathing apparatus.

- Use of personal protective equipment (PPE) minimizes the risk for contact with contaminated materials or individuals. Proper use of advanced forms of PPE requires training, fitting, and an understanding that not all PPE protects against all potential hazards.
- When used inappropriately, PPE becomes a hazard (e.g., dehydration, decreased vision, mobility, and ability to communicate). Some of these hazards result because, while using advanced forms of PPE, the user is unable to eat, drink, or go to the bathroom.
- PPEs are categorized by levels A to D, for the level of safety provided.
    - Level A—Selected when the greatest level of skin, respiratory, and eye protection is required. At this level, maximum protection is provided: a self-contained breathing apparatus, total encapsulating chemical-protective suit, coveralls, undergarments, chemical-resistant boots and gloves, hard hat, and disposable protective suit worn over the encapsulating suit (Fig. 15.6). Highly trained personnel use level A protection in heavily contaminated areas. If you are not wearing this type of protection and you are near an area where level A PPE is being used, get out or do not enter it.
    - Level B—Provides the highest level of respiratory protection but less skin protection. Used by trained responders, this PPE includes a self-contained breathing apparatus; hooded chemical-resistant suit; and face, boot, and glove protection. Level B protection also requires training and fitting.

- Level C—First responders and hospital personnel are trained and fitted to use level C protection, which involves knowing the concentration and type of airborne substance(s) and the criteria for using air-purifying respirators. Level C constitutes the use of full-face or half-mask air-purifying respirators (e.g., N-95 mask), hooded chemical-resistant clothing, and protective gloves and boots. Because of the garment protection worn with levels A, B and C, the user is at risk for dehydration and hyperthermia.
- Level D—Standard work uniforms or work clothes are appropriate and used for nuisance contamination only. The users must wear coveralls and chemical-resistant shoes, and, depending on the contaminant, gloves, goggles, mask, face shield, and hard hats may also be worn. There is no respiratory protection. It is important to implement routine practices when using level D protection. Depending on the circumstances, gown, cap, eye protection, mask, gloves, and shoe covers may be required.
- The most recently labelled level of protection is BioPPE. BioPPE requires the use of standard work clothes along with contact and respiratory protection. Double gloving and an N95 mask (see Chapter 5) or a better respirator are recommended. BioPPE protection is not adequate when caring for patients exposed to toxic chemicals; however, it provides adequate protection against radiological and biological agents.
- Hand hygiene that includes washing with soap and water followed by use of an alcohol gel is important at all levels.

✦ SKILL 15.1   Care of a Patient After Biological Exposure

Bioterrorism involves the intentional use of biological agents to cause illness and death in a population. Adding the agent to food or water and the use of aerosolized agents are common routes of bioterrorism. The use of biological agents is a considerable terrorist threat because they are easy to disperse and can affect large numbers of people at a relatively low cost (Box 15.7). Incubation periods and common initial clinical symptoms make detection of a biological attack difficult. Some biological attacks are unannounced or covert, and the onset of symptoms is delayed by an incubation period (i.e., the time between exposure and onset of symptoms). Differing biological agents have incubation periods from 1 or 2 days to several weeks, during which some of these agents may be transmitted as an infected

patient exposes others. The mode of transmission of the biological agent determines the severity of the disaster. Recognition of bioterrorism is a challenge because early signs and symptoms mimic the flu or produce a rash mistaken for a viral illness (Fig. 15.7 A–B). Sometimes several biological agents are disseminated at the same time, further confusing the issue. To understand how to protect yourself from becoming a victim, you need to understand the mode of transmission and precautions to take for biosafety (Table 15.1).

Delegation and Collaboration

The skill of assessing a patient exposed to a biological agent cannot be delegated to an unregulated care provider (UCP). The nurse directs the UCP to:

- Use appropriate personal protective equipment (PPE) to prevent exposure during care activities.
- Use proper techniques for handling a body after death to prevent contamination.

Equipment

Choice of equipment depends on the route of transmission of the infectious agent. The following is a general list of supplies that might be used in the event of release of the most contagious biological agents:

- Biohazard bags with label
- Soap and water
- 0.5% diluted bleach or an approved germicidal agent
- Negative-pressure room (high-efficiency particulate air [HEPA] filtration may be required) with anteroom
- Clean gloves
- Gown
- Shoe covers
- Head covers
- Mask
- Standard face mask
- N95 mask
- Face shield
- Equipment for physical examination
- Oxygen therapy
- Airway maintenance supplies
- Intravenous therapy supplies

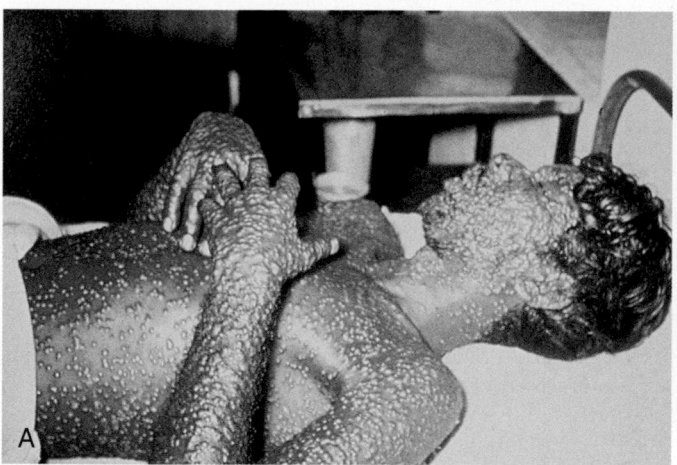
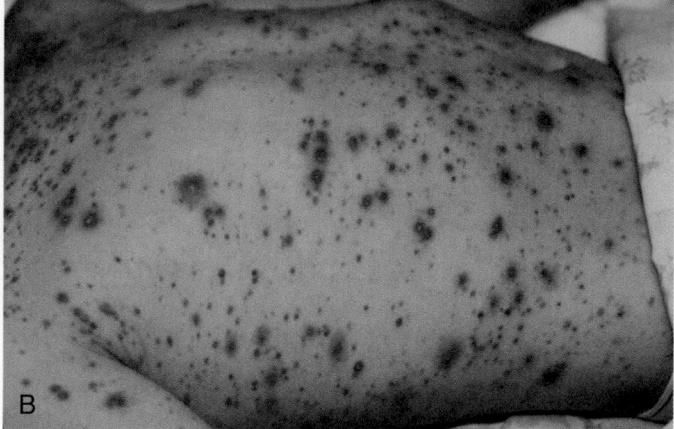

FIG 15.7 Differences in distribution of smallpox versus chickenpox. **A,** Man with smallpox. (*Courtesy CDC/NIP/Barbara Rice.*) **B,** Chickenpox covering patient torso. (*Courtesy David Effron, MD.*)

BOX 15.7

Potential Bioterrorism Agents and Diseases

- Anthrax (*Bacillus anthracis*)
- Botulism (*Clostridium* botulinum toxin)
- Brucellosis (*Brucella* species)
- *Chlamydia psittaci* (psittacosis)
- Ebola virus hemorrhagic fever
- Epsilon toxin of *Clostridium perfringens*
- *Escherichia coli* O157:H7 *(E. coli)*
- Food safety threats (e.g., *Salmonella* species, *E. coli* O157:H7, Shigella)
- Plague *(Yersinia pestis)*

- Q fever (*Coxiella burnetii*)
- Salmonella species (salmonellosis)
- Shigella (Shigellosis)
- Tularemia (*Francisella tularensis*)
- Typhoid fever (*Salmonella* Typhi)
- Variola major (smallpox)
- Vibrio cholerae (cholera)
- Viral hemorrhagic fevers (filoviruses [Ebola, Marburg] and arenaviruses [Lassa, Machupol])
- Water safety threats (e.g., *Vibrio cholerae, Cryptosporidium parvum*)

Data from Centers for Disease Control and Prevention (CDC). (2018). *Bioterrorism agents/diseases*. Retrieved from https://www.emergency.cdc.gov/agent/agentlist.asp.

TABLE 15.1

Summary of Selected Class A Biological Warfare Agents

Disease/Infectious Agent	Form and Incubation/Onset of Symptoms	Untreated Course of Disease		Probable Route of Contamination for Use as a Biological Warfare Agent	Treatment of Mass Casualties	Prophylaxis/ Vaccine
		Early-Onset Symptoms	Late-Onset Symptoms			
Bacterial Biological Agents						
Anthrax *Bacillus anthracis*, a Gram-positive bacillus that can remain stable in spore form	Inhalation or pulmonary (usually within 48 hours but may incubate for up to 60 days)	Febrile flulike symptoms (malaise, low-grade fever, dry cough, and headache)	Severe respiratory distress, hemodynamic failure, and death	Aerosol; no person-to-person transmission	Ciprofloxacin or doxycycline	Ciprofloxacin or, if susceptible, doxycycline; vaccine available but in short supply
	Cutaneous (1–12 days)	Local urticaria; painless papular lesions usually located on head, forearms, or hands	Papular lesions become vesicular, later developing black eschar and edema	Person-to-person transmission with direct contact with skin lesions		
	Gastrointestinal (1–7 days)	Abdominal pain, nausea, vomiting, and diarrhea	Gastrointestinal bleeding, fever; usually followed by toxic sepsis and death	Contaminated food and/or water		
Plague Acute, severe bacterial infection secondary to a Gram-negative bacillus, *Yersinia pestis*	Bubonic Onset of symptoms dependent on route of transmission (1–6 days)	Swollen, tender lymph nodes (most notable femoral and inguinal), high fever, rapid pulse	Hypotension, extreme exhaustion, death	Aerosol and then human-to-human by droplet inhalation	Ciprofloxacin or doxycycline	Ciprofloxacin or doxycycline; no vaccine available at present time
	Pneumonic (1–6 days)	High fever, chills, tachycardia, headache	Fulminate pneumonia (foamy hemoptysis, tachypnea, and dyspnea), sepsis, and death			
Botulism Anaerobic Gram-positive bacillus that produces a potent muscle-paralyzing neurotoxin	Foodborne (12–36 hours)	Nausea, vomiting, diarrhea	Symmetrical cranial nerve paralysis, descending flaccid paralysis (progressive paralysis of arms, respiratory muscles, and legs), and death	Contaminated food	Passive immunization (antitoxin); supportive care	Passive immunization (antitoxin); antitoxin available in short supply
	Inhalational (2 hours–8 days)	No fever, no changes in mental status	Symmetrical cranial nerve paralysis, descending flaccid paralysis (progressive paralysis of arms, respiratory muscles, and legs), and death	Inhalation of aerosolized toxin		
Typhoidal tularemia *Francisella tularensis*, an extremely infectious bacterium	Contaminated water or food or via aerosol distribution (1–14 days)	Flulike symptoms (headache, cough, fever and chills, malaise)	Pharyngeal ulcers, pleuritic chest pain, pneumonia, pericarditis, respiratory failure, sepsis, and death	Inhalation of aerosolized bacteria	Ciprofloxacin or doxycycline	Ciprofloxacin or doxycycline; vaccine available, only limited supply; vaccine offers incomplete protection

Continued

TABLE 15.1

Summary of Selected Class A Biological Warfare Agents—cont'd

Disease/Infectious Agent	Form and Incubation/Onset of Symptoms	Untreated Course of Disease		Probable Route of Contamination for Use as a Biological Warfare Agent	Treatment of Mass Casualties	Prophylaxis/ Vaccine
		Early-Onset Symptoms	Late-Onset Symptoms			
Major Viral Biological Agent of Concern—Smallpox						
Smallpox variola virus	Distribution via airborne droplets, aerosols, and fomites (7–17 days; weaponized smallpox when delivered aerosolized has an incubation period of only 3–5 days)	Acute viral symptoms (high fever, myalgia, headache, and backache)	Continued viral symptoms, high fever, prostration, synchronous onset of rash progressing from macules to papules to vesicles, and eschar formation Vesicles more abundant on extremities and face, and all develop at the same time; pustules appear on palms of hands and soles of feet (unlike chickenpox)	Transmitted person to person by large droplets; therefore, spread may be by inhalation of aerosolized virus, oral secretions, infected human vector exposure, or exposure to contaminated objects	Supportive therapy only (ventilator)	None; vaccine available in short supply

STEP	RATIONALE

ASSESSMENT

1. Perform hand hygiene. Don proper PPE.

2. Identify patient using at least two person-specific identifiers (e.g., name and date of birth or name and medical record number) according to employer policy.

3. Conduct focused health history and physical examination (e.g., skin assessment; pulmonary assessment—oxygen saturation, lung sounds, sputum character; cardiac—heart sounds; gastrointestinal [GI]—nausea, vomiting, diarrhea; neurological—movement of extremities, Glasgow Coma Scale, reflexes). Review history of patient's presenting symptoms and determine if a pattern exists (see Chapter 8).

4. Measure patient's vital signs and include assessment of pain using an appropriate scale (e.g., on a scale of 0 to 10, with 0 being no pain, and 10 worst pain ever).

5. Review results of diagnostic tests and consult with health care provider.

6. Assess patient for health risks (e.g., history of heart disease, pulmonary disease, cancer) that complicate effects of exposure to biological agent.

7. Stay calm. Listen and assess patient's immediate psychological response after exposure. Some patients present with dissociative symptoms (e.g., feeling as though they are "not there" or sensing that everything is outside of the person): disorientation, depression, anxiety, psychosis, and inability to care for self. Even without direct exposure to a biological agent, many individuals, spurred by feelings of fear and doom, present for emergency services.

8. Identify and gather all patient contacts (names, addresses, and phone numbers) before the patient leaves the emergency department (ED).

9. Identify employer resources available (e.g., critical-incident stress-debriefing teams, counsellors, psychiatric/mental health nurse practitioners).

Proper PPE provides safety to personnel and helps prevent spread of the infectious agent to health care providers.

Ensures correct patient. Complies with Accreditation Canada's standards and improves patient safety (Accreditation Canada, 2019).

Symptom identification and clustering data help to accurately determine exposure to type of biological agent and patient's response.

Provides baseline to later evaluate patient's response to therapy.

Initial signs and symptoms of exposure to biological agent suggest common disorders (e.g., flu). Further review of diagnostic findings helps to rule out other common disorders.

Patients with pre-existing medical conditions often require additional treatment or are at greater risk for death.

Aids in providing appropriate crisis intervention and stress management. Remaining calm and projecting confidence while assessing individuals for clinical symptoms reduce anxiety of the ill and worried well as they experience the general sense of panic associated with a biological event.

All patient contacts need to be identified for proper follow-up by the public health department. Often patients will self-triage and transport to the ED.

Expert resources help to assess extent of the psychological impact of disaster.

STEP	RATIONALE

ASSESSMENT

Clinical Decision Point *Consider that a biological event has occurred when large numbers of ill persons present who have unexplained yet similar symptoms; when there are unexplained deaths, particularly among young and healthy populations; when there is an unusual pattern associated with the symptoms (e.g., geographic, seasonal, patient population); when a patient fails to respond to traditional therapy; or when a single patient presents with symptoms suggestive of an uncommon agent (e.g., anthrax or smallpox). Once you suspect a biological event, notify incident command immediately.*

NURSING DIAGNOSES

- Reduced airway clearance
- Inadequate swallowing
- Reduced gas exchange
- Decreased cardiac output
- Acute pain

- Reduced skin integrity
- Acute confusion
- Nausea
- Anxiety/fear
- Post-trauma syndrome

- Potential for imbalanced body temperature
- Potential for imbalanced fluid volume
- Potential for peripheral neurovascular dysfunction

Related factors/Risk factors are individualized on the basis of patient's condition or needs.

PLANNING

1. Expected outcomes following completion of procedure:
   - Patient is comforted.

   - Patient's vital signs return to baseline.

   - Patient's work of breathing decreases.
   - Patient's skin integrity returns to baseline.

   - Patient's level of consciousness (LOC) returns to baseline.

   - Patient's mental health status returns to pretrauma level of functioning.
2. Dispense timely and accurate information: accurate description of agent to which patient is exposed and implications to patient and family.

In some cases, care is only palliative, with comfort as the focus. Do not underestimate the value of *comfort as care.*

When there are no underlying medical conditions and *if* the patient's disease process is responsive to treatment (when available), vital signs will normalize. However, this may take days or weeks.

Indicates improved gas exchange and cardiac output.

Antibiotic and antitoxin therapy will aid in resolution or healing of lesions over time.

Treatment measures restore neurological function and oxygenation status.

Crisis intervention successfully reduces patient's anxiety, fear, and dissociative symptoms.

Information relieves anxiety and fear.

IMPLEMENTATION

1. Continue wearing PPE applied before assessment. Follow transmission-based isolation precautions (see Chapter 5). (See Table 15.1 for route of contamination.) Use strict isolation with smallpox because of its communicability from person to person. Use airborne precautions, contact precautions, and a negative-pressure room for patients suspected of having smallpox.

Reduces transmission of microorganisms and the likelihood of additional secondary sites of contamination.

2. Decontaminate (see emergency policies). If you suspect anthrax, have patient remove clothing and place it in a labelled plastic biohazard bag.
   CAUTION: *Do not pull clothing over patient's head; instead, cut garments off.* Instruct patient to shower thoroughly with soap and water.

Handle clothing minimally to avoid agitation. Showering with soap and water helps decontaminate and reduce exposure (Bower, Henfricks, Pillai, et al., 2015).

3. Administer appropriate antibiotics, antitoxins, or both.

Various biological agents are commonly treated with ciprofloxacin and/or doxycycline.

4. Administer immunizations (in the event of smallpox).

Administration of the smallpox vaccine is the only known method to prevent the development of smallpox in an exposed person. If administered within 4 days of exposure, the vaccine usually prevents smallpox symptoms. If administered 4–7 days after exposure, the vaccine may decrease the severity of the disease (Hussain, 2018).

STEP	RATIONALE

IMPLEMENTATION

5. Administer fluid and nutrition therapy.

Biological agents commonly cause GI disturbances that sometimes result in dehydration.

6. Administer oxygen therapy.

Various biological agents (e.g., pulmonary anthrax) commonly cause respiratory symptoms that result in altered gas exchange.

7. Provide supportive care (e.g., comfort measures, including pain management).

Some victims of a biological attack will not survive; palliative care is essential (see Chapter 17).

8. After leaving patient area, remove most heavily contaminated items first. Peel off gown and gloves, roll inside out, and dispose of them. Perform hand hygiene. Remove face shield from behind and dispose of safely. Remove goggles and mask from behind. Place goggles in container for reprocessing; dispose of mask safely. Perform hand hygiene.

Avoids contamination of self, others, and environment. Reduces transmission of microorganisms.

9. Counsel patient and family about acute and potential long-term psychological effects of exposure. Offer access to trained counselors. Support survivors of a disaster by identifying resources available.

Reaction of patients will include shock, fear, and immobilization. Long-term psychological effects can arise without proper counselling. Social support networks foster coping in the days following a disaster.

Clinical Decision Point *Interprofessional collaboration among health care providers and other rescue workers for an ongoing plan for managing patients exposed to a biological agent while caring for other patients who are already present in the health care facility seeking care for illness unrelated to the current mass casualty incident (MCI).*

EVALUATION

1. Observe for improved airway maintenance, breathing, circulation, LOC, and neurological functioning.

Evaluates patient's response to available treatment and supportive care.

2. Evaluate vital signs and level of pain.

Evaluates patient's response to treatment.

3. Inspect condition of patient's skin; note character of remaining lesions.

Evaluates patient's response to antibiotic therapy.

4. Query patient, "Tell me how you feel right now." Check level of orientation and ability to conduct conversation.

Evaluates patient for changes that suggest either improvement in or deterioration of psychological status.

Unexpected Outcomes	Related Interventions
1. Patient's physical or psychological symptoms progress.	• Notify health care provider. • Notify mental health treatment team. • Remain calm, offer reassurance, and protect self and others from physical harm. • Continue to provide comfort care.
2. Patient death occurs.	• When handling bodies, consider continued risk for contamination; make sure that everyone is fully informed regarding proper procedure.
3. Secondary contamination of rescue workers.	• Rescue workers must immediately report symptoms to a health care provider or nursing supervisor.

Communication and Documentation

- Report suspected cases of a biological incident to health care provider following employer protocol. In the event of an ED exposure to a communicable disease, the department will be locked down immediately. Public health officials (e.g., the public health officer) will determine if the hospital should be locked down.
- Use disaster checklists to quickly document specific data regarding patient status, treatment administered, and response to treatment and comfort measures.
- Report any unexpected outcome to health care provider in charge.

biological event is necessary and includes information about types of biological agents, mode of transmission, symptoms, treatment, and locations of shelters and disaster treatment sites.
- Preparedness includes teaching individuals, families, and communities resilience and the ability to care for themselves when support services are not available or inaccessible.
- Health care providers need an opportunity to debrief after a disaster to help avoid psychological complications such as post-traumatic stress disorder.
- Encourage families to prepare for the unexpected (see Care in the Community).

Special Considerations
Teaching

- Preparation for an MCI goes a long way toward preventing casualties and chaos. Public education of the likelihood of a mass casualty

Pediatric

- Children are one of the most vulnerable populations, and many facets influence the impact of disaster on children. These facets

often include age, sex, family dynamics, and the level of and direct exposure to disaster (Hockenberry & Wilson, 2015).

- Children have both physical and emotional needs during disasters. They often show stress-related symptoms and may have temporary changes in behavior after a disaster (Hockenberry & Wilson, 2015).
- Many disasters result in the need to relocate, which creates stress and unique challenges in children. Stress may be increased by changes in children's cultural, psychological, and social environment. Reactions of their parents and other family members contribute to how well the child will cope with relocation and whether or not they will be able to stay connected with friends and familiar activities (Hockenberry & Wilson, 2015).
- Children are very vulnerable to the adverse effects of environmental chemicals and toxins because (1) kilogram for kilogram children take in larger doses of toxins through food, water, and air; (2) their organ systems are less mature and unable to remove some of the toxins; and (3) their life expectancy is longer, and long-term effects of exposure to toxins is unknown (Hockenberry & Wilson, 2015).
- Disasters disrupt critical infrastructure, and disruption in one sector, for example, electricity, can affect other sectors, such as access to a safe water supply and health care services (Public Safety Canada, 2015c). Outbreaks of communicable diseases have been reported after natural disasters, and children are more likely to develop infections secondary to immature immune systems (Hockenberry & Wilson, 2015).
- Families should be kept together after a disaster. Family togetherness offers reassurance to a child and lessens fears of being abandoned and unprotected (Hockenberry & Wilson, 2015).
- The media has an enormous influence over children and may affect development and behaviour. Encourage parents to limit their children's exposure to media reports of the disaster and to watch television with them whenever possible to clarify information and answer questions (Hockenberry & Wilson, 2015).
- The death of a child is always traumatic; parents may have a compelling need to be present during pediatric resuscitation and at the time of death; ideally you should allow it. It is important for nurses to be present to explain what is happening and facilitate the grieving process (Hockenberry & Wilson, 2015).

Gerontological

- Under disaster conditions triage older persons according to injuries, not age.
- Because older persons often have several concurrent illnesses, exposure to a biological agent often worsens these conditions and results in the need for more immediate care than an initial triage may suggest.
- Older persons are vulnerable during a disaster; they have increased mortality rates and a heightened risk for worse outcomes with increased ED visits after a disaster (Malik, Lee, Doran, et al., 2017).

Care in the Community

- Assemble a disaster kit before disaster strikes. The Canadian Red Cross and Public Safety Canada (2016) offer information on how to assemble a disaster preparedness kit (Box 15.8).

- Individuals with special needs (e.g., hearing impairment, impaired mobility, special diets) and individuals without vehicles require additional planning to be prepared for a disaster.
- Post emergency telephone numbers by the telephone, enter them in smartphone contacts, and teach children how and when to call 9-1-1.
- Family members need to establish a meeting place away from the home in case they cannot stay in their home or cannot reach their home during a disaster.
- Remain isolated and advise friends and relatives not to visit if family members are symptomatic.
- Instruct family to use the appropriate PPE needed to protect the family; this can include sheltering-in-place.
- Maintain strict hand hygiene for both well and symptomatic family members after using the bathroom, before eating and drinking, and after contact with pets.
- When a sick individual's symptoms worsen, transport them to the nearest designated hospital.
- Change a sick person's clothing and bed linens frequently; wash them separately from those of other family members, using any commercial detergent.
- Disinfect surfaces that the symptomatic person comes in contact with. Use an appropriate disinfectant (e.g., Lysol), especially when soiled by blood or other body fluids.
- Family caregivers need to get plenty of rest, drink fluids frequently, and eat a healthy diet. If the caregiver develops symptoms, obtain appropriate medical care immediately.

BOX 15.8

Basic Emergency Kit

- Water (at least 2 litres of water per person per day; minimum 72-hour supply)
- Food that won't spoil (e.g., canned food, energy bars, dried food, peanut butter, rice); replace food in your kit every year
- Manual can opener
- Extra keys to your car and house
- Some cash in small denominations
- A copy of your emergency plan and contact information
- Battery-operated or crank flashlight and radio
- Fresh batteries
- Matches in waterproof container
- Candles
- First-aid kit
- Emergency blanket
- Sanitation and hygiene items (e.g., hand sanitizer, toiletries, toilet paper)
- Cell phone and chargers
- Copies of personal documents (e.g., birth certificates, deed to home, passport)
- Duct tape
- Household chlorine bleach or water-purifying tablets
- Basic tools
- A whistle
- If applicable, medications, infant formula, equipment for people with disabilities, pet supplies

Adapted from Public Safety Canada. (2016). *Emergency kits*. Ottawa, ON: Author. Retrieved from https://www.getprepared.gc.ca/cnt/kts/index-en.aspx.

✦ SKILL 15.2 Care of a Patient After Chemical Exposure

A chemical disaster is the dispersal of a toxic chemical agent into the environment. The mechanism of dispersal is not always known. In fact, the dispersal mechanism, such as an explosion or fire, can be a secondary terrorist attack designed to create greater fatalities. Explosions spread a toxic chemical in uncontrolled directions, creating more victims. Symptoms from chemical exposure are usually apparent within minutes, but some are delayed up to 24 hours. Early recognition of a chemical event is a priority because nurses will need to administer many chemical antidotes quickly. Toxic chemical incidents such as biological events are often unannounced or covert. Terrorists often intend for chemical agents to cause mass casualties and induce fear and mass hysteria.

Chemical events are generally confined to small areas, although larger dispersal of these agents may occur (e.g., via a crop duster). The nature and scale of contamination depends on the state of the agent used (e.g., gas versus liquid), characteristics of the chemical used (e.g., heavy or lighter than air), and where the event occurs (e.g., indoors, where ventilation systems affect dispersal; or outdoors, where wind and velocity affect speed and direction of dispersal). For safety reasons rescue workers should be upwind and uphill from a toxic chemical disaster scene to avoid exposure. The exception is when cyanide gas has been released. Cyanide is lighter than air and thus will travel uphill. Although cyanide has the unique smell of bitter almonds, the presence of this odour is rare among published cases of cyanide poisoning (Parker-Cote, Rizer, Vakkalanka, et al., 2018).

Because symptoms are almost immediate, victims need to be evacuated as quickly as possible from a contaminated zone to a decontamination zone. Appropriate PPE protects rescue workers. Before decontamination, victims are a potential source of contamination for rescue workers. Nurses need to protect themselves against toxic chemical contamination when in contact with a contaminated patient. Secondary contamination is high with toxic chemical incidents. Table 15.2 summarizes chemical warfare agents, presenting symptoms, and untreated course of exposure.

The rapid chemical decontamination of victims of a toxic chemical incident is more important than determining the exact toxic chemical. When rapid decontamination is needed, trained personnel are required. Decontamination is either gross or technical, which generally occurs at a scene. A hospital provides decontamination when a contaminated individual presents for treatment. Interprofessional collaboration is required so that appropriate precautions are used among staff to avoid becoming victims.

Delegation and Collaboration

The skill of assessing and caring for a patient exposed to a chemical agent cannot be delegated to an unregulated care provider (UCP). The nurse directs the UCP to:

- Use appropriate PPE to prevent chemical exposure.
- Use techniques for handling a body after death to prevent contamination.

Equipment

- Decontamination room or area (adult decontamination rooms may not meet the needs of children requiring decontamination; decontamination areas for ambulatory victims may not meet the needs of those who are not ambulatory)
- Scissors or a tool to cut off clothing
- Biohazard bags with labels
- Large volumes of water, decontamination shower (Fig. 15.8)
- Appropriate personal protective equipment (PPE)
- Equipment for physical examination

TABLE 15.2

Summary of Selected Chemical Warfare Agents

Chemical Agent	Onset of Symptoms	Untreated Course of Chemical Exposure
"Lethal" agents— nerve agents (tabun, sarin, soman, and VX)	Symptoms are generally immediate.	Pinpoint pupils and shortly thereafter, salivation, runny nose, dyspnea, chest tightness, nausea, muscle twitching, coma, seizures, and death
"Blood" agents— hydrogen cyanide	Rapid onset of symptoms, though cyanide poisoning is sometimes associated with the smell of bitter almonds.	Death caused by asphyxiation
"Blister" agents— mustard and lewisite	Symptoms may be immediate or delayed.	Skin irritation and blistering
"Choking" agents— phosgene and chlorine	Symptoms can be immediate or delayed up to 24 hours.	Coughing, choking, and disruption in pulmonary function that can lead to death

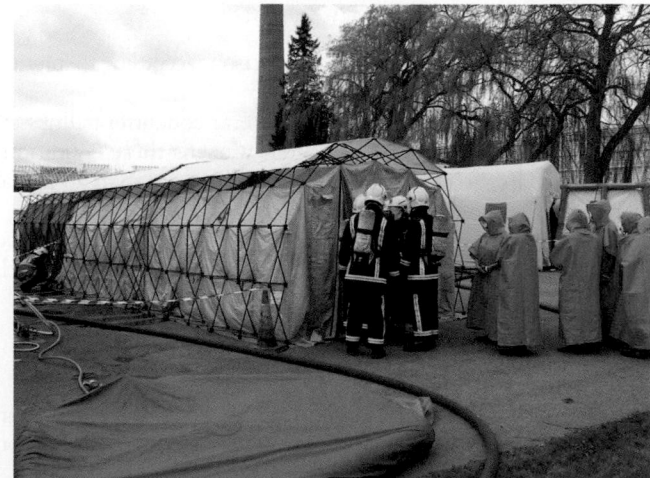

FIG 15.8 Inflatable decontamination shower for ambulatory victims. (*Courtesy Professional Protection Systems, Ltd.*)

STEP	RATIONALE

ASSESSMENT

1. Perform hand hygiene. Don proper PPE.

Provides safety to personnel and helps prevent spread of infectious agent to health care provider.

2. Identify patient using at least two person-specific identifiers (e.g., name and date of birth or name and medical record number) according to employer policy.

Ensures correct patient. Complies with Accreditation Canada's standards and improves patient safety (Accreditation Canada, 2019).

3. Conduct focused health history and physical assessment (see Chapter 8) (e.g., skin assessment; pulmonary assessment—oxygen saturation, lung sounds; cardiac—heart sounds; gastrointestinal—nausea, vomiting) (see Skill 15.1). Observe for presence of liquid on patient's skin, mucous membranes, or clothing and for odour (e.g., chlorine), assessing the condition of skin to determine severity of exposure.

Common conditions present when chemical exposure has occurred. Symptoms vary, depending on type of chemical used.

4. Assess patient for pre-existing medical conditions that will complicate effects of toxic chemical exposure.

These patients will likely require additional treatment and sometimes are at greater risk for death.

Clinical Decision Point *Consider a toxic chemical event when large numbers of ill persons present who have unexplained yet similar symptoms. The primary objective for initial care is decontamination (i.e., the removal of harmful contaminants from the skin surface). This is achieved by removing clothing; scrubbing the skin; and hydrolysis, a process of chemical dilution using large volumes of water.*

5. Remain calm. Listen and assess patient's immediate psychological response after exposure. Some patients present with dissociative symptoms: disorientation, depression, anxiety, psychosis, and inability to care for self. Even without direct exposure to a chemical agent, many individuals, spurred by feelings of fear and doom, will present for emergency services and quickly overwhelm available emergency services.

Aids in being able to provide appropriate crisis intervention and stress management. Remaining calm and projecting confidence reduces anxiety of the ill and worried well as they experience the general sense of panic associated with chemical exposure.

6. Identify employer resources available (e.g., critical-incident stress-debriefing teams, counsellors, psychiatric and mental health nurse practitioners).

Expert resources assess extent of psychological impact of disorders.

NURSING DIAGNOSES

- Reduced airway clearance
- Reduced gas exchange
- Decreased cardiac output
- Inadequate swallowing
- Acute pain

- Reduced skin integrity
- Reduced verbal communication
- Acute confusion
- Anxiety/fear
- Defective oral mucous membrane

- Nausea
- Post-trauma syndrome
- Potential for imbalanced fluid volume
- Potential for peripheral neurovascular dysfunction

Related factors/Risk factors are individualized on the basis of patient's condition or needs.

PLANNING

1. Expected outcomes following completion of procedure:
   - Patient is comforted.

   Because of fatal nature of many chemical agents, the only care available may be palliative.

   - Patient's vital signs return to baseline

   When there are no underlying medical conditions and *if* patient's condition is responsive to treatment (when available), vital signs will return to normal within days or weeks.

   - Patient's work of breathing decreases.

   Indicates improved gas exchange and cardiac output.

   - Patient's skin integrity returns to baseline or no new injury develops.

   Minimizing exposure of skin to chemical agent reduces severity and extent of lesions.

   - Patient's level of consciousness (LOC) returns to baseline.

   Neurological stability is achieved by minimizing exposure to chemical and giving antitoxin quickly.

   - Patient's mental health status returns to a pretrauma level of functioning.

   Crisis intervention successfully reduces patient's anxiety, fear, and dissociative symptoms.

2. Explain care to patient and family, including decontamination and treatment. Explain your role, orient them to location and activities to perform, explain what patient has experienced, and ask, "How are you feeling right now?" Assure them that the health care provider will see them shortly.

Information helps to calm anxiety and fear.

STEP	RATIONALE

IMPLEMENTATION

1. Continue wearing PPE applied during assessment. Prepare for decontamination.	Reduces transmission of and injury from toxic chemicals. Reduces likelihood of secondary toxic chemical contamination to untrained personnel attempting decontamination.

Clinical Decision Point *Only trained personnel using required PPE may decontaminate patients with toxic chemical contamination. Hold victim outside decontamination area until preparations are completed for decontamination. If patient is grossly contaminated, consider decontamination before entry into building.*

2. Provide for patient privacy by closing room curtains or door.	Prevents discomfort and embarrassment when clothing is removed.
3. Decontaminate patient:	
a. Act quickly; avoid touching contaminated parts of clothing as much as possible.	Prevents your own contamination.
b. Remove all of patient's clothing. **CAUTION:** *Do not pull clothing over patient's head; instead, cut garments off.*	Cutting off clothing prevents contamination of head and hair.
c. Use large amounts of soap and water to wash patient thoroughly.	Leads to chemical dilution and, in some cases, prevents patient death.
d. If eyes are burning or vision is blurred, rinse eyes with plain water for 10 to 15 minutes. If patient wears contacts, remove and place with contaminated clothing; do not reinsert in eyes. Wash eyeglasses with soap and water; reapply when completed.	Flushes toxins from eye.
4. Dispose of patient's contaminated clothing in appropriate biohazard bag and seal. Place bag in another plastic bag and seal (see employer policy).	Reduces likelihood of secondary chemical contamination.
5. Initiate treatment for chemical agent using appropriate chemical agent protocol.	Appropriate chemical agent protocol varies with patient exposure, but treatment is based on symptoms—assess breathing, heart rate, perspiration, dizziness, skin tone, and mental status (Public Safety Canada, 2015b).
6. Establish airway if needed; administer oxygen therapy (see Chapter 23).	Various chemical agents commonly cause respiratory problems that will result in altered gas exchange.
7. Control bleeding.	Various chemical agents cause extensive bleeding.
8. Establish intravascular access. Administer fluid and nutrition therapy (see Chapters 29 and 33).	Various chemical agents commonly cause gastrointestinal disturbances that can result in dehydration.
9. Provide supportive care (e.g., comfort measures, including pain management) (see Chapters 16 and 17).	Some victims will not survive; it is essential for the nurse to provide palliative symptom control.
10. Remove most heavily contaminated items first. Peel off gown and gloves, roll inside out, and dispose of them. Perform hand hygiene. Remove face shield from behind and dispose of safely. Remove goggles and mask from behind. Place goggles in container for reprocessing; dispose of mask safely. Perform hand hygiene.	Avoids contamination of self, others, and environment. Reduces transmission of microorganisms.
11. Counsel patient and family on both acute and potential long-term psychological effects of exposure. Offer access to trained counselors.	Reaction of patients to exposure includes shock, immobilization, and fear. Long-term psychological effects can arise without proper counselling.

Clinical Decision Point *Interprofessional collaboration among health care providers and other rescue workers is required for an ongoing plan to manage patients exposed to a toxic chemical agent. You will need to do this while also caring for other patients who are already present in the health care facility seeking care for illness unrelated to the current mass casualty incident (MCI).*

EVALUATION

1. Observe status of airway maintenance, breathing, circulation, LOC, and neurological functioning. Assess vital signs.	Evaluates patient's physical response to available treatment and supportive care.
2. Ask patient to rate pain level on an appropriate pain scale (e.g., scale of 0 to 10, where 0 is no pain and 10 is worst pain ever).	Determines if comfort measures are effective.

STEP	RATIONALE

EVALUATION

3. Inspect condition of skin; note extent of blistering.

Determines extent of healing.

4. Evaluate patient's level of orientation, ability to problem solve, and perception of condition.

Evaluates patient's psychological status and ability to make decisions.

Unexpected Outcomes

1. Secondary contamination of rescue workers occurs.

2. Patient's physical symptoms progress despite appropriate treatment.

3. Patient's psychological symptoms progress despite appropriate treatment. Patient exhibits anxiety, disorientation, and suicidal ideation.

4. Patient death occurs.

Related Interventions

- Rescue workers immediately remove their clothing, scrub their bodies, and use copious amounts of soap and water.
- Contain clothes in appropriate biohazard bags.
- Provide clean clothes.
- Notify health care provider in charge.
- Continue to provide comfort care.

- Notify mental health treatment team.
- Remain calm, offer reassurance, and protect self and others from physical harm.
- Continue to provide comfort measures.
- When handling bodies, there is continued risk for contamination; make sure that everyone is fully informed regarding proper procedures (see Skill 17.2). When delegating preparation of the deceased, always consider the level of training of those managing the body.

Communication and Documentation

- Report suspected cases of a toxic chemical event to health care provider or public health officer.
- Document the patient's status, decontamination and treatment procedures, and response to treatment and comfort measures.
- Report any unexpected outcome to health care provider in charge.

Special Considerations
Teaching

- Preparation for an MCI goes a long way toward preventing casualties and chaos. Public education about the likelihood of a mass casualty chemical event is necessary. This education includes information regarding types of chemical agents, mode of dissemination, symptoms, and treatment.
- Education of the public includes locations of shelters, disaster treatment sites, and how to shelter-in-place (see Box 15.4).
- Preparedness includes teaching individuals, families, and communities resilience and the ability to care for themselves when support services or not available or inaccessible.
- Health care providers need to debrief after a disaster to help avoid psychological complications such as post-traumatic stress disorder.
- See Skill 15.1 for family disaster plan and preparation.

Pediatric

- To avoid becoming a secondary victim, emergency responders need to consider potential contamination of children before picking them up and holding them. Often decontamination consists of providing fresh air and a large volume of low-pressure warm water. Observe children for potential hypothermia, because they are more susceptible.
- Adult decontamination facilities are not always appropriate to meet the needs of children. The special PPE worn by rescue workers may frighten young children. The cleaning process and possible separation from uncontaminated parents will likely cause considerable stress and anxiety. Additional health care workers are often necessary to ensure that adequate decontamination has taken place. Verbal encouragement and praise are effective in facilitating the process.
- See Skill 15.1 for further pediatric considerations.

Gerontological

- See Skill 15.1 for gerontological considerations.

Care in the Community

- Keep upwind and uphill from the release of the toxic chemical unless it is cyanide.
- Use appropriate PPE to protect the family; this includes sheltering-in-place to maximize protection from environmental contamination.
- See Skill 15.1 for further considerations regarding care in the community.

✦ SKILL 15.3 **Care of a Patient After Radiation Exposure**

Radiological events differ from nuclear events. A radiological event is the dispersal of radioactive material via a "dirty bomb," by deliberate contamination of food or water supplies, or over the terrain. A nuclear event involves a device that releases nuclear energy in an explosive manner as a result of a nuclear chain reaction. Radiation affects the body in many ways, depending on the level of exposure. High levels of radiation exposure cause a person to develop acute radiation syndrome (ARS) with symptoms of vomiting, diarrhea, erythema, and changes in blood cell counts (Dörr, Abend, Blakely, et al., 2017).

Radiation comes in a variety of forms. Alpha particles are the least dangerous, travelling only a few centimetres. They do not penetrate materials easily and are harmful only if ingested. An

individual's clothing blocks alpha particles from reaching the skin. Beta particles penetrate a short distance into the skin. Protective clothing is necessary for protection. Gamma rays pose the greatest health risk because the waves penetrate deeply, causing severe burns and internal injury. Lead shielding protects against gamma rays. Blasts caused by a nuclear explosion cause not only injury from radiation exposure but also traumatic injuries and burns. Some victims will present with many combined forms of injury requiring treatment. The sooner symptoms begin to appear, the greater a patient's exposure to the radiation. Early symptoms (i.e., within a few hours) suggest that an individual has received a lethal dose of radiation.

Nuclear incidents usually result in wide destruction requiring specialized equipment and resources at the scene to assess structural damage and levels of radioactivity. Radiological events usually cover much smaller areas, but they are often difficult to define. Specialized equipment and training are required to assess the source of radio-activity, determine the scope of contamination, and perform decontamination. During a nuclear emergency, individuals may be instructed to shelter-in-place. Individuals who were outside during the nuclear emergency are to remove clothes, seal them in a plastic bag, rinse hair and body in a shower, and then don clean clothes from a closed drawer or closet (Public Safety Canada, 2018b).

Delegation and Collaboration

The skill of assessment and care of a patient exposed to a radiological agent cannot be delegated to an unregulated care provider (UCP). The nurse directs the UCP to:

- Use appropriate personal protective equipment (PPE) to prevent exposure.
- Use techniques for handling a body after death to prevent contamination.

Equipment

- Decontamination room or area (adult decontamination rooms do not always meet the needs of children requiring decontamination; decontamination of ambulatory victims will not meet the needs of those who are not ambulatory)
- Scissors or some other tool to cut off clothing
- Clothing containers; type depends on the kind of radiological exposure
- Appropriate PPE for use by personnel in area of radiation release
- Appropriate PPE for health care workers in health care facilities (i.e., surgical masks, N95 masks recommended if available)
- Radiation meter available to survey hands and clothing at frequent intervals
- Equipment for select specimen collection
- Equipment for physical examination

STEP	RATIONALE
ASSESSMENT	
1. Perform hand hygiene. Don proper PPE.	Provides safety to personnel and helps prevent spread of infectious agent to health care provider.
2. Identify patient using at least two person-specific identifiers (e.g., name and date of birth or name and medical record number) according to employer policy.	Ensures correct patient. Complies with Accreditation Canada's standards and improves patient safety (Accreditation Canada, 2019).

Clinical Decision Point *Before assessment a specially trained technician conducts a radiation survey of the patient, initially scanning the face, hands, and feet with a radiation survey instrument. If meter results are positive, a thorough survey (5 to 8 minutes per person) is conducted.*

3. Assess patient's symptoms by performing a focused health history and physical examination (see Skill 15.1).	Symptom identification and clustering data are first steps to determine patient's condition and response to radiation.
4. Measure patient's vital signs and include assessment of pain on an appropriate pain scale (e.g., on a scale of 0 to 10, where 0 is no pain and 10 is worst pain ever).	Provides baseline to later evaluate patient's response to therapy.

Clinical Decision Point *Do not touch a wound if you suspect that radioactive fragments are present.*

5. Assess patient for pre-existing medical conditions that will complicate effects of the radiological exposure. Symptoms of acute radiation syndrome include vomiting, headache, diarrhea, erythema, and changes in blood cell counts (Dörr et al., 2017).	Patients with pre-existing medical conditions can require additional treatment or are at greater risk for death.
6. Determine patient's allergies, specifically allergy for iodine sensitivity.	Patients with iodine sensitivity need to avoid taking potassium iodide, the treatment of choice for radioactive iodine exposure.
7. Assess individual psychological response to radiological event. Some patients present with dissociative symptoms (e.g., feeling as though "not there," sensing that experiences are outside the person): disorientation, depression, anxiety, psychosis, and an inability to care for self. Ask patient, "How do you feel now?" Determine level of orientation, ability to follow conversation.	Allows you to provide appropriate crisis intervention and stress management. Remaining calm and projecting confidence while assessing individuals for clinical symptoms versus feeling of panic go a long way toward reducing anxiety of the ill and worried well as they experience the general sense of panic associated with a radiological event.

STEP	RATIONALE

ASSESSMENT

8. Identify employer resources available (e.g., critical-incident stress-debriefing teams, counselors, psychiatric and mental health nurse practitioners).

Expert resources assess extent of psychological impact of disaster.

Clinical Decision Point *A radiological event is the event most feared by most individuals. Many are uneducated regarding the dangers of and differences among radiation materials. Health care facilities will likely have many anxious, frightened individuals who can potentially create a danger to the environment. Assess individuals for signs of psychological distress. Mental health and well-being after a disaster can deteriorate, causing decreased physical function and increased incidence of illness, and this is an important factor contributing to deterioration of health post disaster (Ohtsuru, Tanigawa, Kumagai, et al., 2015).*

NURSING DIAGNOSES

- Acute pain
- Inadequate fluid volume
- Diarrhea
- Anxiety/Fear
- Nausea
- Potential for post-trauma syndrome
- Potential for infection
- Reduced tissue integrity

Related factors/Risk factors are individualized on the basis of patient's condition or needs.

PLANNING

1. Expected outcomes following completion of procedure:
   - Patient is comforted.
   - Patient is successfully decontaminated.

   - Patient's vital signs return to baseline.

   - Patient is free of nausea and diarrhea.

   - Patient's skin integrity returns to baseline.

   - Patient's immune system (e.g., complete blood count [CBC]) returns to baseline.
   - Patient's work of breathing decreases.
2. Explain care to patient and family. Explain your role, orient to location and activities to perform, explain what patient has experienced, and ask, "How are you feeling right now?" Assure them that the health care provider will see them shortly.

In some cases, the only care that is available is palliative.
Decontamination procedures remove radioactive materials from patient's skin.
When there are no underlying medical conditions and *if the patient's disease process is responsive to treatment (when available), vital signs will return to normal within days or weeks.*
Gastrointestinal (GI) alterations following radiation exposure typically respond to antidiarrheal and antiemetic medications.
Radiological burns are minimized through successful decontamination procedures.
Exposure to radiation is minimized successfully.

Indicates improved gas exchange and cardiac output.
Crisis intervention re-establishes patient's orientation and sense of reality.

IMPLEMENTATION

1. Perform hand hygiene.
2. Continue wearing PPE applied during assessment. Prepare for decontamination. *Only trained personnel use required PPE to decontaminate patients with radiological contamination.*

3. Provide for patient privacy by closing room curtains or door.
4. Decontaminate patient:
   a. Remove patient's clothing.
   b. Wash patient's skin thoroughly with water and soap, taking care not to abrade or irritate the skin. Use tepid decontamination water. Cover wounds with waterproof dressings to avoid spread of radioactivity (Radiation Emergency Medical Management [REMM], 2018).

   c. Have radiation technician resurvey patient after washing. Rewash as necessary.

Reduces transmission of microorganisms.
Reduces likelihood of secondary radiological contamination to untrained personnel attempting decontamination.

Prevents anxiety or embarrassment when clothes are removed.

Normally eliminates up to 90% of contamination.
Use of large amounts of water is critical in decontamination.
Water that is too cold will close pores, and water that is too hot enhances absorption of radioactive materials or can cause a thermal burn (REMM, 2018).

Determines if residual radiation is present.

STEP	RATIONALE

IMPLEMENTATION

d. Isolate and cover any area of skin that is still positive for radiation by using plastic bag or wrap.	Area is washed until no further reduction in contamination is achieved (verified by survey instrumentation) and then covered to reduce exposure of health care workers.
5. Bag and tag patient's contaminated clothing for further evaluation and place in an appropriate biohazard container.	Reduces likelihood of secondary contamination when you use containers designed to contain radiological particles.

Clinical Decision Point *Interprofessional collaboration is required for an ongoing plan to manage patients exposed to radiological materials. You will need to do this while also caring for other patients who are already present in the health care facility seeking care for illness unrelated to the current nuclear or radiological event.*

6. Prepare for possibly obtaining CBC, urinalysis, fecal specimen, and swabs of body orifices (see Chapter 9).	CBC establishes baseline to determine patient's immunological status over time. A health care provider who suspects internal contamination will order collection of urine, feces, and body orifice swabs to analyze for radionuclides.
7. Treat symptoms according to ordinary treatment practices: provide intravenous fluid support, antidiarrheal therapies, antiemetic medications, and potassium iodide tablets.	Patient exposed to radiation is at risk for GI alterations and fluid imbalance. Treatment is directed at minimizing or removing internal contamination (inhalation, ingestion, or absorption through open wounds) (REMM, 2016).
8. Remove most heavily contaminated items first. Peel off gown and gloves, roll inside out, and dispose of them. Perform hand hygiene. Remove face shield from behind and dispose of safely. Remove goggles and mask from behind. Place goggles in container for reprocessing; dispose of mask safely. Perform hand hygiene.	Avoids contamination of self, others, and environment. Reduces transmission of microorganisms.
9. Counsel patient and family on psychological effects of exposure. Offer access to trained counselors.	Reaction of patients to exposure includes shock, immobilization, and fear. Long-term psychological effects can arise without proper counselling.

EVALUATION

1. Observe skin integrity, fluid balance, respiratory and GI status, level of consciousness, and neurological functioning. Look for improvement of other radiological agent-specific symptoms. Evaluate vital signs.	Evaluates patient's physical response to available treatment and supportive care.
2. Monitor CBC and other laboratory tests.	Determines patient's immune response.
3. Evaluate patient's level of consciousness, orientation, and ability to relate events. Ask if patient remembers what has occurred; observe affect.	Determines if psychological status has improved.

Unexpected Outcomes	Related Interventions
1. Secondary contamination of rescue workers occurs.	• Institute appropriate decontamination of worker.
2. Patient's symptoms progress despite appropriate treatment.	• Notify health care provider in charge. • Continue to provide comfort care.
3. Patient's psychological state deteriorates with development of disorientation, suicidal ideation, violence toward others.	• Notify mental health treatment team. • Remain calm, offer reassurance, and protect self and others from physical harm. • Continue to provide comfort care (see Chapter 17).
4. Patient death occurs.	• When handling bodies, consider continued risk for contamination; make sure that everyone is fully informed about proper procedure. • If the deceased is known or suspected to be contaminated, all people handling the body will wear PPE and a personal dosimeter. • When delegating preparation of the deceased, consider the level of training of those managing the body.

Communication and Documentation

- Document patient's status and response to treatment and comfort measures in the patient's chart.
- Report presence of open wound and any suspected radioactive fragment to health care provider in charge.
- Communicate any unexpected outcomes to health care provider.

Special Considerations
Teaching
- See Skill 15.1.

Pediatric
- Children are vulnerable to radiation because (1) their organ systems are more sensitive than those of adults and (2) they have more years of life expectancy over which to develop complications from the radiological exposure.
- See Skills 15.1 and 15.2 for further pediatric considerations.

Gerontological
- Because some older persons have many concurrent illnesses, radiological agents can worsen these conditions and result in the older person needing more immediate care than an initial triage had indicated.
- See Skill 15.1 for further gerontological considerations.

Care in the Community
- When a radiological or nuclear event becomes reality, information could be on the radio, television, or social media sites; listen for special instructions, including appropriate means for maintaining shelter-in-place.
- Keep upwind and uphill from the release of the radioactive materials.
- See Skill 15.1 for further home care considerations.

✦ CLINICAL DEBRIEF

Victims of an explosion at a chemical plant are arriving in the emergency department (ED). Authorities state that the substance is unknown currently, but there were reports by people of a "funny smell" earlier in the day.

1. Which safety measures should the nurses take to avoid exposure to themselves and other patients in the ED?
2. The nurse on the scene has been asked to triage the remainder of victims using the START triage system. Place the following patients in order of highest to lowest priority. A 22-year-old with cyanosis, a respiratory rate of 35, and confusion; a 14-year-old with a diffuse red rash on the extremities; a 56-year-old with controlled bleeding of deep lacerations received from falling debris; a 41-year-old with full-thickness burns on 50% of the body.
3. One of the final victims to arrive in the ED is an 85-year-old man with a history of angina and prostate cancer. The patient lives alone in an apartment in the retirement community; he has audible wheezes on assessment and is able to answer all questions clearly. Vital signs are as follows: P: 96 beats/min, irregular; R: 28 breaths/min; SaO₂: 88%. His electrocardiogram (ECG) on admission to the ED reveals a possible anterior wall myocardial infarction (MI). Using SBAR, show how you would communicate with the health care team about this patient's condition.

✦ REVIEW QUESTIONS

1. The nurse is caring for a patient who had a biological exposure. Which actions can the nurse direct the unregulated care provider (UCP) to complete? *(Select all that apply.)*
   1. Conduct a focused health history.
   2. Handle the body after death.
   3. Review diagnostic test results.
   4. Gather and wear personal protective equipment (PPE).
   5. Administer a decontamination shower.
2. The nurse caring for a patient after radiation exposure suspects that the patient is suffering a psychological response. Which findings led the nurse to suspect a psychological response? *(Select all that apply.)*
   1. Disorientation to place and time
   2. Heightened self-care practices
   3. Depression related to the exposure
   4. Inability to follow a conversation
   5. Planning for a family vacation
3. The nurse is caring for a patient who was exposed to a chemical agent and needs to be decontaminated. Place the following steps in correct order:
   1. Wash patient with soap and water.
   2. Dispose of contaminated clothing.
   3. Remove contaminated clothing.
   4. Administer intravenous (IV) fluids.
   5. Rinse eyes with plain water.
   6. Initiate treatment for chemical agent.

ⓔ *Visit the Evolve site for a complete list of Clinical Debrief and Review Questions answers.*

REFERENCES

Accreditation Canada. (2019). *Required organizational practices handbook—Version 14.* Retrieved from http://www.wrha.mb.ca/quality/files/2019ROPHandbook.pdf

Ben-Ishay, O., Mitaritonno, M., Catena, F., Sartelli, M., Ansaloni, L., & Kluger, Y. (2016). Mass casualty incidents- time to engage. *World Journal of Emergency Surgery,* 11, 8. doi:10.1186/s13017-016-0064-7

Bower, W., Hendricks, K., Pillai, S., Guarnizo, J., & Meaney-Delman, D. (2015). Clinical framework and medical countermeasure use during an anthrax mass-casualty incident. *MMWR Recommendations and Reports,* 64(6), 1–22. doi:10.15585/mmwr.rr6404a1

Brooks, S. K., Dunn, R., Amlôt, R., Greenberg, N., & Rubin, G. J. (2016). Social and occupational factors associated with psychological distress and disorder among disaster responders: A systematic review. *BMC Psychology,* 4(18), 1–13. doi:10.1186/s40359-016-0120

Brooks, S. K., Dunn, R., Amlôt, R., Rubin, G. J., & Greenberg, N. (2017). Social and occupational factors associated with psychological wellbeing among occupational groups affected by disaster: A systematic review. *Journal of Mental Health,* 26(4), 373–384. doi:10.1080/09638237.2017.1294732

Brooks, S. K., Dunn, R., Sage, C. A., Amlôt, R., Greenberg, N., & Rubin, G. J. (2015). Risk and resilience factors affecting the psychological wellbeing of individuals deployed in humanitarian relief roles after a disaster. *Journal of Mental Health,* 24(6), 385–413. doi:10.3109/09638237.2015.1057334

Canadian Centre for Occupational Health and Safety (CCOHS). (2015). *WHMIS 2015—Hazard classes and categories.* Retrieved from http://www.ccohs.ca/oshanswers/chemicals/whmis_ghs/hazard_classes.html

Canadian Nurses Association (CNA). (2012). *Position statement: Emergency preparedness and response.* Ottawa, ON: Author. Retrieved from https://www.cna-aiic.ca/~/media/cna/page-content/pdf-en/ps119_emergency_preparedness_2012_e.pdf?la=en

Canadian Nurses Protective Society (CNPS). (2010). *Professional liability protection in a pandemic.* Ottawa, ON: Author. Retrieved from https://www.cnps.ca/index.php?page=82

Canadian Red Cross. (2019a). *Emergencies and disasters in Canada*. Retrieved from http://www.redcross.ca/how-we-help/emergencies-and-disasters-in-canada

Canadian Red Cross. (2019b). *How we help*. Retrieved from https://www.redcross.ca/how-we-help

Canadian Red Cross. (2019c). *Red Cross stories*. Retrieved from http://www.redcross.ca/about-us/red-cross-stories

Centre for Excellence in Emergency Preparedness (CEEP). (2011). *Position paper on healthcare facility and agency disaster preparedness in Canada*. Retrieved from http://www.ceep.ca/resources/HCF_&_Agency_Preparedness_Position_Paper_-Final.pdf

Community Foundations of Canada. (2017). *When disaster strikes: A guide for community foundations*. Retrieved from https://communityfoundations.ca/wp-content/uploads/2017/12/Disaster_response_toolkit_14.12.17.pdf

Cox, R. (2015). *Measuring community disaster resilience: A review of current theories and practices with recommendations*. A report prepared Public Safety Canada. Ottawa, ON: International Safety Research.

Dörr, H., Abend, M., Blakely, W., et al. (2017). Using clinical signs and symptoms for medical management of radiation casualties—2015 NATO exercise. *Radiation Research*, 187(3), 273–286. doi:10.1667/RR14619.1

Field, J. (2017). What is appropriate and relevant assistance after a disaster? Accounting for culture(s) in the response to Typhoon Haiyan/Yolanda. *International Journal of Disaster Risk Reduction*, 22, 335–344. doi:10.1016/j.ijdrr.2017.02.010

Fu, C., & Underwood, C. (2015). A meta-review of school-based disaster interventions for child and adolescent survivors. *Journal of Child and Adolescent Mental Health*, 27(3), 161–171. doi:10.2989/17280583.2015.1117978

Grolnick, W., Schonfeld, D., Schreiber, M., et al. (2018). Improving adjustment and resilience in children following a disaster: Addressing research challenges. *The American Psychologist*, 73(3), 215–229. doi:10.1037/amp0000181

Hockenberry, M., & Wilson, D. (2015). *Wong's nursing care of infants and children* (10th ed.). St. Louis: Mosby.

Hussain, A. (2018). Smallpox treatment and management. *Medscape*. Retrieved from https://emedicine.medscape.com/article/237229-treatment

Incident Command System (ICS) Canada. (2019). *Incident command system operational description*. Retrieved from http://www.icscanada.ca/en/home.html

Justice Institute of British Columbia & Wilfrid Laurier University. (2015). *The Aboriginal disaster resilience planning guide*. Retrieved from http://www.jibc.ca/news/new-online-resource-launched-strengthen-disaster-resiliency-aboriginal-communities

Kim, H., & Zakour, M. (2017). Disaster preparedness among older adults: Social support, community participation, and demographic characteristics. *Journal of Social Service Research*, 43(4), 498–509. doi:10.1080/01488376.2017.1321081

Malik, S., Lee, D., Doran, K., et al. (2017). Vulnerability of older adults in disasters: Emergency department utilization by geriatric patients after hurricane Sandy. *Disaster Medicine and Public Health Preparedness*, 1–10. doi:10.1017/dmp.2017.44

Ohtsuru, A., Tanigawa, K., Kumagai, A., et al. (2015). Nuclear disasters and health: Lessons learned, challenges, and proposals. *Lancet*, 386, 489–497. doi:10.1016/S0140-6736(15)60994-1

Parker-Cote, J., Rizer, J., Vakkalanka, J., Rege, S., & Holstege, C. (2018). Challenges in the diagnosis of acute cyanide poisoning. *Clinical Toxicology*, 56(7), 609–617. doi:10.1080/15563650.2018.1435886

Public Health Agency of Canada (PHAC). (2005). *Centre for emergency preparedness and response*. Retrieved from https://www.canada.ca/en/public-health/services/emergency-preparedness-response/centre-emergency-preparedness-response.html

Public Health Agency of Canada (PHAC). (2015). *National emergency strategic stockpile*. Ottawa, ON: Author. Retrieved from https://www.canada.ca/en/public-health/services/emergency-preparedness-response/national-emergency-strategic-stockpile.html

Public Safety Canada. (2015a). *All-hazards risk assessment*. Ottawa, ON: Author. Retrieved from https://www.publicsafety.gc.ca/cnt/mrgnc-mngmnt/mrgnc-prprdnss/ll-hzrds-rsk-ssssmnt-en.aspx

Public Safety Canada. (2015b). *Chemical releases*. Ottawa, ON: Author. Retrieved from https://www.getprepared.gc.ca/cnt/hzd/chmclrlss-en.aspx

Public Safety Canada. (2015c). *Enhancing critical infrastructure resiliency*. Ottawa, ON: Author. Retrieved from https://www.publicsafety.gc.ca/cnt/ntnl-scrt/crtcl-nfrstrctr/nhncng-rslnc-en.aspx

Public Safety Canada. (2016). *Emergency kits*. Ottawa, ON: Author. Retrieved from https://www.getprepared.gc.ca/cnt/kts/index-en.aspx

Public Safety Canada. (2017). *An emergency management framework for Canada* (3rd ed.). Ottawa, ON: Author. Retrieved from https://www.publicsafety.gc.ca/cnt/rsrcs/pblctns/2017-mrgnc-mngmnt-frmwrk/index-en.aspx

Public Safety Canada. (2018a). *National public alerting system*. Ottawa, ON: Author. Retrieved from https://www.publicsafety.gc.ca/cnt/mrgnc-mngmnt/mrgnc-prprdnss/ntnl-pblc-lrtng-sstm-en.aspx

Public Safety Canada. (2018b). *Nuclear emergencies*. Ottawa, ON: Author. Retrieved from https://www.getprepared.gc.ca/cnt/hzd/nclrmrgncs-en.aspx

Public Safety Canada. (2018c). *The Canadian disaster database*. Ottawa, ON: Author. Retrieved from https://www.publicsafety.gc.ca/cnt/rsrcs/cndn-dsstr-dtbs/index-en.aspx

Public Safety Canada. (2018d). *The regional resilience assessment program*. Retrieved from https://www.publicsafety.gc.ca/cnt/ntnl-scrt/crtcl-nfrstrctr/crtcl-nfrstrtr-rrap-en.aspx

Radiation Emergency Medical Management (REMM). (2016). *Internal contamination: Via digestive tract (Animation)*. Retrieved from https://www.remm.nlm.gov/contamimage_5.htm

Radiation Emergency Medical Management (REMM). (2018). *Decontamination procedures*. Retrieved from http://www.remm.nlm.gov/ext_contamination.htm

United Nations Office for Disaster Risk Reduction. (2017). *How to make cities more resilient: A handbook for local government leaders*. Retrieved from https://www.unisdr.org/campaign/resilientcities/home/toolkitblkitem/?id=2

World Health Organization (WHO). (2011). *Hospital emergency response checklist: A all-hazards tool for hospital administrators and emergency managers*. Retrieved from http://www.euro.who.int/__data/assets/pdf_file/0008/268766/Hospital-emergency-response-checklist-Eng.pdf

World Health Organization (WHO). (2017). *WHO Toolkit: For the care and support of people affected by complications associated with Zika virus*. Retrieved from http://www.who.int/mental_health/neurology/zika_toolkit/en/

World Health Organization (WHO) & International Council of Nurses (ICN). (2009). *ICN framework of disaster nursing competencies*. Retrieved from http://www.wpro.who.int/hrh/documents/icn_framework.pdf

16 | Pain Assessment and Management

Written by **Patricia A. Potter, RN, MSN, PhD, FAAN, and Monakshi Sawhney, RN(EC), NP(Adult), MN, PhD**

SKILLS AND PROCEDURES

OBJECTIVES

Mastery of content in this chapter will enable the nurse to:
- Understand the components of a pain assessment.
- Assess adverse effects of analgesics.
- Describe how an initial pain assessment allows the nurse to provide a patient basic comfort measures.
- Describe the process for delivering medication through a patient-controlled analgesia (PCA) device.
- Assess a patient receiving epidural analgesia.

- Assess a patient receiving a peripheral nerve block.
- Identify and discuss various nonpharmacological pain-relief measures.
- Assess and implement nonpharmacological measures to relieve pain.
- Evaluate the effectiveness of pain-management techniques.

MEDIA RESOURCES

- evolve http://evolve.elsevier.com/Canada/Perry/clinicalskills/
- Review Questions
- Case Studies

- ▶ Video Clips
- Audio Glossary
- Clinical Debrief and Review Questions Answers

PURPOSE

Pain is the most common reason that people seek health care; yet it is often underrecognized, misunderstood, and inadequately treated. *Pain* is defined as "an unpleasant sensory and emotional experience associated with actual or potential tissue damage or described in terms of such damage" (Merskey & Bogduk, 1994, p. 209). Pain is a biopsychosocial experience that is influenced by biological, psychological, and social factors. *Acute pain* is defined as a response to and experience of unpleasant stimuli. It motivates behaviours to avoid potential or actual tissue damage. It is recent in onset and is self-limiting. Acute pain generally lasts from hours to days or a month after the precipitating event. It resolves as tissue healing occurs (Health Quality Ontario, 2018a; Kent, Tighe, Belfer, et al., 2017). *Chronic pain* is defined as pain that lasts longer than 3 months or past the time of normal tissue healing (Busse, Craigie, Juurilink, et al., 2017). It can impact the person's physical, psychological, and social well-being. Many people in Canada experience chronic pain. Data from a telephone survey of Canadians estimated the prevalence of chronic pain as 18.9% in adults aged 18 years and older (Schopflocher, Taenzer, & Jovey, 2011).

The patient is the only one who knows whether pain is present and what the experience is like. Your role as a nurse is to recognize the unique nature of pain for each patient and help select appropriate therapies. The skills in this chapter emphasize the importance of using critical thinking along with an integrated approach that considers both pharmacological and nonpharmacological therapies in managing a patient's pain.

STANDARDS OF CARE

- Canadian Anesthesiologists' Society, 2018—*Guidelines to the Practice of Anesthesia* (https://www.cas.ca/English/Page/Files/97_Guidelines-2018.pdf)
- Canadian Pain Society (CPS), 2010—*CPS Position Statement* (https://canadianpainsociety.site-ym.com/page/PositionStatement?)
- Health Quality Ontario, 2018a–c—*Opioid Prescribing for Acute Pain; Opioid Prescribing for Chronic Pain; Opioid Use Disorder* (http://www.hqontario.ca/Evidence-to-Improve-Care/Quality-Standards)

- National Pain Centre, 2017—*Canadian Guideline for Opioids for Chronic Non-Cancer Pain* (http://nationalpaincentre.mcmaster.ca/documents/Opioid%20GL%20for%20CMAJ_01may2017.pdf)
- Registered Nurses' Association of Ontario (RNAO), 2013—*Best Practice Guideline: Assessment and Management of Pain* (http://rnao.ca/bpg/guidelines/assessment-and-management-pain)
- Royal College of Anaesthetists, 2010—*Best Practice in the Management of Epidural Analgesia in the Hospital Setting;* (https://www.rcoa.ac.uk/system/files/FPM-EpAnalg2010_1.pdf)

PRINCIPLES FOR PRACTICE

- The Canadian Pain Society's position statement states that patients have the right to access the best pain care possible. This includes the assessment and management of acute, chronic, and cancer pain (Box 16.1).
- Patients' cognitive impairments represent special challenges to pain assessment. Carefully observe a patient's behaviour and nonverbal responses to pain when they are unable to self-report (Box 16.2).
- Pain that patients experience can be acute (transient), chronic (persistent), or both, including cancer and noncancer pain.
- Pain can also be classified as nociceptive or neuropathic. *Nociceptive pain* is defined as pain that occurs as a result of damage to tissues (not nerves) and is due to activation of pain-sensing nerves (Merskey & Bogduk, 1994). Some words that patients use to describe nociceptive pain include *dull, aching, sore,* and *sharp. Neuropathic pain* is defined as pain that occurs as a result of damage from nerves either in the peripheral or central nervous system (Merskey & Bogduk, 1994). Some words that patients

use to describe neuropathic pain include *burning, electric shocks, numb,* and *tingling.*
- The most effective pain management combines pharmacological and nonpharmacological strategies. The classes of analgesics include (1) nonopioids and nonsteroidal anti-inflammatory drugs (NSAIDs), (2) opioids (traditionally called *narcotics*), and (3) adjuvants or coanalgesics (e.g., antidepressants and muscle relaxants) that enhance analgesics or have analgesic properties.
- Implementation of pain management strategies, including the use of nonpharmacological and pharmacological measures in a timely manner, is imperative for optimal relief. Pain is easier to manage before it becomes severe.
- The current approach to acute and chronic pain management is to provide *multimodal analgesia,* which combines drugs with at least two different mechanisms of action and nonpharmacological strategies so pain control can be optimized (Busse et al., 2017; Health Quality Ontario, 2018a, 2018b).
- Practise person-centred care and explore with the patient nonpharmacological (complementary/integrative) strategies to manage pain, which generally do not require a health care provider prescription (check employer policy) and encourage the patient to actively participate in achieving a higher level of comfort and, in some instances, freedom from pain.

BOX 16.1

The Canadian Pain Society's Position Statement

As a chapter of the International Association for the Study of Pain (IASP), the Canadian Pain Society supports the treatment of pain as a basic human right.

Almost all acute and cancer pain can be relieved, and most patients with chronic noncancer pain can be helped. People have a right to access the best care possible for pain, whether this be acute pain, pain caused by cancer, or chronic noncancer pain. Evidence supports that chronic pain is not just a symptom of underlying illness or injury; it is a disease in its own right, with significant changes in complex biological and psychosocial functions.

- Routine assessment is essential for effective management. Pain is a subjective experience involving multiple characteristics, including biological and psychosocial factors, all of which must be considered for comprehensive assessment and management.
- Unrelieved acute pain complicates recovery. Unrelieved pain after surgery or injury results in more complications, longer hospital stays, greater disability, and potentially long-term pain.
- Patients' self-report of pain should be used whenever possible. For patients unable to report pain, a nonverbal assessment method must be used.
- Health care providers have a responsibility to assess pain routinely, to accept patients' pain reports, to document them, and to intervene in order to manage pain.
- The best approach to pain management involves patients, families, and health providers. Patients and families must be informed that they have a right to the best pain care possible and encouraged to communicate the severity of their pain.

From Canadian Pain Society (CPS). (2010). *Position statement* (approved by the Board of Directors Canadian Pain Society, June 4, 2010). Toronto: Author. Retrieved from http://www.canadianpainsociety.ca/?page=PositionStatement.

BOX 16.2

Pain Assessment in Nonverbal Patients

Recommended Assessment Approaches
- Attempt a self-report of pain using simple yes/no responses or vocalizations or a numerical rating scale.
- Search for the potential cause of pain by using physical examination techniques (e.g., palpation).
- Assume that pain is present after ruling out other causes (infection or constipation).
- Identify pathological conditions or procedures that may cause pain.
- Observe patient behaviours (e.g., confusion, pacing, facial expressions, vocalizations, body movements such as guarding) that indicate pain. These vary based on patient's developmental level.
- Ask caregivers or parent for a report on behalf of the patient regarding the patient's pain.
- Attempt an analgesic trial if pathological conditions or procedures that may induce pain are present.

Using a Behavioural Pain Assessment Tool
- Use reliable and valid tools (e.g., Critical Care Pain Observation Tool [CPOT], Pain Assessment Checklist for Seniors with Limited Ability to Communicate [PACSLAC-II], Pain Assessment in Advanced Dementia Scale [PAINAD]) to recognize the presence or absence of pain and provide a rating of pain severity in nonverbal critically ill patients and older persons with impaired cognition (Gelinas, 2016; Horgas, 2017; Tsai, Jeong, & Hunter, 2018).
- Select an appropriate scale for each patient (e.g., visual analogue scale, FACES Scale or FACES Scale–Revised); no one scale is required for all specific groups of patients.
- Vital signs are not sensitive indicators for the presence of pain.

Modified from Gelinas, C. (2016). Pain assessment in the critically ill adult: Recent evidence and new trends. *Intensive and Critical Care Nursing, 34,* 1–11; Herr, K., et al. (2011). *Pain in the nonverbal patient: Position statement with clinical practice recommendations.* The American Society for Pain Management Nursing (ASPMN); Tsai, I. P., Jeong, S. Y., & Hunter, S. (2018). Pain assessment and management for older patients with dementia in hospitals: An integrative literature review. *Pain Management Nursing, 19*(1), 54–71.

PERSON-CENTRED CARE

- Pain management should be person centred, with nurses practising patient advocacy, patient empowerment, compassion, and respect. Caring for patients in pain requires recognition that pain can and should be relieved.
- Teaching the patient and their family about pain treatment and having an attitude of dignity and caring will enable the nurse to individualize a patient's pain control plan.
- Pain is unique to each individual. It is important to recognize all factors influencing a patient's pain and integrate them into an individualized plan for pain management. A timely, factual, and accurate pain assessment requires that the nurse work closely with patients and their families. Be objective, listen carefully, and assess any symptoms that a patient expresses.
- Effective communication and caring are key to gathering all the information needed to accurately determine the character of a patient's pain and its impact. Knowing these factors will help you as a nurse to intervene effectively to manage your patient's pain.
- A patient's culture can influence their recognition of pain, expression of pain, when to seek treatment, and which treatments are desirable (Jin, 2017). Practising person-centred care enables the nurse to choose proper pain assessment tools for completing a culturally sensitive pain assessment.
- Explore a patient's beliefs about pain and discomfort. For example, cultures with a holistic worldview of health and illness mix religious or spiritual aspects, what they consider natural, and the supernatural in their belief systems. Use interpreters to explain pain tools and help patients report their pain as needed.
- The International Nurses Society on Addictions (IntNSA) and the American Society for Pain Management Nursing support the position that every patient with pain, including those with substance-use disorders, has the right to be treated with dignity, respect, and high-quality pain assessment and management (Oliver, Coggins, Compton, et al., 2012).
- When patients with acute pain have pre-existing chronic painful conditions, assessment and management should focus on effective analgesia. This includes the use of pharmacological and non-pharmacological strategies and the prevention of withdrawal (Health Quality Ontario, 2018a).

EVIDENCE-INFORMED PRACTICE

One of the more challenging conditions in pain management is chronic low back pain. In a systematic review by Kamper, Apeldoorn, Smeets, et al. (2015), 41 clinical trials involving patients who had duration of pain of more than 1 year and who often had failed previous treatment were examined. Patients received interprofessional rehabilitation which involved a physical component and one of both of a psychological component or a social or work-targeted component. The strength of the 41 research studies varied in quality. The results showed that:

- Interdisciplinary biopsychosocial rehabilitation interventions were more effective than usual care (moderate-quality evidence) and physical treatments (low-quality evidence) in decreasing pain and disability in people with chronic low back pain.
- For work outcomes, interdisciplinary rehabilitation seems to be more effective than physical treatment but not more effective than usual care.
- A biopsychosocial approach to care is an individual-centred model that considers the person, their health problem, and the social context:

- *Biological* refers to the physical or mental health condition.
- *Psychological* recognizes that personal and psychological factors also influence functioning.
- *Social* recognizes the importance of the social context (e.g., work, family), pressures, and constraints on functioning.

SAFETY GUIDELINES

- Patients who receive opioids (by any route) need to be monitored for signs and symptoms of oversedation and respiratory depression. Excess sedation (difficult to arouse) precedes respiratory depression, especially in opioid-naïve patients (i.e., patients who *are not* receiving opioid analgesics daily) (Chou, Gordon, de Leon-Casasola, et al., 2016; Jarzyna, Jungquist, Pasero, et al., 2016). Use of a standard sedation scale can help prevent respiratory depression as it aids in observing and intervening for oversedation (Box 16.3).
- Monitor activities such as standing, ambulation, and transfer to a chair if the patient has received an opioid. Assess patient's blood pressure, pulse, and respirations before initiating activity.
- If a patient has undergone an outpatient procedure, educate patient and caregiver about precautions: patient cannot drive for 24 hours; caregiver may need to provide help with ambulation or take precautions to make home environment safe.
- Monitor for potential adverse effects of opioid analgesics and recommend or institute supportive measures (e.g., addition of stool softener or high-fibre diet for adverse effect of constipation).
- Epidural analgesia infusion lines should not have any medication ports and should be labelled clearly and identified to prevent accidental connection with tubing of a different type (e.g., intravenous [IV] line, tube feeding, blood infusion line) (Sawhney, 2012; ISMP Canada, 2015). Follow these guidelines:
  - Limit access to epidural lines to health care providers with proper education and competence. There can be serious ramifications of misconnections, infections, occlusions, or misadministration of medications.
  - Trace an epidural catheter line from the access site into the patient's body all the way to the end source of an infusion or capped access port before connecting or reconnecting tubing or administering a medication.
  - Communicate any practice changes, including dressing location, type of tubing and connectors, with all members of the health care team who are providing care to the patient.
- Patients currently receiving opioids for chronic pain require reassessment of any new pain or increased pain (Box 16.4). Use

---

BOX 16.3

Sedation Scale*

S = Sleep, easy to arouse
1 = Awake and alert
2 = Slightly drowsy, easily aroused
3 = Frequently drowsy, arousable, drifts off to sleep during conversation
4 = Somnolent, minimal or no response to physical stimulation
Remember—sedation precedes respiratory depression.

*Many institutional sedation scales include nursing actions to be taken for each level of sedation (Jarzyna et al., 2016).
From Pasero, C., & McCaffery, M. (2011). *Pain assessment and pharmacological management.* St. Louis: Mosby.

Opioid Use Disorder and Pain Treatment

Opioid use disorder is defined as "a problematic pattern of opioid use leading to clinically significant impairment or distress, occurring within a 12-month period" (American Psychiatric Association, 2013, p. 541). It includes 11 criteria:

1. Opioids are taken in larger amounts or over a longer period than was intended.
2. There is a persistent desire or unsuccessful effort to cut down or control opioid use.
3. A great deal of time is spent in activities necessary to obtain or use the opioid or to recover from its effects.
4. There are symptoms of craving, which includes a strong desire or urge to use opioids.
5. Recurrent opioid use results in a failure to fulfill role obligations.
6. Opioid use continues even when the person experiences persistent or recurrent social or interpersonal problems caused or made worse by the effects of opioids.
7. Important social, occupational, or recreational activities are given up or reduced because of opioid use.
8. Recurrent opioid use occurs even in situations in which physical hazards exist.

9. Opioid use continues despite knowing that a persistent or recurring physical or psychological problem, likely to have been caused or made worse by the substance, exists.
10. Tolerance, as defined by either of the following:
    a. A need for increased amounts of opioids to achieve the desired effect.
    b. A diminished effect with continued use of the same amount of an opioid.
11. Withdrawal, as manifested by either of the following:
    a. Opioids (or a closely related substance) are taken to relieve or avoid withdrawal symptoms.
    b. Produced by abrupt cessation, rapid dose reduction, decreasing blood level of an opioid, and/or administration of an antagonist.

Health Quality Ontario (2018c) states that individuals with an opioid use disorder should receive care that is respectful of their rights and dignity and that promotes shared decision making. They should also be treated with the same degree of respect and privacy as any other person. Adequate pain management should not be withheld from a patient for fear of worsening addiction or relapse of addiction (Chou et al., 2016). However, these patients should be monitored carefully.

---

interprofessional collaboration to address pharmacological and nonpharmacological therapies to ensure that all team members are aware of at-home (individualized) dosages and therapies (Busse et al., 2017; Chou et al., 2016).

- Drug–drug interactions, including enhanced or reduced effects or side effects, often occur with the multiple drug use required

by people with chronic pain. This practice is termed *rational polypharmacy* or *multimodal analgesia* (Dale & Stacey, 2016).

- Be knowledgeable about your employer's policy regarding the frequency of pain assessment and timing for follow-up assessments. The first 24 hours a patient is receiving opioids within an acute care facility requires frequent assessment.

✦ SKILL 16.1   Pain Assessment and Basic Comfort Measures

An accurate and comprehensive pain assessment is necessary to identify the nature of pain, the patient's perception of pain, and the effects on their lifestyle, as well as to offer clues regarding the cause of the pain. A thorough assessment enables nurses to arrive at proper nursing diagnoses and select appropriate pain relief therapies. Effectively managing a patient's pain does not necessarily mean eliminating it, but it does mean getting it to an acceptable level for the patient. Pain management requires that the nurse work with the patient to prevent pain whenever possible and identify an acceptable intensity of pain and level of other factors, especially sleep, that allow maximum patient function.

Nurses use the nursing process to recognize distinct and unique differences in patient perceptions and responses to pain. The nursing process offers a guide in providing person-centred care—getting to know a patient and developing an individualized plan of care.

Delegation and Collaboration

Assessment of a patient's pain cannot be delegated to an unregulated care provider (UCP). UCPs may identify to the nurse when a patient

is in pain. The nurse is responsible for completing a pain assessment. UCPs may provide selected nonpharmacological strategies (e.g., back rubs, heat or cold application) as instructed by the nurse and according to employer's policy. The nurse directs the UCP to:

- Eliminate environmental conditions that worsen pain (e.g., an excessively warm, noisy room).
- Provide maximum rest periods for patient; a written schedule for caregivers to follow is ideal.
- Turn and place patients in a position of comfort at least every 2 hours or remind patients to turn themselves. Encourage patient to use a pillow for splinting if needed.
- Observe for and report to the nurse behavioural signs of pain for patients who are unable to self-report (see Box 16.2).
- Screen for pain during patient transfer or other activity that might provoke pain.

Equipment

- Pain rating scale (check employer policy).

STEP	RATIONALE

ASSESSMENT

1. Identify patient using at least two person-specific identifiers (e.g., name and date of birth or name and medical record number) according to employer policy. | Ensures correct patient. Complies with Accreditation Canada's standards and improves patient safety (Accreditation Canada, 2019). |

STEP	RATIONALE

ASSESSMENT

2. Assess patient's risk for pain (e.g., those undergoing invasive procedures, anxious patients, those unable to communicate).

Allows you to anticipate patient's needs and intervene in a timely manner, possibly preventing pain.

3. Ask patient if they are in pain. Observe for nonverbal indicators of pain; ask significant others if they believe patient is in pain. Older persons and patients from various cultures may not admit to having pain. Try using other words, such as *hurt* or *discomfort*, or use a professional interpreter if a language difference exists.

There is no objective test to measure pain.

The patient's self-report of pain is the best way to assess pain (RNAO, 2013). Recognizes that cultural differences exist in how pain is expressed.

4. Perform hand hygiene. Examine site of patient's pain or discomfort when possible. Inspect (discoloration, swelling, drainage), palpate (change in temperature, area of altered sensation, painful area, areas that trigger pain), and assess range of motion of involved joints. Percussion and auscultation can help to identify abnormalities (e.g., underlying mass or lung crackles) and determine cause of pain (see Chapter 8). *When assessing abdomen, always auscultate first and then inspect and palpate.*

Reduces transmission of infection. Reveals nature of pain and directs you toward appropriate interventions.

5. Assess physical, behavioural, and emotional signs and symptoms of pain:

  a. Moaning, crying, whimpering, groaning, vocalizations
  b. Decreased activity
  c. Facial expressions (e.g., grimace, clenched teeth)
  d. Change in usual behaviour (e.g., less active, irritable)
  e. Abnormal gait (e.g., shuffling) and posture (e.g., bent, leaning)
  f. Guarding a body part
  g. Diaphoresis
  h. Changes in sleep patterns
  i. Decreased gastrointestinal (GI) motility, constipation, nausea, and vomiting

  j. Insomnia, anorexia, and fatigue
  k. Depression, hopelessness, anger, fear, social withdrawal

Signs and symptoms may reveal source and nature of pain. Nonverbal responses to pain are useful in assessing pain in patients who are cognitively impaired or nonverbal (RNAO, 2013).

Unrelieved acute pain can cause stimulation of the parasympathetic nervous system, which decreases GI tract activity (Swift, 2018).

Patients with chronic pain often have depression. This combination can increase perception and intensity of pain (Lerman, Rudich, Brill, et al., 2015).

Clinical Decision Point *Physiological responses (e.g., tachycardia, hypertension) to acute pain are of short duration and return to normal within minutes. Be aware that with chronic pain a patient does not usually exhibit physical signs and symptoms. Avoid use of physiological responses alone to determine pain therapy selected, even with acute pain (Pasero & McCaffery, 2011).*

6. Assess characteristics of pain. Follow employer policy regarding frequency of assessment. Use the OPQRSTUV pain assessment.

This acronym guides clinicians in collecting complete information about patient's pain experience (RNAO, 2013).

  a. Onset (e.g., "When did the pain start?")

Identifies when the pain first began.

  b. *Provocative/Palliative* factors (e.g., "What makes your pain better or worse?"). Consider patient's experience with over-the-counter (OTC) medications (including herbal and topical) that help to reduce pain.

Identifies nature and source of pain and what patient does to reduce discomfort. Combination of interventions is often most effective approach to pain relief.

  c. Quality: Use open-ended questions such as "Tell me what your pain feels like."

Helps to determine underlying pain mechanism (e.g., somatic versus neuropathic pain).

  d. *Region/Radiation* (e.g., "Show me everywhere your pain is."). Have patient use finger (if possible) to point out areas of pain.

Identify location of pain and possible causative factors for acute or transient pain.

STEP	RATIONALE

ASSESSMENT

e. Severity: Use valid pain rating scale appropriate to patient's age, language skills, developmental level, culture, and comprehension (see illustrations). Ask patient to rate pain at rest, before any intervention, and when they are moving or engaged in care activity. For patients with dementia or those who have no verbal skills, use observational pain assessment scales such as the Pain Assessment Checklist for Seniors with Limited Ability to Communicate (PACSLAC-II) and the Pain Assessment in Advanced Dementia scale (PAINAD) (Ruest, Bourque, Laroche, et al., 2017).

An appropriate pain rating scale is reliable, is easily understood, and reflects changes in pain intensity

f. Timing: Ask patient if pain is constant, intermittent, continuous, or a combination. Does pain increase during specific times of day, with particular activities, or in specific locations?

Environmental stimuli such as loud noises, bright lights, strong odours, or temperature extremes sometimes alter patient's response to pain.

g. Understanding: What is patient's understanding of the pain and how is it affecting them and their family (e.g., the impact on activities of daily living [ADLs], work, relationships, and enjoyment of life)?

Provides important baseline information to later gauge effectiveness of interventions.

h. Value: Are there any values or beliefs that the patient or family has regarding pain? What are the patient's goals?

This informs person-centred care and helps to better understand any cultural or personal beliefs that impact pain and pain management.

7. Assess patient's health and illness history and type of therapies successfully used to relieve pain (e.g., medications, OTC products, heat and cold therapies).

History provides information for type of therapies to use for patient's specific situation.

Many patients do not mention using OTC products for fear of being criticized or because they do not want them taken away.

8. Assess patient's response to previous pharmacological interventions, especially ability to function (e.g., sleeping, eating, and other ADLs). Determine if any analgesic adverse effects are likely based on medication and patient's previous responses (e.g., itching or nausea).

Determines extent to which therapies have or have not been successful in the past.

Some adverse effects, especially itching that can occur with morphine, are often poorly tolerated by patient and indicate need to identify another analgesic (RNAO, 2013).

9. Assess for allergies to medications, with focus on analgesics.

Some patients with asthma or an allergy to aspirin are also allergic to other nonsteroidal anti-inflammatory drugs (NSAIDs) (Morales, Guthrie, Lipworth, et al., 2015).

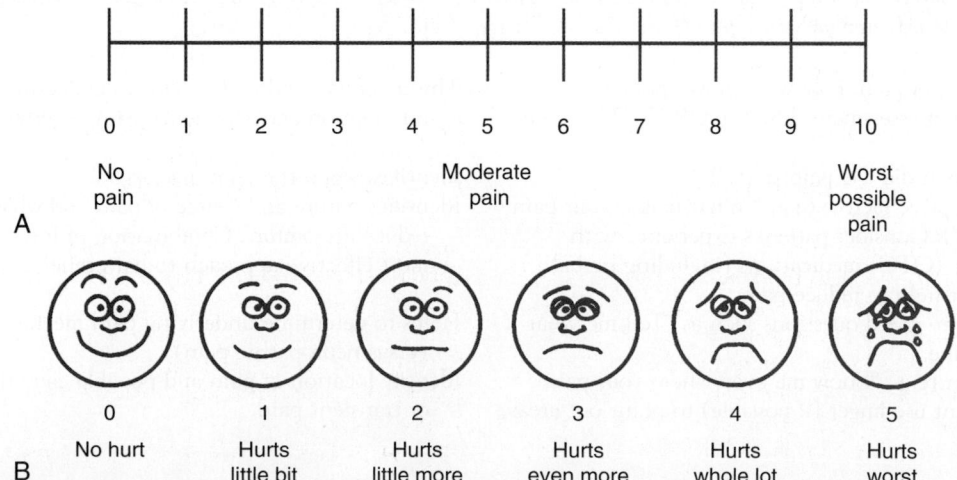

STEP 6d A, Pain rating scale. (From McCaffery, M., & Pasero, C. [1999]. Pain: clinical manual [2nd ed.]. St. Louis: Mosby). **B,** FACES Pain Scale Revised. (From the International Association for the Study of Pain [IASP]. [2001]. FACES pain scale—Revised home. Retrieved from https://www.iasp-pain.org/Education/Content.aspx?ItemNumber=1519.)

STEP	RATIONALE

NURSING DIAGNOSES

- Acute pain
- Reduced stamina
- Anxiety
- Chronic pain

- Insufficient knowledge regarding alternative pain therapies
- Altered sleep pattern
- Fatigue

- Fear
- Reduced physical mobility
- Inadequate coping
- Potential for constipation

Related factors/Risk factors are individualized on the basis of patient's condition or needs.

PLANNING

1. Expected outcomes following implementation of a pain management intervention: • Patient verbalizes full our partial relief from pain	Patient's self-report of pain is single most reliable indicator of pain (RNAO, 2013).
• Patient displays nonverbal behaviours such as relaxed face and absence of squinting.	Nonverbal behaviours can be valid and reliable indicators of pain and pain relief in the cognitively impaired (Herr, Coyne, McCaffery, et al., 2011; RNAO, 2013).
• Patient reports improvement in sleep, nutritional intake, physical activity, and personal relationships.	Adequate pain relief usually permits patient to participate in usual ADLs.
2. Set pain-intensity goal with patient (when able).	Pain is unique to each individual. Patient sets individual goal for tolerable pain severity (RNAO, 2013).

IMPLEMENTATION

1. Perform hand hygiene and apply clean gloves (if indicated).	Reduces transmission of microorganisms.
2. Prepare patient's environment. • Temperature suited to patient	Temperature and sound extremes can enhance patient's perception of pain.
• Sound • Lighting • Eliminate unnecessary interruptions and coordinate care activities; allow for rest.	Bright or very dim lighting can aggravate pain sensation. Fatigue increases pain perception.
3. Teach patient how to use pain rating scale. Explain range of intensity scores and how they relate to measure pain.	Accurate reporting by patient or family improves ongoing pain assessment, treatment, and evaluation.
4. Prepare and administer appropriate pain-relieving medications (nonopioids, opioids, coanalgesic, or multimodal combination) per health care provider's prescription (see Chapter 20). Choice of medication depends on patient's condition. For example, postoperative pain is often treated initially with opioids or acetaminophen and an NSAID (which provide effective nonopioid analgesia for postoperative patients).	Nonopioids are effective for mild-to-moderate pain. Patients with chronic pain are typically prescribed multimodal therapy (more than one type of analgesic) for pain relief.
5. Remove or reduce painful stimuli.	Reduction of pain stimuli and pressure receptors maximizes responses to pain-relieving interventions.
a. Help patient turn and reposition to comfortable position in good body alignment.	Reduces stress on musculoskeletal system.
b. Smooth wrinkles in bed linens.	Reduces pressure and irritation to skin.
c. Loosen constrictive bandages (if appropriate to purpose of bandage) or loosen or remove devices (e.g., blood pressure cuff, elastic hose, or sequential stockings).	Bandage or device encircling extremity can restrict circulation and cause pain (see Chapter 40).
d. Reposition underlying tubes or equipment.	Removes pressure on skin.
e. Use pillows as needed for alignment and positioning support (see illustration)	Helps maintain position that reduces strain on muscles and pressure areas.
6. Teach patient how to splint over painful site using either a pillow or hand.	Splinting reduces pain by minimizing muscle movement at time of stress.
a. Explain purpose of splinting.	Promotes patient's cooperation.
b. Place pillow or blanket over site of discomfort and help patient place hands firmly over area of discomfort (see illustration).	Splinting immobilizes painful area.

STEP	RATIONALE

IMPLEMENTATION

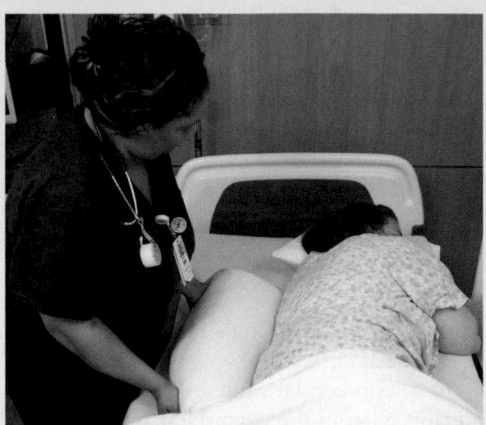

STEP 5e Positioning patient in side-lying lateral position for comfort.

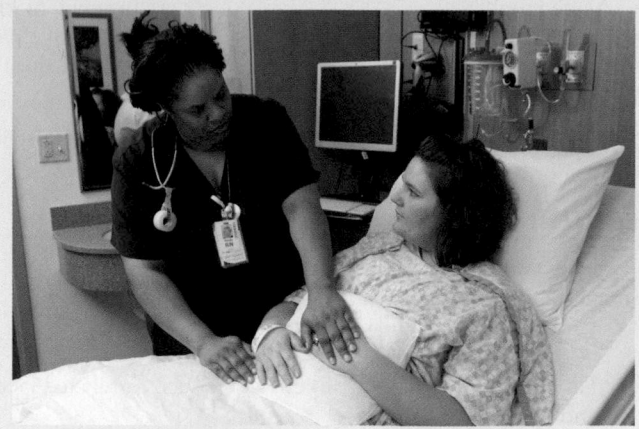

STEP 6b Patient shown how to splint painful area.

c. Have patient hold area firmly while coughing, deep breathing, and turning.	Splinting decreases movement and subsequent pain during activity.
7. Reduce or eliminate emotional factors that increase pain experiences (see Skill 16.5). Use biopsychosocial treatments: cognitive-behavioural and/or behavioural therapies.	Helps patients relax. Thoughts influence feelings, which change perception and behaviours, including a perception of pain relief (Tang, 2018). Psychological approaches to the management of chronic pain emphasize neuromodulation as a long-term therapy (Turk & Gatchel, 2018, p. 313).
a. Offer information that reduces anxiety (e.g., explaining cause of pain, if known).	
b. Offer patient the opportunity to use distraction techniques (e.g., prayer, singing to self, counting) (if appropriate, see Box 16.5).	Serves as form of distraction.
c. Spend time to allow patient to talk about pain and answer questions. Listen attentively.	Conveys caring as part of person-centred care.
8. If used, remove and dispose of gloves. Perform hand hygiene.	Reduces transmission of microorganisms.

EVALUATION

1. Within 1 hour of an intervention (e.g., repositioning or after a medication reaches its peak effect), ask patient to describe level of relief using an intensity scale (e.g., numeric rating scale 0 to 10, with 0 being no pain and 10 being worst pain ever).	Evaluates effectiveness of pain-relieving interventions in timely manner (RNAO, 2013).
2. Compare patient's current pain with personally set pain-intensity goal.	Helps to determine appropriate changes to pain-management plan. Makes patient active participant in care.
3. Compare patient's ability to function and perform ADLs before and after pain interventions.	Contributes to determining effectiveness of pain-relieving interventions, especially in nonverbal patients (RNAO, 2013).
4. Observe patient's nonverbal behaviours.	Determines effectiveness of pain-relieving interventions (Hadjistavropoulos, Herr, Prkachin, et al., 2014).
5. Evaluate for analgesic adverse effects.	Adverse effects of analgesics may be controlled by reducing dose, increasing time intervals, or administering other medications.
6. Use Teach-Back: "We discussed different ways to manage pain. How could you use non-drug ways to manage your pain at home?" Develop a revised teaching plan if the patient is not able to teach back correctly.	Determines patient's level of understanding of instructional topic.

Unexpected Outcomes	Related Interventions
1. Patient verbalizes continued pain that exceeds pain-intensity goal or displays nonverbal behaviour reflecting worsening pain.	• Repeat complete pain assessment. • Implement different nonpharmacological pain-relief measures. • Ask patient and caregivers which alternatives might be helpful. • Notify health care provider.

STEP	RATIONALE

EVALUATION

2. Patient experiences unexpected or adverse reaction to medication.	• Assess unexpected effects on patient. • Notify health care provider immediately. • Be prepared to administer antidote if indicated (e.g., antiemetic, anti-histamine, opioid-reversing agent such as naloxone). • Monitor for effectiveness of antidote; antidote may have shorter half-life than opioid; repeat dose of antidote may be needed. • Complete adverse reaction documentation according to employer policy.

Communication and Documentation

- Document the character of pain before an intervention, the pain-relief therapies used, any patient or family education provided, and patient response to interventions in nurses' notes in electronic health record (EHR) or chart.
- Document your evaluation of patient learning.
- Document inadequate pain relief (not reaching goal), a reduction in patient function, and adverse effects from pain interventions (pharmacological and nonpharmacological) in the EHR or chart. Communicate these findings to the health care provider.

Special Considerations
Teaching

- Review patient's and caregiver's understanding of the pain assessment tool and how to use it when providing pain therapies.
- Explain to patient and caregiver about the behavioural changes that may result from pain (e.g., change in activity level, splinting a body part, decreased social interaction).
- Ask patient and caregiver about fear of addiction, a common primary concern, or other misconceptions that could undermine patient's pain relief (Table 16.1).

Pediatric

- Some children are reluctant to report pain because they have misconceptions about the cause of their pain or they fear the consequences (e.g., another painful procedure or an injection).
- Infants and children experience pain but respond to it differently than adults. Infants and children who do not have the ability to self-report their pain are at risk of having their pain go unrecognized. A valid observational pain assessment tool such as the Face Legs Activity Cry Consolability–revised (FLACC-r), the Children's Hospital of Eastern Ontario Pain Scale (CHEOPS), or the COMORT/COMFORT scale (Andersen, Langius-Eklof, Nakstad, et al., 2017) should be used.
- Parents are helpful when assessing their child's pain and planning pain-relief therapies. Most parents know how their child exhibits pain and which pain-relief interventions have been successful.
- Children with verbal skills can rate their level of pain on the FACES Scale, FACES Pain Scale–Revised, pain rating scale, or Numeric Rating Scale (0–10). The Numeric Rating Scale (0–10) can be used in children over the age of 7 years. With children, 0 = no pain. However, there is no consensus on what 10 should mean. "Most hurt" or "worst hurt you can imagine" are suggestions for defining "10" (Castarlenas, Jensen, von Baeyer, et al., 2017). The absolute value of a pain-intensity score is not as important as the changes in scores in each individual child. In clinical use with children, a change in pain of 2 of 10 (i.e., a change of one face) represents the least change that can be considered clinically

TABLE 16.1

Misconceptions: Barriers to the Assessment and Treatment of Pain

Misconception	Correction
The best judge of the existence and severity of a patient's pain is the health care provider or nurse caring for the patient.	The patient's self-report is the most reliable indicator of the existence and intensity of pain.
Clinicians should use their personal opinions and beliefs about the truthfulness of a patient to determine their true pain status.	Allowing each clinician to act on personal beliefs presents the potential for different pain assessments by different clinicians, leading to different interventions from each clinician. This results in inconsistent and often inadequate pain management. A patient's self-report of pain is the standard for pain assessment.
Visible signs, either physiological or behavioural, always accompany pain and can be used to verify its existence and severity.	Even with severe pain, periods of physiological and behavioural adaptation occur, leading to periods of minimal or no observable signs of pain. Lack of pain expression does not necessarily mean lack of pain.
The pain rating scale preferred for use in daily clinical practice is the visual analogue scale (VAS).	The preferred pain rating scale depends on a patient's cognitive and physical ability, culture, developmental level, and availability, as well as employer policy.
Cognitively impaired older persons are unable to use pain rating scales.	When an appropriate pain rating scale is used and a patient is given sufficient time to process information and respond, many cognitively impaired older persons can use a pain rating scale.
If patients hurt enough, they will tell you.	Patients are often hesitant to report pain for fear of being labelled as complainers, hypochondriacs, or addicts.
Psychosocial interventions alone reduce or alleviate pain.	Nonpharmacological interventions are synergistic with medications but are not a substitute for pharmacological management of pain.

Modified from Pasero, C., & McCaffery, M. (2011). *Pain: Assessment and pharmacological management.* St. Louis: Mosby.

significant when using a FACES Scale–Revised (Tsze, Hirschfeld, von Baeyer, et al., 2015).

- Pharmacological pain support is safe and effective in pediatric patients when the dose is calibrated according to the child's weight; however, recent evidence cautions that this practice may be inappropriate for obese children (Vaughns, 2017).

Gerontological

- Older persons who are able to express themselves can use self-report pain scales. In addition, assessment should include how the pain is affecting function, sleep, appetite, activity, mood, and relationships with others (Booker & Haedtke, 2016).
- Practise person-centred care and take the time required when explaining a pain-assessment scale.
- Pain is not a natural occurrence of aging, although older persons are at risk for experiencing more pain-producing conditions.

- Nonverbal older persons experiencing pain are at high risk of inadequate analgesia (Allione, Pivetta, Pizzolato, et al., 2017). Ensure that your assessment is thorough and evaluate a patient's response critically.

Care in the Community

- Consider home conditions such as type of bed and environmental stimuli. A supportive bed and quiet environment enhance sleep and promote pain management.
- Families are the main support for older persons. Educate them about causes of painful conditions, common misconceptions about use of analgesics, type of pain medications appropriate for the patient, and how to support medication adherence.

✦ SKILL 16.2   Patient-Controlled Analgesia

 Video Clip

Patient-controlled analgesia (PCA) is a method of pain management that permits patients to self-administer analgesic medications (usually opioids, e.g., morphine, hydromorphone, or fentanyl). It is important to understand the analgesics equivalence (equianalgesia) associated with opioids to ensure their safe delivery. For example, hydromorphone is more potent than morphine, and fentanyl is more potent than both morphine and hydromorphone; therefore, the dose delivered to a patient will be adjusted on the basis of the opioid. It is a method of analgesic administration for acute and chronic pain, including conditions such as postoperative pain, cancer, and end-of-life pain. The goal is to maintain a constant plasma level of analgesic. The most common route of using PCA involves intravenous (IV) or subcutaneous drug administration.

PCA devices can be programmed to deliver a patient demand (bolus) dose, a continuous infusion (basal rate), or both. Effectiveness and safety of PCA are dependent on providing a bolus dose that provides analgesia while minimizing adverse effects. Other safety measures include having control limits for the total dosage that can be administered each hour and having a timing control (lockout period) that regulates the minimum interval (e.g., 10 minutes between doses) (Burchum & Rosenthal, 2016).

It is important that patients who will be using PCA understand how, why, and when to self-administer a medication. To receive the preprogrammed bolus dose of analgesic medication the patient must push the applicable button attached to the PCA pump. Monitoring levels of sedation is essential with the use of PCA. This is especially true for most patients who are "opioid naïve" (i.e., those who have never taken opioids for any reason or who have not taken opioids in the past 5 weeks). In addition, oversedation is a risk in patients with obstructive sleep apnea (OSA) (brief cessation of respirations during sleep) or in obese patients with short, thick, necks, who commonly have undiagnosed sleep apnea (Chou et al., 2016). Assessment of patient sedation levels is critical (see Box 16.3).

The advantages of PCA can include achieving more constant serum levels of an opioid and avoiding peaks and troughs of a large

bolus. Patients may report improved satisfaction with pain management related to the ability to control it when they receive their opioid analgesic and the fast onset of the pain medicine. Concerns involving PCA use are patient related, pump failure, or health care provider errors. Patients may misunderstand how PCA therapy works, mistake the PCA button for a nurse call button, or have caregivers operate the demand button. A pump may fail to deliver a drug on demand or have a faulty alarm or low battery. Health care providers may incorrectly program a dose, concentration, or rate. Other errors include failing to clamp or unclamp tubing, improperly loading a syringe or cartridge, failing to monitor for adverse effects or overdose, and not responding to alarms. PCA requires careful monitoring; nurses should never try to operate it without fully understanding the model in use. Many employers require an independent double-check by two nurses when initiating a PCA, changing the dose, or discontinuing the pump medications.

Delegation and Collaboration

The skill of administration of PCA cannot be delegated to an unregulated care provider (UCP). The nurse directs the UCP to:

- Notify the nurse if the patient has a change in health status or increased pain or identifies that someone other than the patient is administering the PCA dose on behalf of the patient.

Equipment

- PCA pump and tubing
- Identification label and time tape (may come attached and completed by pharmacy)
- Needleless connector
- Alcohol swab
- Adhesive tape
- Clean gloves (when applicable)
- Equipment for vital signs and pulse oximeter, or capnography (CO_2) (if available) monitoring equipment

STEP	RATIONALE

ASSESSMENT

1. Check accuracy and completeness of medication administration record (MAR) or computer printout with health care provider's prescription for patient's name, name of medication, dose, frequency of medication (continuous or demand or both), and lockout period. Check medical record for patient's history for drug allergies and typical reactions. Review medication in a drug reference manual.

Health care provider prescription required for administration of opioid medication. Ensures that patient receives right medications.
Avoids placing patient at risk for allergic reaction. Understanding medications before administering them helps prevent medication errors (Adhikari, Tocher, Smith, et al., 2014).

2. Perform hand hygiene. Assess patient's pain (see Skill 16.1). Also assess patient's ability to use the PCA control and their cognitive status for ability to understand purpose of PCA and how to use control device.

Reduces transmission of microorganisms. Reveals source and nature of pain and factors that may increase pain. Determines patient's ability to use PCA safely and correctly.

3. Assess for conditions that predispose patients to adverse effects from opioids. Known, untreated, or unknown OSA poses a significant risk for respiratory depression (Khanna, Sessler, Sun, et al., 2016).

Assessment should be completed before surgery by anaesthesia using the STOP BANG questionnaire (Khanna et al., 2016). Identification of such conditions enables the interprofessional team to take appropriate actions to minimize adverse effects.

4. Apply clean gloves. Assess patency of intravenous (IV) access and surrounding tissue for inflammation or swelling (see Chapter 29).

IV line needs to be patent for safe administration of pain medication. Confirmation of placement of IV catheter and integrity of surrounding tissues ensures that medication is safely administered.

Clinical Decision Point *Be aware that nausea is not an allergic reaction and it can be managed; pruritus alone is not an allergic reaction and is common to opioid use that can be managed.*

5. Assess patient's knowledge and perceived effectiveness of previous pain-management strategies, especially previous PCA use.

Response to pain-control strategies helps identify learning needs and affects patient's willingness to try therapy.

NURSING DIAGNOSES

- Acute pain
- Anxiety
- Chronic pain
- Insufficient knowledge regarding use of PCA
- Fear
- Inadequate coping
- Reduced physical mobility

Related factors are individualized on the basis of patient's condition or needs.

PLANNING

1. Expected outcomes following completion of procedure:
   - Patient verbalizes pain relief.
   - Patient rates pain lower on pain scale.
   - Patient exhibits relaxed facial expression and body position.
   - Patient remains alert and oriented.

   Subjective measure of pain relief.
   Objective measure of pain relief.
   Nonverbal cues of pain relief.

   Indicates freedom from overly sedating effects of opioids. Sleepiness is usually from fatigue and not necessarily a sign of oversedation.

   - Patient increasingly participates in self-care activities.
   - Patient correctly operates PCA device.

   Suggests successful pain relief.
   Demonstrates safe and appropriate use of PCA.

2. Collect appropriate equipment. Draw curtains around patient's bed or close door to room.

   Aids in organization. Maintains patient privacy.

IMPLEMENTATION

1. Perform hand hygiene.

   Reduces transmission of infection.

2. Obtain PCA analgesic (prepared by pharmacy). Check label of medication two times; when removed from storage and when preparing for assembly.

   Follows 10 rights of medication administration to be sure of correct medication. *This is the first and second check for accuracy.*

STEP	RATIONALE

IMPLEMENTATION

3. Identify patient using at least two person-specific identifiers (e.g., name and date of birth or name and medical record number) according to employer policy. Compare identifiers with information on patient's MAR or medical record.

Ensures correct patient. Complies with Accreditation Canada's standards and improves patient safety (Accreditation Canada, 2019).

4. At the patient's side compare MAR or computer printout with name of medication on drug cartridge. Do an independent double-check with another nurse and confirm the prescription and correct setup of PCA. The independent double-check should include verifying the prescription and the device independently and not just examining the existing setup.

Ensures that correct patient receives right medication. *This is the third check for accuracy.*

5. Explain the purpose and demonstrate function of PCA to patient and caregiver as follows:

Reinforces person-centred care and enables patient participation in care and independence in pain control. Preoperative education about PCA therapy improves postoperative pain relief.

   a. Explain type of medication in device.
   b. Explain that self-dosing aids in managing pain prior to repositioning, walking or coughing, and deep breathing.
   c. Explain the safety features of the PCA and that the pump is programmed to deliver a prescribed type and dose of pain medication, lockout interval, and 1- to 4-hour dosage limits. Explain how lockout time prevents overdose.
   d. Demonstrate to patient how to push medication demand button (see illustration). Instruct caregiver to not push PCA button to give medication.
   e. Instruct patient to notify nurse of possible adverse effects, problems in gaining pain relief, changes in severity or location of pain, alarm sounding, or questions.

6. Apply clean gloves. Check the medication vial or medication bag for accurate labelling, and precipitate.

Avoids medication error and injury to patient.

7. Position patient comfortably to be sure that IV or central line site is accessible.

Ensures unimpeded flow of infusion.

8. Insert drug cartridge into infusion device (see illustration) and prime tubing.

Locks system and prevents air from infusing into IV tubing.

9. Attach needleless adapter to tubing adapter of patient-controlled module.

Needed to connect with IV line.

10. Wipe injection port of maintenance IV line vigorously with alcohol or antiseptic for 15 seconds and allow to dry.

Minimizes entry of surface microorganisms during needle insertion, reducing risk of catheter-related bloodstream infection.

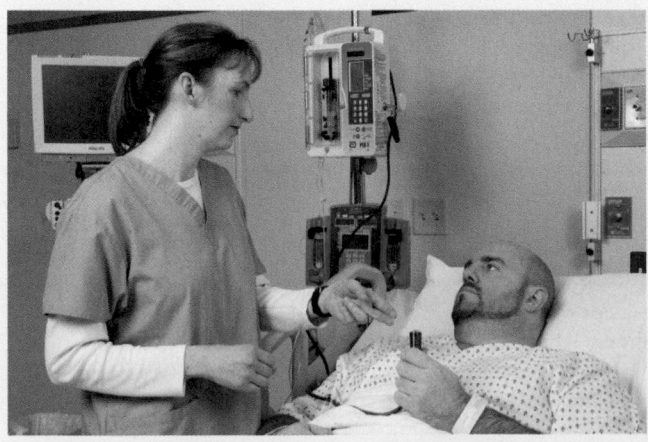

STEP 5d Patient learns how to press PCA device button.

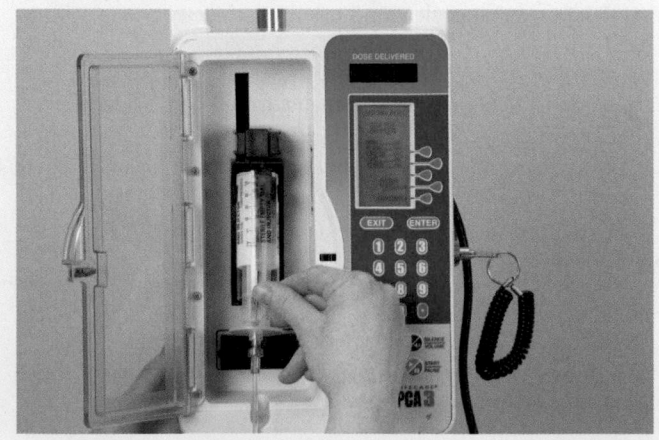

STEP 8 Nurse inserting drug cartridge into PCA device.

STEP	RATIONALE

IMPLEMENTATION

11. Insert needleless adapter into injection port nearest patient (at Y-site of peripheral IV or central line or connect to its own IV site). There should not be a chance to use PCA tubing for administering IV push with another drug.

Establishes route for medication to enter main IV line. Needleless systems prevent needle-stick injuries. Prevents medication interaction and incompatibility.

12. Secure connection and anchor PCA tubing with tape. Label PCA tubing.

Prevents dislodging of needleless adapter from port. Facilitates patient's ability to ambulate. Label prevents error from connecting tubing from different device to PCA.

13. Program computerized PCA pump as prescribed to deliver prescribed medication dose and lockout interval. Have second nurse check setting. (**NOTE**: Recheck with oncoming nurse during shift hand-off to ensure line reconciliation.)

Ensures safe, therapeutic drug administration. With appropriate dose intervals (e.g., 10 minutes), usually an appreciable analgesic effect and/or mild sedation is achieved before patient can access the next dose; thus, there is lower chance for oversedation and respiratory depression.

14. Discard gloves and supplies in appropriate containers. Perform hand hygiene.

Reduces transmission of microorganisms. The Canadian *Controlled Drug and Substances Act* regulates control and dispensation of opioids for all institutions.

15. If patient is experiencing pain, have patient demonstrate use of PCA system; if not, have patient repeat instructions given earlier.

Repeating instructions reinforces learning. Checking patient's understanding through return demonstration helps you determine patient's level of understanding and ability to manipulate device.

16. **To discontinue PCA:**

   a. Check prescription for discontinuation. Obtain necessary information from pump for documentation; note date, time, amount infused, and amount of drug wasted and reason for wastage.

   Two nurses must witness and document the wastage of opioids (formerly called narcotics) to meet the requirements of the *Controlled Drug and Substances Act*.

   b. Perform hand hygiene and apply clean gloves. Turn off pump. Disconnect PCA tubing from primary IV line but maintain IV access.

   Reduces transmission of infection. Ensures continuation of IV infusion.

   c. Dispose of empty cartridge, tubing, and gloves according to employer policy.

EVALUATION

1. Use appropriate pain rating scale to evaluate patient's pain intensity following treatments and procedures according to employer policy.

Determines response to PCA dosing. Documenting "PCA effective" is not an adequate documentation of a patient's pain level.

2. Observe patient for nausea or pruritus.

Common adverse effects of opioid.

3. Monitor patient's level of sedation, vital signs, and pulse oximetry or capnography as per employer policy.

Patient is at highest risk the first 24 hours of use. Excess sedation (difficult to arouse) precedes respiratory depression.

4. Have patient demonstrate dose delivery.

Evaluates skill in use of PCA.

5. Evaluate number of attempts (number of times patient pushed button), delivery of demand doses (number of times drug actually given and total amount of medication delivered in particular time frame), and basal dose if prescribed, following employer policy.

Helps to evaluate effectiveness of PCA dose and frequency in relieving pain. Maintains compliance with *Controlled Drug and Substances Act*.

6. **Use Teach-Back:** "I want to be sure I explained how PCA will help with your pain and how you should use the device. Tell me the steps you will use to activate the PCA." Develop a revised teaching plan if patient is not able to teach back correctly.

Determines patient's level of understanding of instructional topic.

STEP	RATIONALE

EVALUATION

Unexpected Outcomes

1. Patient verbalizes continued or worsening discomfort or displays nonverbal behaviours indicative of pain.

2. Patient is sedated and not easily aroused.

3. Patient unable to manipulate PCA device to maintain pain control.

Related Interventions

- Perform complete pain reassessment.
- Assess for possible complications other than pain.
- Inspect IV site for possible catheter occlusion or infiltration.
- Evaluate number of attempts and deliveries initiated by patient.
- Check that maintenance of IV fluid is running continuously.
- Evaluate pump for operational problems.
- Consult with health care provider.
- Stop PCA.
- Notify health care provider.
- Elevate head of bed 30 degrees unless contraindicated.
- Instruct patient to take deep breaths.
- Apply oxygen at 2 L/min per nasal cannula (if prescribed).
- Assess vital signs, oxygen saturation, and/or capnography.
- Evaluate amount of opioid delivered.
- Ask caregivers if they pressed button without patient's knowledge.
- Review MAR for other possible sedating drugs.
- Prepare to administer an opioid-reversing agent.
- Observe patient frequently.
- Consult with health care provider regarding alternative medication route or possibly a basal (continuous) dose.

Communication and Documentation

- Document the drug, concentration, dose (basal and/or demand), time started, lockout time, amount of IV solution infused, and remaining solution in the electronic health record (EHR) or chart. Use special PCA documentation forms, if available.
- Document findings of the assessment of patient response to analgesia on PCA medication form, in nurses' notes in EHR or chart according to employer policy. This includes vital signs, oximetry or capnography, sedation status, pain rating, and status of vascular access site.
- Document your evaluation of patient learning.

Special Considerations

Teaching

- Provide instructions on how to use PCA prior to starting the PCA pump. If the patient is having surgery, provide education before surgery.
- Encourage patients to push button on the PCA pump before the pain is severe. Teach the patient to use PCA bolus prior to activities or procedures that will increase the pain.
- Explain regimen to caregivers so they can support and coach patient (but not push the bolus button for patient).
- Inform patient of nonpharmacological pain-management strategies that supplement or enhance pharmacological intervention (see Skill 16.5).

Pediatric

- PCA is an effective means of pain control in children who can understand the concept. When selecting children for PCA use,

consider a patient's developmental level, cognitive level, and motor skills. PCA use is safe and effective for patients as young as 5 years old, but is most often used with adolescents (Hayes, Dowling, Peliowski, et al., 2016; Soffin & Liu, 2018). From a developmental perspective, use of PCA is particularly effective with adolescents because it leads to feelings of control.
- Although controversial, some employers have provided specific guidelines and training to allow parents and nurses to push the button for children too young or unable to use the device on their own. When this is allowed, the concept of patient control is negated, and the inherent safety of PCA needs to be monitored (Hockenberry & Wilson, 2015).

Gerontological

- Older persons sometimes appear more sensitive to analgesics and experience more opioid adverse effects (Naples, Gellad, & Hanlon, 2016). Older persons' reduced renal and liver function slows opioid metabolism and excretion. This causes a faster peak effect and a longer duration of action of the opioid. Dosages should be started low and titrated upward slowly until pain relief is achieved (Naples et al., 2016).
- If patient confusion occurs while using PCA, notify health care provider (may need a prescription to lower the dose or lengthen the lockout time). Refusing to provide analgesia is not the answer; confusion may be caused by pain (Pasero & McCaffery, 2011).

◆ SKILL 16.3   Epidural Analgesia

Epidural analgesia is highly effective for controlling acute pain during labour; after surgery; or after trauma to the chest, abdomen, pelvis, or lower limbs. It has the potential to provide excellent pain relief, minimal adverse effects, and high patient satisfaction when compared with other methods of analgesia (Pöpping, Elia, Van Aken, et al., 2014). Patient-controlled epidural analgesia (PCEA) has been shown

to provide excellent control of labour and postoperative pain when compared with intravenous (IV) patient-controlled analgesia (PCA) (Aloia, Bradford, Segraves-Chun, et al., 2017; Freeman, Bloemenkamp, Franssen, et al., 2015). Use of PCEA is safe and efficient, and complications from this technique are rare. Epidural opioids reduce the total amount of opioid medication required to control pain and thus produce fewer opioid-related adverse effects. However, if epidural analgesia is not managed correctly, it can cause serious complications; safe and effective management requires a coordinated interprofessional approach (Bos, Hollmann, & Lirk, 2017).

The epidural space contains a network of vessels, nerves, and fat located between the vertebral column and the dura mater, the outermost meninges covering the spinal cord (Fig. 16.1). Analgesics delivered into this space are distributed by (1) diffusion through the dura mater into the cerebrospinal fluid (CSF), where they act directly on the receptors in the dorsal horn of the spinal cord; (2) blood vessels in the epidural space, where they are delivered systemically; and (3) absorption by fat in the epidural space, creating a depot where the analgesia is slowly released systemically. An analgesic acts by binding to opiate receptors in the dorsal horn of the spinal column, thus blocking pain impulse transmission to the cerebral cortex (Ghelardini, Mannelli, & Bianchi, 2015; Hernandez, Grant, & Wu, 2018).

Opioids and local anaesthetics, separately or in combination, are used in epidural analgesia. Opioids are delivered close to their site of action (central nervous system) and thus require much smaller doses to achieve the same pain relief (Ghelardini et al., 2015). Common opioids via epidural include morphine, hydromorphone, fentanyl, and sufentanil. These opioids differ by their lipophilic "fat-soluble" and hydrophilic "water-soluble" properties, which affect absorption rate and duration of action. Fentanyl and sufentanil are lipophilic, causing them to have a quicker onset and shorter duration of action (2 hours). Morphine and hydromorphone are hydrophilic, resulting in longer onset and duration of action (24 hours) (Hernandez et al., 2018).

The patient is placed in the lateral side-lying or sitting position with the shoulders and hips in alignment and the hips and head flexed during insertion of an epidural catheter. An anaesthesia provider, using sterile technique, typically places a catheter into the epidural space below the second lumbar vertebra, where the

spinal cord ends (Fig. 16.2). However, epidurals may also be placed at the thoracic level of the spinal cord. Temporary or short-term catheters are not sutured in place and exit from the insertion site on the back. A catheter intended for permanent or long-term use is "tunnelled" subcutaneously and exits on the side of the body (Fig. 16.3) or on the abdomen. Tunnelling reduces infection and catheter dislodgement. A sterile occlusive dressing covers the catheter exit site and is secured to the patient. An X-ray film confirms epidural catheter placement.

A health care provider administers epidural medication intermittently via a bolus, or the patient can inject intermittently on demand (PCEA) through a pump. An epidural infusion can also be given continuously via a controlled delivery system such as an implanted infusion pump (Bos et al., 2017). The use of epidural opioids requires astute nursing observation and care; thus, most institutions require specialized training for nurses who will manage epidural analgesia. Nursing students involved in helping with care of patients receiving epidural analgesia must understand all safety principles.

The catheter poses a threat to patient safety because of its anatomical location, its potential for migration through the dura, and its proximity to spinal nerves and vessels. Catheter migration into the subarachnoid space can produce dangerously high medication levels. Frequent complications include hypotension, respiratory depression, motor block, urinary retention, pruritus, and superficial infection around a catheter. ***Do not administer other supplemental opioids or sedatives when patients are on an epidural.*** The combined effect adds to the risk for respiratory depression. In many facilities, anaesthesia providers are the only health care providers who may initiate epidural opioid infusions or administer a medication bolus.

Delegation and Collaboration

The skill of epidural analgesia administration cannot be delegated to an unregulated care provider (UCP).

Equipment

- Clean or sterile gloves.
- Premixed preservative-free epidural analgesic medications as prescribed by health care provider for use in IV infusion pump (usually prepared by pharmacy).
- Clean or sterile gloves.

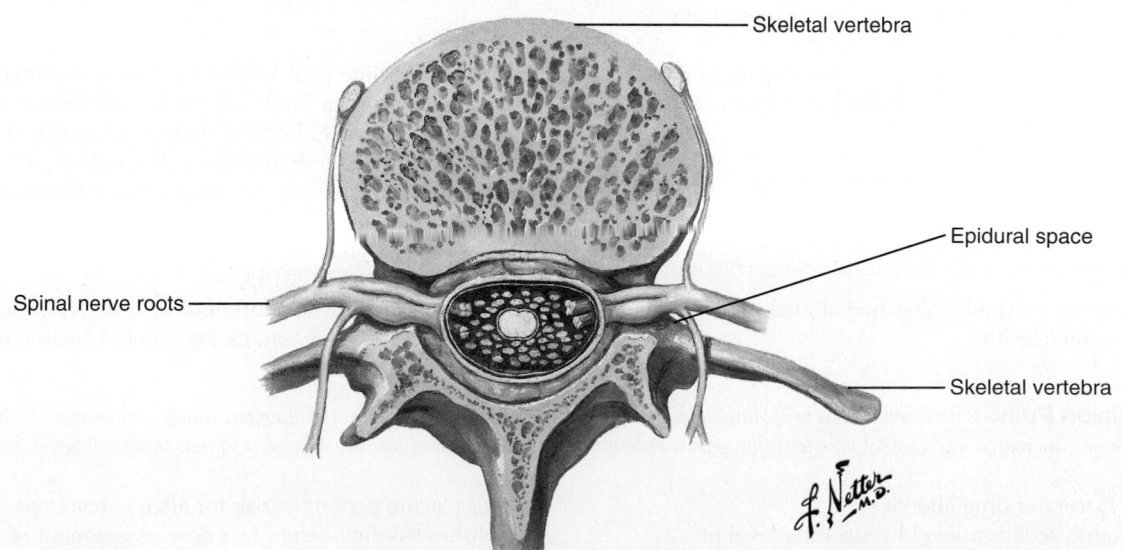

FIG 16.1 Anatomical drawing of epidural space. (*Reprinted from www.netterimages.com ©Elsevier, Inc. All rights reserved.*)

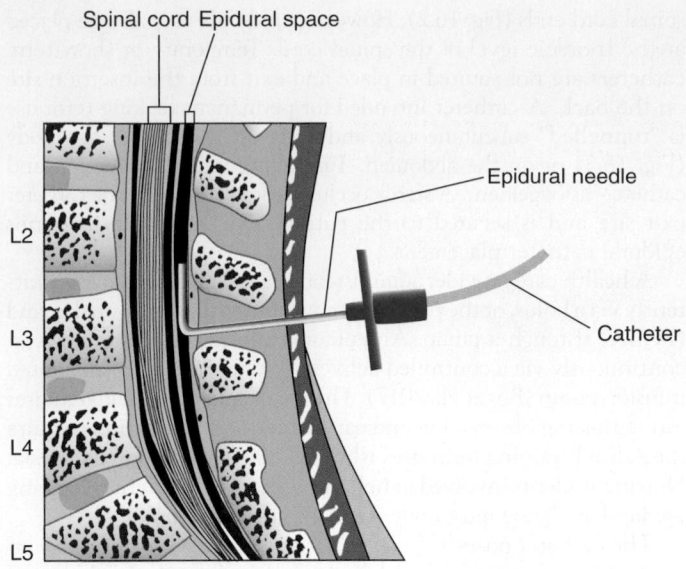

Spinal cord Epidural space

Epidural needle

Catheter

L2

L3

L4

L5

FIG 16.2 Placement of epidural catheter.

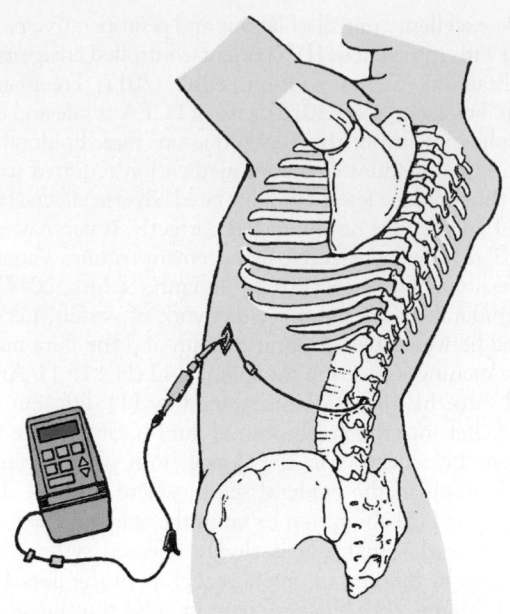

FIG 16.3 Epidural catheter attached to ambulatory infusion pump. *(Image courtesy Astra Zeneca Pharmaceuticals, Wilmington, DE. All rights reserved.)*

- Infusion pump and compatible tubing (do not use Y-ports for infusion; some infusion pumps have colour-coded tubing for intraspinal use).
- Antibacterial filter
- Tape
- Label (for tubing and injection port)
- Equipment for vital signs and pulse oximetry or capnography (see employer policy)

STEP	RATIONALE

ASSESSMENT

1. Assess if patient has completed informed consent and is aware of risk and benefits of epidural analgesia (see employer policy).

Epidural analgesia is a significant procedure that poses risks of serious and potentially fatal complications. Usually, the provider who is placing the epidural will obtain consent.

2. Verify health care provider's prescription against medication administration record (MAR) for name of medication, dosage, route, infusion method (bolus, continuous, or demand), and lockout settings. Recopy or reprint any portion of MAR that is difficult to read.

The prescription sheet is the most reliable source and the only legal record of medications that the patient is to receive. Ensures that right drug is administered to patient.

3. Perform hand hygiene. Assess the patient's pain intensity and pain quality using a valid and reliable pain assessment tool (see Skill 16.1).

Establishes baseline pain level. Cognitively impaired patients or patients for whom English is a second language may have difficulty understanding the therapy, especially if PCEA is used. Nonverbal responses provide baseline pain assessment.

4. Check to see if patient recently received anticoagulants.

Recent anticoagulation may contraindicate the placement of epidural catheter because of inability to apply pressure at insertion site and risk for bleeding (Narouze, Benzon, Provenzano, et al., 2018).

5. Assess if patient routinely takes herbal medications; document complete list.

Some herbal medications interfere with the clotting mechanism (e.g., garlic, Dong Quai, ginkgo biloba) (Narouze et al., 2018).

Clinical Decision Point *Contraindications to epidural analgesia include coagulopathies, abnormal clotting test results, compromised immunity, history of multiple abscesses, increased intracranial pressure, and sepsis. Additional contraindications include skeletal or spinal abnormalities (Chawla, 2017).*

6. Assess for history of drug allergies.

Avoids placing patient at risk for allergic reaction.

7. Assess patient's sedation level by assessing level of wakefulness or alertness, ability to follow commands, and drowsiness (see Box 16.3).

Establishes baseline before first dose. Assessment of sedation level is more reliable for detecting early opioid-induced respiratory depression than decreased respiratory rate. Sedation always precedes respiratory depression from opioids.

STEP	RATIONALE

IMPLEMENTATION

8. Assess rate, pattern, and depth of respirations; pulse oximetry or capnography; blood pressure and temperature (see Chapter 7).

Establishes baseline of circulatory and oxygenation status. Opioids can cause hypotension. Infection is complication of epidurals, reflected by fever.

9. Assess initial motor and sensory function of lower extremities (see Chapter 8). Test sensation to cold in the dermatomes associated with the expected area of sensory block. Assess motor function by having the patient flex both feet and knees and raise each leg off bed. Pay special attention to patients with pre-existing sensory or motor abnormalities.

Establishes baseline. Ongoing monitoring of motor and sensory status ensures that neural blockage is not affecting function (Sawhney, 2012).

Clinical Decision Point *For all patients on PCEA, assess for sensory and motor function before ambulation or transfer.*

10. Perform hand hygiene. Inspect catheter insertion site for redness, warmth, tenderness, swelling, and drainage. Apply sterile gloves when removing occlusive dressing.

Catheter sites are at risk for local infections. Purulent drainage is sign of infection. Clear drainage may indicate CSF leaking from punctured dura. Bloody drainage may indicate that catheter entered blood vessel.

11. Follow catheter tubing and check connection site with epidural tubing. Verify that catheter is secured to patient's skin from back, side, or front. Be sure that catheter is connected securely to IV tubing. Remove gloves and perform hand hygiene.

Prevents catheter dislodgement or migration. Ensures tubing is connected to the correct place. Tubing misconnections cause severe patient injury and death if the wrong medication infuses into the epidural space.

Clinical Decision Point *Note that in most health care settings the pharmacy prepares and provides the medication and infusion bag.*

12. Check patency of epidural tubing. Check infusion pump for proper calibration and operation.

Kinked or clamped tubing interrupts analgesic infusion.

Clinical Decision Point *Note that epidural infusions should be labelled "For Epidural Use Only" (ISMP Canada, 2015). Infusion pumps should be configured specifically for epidural analgesia with preset limits for maximum infusion rate and bolus size; lockout time should be standardized if used for PCEA.*

NURSING DIAGNOSES

- Acute pain
- Anxiety
- Chronic pain
- Reduced stamina
- Insufficient knowledge regarding epidural analgesia
- Reduced physical mobility
- Potential for infection
- Potential for injury

Related factors/Risk factors are individualized on the basis of patient's condition or needs.

PLANNING

1. Expected outcomes following completion of procedure:
   - Patient verbalizes pain relief within 30 to 60 minutes of initiating epidural infusion.

   Indicates that drug and dose are effective in relieving pain, catheter is intact, and equipment is functioning properly in compliance with health care provider's prescription.

   - Patient has no headache during epidural infusion or after discontinuation.

   Indicates that catheter is in epidural space. No CSF leakage.

   - Patient's blood pressure remains within normal range (normotensive), and heart rate remains at or above baseline.

   Indicates absence of some of the circulatory adverse effects of epidural opioids.

   - Patient is alert, oriented, and easily aroused.

   Indicates absence of excessive sedation or oversedation (see Box 16.3).

   - Patient's respirations are regular, of adequate depth, and equal to or greater than 10 breaths/min. Pulse oximetry SpO$_2$ 95% or greater.

   Indicates adequate ventilation and reduced risk for respiratory depression from opioids.

   - Patient voids without difficulty; averages a minimum of 30 mL/h.

   Indicates absence of urinary retention (potential opioid adverse effect).

   - Patient has no or minimal pruritus and no paresthesia of lower extremities.

   Indicates absence of potential adverse effect of epidural medications.

STEP	RATIONALE

PLANNING

- Epidural system remains intact and functioning.

Infusion system is patent; no interruption in medication delivery to epidural space.

2. Explain purpose and function of epidural analgesia and expectations of patient during procedure (e.g., ask patient to call for help before getting out of bed). Demonstrate to patient how to use pump on demand (when appropriate).

Proper explanation enhances patient cooperation and helps with effective results.

3. Place patients receiving epidural analgesia close to the nurses' station.

Ensures close supervision during infusion.

IMPLEMENTATION

1. Identify patient using at least two person-specific identifiers (e.g., name and date of birth or name and medical record number) according to employer policy. Compare identifiers with information on patient's MAR or medical record.

Ensures correct patient. Complies with Accreditation Canada's standards and improves patient safety (Accreditation Canada, 2019).

2. Perform hand hygiene. Follow "10 rights" for administration of medications (see Chapter 20).
   NOTE: *Pharmacy prepares medication for pump.* Check label of medication carefully with MAR or computer printout two times.

Reduces transmission of microorganisms. Ensures safe and appropriate medication administration. *This is the first and second check for accuracy.*

3. When receiving patient during hand-off or when helping during insertion by anaesthesia provider, apply an "epidural line" label to the epidural infusion tubing. Be sure that there are *no Y ports* on tubing. Epidural infusions should be labelled "For Epidural Use Only."

Labelling helps to ensure that analgesic is administered into correct line and the epidural space (ISMP Canada, 2015). Epidural infusion system between pump and patient should be considered closed, with no injection or Y ports.

4. At the bedside compare MAR or computer printout with name of medication on drug container.

This is the third check for accuracy and ensures that right patient receives right medication.

5. Apply clean gloves. Administer infusion: anaesthesia provider typically starts or administers first dose. Thereafter, nurse maintains infusion.

   a. **Continuous infusion:**

Tubing filled with solution and free of air bubbles avoids air embolus.

   (1) Attach container of diluted preservative-free medication to infusion pump tubing and prime tubing (see Chapter 22).

   (2) Insert tubing into infusion pump (see Chapter 22) and attach distal end of tubing to antibacterial filter; then connect to epidural catheter using aseptic technique.

Pump propels fluid through tubing. Filter reduces entrance of microorganisms into infusion line.

   (3) Check infusion pump for proper calibration, setting, and operation. Many facilities require two nurses to check settings as an independent double-check.

Ensures that patient is receiving proper dosing.

   (4) Tape all connections. Start infusion (see Chapter 22).

Taping maintains secure closed system to prevent infection.

   b. Administer bolus dose of analgesic via infusion pump.

Done if the patient is experiencing pain (usually by anaesthesia provider).

   (1) While helping anaesthesia provider, perform Steps 5a(1) to 5a(4). Adjust infusion pump setting for required bolus amount. Initiate pump to deliver prescribed bolus.

Prevents accidental infusion of an overdose.

   c. Administer dose on demand (bolus button) when using PCEA.

Gives patient control over administration of analgesic.

   (1) While helping anaesthesia provider, perform Steps 5a(1) to 5a(4). Set pump for lockout time (as prescribed).

   (2) Have patient initiate demand dose as needed.

6. Explain that nurses will monitor patient's response to epidural analgesic routinely. Also instruct patient on signs or problems to report to nurse (e.g., pruritus, inability to pass urine, change in sensation).

Builds trust to encourage patient to be partner in care.

STEP	RATIONALE

IMPLEMENTATION

7. Keep an IV line patent for 24 hours after epidural analgesia has ended.

Provides route for any emergency medications such as naloxone or lipids.

8. Remove and dispose of gloves. Perform hand hygiene.

Reduces transmission of microorganisms.

9. Before removal of epidural catheter, check for presence of therapeutic anticoagulation. Check employer policy for removal while patient is receiving anticoagulation therapy.

Removal of epidural catheter while patient is anticoagulated increases risk for spinal hematoma because of anticoagulation and inability to compress vessels.

EVALUATION

1. Evaluate patient's pain severity using a valid pain intensity rating scale and evaluate the location and quality of the pain.

Evaluates effectiveness of epidural infusion.

2. Evaluate blood pressure and heart rate; respiratory rate, rhythm, depth, and pattern; pulse oximetry or capnography; and sedation level based on patient's clinical condition. Generally measured more frequently in first 12 hours of infusions (e.g., hourly) (see employer policy), after bolus infusions or changes of infusion rate, and in periods of cardiovascular or respiratory instability (Rowbotham, Cashman, Counsell, et al., 2010).

Oversedation occurs before respiratory depression and should be monitored closely to prevent respiratory depression. Postural hypotension, vasodilation, and heart rate changes may occur from pain or medication adverse effects (Chawla, 2017).

3. Help patient when changing positions.

Protects patient in case of postural hypotension.

4. Evaluate catheter insertion site every 2 to 4 hours for redness, warmth, tenderness, swelling, or drainage. Note character of drainage (e.g., bloody, clear, or purulent). Do not remove dressing unless you are discontinuing the epidural catheter.

Bloody drainage may occur if catheter has migrated into a vessel. Report immediately and treat as emergency (Sawhney, 2012).

5. Inspect epidural site for disruption or displacement of catheter.

Could lead to infusion of medication into higher level of spinal cord.

6. Observe for pruritus, especially of face, head, neck, and torso. Inform patient that this is a side effect but is often not an allergic response.

Pruritus is assessed with opioid use (Thomas, 2017).

7. Observe for nausea and vomiting and presence of headache. Note any nonverbal signs of headache (grimacing, massaging head, positional changes in pain).

Nausea from epidural analgesia worsens by movement. Postdural puncture headache is due to leakage of CSF and low intracranial pressure (Anwari & Hazazi, 2015). The headache is often worse when patient is sitting upright than lying down.

8. Monitor intake and output. Evaluate for bladder distension and urinary frequency or urgency. Consult with health care provider for possible need for intermittent catheterization.

Prevents urinary retention.

9. Evaluate for motor weakness or numbness and tingling of lower extremities (paresthesias).

Reducing epidural dose (per prescription) may help eliminate unwanted motor and sensory deficits (Sawhney, 2012).

10. **Use Teach-Back:** "We discussed the adverse effects or problems that you might have from the epidural medicine that is running. Which effects should you tell me about?" Develop a revised teaching plan if patient or caregiver is not able to teach back correctly.

Determines patient's and caregiver's level of understanding of instructional topic.

Unexpected Outcomes

1. Patient states that pain is still present or has increased. Primary causes are insufficient drug dose or catheter blockage, breakage, or improper position.
2. Patient is sedated or not easily aroused.

Related Interventions

- Check all tubing, connections, medication doses, and pump settings.
- Confer with health care provider on adequacy of medication dose.

- Stop epidural infusion and elevate patient's head of bed 30 degrees (unless contraindicated). *Stay with patient and call for help.*
- Notify health care provider and prepare to administer opioid-reversing agent naloxone per health care provider's prescription.
- Monitor all vital signs, pulse oximetry, capnography, and sedation level continuously until patient is easily aroused.

STEP	RATIONALE

EVALUATION

3. Patient experiences periods of apnea; or respirations are less than 10 breaths/min, shallow, or irregular (check employer policy).

- Instruct patient to take deep breaths.
- Stop epidural infusion, stay with patient, and call for help. Notify health care provider.
- Prepare to administer opioid-reversing agent (naloxone) per health care provider's prescription (see employer policy).
- Monitor at least every 30 minutes until respirations are at least 8 or more per minute and of adequate depth for 2 hours.

4. Patient reports sudden headache. Clear drainage is present on epidural dressing, or more than 1 mL of fluid is aspirated from catheter.

- Stop infusion or bolus dosing. Stay with patient and call for help
- Notify health care provider.

5. Patient experiences minimal urinary output, urinary frequency or urgency, bladder distension, pruritus, or nausea and vomiting.

- Consult with health care provider about reducing dose of opioid and discuss treatment for adverse effects.

Communication and Documentation

- Document drug, dose, method of administration (bolus, demand, or continuous), and time given (if injection) or time begun and ended (if demand or continuous) on appropriate medication record in the electronic health record (EHR) or chart. Specify concentration and diluent.
- With continuous or demand infusion, obtain and document pump readout (frequency according to employer policy).
- Document assessments of patient's status in nurses' notes in EHR or chart and/or on appropriate flow sheet, including vital signs, pulse oximetry/capnography, intake and output, sedation level, pain severity score, neurological status, appearance of epidural site, presence or absence of adverse reactions to medication, and presence or absence of complications resulting from placement and maintenance of epidural catheter.
- Report any adverse reactions or complications to health care provider immediately.
- Document your evaluation of patient and caregiver learning.

Special Considerations
Teaching

- Describe catheter placement and purpose to patient as appropriate. Drawing or showing pictures often helps.
- Teach patient and caregivers the purpose, action, and signs and symptoms of adverse reactions to opioid or local anaesthetic. Teach when and which signs and symptoms to report to a nurse.
- Teach patient to report pain level with acceptable (to patient) pain scale.
- Inform patient of other pain-management strategies that supplement or enhance pharmacological intervention (e.g., imagery, distraction, relaxation) (Chou et al., 2016).
- Some patients may attempt to ambulate without help or overdo other activities. Caution them to call for a nurse to help with any activity until it is determined they are safe to ambulate independently. Explain that the first attempt to ambulate may feel strange secondary to decreased sensation, but motor (leg) function should be unaffected.

Pediatric

- Apply EMLA cream to the epidural site a minimum of 60 minutes before catheter insertion.
- Dosing regimens for children must be adapted for age and weight, with maximum dosage clearly defined to minimize cumulative local anaesthetic toxicity (Rowbotham, Cashman, Counsell, et al., 2010).
- Hourly assessments are recommended, especially in the first 12 hours. There should be regular review of need for infusion, especially after 48 hours (Rowbotham et al., 2010).

Gerontological

- Older persons are at the same risk for complications and medication adverse effects as other adult patients.

Care in the Community

- Patients needing long-term therapy are discharged with a tunnelled catheter. Before considering catheter placement and care in the home, assess patient's fine-motor skills, cognitive ability, and stage of disease and prognosis and the degree of involvement of caregiver (Clarke, 2017).
- Teach patient and caregiver proper dosage and administration of medication. Evaluating patient's technique for catheter care, administering medication, and reinforcing instructions are priorities.
- Teach patient and caregiver aseptic technique for medication administration as needed and for all catheter care procedures, including dressing changes. Instruct patient to change dressing every week (refer to employer policy). Teach signs and symptoms of infection and instruct patient to report to nurse or health care provider immediately should signs and symptoms appear.
- Teach patient and caregiver about signs and symptoms of adverse reactions to medication being used and interventions to alleviate mild adverse effects in the home.
- Provide patient and caregiver phone numbers of health care providers to contact in emergency and resources in the community.

◆ SKILL 16.4 **Peripheral Nerve Blocks for Analgesia**

During surgery for procedures such as hip or knee arthroplasty, shoulder repair or arthroscopy, breast reconstruction, and abdominal surgery some anaesthesiologists and surgeons may administer a single shot or continuous peripheral nerve block (Biswas, Perlas, Ghosh, et al., 2018; Ilfeld, 2017; Sawhney, Median, H., Kashin, et al., 2016). Surgeons may infiltrate local anaesthetics into the wound bed.

When a continuous peripheral nerve block is used, a catheter is put in place close to a nerve. Local anaesthetic is infused into

the catheter through a pump (e.g., bupivacaine or ropivacaine). The local anaesthetic is infused continuously to "bathe" the specific nerve or nerve plexus responsible for pain at the surgical site, thus maintaining analgesia during and after surgery. Patients may still require oral analgesics, but the total dosage is often reduced. Pumps that are used for peripheral nerve blocks may be programmed to deliver a continuous infusion or may include a patient demand or PCA feature.

Assessment of patients who receive peripheral nerve blocks includes assessing pain intensity, location, and quality. The site of the nerve block should be assessed for any bruising or hematoma. If a patient is receiving a continuous peripheral nerve block the site should also be assessed to ensure the infusion catheter is intact (Ilfeld & Mariano, 2018). In patients who undergo upper or lower extremity surgery, assessment also includes checking for sensory and motor block. Patients who have received a lower extremity block are at risk of falling because of the potential motor block they may experience (Crumley Aybar, Median, Kashin, et al., 2016)

Assessment and care of the patient who has received a peripheral nerve block require a coordinated interprofessional approach. With patients undergoing surgery, peripheral nerve blocks are usually initiated preoperatively. Using interprofessional collaboration, the patient is provided with education and prepared for the procedure. After surgery, interprofessional collaboration maximizes patient safety and is used to assess the patient's pain, mobility, and activities of daily living and to provide patient education.

Patients may be discharged home with an ambulatory pump or a disposable pump to deliver local anaesthetics for peripheral nerve blocks. A disposable pump is one-time use only, used for a few days, allowing patients to control their postoperative pain with a local anaesthetic infusion at home. Patients and their caregivers learn how to remove the catheter at home. Nursing care focuses on assessment of catheter site and connections, evaluation of local anaesthetic adverse effects, and patient teaching.

Delegation and Collaboration

The skill of managing local anaesthetic infusion pump analgesia in facilities cannot be delegated to an unregulated care provider (UCP). If the patient is going home with a peripheral nerve block it is important to provide patient and caregiver teaching on how to manage the nerve block.

Equipment

- Pump in place from surgery

Teaching Home Removal of Peripheral Nerve Block Catheter

- Clean gloves
- Sterile 10 × 10–cm (4 × 4–inch) gauze pads
- Band-Aid
- Tape
- Plastic bag

STEP	RATIONALE

ASSESSMENT

1. Identify patient using at least two person-specific identifiers (e.g., name and date of birth or name and medical record number) according to employer policy. Compare identifiers with information on the patient's medication administration record (MAR) or medical record.

   Ensures correct patient. Complies with Accreditation Canada's standards and improves patient safety (Accreditation Canada, 2019).

2. Perform hand hygiene, apply clean gloves, and assess surgical dressing and site of catheter insertion. Dressing should be dry and intact.

   Determines if catheter is placed properly.

3. Be sure that catheter tubing is correctly labelled; then assess catheter connection. Be sure that it is secure. Teach patient and caregiver that if the catheter becomes detached, do *not* reattach or reinsert; instead notify surgeon immediately.

   Reattachment could lead to infection. Tubing misconnections could lead to infusion of inappropriate drugs into surgical wound site.

4. Perform a complete pain assessment (see Skill 16.1).

   Provides baseline to determine efficacy of analgesia.

5. Review surgeon's operative report for position of catheter.

   Confirms catheter location with your own observation

6. Read medication label on device and compare to MAR or health care provider's prescription.

   Provides information regarding type of anaesthetic, concentration, volume, flow rate, date and time prepared.

7. Assess for presence of blood backing up in tubing. If blood is present, stop infusion and notify health care provider. Remove gloves and perform hand hygiene.

   Indicates possible displacement of catheter into blood vessel.

8. Determine level of extremity activity that patient can perform per health care provider's prescriptions.

   Excessive activity can cause catheter displacement.

9. Confirm patient allergies (should be completed preoperatively and intraoperatively). Assess for signs of local anaesthetic toxicity: hypotension, dizziness, tremor, severe itching, swelling of skin or throat, irregular heartbeat, palpitations, confusion, ringing in ears, muscle twitching, numbness around mouth, metallic taste, seizure.

   Early identification of toxicity prevents or lessens possibility of complications. Local anaesthetics can have serious systemic effects (ISMP, 2009).

10. Assess patient's and caregiver's knowledge of infusion pump.

    Assesses level of teaching and support required.

STEP	RATIONALE

NURSING DIAGNOSES

- Acute pain
- Anxiety

- Insufficient knowledge regarding purpose of infusion pump

- Reduced physical mobility
- Potential for infection

Related factors/Risk factors are individualized on the basis of patient's condition or needs.

PLANNING

1. Expected outcomes following completion of procedure:
   - Patient verbalizes full or partial relief from pain.

   - Patient achieves reduction of nonverbal behaviours indicative of pain, such as grimacing, clenching teeth, rocking.
   - Patient moves about in bed, sleeps and eats better, is more active, and communicates easily with family and friends.
   - Patient or caregiver verbalizes correct procedure for catheter removal.

Patient's self-report of pain is single most reliable indicator of pain.
Nonverbal behaviours are valid and reliable indicators of pain in absence of self-report (Naples et al., 2016).

Adequate pain relief allows patient to participate in activities of daily living (ADLs).

IMPLEMENTATION

1. Perform hand hygiene. When repositioning or ambulating patient, use caution.

   Avoids catheter dislodgement.

2. When preparing patient for discharge (depending on type of pump), it may be necessary for you to connect the catheter to a smaller pump for use at home. One example is a pump about the size of a baby bottle. When pump is connected, the balloon inside pump is full of medication, and plunger is all the way to the top. As medication infuses, balloon inside pump shrinks, and plunger goes down.

3. Teach patient or caregiver what to observe and how to prepare for removal of catheter at home (may also be done by community health nurse).
   a. Explain how to perform hand hygiene and apply clean gloves.

   Decreases transmission of microorganisms.

   b. Have patient assume relaxed position in bed or chair with lower extremity in normal alignment.

   Relaxes joint muscles, reducing traction from muscle tension, and provides distraction.

   c. Apply clean gloves and provide clean gloves to patient or caregiver. Have patient or caregiver gently lift adhesive dressing covering catheter insertion site and remove any remaining tape.

   Exposes catheter insertion site.

4. Teach patient or caregiver how to remove catheter.
   a. Explain to patient or caregiver to place 10 × 10–cm (4 × 4–inch) gauze over site, grasp catheter as close as possible to where it enters skin, and gently pull it out with steady motion. This should cause little discomfort or resistance. A small amount of blood or fluid drainage is normal.

   Prevents breakage of catheter.

   b. Instruct patient or caregiver to look for mark (e.g., black dot) on end of catheter tip and hold new sterile gauze using pressure over the site for 2–5 minutes.

   Indicates complete removal of catheter.
   Achieves hemostasis.

   c. Instruct patient or caregiver to wash skin to remove any surgical soap or adhesive near the site and then apply Band-Aid.

   Cleanses insertion site.

   d. Inform patient or caregiver to place catheter in plastic bag, remove and dispose of gloves, and tie bag before discarding in trash. Lastly, instruct patient or caregiver to perform hand hygiene.

   Reduces transmission of microorganisms.

5. Explain to patient that any remaining numbness should go away within 24 hours after catheter is removed.

   Allows patient and caregiver to anticipate progress and recognize problems.

STEP	RATIONALE

IMPLEMENTATION

6. Remind patient or caregiver of follow-up appointment with surgeon.	Increases patient adherence.

EVALUATION

1. Ask patient to rate pain intensity using appropriate scale at both rest and with activity.	Determines patient response to local infusion of medication.
2. Observe for signs of adverse drug reaction and report any signs immediately.	Local analgesics can result in systemic adverse effects if absorbed by veins (Pasero & McCaffery, 2011).
3. Observe patient's position, mobility, relaxation, participation in ADLs, and any nonverbal behaviours.	Indicates successful pain management.
4. Inspect condition of surgical dressing.	Wet dressing indicates possible catheter migration out of wound, especially if drainage is clear.
5. Use Teach-Back: "It is important for you to remove the catheter at home correctly. Explain to me the steps to take to remove the catheter." Develop a revised teaching plan if patient or caregiver is not able to teach back correctly.	Determines patient's and caregiver's level of understanding of instructional topic.

Unexpected Outcomes	**Related Interventions**
1. Patient verbalizes pain intensity greater than previously determined goal or demonstrates nonverbal behaviours indicative of pain. Catheter may be displaced or clogged, or surgical site may be developing complications.	• Check reservoir for presence of medication. • Check patency of tubing. • Notify health care provider.
2. Patient reports symptoms of local anaesthetic adverse reaction (bleeding, arrhythmias, weakness or numbness of affected area, seizure, confusion, infection, drowsiness, ringing in ears), possible hypersensitivity to local anaesthetic, displacement of catheter into vein, or pump failure (releasing too much drug into site).	• Stop infusion (ISMP, 2009). • Notify health care provider.

Communication and Documentation

- Document drug and concentration, date catheter inserted, and type of demand feature (continuous or demand) in MAR in the electronic health record (EHR) or chart.
- Document location of catheter, patient's pain rating, response to anaesthetic, and additional comfort measures given in nurses' notes in EHR or chart.
- Document additional analgesics necessary to control pain on MAR in the EHR or chart.
- Document any adverse reactions to local anaesthetic (ISMP, 2009) in nurses' notes in EHR or chart and report to health care provider.
- Communicate any damp dressing or displaced catheter to surgeon.
- Document your evaluation of patient and caregiver learning.

Special Considerations
Teaching

- Provide preoperative teaching about purpose before patient goes to operating room.
- If pump being used includes a PCA component through the peripheral nerve block catheter, instruct patient to depress button as needed to manage pain.
- Instruct patient to inform nurse if pain exceeds pain-intensity goal because additional oral and/or intravenous analgesics may be administered to manage pain.

Pediatric

- Local continuous infusion pumps have been used for children undergoing orthopaedic surgery. Instruct parents and the child as described under "Care in the Community" considerations. Explain special precautions not to dislodge the catheter.

Gerontological

- Continuous dosing is sometimes administered, but demand doses require a mentally competent adult. In addition, take special precautions to protect the catheter.

Care in the Community

- Instruct patient and caregiver to notify the health care provider immediately if the peripheral nerve block catheter has excessive fluid or bleeding on the dressing occurs; if patient has signs of anaesthetic reaction, including arrhythmias, weakness, or numbness of affected area, seizure, confusion, drowsiness, or ringing in the ears; or if signs of infection develop (redness and tenderness at catheter site, drainage, or fever). Provide written copy of instructions.
- Provide verbal and written instructions regarding how and when to discontinue device when at home.
- Provide instructions regarding any restrictions to extremity movement after surgery.

✦ SKILL 16.5   Nonpharmacological Pain Management

 Video Clip

Effective pain management does not always mean the elimination of pain. A variety of nonpharmacological therapies are available to directly lessen a patient's pain and provide additive relief when analgesics are administered. Nonpharmacological interventions can be used in any health care setting, and there is evidence of their efficacy in providing pain relief (Chou et al., 2016; Health Quality Ontario, 2018a; 2018b). These interventions are used in combination with pharmacological interventions, not in place of them. Nonpharmacological techniques diminish the physical effects of pain, alter a patient's perception of pain, and provide a patient with a greater sense of control.

Nonpharmacological interventions are appropriate for patients who experience anxiety or fear, would like to avoid or reduce pharmacological pain-management interventions, or have inadequate or incomplete pain relief with pharmacological interventions alone. Nurses can help patients manage their pain by teaching them to add a variety of nonpharmacological techniques for self-care (Box 16.5). Patients and families today are more aware of complementary techniques and should be encouraged to continue whatever has helped them. It is important to remember that everyone responds differently, to practise person-centred care, and to encourage patients to try different techniques.

Relaxation and Guided Imagery

Relaxation and guided imagery help to relieve acute and chronic pain, anxiety, and depression. Deep, slow breathing associated with relaxation performed alone or in combination with the focused concentration of guided imagery influences autonomic and pain processing, essential features in the modulation of sympathetic arousal and pain perception (Turk & Gatchel, 2018). Relaxation has been shown to be effective in reducing postoperative pain from upper abdominal surgery and labour pain (Dreyer, Cutshall, Huebner, et al., 2015; Levett, Smith, Bensoussam, et al., 2016). Relaxation and guided imagery provide patients with self-control when pain occurs.

BOX 16.5

Nonpharmacological Strategies for Pain Management*

Relaxation and Power of the Mind
- Self-comfort
- Progressive muscle relaxation
- Biofeedback
- Breathing exercises
- Music relaxation
- Visual imagery

Put Your Body to Work
- Exercise
- Yoga
- Tai chi
- Pacing activities
- Energy conservation
- Body mechanics

Spirituality and Reflection
- Engaging in religious practices (praying)
- Humour
- Setting aside time to focus on what *is*
- Sharing your stress with others
- Journalling

What to Do When Pain Flares
- Cold and hot therapies
- Ball therapy
- Contrast baths
- Massage
- Acupuncture
- Distraction

*Can be used in conjunction with analgesia medications.

In guided imagery, a person draws on personal memories, dreams, and visions to create an image in the mind; concentrates on that image; and gradually becomes less aware of pain. Focus of the imagination helps patients change their perceptions about their disease, treatment, and healing ability, which helps relieve pain, tension, or stress. Choosing images that patients find pleasant requires a careful assessment. Otherwise the nurse may mistakenly describe images of objects or things that a patient fears or dislikes (Giacobbi, Stabler, Stewart, et al., 2015). For example, a scene of rolling waves at the seashore is restful to one patient but may be frightening to another.

Cutaneous Stimulation
Massage

A gentle massage or backrub, a form of cutaneous stimulation, is the application of touch and movement to muscles, tendons, and ligaments without manipulation of the joints. A proper massage not only blocks perception of pain impulses but also helps relax muscle tension and spasm that otherwise might increase pain. Massage therapy can produce a relaxation response that creates a calm state and enhances the ability to rest (Boitor, Gelinas, Richard-Lalonde, et al., 2017). Massage hastens the elimination of wastes stored in muscles, improves oxygenation of tissues, and stimulates the relaxation response in the nervous system. In a meta-analysis of the effect of massage in conjunction with analgesics on pain after thoracic surgery, massage was shown to reduce patients' pain (Boitor et al., 2017). A superficial massage of the back, shoulders, and lower part of the neck is sometimes referred to as a backrub. Offering a backrub after a bath or before a patient prepares for sleep promotes relaxation and comfort. An effective backrub takes 3 to 6 minutes and is an important intervention for decreasing pain and improving sense of well-being. Patients outside of the hospital setting may benefit from massage therapy from a registered massage therapist.

Heat and Cold

Heat and cold applications are placed on the skin to relieve pain and promote healing by improving circulation and reducing edema. The selection of heat versus cold varies with a patient's preference and condition. The application of heat or cold in a facility or home health environment requires a health care provider's prescription. Although the physiological responses to heat and cold differ, superficial heat or cold applications provide comfort in conditions such as muscle spasms, strains, and localized joint pain (see Chapter 41 for a review of warm and cold therapy).

Distraction

Distraction is a technique that diverts an individual's attention away from mild or moderate pain sensation. It can be used alone to manage mild pain or with analgesics to manage brief bouts of severe pain, such as pain related to procedures (Oncology Nursing Society [ONS], 2015; Scheffler, Koranyi, Meissner, et al., 2017). By introducing meaningful stimuli, the nurse helps a patient consciously attend to only one stimulus, thus diverting the attention away from pain. There are internal and external distraction techniques. Internal techniques include having patients count, sing to themselves, pray, or repeat statements in their head, such as "I can cope" (ONS, 2015). External distractions include changing a patient's activity, virtual reality, listening to music, reading, walking, playing

a musical instrument, or watching a comedy program (NIH & NCCIH, 2015; Scheffler et al., 2017). Therapeutic communication with a nurse is another example of distraction. When the distraction is removed, a patient may have a heightened awareness of pain.

Delegation and Collaboration

Assessment of a patient's pain cannot be delegated to an unregulated care provider (UCP). The skill of nonpharmacological pain-management strategies can be delegated, and the nurse directs the UCP by:

- Identifying and explaining which nonpharmacological measures work best for a patient.

- Explaining how to adapt strategies to patient restrictions (e.g., massage in side-lying versus prone position).
- Instructing the UCP to report worsening of a patient's pain.

Equipment

- Pain rating scale
- *Massage:* Lotion or oil (consider aroma therapy lotion), folded sheet, bath towel
- *Relaxation:* Patient's music preference, radio or MP3 or CD player or smartphone
- *Distraction:* Based on patient preference (e.g., reading material, puzzles, video or computer games)

STEP	RATIONALE

ASSESSMENT

1. Assess patient's language level and values they have regarding alternative pain-relief approaches. Identify descriptive terms that you will use when guiding patient through relaxation or guided imagery.

2. Assess character of patient's pain (see Skill 16.1) and review findings to consider cause for pain.

3. Assess facial expressions, nonverbal indications of discomfort (e.g., grimacing, frowning, voice tone), body position and movement (e.g., restlessness, muscle tension), and patient's self-report (see Skill 16.1).

4. Perform hand hygiene, apply gloves when drainage is present. Examine site of patient's pain or discomfort. Include inspection (discoloration, swelling, drainage), palpation (change in temperature, area of altered sensation, painful area, areas that trigger pain), and range of motion of involved joints (if applicable).

5. Assess character of patient's respirations.

6. Review health care provider prescription for pain relief (if required by employer).

7. Assess patient's understanding of pain and willingness to receive nonpharmacological pain-relief measures.

8. Assess preferred patient activities (e.g., puzzles, crocheting or knitting, game on electronic device, board games, music, or relaxation tape).

9. Assess type of image patient would prefer to use in guided imagery.

10. Review any restrictions in patient's mobility or positioning.

Ensures that care is person centred and culturally appropriate. Establishes connection with patient to enhance your ability to guide relaxation.

Establishes baseline to determine effects of intervention. Helps determine if nonpharmacological approaches are appropriate.

Serves as baseline to evaluate effectiveness of pain-relief measures.

Overt signs and symptoms are usually not present with chronic pain. Physical signs and symptoms indicate change in comfort level.

Clinical observations may clarify information from patient. Site of discomfort may direct you to specific types of pain-relief measures.

Establishes baseline. Relaxation techniques focus on breathing.

In some facilities, a prescription is necessary to perform nonpharmacological therapies.

Participation increases effectiveness of pain-relief measure. If patient is reluctant to try activity, provide information about suggested therapy.

Demonstrates person-centred care and improves likelihood of distraction being effective.

Prevents use of image that could frighten patient.

Determines whether massage is appropriate and position to have patient assume.

NURSING DIAGNOSES

- Acute pain
- Anxiety
- Chronic pain
- Reduced stamina

- Insufficient knowledge regarding nonpharmacological methods of pain control

- Inadequate coping
- Powerlessness

Related factors are individualized on the basis of patient's condition or needs.

PLANNING

1. Expected outcomes following completion of procedures:
   - Patient demonstrates and describes pain-relief measures.

Demonstrates patient understanding and learning.

STEP	RATIONALE

PLANNING

- Patient is relaxed and comfortable after technique as evidenced by slow, deep respirations; calm facial expressions; calm tone of voice; relaxed muscles; relaxed posture.

  Nonpharmacological strategies help patient relax and experience less discomfort. Physiological response to relaxation procedures and massage is deep relaxation.

- Patient reports pain relief as assessed by a valid and reliable pain rating scale or tool.

  Patient's subjective report is most reliable indicator of presence of pain.

2. Explain purpose of technique and what you expect of patient during activity. Explain how to use pain rating scale (Skill 16.1).

   Proper explanation of activity enhances patient participation. Accurate reporting of pain by patient improves your evaluation and treatment.

3. Set mutual pain-intensity goal with patient (when able) for rest and during routine care activities.

   Patient sets individual goal for tolerable pain severity.

4. Plan time to perform technique when patient is able to concentrate (e.g., after voiding, awakening from nap).

   Increases opportunity for success.

5. Administer an analgesic 30 minutes before implementing a nonpharmacological therapy.

   Patient is able to gain a level of comfort needed to perform nonpharmacological therapies.

IMPLEMENTATION

1. Perform hand hygiene and prepare patient's environment:

   Reduces transmission of microorganisms.

   - Temperature suited to patient
   - Sound

     Temperature and sound extremes can enhance patient's perception of pain.

   - Lighting

     Bright or very dim lighting can aggravate pain sensation.

   - Minimize interruptions and coordinate care activities; allow for rest.

     Fatigue increases pain perception.

2. **Massage:**

Clinical Decision Point *Massage is contraindicated in cases of muscle, bone, or joint injury; or in bruised, swollen, or inflamed areas.*

   a. Place patient in comfortable position such as prone or side-lying. Have patients with difficulty breathing lie on side of bed with head of bed elevated.

      Enhances relaxation and exposes areas to be massaged.

   b. Adjust bed to comfortable position for you; lower upper side rail on side where you are standing. Drape patient to expose only area that you will massage.

      Ensures proper body mechanics and prevents strain on back.

   c. Turn on music to patient's preference.

      Promotes relaxation.

   d. Ensure that patient is not allergic to lotion; warm lotion in hands or in basin of warm water. **NOTE:** If you massage head and scalp, delay use of lotion until completed.

      Warm lotion is soothing, and warmth helps to produce local muscle relaxation.

   e. Choose stroke technique based on desired effect or body part.

      Ensures fuller relaxation of body part.

Clinical Decision Point *Use very gentle massage with patients who are unable to communicate because they cannot tell you if massage becomes uncomfortable.*

   (1) Effleurage: massaging upward and outward from vertebral column and back again (see illustration).

       Light, gliding stroke used without manipulating deep muscles smooths and extends muscles, increases nutrient absorption, and improves lymphatic and venous circulation.

   (2) Pétrissage: fascicles of muscles are kneaded, lifted, grasped, squeezed, rolled and released (see illustration).

       Kneading tense muscle groups promotes relaxation and stimulates local circulation.

   (3) Friction

       Strong circular strokes bring blood to surface of skin, increasing local circulation and loosening tight muscle groups.

   f. Encourage patient to breathe deeply and relax during massage.

      Potentiates effects of massage.

   g. Standing behind patient, stimulate scalp and temples.

   h. Supporting patient's head, use friction to rub muscles at base of head.

      Strong circular strokes (friction) stimulate local circulation and relaxation.

STEP	RATIONALE

IMPLEMENTATION

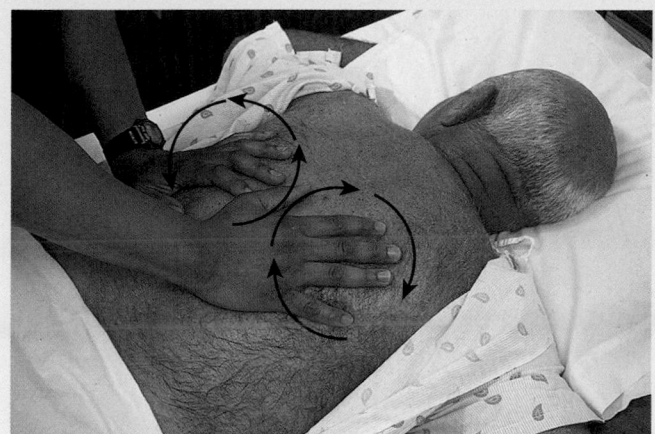

STEP 2e(1) Effleurage.

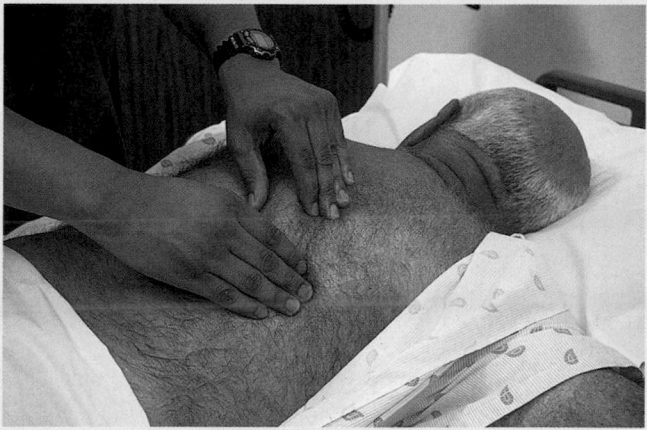

STEP 2e(2) Pétrissage.

i. Reposition if needed. With patient in supine position, massage hands and arms as appropriate.

Releases tension in hands and arms. Hand massage decreases cortisol and increases relaxation (Maratos, Duarte, Barnes, et al., 2017).

    (1) Support hand and apply friction to palm using both thumbs.

    (2) Support base of finger and work each finger in corkscrew-like motion.

    (3) Complete hand massage using effleurage strokes from fingertips to wrist.

    (4) Knead muscles of forearm and upper arm between thumb and forefinger.

Encourages relaxation; enhances circulation and venous return.

j. After determining that patient has no neck injury or condition that contraindicates neck manipulation, massage neck as appropriate:

    (1) Place patient prone unless contraindicated.

Provides access to neck muscles.

    (2) Knead each neck muscle between thumb and forefinger.

Reduces tension that often localizes in neck muscles.

    (3) Gently stretch neck by placing one hand on top of shoulders and other at base of head. Gently move hands away from one another.

Helps relax muscle body.

k. Massage back as appropriate:

Patient with back injury, surgery, or epidural infusion should not receive back massage.

    (1) Assist patient to prone position unless contraindicated; side-lying position is option.

Provides access to muscle groups in back.

    (2) Do not allow hands to leave patient's skin.

Continuous contact with surface of skin is soothing and stimulates circulation to tissues.
Breaking contact with skin can startle patient.

    (3) Apply hands first to sacral area; massage in circular motion. Stroke upward from buttocks to shoulders. Massage over scapulas with smooth, firm stroke. Continue in one smooth stroke to upper arms and laterally along sides of back down to iliac crest (see illustration). Continue massage pattern for 3 minutes.

General, firm pressure applied to all muscle groups promotes relaxation.

    (4) Use effleurage along muscles of spine in upward and outward motion.

Massage follows distribution of major muscle groups.

    (5) Use pétrissage on muscles of each shoulder toward front of patient.

Area often tightens because of tension.

    (6) Use palms in upward and outward circular motion from lower buttocks to neck.

Brings blood to surface of skin.

    (7) Knead muscles of upper back and shoulder between thumb and forefinger.

These muscles are thick and can be massaged vigorously.

STEP	RATIONALE

IMPLEMENTATION

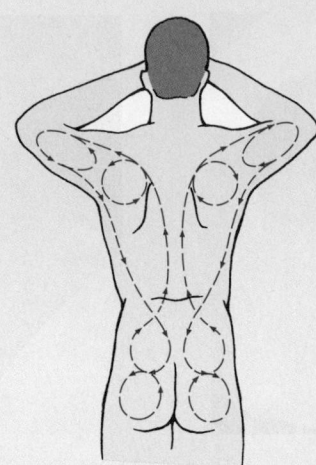

STEP 2k(3) Circular massage of the back.

(8) Use both hands to knead muscles up one side of back and then the other.

(9) End massage with long, stroking effleurage movements. — Most soothing of massage movements.

l. Massage feet as appropriate:

(1) Place patient in supine position. — Returns patient to comfortable anatomical position.

(2) Hold foot firmly. Support ankle with one hand or support sides of foot with each hand while performing massage. — Maintains joint stability and prevents injury during massage.

(3) Make circular motions with thumb and fingers around bones of ankle and top of foot. — All massage strokes help to relax muscles.

(4) Trace space between tendons with firm finger pressure, moving from toe to ankle.

(5) Massage sides and top of each toe.

(6) Use top of fist to make circular motions on bottom of foot.

(7) Knead sides of foot between index finger and thumb.

(8) Conclude with firm, sweeping motions over top and bottom of foot. — Too light strokes may tickle.

m. Tell patient that you are ending massage. — Informs and prepares patient to inhale and exhale deeply.

n. When procedure is complete, instruct patient to inhale deeply and exhale. Caution them to move slowly after resting a few minutes. — Returns patient to more awake and alert state. When deeply relaxed, patient may experience dizziness on arising too rapidly and need time for vessels to redistribute blood supply.

o. Wipe excess lotion or oil from patient's body with bath towel. — Excess lotion or oil can irritate skin and lead to breakdown.

p. Return bed to low position and raise side rails as appropriate when massage is finished. Perform hand hygiene. — Side rails cannot be used as a restraint.

3. Progressive relaxation with deep breathing:

a. Have patient assume comfortable sitting position: sit with feet uncrossed or lie in supine position with small pillow under head. — Maximizes ability to relax.

b. Instruct patient to take several slow, deep, diaphragmatic breaths. It may help to have patient close their eyes. — Increased oxygen lessens anxiety and prevents shortness of breath with relaxation breathing technique. Avoids hyperventilation. Eye closure maintains patient focus on exercise.

STEP	RATIONALE

IMPLEMENTATION

c. Explain as follows: "The air coming in through your nose should move downward into your lower belly. Let your belly expand fully. Now breathe out through your mouth (or your nose, if that feels more natural). Alternate normal and deep breaths several times. Pay attention to how you feel when you breathe in and breathe out normally and when you breathe deeply. Shallow breathing feels tense and constricted, while deep breathing helps you relax."

Patient able to focus on exercise with your coaching. Becoming mindful of how body feels can enhance relaxation.

d. Continue the exercise: "To practice, put one hand on your abdomen, just below your belly button. Feel your hand rise about an inch each time you breathe in and fall about an inch each time you breathe out. Your chest will rise slightly, too, along with your belly. Remember to relax your belly so that each time you breathe in, it expands fully. As you breathe out slowly, let yourself sigh out loud."

Allows patient to master slow, deep breathing.

e. Observe patient and caution against hyperventilation.

Causes patient to eliminate more carbon dioxide than is produced, and consequently results in respiratory alkalosis and an elevated blood pH. Patient becomes dizzy and light-headed.

f. Coach patient to locate any area of muscle tension and alternate tightening and relaxing all muscle groups for 6 to 7 seconds, beginning at feet and working upward toward head.

Relaxation is an integrated response associated with diminished sympathetic nervous system arousal; decreased muscle tension is desired outcome.

  (1) Instruct patient to tighten muscles during inhalation and relax muscles during exhalation.

Relaxation decreases pulse and respiration rates and blood pressure and helps reduce anxiety (Turk & Gatchel, 2018).

  (2) As each muscle group relaxes, ask patient to enjoy relaxed feeling and allow mind to drift and think how nice it is to be relaxed. Have patient breathe deeply.

Allows opportunity to enjoy feelings of relaxation.

  (3) Calmly explain during exercise that patient may feel sensations of tingling, heaviness, floating, or warmth as relaxation occurs.

Prevents anxiety if sensation occurs without warning.

  (4) Have patient continue slow, deep breaths throughout exercise.

  (5) When finished, have patient inhale deeply, exhale, and then initially move about slowly after resting a few minutes.

Returns patient to more awake and alert state. Rising too rapidly can cause dizziness.

4. Guided imagery:

a. Direct patient through guided imagery exercise while having them focus on an image. Example follows:

  (1) Instruct patient to imagine that inhaled air is ball of healing energy.

Developing specific images helps to remove pain perception.

  (2) Imagine that inhaled air travels to area of pain.

Patient's ability to concentrate decreases pain perception.

b. Alternatively, you may direct imagery.

  (1) Ask patient to imagine a pleasant place, such as beach or mountains. Choose an image peaceful for patient.

Directs imagery after selection of restful place.

  (2) Direct patient to experience all sensory aspects of restful place (e.g., for beach: warm breeze, warm sand between toes, warmth of sunshine, rhythmic sound of waves, smell of salt air, gulls gliding and swooping in air).

Helps patient concentrate and relax through stimulation of numerous senses (Turk & Gatchel, 2018, p. 489). Make sure that it is something in their experience, not just yours.

  (3) Direct patient to continue deep, slow, rhythmic breathing.

Promotes relaxation through muscle relaxation.

  (4) Direct patient to count to three, inhale, and open eyes. Suggest that patient move about slowly initially.

STEP	RATIONALE

IMPLEMENTATION

c. Provide patient time to practice exercise without interruption. Practice relaxation tapes are available almost everywhere; libraries are an excellent source.

Guided imagery requires an intense level of concentration that takes time to achieve.

5. Distraction

a. Direct patient's attention away from pain by involving them in a distraction technique.

Redirection of attention can alter emotional or cognitive aspects of pain (Turk & Gatchel, 2018, p. 129).

(1) Music: play selection for approximately 30 minutes in location where patient is comfortable. Set volume or loudness at comfortable level. Use music of patient's choosing. Emphasize listening to rhythm and adjust volume as pain increases or decreases.

Music creates positive psychological outcomes, including decreased anxiety and depression (Turk & Gatchel, 2018, p. 129).

(2) Direct patient to give detailed account of an event or story; describe pleasant memories.

Stress details of event to enhance distraction from painful stimulus.

(3) Provide activity (e.g., puzzle, computer game, reading material) at time when patient is relaxed.

Engagement in activity requires level of comfort for participation.

(4) Engage patient in meaningful conversation; encourage participation of family members and visitors.

Visitors can help direct attention away from mild-to-moderate pain. Rarely is someone in severe pain able to use distraction.

6. Remove and dispose of any supplies. Perform hand hygiene.

Reduces transmission of microorganisms.

EVALUATION

1. Observe character of respirations, body position, facial expression, tone of voice, mood, mannerisms, verbalization of discomfort.

Determines effectiveness of procedure, level of relaxation, degree of pain relief achieved, and which procedures were most effective.

2. Ask patient to use pain rating scale to rate comfort level.

Measures change in pain intensity.

3. Observe patient perform pain-control measures.

Confirms learning.

4. Use Teach-Back: "I want to be sure I explained some techniques for reducing pain without using medication. Tell me what technique you might want to try." Develop a revised teaching plan if patient or caregiver is not able to teach back correctly.

Determines patient's and caregiver's level of understanding of instructional topic.

Unexpected Outcomes

1. Patient is not able to concentrate on technique because pain intensity is unchanged or escalating or demonstrates nonverbal behaviours indicative of pain.

Related Interventions

- Evaluate character of pain and determine if further analgesia is necessary.
- Ensure that environment is conducive to learning and using technique.
- Consult with health care provider on increase in dose or alternate medication.
- Consider different technique or combination of complementary strategies.

Communication and Documentation

- Document in nurses' notes in electronic health record (EHR) or chart patient's assessment findings, procedure and technique(s) used, preparation given to patient, patient's response to procedure or technique, change in overall condition, and further comfort needs related to event. Incorporate pain-relief technique into nursing care plan.
- Communicate patient's response to nonpharmacological interventions to the staff at change of shift or in care plan meeting.
- Document your evaluation of patient and caregiver learning.

- Communicate any unusual responses to techniques (e.g., uncontrolled or aggravated pain or muscle spasms) to health care provider.

Special Considerations
Teaching

- Provide patient information about each nonpharmacological therapy, including purpose, rationale for how pain is relieved, and how patient can maximize benefits. If UCP performs massage, you still need to provide patient education.
- Some techniques require more practice before patients achieve results. Pharmacological intervention is sometimes required to lessen pain so patient can relax.
- Teach patient to rest between periods of activity at home and hospital because fatigue increases pain perception.
- Teach caregiver how to perform massage (if not contraindicated) as part of home care.

Pediatric

- Nonpharmacological pain-management therapies can be used successfully with children. Adapt distraction and relaxation strategies to the developmental level of the child (e.g., use a pacifier for an infant, offer reading or playing a recording of a favorite story for a preschooler, encourage a teenager to listen to music with headphones) (Hockenberry & Wilson, 2015). Play therapists are good resources for appropriate distraction techniques.
- Because children usually have an active imagination, relaxation is often a powerful adjuvant in pain control.

- Parents are very helpful in providing pain relief. For example, they provide comfort by their presence, conversation, and holding and cuddling their child.

Gerontological

- Visual, hearing, cognitive, and motor impairments make it difficult for older persons to be able to effectively use procedures such as distraction, relaxation, or guided imagery. Make certain that glasses, hearing aids, and other assistive devices are in place. Do not assume that complementary techniques will not work among older persons (NIH & NCCIH, 2015).
- Key research and education priorities in pain management in older persons are as follows (Kaasalainen, Zacharias, Hill, et al., 2017):
  - Education includes addressing gaps in education of health care providers, appropriate medication administration, documentation and follow-up, acknowledging opioid use, addressing misconceptions, recognizing impact of culture, and raising public awareness about the impact of pain on older persons.
  - Research includes pain management in long-term care facilities, nonpharmacological interventions, cost versus benefit of pain assessment and management, and system-level issues that impact pain management.

Care in the Community

- Family members need to collaborate in planning time to reduce noise and other stimuli in the home to promote patient's relaxation.

◆ CLINICAL DEBRIEF

A 56-year-old male account executive underwent a colectomy (removal of a portion of colon) this morning. He returns from the operating room with an epidural catheter connected to an epidural pump set to deliver 5 mL/hr of ropivacaine 0.2% with hydromorphone 0.1 mg/mL, with a patient-controlled bolus of 2 mL every 20 minutes prn. The patient has been able to follow instructions and self-administer analgesic doses correctly. The nurse caring for the patient knows to assess for adverse effects of the epidural analgesic.

1. It is approximately 10 hours after surgery, and the patient has not been able to pass urine. The nurse assesses him and scans his bladder and determines there is approximately 500 mL of urine in his bladder. Considering his clinical situation, what could explain the patient's symptoms?
2. His vital signs are BP 132/86 mm Hg, pulse 84 beats/min, regular, R 20 breaths/min, temp 37.6°C. His epidural and surgical dressings are intact. Abdomen is assessed with mild discomfort over bladder due to inability to pass urine. He describes his pain as aching and sometimes sharp and he rates his pain along his abdominal incision as 5/10 on a scale of 0–10. His spouse is visiting and asks if there is a way she can be helpful. Describe ways that his spouse can help promote pain relief. Using SBAR, show how you would communicate with the health care team about this patient.
3. The patient is scheduled to stand up at the bedside within 6 hours of returning from surgery. Describe measures the nurse can institute for him to enhance his ability to safely mobilize and then return to bed more comfortably.

4. On the second day after his surgery, the patient's epidural infusion is discontinued, and he is placed on oral analgesics to manage his pain. Prescriptions: acetaminophen PO 1000 mg q6h, pregabalin PO 25 mg q12h, and hydromorphone 1–3 mg PO q6h prn. The patient's vital signs are stable: BP 125/76, pulse 74 reg, resp 16, temp 37.2°C. Abdomen is assessed and his surgical dressing is intact; the nurse auscultates bowel sounds in all four quadrants. He describes his pain as aching and sometimes sharp and he rates his pain along his abdominal incision as 5/10 on a scale of 0–10. What could the nurse do to help him manage his pain?

◆ REVIEW QUESTIONS

1. The nurse is caring for an older person who has peripheral neuropathy causing ongoing nerve pain. In addition, the patient has discomfort in his back from osteoarthritis. The nurse's assessment reveals that the patient has reduced hearing and is cognitively alert. Which of the following statements accurately describe guidelines for how to select pain-relief therapies for this patient? *(Select all that apply.)*
   1. A cognitive-behavioural strategy would likely not be effective for this patient.
   2. Work with patient to determine the combination of analgesics and/or adjuvants prescribed that is most effective in relieving pain.
   3. Explain to the patient that initial opioid dosages will be high and then tapered down to achieve pain relief.
   4. Be certain that patient's hearing aid is in place before practicing guided imagery.
   5. Plan a quiet time to provide the patient a body massage.

2. The nurse is caring for a patient who is receiving morphine by way of patient-controlled analgesia. The nurse has just completed measuring the patient's respirations and pulse oximetry. The nurse reviews the patient's medical record to identify their risk for oversedation. Which of the following factors increase a patient's risk for oversedation? *(Select all that apply.)*

1. A patient who has received an opioid for pain within the last 2 months
2. A patient who is cognitively impaired
3. A patient who has a history of obstructive sleep apnea
4. A patient who has an allergy to opioids
5. A patient who is opioid naïve

3. Fill in the rationale for each step that explains how to instruct a patient or caregiver in the proper approach for removing a peripheral nerve block catheter in the home.

Step	Rationale
Explain how to perform hand hygiene.	
Have patient or caregiver gently lift the adhesive dressing covering the catheter insertion site and remove any remaining tape.	
Explain to patient or caregiver to grasp the catheter as close as possible to where it enters the skin and gently pull it out.	
Instruct patient or caregiver to hold pressure over the site for 5 minutes, then apply a Band-Aid.	
Explain to patient that any remaining numbness should go away within 24 hours after the catheter is removed.	

(e) *Visit the Evolve site for a complete list of Clinical Debrief and Review Questions answers.*

REFERENCES

Accreditation Canada. (2019). *Required organizational practices handbook—Version 14*. Retrieved from http://www.wrha.mb.ca/quality/files/2019ROPHandbook.pdf

Adhikari, R., Tocher, J., Smith, P., Corcoran, J., & MacArthur, J. (2014). A multi-disciplinary approach to medication safety and the implication for nursing education and practice. *Nurse Education Today*, 34(2), 185–190. doi:10.1016/j.nedt.2013.10.008

Allione, A., Pivetta, E., Pizzolato, E., et al. (2017). Determinants of inappropriate acute pain management in old people unable to communicate verbally in the emergency department. *Turkish Journal of Emergency Medicine*, 17(4), 160–164. doi:10.1016/j.tjem.2017.08.001

Aloia, T., Bradford, K., Segraves-Chun, Y. S., et al. (2017). A randomized controlled trial of postoperative thoracic epidural analgesia versus intravenous patient-controlled analgesia after major hepatopancreatobiliary surgery. *Annals of Surgery*, 266(3), 545–554. doi:10.1097/SLA.0000000000002386

American Psychiatric Association. (2013). *Diagnostic and statistical manual of mental disorders* (5th ed.). Arlington, VA: The Association.

Andersen, R. D., Langius-Eklof, A., Nakstad, B., Bernkler, T., & Jylli, L. (2017). The measurement properties of pediatric observational pain scales: A systematic review of reviews. *International Journal of Nursing Studies*, 73, 93–101. doi:10.1016/j.ijnurstu.2017.05.010

Anwari, J., & Hazazi, A. (2015). Another cause of headache after epidural injection. *Neurosciences : the Official Journal of the Pan Arab Union of Neurological Sciences*, 20(2), 167–169. doi:10.17712/nsj.2015.2.20140769

Biswas, A., Perlas, A., Ghosh, M., et al. (2018). Relative contribution of adductor canal block and intrathecal morphine to analgesia and functional recovery after total knee arthroplasty. *Regional Anesthesia and Pain Medicine*, 43(2), 154–160. doi:10.1097/AAP.0000000000000724

Boitor, M., Gelinas, C., Richard-Lalonde, M., & Thombs, B. D. (2017). The effect of massage on acute postoperative pain in critically and acutely ill adults post-thoracic surgery: Systematic review and meta-analysis of randomized controlled trials. *Heart & Lung : the Journal of Critical Care*, 46(5), 339–346. doi:10.1016/j.hrtlng.2017.05.005

Booker, S., & Haedtke, C. (2016). Controlling pain and discomfort, part 2: Assessment in non-verbal older adults. *Nursing*, 46(5), 66–69. doi:10.1097/01.NURSE.0000480619.08039.50

Bos, E. M. E., Hollmann, M. W., & Lirk, P. (2017). Safety and efficacy of epidural analgesia. *Current Opinion in Anaesthesiology*, 30(6), 736–742. doi:10.1097/ACO.0000000000000516

Burchum, J. R., & Rosenthal, L. D. (2016). *Lehne's pharmacology for nursing care* (9th ed.). St. Louis: Elsevier.

Busse, J., Craigie, S., Juurlink, D. N., et al. (2017). The 2017 Canadian guideline for opioids for chronic non-cancer pain. *Canadian Medical Association Journal*, 198, e659–e666. doi:10.1503/cmaj.170363

Canadian Anesthesiologists' Society. (2018). Guidelines to the practice of anesthesia (revised edition 2018). *Canadian Journal of Anaesthesia = Journal Canadien D'anesthésie*, 65(1), 76–104. doi:10.1007/s12630-017-0995-9

Canadian Pain Society (CPS). (2010). *CPS position statement*. Retrieved from http://www.canadianpainsociety.ca/?page=PositionStatement

Castarlenas, E., Jensen, M. P., von Baeyer, C. L., & Miro, J. (2017). Psychometric properties of the numeric rating scale to assess self-reported pain in children and adolescents: A systematic review. *The Clinical Journal of Pain*, 33, 376–383. doi:10.1097/AJP.0000000000000406

Chawla, J. (2017). Epidural nerve block. *Medscape*. Retrieved from https://emedicine.medscape.com/article/149646-overview#a1

Chou, R., Gordon, D. B., de Leon-Casasola, O. A., et al. (2016). Management of postoperative pain: A clinical practice guideline from the American Pain Society, the American Society of Regional Anesthesia and Pain Medicine, and the American Society of Anesthesiologists' Committee on Regional Anesthesia, Executive Committee, and Administrative Council. *The Journal of Pain : Official Journal of the American Pain Society*, 17(2), 131–157. doi:10.1016/j.jpain.2015.12.008

Clarke, C. (2017). Neuraxial drug delivery for the management of cancer pain: Cost, updates and society guidelines. *Current Opinion in Anaesthesiology*, 30(5), 593–597. doi:10.1097/ACO.0000000000000497

Crumley Aybar, B. L., Gillespie, M. J., Gipson, S. F., Mullaney, C. E., & Tommasino-Storz, M. (2016). Peripheral nerve blocks causing increased risk for fall and difficulty in ambulation for the hip and knee joint replacement patient. *Journal of Perianesthesia Nursing*, 31(6), 504–519. doi:10.1016/j.jopan.2015.01.017

Dale, R., & Stacey, B. (2016). Multimodal treatment of chronic pain. *The Medical Clinics of North America*, 100(1), 55–64. doi:10.1016/j.mcna.2015.08.012

Dreyer, N. E., Cutshall, S. M., Huebner, M., et al. (2015). Effect of massage therapy on pain, anxiety, relaxation, and tension after colorectal surgery: A randomized study. *Complementary Therapies in Clinical Practice*, 21(3), 154–159. doi:10.1016/j.ctcp.2015.06.004

Freeman, L. M., Bloemenkamp, K. W., Franssen, M. T., et al. (2015). Patient-controlled analgesia with remifentanil versus epidural analgesia in labour: Randomised multicentre equivalence trial. *British Medical Journal*, 350, H846. doi:10.1136/bmj.h846

Gelinas, C. (2016). Pain assessment in the critically ill adult: Recent evidence and new trends. *Intensive and Critical Care Nursing*, 34, 1–11. doi:10.1016/j.iccn.2016.03.001. PMID: 27067745.

Ghelardini, C., Mannelli, L., & Bianchi, E. (2015). The pharmacological basis of opioids. *Clinical Cases in Mineral and Bone Metabolism : the Official Journal of the Italian Society of Osteoporosis, Mineral Metabolism, and Skeletal Diseases*, 12(3), 219–221. doi:10.11138/ccmbm/2015.12.3.219

Giacobbi, P. R., Stabler, M. E., Stewart, J., Jaeschke, A. M., Siebert, J. L., & Kelley, G. A. (2015). Guided imagery for arthritis and other rheumatic diseases: A systematic review of randomized controlled trials. *Pain Management Nursing*, 16(5), 792–803. doi:10.1016/j.pmn.2015.01.003

Hadjistavropoulos, T., Herr, K., Prkachin, K. M., et al. (2014). Pain assessment in elderly adults with dementia. *The Lancet. Neurology*, 13, 1216–1227. doi:10.1016/S1474-4422(14)70103-6

Hayes, J., Dowling, J. J., Peliowski, A., Crawford, M. W., & Johnston, B. (2016). Patient-controlled analgesia plus background opioid infusion for postoperative pain in children: A systematic review and meta-analysis of randomized trials. *Anesthesia and Analgesia*, 123(4), 991–1003. doi:10.1213/ANE.0000000000001244

Health Quality Ontario. (2018a). *Opioid prescribing for acute pain*. Toronto: Queen's Printer for Ontario. Retrieved from http://www.hqontario.ca/portals/0/documents/

evidence/quality-standards/qs-opioid-acute-pain-clinician-guide-en.pdf. ISBN 978-1-4868-1407-7.

Health Quality Ontario. (2018b). *Opioid prescribing for chronic pain.* Toronto: Queen's Printer for Ontario. Retrieved from http://www.hqontario.ca/portals/0/documents/evidence/quality-standards/qs-opioid-chronic-pain-clinician-guide-en.pdf. ISBN 978-1-4868-1409-1.

Health Quality Ontario. (2018c). *Opioid use disorder.* Toronto: Queen's Printer for Ontario. Retrieved from http://www.hqontario.ca/portals/0/documents/evidence/quality-standards/qs-opioid-use-disorder-clinician-guide-en.pdf. ISBN 978-1-4868-1405-3.

Hernandez, G. A., Grant, M. C., & Wu, C. L. (2018). Epidural opioids for postoperative pain. In H. T. Benzon, S. N. Raja, S. S. Liu, S. M. Fishman, & S. P. Cohen (Eds.), *Essentials of pain medicine* (4th ed., pp. 129–133). Philadelphia: Elsevier. doi:10.1016/B978-0-323-40196-8.12001-7

Herr, K., Coyne, P., McCaffery, M., Manworren, R., & Merkel, S. (2011). Pain assessment in the patient unable to self-report: Position statement with clinical practice recommendations. *Pain Management Nursing, 12*(4), 230–250. Retrieved from http://www.sockpain.ca/images/pdf/patient_unable_clinical_practice.pdf

Hockenberry, M. J., & Wilson, D. (2015). *Wong's nursing care of infants and children* (10th ed.). St. Louis: Mosby.

Horgas, A. L. (2017). Pain assessment in older adults. *The Nursing Clinics of North America, 52,* 375–385. doi:10.1016/j.cnur.2017.04.006. PMID: 28779820.

Ilfeld, B. (2017). Continuous peripheral nerve blocks: An update of the published evidence and comparison with novel, alternative analgesic modalities. *Anesthesia and Analgesia, 124*(1), 306–334. doi:10.1213/ANE.0000000000001581

Ilfeld, B. M., & Mariano, E. R. (2018). Continuous peripheral nerve blocks. In H. T. Benzon, S. N. Raja, S. S. Liu, S. M. Fishman, & S. P. Cohen (Eds.), *Essentials of pain medicine* (4th ed., pp. 135–146). Philadelphia: Elsevier. doi:10.1016/B978-0-323-40196-8.12001-7

Institute for Safe Medication Practices (ISMP). (2009). *Process for handling elastomeric pain relief balls (On-Q Painbuster and others) requires safety improvements.* ISMP Acute Care Quarterly Action Agenda. Retrieved from https://www.ismp.org/resources/process-handling-elastomeric-pain-relief-balls-q-painbuster-and-others-requires-safety

Institute for Safe Medication Practices (ISMP) Canada. (2015). *Ontario critical incident learning: Resources to sustain incident learning.* Retrieved from https://www.ismp-canada.org/download/ocil/ISMPCONCIL2015-13_IncidentLearning.pdf

Jarzyna, D., Junqquist, C. R., Pasero, C., et al. (2016). American Society for Pain Management Nursing guidelines on monitoring for opioid-induced sedation and respiratory depression. *Pain Management Nursing, 12*(3), 118–145. doi:10.1016/j.pmn.2011.06.008

Jin, M. (2017). *Pain assessment tools used when caring through cultural boundaries: A qualitative systematic literature review.* (Bachelor thesis). Novia University, Finland.

Kaasalainen, S., Zacharias, R., Hill, C., Wickson-Griffiths, A., Hadjistavropoulos, T., & Herr, K. (2017). Advancing the pain management in older adults agenda forward through the development of key research and education priorities: A Canadian perspective. *Canadian Journal of Pain = Revue Canadienne De La Douleur, 1*(1), 171–182. doi:10.1080/24740527.2017.1383139

Kamper, S. J., Apeldoorn, A. T., Smeets, R. J., Ostelo, R. W., Guzman, J., & van Tulder, M. W. (2015). Multidisciplinary biopsychosocial rehabilitation for chronic low back pain: Cochrane systematic review and meta-analysis. *British Medical Journal, 350,* h4. doi:10.1136/bmj.h444

Kent, M. L., Tighe, P. J., Belfer, I., et al. (2017). The ACTTION-APS-AAPM Pain Taxonomy (AAAPT) multidimensional approach to classifying acute pain conditions. *The Journal of Pain, 18*(5), 479–489. doi:10.1016/j.jpain.2017.02.421

Khanna, A., Sessler, D., Sun, Z., et al. (2016). Using the STOP-BANG questionnaire to predict hypoxaemia in patients recovering from noncardiac surgery: A prospective cohort analysis. *British Journal of Anaesthesia, 116*(5), 632–640. doi:10.1093/bja/aew029

Lerman, S. F., Rudich, Z., Brill, S., Shalev, H., & Shahar, G. (2015). Longitudinal associations between depression, anxiety, pain, and pain-related disability in chronic pain patients. *Psychosomatic Medicine, 77*(3), 333–341. doi:10.1097/PSY.0000000000000158

Levett, K. M., Smith, C. A., Bensoussam, A., & Dahlen, H. G. (2016). Complementary therapies for labour and birth study: A randomised controlled trial of antenatal integrative medicine for pain management in labour. *BMJ Open, 6,* e010691. doi:10.1136/bmjopen-2015-010691

Maratos, F., Duarte, J., Barnes, C., McEwan, K., Sheffield, D., & Gilbert, P. (2017). The physiological and emotional effects of touch: Assessing a hand-massage intervention with high self-critics. *Psychiatry Research, 25,* 221–227. doi:10.1016/j.psychres.2017.01.066

Merskey, H., & Bogduk, N. (1994). *Classification of chronic pain* (2nd ed.). Seattle, WA: IASP Press.

Morales, D. R., Guthrie, B., Lipworth, B. J., Jackson, C., Donnan, P. T., & Santiago, V. H. (2015). NSAID-exacerbated respiratory disease: A meta-analysis evaluating prevalence, mean provocative dose of aspirin and increased asthma morbidity. *Allergy, 70*(7), 828–835. doi:10.1111/all.12629

Naples, J., Gellad, W., & Hanlon, J. (2016). Managing pain in older adults: The role of opioid analgesics. *Clinics in Geriatric Medicine, 32*(4), 725–735. doi:10.1016/j.cger.2016.06.006

Narouze, S., Benzon, H. T., Provenzano, D., et al. (2018). Interventional spine and pain procedures in patients on antiplatelet and anticoagulant medications (second edition). Guidelines from the American Society of Regional Anesthesia and Pain Medicine, the European Society of Regional Anaesthesia and Pain Therapy, the American Academy of Pain Medicine, the International Neuromodulation Society, the North American Neuromodulation Society, and the World Institute of Pain. *Regional Anesthesia and Pain Medicine, 43*(3), 225–262. doi:10.1097/AAP.0000000000000700

National Institutes of Health (NIH) & National Center for Complementary and Integrative Health (NCCIH). (2015). *Selected results of the NCCAM funded research on CAM research.* Retrieved from https://nccih.nih.gov/research

National Pain Centre. (2017). *Canadian guideline for opioids for chronic non-cancer pain.* Retrieved from http://nationalpaincentre.mcmaster.ca/documents/Opioid%20GL%20for%20CMAJ_01may2017.pdf

Oliver, J., Coggins, C., Compton, P., et al. (2012). American Society for Pain Management Nursing position statement: Pain management in patients with substance use disorders. *Pain Management Nursing, 13*(3), 169–183. doi:10.1016/j.pmn.2012.07.001

Oncology Nursing Society (ONS). (2015). *Non-medical treatments for pain.* Retrieved from http://www.cancer.org/treatment/treatmentsandsideeffects/physicalsideeffects/pain/non-medical-treatments-for-cancer-pain

Pasero, C., & McCaffery, M. (2011). *Pain assessment and pharmacological management.* St. Louis: Mosby.

Pöpping, D., Elia, N., Van Aken, H. K., et al. (2014). Impact of epidural analgesia on mortality and morbidity after surgery: Systematic review and meta-analysis of randomized controlled trials. *Annals of Surgery, 259*(6), 1056–1067.

Registered Nurses' Association of Ontario (RNAO). (2013). *Assessment and management of pain* (3rd ed.). Toronto, ON: Author. Retrieved from http://rnao.ca/sites/rnao-ca/files/AssessAndManagementOfPain_15_WEB-_FINAL_DEC_2.pdf

Rowbotham, D., Cashman, J., Counsell, D., et al. (2010). *Best practice in the management of epidural analgesia in the hospital setting.* London: Faculty of Pain Medicine of The Royal College of Anaesthetists. Retrieved from https://www.aagbi.org/sites/default/files/epidural_analgesia_2011.pdf

Royal College of Anaesthetists. (2010). *Best practice in the management of epidural analgesia in the hospital setting.* Retrieved from https://www.rcoa.ac.uk/document-store/best-practice-the-management-of-epidural-analgesia-the-hospital-setting

Ruest, M., Bourque, M., Laroche, S., et al. (2017). Can we quickly and thoroughly assess pain with the PACSLAC-II? A convergent validity study in long-term care residents suffering from dementia. *Pain Management Nursing, 18*(6), 410–417. doi:10.1016/j.pmn.2017.05.009

Sawhney, M. (2012). Epidural analgesia: What nurses need to know. *Nursing, 42*(8), 36–42. doi:10.1097/01.NURSE.0000415833.28619.a1

Sawhney, M., Median, H., Kashin, B., et al. (2016). Pain after unilateral total knee arthroplasty: A prospective randomized controlled trial examining the analgesic effectiveness of a combined adductor canal peripheral nerve block with periarticular infiltration versus adductor canal nerve block alone versus periarticular infiltration alone. *Anesthesia and Analgesia, 122*(6), 2040–2046. doi:10.1213/ANE.0000000000001210

Scheffler, M., Koranyi, S., Meissner, W., Strauß, B., & Rosendahl, J. (2017). Efficacy of non-pharmacological interventions for procedural pain relief in adults undergoing burn wound care: A systematic review and meta-analysis of randomized controlled trials. *Burns: Journal of the International Society for Burn Injuries,* doi:10.1016/j.burns.2017.11.019. pii, S0305-4179(17)30659-9.

Schopflocher, D., Taenzer, P., & Jovey, R. (2011). The prevalence of chronic pain in Canada. *Pain Research and Management, 16*(6), 445–450.

Soffin, E. M., & Liu, S. S. (2018). Patient controlled analgesia. In H. T. Benzon, S. N. Raja, S. S. Liu, S. M. Fishman, & S. P. Cohen (Eds.), *Essentials of pain medicine* (4th ed., pp. 117–122). Philadelphia, PA: Elsevier. doi:10.1016/B978-0-323-40196-8.12001-7

Swift, A. (2018). Understanding pain and the human body's response to it. *Nursing Times, 114*(3), 22–26.

Tang, N. K. Y. (2018). Cognitive behavioural therapy in pain and psychological disorders: Towards a hybrid future. *Progress in Neuro-Psychopharmacology and Biological Psychiatry, 87*(Part B), 281–289. doi:10.1016/j.pnpbp.2017.02.023

Thomas, J. (2017). *Clinical guidelines for the care of epidural infusions (adult).* Truro, UK: Royal Cornwall Hospital.

Tsai, I. P., Jeong, S. Y., & Hunter, S. (2018). Pain assessment and management for older patients with dementia in hospitals: An integrative literature review. *Pain Management Nursing*, 19(1), 54–71. doi:10.1016/j.pmn.2017.10.001

Tsze, D. S., Hirschfeld, G., von Baeyer, C. L., Bulloch, B., & Dayan, P. S. (2015). Clinically significant differences in acute pain measured on self-report pain scales in children. *Academic Emergency Medicine : Official Journal of the Society for Academic Emergency Medicine*, 22(4), 415–422. doi:10.1111/acem.12620

Turk, D., & Gatchel, R. (2018). *Psychological approaches to pain management* (3rd ed.). New York: Guilford Press.

Vaughns, J. (2017). *Drug dosing guidelines poor fit for obese patient.* Innovation District. Retrieved from https://innovationdistrict.childrensnational.org/revisit-drug-dosing-guidelines-obese-patients/

17 | Palliative Care

Written by **Holly R.L. Richardson, BScN, MA, PhD**

SKILLS AND PROCEDURES

OBJECTIVES

Mastery of content in this chapter will enable the nurse to:

- Explain the philosophy and principles of an integrated palliative approach to care.
- Differentiate between hospice palliative care and end-of-life care.
- Discuss approaches to goals of care conversations.
- Describe approaches to optimizing comfort and quality of life.

- Describe approaches to psychosocial and spiritual care at the end of life.
- Explain physiological changes typical of impending death.
- Describe the nurse's role in assisting patients and families in grief associated with serious illness and death.
- Describe the process of postmortem care.
- Discuss a nurse's role in facilitating autopsy and organ and tissue donation requests.

MEDIA RESOURCES

- evolve http://evolve.elsevier.com/Canada/Perry/clinicalskills/
- Review Questions

- Case Studies
- Audio Glossary
- Clinical Debrief and Review Questions Answers

PALLIATIVE CARE IN CANADA

Historically, nurses have played a vital role in the care of patients and families facing serious, life-limiting illness and death. The World Health Organization (WHO) defines palliative care as an approach that "improves the quality of life of patients and their families facing the problems associated with life-threatening illness, through the prevention and relief of suffering by means of early identification and impeccable assessment and treatment of pain and other problems, physical, psychosocial and spiritual" (WHO, 2018, para. 1). The specific goals of palliative care are detailed in Box 17.1.

In Canada, the terms *hospice* and *palliative care* are used interchangeably. Unfortunately, both terms are often associated with end-of-life care, leading to an erroneous belief that hospice palliative care (HPC) is relevant only to those in the end stages of a life-limiting illness. This has led to debate about the need to use alternate terms to describe this approach to care. The Canadian Hospice Palliative Care Association (CHPCA), which provides leadership, advocacy, and a national voice for HPC in Canada, endorses the synonymous use of the terms, both of which include end-of-life and bereavement care. Further, the CHPCA states that some may view hospice as community-based rather than hospital-based care. For example, hospice care is often delivered in a limited number of residential hospices (home-like care facilities) that are partially funded through charitable donations (CHPCA, 2019a). People who receive care in residential hospices are often in an advanced stage of illness or nearing the end of life, which may also conflate the term hospice

with end-of-life care. Contrary to this, the Canadian Virtual Hospice (2017) uses the term *hospice* to describe their multitude of online resources to support people and their families at any stage of a life-limiting illness. Despite synonymous use of these terms in Canada, the term *palliative care* has been used by the federal government solely in describing the need for an integrated palliative approach to care, as described below.

HPC is evolving in Canada. Since June 16, 2016, eligible Canadians have had the right to choose medical assistance in dying (MAiD) (Government of Canada, 2016a). When this law was passed, Canadians did not have universal access to quality palliative care, raising concerns that MAiD might be viewed as the only option for some Canadians to relieve their suffering. In response to this gap in essential care, the *Framework on Palliative Care in Canada Act* (Bill C-277) (Government of Canada, 2017) became law on December 12, 2017.

The aims of the *Framework on Palliative Care in Canada Act* are to ensure universal and equitable access to quality palliative care by defining palliative care; identifying health care provider and informal caregiver education needs; supporting palliative care providers; drawing on existing frameworks, strategies, and best practices across the country to inform framework development; doing research and collecting data to evaluate progress in meeting the palliative care needs of Canadians; and evaluating the need for re-establishment of funding for initiatives (Government of Canada, 2017). The CHPCA, in conjunction with the Quality End-of-Life Care Coalition of Canada (QELCCC) and the Canadian federal

government, developed *The Way Forward National Framework: A Roadmap for an Integrated Palliative Approach to Care* (CHPCA, 2015). This is a key document for understanding the direction of hospice palliative care in Canada.

An important aim of an integrated palliative approach is to initiate palliative care early in the course of a life-limiting illness and in all settings, not merely in those that specialize in hospice palliative care. A cultural shift is required where nurses and other health care providers—regardless of setting—must possess and apply basic requisite palliative care competencies. Nurses can advocate for this cultural shift by educating the public and other health care providers. Infographics and videos developed by iPANEL (2012) are tools designed for nurses to facilitate change in their various care areas.

Integrated palliative care is a team-based approach that requires interprofessional collaboration with coordinated communication among team members and also between teams located in various settings (e.g., chronic/acute, primary, specialty, long-term, and home care) to ensure seamless transitions in care (CHPCA, 2015). A palliative care team consists of a variety of professional and essential caregivers, including volunteers and family. Interprofessional collaboration involves understanding the scope and skills of each member and assignment of roles according to the needs of the ill person and family and the availability of team members in the setting of care. Interprofessional collaboration includes, but is not limited to, team rounds where expressed needs of the family are discussed and where team members decide on the best approaches and the appropriate team member(s) to follow up with the family. For example, although nurses may be the first to identify psychosocial and spiritual issues and may provide immediate support, through team discussions or consultations, nurses may draw on the expertise of the social worker, psychologist, or spiritual care provider for follow-up on complex or unresolved issues. Shared documentation records may also facilitate interprofessional collaboration and communication.

Nurses can also identify illness transitions and approaching death and be proactive in assessing for unmet needs. *The Gold Standards Framework Proactive Identification Guide (PIG)* (Thomas, Armstrong Wilson, & GSF Team, 2016), the *Supportive and Palliative Care Indicators Tool (SPICT™)* (University of Edinburgh, 2017), and the *Palliative Performance Scale Version 2 (PPSv2)* (Victoria Hospice, 2001) are useful for determining transitions in care and for predicting the need for an increased focus on a palliative approach or a specialty palliative care consult. Consultation with a specialty palliative care team is another example of interprofessional collaboration, in which a primary or secondary health care team consults a tertiary palliative care team for expert advice or involvement to address complex or unmet needs. An illustration of palliative pathways with varying needs for consultation to specialty palliative care teams can be found in Fig. 17.1.

BOX 17.1

Goals of Palliative Care

- Provide relief from pain and other distressing symptoms.
- Affirm life and regard dying as a natural process.
- Aim to neither hasten nor postpone death.
- Integrate the psychological and spiritual aspects of care.
- Offer a support system to help seriously ill people live as actively as possible until death.
- Offer a support system to help the family cope during the person's illness and in their own bereavement.
- Use interprofessional collaboration to address the needs of ill people and their families, including bereavement counselling, if indicated.
- Enhance quality of life and positively influence the course of illness.
- Apply early in the course of illness in conjunction with other therapies that are intended to prolong life and promote comfort.

Adapted from World Health Organization. (2018). *WHO definition of palliative care*. Retrieved from http://www.who.int/cancer/palliative/definition/en/.

STANDARDS OF CARE

- Canadian Association of Schools of Nursing (CASN), 2011—*Palliative and End-of-Life Care Entry-to-Practice Competencies*

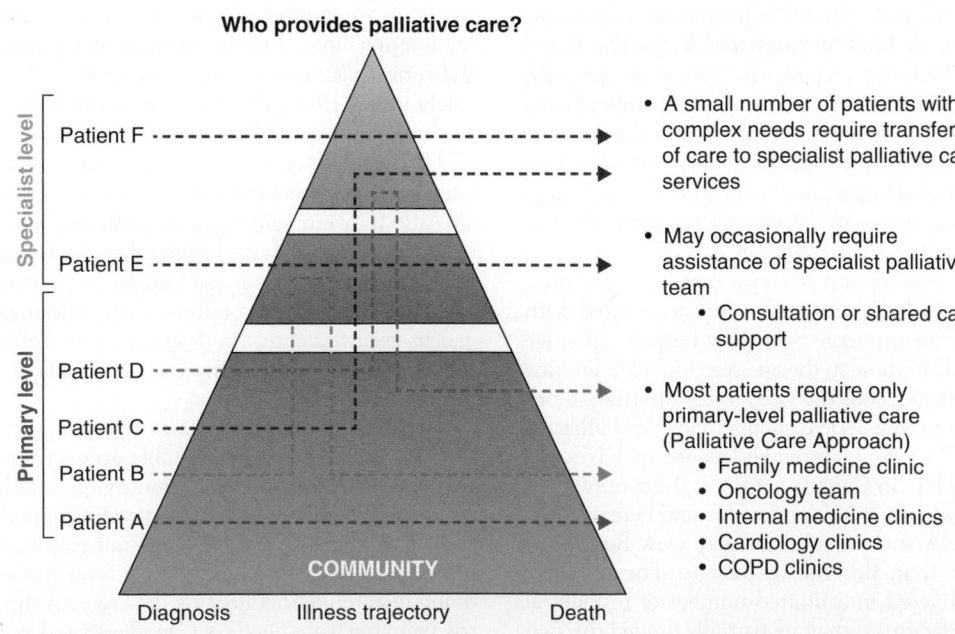

FIG 17.1 Who provides palliative care? *(From Pallium Canada: Used with permission. From K. Downer & D. Marshall. [2016]. The evolving palliative care system in Canada: It's everybody's business [PowerPoint Presentation]. Retrieved from https://www.slideshare.net/CADTH-ACMTS/c6-kathryn-downer)*

and Indicators for Registered Nurses (https://casn.ca/wp-content/uploads/2014/12/PEOLCCompetenciesandIndicatorsEn.pdf)

- Canadian Hospice Palliative Care Nursing Standards Sub-Committee, 2014—CHPCA *Nursing Standards of Practice* (http://acsp.net/media/367211/chpc_ng.standards.2014.14_july_2014.final.pdf)
- Canadian Nurses Association (CNA), 2015—*Respecting Choices in End-of-Life Care: Challenges and Opportunities for RNs* (https://canadian-nurse.com/~/media/canadian-nurse/files/pdf%20en/respecting-choices-in-end-of-life-care.pdf)
- Nova Scotia Health Authority (NSHA), 2017—*The Nova Scotia Palliative Care Competency Framework: A Reference Guide for Health Professionals and Volunteers* (https://library.nshealth.ca/ld.php?content_id=34202519)

PRINCIPLES FOR PRACTICE

Palliative care should be introduced early in the course of a life-limiting illness or frailty and may be provided in conjunction with other life-sustaining treatments, such as surgery and chemotherapy (CHPCA, 2015). A palliative approach to care involves helping ill people achieve an optimal quality of life and to live as actively as possible until death. This approach includes attending to suffering, early recognition and proactive management of pain and symptoms, and identifying when burdens of treatment outweigh benefits or when treatment is misaligned with the ill person's and family's goals and preferences.

The ill person identifies who their family is, which may include those who are not related biologically or through marriage. The family is affected by the illness and death and may also be involved in decision making according to the ill person's wishes or when the ill person lacks capacity to direct care themselves. Family often become informal caregivers in addition to their other roles and responsibilities, resulting in increased risk for caregiver burnout. Nurses need to develop relationships with the ill person's family and develop care plans that include support of the family throughout illness, dying, and bereavement. Developmental needs of children also require special consideration. Therefore, ongoing, holistic assessment of the family along with psychosocial, spiritual, informational, and practical support are needed to maintain family wellness. As end of life approaches, palliative care continues in the facilitation of a peaceful death and in bereavement support for the family that aligns with their spiritual and cultural preferences.

To nurture your capacity as a nurse to remain compassionately engaged with patients and family members, you must also care for yourself physically, spiritually, and emotionally. Explore your own attitudes and beliefs about death and dying and recognize how past experiences with suffering, death, and dying might affect your ability to be emotionally present and provide quality palliative care (NSHA, 2017). Recognize signs of compassion fatigue in self and colleagues and develop strategies to prevent it and cope with personal emotional responses to caring for dying persons and their families. This includes being aware of available psychosocial and spiritual supports (NSHA, 2017).

PERSON-CENTRED CARE

Palliative care is person centred and family centred. The family is the unit of care. The ill person is at the centre of care and should be involved in decision making and care planning as much as they are able and wish to be. As health needs change, revisiting conversations about goals of care promotes dignity and self-determination by enabling the ill person and family to express concerns, feelings, hopes, and wishes; receive relevant information; and lead decision making and care planning according to their preferences (CHPCA, 2015). Nurses may facilitate or be involved in these conversations and provide ongoing compassionate presence and psychosocial and spiritual support during life transitions, including shifts from life-prolonging treatments to a focus on comfort. Goals of care discussions and family decisions should be accurately documented and communicated to the teams involved.

Cultural Safety

Culture affects the meaning of illness, pain, and suffering; how one expresses grief; and ideas about an afterlife. Given the wide range of cultural beliefs, it is important to first engage in self-reflection on your own cultural and personal beliefs about loss and death and explore common end-of-life cultural or religious practices of others. Do not assume an ill person adheres to the practices of their identified culture or religion. Instead, practice cultural humility (Murray, 2016): Be comfortable with not knowing, and engage in respectful curiosity, asking what cultural or spiritual or religious practices are important to the person and family and how to best incorporate these into their plan of care. For further guidance, Rindfleisch (n.d.) has compiled a list of useful assessment tools that can be found at http://projects.hsl.wisc.edu/SERVICE/modules/11/M11_Spiritual_Assessment_Tools.pdf.

When death is near, provide opportunities for families to engage in cultural or religious rites, rituals, or practices that bring peace and meaning to the experience. Interprofessional collaboration may include a consult to an appropriate spiritual care provider, with the family's permission, to ensure that end-of-life rights and rituals are carried out according to cultural and religious needs. See Box 17.2 for a review of select religious and cultural practices near and at the time of death. *Living My Culture* (Canadian Virtual Hospice, 2016) is also a useful resource for exploring palliative and end-of-life needs of a variety of cultural groups.

Practice openness and sensitivity to exploring the unique end-of-life needs and preferences of all families, considering age, gender, sexual orientation, cognitive and physical ability, ethnicity, language, culture, spiritual or religious practices, and preferred life-ways. Family culture also affects communication patterns and roles. Nurses need to understand how families prefer to receive information and the roles they will play in caregiving and decision making.

COMMUNICATION AND COLLABORATIVE CARE PLANNING

Regular and open communication among team members, including the family, is key to providing excellent palliative care. Care coordination and planning requires shared information and decision making and collaborative delivery of care based on family identified needs. The nurse helps identify family needs through conversation and focused assessment and uses the information to contribute to team care planning. Nurses must recognize the need and appropriate timing for conversations and determine the focus and intent when using interprofessional collaboration. Fig. 17.2 illustrates the differences between communication in advance care planning, determining goals of care, and decision making in the moment.

Early initiation of conversations about wishes for future health care begin with development of an advance care plan (ACP). ACPs involve conversations with significant others about values and health care preferences and the appointment of a substitute decision maker (SDM) in advance of events that might result in people being unable to make decisions for themselves. Nurses must understand how an SDM is chosen, or the order of assignment of the SDM if

Select Religious and Cultural Practices Near and at the Time of Death

Indigenous – Allow privacy, time, and space for the gathering of community around the dying person and for ceremonies that may include burning of sacred medicines, if possible. Do not interrupt ceremonies and do not rush to pronounce death or remove the deceased's body. Some Indigenous groups avoid using the deceased's name. Do not refer to the deceased as "the body," but as the person who died. Least interference with the deceased's body may be preferred. If an autopsy is needed, discuss with spiritual advisors or elders about how to do this respectfully (Anderson, n.d.). Organ donation is not prohibited but may be influenced by beliefs about the importance of the deceased's body remaining whole and intact (Davison & Jhangri, 2014). Indigenous people may also adhere to Christian beliefs and practices as a result of colonization. See below for additional information.

Buddhism—People prefer a quiet place for death. Incense may be used. When the person has died, cover the body with a cotton sheet. Leave the deceased's mouth and eyes open. Others should not touch the body. Maintain strict silence after death. Autopsy and organ donation are permitted.

Christianity—Christian denominations have varying practices at time of death. Bible texts may be read near or at the time of death. Protestants may receive the sacraments of Holy Communion or sometimes baptism. Roman Catholics often request sacraments of Penance, Anointing of the Sick, and Holy Communion at the end of life. Many Christian groups offer prayers and anointing and view death as "going home"

to Jesus. There are no prescribed rituals for body preparation, and autopsy and organ donation are usually permissible.

Hinduism—People prefer to die at home or in a quiet setting. Because of a belief in reincarnation, efforts are made to resolve relationships before death. The head of a person nearing death should face the east with a lamp placed near the head. If the dying person is unable to chant a mantra, a family member can chant it into the right ear. Passages from the *Bhagavad Gita* are recited. Family members prefer to wash the body after death and are present to chant, pray, and use incense. Hindus prefer cremation of the body.

Islam—A Muslim reader recites verses from the Qur'an when the person is near death. Family members prepare the body, and non-Muslims should not touch it. Close the person's eyes after death and straighten the arms and legs. Autopsy or organ donation is generally not permissible, except as required by law.

Judaism—Death bed confessional, blessings, and readings from the Torah are traditional in Orthodox Judaism. A family member remains with the body until burial, which takes place within 24 hours, but not on the Sabbath. A family member closes the deceased's eyes on death. Synagogue burial societies may prepare the body, which is wrapped in white linen. Organ donation prohibitions may exist in Orthodox Judaism, but not for all Jews. Autopsies may be considered if organs are not removed.

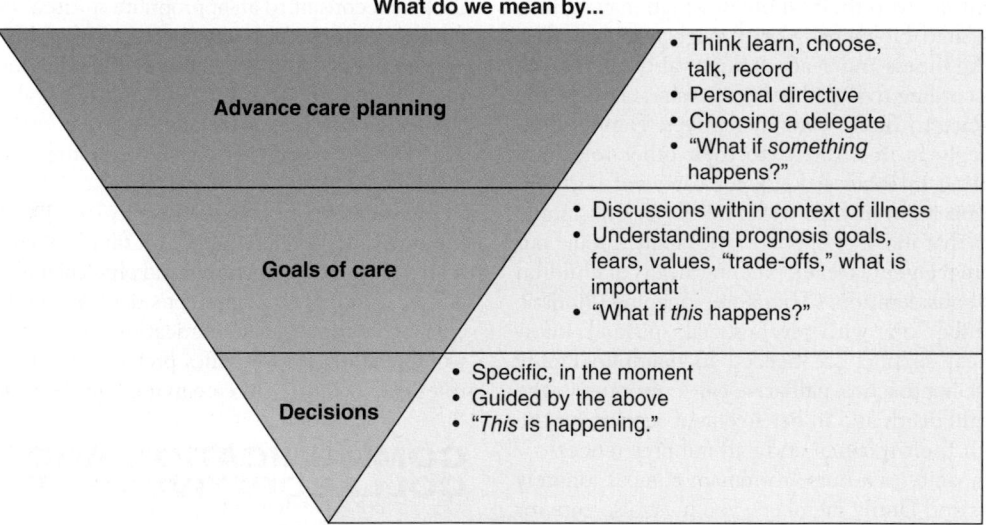

FIG 17.2 How to initiate discussions about serious illness with patients and caregivers (*From Nova Scotia Health Authority [2019]. Conversations about serious illness. Retrieved from https://library.nshealth. ca/SeriousIllness*)

one was not chosen, and support them in their role to make decisions based, as much as possible, on the wishes and preferences of the incapacitated ill or injured person. Nurses should be aware of the associated legal considerations in the province or territory in which they practice.

ACPs can provide a sense of control, prevent unwanted health care interventions, and reduce stress and uncertainty for others when making life-and-death decisions on behalf of an ill or injured person. Note that ACPs may need revisions as health care and life situations change and that the capacity of a patient to make health care decisions may decline as the end of life approaches. Nurses can assist any adult, ill or healthy, to develop an ACP by utilizing the tools developed by CHPCA (2019b), which can be found at

www.advancecareplanning.ca. A copy of the ACP should be placed on the medical record (see employer policy), and the person should be encouraged to provide a copy to the primary care provider and family.

ACPs often include decisions about whether to initiate cardio-pulmonary resuscitation (CPR) (see Chapter 28) or allow natural death (AND). Verbal "do not resuscitate" (DNR) or AND requests should be documented in the medical record according to employer policy and will likely include wishes about the level of care—that is, comfort only or information about when and how to intervene in specific health situations. In instances where a person is in an advanced stage of illness, is frail, or has multiple comorbidities, the outcomes of CPR are often unsuccessful or result in increased suffering

(Andrew, Nehme, Bernard, et al., 2017; Sulzgruber, Sterz, Poppe, et al., 2017). Helping families understand this can alleviate pressure to initiate CPR in these cases and assist in making a decision that is in the best interest of the ill person. Resources for helping families making decisions about CPR can be found at http://www.advancecareplanning.ca/resource/cpr-decision-aids/.

Goals of care conversations take place in the context of illness. They should be initiated early and be revisited whenever health needs change in response to progressing disease or lack of response to treatments. Goals of care conversations begin with understanding what the ill person and family know about the illness and prognosis, how they prefer to receive information, including how much detail, and how they wish to be involved in decision making (You, Fowler, & Heyland, 2014). Informed decision making is based on an understanding of the illness and prognosis while weighing the benefits and burdens of treatment options based on what could happen as the illness progresses. Ariadne Labs (n.d.) provide a serious-illness conversation guide and other resources to assist in facilitating goals of care conversations. Note that ethnicity, religion, and culture influence attitudes toward life-sustaining treatments.

Ongoing conversations about goals of care can prevent the need for decision making in times of crisis and uncertainty (NSHA, 2019). However, despite planning for future possibilities, there are times when decisions need to be made in the moment. These in-the-moment conversations about treatment decisions are guided by the same principles used in goals of care planning.

Ethical and Legal Considerations

Nurses can help to avoid ethical dilemmas by maintaining open communication with the health care team and family about goals of care and suggesting an ethical consult in intractable ethical dilemmas. The CNA's *Respecting Choices in End-of-Life Care: Challenges and Opportunities for RNs* (CNA, 2015) provides guidance with common end-of-life ethical issues. The following is an outline of some of the more common ethical issues in end-of-life care.

Withholding or Withdrawing Treatment

Goals of care conversations often involve decisions to forego initiating medical interventions or to stop treatments that have already begun. Ethically, there is no difference between withholding and withdrawing treatments, although it may be more difficult to discontinue interventions that have been started and are essential to life, for example, mechanical ventilation (Reichlin, 2014). In futile situations, it may help families to weigh benefits and burdens in relation to the ill person's values and quality of life and consider the implications of starting or continuing treatments that prolong life (and perhaps suffering) versus facilitating a peaceful death. Respecting family decisions, despite personal and professional reservations, promotes dignity and prevents distress that can persist into bereavement. In situations where families are not ready to forego initiating treatment not likely to be of benefit, time-limited treatment trials with specific

guidelines for evaluation can be offered. This gives the family the sense of doing everything possible while having time to prepare for the eventual death.

Palliative Sedation and the Principle of Double Effect

Palliative sedation is a legally acceptable means of relieving intractable suffering in the terminally ill by intermittent or continuous administration of sedating medications such as midazolam by a palliative or pain specialist to reduce consciousness. This may be coupled with adjuncts such as continuous opioids to control pain or breathlessness or neuroleptics for delirium (Schildmann, Schildmann, & Kiesewetter, 2015). Although difficult to verify empirically, some argue that palliative sedation hastens death (Rodrigues, Crokaert, & Gastmans, 2018). However, the principle of double effect has been used as ethical justification for palliative sedation for intractable suffering, whether physical, psychological, or existential. It maintains that the nature and intent of the action must be good (i.e., to relieve suffering), that the bad effect must not be the cause of the desired outcome (i.e., hastening death to relieve suffering), that the good effect outweighs the bad effect (i.e., relief of suffering outweighs the risk of hastened death), and that there are no other viable means of achieving the desired effect (Rodrigues et al., 2018). However, controversies remain over issues of autonomy, protection of the vulnerable, and similarities between palliative sedation and assisted dying (Rainone, 2015). Although there are no Canadian best-practice guidelines, the Canadian Society of Palliative Care Physicians (CSPCP) has developed a framework to guide standardization of new and existing policies (Dean, Cellarius, Henry, et al., 2012).

Medical Assistance in Dying (MAiD)

MAiD is legally permissible for eligible Canadians to relieve intractable suffering by intentionally hastening death. Requests for MAiD are rooted in suffering and compromised quality of life. Requests for or questions about MAiD may arise during routine care by the nurse. Responding to requests for MAiD requires an ability to be with suffering and explore its sources while adhering to provincial/territorial laws, regulatory body guidelines, employer policies, and ethical practices. Nurses and other health care providers have the right to conscientiously object to being involved in MAiD on the basis of deeply held personal beliefs and values but must ensure continued quality care until another care provider assumes responsibility. Maintaining confidentiality and gaining permission to share the context of the MAiD request with necessary care providers is of utmost importance. The CNA *Code of Ethics for Registered Nurses* (2017a), the *National Nursing Framework on Medical Assistance in Dying in Canada* (CNA, 2017b), and the *Hospice Palliative Care and Medical Assistance in Dying (MAiD) in Canada* guidelines (CHPCA, 2017) are useful practice resources.

◆ SKILL 17.1   Optimizing Comfort and Quality of Life

Proactive and timely management of symptoms and related distress are key to optimizing comfort and quality of life. Patients living with life-limiting illness experience multiple, complex physical symptoms and often have various emotional, practical, and spiritual concerns. Total pain is a concept introduced by palliative care pioneer Dame Cicely Saunders to describe how physical pain and symptoms are indivisible from the psychosocial, emotional, and spiritual experiences of the person, and how each domain affects

the other (Clark, 2014). Helping begins by understanding the impact of these symptoms and concerns on patients' and their families' lives from their shared and individual points of view. Through careful assessment, nurses can identify needs and provide information and education to enable self-management while drawing on health care team expertise to assist families in taking full advantage of the benefits of palliative care to enhance quality of life.

Delegation and Collaboration

Supportive care for management of symptoms and related distress can be delegated to an unregulated care provider (UCP). However, the nurse must conduct the initial assessments and develop the plan of care. The nurse directs the UCP to:

- Notify the nurse if the ill person reports new symptoms or if existing symptoms worsen or change.
- Provide basic comfort care, such as positioning, room temperature control, hygiene, and mouth care.

- Report possible adverse effects of medications, as instructed by the nurse.
- Speak to unconscious or dying persons, because hearing is the last sense to diminish.

Equipment

- Personal care items most preferred by patient
- Comfort and hygiene products
- Clean gloves

STEP	RATIONALE

ASSESSMENT

1. Identify patient using at least two person-specific identifiers (e.g., name and date of birth or name and medical record number) according to employer policy.

2. Ask patients to describe symptoms in their own words. Use open-ended prompts, such as "Describe your leg pain to me," or "Tell me how you are sleeping since you started taking this medicine."

3. Allow sufficient time for patients to describe their symptoms and encourage them to say more:
   "You've told me about your pain. Do you have pain anywhere else?"
   "Is there anything else bothering you?"
   Use employer-approved pain and symptom assessment tools. The *Edmonton Symptom Assessment Scale (Revised) (ESASr)* (see http://www.gpscbc.ca/sites/default/files/Edmonton%20Symptom%20Assessment%20Scale%20(ESAS-r)%20guidelines-3.pdf)(Watanabe, Nekolaichuk, Beaumont, et al., 2011) is a helpful tool that uses a 0–10 scale to measure the patient's current perception of a myriad of symptoms and includes anterior and posterior body outlines for locating areas of pain. It can be completed by a caregiver, a health care provider, or the ill person, independently or with help. The *Palliative Performance Scale Version Two (PPSv2)* (Victoria Hospice, 2001) is useful for assessing functional ability and as a prognostic tool. It measures the ill person's ability to ambulate, participate in activity or work, perform self-care, and eat or drink, as well as their level of consciousness. It measures each domain in increments of 10, with 0 meaning death and 100 meaning full function. The domain scores are added up and the total is converted to a score out of 100. The final score is reported as a percentage and can be useful in determining when care needs are increasing or when death is approaching.

4. Assess patient's emotional and spiritual health. Does the patient feel anxious, sad, depressed, bored, or understimulated? Ask questions such as "How has your declining health been affecting your life, relationships, sense of self, or well-being?"

5. Assess patient's pain severity using an employer-approved assessment scale and evaluate pain characteristics. Assess behaviour in nonverbal or cognitively impaired patients using an approved assessment tool (see Chapter 16).

Ensures correct patient. Complies with Accreditation Canada's standards and improves patient safety (Accreditation Canada, 2019).

Symptoms are personal perceptions experienced only by the patient (O'Neil-Page, Anderson, & Dean, 2015; Paice, 2015).

Ensures a more complete assessment. Prevents you from making assumptions about patient's symptoms, prematurely stopping the assessment process.

Consistent use of a standard assessment scale helps determine changes in symptoms and evaluate effectiveness of interventions (Paice, 2015).

Tools that can be filled out by the ill person or caregivers enable self-monitoring and care.

Pain and other physical symptoms can cause and be exacerbated by emotional, relational, and spiritual issues. See Cicely Saunders' concept of "total pain" as described above (Clark, 2014).

Consistent use of a standard pain scale helps assess changes in patient pain levels and evaluate effectiveness of pain interventions (Paice, 2015).

STEP	RATIONALE

ASSESSMENT

6. If patient cannot self-report pain, observe for these symptoms (American Cancer Society [ACS], 2016):
  - Noisy breathing—laboured, harsh, or rapid breaths
  - Making pained sounds—including groaning, moaning, or expressing hurt
  - Facial expressions—looking sad, tense, or frightened; frowning or crying
  - Body language—tension, clenched fists, knees pulled up, inflexibility, restlessness, or looking like they are trying to get away from the hurt area
  - Body movement—changing positions to get comfortable but can't

Patients unable to report or verbalize pain show nonverbal signs of pain.

Patients who are nonverbal or cognitively impaired are unable to report pain and are at risk for having their pain go untreated or undertreated. Sometimes behavioural cues such as increased distress, agitation, or changes in activity patterns or interactions with others may indicate underlying pain or other symptoms. Be sure to compare behaviours with typical behaviours for that person (Murray, 2016).

7. Perform hand hygiene.

Reduces transmission of microorganisms.

8. Assess for feeling of breathlessness (does patient feel that they are getting enough air?), respiratory rate, breathing patterns, and lung sounds. Assess for presence of airway secretions.

Dyspnea, air hunger, or shortness of breath results from metabolic or respiratory changes. Near the end of life, Cheyne-Stokes respirations are common and are characterized by alternating periods of apnea and hyperpnea.

9. Observe condition of skin, especially back, heels, and buttocks (see Chapter 8).

Decreased nutrition, hydration, peripheral circulation, and activity level can contribute to skin breakdown.

10. Inspect patient's oral cavity, including mucosa, tongue, and teeth (see Chapter 8).

Dehydration, difficulty swallowing, and inflammation of mouth are common at end of life.

11. Assess bowel function (see Chapter 35).
  a. Determine usual bowel elimination pattern (frequency, character, usual time of day) and effectiveness of usual bowel management routines.
  b. If patient is passing liquid stool, assess for presence of fecal impaction (see employer policy).
  c. Review medication regimens, prescriptions, and over-the-counter medications known to cause constipation (e.g., opioids, antacids).

  d. Identify typical food and fluid intake over 1 week and patient's activity levels.

Patients experience constipation because of decreased fluid and fibre intake, immobility, age, disease processes, or medications such as opioids (Caraccia Economou, 2015). Patients who have diarrhea are at risk for dehydration.

Watery stool leaking around blockage indicates fecal impaction.

Medications can alter bowel elimination patterns. Diarrhea results from infections, diseases, or medications (e.g., antibiotics or chemotherapy). Change in therapy might be necessary.

Oral intake and activity levels influence bowel elimination patterns.

12. Assess urinary elimination (see Chapter 34) and ability to control urination. If incontinent, assess for skin breakdown or patient discomfort.

Urinary incontinence may result from delirium, urinary tract infection, medications, immobility, or severe constipation (Gray & Sims, 2015).

13. Assess patient's appetite, ability to swallow, and for presence of nausea or vomiting. Use standardized tool for assessment if available (American Association of College of Nurses [AACN], 2016).
  a. Consider presence of nausea in patients receiving enteral feedings.

Medications, pain, depression, disease progression, or decreased blood flow to digestive organs near death often contribute to nausea, vomiting, and decreased appetite.

Patients who have decreased consciousness are unable to report nausea.

14. Assess daily food and fluid intake in relation to patient's condition and preferences.

Nutrition screening helps in identifying deficits and allows for interventions to be carried out to improve nutritional status (Shaw & Eldridge, 2015).

15. Use descriptive scale to assess fatigue (e.g., scale with descriptors—none, moderate, severe). Ask if fatigue limits patient's ability to perform desired activities.

Fatigue is the most common symptom of progressive illness and has a profound impact on quality of life (O'Neil-Page et al., 2015).

16. Assess for terminal delirium in patient near death (e.g., confusion, restlessness, and/or agitation, with or without day–night reversal).
  a. Consider if patient has pain, nausea, dyspnea, full bladder or bowel, poor sleep patterns, anxiety, or joint pain from immobility.
  b. Review medical record for hypercalcemia, hypoglycemia, hyponatremia, or dehydration.
  c. Review patient's medications.

Allows you to identify this condition and implement interventions to keep patient safe and decrease patient and family distress (Heidrich & English, 2015).

Risk factors for presence of delirium are common physical problems that need to be treated or ruled out as causative factors.

Metabolic imbalances can cause restlessness or delirium.

Unintended responses to medications result in changed activity states.

STEP	RATIONALE

ASSESSMENT

d. Determine if patient has unresolved emotional or spiritual issues. Refer to spiritual care provider, psychologist, social worker, or other team member, as needed.

Spiritual and emotional distress may contribute to restlessness or increased pain.

NURSING DIAGNOSES

The priority of diagnoses is dependent on the ill person's (or family's) perception of symptoms and whether or not death is near. For example, irregular and noisy breathing and reduced peripheral tissue perfusion evidenced by mottled extremities are normal in the last days and hours of life.

- Inadequate breathing pattern—Less of a priority if expected and not distressing. (See above.)
- Reduced peripheral tissue perfusion—Less of a priority if expected. (See above.)
- Persistent pain
- Acute pain

- Anxiety
- Constipation
- Diarrhea
- Nausea
- Fatigue—The person may rate this as very distressing, and therefore it may be a greater priority
- Reduced stamina

- Total urinary incontinence
- Bowel incontinence
- Inadequate hydration of oral mucous membranes
- Inadequate swallowing
- Potential for constipation

Related factors/Risk factors are individualized on the basis of patient's condition or needs.

PLANNING

1. Expected outcomes following completion of procedure:
- Patient reports acceptable level of pain.
- Patient reports feeling warm and comfortable.

- Patient reports comfortable eating and drinking patterns.

- Patient has soft, formed bowel movements.
- Skin remains free of irritation or breakdown.

- Patient is not restless.
- Patient reports less distress from fatigue.

- Patient experiences less respiratory distress.

Indicates pain control.
Warming interventions help reverse effects of reduced peripheral circulation.
Optimal food and fluid intake are based on patient preferences and comfort.
Indicates adequate bowel function and peristaltic activity.
Interventions to protect skin from immobility and bowel or urinary incontinence are effective.
Therapies have calming effect.
Energy conservation methods are effective; patient adjusts to changes in activity level.
Patient is less apprehensive and breathes easily.

IMPLEMENTATION

1. Perform hand hygiene.
2. Provide pain relief. Use a multimodal approach.

Reduces transmission of microorganisms.
Nonpharmacological measures supplement pain medication and can increase patient comfort (Paice, 2015).

a. Administer prescribed analgesics and adjuvants. Confer with the prescriber and recommend an around-the-clock (ATC) dosing schedule, especially if pain is anticipated for most of the day. A variety of extended- or controlled-release oral opioid formulations (dosing intervals of 8, 10, 12, or 24 hours) and transdermal patches (72 hours) are effective.

Opioids should be given on a fixed dosage schedule ATC rather than prn, with doses given before pain returns (Burchum & Rosenthal, 2016). An ATC medication lessens the severity of end-of-dose pain, allowing a patient to sleep through the night and reduce "clock watching" for the next dose. Extended-release medications maintain constant serum opioid concentration, minimizing toxic and subtherapeutic concentrations (Burchum & Rosenthal, 2016).

b. Draw on team expertise and utilize pharmacological as well as nonpharmacological and complementary and alternative medicine (CAM) approaches where appropriate (e.g., massage, acupuncture, music therapy, mind/body approaches) (see Chapter 16).

Use of complementary therapies can help alleviate symptoms and related suffering and give patients and families a sense of self-efficacy (Kravits, 2015).

c. Provide patient and family education on causes and patterns of pain and safety of opioid use and explain interventions.

Encourages patient autonomy and reduces emotional distress, clarifying misinformation about opioid therapies.

STEP	RATIONALE

IMPLEMENTATION

d. Reassess patient's pain 1 hour after administration of pain medication or complementary therapy.

To determine if desired effect of medication or complementary treatment was achieved; if patient has reduced pain level.

3. Provide general comfort measures.

   a. Provide bath and skin care based on patient's preferences and hygiene needs (see Chapter 18). **NOTE:** Daily baths are not always desired or necessary at end of life if they cause discomfort, fatigue, or increased pain.

Clean skin promotes comfort and reduces risk of skin breakdown.

   b. Provide eye care and use artificial tears in patients with decreased consciousness (see Chapter 19).

Eye irritation causes pain. Blink reflex diminishes near death, causing drying of cornea.

   c. Reposition every 2 hours if on a regular mattress or every 4 hours if using a pressure-relieving mattress according to the person's goals of care and wishes and be sure to premedicate if movement causes pain (Scarborough, 2016). Do not position on tubes or other objects. Keep skin clean and dry. Use a pH-balanced cleanser instead of soap and keep skin moisturized. Also ensure adequate hydration and nutrition according to goals of care and wishes (Scarborough, 2016).

Prolonged, even slight pressure from weight of patient's body or objects causes skin injury. There is significant risk for pressure injuries in older persons, in those with inadequate hydration and nutrition, and especially in the last couple of weeks before death, due to physiological shutdown (Scarborough, 2016). In advanced states of illness or frailty, some wounds cannot be healed, although control of pain, odour, and exudate can prevent reduced quality of life (Scarborough, 2016)

4. Provide oral hygiene after meals and at bedtime while patient is awake and more frequently in mouth-breathing or unconscious patients (see Chapter 18).

Oral mucosa integrity is needed for normal swallowing and to minimize anorexia and malnutrition. Mouth rinses remove oral debris and clean the mouth. Dehydration develops as patient experiences metabolic changes and fluid intake declines.

   a. Use antifungal oral rinses as prescribed or sodium bicarbonate or normal saline rinses.

Patients near death breathe through the mouth, which dries oral mucosa.

   b. Moisten lips with nonpetroleum balm.

Prevents skin breakdown.

5. Initiate bowel management regimen to reduce risk for constipation or diarrhea.

Interventions improve peristalsis in constipation, soften fecal mass, and decrease abdominal discomfort (Clark & Currow, 2014; Santucci & Battista, 2015).

   a. Give patients whatever fluids they enjoy if medically tolerated. Near end of life, patient may refuse fluids. Do not force fluid intake.

Decreased blood flow to intestines at end of life causes lack of appetite and anorexia.

   b. Encourage regular physical activity (e.g., walking) if tolerated.

   c Administer daily stool softener or laxative, especially in patients using opioids for pain management.

   d. In case of diarrhea, provide low-residue diet; treat infections or discontinue medications if possible. Administer antidiarrheal medications. Patients with persistent diarrhea require rigorous skin care to promote comfort and prevent skin breakdown.

Treatments reduce incidence and severity of diarrhea, which can lead to dehydration.

6. Manage urinary incontinence with intervention appropriate for patient's conditions (e.g., condom catheter, adult incontinence pads [see Chapter 34]).

Urinary output declines near death, making it possible to manage incontinence without an in-dwelling catheter.

Clinical Decision Point *Consider an in-dwelling catheter only if skin integrity, patient preference, or fatigue from bed changes becomes an issue.*

7. Offer patient favourite foods in amount and at time they desire. Do not overly encourage patient to eat.

Patients may be experiencing gastrointestinal (GI) distress, dry mouth, or other symptoms related to their disease process, which may contribute to decreased oral intake. In addition, patients nearing final hours of life decrease their oral intake as a result of slowing of bodily functions or altered level of consciousness (Gillespie & Raftery, 2014).

   a. Treat nausea by administering antiemetics intravenously or rectally as prescribed. As nausea subsides, offer clear liquids and ice chips. Avoid caffeinated liquids, milk, and fruit juices.

GI mucosa tolerates clear liquids more readily. Certain liquids increase stomach acidity.

STEP	RATIONALE

IMPLEMENTATION

8. Manage fatigue.

   Taking rest breaks during activity will help conserve energy. Tired patients need help and monitoring to ensure patient safety.

   a. Help patient identify valued or desired tasks and preferred time of day to perform tasks and determine how to conserve energy for only those tasks. Help with activities of daily living. Eliminate extra steps in activities.

   b. Explain care activities before performing them and include patient in setting daily schedule.

   Minimizes anxiety and maintains patient's autonomy and involvement.

   c. Discuss with patient easy ways to incorporate exercise (e.g., yoga, walking, biking, and swimming) into daily activities.

   Research has shown that physical activity seems to improve quality of life for people throughout chronic illness, including at the end of life (Wilson, & Michael, 2015).

9. Support patient's breathing efforts.

   a. Position for comfort in semi-Fowler's or Fowler's position.

   Promotes maximal ventilation, lung expansion, and drainage of secretions.

   b. Elevate head to facilitate postural drainage. Turn from side to side to mobilize and drain secretions. Suction only if necessary.

   Deep airway suctioning causes discomfort and is not effective in reducing airway noise or secretion clearance (Bailey & Harmon, 2018).

   c. Provide prescribed antimuscarinic medications.

   Anticholinergic (which are antimuscarinic) medications reduce saliva and excessive secretions, thus decreasing noisy respirations (Dudgeon, 2015), but they should be initiated early to be effective (Murray, 2016).

   d. Stay with patients experiencing dyspnea or air hunger. Use interventions that patients perceive as relieving their shortness of breath (choice of oxygen-delivery modes, fan near face, body position). Administer opioids or anxiolytics as prescribed. Benzodiazepines may also be administered for anxiety related to dyspnea. Keep room cool with low humidity.

   Sharing control with patients reduces anxiety that contributes to feelings of air hunger. Morphine is the medication of choice for dyspnea, decreasing respiratory rate, and decreasing anxiety (Dudgeon, 2015).

10. Manage restlessness.

    a. Keep patient's room quiet with soft lighting and at comfortable temperature. Offer caregivers the opportunities to maintain close contact. Encourage use of soft music, prayer, or reading from patient's favourite book.

    Reduces unnecessary external stimulation and provides comforting space. Privacy allows caregivers the chance to provide verbal assurances and touch; physical touch may provide comfort and reassurance (Murray, 2016).

    b. Use least-sedating pharmacological options to control restlessness. Consult with health care team about titrating a medication (e.g., lorazepam). Discontinue all nonessential medication. Use subcutaneous, transdermal, sublingual, or rectal medication delivery routes.

    Reduces delirium without making patient unconscious. Control of restlessness relieves family's concern that patient is in pain, distress, or danger. Determine cause of delirium, if possible, to decrease use of medication (Bailey & Harmon, 2018).

11. Manage anxiety.

    a. Provide counselling and supportive therapy. Consult with prescribing health care provider for benzodiazepines, the medications of choice. Offer available counselling services (e.g., spiritual care, psychologist, social worker).

    Counselling improves patient and family understanding of the disease and its expected course and is used to identify strengths and coping strategies.

Clinical Decision Point *Caution: The use of benzodiazepines in very old persons can result in a paradoxical agitation.*

EVALUATION

1. Ask patient to rate pain using an employer-approved assessment scale and evaluate pain characteristics. Assess behaviour in nonverbal or cognitively impaired patients using an approved assessment tool (see Chapter 16).

   Determines extent of pain relief.

2. Ask patient to describe mouth comfort, and inspect oral cavity.

   Evaluates condition of oral cavity and ability to chew, swallow, and speak.

3. Evaluate frequency of defecation; after patient defecates, inspect feces.

   Determines status of bowel function and character of stool.

STEP	RATIONALE

EVALUATION

4. Observe skin condition.

Determines if skin tears or areas of pressure or maceration are present.

5. Ask patient to rate fatigue (scale from none to moderate to severe or ESASr) and compare with baseline. Observe for fatigue or shortness of breath when patient performs activities.

Determines if patient is less distressed with activity.

6. Observe patient's respiratory patterns and ask if breathing is easy and comfortable.

Determines if respiratory distress is relieved.

7. Observe patient's behaviour or ask caregiver to report on it. Note level of restlessness.

Determines level of comfort and extent of restlessness.

8. **Use Teach-Back:** "I want to be sure I explained that we want to control your pain, and this requires you to describe it. Tell me what the numbers on the pain scale mean. Tell me when is a good time to let me know about your pain before it gets too severe." Develop a revised teaching plan if patient or caregiver is not able to teach back correctly.

Determines patient's and caregiver's level of understanding of instructional topic.

Unexpected Outcomes

1. One or several symptoms remain unresolved, with patient reporting little or no relief.
2. Patient becomes anxious, fearful, or exhausted as a result of continued symptoms.

Related Interventions

- Increase frequency of or change an intervention.
- Try combination therapies.
- Give patient therapy choices and try different interventions.
- Elicit support from other team members, for example, spiritual care, psychology, social work.
- Explain goals of therapies and possible reasons for symptoms.
- Answer call lights quickly and explain plan of care throughout the day.

Communication and Documentation

- Document detailed description of patient symptoms in nurses' notes in electronic health record (EHR) or chart and/or appropriate flow sheets. Use consistent descriptors for comparison over time.
- Document your evaluation of patient and caregiver learning.
- Document type of interventions used and patient's response in nurses' notes in EHR or chart. Note successful interventions in the care plan.
- Report unexpected new symptoms or uncontrolled existing symptoms to health care provider and team.

Special Considerations
Teaching

- Involve the patient and caregivers in planning and care giving. With proper instruction, they can perform most symptom-management interventions, perform personal care (e.g., bathing, oral hygiene), and administer medications and treatments in the home setting.

Pediatric

- Teach parents how to recognize and assess pain in a nonverbal child.
- Be honest and use developmentally appropriate language to keep children informed of changes in their own or their loved one's illness.
- Maintain routines and usual childhood activities as much as possible.
- Encourage involvement of children in care giving on the basis of their ability, needs, and readiness (Hockenberry & Wilson, 2015).

Gerontological

- Include older persons in conversations and accommodate communication limits (e.g., hearing deficits).
- Older persons need companionship and maintenance of self-esteem. Detached caregiver behaviours such as being slow to respond to physical discomforts, failing to keep room odour free, and speaking in hushed tones of voice are often perceived by the person as abandonment. Encourage a family member, friend, sitter, or hospice volunteer to stay with the patient during the night. Some older persons who have developed a lifestyle around aloneness prefer solitude. Demonstrate person-centred care by being sensitive to patient's preferences (Touhy, Jett, Boscart, et al., 2019).
- Assessing and addressing pain in an older person who is cognitively impaired or nonverbal is sometimes difficult and involves proactive symptom management.
- Patients at the end of life or with dementia lose their capacity to report adverse effects, call for help, evaluate treatments, or make decisions. Among the risks is poor symptom management and patient falls. Use effective communication with those with cognitive impairment and be aware of likely causes of anxiety, fear, and resistance to care when carrying out interventions (Regan, Tapley, & Jolley, 2014). Ensure safety measures are in place.

Care in the Community

- Prevent caregiver fatigue by recommending that family members monitor their own energy levels and request respite care when they need relief. Suggest resources for help with meals, shopping, or staying with the patient while family goes out. Information about "patient benefits" and "caregiver and survivor benefits" to support palliative care in the community can be found by

TABLE 17.1

Physical Signs and Symptoms in the Final Stages of Dying

Physical Signs and Symptoms	Rationale	Intervention
Coolness, colour, and temperature change in hands, arms, feet, and legs; mottling of legs; perspiration	Peripheral circulation diminished as blood shunts to vital organs Patient may feel cool to touch, but core temperature normal	Place socks on feet. Cover with light blanket. Do not use electric blanket because person is unable to report excess heat.
Increased sleeping	Decreased energy, psychological withdrawal, medications	Spend time with person; hold their hand. Speak to person, even if there is no response. Maintain compassionate presence with the person and family. This in itself can be very therapeutic.
Disorientation, confusion of time, place, person	Metabolic changes, medications, changing sleep–wake cycles, decreased oxygenation	Identify self by name; reorient person to time and place. Decrease environmental stimuli.
Incontinence of bladder and/or bowel	Decreased muscle tone and consciousness	Change bedding as appropriate. Use bed pads; try not to use in-dwelling catheters.
Upper airway secretions; noisy respirations	Decreased cough reflex, inability to expectorate secretions or clear throat, relaxation of glottis, decreased muscle tone	Elevate head with pillow or raise head of bed; turn head to side to drain secretions. Suction minimally. Administer anticholinergics as prescribed.
Restlessness	Metabolic changes and decrease in oxygen to brain	Calm patient by speech and action; reduce light, rub back, stroke arms, or read aloud. Do not use restraints.
Decreased intake of food and fluids, nausea	Blood shunted away from gastrointestinal (GI) tract, causing decreased GI motility and anorexia; ketosis	Do not force patient to eat or drink; give ice chips or popsicles if desired. Provide mouth care.

Modified from Touhy, T. A., Jett, K. F., Boscart, V., & McCleary, L. (2019). *Ebersole and Hess' gerontological nursing and healthy aging* (2nd Canadian ed.). Toronto: Elsevier Canada.

searching these terms on the Canadian Virtual Hospice (2017) website. Additional resources for Indigenous peoples can be found under "Home and Community Care" on the Government of Canada (2016b) website. Volunteers are also an integral part of the palliative care team and can provide additional support to families in the community, such as transportation and visiting to enable family to go out, among other things.

END-OF-LIFE CARE

Nurses need to recognize a patient's transition to the end-of-life and active dying phases and communicate to the patient and family the expectation of imminent death. The *Palliative Performance Scale Version Two (PPSv2)* (Victoria Hospice, 2001) may be useful in determining when death is nearing. This is a good time to revisit conversations about preferences for end-of-life care.

Allow young children to visit a dying parent or grandparent if desired. Encourage parents to express their concerns about how to talk about death and loss with their child. Do not use euphemisms to describe death to children. Instead, use the words *die*, *dying*, or *died*. Offer resources such as story books to help parents explain death to children. Helpful resources can be found on the Canadian Virtual Hospice (2017) website at http://www.virtualhospice.ca/.

Care in the Community

If a home death is planned, help families to prepare for this. Ensure presence of all necessary equipment as well as a medication kit containing common medications needed for symptom management at the end of life. Ensure that there is a plan in place for the pronouncement of death and removal of the body from the home (NSHA, 2017).

For expected home deaths, a letter can be written by the physician, or nurse practitioner in some provinces, informing the coroner/medical examiner's office and the funeral home of the expected death. If this is in place, there is no law regarding who can pronounce a death. If an expected death occurs in a hospital, long-term care, or other facility, the nurse should adhere to employer policy on pronouncement of death (Canadian Medical Protective Society [CMPS], 2016). For home deaths, advise the family not to call emergency responders at the time of death, to avoid invoking procedures necessary to investigate unexpected or suspicious deaths.

Educate the patient and family members about signs of imminent death, what to expect, and how to recognize and attend to discomfort (Table 17.1). Ensure that the family has access to 24/7 support if at home (Murray, 2016). Educating a person and family about what to expect during the final days or hours can alleviate anxiety and promote a more positive death experience for all involved (Dosser & Kennedy, 2014; Moir, Roberts, Martz, et al., 2015). Consider the type of support that family members will need at the time of death and make arrangements. *Considerations for a Home Death*, found on the Canadian Virtual Hospice website (Stenekes & Streeter, 2017), and Victoria Hospice's (n.d.) *Psychosocial Assessment* tool are useful resources.

◆ SKILL 17.2 **Care of a Person's Body After Death**

At the time of death, nurses provide compassionate care to patients and family members through their presence, by offering information, guidance, and support, and by facilitating communication. In addition, nurses provide postmortem care (i.e., care of the body after death) in a dignified, respectful manner, consistent with a patient's religious and cultural practices and the local law (National

Consensus Project [NCP] for Quality Palliative Care, 2013). Box 17.2 outlines some religious and cultural practices that influence how to care for a person's body near or after death.

Organ donation is another important nursing consideration near the time of death that is influenced by cultural or religious beliefs and legislation. While the Canadian government is responsible for ensuring the safety of donated organs, provinces and territories have specific guidelines and procedures as well as laws regarding consent. Explicit, rather than presumed, consent is required in Canada, and donors can give prior consent by indicating this on their health card or driver's license or through a registry. In the absence of prior consent, the next-of-kin can give consent. Even with prior consent of the donor, agreement of the family is sought before organ procurement (Norris, 2018).

In the case of vital organ donation (e.g., heart, lungs, liver, pancreas, small bowel, or kidneys), a patient must remain on life support until the organs are surgically removed. A nurse's role in organ procurement includes helping to identify potential organ donors, providing care for the donor's body, and caring for the family throughout the donation process (Findlater & Thomson, 2018; Matzo & Hill, 2014). Family members often need help understanding what "brain death" means (i.e., the irreversible absence of all brain function, including the brainstem) for a person who has died. Patients appear to still be alive because life support keeps the deceased's organs functioning until they can be retrieved. Tissues such as eyes, bone, and skin are retrieved from deceased patients not on life support. Because of the sensitive nature of making requests for organ donation, professionals educated in organ procurement often assume that responsibility. They inform family members of their options for donation and inform them that donation does not delay funeral arrangements.

Nurses may facilitate the organ donation request by providing a private place and helping to identify the SDM to be involved in the request. Sometimes nurses notify the local donor registry to determine if a patient qualifies for organ donation because certain medical conditions prohibit donation. Nurses also reinforce explanations of the donation procedure and inform the family about how the deceased's body will be cared for. Above all, nurses must honour the family's cultural and religious practices and support their final decision. Donor families often report that donating organs helped them in their grief and that they felt positive about the experience.

The second procedure of legal and medical significance often performed after a death is an autopsy, or postmortem examination.

An autopsy, the surgical dissection of a body after death, helps determine the exact cause and circumstances of a death, discovers the pathway of a disease, or provides research data. It is not performed in every death. Provincial laws determine when autopsies are required, but they are usually performed in circumstances of unexpected, unexplained deaths (e.g., when death occurs within 24 hours of hospital admission; unexpected death in the home) and deaths resulting from accidents or drugs (Statistics Canada, 2015).

Certification of death and completion of the death certificate are also guided by provincial/territorial legislation and should be completed as soon as possible after the death. Physicians, and in some regions, certified nurse practitioners who have knowledge of the person's illness leading up to the death can complete the death certificate in nonreportable cases. Each province/territory uses either the coroner or medical examiner's system to determine the process for investigation and which deaths are considered reportable (CMPS, 2016; Statistics Canada, 2015).

Delegation and Collaboration

The skill of caring for a body after death can be delegated to an unregulated care provider (UCP). However, it is often easier for the nurse and UCP to work together in providing postmortem care. The nurse directs the UCP to:

- Follow employer policy and the law in cases of autopsy or organ and tissue donation.
- Honour family cultural or religious rituals when performing postmortem care.
- Handle the body with dignity and respect for privacy.

Equipment

- Clean gloves and isolation gown
- Plastic bag for hazardous waste disposal
- Washbasin, washcloth, warm water, and bath towel
- Clean gown or disposable gown for body as indicated by employer policy
- Shroud kit with name tags
- Syringes for removing urinary catheter
- Scissors
- Small pillow or towel
- Paper tape, gauze dressings
- Paper bag, plastic bag, or other suitable receptacle for patient's belongings to be returned to family members
- Valuables envelope

STEP	RATIONALE

ASSESSMENT

1. Ask the responsible health care provider to establish the time of death and determine the need for an autopsy. If an autopsy is planned or a possible crime is involved, use special precautions to preserve evidence (see local law and employer policy).

Validates the patient's death. Autopsy can determine cause of death and reveal more about a disease. When an autopsy is not required by law, a patient's legal representative and the health care provider or designated requester must complete and sign an autopsy consent form (Calgary Laboratory Services, 2019).

2. Determine if family members or significant others are present and if they have been informed of the death. Identify patient's surrogate (next of kin or durable power of attorney [DPOA]).

Verifies that family has been notified of patient's death, to avoid inappropriate communication of this sensitive information.

3. Determine if patient's surrogate has been asked about organ and tissue donation and validate that a donation request form has been signed. Notify organ request team as per policy.

Federal guidelines require documentation that explicit consent has been given (Norris, 2018).

STEP	RATIONALE

ASSESSMENT

4. Provide family members and friends a private place to gather. Allow them time to ask questions (including those about medical care) or discuss grief.

Creates safe environment for grieving family. Questions provide information about how they are coping with loss and their needs.

5. Ask family members if they have requests for preparation or viewing of the body (e.g., washing the body, positioning of body, special clothing, shaving). Determine if they wish to be present or help with care of the body.

Respects individuality of patient and family and supports their right to having cultural or religious values and beliefs upheld. Provides closure for those who wish to help with body preparation (Hadders, Paulson, & Fougner, 2014).

6. Contact support person (e.g., spiritual care, social work) to stay with family members not helping to prepare the body. Implement in timely manner a bereavement care plan after patient's death when family remains the focus of care (NCP, 2013).

Provides family support during an emotional time.

7. Consult health care provider's prescription for special care directives or specimens that are to be collected.

Specimens may be used in determining cause of death.

8. Perform hand hygiene; apply clean gloves, gown, or protective barriers.

Reduces transmission of microorganisms.

9. Assess general condition of the body and note presence of dressings, tubes, and medical equipment. (If leaving room at this time, remove personal protective equipment and perform hand hygiene.)

Validates if tissue damage was present before postmortem care.

NURSING DIAGNOSES

For patients:
- Potential for impaired skin integrity

For family members and significant others:
- Inadequate coping
- Compromised family coping
- Potential for complicated grief
- Powerlessness
- Insufficient knowledge regarding organ donation
- Grieving

Related factors/Risk factors are individualized on the basis of the patient's, family's, and significant others' needs.

PLANNING

1. Expected outcomes following completion of procedure:
   - Body is free of new skin damage.

   Careful handling of body prevents lacerations, bruises, or abrasions during postmortem care.

   - Family and significant others are able to express grief.

   Family and significant others feel supported through their loss.

Clinical Decision Point *Immediately after death and before proceeding with other activities, place the deceased's body in a supine position and straighten the limbs (Horst, 2017). This will prevent livor mortis from occurring in the face and other areas visible to the family during viewing. Livor mortis is purplish discoloration of skin due to pooling of blood in dependent areas that occurs within 30 minutes after death and that can last up to 12 hours (Claridge, 2017). Proper positioning also prevents unnatural alignment of the body prior to rigor mortis, which is the stiffening of the body that occurs within about 2 hours of the death and lasts for about 36–48 hours (Claridge, 2017). A pillow may be used (Henry & Wilson, 2012) in preparation for family viewing if needed.*

2. Position patient supine in bed, arms at sides, in a private room if possible. If patient has a roommate, explain and move roommate to another location temporarily.

Provides staff with larger area for postmortem care and for family members to gather in a private setting.

Clinical Decision Point *It is best practice to carry out "personal care after death" within 2 to 4 hours of death to preserve the deceased's appearance, condition, dignity, and ability to donate tissue (Henry & Wilson, 2012, p. 9).*

3. As soon as possible, a patient's death must be certified by someone in authority (e.g., physician, or in some jurisdictions, a certified nurse practitioner). This person completes forms certifying the cause, time, and place of death. The legal form is necessary for life insurance and financial and property issues.

These steps make it possible for an official death certificate to be prepared.

STEP	RATIONALE

PLANNING

4. Direct UCP to gather needed equipment and arrange at bedside.

Because this is often an emotional time for family members, organized, efficient care is important.

IMPLEMENTATION

1. Help family members notify others of the death. Promptly notify the mortuary, as chosen by the family, and discuss plans for postmortem care.

Following a death, grieving persons have difficulty focusing on details and often need guidance. Being informed increases a sense of control.

2. If patient has made tissue donation, consult employer policy for guidelines related to care of the body.

Retrieval of tissues (e.g., eyes, bone, skin) may require special procedures.

3. Perform hand hygiene; apply clean gloves, gown, or protective barriers.

Reduces transmission of microorganisms.

Clinical Decision Point *If caregivers are helping in postmortem care, ensure they wear a gown and gloves to protect them from body fluids.*

4. Identify patient using at least two person-specific identifiers (e.g., name and date of birth or name and medical record number) according to employer policy. Tag the body and leave tag on body as directed by employer policy.

Ensures correct patient. Complies with Accreditation Canada's standards and improves patient safety (Accreditation Canada, 2019).

5. Remove in-dwelling devices (e.g., urinary catheter, endotracheal tube). Disconnect and cap off (no need to remove) intravenous lines. *Do not remove in-dwelling devices in cases of autopsy* (follow employer policy).

Creates normal appearance for family viewing of body. Removing intravenous catheters allows fluids to leak. Removal of tubes and lines is contraindicated if an autopsy is planned.

6. Clean the mouth and clean and replace dentures as soon as possible (Henry & Wilson, 2012). If dentures cannot be replaced, send them with body in clearly labeled denture cup and transport with body to mortuary. If culturally appropriate, close mouth with rolled-up towel under chin.

Gives face more natural appearance. If dentures are not replaced, it can be very difficult later for workers at funeral home to place dentures.

7. Place small pillow under head or position according to cultural preferences. Do not tie hands together on top of body. Check employer policy regarding need to secure hands and feet. Use only circular gauze bandaging on body.

Patient appears natural. Weight of limp arms causes skin damage and discoloration if hands are tied. Some employers require securing limbs to prevent tissue damage when body is being moved.

8. Close eyes by applying light pressure for 30 seconds. Use saline-moistened gauze if corneal or eye donation is to take place (Henry & Wilson, 2012). Some cultures prefer that eyes remain open.

Closed eyes convey to some people a more peaceful and natural appearance. Gauze prevents corneal drying.

9. Groom and arrange hair into preferred style, if known. Remove any clips, hairpins, or rubber bands. Do not shave patient. Some faith groups prohibit shaving.

Hard objects damage or discolour face and scalp. Shaving too soon after death can cause bruising, so this is done by the funeral director. Explain this to the family if they request shaving (Henry & Wilson, 2012).

10. Wash soiled body parts. Some cultural practices require that family members clean the body (see Box 17.2).

Prepares body for viewing and reduces odours. Mortuary personnel provide complete bath.

11. Remove soiled dressings and replace with clean dressings, using paper tape or circular gauze bandaging.

Changing dressings controls odours and creates more acceptable appearance. Paper tape minimizes skin damage when tape is removed.

Clinical Decision Point *Turning a recently dead body to the side sometimes causes the flow of exhaled air. This is a normal event and not a sign of life.*

12. Place absorbent pad under buttocks.

Relaxation of sphincter muscles at time of death causes release of urine or feces.

13. Place clean gown on body. Some employers require gown removal before placing body in shroud.

Provides privacy and prepares body for viewing.

14. Identify personal belongings that stay with body and those to be given to family.

Prevents loss of valuable or meaningful property.

STEP	RATIONALE

IMPLEMENTATION

15. If family requests viewing, respect individual cultural practices. Otherwise, place clean sheet over body up to chin with arms outside covers. Remove medical equipment from room. Provide soft lighting and chairs.

Maintains respect for patient and those viewing body. Prevents exposure of body parts. Removing medical equipment provides more peaceful, natural setting.

16. Allow family time alone with body and encourage them to say goodbye with religious rituals and in a culturally appropriate manner. Some families want time to sit quietly with the body, console each other, and share memories (National Institute on Aging [NIA], 2017). Some cultural practices include maintaining silence at the time of death, whereas others express grief with intense emotional displays, loud wailing, or "falling out." Do not rush any grieving process.

Compassionate care provides family members with a meaningful experience during the phase of grief. Ensure privacy and a safe environment. Provide chair at bedside for family member who might collapse.

17. After viewing, remove linens and gown per employer policy. Place body in shroud provided by the employer (Fig. 17.3).

Shroud protects injury to skin, avoids exposure of body, and provides barrier against potentially contaminated body fluids.

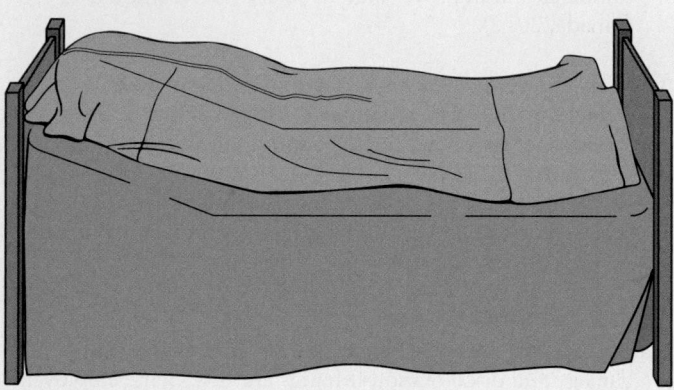
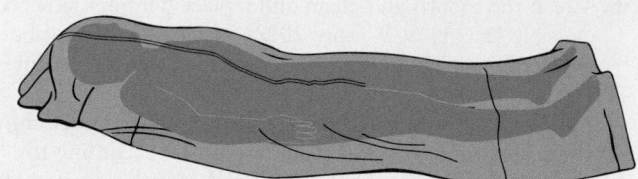

FIG 17.3 Body in shroud.

18. Place identification label on outside of shroud if required by employer policy. Follow employer policy for marking a body that poses an infectious risk to others. Remove and dispose of personal protective equipment and perform hygiene.

Ensures proper identification of body. Reduces exposure of morgue and mortuary staff to contamination.

19. Arrange prompt transportation of body to the mortuary. If you anticipate a delay, transport body to the morgue. If the death occurred at home, inform the family of proper positioning and that a cool room temperature will help maintain the condition of the body.

Mortuary personnel get best results if embalming occurs before full rigor mortis (i.e., stiffening of body after death) occurs.

EVALUATION

1. Observe family members', friends', and significant others' response to the loss.

The need for referral or help is based on evaluation of person's unique response to loss.

2. Note appearance and condition of patient's skin during preparation of the body.

Provides information for postmortem care documentation.

Unexpected Outcomes

1. A family member becomes immobilized with grief and has difficulty functioning.
2. A grieving person becomes agitated and threatens or strikes out against others.

Related Interventions

- Enlist the help of a family member or trusted friend to provide direction and support.
- Call for assistance from a psychiatric nurse practitioner, spiritual care provider, or social worker who has a relationship with the family.
- Enlist help from security staff or crisis intervention professional if safety is a concern.

Communication and Documentation

- Document time of death in the nurses' notes in electronic health record (EHR) or chart, describe any resuscitative measures taken (if applicable), and note the name of the professional certifying the death.
- Document any special preparation of the body for autopsy or organ/tissue donation. Note whom you called and who made the request for organ/tissue donation.
- Document names of mortuary and names of family members consulted at the time of death and their relationship to the deceased.
- Document on appropriate form personal articles left on the body (e.g., teeth or glasses), jewellery taped to skin, or tubes and lines left in place. Note how valuables and personal belongings were handled and who received them. Secure signatures as required by employer policy.
- Document time the body was transported and its destination. Note the location of body identification tags.

Special Considerations
Pediatric

- Offer family members, especially parents, opportunities to be with the child throughout the dying process and help with body preparation.

- Parents frequently want to hold their child's body after death. Parents of deceased newborns often want a memento of their baby (e.g., picture, article of clothing, footprint, or lock of hair). Make every effort to honour parent requests.

Gerontological

- Some older people have very small families and surviving circles of friends. Nurses and other care providers are sometimes the only human presence during death. Arrange for someone to be with the person when death is imminent.

End-of-Life Care in the Community

- After death in the home, follow employer guidelines for body preparation and transfer and for disposal of durable medical equipment (e.g., tubing, needles, syringes), soiled dressings or linens, and medications. Instruct family members in safe and proper handling and disposal of medical waste.

◆ **SKILL 17.3**   **Supporting Ill Persons and Families in Grief**

Grief experiences in situations of serious illness and at the end of life have profound physical, psychological, social, and spiritual effects on dying people, family members, friends, and caregivers. The grief associated with serious illness or death arises from fear of the unknown, pain, sadness about leaving loved ones behind, loss of control, or unresolved guilt.

Hospitalization, chronic illness, and disability involve multiple losses. Hospitalized people lose privacy and control over normal routines. With chronic illness, a person's body no longer functions as it once did, leading to a loss of self-esteem and social roles. Disability and threat of end of life creates financial insecurity and often threatens interpersonal relationships. Death separates people from the physical presence of a person in their lives. Family and friends may also grieve these cumulative losses, whether related to the loss of the person they once knew and the roles they played in their lives, witnessing decline and suffering, or the ultimate loss through death itself. The family is the unit of care throughout the illness and becomes the sole focus of care following the death.

Grief

Grief is the emotional response to a loss, based on personal experiences, psychological makeup, cultural expectations, and family and spiritual beliefs. Losses at the end of life may be financial, physical, emotional, social, or spiritual. Examples of these losses include role changes, altered self-image, or loss of income or relationships. The depth and duration of grief (e.g., one's inner emotional response to loss) depend on the type of loss and the person's perception of it. Coping with grief involves a period of mourning (e.g., the outward, social expressions of grief and the behaviours associated with loss) (Corless, 2015). Mourning behaviours and rituals help grieving individuals adapt to loss, receive social support, adjust expectations, and go forward in life. Most mourning rituals are culturally influenced, learned behaviours. Bereavement is the "state of having lost a significant other" and is the socially recognized period in which those legally or biologically closest to the deceased attend to personal and practical matters related to the death (Corless, 2015, p. 487).

As a nurse, supporting the bereft begins with being compassionately present and assessing the family for bereavement risks. The *Bereavement Risk Assessment Tool (BRAT)* (Victoria Hospice, 2008) is a useful resource for assessing risk for difficult or complicated bereavement and to predict the possible need for additional follow-up or resources to support a grieving family (Murray, 2016). It is also important to understand various types of grief. Normal or uncomplicated grief is evidenced by a variety of physical, cognitive, emotional, and behavioural responses that are as varied as the individuals experiencing them. Some people do not report feeling distressed or depressed, and others feel distressed for a lifetime without negative consequences. Grieving people may also need reassurance that their responses are common reactions to loss. For example, it is not uncommon for family members to feel the presence of the deceased person and to yearn for their return (Corless, 2015). An uncomplicated grief experience often helps a person mature and develop life perspective, although some people may prefer not to process the emotional experience of grief and focus instead on resilience, growth, or positive outcomes after a loss.

Anticipatory grief is an unconscious process that occurs before an actual loss or death and involves gradual disengagement from what is being lost. For example, if a dying process is lengthy, the person and family prepare for death before it occurs and sometimes, but not always, display fewer common grief responses at the time of death (Corless, 2015).

Complicated grief is characterized by prolonged and intense emotional distress related to loss that may interfere with daily functioning. Criteria for a person experiencing complicated grief may include denial, repression, or avoidance of the loss and associated pain or intense preoccupation with or yearning for the deceased (Corless, 2015). Timelines and criteria for differentiating between

a brief depressive episode related to complicated or even normal grief and a major depressive episode vary. For example, the bereavement clause was removed from the *Diagnostic and Statistical Manual of Mental Disorders*, 5th edition (American Psychiatric Association, 2013), leading to earlier intervention in grief responses that meet the criteria for a major depressive episode. This has led to concerns about the medicalization of a normal human response to loss.

Use evidence-informed tools, such as the BRAT, to assess for depression and refer for follow-up and counselling as needed. Although distinguishing between a brief, bereavement-related depressive episode and major depression may be difficult, research indicates that people experiencing a bereavement-related depressive episode are less likely than those with non-bereavement-related depression to feel worthless, to withdraw from others, to engage in social conflict, to self-medicate, to have thoughts of suicide or want to die, or to feel distress (McCabe, & Christopher, 2016).

Use basic knowledge of grief responses to support patients and their families and to address other common psychosocial and spiritual symptoms at the end of life. Families and friends may talk openly about a person's approaching death, and others may choose not to acknowledge it. Health care providers, depending on their own personal and cultural understandings of grief and death, often avoid initiating conversations on these difficult topics. Provide opportunities for discussion, paying close attention to a person's response and indications of a desire to talk further.

Delegation and Collaboration

The skills of assessing patients' or family members' grief reactions and designing appropriate interventions cannot be delegated to an unregulated care provider (UCP). The nurse directs the UCP to:

- Inform the nurse when a patient or family member exhibits behaviour commonly associated with grief (e.g., crying, anger, withdrawal).
- Form supportive relationships with patients and families and inform the nurse when patients or family members have questions or concerns.
- Alert the nurse to the arrival of family members so the nurse can discuss the plan of care and offer support.

STEP	RATIONALE

ASSESSMENT

1. Sit near patient in a quiet, private location. Centre yourself and establish quiet, compassionate presence. Establish eye contact. Be aware that use of sustained eye contact in some cultures conveys disrespect or may cause discomfort.

A willingness to be present with another in their suffering expresses compassion and offers opportunities for healing (Borneman & Brown-Saltzman, 2015). Privacy protects confidentiality and promotes a sense of safety for patient when expressing thoughts and emotions.

2. Consider the influence of patient's cultural background on communication. Apply principles of plain language and health literacy during assessment (NCP, 2013).

Individual differences influence patient's grief response and communication style (Corless, 2015).

3. Listen carefully to patient's story. Observe patient responses. Use open communication. As a nurse, listen carefully to understand the significance of a loss to a patient or family member, identify concerns, and assess their ability to sustain hope and move forward in life.

Develops trust in a caring relationship. Actively listening to patient's concerns and verbalizing patient's needs convey empathy and compassion (Doherty & Thompson, 2014).

4. Determine meaning of the loss to patient: its type, suddenness, and when it occurred. Use open-ended questions such as:
   - "Tell me how your loss affects your family."
   - "You said your illness was unexpected. Describe how that made you feel?"

The type, meaning, suddenness, and time elapsed since the loss influence the grief experience and coping methods.

5. Combine knowledge of grief theory and responses with observation of patient behaviours. Validate observations by sharing them with patient; paraphrase, clarify, or summarize, as in the following examples:
   - "You've mentioned several times that you feel hopeless."
   - "It seems that this is hard for you to talk about."
   - "You look sad. Is there something in particular that brought on your tears?"

Use information about grief theory and common grief responses to guide discussion, not to judge patient's responses. Confirms accuracy of your observations and validates patient's feelings. Prompts patient to continue.

6. Encourage patient to describe the loss and its impact on daily life (e.g., "You said your diagnosis changed your life forever. Tell me more").

Listening to patient's description helps to minimize assumptions.

7. Ask patient to describe the coping strategies that they use most often in difficult times (e.g., "What or who helps you in times of crisis?").

Familiar, effective coping strategies are often helpful in the current crisis, loss, or grief experience.

8. Assess caregivers' unique needs and resources. Note if patient receives care at home and who gives the care.

Illness significantly affects caregiver and family relationships. Although they experience similar issues, their needs may differ.

STEP	RATIONALE

ASSESSMENT

9. Assess patient's spiritual needs, beliefs, and resources. Focus on aspects likely to be involved (e.g., trust, feelings of connectedness, life meaning and purpose, faith/belief, and hope). The *FICA Spiritual History Tool* is a helpful resource (Puchalski, 2014).

Identifies patient's spiritual beliefs and values. Enables patient autonomy by identifying beliefs and preferences for care or rituals related to faith or spirituality. Offers a greater understanding of patient's culture and values, leading to patient-centred care (Hodge, 2015).

NURSING DIAGNOSES

- Inappropriate denial
- Hopelessness
- Compromised family coping
- Death anxiety
- Anxiety

- Fear
- Potential for complicated grieving
- Potential for spiritual distress
- Potential for caregiver role strain
- Readiness for enhanced hope

- Readiness for enhanced coping
- Readiness for enhanced family coping
- Grieving

Related factors/Risk factors are individualized on the basis of patient's condition or needs.

PLANNING

1. Expected outcomes following completion of procedures:
   - Patient maintains relationships with significant people.
   - Patient expresses grief in keeping with their cultural and religious practices.
   - Patient uses effective coping strategies.
   - Patient maintains normal life routines.

Patient in grief or loss retains connections with social network.
Patient receives support necessary to retain cherished values and ways of being.
Patient identifies sense of relief and peace.
Patient adjusts to life-changing circumstances and maintains sense of control.

IMPLEMENTATION

1. Show an empathic understanding of patient's strengths and needs. Provide compassionate presence.
2. Offer information about patient's illness and treatment. Clarify misunderstandings or misinformation. Use culturally appropriate language and simple terms.
3. Encourage patient to sustain relationships with others to help maintain independence and receive necessary help. Include patient-identified support people in discussions.
4. Help patient achieve short-term goals (e.g., symptom relief, task completion, resolution of relational problems).
5. Provide frequent opportunities for patient and family members to express their fears and concerns. Be attentive to expressions of intense emotions.
6. Educate and support patient and family. Discuss procedures, plan of care, and anticipated changes. Use interprofessional collaboration as appropriate to support patient's needs and preferences.
7. Instruct patient in relaxation strategies: mindfulness-based stress reduction, guided imagery, meditation, hand massage, healing touch (see Chapter 16).
8. Encourage visits with loved ones, life review with stories or photographs, or projects such as organizing photo albums or journal writing.
9. Facilitate patient's religious/spiritual practices and connections with religious community. Use prayer or music and provide a listening presence. Make a referral to a spiritual-care provider if appropriate.

Promotes nurse–patient trust, caring, compassion, and empathy (Doherty & Thompson, 2014).
Misunderstanding adds to patient's uncertainty, anxiety, and suffering.

Affiliation with others offers support and helps patient stay engaged in life.

Helping patients identify and meet their personal goals contributes to their quality of life.
Emotions change quickly and frequently during stress and complicate communication for nurses and patients.

Provides emotional support and comfort, decreases anxiety, and allows patient to rest. Advocating for patient encourages patient autonomy and incorporates patient preferences into plan of care (Arbour & Wingard, 2014).
Complementary therapies have been shown in select cases to relieve anxiety and effectively reduce stress, thus providing useful coping strategies (Stomski, Petterson, Kristjanson, et al., 2018).
Reviewing positive and negative events in one's life allows a person to find meaning in their experiences, resolve conflicts, and come to a place of acceptance (Keall, Clayton, & Butow 2015).
Spiritual interventions help patients maintain hope and connect with the core of their identity. Spiritual interventions can decrease anxiety, promote a sense of peace, and help patients find meaning in their life (Goncalves, Lucchetti, Menezes, et al., 2017).

STEP	RATIONALE

EVALUATION

1. Note patient descriptions of relationships and activities with others.
2. Observe patient's behaviours during ongoing interactions.
3. Elicit patient perceptions of benefit gained from use of coping interventions.
4. Discuss progress toward performing routine activities at home.

Provides information on extent to which patient retains relational ties.
Demonstrates patient's ability to express grief and coping.
Evaluates efficacy of interventions.

Evaluates patient's achievement of desired goals or need for goal revision.

Unexpected Outcomes
1. Patient does not acknowledge loss and shows signs of extreme sorrow, anger, withdrawal, or denial.
2. Family and patient relationships do not give patient needed support.

Related Interventions
- Consider referral to grief specialist professional (e.g., nurse practitioner, psychologist, spiritual-care provider, social worker).
- Share and validate observations of family strain or patient concern over family interactions.
- Consider family–patient discussion with health care team.

Communication and Documentation

- Document interventions used to support patient coping and note patient's verbal and nonverbal responses in nurses' notes in electronic health record (EHR) or chart.
- Report patient's grief reactions to members of the interprofessional team, noting behaviours that affect health outcomes such as treatment refusals or prolonged inactivity.

Special Considerations
Teaching

- Give caregivers and family members basic information about common grief responses and how to offer support. Coach them on ways to provide physical, emotional, and spiritual support to patient and one another (e.g., providing basic hygiene, listening attentively, avoiding false reassurances, allowing for the expression of difficult emotions, talking about normal family activities).

Pediatric

- Children's understanding of death is influenced by age and developmental level and differs from that of adults. Respect parents' wishes about when and what to tell children about illness or death. When discussing sensitive topics with children, encourage parents to offer caring explanations at a level a child is able to understand. Avoid using euphemisms for death. Instead, use the words *die* or *died* to prevent confusion, especially among young children.
- Play therapy or drawing helps children express thoughts, emotions, or fears about illness or death.
- Be alert to all family members' grief reactions because they may feel guilt, resentment, or helplessness with the illness or death of a sibling, child, or grandchild. Facilitate communication with family members who must be separated from the child.
- Surrogate decision makers, usually the parents, need to make health care decisions for infants and young children. Some decisions are difficult because outcomes in children are often unpredictable.

Gerontological

- Losing a spouse after a long and satisfying relationship is very difficult and is essentially a loss of self. The mourning is as much for oneself as for the individual (Touhy et al., 2019).
- Intense grief may cause a temporary decrease in cognitive function that can manifest as confusion (Touhy et al., 2019).
- Many older persons have coexisting medical conditions that add to their symptom burden. They also have lived long enough to have experienced cumulative losses, including members of their family and community, which complicates their grief experience.

✦CLINICAL DEBRIEF

You are caring for an older adult male who is hospitalized for abdominal pain, anorexia, weight loss, and weakness. He was treated 10 years earlier for prostate cancer. Test results now confirm that he has a large tumour in his abdomen and the cancer has spread to the lymph nodes. No medical interventions are available to cure his disease. When you enter the room, the patient tells you in an angry voice that he wants to transfer to a different hospital where people will help him fight his cancer.
1. Which approaches should you use in response to his statement?
2. The next day the patient reports mild abdominal pain and mentions that he has not had a bowel movement for 3 days. His partner reports to you that he has not had anything to eat or drink for 24 hours.

a. What might be the cause of the patient not having a bowel movement?
b. List three interventions to provide.
3. Four weeks later you take care of this patient again. His symptoms include weight loss, anorexia, worsening abdominal pain, depression, and anxiety. His partner tells you that the nurse practitioner asked them if they would be open to a consult to the specialist palliative care team. His partner says to you, "I'm still not sure if palliative care would be best for us." Which key points would you include in a discussion with the patient and partner about palliative care? Using SBAR, show how you would communicate your assessment with the other health care providers.

✦ REVIEW QUESTIONS

1. The nurse is caring for a patient with cancer who has been admitted to the palliative care unit. What are the goals of palliative care? *(Select all that apply.)*
   1. Physical symptom management
   2. Facilitating maintenance of cultural and spiritual preferences
   3. Curative care
   4. Extending life as long as possible
   5. Providing a dignified death
   6. Improving quality of life

2. A nurse suggests that a patient receive a consult to a specialist palliative care team for symptom management related to anxiety and increasing pain. A family member asks the nurse if this means that the patient is dying. What should the nurse tell the patient and family about the care the patient is receiving? *(Select all that apply.)*
   1. Palliative care and end-of-life care are the same thing.
   2. Palliative care is for any patient, any time with any chronic disease, in any setting.
   3. A specialty palliative care team helps regular caregivers manage complex symptoms.
   4. Palliative care interventions relieve suffering and the symptoms of illness and treatment.

3. A nurse has the responsibility of managing a deceased patient's postmortem care. Arrange the steps for postmortem care in the proper order.
   1. Bathe the deceased's body.
   2. Collect any needed specimens.
   3. Remove all drains and in-dwelling tubes.
   4. Position the body for family visit and viewing.
   5. Speak to the family members about their possible participation.
   6. Confirm that request for organ/tissue donation and/or autopsy has been made.
   7. Notify a support person (e.g., spiritual-care provider, bereavement specialist) for the family.
   8. Accurately tag the body, indicating deceased's identity and safety issues regarding infection control.

ⓔ *Visit the Evolve site for a complete list of Clinical Debrief and Review Questions answers.*

REFERENCES

Accreditation Canada. (2019). *Required organizational practices handbook—Version 14.* Retrieved from http://www.wrha.mb.ca/quality/files/2019ROPHandbook.pdf

American Association of Colleges of Nursing (AACN). (2016). *Competencies and recommendations for educating undergraduate nursing students: Preparing nurses to care for the seriously ill and their families.* Retrieved from https://www.aacnnursing.org/Portals/42/ELNEC/PDF/New-Palliative-Care-Competencies.pdf

American Cancer Society (ACS). (2016). *Physical symptoms in the last 2 to 3 months of life.* Retrieved from http://www.cancer.org/treatment/nearingtheendoflife/nearingtheendoflife/nearing-the-end-of-life-physical-symptoms

American Psychiatric Association. (2013). *Diagnostic and statistical manual of mental disorders* (5th ed.). Washington, DC: Author.

Anderson, I. (n.d.). *Indigenous perspectives on death and dying. Ian Anderson continuing education program in end-of-life care* [PPT]. Retrieved from http://www.cpd.utoronto.ca/endoflife/PPT%20Indigenous%20Perspectives.pdf

Andrew, E., Nehme, Z., Bernard, S., & Smith, K. (2017). The influence of comorbidity on survival and long-term outcomes after out-of-hospital cardiac arrest. *Resuscitation, 110,* 42–47. doi:10.1016/j.resuscitation.2016.10.018

Arbour, R., & Wiegand, D. (2014). Self-described nursing roles experienced during care of dying patients and their families: A phenomenological study. *Intensive Critical Care Nursing, 30*(4), 211–218.

Ariadne Labs. (n.d.). *Serious illness care resources* [Website]. Boston, MA: Author. Retrieved from https://www.ariadnelabs.org/areas-of-work/serious-illness-care/resources/#Downloads&%20Tools

Bailey, F., & Harmon, S. (2018). Palliative care: The last hours and days of life. *UpToDate.* Retrieved from http://www.uptodate.com/contents/palliative-care-the-last-hours-and-days-of-life

Borneman, T., & Brown-Saltzman, K. (2015). Meaning in illness. In B. R. Ferrell, N. Coyle, & J. Paice (Eds.), *Textbook of palliative nursing* (4th ed.). New York: Oxford University Press.

Burchum, J. R., & Rosenthal, L. D. (2016). *Lehne's pharmacology for nursing care* (9th ed.). St. Louis: Elsevier.

Calgary Laboratory Services. (2019). *Autopsy information for next of kin.* Retrieved from http://www.calgarylabservices.com/lab-services-guide/anatomic-cytopathology/autopsy/autopsy-information-next-of-kin.aspx

Canadian Association of Schools of Nursing (CASN). (2011). *Palliative and end-of-life care entry-to-practice competencies and indicators for registered nurses.* Ottawa, ON: Author. Retrieved from https://casn.ca/wp-content/uploads/2014/12/PEOLCCompetenciesandIndicatorsEn1.pdf

Canadian Hospice Palliative Care Association (CHPCA). (2015). *The way forward national framework: A roadmap for an integrated palliative approach to care.* Retrieved from http://www.hpcintegration.ca/media/60044/TWF-framework-doc-Eng-2015-final-April1.pdf

Canadian Hospice Palliative Care Association (CHPCA). (2017). *Hospice palliative care and medical assistance in dying (MAiD) in Canada: How will they co-exist? Guidance for health care professionals.* Retrieved from http://www.chpca.net/media/540325/chpca-maid-booklet-eng-12page-final-web.pdf

Canadian Hospice Palliative Care Association (CHPCA). (2019a). *FAQs.* Retrieved from http://www.chpca.net/family-caregivers/faqs.aspx

Canadian Hospice Palliative Care Association (CHPCA). (2019b). *Who will speak for you?* Retrieved from http://www.advancecareplanning.ca

Canadian Hospice Palliative Care Nursing Standards Sub-Committee. (2014). *Canadian hospice palliative care nursing standards of practice.* Retrieved from http://acsp.net/media/367211/chpc_ng.standards.2014.14_july_2014.final.pdf

Canadian Medical Protective Society (CMPS). (2016). *Completing medical certificates of death: Who's responsible?* Retrieved from https://www.cmpa-acpm.ca/en/advice-publications/browse-articles/2016/completing-medical-certificates-of-death-who-s-responsible

Canadian Nurses Association (CNA). (2015). *Respecting choices in end-of-life care: Challenges and opportunities for RNs.* Ottawa, ON: Author. Retrieved from https://canadian-nurse.com/~/media/canadian-nurse/files/pdf%20en/respecting-choices-in-end-of-life-care.pdf

Canadian Nurses Association (CNA). (2017a). *Code of ethics for registered nurses.* Ottawa, ON: Author. Retrieved from https://cna-aiic.ca/~/media/cna/page-content/pdf-en/code-of-ethics-2017-edition-secure-interactive.pdf?la=en

Canadian Nurses Association (CNA). (2017b). *National nursing framework on medical assistance in dying in Canada.* Retrieved from https://www.cna-aiic.ca/~/media/cna/page-content/pdf-en/cna-national-nursing-framework-on-maid.pdf?la=en

Canadian Virtual Hospice. (2016). *Living my culture* [website]. Retrieved from http://livingmyculture.ca/culture/

Canadian Virtual Hospice. (2017). [*Home page*]. Retrieved from http://www.virtualhospice.ca/en_US/Main+Site+Navigation/Home.aspx

Caraccia Economou, D. (2015). Bowel management: Constipation, diarrhea, obstruction, and ascites. In B. R. Ferrell, N. Coyle, & J. Paice (Eds.), *Textbook of palliative nursing* (4th ed.). New York: Oxford University Press.

Claridge, J. (2017). *Rigor mortis and lividity* [website]. Retrieved from http://www.exploreforensics.co.uk/rigor-mortis-and-lividity.html

Clark, D. (2014, September 25). *'Total pain': The work of Cicely Saunders and the maturing of a concept.* Retrieved from http://endoflifestudies.academicblogs.co.uk/total-pain-the-work-of-cicely-saunders-and-the-maturing-of-a-concept/

Clark, K., & Currow, D. (2011). Advancing research into symptoms of constipation at the end of life. *International Journal of Palliative Nursing, 20*(8), 370–372. doi:10.12968/ijpn.2014.20.8.370

Corless, I. B. (2015). Bereavement. In B. R. Ferrell, N. Coyle, & J. Paice (Eds.), *Textbook of palliative nursing* (4th ed.). New York: Oxford University Press.

Davison, S. N., & Jhangri, G. S. (2014). Knowledge and attitudes of Canadian First Nations people toward organ donation and transplantation: A quantitative and qualitative analysis. *American Journal of Kidney Diseases, 64*(5), 781–789. doi:10.1053/j.ajkd.2014.06.029

Dean, M. M., Cellarius, V., Henry, B., Oneschuk, D., & Librach, S. L. (2012). Framework for continuous palliative sedation therapy (CPST) in Canada. *Journal of Palliative Medicine, 15*(8), 870–879. doi:10.1089/jpm.2011.0498

Doherty, M., & Thompson, H. (2014). Enhancing person-centered care through the development of a therapeutic relationship. *British Journal of Community Nursing*, 19(10), 504–507. doi:10.12968/bjcn.2014.19.10.502

Dosser, I., & Kennedy, C. (2014). Improving family caregivers' experiences of support at the end of life by enhancing communication: An action research study. *International Journal of Palliative Nursing*, 20(12), 608–616. doi:10.12968/ijpn.2014.20.12.608

Dudgeon, D. (2015). Dyspnea, terminal secretions, and cough. In B. R. Ferrell, N. Coyle, & J. Paice (Eds.), *Textbook of palliative nursing* (4th ed.). New York: Oxford University Press.

Findlater, C., & Thomson, E. (2018). Organ donation and management of the potential organ donor. *Anesthesia and Intensive Care Medicine*, 19(10), 527–533. doi:10.1016/j.mpaic.2015.04.013

Gillespie, L., & Raftery, A. (2014). Nutrition in palliative and end-of-life care. *British Journal of Community Nursing*, 19(Sup7).

Goncalves, J., Lucchetti, G., Menezes, P., & Vallada, H. (2017). Complementary religious and spiritual interventions in physical health and quality of life: A systematic review of randomized controlled clinical trials. *PlosOne*, 12(10), e0186539. doi:10.1371/journal.pone.0186539

Government of Canada. (2016a). *Bill C-14: An Act to amend the Criminal Code and to make related amendments to other Acts (medical assistance in dying)*. Ottawa: Public Works and Government Services Canada. Retrieved from http://www.parl.ca/DocumentViewer/en/42-1/bill/C-14/royal-assent. (2016). 1st Reading, April 14, 2016, 42nd Parliament, 1st Session.

Government of Canada. (2016b). *Home and community care*. Retrieved from https://www.canada.ca/en/indigenous-services-canada/services/first-nations-inuit-health/health-care-services/home-community-care.html

Government of Canada. (2017). *Bill C-277: Framework on Palliative Care in Canada Act*. Ottawa: Public Works and Government Services Canada. Retrieved from http://www.parl.ca/DocumentViewer/en/42-1/bill/C-277/royal-assent. (2017). 1st Reading, May 30, 2016, 42nd Parliament, 1st Session.

Gray, M., & Sims, T. (2015). Urinary tract disorders. In B. R. Ferrell, N. Coyle, & J. Paice (Eds.), *Textbook of palliative nursing* (4th ed.). New York: Oxford University Press.

Hadders, H., Paulson, B., & Fougner, V. (2014). Relatives' participation at the time of death: Standardisation in pre- and post-mortem care in a palliative medical unit. *European Journal of Oncology Nursing*, 18(2), 159–166. doi:10.1016/j.ejon.2013.11.004

Heidrich, D. E., & English, N. K. (2015). Delirium, confusion, agitation, and restlessness. In B. R. Ferrell, N. Coyle, & J. Paice (Eds.), *Textbook of palliative nursing* (4th ed.). New York: Oxford University Press.

Henry, C., & Wilson, J. (2012). Personal care at the end of life and after death. *Nursing Times*, 108. Retrieved from https://www.nursingtimes.net/clinical-archive/end-of-life-and-palliative-care/personal-care-at-the-end-of-life-and-after-death/5044559.article

Hockenberry, M. J., & Wilson, D. (2015). *Wong's nursing care of infants and children* (10th ed.). St. Louis: Mosby.

Hodge, D. R. (2015). Administering a two-stage spiritual assessment in healthcare settings: A necessary component of ethical and effective care. *Journal of Nursing Management*, 23(1), 27–38. doi:10.1111/jonm.12078

Horst, G. R. (2017, December). *Care of the body after death*. Retrieved from http://www.virtualhospice.ca/en_US/Main+Site+Navigation/Home/Topics/Topics/Final+Days/Care+of+the+Body+After+Death.aspx

iPANEL. (2012). *Initiative for a palliative approach in nursing: Evidence and leadership* [website]. Retrieved from http://www.ipanel.ca/

Keall, R. M., Clayton, J. M., & Butow, P. N. (2015). Therapeutic life review in palliative care: A systematic review of quantitative evaluations. *Journal of Pain and Symptom Management*, 49(4), 747–761. doi:10.1016/j.jpainsymman.2014.08.015

Kravits, K. (2015). Complementary and alternative therapies in palliative care. In B. R. Ferrell, N. Coyle, & J. Paice (Eds.), *Textbook of palliative nursing* (4th ed.). New York: Oxford University Press.

Matzo, M., & Hill, J. (2014). Peri-death nursing care. In M. Matzo & D. Sherman (Eds.), *Palliative care nursing: Quality care at the end of life* (4th ed.). New York: Springer.

McCabe, P. J., & Christopher, P. P. (2016). Symptom and functional traits of brief major depressive episodes and discrimination of bereavement. *Depression and Anxiety*, 33(2), 112–119. doi:10.1002/da.22446

Moir, C., Roberts, R., Martz, K., Perry, J., & Tivis, L. J. (2015). Communicating with patients and their families about palliative and end-of-life care: Comfort and educational needs of nurses. *International Journal of Palliative Nursing*, 21(3), 109–112. doi:10.12968/ijpn.2015.21.3.109

Murray, K. (2016). *Essentials in hospice and palliative care: A practical resource for every nurse*. Victoria, BC: Life and Death Matters.

National Consensus Project (NCP) for Quality Palliative Care. (2018). *Clinical practice guidelines for quality palliative care* (4th ed.). Retrieved from https://www.nationalcoalitionhpc.org/wp-content/uploads/2018/10/NCHPC-NCPGuidelines_4thED_web_FINAL.pdf

National Institute on Aging (NIA). (2017). *What to do after someone dies*. Retrieved from https://www.nia.nih.gov/health/publication/end-life-helping-comfort-and-care/things-do-after-someone-dies

Norris, S. (2018). Consent for organ donation in Canada. *Library of Parliament*. Retrieved from https://hillnotes.ca/2018/01/23/consent-for-organ-donation-in-canada/

Nova Scotia Health Authority (NSHA). (2017). *The Nova Scotia Palliative Care Competency Framework: A reference guide for health professionals and volunteers*. Halifax, NS: Author. Retrieved from https://library.nshealth.ca/ld.php?content_id=34202519

Nova Scotia Health Authority (NSHA). (2019). *Conversations about serious illness*. Retrieved from https://library.nshealth.ca/SeriousIllness

O'Neil-Page, E., Anderson, P. R., & Dean, G. E. (2015). Fatigue. In B. R. Ferrell, N. Coyle, & J. Paice (Eds.), *Textbook of palliative nursing* (4th ed.). New York: Oxford University Press.

Paice, J. (2015). Pain at the end of life. In B. R. Ferrell, N. Coyle, & J. Paice (Eds.), *Textbook of palliative nursing* (4th ed.). New York: Oxford University Press.

Puchalski, C. M. (2014). The FICA spiritual history tool #274. *Journal of Palliative Medicine*, 17(1), 105–106. doi:10.1089/jpm.2013.9458

Rainone, F. (2015). Palliative sedation: Controversies and challenges. *Progress in Palliative Care*, 23(3), 153–162. doi:10.1179/1743291X15Y.0000000004

Regan, A., Tapley, M., & Jolley, D. (2014). Improving end-of-life care for people with dementia. *Nursing Standards*, 28(48), 37–43. doi:10.7748/ns.28.48.37.e8760

Reichlin, M. (2014). On the ethics of withholding and withdrawing medical treatment. *Multidisciplinary Respiratory Medicine*, 9(1), 39. doi:10.1186/2049-6958-9-39

Rindfleisch, J. A. (n.d.). *Whole health: Change the conversation. Spiritual assessment tools*. Retrieved from http://projects.hsl.wisc.edu/SERVICE/modules/11/M11_Spiritual_Assessment_Tools.pdf

Rodrigues, P., Crokaert, J., & Gastmans, C. (2018). Palliative sedation for existential suffering: A systematic review of argument-based ethics literature. *Journal of Pain and Symptom Management*, 55(6), 1577–1590. doi:10.1016/j.jpainsymman.2018.01.013

Santucci, G., & Battista, V. (2015). Methylnaltrexone for opioid-induced constipation in patients at the end of life. *International Journal of Palliative Nursing*, 21(4), 162–164. doi:10.12968/ijpn.2015.21.4.162

Scarborough, P. (2016). *Palliative wound care: Balancing the burdens and benefits for patients on hospice care* [PowerPoint slides]. Retrieved from http://cchospice.org/wp-content/uploads/2016/09/G4-Palliative-Wound-Care.pdf

Schildmann, E. K., Schildmann, J., & Kiesewetter, I. (2015). Medication and monitoring in palliative sedation therapy: A systematic review and quality assessment of published guidelines. *Journal of Pain and Symptom Management*, 49(4), 734–746. doi:10.1016/j.jpainsymman.2014.08.013

Shaw, C., & Eldridge, L. (2015). Nutritional considerations for the palliative care patient. *International Journal of Palliative Nursing*, 21(1), 7–8, 10, 12–15. doi:10.12968/ijpn.2015.21.1.7

Statistics Canada. (2015). *Canadian coroner and medical examiner database: Annual report*. Retrieved from https://www.statcan.gc.ca/pub/82-214-x/2012001/int-eng.htm#cl

Stenekes, S., & Streeter, L. (2017). *Considerations for a home death*. Retrieved from http://www.virtualhospice.ca/en_US/Main+Site+Navigation/Home/Topics/Topics/Decisions/Considerations+for+a+Home+Death.aspx

Stomski, N., Petterson, A., Kristjanson, L., et al. (2018). The effect of self-selected complementary therapies on cancer patients' quality of life and symptom distress: A prospective cohort study in an integrative oncology setting. *Complementary Therapies in Medicine*, 37, 1–5. doi:10.1016/j.ctim.2018.01.006

Sulzgruber, P., Sterz, F., Poppe, M., et al. (2017). Age-specific prognostication after out-of-hospital cardiac arrest—The ethical dilemma between 'life-sustaining treatment' and 'the right to die' in the elderly. *European Heart Journal: Acute Cardiovascular Care*, 6(2), 112–120. doi:10.1177/2048872616672076

Thomas, K., & Armstrong Wilson, P., GSF Team. (2016). *The gold standards framework proactive identification guidance (PIG)* (6th ed.). National Gold Standards Framework Centre in End of Life Care. Retrieved from https://www.goldstandardsframework.org.uk/cd-content/uploads/files/PIG/NEW%20PIG%20-%20%20%202020.1.17%20KT%20vs17.pdf

Touhy, T. A., Jett, K. F., Boscart, V., & McCleary, L. (2019). *Ebersole and Hess' gerontological nursing and healthy aging* (2nd Canadian ed.). Toronto, ON: Elsevier Canada.

University of Edinburgh. (2017). *Supportive and palliative care indicators tool (SPICT™)*. Retrieved from https://www.spict.org.uk/

Victoria Hospice. (2001). *Palliative performance scale version 2 (PPSv2)*. Retrieved from https://www.victoriahospice.org/i-am-health-care-professional/clinical-tools

Victoria Hospice. (2008). *Bereavement risk assessment tool (BRAT)*. Retrieved from https://www.victoriahospice.org/i-am-health-care-professional/clinical-tools

Victoria Hospice. (n.d.). *Psychosocial assessment*. Retrieved from https://www.victoriahospice.org/i-am-health-care-professional/clinical-tools

Watanabe, S. M., Nekolaichuk, C., Beaumont, C., Johnson, L., Myers, J., & Strasser, F. (2011). A multi-centre comparison of two numerical versions of the Edmonton Symptom Assessment System in palliative care patients. *Journal of Pain Symptom Management*, 41, 456–468.

Wilson, D. J., & Michael, K. (2015). Rehabilitation and palliative care. In B. R. Ferrell, N. Coyle, & J. Paice (Eds.), *Textbook of palliative nursing* (4th ed.). New York: Oxford University Press.

World Health Organization. (2018). *WHO definition of palliative care*. Geneva: Author. Retrieved from http://www.who.int/cancer/palliative/definition/en/

You, J., Fowler, R. A., & Heyland, D. K. (2014). Just ask: Discussing goals of care with patients in hospital with serious illness. *Canadian Medical Association Journal*, 186(6), 425–432. doi:10.1503/cmaj.121274

18 | Personal Hygiene and Bed Making

Written by **Jennifer Painter, MSN, APRN, CNS, RN-BC, OCN, AOCNS; and Ashley Crane, RN, MN**

OBJECTIVES

Mastery of content in this chapter will enable the nurse to:
- Discuss clinical guidelines to use for providing personal hygiene to patients.
- Identify principles of aseptic technique applied while administering a bed bath.
- Administer a complete bed bath.
- Explain precautions to take when assisting patients with a tub bath or shower.
- Discuss precautions for minimizing transmission of infection during hygienic care.
- Identify clinical guidelines to follow when administering oral hygiene.

- Explain differences in providing oral hygiene for dependent patients and that for unconscious patients.
- Identify clinical guidelines for administering hair, nail, and foot care.
- Comb, brush, and shampoo the hair of a bed-bound patient.
- Shave a patient safely.
- Identify risk factors for foot and nail problems.
- Safely administer nail care.
- Change the linen on an unoccupied bed and on an occupied bed.

MEDIA RESOURCES

- **evolve** http://evolve.elsevier.com/Canada/Perry/clinicalskills/
- Review Questions
- Case Studies

- ▶ Video Clips
- Audio Glossary
- Clinical Debrief and Review Questions Answers

PURPOSE

Hygiene is important for promoting and preserving physical and mental health. When the nurse delivers hygiene to a patient, it is an excellent time to discuss health-related concerns, perform a physical assessment, and provide patient education. Providing personal hygiene is also necessary for an individual's comfort, safety, and sense of well-being.

STANDARDS OF CARE

- Accreditation Canada, 2019—*Required Organizational Practices Handbook—Version 14* (http://www.wrha.mb.ca/quality/files/2019ROPHandbook.pdf
- Agency for Healthcare Research and Quality (AHRQ), 2013a—*Bathing the Patient With Dementia*
- Canadian Dental Association, 2019d—*Your Oral Health* (https://www.cda-adc.ca/en/oral_health/index.asp)

- Wound Care Canada, 2017—*Foundations of Best Practice for Skin and Wound Management* (https://www.woundscanada.ca/health-care-professional/resources-health-care-pros/12-healthcare-professional/110-supplements)

PRINCIPLES FOR PRACTICE

- Regular bathing of all patients is essential to maintaining skin integrity by promoting circulation and hydration.
- When bathing people with dementia, it is important to balance the need for patient independence and privacy with the requirement to ensure that the patient is safe (Alzheimer Society Canada [ASC], 2017).
- When providing patient hygiene, maintain a patient's privacy and comfort and encourage patients to participate in their hygiene care.

PERSON-CENTRED CARE

- As a nurse, always convey sensitivity and respect for a patient's personal cultural beliefs and habits in the way you provide hygiene. For example, modesty is very important for Muslims. They prefer a health care provider of the same sex and for the provider to request permission before uncovering any part of the body (Rassool, 2015).
- Skin problems cause changes that affect a patient's appearance and body image. Be sensitive to a patient's feelings while caring for skin problems.
- It is important to know if a patient's ethnicity requires certain customs to be followed in the way personal hygiene is performed.
- Be sure to take each patient's preferences into consideration when providing hygiene. Simply asking patients about their preferences (e.g., products to use, best time to perform aspects of hygiene) can create a more trusting and nurturing environment.
- Have an awareness of cultural considerations and assess the patient's self-care ability to provide culturally sensitive person-centered care.
- Some patients living with dementia have apprehension about and possibly fear bathing (ASC, 2017). The dignity of patients with dementia can be preserved by shifting the focus of care from tasks of bathing to needs and abilities of the person—practise person-centred care and make the bathing experience as pleasant for the patient as possible.

EVIDENCE-INFORMED PRACTICE

- Recent evidence supports the use of daily bathing with chlorhexidine gluconate (CHG) to reduce the rate of health care–associated infections (HAIs). CHG should not be used for patients with an allergy to CHG, for bathing above the jawline to avoid exposure to mucous membranes, and on areas of skin breakdown (Noto, Domenico, Byrne, et al., 2015).
- Results from multiple studies conducted in long-term acute care facilities and in both medical and surgical intensive care units support daily bathing with 2% CHG (cloths or in bath water) as it substantially reduces colonization and bloodstream HAIs, including methicillin-resistant *Staphylococcus aureus* (MRSA) and vancomycin-resistant *Enterococcus* (VRE) infections (Lowe, Lloyd-Smith, Sidhu, et al., 2017; Raines & Rosen, 2016).
- A systematic review and meta-analysis confirmed that 2% CHG reduces central line–associated bloodstream infections (CLABSIs) (Shah, Schwartz, Luna, et al., 2016). CHG-impregnated bathing cloths are more expensive than using CHG solution in bath water; however, both methods of bathing are effective. If using CHG solution in bath water, it is important to reserve a bath basin only for bathing and not for storage. Bathing should be provided daily. Use of CHG-impregnated bathing cloths is well tolerated by the skin and is effective against a wide spectrum of Gram-positive and Gram-negative bacteria, including MRSA.

SAFETY GUIDELINES

- Patients who are totally dependent on someone else require help with personal hygiene or must learn or adapt to new hygiene techniques. When providing personal hygiene, important safety principles to follow are prevention of infection and of patient injury.
- Keep all personal-hygiene care items within a patient's reach. When the head of the bed is raised, the bedside stand is usually not within easy reach and must be moved forward. If a patient must leave the bed to go to the bathroom, be sure that there is a clear pathway to prevent falls.
- Use clean gloves when you anticipate contact with nonintact skin or mucous membranes or when there is or may likely be contact with drainage, secretions, excretions, or blood. Additional precautions requiring other personal protective equipment (PPE) may be necessary, depending on the patient's condition (see Chapter 5).
- To reduce the risk of infection, always perform hygiene measures moving from cleanest to less clean or dirty areas. This often requires a change of gloves and performing hand hygiene during care activities.
- When using water or solutions for hygiene care, be sure to test the solution temperature to prevent burn injury. This is especially important for patients with reduced sensation, such as those with diabetes mellitus, peripheral neuropathy, or spinal cord injury. It is also important for patients who are unable to communicate.
- To avoid injury when performing hygiene care, use principles of body mechanics and safe patient handling (see Chapter 11) and assess the patient's ability to participate in care by using an appropriate assessment tool (e.g., Mini-Mental State Examination [MMSE], Barthel ADL Index, Functional Independence Measure [Mlinac & Feng, 2016]).
- The nurse is responsible and accountable for assessing and evaluating a patient before and after care to detect unexpected outcomes and to give proper direction to unregulated care providers (UCPs) when delegating hygiene care.
- Monitor laboratory findings such as coagulation studies before administering oral care to prevent bleeding.

THE SKIN

The skin is the largest organ in the human body; it protects the body from heat, light, injury, and infection. It serves to (1) help regulate body temperature; (2) store water, vitamin D, and fat; (3) help sense pain and other stimuli; and (4) prevent the entry of bacteria. Three primary layers make up the skin: the epidermis, dermis, and subcutaneous tissue. The skin covers the entire surface of the body and is continuous with mucous membranes of the mouth, eyes, ears, nose, vagina, and rectum. Thorough hygiene is essential for the integrity and function of each skin layer.

The epidermis, or outer skin layer, is the first line of defense against external injury and infection. Sebum, secreted from hair

follicles from sebaceous glands, provides an acidic coating. This acidic coating protects the epidermis against penetration by chemicals and microorganisms. It also minimizes loss of water and plasma proteins.

Two types of sweat glands, the eccrine and apocrine glands, are distributed over the surface of the skin. Eccrine glands secrete a watery fluid (sweat) that helps control temperature through evaporation. The apocrine glands secrete sweat in the axillary and genital areas. Bacterial decomposition of sweat from the apocrine glands causes body odour.

The subcutaneous tissue layer contains blood vessels, nerves, lymph tissue, and loose connective tissue filled with fat cells. Fatty tissue insulates the body. Subcutaneous tissue also provides support for upper skin layers.

Bacteria reside on the outer surface of the skin. The resident bacteria are normal flora that do not cause disease but prevent disease-causing microorganisms from reproducing. Because a part of the skin is usually exposed to environmental irritants and is an active organ sensitive to physiological changes within the body, some skin problems commonly occur (Table 18.1).

THE MOUTH

The oral cavity, which is lined with a normally moist and intact light pink mucous membrane, contains the teeth and gums. The membranous lining protects underlying organs; secretes mucus to keep the oral cavity lubricated; and absorbs water, salts, and other solutes. Saliva, a clear viscous fluid secreted by the mucous and

TABLE 18.1

Common Skin Problems

Problem	Characteristics	Implications	Interventions
Dry skin	Flaky, rough texture caused by lack of moisture in outer stratum corneum, resulting in less pliable epidermis; most common on anterior surfaces of lower legs, knees, elbows, and backs of hands	Skin may crack, bleed, and become inflamed. As a result, redness, pruritus, and discomfort may develop.	Effective treatment of dry skin does not include limiting frequency of bathing but lies in bathing with warm, not hot, water and use of moisturizers (nonpetroleum). Use super-fatted soap (e.g., Dove) for cleaning. Rinse body of all soap well because residue left can cause irritation and breakdown. Add moisture to air through use of humidifier. Increase fluid intake when skin is dry.
Acne *(From James, W. D., et al. [2007]. Andrew's diseases of the skin: Clinical dermatology [10th ed.]. Philadelphia: Saunders.)*	Inflammatory, papulopustular skin eruption, usually involving bacterial breakdown of sebum; appears on face, neck, shoulders, and back	Infected material within pustule can spread if area is squeezed or picked. Permanent scarring can result.	Wash hair and skin each day with warm water and soap to remove oil. Use cosmetics sparingly because oily cosmetics or creams accumulate in pores and tend to make condition worse. Implement necessary dietary restrictions by eliminating foods found to aggravate condition. Use prescribed topical antibiotics for severe acne.
Hirsutism *(From Goyal, D., et al. [2010]. Coffin-Siris syndrome with Mayer-Rokitansky-Küster-Hauser syndrome: A case report. Journal of Medical Case Reports, 4, 354.)*	Excessive growth of body and facial hair, especially in women	May cause negative body image by giving female a male appearance.	Shaving is safest method to remove hair. Electrolysis and laser permanently remove hair. Tweezing and bleaching are temporary.

TABLE 18.1

Common Skin Problems—cont'd

Problem	Characteristics	Implications	Interventions
Skin rashes 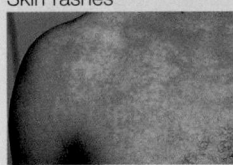	Skin eruption that results from overexposure to sun or moisture or from allergic reaction; may be flat or raised, localized or systemic, pruritic or nonpruritic	If skin is continually scratched, inflammation and infection may occur. Rashes also cause discomfort.	Wash area thoroughly and apply antiseptic spray or lotion to prevent further itching and aid healing process. Warm or cold soaks may relieve inflammation.
Contact dermatitis 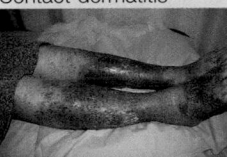 *(From Lewis, S.L., et al. [2011]. Medical-surgical nursing: assessment and management of clinical problems, [8th ed.]. St. Louis: Mosby.)*	Acute or chronic eczematous rash characterized by abrupt onset with well-defined geometric margins of erythema, pruritus, pain, and appearance of scaly, oozing lesions; appears on head, neck, scalp, hands, legs, dorsum of feet, and trunk	Dermatitis is often difficult to eliminate because the person is usually in continual contact with substance causing skin reaction. Substance may be hard to identify.	Identify and avoid contributing agents (e.g., cleaners, poison ivy or oak, cosmetics, latex, shoes/rubber). Treatment consists of removing contributing agent, if identified, and applying over-the-counter topical steroids or calamine lotion. In some cases, steroids may be prescribed. Patients may also find comfort with tepid baths.
Abrasion 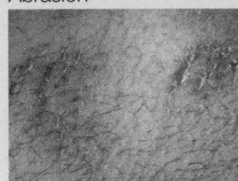 *(From Cottran, S. R., et al. From the teaching collection of the Department of Dermatology, University of Texas, Southwestern Medical School, Dallas.)*	Scraping or rubbing away of epidermis may result in localized bleeding and later weeping of serous fluid	Infection occurs easily as result of loss of protective skin layer.	Nurses should keep nails short and not wear jewellery when providing care, to avoid patient injury. Wash abrasions with mild soap and water. Dressing or bandage could increase risk for infection because of retained moisture.

salivary glands of the mouth, helps to prevent dental caries and plaque formation and lubricates the oral cavity. Lubrication of the oral cavity aids in chewing and swallowing. Saliva provides a means for removing cellular and bacterial debris that can cause infection, particularly fungal infection (Villa, Connell, & Abati, 2015). Hyposalivation results in dry mouth, or xerostomia, and affects taste, swallowing, digestion, nutrition, and denture fit (Villa et al., 2015).

The teeth are organs of chewing, or mastication. Dentin, a hard, ivorylike substance that surrounds the pulp cavity, forms the major part of a tooth (Fig. 18.1). A layer of enamel, visible in the oral cavity, covers the upper part of the tooth, or crown. The periodontal membrane, just below the gum margins, surrounds the tooth root and holds it firmly in place. A tooth receives its blood, lymph, and nerve supply from the base of the tooth socket within the jaw. Healthy teeth are smooth, shiny, and properly aligned.

The gums, or gingivae, are mucous membranes with underlying supportive fibrous tissue. They encircle the necks of erupted teeth to hold them firmly in place. The gums normally are pink, moist, firm, and relatively inelastic.

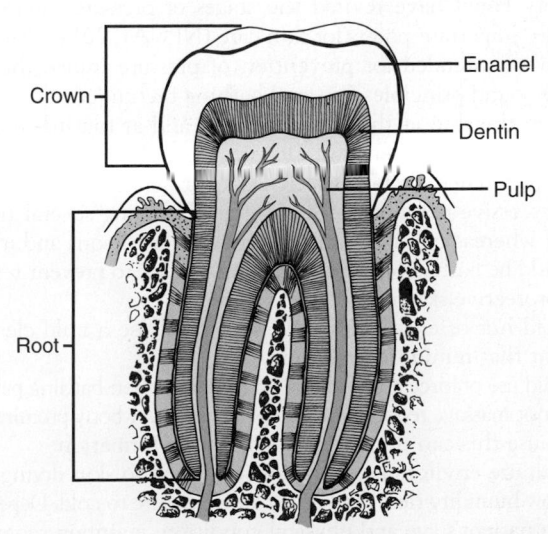

FIG 18.1 Normal tooth.

EYES, EARS, AND HAIR

Hair grows from follicles located within the dermis of the skin (Fig. 18.2). Tiny blood vessels supply nourishment for each follicle for normal hair growth. Each hair has a shaft extending from the follicle. Sebaceous glands secrete the oily substance (i.e., sebum) into each follicle, which lubricates the hair and scalp. The hair shaft is normally shiny and pliant and is not excessively oily, dry, or brittle. The primary function of hair is to act as the first line of protection. For example, hair protects the scalp from injury. Eyebrows and eyelashes protect the eyes from foreign particles. Personal hygiene related to the eyes and ears is covered in Chapter 19.

Special hair-care practices focus on care for scalp, axilla, and pubic areas. Hair growth, distribution, and pattern are indicators of a person's health status. Hormonal changes, emotional and physical stress, aging, intake of toxins (e.g., arsenic, cocaine), gender, ethnicity, nutrition, infection, and certain diseases affect hair characteristics. A person's appearance and sense of well-being often depend on the way the hair looks and feels. Illness or disability sometimes prevents patients from maintaining daily hair care.

THE NAILS

The nails are epithelial tissues that grow from the root of the nail bed, located in the skin at the nail groove. A normal, healthy nail

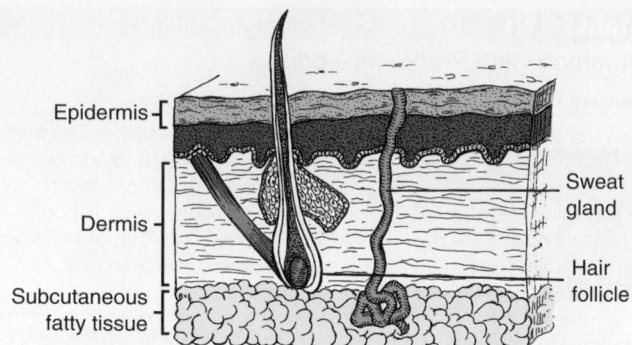

FIG 18.2 Cross-section of hair follicle and supporting structures.

is transparent, smooth, and convex, with a pink nail bed and translucent white tip. A normal colour indicates adequate oxygenation to peripheral tissues. Pigment deposits or bands are common in nail beds of patients with dark skin. The feet and nails require special care to prevent infection, odour, and injury. Problems typically result from abuse or poor care. Foot pain can often change a walking gait, causing strain on different muscle groups.

✦ SKILL 18.1   Complete or Partial Bed Bath

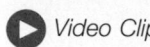 *Video Clip*

Bathing removes sweat, oil, dirt, and microorganisms from the skin. It also stimulates circulation and provides a refreshed and relaxed feeling. For some patients, a bath is a time for socialization and pleasure, especially for those who are bedridden or seriously disabled. It is important to encourage patients to actively participate in bathing, while being mindful of any limitations they may have and ensuring a safe environment (see Chapter 14).

Wound Care Canada highlights the importance of skin care in the prevention and management of pressure injuries and the essential role of interprofessional collaboration in maintaining skin integrity (Norton, Parslow, Johnston, et al., 2018). The National Pressure Ulcer Advisory Panel (NPUAP) and The European Pressure Ulcer Advisory Panel have revised the stages of pressure injuries and redefined important points for skin care (NPUAP, 2014). Although these were intended for prevention of pressure injury, they also provide sound principles for good bathing techniques.

- Clean the skin at the time of soiling and at routine intervals. Individualize frequency of cleaning according to patient need and preference. Problems such as incontinence, wound drainage, or excessive diaphoresis often require bathing several times a day; whereas other patients, such as older persons and infants, should be bathed only once or twice a week to prevent removal of protective skin oils.
- Avoid hot or excessively cold water and use a mild cleansing agent that minimizes irritation.
- Avoid use of force and friction on the skin when bathing patients. Do not massage reddened areas, especially over bony prominences, because this can promote pressure injury formation.
- Minimize environmental factors that lead to skin drying, such as low humidity (less than 40%) and exposure to cold. Depending on a patient's age and physical condition, maintain room temperature between 20° and 23°C (68° and 74°F). Infants, older

persons, and acutely ill patients may need a warmer temperature. However, certain critically ill patients require cooler room temperatures to lower the metabolic demands of the body. Controlling drafts and eliminating lingering odours from draining wounds, vomitus, bedpans, or urinals also improve a patient's comfort.

- Use bathing as a time to interact with and assess a patient. When giving a complete bath, perform a physical assessment of all body systems and discuss issues of concern for a patient.
- During bathing help patients through normal joint range-of-motion (ROM) exercises to promote circulation and joint integrity.
- For patients who tire easily, consider giving a partial instead of complete bed bath.
- There are two categories of baths: cleansing and therapeutic. Cleansing baths include the bed bath, tub bath, sponge bath at the sink, shower, and prepackaged disposable bed bath (Box 18.1). The type of cleansing bath to use depends on the assessment of a patient's physical capabilities and the degree of hygiene required. When a person is unable to perform personal care because of illness or disability, the nurse is responsible for helping with bathing. The nurse can also clean and groom the patient's hair, shave a patient, and clean the nails during or immediately after a bath.

Health care providers generally prescribe therapeutic baths for a specific effect, such as soothing the skin or promoting the healing process. Types of therapeutic baths include the following:

- *Sitz bath:* Cleans and reduces pain and inflammation of perineal and anal areas. It is used for patients who have undergone rectal or perineal surgery or childbirth or who have local irritation from hemorrhoids or fissures. A patient sits in a special tub or basin (see Chapter 41).

Types of Baths

- **Complete bed bath:** Bath administered to totally dependent patient in bed.
- **Partial bed bath:** Bed bath that consists of bathing only body parts that would cause discomfort if left unbathed, such as the hands, face, axilla, and perineal area. Partial bath also includes washing the back and providing a back rub. Dependent patients in need of partial hygiene or self-sufficient bedridden patients who are unable to reach all body parts receive a partial bed bath.
- **Sponge bath at the sink:** Involves bathing from a bath basin or sink with patient sitting in a chair. The patient is able to perform part of the bath independently. The nurse helps with hard-to-reach areas.
- **Tub bath:** Involves immersion in a tub of water that allows more thorough washing and rinsing than a bed bath. Patients may require nurse's help. Some facilities have tubs equipped with lifting devices that facilitate positioning dependent patients in the tub.
- **Shower:** Patient sits or stands under a continuous stream of water. The shower provides more thorough cleaning than a bed bath but can be tiring.
- **Disposable bed bath/travel bath:** The bag bath contains several soft, nonwoven cotton cloths that are premoistened in no-rinse solution and are heated before use. The bag bath offers an alternative because of the ease of use, reduced time bathing, and patient comfort (Nøddeskou, Hemmingsen, & Hørdam, 2015).

- *Medicated bath (addition of over-the-counter, herbal, or health care provider–prescribed ingredient to bath):* Relieves skin irritation and creates an antibacterial and drying effect.

Perineal care (see Procedural Guideline 18.1) involves thorough cleaning of a patient's external genitalia and surrounding skin. A patient routinely receives perineal care during a bath. However, patients at risk for acquiring an infection need more frequent perineal care, such as those who have incontinence-associated dermatitis (IAD) or an in-dwelling Foley catheter or who are postpartum or recovering from rectal or genital surgery.

Delegation and Collaboration

Assessment of the patient's skin, pain level, and ROM cannot be delegated to an unregulated care provider (UCP). Bathing is a fundamental nursing skill and responsibility of a registered nurse (RN)/licensed (registered) practical nurse and provides many opportunities for patient assessment. This skill may be delegated to a UCP. The nurse instructs the UCP about:
- Not massaging reddened skin areas during bathing.
- Contraindications to soaking a patient's feet.
- Reporting any signs of impaired skin integrity to the nurse.
- Proper ways to position male and female patients with musculoskeletal limitations or an in-dwelling Foley catheter or other equipment (e.g., intravenous [IV] tubing).

Equipment

- Washcloths and bath towels
- Bath blanket
- Bar or liquid soap, or 120 mL bottle of 4% chlorhexidine gluconate (CHG) (dispensed in a single bath-size bottle)
- Toiletry items (deodorant, lotion)
- Disposable wipes
- Warm water
- Clean hospital gown or patient's own pajamas or gown
- Laundry bag
- Clean gloves
- Washbasin
- Eye patch/shield and nonallergenic tape (for unconscious patient)

STEP	RATIONALE

ASSESSMENT

1. Identify patient using at least two person-specific identifiers (e.g., name and date of birth or name and medical record number) according to employer policy.

   Ensures correct patient. Complies with Accreditation Canada's standards and improves patient safety (Accreditation Canada, 2019).

2. Perform hand hygiene. Assess room environment for safety (e.g., check room for spills; make sure that equipment is working properly and that bed is in locked, low position).

   Reduces transmission of microorganisms.

   Identifies safety hazards in patient environment that could cause or potentially lead to harm (Public Health Agency of Canada [PHAC], 2015).

3. Assess patient's fall risk status (if partial bathing out of bed or self-bath is to be performed) (see Chapter 14).

   Allows you to anticipate needed precautions, such as having patient sit on chair in front of basin.

4. Assess patient's tolerance for bathing: activity tolerance, comfort level, musculoskeletal function, and presence of shortness of breath.

   Determines patient's ability to perform or tolerate bathing and type of bath to administer (e.g., tub bath, bed bath).

5. Assess patient's cognitive (Mini-Mental State Examination [MMSE]) and functional status (e.g., Barthel's index covers nine domains [feeding, bathing, grooming, dressing, bowel, bladder, toilet, transfers, mobility, and stairs]; Functional Independence Measure [more comprehensive and includes domains of social cognition and communication]) to assess self-care ability (Mlinac & Feng, 2016). For patients with suspected dementia, observe behaviour, especially after telling patient it is bath time; do they become agitated?

   Every person entering a long-term care setting should be formally assessed for cognitive and functional status according to employer policy. Functional status assesses a patient's capacity for self-bathing and how much supervision or help is needed to accomplish daily ADL tasks. Every attempt should be made to avoid bathing people against their will (AHRQ, 2013a).

Clinical Decision Point *Patients with dementia may become agitated. Observe for behaviours such as restlessness, yelling, and fighting with caregivers.*

STEP	RATIONALE

ASSESSMENT

6. Assess patient's visual status, ability to sit without support, hand grasp, ROM of extremities (see Chapter 8).

Further determines degree of help needed for bathing.

7. Assess for presence and position of external medical device or equipment (e.g., IV line or oxygen tubing).

Affects how you will position patient and plan bathing activities.

8. Assess patient's usual bathing routine (ASC, 2017): How often does the person bathe? Usually shower or bath? What time of day? Does the person use any special products, robes, towels, or equipment during bathing (e.g., scented soaps, music, back brush, or sponge) to make the experience more enjoyable? Is the person concerned about loss of privacy?

Demonstrates person-centred care and encourages patient to participate in self-care. Promotes patient's comfort and willingness to cooperate. Using a patient's established routine may reduce agitation in a patient with dementia.

9. Ask if patient has noticed any problems related to condition of skin and genitalia.

Provides information to direct physical assessment of skin and genitalia during bathing. Also influences selection of skin-care products.

10. Before or during bath, assess condition of patient's skin. Note presence of dryness, indicated by flaking, redness, scaling, and cracking or excessive moisture, inflammation, or pressure injuries (see Chapter 39).

Provides baseline for comparison of skin integrity over time.

11. Identify risks for skin impairment: older age, immobilization, reduced sensation, nutrition and hydration, excess skin moisture or drainage, shear or friction on skin, vascular insufficiencies, presence of external devices. *Option:* Use a pressure injury assessment tool (e.g., Braden Scale; see Chapter 39).

Risk factors increase the likelihood of injury to the skin because of pressure, impaired tissue synthesis, softening of or friction on tissues, and impaired circulation.

12. Assess patient's comfort on a 0-to-10 pain scale (with 0 being no pain, and 10 being the worst pain ever experienced).

Bath can soothe and comfort patient. Provides baseline measure.

13. Assess patient's knowledge and perceptions of the importance of skin hygiene, preventive measures to take, and common skin problems encountered (see Table 18.1).

Determines patient's willingness to learn and type of instruction required.

14. Review medical record for prescriptions for specific precautions concerning patient's movement or positioning and whether there is a prescription for a therapeutic bath. Note and confirm with patient any allergies or sensitivities to bath products.

Prevents accidental injury to patient during bathing activities. Determines level of help that patient needs. Prevents allergic reactions to hygiene products during bathing.

NURSING DIAGNOSES

- Bathing/self-care deficit
- Reduced stamina
- Reduced physical mobility

- Reduced skin integrity
- Inadequate knowledge regarding skin care

- Potential for impaired skin integrity
- Potential for infection

Related factors are individualized on the basis of patient's condition or needs.

PLANNING

1. Expected outcomes following completion of procedure:
   - Skin is free of excretions, drainage, or odour.
   - Skin shows decreased redness, cracking, flaking, and scaling.
   - Joint ROM remains same or improves from previous measurement.
   - Patient expresses sense of comfort and relaxation.
   - Patient tolerates bath without fatigue or chilling.

   - Patient describes benefits and techniques of proper hygiene and skin care.

Skin is clean.

Indicates reduction in skin dryness.

Repeated ROM exercise during bathing helps prevent contractures and promotes joint movement.

Bath relaxes patient and removes sources of discomfort.

Fatigue during bathing indicates worsening of chronic cardiopulmonary conditions.

Demonstrates learning with ability to repeat back to demonstrate understanding.

STEP	RATIONALE

PLANNING

2. Explain procedure and ask patient for suggestions on how to prepare supplies. If partial bath, ask how much of bath patient wishes to complete.

Promotes patient's cooperation, participation, and promotion of self-care as appropriate.

3. Adjust room temperature and ventilation, close room doors and windows, and draw room divider curtain.

Warm room that is free of drafts prevents rapid loss of body heat during bathing. Privacy provides for patient's mental and physical comfort.

4. Prepare equipment and place supplies on bedside table. If it is necessary to leave room, be sure that call light is within patient's reach, bed is in low position, and wheels are locked.

Avoids interrupting procedure or leaving patient unattended to retrieve missing equipment. Provides for patient safety.

Clinical Decision Point *Never leave the bedside without ensuring that the appropriate number of side rails have been raised (see employer policy). The number of side rails depends on the patient's fall risk assessment; however, having all side rails raised may be considered a restraint if the patient is unable to lower the rail.*

IMPLEMENTATION

1. Offer patient bedpan or urinal. Apply clean gloves to help patient as needed. Provide toilet tissue and dispose of any excrement properly. Dispose of gloves if applied and perform hand hygiene. Provide patient towel and moist washcloth.

Patient feels more comfortable after voiding. Prevents interruption of bath.

2. Perform hand hygiene. If patient has nonintact skin or skin is soiled with drainage, excretions, or body secretions, apply new pair of clean gloves before beginning bath.

Reduces transmission of microorganisms.

3. Raise bed to comfortable working height. Lower side rail closest to you and help patient assume comfortable supine position, maintaining body alignment. Bring patient toward side closest to you (staying supine).

Aids access to patient. Maintains patient's comfort throughout procedure. Uses proper body mechanics, thus minimizing strain on back muscles. If patient is overweight, get help from another caregiver or use lift device for positioning (see Chapter 11).

4. Place bath blanket over patient. Have patient hold top of bath blanket and remove top sheet from under bath blanket without exposing patient. Place soiled linen in laundry bag.

Blanket provides warmth and privacy.
Take care to avoid linen contacting uniform.

5. Remove patient's gown or pajamas.

Provides full exposure of body parts during bathing.

   a. If gown has snaps on sleeves, simply unsnap and remove gown without pulling IV tubing (if present).

   b. If gown has no snaps and if an extremity is *injured* or has reduced mobility, begin removal from *unaffected* side first.

Undressing unaffected side first allows easier manipulation of gown over body part with reduced ROM.

   c. If patient has an IV line and gown with no snaps, remove gown from arm *without* IV line first. Then remove gown from arm with IV line (see illustration A). Pause IV fluid infusion by pressing appropriate sensor on IV pump. Remove IV tubing from pump; use regulator to slow IV infusion. Remove IV bag from pole (see illustration B) and slide IV bag and tubing through arm of patient's gown (see illustration C). Rehang IV bag (see illustration D), reconnect tubing to pump, open regulator clamp, and restart IV fluid infusion by pressing appropriate sensor on IV pump. If IV fluids are infusing by gravity, check IV flow rate and regulate if necessary. *Do not disconnect IV tubing to remove gown.*

Manipulation of IV tubing and bag can disrupt IV infusion flow rate.

6. Raise side rail. Lower bed temporarily to lowest position and raise on return after you fill wash basin two-thirds full with warm water. Place basin along with supplies on over-bed table and position over patient's bed. Check water temperature by placing your forearm in the water or by using a handheld thermometer, and have patient place fingers in water to ensure it is not too hot or too cool.

Raising side rail and lowering bed maintains patient's safety. Warm water promotes comfort, relaxes muscles, and prevents unnecessary chilling. Use of over-bed table allows you to move to opposite side of bed without having to move equipment. Test water temperature to prevent burns to skin.

STEP	RATIONALE

IMPLEMENTATION

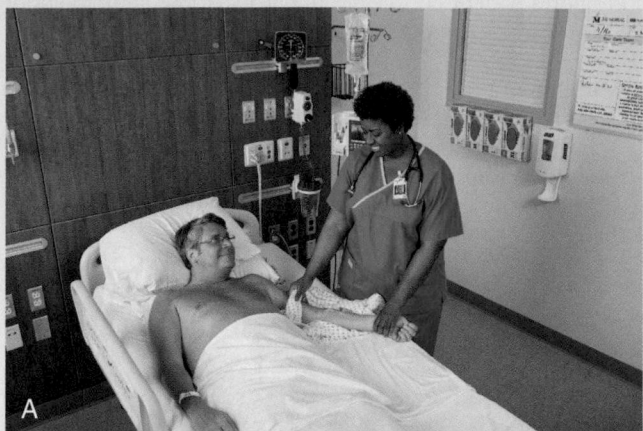
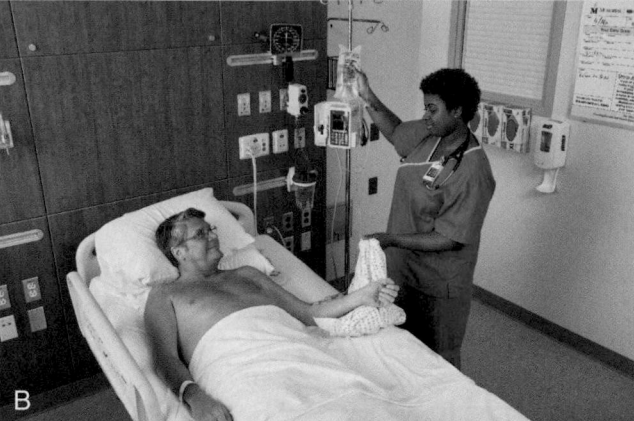
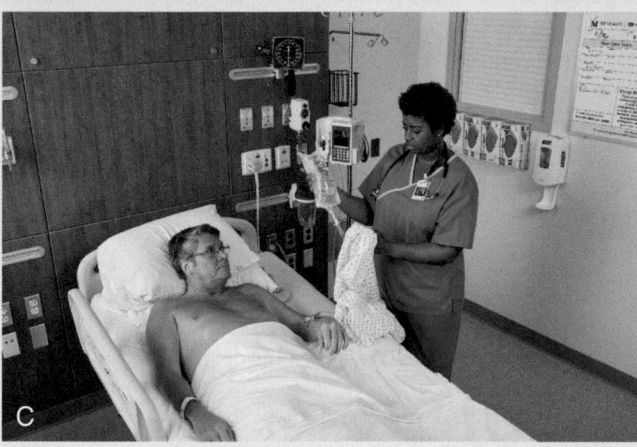
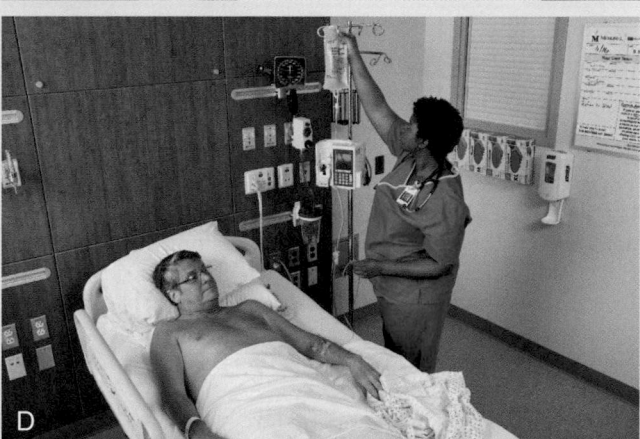

STEP 5c A, Remove patient's gown. **B,** Remove IV bag from pole. **C,** Slide IV tubing and bag through arm of patient's gown. **D,** Rehang IV bag.

7. Lower side rail. Remove pillow (if tolerated). Raise head of bed 30 to 45 degrees if allowed. Place bath towel under patient's head. Place second bath towel over patient's chest.

8. Wash face.

Removal of pillow makes it easier to wash patient's ears and neck. Placement of towels prevents soiling of bed linen and bath blanket.

Clinical Decision Point *Do not use bath water with 4% liquid CHG added or 2% CHG bathing cloths (see Procedural Guideline 18.2) on the eyes or face (AHRQ, 2013b).*

a. Inquire if patient is wearing contact lenses. You may choose to remove at this time.

Prevents accidental injury to eyes.

b. Form a mitt with washcloth (see illustration); immerse in water and wring thoroughly.

Mitt retains water and heat better than loosely held washcloth; keeps cold edges from brushing against patient and prevents splashing.

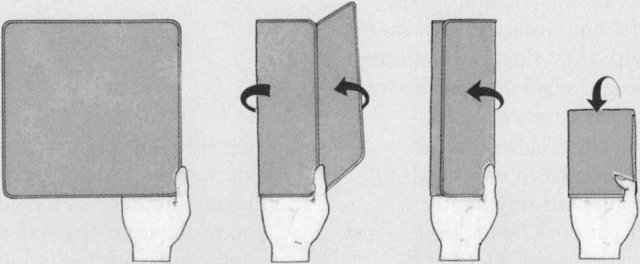

STEP 8b Steps for folding washcloth to form a mitt.

STEP	RATIONALE

IMPLEMENTATION

c. Wash patient's eyes with plain warm water, using a clean area of cloth for each eye and bathing from inner to outer canthus (see illustrations). Soak any crusts on eyelid for 2 to 3 minutes with warm, damp cloth before attempting removal. Dry around eyes thoroughly but gently.

Soap irritates eyes. Use of separate sections of mitt reduces infection transmission. Bathing eye gently from inner to outer canthus prevents secretions from entering nasolacrimal duct. Pressure causes internal injury.

d. Ask if patient prefers to use soap on face. Otherwise wash, rinse, and dry forehead, cheeks, nose, neck, and ears without using soap. Ask men if they want to be shaved (see Procedural Guideline 18.4).

Soap tends to dry face, which is exposed to air more than other body parts.

e. Provide eye care for unconscious patient.

Patients who are unconscious have lost the normal protective corneal reflex of blinking, increasing the risk for corneal drying, abrasions, and eye infection.

(1) Instill eye drops or ointment per health care provider's prescription (see Chapter 19).

(2) In the absence of blink reflex, keep eyelids closed. Close eye gently, using back of your fingertip, before placing eye patch or shield. Place tape over patch or shield. Do not tape eyelid.

When blink reflex is absent, patient loses a protective mechanism. Keeping eyelids closed maintains eye moisture and prevents injury.

9. Wash upper extremities and trunk. *Option:* Change bath water at this time. Prepare contents of a full 120-mL bottle of 4% CHG with 3.8 L of water or use no-rinse 2% CHG cloths (Alserehi, Filippell, Emerick, et al., 2018; Supple, Kumaraswami, Kundrapu, et al., 2015).

Evidence shows that CHG use in daily bathing can reduce incidence of hospital-acquired infections (Lowe et al., 2017; Shah et al., 2016). CHG reduces bacteria for up to 24 hours and prevents infection (Alserehi et al., 2018).

Clinical Decision Point *When using CHG use one washcloth or wipe for washing each major body part. Then dispose of cloth and use a new cloth for the next body part (Raines & Rosen, 2016). Dipping cloth back into basin contaminates solution and makes CHG less effective. Do not rinse after bathing with CHG solution. Allow CHG to dry on the skin to achieve antimicrobial effects.*

a. Remove bath blanket from patient's arm that is closest to you. Place bath towel lengthwise under arm and wash using long, firm strokes from distal to proximal (fingers to axilla).

Long, firm strokes promote venous return.

b. Raise and support arm above head (if possible) to wash axilla, rinse, and dry thoroughly (see illustration). Apply deodorant to underarms as needed or desired.

Movement of arm exposes axilla and exercises normal ROM of joint. Deodorant controls body odour.

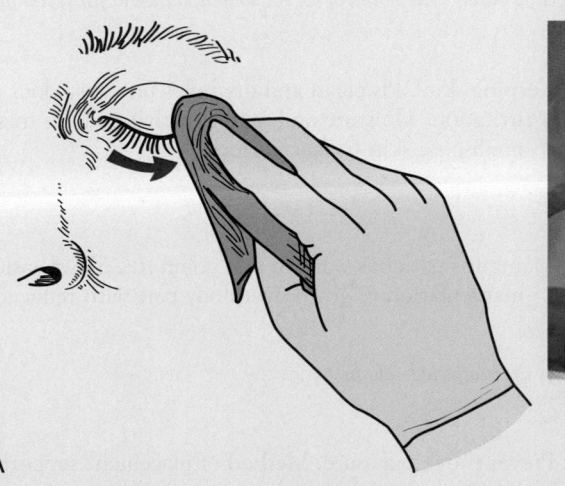
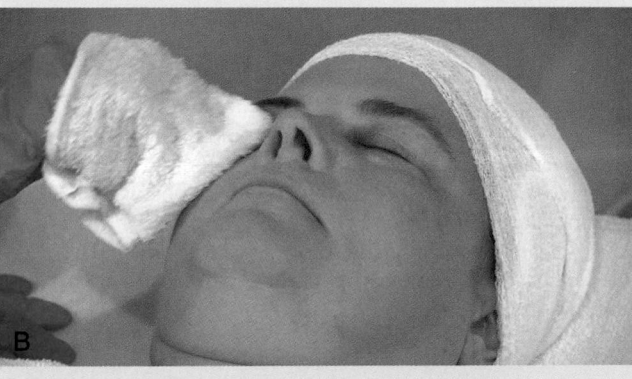

STEP 8c Wash eye from inner to outer canthus. **A,** Direction for cleaning eye. **B,** Washing eye from inner to outer canthus.

STEP	RATIONALE

IMPLEMENTATION

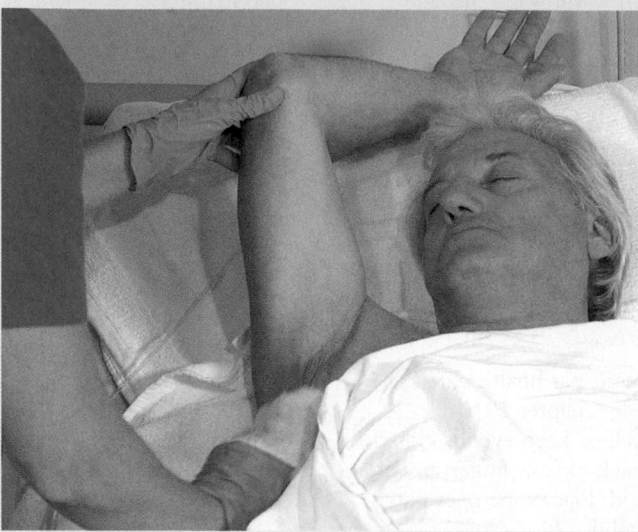

STEP 9b Position of patient's arm for washing axilla.

c. Move to other side of bed and repeat steps with other arm.

d. Cover patient's chest with bath towel and fold bath blanket down to umbilicus. Bathe chest with long, firm strokes. Take special care with skin under female patient's breasts, lifting breast upward if necessary while bathing underneath breast. Rinse if using soap and water and dry well.

Draping prevents unnecessary exposure of body parts. Towel maintains warmth and privacy. Secretions and dirt collect easily in areas of tight skinfolds. Skin under breasts is vulnerable to excoriation if not kept clean and dry.

10. Wash hands and nails.

a. Fold bath towel in half and lay it on bed beside patient. Place basin on towel. Immerse patient's hand in water. Allow hand to soak for 3 to 5 minutes before cleaning fingernails (see Skill 18.4). **NOTE:** Do not soak fingers of patient with diabetes mellitus. Remove basin and dry hand well. Repeat for other hand.

Soaking softens cuticles and calluses of hand, loosens debris beneath nails, and enhances feeling of cleanliness. Thorough drying removes moisture from between fingers. Soaking hands of patient with diabetes mellitus can lead to maceration and risk for infection.

11. Check temperature of bath water and change water if necessary; otherwise continue.

Warm water maintains patient's comfort.

Clinical Decision Point *If using CHG solution in bath water, do not discard water. One bottle of CHG soap is sufficient for a complete bath.*

12. Wash abdomen.

a. Place bath towel lengthwise over chest and abdomen. (You may need two towels.) Fold bath blanket down to just above pubic region. Bathe, rinse, and dry abdomen with special attention to umbilicus and skinfolds of abdomen and groin. Keep abdomen covered between washing and rinsing. Dry well.

Keeping skinfolds clean and dry helps prevent odour and skin irritation. Moisture and sediment that collects in skinfolds predispose skin to maceration.

b. Apply clean gown or pajama top by dressing affected side first. *Option:* You may omit this step until completion of bath.

Maintains patient's warmth and comfort. Allows easier manipulation of gown over body part with reduced ROM.

Clinical Decision Point *If one extremity is injured or immobilized, always dress affected side first.*

13. Wash lower extremities.

a. Cover chest and abdomen with top of bath blanket. Expose near leg by folding blanket toward midline. Be sure that other leg and perineum remain draped. Place bath towel under leg as you support patient's knee and ankle.

Prevents overexposure. Method of placement supports patient's joint.

STEP	RATIONALE

IMPLEMENTATION

b. Wash leg using long, firm strokes from ankle to knee and knee to thigh (see illustration). Assess condition of extremities.

Promotes circulation and venous return. Assessment is key to identifying signs and symptoms of venous thrombosis.

Clinical Decision Point *During the bath assess for signs of warmth, redness, swelling, tenderness, and pain in the lower extremities because these might be early signs of a venous thromboembolism.*

c. Clean foot, making sure to bathe between toes. Dry toes and feet completely.

d. Raise side rail; remove towel; move to opposite side of bed, lower side rail, place dry towel under second leg, and repeat Steps 13b and 13c for other leg and foot. Apply a light layer of moisturizing lotion to both feet. When finished, remove used towel.

Secretions and moisture are often present between toes, predisposing patient to maceration and skin breakdown.
Moisturizers are effective in reducing dry skin; however, in excess they can cause maceration.

e. Cover patient with bath blanket, raise side rail, and change bath water (if using plain soap and water).

Decreased bath water temperature causes chilling. Clean water reduces microorganism transmission.

14. Wash back.

a. Apply clean gloves (if not already applied). Lower side rail. Help patient assume prone or side-lying position, using safe patient-handling techniques (see Chapter 11) (as applicable). Place towel lengthwise along patient's side.

Exposes back and buttocks for bathing.

b. If fecal material is present, enclose in fold of underpad or toilet tissue and remove with disposable wipes.

Skinfolds near buttocks and anus may contain fecal secretions and microorganisms.

c. Keep patient draped by sliding bath blanket over shoulders and thighs during bathing. Wash, rinse, and dry back from neck to buttocks with long, firm strokes. Pay special attention to folds of buttocks and anus.

Maintains warmth and prevents unnecessary exposure.

d. Clean buttocks and anus, washing front to back (see illustration). Clean, rinse, and dry area thoroughly. If needed, place clean, absorbent pad under patient's buttocks.

Cleaning buttocks after back prevents contamination of water.

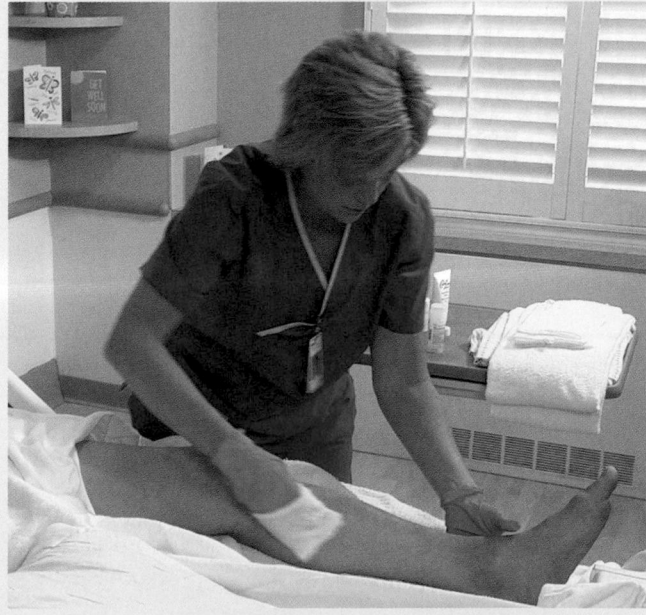

STEP 13b Washing patient's leg.

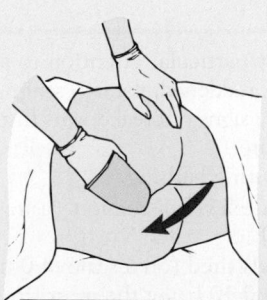

STEP 14d Clean buttocks and anus, washing front to back.

STEP	RATIONALE

IMPLEMENTATION

15. While patient is supine, provide perineal care (see Procedural Guideline 18.1).

Clinical Decision Point *At end of bath, if you have used 4% CHG solution, skin may feel sticky for a few minutes. Do NOT wipe off. Allow to air dry (AHRQ, 2013b).*

16. Massage back if patient desires. — Promotes patient relaxation.

17. Clean and file nails as needed (check employer policy) (see Skill 18.4).

18. Apply body lotion to skin and topical moisturizing agents to dry, flaky, reddened, or scaling areas. **NOTE:** If using CHG solution for bathing, only use a product compatible with CHG (AHRQ, 2013b). — Dry skin results in reduced pliability and cracking. Moisturizers help to prevent skin breakdown.

Clinical Decision Point *Massage may be contraindicated in the presence of acute inflammation, over bony prominences, and where there is the possibility of damaged blood vessels or fragile skin (Westman & Blaisdell, 2016). Massage of the legs is also contraindicated because of the possible presence of a blood clot, which could become dislodged.*

19. Remove and dispose of gloves and perform hand hygiene before helping patient complete grooming (e.g., combing hair, shaving). — Reduces transmission of microorganisms. Promotes patient's body image.

20. Check function and position of external devices (e.g., in-dwelling catheters, nasogastric tubes, IV tubes, braces). — Ensures that bathing activities did not disrupt systems.

21. Replace top bed linen by pulling sheet and bedspread from foot of bed to cover patient before removing bath blanket. Apply gloves if linen is soiled. *Option:* Make occupied bed at this time (see Procedural Guideline 18.6). — Maintains patient warmth and privacy.

22. Place bed in low, locked position and raise appropriate number of side rails so they do not restrain patient from exiting bed safely. Make sure that patient is in comfortable position with call light and personal possessions in reach. — Maintains patient safety. Reaching for call light or personal items can lead to a fall.

23. Disinfect/rinse and dry bed basin according to employer policy. This is especially important if using CHG solution. DO NOT use basin for CHG as storage container for supplies — Reduces transmission of micro-organisms. Evidence has shown that basins are frequently contaminated with microbes and are a possible source for the spread of health care-associated infections (Lowe et al., 2017).

24. Perform hand hygiene and leave room. — Reduces transmission of microorganisms.

EVALUATION

1. Observe skin; pay particular attention to areas that were previously soiled, reddened, flaking, scaling, or cracking or that showed early signs of breakdown. Inspect areas normally exposed to pressure. — Bathing should leave skin clean and clear. If there are signs of skin irritation (e.g., redness, blistering), take steps to reduce pressure.

2. Observe ROM during bathing. — Measures joint mobility.

3. Ask patient to rate level of comfort (using an appropriate pain rating scale). — Determines changes in level of comfort during bathing.

4. Ask if patient feels tired (on a scale of 0 to 10, with 0 being not tired at all and 10 being the most tired ever). — Measures tolerance to bathing activity.

STEP	RATIONALE

EVALUATION

5. Use Teach-Back: "I want to be sure I explained the importance of keeping your skin clean, especially while in the hospital. Tell me why we want to bathe you daily." Develop a revised teaching plan if patient or caregiver is not able to teach back correctly.

Determines patient's and caregiver's level of understanding of instructional topic.

Unexpected Outcomes	Related Interventions
1. Areas of excessive dryness, rashes, irritation, or pressure injury appear on skin.	• Review employer skin-care policy regarding special cleansing and moisturizing products. • If using CHG soap, it may become necessary to reduce frequency of bathing. Sensitivity to CHG is rare. • Limit frequency of complete baths. • Complete pressure injury assessment (see Chapter 39). • Institute turning and positioning measures to keep patient off pressure injury. • Obtain special bed surface if patient is at risk for skin breakdown. • Notify health care provider and/or obtain wound consultation.
2. Patient becomes excessively tired and unable to cooperate or participate in bathing.	• Reschedule bathing to a time when patient is more rested. • Patients with cardiopulmonary conditions and breathing difficulties require pillow or elevated head of bed during bathing. • Notify health care provider about changes in patient's fatigue level. • Perform hygiene measures in stages between scheduled rest periods.
3. Patient seems unusually restless or expresses discomfort.	• Use less stressful method of bathing, such as a disposable bath (see Procedural Guideline 18.2). • Consider analgesia before bathing. • Schedule rest periods before bathing.

Communication and Documentation

- Document procedure, observations (e.g., breaks in skin, inflammation, or areas of pressure injury), level of patient participation, and how the patient tolerated procedure in nurses' notes in electronic health record (EHR) or chart.
- Report evidence of alterations in skin integrity, break in suture line, or increased wound secretions to nurse in charge or health care provider. Patient may require special skin care.
- Document your evaluation of patient and caregiver learning.

Special Considerations
Teaching

- Teach patients how to inspect surfaces between skinfolds and explain the signs of irritation or breakdown. Use simple language.
- Consider the need to include a caregiver in learning the bathing process. Plan for a return demonstration.

Pediatric

- Some adolescents require or prefer more frequent bathing as a result of more active sebaceous glands.
- Young adolescent girls should learn basic perineal hygiene measures and know why they are predisposed to urinary tract infections.
- To maintain safety when bathing children, they must be supervised at all times, and water temperature should be checked with your elbow or wrist to ensure that it is not too hot (Canadian Paediatric Society, 2015).

Gerontological

- Older persons with incontinence need meticulous skin care to reduce incontinence-associated dermatitis (IAD) and the risk

of infection. The use of barrier creams is sometimes recommended to keep the skin intact and free from infections.

- If patients have signs of dementia, caregiver behaviour, especially 5 seconds before a bath, may be considered by the patient to be an assault. Behaviours that trigger agitation include confrontational communication; invalidation of the patient's feelings; absence of personal restraint; touching feet, axilla, or perineal area; non–bath-related communications; and failing to prepare the patient for the bath (AHRQ, 2013a).
- When giving a patient with dementia a bath, follow these guidelines (ASC, 2017):
  - Practise person-centred nursing care and maintain the patients' normal routine as much as possible.
  - Provide adequate lighting and prepare the bath ahead of time.
  - Encourage toileting prior to bathing to reduce the chances of incontinence in the bath.
  - Do not rush, and speak in a low pleasant voice, giving information before and all through the bathing process. Offer support and encouragement.
  - If agitation occurs, use distraction; bring up a pleasant topic; or use other distraction such as music, singing, holding an object, or eating.
  - Concentrate on the person's feelings and reactions. Pay attention and do not converse with others.

Care in the Community

- Type of bath chosen depends on assessment of the home, availability of running water, and condition of bathing facilities.
- In the home, set up equipment according to patient's established routines.

- Patients at risk for falls may benefit from the following:
  - Installation of grab bars in shower
  - Adhesive strips applied to shower or tub floor
  - Addition of a shower chair or placement of a chair or stool

Long-Term Care

- Tubs in long-term care settings frequently come equipped with electronic thermometers to measure water temperature. The tubs also have hydraulic lifts to help residents into the tub.

PROCEDURAL GUIDELINE 18.1 *Perineal Care*

Perineal care involves thorough cleaning of the patient's external genitalia and surrounding skin. A patient routinely receives perineal care during a complete bed bath (see Skill 18.1). However, patients who have fecal or urinary incontinence, an in-dwelling Foley catheter, or rectal or genital surgery may need more frequent perineal care. This is especially important for patients with in-dwelling Foley catheters, in the effort to reduce catheter-associated urinary tract infection (CAUTI). Wear clean gloves during perineal care because of the risk of contact with infectious organisms present in fecal, urinary, or vaginal secretions. To avoid embarrassment, always act in a professional and sensitive manner and provide patient privacy at all times.

Delegation and Collaboration
The skill of perineal care can be delegated to an unregulated care provider (UCP). The nurse instructs the UCP to:
- Avoid any physical restriction that affects proper positioning of patient.
- Properly position a patient with an in-dwelling Foley catheter.
- Inform the nurse of any perineal drainage, excoriation, or rash observed.

Equipment
- Washcloths, bath towels, and bath blanket
- Cleaning product for bath (chlorhexidine gluconate [CHG] cloths can be used for perineal and catheter care; however, some facilities do not use CHG because of concern over risk of mucosal irritation (see employer policy)
- Disposable wipes and wash basin
- Warm water
- Laundry bag
- Waterproof pad or bedpan
- Clean gloves
- Additional supplies when perineal care is provided other than during a bath: cotton balls or swabs, solution bottle or container filled with warm water or prescribed rinsing solution, waterproof bag

Procedural Steps
1. Identify patient using at least two person-specific identifiers (e.g., name and date of birth or name and medical record number), according to employer policy (Accreditation Canada, 2019).
2. Assess environment for safety (e.g., check room for spills, make sure that equipment is working properly and that bed is in locked, low position).
3. Assemble supplies. Provide privacy and explain procedure and importance in preventing infection.
4. Perform hand hygiene. Apply clean gloves. Place basin with warm water and cleansing solution on over-bed table.
5. **Perineal care for a female:**
   a. If patient can manoeuvre and handle washcloth, allow her to clean perineum on her own.

b. Help patient assume dorsal recumbent position. Note restrictions or a limitation in patient's positioning. Position waterproof pad under patient's buttocks.
c. Drape patient with bath blanket placed in shape of a diamond.
d. Fold both outer corners of bath blanket up around patient's legs onto abdomen and under hip (see illustration). Lift lower tip of bath blanket when you are ready to expose the perineum.

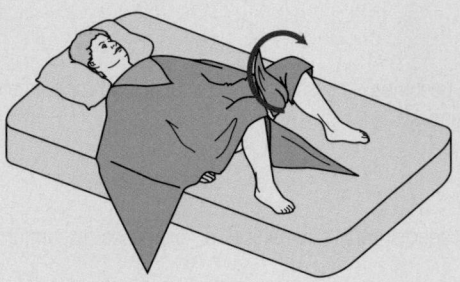

STEP 5d Drape patient for perineal care.

e. Wash and dry patient's upper thighs. (**NOTE:** If employer uses CHG solution for perineal care, do not rinse; allow to dry.)
f. Wash labia majora. Use nondominant hand to gently retract labia from thigh. Use dominant hand to wash carefully in skinfolds. Wipe in direction from perineum to rectum (front to back). Repeat on opposite side using separate section of washcloth or new washcloth. Rinse and dry area thoroughly.
g. Gently separate labia with nondominant hand to expose urethral meatus and vaginal orifice. With dominant hand, wash downward from pubic area toward rectum in one smooth stroke (see illustration). Use separate section of cloth for each stroke. Clean thoroughly over labia minora, clitoris, and vaginal orifice. Avoid tension on in-dwelling catheter if present and clean area around it thoroughly.

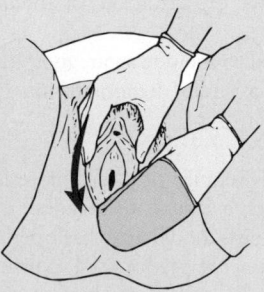

STEP 5g Clean from perineum to rectum (front to back).

h. Rinse and dry area thoroughly, using front-to-back method.
i. If patient uses bedpan, pour warm water over perineal area and dry thoroughly. (Exception: do not rinse if using CHG.)

PROCEDURAL GUIDELINE 18.1 *Perineal Care—cont'd*

j. Fold lower corner of bath blanket back between patient's legs and over perineum. Ask patient to lower legs and assume comfortable position.

6. **Perineal care for a male:**

   a. If patient is able to manoeuvre and handle washcloth, allow him to clean perineum on his own.

   b. Help patient to supine position. Note restriction in mobility.

   c. Fold lower half of bath blanket up to expose upper thighs. Wash and dry thighs.

   d. Cover thighs with bath towels. Raise bath blanket to expose genitalia. Gently raise penis and place bath towel underneath. Gently grasp shaft of penis. If patient is uncircumcised, retract foreskin. If patient has an erection, defer procedure until later.

   e. Wash tip of penis at urethral meatus first. Using circular motion, clean from meatus outward (see illustration). Discard washcloth and repeat with clean cloth until penis is clean. Rinse and dry gently and thoroughly. (Exception: do not rinse if using CHG.)

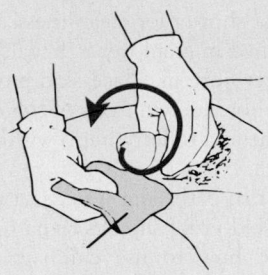

STEP 6e Use circular motion to clean tip of penis.

f. Return foreskin to its natural position.

Clinical Decision Point *After administering male perineal care for uncircumcised males, make sure that foreskin is in its natural position. This position is extremely important in patients with decreased sensation in their lower extremities. Tightening foreskin around shaft of penis causes local edema and discomfort and, if not corrected, may cause permanent urethral damage.*

g. Take a new washcloth and gently clean shaft of penis and scrotum by having patient abduct legs. Pay special attention to underlying surface of penis. Lift scrotum carefully and wash underlying skinfolds. Rinse and dry thoroughly. (Exception: do not rinse if using CHG.)

h. Fold bath blanket back over patient's perineum and help him to comfortable position.

7. For both female and male patient, avoid placing tension on an in-dwelling catheter, if present, and clean around it thoroughly during procedure.

8. Observe perineal area for any irritation, redness, or drainage that persists after perineal hygiene.

9. Dispose of gloves and used supplies in proper receptacles and perform hand hygiene.

10. **Use Teach-Back:** "We talked about how to wash your genital area to reduce the chance of infection. Describe for me how to wash your genital area." Develop a revised teaching plan if patient or caregiver is not able to teach back correctly.

PROCEDURAL GUIDELINE 18.2 *Use of Disposable Bed Bath, Tub, or Shower*

The use of disposable washcloths impregnated with an antiseptic solution such as chlorhexidine gluconate (CHG) is more common now in acute care hospitals, especially critical care settings. However, the cloths can be used in any setting. CHG cloths should be used for all bathing purposes, including once-a-day full-body bathing, incontinence care, or any other reasons for additional cleaning (AHRQ, 2013b). CHG replaces soap and water baths; thus, the cloths should not be used as a "top coat" after bathing. Rather, CHG cloths clean and remove bacteria, and the antiseptic binds to the skin for persistent antibacterial activity lasting 24 hours (AHRQ, 2013b).

Although showers are available to patients in acute care, tub and shower bathing are more common in long-term care settings. When patients use a tub or shower, follow guidelines to maintain patient safety to prevent falls.

Delegation and Collaboration

The skill of bathing in a tub or shower or using disposable cloths for bathing can be delegated to an unregulated care provider (UCP). The nurse instructs the UCP to:

- Not massage reddened skin areas during bathing.
- Properly position male and female patients with musculoskeletal limitations or an in-dwelling Foley catheter or other equipment (e.g., intravenous tubing).

- Report changes in skin or perineal area or signs of impaired skin integrity to the nurse.

Equipment

- Washcloths and bath towels (for tub or shower), bath blanket, cleaning product, toiletry items (deodorant, lotion), disposable wipes, clean hospital gown or patient's own pajamas or gown, laundry bag
- Prepackaged, disposable bathing cloths
- Clean gloves

Procedural Steps

1. Identify patient using at least two person-specific identifiers (e.g., name and date of birth or name and medical record number) according to employer policy (Accreditation Canada, 2019).

2. Assess environment for safety (e.g., check room for spills; make sure that equipment is working properly; check that bed is in locked, low position) and provide privacy.

3. Assess degree of help patient will need for bathing, risk for falling (e.g., ability to stand, get into a tub), patient's risk for skin breakdown, and presence of allergy or sensitivity to bathing solution (e.g., CHG) (see Skill 18.1).

4. Perform hand hygiene and apply clean gloves.

Continued

PROCEDURAL GUIDELINE 18.2 *Use of Disposable Bed Bath, Tub, or Shower—cont'd*

5. Arrange supplies and toiletry items at bedside if using bathing cloths; otherwise prepare supplies and equipment in patient's bathroom or a shower room.
6. **Bathing cloths:** (This procedure follows the AHRQ [2013b] universal bathing protocol for decolonization, used commonly in critical care and acute care hospitals.)
   a. Adjust room temperature and ventilation, close room doors and windows, and draw room divider curtain.
   b. Position patient supine or in a position of comfort. Use a bath blanket to drape areas of body not being cleaned as bath proceeds (see Skill 18.1).
   c. Help patient remove old gown (see Skill 18.1).
   d. *Option:* Warm package of bathing cloths in a microwave, following package directions. Do not use a microwave that is used for food preparation. The cleaning pack contains six premoistened cloths.

Clinical Decision Point *Check temperature of cloth after warming and have patient check as well to prevent burns to the skin.*

   e. Wash patient's face and eyes with plain warm water (see Skill 18.1).
   f. Use all six bathing cloths in the following order (see illustration), positioning and using drapes as described in Skill 18.1 (AHRQ, 2013b):
   g. Firmly massage skin with CHG cloth. Tell patient that the skin may feel sticky for a few minutes.

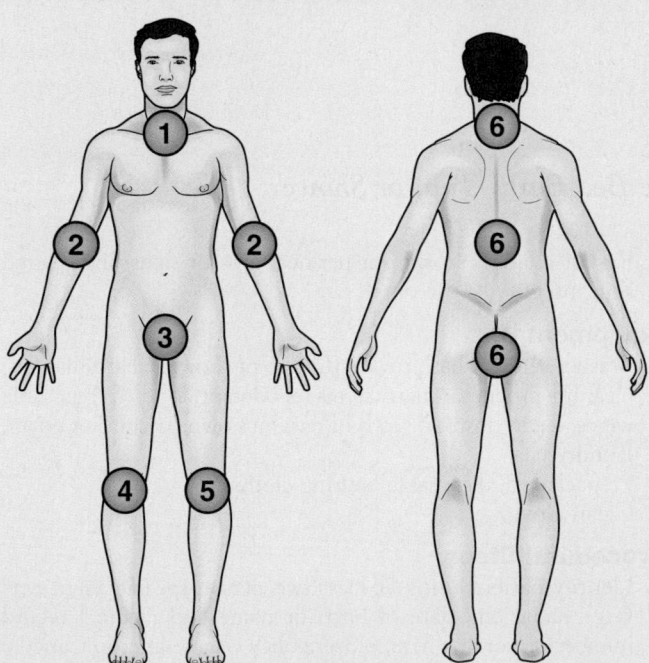

STEP 6f Order for use of six bathing cloths.
(1) Cloth 1: Neck, shoulders, and chest
(2) Cloth 2: Both arms, both hands, web spaces, and axilla
(3) Cloth 3: Abdomen and groin/perineum
(4) Cloth 4: Right leg, right foot, and web spaces
(5) Cloth 5: Left leg, left foot, and web spaces
(6) Cloth 6: Back of neck, back, and buttocks.

   h. Ensure thorough cleaning of soiled areas such as the neck, skinfolds, and perineal areas. CHG is safe to use on perineal areas, including external mucosa. It is also safe for superficial wounds, including stage 1 and stage 2 decubitus pressure injuries (AHRQ, 2013b).
   i. Do NOT rinse, wipe off, or dry with another cloth. Allow to air dry (AHRQ, 2013b).
   j. CHG cloths have built-in moisturizers. Skin may feel sticky for a few minutes.
   k. If additional moisturizer is needed, use only CHG-compatible products.
   l. Dispose of leftover cloths, help patient to comfortable position, and assist in applying clean gown.
7. **Tub bath or shower:**
   a. Assess patient's fall risk status; consider patient's physical ability to stand, get into tub, and review prescriptions for precautions concerning their movement or positioning. A health care provider's prescription usually is needed for tub bath or shower.
   b. Schedule use of shower or tub.
   c. Check tub or shower for cleanliness. Use cleaning techniques outlined in employer policy. Place rubber mat on tub or shower bottom. Place skid-proof disposable bath mat or towel on floor in front of tub or shower.
   d. Place hygiene and toiletry items within easy reach of tub or shower.
   e. Help patient to bathroom if necessary. Have them wear a robe and skid-proof slippers to bathroom.
   f. Demonstrate how to use call signal for help. Place "occupied" sign on bathroom door. Close door.
   g. Fill bathtub halfway with warm water. Check temperature of bath water, have patient test it, and adjust it if it is too warm or too cold. Explain which faucet controls hot water.

Clinical Decision Point *Do not use bath oil in tub water because this can cause slipping and resultant fall.*

   h. If patient is taking shower, turn shower on and adjust water temperature before they enter the shower stall. Use shower seat or tub chair if available (see illustration).

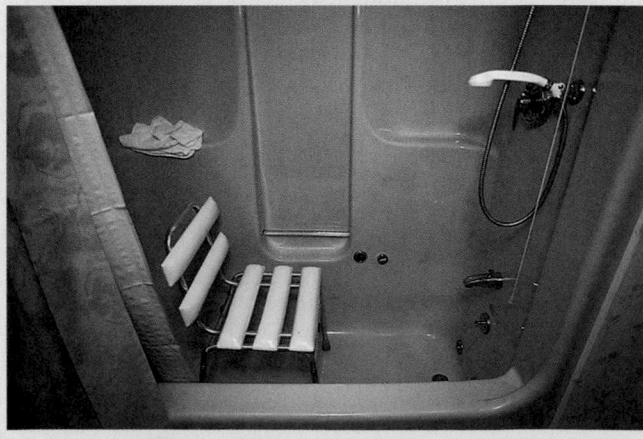

STEP 7h Shower seat for patient safety.

PROCEDURAL GUIDELINE 18.2 *Use of Disposable Bed Bath, Tub, or Shower—cont'd*

i. Tell patient that you will not allow them to remain in tub longer than 20 minutes. Provide privacy for patient and check on patient every 5 minutes, if patient health status indicates that it is safe to leave them alone. Remove and dispose of gloves; perform hand hygiene.

j. Apply clean gloves. Return to bathroom when patient signals, and knock before entering.

k. For patient who is unsteady, drain tub of water before they attempt to get out. Place bath towel over patient's shoulders. Help them get out of tub as needed and help with drying. If possible, have a shower chair available for patient to sit.

l. Help patient as needed to don clean gown or pajamas, slippers, and robe. (In home, extended care, or rehabilitation setting, encourage patient to wear regular clothing.)

m. Help patient to room and to comfortable position in bed or chair. Leave call light in reach.

n. Clean tub or shower according to employer policy. Remove soiled linen and place in dirty laundry bag. Discard disposable equipment in proper receptacle. Place "unoccupied" sign on bathroom door. Return supplies to storage area.

o. Remove and dispose of gloves. Perform hand hygiene.

8. Evaluate condition of patient's skin. Pay attention to areas that were previously soiled, reddened, flaking, scaling, or showing signs of breakdown.

9. Ask patient to rate level of fatigue and comfort.

✦ SKILL 18.2   Oral Hygiene

Maintenance of daily oral hygiene, including brushing, flossing, and rinsing, is essential for the prevention and control of plaque-associated oral diseases. In addition to preventing inflammation and infection, oral hygiene in general promotes comfort, ease of swallowing for better food intake, and verbal communication. Brushing cleans the teeth of food particles, plaque (the cause of dental caries), and bacteria; massages the gums; and relieves discomfort from unpleasant odours and tastes. Flossing removes tartar that collects at the gum line. Rinsing removes dislodged food particles and excess toothpaste.

When a patient becomes ill, many factors influence the need for oral hygiene. Offer oral hygiene help as required, from preparing needed supplies to actually brushing a patient's teeth. Plan the frequency of care on the basis of a patient's clinical condition and the condition of their oral cavity. For example, a stroke patient who has difficulty swallowing may require care as often as every 4 hours; a patient on a ventilator will require special care to reduce the chances of developing ventilator-associated pneumonia (VAP) (see Skill 18.3).

In addition to recommendations for the general population, there are oral-care regimens designed to relieve discomfort and facilitate healing of chemotherapy- and radiation therapy–related mucositis, stomatitis, and xerostomia. These types of oral lesions are very painful and interfere with a patient's nutrition. Specific regimens are discussed later in this chapter.

Delegation and Collaboration

The skill of oral hygiene (including tooth brushing, flossing, and rinsing) can be delegated to an unregulated care provider (UCP). However, the nurse is responsible for assessing the patient's gag reflex to determine if the patient is at risk for aspiration. The gag reflex is triggered when an object touches the back of the mouth, causing contraction of muscles in the throat. The nurse instructs the UCP about:

- Types of changes in oral mucosa (e.g., presence of lesions or open areas) for which to observe and report to the nurse.
- Reporting patient's complaints of pain or occurrence of bleeding during oral care.
- Being aware of special precautions such as aspiration precautions, including:
  - Keeping head of bed (HOB) raised 30 to 45 degrees (not lower).
  - Explaining need to report excessive coughing or choking during procedure.
- Not flossing when a patient has a bleeding tendency.

Equipment

- Soft-bristled toothbrush (hard-bristle toothbrush damages enamel and gums)
- Nonabrasive fluoride toothpaste or dentifrice
- Dental floss
- Chlorhexidine gluconate (CHG) 0.12% (*optional*, see employer policy)
- Tongue depressor
- Penlight
- Water glass with cool water, straw
- Normal saline or an essential oil–antiseptic mouth rinse (*optional*)
- Emesis basin
- Bath towels to place over patient's chest; paper towels
- Clean gloves
- *Option:* Moisturizing lubricant for lips

STEP	RATIONALE

ASSESSMENT

STEP	RATIONALE
1. Identify patient using at least two person-specific identifiers (e.g., name and date of birth or name and medical record number) according to employer policy.	Ensures correct patient. Complies with Accreditation Canada's standards and improves patient safety (Accreditation Canada, 2019).
2. Assess environment for safety (e.g., check room for spills; make sure that equipment is working properly and that bed is in locked, low position).	Identifies safety hazards in patient environment that could cause or potentially lead to harm (PHAC, 2015).

STEP	RATIONALE

ASSESSMENT

3. Perform hand hygiene and apply clean gloves.

Reduces transmission of microorganisms in blood or saliva.

4. Instruct patient not to bite down during assessment of oral cavity. Using a penlight and tongue depressor, inspect integrity of lips, teeth, buccal mucosa, gums, palate, and tongue (see Chapter 8).

Determines status of patient's oral cavity and extent of need for oral hygiene. Provides baseline to determine change after hygiene.

5. Identify presence of common oral problems.

Helps determine type of hygiene and information that patient requires for self-care.

   a. *Dental caries:* Chalky-white discolouration of tooth or presence of brown or black discolouration

   b. *Gingivitis:* Inflammation of gums

   May indicate periodontal disease.

   c. *Periodontitis:* Receding gum lines, inflammation, gaps between teeth

   May indicate periodontal disease.

   d. *Halitosis:* Bad breath

   May indicate periodontal disease.

   e. *Cheilosis:* Cracking lips

   f. *Stomatitis:* Inflammation of mouth tissues or structures

   g. *Mucositis:* Inflammation of oral mucous membrane

   h. Dry, cracked, coated tongue

6. Remove gloves and perform hand hygiene.

Prevents transmission of microorganisms.

7. Review medical record and assess patient's risk for oral hygiene problems:

Certain conditions increase likelihood of impaired oral cavity integrity and need for preventive care.

   a. Dehydration: Inability to take fluids or food by mouth; health care provider's prescription prohibiting food or fluids by mouth (NPO) for a procedure or because of patient's condition. It is extremely important to perform regular oral care when a patient is NPO.

   Causes excess drying and fragility of mucous membranes and lips; increases accumulation of thick secretions on tongue and gums.

   b. Presence of nasogastric or oxygen tubes; mouth breathers

   Causes drying of mucosa.

   c. Chemotherapeutic medications

   Medications kill rapidly multiplying cells, including sloughing of normal cells lining oral cavity. Mucositis with ulcers and inflammation can develop.

   d. Radiation therapy to head and neck

   Reduces salivary flow and lowers pH of saliva; leads to stomatitis and tooth decay (National Cancer Institute [NCI], 2016).

   e. Presence of artificial airway (e.g., endotracheal tube)

   Tube irritates gums and mucosa. Excess secretions accumulate on teeth and tongue.

   f. Blood-clotting disorders (e.g., leukemia, aplastic anemia)

   Predisposes to inflammation and bleeding of gums.

   g. Oral surgery, trauma to mouth

   Break in mucosa increases risk for infection. Vigorous brushing can disrupt suture lines.

   h. Aging

   With advancing age mucosa becomes thin and less elastic.

   i. Chemical injury

   Results from irritants such as alcohol, tobacco, acidic foods, or adverse effects of medications (e.g., antibiotics, steroids, antidepressants).

   j. Diabetes mellitus

   Prone to dryness of mouth, gingivitis, periodontal disease, and loss of teeth.

8. Determine patient's oral hygiene practices.

Identifies errors in patient's technique, deficiencies in preventive oral hygiene, patient's level of knowledge regarding dental care.

   a. Frequency of tooth brushing and flossing

   The Canadian Dental Association (CDA) (2012b; 2019b) recommends brushing teeth at least twice a day with CDA-approved fluoridated toothpaste and once-a-day flossing.

   b. Type of toothpaste, dentifrice, and mouth rinse used (assess if chlorhexidine is indicated for use)

   Mouthwashes and oral-care products with CDA seal of recognition demonstrate oral health benefits (CDA, 2019c).

   c. Last dental visit and frequency of visits

   The CDA recommends regular dental visits; however, frequency of visits can vary for each patient and should be determined by their dentist (CDA, 2012c).

9. Assess patient's ability to grasp and manipulate toothbrush.

Determines level of help required from nurse. Some older patients or people with musculoskeletal or nervous system alterations are unable to hold toothbrush with a firm grip or manipulate brush. Large-handled toothbrushes or a toothbrush handle pushed through a small rubber ball may be of help.

STEP	RATIONALE

NURSING DIAGNOSES

- Bathing/self-care deficit
- Impaired oral mucous membrane
- Deficient knowledge regarding oral hygiene care
- Risk for infection

Related factors are individualized on the basis of patient's condition or needs.

PLANNING

1. Expected outcomes following completion of procedure:
   - Patient expresses feeling of mouth cleanliness.
   - Oral cavity structures have normal characteristics:
   - Oral mucosa is moist, intact, and of normal colour.
   - Gums are pink, firm, and adherent to neck of teeth.
   - Teeth are clean, smooth, and shiny.
   - Tongue is pink and without secretions or coating.
   - Patient describes correct oral hygiene techniques.
   - Patient makes choices regarding hygiene procedure and helps by flossing and brushing.
2. Gather equipment and supplies at bedside.

3. Explain procedure to patient and discuss preferences regarding use of hygiene aids.

Hygiene measures remove secretions and thickened mucosa. Hygiene measures maintain integrity of teeth and healthy oral mucosa.

Demonstrates understanding of instruction.
Patient is able to manage self-care.

Avoids interrupting procedure or leaving patient unattended to retrieve missing equipment.
Some patients feel uncomfortable about having nurse care for their basic needs. Patient involvement with procedure minimizes anxiety.

IMPLEMENTATION

1. Perform hand hygiene. Close room doors and draw room divider curtain.
2. Arrange supplies on bedside table so they are within easy reach.
3. Raise bed to comfortable working height. Raise HOB to at least semi-Fowler's position (unless contraindicated) and lower side rail. Move patient or help patient move close to side from which you choose to work. A side-lying position can be used.
4. Place towel over patient's chest.
5. Perform hand hygiene. Apply clean gloves.
6. Apply toothpaste to brush bristles. Hold brush over emesis basin. Pour small amount of water over toothpaste.
7. Patient may help by brushing. Hold toothbrush bristles at 45-degree angle to gum line (see illustration). Be sure that tips of bristles rest against and penetrate (gently) under gum line. Brush inner and outer surfaces of upper and lower teeth by brushing from gum to crown of each tooth. Clean biting surfaces of teeth by holding top of bristles parallel with teeth and brushing gently back and forth (see illustration). Brush sides of teeth by moving bristles back and forth (see illustration).

Reduces transmission of microorganisms. Privacy ensures patient's mental and physical comfort.
Creates organized workspace.

Raising bed and positioning patient promote good body mechanics and prevent nurse from having muscle strain. Semi-Fowler's position helps prevent patient from choking or aspirating. **NOTE:** If patient is overweight, use safe handling techniques (see Chapter 11).
Prevents soiling of patient's gown.
Prevents transmission of microorganisms in body fluids.
Moisture aids in distribution of toothpaste over tooth surfaces.

Angle allows brush to reach all tooth surfaces and clean under gum line where plaque and tartar accumulate. Back-and-forth motion loosens food particles caught between teeth and along chewing surfaces.

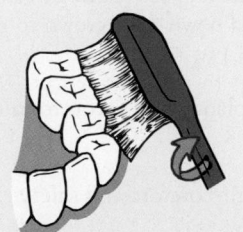 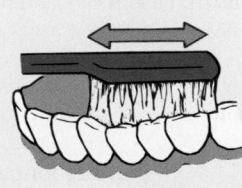 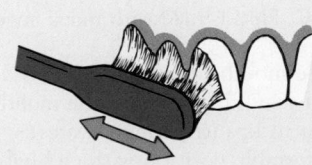

STEP 7 Directions of brush for tooth brushing.

STEP	RATIONALE

IMPLEMENTATION

8. Have patient hold brush at 45-degree angle and lightly brush over surface and sides of tongue (see illustration). Avoid initiating gag reflex.

Microorganisms collect and grow on surface of tongue and contribute to bad breath. Gagging may cause aspiration of toothpaste.

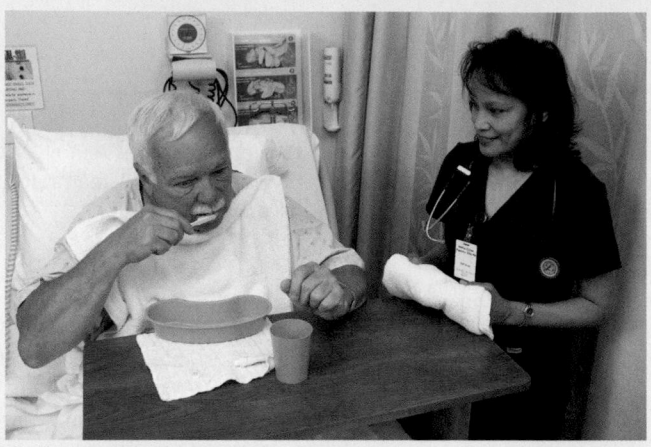

STEP 8 Nurse observes patient's tooth-brushing technique, including brushing of tongue.

9. Allow patient to rinse mouth thoroughly with water by taking several sips of water (may use straw), swishing water across all tooth surfaces, and spitting into emesis basin. Use this time to observe patient's brushing technique and teach importance of brushing teeth twice a day.

Rinsing removes food particles.

10. Have patient rinse teeth with antiseptic mouthwash for 30 seconds. Then have them spit rinse into emesis basin.

The CDHA recommends that oral rinsing with a commercially available mouthwash, as a complement to brushing and flossing, helps reduce plaque and gingival inflammation in adults (Asadoorian, 2017).

11. Help to wipe patient's mouth.

Promotes sense of comfort.

12. Allow patient to floss. Floss between all teeth. Hold floss against tooth while moving it up and down sides of teeth. Instruct patient in importance of daily flossing (see illustrations).

Flossing once daily removes plaque and decay-causing bacteria between teeth and under gum line, preventing gum disease.

Immunocompromised patients are sometimes on precautions that prohibit use of floss or Waterpiks because of dislodging bacteria and possible bleeding of gums.

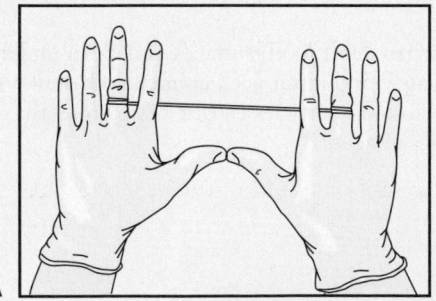 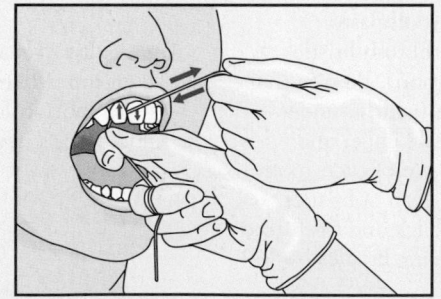 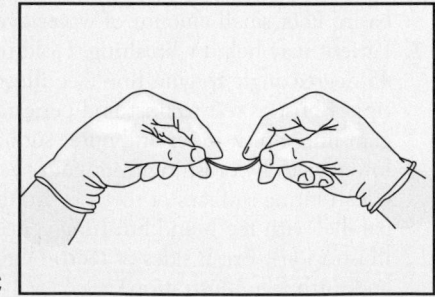

STEP 12 Flossing. **A,** Dental floss is held between middle fingers to floss upper teeth. **B,** Floss is moved in up-and-down motions between teeth. Floss is moved up and down from crown to gum line. **C,** Floss is held with index fingers to floss lower teeth.

13. Allow patient to rinse mouth thoroughly with cool water and spit into emesis basin. Help to wipe the mouth. Apply moisturizing lubricant to lips (if patient desires).

Rinsing removes plaque and tartar from oral cavity.

14. Help patient to comfortable position with call light in reach, remove emesis basin pend over-bed table, raise side rail if appropriate, and lower bed to original position.

Provides for patient comfort and safety.

STEP	RATIONALE

IMPLEMENTATION

15. Wipe off bedside table, discard soiled linen in dirty laundry bag, remove soiled gloves, and return equipment to proper place.

Proper disposal of soiled equipment prevents spread of infection.

16. Perform hand hygiene.

Reduces transmission of microorganisms.

EVALUATION

1. Ask patient if any area of oral cavity feels uncomfortable or irritated.

Pain indicates need for further inspection for possible breaks in oral mucosa or identification of stomatitis or infection.

2. Apply clean gloves and inspect condition of oral cavity. Perform hand hygiene.

Determines effectiveness of hygiene and rinsing.

3. Observe patient brushing and flossing.

Evaluates patient's ability to demonstrate correct technique.

4. **Use Teach-Back:** "We discussed what is important for taking proper care of your teeth and gums. Tell me how often you should brush your teeth and what to use." Develop a revised teaching plan if patient or caregiver is not able to teach back correctly.

Determines patient's and caregiver's level of understanding of instructional topic.

Unexpected Outcomes

1. Mucosa is dry and inflamed. Tongue has thick coating.

2. Cheilosis—Dry, cracked lips

3. Gum margins are retracted from teeth, with localized areas of inflammation. Bleeding occurs around gum margins.

4. Mucosa becomes inflamed from repeated chemotherapy administration, and a lesion from sloughing of tissue develops. These conditions can also be caused by radiation therapy used to treat head and neck cancers.

Related Interventions

- Increase patient's hydration.
- Increase frequency of oral care, focusing on tongue brushing.
- Apply moisturizing lubricant to patient's lips.
- Report findings because patient may have an underlying bleeding tendency.
- Switch to softer-bristled toothbrush or sponge toothette.
- Avoid vigorous brushing and flossing.
- Determine best-practice oral regimen for mucositis and stomatitis. Common regimens used to promote healing and comfort include:
- Use fluoride toothpaste.
- Use one of the following rinses made with salt and/or baking soda (NCI, 2016):
- 5 mL (1 tsp) salt in 1 L (4 cups) of water
- 5 mL (1 tsp) baking soda in 250 mL (1 cup) of water
- 2.5 mL (½ tsp) salt and 30 mL (2 tbsp) baking soda in 1 L (4 cups) of water
- An antibacterial rinse two to four times a day for gum disease; rinse for 1 to 2 minutes
- If dry mouth (xerostomia) and hyposalivation occur, additional rinses to increase moisture may be used. Brushing and gentle flossing should be continued as well.

Communication and Documentation

- Document procedure on basic care checklist in nurses' notes in electronic health record (EHR) or chart.
- Record condition of oral cavity in nurses' notes in EHR or chart.
- Document your evaluation of patient and caregiver learning.
- Report bleeding, pain, or presence of lesions to nurse in charge or health care provider.

Special Considerations
Teaching

- Educate patients about methods to prevent tooth decay (e.g., reduce intake of carbohydrates, especially sweet, sticky snacks between meals; brush within 30 minutes of eating sweets; rinse mouth thoroughly with water or alcohol-free antiseptic mouth rinse; use fluoride toothpaste). Use simple language and available teaching materials at proper literacy level.

- Educate patients to visit a dentist regularly (based on dentist's recommendations) for professional cleaning and oral examination; frequency of visits varies for each patient and should be determined by their dentist (CDA, 2012c).
- When teaching special oral-care regimens, include caregiver.
- Avoid mints if conditions of the mouth are associated with ulcerations of the oral mucosa.

Pediatric

- Every infant should receive an oral-health risk assessment from their primary health care provider or qualified health care provider within 6 months of the eruption of the first tooth or by 12 months of age (CDA, 2012a).
- Oral hygiene measures should be started before a child has a tooth. The goal is to wipe gums and teeth. Tooth brushing should be performed for children by a parent twice daily, using a soft

toothbrush of age-appropriate size and the correct amount of fluoridated toothpaste (CDA, 2019a).

- Children under 3 years should have their teeth brushed by an adult. Using fluoridated toothpaste is determined by level of risk of developing tooth decay. If a child is low risk, their teeth can be brushed with a toothbrush moistened with water. Otherwise, a minimal amount (size of grain of rice) of fluoridated toothpaste can be used. For children age 3 to 6 years, a small amount (size of a green pea) of fluoridated toothpaste is recommended (CDA, 2019a).

- Teach parents that infants should not be put to bed with a bottle; this causes tooth decay and ear infections. Limit snacks to three or four per day. Avoid giving sugary snacks and drinks and sticky candy.

Gerontological

- A number of normal age-related changes occur in the oral cavity. Thinning of the oral mucosa and decreased vascularity of the gingivae predispose older persons to injury and periodontal disease. Loss of tissue elasticity and decreased mass and strength of the muscles make chewing more difficult. Loss of the alveolar bone can loosen natural teeth.

- The number of taste buds declines with advancing age. In an attempt to enhance the taste of food, some older persons choose

salty and sugary foods, which erode tooth enamel and expose dentin.

- It is recommended that an adult not smoke, chew tobacco, or use snuff. Smoking may impair blood flow to the gums, reducing the amount of oxygen and nutrients to the tissues and making them more vulnerable to infection. Chemicals in tobacco smoke cause inflammation and cell damage and can weaken the immune system. Nicotine is toxic to cells that make new connective tissue and also increases the production of an enzyme that breaks down tissue (National Institute of Dental and Craniofacial Research, 2018).

- Some older persons may find it difficult to maintain good oral hygiene with flossing and brushing because of decreased dexterity and decreasing eyesight.

Care in the Community

- During the initial home visit, document the condition of a patient's mouth, teeth, and gums, as part of a comprehensive health assessment, thus providing a baseline for assessing the patient's ability to comply with special diets and fluid intake and carry out oral hygiene practices.

PROCEDURAL GUIDELINE 18.3 *Care of Dentures*

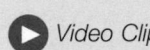 *Video Clip*

Oral bacteria from multiple strains and *Candida* species are found on acrylic dentures (Villa et al., 2015). Encourage patients who wear dentures to continue to care for them and provide this care as frequently as with natural teeth. Loose dentures can cause discomfort and make it difficult for patients to chew food and speak clearly. Routine denture care reduces the risk for gingival infection. Offer dental care after every meal and before a patient goes to bed. Some patients are unable to care for their dentures, and nurses become responsible for providing denture and oral care. Dentures are a patient's personal property; be sure to handle them with care because they are easy to break. Reinsert them as soon as possible. Note that it is common for patients to choose to not wear their dentures during an acute illness.

Delegation and Collaboration

The skill of denture care can be delegated to an unregulated care provider (UCP). The nurse instructs the UCP to:

- Not use hot or excessively cold water when caring for dentures.
- Inform the nurse if there are cracks in dentures.
- Inform the nurse if the patient has any oral discomfort.

Equipment

- Soft-bristled toothbrush or denture toothbrush
- Denture dentifrice or denture paste (regular toothpaste may be abrasive to dentures), denture adhesive (*optional*)
- Glass of water
- Emesis basin or sink
- 10 × 10–cm (4 × 4–inch) gauze
- Washcloth
- Denture cup (for storage)
- Clean gloves

Procedural Steps

1. Identify patient using at least two person-specific identifiers (e.g., name and date of birth or name and medical record number) according to employer policy (Accreditation Canada 2019).
2. Assess environment for safety (e.g., check room for spills; make sure that equipment is working properly, and that bed is in locked, low position).
3. Perform hand hygiene.
4. Assess patient to ensure dentures fit and for any gum or mucous membrane tenderness or irritation. Ask patient about denture care and product preferences.
5. Determine if patient has necessary dexterity to clean dentures independently or requires help.
6. Position patient comfortably sitting up in bed or help them walk from bed to chair placed in front of sink.
7. Fill emesis basin with tepid water. (If using sink, place washcloth in bottom of sink and fill sink with approximately 2.5 cm [1 inch] of water.)
8. Apply clean gloves.
9. Ask patient to remove dentures. If patient is unable to do this independently, grasp upper plate at front with thumb and index finger wrapped in gauze and pull downward. Gently lift lower denture from jaw and rotate one side downward to remove from patient's mouth. Place dentures in emesis basin or sink lined with washcloth and 2.5 cm (1 inch) of water.
10. Apply cleaning agent to brush and brush surfaces of dentures (see illustration). Hold dentures close to water. Hold brush horizontally and use back-and-forth motion to clean biting surfaces. Use short strokes from top of denture to biting surfaces to clean outer teeth surfaces. Hold brush vertically and use short strokes to clean inner teeth surfaces. Hold brush

PROCEDURAL GUIDELINE 18.3 *Care of Dentures—cont'd*

horizontally and use back-and-forth motion to clean under-surface of dentures (see Skill 18.2).

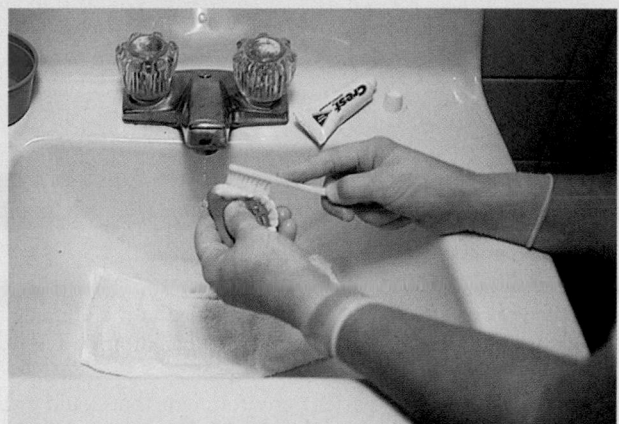

STEP 10 Brushing surface of dentures.

11. Rinse thoroughly in tepid water. If water is too cold, dentures can crack. If it is too hot, dentures can become warped and no longer fit.

12. Some patients use an adhesive to seal dentures in place. Apply a thin layer to undersurface before inserting.

13. If patient needs help with inserting dentures, moisten upper denture and press firmly to seal it in place. Insert moistened lower denture (if applicable). Ask if dentures feel comfortable.

14. Some patients prefer to store their dentures to give gums a rest and reduce risk for infection. Store in tepid water in enclosed, labelled denture cup. Keep denture cup in a secure place labelled with patient's name to prevent loss when not worn (e.g., at night, during surgery).

15. Dispose of supplies. Remove and discard gloves and perform hand hygiene.

16. Return patient to a comfortable position. Leave call light in reach.

♦ SKILL 18.3 Performing Mouth Care for an Unconscious or Debilitated Patient

Unconscious or debilitated patients pose challenges because of their risk for alterations of the oral cavity from drying of the mucous membrane, thickened secretions, and the inability to eat or drink. They are susceptible to infection because of the change in the normal flora of the oral cavity and at risk for infection because of increased plaque formation from the dryness of the mouth and decreased salivation. Dryness of the oral mucosa is also caused by mouth breathing and oxygen therapy. Respiratory secretions often are thick and place patients at risk for ineffective airway clearance, requiring oral suction (see Chapter 25). Debilitated patients are also at risk for aspiration. Although saliva production is decreased, saliva is present and can pool in the back of the oral cavity, which is a contributing factor for aspiration in patients with reduced gag reflexes. The secretions in the oral cavity change very rapidly to Gram-negative pneumonia–producing bacteria if aspiration occurs.

The critically ill patient with an endotracheal tube who is on mechanical ventilation is at risk for ventilator-associated pneumonia (VAP). Once intubated, an endotracheal tube causes a bypass of normal airway defenses, which also causes a rapid change in the normal oral flora (Centers for Disease Control and Prevention [CDC], 2017b). Some patients require mouth care as often as every 1 to 2 hours until the mucosa returns to normal. Proper hygiene requires keeping the mucosa moist and removing secretions as they accumulate in the back of the throat. The Canadian Patient Safety Institute (CPSI) has recommended using chlorhexidine gluconate (CHG) as part of daily oral care every 12 hours (CPSI, 2016) in critically ill patients. Many hospitals use an oral-care bundle to reduce incidence of VAP, including oral care and decontamination with chlorhexidine every 12 hours, and keeping the head of bed (HOB)

elevated 30 to 45 degrees or more unless contraindicated to prevent aspiration of oral secretions. Check employer policy regarding use of CHG in oral care.

Because many debilitated patients have either a reduced or absent gag reflex as a result of change in consciousness or a neurological injury, providing oral care requires protecting patients from choking and aspiration. The safest technique is to have two nurses provide care. One nurse provides oral care while another nurse suctions oral secretions, as necessary, with a Yankauer suction tip (see Chapter 25). A UCP may assist the nurse with oral care and suctioning. It is important to evaluate the level and frequency of oral care on a daily basis during assessment of the oral cavity. Routine suctioning of the mouth and pharynx is required to manage oral secretions to reduce the risk for aspiration.

Delegation and Collaboration

The skill of providing oral hygiene to an unconscious or debilitated patient can be delegated to a UCP. The nurse is responsible for assessing a patient's gag reflex. The nurse instructs the UCP to:

- Have another nurse help the UCP and properly position patient for mouth care.
- Be aware of special precautions, such as aspiration precautions.
- Use an oral suction catheter for clearing oral secretions (see Skill 25.1).
- Report signs of impaired integrity of oral mucosa to the nurse.
- Report any bleeding of mucosa or gum or excessive coughing or choking to the nurse.

Equipment

- Small pediatric, soft-bristled toothbrush, toothette sponges, or suction toothbrushes for patients for whom brushing is contraindicated
- Antibacterial solution per organization protocol (e.g., CHG)
- Fluoride toothpaste
- Water-based mouth moisturizer
- Tongue blade

- Penlight
- Oral suction equipment
- Oral airway (uncooperative patient or patient who shows bite reflex)
- Water-soluble lip lubricant
- Water glass with cool water
- Face and bath towel
- Emesis basin
- Clean gloves

STEP	RATIONALE

ASSESSMENT

1. Identify patient using at least two person-specific identifiers (e.g., name and date of birth or name and medical record number) according to employer policy.	Ensures correct patient. Complies with Accreditation Canada's standards and improves patient safety (Accreditation Canada, 2019).
2. Assess environment for safety (e.g., check room for spills; make sure that equipment is working properly and that bed is in locked, low position).	Identifies safety hazards in patient environment that could cause or potentially lead to harm (PHAC, 2015).
3. Perform hand hygiene and apply clean gloves.	Reduces transmission of microorganisms in blood or saliva.
4. Assess for presence of gag reflex by placing tongue blade on back half of tongue.	Helps in determining aspiration risk.

Clinical Decision Point *Patients with impaired gag reflex still require oral care; however, they have a higher risk for aspiration. Keep suction equipment available when caring for patients who are at risk for aspiration.*

5. Inspect condition of oral cavity (see Chapter 8).	Determines condition of oral cavity and need for hygiene. Establishes baseline to show improvement following oral care.
6. Remove gloves. Perform hand hygiene.	Prevents transmission of infection.
7. Assess patient's risk for oral hygiene problems (see Skill 18.2).	Certain conditions increase likelihood of alterations in integrity of oral cavity mucosa and structures, necessitating more frequent care.
8. Assess patient's respirations or oxygen saturation.	Helps in early recognition of aspiration.

NURSING DIAGNOSES

- Impaired oral mucous membrane
- Risk for aspiration
- Risk for infection

Related factors are individualized on the basis of patient's condition or needs.

PLANNING

1. Expected outcomes following completion of procedure: • Oral cavity structures have normal characteristics: buccal mucosa and tongue are pink, moist, and intact; gums are moist and intact; teeth are clean, smooth, and shiny; tongue is pink and without coating; lips are moist, smooth, and without cracks.	Degree of improvement in condition of oral cavity following oral hygiene depends on extent of secretions or changes that existed before care.
• Debilitated patient expresses feeling of mouth cleanliness.	Comfort achieved.
• Oropharynx remains clear of secretions.	Secretions removed, thus avoiding aspiration.
2. Gather equipment and supplies at bedside.	Avoids interrupting procedure or leaving patient unattended to retrieve missing equipment.
3. Explain procedure to patient or caregiver if present.	Even debilitated or intubated patients are usually able to hear. Explanation can reduce anxiety.

IMPLEMENTATION

1. Pull curtain around bed or close room door.	Provides privacy.
2. Perform hand hygiene and apply clean gloves.	Reduces transfer of microorganisms.

STEP	RATIONALE

IMPLEMENTATION

3. Place towel on over-bed table and arrange equipment. If needed, turn on suction machine and connect tubing to suction catheter.

Prevents soiling of tabletop. Equipment prepared in advance ensures smooth, safe procedure. Supplies within reach create organized workspace.

4. Raise bed to appropriate working height; lower side rail. Unless contraindicated (e.g., head injury, neck trauma), position patient in Sims' or side-lying position. Turn patient's head toward mattress in dependent position with HOB elevated at least 30 degrees.

Use of good body mechanics with bed in high position prevents injury.
Allows secretions to drain from mouth instead of collecting in back of pharynx. Prevents aspiration. If patient is overweight, follow safe handling techniques for positioning (see Chapter 11).

5. Place towel under patient's head and emesis basin under chin.

Prevents soiling of bed linen.

6. Remove dentures or partial plates if present.

Allows for thorough cleaning of prosthetics later. Provides clearer access to oral cavity.

7. If patient is uncooperative or having difficulty keeping mouth open, insert an oral airway. Insert upside down and turn airway sideways and over tongue to keep teeth apart. Insert when patient is relaxed, if possible. Do not use force.

Prevents patient from biting down on nurse's fingers and provides access to oral cavity.

Clinical Decision Point *Never place fingers into the mouth of an unconscious or debilitated patient as this may occlude the airway. Also, the normal response is to bite down.*

8. Clean mouth using brush moistened in water. Apply toothpaste or use antibacterial solution first to loosen crusts. Hold toothbrush bristles at 45-degree angle to gum line. Be sure that tips of bristles rest against and penetrate gently under gum line. Brush inner and outer surfaces of upper and lower teeth by brushing from gum to crown of each tooth; clean biting surfaces of teeth by holding top of bristles parallel with teeth and brushing gently back and forth (see Skill 18.2). Brush sides of teeth by moving bristles back and forth. Use toothette sponge if patient has bleeding tendency or use of toothbrush is contraindicated. Suction any accumulated secretions. Moisten brush with clear water or CHG solution to rinse. Clean lips and mucosa with toothette (see illustration). Use brush or toothette to clean roof of mouth, gums, and inside cheeks. Gently brush tongue but avoid stimulating gag reflex (if present). Repeat rinsing several times and use suction to remove secretions. Use towel to dry off lips.

Brushing action removes food particles between teeth and along chewing surfaces and crusts for mucosa. Do not use commercial swabs because they do not clean teeth. Repeated rinsing removes all debris and helps to moisten mucosa.
Suction removes secretions and fluids that collect in posterior pharynx, thus reducing aspiration risk.

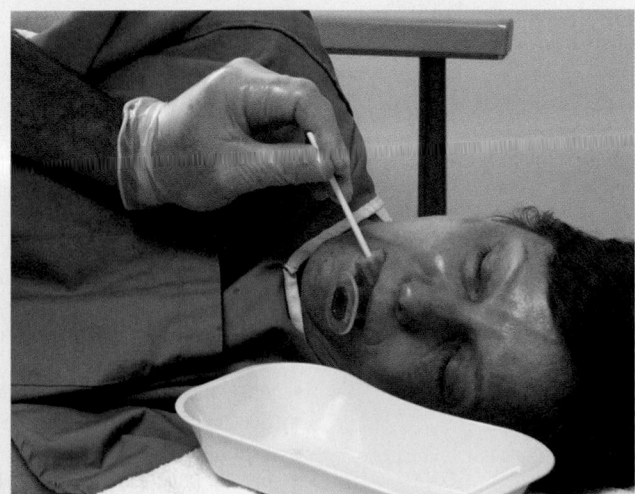

STEP 8 Cleaning lips and mucosa around oral airway with toothette.

STEP	RATIONALE

IMPLEMENTATION

9. Apply thin layer of water-soluble moisturizer to lips (see illustration).

Lubricates lips to prevent drying and cracking.

10. Inform patient that procedure is completed. Return patient to comfortable and safe position.

Provides meaningful stimulation to unconscious or less-responsive patient.

11. Raise side rails as appropriate and return bed to locked, low position. Leave call light in reach.

Reduces risk of falls from bed.

12. Clean equipment and return to its proper place. Place soiled linen in dirty laundry bag.

Proper disposal of soiled equipment prevents spread of infection.

13. Remove and dispose of gloves in proper receptacle and perform hand hygiene.

Reduces transmission of microorganisms.

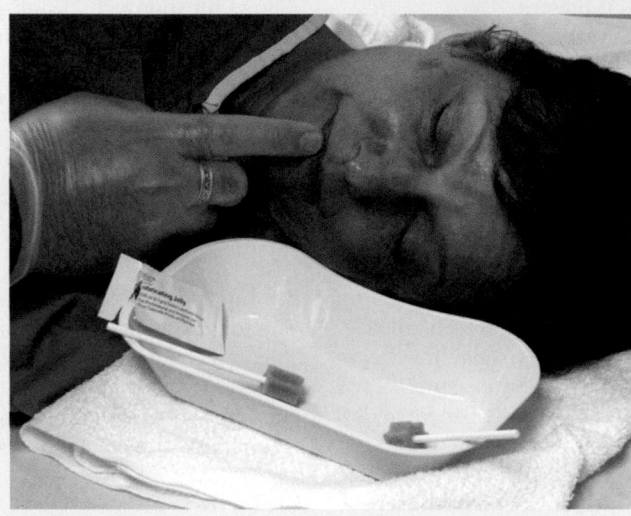

STEP 9 Application of water-soluble moisturizer to lips.

EVALUATION

1. Apply clean gloves and use tongue blade and penlight to inspect oral cavity.

Determines efficacy of cleaning. Once thick secretions are removed, underlying inflammation or lesions may be revealed.

2. Ask debilitated patient if mouth feels clean.

Evaluates level of comfort.

3. Use Teach-Back: "I explained what is needed to reduce your spouse's risk of choking on secretions in his throat. Tell me the ways you will prevent him from choking when you give mouth care at home." Develop a revised teaching plan if patient or caregiver is not able to teach back correctly.

Determines patient's and caregiver's level of understanding of instructional topic.

Unexpected Outcomes

1. Secretions or crusts remain on mucosa, tongue, or gums.
2. Localized inflammation or bleeding of gums or mucosa is present.

Related Interventions

- Provide more frequent oral hygiene.
- Provide more frequent oral hygiene with toothette sponges.
- Apply water-based mouth moisturizer to provide moisture and maintain integrity of oral mucosa.
- Chemotherapy and radiation can cause mucositis (inflammation of mucous membranes in mouth) because of sloughing of epithelial tissue. Room-temperature saline rinses, bicarbonate and sterile water rinses, and oral care with a soft-bristled toothbrush decrease severity and duration of mucositis.

3. Lips are cracked or inflamed.
4. Patient aspirates secretions.

- Apply moisturizing gel or water-soluble lubricant to lips more often.
- Suction oral airway as secretions accumulate to maintain airway patency (see Chapter 25).
- Elevate patient's HOB to facilitate breathing.
- If aspiration is suspected, notify health care provider. Using interprofessional collaboration, prepare patient for chest X-ray film examination.

Communication and Documentation

- Document procedure, appearance of oral cavity, presence of gag reflex, and patient's response to procedure in medical record in nurses' notes in electronic health record (EHR) or chart.
- Document your evaluation of patient and caregiver learning.
- Report any unusual findings (e.g., bleeding, ulceration, choking response) to nurse in charge or health care provider.

Special Considerations
Teaching

- It is important that caregivers understand how to provide good oral care when required for a patient in the home. Instruction in how to perform mouth care is necessary so the caregiver understands how to protect the patient from aspirating while thoroughly cleaning oral cavity. Use the teach-back technique by observing caregiver perform mouth care procedure effectively or asking them to describe the procedure.

Care in the Community

- Irrigate oral cavity with bulb syringe; if unavailable, substitute gravy baster or large syringe. Caution caregiver against instilling a large amount of water or rinsing agent in the oral cavity because of the risk of aspiration. Observe caregiver irrigate oral cavity.
- Encourage caregiver to clean patient's mouth at least twice a day. If patient breathes through mouth, a soft-bristled toothbrush moistened and used every 1 to 2 hours will keep mouth moist and fresh.

PROCEDURAL GUIDELINE 18.4 *Hair Care—Combing and Shaving*

A person's comfort, appearance, and sense of well-being can be influenced by how the hair looks and feels. Brushing, combing, and shaving are basic hygiene measures for all patients unable to provide their own self-care. Most long-term care facilities have beauty shops where patients can go for professional hair care. An immobilized patient's hair soon becomes tangled if not brushed or combed regularly. Dressings may leave sticky adhesive, blood, or antiseptic solutions on the hair. Diaphoresis leaves hair oily and unmanageable. Proper hair care is important to a person's body image.

Certain chemotherapy medications and radiation therapy cause loss of hair (alopecia). Many patients choose to wear a wig; however, some choose to wear hair scarves or turbans. Table 18.2 describes common hair and scalp conditions and nursing interventions.

Dependent patients with beards or mustaches need help keeping facial hair clean, especially after eating. Shaving facial hair is a task most men prefer to do for themselves daily. Because some religions and cultures forbid cutting or shaving any body hair, it is important to obtain consent from these patients. Make sure to be aware if patients are at risk for bleeding before shaving.

Delegation and Collaboration

The skills of combing and shaving can be delegated to an unregulated care provider (UCP). The nurse instructs the UCP to:

- Properly position a patient with head or neck mobility restrictions.
- Report how the patient tolerated the procedure and any concerns (e.g., neck pain).
- Use an electric razor for any patient at risk for bleeding tendencies.

Equipment
Hair Care
- Wide-tooth comb and hairbrush

TABLE 18.2

Hair and Scalp Problems

Characteristics	Implications	Interventions
Dandruff—Scaling of scalp accompanied by itching; in severe cases dandruff on eyebrows	Dandruff causes embarrassment; if it enters eyes, conjunctivitis may develop.	Shampoo regularly with medicated shampoo; in severe cases obtain health care provider's advice.
Ticks—Small grey-brown parasites that burrow into skin and suck blood	Ticks transmit several diseases, including Rocky Mountain spotted fever, Lyme disease, and tularemia.	Do not pull ticks from skin because sucking apparatus remains and may become infected; placing drop of oil on tick or covering it with petrolatum eases removal; oil suffocates tick.
Pediculosis capitis (head lice)—Tiny grey-brown white parasitic insects that attach to hair strands; about size of a sesame seed; nits or eggs look like oval particles attached at an angle to hair shaft; bites or pustules may be observed behind ears and at hairline	Head lice are difficult to remove and if not treated, may spread to furniture and other people.	Check entire scalp. Use medicated shampoo for eliminating lice or permethrin (Nix), available as a crème rinse. *Caution against use of products containing lindane because the ingredient is toxic and known to cause adverse reactions* (National Pediculosis Association, 2019). Remove patient's clothing before treatment and apply new clothing following treatment. Repeat treatment according to product directions. Check hair for nits and comb with nit comb for 2 to 3 days until sure all lice and nits have been removed. Manual removal of lice is the best option when treatment has failed. Vacuum infested areas of home. Wash linens in hot water and dry for at least 30 minutes.

Continued

PROCEDURAL GUIDELINE 18.4 *Hair Care—Combing and Shaving—cont'd*

TABLE 18.2

Hair and Scalp Problems—cont'd

Characteristics	Implications	Interventions
Pediculosis corporis (body lice)—Tend to cling to clothing; thus, may not be easily seen; suck blood and lay eggs on clothing and furniture	Patient itches constantly; scratches on skin may become infected; hemorrhagic spots may appear on skin where lice are sucking blood. It may spread to other people.	Patient should bathe or shower thoroughly; after skin is dried, apply lotion for eliminating lice; after 12 to 24 hours another bath or shower should be taken; bag infested clothing or linen until laundered. Vacuum items that cannot be washed.
Pediculosis pubis (crab lice)—Found in pubic hair; grey-white with red legs	Lice may spread through bed linen, clothing, furniture, or sexual contact.	Shave hair of affected area; clean as for body lice; if lice were sexually transmitted, partner must be notified.
Hair loss (alopecia)—Balding patches in periphery of hairline; hair becomes brittle and broken; caused by diseases, medication adverse effects, and improper use of hair-care products and hair-styling devices	Patches of uneven hair growth and loss alter patient's appearance.	Offer patients access to scarves, hairpieces, or wigs. Stop hair-care practices that damage hair.

Shaving With Razor
- New disposable or electric razor
- Clean gloves
- Bath towel(s), mirror, washcloth, washbasin
- Shaving cream or soap, aftershave lotion (if patient desires and it is not contraindicated)

Mustache Care
- Scissors, brush or comb
- Bath towel
- Gooseneck lamp or overhead light

Procedural Steps
1. Identify patient using at least two person-specific identifiers (e.g., name and date of birth or name and medical record number) according to employer policy (Accreditation Canada, 2019).
2. Perform hand hygiene. Inspect condition of hair and scalp. Inspect for presence of any infestation (e.g., pediculosis). **NOTE:** Apply clean gloves and gown if infestation is suspected; discard gloves and perform hand hygiene after inspection.
3. Assess patient's hair-care and shaving product preferences (e.g., shampoo, aftershave lotion, skin conditioner).
4. Assess if patient has bleeding tendency. Review medical history, medications, and laboratory values (e.g., platelet count, anticoagulation studies).

Clinical Decision Point *Have any patient on anticoagulants or who has low platelets use an electric razor.*

5. Assess patient's ability to manipulate comb, brush, or razor.
6. Gather equipment and supplies at patient's bedside. Explain your intent to provide hair or beard care. Ask patient to explain during procedure steps what they will use to comb hair or shave. Ask patient to indicate if they are uncomfortable during the procedure.
7. Position patient sitting in chair or up in bed with head elevated 45 to 90 degrees (as tolerated).
8. Provide privacy; close door or pull curtain. Arrange supplies at bedside table and adjust lighting.
9. Perform hand hygiene and apply clean gloves if necessary.

10. **Combing and brushing hair:**
    a. Part hair into two sections and then separate it into two more sections (see illustrations).

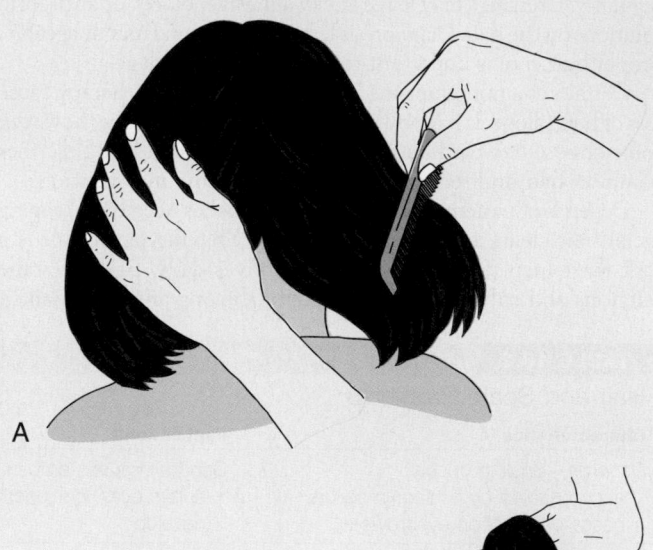

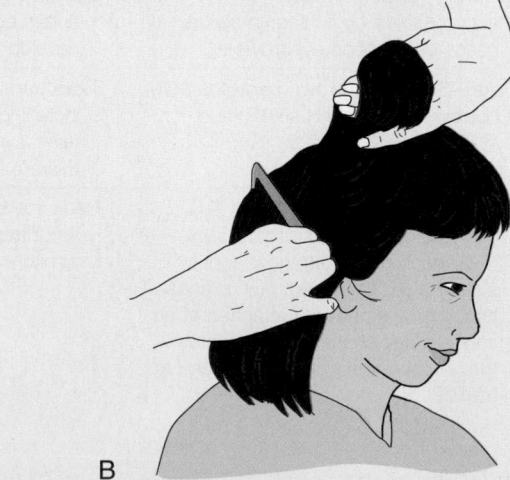

STEP 10a Parting hair. **A,** Part hair down the middle and divide it into two main sections. **B,** Part main section into two smaller sections.

PROCEDURAL GUIDELINE 18.4 *Hair Care—Combing and Shaving—cont'd*

b. Brush or comb from scalp toward hair ends.

c. Moisten hair lightly with water, conditioner, or alcohol-free detangle product before combing.

d. Move fingers through hair to loosen any larger tangles.

e. Using a wide-tooth comb, start on either side of head and insert comb with teeth upward to hair near scalp. Comb through hair in circular motion by turning wrist while lifting up and out. Continue until all hair is combed through and comb into place to shape and style.

11. Shaving with disposable razor:

a. Place bath towel over patient's chest and shoulders.

b. Run warm water in washbasin. Check water temperature.

c. Place washcloth in basin and wring out thoroughly. Apply cloth over patient's entire face for several seconds.

d. Apply approximately 0.6 cm ($\frac{1}{4}$ inch) shaving cream or soap to patient's face. Smooth cream evenly over sides of face, on chin, and under nose.

e. Hold razor in dominant hand at 45-degree angle to patient's skin. Begin by shaving across one side of patient's face using short, firm strokes in direction that hair grows (see illustration). Use nondominant hand to gently pull skin taut while shaving. Ask patient if he feels comfortable.

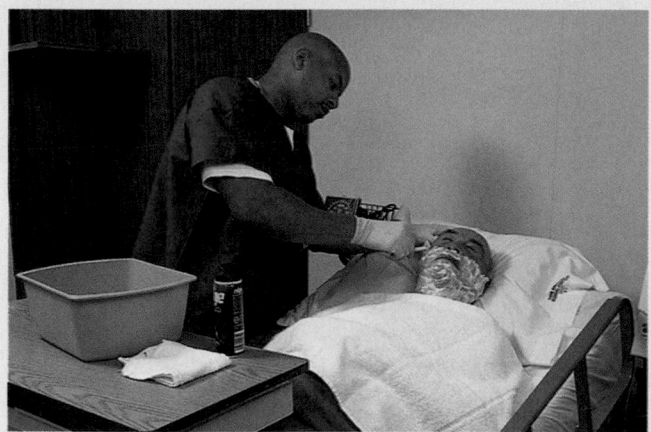

STEP 11e Shaving patient using short, firm strokes.

f. Dip razor blade in water because shaving cream accumulates on edge of blade.

g. After all facial hair is shaved, rinse face thoroughly with warm, moistened washcloth.

h. Dry face thoroughly and apply aftershave lotion if desired. Remove towel.

12. Shaving with electric razor:

a. Place bath towel over patient's chest and shoulders.

b. Apply skin conditioner or preshave preparation.

c. Turn razor on and begin by shaving across side of face. Gently hold skin taut while shaving over surface of skin. Use gentle downward stroke of razor in direction of hair growth.

d. After completing shave, remove towel and apply aftershave lotion as desired unless contraindicated.

13. Mustache and beard care:

a. Place bath towel over patient's chest and shoulders.

b. If necessary, gently comb mustache or beard.

c. Allow patient to use mirror and direct areas to trim with scissors.

d. After completing, remove towel.

14. Help patient assume desired comfortable position. Leave call light in reach.

15. Return reusable equipment to proper place. Discard soiled linen in dirty laundry bag. Perform hand hygiene.

16. Ask patient how the hair and scalp feel.

17. Inspect condition of shaved area and skin underneath beard or mustache. Look for areas of localized bleeding from cuts and areas of dryness.

18. Ask patient if face feels clean and comfortable.

19. **Use Teach-Back:** "I want to be sure I explained to you the risks of using a regular razor at home. Tell me what type of razor you should use and why this is important. Tell me the things to watch for with a bleeding tendency." Develop a revised teaching plan if patient or caregiver is not able to teach back correctly.

PROCEDURAL GUIDELINE 18.5 *Hair Care—Shampooing*

The frequency of shampooing depends on the condition of the hair and a person's daily routines and cultural preferences. Dry hair, which commonly results from aging and protein deficiency, requires less frequent shampooing than oily hair. In some health care facilities, the nurse needs a health care provider's prescription to shampoo a patient who is dependent or has limited mobility because it is challenging to find ways to shampoo the hair without causing injury to a patient's neck.

Remind hospitalized patients that more frequent shampooing is necessary when they remain in bed for extended periods of time, have excessive perspiration, or undergo treatments that leave blood or solutions in the hair. Two types of shampooing are available for patients: (1) traditional shampoo and water, or (2) a disposable

dry shampoo cap. Patients who are able to sit in a chair in front of a sink can be shampooed. Make sure that a patient's condition does not contraindicate neck hyperextension. Exercise caution with patients who have suffered neck injuries, because flexion and hyperextension of the neck could cause further injury. In addition, patients with positional vertigo are not able to tolerate neck hyperextension if it increases their dizziness. A folded towel placed under the neck on the edge of the sink provides added comfort.

If a patient cannot sit in a chair or be transferred to a stretcher, shampoo the hair with the patient in bed, using traditional shampoo and water or a disposable shampoo product.

Continued

PROCEDURAL GUIDELINE 18.5 *Hair Care—Shampooing—cont'd*

Delegation and Collaboration

The skill of shampooing the hair of bed-bound patients and the use of a disposable shampoo product can be delegated to an unregulated care provider (UCP). The nurse instructs the UCP about:

- Proper way to position a patient with a head or neck mobility restriction.
- Knowledge of care for lice, stressing steps to take to prevent transmission to other patients.

Equipment

- Bath towels
- Clean gloves; clean gown (*optional*) (if patient has known head lice)
- Clean comb and brush

Regular Shampoo

- Washcloth
- Shampoo, hair conditioner (*optional*), hydrogen peroxide (*optional*)
- Water pitcher with warm water
- Plastic shampoo board, wash basin
- Bath blanket, waterproof pad
- Hydrogen peroxide and saline (*optional*)

Disposable Shampoo

- Disposable shampoo cap product

Procedural Steps

1. Identify patient using at least two person-specific identifiers (e.g., name and date of birth or name and medical record number) according to employer policy (Accreditation Canada, 2019).
2. Inspect condition of hair and scalp before beginning shampoo. This determines if special shampoos or treatments are necessary (e.g., dandruff, lice, removal of blood). If draining head wounds are suspected, apply clean gloves. If lice are present, wear disposable gown in addition to gloves (National Pediculosis Association, 2019).
3. Review medical record to determine that there are no contraindications to the procedure. Check employer policy for health care provider prescriptions as needed. Certain medical conditions, such as head and neck injuries, spinal cord injuries, and arthritis, place a patient at risk for injury during shampooing because of positioning and manipulation of the patient's head and neck.
4. Assess environment for safety (e.g., check room for spills; make sure that equipment is working properly and that bed is in locked, low position) (PHAC, 2015).
5. Explain procedure to patient, using simple language.
6. Perform hand hygiene. Assemble equipment at bedside, including pitcher with warm water.
7. Provide privacy by closing room door or curtain dividers. Raise bed to comfortable working height and lower side rail on side where you will stand.
8. **Shampooing bed-bound patient with shampoo board:**
   a. Apply clean gloves. Place waterproof pad under patient's shoulders, neck, and head.
   b. Position patient supine with head and shoulders at top edge of bed. Place shampoo board under patient's head and

washbasin under end of trough spout (see illustration). Be sure that trough spout extends beyond edge of mattress.

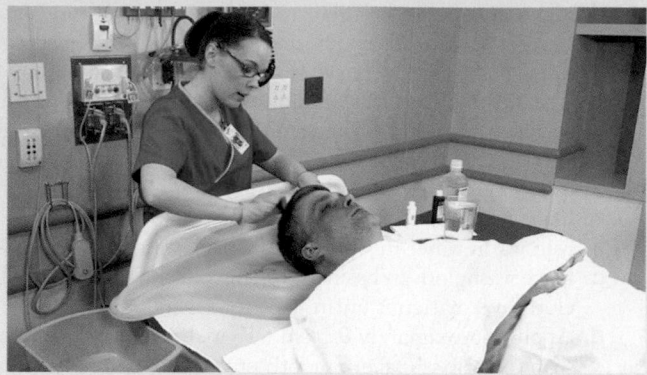

STEP 8b Patient positioned over shampoo board.

   c. Place rolled towel under patient's neck and bath towel over patient's shoulders.
   d. Brush and comb patient's hair.
   e. Ask patient to hold towel or washcloth over eyes.
   f. Test water temperature. Slowly pour water from pitcher over hair until it is completely wet (see illustration). If hair contains matted blood, apply hydrogen peroxide to dissolve clots and rinse with saline. Apply small amount of shampoo.

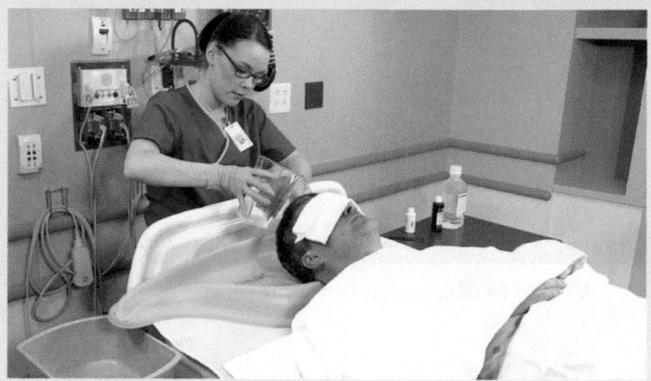

STEP 8f Nurse pouring water over patient's hair.

   g. Work up lather with both hands. Start at hairline and work toward back of neck. Lift head slightly with one hand to wash back of head. Shampoo sides of head. Massage scalp by applying pressure with fingertips.
   h. Rinse hair with water. Make sure that water drains into basin. Repeat rinsing until hair is free of soap. (If you need to refill pitcher, raise side rail when leaving bedside.)
   i. Apply conditioner or crème rinse if requested and rinse hair thoroughly.
   j. Wrap patient's head in bath towel. Dry face with cloth used to protect eyes. Dry off any moisture along neck or shoulders.

PROCEDURAL GUIDELINE 18.5 *Hair Care—Shampooing—cont'd*

k. Dry patient's hair and scalp. Use second towel if first one becomes saturated.

l. Comb hair to remove tangles and dry with dryer if desired.

m. Apply oil preparation or conditioning product to hair if desired by patient.

n. Variation for patients with coarse, curly hair: Condition hair after washing. To untangle hair, use wide teeth of comb. Beginning at nape of neck, comb small subsections of hair, starting at hair ends. Continue to work through small sections until hair is free of tangles.

o. Help patient to comfortable position and complete styling of hair. Leave call light in reach.

p. Dispose of supplies. Store reusable supplies. Remove gloves and perform hand hygiene.

9. Shampooing with disposable shampoo product:

a. Patient can be sitting on chair or in bed. Apply clean gloves.

b. Comb hair to remove any tangles or debris.

c. Open package, apply cap, and secure all hair beneath cap (see illustration).

d. Massage head through cap. Check fitting around head to maintain correct fit.

e. Massage 2 to 4 minutes according to directions on package; additional time may be required for longer hair or hair matted with blood.

f. Discard cap in garbage; do not dispose of in toilet because it may clog plumbing.

g. If patient desires, towel dry hair. Brush or comb patient's hair.

h. Remove gloves. Perform hand hygiene.

i. Help patient to comfortable position with call light in reach.

10. Inspect condition of hair and scalp.

11. Use Teach-Back: "During the shampoo we discussed ways to reduce risk of getting exposed to lice in your home. Tell me three ways to reduce the chance of exposing yourself and others to lice." Develop a revised teaching plan if patient or caregiver is not able to teach back correctly.

STEP 9c Patient wearing disposable shampoo cap.

↓ SKILL 18.4 Performing Nail and Foot Care

The best time to provide nail and foot care is during a patient's daily bath. Many facilities require a health care provider's prescription before the nurse can trim nails, and some require special certification to provide nail care (check employer policy). Feet and nails often require special care to prevent infection, odours, pain, and injury to soft tissues. Often people are unaware of foot or nail problems until discomfort or pain occurs. Common foot and nail problems are presented in Table 18.3. For proper foot and nail care, instruct patients to protect the feet from injury, keep them clean and dry, and wear appropriate footwear. Instruct patients how to properly inspect the feet for lesions, dryness, or signs of infection. To maintain and promote foot and nail health,

patients should visit a podiatrist when necessary. This is especially important for patients with foot disorders, peripheral vascular diseases (PVDs), or diabetes mellitus; older persons; and patients who are immunocompromised.

Patients most at risk for developing serious foot problems are those with peripheral neuropathy and PVD. These two disorders, commonly found in patients with diabetes mellitus, cause a reduction in blood flow to the extremities and a loss of sensory, motor, and autonomic nerve function. As a result, a patient is unable to feel heat and cold, pain, pressure, and positioning of the foot or feet. The reduction in blood flow impairs healing and promotes risk for infection. The development of diabetic foot ulcers has three

TABLE 18.3

Common Foot and Nail Problems

Condition	Characteristics	Implications	Interventions
Callus 	Thickened part of epidermis, consisting of mass of horny, keratotic cells; usually flat, painless, and found on undersurface of foot or palm of hand; caused by local friction or pressure	Foot calluses may cause discomfort when wearing tight-fitting shoes.	Refer patient to podiatrist; do not self-treat. Use of orthotic devices cushions and redistributes weight and pressure off calluses.
Corns 	Keratosis caused by friction and pressure from shoes; mainly on toes, over bony prominence; usually cone-shaped, round, and raised; calluses with painful core	Conical shape compresses underlying dermis, making it thin and tender. Pain is aggravated by tight-fitting shoes. Patients may suffer alteration in gait because of pain.	Refer patient to podiatrist. Avoid use of oval corn pads, which increase pressure on toes. Use wider, softer shoes.
Plantar warts 	Fungating lesions on sole of foot caused by papillomavirus	Warts may be contagious, are painful, and make walking difficult.	Refer patient to podiatrist.
Athlete's foot (tinea pedis) 	Fungal infection of foot; scaliness and cracking of skin between toes and on soles of feet; small blisters containing fluid may appear, apparently induced by constricting footwear	Athlete's foot can spread to other body parts, especially hands. It is contagious and frequently recurs.	Feet should be well ventilated. Drying feet well after bathing and applying powder help prevent infection. Wearing clean socks or stockings reduces incidence. Health care provider may prescribe application of griseofulvin, miconazole nitrate, or tolnaftate.
Ingrown nails 	Toenail or fingernail growing inward into soft tissue around nail; results from improper nail trimming, poor shoe fit, or heredity	Ingrown nails can cause localized pain when pressure is applied.	Treatment is frequent warm soaks *(exception: patient with diabetes mellitus)* in antiseptic solution and removal of part of nail that has grown into skin. Teach patient proper nail-trimming techniques. Refer to podiatrist.
Paronychia 	Inflammation of tissue surrounding nail after hangnail or other injury; occurs in people who frequently have their hands in water; common in patients with diabetes mellitus	Area can become infected.	Treatment is warm compresses or soaks *(exception: patient with diabetes mellitus)* and local application of antibiotic ointments. Paronychia can be prevented by careful manicuring.
Foot odours	Result of excess perspiration promoting microorganism growth and possibly faulty foot hygiene or improper footwear	Excess perspiration causes discomfort.	Frequent washing, use of foot deodorants and powders, and clean footwear prevent or reduce this problem.

contributing factors: (1) peripheral neuropathy (changes in the function and efficiency of the nerves), (2) ischemia (decrease in the blood flow related to plaque formation in arteries), and (3) a pivotal event (trauma caused by banging the toe or stepping on a foreign object). If foot ulcers do not heal, they can become infected quickly and lead to gangrene and subsequent amputation.

Delegation and Collaboration

The skill of nail and foot care of patients *without diabetes mellitus* or *circulatory compromise* can be delegated to an unregulated care provider (UCP). The nurse instructs the UCP about:

- Not trimming patient's nails (unless permitted by employer policy or health care provider prescription).

- Special considerations for patient positioning.
- Reporting any breaks in skin, redness, numbness, swelling, or pain to the nurse.

Equipment

- Washbasin
- Emesis basin
- Washcloth and towel
- Nail clippers (check employer policy)
- Soft nail or cuticle brush
- Plastic applicator stick
- Emery board or nail file
- Body lotion
- Disposable bath mat
- Clean gloves

STEP	RATIONALE

ASSESSMENT

1. Identify patient using at least two person-specific identifiers (e.g., name and date of birth or name and medical record number) according to employer policy.	Ensures correct patient. Complies with Accreditation Canada's standards and improves patient safety (Accreditation Canada, 2019).
2. Assess environment for safety (e.g., check room for spills; make sure that equipment is working properly and that bed is in locked, low position).	Identifies safety hazards in patient environment that could cause or potentially lead to harm (PHAC, 2015).
3. Perform hand hygiene and apply clean gloves. Inspect all surfaces of fingers, toes, feet, and nails. **NOTE:** *This can be done during the bath.* Pay close attention to areas of dryness, inflammation, or cracking. Also inspect areas between toes and on heels and soles of feet. Inspect socks for stains.	Integrity of feet and nails determines frequency and level of hygiene required. Heels, soles, and sides of feet are prone to irritation from ill-fitting shoes. Socks may become stained from bleeding or draining ulcer.
4. Assess circulation to extremities bilaterally: Inspect colour of skin; palpate temperature of toes, feet, and fingers and capillary refill of nails; palpate radial and ulnar pulse of each hand and dorsalis pedis pulse of foot; note character and symmetry of pulses (see Chapters 7 and 8). Remove gloves and perform hand hygiene.	Extremities should always be assessed bilaterally to check for symmetry. Weak or absent pulses, pallor, decreased capillary refill and temperature are all signs of peripheral artery disease (PAD), which occurs when blood vessels in legs are narrowed or blocked by fatty deposits and blood flow to feet and legs decreases. Swelling, pain, and varicose veins indicate venous insufficiency (Henke, 2017).
5. Observe patient's walking gait (when appropriate). Have patient walk down the hall or walk in a straight line while wearing comfortable shoes or slippers (if able). Ask if patient has pain when walking (use pain scale).	Alterations in bony structures of feet may cause pain, imbalance, and unsteady gait.
6. Ask if patient has history of leg pain on walking that is relieved with rest.	Claudicating pain is related to ischemia with diabetic and neuropathic disorders.
7. Ask if patient uses nail polish and polish remover frequently.	Chemicals in these products cause excessive dryness of nails.
8. Assess type of footwear patient wears: Does patient wear socks? Compression hose? Are shoes tight or ill fitting? Are garters or knee-high nylons worn? Is footwear clean?	Some types of shoes and footwear predispose patient to foot and nail problems (e.g., infection, areas of friction, ulcerations).
9. Identify patient's risk for foot or nail problems.	Certain conditions increase likelihood of foot or nail problems (e.g., diabetes mellitus, immunocompromised).
a. Older person	Poor vision, lack of coordination, or inability to bend over contributes to difficulty in performing foot and nail care. Normal physiological changes of aging can result in brittle nails. Discoloured, thickened, and deformed nails can indicate infection, fungus, or disease (CDC, 2017a).
b. Diabetes mellitus	Vascular changes reduce blood flow to peripheral tissues. Break in skin integrity places patient with diabetes mellitus at high risk for skin infection.
c. Heart failure, renal disease	Both conditions increase tissue edema, particularly in dependent areas (e.g., feet). Edema reduces blood flow to neighbouring tissues.
d. Cerebrovascular accident (stroke)	Presence of residual foot or leg weakness or paralysis results in altered walking patterns. Altered gait pattern causes increased friction and pressure on feet.
10. Assess for use of home remedies.	It is always a good idea to evaluate a patient's self-care routine. Patient's personal care practices may overlap or clash with prescribed medical treatment. Collaborate with patient when possible to ensure best outcome possible.

STEP	RATIONALE

ASSESSMENT

a. Over-the-counter (OTC) liquid preparations to remove corns or warts

Patients with diabetes mellitus or circulatory insufficiency should seek professional treatment and avoid self-treating.

b. Cutting corns or calluses with razor blade or scissors

Carries risk for cutting skin, which can lead to infection.

c. Use of oval corn pads

May exert pressure on toes, thereby decreasing circulation to surrounding tissues. Seek professional treatment.

d. Application of adhesive tape

Skin of older person is thin and delicate and prone to tearing when adhesive tape is removed.

11. Assess patient's ability to care for nails or feet: visual alterations, fatigue, and musculoskeletal weakness.

Extent of patient's ability to perform self-care determines degree of help required from nurse and need to educate caregiver.

NURSING DIAGNOSES

- Bathing/self-care deficit
- Reduced physical mobility
- Reduced skin integrity

- Reduced tissue perfusion
- Inadequate knowledge regarding foot and nail care

- Potential for infection

Related factors are individualized on the basis of patient's condition or needs.

PLANNING

1. Expected outcomes following completion of procedure:
- Nails are smooth. Cuticles and tissues surrounding nail are clear and of normal colour. Surfaces of feet are smooth.

Excess skin layers are removed. Nail integrity and cleanliness are maintained.

- Patient walks freely, without pain or unusual gait.

Foot care removes excess skin layers or shortens nails so that patient can walk more comfortably.

- Patient explains or demonstrates nail care correctly.

Patient learns self-care skill.

2. Gather equipment and supplies at bedside on over-bed table.

Avoids interrupting procedure or leaving patient unattended to retrieve missing equipment.

3. Explain procedure to patient, including fact that proper soaking of nails on hands requires several minutes in warm water. Exception: Patients with diabetes mellitus do not soak hands or feet.

Patient must be willing to place fingers in basin for up to 10 minutes. Patient may become anxious or tired.

4. Obtain health care provider's prescription for cutting nails (check employer policy). Obtaining prescription for podiatry consultation should be initiated if patient has diabetes mellitus, PAD, or PVD.

Patient's skin may be cut accidentally. Certain patients are more at risk for infection, depending on their medical condition.

A podiatrist should assess and develop a regular schedule for nail care for patients with vascular insufficiency or peripheral neuropathy.

IMPLEMENTATION

1. Perform hand hygiene and apply clean gloves.

Reduces transmission of infection.
Easy access to equipment prevents delays.

2. Pull curtain around bed or close room door to provide privacy.

Maintaining patient's privacy reduces anxiety.

3. Help ambulatory patient sit in chair and place disposable bath mat on floor under patient's feet. Help bed-bound patient to supine position with head of bed elevated 45 degrees and place waterproof pad on mattress (keep side rail up until ready to begin).

Sitting in chair facilitates immersing feet in basin. Bath mat protects feet from exposure to soil or debris.

4. Fill washbasin with warm water. Test water temperature. Place basin on floor or lower side rail and then place basin on pad on mattress. Have patient immerse feet. If patient has diabetes mellitus, peripheral neuropathy, or PVD, go to Step 13 to begin foot care.

Prevents accidental burns to patient's skin.

Clinical Decision Point *Patients who have diabetes mellitus, peripheral neuropathy, or PVD should not soak their hands and feet because of the increased risk of maceration that makes skin susceptible to infection.*

STEP	RATIONALE

IMPLEMENTATION

5. Adjust over-bed table to low position and place it over patient's lap.

Easy access prevents accidental spills.

6. Fill emesis basin with warm water and place basin on towel on over-bed table. Test water temperature.

Warm water softens fingernails and thickened epidermal cells. Prevents accidental burns to patient's skin.

7. Instruct patient to place fingers in emesis basin and arms in comfortable position.

Prolonged positioning causes discomfort unless normal anatomical alignment is maintained.

8. Allow feet and fingernails to soak 5 to 10 minutes. If patient has diabetes mellitus, peripheral neuropathy, or PVD, skip this step and go straight to Step 9.

Goal is to soften debris beneath nails so it can be removed easily.

9. Clean gently under fingernails with end of plastic applicator stick while fingers are immersed (see illustration).

Removes debris under nails that harbours microorganisms.

10. Use soft cuticle brush or nailbrush to clean around cuticles to decrease overgrowth.

Nailbrush helps to prevent inflammation and injury to cuticles. The cuticle slowly grows over the nail and must be pushed back with a soft nail brush regularly.

11. Remove emesis basin and dry fingers thoroughly.

Thorough drying impedes fungal growth and prevents maceration of tissues.

Clinical Decision Point *Check employer policy for appropriate process for cleaning beneath nails. Do not use an orange stick or end of cotton swab; these may splinter and can cause injury.*

12. *Check employer policy on nail care regarding filing and trimming.* Trim nails straight across at level of finger or follow curve of finger, ensuring that you do not cut down into nail grooves (see illustration). Use disposable emery board and file nail to ensure that there are no sharp corners.

Trimming straight across avoids skin overgrowth at nail edges, which can lead to ingrown nails or infection.
Filing nail straight across to eliminate sharp nail edges minimizes risk that nail can injure the adjacent finger.

13. Move over-bed table away from patient. Begin foot care by scrubbing callused areas of feet with washcloth.

Provides easier access to feet. Friction removes dead skin layers.

14. Clean between toes with washcloth.

15. Dry feet thoroughly and trim or cut toenails (see Step 12).

Moisture can cause skin maceration.

16. Apply lotion to feet and hands. Rub in thoroughly. Do not leave excess lotion between toes.

Lotion lubricates dry skin by helping to retain moisture.

17. Help patient back to bed and into comfortable, safe position, leaving call light within reach.

18. Sanitize or dispose of equipment according to employer policy. Emery boards should be disposable. Dispose of soiled linen in dirty laundry bag. Remove gloves and perform hand hygiene.

Reduces transmission of infection.

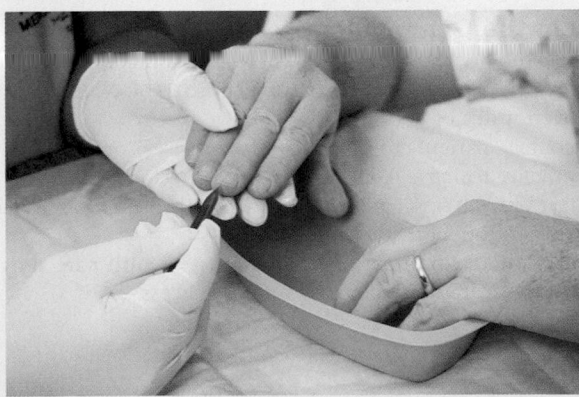

STEP 9 Clean under fingernails.

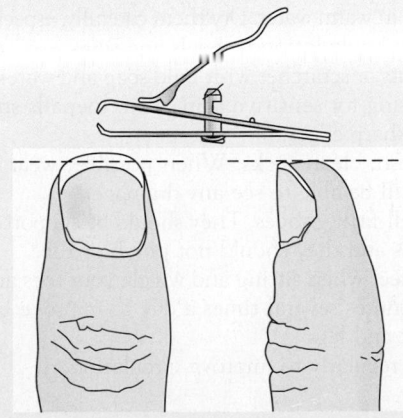

STEP 12 Trim nails straight across when using nail clipper.

STEP	RATIONALE

EVALUATION

1. Inspect nails, areas between fingers and toes, and surrounding skin surfaces.
2. If possible, have patient stand and walk and rate any pain.

3. Observe patient's walk after foot and nail care.
4. **Use Teach-Back:** "We discussed how to prevent infection in the skin around your nails. This is important because you have diabetes. Tell me the tips you should follow to protect your feet from infection." Develop a revised teaching plan if patient or caregiver is not able to teach back correctly.

Inspection enables you to evaluate condition of skin and nails and allows you to note any remaining rough nail edges.
Evaluates if nail care removed excess skin or uneven nail surfaces that can cause discomfort.
Evaluate level of comfort and mobility achieved.
Determines patient's and caregiver's level of understanding of instructional topic.

Unexpected Outcomes	Related Interventions
1. Cuticles and surrounding tissues are inflamed and tender to touch.	• Repeat nail care. • Evaluate need for antifungal cream.
2. Localized areas of tenderness occur on feet with calluses or corns at point of friction.	• Change in footwear or corrective foot surgery may be needed for permanent improvement in calluses or corns. • Refer patient to podiatrist.
3. Ulcerations involving toes or feet may remain.	• Institute wound care policies (see Chapter 39). • Consult with wound care specialist and/or podiatrist. • Increase frequency of assessment and hygiene.

Communication and Documentation

- Document procedure and observations of condition of nails and skin around nails in medical record in nurses' notes in electronic health record (EHR) or chart.
- Report any areas of discomfort, breaks in skin, or ulcerations to nurse in charge or health care provider.
- Document your evaluation of patient and caregiver learning.

Special Considerations
Teaching

- Use a variety of teaching formats regarding foot and nail care (e.g., brochures, videos, DVDs, websites) that are consistent with patient's health literacy level. Instruct patient not to walk barefoot or use corn or callus products. Include caregiver in foot and nail care education.
- Instruct a patient with diabetes mellitus, peripheral neuropathy, or PVD to do the following (Diabetes Canada, 2019):
  - Inspect your feet daily to make sure there are no cuts, cracks, ingrown toenails, or blisters. Use a mirror to see the bottom of your feet, or ask someone to check them for you. Wash your feet in warm water. Dry them carefully, especially between the toes. Apply lotion to heels and soles.
  - Clean cuts or scratches with mild soap and water. Cover with dry dressing for sensitive skin. Trim toenails straight across and file sharp edges.
  - Wear fresh, clean socks. When possible, wear white socks, as you will be able to see any drainage.
  - Wear well-fitting shoes. They should be supportive and have low heels and they should not pinch or rub.
  - Elevate feet when sitting and wiggle your toes and ankles for a few minutes several times a day to improve blood flow in your feet and legs.
  - Exercise regularly to improve circulation.

- See more at http://www.diabetes.ca/diabetes-and-you/healthy-living-resources/foot-care/a-step-towards-good-health.

Pediatric
- Teach a parent how to assess a child's nails and trim them to prevent the child from scratching the skin.
- Use appropriate-size clippers for infants and small children (check employer policy). *Do not use scissors*.

Gerontological
- Changes in aging skin include thinning of epidermis and subcutaneous fat and dryness because of decreased activity of oil and sweat glands. These changes are often evident in the feet. In addition, nails become discoloured, thickened, deformed, and brittle.
- PVD, peripheral neuropathy, and long periods of limited exercise or bed rest impact balance, stability, and sensory impairment, resulting in impaired mobility.
- Older persons may lose the dexterity and coordination needed to trim nails regularly.

Care in the Community
- Assess the home for any areas where a person could accidentally injure the feet, such as rugs, objects that block pathways, or uneven walks or flooring.
- Encourage patients to not go barefoot or wear open-toed shoes.
- *Alternative therapy:* Apply moleskin to friction areas of the foot or feet or wrap small pieces of lamb's wool around toes to reduce irritation from corns or bunions.
- Place contact information of podiatrist, health care provider, and home care nurse close by for easy access.

PROCEDURAL GUIDELINE 18.6 *Making an Occupied Bed*

The hospital bed is the piece of equipment a patient uses most. It should be comfortable, safe, and adaptable to various positions. The typical hospital bed consists of a firm mattress on a metal frame that can be raised or lowered horizontally. The frame is divided into three sections so that the operator can raise and lower the head and foot of the bed separately and incline the entire bed with the head up or down. Table 18.4 shows common bed positions. Each bed sits on four casters that allow health care workers to move it easily. Each caster may have a brake to make sure the bed is stationary. Beds have side rails (adjustable metal frames) that can be raised or lowered by pushing or pulling a knob located on both sides of the bed. Research shows that the risk for patient falls is greater when side rails on both sides of a bed are raised, because patients try to climb over the rails to exit the bed. Raising only one rail (when there are only two) or three (when there are four rails) gives patients an exit to move independently.

At times, it is necessary to make a bed that is occupied by a patient who cannot tolerate being out of bed. If a patient is confined to bed, the bed should be made in a way that conserves time and the patient's energy. A patient's weight, ability to move and turn, pain acuity, and restrictions related to clinical condition or treatment all affect the number of individuals who need to be involved in making an occupied bed. It is essential to use safe patient-handling techniques when turning and positioning a patient over bed linen (see Chapter 11). In cases in which a patient experiences severe pain, an analgesic administered 30 to 60 minutes before making a bed can control pain and maintain comfort.

Even though a patient is unable to get out of bed, encourage self-help as much as possible. For example, if patients can turn, help in moving up in bed, or hold top sheets during application, have them do so. These activities help maintain a patient's strength and mobility and allow participation in hygiene care.

Delegation Considerations

The skill of making an occupied bed can be delegated to an unregulated care provider (UCP). The nurse instructs the UCP about:

- Any position or activity restrictions that apply.
- Looking for wound drainage or loosened equipment that might be found in the bed linens.
- When to obtain help from other caregivers for positioning a patient during linen change and the importance of using good body mechanics and supporting patient alignment.

TABLE 18.4

Common Bed Positions

Position		Description	Uses
Fowler's	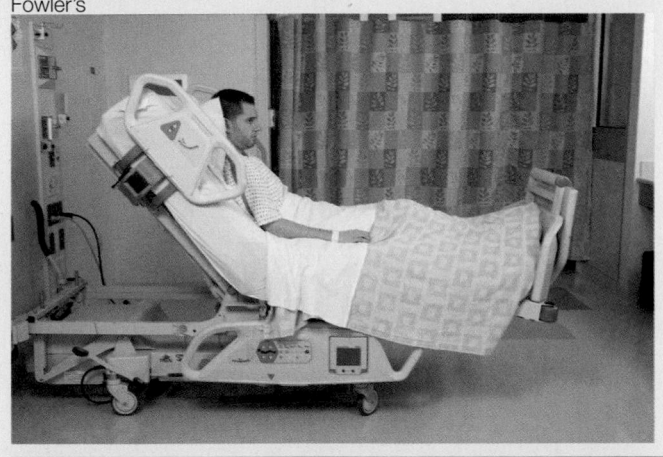 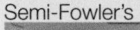	Head of bed raised to angle of 45 to 90 degrees; semi-sitting position; foot of bed may also raise at knee	Preferred while patient eats; used during nasogastric tube insertion and nasotracheal suction; promotes lung expansion
Semi-Fowler's	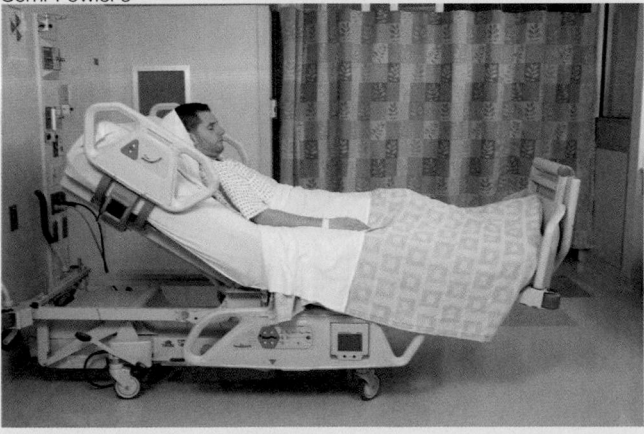	Head of bed raised approximately 30 to 45 degrees; incline less than Fowler's position; foot of bed may also raise at knee	Promotes lung expansion; relieves strain on abdominal muscles Used when patients receive gastric feedings, to reduce risk for aspiration

Continued

PROCEDURAL GUIDELINE 18.6 *Making an Occupied Bed—cont'd*

TABLE 18.4

Common Bed Positions—cont'd

Position	Description	Uses
Trendelenburg's 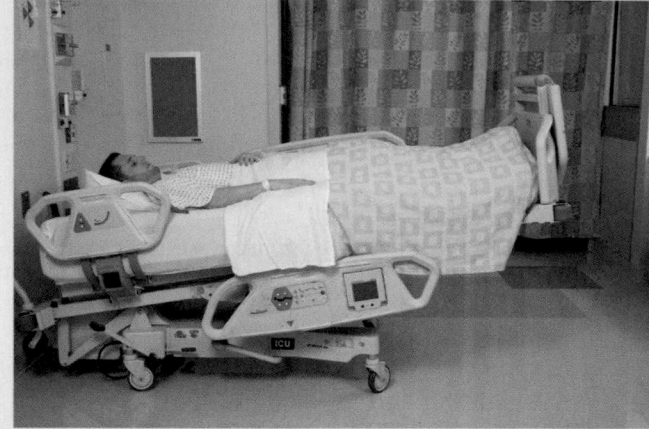	Entire bedframe tilted with head of bed down	For postural drainage; facilitates venous return in patients with poor peripheral perfusion
Reverse Trendelenburg's 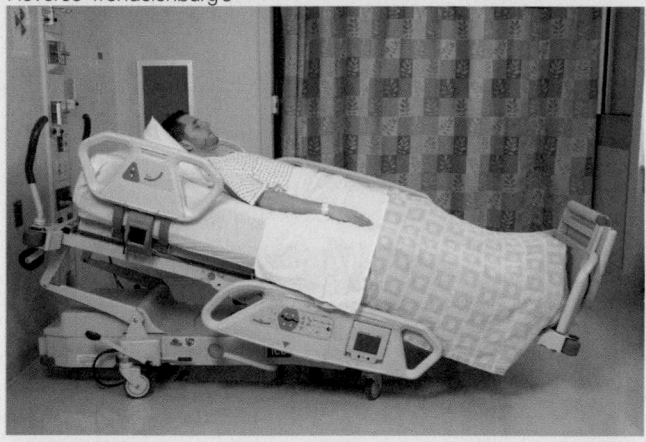	Entire bedframe tilted with foot of bed down	Used infrequently; promotes gastric emptying and prevents esophageal reflux
Supine or flat 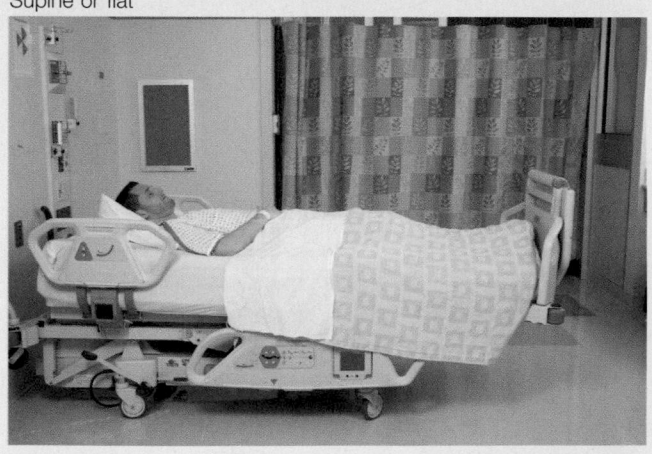	Entire bedframe horizontally parallel with floor	For patients with vertebral injuries and in cervical traction; position used for patients who are hypotensive and generally preferred by patients for sleeping

PROCEDURAL GUIDELINE 18.6 *Making an Occupied Bed—cont'd*

- Using special precautions (e.g., aspiration precautions [see Chapter 31] or positioning for tube-feeding infusion [see Chapter 32]) when positioning a patient during bed making.

Equipment
- Linen bags
- Mattress pad (change only when soiled)
- Bottom sheet (flat or fitted)
- Drawsheet (*optional*)
- Top sheet, blanket, bedspread, pillowcases
- Waterproof pads (*optional*)
- Clean gloves (if linen is soiled or there is risk of exposure to body fluids)
- Antiseptic cleanser
- Washcloth

Procedural Steps
1. Review medical record and assess restrictions in mobility or positioning of patient.
2. Organize supplies and close room door or divider curtain to provide privacy.
3. Assess environment for safety (e.g., check room for spills; make sure that equipment is working properly and that bed is in locked position and appropriate number of side rails are raised).
4. Perform hand hygiene. Apply clean gloves if patient has been incontinent or if drainage is present on linen.
5. Explain procedure to patient, noting that patient will be asked to turn over layers of linen.
6. Raise bed to a comfortable working height; lower head of bed (HOB) as tolerated, keeping patient comfortable. Remove call light.

Clinical Decision Point *If patient is on aspiration precautions or receiving tube feeding, maintain HOB no lower than 30 degrees.*

7. Lower side rail on side where you are standing. Loosen all top linen. Remove bedspread and blanket separately, leaving patient covered with top sheet. If blanket or spread is soiled, place in linen bag. If to be reused, fold into square and place over back of chair.
8. Cover patient with clean bath blanket by unfolding it over top sheet. Have patient hold top edge of bath blanket or tuck blanket under shoulders. Grasp top sheet under bath blanket at patient's shoulders and bring sheet down to foot of bed. Remove sheet and discard in dirty laundry bag.
9. Position patient on far side of bed, turned onto side and facing away from you. **NOTE:** This is when another caregiver can help you by standing at bedside across from you. Encourage patient to use side rail to turn. Adjust pillow under patient's head.
10. Assess to make sure that there is no tension on any external medical devices.
11. Loosen bottom linens, moving from head to foot. Fanfold or roll any cloth pads, drawsheet (if present), and bottom sheet (in that order) toward patient. Tuck edges of old linen just under patient's buttocks, back, and shoulders (see illustration). Do not fanfold mattress pad (if it is to be reused). Remove any disposable pads and discard in receptacle.

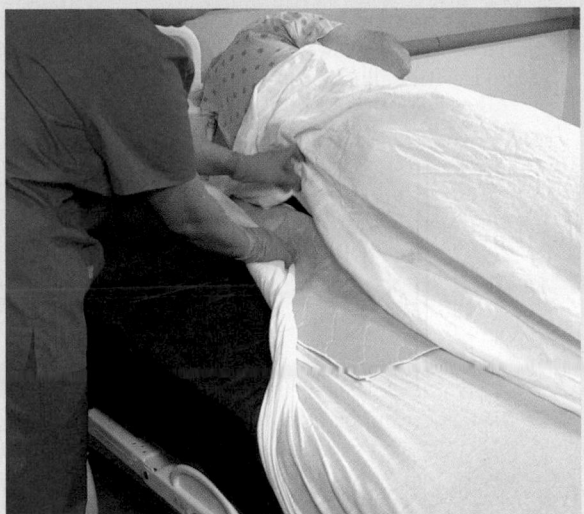

STEP 11 Tuck all soiled linen from one side of bed alongside patient's back.

12. Clean, disinfect, and dry mattress surface if it is soiled or has moisture (see employer policy).
13. Apply clean linens to the exposed half of bed in separate layers. When needed, start with a new mattress pad by placing it lengthwise with centre crease in middle of bed. Fanfold pad to centre of bed alongside patient. Repeat process with bottom sheet.
14. Pull new fitted sheet smoothly over mattress corner at top and bottom of bed. If using a flat sheet, allow edge of sheet to hang about 25 cm (10 inches) over mattress edge at head of bed. Be sure that lower hem of bottom flat sheet lies seam down and with bottom edge of mattress.
15. If bottom sheet is flat, mitre top corner at HOB. Face HOB diagonally. Place hand away from HOB under top corner of mattress, lift, and with other hand tuck edge of bottom sheet smoothly under mattress so side edges of sheet above and below mattress meet when brought together.
16. If bottom sheet is flat, mitre top corner at HOB.
    a. Face HOB diagonally. Place hand away from HOB under top corner of mattress, near mattress edge, and lift.
    b. With other hand, tuck top edge of bottom sheet smoothly under mattress so side edges of sheet above and below mattress meet when brought together.
    c. To mitre a corner, pick up top edge of sheet at about 45 cm (18 inches) from top end of mattress (see illustration).

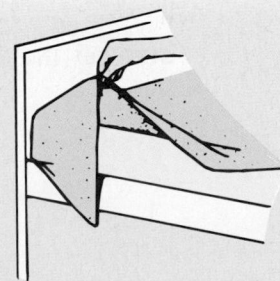

STEP 16c Top edge of sheet picked up.

Continued

PROCEDURAL GUIDELINE 18.6 *Making an Occupied Bed—cont'd*

d. Lift sheet and lay it on top of mattress to form a neat triangular fold with lower base of triangle even with mattress side edges (see illustration).

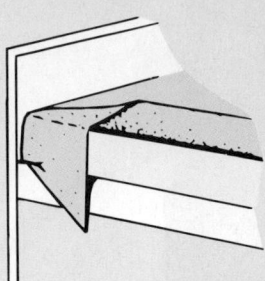

STEP 16d Sheet on top of mattress in a triangular fold.

e. Tuck lower edge of sheet, which is hanging free below the mattress, under the mattress. Tuck with palms down, without pulling triangular fold.

f. Hold part of sheet covering side of mattress in place with one hand (see illustrations). With other hand pick up top of triangular linen fold and bring it down over side of mattress. Tuck under mattress with palms down without pulling fold (see illustration).

17. Tuck remaining part of sheet under mattress, moving toward foot of bed. Keep linen smooth.

18. Place new drawsheet along middle of bed lengthwise. Fanfold or roll drawsheet on top of clean bottom sheet. Tuck under patient's buttocks and torso without touching old linen.

19. Add waterproof pad (absorbent side up) over drawsheet with seam side down. Fanfold toward patient. Continue to keep clean and soiled linen separate. Also keep linen under patient as flat as possible because patient will need to roll over old and new layers of linen when you are ready to make other side of bed.

20. Advise patient that they will be rolling over a thick layer of linens. Keeping patient covered, ask patient to roll toward you slowly over layers of linen and to not raise the hips (see illustration). Stress the need to roll while staying aligned.

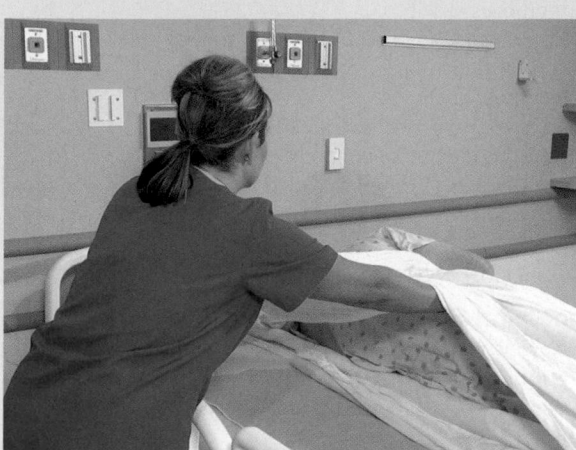

STEP 20 Patient begins rolling over layers of linen.

21. Now raise side rail and move to opposite side of bed. Option: The caregiver helping you can help position patient. Have patient roll away from you toward other side of bed, over all of the folds of linen. Again, have patient keep hips still.

22. Loosen edges of soiled linen from under mattress. Remove soiled linen by folding into a bundle or square.

23. Hold linen away from your body and place it in laundry bag.

24. Clean, disinfect, and dry other half of mattress as needed.

25. Pull clean, fanfolded or rolled mattress pad; sheet; drawsheet; and pad out from beneath patient toward you. Smooth all linen out over mattress from head to foot of bed. Help patient roll back to supine position, and reposition pillow.

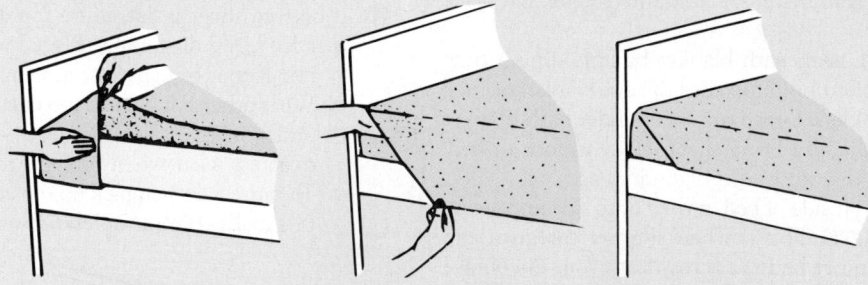

STEP 16f Triangular fold placed over side of mattress; sheet tucked under mattress.

PROCEDURAL GUIDELINE 18.6 *Making an Occupied Bed—cont'd*

26. If bottom sheet is fitted, pull corners over mattress edges. If flat sheet is used, mitre top corner of bottom flat sheet (see Steps 16a–f).
27. Facing side of bed, grasp remaining edge of bottom flat sheet. Lean back slightly, keep back straight, and pull while tucking excess linen under mattress from HOB to foot of bed. Avoid lifting mattress during tucking.
28. Smooth fanfolded drawsheet over bottom sheet (tucking is optional). Smooth waterproof pads, making sure that bed surface is wrinkle free.
29. Place top sheet over patient with vertical centrefold lengthwise down middle of bed and with seam side of hem facing up. Open sheet out from head to foot and unfold over patient. Be sure that top edge of sheet is even with top edge of mattress.
30. Place clean or reused bed blanket on bed over patient. Make sure that top edge is parallel with top edge of sheet and 15 to 20 cm (6 to 8 inches) from edge of top sheet. Raise side rail.
31. Go to other side of bed. Lower side rail. Spread sheet and blanket out evenly.
32. Have patient hold onto sheet and blanket while you remove bath blanket; discard in linen bag.
33. Make cuff by turning edge of top sheet down over top edge of blanket.
34. Make horizontal toe pleat; stand at foot of bed and fanfold in sheet and blanket 5 to 10 cm (2 to 4 inches) across bed. Pull sheet and blanket up from bottom to make fold approximately 15 cm (6 inches) from bottom edge of mattress.
35. Standing at side of bed, tuck in remaining part of sheet and blanket under foot of mattress. Tuck top sheet and blanket together. Be sure that toe pleats are not pulled out.
36. Make modified mitred corner with top sheet and blanket. Follow Steps 16a–f. After making triangular fold, do not tuck tip of triangle (see illustration).

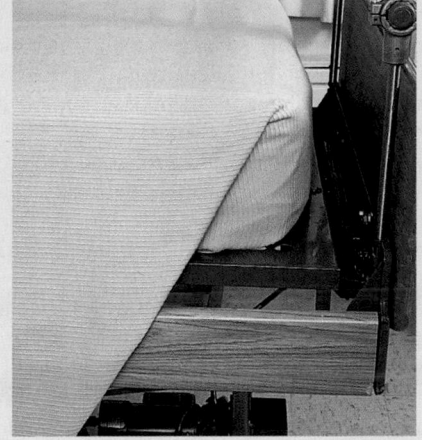

STEP 36 Modified mitred corner.

37. Go to other side of bed. Repeat Steps 35 and 36.
38. Change pillowcase. Have patient raise head. While supporting neck with one hand, remove pillow. Allow patient to lower head. Remove soiled case and place in linen bag. Grasp clean pillowcase at centre of closed end. Gather case, turning it inside out over the hand holding it. With the same hand, pick up middle of one end of pillow. Pull pillowcase down over pillow with other hand. Do not hold pillow against your uniform. Be sure that pillow corners fit evenly into corners of case. Reposition pillow under patient's head.
39. Place call light within patient's reach on bedrail or pillow; return bed to locked, low position; and raise side rail (as needed).
40. Place all linen in dirty laundry bag. Remove and dispose of gloves.
41. Arrange and organize patient's room and perform hand hygiene.
42. During procedure inspect skin for areas of irritation. Observe patient for signs of fatigue, dyspnea, pain, or other sources of discomfort.

PROCEDURAL GUIDELINE 18.7 *Making an Unoccupied Bed*

A bed may be made with the patient out of the bed (unoccupied) or in the bed (occupied). In some settings bed linen is not changed every day; however, any wet or soiled linen must always be changed promptly. Moisture on bed linen can easily lead to skin breakdown. An unoccupied bed is one left open with the top sheets fanfolded down. A postoperative surgical bed is prepared for patients returning from the operating room (OR) or procedural area. The bed is left with the top sheets fanfolded lengthwise and not tucked in, to facilitate a patient's transfer from a stretcher. A closed bed, which is made with the top sheets pulled up to the head of the bed, is made by the housekeeping department after a patient is discharged and the bed is cleaned.

Delegation and Collaboration

The skill of making an unoccupied bed can be delegated to an unregulated care provider (UCP). The nurse instructs the UCP about:

- Position or activity restrictions that apply to patient's ability to get out of and back into bed.
- The type of special linen to use if patient is on an airflow mattress.

Equipment

- Linen/laundry bags
- Mattress pad (change only when soiled)
- Bottom sheet (flat or fitted)
- Drawsheet (*optional*)
- Waterproof pads (*optional*)
- Top sheet, blanket, spread, pillowcases
- Clean gloves (if linen is soiled or if there is risk of exposure to body fluids)
- Antiseptic cleanser
- Washcloth

Continued

PROCEDURAL GUIDELINE 18.7 *Making an Unoccupied Bed—cont'd*

Procedural Steps

1. Perform hand hygiene. Arrange supplies at beside.
2. Assess environment for safety (e.g., check room for spills; make sure that equipment is working properly and that bed is in locked, low position).
3. Pull room divider curtain or close room door to provide privacy. Follow steps for transferring patient to bedside chair or recliner (see Chapter 11).
4. Lower remaining side rails on bed and raise bed to comfortable working position.
5. Apply clean gloves if linen is soiled with body fluids. Remove all linen, hold away from uniform, and place in laundry bag. Avoid shaking or fanning linen.
6. Straighten mattress and wipe off any moisture with a washcloth moistened in antiseptic solution (consult employer's housekeeping guidelines). Dry thoroughly.
7. Apply all bottom linen on one side of bed before moving to opposite side.
   a. For fitted sheet: Make sure that fitted sheet is placed smoothly over mattress and top and bottom mattress edge. Fit corners on one end and then the other.
   b. For flat sheet: Place sheet over mattress. Allow about 25 cm (10 inches) to hang over side mattress edge. Lower hem of sheet should lie seam down, even with bottom edge of mattress. Pull remaining top part of sheet over top edge of mattress. While standing at head of bed, mitre top corner of bottom sheet (see Procedural Guideline 18.6, Step16a–f). Tuck remaining part of flat bottom sheet under mattress.
   c. *Optional:* Apply drawsheet and/or waterproof pad laying centrefold along middle of bed lengthwise. Smooth drawsheet/pad over mattress. Tuck excess edge of drawsheet under mattress, keeping palms down.
8. Move to opposite side of bed. Repeat Step 7.
9. Place top sheet over bed with vertical centrefold lengthwise down middle of bed. Open sheet out from head to foot, being sure that top edge of sheet is even with top edge of mattress. *Optional:* Spread a blanket or bedspread evenly over top sheet in same fashion.
10. Standing on one side at foot of bed, lift mattress corner slightly with one hand and with other hand tuck top sheet and blanket or spread under mattress.
11. Make modified mitred corner with top sheet, blanket, and spread. After making triangular fold, leave tip of triangle untucked (see Procedural Guideline 18.6, Step 36).
12. Make cuff by turning edge of top sheet down over top edge of blanket and spread.
13. Standing on one side at foot of bed, lift mattress corner slightly with one hand and with other hand tuck top sheet, blanket, and spread under mattress. Be sure that toe pleats are not pulled out.
14. Make modified mitred corner with top sheet, blanket, and spread. After making triangular fold, do not tuck tip of triangle (see Procedural Guideline 18.6, Step 36).
15. Go to other side of bed. Spread sheet, blanket, and spread out evenly. Make cuff with top sheet and blanket (closed bed). Make modified corner at foot of bed. Alternatively, fanfold sheet, blanket, and spread at foot of bed, with top layer ready to be pulled up (this leaves an open bed). *Optional:* Make horizontal toe pleat; stand at foot of bed and fanfold in sheet 5 to 10 cm (2 to 4 inches) across bed. Pull sheet up from bottom to make fold approximately 15 cm (6 inches) from bottom edge of mattress.
16. Apply clean pillowcase.
17. Place call light within patient's reach on bedrail or pillow and return bed to lowest position, allowing for patient transfer. Help patient to bed.
18. Place linen bag in dirty laundry bag. Remove and dispose of gloves.
19. Arrange and organize patient's room and perform hand hygiene.

◆ CLINICAL DEBRIEF

A 78-year-old male has a 3-year history of type 1 diabetes mellitus and hypertension. He was just discharged after 5 days of hospitalization with diagnoses of healing right-heel ulcer and controlled hypertension. His discharge summary notes that he requires help with daily dressing changes for the ulcer. He lives alone and is able to perform all routine activities of daily living (ADLs). During the initial home visit his vital signs were as follows: temp 37°C, pulse 86 beats/min, BP 135/85 mm Hg, respiratory rate 30 breaths/min. The community health nurse noted a right-heal ulcer 2 cm × 2 cm (0.8 × 0.8 inch); no drainage was noted. A 10 ×10 cm (4 ×4 inch) dressing was applied, covered, and wrapped with gauze cling wrap. The nurse assessed that, although the patient understands the need for the daily dressing changes, he is not able to state which precautions are needed to prevent any recurrence.

1. List three actions that he should follow for maintaining good foot care.
2. The nurse is caring for a patient with diabetes mellitus. Which factor places the patient at risk for oral problems?
   1. Break in mucosa and disruption of suture lines with vigorous brushing.
   2. Mucosa becomes thin and less elastic.
   3. Irritation of oral mucosa.
   4. Dryness of mouth with gingivitis.
3. Using SBAR, show how would you communicate with the health care team about this patient's status.

◆ REVIEW QUESTIONS

1. The nurse is caring for a critically ill patient with an endotracheal tube who is on mechanical ventilation. Which of the following reasons places the patient at risk for ventilator-associated pneumonia (VAP)? *(Select all that apply.)*
   1. The mucous inside the artificial airway grows Gram-negative bacteria.
   2. An endotracheal tube bypasses normal airway defenses, leading to a change in the normal oral flora.
   3. A critically ill patient often has a reduced gag reflex.

4. Presence of an endotracheal tube makes it impossible to suction oral secretions.
5. Critically ill patients have an abnormal amount of mucosa released in the oral cavity.

2. Which of the following actions are steps used when making an unoccupied bed? *(Select all that apply.)*
   1. Raise bed to working height.
   2. Wear clean gloves at all times.
   3. Apply all bottom linen on one side of bed before moving to opposite side.
   4. Remove soiled linen and place on the floor.
   5. Tuck top sheet and blanket in at bottom of bed using a modified mitred corner.
   6. Keep top blanket at head of bed when procedure is completed.
   7. Make horizontal toe pleat with all top layers of linen.

3. Place the following steps for providing oral care to a debilitated patient in the correct order.
   1. Remove dentures or partial plates if present.
   2. Apply thin layer of water-soluble moisturizer to lips.
   3. Perform hand hygiene and apply clean gloves.
   4. Brush inner and outer surfaces of upper and lower teeth by brushing from gum to crown of each tooth; then clean biting surfaces of teeth.
   5. If needed, turn on suction machine and connect tubing to suction catheter.
   6. Position patient in side-lying position with head turned toward mattress in dependent position.
   7. If patient is uncooperative or having difficulty keeping mouth open, insert an oral airway.

ⓔ *Visit the Evolve site for a complete list of Clinical Debrief and Review Questions answers.*

REFERENCES

Accreditation Canada. (2019). *Required organizational practices handbook—Version 14.* Retrieved from http://www.wrha.mb.ca/quality/files/2019ROPHandbook.pdf.

Agency for Healthcare Research and Quality (AHRQ). (2013a). *National guideline clearinghouse: Bathing persons with dementia.* Retrieved from http://ahrqguideline.careset.com/www.guideline.gov/bathing-persons-with-dementia#main-content.

Agency for Healthcare Research and Quality (AHRQ). (2013b). *Universal ICU decolonization: An enhanced protocol.* Retrieved from http://www.ahrq.gov/professionals/systems/hospital/universal_icu_decolonization/universal-icu-ape4.html.

Alserehi, H., Filippell, M., Emerick, M., et al. (2018). Chlorhexidine gluconate bathing practices and skin concentrations in intensive care unit patients. *American Journal of Infection Control, 46*(2), 226–228. doi:10.1016/j.ajic.2017.08.022.

Alzheimer Society Canada (ASC). (2017). *Bathing.* Retrieved from http://alzheimer.ca/en/Home/Living-with-dementia/Day-to-day-living/Personal-care/Bathing.

Asadoorian, J. (2017). Therapeutic oral rinsing with non-commercially available products: Position paper and statement from the Canadian Dental Hygienists Association, part 2. *Canadian Journal of Dental Hygiene, 51*(1), 30–41.

Canadian Dental Association (CDA). (2012a). *CDA position on first visit to the dentist.* Retrieved from https://www.cda-adc.ca/en/about/position_statements/firstvisit/.

Canadian Dental Association (CDA). (2012b). *CDA position on use of fluorides in caries prevention.* Retrieved from http://www.cda-adc.ca/en/about/position_statements/fluoride/.

Canadian Dental Association (CDA). (2012c). *Frequency of dental care.* Retrieved from https://www.cda-adc.ca/en/about/position_statements/frequencyofcare/.

Canadian Dental Association (CDA). (2019a). *Dental care for children: Cleaning teeth.* Retrieved from https://www.cda-adc.ca/en/oral_health/cfyt/dental_care_children/cleaning.asp.

Canadian Dental Association (CDA). (2019b). *Flossing & brushing.* Retrieved from http://www.cda-adc.ca/en/oral_health/cfyt/dental_care_seniors/flossing_brushing.asp.

Canadian Dental Association (CDA). (2019c). *Oral health articles, oral health: An important piece of your overall health.* Retrieved from http://www.cda-adc.ca/en/about/media_room/health_month/publicity/oral_health_articles.asp.

Canadian Dental Association (CDA). (2019d). *Your oral health.* Retrieved from https://www.cda-adc.ca/en/oral_health/index.asp.

Canadian Paediatric Society. (2015). *Caring for kids: Keep your baby safe.* Retrieved from https://www.caringforkids.cps.ca/handouts/keep_your_baby_safe.

Canadian Patient Safety Institute (CPSI). (2016). *Ventilator-associated pneumonia (VAP).* Retrieved from http://www.patientsafetyinstitute.ca/en/Topic/Pages/Ventilator-Associated-Pneumonia-(VAP).aspx.

Centers for Disease Control and Prevention (CDC). (2017a). *Fungal nail infections.* Retrieved from https://www.cdc.gov/fungal/nail-infections.html.

Centers for Disease Control and Prevention (CDC). (2017b). *Oral and dental health.* Retrieved from http://www.cdc.gov/nchs/fastats/dental.htm.

Diabetes Canada. (2019). *A step towards good health.* Retrieved from https://www.diabetes.ca/diabetes-and-you/healthy-living-resources/foot-care/a-step-towards-good-health.

Henke, P. (2017). *Chronic venous insufficiency.* Society for Vascular Surgery (SVS). Retrieved from https://vascular.org/patient-resources/vascular-conditions/chronic-venous-insufficiency.

Lowe, C. F., Lloyd-Smith, E., Sidhu, B., et al. (2017). Reduction in hospital-associated methicillin-resistant *Staphylococcus aureus* and vancomycin-resistant *Enterococcus* with daily chlorhexidine gluconate bathing for medical inpatients. *American Journal of Infection Control, 45*(3), 255–259. doi:10.1016/j.ajic.2016.09.019.

Mlinac, M., & Feng, M. (2016). Assessment of activities of daily living, self-care, and independence. *Archives of Clinical Neuropsychology, 31*(6), 506–516. doi:10.1093/arclin/acw049.

National Cancer Institute (NCI). (2016). *Oral complications of chemotherapy and head/neck radiation (PDQ)—Patient version.* Retrieved from http://www.cancer.gov/cancertopics/pdq/supportivecare/oralcomplications/Patient.

National Institute of Dental and Craniofacial Research. (2018). *Older adults and oral health.* Retrieved from http://www.nidcr.nih.gov/oralhealth/OralHealthInformation/OlderAdults/.

National Pediculosis Association. (2019). *Welcome to HeadLice.org.* Retrieved from http://www.headlice.org/index.html.

National Pressure Ulcer Advisory Panel (NPUAP). (2014). *Prevention and treatment of pressure ulcers: Quick reference guide.* Retrieved from http://www.npuap.org/wp-content/uploads/2014/08/Quick-Reference-Guide-DIGITAL-NPUAP-EPUAP-PPPIA-Jan2016.pdf.

Nøddeskou, L. H., Hemmingsen, L. E., & Hørdam, B. (2015). Elderly patients' and nurses' assessment of traditional bed bath compared to prepacked single units—Randomized control trial. *Scandinavian Journal of Caring Sciences, 29*(2), 347–352. doi:10.1111/scs.12170.

Norton, L., Parslow, N., Johnston, D., et al. (2018). *Foundations of best practice for skin and wound management. Best practice recommendations for the prevention and management of pressure injuries.* Retrieved from https://www.woundscanada.ca/docman/public/health-care-professional/bpr-workshop/172-bpr-prevention-and-management-of-pressure-injuries-2/file.

Noto, M. J., Domenico, H. J., Byrne, D. W., et al. (2015). Chlorhexidine bathing and health care-associated infections: A randomized clinical trial. *Journal of American Medical Association, 313*(4), 369–378. doi:10.1001/jama.2014.18400.

Public Health Agency of Canada (PHAC). (2015). *You can prevent falls!* Retrieved from https://www.canada.ca/content/dam/phac-aspc/migration/phac-aspc/seniors-aines/alt-formats/pdf/publications/public/injury-blessure/prevent-eviter/prevent-eviter-e.pdf.

Raines, K., & Rosen, K. (2016). The effect of chlorhexidine bathing rates of nosocomial infections among the critically ill population: An analysis of current research and recommendations for practice. *Dimensions of Critical Care Nursing, 35*(2), 84–91. doi:10.1097/DCC.0000000000000165.

Rassool, G. H. (2015). Cultural competence in nursing Muslim patients. *Nursing Times, 111*(14), 12–15. doi:01.04.15.

Shah, H. N., Schwartz, J. L., Luna, G., & Cullen, D. L. (2016). Bathing with 2% chlorhexidine gluconate: Evidence and costs associated with central line–associated bloodstream infections. *Critical Care Nursing Quarterly, 39*(1), 42–50. doi:10.1097/CNQ.0000000000000096.

Supple, L., Kumaraswami, M., Kundrapu, S., et al. (2015). Chlorhexidine only works if applied correctly: Use of a simple colorimetric assay to provide monitoring and feedback on effectiveness of chlorhexidine application. *Infection Control and Hospital Epidemiology, 36*(9), 1095–1097. doi:10.1017/ice.2015.124.

Villa, A., Connell, C. L., & Abati, S. (2015). Diagnosis and management of xerostomia and hyposalivation. *Therapeutics and Clinical Risk Management, 5*(11), 45–51. doi:10.2147/TCRM.S76282.

Westman, K., & Blaisdell, C. (2016). Many benefits, little risk: The use of massage in nursing practice. *American Journal of Nursing, 116*(1), 34–39.

Wound Care Canada. (2017). *Foundations of best practice for skin and wound management.* Retrieved from https://www.woundscanada.ca/health-care-professional/resources-health-care-pros/12-healthcare-professional/110-supplements.

19 | Care of the Eye and Ear

Written by **Anne Griffin Perry, RN, MSN, EdD, FAAN, and Shelley L. Cobbett, RN, GnT, MN, EdD**

SKILLS AND PROCEDURES

OBJECTIVES

Mastery of content in this chapter will enable the nurse to:

- Explain safety guidelines used in the care of eye and ear prostheses.
- Identify person-centred care guidelines used in caring for eye and ear prostheses.
- Correctly remove, store, clean, and insert a contact lens.
- Correctly perform eye and ear irrigations.
- Describe techniques that determine whether a hearing aid functions properly.
- Correctly remove, clean, and reinsert a hearing aid.

MEDIA RESOURCES

- evolve http://evolve.elsevier.com/Canada/Perry/clinicalskills/
- Review Questions
- Audio Glossary
- Clinical Debrief and Review Questions Answers

PURPOSE

Vision and hearing are two special senses that help people carry out all daily and recreational activities. Risks to a patients' eye or ear structures or function can alter independence, safety, body image, and self-confidence. The skills in this chapter show how to help patients protect their vision and hearing and use artificial sensory devices correctly to replace or restore sensory function.

STANDARDS OF CARE

- Canadian Academy of Audiology, 2015–2016—*Reports, Guidelines, and Position Statements* (https://canadianaudiology.ca/professional-resources/guidelines-and-position-statements/)
- Canadian Association of Optometrists (CAO), n.d.—*Frequency of Eye Examinations* (https://opto.ca/health-library/frequency-of-eye-examinations)
- Canadian Hearing Society, 2019—*Programs and Services* (http://www.chs.ca/programs-and-services)

PRINCIPLES FOR PRACTICE

- Meaningful sensory stimuli help people learn about their environment.
- Receiving and understanding environmental stimuli promote healthy functioning.
- Alteration in a patient's vision and hearing affects health literacy, independence, and adherence to medical and pharmacological therapies.
- Artificial sensory aids can restore some vision and hearing loss. However, these aids must fit and work properly for patients to function optimally in their environments.
- When caring for patients who use aids to help with visual or auditory loss, it is important that the nurse and the health care team, along with the patient and their family, understand how to clean and care for these aids. Breakage or loss of an aid is expensive.

PERSON-CENTRED CARE

- When a patient is without visual or hearing devices, communication is altered, and the patient is isolated socially and becomes more dependent (Mick, Parfyonov, Wittich, et al., 2018).
- The noises within hospitals, rehabilitation centres, and skilled nursing facilities make hearing difficult. Hard flooring surfaces, medical equipment, televisions, and the constant need to speak with other health care providers all produce noise.

- Hearing-impaired patients need time to adjust to their hearing aid. For example, increased background noise makes hearing with an aid even more difficult. The noisy environments of hospitals and other health care facilities further contribute to adjustment to hearing aids (Mick et al., 2018).
- When a patient has auditory impairments, the increased background noise in an unfamiliar environment often makes a patient more anxious and decreases their ability to adjust to new surroundings.
- As a nurse, at times you can use touch to get the attention of a patient with severe visual loss or decreased hearing. Practise person-centred care and ask patients if touch is acceptable.
- Understand the cause of a person's sensory loss and then determine the patient's own perception of the reason for the loss.
- Identify a patient's usual practices in using and maintaining sensory assistive devices.

EVIDENCE-INFORMED PRACTICE

Dual sensory impairment (DSI), the concurrent losses in vision and hearing, has the potential to cause a decline in cognitive function or contribute to acute confusion or depression and increased mortality risk (Mick et al., 2018).

- DSI in rehabilitation or long-term care settings affects a patient's independence, socialization, and success in using assistive devices and rehabilitation services (Tremblay, 2015).
- There is mounting evidence that there are central effects of biological aging and peripheral pathology that affect a person's neural detection of sound, which occurs as early as middle age (Tremblay, 2015). Older persons often do not seek sufficient screening and early intervention (Yuan, Sun, Sang, et al., 2017).
- Identify patients at risk for hearing impairments: male over age 65, male or female over age 75, resident in nursing facility, existing visual impairment, chronic ear infection, prolonged exposure to loud noises, and use of ototoxic medication (Heine & Browning, 2015).
- Vision loss includes people who are blind or partially blind: no sight from birth, "legally blind" (best corrected visual acuity of ≤20/200 and/or a visual field <20 degrees). Vision loss can include other forms of impairment, such as nystagmus that reduces vision and depth perception (Canadian National Institute for the Blind [CNIB], 2018).
- Involving patients with DSI in volunteer work has been shown to result in fewer depressive symptoms compared to people without sensory loss who volunteer (White, 2015).
- Patients with DSI have unique communication needs that require a thorough assessment (Mick et al., 2018).

SAFETY GUIDELINES

- As a nurse, whenever you care for patients with sensory alterations, safety is a priority. Anticipate how the sensory alteration places a patient at risk for injury (e.g., ability to manoeuvre through home, climb stairs, and respond to alarms).
- Select interventions based on the type of sensory loss, patient preference, and patient safety.
- Interprofessional collaboration related to the plan of care for a patient with sensory alterations is beneficial to maximize patient safety and ensure optimal patient care.
- Orient the patient to any new environment or changes within an existing environment to minimize safety hazards (e.g., visual loss affects a patient's ability to see the edge of the stairs). In addition, educate caregivers about the best way to help the patient adapt to sensory loss.
- When patients have visual impairments, they may have difficulty with tasks requiring visual detail (e.g., reading prescriptions or syringe scales). Visual impairment can increase the risk of improper administration of medications in the home setting. In addition, certain eye conditions such as cataracts and macular degeneration cause a patient difficulty when adjusting to changes in contrast and brightness.
- Provide additional time for patients with hearing loss to ask repeated questions about their care or upcoming procedure.
- If a patient must sign a consent form for a procedure or surgery, be sure to have a method to verify that the patient read, heard, and understood the procedure.

PROCEDURAL GUIDELINE 19.1 *Eye Care for Unconscious Patients*

Unconscious patients do not have the natural protective mechanisms of blinking and eye lubrication to protect the cornea. Critically ill patients often develop ocular surface disorders such as exposure keratopathy. Critically ill patients are often on mechanical ventilators and thus heavily sedated, which alters the normal blinking reflex (Alansari, Hijazi, & Maghrabi, 2015).

The blinking reflex flushes debris out of the eye. When patients are heavily sedated or in a coma, tear production is reduced, thus decreasing the normal lubrication of the corneal surface. Tears maintain a moist environment, lubricate the eyes, wash away foreign material and cell debris, prevent organisms from adhering to the ocular surface, and transport oxygen to the outer eye surface. When a patient's normal protective eye mechanisms are not effective, eye care is a must. Left unprotected, damage to the cornea can occur. This damage ranges from corneal scarring, infection, premature cataract formation, to vision changes. Simple eye hygiene measures such as moisture chambers, lubrication, and corneal surface protection are the best interventions to decrease the risk for or prevent damage to the cornea (Taheri-Kharameh, 2017).

Delegation and Collaboration

The skill of providing basic eye care for a comatose patient can be assigned to an unregulated care provider (UCP). However, it is the nurse's responsibility to assess a patient's eyes and administer the sterile lubricant. The nurse instructs the UCP to:

- Adapt the skill for specific patients (e.g., using skin-sensitive tape to affix eye pads).
- Immediately report any eye drainage or irritation to the nurse for further assessment.

Equipment

- Clean gloves
- Warm water
- Normal saline solution

Continued

PROCEDURAL GUIDELINE 19.1 *Eye Care for Unconscious Patients—cont'd*

- Clean washcloth
- Cotton balls
- Eye pads or patches
- Paper tape
- Eyedropper bulb syringe
- Sterile lubricant or eye preparations as prescribed
- *Option:* A moisture chamber (e.g., polyethylene covers, swimming goggles, shields, pads, or eye patch seals off the eye from the environment [Taheri-Kharameh, 2017]) may also be used; verify with employer policy.

Procedural Steps

1. Perform hand hygiene.
2. Observe patient's eyes for drainage, irritation, redness, and lesions. Apply clean gloves if drainage is present.
3. Always explain each step of the procedure. It is unknown how much an unconscious patient can hear; thus, it is important to continually orient a patient to any procedure.
4. Assess for blink reflex (see Chapter 8).
5. Examine the pupils; determine if pupils are equal and round and react to light and accommodation (PERRLA) (see Chapter 8).
6. Observe patient's eye movements, noting symmetry of movement.
7. Explain procedure to patient and caregiver.

8. Position patient in supine position.
9. Use clean washcloth or cotton balls moistened with warm water or saline and gently wipe each eye from inner to outer canthus. Use a separate, clean cotton ball or corner of the washcloth for each eye.

Clinical Decision Point *Be sure water is warm and not hot, to avoid damaging eye.*

10. Use an eyedropper to instill the prescribed lubricant (e.g., saline, methylcellulose, liquid tears) as prescribed, wiping away any excess lubricant.
11. If the blink reflex is absent, gently close patient's eyes and apply eye patches or pads. Secure patch, being careful not to tape patient's eyes.
12. Dispose of excess material, remove gloves, and perform hand hygiene.
13. Remove eye pads or patches every 4 hours or as prescribed and observe condition of patient's eyes for drainage, irritation, redness, and lesions.
14. Document findings on flow sheet or in nurses' notes in electronic health record (EHR) or chart.
15. Notify health care provider if signs of irritation or infection are present.

PROCEDURAL GUIDELINE 19.2 *Taking Care of Contact Lenses*

A contact lens is a thin, concave disk that fits directly over the cornea of the eye. It is transparent over at least the pupil and may be colourless or tinted. Contact lenses correct refractive errors of the eye or abnormalities in the shape of the cornea that distort vision. They are relatively easy to apply and remove.

Today, rigid gas permeable (RGP) and soft contact lenses are available. RGP lenses are smaller than the soft lenses, and initial awareness of the lens is present; total comfort usually occurs within a couple of weeks. RGP lenses are removed at the end of the day. Daily disposable soft contact lenses are made of a flexible hydrogel plastic and cover the entire cornea and a small rim of the sclera. Contact lenses must accommodate patient needs for comfort, vision correction, and convenience and must be prescribed by an eye care professional (CAO, 2017). Usually, if a patient is not able to provide self-care related to contact lenses while hospitalized, the patient will wear eyeglasses.

It is important to remember that all lenses must be removed periodically to prevent infection and corneal damage and that proper cleaning is necessary before reinserting a lens. As contact lenses are worn, secretions and foreign matter adhere to the lens surface (CAO, 2017). It is extremely important to determine whether patients wear contact lenses, particularly when they are admitted to hospitals or agencies in unresponsive or confused states. If a seriously ill patient is wearing contact lenses and this fact goes undetected, severe corneal injury can result.

Delegation and Collaboration

The skill of taking care of contact lenses can be assigned to an unregulated care provider (UCP). However, it is the nurse's responsibility to assess a patient's eyes. The nurse directs the UCP to:

- Know a patient's specific type of contact lens, including cleaning solutions and routine, wear schedule, storage, and replacement schedule.
- Report immediately to the nurse any eye pain or discomfort, redness, swelling, tearing, or drainage.
- Carefully handle the lens to prevent damage and injury.

Equipment

- Bath towels or waterproof pads
- Sterile saline solution
- Sterile lens care solution(s) for cleaning, disinfecting, and rinsing
- Sterile wetting or conditioning solution (depends on care regimen)
- Sterile enzyme solution (depends on care regimen)
- Flashlight or penlight
- Clean lens storage container
- Suction cup (*optional*)
- Powder-free, clean gloves

Procedural Steps

1. Identify patient using at least two person-specific identifiers (e.g., name and date of birth or name and medical record number) according to employer policy (Accreditation Canada, 2019).
2. Inspect patient's eyes or ask patient if contact lens is in place.

Clinical Decision Point *If a patient is unconscious or confused, the nurse must assess for presence of contact lenses, which are often difficult to detect if they are colourless (not tinted).*

PROCEDURAL GUIDELINE 19.2 *Taking Care of Contact Lenses—cont'd*

3. Determine if patient can manipulate and hold contact lenses and if glasses are available for periods when contacts are not in use. Determine patient's usual routine for wearing, cleaning, and storing lenses.
4. Assess patient for any unusual visual signs or symptoms (e.g., change in visual acuity, blurred vision, halos, photophobia).
5. Review types of medication prescribed for patient: sedatives, hypnotics, muscle relaxants, antihistamines, or another medication that decreases blink reflex and subsequent lubrication of cornea.
6. Explain procedure to patient.
7. Perform hand hygiene.
8. Verify expiration date of all solutions and assemble equipment at bedside.
9. Be sure that your fingernails are short and smooth.
10. Position patient in supine or high-Fowler's position in bed.
11. Apply clean gloves. Place towel just below patient's face.
12. **Removing lenses:**
    a. Removal of soft lens: Follow Steps (1) through (6) for each eye.
       (1) If you are unable to visualize the lens, shine a penlight or flashlight sideways onto the eye to locate the position of the lens.
       (2) Add 2 or 3 drops of sterile saline solution to patient's eye.
       (3) If possible, ask patient to look straight ahead. Retract lower eyelid and expose lower edge of lens.
       (4) Use pad of index finger to slide lens off cornea down onto lower sclera (white of the eye).
       (5) Pull upper eyelid down gently with thumb of other hand and compress lens slightly between thumb and index finger.
       (6) Gently pinch lens and lift out without allowing edges to stick together. Place lens in storage case.

Clinical Decision Point *If lens edges stick together, place lens in palm and soak thoroughly with sterile saline solution. Gently roll lens with index finger in back-and-forth motion. If necessary, soak lens in storage solution, which may return lens to normal shape.*

    b. Removal of hard lenses: Follow Steps (1) through (6) for each eye.
       (1) Inspect the eye to be sure that lens is positioned directly over the cornea. If you are unable to visualize the lens, shine a penlight or flashlight sideways onto the eye to locate position of the lens.

Clinical Decision Point *If lens is not positioned directly over the cornea, have patient close eyelid, place index and middle fingers of one hand on eyelid just beside the lens and beneath, and gently attempt to massage lens back into place. If lens cannot be repositioned, an immediate referral to an ophthalmologist is needed.*

       (2) Place index finger on outer corner of patient's eye and gently draw skin back toward ear.
       (3) Ask patient to blink. Do not release pressure until blink is completed.

Clinical Decision Point *For patients unable to open eye or blink on command, use a lens suction cup to remove lens from eye. Gently apply suction cup to lens surface and lift out.*

       (4) If lens does not dislodge, gently retract eyelid beyond edge of lens. Press lower eyelid gently against lower edge of lens to dislodge lens.
       (5) Allow both eyelids to close slightly and grasp lens as it rises from the eye. Cup lens in hand.
       (6) Inspect lens to be sure that it is intact. Place it in storage container.
    c. After lenses are removed, inspect eye for redness, pain, or swelling of eyelids or conjunctiva; discharge; or excess tearing.
13. **Cleaning and storage:** Typical cleaning and disinfecting of contact lenses (verify specific method for lenses):
    a. Apply 1 or 2 drops of cleaning solution to lens in palm of hand. Using index finger (soft lenses) or little finger (rigid lenses), rub lens gently but thoroughly on both sides for 20 to 30 seconds.
    b. Holding lens over emesis basin, rinse thoroughly with recommended rinsing solution.

Clinical Decision Point *Only use solutions for cleaning and disinfecting that have been prescribed (CAO, 2017). Do not use tap or bottled water. Follow prescriber's instructions and schedules.*

    c. Place lens in proper storage case compartment: "R" for right lens and "L" for left. Rigid lenses are placed inside up.
    d. Fill with recommended disinfectant or storage solution.
    e. Secure cover(s) over storage case. Label case with patient's name, identification number, and room number.
14. **Inserting lenses:**
    a. Inserting a soft lens: Follow Steps (1) through (5) for each eye.
       (1) Remove right lens from storage case and rinse with recommended rinsing solution; inspect lens for foreign materials, tears, and other damage.
       (2) Hold lens on tip of index finger of dominant hand with concave side up.
       (3) Inspect lens from side at eye level to ensure that it is not inverted (see illustration).

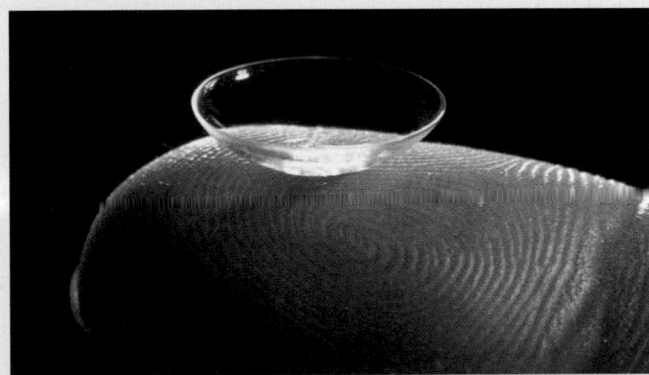

STEP 14a(3) Correct position of soft lens before insertion.

Continued

PROCEDURAL GUIDELINE 19.2 *Taking Care of Contact Lenses—cont'd*

(4) Using middle or index finger of opposite hand, retract upper lid until iris is exposed (see illustration). Using middle finger of hand holding the lens, pull down lower lid.

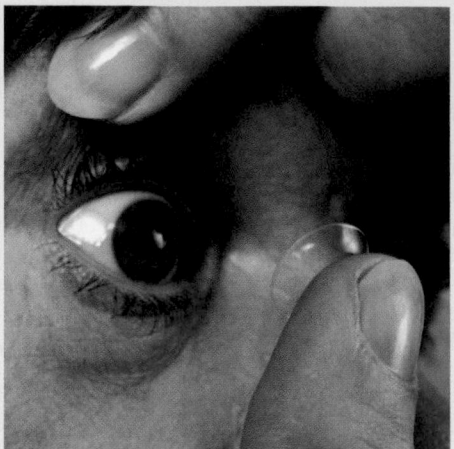

STEP 14a(4) Correct position of hands for soft lens insertion.

(5) Instruct patient to look straight ahead and focus on an object in the distance. Gently place lens directly on cornea and release lids slowly, starting with lower lid.

b. Inserting a rigid lens: Follow Steps (1) through (6) for each eye.

(1) Remove right lens from storage case; attempt to lift lens straight up.

(2) Hold lens on tip of index finger of dominant hand with concave side up.

(3) Inspect lens to ensure that it is moist, clean, clear, and free of chips or cracks.

(4) Wet lens surfaces with a few drops of prescribed wetting solution.

(5) Using middle finger of hand holding lens, pull down lower lid (see illustration).

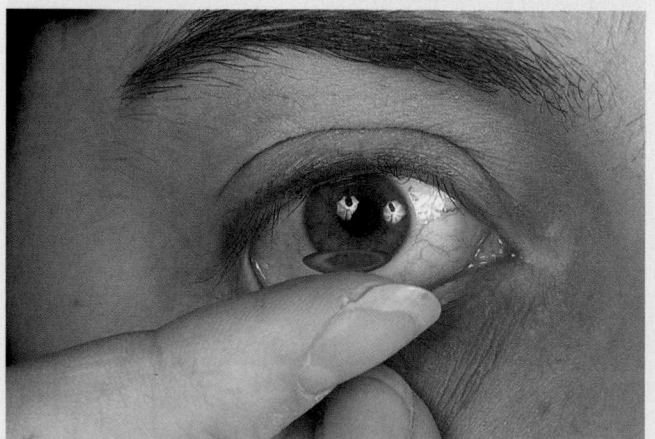

STEP 14b(5) Hand position for rigid lens insertion.

(6) Instruct patient to look straight ahead and focus on an object in the distance (see illustration). Gently place lens directly on cornea and release lids slowly, starting with lower lid.

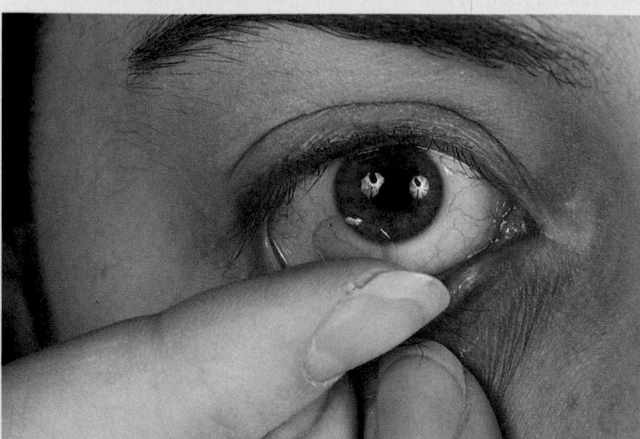

STEP 14b(6) Instruct patient to look straight ahead and focus on an object in the distance.

(a) Ask patient to close eyes briefly and avoid blinking.

15. Inspect eye to ensure that lens is on cornea.

Clinical Decision Point *If lens is on sclera rather than cornea, ask patient to slowly close eye and look toward the lens. Gentle pressure on the eyelid may help to centre the lens on the cornea. Ask patient to blink a few times.*

16. Ask patient to cover other eye with hand and report if vision is clear and lens is comfortable.

17. Repeat procedure to insert lens in other eye.

18. Discard solution from storage case and rinse case thoroughly with sterile lens storage solution. Sterilize or replace case as recommended by manufacturer. Allow case to air dry. Dispose of towel, remove gloves, and perform hand hygiene.

19. Ask patient if lens feels comfortable after removal and reinsertion of lenses.

20. Ask patient if there is blurred vision, pain, or foreign body sensation.

21. Observe eye for drainage or redness.

22. **Use Teach-Back:** "I want to be sure you understand how to clean your contact lenses. Describe for me the way to clean your lenses." Develop a revised teaching plan if patient or caregiver is not able to teach back correctly.

◆ SKILL 19.1 Eye Irrigation

Chemical injuries to the eye are often work related, caused by common household cleaning solutions or other fumes and aerosols. Acid burns such as bleach, toilet cleaners, and battery fluid cause a haze on the cornea, which often clears, and there is a good chance of recovery. Alkaline burns such as lye, ammonia, and dishwasher detergent often cause permanent injury to the eye. Alkaline burns cause very rapid, irreversible damage (Mashige, 2016). A chemical injury to the eye is an emergency and requires flushing the eye with copious amounts of irrigation fluid. Cool tap water is recommended because it is effective, is immediately available for first aid, and initially helps to dilute the concentration of the chemical. Tap water irrigation is also used in emergency situations when a foreign object has entered the eye. It is important to flush out the eye with clean water or saline while seeking medical care (Fig. 19.1). Irrigate immediately with copious amounts of cool water, saline, or lactated Ringer's solution for at least 20–30 minutes to minimize corneal damage (Mangan, 2015, 2016). If the person wears a contact lens that did not wash out with the irrigation, have them try to remove the lens. The goal in treating ocular chemical injury is to prevent or reduce visual loss caused by the burn (Mashige, 2016).

Delegation and Collaboration

The skill of eye irrigation cannot be delegated to an unregulated care provider (UCP). The nurse directs the UCP to:

- Report any patient complaint of discomfort or excess tearing following irrigation.

Equipment

- Emergency: Cool tap water
- Prescribed irrigating solution: volume usually 30 to 180 mL at 32° to 38°C (90° to 100°F) (For chemical flushing, use normal saline or lactated Ringer's solution in large volume to provide continuous irrigation over 15 minutes.)
- pH test strip
- Sterile basin or bag of solution
- Curved emesis basin
- Waterproof pad or towel
- 10 × 10–cm (4 × 4–inch) gauze pads
- Soft bulb syringe, eyedropper, or intravenous (IV) tubing
- Clean gloves
- Penlight
- Medication administration record (MAR)

STEP	RATIONALE

ASSESSMENT

1. In acute emergent situations: Use copious amounts of clear, cool water (normal saline, or lactated Ringer's if quickly available) to flush eyes for at least 20–30 minutes. Sometimes irrigating volume ≥20 L is required (Mangan, 2015). — Minimizes corneal damage (Mashige, 2016).

2. If not an immediate emergency, identify patient using at least two person-specific identifiers (e.g., name and date of birth or name and medical record number) according to employer policy. — Ensures correct patient. Complies with Accreditation Canada's standards and improves patient safety (Accreditation Canada, 2019).

Clinical Decision Point *When eye irrigation is an emergency treatment for a chemical burn, follow employer protocol (i.e., usually copious eye irrigation with cool water, normal saline, or lactated Ringer's solution). When possible, determine the chemical. However, do not stop to obtain a history or an eye examination. Irrigation is the immediate treatment; delays in irrigation by as little as 20 seconds have been associated with more severe injury in alkaline burns. Once the acute phase is over, an irrigation solution that buffers alkali or acid chemical is then selected, and further examination of the eye is possible (Mashige, 2016).*

3. Review health care provider's medication prescription, including solution to be instilled and affected eye(s) (right, left, or both) to receive irrigation. — Ensures safe and correct administration of irrigant.

4. Obtain history of injury to assess reason for eye irrigation (e.g., type of injury, when it occurred). — Determines amount and type of solution and immediacy of need for treatment.

5. Determine patient's ability to open affected eye. — Spasm of the eyelid or pain makes opening the eye difficult. Local anaesthetics such as proparacaine or tetracaine cause topical numbness and are used before eye examination procedures.

6. If time permits, do a complete eye examination, including determining if pupils are equal and round and react to light and accommodation (PERRLA) (see Chapter 8). Have patient look in all directions to determine if there are any visible foreign bodies. — Provides baseline information and determines presence of any foreign bodies.

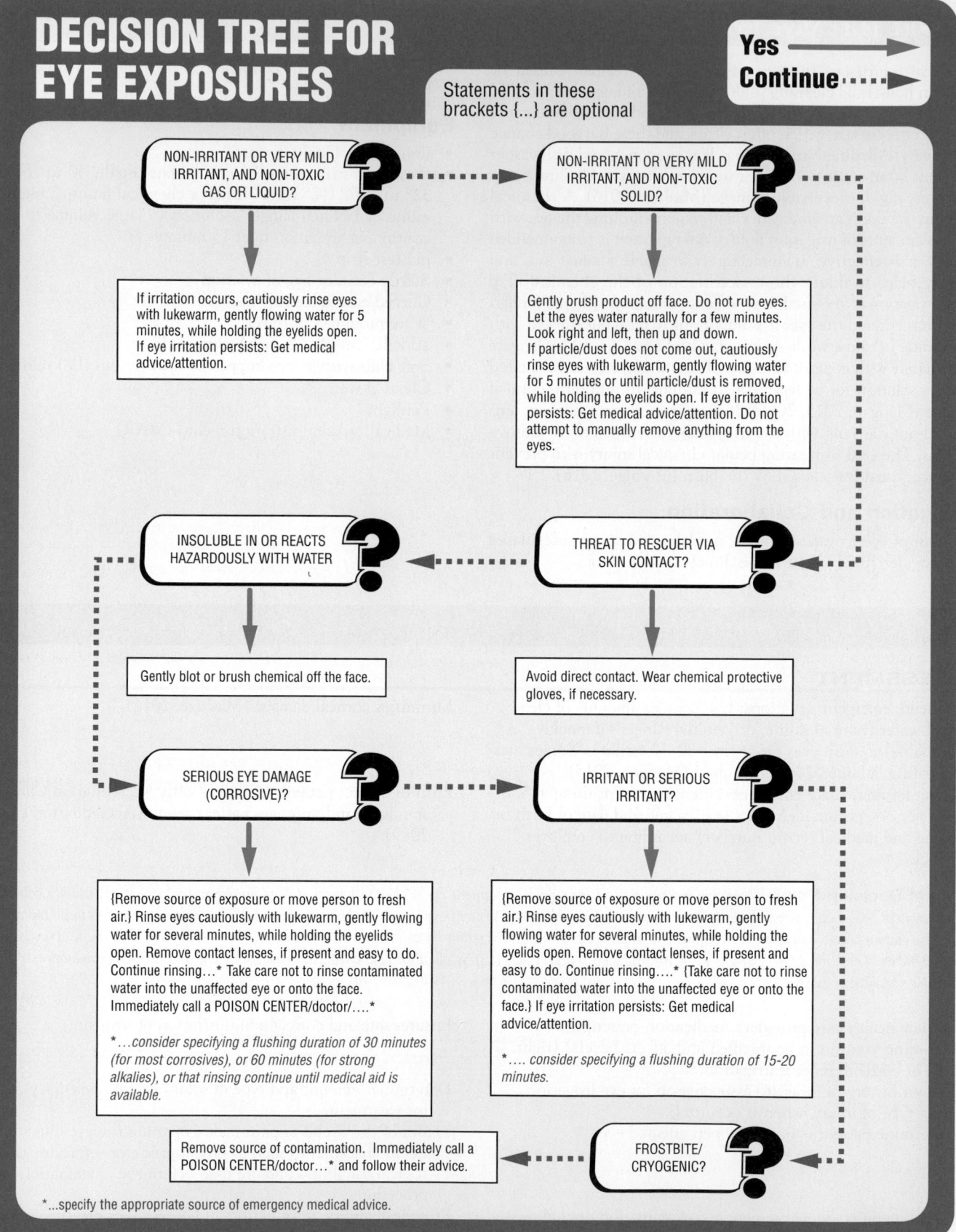

FIG 19.1 Decision tree for eye exposures. (*From Canadian Centre for Occupational Health and Safety* [CCOHS]. [2012]. *The Safety Data Sheet—A Guide to First-Aid Recommendations. Retrieved from* http://www.ccohs.ca/products/publications/firstaid/eye.pdf)

STEP	RATIONALE

ASSESSMENT

7. Observe eye for redness, excessive tearing, discharge, and swelling. Ask patient about symptoms of itching, burning, pain, blurred vision, or photophobia.

   Establishes baseline signs and symptoms.

8. Ask patient to rate level of pain using an appropriate pain rating scale (e.g., on a scale of 0 to 10, with 0 being no pain, and 10 being the worst pain ever).

   Establishes baseline for level of pain. Adequate pain control is essential to a more complete eye examination by an ophthalmologist (Mashige, 2016).

9. Assess patient's ability to cooperate.

   Determines level of assistance needed.

NURSING DIAGNOSES

- Acute pain
- Eyelid edema
- Potential for infection
- Potential for injury

Related factors/Risk factors are individualized on the basis of patient's condition or needs.

PLANNING

1. Expected outcomes following completion of procedure:
   - Patient demonstrates minimal anxiety during and after irrigation.

     Potential for anxiety and pain is high during emergency.

   - Patient verbalizes reduced pain, burning, or itching and improved visual acuity after irrigation.

     Reflects effectiveness of procedure in removing irritant.

   - Patient maintains normal pupillary reaction and eye movement after irrigation.

     Reflects effectiveness of procedure in minimizing exposure to irritant and preventing eye damage.

2. Discuss procedure with patient.

   Decreases patient anxiety.

3. Check accuracy and completeness of each MAR with health care provider's written prescription. Check patient's name, irrigation solution name and concentration, route of administration, and time for administration. Compare MAR with label of eye irrigation solution.

   The prescription sheet is the most reliable source and only legal record of drugs or procedure that patient is to receive. Ensures that patient receives correct medication.

4. Assemble supplies at bedside.

   Provides easy access to supplies.

5. Help patient to side-lying position on side of affected eye. Turn head toward affected eye. If both eyes are affected, place patient supine for simultaneous irrigation of both eyes.

   Position facilitates flow of solution from inner to outer canthus, preventing contamination of unaffected eye and nasolacrimal duct.

IMPLEMENTATION

1. Perform hand hygiene. Apply clean gloves.

   Reduces transmission of microorganisms. Protects hands from chemical irritants.

2. Remove any contact lens, if possible (see Procedural Guideline 19.2). Remove gloves after contact lens is removed. Reapply new gloves.

   Prompt removal of lenses is needed to safely and completely irrigate foreign substances from patient's eyes. Removal of gloves following contact lens removal prevents reintroduction of chemical transferred from lens to glove.

Clinical Decision Point *In an emergency such as first aid for a chemical burn, do not delay by removing patient's contact lens before irrigation. Do not remove lens unless rapid swelling is occurring. Flush eye from the inner to outer canthus with cool tap water immediately (Mangan, 2015).*

3. Explain to patient that eye can be closed periodically and that no object will touch it.

   Informing patients what to expect decreases anxiety and reassures them.

4. Place towel or waterproof pad under patient's face and curved emesis basin just below patient's cheek on side of affected eye.

   Catches irrigation fluid.

5. Using gauze moistened with prescriber's solution (or normal saline), gently clean visible secretions or foreign material from eyelid margins and eyelashes, wiping from inner to outer canthus.

   Minimizes transfer of material into eye during irrigation. Prevents secretions from entering nasolacrimal duct.

STEP	RATIONALE

IMPLEMENTATION

6. Explain next steps to patient and encourage relaxation:
    a. With gloved finger gently retract upper and lower eyelids to expose conjunctival sacs.

Retraction minimizes blinking and allows irrigation of conjunctiva.

    b. To hold lids open, apply gentle pressure to lower bony orbit and bony prominence beneath eyebrow. Do not apply pressure over eye.

7. Hold irrigating syringe, dropper, or IV tubing approximately 2.5 cm (1 inch) from inner canthus.

Direct contact with irrigation equipment may injure eye.

8. Ask patient to look toward brow. Gently irrigate with steady stream toward lower conjunctival sac, moving from inner to outer canthus (see illustration).

Minimizes force of stream on patient's cornea. Flushes irritant out and away from the other eye and nasolacrimal duct.

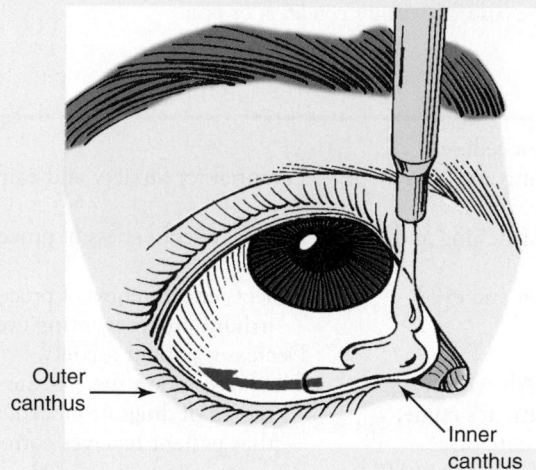

Outer canthus

Inner canthus

STEP 8 Irrigation of eye from inner to outer canthus.

9. Reinforce importance of procedure and encourage patient by using calm, confident, soft voice.

Reduces anxiety.

10. Allow patient to blink periodically.

Lid closure moves secretions from upper conjunctival sac.

11. Continue irrigation with prescribed solution volume or time or until secretions are cleared. (NOTE: In emergent situation: An irrigation of 20–30 minutes or more is needed to flush chemicals.)

Assessment of eye secretion pH may be necessary if eye was exposed to an acidic or basic solution during injury (Mangan, 2015).

12. Blot excess moisture from eyelids and face with gauze or towel.

13. Dispose of soiled supplies, remove gloves, and perform hand hygiene.

Reduces transmission of microorganisms.

EVALUATION

1. Observe for verbal and nonverbal signs of anxiety during irrigation.

Verifies that patient is adequately comforted.

2. Assess patient's comfort level after irrigation.

Verifies effective removal of irritant.

3. Inspect eye for movement and to determine if PERRLA.

Impaired reaction to light, accommodation, or movement may indicate injury.

4. Ask patient about improved visual acuity. Have patient read written material.

Corneal damage from irritant can result in altered visual acuity (e.g., blurred vision, cloudiness).

5. **Use Teach-Back:** "I want to be sure I explained why it is important that I clean your eyes this way. Tell me the purpose of cleaning your eyes in this manner." Develop a revised teaching if patient and caregiver are not able to teach back correctly.

Determines patient's and caregiver's level of understanding rationale for eye irrigation.

STEP	RATIONALE

EVALUATION

Unexpected Outcomes

1. Anxiety.

2. Patient has pain or foreign body sensation in eye following irrigation, excessive tearing, or photophobia.

Related Interventions

- Reinforce rationale for irrigation.
- Allow patient to close eye periodically during irrigation.
- Instruct patient to take slow, deep breaths.
- Advise patient to close eye and avoid eye movement.
- Immediately notify health care provider or eye care practitioner.

Communication and Documentation

- Document in nurses' notes in electronic health record (EHR) or chart the condition of eye and patient's report of pain and visual symptoms. Record amount and type of irrigation in patient's MAR.
- Document your evaluation of patient and caregiver learning.
- Report continuing symptoms of pain or blurred vision.

Caring for a Patient With a Prosthetic Eye

- Prosthetic eyes are made from various materials. In the past, glass was the most common material but is rarely used today, with poly methyl-methacrylate being most common because of its durability, availability, and minimal cost (Cafiero-Chin, Marques, & Danz, 2015).
- A detailed history is required related to the patient's wearing habits, how often the prosthesis is used, and in which manner the prosthesis is to be removed and cleaned.
- Removal of the prosthetic device is similar to removal of a hard contact lens. A small suction device can be used or it can be removed manually. When removing manually, the prosthesis should be pushed up over the lower eyelid, allowing the device to slip out from the bottom (Cafiero-Chin et al., 2015).
- To replace the prosthesis, the top is inserted first by pushing up under the upper eyelid and sliding the lower portion under the lower eye lid (Cafiero-Chin et al., 2015).

Special Considerations
Teaching

- Help patient identify potential hazards at home and work and steps to take to prevent accidents. Personal protective eyewear, such as goggles, face shields, safety glasses, or full-face respirators, must be used when an eye hazard exists. The eye protection chosen for specific work situations depends on the nature and extent of the hazard, the circumstances of exposure, other protective equipment used, and personal vision needs (Canadian Centre for Occupational Health and Safety [CCOHS], 2019).
- Review first-aid procedures for eye emergencies with patient and caregiver.
- Instruct patient to not press or rub an injured eye.
- Instruct patient to consult with ophthalmologist before reinserting contact lens.

Pediatric

- A child with a foreign body or chemical in the eye may panic. It may be necessary to restrain the child to safely and quickly irrigate the eye.

Care in the Community

- With chemical-splash eye injuries, a home shower or garden hose can be used to immediately irrigate the eye(s) for a minimum of 20 to 30 minutes (see Fig. 19.1) prior to going to the emergency department (Mangan, 2015).
- If the injury occurred in the workplace, refer to the MSDS (material safety data sheet) if available (Mangan, 2015).

◆ SKILL 19.2 Ear Irrigation

The common indications for irrigation of the external ear are presence of foreign bodies, local inflammation, and buildup of cerumen (ear wax) in the ear canal. The procedure is not without potential hazards. Usually irrigations are performed with liquid warmed to body temperature to avoid vertigo or nausea in patients. Ear irrigations are effective when the use of commercial drops is unsuccessful in removing cerumen buildup (Harkin, 2015). The greatest danger during ear irrigation is trauma to the tympanic membrane by forcing irrigant into the ear canal under pressure. Damage to the external auditory meatus may occur by scratching the lining of the canal if a patient suddenly moves or if there is inadequate control of the irrigating syringe. Drying the ear improperly may lead to acute otitis externa (infection of the outer ear).

Ear emergencies can include the presence of foreign bodies, insect bites, or percussion injuries. In addition, a patient can have damage from inside the ear, which includes blood and drainage. Sometimes the cause of bloody drainage may be the result of a head or neck injury. If a head or neck injury is suspected, immobilize the patient. Cover the outside of the ear with a sterile dressing (if available), get medical help immediately, and do not irrigate the ear. In addition, do not irrigate the ear if an object is present in the canal; there is a history of ruptured tympanic membrane; or a patient has otitis externa, previous ear surgery (e.g., mastoidectomy), or very hard cerumen (Wyk, 2017).

Delegation and Collaboration

The skill of administering ear irrigation cannot be delegated to an unregulated care provider (UCP). The nurse directs the UCP to:

- Immediately report any potential side effects of ear irrigation (e.g., pain, drainage, dizziness).
- Help a patient when ambulating because some light-headedness may be present, which increases a patient's risk for falling.

Equipment

- Clean gloves
- Otoscope (optional)

- Irrigation or bulb syringe
- Basin for irrigating solution (Use sterile basin if sterile irrigating solution is used [when tympanic membrane is ruptured].)
- Emesis basin for drainage or irrigating solution exiting the ear
- Towel
- Cotton balls or 10 × 10–cm (4 × 4–inch) gauze
- Prescribed irrigating solution warmed to body temperature, or mineral oil, over-the-counter softener
- Medication administration record (MAR) (print or electronic)

STEP	RATIONALE

ASSESSMENT

1. Identify patient using at least two person-specific identifiers (e.g., name and date of birth or name and medical record number) according to employer policy. Compare identifiers with information on patient's MAR or medical record.

Ensures correct patient. Complies with Accreditation Canada's standards and improves patient safety (Accreditation Canada, 2019).

2. Review health care provider's medication prescription, including solution to be instilled and affected ear(s). **NOTE:** Abbreviations AU for right ear, AS for left ear, and AD for both ears, are no longer acceptable (Institute for Safe Medication Practices [ISMP] Canada, 2018); specific ears are to be written out.

Ensures safe and correct administration of medication.

3. Review medical record for history of ruptured tympanic membrane, placement of myringotomy tubes, or surgery of the auditory canal.

These conditions contraindicate irrigation.

4. Inspect pinna and external auditory meatus for redness, swelling, drainage, abrasions, and presence of cerumen or foreign objects.

Findings provide baseline to monitor effects of medication or solution.

   a. Always attempt to remove foreign objects in ear by first simply straightening ear canal.

This may cause object to fall out.

Clinical Decision Point *If vegetable matter such as a dried bean or pea is occluded in the canal, do not perform irrigation. The material can swell on contact with water and cause further damage to the canal (Harkin, 2015; Hockenberry & Wilson, 2015).*

5. Use otoscope to inspect deeper parts of auditory canal and tympanic membrane. **Caution:** Do not push an object further into the ear canal.

Verifies if tympanic membrane is intact.

6. Ask if patient is experiencing pain, using a scale of 0 to 10 (where 0 is no pain, and 10 is the worst pain ever experienced).

Pain is symptomatic of external ear infection or inflammation.

7. Note patient's ability to hear clearly.

Occlusion of auditory canal by cerumen or foreign object can impair hearing.

8. Review patient's knowledge of purpose for irrigation and normal care of ears.

May indicate need for instruction regarding hygiene.

NURSING DIAGNOSES

- Pain (acute or chronic)
- Insufficient knowledge regarding purpose for irrigation
- Potential for injury

Related factors/Risk factors are individualized on the basis of patient's condition or needs.

STEP	RATIONALE

PLANNING

1. Expected outcomes following completion of procedure:
- Patient denies pain during instillation.
- Patient demonstrates hearing conversation more clearly in affected ear.
- Patient can discuss purpose of irrigation and describe correct ear-care techniques.
- Patient's canal is clear of cerumen, foreign material, and discharge.

Fluid is properly instilled.
Obstruction in ear canal is resolved.

Feedback reflects patient's learning.

Inflammation, irritation, and occlusion of canal are relieved.

2. Check accuracy and completeness of each MAR with health care provider's written medication or procedure prescription. Check patient's name, drug name and dosage, route of administration, and time for administration. Compare MAR with label of ear irrigation solution.

The prescription sheet is the most reliable source and only legal record of drugs or procedure that patient is to receive. Ensures that patient receives correct medication.

3. If patient is found to have impacted cerumen, instill 1 or 2 drops of mineral oil or over-the-counter softener into ear twice a day for 2 to 3 days before irrigation.

Loosens cerumen and ensures easier removal during irrigation.

4. Explain procedure. Prepare patient that irrigation may cause sensation of dizziness, ear fullness, and warmth.

Prepares patient to anticipate effects of irrigation and promotes cooperation.

IMPLEMENTATION

1. Perform hand hygiene and arrange supplies at bedside.

Reduces transfer of microorganisms; helps nurse perform procedure smoothly.

2. Close curtain or room door.

Maintains privacy.

3. Help patient to sitting or lying position with head turned toward affected ear. Place towel under patient's head and shoulder, and have patient, if able, hold emesis basin under affected ear.

Position minimizes leakage of fluids around neck and facial area. Solution will flow from ear canal to basin.

4. Pour prescribed irrigating solution into basin. Check temperature of solution by pouring small drop on your inner forearm.
NOTE: If sterile irrigating solution is used, sterile basin is required.

5. Apply clean gloves. Gently clean auricle and outer ear canal with gauze or cotton balls. Do *not* force drainage or cerumen into ear canal.

Prevents infected material from re-entering ear canal. Forceful instillation of solution into occluded canal can cause injury to eardrum.

6. Fill irrigating syringe with solution (approximately 50 mL).

Enough fluid is needed to provide a steady irrigating stream.

7. For adults and for children over 3 years old, gently pull pinna up and back. In children age 3 years or younger, pinna should be pulled down and back (Hockenberry & Wilson, 2015). Adults can lie supine. Place tip of irrigating device just inside external meatus. Leave space around irrigating tip and canal.

Pulling pinna straightens external ear canal. Prevents obstruction of canal with device, which can lead to increased pressure on tympanic membrane.

8. Slowly instill irrigating solution by holding tip of syringe 1 cm (½ inch) above opening to ear canal. Direct fluid toward superior aspect of ear canal. Allow it to drain out into basin during instillation. Continue until canal is cleaned or solution is used (see illustration).

Slow instillation prevents buildup of pressure in ear canal and ensures contact of solution with all canal surfaces.

STEP	RATIONALE

IMPLEMENTATION

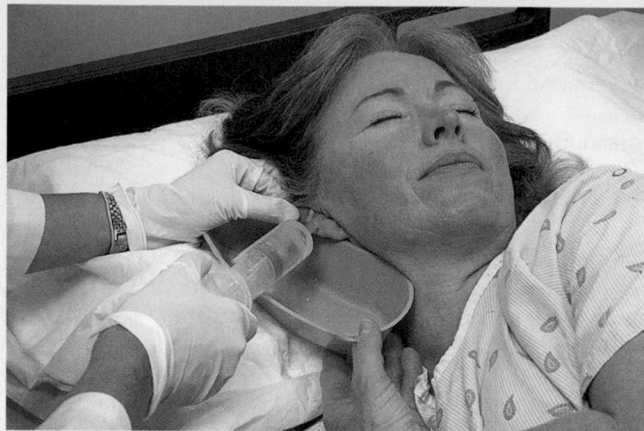

STEP 8 Tip of syringe does not occlude ear canal during irrigation.

9. Maintain flow of irrigation in steady stream until pieces of cerumen or exudate flow from canal.

Constant flow of fluid loosens cerumen.

10. Periodically ask if patient is experiencing pain, nausea, or vertigo.

Symptoms indicate that irrigating solution is too hot or too cold or instilled with too much pressure.

11. Drain excessive fluid from ear by having patient tilt head toward affected side.

Excess fluid may promote microorganism growth if not drained.

12. Dry outer ear canal gently with cotton ball. Leave cotton ball in place for 5 to 10 minutes.

Drying prevents buildup of moisture that can lead to otitis externa.

13. Help patient to sitting position.

Maintains comfort.

14. Remove gloves, dispose of supplies, and perform hand hygiene.

Reduces transmission of infection.

EVALUATION

1. Ask patient if pain is noted during instillation of solution.

Fluid instilled improperly under pressure causes discomfort.

2. Ask patient about sensations of light-headedness or dizziness.

Instillation of fluid into ear can cause some light-headedness or dizziness, which can put patient at risk for falling.

3. Reinspect condition of meatus and canal.

Determines if solution relieves symptoms and removes foreign materials.

4. Assess patient's hearing acuity.

Determines if hearing is improved.

5. **Use Teach-Back:** "I want to be sure you understand how to safely insert the syringe to clean an ear. Show me how you would do this for your mother." Develop a revised teaching plan if caregiver is not able to teach back correctly.

Determines caregiver's level of understanding of instructional topic.

Unexpected Outcomes

1. Patient indicates increased ear pain during irrigation.

2. Ear canal remains occluded with cerumen.

3. Foreign body remains in ear canal.

Related Interventions

• Rupture of eardrum may have occurred. Stop irrigations and notify health care provider immediately.
• Repeat irrigation.
• Referral to auditory specialist if foreign object remains after irrigation.

Communication and Documentation

• Document the procedure, amount of solution instilled, time of administration, and ear receiving irrigation on flow sheet or in nurses' notes in electronic health record (EHR) or chart.

• Document your evaluation of patient and caregiver learning.
• Document appearance of external ear and patient's hearing acuity on flow sheet or in nurses' notes in EHR or chart.
• Report adverse effects or patient response and/or withheld drugs to nurse in charge or health care provider.

Special Considerations
Teaching
- Instruct patient that cerumen has an antibacterial effect that maintains an acid pH in the auditory canal.
- Instruct patients to clean ears daily with a washcloth, soap, and warm water.
- Warn patients against placing objects (including cotton swabs) in ears.

Pediatric
- When cleaning the ear of a small child, be certain that child's head is immobilized to prevent puncturing eardrum. It may be necessary to have child's parent or staff participate (Hockenberry & Wilson, 2015).

Care in the Community
- Instruct patient to use a clean bulb syringe for irrigation. Mineral oil drops or over-the-counter otic preparations can help with removal of cerumen.

✦ SKILL 19.3 Care of Hearing Aids

Hearing is vital for normal communication and orientation to sounds in the environment. Hearing impairment is most common in older persons. Many patients do not seek professional help for this impairment, nor do they consistently wear aids (Yuan et al., 2017). According to Statistics Canada (2016), 40% of adults aged 20–79 have at least slight hearing loss in one or both ears; persons aged 60–79 were 78% more likely to have hearing loss than younger adults; and males have a higher incidence of hearing loss than females.

Initially a person with hearing loss may deny the condition or think that there is a stigma attached to the actual hearing loss or the need for a hearing aid (Mashige, 2016). Any hearing loss has social implications, and the person may not engage in social activities. In addition, in social situations people with a hearing aid often believe that, once their aid is observed, conversation occurs "around them" (Mashige, 2016). There are also many safety considerations. Not only do people with hearing loss have difficulty hearing car horns and emergency sirens, they also have difficulty understanding patient education and, as a result, may not manage their symptoms or therapies safely.

When a patient has a hearing aid, the nurse's role is to understand how it functions and how to help the patient care for it. It is the role of a hearing professional to determine which type of aid the patient needs and how to establish the best auditory settings for each individual patient (CAA, 2015). For people with hearing loss, a proper hearing aid improves the ability to hear and understand spoken words. Several styles of hearing aids are currently available to patients (Table 19.1). Hearing aids amplify sound so it is heard at a more effective level. All hearing aids have four basic components:

1. A microphone, which receives and converts sound into electrical signals
2. An amplifier, which increases the strength of the electrical signal
3. A receiver, which converts the strengthened signal back into sound
4. A power source (batteries)

Hearing aids do not all work the same. The two main types of electronic hearing aids are analogue and digital. Analogue technology converts sound waves into electrical waves, which are amplified. These are custom built to meet the needs of the user and programmed by the manufacturer according to the specifications of the audiologist. Digital technology converts sound waves into numerical codes. The aid is programmed to amplify some frequencies more than others. Digital technology allows the hearing aid to communicate with a number of external devices, including smartphones and Bluetooth technology (Chasin, 2018).

It is a challenge to adjust one's communication style to accommodate a patient with a hearing impairment. Practise person-centred care using the patient as a resource for identifying the communication techniques that are most helpful for that person. Be sure that a patient can see your face; speak slowly in a normal tone; and rephrase rather than repeat if they cannot understand you. Also remember that a patient may be unable to hear alerts, such as fire alarms or overhead announcements.

Delegation and Collaboration

This skill of caring for a hearing aid can be delegated to an unregulated care provider (UCP). The nurse directs the UCP to:
- Report ear pain, inflammation, drainage, odour, or changes in hearing.
- Identify alternative ways to communicate with a patient while the aid is not in use.
- Learn how to carefully handle the aid to prevent damage or injury.

Equipment
- Soft towel and washcloth
- Facial tissues
- Brush or wax loop
- Storage case
- Warm water and soap
- Spare battery, size depends on aid (*optional*)
- Clean gloves (if drainage present)

STEP	RATIONALE

ASSESSMENT

STEP	RATIONALE
1. Identify patient using at least two person-specific identifiers (e.g., name and date of birth or name and medical record number) according to employer policy.	Ensures correct patient. Complies with Accreditation Canada's standards and improves patient safety (Accreditation Canada, 2019).

TABLE 19.1

Types of Hearing Aids

Type	Advantages	Disadvantages	Cautions
In-the-ear (ITE) hearing aids fit completely in the outer ear and are used for mild-to-severe hearing loss. 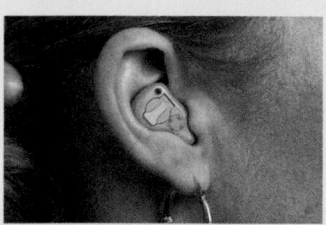	Design of the aid can improve sound transmission through telephone calls. Some ITEs have a *telecoil,* which is a magnetic circuit that allows users to receive sound through the circuitry of the hearing aid instead of the microphone.	ITE aids are damaged by cerumen and ear drainage, and their small size can cause adjustment problems and feedback. They cannot be used with many assistive listening devices.	Not usually worn by children because the casings need to be replaced as the ear grows
Behind-the-ear (BTE) hearing aids are worn behind the ear and are connected to a plastic ear mould that fits inside the outer ear. Used for mild-to-profound hearing loss. 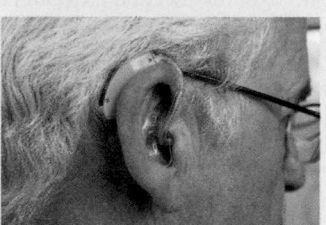	Sound travels through the ear mould into the ear. Useful for persons with chronic ear infections, excess cerumen or small ear canals. Can be used with a variety of other assistive devices.	Poorly fitting BTE ear moulds can cause feedback, a whistling sound caused by the fit of the hearing aid.	May not be appropriate for children or adults who are active in sports because of potential for damage of the device
Open-fit hearing aids are customized to fit the size and shape of the ear canal and are best used for persons with mild to moderate high-frequency hearing loss. 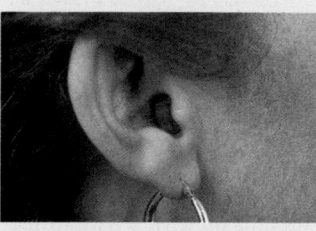	Amplifier and electronics can sit behind the ear, and a slim tube with a small tip is placed in the ear canal.	Because of their small size, canal aids may be difficult for the user to adjust and remove and may not be able to hold additional devices such as a telecoil.	Expensive and not recommended for children Can also be damaged by cerumen and ear drainage
Contralateral routing of signal (CROS) is designed for persons with one ear that is unaidable.	Microphone is placed on the unaidable ear and sound is routed to a hearing aid in the other ear.	Does not fully restore ability to localize sounds in space but provides useful sound information to the person.	CROS can be used in children, depending on their age and environment.

Data from Canadian Academy of Audiology (CAA). (2015). *Hearing aids, implants and other devices.* Retrieved from https://canadianaudiology.ca/for-the-public/hearing-aids-and-implants/#what-kinds-of-hearing-aids-are-there; National Institute on Deafness and Other Communication Disorders (NIDCD). (2013). *Hearing aids.* Retrieved from http://www.nidcd.nih.gov/health/hearing/pages/hearingaid.aspx#hearingaid_01.

STEP	RATIONALE

ASSESSMENT

2. Determine whether patient can hear clearly with hearing aid, by talking slowly and clearly in normal tone of voice.

Inability to hear may indicate a problem with the hearing aid or battery or that the particular model is no longer effective for patient.

3. Ask if patient is able to manipulate and hold hearing aid, or, preferably, observe patient insert aid independently.

Determines level of assistance required in care.

STEP	RATIONALE

ASSESSMENT

4. Assess if hearing aid is working by removing it from patient's ear. Close battery case and turn volume slowly to high. Cup hand over hearing aid. If you hear a squealing sound (feedback), it is working. If no sound is heard, replace batteries and test again.

May indicate malfunctioning of hearing aid.

5. Determine patient's usual hearing aid–care practices.

Provides information as to how patient cares for device, and identifies patient preferences.

6. Assess patient for any unusual physical or auditory signs or symptoms (pain, itching, redness, discharge, odour, tinnitus, decreased acuity). If hearing is reduced, ask: when did this start, is it present all the time, does the quality of hearing acuity change with male or female voices, adult or children's voices?

May indicate injury, infection, or cerumen accumulation.

7. Inspect ear mould for cracked or rough edges.

Poorly fitting hearing aids cause irritation or discomfort to external ear canal.

8. Inspect for accumulation of cerumen around aid and plugging of opening in aid.

Cerumen can block sound reception (Harkin, 2015; White, 2015).

9. Assess patient's knowledge of and routines for cleaning and caring for hearing aid.

Determines adherence to and knowledge of self-care.

NURSING DIAGNOSES

- Reduced verbal communication
- Insufficient knowledge regarding hearing aid care
- Potential for injury
- Potential for situational low self-esteem

Related factors/Risk factors are individualized on the basis of patient's condition or needs.

PLANNING

1. Expected outcomes following completion of procedure:
- Patient verbalizes comfort after removal and reinsertion of hearing aid.

Hearing aid is removed or inserted properly and positioned correctly.

- Patient responds appropriately to normal conversation and environmental sounds.

Hearing aid and batteries are operational. Aid is secure and unobstructed.

- Patient demonstrates proper care of hearing aid.

Learning is achieved.

2. Discuss procedure with patient. Explain all steps before removing aid.

Patient can help in planning by explaining additional tips for care. Patient may be confused or anxious if verbal instructions are given after removal of hearing aid.

3. Assemble supplies at bedside. Place towel over work area.

Provides easy access to supplies. Towel catches hearing aid if accidentally dropped and avoids breakage.

4. Have patient assume supine, side-lying, or sitting position in bed or chair.

Provides easy access for nurse. Promotes patient comfort.

IMPLEMENTATION

1. Perform hand hygiene and apply clean gloves if patient has ear drainage.

Reduces transmission of microorganisms.

2. Removing and cleaning hearing aid(s):

a. Patient or nurse turns hearing aid(s) volume off, usually by turning volume control to left. Then grasp aid securely and gently remove device following natural ear contour.

Prevents feedback (whistling) during removal. Prevents dropping hearing aid. Prevents injury to ear.

Clinical Decision Point *Some hearing aids, such as the completely-in-canal (CIC) device, do not have a volume control but are turned off by opening the battery door. Other aids have the volume control located on the remote. Be sure that the patient knows the importance of having the volume turned off when the aid is not in use.*

STEP	RATIONALE

IMPLEMENTATION

b. Hold aid over towel and wipe exterior with tissue to remove cerumen.	Prevents breakage or damage if aid is dropped. Cerumen may irritate canal and interfere with fit.
c. Inspect all openings in aid for accumulated cerumen. Carefully remove cerumen with wax loop or other device supplied with hearing aid.	Cerumen may block sound from receiver. It may also block pressure equalization channel and create feeling of ear pressure.

Clinical Decision Point *The pressure equalization channel is a tiny hole through the entire length of the ear mould and should be clear for the entire length. The receiver points into the ear through another opening. It is easily damaged. NEVER insert anything into the receiver port!*

d. Inspect ear mould for rough edges or any frays in cords.	May irritate ear canal.
e. Open battery door, place hearing aid in labelled storage container, and allow it to air dry.	Allows drying of internal components. Protects against breakage and loss.
f. Assess ear for redness, tenderness, discharge, or odour.	Signs may indicate injury or infection.
g. Repeat procedure for other hearing aid if bilateral.	
h. Place towel beneath patient's ear(s). Wash ear canal(s) with washcloth moistened in soap and water. Rinse and dry.	Absorbs excess water. Removes cerumen from ear canal. Removes soap residue and water that may harbour microbes or damage aid.
i. Dispose of towels, remove gloves, and perform hand hygiene.	Reduces transmission of microorganisms.
j. If storing hearing aid(s), place each in dry storage case with desiccant material. Label case with patient's name and room number. If there is more than one aid, note right or left. Indicate in patient's medical record where aid is stored.	Protects hearing aid against damage, moisture, and breakage. Documents how and where hearing aid is stored.
3. Inserting hearing aid(s):	
a. Remove hearing aid(s) from storage case and check battery (see assessment). Check that volume is off.	
b. Identify hearing aid as either right (marked "R" or red colour coded) or left (marked "L" or blue colour coded).	Proper orientation prevents damage and injury.
c. When possible, allow patient to insert aid. Otherwise, hold hearing aid with thumb and index finger of dominant hand so canal (long part with holes) is at bottom. Insert pointed end of ear mould into ear canal. Follow natural ear contours to guide aid into place.	Prevents dropping of aid. Proper positioning prevents injury. Pulling on ear may distort canal and make insertion more difficult.
d. Anchor any separate pieces, as in case of behind-the-ear (BTE) aid or body aid.	Prevents pieces from falling and breaking.
e. Adjust or have patient adjust volume gradually to comfortable level for talking to patient in regular voice 0.9 to 1.2 metres (3 to 4 feet) away. Rotate volume control toward nose to increase volume and away from nose to decrease volume.	Gradual adjustment prevents discomfort and injury to ear.
f. Repeat insertion for other hearing aid, if bilateral.	
g. Close and store case. Remove and dispose of gloves. Perform hand hygiene.	Preserves desiccant. Prevents loss. Reduces transmission of microorganisms.

EVALUATION

1. Ask patient to rate level of comfort after removal or insertion.	Verifies proper technique and positioning.
2. Observe patient during normal conversation and in response to environmental sounds.	Verifies that aid is operational, correctly positioned, unobstructed, and effective.
3. Use Teach-Back: "I want to be sure you understand what I showed you about how to remove, clean, and reinsert your father's hearing aid. Let's take time now so you can show me how to do it." Develop a revised teaching plan if caregiver is not able to teach back correctly.	Determines patient's and caregiver's level of understanding of instructional topic.

STEP	RATIONALE

EVALUATION

Unexpected Outcomes	Related Interventions
1. Patient is unable to hear conversations or environmental sounds. Patient's verbal responses are inappropriate.	• Check function, type, and placement of battery and replace it if indicated. • Increase volume if adjustable. • Inspect aid and ear canal for cerumen blockage. • Refer to audiologist for reassessment.
2. Patient experiences discomfort or pain, inflammation, drainage, or odour from affected ear.	• Remove aid and inspect for sharp or rough edges. Refer to provider for repair. • Assess ear for signs of injury or infection. • Confirm correct R or L placement. Reposition hearing aid.

Communication and Documentation

- Document removal of hearing aid, storage location if not reinserted after cleaning, and patient's preferred communication techniques on flow sheet or in nurses' notes in electronic health record (EHR) or chart. If family takes aid home, be sure that this information is documented.
- Document your evaluation of patient and caregiver learning.
- Report any signs or symptoms of infection or injury or sudden decrease in hearing acuity.

Special Considerations
Teaching

- Instruct family that batteries are toxic if swallowed and to keep them away from pets and children.
- Patients should insert the aid after their hair is dried and any hair spray applied. Heat from the hair dryer or perfumes and hair spray can damage the aid.
- Dogs in particular and cats are attracted to the smell of used hearing aids. Advise patient to protect the hearing aids and their pets by properly storing the aids out of reach.
- Encourage patients to identify helpful communication tips and teach them to others. Many patients find facial cues informative. Speakers must:
  1. Face patient, stay within 0.9 to 1.2 metres (3 to 4 feet) away, and keep hands away from mouth.
  2. Get patient's attention before speaking.
  3. Rephrase rather than repeat when a patient cannot understand.
  4. Reduce background noise or move to a quiet area.

Pediatric

- Children are more often fitted with BTE hearing aids because the ear canal is still growing.
- The aid is made less conspicuous with hair styling or becomes a statement of fashion and personality with a brightly coloured or transparent case.
- Children need help to prevent acoustic feedback (whistling), which they are unable to hear. This is usually eliminated by removing and reinserting the device and making sure that no hair is caught between the ear mould and canal or lowering the volume of the device (Hockenberry & Wilson, 2015).

Gerontological

- Advise patient to protect the hearing aid from water, alcohol, hair spray or cologne, perspiration, rain, and snow and to avoid exposing it to extremes of temperature.
- Encourage patient to store hearing aids and batteries with desiccant or in an electronic dryer to prolong aid's life, minimize repairs, and preserve batteries.
- The small size of some hearing aids may make them difficult to manipulate, particularly for individuals with decreased dexterity or visual acuity. Consult an audiologist to identify an aid that accommodates a patient's particular need.

Care in the Community

- Determine presence and willingness of caregiver to perform necessary care of hearing aid if required.
- Assess patient's home and determine need for special precautions given patient's hearing status.

◆ CLINICAL DEBRIEF

A 68-year-old married man and his wife have two grown children who are married with children. He has worn bilateral in-the-ear (ITE) hearing aids for the last 10 years. He knows how to care for his aids. He is comfortable and satisfied with them. When the aids are working well, he notes that he hears his family and coworkers clearly, has minimal distortion in large gatherings, and is able to distinguish emergency sirens and car horns when he is driving. Three weeks ago, he had an upper respiratory tract infection, and since that time both he and his wife have noticed changes in his hearing acuity. He is now visiting his primary care clinic to see what can be done with his hearing before he goes back to the audiologist.

1. He thinks that he has diminished hearing in the left ear and senses drainage from that ear. Which assessments should the nurse complete?
2. Their preschool- and school-age grandchildren visit frequently and are curious about the hearing aids. Neither the patient nor his wife

remembers any patient education regarding hearing aid safety related to young children. What will the nurse include in a teaching session regarding hearing aid safety?

3. During assessment of the left ear the nurse identifies excessive wax, purulent drainage, and a cloudy tympanic membrane. Using SBAR (*Situation, Background, Assessment,* and *Recommendation*), communicate this information to the health care team.

◆ REVIEW QUESTIONS

1. The nurse decides to check the functioning of the hearing aid. Place the following steps in appropriate order for cleaning the hearing aid.
   a. Wash ear canal.
   b. Place hearing aid in storage case.
   c. Perform hand hygiene and apply clean gloves.
   d. Grasp aid securely and remove from ear following natural ear contour.
   e. Use brush to clean holes in aid.
   f. Have patient turn hearing aid volume off.

2. Which important nursing responsibilities pertain to eye irrigations? *(Select all that apply.)*
   1. Irrigating the eye immediately in emergent situations
   2. Removing dried secretions with moistened gauze
   3. Gently securing the eyelids with paper tape
   4. Checking for the pupillary response
   5. Preventing injury to the patient's corneas

3. When caring for a patient who is hearing impaired, which approaches best facilitate comunication? *(Select all that apply.)*
   1. Speaking slightly more loudly than usual
   2. Speaking slightly more slowly using a normal tone
   3. Standing so patient can see the nurse's face
   4. Rephrasing rather than repeating
   5. Using hand gestures to help explain what is being said

ⓔ *Visit the Evolve site for a complete list of Clinical Debrief and Review Questions answers.*

REFERENCES

Accreditation Canada. (2019). *Required organizational practices handbook—Version 14*. Retrieved from http://www.wrha.mb.ca/quality/files/2019ROPHandbook.pdf

Alansari, M., Hijazi, M., & Maghrabi, K. (2015). Making a difference in eye care of the critically ill patients. *Journal of Intensive Care Medicine*, 30(6), 7. doi:10.1177/0885066613510674

Cafiero-Chin, M., Marques, C., & Danz, H. (2015). Ocular prosthesis: Indications to management. *Canadian Journal of Optometry*, 77(2), 24–32.

Canadian Academy of Audiology (CAA). (2015). *Hearing aids, implants and other devices*. Retrieved from https://canadianaudiology.ca/for-the-public/hearing-aids-and-implants/#what-kinds-of-hearing-aids-are-there

Canadian Academy of Audiology (CAA). (2015–2016). *Reports, guidelines, and position statements*. Retrieved from https://canadianaudiology.ca/professional-resources/guidelines-and-position-statements/

Canadian Association of Optometrists (CAO). (n.d.). *Frequency of eye examinations*. Retrieved from https://opto.ca/health-library/frequency-of-eye-examinations

Canadian Association of Optometrists (CAO). (2017). *Contact lens*. Retrieved from https://opto.ca/health-library/wear-care-for-contact-lenses

Canadian Centre for Occupational Health and Safety (CCOHS). (2019). *Eye and face protectors*. Retrieved from https://www.ccohs.ca/oshanswers/prevention/ppe/glasses.html; http://www.chs.ca/programs-and-services

Canadian Hearing Society. (2019). *Programs and services*. Retrieved from http://www.chs.ca/programs-and-services

Canadian National Institute for the Blind (CNIB). (2018). *What is blindness?* Retrieved from https://cnib.ca/en/sight-loss-info/blindness/what-blindness?region=ns

Chasin, M. (2018). Hearing aids–From here to eternity and beyond: An article written for the hard of hearing consumer and their family. *Canadian Audiologist*, 5(2), 1.

Harkin, H. (2015). Ear care and irrigation with water: An update. *Practice Nurse*, 45(7), 24.

Heine, C., & Browning, C. (2015). The dual sensory loss in older persons: A systematic review. *The Gerontologist*, 55(5), 913–928. doi:10.1093/geront/gnv074

Hockenberry, M. J., & Wilson, D. (2015). *Wong's nursing care of infants and children* (10th ed.). St. Louis: Mosby.

Institute for Safe Medication Practices (ISMP) Canada. (2018). *Do not use. Dangerous abbreviations, symbols and dose designations*. Retrieved from https://www.ismp-canada.org/download/ISMPCanadaListOfDangerousAbbreviations.pdf

Mangan, R. (2015). Quickly douse chemical burns. *Review of Optometry*, 152(2), 22–25.

Mashige, K. (2016). Chemical and thermal ocular burns: A review of causes, clinical features and management protocols. *South African Family Practice*, 58(1), 1–4. doi:10.1080/20786190.2015.1085221

Mick, P., Parfyonov, M., Wittich, W., Phillips, N., & Picenhora-Fuller, M. (2018). Associations between sensory loss and social networks, participation, support, and loneliness. Analysis of the Canadian longitudinal study on aging. *Canadian Family Physician*, 64, e33–e41.

Statistics Canada. (2016). *Health fact sheets. Hearing loss of Canadians, 2012 to 2015*. Ottawa, ON: Author.

Taheri-Kharameh, Z. (2017). Eye care in the intensive care patients: An evidence-based review. *BMJ Open*, 7(Suppl. 1), A65. doi:10.1136/bmjopen-2016-015415.177

Tremblay, K. L. (2015). The ear-brain connection: Older ears and older brains. *American Journal of Audiology*, 24(2), 117–120. doi:10.1044/2015_AJA-14-0068

White, S. (2015). Practical implementation tips: Dual sensory loss. *Practice Guideline*, 18(6), 30.

Wyk, F. (2017). Cerumen impaction removal. *Medscape*. Retrieved from https://emedicine.Medscape.com/article/1413546-overview#a3

Yuan, J., Sun, Y., Sang, S., Pham, J., & Kong, W. (2017). The risk of cognitive impairment associated with hearing function in older adults: A pooled analysis of data from eleven studies. *Scientific Reports*, 8(1), 2137. doi:10.1038/s41598-018-20496-w

20 | Safe Medication Preparation

Written by **Wendy R. Ostendorf, RN, MS, EdD, CNE, and Shelley L. Cobbett, RN, GnT, MN, EdD**

OBJECTIVES

Mastery of content in this chapter will enable the nurse to:

- Discuss nursing roles and responsibilities in medication administration.
- Discuss the Canadian Patient Safety Institute Goals of the Medication Safety Action Plan.
- Discuss factors that contribute to medication errors.
- Differentiate among different types of medication actions.
- List and discuss the 10 rights of medication administration.
- Identify the system of measurement for a given prescribed medication.

- Accurately calculate medication doses.
- Describe the safety features of medication delivery systems.
- Identify guidelines for safe administration of medications.
- Implement nursing actions to prevent medication errors.
- Discuss medication error disclosure requirements.
- Discuss methods used to educate patients about prescribed medications.

MEDIA RESOURCES

- evolve http://evolve.elsevier.com/Canada/Perry/clinicalskills/
- Review Questions
- Case Studies

- Audio Glossary
- **NSO** Nursing Skills Online
- Clinical Debrief and Review Questions Answers

PURPOSE

Safe and accurate medication administration is a challenging and important nursing responsibility. All professional nurses need to understand the implications involved in medication administration. Safe medication administration requires good judgement, critical thinking, and clinical decision-making skills. This includes thorough patient assessment and an understanding of pharmacotherapeutics, pharmacokinetics, growth and development, nutrition, and mathematics.

STANDARDS OF CARE

- Accreditation Canada, 2019—*Required Organizational Practices Handbook—Version 14* (http://www.wrha.mb.ca/quality/files/2019 ROPHandbook.pdf)
- Canadian Patient Safety Institute (CPSI), 2014—*Medication Safety Action Plan* (http://www.patientsafetyinstitute.ca/en/About/ PatientSafetyForwardWith4/Documents/A%20Medication%20 Safety%20Action%20Plan.pdf); 2016—*Medication Safety* (http:// www.patientsafetyinstitute.ca/en/About/PatientSafety ForwardWith4/pages/medication-safety.aspx)
- Institute for Safe Medication Practices Canada (ISMP), 2014–2019—*Oral Dosage Forms That Should Not be Crushed; Do Not Use. Dangerous Abbreviations, Symbols, and Dose Designations; High-Alert Medications in Acute Care; Preventable Medication Errors—Look-Alike/Sound-Alike Drug Names; Key Elements of Safe Medication Use; Canadian Medication Incident Reporting and Prevention System (CMIRPS) Program* (https://www.ismp-canada.org/ publications.htm)
- Provincial Nursing Association Medication Guidelines, for example:
  - College of Registered Nurses of British Columbia (CRNBC) (2019)—*Medication Administration* (https://www.crnbc.ca/ Standards/PracticeStandards/Pages/medicationadmin.aspx)
  - College of Registered Nurses of Nova Scotia (CRNNS) (2017)—*Medication Guidelines for Registered Nurses* (https:// crnns.ca/wp-content/uploads/2015/05/Medication-Guidelines.pdf)

PRINCIPLES FOR PRACTICE

Pharmacological Concepts

Medication Names

NSO *Nursing Skills Online Safe Medication Preparation Module 5 / Lesson 1*

Some medications have as many as three different names. The chemical name describes the drug composition and molecular structure, such as N-acetyl-para-aminophenol, commonly known as Tylenol. It is rarely used in clinical practice. A manufacturer who first develops a medication provides the generic name (e.g., acetaminophen is the generic name for Tylenol). The generic name is the name that is listed in official publications such as the *Health Canada's Drug Product Database* or the *RxTx Database* (formerly the *Canadian Compendium of Pharmaceuticals and Specialties* [CPS]). A medication trade name or brand name is used to market the medication. The trade name has the symbol ™ at the upper right of the name, indicating a manufacturer trademark of the name (e.g., Tempra™, Tylenol™).

Many companies choose brand and generic names that are easy to remember, and they can be very similar, which contributes to medication errors. ISMP Canada (2014) has identified several problematic medications with similar names and spelling, such as Celebrex for arthritis and Celexa for depression; Lamictal for epilepsy and Lamisil for fungal infections; Losec for ulcers and Lasix for fluid retention. Another measure to help address the confusion around medications having similar names includes the use of TALL-man lettering (ISMP, 2016). This measure uses capital letters in specific parts of a word and helps distinguish dissimilarities in medication names; for example, TEGretol (for seizures) can be confused with TRENtal, which is prescribed for intermittent claudication; but the TALL-man letters emphasize the difference in the medication name.

The physical appearances of some medications with similar colour, size, and shape have led to medication errors. Generic medications are often prescribed as a more cost-efficient substitution for brand-name medications. However, there may be dramatic differences in appearance of generic medications, depending on the manufacturer (Fraser, Albaum, Tadrous, et al., 2015). Patients may be confused as to why their medication has a different colour or shape when the prescription is refilled. However, medications are found under a variety of different names, and as a nurse you must be careful to obtain the exact name and spelling before administering a medication.

Classification

Medications with similar characteristics are categorized by their class. Medication classification indicates the effect of a medication on a body system, the symptoms the medication relieves, or the desired effect of the medication. For example, patients with type 2 diabetes mellitus often take oral hypoglycemic medications to control their blood glucose levels. The sulfonylureas are one classification of 11 medications used to treat hyperglycemia. Some medications are part of more than one class. For example, aspirin is an analgesic, antipyretic, and anti-inflammatory medication.

Medication Forms

Medications are available in a variety of forms or preparations. The form of the medication determines its route of administration. The composition of a medication influences its absorption and metabolism. Many medications are made in several forms, such as tablets, caplets, or suppositories. When administering a medication, be certain to use the proper form (Table 20.1).

Pharmacokinetics

A medication must enter a patient's body; be absorbed and distributed to cells, tissues, or a specific organ; and then alter physiological function to be therapeutic. *Pharmacokinetics* is the study of how medications enter the body, reach their site of action, are metabolized, and exit the body. Understanding pharmacokinetics allows you to properly time medication administration, select an administration route, and judge a patient's response to medications. *Absorption* is the passage of medication molecules into the blood from the site of administration. Factors that influence the rate of absorption include the administration route, ability of a medication to dissolve, blood flow to the administration site, body surface area, and lipid solubility of a medication (Table 20.2). After a medication is absorbed, it is distributed to tissues and organs and finally to the site of medication action. The rate and extent of distribution depend on circulation, cell membrane permeability, and protein binding. Poor perfusion (e.g., heart failure) alters medication distribution. A medication must pass through biological membranes to reach certain organs. Some membranes are barriers to the passage of medications. For example, the blood–brain barrier allows only fat-soluble medications to pass into the brain and cerebrospinal fluid. The degree to which

TABLE 20.1	

Forms of Medication

Form	Description
Medication Forms Commonly Prepared for Administration by Oral Route	
Solid Forms	
Caplet	Shaped like a capsule and coated for ease of swallowing
Capsule	Medication encased in a gelatin shell
Tablet	Powdered medication compressed into a hard disk or cylinder; in addition to primary medication, contains binders (adhesive to allow powder to stick together), disintegrators (to promote table dissolution), lubricants (for ease of manufacturing), and fillers (for convenient tablet size)
Enteric coated	Coated tablet that does not dissolve in stomach; coating dissolves in intestine, where medication is absorbed
Liquid Forms	
Elixir	Clear fluid containing water and alcohol; often sweetened
Extract	Concentrated medication form made by removing the active part of the medication from its components. Extracts are prepared as a syrup or dried form of pharmacologically active medication, usually made by evaporating solution
Aqueous solution	Substance dissolved in water and syrups
Aqueous suspension	Finely dissolved medication particles in liquid medium must be shaken; when left standing, particles settle to bottom of container
Syrup	Medication dissolved in concentrated sugar solution
Tincture	Alcohol extract from plant or vegetable
Other Oral Forms and Terms Associated With Oral Preparations	
Troche (lozenge)	Flat, round tablet that dissolves in mouth to release medication; not meant for ingestion
Aerosol	Aqueous medication sprayed and absorbed in mouth and upper airway; not meant for ingestion
Sustained release	Tablet or capsule that contains small particles of a medication coated with material that provides medication over an extended period of time
Controlled release	Medication that maintains constant levels in blood or tissue and promotes localization of the medication at a specific site; its release follows a specific, predetermined pattern
Medication Forms Commonly Prepared for Administration by Topical Route	
Ointment (salve or cream)	Semisolid, externally applied preparation, usually containing one or more medications
Liniment	Usually contains alcohol, oil, or soapy emollient applied to skin
Lotion	Semiliquid suspension that usually protects, cools, or cleans skin
Paste	Medication preparation that is thicker than ointment; absorbed through skin more slowly than ointment; often used for skin protection
Transdermal patch or disk	Medicated disk or patch embedded with medication that is applied to skin Medication absorbed through skin over a designated period of time (e.g., 24 hours)
Medication Forms Commonly Prepared for Administration by Parenteral Route	
Solution	Sterile preparation that contains water or normal saline with one or more dissolved compounds
Powder	Sterile particles of medication that are dissolved in a sterile liquid (e.g., water, normal saline) before administration
Medication Forms Commonly Prepared for Instillation Into Body Cavities	
Suppository	Solid dosage form mixed with gelatin and shaped in form of a pellet for insertion into body cavity (rectum or vagina) (Suppository melts when it reaches body temperature and is then absorbed.)
Intraocular disk	Small, flexible oval (similar to a contact lens) consisting of two soft outer layers and a middle layer containing medication; slowly releases medication when moistened by ocular fluid

medications bind to serum proteins such as albumin affects distribution. Most medications bind to albumin to some extent. When this happens, they are unable to exert pharmacological activity. Only the unbound, or "free," medication is active. Older persons and patients with liver disease or malnutrition have reduced albumin, which increases their risk for medication toxicity.

After a medication reaches its site of action, it is metabolized into a less active or inactive form. Biotransformation occurs under the influence of enzymes that detoxify, degrade (break down), and remove biologically active chemicals. Most biotransformation occurs in the liver, although the lungs, kidneys, blood, and intestines also play a role. Patients (e.g., older persons and those living with chronic

TABLE 20.2

Medication Absorption

Absorption Factor	Physiological Effects
Route of administration	Topical applications on skin absorb slowly. Medications applied to mucous membranes and respiratory airways absorb quickly. Oral medications pass through the gastrointestinal tract and absorb slowly. The intravenous route produces the most rapid absorption because the medication is available immediately when it enters the systemic circulation.
Ability to dissolve	Solutions and liquid suspensions absorb more readily than tablets or capsules. Acidic medications pass through the gastric mucosa rapidly and absorb rapidly, whereas basic medications (pH greater than 7.0) do not absorb before reaching the small intestine.
Blood flow	When the administration site contains a rich blood supply, medications absorb rapidly.
Body surface area	A medication in contact with a large surface area (e.g., small intestine) absorbs faster than one in contact with smaller surface area (e.g., stomach).
Lipid solubility	Medications that are highly lipid soluble absorb more readily.

disease) are at risk for medication toxicity if their organs cannot metabolize medications effectively.

The final aspect of pharmacokinetics is *excretion*, the process by which medications exit the body through the lungs, exocrine glands, bowel, kidneys, and liver. The chemical makeup of a medication determines the organ of excretion. For example, gaseous and volatile compounds such as alcohol and nitrous oxide exit through the lungs. The site of excretion poses implications for nursing care. For example, when medications exit through sweat glands, the nurse needs to provide skin care to reduce irritation. Nurses must know if a medication is excreted through the intestines because the administration of laxatives or enemas increases peristalsis, accelerates excretion, and thus lessens the time for medication effects. When patients have reduced renal function, they are at risk for medication toxicity since kidneys are the main organs for medication excretion.

Pharmacotherapeutics

Pharmacotherapeutics is the study of the therapeutic uses and effects of medications. Medications vary in the way they act and their types of action. Patients do not always respond in the same way to each successive dose of a medication. Sometimes the same medication causes very different responses in different patients. Therefore, it is essential to understand all the effects that medications have on patients.

Therapeutic Effects

Each medication has a therapeutic effect (i.e., the intended or desired physiological response of a medication). For example, morphine sulphate, an analgesic, is administered to relieve a patient's pain. Sometimes a single medication has many therapeutic effects. For example, aspirin relieves pain and reduces fever and tissue inflammation. Knowing the desired therapeutic effect for each medication allows the nurse to provide patient education and accurately evaluate its desired effect.

Adverse Effects

Adverse drug events or effects (ADEs) are unintended, undesirable, and often unpredictable. Although sometimes they are apparent immediately, unfortunately, they often take weeks or months to develop. Early clinical recognition is the important first step in identification. ADEs range from mild (e.g., rashes or photosensitivity to light) to potentially fatal (anaphylaxis). Prompt recognition and reporting of ADEs prevent serious injury to patients. Always assess

patients who may be at high risk for an ADE, such as pregnant women and patients with chronic disorders (e.g., hypertension, epilepsy, heart disease, psychoses) (Burchum & Rosenthal, 2016). According to Accreditation Canada (2017), there are three patient safety incident categories: harmful incidents (which replaced the term *adverse or sentinel events*), no-harm incidents, and near misses. Health care providers are encouraged to report patient safety incidents to Health Canada's Adverse Reaction and Medical Device Problem Reporting Program as part of Canada's Vigilance Program, CIHI's National System for Incident Reporting, ISMP Canada, and the World Health Organization's Global Patient Safety Alerts.

Side Effects

Every medication has the potential for harm. No medication is totally safe and absolutely free of nontherapeutic effects. Side effects are predictable and often unavoidable secondary effects produced at a usual therapeutic medication dose. They are either harmless or cause injury. The intensity of side effects is often dose dependent. If the side effects are serious enough to outweigh the benefits of the therapeutic action of a medication, the health care provider will likely discontinue the medication. Patients commonly stop taking medications because of side effects such as anorexia, nausea, vomiting, dizziness, drowsiness, dry mouth, constipation, and diarrhea. Report any side effect to the health care provider to ensure that it is not incorrectly interpreted as a more serious adverse reaction. Health care providers report side effects to Health Canada with the online Side Effect Reporting Form, as part of Canada's Vigilance Program. The *Protecting Canadians From Unsafe Drugs Act* (Vanessa's Law) was passed in November 2014 and was the basis for a regulatory initiative for mandatory reporting of serious adverse drug reactions and medical incidents, "Forward Regulatory Plan 2018–2020" (Health Canada, 2018). Proposed amendments to the Food and Drug Regulations and Medical Device Regulations will identify applicable health care institutions for mandatory reporting, types of reportable incidents, applicable therapeutic products and databases, and timelines for reporting (Health Canada, 2018).

Toxic Effects

Toxic effects develop after prolonged intake of a medication or when a medication accumulates in the blood because of impaired metabolism or excretion. Excess amounts of a medication within the body sometimes have lethal effects, depending on the action of the medication. For example, toxic levels of morphine, an opioid, cause severe respiratory depression and death. Antidotes are available

TABLE 20.3

Mild Allergic Reactions

Symptom	Description
Urticaria (hives)	Raised, irregularly shaped skin eruptions with varying sizes and shapes; reddened margins and pale centres
Rash	Small, raised vesicles that are usually reddened; often distributed over the entire body
Pruritus	Itching of the skin; accompanies most rashes
Rhinitis	Inflammation of mucous membranes lining the nose, causing swelling and a clear watery discharge

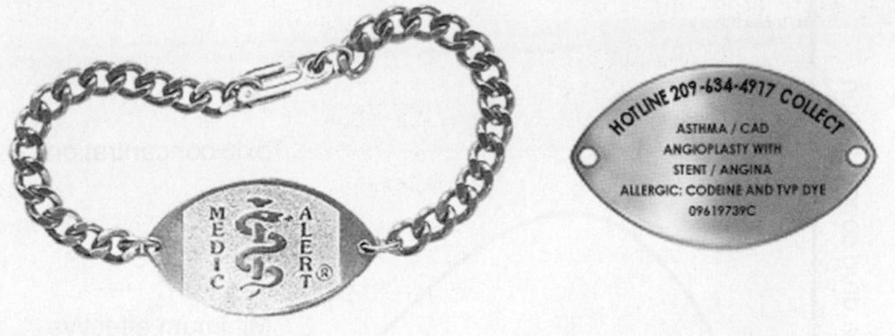

FIG 20.1 Medical Alert bracelet. (*From Potter, P. A., Perry, A. G., Stockert, P. A., Hall, A. M., Astle, B. J., & Duggleby, W. [Eds.]. [2019]. Canadian Fundamentals of Nursing [6th ed., Fig. 34-2]. Toronto: Elsevier Canada.*)

to treat specific types of medication toxicity. For example, naloxone, an opioid antagonist, reverses the effects of opioid toxicity.

Idiosyncratic Reactions

An idiosyncratic reaction is an unpredictable effect in which a patient overreacts or underreacts to a medication or has a reaction different from normal. Predicting which patients will have an idiosyncratic response is impossible. For example, lorazepam is an anti-anxiety medication that may cause agitation and delirium when given to an older person.

Allergic Reactions

Allergic reactions also are adverse unpredictable responses to a medication. Exposure to an initial dose of a medication causes a patient to become sensitized immunologically. The medication acts as an antigen, which causes antibodies to be produced. With repeated administration a patient develops an allergic response to the medication, its chemical preservatives, or a metabolite. An allergic reaction ranges from mild to severe, depending on the patient and the medication (Table 20.3). Among the different classes of medications, antibiotics cause a high incidence of allergic reactions. Severe or anaphylactic reactions, which are life threatening, are characterized by sudden constriction of bronchiolar muscles, edema of the pharynx and larynx, severe wheezing, and shortness of breath. Some patients become severely hypotensive, necessitating emergency resuscitation measures.

It is common practice for hospitalized patients with known medication allergies to have their allergy information recorded in a clearly identifiable place. This allows all caregivers to be aware of each patient's allergies. In many facilities this information is recorded in a special section of the electronic health record (EHR), on the front of a patient's hard-copy medical record or chart, in the medication administration record (MAR), or on a specially designed label that is applied to the front of a patient's chart. Patients also receive colour-coded allergy identification bands to wear around the wrist. *Always record a patient's allergies in the MAR.* Patients who are cared for in other settings (e.g., home or community clinics) and have a known history of an allergy to a medication or substance should wear an Medic-Alert bracelet or medal, which alerts all health care providers to these allergies in case a patient is found unconscious or is unable to communicate (Fig. 20.1). It is often common that patients list having an allergy to a medication when it is not a true allergy but rather a severe side effect or an ADE. It is important for the nurse to be aware of the difference between a true allergy and a side effect. Ask the patient which type of reaction they experienced and offer them examples, such as nausea versus hives.

Medication Tolerance and Dependence

Medication tolerance occurs over time. It is usually noted clinically when patients receive the same medication for long periods and require higher doses to produce the desired therapeutic effect. Medications known to produce tolerance include opium alkaloids (e.g., morphine), nitrates, and ethyl alcohol. Patients hospitalized for acute episodes of illness usually do not develop tolerance. It may take a month or longer for tolerance to occur.

Medication tolerance is not the same as medication dependence. Two types of medication dependence exist: psychological (or addiction) or physiological. In psychological dependence a patient desires the medication for benefit other than the intended effect. Physiological dependence is a physiological adaptation to a medication that manifests itself by intense physical disturbance when the medication is withdrawn. When patients receive medications for a short term, such as for postoperative pain, dependence is rare. If a patient is dependent on alcohol, a higher-than-usual medication dose is necessary for the desired effect of the medication.

Medication Interactions

When one medication modifies the action of another medication, a medication interaction occurs. Medication interactions are common in individuals taking many medications. Some medications increase or diminish the action of other medications and alter the way in which another medication is absorbed, metabolized, or eliminated from the body. When two medications have a synergistic effect, their combined effect is greater than the effect of one medication given separately. For example, alcohol is a central nervous system depressant that has a synergistic effect with antihistamines, antidepressants, and opioids. Sometimes a medication interaction is the desired effect. Health care providers often combine medications to create an interaction that has a therapeutic effect. For example, a patient with hypertension may receive several medications such as diuretics and vasodilators, which act together to control the blood pressure when one medication alone is not effective.

Medication Dose Responses

A medication undergoes absorption, distribution, metabolism, and excretion after administration. Medications take time to enter the bloodstream, except when administered intravenously. When a medication is prescribed, the goal is a constant blood level within a safe therapeutic range. The minimum effective concentration (MEC) is the plasma level of the medication below which the effect of the medication does not occur. The toxic concentration is the level at which toxic effects occur. The safe therapeutic range is between the MEC and the toxic concentration (Fig. 20.2). When a medication is administered repeatedly, its serum level fluctuates

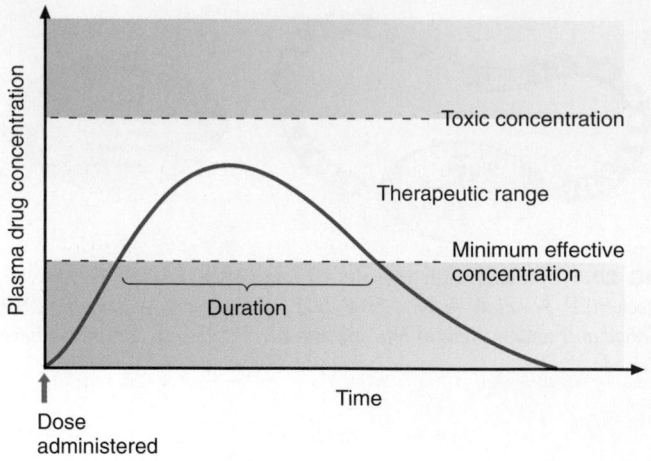

FIG 20.2 The therapeutic range of medication occurs between the minimum effective concentration and the toxic concentration. (*From Burchum, J., & Rosenthal, L. [2016]. Lehne's pharmacology for nursing care [9th ed.]. St. Louis: Saunders.*)

TABLE 20.4	
Routes of Medication Administration	
Route	**Description**
Nonparenteral	
Oral, buccal	By mouth/mucous membrane
Sublingual	Under the tongue
Topical	On the skin (as a cream or patch) and eyedrops/eardrops
Suppository	Into the rectum or vagina
Parenteral	
Intramuscular (IM)	Into a muscle
Subcutaneous (SUBCUT)	Into the subcutaneous tissue of the skin
Intradermal (ID)	Into the dermis of the skin
Epidural	Into the epidural space
Intravenous (IV)	Into a vein

between doses. The highest level is called the *peak concentration,* and the lowest level is called the *trough concentration.* After peaking, the serum concentration falls progressively. With intravenous (IV) infusions, the peak concentration occurs quickly, but the serum level also begins to fall immediately. Some medication doses (e.g., vancomycin or gentamicin) are based on peak and trough serum levels. A patient's trough level is drawn as a blood sample 30 minutes before administering the medication, and the peak level is drawn whenever the medication is expected to reach its peak concentration. The results of the blood test reveal if the medication is reaching its therapeutic blood level.

All medications have a biological half-life, which is the time it takes for excretion processes to lower the serum medication concentration by half. To maintain a therapeutic plateau, a patient needs to receive regular fixed doses. For example, pain medications are most effective for some cancer patients when they are given around the clock (ATC) rather than when a patient intermittently complains of pain, because the body maintains an almost constant level of pain medication (Burchum & Rosenthal, 2016). After an initial medication dose, the patient receives each successive dose when the previous dose reaches its half-life. The patient and nurse need to follow regular dosage schedules and administer prescribed doses at correct intervals. Know the following time intervals of medication action to anticipate the effect of a medication:

- *Onset of medication action:* Time it takes after a medication is administered for it to produce a response
- *Peak action:* Time it takes for a medication to reach its highest effective peak concentration
- *Trough:* Minimum blood serum concentration of medication reached just before the next scheduled dose
- *Duration of action:* Length of time during which a medication is present in a concentration great enough to produce a therapeutic effect
- *Plateau:* Blood serum concentration reached and maintained after repeated, fixed doses

Routes of Administration

The route prescribed for administering a medication (Table 20.4) depends on its properties and desired effect and on a patient's physical and mental condition. Because of what a nurse knows about each patient, the nurse needs to collaborate with a health care provider

in determining the best route for a patient's medical condition. Table 20.5 summarizes the factors that influence the choice of administration routes.

Medication Distribution

Health care providers (e.g., physicians, pharmacists, Registered nurses) write medication prescriptions, pharmacists dispense medications, and nurses verify and deliver medications to patients. *Verification* is the three-system check to ensure safe medication administration. The first check is the health care provider prescribing the right drug for the right purpose. The pharmacist is the second check to ensure that the medication is appropriate and prescribed correctly and then provided to the unit correctly. Finally, the nurse verifies the medication before administration with the three checks for accuracy to be sure that it is appropriate and prescribed correctly.

A number of technologies for medication distribution have the potential for reducing medication errors and ADEs. These technologies include computerized provider order entry (CPOE), automated dispensing system (ADS), and bar coding (Shah, Lo, Babich, et al., 2016).

Computerized Provider Order Entry

CPOE is a system that allows health care providers to enter orders (prescriptions) for medications electronically, eliminating the need for written prescriptions. CPOE increases the accuracy and legibility of medication orders, creates evidence-informed order sets, and strengthens nursing documentation and coordination of care (Lin, Chan, Mohindra, et al., 2017). Decision support software integrated into a CPOE system allows for automatic medication allergy checks, dosage indications, baseline laboratory result checks, and identification of potential medication interactions. When a health care provider enters a prescription through CPOE, the information immediately transmits to the pharmacy and ultimately to the patients' MAR without the need for written transcription.

Distribution Systems

Systems for storing and distributing medications vary. Facilities providing nursing care have special areas for stocking and dispensing medications. Special medication rooms, portable locked carts, computerized medication cabinets, and individual storage units next to patients' rooms are examples of storage areas used. Medication storage areas must be locked when unattended.

TABLE 20.5

Factors Influencing Choice of Administration Routes

Advantages	Disadvantages/Contraindications
Oral, Buccal, Sublingual Routes	
Routes are easy and comfortable to administer, convenient, economical; may produce local or systemic effects; and rarely cause anxiety for patient.	Routes are avoided when patient has alterations in GI function (e.g., nausea and vomiting), with reduced GI motility (after general anaesthesia or bowel inflammation), and with surgical resection of part of GI tract.
	Gastric secretions destroy some medications. Oral administration is contraindicated in patients who are NPO and unable to swallow (e.g., patients with neuromuscular disorders, esophageal strictures, and mouth lesions).
	Do not give oral medications when patient has gastric suction or before certain diagnostic tests or surgery.
	An unconscious or confused patient is unable or unwilling to swallow or hold sublingual medication under tongue or buccal medication in cheek.
	Oral medications sometimes irritate lining of GI tract, discolour teeth, or have an unpleasant taste.
Subcutaneous, Intramuscular, Intravenous, Intradermal, Epidural Routes	
Routes provide means of administration when oral medications are contraindicated. More rapid absorption occurs than with topical or oral routes.	There are risks for introducing infection, and medications are expensive. Some patients experience pain from repeated needle-sticks. Avoid subcutaneous, IM, and ID routes in patients with bleeding tendencies.
	There is risk for tissue damage with subcutaneous injections.
IV infusion provides medication delivery when patient is critically ill or long-term therapy is necessary. If peripheral perfusion is poor, IV route is preferred over injections.	IV and IM routes have higher absorption rates, thus placing patients at higher risk for reactions.
Epidural provides excellent pain control.	It limits mobility during administration, and there is risk for infection.
Skin	
Topical	
Topical skin applications provide primarily local effect. Route is usually painless. Limited side effects occur.	Extensive applications often require dressings that are bulky for a patient when manoeuvring.
	Do not apply to skin if abrasions are present, unless that is the reason for order.
	Medications can be absorbed by person applying them if gloves are not worn.
Transdermal	
Transdermal applications provide prolonged systemic effects with limited side effects.	Application leaves oily or pasty substance on skin and may soil clothing. Some patients have sensitivity to adhesive.
Mucous Membranes (Includes Eyes, Ears, Nose, Vaginal, Rectal, Buccal, and Sublingual Routes)	
Therapeutic effects are provided by local application to involved sites. Aqueous solutions are readily absorbed and capable of causing systemic effects.	Mucous membranes are highly sensitive to some medication concentrations.
	Insertion of rectal and vaginal medications often causes embarrassment.
Mucous membranes provide route of administration when oral medications are contraindicated.	Rectal suppositories are contraindicated if patients have had rectal surgery or if active rectal bleeding is present.
	If eardrum is ruptured, otic medications are usually contraindicated.
Inhalation	
Inhalation provides rapid relief for local respiratory problems. An inhaled form of insulin is also available. Route provides easy access for introduction of general anaesthetic gases.	Some local agents cause serious systemic effects.
	If patients are unable to administer inhaler correctly, medication is ineffective.
	Inhalation is difficult to learn for older persons and children.
Intraocular Disk	
Route is advantageous in that it does not require frequent administration (e.g., as for eyedrops). Patient can also wear disk when sleeping or swimming. Dry eyes do not affect medication delivery.	Local reactions such as tearing, itching, or redness of the eyes occur.
	Patient needs to know how to insert disk into and remove from eye.
	Medication is often expensive.
	Medication is contraindicated in patients with eye infections.

GI, Gastrointestinal; *ID,* intradermal; *IM,* intramuscular; *IV,* intravenous; *NPO,* nothing by mouth.

Unit Dose

A unit-dose system uses an ADS or cart containing a drawer with a 24-hour supply of medications for each patient. Each drawer has a label with the name of the patient and the designated room. The unit dose is the prescribed dose of medication that the patient receives at one time. Each medication form is wrapped in a foil or paper container separately. Liquid doses come in prepackaged foil or plastic cups (e.g., for use in long-term care or the home setting). The cart also contains limited amounts of stock medication for special situations. At a designated time each day, the pharmacist or a pharmacy technician refills the drawers in the cart with a fresh supply. Controlled substances are not in the individual patient drawer; they are in a larger locked drawer to keep them secure. A unit-dose system is designed to reduce the number of medication errors and saves steps in dispensing medications.

Automated Medication Dispensing System

ADSs are variations of unit-dose and floor stock systems (Fig. 20.3). The systems within the health care facility are networked with one another and with other computer systems in the facility (e.g., computerized medical record). ADSs control the dispensing of all medications, including opioid narcotics. Each nurse has a security code, which allows access to the system. If an employer uses a system that requires bioidentification, the nurse has to place their finger on a screen to access the computer. Once logged onto the ADS, the nurse selects a patient's name and medication profile. Then the nurse selects the medication, dosage, and route from a list displayed on the computer screen. The system opens the medication drawer or dispenses the medication to the nurse and records the event. If the system is connected to the patient's EMR, information about the medication (e.g., name, dose, time) and the name of the nurse who retrieved it from the ADS are recorded. There is evidence of an increase in reported medication errors with use of the system and a reduction in dispensing errors through the use of alerts that are embedded within the clinical decision support system (Shah et al., 2016).

The bar code medication administration (BCMA) system is often used to identify the patient, the medication, and the identification tag of the nurse administering the medication before recording this information in the patient's EMR. Facilities that implement ADS with BCMA often reduce the incidence of medication errors.

Special Handling of Controlled Substances

As a nurse you are responsible for following legal regulations when administering controlled substances (e.g., opioids). Violations of the *Controlled Drug and Substances Act* may result in fines, imprisonment, and loss of license. Facilities have policies for the proper storage and distribution of controlled substances (Box 20.1). Many facilities use computerized systems for medication access and distribution.

Bar Coding

EHR technology is used to improve patient care quality and coordination by providing health care providers easier access to patient information in a secure format. The use of electronic bar codes on medication labels and packaging has the potential to improve patient safety in a number of ways. Bar codes electronically link with a hospital computer system. A patient's MAR entered into the computer database and encoded in the patient's wristband is accessible to a nurse through a handheld device. The device scans the patient's wristband and then displays the MAR. When administering a medication, the nurse scans the bar code on the medication and the patient's medical record number on the wristband. The computer processes the scanned information, charts it, and updates the patient's MAR record appropriately. The use of bar codes improves accuracy of patient identification, provides alert to potential medication error, and improves medical record keeping.

Systems of Medication Measurement

NSO *Nursing Skills Online Safe Medication Preparation Module 5 / Lesson 3*

The proper administration of medication depends on the nurse's ability to compute medication doses accurately and measure medications correctly. A careless mistake in placing a decimal point or adding a zero to a dosage can lead to fatal errors. The health care provider and patient depend on nurses to check doses before administering medications. The most common medication measurement system is the metric system, although sometimes household systems of measurement (e.g., 1 cup, 1 teaspoon) are used.

Metric System

As a decimal system the metric system is the most logically organized of the measurement systems. Metric units are easy to convert and compute through simple multiplication and division. Each basic unit of measure is organized into units of 10. Multiplying or dividing

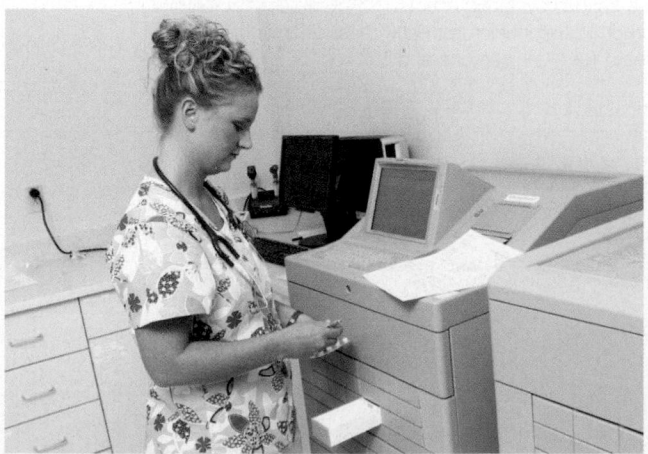

FIG 20.3 Automated medication dispensing system.

BOX 20.1

Guidelines for Safe Opioid Administration and Control

- All controlled drugs and substances are stored in a securely locked, substantially constructed cabinet (i.e., ADS) or a locked room.
- Authorized nurses carry a set of keys or an individual computer entry code for the ADS.
- An inventory record is used each time a controlled substance is dispensed. Records are often kept electronically and provide an accurate ongoing account of the medications used, wasted, and remaining. If you find a discrepancy, correct and report it immediately.
- Use a special inventory record to document a patient's name, date, name of medication, dose, time of medication administration, and signature of nurse dispensing the medication.
- A second nurse witnesses disposal of the unused part if a nurse gives only part of a dose of a controlled substance. Computerized systems record the nurses' names electronically. If paper records are kept, both nurses sign their names on the form. Follow employer policy for appropriate waste of opioids. Do not place wasted part of medications in sharps containers.

ADS, Automated dispensing system.

by 10 forms secondary units. In multiplication the decimal point moves to the right; in division the decimal moves to the left. For example:

$$10 \text{ mg} \times 10 = 100 \text{ mg}$$
$$10 \text{ mg} \div 10 = 1 \text{ mg}$$

The basic units of measure in the metric system are the metre (length), the litre (volume), and the gram (weight). For medication calculations you will primarily use volume and weight units. In the metric system lowercase or capital letters designate the basic units and subdivisions of units:

Gram = g or Gm
Litre = l or L
Milligram = mg
Millilitre = mL
Microgram = mcg (do NOT use μg [ISMP, 2018a])

When writing medication dosages in metric units, health care providers and nurses use either fractions or multiples of a unit. Convert fractions to decimals:

500 mg or 0.5 g, not ½ g

10 mL or 0.01 L, not 1/100 L

Many actual or potential medication errors happen with the use of fractions or decimal points. Use practice standards when medications are prescribed in fractions to prevent errors. For example, never use a trailing zero (e.g., 1.0 mg) and always include a zero before a decimal point (e.g., 0.1 mL) (ISMP, 2018a).

Household Measurement

Household measures are familiar to most people, but these are no longer recommended for medication administration because of the variability in the size of household utensils. Household measures include drops, teaspoons, tablespoons, and cups for volume and ounces and pounds for weight. A transition period may be necessary during which the household measure can be listed in parentheses immediately following the metric measure (e.g., 5 mL [one teaspoon]). To calculate medications accurately, you need to know common equivalents of metric and household units (Table 20.6).

Solutions

Solutions of various concentrations are used for injections, irrigations, and infusions. A solution is a given mass of solid substance dissolved in a known volume of fluid or a given volume of liquid dissolved in a known volume of another fluid. Solutions are available in units of mass per units of volume (e.g., g/mL or g/L). The concentration of a solution can also be expressed as a percentage. A 10% solution is 10 g of solid dissolved in 100 mL of solution. A proportion also expresses concentrations. A 1/1000 solution represents a solution containing 1 g of solid in 1000 mL of liquid or 1 mL of liquid mixed with 1000 mL of another liquid.

PERSON-CENTRED CARE

- A nurse's responsibility when administering medications safely must include interprofessional collaboration and effective communication with health care team members and caregivers.

TABLE 20.6

Equivalents of Measurement

Metric	Household
1 mL	15 drops (gtt)
5 mL	1 teaspoon (tsp)
15 mL	1 tablespoon (tbsp)
30 mL	1 fluid ounce
240 mL	1 cup (c)
480 mL (approximately 500 mL)	1 pint (pt)
960 mL (approximately 1 L)	1 quart (qt)
3840 mL (approximately 4 L)	1 gallon (gal)

- Patients are an important resource for understanding the knowledge they have about their medications, their perceptions about the effects of medications, and their expectations for treatment.
- Consider factors that influence patient's abilities to communicate effectively, such as anxiety, pain, hearing, or their cultural background. Person-centred therapeutic communication is essential to nursing practice and critical in safe medication administration.
- A new scientific field, *pharmacogenetics*, involves the study of the genetic influence on medication response that occurs from inherited metabolic defects or deficiencies. The most common mechanism of genetic influence on medications is the alteration in medication metabolism. The outcome is either a reduced benefit or increased toxicity of the medication (Burchum & Rosenthal, 2016). As a nurse you cannot detect a genetic abnormality. However, you can learn to become aware of cultural differences in medication responses to better monitor medication therapy.
- Culturally a patient's values and beliefs affect medication response.
- A patient's level of education, prior experience with medication therapy, and the caregiver's influence on actions significantly influence medication adherence. For example, in some cultures it is not acceptable to complain about gastrointestinal problems; thus it is common for patients not to report nausea, vomiting, and bowel changes related to medication use.
- Use of herbal and homeopathic remedies in some cultures alters response to a medication.
- Ethnicity needs to be considered when medications are prescribed and administered.

Safe Medication Administration

Standards are actions that help ensure safe nursing practice. Standards for medication administration are set by health care facilities, the nursing profession, and other organizations (Box 20.2). Most facilities have procedure manuals that contain policies about which medications nurses can and cannot deliver. The types and dosages that nurses may administer often vary from unit to unit within a facility. Provincial/territorial professional nursing association standards apply to the activity of safe medication administration. As a nurse, to prevent medication errors, ensure effective interprofessional collaboration and follow the rules of medication administration (which range in the literature from the 5 to 10 rights [Rohde & Domm, 2017]) consistently every time you administer medications. Many medication errors are linked in some way to an inconsistency in adhering to the 10 rights:

1. Right patient
2. Right dose

BOX 20.2

Safe Medication Practices

- Accurate patient (client) identification using at least two person-specific identifiers (two patient identifiers) (neither can be patient's room number) when providing care, treatment (e.g., medications), or services.
- Improve the effectiveness of communication among caregivers (e.g., use of SBAR).
- Verbal or telephone prescriptions require a verification "repeat-back" of the complete order or test result by the person receiving the prescription/test result.
- Standardize a "Do-Not-Use" list of abbreviations, acronyms, symbols, and dose designations.
- Improve the safety of using medications.
- Identify and at a minimum annually review a list of look-alike/sound-alike medications used by the organization.
- Before a procedure, label all medications and medication containers (e.g., syringes) that are not labelled. Do this in areas where medicines and supplies are set up, such as on and off the sterile field in perioperative and other procedural settings. Labels include medication name, strength, amount, expiration date when not used within 24 hours, and expiration time when expiration occurs in less than 24 hours.
- Take extra care with patients who take anticoagulants. Use only oral unit-dose products and premixed infusions. When heparin is administered intravenously and continuously, use programmable infusion pumps.
- Maintain and communicate accurate patient medication information.
- Accurately and completely reconcile medications across the continuum of care.
- There is a process for comparing the patient's current medications with those prescribed for the patient while under the care of the health care facility.
- Communicate a complete list of the patient's medications to the next provider of service when a patient is referred or transferred to another setting, service, or level of care. Also provide the complete list to the patient on discharge from the facility.
- Practise person-centred care and encourage patients' active involvement in their own care.

Modified from Accreditation Canada. (2017). *Medication management standards*. Retrieved from https://store.accreditation.ca/products/medication-management-standards and Institute for Safe Medication Practices (ISMP). (2017). *2018–2019 targeted medication safety best practices for hospitals*. Retrieved from http://www.ismp.org/tools/bestpractices/TMSBP-for-Hospitals.pdf)

3. Right medication
4. Right route
5. Right time
6. Right education
7. Right to refuse
8. Right assessment
9. Right evaluation
10. Right documentation

Right Medication

At the time of admission, when transferring to a different unit, and when discharging patients from a hospital, the nurse needs to assess their medication regimen, especially if they were admitted to the hospital because of a problem with medication self-administration. A strategy to reduce medication errors at transition points is the process of medication reconciliation. Medication reconciliation is a three-step process: the health care team (1) works with the patient and/or caregiver to generate a best possible medication history (BPMH), (2) identifies and resolves medication discrepancies, and

BOX 20.3

Guidelines for Verbal, Telephone, Text, and Email Prescriptions

- Only employer-authorized staff receive and record prescriptions that are not written.
- Clearly identify patient's name, room number, and diagnosis.
- Although increasing numbers of health care providers are using mobile devices to communicate prescriptions, this type of communication is discouraged, given the risk of violation of confidential health information and incomplete communication of patient status (CRNNS, 2017). Always refer to your employer's policy related to prescriptions received via a mobile device.
- Telephone orders for chemotherapy are not accepted unless they address holding or discontinuing the medication.
- **Repeat back** all verbal and telephone prescriptions to health care provider.
- Use clarification questions to avoid misunderstandings.
- Document either "verbal order" or "telephone order," including date and time, name of patient, and complete prescription; write the name of the health care provider and sign your name.
- Follow employer policies; some require documentation of the "repeat-back" or two nurses to review and sign telephone or verbal prescriptions.
- Health care provider co-signs the prescription within the time frame required by the facility (usually 24 hours; verify employer policy).

(3) communicates a complete and accurate list of medications (Accreditation Canada, 2017). Patients often leave the hospital with a basic knowledge of their medications but are unable to safely self-administer them once they return home. When patients enter a health care facility, it is critical for health care providers to have an accurate list of the medications patients are currently prescribed to take and any over-the-counter (OTC) medications being used.

A medication prescription is required for every medication that the nurse administers to a patient. Some health care providers write prescriptions by hand in a patient's chart. However, many agencies use CPOE, eliminating the need for handwritten prescriptions and enhancing patient safety (Lin et al., 2017). Regardless of how a prescription is received, the nurse needs to compare the health care provider's orders with the MAR or electronic MAR (eMAR) when the medication is prescribed initially. Nurses verify medication information whenever new MARs are written or distributed or when patients transfer from one nursing unit or health care setting to another (Accreditation Canada, 2017).

ISMP (2018a) published a list of *Dangerous Abbreviations, Symbols, and Dose Designations* to increase patient safety (see Box 4.2). Nurses are responsible for using correct abbreviations and verifying that the prescription was transcribed accurately.

Medication Prescriptions (Orders). Nurses must have a medication prescription before administering medications to a patient. Verbal and telephone prescriptions may occur when written or electronic communication between the health care provider and nurse is not possible. When nurses receive a verbal or telephone prescription, they write or enter the information on the health care provider's prescription sheet. The nurse then repeats back the prescription for verification and documents that the repeat-back occurred. The name of the health care provider and the nurse's signature are included. The health care provider will countersign the order at a later time, usually within 24 hours after making it (see employer policy). Box 20.3 provides guidelines for safely taking verbal or telephone prescriptions for medications.

Common types of medication prescriptions based on frequency and/or urgency of medication administration include prn and single

(one-time) prescriptions, which include stat and now prescriptions. Each prescription needs to include the patient's name, date prescribed, medication name, strength and dosage, route, dose frequency, and time(s) of administration. Standing prescriptions and prescriptions to resume previous medications are no longer supported as best practice (Accreditation Canada, 2017) and have been replaced with preprinted or electronic order sets and protocols (College and Association of Registered Nurses of Alberta [CARNA], 2015/2018). Order sets provide the prescriber with a choice of medications or treatments that apply to a specific patient population. The ISMP has established guidelines for the development of standardized order sets. A protocol guides clinical decision making related to prescriptions or interventions for specific health care issues.

A medication can be prescribed to be given only when a patient requires or requests it (i.e., prn). The nurse must assess a patient thoroughly to determine whether they need the medication. A prn prescription usually has a minimum interval set for the time of administration.

Single (one-time) prescriptions are common for preoperative medications or medications given before diagnostic procedures. The medication is prescribed to be given only once at a specified time. A stat prescription means that a single dose of medication is given immediately and only once. Stat prescriptions are used for emergencies when a patient's condition changes suddenly. A now prescription is more specific than a one-time prescription and is used when a patient needs a medication quickly but not as soon as a stat prescription. When nurses receive a now prescription, they have up to 90 minutes to give the medication (see employer policy). Range prescriptions are used when a patient's need for medication varies but there continue to be concerns about providing enough guidance to nurses while still allowing them to address the individual needs of a patient (Accreditation Canada, 2017). An example of a poorly written range prescription is "give morphine sulphate 2 to 6 mg IV push every 2 to 4 hours prn for pain." This prescription is not specific with regard to guidelines needed to give a correct dose. A range prescription must provide objective measures for nurses to use to determine the correct dose. An example of a clearly written range prescription is "give acetaminophen 325 mg–650 mg every 4 hours prn pain. For pain rated as 1–5, 325 mg; for pain rated as 5–10, 650 mg." A range prescription should include specific indications (e.g., pain-rating score, temperature level). Once a dosage is chosen and administered with a range order, the nurse cannot use any portion of the remainder of the range dose within that same time frame (CARNA, 2015/2018).

As a nurse, once you determine that information on the patient's MAR is accurate, use the MAR to prepare and administer medications. When preparing medications from bottles or containers, *compare the label of the medication container with the MAR three times:* (1) before removing the container from the supply drawer or shelf, (2) as the amount of medication prescribed is removed from the container, and (3) at the patient's bedside before administering the medication to the patient. Always prepare medications from clearly labelled containers (Accreditation Canada, 2017). With unit-dose prepackaged medications, check the label with the MAR when taking medications out of the medication-dispensing system. Finally, verify all medications at the patient's bedside with the patient's MAR and use at least two person-specific identifiers before giving the patient any medications (Accreditation Canada, 2019).

If a patient questions a medication, stop and recheck to be certain that there is no mistake. An alert patient or caregiver will know whether a medication is different from those received before. In most cases the medication prescription has been changed, or the medication is manufactured by a different company than the patient has been using at home. However, attention to a patient's question is how errors are identified and prevented.

Right Dose

The unit-dose system is designed to minimize errors. When a medication is prepared from a larger volume or strength than needed or when the health care provider prescribes a system of measurement different from that which the pharmacist supplies, the chance of error increases. After calculating the doses of high-risk medications such as insulin or warfarin, the nurse needs to compare the calculation with one done independently by a second nurse. This is especially important if it is an unusual calculation or involves a potentially toxic medication.

After calculating doses, prepare medications accurately. Use syringes and sealed droppers when it is necessary to measure medications accurately. For example, ISMP (2017) recommends the use of an oral syringe that measures in millilitres (mL). If an oral solution is available only in a bulk size (such as a bottle) or if the patient-specific dose is less than the unit dose amount (e.g., dose is 3 mL when the unit dose product is 5 mL), the pharmacy should prepare the patient-specific dose in an oral syringe (or cup) and dispense it to the unit (ISMP, 2017). Nurses are no longer encouraged to pour medications into graduated cups, because of the risk of medication errors. When preparing medication in an oral syringe, draw up the medication slowly to prevent air bubbles from entering the syringe. Air displaces the medication and leads to inaccurate doses. For the home, the ISMP is now recommending that the patient or caregiver be provided an oral syringe or dosing cup that accurately measures the medication.

Medication errors can occur when pills need to be split. Studies show that the accuracy of split tablets is questionable, even if a tablet is scored (ISMP, 2006). In addition, in the home setting patients may assume that tablets in containers have already been split when they have not, or split them again when they have been split already (ISMP, 2006).

To promote patient safety in some inpatient settings, pharmacists split medications, label and package them, and return them to the nurse for administration. Because pill splitting can be problematic in the home, it is important to determine if a patient has the manual dexterity or visual acuity to split tablets. If possible, determine if their pharmacy can split the pill or encourage the health care provider to order medications that do not require splitting.

Tablets are sometimes crushed and mixed with food. Be sure to clean the crushing device completely before crushing the tablet. Remnants of previously crushed medications increase concentration of the medication or result in a patient receiving part of an unprescribed medication. Mix crushed medications with very small amounts of food or liquid. Do not use a patient's favorite foods or liquids because medications alter their taste and decrease the patient's desire for them. This is especially a concern for pediatric patients. *Always check to determine whether a medication can be crushed* (see Chapter 21). Some medications (e.g., enteric-coated or slow-release) have special coatings to prevent them from being absorbed too quickly. These medications should not be crushed. Refer to the "Do Not Crush List" (ISMP, 2018d) to ensure that a medication is safe to crush.

Right Patient

Medication errors often occur because one patient gets a medication intended for another patient. Therefore, a key step in administering medications safely is being sure to give the right medication to the right patient. It is difficult to remember every patient's name and face. Before giving a medication to a patient, always use at least

two person-specific identifiers (Accreditation Canada, 2019). Acceptable patient identifiers include the patient's name, an identification number assigned by a health care facility such as the medical record number, or date of birth. Do not use a patient's room number as an identifier. The required identification process mandates collecting patient identifiers reliably when a patient is first admitted to a health care facility. Once identifiers are assigned to a patient (e.g., putting identifiers on an armband and placing the armband on the patient), a nurse uses them to match the patient with the patient name on the MAR.

To identify a patient correctly in an acute care setting, at the patient's bedside compare the patient identifiers on the MAR with those on their identification bracelet (Fig. 20.4). Asking patients to state their full name and identification information provides a third way to verify that you as the nurse are giving medications to the right patient. If an identification bracelet becomes smudged or illegible or is missing, get a new one for the patient. In health care settings where patients do not have an identification bracelet (e.g., long-term care facility), nurses must adhere to best medication practice and use a system to verify the patient's identification with at least two person-specific identifiers, such as resident picture, before administering medications.

In addition to using two person-specific patient identifiers, some facilities use a wireless bar-code scanner to help identify the right patient (Fig. 20.5). This system requires the nurse to scan a personal bar code that is commonly placed on the nurse's name badge first. Then a bar code is scanned from the single-dose medication package. Finally, the nurse scans the patient's armband. All of this information is stored in the computer for documentation purposes. The system helps prevent medication errors because it provides another step to ensure that the right patient receives the right medication.

Right Route

The health care provider's prescription must designate a route of administration. If the route of administration is missing or if the specified route is not the recommended route, consult the health care provider immediately. Recent evidence shows that medication errors involving the wrong route are common. For example, enteral and parenteral medications may become confused in the pediatric setting where liquid medications are frequently given orally. When oral medications are prepared in parenteral syringes, there is an increased risk of giving an oral medication through the parenteral route (ISMP, 2017). The injection of a liquid intended for oral use produces local complications such as sterile abscess or fatal systemic effects. Medication companies label parenteral medications "for injectable use only." Label the syringe after preparing a medication, include the location if appropriate (e.g., right eye), and always use different syringes for enteral and parenteral medication administration (ISMP, 2017).

Right Time

Safe medication administration involves adherence to prescribed doses and dosage schedules. Some facilities set schedules for medication administration. However, nurses are able to alter this schedule based on knowledge about a medication. For example, at some facilities medications that are taken once a day are given at 9:00 AM. However, if a medication works best when given at bedtime, the nurse administers it before the patient goes to sleep. In addition, acute care agencies use guidelines from the ISMP and Accreditation Canada (2017) to determine safe, effective, and timely administration of scheduled medications. Facilities need clear policies to determine which medications are not eligible for scheduled dosing times and must be given at precise times (e.g., stat doses, first-time or loading doses, one-time doses). Time-sensitive medications require standardized administration schedules (Accreditation Canada, 2017). With time-sensitive medications (e.g., antibiotics, anticoagulants, insulin), early or delayed administration of maintenance doses of more than 30 minutes before or after the scheduled dose will most likely cause harm or result in subtherapeutic responses in a patient. Non–time-sensitive medications include medications in which the timing of administration most likely will not affect the desired effect of the medication if the medication is given 1 to 2 hours before or after its scheduled time. Thus, nurses need to administer time-sensitive–scheduled medications at a precise time or within

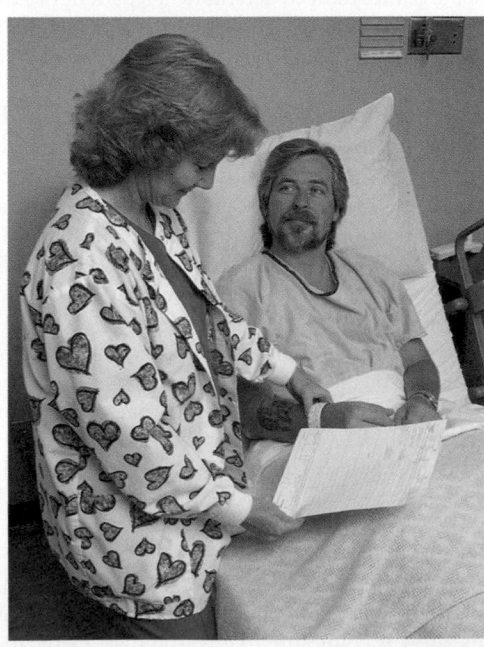

FIG 20.4 Before administering any medications, check patient's identification and allergy bracelets.

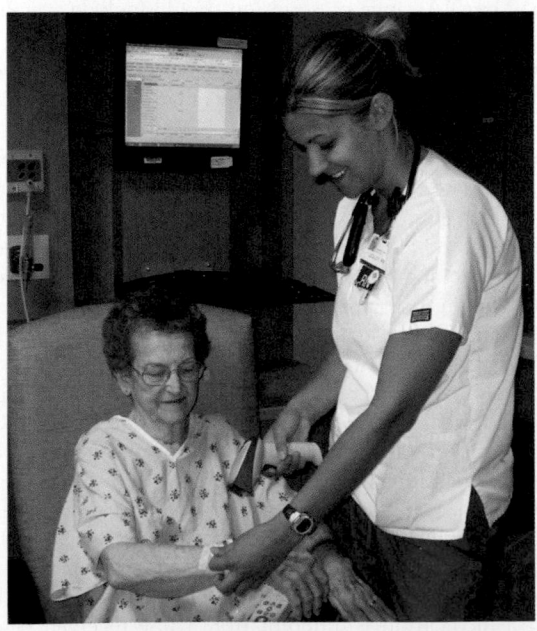

FIG 20.5 Nurse using bar-code scanner to identify patient during medication administration.

30 minutes before or after the scheduled time. Medications identified as non–time-sensitive are administered within 1 to 2 hours of their scheduled time. Nurses must know their employer's policies about the timing of medications to ensure that they administer medications at the right time (ISMP, 2011).

Nurses must also know why a medication is prescribed for a certain time of the day and whether they are able to alter the time schedule. For example, two medications are prescribed, one q8h (every 8 hours) and the other 3 times per day. Both medications are scheduled 3 times a day over 24 hours. The health care provider intends for the nurse to give the q8h medication as time-sensitive to maintain its therapeutic blood levels. In contrast, the nurse needs to give the other medication during the waking hours. Each facility has a recommended time schedule for medications prescribed at frequent intervals.

Nurses need to give priority to medications that must act at certain times. For example, give insulin at a precise interval before a meal. Give antibiotics on time to maintain therapeutic blood levels. Some medications require the nurse's clinical judgement to determine the proper time for administration. Administer a prn sleeping medication when the patient is ready for bed. Always document whenever there is a call to the patient's health care provider to obtain a change in a medication prescription.

When preparing patients for discharge, help them plan schedules based on preferred medication intervals, pharmacokinetics of the medication, and the patient's daily schedule. For patients who have difficulty remembering when to take medications, make a chart that lists the times when they should take each medication or prepare a special container to hold each timed dose.

Right Documentation

Accurate documentation allows nurses and other health care providers to communicate with one another and improves medication safety. Many medication errors result from inaccurate documentation. Therefore, always document accurately at the time of administration and verify any inaccurate documentation before administering medications. To ensure the right documentation, first make sure that the information on the patient's MAR corresponds exactly with the health care provider's prescription and the label on the medication container. Written prescriptions and medication forms must include the patient's name; the name of the prescribed medication; and the medication dosage, route, and frequency. If there is any question about a medication prescription because it is incomplete, illegible, vague, or not understood, contact the health care provider before administering the medication. Nurses have a duty to question a medication prescription that is unclear or unusual (Canadian Nurses Protective Society [CNPS], 2007).

Nurses should never document that they have administered a medication until they have actually given it. They need to document the name of the medication, the dose, the time of administration, and the route on the patient's MAR as soon as it is administered.

Also document the site of any injections and the patient's response to medications. Document the response to medications, such as therapeutic or if ADEs or side effects occur. For example, if pain medication is administered, as the nurse you must reassess and document if the medication was effective in controlling pain. Your efforts to ensure proper documentation help provide safe care.

Right Education

Prior to administering a medication, it is important for the nurse to inform the patient of what the medication is, its desired effects, and any patient side effects. The nurse should also ask the patient if they have any known allergies.

Right to Refuse

A patient (or legal guardian) has the right to refuse any medication. The nurse should inform the patient or guardian of the consequences of not receiving the prescribed medication. The nurse needs to verify that the information is understood using teach-back techniques, and develop a revised teaching plan if the patient (or guardian) is not able to correctly identify the consequences of not taking the medication. The nurse must notify the health care provider that the prescribed medication has been refused, and document the refusal of the medication, the teaching that was completed related to the consequences of not taking the medication, and that the health care provider has been notified.

Right Assessment

Prior to administering a medication, the nurse should properly assess the patient to determine that the medication is safe and appropriate. For example, when administering toloxin, the nurse needs to assess the patient's pulse; if the pulse is below 60 beats/min (50 beats/min in some facilities—always check employer policy), the nurse must withhold the dose. If a medication is unsafe or inappropriate to administer, the nurse is to notify the health care provider who prescribed the medication. The nurse documents that the medication was not administered, the reason why it was not administered, and that the health care provider was notified.

Right Evaluation

After the medication has been administered, the nurse should assess the patient for any side effects or ADEs, as well as for effectiveness of the medication. For example, when medicating a patient for pain, it is important for the nurse to reassess the patients' pain 30–45 minutes after administering the medication. The nurse should compare the patient's premedication status with postmedication status and document the patient's response to the medication.

Medication Preparation

It is legally advisable to administer only the medications that you as the nurse prepare. Administering a medication prepared by another health care provider increases the opportunity for errors. You must perform several steps before actual administration of medications, including interpreting medication labels, converting measurement units within a system or between systems, and calculating medication doses. The importance of checking similar names and verifying the correct medication cannot be overemphasized.

Interpreting Medication Labels

Medication labels include several basic pieces of information: the trade name of the medication in large letters, the generic name in smaller letters, the form of the medication, the dosage, the expiration date, the lot number, and the name of the manufacturer (Fig. 20.6). The trade name given by the manufacturer often suggests the action of the medication, and the generic name is the chemical name.

Clinical Calculation

To administer medications safely, nurses use their mathematics skills to safely calculate dosages and mix solutions. This skill is important because medications are not always dispensed in the unit of measure in which they are prescribed. Medication companies package and bottle medications in standard dosages. For example, a patient's health care provider prescribes 20 mg of a medication that is packaged in 40-mg vials. The nurse is responsible for converting available units of volume and weight to the desired doses. Therefore, the nurse needs to be aware of approximate equivalents in all major measurement systems and make use of conversion tables. In addition

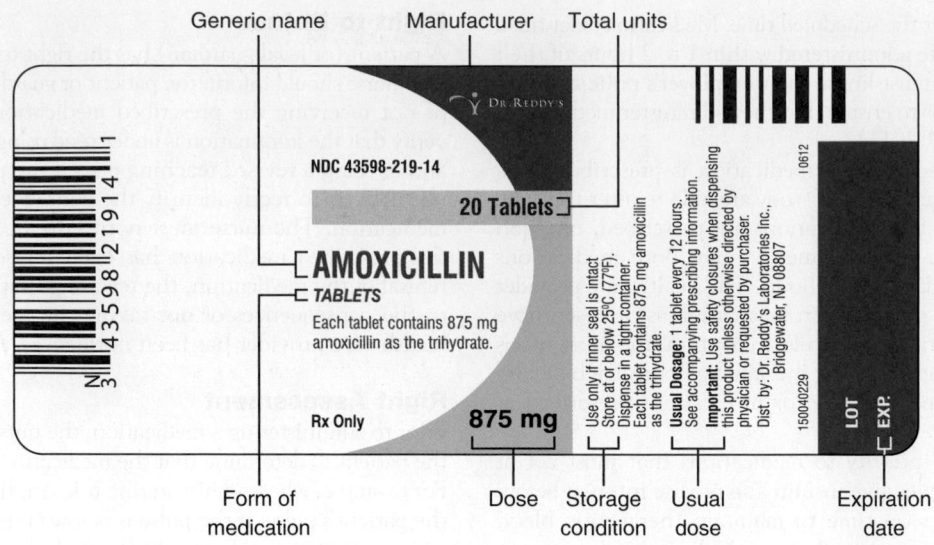

Generic name Manufacturer Total units

Form of medication Dose Storage condition Usual dose Expiration date

FIG 20.6 Interpreting medication label. (*Courtesy Dr. Reddy's Laboratories, Inc.*)

BOX 20.4

Formula Method

$$\frac{D}{H} = V = \text{Amount to give}$$

D is the desired dose or the dose prescribed (e.g., 250 mg of penicillin PO 4 times daily).

H is the medication dose on hand or available for use. The dose is on the medication label (e.g., penicillin tablets 250 mg each).

V is the volume (liquid) or vehicle (number of tablets, capsules) that delivers the available dose.

NOTE: The desired dose (D) and the on-hand dose (H) must be in the same unit of measurement. If they are in different units, you must convert them before completing the formula.

BOX 20.5

Dimensional Analysis

Use the following steps to solve medication problems using dimensional analysis:

1. Identify the unit of measure that you need to administer. For example, if you are giving a pill, you will usually be giving a tablet or a capsule; for parenteral or oral medications, the unit is millilitre.
2. Estimate the answer in your mind.
3. Place the name or appropriate abbreviation for *x* on the left side of the equation (e.g., *x* tab, *x* mL).
4. Place available information from the problem in a fraction format on the right side of the equation. Place the abbreviation or unit that matches what you are going to administer (determined in Step 1) in the numerator.
5. Look at the medication prescription and add other factors into the problem. Set up the numerator so it matches the unit in the previous denominator.
6. Cancel out like units of measurement on the right side of the equation. You should end up with only one unit left in the equation, and it should match the unit on the left side of the equation.
7. Reduce to the lowest terms if possible and solve the problem or solve for *x*. Label your answer.
8. Compare your estimate from Step 2 with your answer in Step 7.

---

to medication administration, nurses use volume and weight conversions in a variety of other nursing activities, including converting fluid ounces to millilitres to measure intake and output (I&O) or converting volume equivalents to calculate IV flow rates.

Conversions Within One System. Converting measurements within one system is relatively easy; simply divide or multiply in the metric system. For example, to change milligrams to grams, divide by 1000 or move the decimal three points to the left.

$$1000 \text{ mg} = 1 \text{ g}$$

$$350 \text{ mg} = 0.35 \text{ g}$$

To convert litres to millilitres, multiply by 1000 or move the decimal three points to the right.

$$1 \text{ L} = 1000 \text{ mL}$$

$$0.25 \text{ L} = 250 \text{ mL}$$

Dosage Calculations. Dosage calculations are necessary when the dose on the medication label differs from the dose prescribed. There are several dose-calculation methods, including formula (Box 20.4), dimensional analysis (Box 20.5), and ratio and proportion

(Box 20.6). The most common methods are ratio-proportion or use of a formula.

The Formula Method. Dose prescribed: Gentamicin 50 mg IM

Medication available: 100 mg in 1 mL

Step 1.

$$\frac{\text{Dose prescribed}}{\text{Dose on hand}} \times \text{Amount on hand} = \text{Amount to administer}$$

Step 2. Calculate your answer:

$$\frac{50 \text{ mg}}{100 \text{ mg}} \times 1 \text{ mL} \times = 0.5 \text{ mL}$$

Dimensional Analysis Method. This method is used when the dose prescribed has the same label as the dose available.

The Ratio-and-Proportion Method

1. The numbers in a ratio are separated by a colon (:).
2. A proportion is an equation that has two ratios of equal value.
3. The first and last numbers are called the *extremes*. The second and third numbers are called the *means*.
4. Write a proportion in one of three ways:
   a. 1 : 2 = 5 : 10
   b. 1 : 2 :: 5 : 10
   c. $\frac{1}{2} = \frac{5}{10}$
5. Make sure that all the terms are in the same unit or system of measurement.
6. Label all the terms in the proportion.
7. Place the ratio you know (e.g., information on the medication label) first.
8. Put the terms of the ratio in the same sequence (e.g., mg : mL = mg : mL).
9. Cross-multiply the means and the extremes and then divide both sides by the number for the *x* to obtain the dosage.
10. Always label the answer.

Dose prescribed: Salazopyrin po 0.5 g

Tablets available: 0.25 g per tablet

Step 1. The starting factor is 0.5 g.

The answer label is tablets (i.e., how many tablets should be given?)

Step 2. Formulate the conversion equation:

The equivalent needed is 1 tablet = 0.25 g.

$$\frac{0.5\,g}{1} \times \frac{1\,tab}{0.25\,g} = tabs$$

Cancel labels (g). **NOTE:** If properly written, all labels except the answer label will cancel.

Step 3. Solve the equation. Reduce the numerical values and multiply the numerators and denominators.

Ratio-and-Proportion Method. A ratio indicates the relationship between two numbers.

Dose prescribed: Phenytoin solution 100 mg po

Medication available: 125 mg/5 mL

Step 1. Set up the proportion:

$$\frac{125\,mg}{5} \times \frac{100\,mg}{x\,mL}$$

Step 2. Cross-multiply the equation:

$$125x = 100 \times 5$$
$$125x = 500$$

Step 3. Divide both sides by the number before *x*:

$$\frac{125x}{125} = \frac{500}{125}$$
$$x = \frac{500}{125}$$
$$x = 4\,mL$$

Pediatric Doses. Calculating children's medication doses requires caution (Hockenberry & Wilson, 2015). Evidence shows that children are at risk for experiencing an ADE as a result of their metabolic rate (Burchum & Rosenthal, 2016). Factors contributing to errors include workload, distractions, and lack of knowledge (Gann, 2015). The child's age, weight, and maturity of body systems all affect the ability to metabolize and excrete medication. Other

Safe Medication Administration in Older Persons

- Consult with the health care provider to keep the medication plan as simple as possible (Burchum & Rosenthal, 2016).
- Keep instructions clear and simple and provide written materials in large print (Burchum & Rosenthal, 2016).
- Teach the complications and interactions of all over-the counter medications (Accreditation Canada, 2017).
- Teach the older person to set up a daily or weekly schedule for medications using memory aids such as a calendar (Verloo, Chiolero, Kiszio, et al., 2017). Have a caregiver help with medication administration, as needed.
- Reduce the chance of errors by colour coding or labelling medication bottles (Verloo et al., 2017).
- Include patient's support person or caregiver in any type of instruction.
- Evaluate teaching by having patient teach back instructions.

factors that influence medication dosages in children include the difficulty in evaluating the desired effect and the hydration status of the child. In most cases the health care provider will calculate the dose for a child before prescribing the medication. However, it is the nurse's responsibility to be aware of the safe dosage range for any medication administered, and the nurse should recheck and/ or recalculate to confirm the correct dose. Different formulas and methods are used to calculate medication doses in children. The two most common methods of calculating pediatric dosages are based on the child's weight or body surface area (BSA). Refer to a pediatric pharmacology resource, a pharmacist, or the health care provider if you have to calculate a medication based on BSA. Most of the time you calculate medications based on the child's weight.

Older Person Dosages. Older persons also require special consideration during medication administration (Box 20.7). The changes of aging alter pharmacokinetics. In addition to physiological changes of aging, behavioural and social and economic issues influence the older person's use of medications.

A common problem for older persons is polypharmacy. There is no consensus definition for polypharmacy, although the common definitions include five or more concurrent medications or the mixing of nutritional or herbal supplements with medications (Burchum & Rosenthal, 2016). Older persons experience polypharmacy when they seek relief from a variety of symptoms (e.g., constipation, insomnia, pain) and see multiple health care providers. When determining polypharmacy, nurses must review all older persons' prescribed medications and all other supplements and OTC medications. Polypharmacy increases the risk for patient safety incidents and interactions with other medications.

The entire health care team shares the responsibility of reducing or eliminating the risk factors associated with medication regimens that older persons receive. Safety precautions include assessing a patient's health status, current medication regimen (including OTC medications and herbal products), the reason for existing and proposed medications, and any environmental factors that influence accurate and safe medication administration by the patient and caregiver(s). Refer to ISMP Canada's Beers List (https:// www.ismp-canada.org/beers_list/#l=qone) for a list of potentially inappropriate medications for older persons.

EVIDENCE-INFORMED PRACTICE

Many medication errors occur when nurses become distracted or lose focus during medication administration or fail to follow

best-practice protocols and procedures related to medication administration (Accreditation Canada, 2017). Research reveals that $397 million is spent every year in Canada as a result of preventable adverse events (CPSI, n.d.). Nurses become interrupted while accessing dispensing systems, depositing medications into delivery containers, and confirming prescriptions on computer screens. The majority of distractions have been identified as a result of interruptions by patients, family and friends of the patient, or other interprofessional team members (Yoder, Schadewald, & Dietrich, 2015). Nurses need systems in place to avoid distractions to help prevent medication errors, including:

- Wearing a medication safety vest, sash, or red apron
- Using visible medication preparation signs
- Medication administration checklists
- Staff and patient education
- Establishing no-interruption zones (NIZs) defined by a red tape outline around the medication ADS

NURSING PROCESS

Application of the nursing process ensures that critical thinking and clinical judgement are integrated into a patient's care. As a nurse your role extends beyond simply giving medications to a patient. You are also responsible for understanding why your patient is receiving the medication; monitoring patients' responses to medications; providing education to patients and caregivers; and informing health care providers when medications are effective, ineffective, or no longer necessary.

Assessment

As a nurse, before administering medications, perform a physical assessment, which will reveal physical findings for any indications or contraindications for medication therapy (e.g., inability to swallow because of mucositis). Be sure to also assess the patient's sensory, motor, and cognitive functions to determine if the patient can prepare and administer medications at home. Continue your assessment by determining if the patient has a history of medication allergies. When assessing for medication allergies, you must differentiate between actual allergic reactions, which can be life threatening, and medication sensitivities, which are uncomfortable side effects. In an acute care setting, patients with allergies wear identification bands that list each medication allergy. All allergies and types of reactions are noted on the patient's admission notes, medication records, and history and physical examination. *Never give a patient a medication when there is a known allergy.*

Your assessment also involves identifying medications that a patient takes every day at home, including prescriptions, OTC preparations, and herbal supplements. Determine how long the patient has taken each medication, current dosage schedule, and whether they have had any adverse effects to any of the medications. The patient should know the name, purpose, dosage, route, and side effects of medications and supplements that are being taken. Often patients take many medications and carry a list that includes this information. Patients have different levels of understanding. One patient may describe a diuretic as a "water pill," whereas another describes it as a medication to minimize swelling and lower blood pressure. Practise person-centred care and assess the patient's level of knowledge to determine the need for teaching. If a patient is unable to understand or remember pertinent information, it may be necessary to involve a caregiver.

Complete appropriate assessments, which may include vital signs, laboratory data, and the nature and severity of symptoms. If data contraindicate medication administration, withhold the medication

and notify the health care provider. When in doubt about medication information, check available medication references or the pharmacy.

Planning

During planning organize nursing activities to ensure the safe administration of medications. Current evidence shows that distractions or hurrying during preparation for medication administration increases the risk for medication errors (Yoder et al., 2015). The following are general goals of medication administration:

- Patient achieves therapeutic effect of the prescribed medication.
- There are no patient complications related to the prescribed medication.
- Patient and caregiver understand medication therapy.
- Patient and caregiver self-administer medication safely (when appropriate).

Implementation

Nursing interventions focus on safe and effective medication administration. This includes careful medication preparation, accurate and timely administration, and patient education.

Preadministration Activities

1. Identify the medication action, purpose, side effects, and nursing implications for administering and monitoring. Ensure that the medication prescription has not expired. Follow employer policy for prescription renewal.
2. Minimize distractions during medication preparation (e.g., discussion with staff, phone call, pager), close the door of the medication room or post "Do Not Disturb" signage, and do not perform other tasks while preparing a medication. Do not allow interruptions.
3. Make sure that the information on the medication computer sheet or MAR corresponds exactly with the health care provider's written prescription and with the medication container label. Do not interpret illegible handwriting; clarify with health care provider.
4. Read the label on the medication container and compare it with the MAR *at least 3 times:* before removing the container from the supply drawer, when preparing the medication, and just before administering the medication to the patient.
5. Double-check all calculations and other high-risk medication administration processes (e.g., insulin, patient-controlled analgesia) and verify with another nurse.
6. Review any preadministration assessments (e.g., vital signs, review of laboratory results).
7. Use good hand-hygiene technique. Avoid touching tablets and capsules. Use sterile technique for parenteral medications. Wear clean gloves when administering parenteral medications and certain topical medications.
8. Administer only those medications that you personally prepare. Do not ask another person to administer medications that you prepare. Keep medications secure.
9. When preparing medications, be sure that the label is clear and legible and that the medication is mixed properly; has not changed in colour, clarity, or consistency; and has not expired.
10. Keep tablets and capsules in their wrappers and open them at the patient's bedside. This allows you to review each medication with the patient. If a patient refuses medication, there will be no question which one was withheld.
11. Health Canada (2016) has a standard for labelling syringes, including before a procedure labelling all medicines that are not labelled (e.g., medicines in syringes and basins) and

using ink that is resistant to isopropyl or ethyl alcohol. This should be done in the area where medicines and supplies are set up.

Medication Administration

1. Follow the *10 rights* of medication administration.
2. Educate the patient about the name, purpose, action, and common side effects of each medication. Evaluate their knowledge of the medication and provide appropriate teaching using teach-back technique.
3. Stay with the patient until the medication is taken. Provide help as necessary. Do not leave medication at the bedside without a health care provider's prescription. For example, some patients may take their own vitamins while in the hospital.
4. Respect the patient's right to refuse a medication. If the medication wrapper remains intact, return the medication to the patient's unit-dose drawer. When medication is refused, determine the reason and take action accordingly.

Postadministration Activities

1. Record medications immediately after administration (see employer policy). Include the medication name, dose, route, time, and your signature.
2. Document preassessment as required (e.g., blood pressure measurement before antihypertensives).
3. Document postassessment data pertinent to patient's response. This is especially important when giving prn medications.
4. If a patient refuses a medication, document that it was not given, the reason for refusal, patient education provided and when you notified the health care provider.

Evaluation

After you administer a medication, consider how the medication is expected to affect the patient and evaluate their condition and response to it. Look for therapeutic and adverse effects. If adverse effects develop, you need to recognize the clinical signs and respond quickly:

1. Monitor for evidence of therapeutic effects, side effects, and adverse drug events. This includes monitoring physical response (e.g., heart rhythm, blood pressure, urine output, or laboratory results).
2. When a medication is given for relief of symptoms, ask the patient to report if symptoms have diminished or been relieved. For example, complete a pain assessment after medication is administered (e.g., 30 minutes after medicating for pain).
3. Observe injection sites for bruises, inflammation, localized pain, numbness, or bleeding.
4. Evaluate that patient and caregiver understand purpose of medication therapy, dose regimens, and ability to self-administer medication by using teach-back techniques.

REPORTING MEDICATION ERRORS

Medication errors often harm patients because of inappropriate medication use. Errors include inaccurate prescribing; administering the wrong medication, by the wrong route, and in the wrong time interval; and administering extra doses or failing to administer a medication. Medication errors are related to professional practice, health care product design, or procedures and systems such as product labelling and distribution. When an error occurs, the patient's safety and well-being become the top priority. A nurse assesses and examines the patient's condition and notifies the health care provider of the incident as soon as possible. Once the patient is stable, the nurse reports the incident to the appropriate person in the facility (e.g., manager or supervisor).

As a nurse, you are professionally responsible and ethically accountable to report all medication errors (harmful incidents, no-harm incidents, or near misses). A written report is completed usually within 24 hours of an incident (see employer policy). This report (e.g., incident report, adverse event report) is an internal audit tool and not a permanent part of the medical record. To legally protect interprofessional team members and the facility, do not refer to this report in the nurses' notes in the EHR or chart. Facilities use these reports to track patterns and initiate performance improvement programs as needed. Depending on the circumstances and the severity of the outcome, the nurse or facility may be responsible for reporting the incident to Canada's Vigilance Program and ISMP Canada (ISMP, 2019).

As a nurse, you should feel comfortable in reporting an error and not fear repercussions from managerial staff. The consequences of a medication error depend on several factors, including previous work performance, consequences to the patient, and the nurse's response to the error. Outcomes of reporting an error include a patient safety or quality improvement review, employee discipline, professional discipline, and/or a civil lawsuit (CNPS, 2007). Even when a patient suffers no harm from a medication error, the facility can still learn why the mistake occurred and what to do in the future to avoid similar errors. Most medication errors can be avoided by applying the principles of the 10 rights of medication administration (CNPS, 2007). There are strategies that you can implement to prevent medication errors (Box 20.8).

MEDICATION ERROR DISCLOSURE

Patient and family disclosure of medication errors is based on principles of patient safety, openness, transparency, accountability, and compassion (CPSI, 2011). Accreditation Canada (2019) has a Required Organizational Practice (ROP) for disclosure, called *Patient Safety Incident Disclosure* (formerly called *adverse or sentinel events disclosure*). Facilities must implement a formal and transparent policy and process of disclosure to patients, which include support mechanisms for patients, families, and care of interprofessional health team members. Under Canada's Constitution, each province/territory is responsible for its own liability laws. The first Canadian *Apology Legislation* was passed in 2006 by British Columbia (MacDonald & Attaran, 2009). Since that time, other provinces have followed suit. Be familiar with the apology legislation in the province or territory in which you practise nursing, as well as your employer-specific policies. Current literature; national and international best practices; and ethical, professional, and legal considerations all support open and honest disclosure of patient safety incidents (CPSI, 2011). Disclosing a patient safety incident to the patient and family demonstrates respect and person-centred care and facilitates safe and appropriate clinical care.

PATIENT AND CAREGIVER TEACHING

A well-informed patient is more likely to take medications correctly. However, many patients have limited health literacy, meaning that they do not understand how to read medication labels and calculate doses. Nurses also care for patients who do not speak English. Thus any education requires a person-centred approach to assess a patient's learning needs and abilities.

Nurses need to provide person-centred teaching according to patient preference, using visual aids, instructional booklets written

Steps to Prevent Medication Errors

- Always follow the 10 rights of medication administration.
- Only prepare medications for one patient at a time.
- Be sure to read labels at least three times (comparing MAR with label): When removing medication from storage, before taking to patient's room, before giving medication.
- Use at least two person-specific identifiers every time you administer medications (e.g., patient name, date of birth, hospital number).
- Do not allow any other activity to interrupt administration of medication to a patient (e.g., phone call, pager, discussion with other staff).
- Double-check all calculations and other high-risk medication administration processes (e.g., patient-controlled analgesia) and verify with another nurse.
- Do not interpret illegible handwriting; clarify with the health care provider.
- Question unusually large or small doses.
- Document all medications as soon as they are given.
- When you have made or discovered an error, reflect on what went wrong and ask how you could have prevented it. Complete a written report per employer policy.
- Evaluate the context or situation in which a medication error occurred. This helps to determine if nurses have the necessary resources for safe medication administration.
- When repeated medication errors occur within a work area, identify and analyze the factors that may have caused the errors and take corrective action.
- Attend in-service programs on the medications you commonly administer.
- Ensure that you are well rested when caring for patients. Nurse fatigue is associated with increased medication errors (Dykstra, Sendelbach, & Steege, 2016).
- Practise person-centred care when administering medications. Address patients' concerns about medications before administering them (e.g., concerns about their appearance or side effects).
- Follow established employer policies and procedures when using technology to administer medications (e.g., ADS and bar-code scanning). Medication errors occur when nurses "work around" the technology (e.g., override alerts without thinking about them) (Seaman & Erlen, 2015).

ADS, automated dispensing system; *MAR,* medication administration record.

in simple language or the patient's language, video recordings or DVDs, or online resources. When teaching patients about their medications, include people identified as being significant to the patient's recovery (e.g., family members, caregivers, or home care providers).

When providing patient teaching, begin instruction as soon as possible so you can have several teaching sessions. It is ideal to use instructional materials written no higher than a sixth-grade reading level. Provide instructions written in the patient's language, if available. When providing instruction, have the patient or caregiver repeat the name and use for each medication plus the dosing instructions. Current recommendations suggest the use of teach-back as a method to confirm patient learning and improve health care provider education (Nouri & Rudd, 2015). Have the patient explain the topic you taught them so you can confirm understanding. Have the patient demonstrate preparation of each medication. Provide time to discuss problem scenarios (e.g., side effects develop or a syringe becomes contaminated) to ensure that the patient is aware of what to do should something go wrong. Determine if the patient requires an adherence aid or memory cue. This is especially important among older persons. If the patient speaks another language, have a professional interpreter available during instruction. Do not use a family member as an interpreter. Medication dose containers organized by the hours and days of the week are very useful. In the event that patients miss a dose of medication, they need to know how to adjust their medication schedule safely.

Evaluating the effectiveness of teaching ensures that a patient can administer medications in a safe manner. One method of evaluating patient understanding is to create medication cards with the generic and trade names of the medication on the front of the card and all pertinent medication information on the back of the card. Another method is to have patients read labels on prepared medications. Remember that medication bottles often have fine print and are difficult to read for the patient with impaired vision. Have the pharmacy prepare large-print labels when appropriate. If the patient correctly identifies the name of the medication, ask the following questions:

- Why are you taking this medication?
- How often do you take this medication and at what time of day?
- What side effects can occur with this medication?
- If this side effect occurs, what are you going to do about it?

Be sure to also assess the patient's sensory, motor, and cognitive functions (e.g., ability to open medication bottles). Impairments may affect the patient's ability to safely self-administer medications, and caregivers or community health workers may need to help with medication administration. Many self-help devices are also available for purchase (e.g., pill boxes with times displayed and electronic dispensers).

◆ CLINICAL DEBRIEF

A 72-year-old male patient visits the medical clinic 1 month after a myocardial infarction (heart attack). He denies any chest pain since his angioplasty, which involved insertion of a stent into one of his coronary arteries to dilate the artery and improve blood flow to the heart. He is currently taking an antidepressant, a thyroid supplement, a stool softener, and a cardiac medication (beta-adrenergic blocker). In addition, he takes melatonin, an herbal preparation for sleep. The health care provider has recently revised the cardiac medication to metoprolol. He is now instructed to take 75 mg by mouth twice daily. The nurse notes that the medication is available in 150-mg tablets. The patient tells the clinic nurse that he has experienced some weakness and dizziness over the past week.

1. Which of the medications taken by the patient are likely to cause weakness and dizziness? Which nursing interventions should be included if he is experiencing these issues?
2. What might the health care provider who prescribed the medication do after receiving the nurse's report of the patient's weakness and dizziness? Use one of the methods provided to calculate the number of tablets of medication to administer.
3. As the nurse, which factors would be important for you to assess so the patient may take the 75-mg dose safely? Using SBAR, show how you would communicate with the health care team about this patient.

✦ REVIEW QUESTIONS

1. The health care provider has written the following prescriptions. Which prescriptions do you need to clarify before administering the medication? (Select all that apply and provide rationale for your answers. Rewrite the prescription so it follows the ISMP current medication prescription safety guidelines.)

1. Timoptic .25% solution 1 drop OD bid
2. Metoprolol 12.50 mg qd
3. Insulin glargine 6 u SC twice a day
4. Enalapril 2.5 mg. PO three times a day; hold for systolic blood pressure <100

2. An older person states that she cannot see her medication bottles clearly to determine when to take her prescription. What should the nurse do? *(Select all that apply.)*

1. Provide a pill-dispensing system that allows the patient or caregiver to prepare medications for each day of the week.
2. Provide larger, easier-to-read labels on medication bottles.
3. Tell the patient what is in each container of medication.
4. Have a caregiver administer the medication.
5. Use teach-back to ensure that patient knows what medication to take and when.

3. The nurse must take a verbal order during an emergency on the unit. Which of the following guidelines can be used for taking verbal or telephone orders? *(Select all that apply.)*

1. Only authorized staff receive and record verbal or telephone orders. Facility identifies in writing the staff who are authorized.
2. Clearly identify patient's name, room number, and diagnosis.
3. Repeat back all orders to health care provider.
4. Use clarification questions to avoid misunderstandings.
5. Write "verbal order" or "telephone order," including date and time, name of patient, and complete prescription; write the name of the health care provider and sign the entry.

ⓔ *Visit the Evolve site for a complete list of Clinical Debrief and Review Questions answers.*

REFERENCES

Accreditation Canada. (2017). *Medication management standards.* Retrieved from https://store.accreditation.ca/products/medication-management-standards

Accreditation Canada. (2019). *Required organizational practices handbook—Version 14.* Retrieved from http://www.wrha.mb.ca/quality/files/2019ROPHandbook.pdf

Burchum, J., & Rosenthal, L. (2016). *Lehne's pharmacology for nursing care* (9th ed.). St. Louis: Saunders.

Canadian Nurses Protective Society (CNPS). (2007). Medication errors. *InfoLaw, 5*(2), 2.

Canadian Patient Safety Institute (CPSI). (n.d.). *The economics of patient safety in acute care. A technical report.* Retrieved from http://www.patientsafetyinstitute.ca/en/toolsResources/Research/commissionedResearch/EconomicsofPatientSafety/Documents/Economics%20of%20Patient%20Safety%20-%20Acute%20Care%20-%20Final%20Report.pdf

Canadian Patient Safety Institute (CPSI). (2011). *Canadian disclosure guidelines: Being open with patients.* Edmonton, AB: Author.

Canadian Patient Safety Institute (CPSI). (2014). *Medication safety action plan.* Retrieved from http://www.patientsafetyinstitute.ca/en/About/PatientSafetyForwardWith4/Documents/A%20Medication%20Safety%20Action%20Plan.pdf

Canadian Patient Safety Institute (CPSI). (2016). *Medication safety.* Retrieved from http://www.patientsafetyinstitute.ca/en/About/PatientSafetyForwardWith4/pages/medication-safety.aspx

College and Association of Registered Nurses of Alberta (CARNA). (2015/2018). *Medication guidelines.* Retrieved from http://www.nurses.ab.ca/content/dam/carna/pdfs/DocumentList/Guidelines/MedicationGuidelines_Mar2015.pdf

College of Registered Nurses of British Columbia (CRNBC). (2019). *Medication administration.* Retrieved from https://www.crnbc.ca/Standards/PracticeStandards/Pages/medicationadmin.aspx

College of Registered Nurses of Nova Scotia (CRNNS). (2017). *Medication guidelines for registered nurses.* Retrieved from https://crnns.ca/wp-content/uploads/2015/05/Medication-Guidelines.pdf

Dykstra, J., Sendelbach, D., & Steege, L. (2016). Fatigue in float nurses: Patient, nurse, task, and environmental factors across unit work systems. *Proceedings of the Human Factors and Ergonomics Society 2016 Annual Meeting, 60*(1), 623–627. doi:10.1177/1541931213601142

Fraser, L., Albaum, J., Tadrous, M., Burden, A., Shariff, S., & Cadarette, S. (2015). Patterns of use for brand-name versus generic oral bisphosphonate drugs in Ontario over a 13-year period: A descriptive study. *CMAJ Open, 3*(1), E91–E96. doi:10.9778/cmajo.2014-0090

Gann, M. (2015). How informatics nurses use bar-code technology to reduce medication errors. *Nursing, 45*(3), 60–66. doi:10.1097/01.NURSE.0000458923.18468.37

Health Canada. (2016). *Good label and package practices guide for prescription drugs.* Ottawa, ON: Author. Retrieved from https://www.canada.ca/content/dam/hc-sc/migration/hc-sc/dhp-mps/alt_formats/pdf/pubs/medeff/guide/2016-label-package-practices-pratiques-etiquetage-emballage-rx/glppg-gbpee-rx-eng.pdf

Health Canada. (2018). *Regulatory initiative: Mandatory reporting of serious adverse drug reactions and medical device incidents by health care institutions—Forward regulatory plan 2018–2020.* Retrieved from https://www.canada.ca/en/health-canada/corporate/about-health-canada/legislation-guidelines/acts-regulations/forward-regulatory-plan/2017-2019/adverse-drug-reactions.html

Hockenberry, M. J., & Wilson, D. (2015). *Wong's nursing care of infants and children* (10th ed.). St. Louis: Mosby.

Institute for Safe Medication Practices (ISMP). (2006). *Tablet splitting: Do it only if you "half" to, and then do it safely.* Retrieved from https://www.ismp.org/resources/tablet-splitting-do-it-only-if-you-half-and-then-do-it-safely

Institute for Safe Medication Practices (ISMP). (2011). *Guidelines for timely administration of scheduled medications (acute).* Retrieved from https://www.ismp.org/guidelines/timely-administration-scheduled-medications-acute

Institute for Safe Medication Practices Canada (ISMP). (2014). *Preventable medication errors—Look-alike/sound-alike drug names.* Retrieved from https://www.ismp-canada.org/download/PharmacyConnection/PC2014-02-Spring_LookalikeSoundalike.pdf

Institute for Safe Medication Practices Canada (ISMP). (2016). *Drug labelling and the application of TALLman lettering project report.* Retrieved from https://www.ismp-canada.org/download/TALLman/TALLmanLettering-ProjectReport.pdf

Institute for Safe Medication Practices (ISMP). (2017). *2018–2019 Targeted medication safety best practices for hospitals.* Retrieved from https://www.ismp.org/sites/default/files/attachments/2017-12/TMSBP-for-Hospitalsv2.pdf

Institute for Safe Medication Practices Canada (ISMP). (2018a). *Do not use. Dangerous abbreviations, symbols, and dose designations.* Retrieved from https://www.ismp-canada.org/download/ISMPCanadaListOfDangerousAbbreviations.pdf

Institute for Safe Medication Practices (ISMP). (2018b). *High-alert medications in acute care.* Retrieved from https://www.ismp.org/recommendations/high-alert-medications-acute-list

Institute for Safe Medication Practices (ISMP). (2018c). *Key elements of safe medication use.* Retrieved from https://www.ismp.org/ten-key-elements

Institute for Safe Medication Practices (ISMP). (2018d). *Oral dosage forms that should not be crushed.* Retrieved from https://www.ismp.org/recommendations/do-not-crush

Institute for Safe Medication Practices Canada (ISMP). (2019). *Canadian Medication Incident Reporting and Prevention System (CMIRPS) program.* Retrieved from https://www.ismp-canada.org/cmirps/

Lin, K., Chan, K., Mohindra, R., Milne, K., Thoma, B., & Bond, C. (2017). SGEM hot off the press: Computer provider order entry (CPOE) and emergency department flow. *CJEM, 19*(2), 147–153. doi:10.1017/cem.2017.7

MacDonald, N., & Attaran, A. (2009). Medical errors, apologies and apology laws. *CMAJ : Canadian Medical Association Journal = Journal de l'Association Medicale Canadienne, 180*(1), 11. doi:10.1503/cmaj.081997

Nouri, S., & Rudd, R. (2015). Health literacy in the "oral exchange": An important element of patient provider communication. *Patient Education and Counseling, 98*(5), 565–571. doi:10.1016/j.pec.2014.12.002

Rohde, E., & Domm, E. (2017). Nurses' clinical reasoning practices that support safe medication administration: An integrative review of the literature. *Journal of Clinical Nursing, 17*(3–4), e402–e412. doi:10.1111/jocn.14077

Seaman, J., & Erlen, J. (2015). Workarounds in the workplace: A second look. *Orthopaedic Nursing, 34*(4), 235–240. doi:10.1097/NOR.0000000000000161

Shah, K., Lo, C., Babich, M., Tsao, N., & Bansback, N. (2016). Bar code medication administration technology: A systematic review of impact on patient safety when used with computerized prescriber order entry and automated dispensing devices. *The Canadian Journal of Hospital Pharmacy, 69*(5), 394–402.

Verloo, H., Chiolero, A., Kiszio, B., Kampel, T., & Santschi, V. (2017). Nurse interventions to improve medication adherence among discharged older adults: A systematic review. *Age and Ageing, 46*(5), 747–754. doi:10.1093/ageing/afx076

Yoder, M., Schadewald, D., & Dietrich, K. (2015). The effect of a safe zone on nurse interruptions, distractions, and medication administration errors. *Journal of Infusion Nursing, 38*(2), 140–151. doi:10.1097/NAN.0000000000000095

21 | Nonparenteral Medications

Written by **Anne Griffin Perry, RN, MSN, EdD, FAAN, and Nicole Lewis-Power, RN, MN, PhD(c)**

OBJECTIVES

Mastery of content in this chapter will enable the nurse to:
- Describe common principles to follow in the administration of medications.
- Discuss patient-centred practices to use to improve a patient's medication adherence.
- Safely and correctly administer a medication by oral, enteral, and topical routes.
- Identify guidelines for administering oral, enteral, and topical medications.
- Describe factors to assess before administering medications.
- Differentiate types of topical administrations that require sterile technique and those that require clean medical aseptic technique.
- Instruct patients in the proper use of a metered-dose inhaler (MDI), a dry powder inhaler (DPI), and small-volume nebulizer.
- Identify conditions contraindicating the administration of medications by various oral and topical routes.
- Prepare a teaching plan regarding medication use for a selected patient.

MEDIA RESOURCES

- evolve http://evolve.elsevier.com/Canada/Perry/clinicalskills/
- Review Questions
- Audio Glossary
- ▶ Video Clips
- **NSO** Nursing Skills Online
- Clinical Debrief and Review Questions Answers

PURPOSE

Administration of nonparenteral medications includes those that are given orally, enterally, and topically. Nonparenteral medications exclude any medication administered via an injection or intravenous infusion. The nonparenteral route chosen depends on the properties and desired effects of the medication and the physical and mental condition of a patient. There are many reasons why it may be necessary to change from one route to another. When this occurs, the nurse is responsible for consulting with a health care provider for a prescription or conferring with the pharmacist to safely meet a patient's needs.

STANDARDS OF CARE

- Accreditation Canada, 2019—*Required Organizational Practices Handbook—Version 14* (http://www.wrha.mb.ca/quality/files/2019ROPHandbook.pdf)
- Institute for Safe Medication Practices (ISMP), 2011—*Guidelines for Timely Administration of Scheduled Medications (Acute)* (https://www.ismp.org/guidelines/timely-administration-schedule d-medications-acute)
- Institute for Safe Medication Practices (ISMP), 2015—*List of Confused Drug Names* (https://www.ismp.org/recommendations/confused-drug-names-list)

- Institute for Safe Medication Practices (ISMP), 2017—2018–2019 *Targeted Medication Safety Best Practices for Hospitals* (https://www.ismp.org/sites/default/files/attachments/2017-12/TMSBP-for-Hospitalsv2.pdf)
- Institute for Safe Medication Practices Canada (ISMP), 2018a—*Do Not Use. Dangerous Abbreviations, Symbols, and Dose Designations* (https://www.ismp-canada.org/download/ISMPCanadaListOfDangerousAbbreviations.pdf)
- Institute for Safe Medication Practices (ISMP), 2018b—*Oral Dosage Forms That Should Not be Crushed* (https://www.ismp.org/recommendations/do-not-crush)

PRINCIPLES FOR PRACTICE

- The major principle of practice with nonparenteral medication administration is patient safety (see Safety Guidelines).
- The oral route (by mouth) is the easiest and most desirable way to administer medications.
- Topical administration of medications involves applying medications directly to skin or mucous or tissue membranes. See Box 21.1 for examples of topical medication routes.
- Medications are applied to the skin by spraying, painting, or spreading medication over a localized area. Transdermal patches (adhesive-backed medicated disks) applied to the skin provide a continuous release of medication over several hours or days.
- Medications applied to membranes such as the cornea of the eye or the rectal mucosa are absorbed quickly because of the vascularity of the membrane and can also have systemic effects. In addition, nurses can experience systemic effects of a topical medication if they do not wear clean gloves.

PERSON-CENTRED CARE

- An excellent time to provide patient education is during medication administration. The nurse must assess the patient's and caregiver's health literacy, health beliefs, and cultural practices.
- The goal of patient education is to improve patient adherence to medication regimens. Patients fail to adhere to medication regimens because of patient, medication, and health care provider issues. Patient issues include medication knowledge, health literacy, and financial limitations. Clear, concise, and, at times, one-on-one patient education can improve adherence to medication, which in turn improves patient outcomes (Ari, 2015).

BOX 21.1

Examples of Topical Medication Routes

1. *Sublingual:* Medication placed under the tongue; is dissolvable
2. *Buccal:* Medication placed between the upper or lower molar teeth and cheek area; is dissolvable
3. *Direct application to skin or mucosa:* Lotion, ointment, cream, powder, foam, spray, patch, and disk
4. *Direct application to mucous membrane:* Eyedrops, gargling, swabbing the throat; *Spraying:* Instillation into nose or throat
5. *Inhalation of medicated aerosol spray:* Distributes medication throughout the nasal passages and the tracheobronchial airway; two types of devices designed for this purpose: metered-dose inhalers (MDIs) and small-volume nebulizers
6. *Inhalation of dry powder medication:* Distributes medication in powder form throughout the tracheobronchial airway; device designed for this purpose: dry powder inhaler (DPI)
7. *Inserting medication into a body cavity:* Rectal or vaginal suppositories, vaginal creams, or foams

---

- Print materials used for instruction should be written at an appropriate reading level (e.g., grade 6) and delivered in a manner that meets individual patient needs such as visual impairment or hearing or cognitive impairments. Involve caregivers in the education sessions because they may be the ones administering medications.
- Cognitive impairment and depression have an effect on health literacy. Individualized patient education techniques that simplify tasks and patient roles may help to overcome cognitive load and suboptimal performance in self-medication administration (Soones, Lin, Wolf, et al., 2017).
- Medication issues related to medication nonadherence include complex medication regimens and medication discrepancies. Health care provider issues include poor instruction, inappropriate prescriptions, and lack of provider knowledge about adherence. Patients need explanations about the purpose of medications, benefits, expected effects, and how to plan a daily schedule.
- Health beliefs vary by culture and influence how patients manage and respond to medication therapy. Differences in values, attitudes, and beliefs affect a patient's adherence to medication therapy. For example, herbal remedies and alternative therapies may be common practice in some cultures and interfere with prescribed medications. It is also important to consider cultural influences on medication response, metabolism, and side effects if a patient is not responding to medication therapy as expected. For example, certain cultural food preferences may have food–medication interactions.
- Vegetarian diets can affect warfarin or medications for glycemic control. A change in the medication may be necessary by the prescriber, or the patient may need counselling about how to change their dietary patterns.

EVIDENCE-INFORMED PRACTICE

- Medication competency is a skill that all nurses must possess to improve the quality and safety of medication administration. When nurses follow guidelines such as the 10 rights of medication administration (see Chapter 20) and the ISMP Canada guidelines for timely administration, correct crushing and splitting of pills, avoiding confusing abbreviations, and double-checking for sound-alike medications, medication errors are reduced (ISMP, 2011, 2015, 2018a, 2018b).
- Knowledge of technology and nurse competencies is essential to increase patient safety and promote best practices (Liston & McKinnon, 2017).
- Use of bar code medication administration (BCMA) or automated dispensing medication cabinets (e.g., Pyxis) helps ensure verification of the right patient and that the right medication, right dose, and right route are used and at the right time, in the presence of medication administration technology, and helps to reduce medication errors (Risør, Lisby, & Sørensen, 2018; Shah, Lo, Babich, et al., 2016)
- Evidence suggests that a quiet environment free of distractions and interruptions allows the nurse to focus when preparing medications. Thus having a medication zone free of distractions, clutter, and interruptions helps reduce the risk for medication errors (Yoder, Schadewald, & Dietrich, 2015).
- Nurses need to follow best practices for calculating medication doses, double-check the calculations, and *not* administer medication if the dosage appears incorrect (Douglass, Elder, Watson, et al., 2018). They should follow employer policy for medication calculations for the very young or high-risk medications (e.g., cardiotonics, insulin, and some opioid medications).

- Best-practice guidelines for safe medication administration require critical thinking, clinical decision-making competency, and theoretical and clinical practice competency. Medication administration is not a routine nursing action; nurses must adhere to the 10 rights of medication administration at all times to ensure patient safety. As a nurse you must think critically about the medications you are giving. Ask yourself: "Is the medication still appropriate for the patient's condition, or do I need to contact the health care provider?" "This pill looks different. I need to verify with pharmacy" (Flynn, Evanish, Fernald, et al., 2016).

SAFETY GUIDELINES

- Safe medication administration requires nurses to follow the 10 rights of medication administration for all nonparenteral medications. Nurses should also know the ISMP (2017) guidelines, medication actions and interactions, potential side effects and adverse effects, and how to safely administer medication through various nonparenteral routes. When the 10 rights are not followed, negative and sometimes harmful effects can occur. For example, administering medications to the wrong client can result in major health consequences (e.g., the client could develop hypoglycemia if insulin is administered), as can giving a patient an incorrect dose (e.g., too much morphine could cause respiratory depression).
- Assess a patient's sensory function, including sight, hearing, touch, and physical coordination and dexterity. Sensory function and coordination deficits impair a patient's ability to see medications, read labels at home, and discriminate one medication from another. Coordination and dexterity impairments reduce a patient's ability to open prescription bottles and dispense the correct dosage.
- Patients often receive more than one oral medication at a time. It is important to evaluate each medication for potential medication–medication or medication–food interactions. When

unsure, consult with a pharmacist to clarify the risk of an interaction and determine the measure to reduce it.
- Some medications require double-checks by two nurses to ensure that the right medication and right dose (always check employer policy as to which medications require double-checks by two nurses) are given. Double-checks are carried out for high-risk medications (e.g., insulin), in pediatric settings, and for chemotherapy medications (Schwappach, Pfeiffer, & Taxis, 2016).
- Nurses must always assess for medication allergies. If the patient reports having an allergy, ask about the type of reaction that occurred.
- Evaluate if the patient can take medication with food. In most cases the presence of food in the stomach delays medication absorption. However, some medications must be taken before meals, and others may need to be taken with meals. Some medications irritate the stomach lining and need to be taken with food.
- For all medications administered, review the prescription for the patient's name, medication, dosage, route, and time of administration.
- Use the correct equipment for administering all medications. For example, when delivering liquid medications, use only unit dose containers dispensed by the pharmacy (ISMP, 2017).
- For all medications administered, gather information pertinent to the medication(s) prescribed: purpose, normal dosage and route, common side effects, time of onset and peak, contraindications, and nursing implications.
- Determine if medications require any specific nursing actions (e.g., obtaining vital signs, medication levels, or electrolytes) before administration.
- Prepare the patient for discharge by instructing them in self-administration techniques, as appropriate. Include caregivers if possible.
- Check the expiration date for all medications.

✦ SKILL 21.1 Administering Oral Medications

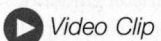 *Video Clip* **NSO** *Nursing Skills Online Administration of Nonparenteral Medications Module 6 / Lesson 1*

Patients are usually able to ingest or self-administer oral medications with few problems. If oral medications are contraindicated (e.g., inability to swallow, gastric suction), it is important to take precautions to protect patients from aspiration (see Skill 31.3). Nurses usually prepare medications in areas designed for medication preparation or at unit-dose carts.

The form or preparation of an oral medication affects how well it is absorbed after it is ingested. Liquids are absorbed faster than tablets or capsules and are usually absorbed in the stomach. Give an oral medication with a meal if its absorption is enhanced by food in the stomach. Some medications must be taken between meals, 2 to 3 hours later (Burchum & Rosenthal, 2016). When administering multiple oral medications, give oral medications before sublingual and buccal medications. Use interprofessional collaboration (e.g., pharmacist) for further guidance as required.

Other oral medications are absorbed in the intestinal tract. Enteric-coated preparations resist being dissolved by gastric juices. The enteric coating protects the stomach lining from irritation by the medication. These preparations are absorbed in the small intestine. Never crush or split an enteric-coated medication. Crushing or splitting these preparations causes the medication to be released too early; the medication may become inactive in the stomach or fail to reach the intended site of action (ISMP, 2018b).

Delegation and Collaboration

The skill of administering oral medications may be delegated to an unregulated care provider (UCP) in some jurisdictions, for example, in the home setting (always check employer policy). The nurse instructs the UCP about:
- Potential adverse effects of medications and to report their occurrence.
- Informing the nurse if the patient's condition changes or worsens (e.g., pain, itching, or rash) after medication administration.

Equipment

- Medication administration record (MAR) (electronic or printed)
- Automated, computer-controlled medication-dispensing system or unit-dose medication cart
- Oral syringes marked "oral use only"
- Glass of water, juice, or preferred liquid and drinking straw
- Device for crushing or splitting tablets (*optional*)
- Paper towels
- Clean gloves (if handling an oral medication) **NOTE:** Gloves must be worn when administering an oral chemotherapy medication.
- Medication cup

STEP	**RATIONALE**

ASSESSMENT

1. Check accuracy and completeness of each MAR with health care provider's medication prescription. Check patient's name and medication name, dosage, and route and time of administration. Clarify incomplete or unclear prescriptions with health care provider before administration.

The health care provider's prescription is the most reliable source and only legal record of medications that patient is to receive. It ensures that patient receives correct medication (Basukala, Mehrotra, & Devarakonda, 2017). Handwritten MARs are a source of medication errors (Basukala et al., 2017).

2. Review pertinent information related to medication, including action, purpose, normal dose and route, adverse effects, time of onset and peak action, and nursing implications.

Allows you to anticipate effects of medication and observe patient's response.

3. Assess for any contraindications to patient receiving oral medication, including being on NPO status, inability to swallow, nausea/vomiting, bowel inflammation, reduced peristalsis, recent gastrointestinal (GI) surgery, gastric suction, and decreased level of consciousness (LOC). Notify health care provider if any contraindications are present.

Alterations in GI function can interfere with medication absorption, distribution, and excretion. Giving oral medications to patients with impaired swallowing or decreased LOC increases their risk for aspiration (Leder, Suiter, Agogo, et al., 2016; Schiele, Penner, Schneider, et al., 2015). Patients with GI suction do not receive actions of oral medications because the medications are suctioned from the GI tract before they are absorbed.

4. Assess risk for aspiration using a dysphagia screening tool if available (see Skill 31.3). Protect patient from aspiration by assessing swallowing ability (Box 21.2).

Aspiration occurs when food, fluid, or medication intended for GI administration is inadvertently administered into the respiratory tract. Patients with altered ability to swallow are at higher risk for aspiration (Leder et al., 2016; Schiele et al., 2015).

5. Assess patient's medical, medication, and diet history and history of allergies. List any medication allergies on each page of MAR (in red ink) and prominently display on patient's medical record. When allergies are present, patient should wear an allergy bracelet.

Information reflects patient's need for and potential responses to medication. Information reveals potential food and medication interactions. Communication of allergies is essential for safe, effective patient care.

6. Gather and review physical assessment findings and laboratory data that influence medication administration, such as vital signs and results of renal and liver function studies.

Data may reveal need to contraindicate medication administration. Renal and liver function status affects metabolism and excretion of medications (Burchum & Rosenthal, 2016).

7. Assess patient's knowledge regarding health and medication use, medication schedule, and ability to prepare medications.

Determines patient's need for medication education and guidance needed to achieve medication adherence (e.g., involvement of caregiver).

8. Assess patient's preference for fluids and determine if medications can be given with these fluids. Maintain fluid restrictions as prescribed.

Some fluids interfere with medication absorption (e.g., dairy products affect tetracycline). Offering fluids during medication administration is an excellent way to increase patient's fluid intake. Fluids ease swallowing and facilitate absorption from the GI tract. However, fluid restrictions exist; skillful planning of fluid intake must coordinate with medication times and type of medications.

BOX 21.2

Protecting the Patient From Aspiration

- Assess patient's ability to swallow and cough and check for presence of gag reflex.
- Prepare oral medication in form that is easiest to swallow.
- Allow patient to self-administer medications if possible.
- If patient has unilateral (one-sided) weakness, place medication in stronger side of mouth.
- Administer pills one at a time, ensuring that each medication is properly swallowed before next one is introduced.

- Thicken regular liquids or offer fruit nectars if patient cannot tolerate thin liquids.
- Avoid straws because they decrease control patient has over volume intake, which increases risk of aspiration.
- Have patient hold and drink from a cup if possible.
- Time medications to coincide with meals or when patient is well rested and awake, if possible.
- Administer medications using another route if risk of aspiration is severe.

STEP	RATIONALE

NURSING DIAGNOSES

- Inadequate swallowing
- Inadequate knowledge regarding medications and medication administration
- Readiness for enhanced self-health management
- Potential for nonadherence
- Potential for aspiration

Related factors/Risk factors are individualized on the basis of patient's condition or needs.

PLANNING

1. Expected outcomes following completion of procedure:
   - Patient responds appropriately to desired medication effect within period of onset of medication action.
   - Patient denies any GI discomfort or symptoms of alterations.
   - Patient explains purpose of medication and medication dosage schedule.

   Medication has exerted its therapeutic action.

   Oral medications can irritate GI mucosa.

   Demonstrates understanding of medication therapy.

2. Explain procedure to patient. Be specific if patient wishes to self-administer medications.

   Makes patient a participant in care, which minimizes anxiety. Begins patient teaching regarding medications. Prepares patient to self-administer medication, which increases feelings of independence.

3. Collect appropriate equipment and MAR.

   Promotes time management and efficiency when preparing medications for all patients.

4. Plan preparation of medication to avoid interruptions and distractions. Do not take phone calls or talk with others (see employer policy).

   Interruptions contribute to occurrence of medication administration errors (Yoder et al., 2015).

IMPLEMENTATION

1. Prepare medications.
   a. Perform hand hygiene.

   Reduces transfer of microorganisms.

   b. Arrange medication tray and cups in medication preparation area or move medication cart to position outside patient's room.

   Organization of equipment saves time and reduces error.

   c. Log on to automated dispensing system (ADS) or unlock medicine drawer or cart.

   Medications are safeguarded when locked in cabinet, cart, or ADS.

   d. Prepare medications for *one patient at a time*. Follow the 10 rights of medication administration. Keep all pages of MARs or computer printouts for one patient together or look at only one patient's medication administration computer screen.

   Prevents preparation errors.

   e. Select correct medication from ADS, unit-dose drawer, or stock supply. Compare name of medication on label with MAR or computer printout (see illustration). Exit ADS after removing medication(s).

   Reading label and comparing it against transcribed prescription reduces errors. Exiting ADS ensures that no one else can remove medications using your identity. *This is the first check for accuracy.*

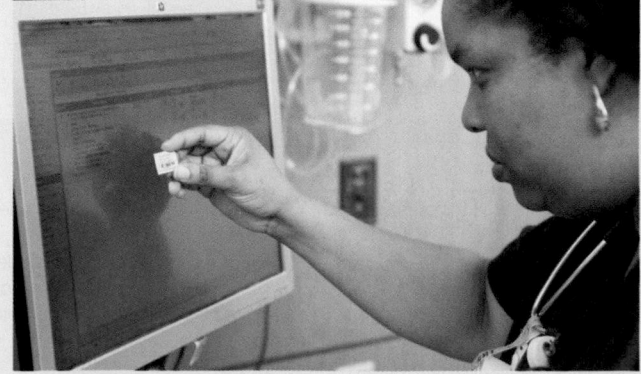

STEP 1e Nurse compares label of medication with transcribed medication prescription on computerized MAR.

STEP	RATIONALE

IMPLEMENTATION

f. Check or calculate medication dose as necessary. Double-check any calculation. Check expiration date on all medications and return outdated medication to pharmacy.

Double-checking pharmacy calculations reduces risk for error. Employer policy may require you to check calculations of certain medications (e.g., insulin) with another nurse (ISMP, 2013; Schwappach et al., 2016). Expired medications may be inactive or harmful to patient.

g. If preparing a controlled substance, check record for previous medication count and compare current count with available supply. Controlled medications may be stored in computerized locked cart (see Chapter 20).

Controlled substance laws require nurses to carefully monitor and count dispensed narcotics.

h. Prepare solid forms of oral medications.

(1) To prepare unit-dose tablets or capsules, place packaged tablet or capsule directly into medication cup without removing wrapper. Administer medications only from containers with labels that are clearly marked. Double check medication label with patient MAR.

Wrappers maintain cleanliness and identify medication name and dose, which can facilitate teaching.
This is the second check for accuracy.

(2) When using a blister pack, "pop" medications through foil or paper backing into a medication cup.

Packs provide a 1-month supply, with each "blister" usually containing a single dose.

(3) If it is necessary to give half the dose of medication, pharmacy should split, label, package, and send medication to unit. If you need to split a medication, cut with a clean pillating device. Tablets that can be cut in half must be prescored (i.e., have a manufactured line that traverses the centre of the tablet).

In health care agencies, only pharmacy should split tablets to ensure patient safety (Food and Drug Administration [FDA], 2017). Reduces contamination of tablet.

(4) Place all tablets or capsules that patient will receive in one medicine cup, except for those requiring preadministration assessments (e.g., pulse rate or blood pressure). Place those medications in separate, additional cup with wrapper intact.

Keeping medications that require preadministration assessments separate from others serves as reminder and makes it easier to withhold medications as necessary.

(5) If patient has difficulty swallowing and liquid medications are not an option, use a pill-crushing device. Clean device before using. Place medicine between two cups, and grind and crush (see illustration). Mix ground tablet in small amount (teaspoon) of soft food (custard or applesauce).

Large tablets are often difficult to swallow. Ground tablet mixed with palatable soft food is usually easier to swallow.

Clinical Decision Point *Not all medications can be crushed safely (e.g., capsules, enteric-coated pills). Use interprofessional collaboration (e.g., pharmacist) or the ISMP (2018b) Do Not Crush List when unsure if a medication can be crushed safely.*

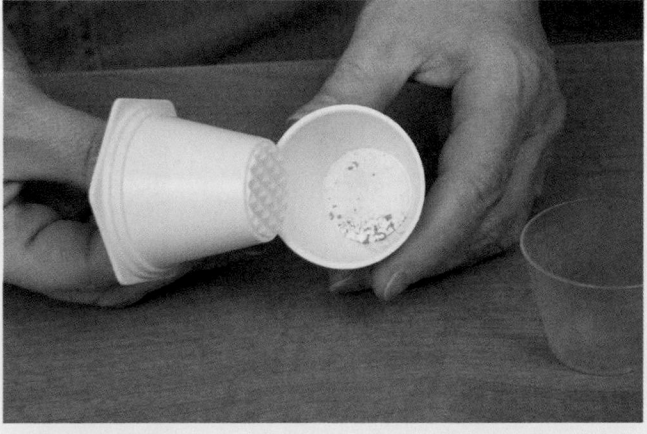

STEP 1h(5) Crushing tablet with pill-crushing device.

STEP	RATIONALE

IMPLEMENTATION

i. Prepare liquids.

(1) Use unit-dose container with correct amount of medication. Gently shake container. Administer medication packaged in a single-dose cup directly from the single-dose cup. Double check medication label with patient MAR. Do not pour medicine into another cup. Check expiration date.

Using unit-dose container with correct dosage of medication provides most accurate dose of medication (ISMP, 2017). Shaking container ensures that medication is mixed before administration.
This is the second check for accuracy.

Clinical Decision Point *On the basis of current best practice (ISMP, 2017b), liquid medications that are not available or are not in correct dose in a unit-dose container should be dispensed by the pharmacy in special oral syringes marked "Oral Use Only." These syringes do not connect to any type of parenteral (e.g., intravenous [IV]) tubing. In addition, current evidence shows that liquid measuring devices on patient care units result in inaccurate dosing. Having oral medications prepared in the pharmacy ensures that you give the most accurate dose possible of a medication and prevents parenteral administration of oral medications.*

(2) Administer medications in only oral use syringes prepared by pharmacy (see illustration). *Do not* use hypodermic syringe or syringe with needle or syringe cap (see Chapter 20).

(3) Gently shake container. If medication is in a multidose bottle, remove bottle cap from container, and place cap upside down on work surface.

(4) Hold bottle with label against palm of hand while pouring.

(5) Hold medication cup at eye level and fill to desired level on scale. Scale should be even with fluid level at its surface or base of meniscus.

(6) Discard any excess liquid into sink. Wipe lip and neck of bottle with paper towel and recap bottle.

(7) For doses of liquid medications less than 10 mL, draw liquid into a calibrated oral syringe.

Only use syringes specifically designed for oral use when administering liquid medications. If using hypodermic syringes, the medication may be administered parenterally accidentally; or the syringe cap or needle, if not removed from the syringe before administration, may become dislodged and accidentally aspirated during administration of oral medications (ISMP, 2017b).
Allows more accurate measurement of small amounts.

j. Check the medication label one more time before returning stock containers or unused unit-dose medications to shelf or drawer. Label medication cups and poured medications with patient's name before leaving medication preparation area. Never leave medications unattended.

Ensures that correct medications are prepared for correct patient.
This is the third check for accuracy.

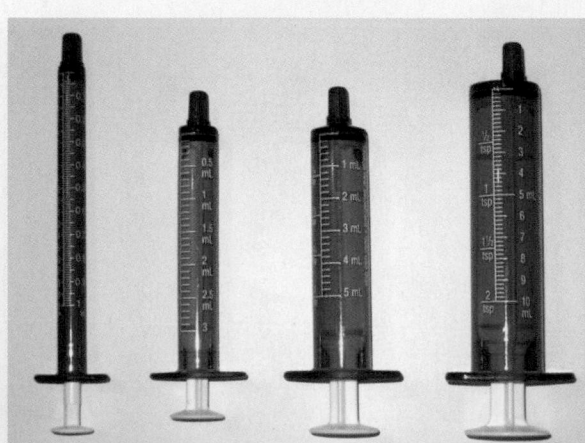

STEP 1i(2) Use special oral medication syringes to prepare small amounts of liquid medications.

STEP	RATIONALE

IMPLEMENTATION

2. Administer medications.

a. Take medication(s) to patient at correct time (see employer policy). Medications that require exact timing include stat, first-time or loading doses, and one-time doses. Give time-critical scheduled medications (e.g., antibiotics, anticoagulants, insulin, anticonvulsants, immunosuppressive medications) at exact time prescribed (no later than 30 minutes before or after scheduled dose). Give non–time-critical scheduled medications within a range of 1 or 2 hours of scheduled dose, according to employer policy (ISMP, 2011). During administration, apply 10 rights of medication administration. Perform hand hygiene.

Employers must adopt medication administration policy and procedure for timing of medication administration that considers nature of the prescribed medication, specific clinical application, and patient needs. Time-critical scheduled medications are those for which early or delayed administration of maintenance doses of greater than 30 minutes before or after the scheduled dose may cause harm or result in substantial suboptimal therapy or pharmacological effect. Non–time-critical medications are those for which early or delayed administration within a specified range of either 1 or 2 hours should not cause harm or result in substantial suboptimal therapy or pharmacological effect (ISMP, 2011).

b. Identify patient using at least two person-specific identifiers (e.g., name and date of birth or name and medical record number) according to employer policy. Compare identifiers with information on patient's MAR or medical record and ID band. Replace missing or faded ID bands.

Ensures correct patient. Complies with Accreditation Canada's standards and improves patient safety (Accreditation Canada, 2019).

c. At patient's bedside, again compare MAR or computer printout with names of medications on medication labels and patient name. Ask patient if they have allergies.

Ensures that the right patient receives correct medication. Confirms patient's allergy history.

d. Explain the purpose of each medication, action, and most common possible adverse effects. Allow sufficient time for patient to ask questions.

Patient has the right to be informed, and patient understanding of each medication improves adherence to medication therapy.

e. Perform necessary preadministration assessment (e.g., blood pressure, pulse) for specific medications. Ask patient if they have allergies.

Determines whether specific medications should be withheld at that time. Confirms patient's allergy history.

Clinical Decision Point *If patient expresses concern regarding accuracy of a medication, do not give the medication. Explore patient's concern and verify health care provider's prescription before administering. Listening to patient's concerns may prevent a medication error.*

f. Help patient to sitting or Fowler's position. Use side-lying position if they are unable to sit. Have patient stay in this position for 30 minutes after administration.

Decreases risk for aspiration during swallowing.

g. *For tablets:* Patient may wish to hold solid medications in hand or cup before placing in mouth. Offer water or preferred liquid to help patient swallow medications.

Patient can become familiar with medications by seeing each medication. Choice of fluid can improve fluid intake.

Clinical Decision Point *If administering an oral chemotherapy medication, administer it from the cup directly into the patient's mouth or apply gloves before handling pill or tablet. Never use bare hands to touch a chemotherapy medication, as residue can be absorbed through your skin (Dana Farber Cancer Institute, 2015).*

h. *For orally disintegrating formulations (tablets or strips):* Remove medication from packet just before use. Do not push tablet through foil. Place medication on top of patient's tongue. Caution against chewing it.

Orally disintegrating formulations begin to dissolve when placed on tongue. Water is not needed. Careful removal from packaging is necessary because tablets and strips are thin and fragile.

i. *For sublingually administered medications:* Have patient place medication under tongue and allow it to dissolve completely (see illustration). Caution patient against swallowing tablet.

Medication is absorbed through blood vessels of undersurface of tongue. If swallowed, it is destroyed by gastric juices or rapidly detoxified by the liver, preventing therapeutic blood level.

j. *For buccal administered medications:* Have patient place medication in mouth against mucous membranes of cheek and gums until it dissolves (see illustration).

Buccal medications act locally or systemically as they are swallowed in saliva.

Clinical Decision Point *Avoid administering anything by mouth until orally disintegrating buccal or sublingual medication is completely dissolved.*

k. *For powdered medications:* Mix with liquids at bedside and give to patient to drink.

When prepared in advance, powdered medications thicken; some even harden, making swallowing difficult.

STEP	RATIONALE

IMPLEMENTATION

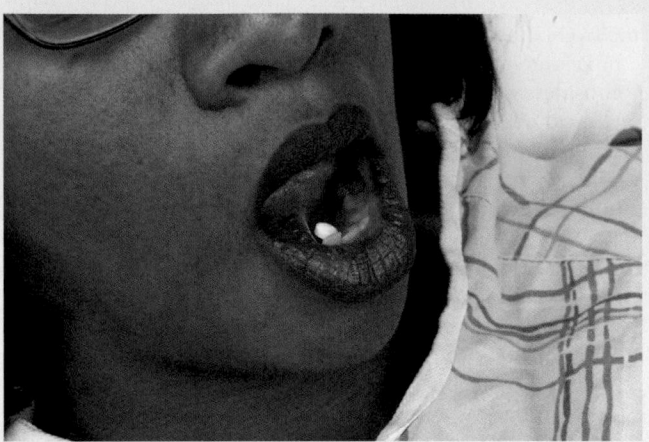

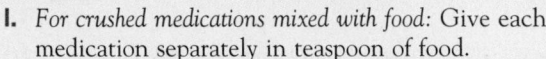

STEP 2i Proper placement of sublingual tablet in sublingual pocket.

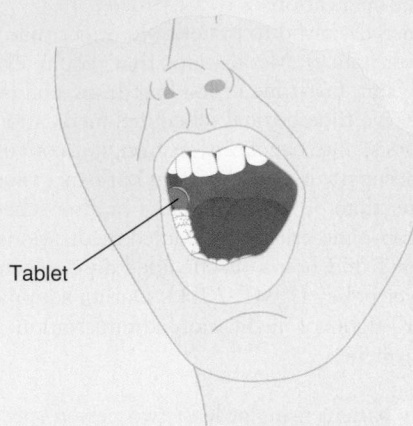

STEP 2j Buccal administration of tablet.

l. *For crushed medications mixed with food:* Give each medication separately in teaspoon of food.

Ensures that patient swallows all of medicine.

m. *For lozenge:* Caution patient against chewing or swallowing lozenges.

Lozenges act through slow absorption through oral mucosa, not gastric mucosa.

n. *For effervescent medication:* Add tablet or powder to glass of water. Administer immediately after dissolving.

Effervescence improves unpleasant taste and often relieves GI problems.

o. If patient is unable to hold medications, place medication cup to lips and gently introduce each medication into mouth one at a time. A spoon can also be used to place pill in patient's mouth. Do not rush or force medications.

Administering a single tablet or capsule eases swallowing and decreases risk for aspiration.

Clinical Decision Point *If tablet or capsule falls to the floor, discard it and repeat preparation. Medication is contaminated.*

p. Stay until patient swallows each medication completely or takes it by the prescribed route. Ask patient to open mouth if uncertain whether medication has been swallowed.

Ensures that patient receives prescribed dose. If left unattended, patient may not take dose or may save medications, causing health risks.

q. For highly acidic medications (e.g., aspirin), offer patient a nonfat snack (e.g., crackers) if not contraindicated by their condition.

Reduces gastric irritation. Fat content of foods may delay medication absorption.

3. Help patient return to position of comfort.

Maintains patient's comfort.

4. Dispose of soiled supplies and perform hand hygiene. Return cart to medication room if used. Clean work area.

Reduces spread of microorganisms.

5. Replenish stock such as cups and straws, return cart to medication room, and clean work area.

Enhances efficiency and reduces transfer of microorganisms.

EVALUATION

1. Return to bedside to evaluate patient's response to medications at times that correlate with onset, peak, and duration of medication.

Evaluates therapeutic benefit of medication and helps to detect onset of adverse effects or allergic reactions. Sublingual medications act in 15 minutes; most oral medications act in 30 to 60 minutes.

STEP	RATIONALE

EVALUATION

2. Ask patient or caregiver to identify medication name and explain purpose, action, dose schedule, and potential side effects.

Determines level of knowledge gained by patient and caregiver.

3. Use Teach-Back: "I want to be sure I showed you how to use your sublingual nitroglycerin. Show me where you will place your pill in your mouth." Develop a revised teaching plan if patient or caregiver is not able to teach back correctly.

Determines patient's and caregiver's level of understanding of instructional topic.

Unexpected Outcomes	Related Interventions
1. Patient exhibits adverse effects (e.g., side effect, toxic effect, allergic reaction).	• Notify health care provider and pharmacy. • Withhold further doses. • Assess vital signs. • Symptoms such as urticaria, rash, pruritus, rhinitis, and wheezing may indicate an allergic reaction and need for emergency medications. • Add allergy information to patient's medical record.
2. Patient refuses medication.	• Assess why patient is refusing medication. • Provide further instruction • Do not force patient to take medications. • Notify health care provider.
3. Patient is unable to explain medication information.	• Further assess patient's or caregiver's knowledge of medications and guidelines for medication safety. • Further instruction or different approach to instruction is necessary.

Communication and Documentation

- Document medication, dose, route, and time administered on patient's MAR immediately after administration, not before. Include initials or signature.
- Document patient's response to medication, patient teaching, and validation of patient's understanding on flow sheet or in nurses' notes in electronic health record (EHR) or chart.
- If medication is withheld or refused, document reason on flow sheet or in nurses' notes in EHR or chart and follow employer policy for noting withheld doses.
- Report adverse effects, patient response, and/or withheld medications to nurse in charge or health care provider. Depending on medication, immediate health care provider notification may be required.

Special Considerations
Teaching

- Instruct patient and caregiver about specific information pertaining to medication regimen (purpose, action, dose, dosage intervals, adverse effects, foods to avoid or take with medications).
- If patient is taking multiple medications, consider recommending a dose organizer. Use interprofessional collaboration (e.g., pharmacist) to assist patients to organize their medications and consider the use of blister packs with the times for administration highlighted.
- All patients should learn the basic guidelines for medication safety in the home (see Skill 42.3).

Pediatric

- Liquid forms of medication are safer to swallow to avoid aspiration of small pills.
- Children refuse bitter or distasteful oral preparations. Mix the medication with a small amount (about 5 mL) of a sweet-tasting substance such as jam, applesauce, sherbet, ice cream, or fruit puree.

Do not use honey for infants because of the risk of botulism. Offer the child juice or a flavoured ice pop after medication administration. Do not place medication in an essential food item such as milk or formula; the child may refuse the food at a later time.
- Measure liquid medications with a plastic calibrated oral dosing syringe or a spoon. Using interprofessional collaboration, nurses and pharmacists can teach parents how to draw up liquid medications prior to discharge.

Gerontological

- Physiological changes of aging influence how oral medications are distributed, absorbed, and excreted. Common changes include loss of elasticity in oral mucosa; reduction in parotid gland secretion, causing dry mouth; delayed esophageal clearance; impaired swallowing; reduction in gastric acidity and stomach peristalsis; increased susceptibility to highly acidic medications; reduced liver function, resulting in altered medication metabolism; and reduced renal function and colon motility, slowing medication excretion (Touhy, Jett, Boscart, et al., 2019). Both altered medication metabolism and excretion may lead to medication toxicity (Burchum & Rosenthal, 2016).
- Give medications with a full glass of water (unless restricted) to aid passage of the medication. Give patient time to swallow.
- Patients may have several health problems or chronic conditions requiring the use of multiple medications, often prescribed by different health care providers. Polypharmacy creates a high risk for medication interactions and adverse reactions (Burchum & Rosenthal, 2016).

Care in the Community

- When measuring liquid medications at home, instruct patients and caregivers how to accurately use a dosing cup to administer medications in the home (see Chapter 20).
- See Skills 42.3 and 43.6.

Patients who have enteral feeding tubes are unable to receive food or medications by mouth. Nasogastric feeding tubes generally are small-bore tubes that are inserted into the stomach via one of the nares (see Chapter 32). For long-term enteral feedings, a percutaneous endoscopic gastrostomy (PEG) tube or a jejunostomy tube may be inserted surgically. *Do not administer medications into nasogastric tubes that are inserted for decompression.*

In addition to administering the correct medication, it is important that the enteral access connector be appropriate for the type of enteral tube (Lord, 2018). These devices are not compatible with Luer or needleless connectors. They are designed for specific enteral feeding tubes. The goal of these new access connectors is to reduce enteral tube misconnections and medication errors (Guenther, 2015).

Preferably, medications administered by enteral tubes should be in liquid form. However, when the liquid form of the medication is not available, you need to prepare an oral medication tablet or capsule by crushing or dissolving it. Facility pharmacies may be able to provide the prescribed medication in a liquid suspension, which does not affect its effectiveness (Salmon, Pont, Chevallard, et al., 2013). However, *do not crush* sublingual, sustained-release, chewable, long-acting, capsules or enteric-coated medications. Use interprofessional collaboration (e.g., pharmacist) to confirm whether you can crush or dissolve a medication. Always verify correct placement of a nasogastric tube before administering medications (see Skill 32.2).

Delegation and Collaboration

The skill of administering medications by enteral feeding tubes cannot be delegated to an unregulated care provider (UCP). The nurse instructs the UCP to:
- Keep the head of the bed elevated a minimum of 30 degrees (preferably 45 degrees) for 1 hour after medication administration (follow employer policy).

- Report immediately to the nurse coughing, choking, gagging, or drooling of liquid or dissolved pills.
- Report to the nurse occurrence of possible medication adverse effects (specific to medication).

Equipment
- Medication administration record (MAR) (electronic or printed)
- Appropriate medication syringe or 60-mL Asepto syringe for large-bore tubes only
- Enteral-only connector (ENFit) designed to fit the specific enteral tube (Fig. 21.1)
- Gastric pH test strip (scale of 1 to 11)
- Graduated container
- Medication to be administered
- Pill crusher if medication in tablet form
- Water or sterile water for immunocompromised patients
- Tongue blade or straw to stir dissolved medication
- Clean gloves
- Stethoscope and pulse oximeter (for evaluation)

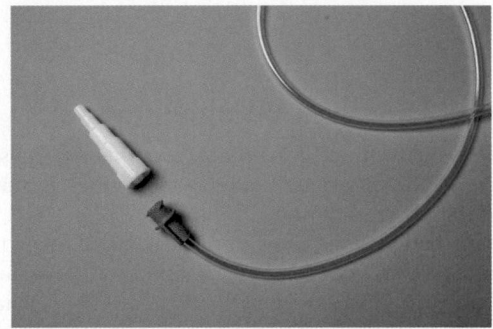

FIG 21.1 Enteral connector.

STEP	RATIONALE

ASSESSMENT

1. Check accuracy and completeness of each MAR with health care provider's medication prescription. Check patient's name, medication name and dosage, route of administration, and time for administration. Clarify incomplete or unclear prescriptions with health care provider before administration.

2. Review pertinent information related to medication, including action, purpose, normal dose and route, adverse effects, time of onset and peak action, and nursing implications.

3. Assess for any contraindications to receiving enteral medications, including presence of bowel inflammation, reduced peristalsis, recent gastrointestinal (GI) surgery, and gastric suction that cannot be turned off.

4. Assess patient's medical, medication, and diet history and history of allergies. List patient's food and medication allergies on each page of the MAR and prominently display it on the patient's medical record per employer policy. When patient has allergy, provide allergy bracelet. If you identify contraindications, withhold medication and inform health care provider.

The health care provider's prescription is the most reliable source and only legal record of medications that patient is to receive. Ensures that patient receives correct medication (Basukala et al., 2017). Handwritten MARs are a source of medication errors (Basukala et al., 2017).

Allows you to anticipate effects of medication and observe patient's response.

Alterations in GI function can interfere with medication absorption, distribution, and excretion. Patients with GI suction do not benefit from medication because it may be suctioned from the GI track before it is absorbed.

Information reflects patient's need for and potential responses to medications. Information also indicates potential food and medication interactions. Some medications may require tube feeding to be stopped for an hour before and 2 hours after dose (Burchum & Rosenthal, 2016). Communication of allergies is essential for safe, effective care.

STEP	RATIONALE

ASSESSMENT

5. For postoperative patient, review postoperative prescriptions for type of enteral tube care.

Manipulation and irrigation of tube or instillation of medications may be contraindicated.

6. Gather and review physical assessment data (e.g., bowel sounds, abdominal distension) and laboratory data (e.g., renal and liver function) that may influence medication administration.

Physical examination findings or laboratory data may contraindicate medication administration.

7. Check with pharmacy for availability of liquid preparation for patient's medications. Prescriber may need to change dosage form.

When possible, liquid formulation of the medication is the best option. The employer pharmacy may have the ability to provide a liquid preparation that is compatible with the enteral nutrition formula.

8. Before administration of enteral medications, verify placement of feeding tube (see Skill 32.2) and determine that tube is placed in the stomach or small intestine correctly.

Reduces risk for aspiration.
Ensures that point of medication absorption is not bypassed by feeding tube. For example, some medications (e.g., antacids) are absorbed in the stomach. If the patient's tube is placed in the intestines, these medications are not absorbed because the stomach is bypassed by the tube (McIntyre & Monk, 2014).

NURSING DIAGNOSES

- Inadequate swallowing
- Inadequate feeding and/or self-care
- Potential for aspiration

Related factors/Risk factors are individualized on the basis of patient's condition or needs.

PLANNING

1. Expected outcomes following completion of procedure:
   - Patient experiences desired medication effect within period of onset of medication.

   Medication has exerted its therapeutic action.

   - Patient's feeding tube remains patent after administration of medication.

   Patent enteral tube indicates passage of medication into stomach, ensuring proper absorption. If tube becomes blocked, administration of other medications and feedings is not possible.

   - Patient does not aspirate during or after medication administration.

   Patient safety in medication administration is maintained.

2. Collect appropriate equipment and MAR.

   Ensures time management and efficiency.

IMPLEMENTATION

1. Perform hand hygiene. Prepare medications for instillation into feeding tube (see Skill 21.1). Check medication label against MAR two times (when removing medication from drawer/cabinet and prior to preparing medication for administration). Fill graduated container with 50 to 100 mL of tepid water. Use sterile water for immunocompromised or critically ill patients (Allen, 2015; White & Bradman, 2015).

These are the first and second checks for accuracy. Preparation process ensures that right patient receives right medication. Tepid water prevents abdominal cramping, which can occur with cold water.

Clinical Decision Point *Whenever possible, use liquid medications instead of crushed tablets. If you have to crush tablets, flush the tubing before and after the medication administration to prevent the medication from adhering to the inside of the tube. In addition, make sure that concentrated medications are thoroughly diluted. Never add crushed medications directly to a tube feeding (White & Bradman, 2015).*

   a. *Tablets:* Crush each tablet into a fine powder, using pill-crushing device or two medication cups (see Skill 21.1). Dissolve each tablet in separate cup of 30 mL of warm water.

   Fine powder dissolves more easily, reducing chance of occluding feeding tube.

STEP	RATIONALE

IMPLEMENTATION

b. *Capsules:* Ensure that contents of capsule (granules or gelatin) can be expressed from covering (consult with pharmacist). Apply gloves and open capsule or pierce gel cap with sterile needle and empty contents into 30 mL of warm water (or solution designated by manufacturer). Gel caps dissolve in warm water, but this may take 15 to 20 minutes.

Ensures that contents of capsules are in solution to prevent occlusion of tube.

c. Prepare liquid medication according to Skill 21.1.

2. Take medication(s) to patient at correct time (see employer policy). Medications that require exact timing include stat, first-time or loading doses, and one-time doses. Give time-critical scheduled medications (e.g., antibiotics, anticoagulants, insulin, anticonvulsants, immunosuppressive) at exact time prescribed (no later than 30 minutes before or after scheduled dose). Give non–time-critical scheduled medications within a range of 1 or 2 hours of scheduled dose, according to employer policy (ISMP, 2011). During administration, apply 10 rights of medication administration. Perform hand hygiene.

Hospitals must adopt medication administration policy and procedure for timing of medication administration that considers nature of the prescribed medication, specific clinical application, and patient needs. Time-critical scheduled medications are those for which early or delayed administration of maintenance doses of greater than 30 minutes before or after the scheduled dose may cause harm or result in substantial suboptimal therapy or pharmacological effect. Non–time-critical medications are those for which early or delayed administration within a specified range of either 1 or 2 hours should not cause harm or result in substantial suboptimal therapy or pharmacological effect (ISMP, 2011).

3. Identify patient using at least two person-specific identifiers (e.g., name and date of birth or name and medical record number) according to employer policy. Compare identifiers with information on patient's MAR or medical record and ID band. Replace missing or faded ID bands.

Ensures correct patient. Complies with Accreditation Canada's standards and improves patient safety (Accreditation Canada, 2019).

4. At patient's bedside again compare MAR or computer printout with names of medications on medication labels and patient name. Ask patient if they have allergies.

Ensures that the right patient receives correct medication. Confirms patient's allergy history.

5. Explain procedure to patient and discuss purpose of each medication, action, and possible adverse effects. Allow patient to ask any questions about the medications.

Helps patient be a participant in care, which minimizes anxiety. Patient has right to be informed, and patient's understanding of each medication improves adherence to medication therapy. Begins patient teaching regarding medications.

6. Assist patient to sitting position. Elevate head of bed to minimum of 30 degrees and preferably 45 degrees (unless contraindicated) or sit patient up in a chair (Schiele et al., 2015).

Reduces risk for aspiration, keeping head above stomach.

7. If continuous enteral tube feeding is infusing, adjust infusion pump setting to hold tube feeding. If the patient needs to take the medication on an empty stomach or if the medication is not compatible with the feeding solution, stop the feeding 15 to 30 minutes before medication administration.

Feeding solution should not infuse while residuals are checked or while medications are administered. The presence of a feeding solution may impede medication absorption (Klang, McLymont, & Ng, 2013).

8. Apply clean gloves. Check placement of feeding tube (see Skill 32.2) by observing gastric contents and checking pH of aspirate contents. *Gastric pH less than 5.0 is a good indicator that tip of tube is correctly placed in stomach* (Clifford, Heimall, Brittingham, et al., 2015).

Ensures proper tube placement and reduces risk of introducing fluids into respiratory tract.

9. Check for gastric residual volume (GRV). Draw up 10 to 30 mL of air into a 60-mL syringe and connect syringe to feeding tube. Flush tube with air and pull back slowly to aspirate gastric contents (see illustration). Determine GRV using either scale on syringe or a graduate container. Return aspirated contents to stomach unless a single GRV exceeds 250 mL (see employer policy). When GRV is excessive, hold medication and contact health care provider. The frequency of determining GRV may vary; check your employer's policy.

Large residuals indicate delayed gastric emptying and put patient at increased risk for aspiration (Malone, 2014).

STEP	RATIONALE

IMPLEMENTATION

10. Irrigate the tubing.

   a. Pinch or clamp enteral tube and remove syringe. Draw up 30 mL of water into syringe. Reinsert tip of syringe into tube, release clamp, and flush tubing. Clamp tube again and remove syringe.

Pinching or clamping tubing prevents leakage or spillage of stomach contents. Flushing ensures that tube is patent.

   b. Using the appropriate enteral connector (see Fig. 21.1), attach to enteral tube.

Standardization of connector tubing improves patient safety. Tubing standards are designed to reduce tubing misconnections that can result in patient injury (Lord, 2018).

Clinical Decision Point *Verify that the connector meets the ISO tubing connector standards. Do not attach the enteral tubing to a standardized Luer syringe or needleless device (Guenther, 2015).*

11. Remove bulb or plunger of syringe and reinsert syringe into tip of feeding tube.

Removal of bulb or plunger prepares syringe for delivery of medications.

12. Administer dose of first liquid or dissolved medication by pouring into syringe (see illustration). Allow to flow by gravity.

Clinical Decision Point *Sometimes it is necessary to transfer oral medications into a medication cup for enteral administration. If medication does not flow freely, raise the height of the syringe to increase the rate of flow or try having the patient change position slightly because the end of the feeding tube may be against the gastric mucosa. If these measures do not improve the flow, a gentle push with bulb of Asepto syringe or plunger of the syringe may facilitate flow of fluid.*

   a. If giving only one dose of medication, flush tubing with 30 to 60 mL of water after administration.

Maintains patency of enteral tube and ensures that medication passes through tube to stomach (White & Bradman, 2015).

   b. To administer more than one medication, give each separately and flush between medications with 15 to 30 mL of water.

Allows for accurate identification of medication if dose is spilled. In addition, some medications may be incompatible, and giving medication separately followed by a flush solution decreases the risk for medication incompatibilities (White & Bradman, 2015).

   c. Follow last dose of medication with 30 to 60 mL of water.

Maintains patency of enteral tube and ensures passage of medication into stomach (White & Bradman, 2015).

13. Clamp proximal end of feeding tube if tube feeding is not being administered and cap end of tube.

Prevents air from entering stomach between medication doses.

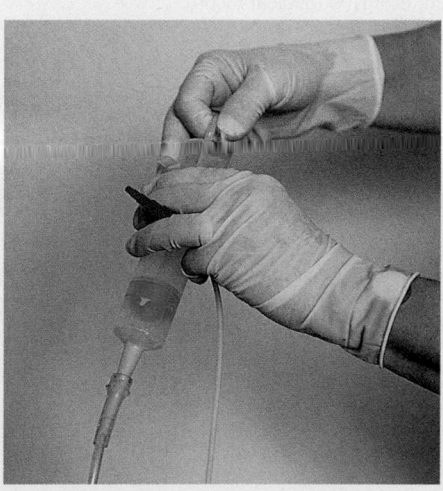

STEP 9 Aspirate stomach contents for residual volume.

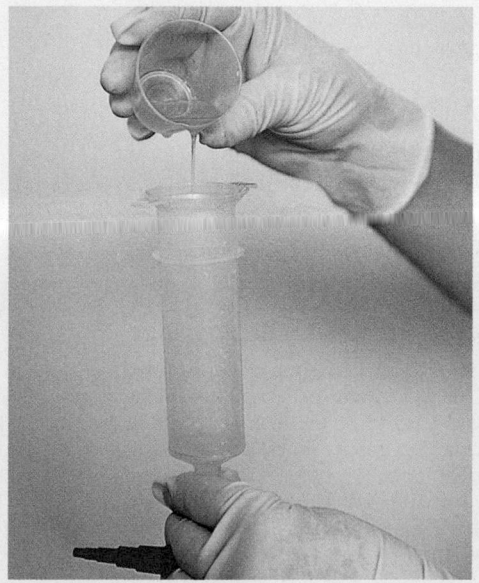

STEP 12 Pour liquid medication into syringe.

STEP	RATIONALE

IMPLEMENTATION

14. When continuous tube feeding is being administered by infusion pump, follow medication administration. If medications are not compatible with feeding solution, hold feeding for additional 30 to 60 minutes (White & Bradman, 2015).

Allows for adequate absorption of medication and avoids potential medication–food interaction between medication and enteral feeding (White & Bradman, 2015).

15. Help patient to comfortable position and keep head of bed elevated for 1 hour (see employer policy).

Reduces risk of aspiration.

16. Dispose of soiled supplies, rinse graduated container and syringe with tap water, remove and dispose of gloves, and perform hand hygiene.

Reduces spread of microorganisms.

EVALUATION

1. Observe patient for signs of aspiration, such as choking, gurgling, gurgling speech, breath sounds, and difficulty breathing.

Provides for prompt intervention if aspiration has occurred.

2. Return within 30 minutes to evaluate patient's response to medications.

Monitoring patient's response evaluates therapeutic benefit of medication and helps detect onset of adverse effects or allergic reactions.

3. Use Teach-Back: "I want to be sure I explained clearly why your father must take his medications through his feeding tube. Tell me why he is receiving his medications through his feeding tube." Develop a revised teaching plan if caregiver is not able to teach back correctly.

Determines caregiver's level of understanding of instructional topic.

Unexpected Outcomes

1. Patient exhibits signs of aspiration, including respiratory distress, changes in vital signs, or changes in oxygen saturation.

2. Patient does not receive medication because of blocked enteral tube.

3. Patient exhibits adverse effects or allergic reaction.

Related Interventions

- Stop all medications/fluids through feeding tube.
- Elevate head of bed and stay with patient.
- Assess vital signs and breath sounds while another staff member notifies health care provider.
- For newly inserted tube, notify health care provider and obtain X-ray film confirmation of placement.
- Requires interventions to unclog tube to ensure medication delivery (Box 21.3).
- Withhold further doses.
- Always notify health care provider and pharmacy when patient exhibits adverse effects.
- Symptoms such as urticaria, rash, pruritus, rhinitis, and wheezing indicate allergic reaction.
- Enter patient allergy in medical record.

BOX 21.3

Unclogging a Blocked Feeding Tube

- Prevent tube from becoming blocked by flushing it with at least 15 to 30 mL of tepid water before and after administering each dose of medication, 30 to 60 mL after last dose of medication, before and after checking gastric residual volumes, and every 4 to 12 hours around the clock (refer to employer policies).
- Gently flush tube with large-bore syringe and warm water. Do not use small-bore syringe because this exerts too much pressure and may rupture tube.

- If irrigation with water is not effective, obtain a prescription for a pancrelipase tablet and follow manufacturer guidelines for tube irrigation. In addition, a declogging stylus may be used (see employer policy).
- The tube may have to be removed, and a new one inserted if the medication is urgent.

Modified from Blumenstein, I., Shastri, Y. M., & Stein, J. (2014). Gastroenteric tube feeding: Techniques, problems and solutions. *World Journal of Gastroenterology,* 20(26), 8505. doi:10.3748/wjg.v20.i26.8505.

Communication and Documentation

- Document in nurses' notes in electronic health record (EHR) or chart the method used to check placement of enteral tube, GRV, and pH of stomach aspirate.
- Document actual time that each medication was administered on MAR immediately after administration, not before. Include initials or signature.
- Document patient's response to medication, patient teaching, and validation of patient understanding on flow sheet or in nurses' notes in EHR or chart.
- Document total amount of water used for medication administration on proper intake and output (I&O) form.
- Report and document adverse effects, patient response, and/or withheld medications to nurse in charge or health care provider.

Special Considerations
Teaching

- Teach patient or caregiver how to store medications and tube-feeding supplements (see Chapter 32).
- Demonstrate to patient or caregiver how to prepare medications, including crushing them if appropriate.
- Demonstrate to patient or caregiver how to verify correct placement of tube.
- Teach patient or caregiver the importance of consistent flushing of feeding tube before and after medication administration.

Pediatric

- Volumes for instillation of medications or for irrigation of enteral tubes should be small enough to clear tubing (Perry, Hockenberry, Lowdermilk, et al., 2017).

✦ SKILL 21.3 Applying Topical Medications to the Skin

▶ *Video Clip* **NSO** *Nursing Skills Online Administration of Nonparenteral Medications Module 6 / Lesson 3*

Topical administration of medication involves applying medications locally to the skin, mucous membranes, or tissues. Topical medications such as lotions, transdermal patches, pastes, and ointments primarily produce local effects; but they can create systemic effects if absorbed through the skin. Systemic effects are more likely to occur if the skin is thin, medication concentration is high, contact with the skin is prolonged, or the medication is applied to skin that is not intact. In addition, skin hydration and environmental humidity affect percutaneous absorption of a medication. An increase in skin hydration increases absorption (Lawton, 2013). Apply topical medications using gloves and applicators to protect from accidental exposure. Skin encrustations and dead tissue harbour microorganisms and block contact of medications with the affected tissue or membrane.

Never apply new medication over a previously applied medication because it will decrease the therapeutic benefit to a patient. Always clean the skin or wound thoroughly before applying a new dose of a topical medication. Apply each type of medication, whether an ointment, lotion, powder, or patch, in a specific way to ensure proper penetration and absorption (Lawton, 2013).

Delegation and Collaboration

The skill of administering most topical medications, including skin patches, cannot be delegated to an unregulated care provider (UCP).

However, some facilities (e.g., long-term care) may allow UCPs to apply some forms of topical medications (e.g., skin barriers) to irritated skin or for the protection of the perineum during morning or perineal care. Check employer policies. The nurse instructs the UCP to:
- Report immediately to the nurse any patient skin irritation, burning, blistering, or increased itching.
- Not apply any dressing over the topical medication unless instructed to do so.

Equipment

- Medication administration record (MAR) (electronic or printed)
- Clean gloves (for intact skin) or sterile gloves (for nonintact skin)
- Cotton-tipped applicators or tongue blades (*optional*)
- Prescribed medication (powder, cream, lotion, ointment, spray, patch)
- Basin of warm water, washcloth, towel, nondrying soap
- Sterile dressing, tape (if needed)
- Felt-tip pen (*optional*)
- Plastic wrap, transparent dressing (if prescribed) (*optional*)

STEP	RATIONALE
ASSESSMENT	
1. Check accuracy and completeness of each MAR with health care provider's medication prescription. Check patient's name, medication name and dosage, route of administration, and time for administration. Clarify incomplete or unclear prescriptions with health care provider before administration.	The prescription sheet is the most reliable source and only legal record of medications that patient is to receive. It ensures that patient receives correct medications (Basukala et al., 2017). Handwritten MARs are a source of medication errors (Basukala et al., 2017).
2. Review pertinent information related to medication, including action, purpose, normal dose and route, adverse effects, time of onset and peak action, and nursing implications.	Allows you to anticipate effects of medication and observe patient's response.

STEP	RATIONALE

ASSESSMENT

3. Assess condition of skin or membrane where medication is to be applied (see Chapter 8). If there is an open wound, perform hand hygiene and apply clean gloves. First wash site thoroughly with mild, nondrying soap and warm water, rinse, and dry. Be sure to remove any previously applied medication or debris. Also remove any blood, body fluids, secretions, or excretions. Assess for symptoms of skin irritation such as pruritus or burning. Remove gloves when finished. Perform hand hygiene.

Cleaning site thoroughly promotes proper assessment of skin surface. Assessment provides baseline to determine change in condition of skin after therapy. Application of certain topical medications can lessen or aggravate these symptoms.

Cleaning removes any residual medication from the previous dose, which reduces potential adverse medication reactions or skin irritation (Cohen, 2013).

4. Assess patient's medical and medication history and history of allergies (including latex and topical medication). Ask if patient has had reaction to a cream or lotion applied to skin. List medication allergies on each page of the MAR and display it prominently on the patient's medical record per employer policy. When patient has allergy, provide allergy bracelet.

Information reflects patient's need for and potential responses to medications. Allergic contact dermatitis is relatively common and can worsen dermatological (skin) condition. In addition, some patients may be allergic to preservatives or fragrances in topical medications. Latex allergy requires use of nonlatex gloves. Communication of allergies is essential for safe and effective care.

5. Determine amount of topical medication required for application by assessing skin site, reviewing health care provider's prescription, and reading application directions carefully (a thin, even layer is usually adequate).

An excessive amount of topical medication can irritate skin chemically, negate effectiveness of medication, and/or cause adverse systemic effects such as decreased white blood cell (WBC) counts.

6. Assess patient's knowledge of action and purpose of medication being given, application schedule, and willingness to adhere to medication regimen.

Reveals patient's level of understanding and whether instruction is necessary.

7. Determine if patient or caregiver is physically able to apply medication by assessing grasp, hand strength, reach, and coordination.

Necessary if patient is to self-administer medication at home.

NURSING DIAGNOSES

- Inadequate knowledge regarding medication and medication application
- Pain (acute or chronic)
- Reduced physical mobility
- Reduced skin integrity
- Readiness for enhanced self-health management
- Potential for infection

Related factors/Risk factors are individualized on the basis of patient's condition or needs.

PLANNING

1. Expected outcomes following completion of procedure:
   - Patient is able to identify medication and describe action, purpose, dose, adverse effects, and schedule of medication.

   Demonstrates learning.

   - Patient is able to apply medication without help on prescribed schedule.

   Demonstrates learning and adherence.

   - With repeated applications, skin becomes clear, without inflammation or drainage from lesions.

   Existing lesions heal and/or disappear as result of therapeutic action of medication.

2. Collect appropriate equipment and MAR.

   Ensures time management and efficiency.

IMPLEMENTATION

1. Perform hand hygiene. Prepare medications for application. Check label of medication against MAR two times (when removing medication from drawer/cabinet and prior to preparing medication for administration; see Skill 21.1). Preparation usually involves taking bottle or tube of lotion, cream, ointment, or patch out of storage and to patient's room. Check expiration date on container.

Reduces transmission of infection. *These are the first and second checks for accuracy.* Process ensures that right patient receives right medication.

STEP	RATIONALE

IMPLEMENTATION

2. Take medication(s) to patient at correct time (see employer policy). Medications that require exact timing include stat, first-time or loading doses, and one-time doses. Give time-critical scheduled medications (e.g., antibiotics, anticoagulants, insulin, anticonvulsants, immunosuppressive medications) at exact time prescribed (no later than 30 minutes before or after scheduled dose). Give non–time-critical scheduled medications within a range of 1 or 2 hours of scheduled dose, according to employer policy (ISMP, 2011). During administration, apply 10 rights of medication administration. Close room curtain or door. Perform hand hygiene.

Agencies must adopt medication administration policies for timing of medication administration that considers nature of the prescribed medication, specific clinical application, and patient needs. Time-critical scheduled medications are those for which early or delayed administration of maintenance doses of greater than 30 minutes before or after the scheduled dose may cause harm or result in substantial suboptimal therapy or pharmacological effect. Non–time-critical medications are those for which early or delayed administration within a specified range of either 1 or 2 hours should not cause harm or result in substantial suboptimal therapy or pharmacological effect (ISMP, 2011).

3. Help patient to comfortable position. Arrange supplies at bedside.

Allows easy access to application site.

4. Identify patient using at least two person-specific identifiers (e.g., name and date of birth or name and medical record number) according to employer policy. Compare identifiers with information on patient's MAR or medical record and ID band. Replace missing or faded ID bands.

Ensures correct patient. Complies with Accreditation Canada's standards and improves patient safety (Accreditation Canada, 2019).

5. At patient's bedside again compare MAR or computer printout with names of medications on medication labels and patient name. Ask patient if they have allergies.

Ensures that the right patient receives correct medication. Confirms patient's allergy history.

6. Explain procedure to patient and discuss purpose of each medication, action, and possible adverse effects. Allow patient to ask any questions about the medications.

Demonstrates person-centred care, which minimizes anxiety. Patient has the right to be informed, and their understanding of each medication improves adherence to medication therapy. Begins patient teaching regarding medications.

7. If skin is broken, apply sterile gloves. Otherwise apply clean gloves.

Reduces spread of microorganisms.

8. Apply topical creams, ointments, and oil-based lotions.

   a. Expose affected area while keeping unaffected areas covered.

   Provides visualization for application and protects privacy.

   b. Wash, rinse, and dry affected area before applying medication if not done earlier (see Assessment, Step 3).

   Cleaning removes microorganisms from remaining debris and any surface medication.

   c. If skin is excessively dry and flaking, apply topical medication while skin is still damp.

   Increased skin hydration and surface humidity enhance absorption of topical medication (Lawton, 2013).

   d. After washing, remove gloves, perform hand hygiene, and apply new clean or sterile gloves.

   Sterile gloves are used when applying medications to open, noninfectious skin lesions. Changing gloves prevents cross-contamination of infected or contagious lesions. Gloves also protect you from topical absorption of the medication and subsequent medication effects (Lawton, 2013).

   e. Place required amount of medication in palm of gloved hand and soften by rubbing briskly between hands.

   Softening topical medications makes it easier to spread on skin.

   f. Tell patient that initial application of medications may feel cold. Once medication is softened, spread it evenly over skin surface, using long, even strokes that follow direction of hair growth. Do not vigorously rub skin. Apply to thickness specified by manufacturer instructions.

   Ensures even distribution and sufficient dosage of medication. Technique prevents irritation of hair follicles.

   g. Explain to patient that skin may feel greasy after application.

   Ointments often contain oils.

9. Technique for applying antianginal (nitroglycerin) ointment.

   a. Remove previous dose paper. Fold used paper containing any residual medication with used sides together and dispose of it in biohazard garbage container. Wipe off residual medication with tissue.

   Prevents overdose that can occur with multiple-dose papers left in place. Proper disposal protects you and others from accidental exposure to medication.

   b. Write date, time, and your initials on new application paper.

   Label provides reference to prevent missing doses.

STEP	RATIONALE

IMPLEMENTATION

c. Antianginal (nitroglycerin) ointments are usually prescribed in inches and can be measured on small sheets of paper marked off in 1.25 cm (1/2 inch) markings. Unit-dose packages are available. Apply desired number of inches of ointment to paper-measuring guide (see illustration).

Ensures correct dose of medication.

Clinical Decision Point *Unit-dose packages are available.* **NOTE:** *One package equals 2.5 cm (1 inch); smaller amounts should not be measured from this package.*

d. Select new application site, rotate sites: apply nitroglycerin to chest area, back, abdomen, or anterior thigh (Burchum & Rosenthal, 2016). Do not apply on nonintact skin or hairy surfaces or over scar tissue.

Application sites are rotated to reduce skin irritation. Application on nonintact skin may result in increased absorption of medication. Application on hairy surfaces or scar tissue may decrease absorption (Burchum & Rosenthal, 2016).

e. Apply ointment to skin surface by holding edge or back of paper-measuring guide and placing ointment and wrapper directly on skin (see illustration). Do not rub or massage ointment into skin.

Minimizes chance of ointment covering gloves and later touching nurse's hands. Medication is designed to absorb slowly over several hours; massaging increases absorption rate.

f. Secure ointment and paper with transparent dressing or strip of tape. Apply dressing or plastic wrap only when instructed by pharmacy (Lawton, 2013).

Prevents staining of clothing or inadvertent removal of medication. Covering topical medications with dressing or plastic wrap increases heat and skin humidity and rate of absorption of medication (Cohen, 2013; Lawton, 2013).

10. Technique for applying transdermal patches (e.g., analgesic, nicotine, nitroglycerin, estrogen).
a. If old patch is present, remove it and clean area. Be sure to check between skinfolds for patch.

Failure to remove old patch can result in overdose. Many patches are small, clear, or flesh coloured and can be easily hidden between skinfolds. Cleaning removes residual medication traces of previous patch.

b. Dispose of old patch by folding in half with sticky sides together. Some facilities require patch to be cut before disposal (see employer policy). Dispose of it in biohazard garbage bag.

Proper disposal prevents accidental exposure to medication.

c. Date and initial outer side of new patch before applying it and note time of administration. Use soft-tip or felt-tipped pen.

Visual reminder prevents missing or extra doses. Ballpoint pen damages patch and alters medication delivery.

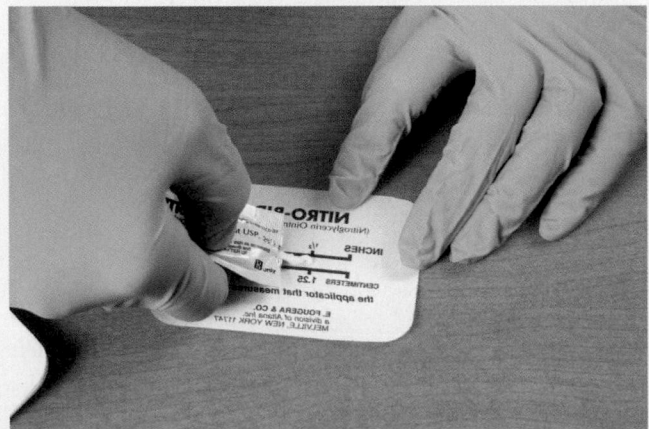

STEP 9c Ointment spread in centimetres/inches over measuring guide.

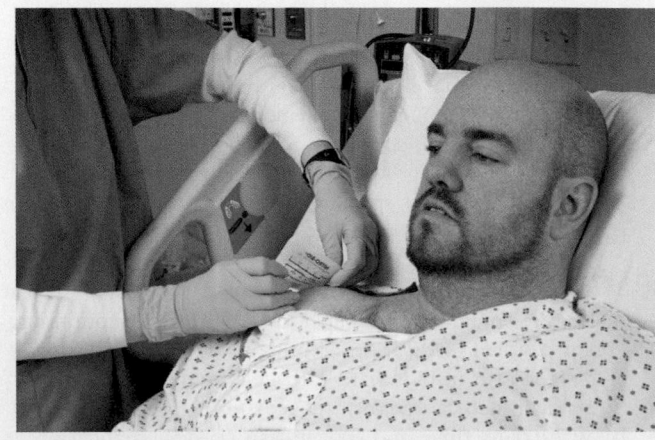

STEP 9e Nurse applies wrapper with medication to patient's skin.

STEP	RATIONALE

IMPLEMENTATION

d. Choose a new site that is clean, intact, dry, and free of hair. Some patches have specific instructions for placement locations (e.g., Testoderm patches are placed on scrotum; a scopolamine patch is placed behind the ear; *never apply* an estrogen patch to breast tissue or waistline). Do not apply patch on skin that is oily, burned, cut, or irritated in any way.	Ensures complete medication absorption. Estrogen patches should never be placed on the breast, genitals, or other reproductive organs. There is a risk for systemic absorption of the hormone, which can increase patient's risk for breast, testicular, or ovarian cancers (Cohen, 2013).
e. Carefully remove patch from its protective covering by pulling off liner. Hold patch by edge without touching adhesive edges.	Touching only edges ensures that patch will adhere to the skin and that medication dose has not changed. Removing protective covering allows medication to be absorbed through skin.
f Apply patch. Hold palm of one hand firmly over patch for 10 seconds. Make sure that it sticks well, especially around edges. Apply overlay if provided with patch.	Adequate adhesion prevents loss of patch, which results in decreased dose and effectiveness.

Clinical Decision Point *Never apply heat, such as with a heating pad, over a transdermal patch because this results in an increased rate of absorption with potentially serious adverse effects (Cohen, 2013; Lawton, 2013).*

g. Do not apply patch to previously used sites for at least 1 week.	Rotation of site reduces skin irritation from medication and adhesive (Lawton, 2013).
h. Instruct patient that transdermal patches are never to be cut in half; a change in dose would require prescription for new strength of transdermal medication.	Cutting transdermal patch in half would alter intended medication delivery of transdermal system, resulting in inadequate or altered medication levels.

Clinical Decision Point *It is recommended to have a daily "patch-free" interval of 10 to 12 hours because tolerance develops if patches are used 24 hours a day every day (Burchum & Rosenthal, 2016). Apply a new patch each morning, leave in place for 12 to 14 hours, and remove in the evening. This applies only to certain types of patches; for example, pain patches should not have a "patch-free" break to ensure consistent pain management.*

i. Instruct patient to always remove old patch and clean skin before applying new one. Patients should not use alternative forms of medication when using patches. For example, patients should not apply nitroglycerin ointment in addition to patch unless specifically prescribed to do so by their health care provider.	Use of patch with additional or alternative medication preparation can result in toxicity or other adverse effects.
11. Technique for administering aerosol sprays (e.g., local anaesthetic sprays).	
a. Shake container vigorously. Read container label for distance recommended to hold spray away from area, usually 15 to 30 cm (6 to 12 inches).	Mixing ensures delivery of fine, even spray. Proper distance ensures that fine spray hits skin surface. Holding container too close results in thin, watery distribution.
b. Ask patient to turn face away from spray or briefly cover face with towel while spraying neck or chest.	Prevents inhalation of spray.
c. Spray medication evenly over affected site (in some cases, time spray for a period of seconds).	Ensures that affected area of skin is covered with thin spray.
12. Technique for applying suspension-based lotion:	
a. Shake container vigorously.	Mixes powder throughout liquid to form well-mixed suspension.
b. Apply small amount of lotion to small gauze dressing or pad and apply to skin by stroking evenly in direction of hair growth.	Method of application leaves protective film of powder on skin after water base of suspension dries. Technique prevents irritation to hair follicles.
c. Explain to patient that area will feel cool and dry.	Water evaporates to leave thin layer of powder.
13. Technique for applying powder:	
a. Be sure that skin surface is thoroughly dry. With your nondominant hand, fully spread apart any skinfolds such as between toes or under axilla and dry with towel.	Minimizes caking and crusting of powder. Fully exposes skin surface for application.
b. If area of application is near face, ask patient to turn face away from powder or briefly cover face with towel.	Prevents inhalation of powder.
c. Dust skin site lightly with dispenser so area is covered with fine, thin layer of powder. *Option:* Cover skin area with dressing if prescribed by health care provider.	Thin layer of powder has slight lubricating properties, which reduces friction and promotes drying (Burchum & Rosenthal, 2016).

STEP	RATIONALE

IMPLEMENTATION

14. Help patient to comfortable position, reapply gown, and cover with bed linen as desired.

Provides for patient's sense of well-being.

15. Dispose of soiled supplies in receptacle especially designated for such articles, remove and dispose of gloves, and perform hand hygiene.

Keeps patient's environment neat and reduces spread of infection and residual medication to others.

EVALUATION

1. Inspect condition of skin between applications.

Determines if skin condition is improving or verifies that skin is intact and not irritated.

2. Have patient keep diary of doses taken.

Confirms adherence to prescribed therapy.

3. Observe patient or caregiver apply topical medication.

Return demonstration measures learning.

4. Use Teach-Back: "I want to be sure I explained the action of the dose of medicine you are taking and the side effects of cortisone cream medication. In your own words, tell me how the medication works, your correct dose, and any side effects." Develop a revised teaching plan if patient or caregiver is not able to teach back correctly.

Determines patient's and caregiver's level of understanding of instructional topic.

Unexpected Outcomes

1. Skin site appears inflamed and edematous with blistering and oozing of fluid from lesions. These signs indicate subacute inflammation or eczema that can develop if skin lesions are getting worse.
2. Patient is unable to explain information about medication or does not administer as prescribed.
3. Patient continues to complain of tenderness and/or pruritus. Can indicate slow or impaired healing.

Related Interventions

- Hold medication.
- Notify health care provider; alternative therapies may be needed.

- Identify possible reasons for nonadherence and explore alternative approaches or options.
- Notify health care provider; alternative therapies may be needed.

Communication and Documentation

- Document actual time that each medication was administered, type of medication applied, strength, and site of application in MAR immediately after administration, not before. Include initials or signature.
- Document patient's response to medication, patient teaching, and validation of patient's understanding on flow sheet or in nurses' notes in electronic health record (EHR) or chart.
- Document condition of skin before each application on flow sheet or in nurses' notes in EHR or chart.
- Report adverse effects and patient response and/or withheld medications to nurse in charge or health care provider. Depending on medication, immediate health care provider notification may be required.

Special Considerations
Teaching

- Instruct patient and caregiver to:
  - Not apply to irritated or damaged skin.
  - Not use heating pads, hot water bottle, or warm compresses over medication.
  - Only use a bandage or plastic wrap if instructed by a pharmacist.
  - Use medication exactly as prescribed.
  - Contact health care provider if medication comes in contact with eyes or other mucous membranes such as the mouth.
- Instruct patients to use only warm-water rinse without soap for cleaning inflamed skin.
- If a transdermal patch loosens or falls off before the next scheduled dose, refer to your health care provider's instructions or the manufacturer's instructions, according to the drug that is being administered transdermally. In general, for a loose patch, use the palm of your hand to press the patch back onto the skin (Murrell, 2018). If one edge of the patch becomes loose, use tape of a sticky adhesive film to secure the loose edge (Murrell, 2018). If the patch falls off, do not reapply it but apply a new one, either immediately or at the next scheduled dose, depending on the medication.

Gerontological

- Changes in the skin of an older person include increased fragility, wrinkling, dryness, flaking, and increased tendency to bruise. Be aware of these changes when applying topical medications to ensure proper application.

Care in the Community

- Instruct patient to wrap applicators, used patches, and similar materials and dispose of them into cardboard or plastic disposable containers. Careful disposal is necessary to ensure the safety of patient, other adults, pets, and children.

◆ SKILL 21.4 Administering Ophthalmic Medications

▶ *Video Clip* **NSO** *Nursing Skills Online Administration of Nonparenteral Medications Module 6 / Lesson 4*

Common eye (ophthalmic) medications are in the form of drops and ointments, including over-the-counter preparations such as artificial tears and vasoconstrictors. However, many patients receive prescribed ophthalmic medications for eye conditions such as glaucoma and infection and following cataract extraction. In addition, there is a third type of delivery system, the intraocular disk. Medications delivered by disk resemble a contact lens; but the disk is placed in the conjunctival sac, not on the cornea, and it remains in place for up to 1 week.

The eye is the most sensitive organ to which medications are applied. The cornea is richly supplied with sensitive nerve fibres. Care must be taken to prevent instilling medication directly onto the cornea. The conjunctival sac is much less sensitive and thus a more appropriate site for medication instillation.

Any patient receiving topical eye medications should learn correct self-administration of the medication, especially patients with glaucoma, who must often undergo lifelong medication administration for control of their disease. The nurse can easily instruct patients while administering medications. Caregivers often administer eye medications when patients are unable to manipulate applicators (e.g., arthritis or neurological condition), immediately after eye surgery, and when a patient's vision is so impaired that it is difficult to assemble needed supplies and handle applicators correctly.

Delegation and Collaboration

The skill of administering ophthalmic medications cannot be delegated to an unregulated care provider (UCP). The nurse instructs the UCP about:

- The specific potential adverse effects of medications and to report their occurrence.
- The potential for temporary burning or blurring of vision after administration of eye medications.

Equipment

- Medication administration record (MAR) (electronic or printed)
- Appropriate medication (eyedrops with sterile eyedropper, ointment tube, medicated intraocular disk)
- Clean gloves

Eyedrops/Ointment

- Cotton ball or tissue
- Wash basin filled with warm water and washcloth
- Eye patch and tape *(optional)*

STEP	RATIONALE

ASSESSMENT

1. Check accuracy and completeness of each MAR with health care provider's medication prescription. Check patient's name, medication name and dosage, route (one or both eyes), and time for administration. Clarify incomplete or unclear prescriptions with health care provider before administration.

The prescription sheet is the most reliable source and only legal record of medications that patient is to receive. Ensures that patient receives correct medications (Basukala et al., 2017).

Handwritten MARs are a source of medication errors (Basukala et al., 2017).

2. Review pertinent information related to medication, including action, purpose, normal dose and route, adverse effects, time of onset and peak action, and nursing implications.

Allows you to anticipate effects of medication and observe patient's response.

3. Assess condition of external eye structures (see Chapter 8). This may be done just before medication instillation (if drainage is present, apply clean gloves).

Provides baseline to determine if local response to medications occurs. Also indicates need to clean eye before medication application.

4. Determine whether patient has any symptoms of eye discomfort or visual impairment.

Certain eye medications act to either lessen or increase these symptoms.

5. Assess patient's medical and medication history and history of allergies (including latex). List medication allergies on each page of the MAR and prominently display it on the patient's medical record per employer policy. When patient has allergy, provide allergy bracelet.

Factors influence how certain medications act. Reveals patient's need for and likely response to medication. Communication of allergies is essential for safe and effective care.

6. Assess patient's level of consciousness (LOC) and ability to follow directions.

If patient becomes restless or combative during procedure, greater risk for accidental eye injury exists.

STEP	RATIONALE

ASSESSMENT

7. Assess patient's knowledge regarding medication therapy and desire to self-administer medication.

Indicates need for health teaching. Motivation influences teaching approach.

8. Assess patient's ability to manipulate and hold dropper or ocular disk.

Reflects patient's ability to learn to self-administer medication.

NURSING DIAGNOSES

- Inadequate knowledge regarding medication and self-administration
- Pain (acute or chronic)
- Reduced physical mobility
- Readiness for enhanced self-health management
- Potential for injury

Related factors/Risk factors are individualized on the basis of patient's condition or needs.

PLANNING

1. Expected outcomes following completion of procedure:
   - Patient experiences desired effect of medication.
   - Patient denies discomfort.
   - Patient experiences no adverse effects, and symptoms (e.g., irritation) are relieved.
   - Patient can discuss information about medication and technique correctly.
   - Patient demonstrates self-instillation of eyedrops.
2. Collect appropriate equipment and MAR.

Medication is administered correctly without injury to patient.
Medication is administered correctly without injury to patient.
Medication is distributed and absorbed properly.

Demonstrates learning.

Demonstrates learning.
Ensures time management and efficiency.

IMPLEMENTATION

1. Perform hand hygiene and prepare medications for instillation. Check label of medication against MAR two times (when removing medication from drawer/cabinet and prior to preparing medication for administration; see Skill 21.1). Preparation usually involves taking eyedrops out of refrigerator and rewarming to room temperature before administering to patient. Check expiration date on container.

Reduces transmission of infection. Warming eyedrops reduces eye irritation.
These are the first two checks for accuracy. Process ensures that right patient receives right medication.

2. Take medication(s) to patient at correct time (see employer policy). Medications that require exact timing include stat, first-time or loading doses, and one-time doses. Give time-critical scheduled medications (e.g., antibiotics, anticoagulants, insulin, anticonvulsants, immunosuppressive medications) at exact time prescribed (no later than 30 minutes before or after scheduled dose). Give non–time-critical scheduled medications within a range of 1 or 2 hours of scheduled dose, according to employer policy (ISMP, 2011). During administration, apply 10 rights of medication administration. Perform hand hygiene.

Employers must adopt medication administration policies for timing of medication administration that considers nature of the prescribed medication, specific clinical application, and patient needs. Time-critical scheduled medications are those for which early or delayed administration of maintenance doses of greater than 30 minutes before or after the scheduled dose may cause harm or result in substantial suboptimal therapy or pharmacological effect. Non–time-critical medications are those for which early or delayed administration within a specified range of either 1 or 2 hours should not cause harm or result in substantial suboptimal therapy or pharmacological effect (ISMP, 2011).

3. Help patient to comfortable sitting position. Arrange supplies at bedside.

Ensures an organized procedure.

4. Identify patient using at least two person-specific identifiers (e.g., name and date of birth or name and medical record number) according to employer policy. Compare identifiers with information on patient's MAR or medical record and ID band. Replace missing or faded ID bands.

Ensures correct patient. Complies with Accreditation Canada's standards and improves patient safety (Accreditation Canada, 2019).

5. At patient's bedside again compare MAR or computer printout with names of medications on medication labels and patient name. Ask patient if they have allergies.

Ensures that the right patient receives correct medication. Confirms patient's allergy history.

STEP	RATIONALE

ASSESSMENT

6. Explain procedure to patient and sensations to expect. Discuss purpose of each medication, action, and possible adverse effects. Allow patient to ask any questions about the medications. Patients who self-instill medications may be allowed to give drops under nurse's supervision (check employer policy). Tell patients receiving eyedrops (mydriatics) that vision will be blurred temporarily and sensitivity to light may occur.

Helps patient be a participant in care, which minimizes anxiety. Patient has the right to be informed, and patient's understanding of each medication improves adherence to medication therapy. Begins patient teaching regarding medications.

Clinical Decision Point *Instruct and reinforce that patient should not drive or operate machinery or perform any activity that requires clear vision until vision and sensitivity to light return to normal.*

7. Instill eye medications.

If administering more than one eye medication, wait 10 minutes in between medications to ensure that the first medication has had time to absorb and that the second medication does not wash out the first one. Eye ointments should be applied last.

a. Apply clean gloves. Ask patient to lie supine or sit back in chair with head slightly hyperextended, looking up.

Position provides easy access to eye for medication instillation and minimizes drainage of medication into tear duct.

Clinical Decision Point *Do not hyperextend the neck of a patient with cervical spine injury.*

b. If drainage or crusting is present along eyelid margins or inner canthus, gently wash away. Soak any dried crusts with warm, damp washcloth or cotton ball over eye for several minutes. Always wipe clean from inner to outer canthus (see illustration). Remove gloves and perform hand hygiene.

Soaking allows easy removal of crusts without applying pressure to eye. Cleaning from inner to outer canthus avoids entrance of microorganisms into lacrimal duct (Burchum & Rosenthal, 2016).

c. Explain that there might be temporary burning sensation from drops.

Corneas are highly sensitive.

d. Instill eyedrops.

(1) *Option:* Apply clean gloves if eye drainage present. Hold clean cotton ball or tissue in nondominant hand on patient's cheekbone just below lower eyelid.

Prevents transmission of infection. Cotton or tissue absorbs medication that escapes eye.

(2) With tissue or cotton ball resting below lower lid, gently press downward with thumb or forefinger against bony orbit, exposing conjunctival sac. Never press directly against patient's eyeball.

Prevents pressure and trauma to eyeball and prevents fingers from touching eye.

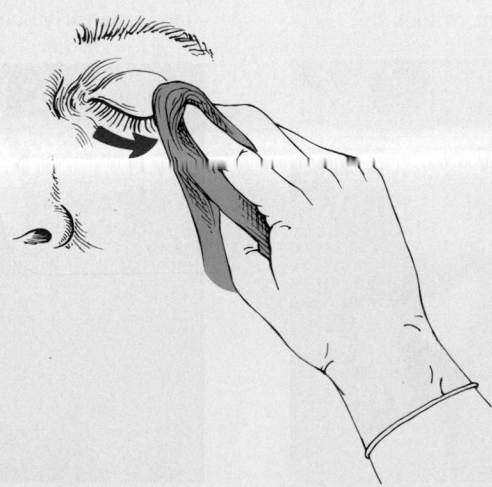

STEP 7b Clean eye, washing from inner to outer canthus before administering drops or ointment.

STEP	RATIONALE

IMPLEMENTATION

(3) Ask patient to look at ceiling. Rest dominant hand on patient's forehead; hold filled medication eyedropper approximately 1 to 2 cm (approximately ¼ to ½ inch) above conjunctival sac.

Action moves cornea up and away from conjunctival sac and reduces blink reflex. Prevents accidental contact of eyedropper with eye and reduces risk of injury and transfer of microorganisms to dropper (ophthalmic medications are sterile).

(4) Drop prescribed number of drops into conjunctival sac (see illustration).

Conjunctival sac normally holds 1 or 2 drops. Provides even distribution of medication across eye.

(5) If patient blinks or closes eye, causing drops to land on outer lid margins, repeat procedure.

Therapeutic effect of medication is obtained only when drops enter conjunctival sac.

(6) When administering drops that may cause systemic effects, apply gentle pressure to patient's nasolacrimal duct with clean tissue for 30 to 60 seconds over each eye, one at a time (see illustration). Avoid pressure directly against patient's eyeball.

Prevents overflow of medication into nasal and pharyngeal passages. Prevents absorption into systemic circulation (Shaw & Lee, 2017).

(7) After instilling drops, ask patient to close eyes gently.

Helps distribute medication. Squinting or squeezing eyelids forces medication from conjunctival sac (Shaw & Lee, 2017).

e. Instill ophthalmic ointment.

(1) *Option:* Apply clean gloves if eye drainage is present. Holding applicator above lower lid margin, apply thin ribbon of ointment evenly along inner edge of lower eyelid on conjunctiva (see illustration) from inner to outer canthus.

Reduces transmission of infection. Distributes medication evenly across eye and lid margin.

(2) Have patient close eye and rub lid lightly in circular motion with cotton ball if not contraindicated. Avoid placing pressure directly against patient's eyeball.

Further distributes medication without traumatizing eye.

(3) If excess medication is on eyelid, gently wipe it from inner to outer canthus.

Promotes comfort and prevents trauma to eye.

(4) If patient needs an eye patch, apply clean one by placing it over affected eye so entire eye is covered. Tape securely without applying pressure to eye.

Clean eye patch reduces risk of infection.

f. Insert intraocular disk.

(1) Apply clean gloves. Open package containing disk. Gently press your fingertip against disk so it adheres to your finger. It may be necessary to moisten gloved finger with sterile saline. Position convex side of disk on your fingertip.

Allows you to inspect disk for damage or deformity.

(2) With your other hand gently pull patient's lower eyelid away from eye. Ask patient to look up.

Prepares conjunctival sac for receiving medicated disk and moves sensitive cornea away.

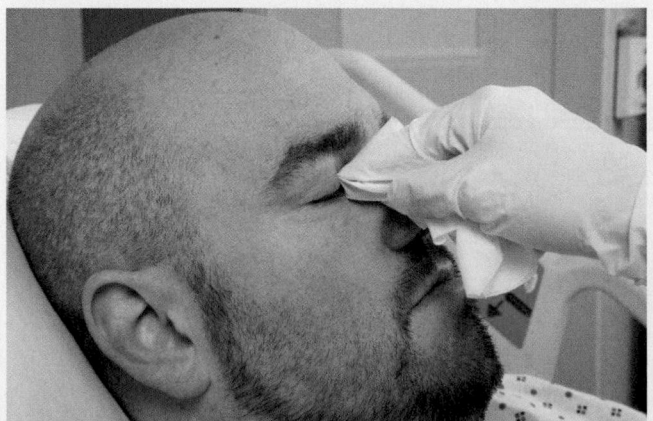

STEP 7d(6) Apply gentle pressure against nasolacrimal duct after giving eye medications.

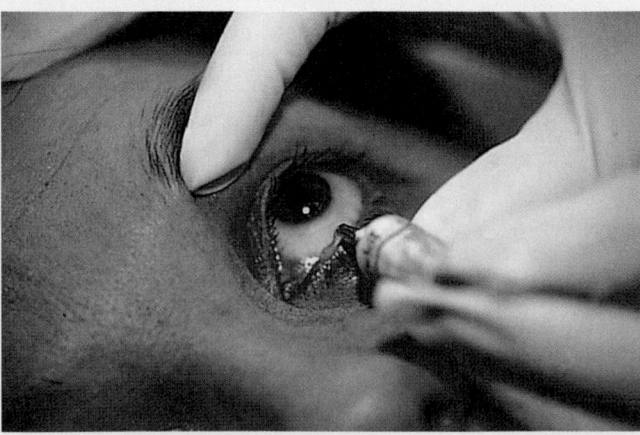

STEP 7e(1) Nurse applies ointment along inner edge of lower eyelid from inner to outer canthus.

STEP	RATIONALE

IMPLEMENTATION

    (3) Place disk in conjunctival sac so it floats on sclera between iris and lower eyelid (see illustration).   Ensures delivery of medication.

    (4) Pull patient's lower eyelid out and over disk (see illustration). You should not be able to see disk at this time. Repeat if you can see disk.   Ensures accurate medication delivery.

8. After administering eye medications, remove and dispose of gloves and soiled supplies; perform hand hygiene.   Reduces spread of microorganisms.

9. Remove intraocular disk.

    a. Perform hand hygiene and apply clean gloves. Gently pull downward on lower eyelid using your nondominant hand.   Exposes disk.

    b. Using forefinger and thumb of your dominant hand, pinch disk and lift it out of patient's eye (see illustration).

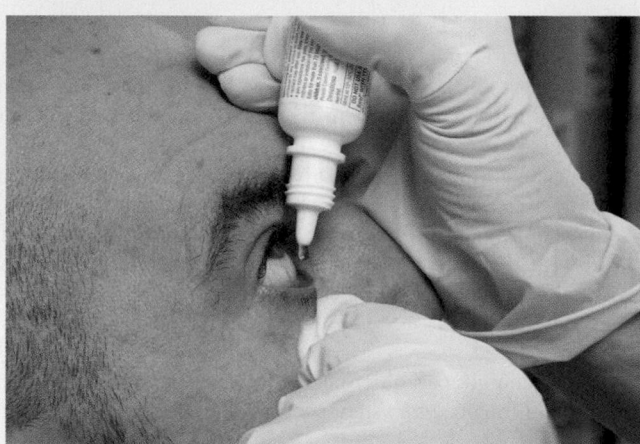

STEP 7d(4) Hold eyedropper over lower conjunctival sac.

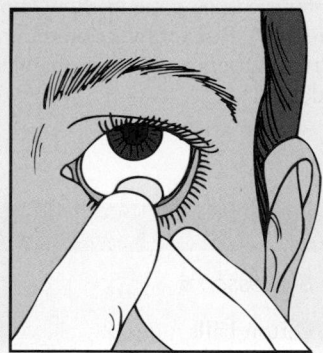

STEP 7f(3) Place intraocular disk in conjunctival sac between iris and lower eyelid.

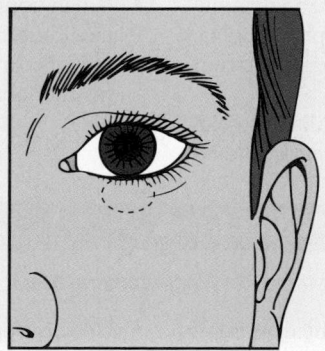

STEP 7f(4) Gently pull patient's lower eyelid over disk.

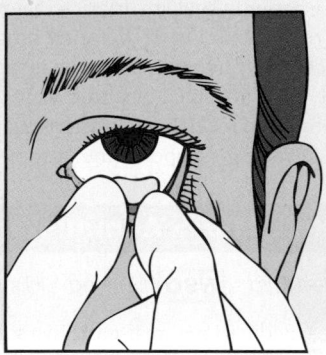

STEP 9b Carefully pinch disk to remove it from patient's eye.

EVALUATION

1. Observe response to medication by assessing visual changes, asking if symptoms are relieved, and noting any adverse effects or discomfort felt.   Evaluates effects of medication.

2. Ask patient to discuss purpose of medication, action, adverse effects, and technique of administration.   Determines patient's level of understanding.

3. Use Teach-Back: "I want to be sure I showed you how to insert the eye disk. Show me how to insert it into your left eye." Develop a revised teaching plan if patient or caregiver is not able to teach back correctly.   Determines patient's and caregiver's level of understanding of instructional topic.

STEP	RATIONALE

EVALUATION

Unexpected Outcomes

1. Patient complains of burning or pain or experiences local adverse effects (e.g., headache, bloodshot eyes, local eye irritation). Medication concentration and patient's sensitivity both influence chances of adverse effects developing.
2. Patient experiences systemic effects from drops (e.g., increased heart rate and blood pressure from epinephrine, decreased heart rate and blood pressure from timolol).
3. Patient is unable to explain medication information or steps for taking eyedrops and/or has trouble manipulating dropper.

Related Interventions

- Eyedrops may have been instilled onto cornea, or dropper touched surface of eye.
- Notify health care provider for possible adjustment in medication type and dosage.
- Notify health care provider immediately.
- Remain with patient. Assess vital signs.
- Withhold further doses.
- Repeat instructions and include caregiver as appropriate. Include return demonstration.

Communication and Documentation

- Document medication, concentration, dose or strength, number of drops, site of application (left, right, or both eyes), and time of administration on MAR immediately after administration, not before. Include initials or signature.
- Document patient teaching and validation of patient's understanding on flow sheet or in nurses' notes in electronic health record (EHR) or chart.
- Document objective data related to tissues involved (e.g., redness, drainage, irritation), any subjective data (e.g., pain, itching, altered vision), and patient's response to medications. Note any adverse effects experienced on flow sheet or in nurses' notes in EHR or chart.
- Report adverse effects and patient response and/or withheld medications to nurse in charge or health care provider. Depending on medication, immediate health care provider notification may be required.

Special Considerations

Teaching

- Warn patients that mydriatics (agent used to dilate the pupils) temporarily blur vision. Wearing sunglasses reduces photophobia. If necessary, have patient make arrangements for transportation home from an office or clinic visit.
- Patients who receive medications that paralyze the ciliary muscles of the eye (e.g., scopolamine, atropine, and cycloplegics) should

not drive or attempt to perform any activity that requires acute vision after receiving medication.

Pediatric

- Infants often clench the eyes tightly to avoid eyedrops. Place the drops at the nasal corner where the lids meet with the infant supine. When the infant opens the eye, the medication will flow into it.
- If the eye ointment is to be given once a day, administer at bedtime because it will blur the child's vision (Perry et al., 2017).
- When parents are present, have them gently hold the child's head with the child in their lap, when appropriate. Keep the child's hands away from the eyes.

Gerontological

- Before discharging an older person, evaluate patient's ability to perform all the necessary steps for the administration of eyedrops and ointments.

Care in the Community

- When using over-the-counter eyedrops, patients should not share medications with other caregivers. Risk for infection transmission is high. In addition, instruct patients to follow manufacturer instructions carefully for dosing.

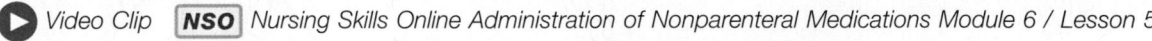

✦ SKILL 21.5   Administering Ear Medications

▶ *Video Clip* **NSO** *Nursing Skills Online Administration of Nonparenteral Medications Module 6 / Lesson 5*

Ear (otic) medications are usually in a solution and instilled by drops. When administering ear medications, be aware of certain safety precautions. Internal ear structures are very sensitive to temperature extremes; administer eardrops at room temperature. Instilling cold drops can cause vertigo (severe dizziness) or nausea and debilitate a patient for several minutes. Although structures of the outer ear are not sterile, use sterile drops and solutions in case the eardrum is ruptured. A final safety precaution is to avoid forcing any solution into the ear. Do not occlude the ear canal with a medicine dropper because this can cause pressure within the canal during instillation and subsequent injury to the eardrum. If you follow these precautions, instillation of eardrops is a safe and effective therapy.

Equipment

- Medication administration record (MAR) (electronic or printed)
- Medication bottle with dropper

- Cotton-tipped applicator, cotton balls
- Clean gloves if drainage is present

Delegation and Collaboration

The skill of administering ear medications cannot be delegated to an unregulated care provider (UCP). The nurse instructs the UCP about:

- Potential adverse effects of medications and to report their occurrence.
- The potential for dizziness or irritation after administration of ear medications.

STEP	RATIONALE

ASSESSMENT

1. Check accuracy and completeness of each MAR with health care provider's medication prescription. Check patient's name, medication name and dosage, route, and time for administration. Clarify incomplete or unclear prescriptions with health care provider before administration.

The prescription sheet is the most reliable source and only legal record of medications that patient is to receive. It ensures that patient receives correct medications (Basukala et al., 2017). Handwritten MARs are a source of medication errors (Basukala et al., 2017).

2. Review pertinent information related to medication, including action, purpose, normal dose and route (one or both ears), adverse effects, time of onset and peak action, and nursing implications.

Allows you to anticipate effects of medication and observe patient's response.

3. Assess condition of external ear structures (see Chapter 8). This may be done just before medication instillation (if drainage is present, apply clean gloves).

Provides baseline to determine if local response to medications occurs. Also indicates need to clean ear before medication application.

4. Determine whether patient has any symptoms of ear discomfort or hearing impairment.

Certain ear medications act to either lessen or increase these symptoms. Occlusion of external ear canal by swelling, drainage, or cerumen can impair hearing acuity and cause pain.

5. Assess patient's medical and medication history and history of allergies (including latex). List medication allergies on each page of the MAR and prominently display it on the patient's medical record per employer policy. When patient has allergy, provide allergy bracelet.

Factors influence how certain medications act. Reveals patient's need for medication.

Communication of allergies is essential for safe and effective care.

6. Assess patient's level of consciousness (LOC) and ability to follow directions.

If patient becomes restless or combative during procedure, greater risk for accidental ear injury exists.

7. Assess patient's knowledge regarding medication therapy and desire to self-administer medication.

Indicates need for health teaching. Motivation influences teaching approach.

8. Assess patient's ability to manipulate and hold ear dropper.

Reflects patient's ability to learn to self-administer medication.

NURSING DIAGNOSES

- Insufficient knowledge regarding medication and self-administration
- Pain (acute or chronic)
- Reduced physical mobility
- Readiness for enhanced self-health management
- Potential for injury

Related factors/Risk factors are individualized on the basis of patient's condition or needs.

PLANNING

1. Expected outcomes following completion of procedure:
   - Patient experiences desired effect of medication.
   - Patient denies discomfort.
   - Patient experiences no adverse effects, and symptoms (e.g., dizziness, ear irritation) are relieved.
   - Patient can discuss information about medication and technique correctly.
   - Patient demonstrates self-instillation of eardrops.
2. Collect appropriate equipment and MAR.

Medication is administered correctly without injury to patient.
Medication is administered correctly without injury to patient.
Medication is distributed and absorbed properly.

Demonstrates learning.

Demonstrates learning.
Ensures time management and efficiency.

IMPLEMENTATION

1. Perform hand hygiene and prepare medications for instillation. Check label of medication against MAR two times (when removing medication from drawer/cabinet and prior to preparing medication for administration; see Skill 21.1). Preparation usually involves taking eardrops out of refrigerator and rewarming to room temperature before administering to patient. Check expiration date on container.

Hand hygiene reduces transmission of infection. Ear structures are very sensitive to temperature extremes. Cold may cause vertigo and nausea.
These are the first two checks for accuracy. Process ensures that right patient receives right medication at the right time.

STEP	RATIONALE

IMPLEMENTATION

2. Take medication(s) to patient at correct time (see employer policy). Medications that require exact timing include stat, first-time or loading doses, and one-time doses. Give time-critical scheduled medications (e.g., antibiotics, anticoagulants, insulin, anticonvulsants, immunosuppressive medications) at exact time prescribed (no later than 30 minutes before or after scheduled dose). Give non–time-critical scheduled medications within a range of 1 or 2 hours of scheduled dose, according to employer policy (ISMP, 2011). During administration apply 10 rights of medication administration. Perform hand hygiene.

Hospitals must adopt medication administration policy and procedure for timing of medication administration that considers nature of the prescribed medication, specific clinical application, and patient needs. Time-critical scheduled medications are those for which early or delayed administration of maintenance doses of greater than 30 minutes before or after the scheduled dose may cause harm or result in substantial suboptimal therapy or pharmacological effect. Non–time-critical medications are those for which early or delayed administration within a specified range of either 1 or 2 hours should not cause harm or result in substantial suboptimal therapy or pharmacological effect (ISMP, 2011).

3. Arrange supplies at bedside.

4. Identify patient using at least two person-specific identifiers (e.g., name and date of birth or name and medical record number) according to employer policy. Compare identifiers with information on patient's MAR or medical record and ID band. Replace missing or faded ID bands.

Ensures correct patient. Complies with Accreditation Canada's standards and improves patient safety (Accreditation Canada, 2019).

5. At patient's bedside again compare MAR or computer printout with names of medications on medication labels and patient name. Ask patient if they have allergies.

Ensures that the right patient receives correct medication. Confirms patient's allergy history.

6. Explain procedure to patient and sensations to expect. Discuss purpose of each medication, action, and possible adverse effects. Allow patient to ask any questions about the medications. Patients who self-instill medications may be allowed to give drops under nurse's supervision (check employer policy).

Helps patient be a participant in care, which minimizes anxiety. Patient has the right to be informed, and patient's understanding of each medication improves adherence to medication therapy. Begins patient teaching regarding medications.

7. Position patient on side (if not contraindicated) with ear to be treated facing up, or patient may sit in chair or at bedside. Stabilize patient's head with their own hand. *Option:* Apply clean gloves if ear drainage is present.

Facilitates distribution of medication into ear.

8. Straighten ear canal by pulling pinna up and back to 10 o'clock position (adult, or child older than age 3) (see illustration) or down and back to 6 to 9 o'clock position (child under age 3).

Straightening ear canal provides direct access to deeper ear structures. Anatomical differences in younger children and infants necessitate different methods of positioning canal (Perry et al., 2017).

9. If cerumen or drainage occludes outermost part of ear canal, wipe out gently with cotton-tipped applicator (see illustration). Take care not to force cerumen into canal.

Cerumen and drainage harbour microorganisms and can block distribution of medication into canal. Occlusion blocks sound transmission.

10. Instill prescribed drops holding dropper 1 cm (about ½ inch) above ear canal.

Avoiding contact with external ear canal prevents contamination of dropper, which could contaminate medication in container.

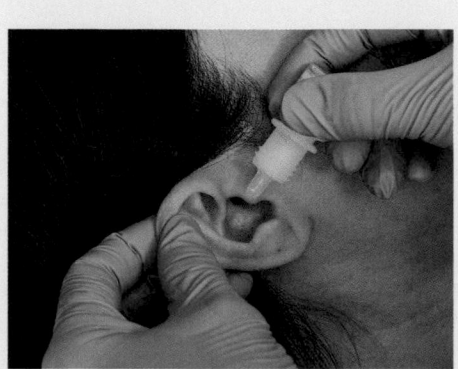

STEP 8 Pull pinna up and back for adults and for children older than 3 years.

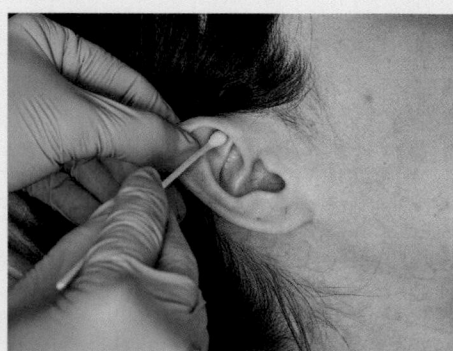

STEP 9 Always clean only outer canal. Do not push cerumen or secretions into ear.

STEP	RATIONALE

IMPLEMENTATION

11. Ask patient to remain in side-lying position for a few minutes. Apply gentle massage or pressure to tragus of ear with finger (see illustration).

Allows complete distribution of medication. Pressure and massage move medication inward.

12. If prescribed, gently insert part of cotton ball into outermost part of canal. Do not press cotton into canal.

Prevents escape of medication when patient sits or stands.

13. Remove cotton after 15 minutes. Help patient to comfortable position after drops are absorbed.

Allows time for medication distribution and absorption.

14. Dispose of soiled supplies in proper receptacle, remove and dispose of gloves, and perform hand hygiene.

Reduces spread of microorganisms.

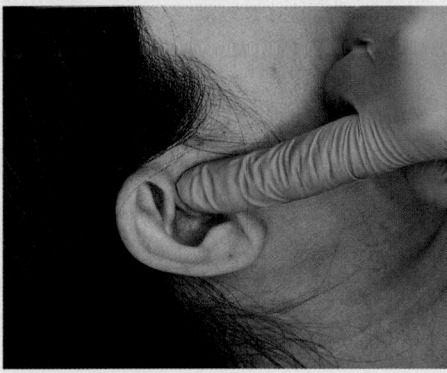

STEP 11 Nurse applies gentle pressure to tragus of ear after instilling drops.

EVALUATION

1. Observe response to medication by assessing hearing changes, asking if symptoms are relieved, and noting any adverse effects or discomfort felt.

Evaluates effects of medication.

2. Ask patient to discuss purpose of medication, action, adverse effects, and technique of administration.

Determines patient's level of understanding.

3. **Use Teach-Back:** "I want to be sure I clearly showed you how to administer eardrops. Let's take this time we have, and show me how to place eardrops in your right ear." Develop a revised teaching plan if patient or caregiver is not able to teach back correctly.

Determines patient's and caregiver's level of understanding of instructional topic.

Unexpected Outcomes

Ear canal remains inflamed, swollen, tender to palpation. Drainage is present.

Patient's hearing acuity does not improve.

Related Interventions
- Hold next dose.
- Notify health care provider for possible adjustment in medication type and dosage.
- Notify health care provider.
- Cerumen may be impacted, requiring ear irrigation.

Communication and Documentation

- Document medication, concentration, dose or strength, number of drops, site of application (left, right, or both ears), and time of administration on MAR immediately after administration, not before. Include initials or signature.
- Document patient teaching and validation of patient's understanding on flow sheet or in nurses' notes in electronic health record (EHR) or chart.

- Document objective data related to tissues involved (e.g., drainage, tenderness, irritation), any subjective data (e.g., ear pain, ringing in ears, change in hearing acuity), and patient's response to medications. Note any adverse effects experienced in nurses' notes in EHR or chart.
- Report adverse effects and patient response and/or withheld medications to nurse in charge or health care provider. Depending on medication, immediate health care provider notification may be required.

Pediatric

- Insert cotton pledgets (small wads of absorbent cotton) loosely into ear canal to prevent medication from flowing out. To prevent cotton from absorbing medication, premoisten it with a few drops of medication (Perry et al., 2017).

- Ensure that parents are taught how to correctly administer the eardrops (e.g., for children under 3, gently pull the pinna downward and straight back).
- Teach parents of children with frequent otitis media the signs of hearing loss and the need for follow-up care.

♦ SKILL 21.6 Administering Nasal Instillations

Patients with nasal sinus problems may receive medications by spray, drops, or tampons. The most commonly administered form of nasal instillation is a decongestant spray or drops used to relieve sinus congestion and cold symptoms. Many over-the-counter (OTC) nasal preparations contain sympathomimetic medications (e.g., Neo-Synephrine). These medications are relatively safe when administered nasally because only small doses are needed. However, the medications can enter the systemic circulation by way of the nasal mucosa or by the gastrointestinal tract if an excess amount is swallowed, causing restlessness, nervousness, tremors, or insomnia in some patients. Long-term use of decongestant nasal spray can worsen nasal congestion because of a rebound effect. Nasal sprays are easy for a patient to self-administer. Health care providers treat severe nosebleeds by placing nasal packing or tampons, which are treated with epinephrine to slow bleeding.

Delegation and Collaboration

The skill of administering nasal instillations cannot be delegated to an unregulated care provider (UCP). The nurse directs the UCP about:

- Potential adverse effects of medications and to report their occurrence to the nurse.
- Reporting any bloody nasal drainage to the nurse.

Equipment

- Medication administration record (MAR) (electronic or printed)
- Prepared medication with clean dropper or spray container
- Facial tissue
- Small pillow (*optional*)
- Washcloth (*optional*)
- Clean gloves

STEP	RATIONALE

ASSESSMENT

1. Check accuracy and completeness of each MAR with health care provider's medication prescription. Check patient's name, medication name and dosage, route (which sinus), and time for administration. Clarify incomplete or unclear prescriptions with health care provider before administration.

The prescription sheet is the most reliable source and only legal record of medications that patient is to receive. It ensures that patient receives the correct medications (Basukala et al., 2017).
Handwritten MARs are a source of medication errors (Basukala et al., 2017).

2. Review pertinent information related to medication, including action, purpose, normal dose and route, adverse effects, time of onset and peak action, and nursing implications.

Allows you to anticipate effects of medication and observe patient's response.

3. Assess patient's medical history (e.g., hypertension, heart disease, diabetes, and hyperthyroidism), medication history, and history of allergies. List medication allergies on each page of the MAR and prominently display it on the patient's medical record per employer policy. When patient has allergy, provide allergy bracelet.

These conditions contraindicate use of decongestants that stimulate central nervous system. Communication of allergies is essential for safe and effective care.

4. Perform hand hygiene. Use penlight and inspect condition of nose and sinuses (see Chapter 8). Palpate sinuses for pain or tenderness. Note type of drainage if present.

Provides baseline to monitor effects of medication. Presence of discharge interferes with medication absorption. Clear nasal discharge indicates sinus problem. Yellow or greenish discharge indicates infection.

5. Assess patient's knowledge regarding use of nasal instillations, technique for instillation, and willingness to learn self-administration.

Requires health teaching regarding use of medications. Motivation influences teaching approach.

NURSING DIAGNOSES

- Insufficient knowledge regarding medication action and purpose
- Pain (acute or chronic)
- Readiness for enhanced self-health management
- Potential for injury

Related factors/Risk factors are individualized on the basis of patient's condition or needs.

STEP	RATIONALE

PLANNING

1. Expected outcomes following completion of procedure:
  • Patient can breathe without difficulty through nose.
  • Patient's nasal sinuses are clear, moist, pink, and without drainage after repeated instillations (applies to anti-infective medications).
  • Patient can explain purpose of medication and administers nasal instillations correctly.

2. Collect appropriate equipment and MAR.

Nasal congestion has been relieved.
Inflammation of mucosa has been relieved.

Feedback reflects patient's learning.

Ensures time management and efficiency.

IMPLEMENTATION

1. Perform hand hygiene and prepare medications for instillation. Check label of medication against MAR two times (when removing medication from drawer/cabinet and prior to preparing medication for administration; see Skill 21.1). Preparation usually involves taking nasal drops or sprays out of storage and into patient's room. Check expiration date on container.

2. Take medication(s) to patient at correct time (see employer policy). Medications that require exact timing include stat, first-time or loading doses, and one-time doses. Give time-critical scheduled medications (e.g., antibiotics, anticoagulants, insulin, anticonvulsants, immunosuppressive medications) at exact time prescribed (no later than 30 minutes before or after scheduled dose). Give non–time-critical scheduled medications within a range of 1 or 2 hours of scheduled dose, according to employer policy (ISMP, 2011). During administration, apply 10 rights of medication administration. Perform hand hygiene.

3. Identify patient using at least two person-specific identifiers (e.g., name and date of birth or name and medical record number) according to employer policy. Compare identifiers with information on patient's MAR or medical record and ID band. Replace missing or faded ID bands.

4. At patient's bedside again compare MAR or computer printout with names of medications on medication labels and patient name. Ask patient if they have allergies.

5. Explain procedure to patient and sensations to expect. Discuss purpose of each medication, action, and possible adverse effects. Allow patient to ask any questions about medications. Patients who self-instill medications may be allowed to give drops under nurse's supervision (check employer policy). Tell patients receiving nasal instillation that they may experience burning or stinging of mucosa or choking sensation as medication trickles into throat.

6. Arrange supplies and medications at bedside. Apply clean gloves (if drainage is present).

7. Gently roll or shake container. Instruct patient to clear or blow nose gently unless contraindicated (e.g., risk of increased intracranial pressure or nosebleed).

8. Administer nose drops.
  a. Help patient to upright position (Giallourakis, 2016).
    (1) For access to posterior pharynx, tilt patient's head backward.

These are the first two checks for accuracy. Process ensures that right patient receives right medication at the right time.

Hospitals must adopt medication administration policy and procedure for timing of medication administration that considers nature of the prescribed medication, specific clinical application, and patient needs. Time-critical scheduled medications are those for which early or delayed administration of maintenance doses of greater than 30 minutes before or after the scheduled dose may cause harm or result in substantial suboptimal therapy or pharmacological effect. Non–time-critical medications are those for which early or delayed administration within a specified range of either 1 or 2 hours should not cause harm or result in substantial suboptimal therapy or pharmacological effect (ISMP, 2011).

Ensures correct patient. Complies with Accreditation Canada's standards and improves patient safety (Accreditation Canada, 2019).

Ensures that the right patient receives correct medication. Confirms patient's allergy history.

Helps patient be a participant in care, which minimizes anxiety. Patient has the right to be informed, and patient's understanding of each medication improves adherence to medication therapy. Begins patient teaching regarding medications.

Reduces spread of microorganisms; ensures smooth, orderly procedure.

Ensures distribution of medication. Allows medication to reach sinuses.

Proper positioning provides access to specific nasal passages.

STEP	RATIONALE

IMPLEMENTATION

(2) For access to ethmoid or sphenoid sinus, tilt head back over edge of bed or place small pillow under patient's shoulder and tilt head back (see illustration).

(3) For access to frontal and maxillary sinus, tilt head back over edge of bed or pillow with head turned toward side to be treated (see illustration). | Position allows medication to drain into affected sinus.

b. Support patient's head with nondominant hand. | Prevents straining neck muscles.

c. Instruct patient to breathe through mouth. | Mouth breathing reduces chance of aspirating nasal drops into trachea and lungs.

d. Hold dropper 1 cm (about ½ inch) above nares and instill prescribed number of drops toward midline of ethmoid bone. | Avoids contamination of dropper. Instilling toward ethmoid bone facilitates distribution of medication over nasal mucosa.

e. Have patient remain in supine position 5 minutes. | Prevents premature loss of medication through nares.

f. Offer facial tissue to blot runny nose but caution patient against blowing nose for several minutes. | Provides comfort but allows for absorption of medication.

9. Administer nasal spray.

a. Help patient into upright position with head tilted slightly forward. | Proper positioning permits medication spray to reach nasal passages.

b. Instruct or assist patient to insert tip of nasal spray into appropriate nares and occlude other nostril with finger (see illustration). Point spray tip toward side and away from centre of nose (Giallourakis, 2016). | Allows for proper administration of medication.

c. Have patient spray medication into nose while inhaling. Help them remove nozzle from nose and instruct to breathe out through mouth. | Allows for proper administration and distribution of nasal medication as high into nasal passages as possible.

d. Offer facial tissue to blot runny nose but caution patient against blowing nose for several minutes. | Provides comfort but allows for absorption of medication.

Clinical Decision Point *Some medications are designed for one spray per dose. Examples include calcitonin, desmopressin, and sumatriptan. It is essential to ensure that the patient understands the correct number of sprays to use per dose to prevent overdosing.*

10. Help patient to a comfortable position after medication is absorbed. | Restores comfort.

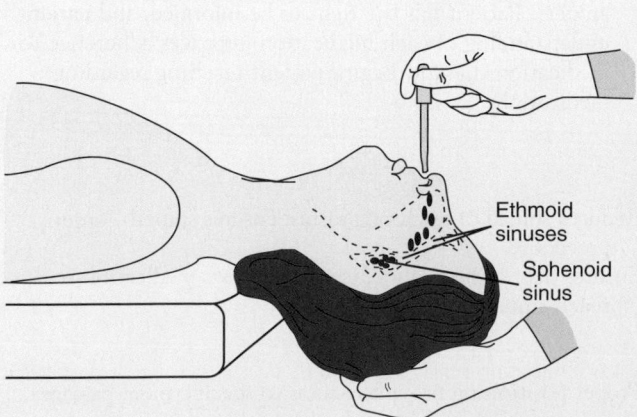

STEP 8a(2) Position for instilling nose drops into ethmoid or sphenoid sinus.

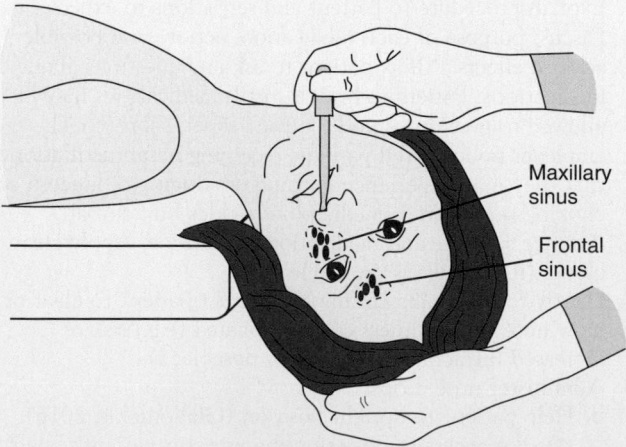

STEP 8a(3) Position for instilling nose drops into frontal and maxillary sinus.

STEP	RATIONALE

IMPLEMENTATION

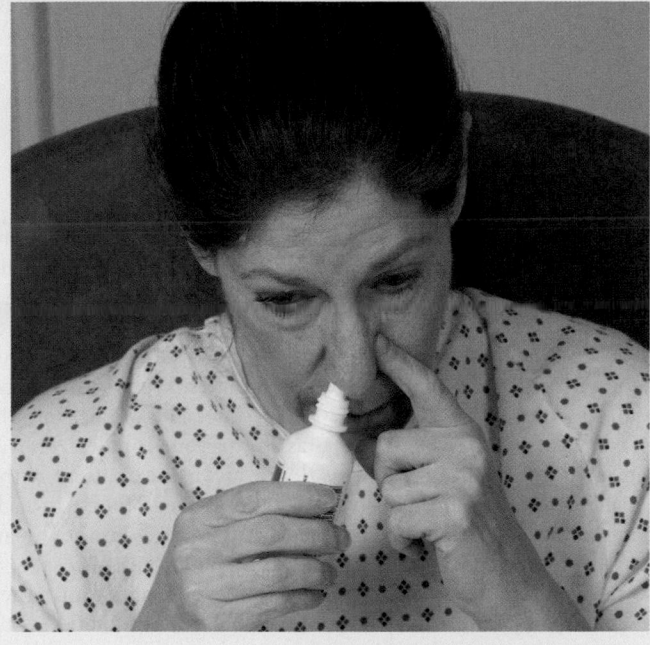

STEP 9b Occlude other nostril before self-administering nasal spray.

11. Dispose of soiled supplies, remove and dispose of gloves, and perform hand hygiene.	Reduces spread of microorganisms.

EVALUATION

1. Observe patient for onset of adverse effects 15 to 30 minutes after administration.	Medications absorbed through mucosa can cause systemic reaction.
2. Ask if patient can breathe through nose after decongestant administration. It may be necessary to have patient occlude one nostril at a time and breathe deeply.	Determines effectiveness of decongestant medication.
3. Reinspect condition of nasal passages between instillations.	Condition of mucosa reveals response to medication.
4. Ask patient to describe risks of overuse of decongestants and methods for administration.	Feedback ensures that patient can self-administer medications properly.
5. Have patient demonstrate self-medication.	Feedback demonstrates learning.
6. **Use Teach-Back:** "I want to be sure I explained the importance of not overusing your nasal spray. Explain to me why it is important not to overuse nasal sprays." Develop a revised teaching plan if patient or caregiver is not able to teach back correctly.	Determines patient's and caregiver's level of understanding of instructional topic.

Unexpected Outcomes

1. Patient is unable to breathe easily through nasal passages. Mucosa appears swollen, and congestion is unrelieved, possibly because of rebound effect.
2. Nasal mucosa remains inflamed and tender, with discharge from nares.
3. Patient indicates sinus headache. Sinuses remain congested.

Related Interventions

- Stop medication use.
- Notify health care provider and consider alternative therapy.
- Consider alternative therapy.
- Consider alternative therapy.

Communication and Documentation

- Document medication name, concentration, number of drops, nares into which medication was instilled, and actual time of administration on MAR immediately after administration, not before. Include initials or signature.

- Document patient's response to medication, patient teaching, and validation of patient's understanding on flow sheet or in nurses' notes in electronic health record (EHR) or chart.
- Report any unusual systemic or adverse effects and patient response and/or withheld medications to nurse in charge or health care provider.

Special Considerations
Teaching
• Instruct patients that each caregiver should have a different dropper or spray applicator. Instruct patients to wash or rinse applicators after each use.
• Use OTC nasal sprays or nose drops for only one illness; bottles easily become contaminated with bacteria.

• Overuse of nasal sprays and drops can cause rebound sinus congestion, resulting in sinus pain and headache.

Pediatric
• Infants are nose breathers, and the possible congestion caused by nasal medications may inhibit their sucking. Administer nose drops if prescribed 20 to 30 minutes before feedings (Perry et al., 2017).

✦ SKILL 21.7   Using Metered-Dose Inhalers (MDIs)

NSO *Nursing Skills Online Administration of Nonparenteral Medications Module 6 / Lesson 6*

Medications administered with handheld inhalers are dispersed through an aerosol spray, mist, or powder that penetrates the airways. For aerosol medication administration, some aerosols are administered by connecting to the wall outlet—either medical air or oxygen. When to use medical air or oxygen will depend on employer policy and the patient population (e.g., a patient with chronic obstructive pulmonary disease [COPD] would require medical air, whereas a pediatric patient would require oxygen). Pressurized metered-dose inhalers (pMDIs), breath-actuated metered-dose inhalers (BAIs), and dry powder inhalers (DPIs) deliver medications that produce local effects such as bronchodilation. Some of these medications are absorbed rapidly through the pulmonary circulation and create systemic side effects (e.g., albuterol may cause palpitations, tremors, and tachycardia). Patients who receive medications by inhalation frequently suffer from asthma and chronic respiratory disease. Medications administered by inhalation provide control of airway hyperactivity or bronchial constriction. Because patients depend on these medications for disease control, patient education is vital for correct use of inhalers and to ensure effectiveness of inhaled medications.

An MDI is a small, handheld device that disperses medication into the airways through an aerosol spray or mist by activation of a propellant. Dosing is usually achieved with 1 or 2 puffs. DPIs deliver inhaled medication in a fine powder formulation to the respiratory tract (see Procedural Guideline 21.1). The deeper passages of the respiratory tract provide a large surface area for medication absorption, and the alveolar-capillary network absorbs medication rapidly.

An MDI delivers a measured dose of the medication with each push of a canister. Approximately 2.3 to 4.5 kg (5 to 10 lb) of pressure is needed to activate the aerosol. This is difficult for some older patients because hand strength diminishes with age. Because use of an MDI requires coordination during the breathing cycle, many patients spray only the back of their throats and fail to receive a full dose. The inhaler must be depressed to expel medication just as the patient inhales. This ensures that medication reaches the lower airways. A patient with poor coordination may need to use a spacer device or a BAI to administer the medication properly. A spacer device decreases the amount of medication deposited into the oropharyngeal mucosa. Some spacers have a one-way valve that activates on inhalation, thereby removing the need for good hand–breath coordination (Burchum & Rosenthal, 2016). Box 21.4 summarizes common problems that occur when using an inhaler.

Delegation and Collaboration
The skill of administering MDIs cannot be delegated to an unregulated care provider (UCP). The nurse instructs the UCP about:
• Potential adverse effects of medications and to report their occurrence to the nurse.
• Reporting breathing difficulty (e.g., paroxysmal or sustained coughing, audible wheezing) to the nurse.

Equipment
• Medication administration record (MAR) (electronic or printed)
• Inhaler device with medication canister (MDI or DPI) (Fig. 21.2, A–C)
• Spacer device such as AeroChamber or InspirEase (*optional*)
• Facial tissues (*optional*)
• Stethoscope
• Peak flowmeter (*optional*)

BOX 21.4

Common Problems in Using an Inhaler

• *Not taking the medication as prescribed:* Taking either too much or too little.
• *Incorrect activation:* This usually occurs through pressing the canister *before* taking a breath. These actions should be done simultaneously so that the medication can be carried down to the lungs with the breath.
• *Forgetting to shake the inhaler:* The medication is in a suspension; therefore, particles may settle. If the inhaler is not shaken, it may not deliver the correct dose of the medication.
• *Not waiting long enough between puffs:* A delay between puffs is needed before taking a second puff; otherwise an incorrect dose may be delivered, or the medication may not penetrate into the lungs.
• *Failure to clean the valve:* Particles may jam the valve in the mouthpiece unless it is cleaned occasionally. This is a frequent cause of failure to get 200 puffs from one inhaler.
• *Failure to observe whether the inhaler is actually releasing a spray:* If it is not, this should be checked with the pharmacist.
• *Failure to recognize when the canister is empty:* This occurs when the metered-dose inhaler has no built-in dose counter or instructions in dose counting.

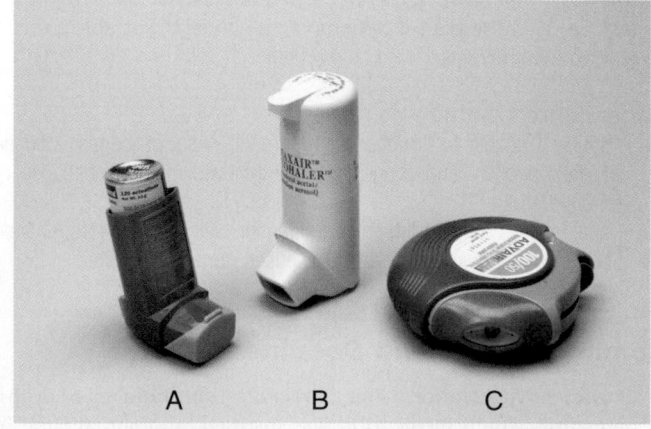

FIG 21.2 Types of inhalers. **A,** Metered-dose inhaler (MDI). **B,** Breath-actuated inhaler (BAI). **C,** Dry powder inhaler (DPI).

STEP	RATIONALE

ASSESSMENT

1. Check accuracy and completeness of each MAR with health care provider's medication prescription. Check patient's name, medication name and dosage, route, and time for administration. Clarify incomplete or unclear prescriptions with health care provider before administration.

The prescription sheet is the most reliable source and only legal record of medications that patient is to receive. It ensures that patient receives correct medications (Basukala et al., 2017).

Handwritten MARs are a source of medication errors (Basukala et al., 2017).

2. Review pertinent information related to medication, including action, purpose, normal dose and route, adverse effects, time of onset and peak action, and nursing implications.

Allows you to anticipate effects of medication and observe patient's response.

3. Assess patient's medical and medication history and history of allergies. List medication allergies on each page of the MAR and prominently display it on the patient's medical record per employer policy. When patient has allergy, provide allergy bracelet.

Factors influence how certain medications act. Reveals patient's need for medication.

Communication of allergies is essential for safe and effective care.

4. Assess respiratory pattern and auscultate breath sounds (see Chapter 8). Also assess exercise tolerance; does patient develop shortness of breath easily?

Establishes baseline of airway status for comparison during and after treatment.

5. Assess patient's ability to hold, manipulate, and depress canister and inhaler.

Any impairment of grasp or presence of hand tremors interferes with patient's ability to depress canister within inhaler. Spacer device is often necessary.

6. If patient was previously instructed in self-administration, have them demonstrate how to use the device.

Often patients who have adequate understanding of how to use an inhaler forget the procedure. Ongoing assessment of inhaler technique identifies areas for further education and reinforcement (Ari, 2015).

7. Assess patient's readiness and ability to learn (e.g., asks questions about medication; is alert; participates in own care; is not fatigued, in pain, or in respiratory distress).

One-on-one patient assessment prepares patient for self-management and greater adherence to inhaler use (Ari, 2015). In some situations, mental or physical limitations affect patient's ability to learn and methods used for instruction.

8. Assess patient's knowledge and understanding of disease and purpose and action of prescribed medications.

Knowledge of disease is essential for patient to realistically understand use of inhaler.

NURSING DIAGNOSES

- Inadequate breathing pattern
- Reduced gas exchange
- Reduced stamina

- Anxiety
- Insufficient knowledge regarding use of MDI

- Ready for enhanced self-health management
- Potential for injury

Related factors/Risk factors are individualized on the basis of patient's condition or needs.

PLANNING

1. Expected outcomes following completion of procedure:
  - Patient correctly self-administers a metered dose.
  - Patient describes proper time during respiratory cycle to inhale and spray and number of inhalations for each administration.
  - Patient's breathing pattern improves, and lung sounds indicate that airways are less restrictive.

2. Collect appropriate equipment and MAR.

Demonstrates learning.

Demonstrates learning and ensures correct administration of medication

Demonstrates therapeutic effect of medication in improving gas exchange.

Ensures time management and efficiency.

IMPLEMENTATION

1. Perform hand hygiene and prepare medications for inhalation. Check label of medication against MAR two times (when removing medication from drawer/cabinet and prior to preparing medication for administration; see Skill 21.1). Preparation usually involves taking inhaler device out of storage and into patient's room. Check expiration date on container.

These are the first two checks for accuracy. Process ensures that right patient receives right medication at the right time.

STEP	RATIONALE

IMPLEMENTATION

2. Take medication(s) to patient at correct time (see employer policy). Medications that require exact timing include stat, first-time or loading doses, and one-time doses. Give time-critical scheduled medications (e.g., antibiotics, anticoagulants, insulin, anticonvulsants, immunosuppressive medications) at exact time prescribed (no later than 30 minutes before or after scheduled dose). Give non–time-critical scheduled medications within a range of 1 or 2 hours of scheduled dose, according to employer policy (ISMP, 2011). During administration apply 10 rights of medication administration. Perform hand hygiene.

Hospitals must adopt medication administration policy and procedure for timing of medication administration that considers nature of the prescribed medication, specific clinical application, and patient needs. Time-critical scheduled medications are those for which early or delayed administration of maintenance doses of greater than 30 minutes before or after the scheduled dose may cause harm or result in substantial suboptimal therapy or pharmacological effect. Non–time-critical medications are those for which early or delayed administration within a specified range of either 1 or 2 hours should not cause harm or result in substantial suboptimal therapy or pharmacological effect (ISMP, 2011).

3. Identify patient using at least two person-specific identifiers (e.g., name and date of birth or name and medical record number) according to employer policy. Compare identifiers with information on patient's MAR or medical record and ID band. Replace missing or faded ID bands.

Ensures correct patient. Complies with Accreditation Canada's standards and improves patient safety (Accreditation Canada, 2019).

4. At patient's bedside again compare MAR or computer printout with names of medications on medication labels and patient name. Ask patient if they have allergies.

Ensures that the right patient receives correct medication. Confirms patient's allergy history.

5. Explain procedure to patient. Be specific if patient wishes to self-administer medication. Explain where and how to set up at home. Discuss purpose of each medication, action, and possible adverse effects. Allow patient to ask any questions about the medications. Explain what a metered dose is and how to administer. Warn about overuse of inhaler and side effects.

Helps patient be a participant in care, which minimizes anxiety. Patient has the right to be informed, and patient's understanding of each medication improves adherence to medication therapy. Begins patient teaching regarding medications.

6. Allow adequate time for patient to manipulate inhaler, canister, and spacer device (if provided). Explain and demonstrate how canister fits into inhaler.

Patient must be familiar with how to use equipment.

Clinical Decision Point *If using an MDI that is new or has not been used for several days, push a "test spray" into the air to prime the device before using. This ensures that the MDI is patent and the metal canister is positioned properly.*

7. Explain and demonstrate steps for administering MDI without spacer.

Simple one-on-one instruction and demonstration of step-by-step administration allows patient to ask questions at any point during procedure and increases patient adherence to inhaler use (Ari, 2015).

   a. Remove mouthpiece cover from inhaler after inserting MDI canister into holder.

   b. Shake inhaler well for 2 to 5 seconds (five or six shakes).

Ensures mixing of medication in canister.

   c. Hold inhaler in dominant hand.

   d. Have patient stand or sit and instruct them to position inhaler in one of two ways:

      (1) Have patient place the mouthpiece in the mouth between the teeth and over the tongue, aimed toward back of throat, with lips closed tightly around it. Do not block the mouthpiece with the teeth or tongue (see illustration).

Ensures proper fit to inhale medication.

      (2) Position mouthpiece 2.5 to 5 cm (1 to 2 inches) in front of widely opened mouth (see illustration), with opening of inhaler toward back of throat. Lips should not touch inhaler.

Directs aerosol spray toward airway. This is best way to deliver medication without a spacer.

   e. While holding the mouthpiece away from the mouth, have patient take deep breath and exhale completely.

Empties lung volume and prepares airway to receive medication.

STEP	RATIONALE

IMPLEMENTATION

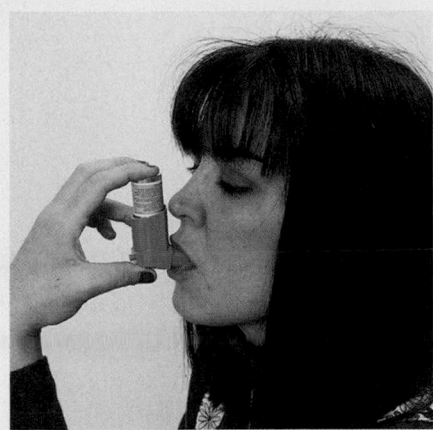

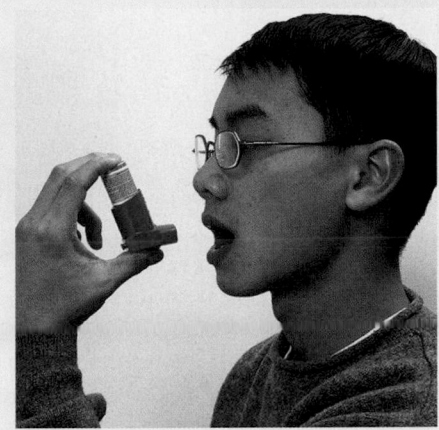

STEP 7d(1) Patient opens lips and places inhaler mouthpiece in mouth with opening toward back of throat.

STEP 7d(2) Patient positions inhaler mouthpiece 2 to 4 cm (1 to 2 inches) from widely open mouth. This is considered the best way to deliver medication without a spacer.

---

f. With inhaler positioned, have patient hold it with thumb at mouthpiece and index and middle fingers at top. This is a three-point or bilateral hand position.

Hand position ensures proper activation of MDI and distribution of dosage (Burchum & Rosenthal, 2016).

g. Instruct patient to tilt head back slightly and inhale slowly and deeply through mouth for 3 to 5 seconds while depressing canister fully.

Medication is distributed to airways during inhalation.

h. Have patient hold breath for about 10 seconds.

Allows tiny drops of aerosol spray to reach deeper branches of airways.

i. Remove MDI from mouth before exhaling and exhale slowly through nose or pursed lips.

Keeps small airways open during exhalation.

8. Explain and demonstrate steps to administer MDI using spacer device.

Simple one-on-one instruction and demonstration of step-by-step administration allows patient to ask questions at any point during procedure and increases patient adherence to inhaler use (Ari, 2015).

a. Remove mouthpiece cover from MDI and mouthpiece of spacer device.

Inhaler fits into end of spacer device.

b. Shake inhaler well for 2 to 5 seconds (five or six shakes).

Ensures mixing of medication in canister.

c. Insert MDI into end of spacer device.

Spacer device traps medication released from MDI; patient then inhales medication from device. These devices improve delivery of correct dose of inhaled medication (Momeni, Nokhodchi, Ghanbarzadeh, et al., 2016)

d. Instruct patient to place spacer device mouthpiece in mouth and close lips. Do not insert beyond raised lip on mouthpiece. Avoid covering small exhalation slots with lips.

Medication should not escape through mouth.

e. Have patient breathe normally through spacer device mouthpiece (see illustration).

Allows patient to relax before delivering medication.

f. Instruct patient to depress medication canister, spraying one puff into spacer device.

Device contains fine spray and allows patient to inhale more medication. The spacer increases medication delivery and deposition of the medication on the oropharyngeal mucosa (Burchum & Rosenthal, 2016).

g. Patient breathes in slowly and fully (for 5 seconds).

Ensures that particles of medication are distributed to deeper airways.

h. Instruct patient to hold full breath for 10 seconds.

Ensures full medication distribution.

9. Instruct patient to wait 20 to 30 seconds between inhalations (if same medication) or 2 to 5 minutes between inhalations (if different medications).

Medications must be inhaled sequentially. Always administer bronchodilators before steroids so dilators can open airway passages (Burchum & Rosenthal, 2016).

STEP	RATIONALE

IMPLEMENTATION

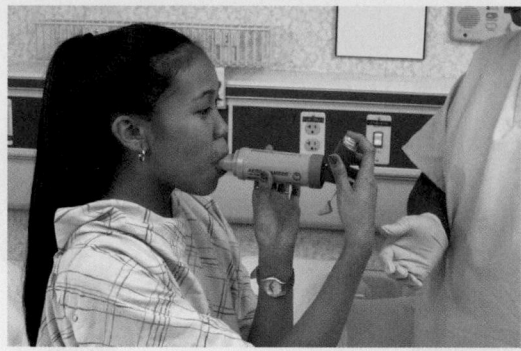

STEP 8e Using spacer device with an MDI.

10. Instruct patient to not repeat inhalations before next scheduled.

Medications are prescribed to be delivered at intervals during the day to provide constant medication levels and minimize adverse effects. Beta-adrenergic MDIs are used either on an "as needed" basis or regularly every 4 to 6 hours.

11. Warn patients that they may feel gagging sensation in throat caused by droplets of medication on pharynx or tongue.

This occurs when medication is sprayed and inhaled incorrectly.

12. Instruct patient to rinse mouth with warm water about 2 minutes after last dose and then spit water out.

Steroids may alter normal flora of oral mucosa and lead to development of fungal infection. Rinsing out patient's mouth reduces risk of fungal infection (Ari, 2015).

13. Clean the MDI.

Removes residual medication and reduces spread of microorganisms.

a. For daily cleaning, instruct patient to remove medication canister, rinse inhaler and cap with warm running water, and be sure that inhaler is completely dry before reuse. Patient should not get valve mechanism of canister wet.

Water damages valve mechanism of canister.

b. Instruct patient to clean mouthpiece twice a week with a mild dishwashing soap, rinse it thoroughly, and dry it completely before storage.

14. Ask if patient has any questions.

Clarifies misconceptions or misunderstanding and provides opportunity for further patient education (Ari, 2015).

15. Help patient to comfortable position and perform hand hygiene.

Reduces spread of microorganisms and promotes patient comfort.

EVALUATION

1. Auscultate patient lungs, listen for abnormal breath sounds, and obtain peak flow measures if prescribed.

Determines patient response to medication.

2. Have patient explain and demonstrate steps in use and cleaning of inhaler.

Return demonstration provides feedback for measuring patient's learning.

3. Ask patient to explain medication schedule and dose of medication.

Improves likelihood of adherence to therapy.

4. Ask patient to describe adverse effects of medication and criteria for calling health care provider.

Allows patient to recognize signs of overuse and need to seek medical support when medications are ineffective.

5. **Use Teach-Back:** "I want to be sure I clearly showed you how to use your inhaler. Show me how you will use the inhaler to take your medicine." Develop a revised teaching plan if patient or caregiver is not able to teach back correctly.

Determines patient's and caregiver's level of understanding of instructional topic.

STEP	RATIONALE

EVALUATION

Unexpected Outcomes

1. Patient's respirations are rapid and shallow; breath sounds indicate wheezing.

2. Patient needs bronchodilator more than every 4 hours (may indicate respiratory problem).
3. Patient experiences cardiac dysrhythmias (light-headedness, syncope), especially if receiving beta-adrenergic medications.

Related Interventions

- Evaluate vital signs and respiratory status.
- Notify health care provider.
- Reassess type of medication and/or delivery method.
- Reassess type of medication and delivery methods needed.
- Notify health care provider.
- Withhold all further doses of medication.
- Evaluate cardiac and pulmonary status (see Chapter 8).
- Notify health care provider for reassessment of type of medication and delivery method.

Communication and Documentation

- Document medication administered, dose or strength, route, number of inhalations, and actual time administered on MAR immediately after administration, not before. Include initials or signature.
- Document patient teaching and validation of patient's understanding on flow sheet or in nurses' notes in electronic health record (EHR) or chart.
- Document on flow sheet or in nurses' notes in EHR or chart patient's response to MDI (e.g., breath sounds), evidence of adverse effects (e.g., arrhythmia, feelings of anxiety), and ability to use MDI.
- Report adverse effects and patient response and/or withheld medications to nurse in charge or health care provider.

Special Considerations

Teaching

- Allow for one-on-one supervised practice of the procedures. Patients may have difficulty timing an inhalation with activation of the medication canister without repeated instruction (Ari, 2015).
- Teach patient to keep track of the number of inhalations in the MDI (Box 21.5).
- Teach patients to use small, handheld peak flowmeters to monitor response to therapy when inhalers are prescribed (Barrons, Pegram

& Borries, 2011). A peak flowmeter measures the peak expiratory flow rate (PEFR), which is a person's maximum speed of expiration (Box 21.6).
- Teach patient to rinse their mouth with water after the use of inhalers.

Pediatric

- A spacer is of benefit to young children because they have difficulty coordinating inhaler activation and inhaling (Perry et al., 2017).
- Educate child and parent about the need to use the inhaler during school hours. Help family find resources within the school or day care facility. Many school systems do not permit self-administration of MDIs. Follow school policy regarding having the MDI available for use during school hours. A health care provider's prescription may be necessary.

Gerontological

- Older persons may be unable to depress medication canisters because of weakened grasp or inability to coordinate actuation of the canister with inhalation. The use of a spacer device may be helpful.

Care in the Community

- Remind patients to carry prescribed inhalers to use as immediate treatment in case of an acute asthma attack.

BOX 21.5

Counting Doses in a Metered-Dose Inhaler

Most metered-dose inhalers (MDIs) currently do not have automatic dose counters. Patients need to keep careful track of the number of inhalations used in their MDIs. Failure to do so may result in patients using an empty inhaler during an acute exacerbation of a respiratory problem. To track doses:

- Note first day of use on a calendar.
- Note number of inhalations in the canister (e.g., 200 inhalations per MDI).
- Note number of inhalations used per day (e.g., 2 inhalations a day three times a day equals 6 inhalations per day).
- Divide the total number of inhalations in the canister by the number of inhalations needed per day to determine the number of days that the inhaler should last (e.g., 200 inhalations divided by 6 inhalations per day equals approximately 33 days of three times-a-day dosing).
- Mark on a calendar the date the inhaler will be empty and obtain a refill of the inhaler a few days before this target date.

BOX 21.6

How to Use a Peak Flowmeter

1. Move the marker to the bottom of the numbered scale and connect the mouthpiece to the peak flowmeter.
2. Have patient stand up if able.
3. Have patient take a deep breath, filling the lungs completely.
4. Have the patient place the lips tightly around the mouthpiece of the flowmeter and then blow as hard and as fast as possible with a single breath.
5. Note the final position of the marker. This is the patient's peak flow rate.
6. Have the patient repeat the steps blowing into the peak flowmeter two more times. Record the highest reading of the three.

PROCEDURAL GUIDELINE 21.1 *Using Dry Powder–Inhaled (DPI) Medications*

Dry powder inhalers (DPIs) hold dry powder medication and create an aerosol when the patient inhales through a reservoir that contains the medication. In contrast with the metered-dose inhaler (MDI), a DPI has no propellant. DPIs require less manual dexterity; and because the device is breath activated, there is no need to coordinate puffs with inhalation. Compared with MDIs, DPIs deliver more medication to the lungs (Burchum & Rosenthal, 2016). A DPI does not require a spacer. Medication inside a DPI can clump if the patient lives in a humid climate. Some patients cannot inhale fast enough to administer the entire dose of medication.

Delegation and Collaboration

The skill of administering DPI medications cannot be delegated to an unregulated care provider (UCP). The nurse directs the UCP about:

- Potential adverse effects of medications and to report their occurrence to the nurse.
- Reporting paroxysmal coughing, audible wheezing, and patient's report of breathlessness or difficulty breathing to the nurse.

Equipment

- Medication administration record (MAR) (electronic or printed)
- DPI (see Fig. 21.2 C)
- Stethoscope
- Wash basin or sink with warm water
- Facial tissues *(optional)*

Procedural Steps

1. Check accuracy and completeness of each MAR with health care provider's medication prescription. Check patient's name, medication name and dosage, route (which sinus), and time for administration. Clarify incomplete or unclear prescriptions with health care provider before administration.
2. Review pertinent information related to medication, including action, purpose, normal dose and route, adverse effects, time of onset and peak action, and nursing implications.
3. Assess patient's medical and medication history and history of allergies. List medication allergies on each page of the MAR and prominently display it on the patient's medical record per employer policy. When patient has allergy, provide allergy bracelet.
4. Assess respiratory pattern and auscultate breath sounds (see Chapter 8).
5. Assess patient's knowledge of medication and readiness to learn (e.g., asks questions about medication, requests education in use of DPI, is mentally alert, participates in own care).
6. Assess patient's ability to learn. Patient should not be fatigued, in pain, or in respiratory distress; assess level of understanding of technical vocabulary terms.
7. Determine patient's ability to hold, manipulate, and activate DPI.
8. If previously instructed in self-administration of DPI, assess patient's technique in using it.
9. Perform hand hygiene, prepare medication for inhalation, and check label on inhaler against MAR three times (when removing medication from drawer/cabinet, prior to preparing

medication for administration, and prior to returning medication container to drawer or discarding one-time use vial; see Skill 21.1). Preparation usually involves taking inhaler device out of storage and into patient's room. *These are the three checks for accuracy. Check expiration date on container.*

10. Take medication to patient at correct time (see employer policy). Give medications that require exact or precise timing when prescribed, give time-critical medications at time prescribed (no later than 30 minutes before or after), and give non–time-critical medications within 1 or 2 hours of scheduled dose (ISMP, 2011) (see employer policy). During administration apply 10 rights of medication administration. Perform hand hygiene.
11. Identify patient using at least two person-specific identifiers (e.g., name and date of birth or name and medical record number) according to employer policy. Compare identifiers with information on patient's MAR or medical record.
12. At patient's bedside again compare MAR or computer printout with names of medications on medication labels and patient name. Ensures that the right patient receives the correct medication. Ask patient if they have allergies.
13. Explain procedure and discuss purpose of each medication, action, and possible adverse effects. Allow patient to ask any questions about the medications. Explain what a DPI is and how to administer. Warn about overuse of inhaler and adverse effects.
14. If DPI has an external counter, note number indicated to determine doses remaining. Otherwise use technique in Box 21.5 for counting doses.
15. Prepare DPI for administration. Perform hand hygiene. Some DPIs require loading medication before administration; some require rotation of a lever to load medication or insert a capsule; and some require insertion of a disk into inhaler device. Follow manufacturer specific instructions.

Clinical Decision Point *The patient's inhaled breath pulls the medication into the airway. DPIs may differ as to how fast the patient should inhale the medication; consult specific instructions of manufacturer. In addition, do not shake DPI because powdered medication may spill out of device.*

16. Have patient exhale fully and then place lips over mouthpiece of DPI and inhale quickly and as deeply as possible. Remove inhaler from mouth as soon as inhalation is complete.
17. Have patient hold breath for 10 seconds or as long as possible and then exhale. Do not exhale into DPI.
18. Instruct patients that, unlike with other inhaled medications, they may not taste or feel the dry powder or there may be a slight sweet taste.
19. After using DPI, have patient rinse mouth with warm water and spit it out to reduce throat irritation and prevent oral candidiasis.
20. Return DPI to closed position or remove loaded capsule or disk if necessary. If an external counter is present, note number, which should be one less than the number in Step 14.

PROCEDURAL GUIDELINE 21.1 *Using Dry Powder–Inhaled (DPI) Medications—cont'd*

21. Have patient demonstrate use of DPI at next scheduled dose. Ask them to discuss purpose, action, and adverse effects of medication.

22. Auscultate breath sounds, evaluate respiratory rate, and ask patient about their ease of breathing.

23. Record medication, dose or strength, route, number of inhalations, and time administered on MAR immediately after administration, not before. Include initials or signature.

24. Record patient teaching and validation of patient's understanding in nurses' notes in electronic health record (EHR) or chart.

25. Use Teach-Back: "I want to be sure I explained how often you need to use this DPI medication. Tell me when you will use this medication." Develop a revised teaching plan if patient or caregiver is not able to teach back correctly.

◆ SKILL 21.8   Using Small-Volume Nebulizers

Nebulization is a process of adding medications or moisture to inspired air by mixing particles of various sizes with air. Adding moisture to the respiratory system through nebulization improves clearance of pulmonary secretions. Medications such as bronchodilators, mucolytics, and corticosteroids are often administered by nebulization.

Small-volume nebulizers convert a medication solution into a mist that is then inhaled by a patient into his or her tracheobronchial tree. The droplets in the mist are much finer than those created by metered-dose inhalers (MDIs) or dry powder inhalers (DPIs). A face mask or a mouthpiece held between the teeth delivers a nebulized mist. A nebulized medication is designed to create a local effect, but it can be absorbed into the bloodstream through the alveoli. As a result, systemic effects from the medication may occur.

Delegation and Collaboration

In many health care facilities, a respiratory therapist performs the skill of administering medications by nebulizer. The nurse must be aware of the type and actions of the inhaled medication that the patient is receiving. The skill of administering medications by nebulizer cannot be delegated to an unregulated care provider (UCP). The nurse instructs the UCP about:

- Potential adverse effects of medications and to report their occurrence to the nurse.
- Reporting paroxysmal coughing, ineffective breathing patterns, and other respiratory difficulties to the nurse.

Equipment

- Medication administration record (MAR) (electronic or printed)
- Medication prescribed and diluent (if needed)
- Medicine dropper or syringe
- Nebulizer bottle and tubing assembly
- Small-volume nebulizer machine (often called *handheld nebulizer* or *nebulizer*)
- Pulse oximeter and peak flow device
- Stethoscope
- *Option:* nose clip

STEP	RATIONALE

ASSESSMENT

1. Check accuracy and completeness of each MAR with health care provider's medication prescription. Check patient's name, medication name and dosage, route, and time for administration. Clarify incomplete or unclear prescriptions with health care provider before administration.

The prescription sheet is the most reliable source and only legal record of medications that patient is to receive. It ensures that patient receives correct medications (Basukala et al., 2017).

Handwritten MARs are a source of medication errors (Basukala et al., 2017).

2. Review pertinent information related to medication, including action, purpose, normal dose and route, adverse effects, time of onset and peak action, and nursing implications.

Allows you to anticipate effects of medication and observe patient's response.

3. Assess patient's medical and medication history and history of allergies. List medication allergies on each page of the MAR and prominently display it on the patient's medical record per employer policy. When patient has allergy, provide allergy bracelet.

These factors influence how certain medications act. Information also reflects patient's need for medications and risk for adverse effects. Communication of allergies is essential for safe and effective care.

4. Assess patient's grasp and ability to assemble, hold, and manipulate nebulizer equipment.

Any impairment of cognition or grasp or the presence of hand tremors affects patient's ability to use equipment.

5. Assess pulse, respirations, breath sounds, pulse oximetry, and peak flow measurement (if prescribed) before beginning treatment.

Establishes baseline for comparison during and after treatment.

STEP	RATIONALE

ASSESSMENT

6. Assess patient's knowledge of medication and readiness to learn (e.g., patient asks questions about medication, requests education in use of nebulizer, is mentally alert, participates in own care).

Determines level of instruction needed to assume self-administration.

7. Assess patient's ability to learn. Patient should not be fatigued, in pain, or in respiratory distress; assess level of understanding of technical vocabulary terms.

Determines best time to provide instruction and techniques to use.

8. Assess patient's ability to manipulate nebulizer mouthpiece and tubing.

Presence of mobility restrictions indicates need for assistance.

NURSING DIAGNOSES

- Reduced gas exchange
- Inadequate breathing pattern
- Reduced stamina

- Anxiety
- Insufficient knowledge regarding use of nebulizers

- Readiness for enhanced self-health management
- Potential for injury

Related factors/Risk factors are individualized on the basis of patient's condition or needs.

PLANNING

1. Expected outcomes following completion of procedure:
   - Patient's breathing pattern is effective.
   - Patient's oxygen saturation level is adequate.
   - Patient describes adverse effects of medication and criteria for calling health care provider (e.g., low peak flow rate).
   - Patient demonstrates self-administration of nebulized dose of medication correctly.
2. Collect appropriate equipment and MAR.

Demonstrates therapeutic effect of medication.
Demonstrates therapeutic effect of medication.
Increases likelihood of adherence to therapeutic regimen.

Demonstrates proper administration of medication and documents learning.
Ensures time management and efficiency.

IMPLEMENTATION

1. Perform hand hygiene and prepare medications for inhalation. Check label of medication against MAR two times (when removing medication from drawer/cabinet and prior to preparing medication for administration; see Skill 21.1). Preparation usually involves taking medication vial out of storage and taking to patient's room. Check expiration date on container.

These are the first two checks for accuracy. Process ensures that right patient receives right medication at the right time.

2. Take medication(s) to patient at correct time (see employer policy). Medications that require exact timing include stat, first-time or loading doses, and one-time doses. Give time-critical scheduled medications (e.g., antibiotics, anticoagulants, insulin, anticonvulsants, immunosuppressive medications) at exact time prescribed (no later than 30 minutes before or after scheduled dose). Give non–time-critical scheduled medications within a range of 1 or 2 hours of scheduled dose, according to employer policy (ISMP, 2011). During administration, apply 10 rights of medication administration. Perform hand hygiene.

Hospitals must adopt medication administration policy and procedure for timing of medication administration that considers nature of the prescribed medication, specific clinical application, and patient needs. Time-critical scheduled medications are those for which early or delayed administration of maintenance doses of greater than 30 minutes before or after the scheduled dose may cause harm or result in substantial suboptimal therapy or pharmacological effect. Non–time-critical medications are those for which early or delayed administration within a specified range of either 1 or 2 hours should not cause harm or result in substantial suboptimal therapy or pharmacological effect (ISMP, 2011).

3. Identify patient using at least two person-specific identifiers (e.g., name and date of birth or name and medical record number) according to employer policy. Compare identifiers with information on patient's MAR or medical record and ID band. Replace missing or faded ID bands.

Ensures correct patient. Complies with Accreditation Canada's standards and improves patient safety (Accreditation Canada, 2019).

4. At patient's bedside again compare MAR or computer printout with names of medications on medication labels and patient name. Ask patient if they have allergies.

Ensures that the right patient receives correct medication. Confirms patient's allergy history.

STEP	RATIONALE

IMPLEMENTATION

5. Explain procedure to patient. Be specific if patient wishes to self-administer medication. Discuss purpose of each medication, action, and possible adverse effects. Allow patient to ask any questions about the medications. Explain how to assemble nebulizer and proper use.

Helps patient be a participant in care, which minimizes anxiety. Patient has right to be informed, and patient's understanding of each medication improves adherence to medication therapy. Begins patient teaching regarding medications (Ari, 2015).

6. Assemble nebulizer equipment per manufacturer directions.

Assembly may vary slightly with different manufacturers. Proper assembly ensures safe delivery of medication.

7. Add prescribed medication by pouring medicine into nebulizer cup. (*Option:* You may use a medicine dropper or syringe to instill medication.)

Ensures proper dose and delivery of prescribed medication.

8. Attach top to nebulizer cup and be sure that it is secure. Then connect cup to mouthpiece or face mask.

Prevents loss of medication.

9. Connect tubing to both aerosol compressor and nebulizer cup.

Ensures aerosol delivery to mouthpiece.

10. Have patient hold mouthpiece between lips with gentle pressure, but be sure lips are sealed (see illustration).

Prevents escape of nebulized medication.

   a. If patient is an infant, child, or tired adult or unable to follow instructions, use face mask.

Use of face mask does not require patient to remember to hold mouthpiece correctly. Correct delivery ensures sufficient deposition of medication.

   b. Use special adapters for patients with tracheostomy.

Promotes greater deposition of medication in airways.

11. Turn on small-volume nebulizer machine and ensure that a sufficient mist begins to flow.

Verifies that equipment is working properly during delivery of medication.

12. Instruct patient take deep breath, slowly, to a volume slightly greater than normal. Encourage brief, end-inspiratory pause for about 2 to 3 seconds; then have patient exhale passively. *Option:* If needed, use a nose clip so patient breathes only through the mouth (Medline Plus, 2014).

Improves effectiveness of medication.

   a. If patient is dyspneic, encourage them to hold every fourth or fifth breath for 5 to 10 seconds.

Maximizes effectiveness of medication.

   b. Remind patient to repeat breathing pattern until medication is completely nebulized. This usually takes about 10 to 15 minutes (Medline Plus, 2019).

Maximizes effectiveness of medication.

     (1) Some health care providers prescribe time limit as length of treatment rather than waiting for medication to completely nebulize.

   c. Tap nebulizer cup occasionally during and toward end of treatment.

Releases droplets that are clinging to side of cup, thus allowing for renebulization of solution.

   d. Monitor patient's pulse during procedure, especially if beta-adrenergic bronchodilators are used.

Enables you to observe for potential adverse effects of medications.

13. When medication is completely nebulized, turn off machine. Rinse nebulizer cup per employer policy. Dry completely and store tubing assembly per employer policy.

Proper storage reduces transfer of microorganisms.

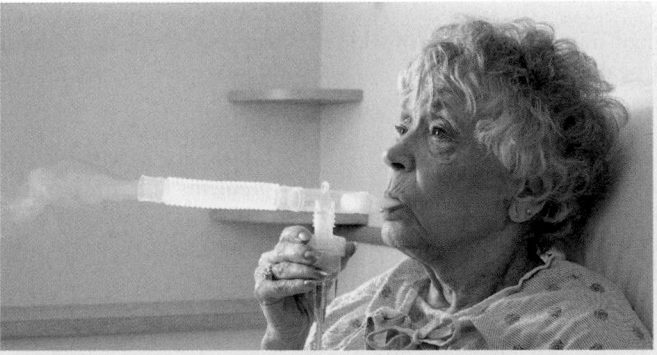

STEP 10 Nebulizer mouthpiece placed between patient's lips.

STEP	RATIONALE

IMPLEMENTATION

14. If steroids are nebulized, instruct patient to rinse mouth and gargle with warm water after nebulizer treatment. Have patient spit out solution.

Removes medication residue from oral cavity and helps to prevent oral candidiasis, a possible adverse effect of inhaled steroid therapy.

15. After nebulizer treatment is complete, have patient take several deep breaths and cough to expectorate mucus.

Nebulized medication is often prescribed to open airways and promote expectoration of mucus.

16. Help patient to comfortable position and perform hand hygiene.

Reduces spread of microorganisms and promotes patient comfort.

EVALUATION

1. Assess patient's respirations, breath sounds, cough effort, sputum production, pulse oximetry, and peak flow measures if prescribed.

Determines status of breathing pattern and adequacy of ventilation/gas exchange. Allows comparison with baseline data and evaluation of effectiveness of procedure.

2. Ask patient to explain medication schedule.

Improves likelihood of adherence to therapy.

3. Ask patient to describe adverse effects of medication and criteria for calling health care provider.

Allows patient to recognize signs of overuse and need to seek medical support when medications are ineffective.

4. Use Teach-Back: "I want to be sure I was clear about how to put together the nebulizer and add medications. Show me the steps for assembling the nebulizer and adding medications." Develop a revised teaching plan if patient or caregiver is not able to teach back correctly.

Determines patient's and caregiver's level of understanding of instructional topic.

Unexpected Outcomes

1. Patient's breathing pattern is ineffective; respirations are rapid and shallow; breath sounds indicate wheezing.
2. Patient experiences paroxysms of coughing. Aerosolized particles can irritate posterior pharynx.
3. Patient experiences cardiac dysrhythmias (light-headedness, syncope), especially if receiving beta-adrenergics.

Related Interventions

- Reassess type of medication and/or delivery method.
- Notify health care provider.
- Reassess type of medication and/or delivery method.
- Notify health care provider.
- Withhold all further doses of medication. Assess vital signs.
- Notify health care provider for reassessment of type of medication and delivery method.

Communication and Documentation

- Document medication, dose and strength, route, length of treatment, and time administered on MAR immediately after administration, not before. Include initials or signature.
- Document patient teaching and validation of patient's understanding on flow sheet or in nurses' notes in electronic health record (EHR) or chart.
- Document patient's response to treatment on flow sheet or in nurses' notes in EHR or chart.
- Report adverse effects and patient response and withheld medications to nurse in charge or health care provider.

Special Considerations
Teaching

- Teach patient not to store medication in nebulizer for later use.
- Advise patients taking long-acting beta-agonists about possible adverse effects, including nervousness, restlessness, tremor, headache, nausea, rapid or pounding heart rate, and dizziness.
- Teach patients how to use small, handheld peak flowmeters to monitor response to therapy when inhaled medications are prescribed (Barrons, Pegram, & Borries, 2011) (see Box 21.6).

Pediatric

- Use a mask for the nebulizer treatment if child is too young to hold mouthpiece correctly for the duration of the treatment (Perry et al., 2017).
- Instruct child to breathe normally with mouth open to provide a direct route to the airways for the medication.
- Educate child and parent about the need to use the nebulizer during school or day care hours. Help family find resources within the school or day care facility. Follow school policy regarding having the nebulizer and medication available for use during school hours. A health care provider's prescription may be necessary.

Gerontological

- Older persons with a weak grasp, hand tremors, or coordination problems may not be able to manipulate or hold a nebulizer. In some situations an aerosol mask would be more beneficial, for example, an older patient with Parkinson's disease.

Care in the Community

- When at home, nebulizer parts should be rinsed after each use with clear water and air dried (Medline Plus, 2019). Do not store nebulizer parts until completely dry.

✦ SKILL 21.9 Administering Vaginal Instillations

NSO *Nursing Skills Online Administration of Nonparenteral Medications Module 6 / Lesson 7*

Female patients who develop vaginal infections often require topical application of anti-infective medications. Vaginal medications are available in foam, jelly, cream, or suppository form. Medicated irrigations or douches can also be given. However, their excessive use can lead to vaginal irritation.

Vaginal suppositories are oval shaped and come individually packaged in foil wrappers. They are larger and more oval than rectal suppositories (Fig. 21.3). Storage in a refrigerator prevents the solid suppositories from melting. A suppository is inserted into the vagina with an applicator or a gloved hand. After insertion, body temperature causes the suppository to melt for effective medication distribution. Foam, jellies, and creams can be inserted with an inserter or applicator. Patients often prefer administering their own vaginal medications, and they should be given privacy to do so. Offer the patient a perineal pad to wear after medication instillation to collect excess drainage. Because vaginal medications are frequently given to treat infection, any discharge is often foul smelling. Follow good aseptic technique and offer patient frequent opportunities for perineal hygiene (see Procedural Guideline 18.1).

Delegation and Collaboration

The skill of administering vaginal medications cannot be delegated to an unregulated care provider (UCP). The nurse instructs the UCP about:

- Potential adverse effects of medications and to report their occurrence to the nurse.
- Reporting any change in comfort level or new or increased vaginal discharge or bleeding to the nurse.

Equipment

- Medication administration record (MAR) (electronic or printed)
- Vaginal cream, foam, jelly, tablet, suppository, or irrigating solution
- Applicators (Fig. 21.4) (if needed)
- Clean gloves
- Tissues

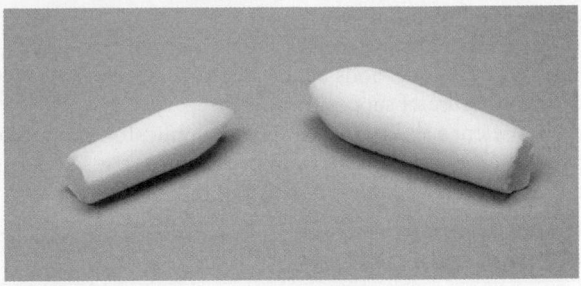

FIG 21.3 Vaginal suppositories *(right)* are larger and more oval than rectal suppositories *(left)*.

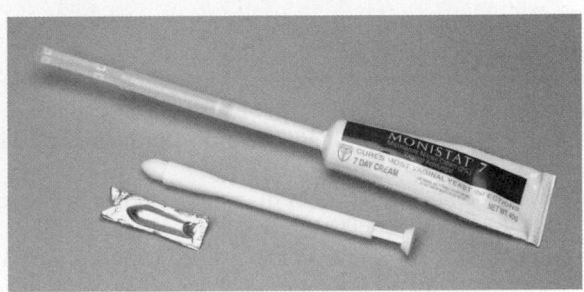

FIG 21.4 From top: Vaginal cream with applicator, applicator, and vaginal suppository. *(From Lilley, L. L., et al. [2011]. Pharmacology and the nursing process [6th ed.]. St. Louis: Mosby.)*

- Towels, washcloths, or both
- Perineal pad; drape or sheet
- Water-soluble lubricants
- Bedpan
- Irrigation or douche container (if needed)
- *Option:* Gooseneck lamp

STEP	RATIONALE

ASSESSMENT

1. Check accuracy and completeness of each MAR with health care provider's medication prescription. Check patient's name, medication name and dosage, route, and time for administration. Clarify incomplete or unclear prescriptions with health care provider before administration.

   The prescription sheet is the most reliable source and only legal record of medications that patient is to receive. It ensures that patient receives correct medications (Basukala et al. 2017). Handwritten MARs are a source of medication errors (Basukala et al., 2017).

2. Review pertinent information related to medication, including action, purpose, normal dose and route, adverse effects, time of onset and peak action, and nursing implications.

   Allows you to anticipate effects of medication and observe patient's response.

3. Assess patient's medical and medication history and history of allergies. List medication allergies on each page of the MAR and prominently display it on the patient's medical record per employer policy. When patient has allergy, provide allergy bracelet.

   These factors influence how certain medications act. Information also reflects patient's need for medications and risk for adverse effects. Communication of allergies is essential for safe and effective care.

4. Perform hand hygiene and apply clean gloves. During perineal care, inspect condition of vaginal tissues; note if drainage is present. Remove gloves and perform hand hygiene.

   Prevents transmission of microorganisms. Identifies symptoms of vaginal irritation or infection.

STEP	RATIONALE

ASSESSMENT

5. Ask if patient is experiencing any symptoms of pruritus, burning, or discomfort.

Identifies symptoms of vaginal irritation or infection.

6. Review patient's knowledge of medication and readiness to learn (e.g., asks questions about medication, requests education in use of suppository).

Indicates need for health teaching. Understanding influences adherence to therapy.

7. Assess patient's ability to manipulate applicator, suppository, or irrigation equipment and to properly position self to insert medication (may be done just before insertion).

Presence of mobility restrictions indicates need for help.

NURSING DIAGNOSES

- Insufficient knowledge regarding vaginal medication administration
- Pain (acute or chronic)
- Reduced functional mobility
- Potential sexual dysfunction

Related factors/Risk factors are individualized on the basis of patient's condition or needs.

PLANNING

1. Expected outcomes following completion of procedure:
   - Vaginal tissues are pink and smooth. Genitalia are clear and without discharge.

   Tissues take on normal characteristics.

   - Patient denies symptoms of discomfort and expresses relief from symptoms of infection or inflammation. Small amount of discharge the colour of medication is present.

   Inflammation or infection has resolved. When suppository or cream becomes distributed, small amount may escape from vaginal orifice.

   - Patient can discuss information about prescribed medication.

   Feedback reflects patient's learning.

   - Patient demonstrates self-administration of suppository, medication, or irrigation.

   Demonstrates learning.

2. Collect appropriate equipment and MAR.

Ensures time management and efficiency.

IMPLEMENTATION

1. Perform hand hygiene. Prepare suppository for administration. Check label of medication against MAR two times (when removing medication from drawer/cabinet and prior to preparing medication for administration; see Skill 21.1). Preparation usually involves taking suppository out of refrigerator and taking to patient's room. Check expiration date on container.

These are the first two checks for accuracy. Process ensures that right patient receives right medication.

2. Take medication(s) to patient at correct time (see employer policy). Medications that require exact timing include stat, first-time or loading doses, and one-time doses. Give time-critical scheduled medications (e.g., antibiotics, anticoagulants, insulin, anticonvulsants, immunosuppressive medications) at exact time prescribed (no later than 30 minutes before or after scheduled dose). Give non–time-critical scheduled medications within a range of 1 or 2 hours of scheduled dose, according to employer policy (ISMP, 2011). During administration, apply 10 rights of medication administration. Perform hand hygiene.

Hospitals must adopt medication administration policy and procedure for timing of medication administration that considers nature of the prescribed medication, specific clinical application, and patient needs. Time-critical scheduled medications are those for which early or delayed administration of maintenance doses of greater than 30 minutes before or after the scheduled dose may cause harm or result in substantial suboptimal therapy or pharmacological effect. Non–time-critical medications are those for which early or delayed administration within a specified range of either 1 or 2 hours should not cause harm or result in substantial suboptimal therapy or pharmacological effect (ISMP, 2011).

3. Identify patient using at least two person-specific identifiers (e.g., name and date of birth or name and medical record number) according to employer policy. Compare identifiers with information on patient's MAR or medical record and ID band. Replace missing or faded ID bands.

Ensures correct patient. Complies with Accreditation Canada's standards and improves patient safety (Accreditation Canada, 2019).

4. At patient's bedside again compare MAR or computer printout with names of medications on medication labels and patient name. Ask patient if they have allergies.

Ensures that the right patient receives correct medication. Confirms patient's allergy history.

STEP	RATIONALE

IMPLEMENTATION

5. Explain procedure to patient. Be specific if patient plans to self-administer medication. Discuss purpose of each medication, action, and possible adverse effects. Allow patient to ask any questions about the medications. Explain procedure if patient plans to self-administer medication.

Helps patient be a participant in care, which minimizes anxiety. Patient has right to be informed, and patient's understanding of each medication improves adherence to medication therapy. Begins patient teaching regarding medications.

6. Arrange supplies at bedside and apply clean gloves. Close door or pull curtain.

Reduces transfer of microorganisms.

7. Have patient void (using bathroom facilities or bedpan). Help her lie in dorsal recumbent position. Patients with restricted mobility in knees or hips may lie supine with legs abducted.

Voiding prevents passing of urine during insertion of suppository. Position provides easy access to and good exposure of vaginal canal. Dependent position also allows suppository to completely dissolve in vagina.

8. Keep abdomen and lower extremities draped.

Minimizes patient's embarrassment by limiting exposure.

9. Be sure that vaginal orifice is well illuminated by room light. Otherwise position portable gooseneck lamp.

Proper insertion requires visualization of external genitalia if not self-administered.

10. Insert vaginal suppository.

   a. Remove suppository from wrapper and apply liberal amount of water-soluble lubricant to smooth or rounded end (see illustration). Be sure that suppository is at room temperature. Lubricate gloved index finger of dominant hand.

Lubrication reduces friction against mucosal surfaces during insertion. Use of petroleum jelly may leave residue that harbours bacteria and yeast fungi.

   b. With nondominant gloved hand gently separate labial folds in front-to-back direction.

Exposes vaginal orifice.

   c. With dominant gloved hand insert rounded end of suppository along posterior wall of vaginal canal the entire length of finger (7.5 to 10 cm [3 to 4 inches]) (see illustration).

Proper placement of suppository ensures equal distribution of medication along walls of vaginal cavity.

   d. Withdraw finger and wipe away remaining lubricant from around orifice and labia with tissue or cloth.

Maintains comfort.

11. Apply cream or foam.

   a. Fill cream or foam applicator following package directions.

Dose is based on volume in applicator.

   b. With nondominant gloved hand gently separate labial folds.

Exposes vaginal orifice.

   c. With dominant gloved hand gently insert applicator approximately 5 to 7.5 cm (2 to 3 inches). Push applicator plunger to deposit medication into vagina (see illustration).

Allows equal distribution of medication along vaginal walls.

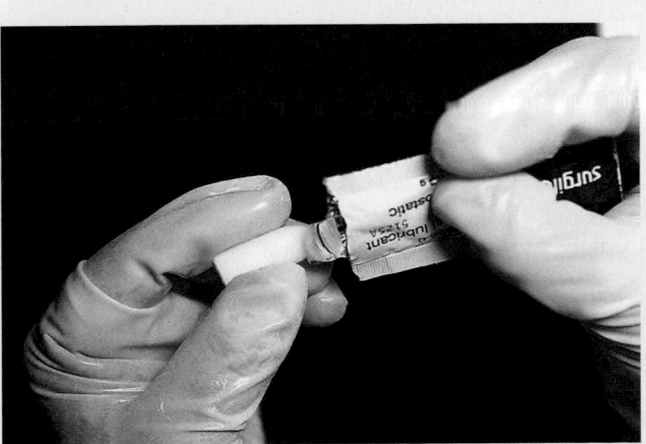

STEP 10a Lubricate tip of suppository.

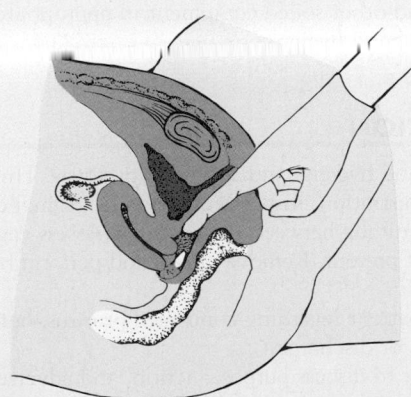

STEP 10c Angle of vaginal suppository insertion.

STEP	RATIONALE

IMPLEMENTATION

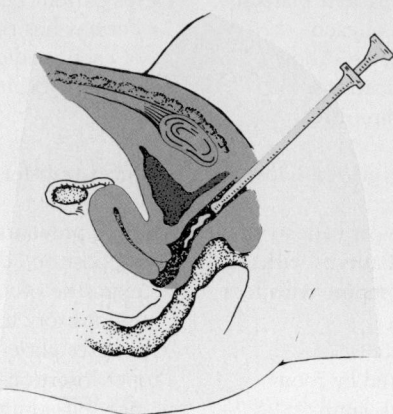

STEP 11c Applicator inserted into vaginal canal. Plunger pushed to instill medication.

d. Withdraw applicator and place on paper towel. Wipe off residual cream from labia or vaginal orifice with tissue or cloth.	Maintains patient comfort.
12. Administer irrigation or douche, if prescribed.	
a. Place patient on bedpan with absorbent pad underneath.	Allows hips to be higher than shoulders and solution to reach posterior wall of vagina. Bedpan collects solution.
b. Be sure that irrigation or douche fluid is at body temperature. Run fluid through container nozzle (priming the tubing).	Body temperature promotes patient comfort. Priming tubing removes air and moistens nozzle tip.
c. Gently separate labial folds and direct nozzle toward sacrum, following floor of vagina.	Correct angle allows nozzle access into vagina.
d. Raise container approximately 30 to 50 cm (12 to 20 inches) above level of vagina. Insert nozzle 7 to 10 cm (3 to 4 inches). Allow solution to flow while rotating nozzle. Administer all irrigating solution.	Rotating nozzle allows irrigation of all areas in vagina.
e. Withdraw nozzle and help patient to comfortable sitting position.	Remaining solution drains by gravity.
f. Allow patient to remain on bedpan for a few minutes. Clean perineum with soap and water.	Ensures that all solution drains from vagina. Provides comfort for patient.
g. Help patient off bedpan. Dry perineal area.	Provides comfort.
13. Instruct patient who received suppository, cream, or tablet to remain on her back for at least 10 minutes.	Allows melting and spreading of medication throughout vaginal cavity and prevents loss through vaginal orifice.
14. If using an applicator, wash with soap and warm water, rinse, air dry, and then store for future use.	Vaginal cavity is not sterile. Soap and water help to remove bacteria and residual cream from applicator.
15. Offer perineal pad when patient resumes ambulation.	Provides patient comfort.
16. Discard gloves by turning them inside out and dispose of them and other soiled equipment in appropriate receptacle. Perform hand hygiene.	Reduces spread of microorganisms.

EVALUATION

1. Perform hand hygiene and apply clean gloves. Thirty minutes after administration, inspect condition of vaginal canal and external genitalia between applications. Assess vaginal discharge if present. Remove gloves and perform hand hygiene.	Determines whether vaginal medication effectively reduced irritation or inflammation of tissues.
2. Question patient regarding continued pruritus, burning, discomfort, or discharge.	Determines whether symptoms are relieved.
3. Ask patient to discuss purpose, action, and adverse effects of medication.	Reflects patient's understanding of medication therapy.

STEP	RATIONALE

EVALUATION

4. Use Teach-Back: "I want to be sure I explained how to use the vaginal cream applicator. Tell me how you will draw the correct amount of cream into the applicator." Develop a revised teaching plan if patient or caregiver is not able to teach back correctly.

Determines patient's and caregiver's level of understanding of instructional topic.

Unexpected Outcomes	Related Interventions
1. Patient reports localized pruritus and burning.	• Results of infection or inflammation but may be possible adverse effects of some medications (e.g., miconazole).
	• Monitor symptoms; report to health care provider.
2. Patient is unable to discuss medication therapy correctly.	• Repeat instructions or assess if patient can learn.
	• Include caregiver when appropriate.
3. Patient is unable to self-administer medications.	• Reinstruction is necessary.

Communication and Documentation

- Document medication (or solution if vaginal instillation), dose, type of instillation, and time administered on MAR immediately after administration, not before. Include initials or signature.
- Document patient response to medication, patient teaching, and validation of understanding and ability to self-administer medication on flow sheet or in nurses' notes in electronic health record (EHR) or chart.
- Report to health care provider if patient states that symptoms do not disappear, or symptoms get worse.
- Report adverse effects and patient response and/or withheld medications to supervisor or health care provider.

Special Considerations
Teaching

- Encourage patient to take *all* the medication as prescribed, for the prescribed amount of time, to ensure effectiveness of the treatment.

- Female patients taking antifungal medications for the treatment of vaginal infections should abstain from sexual intercourse until the treatment is completed and the infection is resolved. They should be told to continue to take the medication even if actively menstruating. Patients should notify the health care provider if symptoms persist past the treatment time period (Burchum & Rosenthal, 2016).
- Many females prefer to self-administer vaginal irrigations and medications. These procedures may be self-administered while patient is sitting on the toilet. Ensure that patient is able to perform the procedure correctly.

Gerontological

- Older persons may have difficulty manipulating suppository, applicator, or irrigating equipment. If so, a caregiver may need instruction on how to administer the medication.

◆ SKILL 21.10 Administering Rectal Suppositories

NSO *Nursing Skills Online Administration of Nonparenteral Medications Module 6 / Lesson 7*

A rectal suppository is a form of medication that acts when it melts and is absorbed into the rectal mucosa. Rectal medications exert either local effects on gastrointestinal (GI) mucosa (e.g., promoting defecation) or systemic effects (e.g., relieving nausea or providing analgesia). The rectal route is not as reliable as oral or parenteral routes in terms of medication absorption and distribution. However, the medications are relatively safe because they rarely cause local irritation or adverse effects. Rectal medications are contraindicated in patients with recent surgery on the rectum, bowel, or prostate gland; rectal bleeding or prolapse; and very low platelet counts (Burchum & Rosenthal, 2016).

Rectal suppositories are thinner and more bullet-shaped than vaginal suppositories (see Fig. 21.3). The rounded end prevents anal trauma during insertion. When administering a rectal suppository, placing it past the internal anal sphincter and against the rectal mucosa is important. Improper placement can result in expulsion of the suppository before the medication dissolves and is absorbed into the mucosa. If a patient prefers to self-administer a suppository, give specific instructions so the medication is deposited correctly. Do not cut the suppository into sections to divide the dosage; the active medication may not be distributed evenly within

the suppository, and the result may be an inaccurate dose (Burchum & Rosenthal, 2016)

Delegation and Collaboration

The skill of rectal medication administration cannot be delegated to an unregulated care provider (UCP). The nurse instructs the UCP about:

- Reporting expected fecal discharge or bowel movement to the nurse.
- Potential adverse effects of medications and to report their occurrence to the nurse.
- Informing the nurse of any rectal pain or bleeding.

Equipment

- Medication administration record (MAR) (electronic or printed)
- Rectal suppository
- Water-soluble lubricating jelly
- Clean gloves
- Tissue
- Drape

STEP	RATIONALE

ASSESSMENT

1. Check accuracy and completeness of each MAR with health care provider's medication prescription. Check patient's name, medication name and dosage, route, and time for administration. Clarify incomplete or unclear prescriptions with health care provider before administration.

The prescription sheet is the most reliable source and only legal record of medications that patient is to receive. It ensures that patient receives correct medications (Basukala et al., 2017).

Handwritten MARs are a source of medication errors (Basukala et al., 2017).

2. Review pertinent information related to medication, including action, purpose, normal dose and route, adverse effects, time of onset and peak action, and nursing implications.

Allows you to anticipate effects of medication and observe patient's response.

3. Review patient's medical history for history of rectal surgery or bleeding, cardiac problems, history of allergies, and medication history. List medication allergies on each page of the MAR and prominently display it on the patient's medical record per employer policy. When patient has allergy, provide allergy bracelet.

Conditions may contraindicate use of suppository. Communication of allergies is essential for safe and effective care.

4. Review any presenting signs and symptoms of GI alterations (e.g., constipation or diarrhea).

Conditions indicate use of suppository.

5. Assess patient's ability to hold suppository and position self to insert medication.

Mobility restriction indicates need for nurse to help with medication administration.

6. Review patient's knowledge of purpose of medication therapy and interest in self-administering suppository.

Indicates need for health teaching. Level of motivation influences teaching approach.

NURSING DIAGNOSES

- Pain (acute or chronic)
- Reduced functional ability
- Constipation

- Insufficient knowledge regarding suppository administration

- Ready for enhanced self-health management

Related factors/Risk factors are individualized on the basis of patient's condition or needs.

PLANNING

1. Expected outcomes following completion of the procedure:
- Patient reports relief or reduction in symptoms for which medication is prescribed.

Medication acts effectively.

- Patient describes purpose of medication.

Feedback reflects patient's learning.

- Patient demonstrates self-administration of rectal suppository.

Demonstrates learning.

2. Collect appropriate equipment and MAR.

Ensures time management and efficiency.

IMPLEMENTATION

1. Perform hand hygiene and prepare suppository for administration. Check label of medication against MAR two times (when removing medication from drawer/cabinet and prior to preparing medication for administration; see Skill 21.1). Check expiration date on container.

These are the first two checks for accuracy. Process ensures that right patient receives right medication at the right time.

2. Take medication(s) to patient at correct time (see employer policy). Medications that require exact timing include stat, first-time or loading doses, and one-time doses. Give time-critical scheduled medications (e.g., antibiotics, anticoagulants, insulin, anticonvulsants, immunosuppressive medications) at exact time prescribed (no later than 30 minutes before or after scheduled dose). Give non–time-critical scheduled medications within a range of 1 or 2 hours of scheduled dose, according to employer policy (ISMP, 2011). During administration, apply 10 rights of medication administration. Perform hand hygiene.

Hospitals must adopt medication administration policy and procedure for timing of medication administration that considers nature of the prescribed medication, specific clinical application, and patient needs. Time-critical scheduled medications are those for which early or delayed administration of maintenance doses of greater than 30 minutes before or after the scheduled dose may cause harm or result in substantial suboptimal therapy or pharmacological effect. Non–time-critical medications are those for which early or delayed administration within a specified range of either 1 or 2 hours should not cause harm or result in substantial suboptimal therapy or pharmacological effect (ISMP, 2011).

STEP	RATIONALE

IMPLEMENTATION

3. Identify patient using at least two person-specific identifiers (e.g., name and date of birth or name and medical record number) according to employer policy. Compare identifiers with information on patient's MAR or medical record and ID band. Replace missing or faded ID bands.

Ensures correct patient. Complies with Accreditation Canada's standards and improves patient safety (Accreditation Canada, 2019).

4. At patient's bedside again compare MAR or computer printout with names of medications on medication labels and patient name. Ask patient if they have allergies.

Ensures that the right patient receives correct medication. Confirms patient's allergy history.

5. Explain procedure to patient. Be specific if patient wishes to self-administer medication. Discuss purpose of each medication, action, and possible adverse effects. Allow patient to ask any questions about the medications. Explain procedure if patient plans to self-administer medication.

Helps patient be a participant in care, which minimizes anxiety. Patient has the right to be informed, and patient's understanding of each medication improves adherence to medication therapy. Begins patient teaching regarding medications.

6. Arrange supplies at bedside and apply clean gloves. Close room curtain or door.

Reduces transfer of microorganisms. Maintains privacy and minimizes embarrassment.

7. Help patient assume left side-lying Sims' position with upper leg flexed upward.

Position exposes anus and relaxes external anal sphincter. Left side-lying Sims' position lessens likelihood of suppository or feces being expelled.

8. If patient has mobility impairment, help into lateral position. Obtain help to turn patient and use pillows under upper arm and leg.

Provides support during procedure and patient comfort.

9. Keep patient draped with only anal area exposed.

Maintains privacy and facilitates relaxation.

10. Examine condition of anus externally. *Option:* Palpate rectal walls as needed (e.g., if impaction is suspected) (see Chapter 8). If you palpate rectal walls, dispose of gloves by turning them inside out and placing them in proper receptacle if they become soiled. Otherwise keep gloves on your hands and proceed to Step 12.

Determines presence of active rectal bleeding. Palpation determines whether rectum is filled with feces, which interferes with suppository placement. Reduces spread of infection.

Clinical Decision Point *Do not palpate patient's rectum if there is a recent history of rectal surgery. A suppository is contraindicated in the presence of active rectal bleeding and diarrhea (Burchum & Rosenthal, 2016).*

11. Perform hand hygiene and apply new pair of clean gloves (if previous gloves were soiled and discarded).

Minimizes contact with fecal material to reduce transmission of infection.

12. Remove suppository from foil wrapper and lubricate rounded end with water-soluble lubricant. Lubricate gloved index finger of dominant hand. If patient has hemorrhoids, use liberal amount of lubricant and touch area gently.

Lubrication reduces friction as suppository enters rectal canal.

13. Ask patient to take slow, deep breaths through mouth and relax anal sphincter.

Forcing suppository through constricted sphincter causes pain.

14. Retract patient's buttocks with nondominant hand. With gloved index finger of dominant hand, insert suppository gently through anus, past internal sphincter, and against rectal wall, 10 cm (4 inches) in adults (see illustration) or 5 cm (2 inches) in infants and children. You should feel rectal sphincter close around your finger.

Suppository needs to be against rectal mucosa for eventual absorption and therapeutic action.

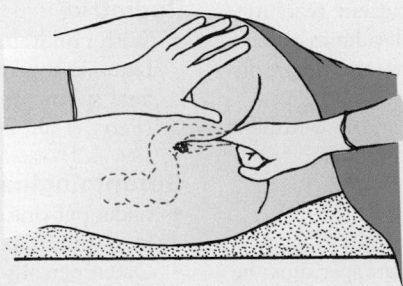

STEP 14 Insert rectal suppository past sphincter and against rectal wall.

STEP	RATIONALE

IMPLEMENTATION

Clinical Decision Point *Do not insert suppository into a mass of fecal material; this will reduce effectiveness of medication.*

15. *Option:* A suppository may be given through a colostomy (not ileostomy) if prescribed. Patient should lie supine. Use small amount of water-soluble lubricant for insertion.
16. Withdraw finger and wipe patient's anal area.   Provides comfort.
17. Ask patient to remain flat or on side for 5 minutes.   Prevents expulsion of suppository.
18. Discard gloves by turning them inside out and dispose of   Reduces transfer of microorganisms.
    them and used supplies in appropriate receptacle. Perform
    hand hygiene.
19. If suppository contains laxative or fecal softener, place call   Ability to call for help provides patient with sense of control
    light within reach so patient can obtain help to reach   over elimination.
    bedpan or toilet.
20. If suppository was given for constipation, remind patient   Allows staff to evaluate results of suppository.
    not to flush commode after bowel movement.

EVALUATION

1. Return to bedside within 5 minutes to determine if   Determines if medication is distributed properly. Reinsertion may
   suppository was expelled.   be necessary.
2. Ask if patient experienced localized anal or rectal discomfort Determines whether insertion of suppository was irritating.
   during insertion.
3. Evaluate patient at time of peak medication effect for relief of Determines effectiveness of medication.
   symptoms for which medication was prescribed.
4. **Use Teach-Back:** "I want to be sure I explained clearly to   Determines patient's and caregiver's level of understanding of
   you how to insert a rectal suppository. Describe the steps you   instructional topic.
   take to insert the suppository." Develop a revised teaching
   plan if patient or caregiver is not able to teach back correctly.

Unexpected Outcomes	Related Interventions
1. Patient's symptoms are unrelieved.	• Explore alternative therapy.
2. Patient experiences decreased heart rate during rectal suppository insertion.	• Unintended vagal stimulation may occur, resulting in bradycardia in some patients.
	• Monitor heart rate of patient. Rectal route may not be suitable for certain cardiac conditions.
3. Patient reports rectal pain during insertion.	• Suppository may need more lubrication.
	• Rectal route may not be suitable; assess and notify health care provider.

Communication and Documentation

- Document the medication, dosage, route, and actual time and date of administration on MAR immediately after administration, not before. Include initials or signature.
- Document patient response to medication, patient teaching, and validation of patient understanding and self-administration of suppository on flow sheet or in nurses' notes in electronic health record (EHR) or chart.
- Report adverse effects and patient response and/or withheld medication to nurse in charge or health care provider.

Special Considerations
Teaching

- Be certain that patient is aware that the foil wrapper must be removed before insertion and that the suppository is to be inserted rectally and not taken orally. If patient chooses to self-administer

suppositories or if a caregiver plans to administer, teach principles and techniques of infection control to prevent contact with and spread of fecal material.

Pediatric

- With children, it is often necessary to gently hold or tape the buttocks together for 5 to 10 minutes to relieve pressure on the anal sphincter until the urge to expel the suppository is gone (Perry et al., 2017).

Gerontological

- Older persons with loss of sphincter control may have difficulty retaining suppository.
- Older persons may have difficulty manipulating suppository, applicator, or irrigating equipment. If so, a caregiver may need instruction on how to insert the medication.

◆ CLINICAL DEBRIEF

A 75-year-old homemaker is hospitalized for 3 days with a diagnosis of dehydration, following a week of gastroenteritis. She has a history of hypertension, asthma, angina (heart pain), and osteoarthritis in her hands. She also has an abscess on her right calf that was caused by an infected bug bite. Her medications include:

- Hydrochlorothiazide 25 mg every morning by mouth (PO) (diuretic)
- Diltiazem SR capsule, 60 mg twice a day PO (calcium channel blocker)
- Salbutamol MDI 2 puffs four times a day (inhaled bronchodilator)
- Bacitracin topical ointment (500 units/g) applied topically to wound twice a day (antibiotic)
- Nitroglycerin transdermal patch, 0.2 mg/hr, one each morning topically (nitrate)
- Nitroglycerin sublingual tablets, 400 mcg, as needed for chest pain (nitrate)

1. She is discharged and has a community nurse follow-up. On initial history she tells the nurse that she sometimes feels dizzy when she changes position. She also complains of a cough. The nurse decides to do a cardiopulmonary assessment first. While listening to her breath sounds, the nurse notes that she has three nitroglycerin transdermal patches on her chest. What should the nurse do first?

2. While inspecting her abscess, the nurse finds that there is a thick crust of old medication on the wound. She explains, "I don't like to waste the medication that is already there, so I just put the new medicine on top of it." How should the nurse intervene?

3. The nurse returns to the home 2 days later and notices that she is still not cleaning the wound and that the wound is larger (3 × 5 cm [1.25 × 2 inches]), is blistered, and has yellow, foul-smelling drainage. Using SBAR, show how to communicate with other community care nurses for this patient.

◆ REVIEW QUESTIONS

1. A patient is to receive medications through a small-bore nasogastric feeding. Which nursing actions are appropriate? *(Select all that apply.)*
   1. Verifying tube placement after medications are given
   2. Mixing all medications together and giving all at once
   3. Using an enteral tube syringe to administer medications
   4. Flushing the tube with 30 to 60 mL of water after the last dose of medication
   5. Checking for gastric residual before giving the medications
   6. Keeping the head of the bed elevated 30 to 60 minutes after the medications are given

2. The nurse is caring for a patient who is receiving nitroglycerin ointment. Which nursing interventions are most appropriate to protect the nurse against accidental exposure? *(Select all that apply.)*
   1. Cleaning skin thoroughly before applying the next dose of medication
   2. Wearing gloves when applying the ointment
   3. Using the appropriate applicator to apply the medication
   4. Drawing blood to test for therapeutic medication values
   5. Wearing gloves to discard used ointment wrappers
   6. Performing hand hygiene immediately after medication application

3. A nurse is administering a metered-dose inhaler (MDI) with a spacer to a patient with chronic obstructive pulmonary disease. Place the steps of the procedure in the correct order.
   1. Insert MDI into end of spacer.
   2. Perform a respiratory assessment.
   3. Remove mouthpiece from MDI and spacer device.
   4. Place spacer mouthpiece into patient's mouth and instruct patient to close lips around it.

5. Depress medication canister, spraying 1 puff into spacer device.
6. Shake inhaler for 2 to 5 seconds.
7. Instruct patient to hold breath for 10 seconds.
8. Instruct patient to breathe in slowly through mouth for 3 to 5 seconds.

ⓔ *Visit the Evolve site for a complete list of Clinical Debrief and Review Questions answers.*

REFERENCES

Accreditation Canada. (2019). *Required organizational practices handbook—Version 14.* Retrieved from http://www.wrha.mb.ca/quality/files/2019ROPHandbook.pdf

Allen, S. M. (2015). As a flushing agent for enteral nutrition, does sterile water compared with tap water affect associated risk of infection in critically ill patients? *Alabama Nurse, March-April-May,* 5.

Ari, A. (2015). Patient education and adherence to aerosol therapy. *Respiratory Care,* 60(6), 941–957. doi:10.4187/respcare.03854

Barrons, R., Pegram, A., & Borries, A. (2011). Inhaler device selection: Special considerations in elderly patients with chronic obstructive pulmonary disease. *American Journal of Health-System Pharmacy,* 68(13), 1221–1232. doi:10.2146/ajhp100452

Basukala, S., Mehrotra, S., & Devarakonda, S. (2017). Medication errors in outpatient setting of a tertiary care hospital: Classification and root cause analysis. *International Journal of Basic & Clinical Pharmacology,* 4(6), 1235–1240. doi:10.18203/2319-2003.ijbcp20151365

Burchum, J. R., & Rosenthal, L. D. (2016). *Lehne's pharmacology for nursing care* (8th ed.). Philadelphia: Saunders.

Clifford, P., Heimall, L., Brittingham, L., & Finn Davis, K. (2015). Following the evidence: Enteral tube placement and verification in neonates and young children. *Journal of Perinatal and Neonatal Nursing,* 29(2), 149–161. doi:10.1097/JPN.0000000000000104

Cohen, H. (2013). Prevent adverse medication events from topical medications. *Nursing,* 43(7), 68–69. doi:10.1097/01.NURSE.0000429812.64600.bf

Dana Farber Cancer Institute. (2015). *Five things you need to know about oral chemotherapy.* Retrieved from http://blog.dana-farber.org/insight/2015/03/five-things-you-need-to-know-about-oral-chemotherapy/

Douglass, A. M., Elder, J., Watson, R., et al. (2018). A randomized controlled trial on the effect of a double check on the detection of medication errors. *Annals of Emergency Medicine,* 71(1), 74–82. doi:10.1016/j.annemergmed.2017.03.022

Flynn, F., Evanish, J. Q., Fernald, J. M., Hutchinson, D. E., & Lefaiver, C. (2016). Progressive care nurses improving patient safety by limiting interruptions during medication administration. *Critical Care Nurse,* 36(4), 19–35. doi:10.4037/ccn2016498

Food and Drug Administration (FDA). (2017). *Tablet splitting.* Retrieved from https://www.fda.gov/ForConsumers/ConsumerUpdates/ucm265754.htm

Giallourakis, A. (2016). *Nasal sprays work best when you use them correctly—Here's how.* Retrieved from https://health.clevelandclinic.org/nasal-sprays-work-best-when-you-use-them-correctly-heres-how/

Guenther, P. (2015). New enteral connectors: Raising awareness. *Nutrition in Clinical Practice,* 29(5), 612–614. doi:10.1177/0884533614543330

Institute for Safe Medication Practices (ISMP). (2011). *Guidelines for timely administration of scheduled medications (acute).* Retrieved from https://www.ismp.org/guidelines/timely-administration-scheduled-medications-acute

Institute for Safe Medication Practices (ISMP). (2013). Independent double checks: Undervalued and misused. *ISMP Medication Safety Alert,* 18(12).

Institute for Safe Medication Practices (ISMP). (2015). *List of confused drug names.* Retrieved from https://www.ismp.org/recommendations/confused-drug-names-list

Institute for Safe Medication Practices (ISMP). (2017). *2018–2019 Targeted medication safety best practices for hospitals.* Retrieved from https://www.ismp.org/sites/default/files/attachments/2017-12/TMSBP-for-Hospitalsv2.pdf

Institute for Safe Medication Practices Canada (ISMP). (2018a). *Do not use. Dangerous abbreviations, symbols, and dose designations.* Retrieved from https://www.ismp-canada.org/download/ISMPCanadaListOfDangerousAbbreviations.pdf

Institute for Safe Medication Practices (ISMP). (2018b). *Oral dosage forms that should not be crushed.* Retrieved from https://www.ismp.org/recommendations/do-not-crush

Klang, M., McLymont, V., & Ng, N. (2013). Osmolality, pH, and compatibility of selected oral liquid medications with an enteral nutrition product. *JPEN. Journal of Parenteral and Enteral Nutrition,* 37(5), 689–694. doi:10.1177/0148607112471560

Lawton, S. (2013). Safe and effective application of topical treatments to the skin. *Nursing Standard,* 23(42), 50–56.

Leder, S. B., Suiter, D. M., Agogo, G. O., & Cooney, L. M., Jr. (2016). An epidemiologic study on ageing and dysphagia in the acute care geriatric-hospitalized population: A replication and continuation study. *Dysphagia*, 31(5), 619–625. doi:10.1007/s00455-016-9714-x

Liston, J., & McKinnon, T. (2017). Self-assessment of perceived informatics competencies among staff nurses at Sutter Maternity and Surgery Hospital. *Journal of Informatics Nursing*, 2(1), 12–16.

Lord, L. (2018). Enteral access devices: Types, function, care and challenges. *Nutrition in Clinical Practice*, 33(1), 16–38. doi:10.1002/ncp.10019

Malone, A. (2014). Clinical guidelines from the American Society for Parenteral and Enteral Nutrition: Best practices recommendations for patient care. *Journal of Infusion Nursing*, 37(3), 179–184. doi:10.1097/NAN.0000000000000035

McIntyre, C. M., & Monk, H. M. (2014). Medication absorption considerations in patient with postpyloric enteral feeding tubes. *American Journal of Health-System Pharmacy*, 71(7), 549–556. doi:10.2146/ajhp130597

Medline Plus, US National Library of Medicine. (2019). *How to use a nebulizer.* Retrieved from https://www.nlm.nih.gov/medlineplus/ency/patientinstructions/000006.htm

Momeni, S., Nokhodchi, A., Ghanbarzadeh, S., & Hamishehkar, H. (2016). The effect of spacer morphology on the aerosolization performance of metered-dose inhalers. *Advanced Pharmaceutical Bulletin*, 6(2), 257–260. doi:10.15171/apb.2016.035

Murrell, D. (2018). *How to apply a transdermal patch.* Retrieved from https://www.healthline.com/health/general-use/how-to-use-transdermal-patch

Perry, S. E., Hockenberry, M. J., Lowdermilk, D. L., Wilson, D., Keenan-Lindsay, L., & Sams, C. A. (2017). *Maternal child nursing care in Canada* (2nd ed.). Toronto: Elsevier Canada.

Risør, B. W., Lisby, M., & Sørensen, J. (2018). Complex automated medication systems reduce medication administration errors in a Danish acute medical unit. *International Journal for Quality in Health Care*, doi:10.1093/intqhc/mzy042

Salmon, D., Pont, E., Chevallard, H., et al. (2013). Pharmaceutical and safety considerations of tablet crushing in patients undergoing enteral intubation. *International Journal of Pharmaceuticals*, 443(1–2), 146–153. doi:10.1016/j.ijpharm.2012.12.038

Schiele, J. T., Penner, H., Schneider, H., et al. (2015). Swallowing tablets and capsules increases the risk of penetration and aspiration in patients with stroke-induced dysphagia. *Dysphagia*, 30(5), 571–582. doi:10.1007/s00455-015-9639-9

Schwappach, D. L. B., Pfeiffer, Y., & Taxis, K. (2016). Medication double-checking procedures in clinical practice: A cross-sectional survey of oncology nurses' experiences. *BMJ Open*, 6(6), e011394. doi:10.1136/bmjopen-2016-011394

Shah, K., Lo, C., Babich, M., Tsao, N. W., & Bansback, N. J. (2016). Bar code medication administration technology: A systematic review of impact on patient safety when used with computerized prescriber order entry and automated dispensing devices. *Canadian Journal of Hospital Pharmacy*, 69(5), 394–402.

Shaw, M., & Lee, A. (2017). *Ophthalmic nursing* (5th ed.). Boca Raton, FL: Taylor and Francis Group.

Soones, T. N., Lin, J. L., Wolf, M. S., et al. (2017). Pathways linking health literacy, health beliefs, and cognition to medication adherence in older with asthma. *Journal of Allergy and Clinical Immunology*, 139(3), 804–809. doi:10.1016/j.jaci.2016.05.043

Touhy, T. A., Jett, K. F., Boscart, V., & McCleary, L. (2019). *Ebersole and Hess' gerontological nursing and healthy aging* (2nd Canadian ed.). Toronto, ON: Elsevier Canada.

White, R., & Bradnam, V. (2015). *Handbook of medication administration via enteral feeding tubes.* London, UK: Pharmaceutical Press.

Yoder, M., Schadewald, D., & Dietrich, K. (2015). The effect of a safe zone on nurse interruptions, distractions, and medication administration errors. *Journal of Infusion Nursing*, 38(2), 140–151. doi:10.1097/NAN.0000000000000095

22 | Parenteral Medications

Written by **Wendy R. Ostendorf, RN, MS, EdD, CNE; and Maureen MacInnis-Wheatley, RN, MN**

SKILLS AND PROCEDURES

OBJECTIVES

Mastery of content in this chapter will enable the nurse to:
- Correctly prepare injectable medications from a vial and an ampoule.
- Identify advantages, disadvantages, and risks of administering medications by each parenteral route.
- Evaluate the effectiveness and outcomes of administering medications by each parenteral route.
- Explain the importance of selecting the proper-size syringe and needle for an injection.
- Discuss factors to consider when selecting injection sites.

- Identify the anatomical landmarks used to locate each site.
- Discuss ways to promote patient comfort while administering an injection.
- Correctly administer intradermal, subcutaneous, and intramuscular injections.
- Initiate, maintain, and discontinue a continuous subcutaneous infusion.
- Compare the risks of three different intravenous routes.
- Correctly administer an intravenous medication by intravenous piggyback, intermittent infusion, or bolus.

MEDIA RESOURCES

- **evolve** http://evolve.elsevier.com/Canada/Perry/clinicalskills/
- Review Questions
- ▶ Video Clips

- Audio Glossary
- **NSO** Nursing Skills Online
- Clinical Debrief and Review Questions Answers

PURPOSE

Medications administered by the *parenteral* route enter body tissues and the circulatory system by injection. Injected medications are more quickly absorbed than oral medications. Parenteral routes are used when patients are vomiting or cannot swallow, when rapid onset of a medication is needed, or when patients are NPO (nothing by mouth). These medication administration procedures are invasive and thus pose greater risks than those associated with administering nonparenteral medications (see Chapter 21).

The four most common routes for parenteral administration are described in this chapter:
1. *Subcutaneous (SUBCUT) injection:* Injection into tissues just under the dermis of the skin
2. *Intramuscular (IM) injection:* Injection into the body of a muscle

3. *Intradermal (ID) injection:* Injection into the dermis just under the epidermis
4. *Intravenous (IV) injection or infusion:* Injection into a vein

STANDARDS OF CARE

- Accreditation Canada, 2019—*Required Organizational Practices Handbook—Version 14* (http://www.wrha.mb.ca/quality/files/2019ROPHandbook.pdf)
- Canadian Nurses Association (CNA), 2017—*Code of Ethics for Registered Nurses* (https://cna-aiic.ca/~/media/cna/page-content/pdf-en/code-of-ethics-2017-edition-secure-interactive)
- Infusion Nurses Society (INS), 2016—*Infusion Therapy Standards of Practice* (https://www.ins1.org/default.aspx)

- Institute for Safe Medication Practices (ISMP), 2011—*Guidelines for Timely Administration of Scheduled Medications (Acute)* (http://www.ismp.org/Tools/guidelines/acutecare/tasm.pdf)
- Institute for Safe Medication Practices (ISMP), 2012—*Side Tracks on the Safety Express. Interruptions Lead to Errors and Unfinished. Wait, What Was I Doing?* (http://www.ismp.org/newsletters/acutecare/showarticle.aspx?id=37)
- Institute for Safe Medication Practices (ISMP), 2015—*Safe Practice Guidelines for Adult IV Push Medications.* (https://www.ismp.org/sites/default/files/attachments/2017-11/ISMP97-Guidelines-071415-3.%20FINAL.pdf)
- Institute for Safe Medication Practices (ISMP), 2017b—*Targeted Medication Safety Best Practices for Hospitals* (https://www.ismp.org/sites/default/files/attachments/2019-01/TMSBP-for-Hospitalsv2.pdf)
- Professional Practice Standards set by provincial and territorial nursing associations

PRINCIPLES FOR PRACTICE

- When managing a patient's medications, communicate clearly with the health care team, assess and incorporate the patient's priorities of care and preferences, and use the best evidence when making decisions about patient care.
- Use technology (e.g., bar scanning, electronic medication administration record [MAR]) that is available in the facility when preparing and giving medications.
- Educate patients and caregivers about each medication they take while you are administering medications. Patients often can identify inappropriate medications. Make sure that you answer all questions before administering medications.
- Minimize a patient's discomfort when giving an injection:
  - Use sharp, bevelled needles in the shortest length and smallest gauge possible.
  - Change the needle after drawing up the medication.
  - Position and flex a patient's limbs to reduce muscular tension.
  - Divert the patient's attention away from the injection procedure.
  - Apply a vapocoolant spray (e.g., Flouri-Methane spray) or topical anaesthetic (e.g., EMLA cream) to an injection site before giving a medication, when possible, or place wrapped ice on the site for a minute before injection.

PERSON-CENTRED CARE

- Research shows that ethnicity, genetics, and culture may influence a patient's drug response, pharmacokinetics, and pharmacodynamics, and patient adherence and understanding (Burchum & Rosenthal, 2016; Giger, 2017; Tantisira & Weiss, 2019).
- Knowledge about variations in therapeutic dose and adverse effects is essential in administering medications to different ethnic groups. Some patients experience a therapeutic response at a different dosage than recommended and require careful monitoring.
- As a nurse you need skill in communicating with and educating diverse patient populations. For example, if a patient values patience and modesty, make your questions specific and take time when assessing their knowledge about adverse drug effects.
- Cultural assessment also yields information about dietary preferences, tobacco and alcohol use, and use of herbal remedies that affect drug action and response.
- Practising person-centred care ensures that cultural context is considered when planning education for patients and families (Burchum & Rosenthal, 2016).

EVIDENCE-INFORMED PRACTICE

IM injection technique has been modified over the past several years in response to evidence and research about best practices for patient assessment and site selection. In the past, site selection was not evidence informed, and needle selection was based on nursing preference and ritualistic practice (Greenway, 2014). There is now enough consensual evidence to develop guidelines for administration of IM injections. Based on this evidence:

- Select needle size based on patient gender, weight and body mass index, condition, site, drug, and volume.
- Make the ventrogluteal site the first choice for all IM injections, unless contraindicated in a specific patient, because this site has reduced risks of nerve or muscle injury.
- Assess the skin and the patient's condition before and after an IM injection.
- Inject at 90 degrees, dartlike, to the hub of the needle and inject at 1 mL per 10 seconds.
- Wait at least 10 seconds before withdrawing the needle.

SAFETY GUIDELINES

Patient safety in administering medication involves following the 10 rights of medication administration (see Chapter 20). Follow these guidelines to ensure safe medication administration:

- Be vigilant during medication administration. Avoid distractions while preparing an injection.
- Create no-interruption zones (NIZ) by placing red tape or tile borders on the floor around medication carts. Nurses standing in these zones are not to be interrupted (ISMP, 2012).
- Ensure that patients receive the appropriate medications. Know why the patient is receiving each medication; know what you need to do before, during, and after medication administration; and evaluate the effectiveness of medications and any adverse effects after administration.
- Verify that the medications have not expired.
- Follow best practice guidelines for timing of medication administration.
  - Medications that require exact timing include stat, first-time, or loading doses, and one-time doses.
  - *Time-critical medications* are drugs that may cause harm or result in substantial suboptimal therapy or pharmacological effect if not administered at the scheduled time (must be given no later than 30 minutes before or after the scheduled dose) (e.g., antibiotics, insulin, anticoagulants, anticonvulsants, immunosuppressive agents).
  - *Non–time-critical medications* are drugs that should not cause harm or result in substantial suboptimal therapy or pharmacological effect if given within a range of 1 or 2 hours of the scheduled time (ISMP, 2011).
- Use at least two person-specific identifiers before administering medications and check against the MAR. Follow employer policy for patient identification (Accreditation Canada, 2019).
- Clarify unclear medication prescriptions and ask for help whenever you are uncertain about a prescription or calculation. Consult with other health care team members and be sure that you have resolved all concerns related to medication administration before preparing and giving medications.
- Follow all policies related to use of the technology and do not use "work-arounds." Nurses who use "work-arounds" fail to follow employer policies during medication administration in an attempt to get medications administered to patients in a timelier manner.

- Use strict aseptic technique during medication preparation and administration (Table 22.1).
- The nurse usually cannot delegate medication administration. Ensure that you follow standards set by the legislation in your province or territory and employer policy.
- Insert the needle at the proper angle, smoothly, and quickly (Fig. 22.1). Do not hesitate. Then, slowly push the needle into tissue.
- Inject the medication slowly (1 mL/10 seconds), but smoothly.
- Hold the syringe steady once the needle is in the tissue to prevent tissue damage.
- Withdraw the needle smoothly at the same angle used for insertion.
- Gently apply an antiseptic pad (e.g., alcohol) or dry gauze pad to the site.
- Apply gentle pressure at the injection site.
- Rotate injection sites to prevent the formation of indurations and abscesses

TABLE 22.1

Preventing Infection During an Injection

Principle	Technique
Prevent contamination of solution	Ampoules should not sit open, and medication should be removed quickly.
Prevent needle contamination	Avoid letting needle touch contaminated surface (e.g., outer edges of ampoule or vial, outer surface of needle cap, your hands, countertop, or table surface). Change the needle after drawing up the medication. Avoid touching length of plunger or inner part of barrel. Keep tip of syringe covered with cap or needle.
Prepare skin	Wash skin soiled with dirt, drainage, or feces with soap and water. Use friction and a circular motion while cleaning with an antiseptic swab. Swab from centre of site and move outward in a 5-cm (2-inch) radius.
Reduce transfer of microorganisms	Perform hand hygiene for a minimum of 15 seconds.

Needle-Stick Prevention

The most frequent route of exposure to bloodborne disease for health care workers is from needle-stick injuries (Canadian Centre for Occupational Health and Safety [CCOHS], 2019; Public Health Agency of Canada [PHAC], 2013). These injuries occur when health care workers recap needles, mishandle intravenous (IV) lines and needles, or leave needles at a patient's bedside. However, the implementation of safe needle devices can prevent needle-sticks (CCOHS, 2019) (see Fig. 22.2, C). Occupational Health and Safety legislation varies from one province/territory to another. In practice settings where these safety devices are not available, nurses should lobby for their implementation as evidence-informed best practice.

A sharp (needle, lancet) with engineered sharps injury protection (SESIP) is a device designed to prevent needle-sticks. One type of SESIP is a blunt-end cannula; another is a safety syringe equipped with a plastic guard or sheath that slips over the needle as it is withdrawn from the skin (Fig. 22.2, A–C). The guard immediately covers the needle, eliminating the chance for a needle-stick injury. A variety of other SESIP devices are found in needleless IV line connection systems (see Chapter 29). Box 22.1 lists recommendations to reduce the risk of needle-stick injuries.

Special puncture- and leak-proof containers are available for the disposal of sharps. Containers are made so only one hand needs to be used when disposing of an uncapped needle. In addition, containers must stand upright, not be allowed to overfill, and be coloured red or labelled with a biohazard symbol (Fig. 22.3).

Equipment

The appropriate size of the syringe, and length and gauge of the needle, is determined on the basis of the volume of solution prescribed, medication route, type of medication prescribed, viscosity of the medication, and patient body size, age, and gender for intramuscular injections. To ensure a constant and accurate delivery of medication, use electronic infusion pumps to deliver IV or continuous subcutaneous infusions.

Syringes

Syringes are single use, disposable, and either Luer-Lok or non–Luer-Lok. The design of the syringe tip influences the name. Syringes come with or without a sterile needle and with a needleless SESIP device. The parts of a syringe are shown in (Fig. 22.4). Non–Luer-Lok

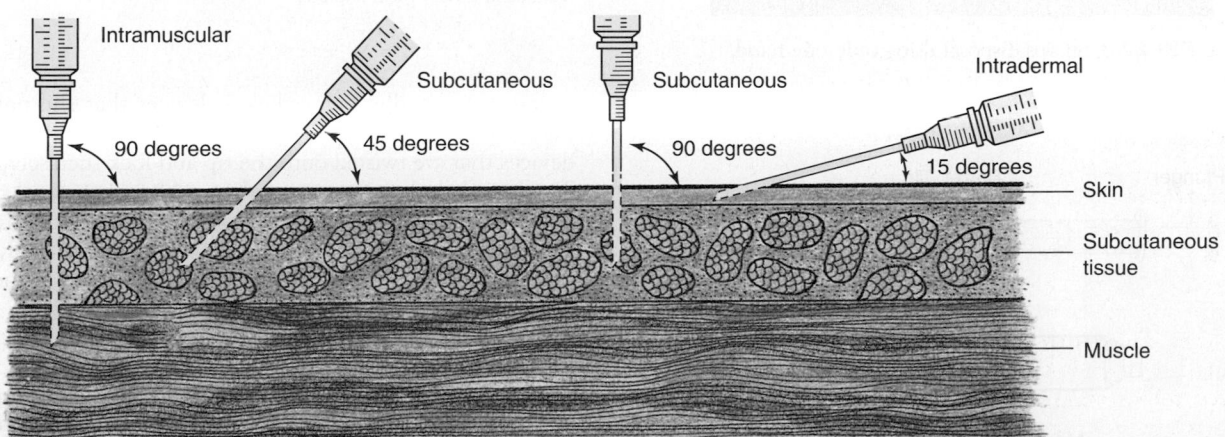

FIG 22.1 Comparison of angles of insertion of intramuscular (90 degrees), subcutaneous (45 or 90 degrees), and intradermal (15 degrees) injections.

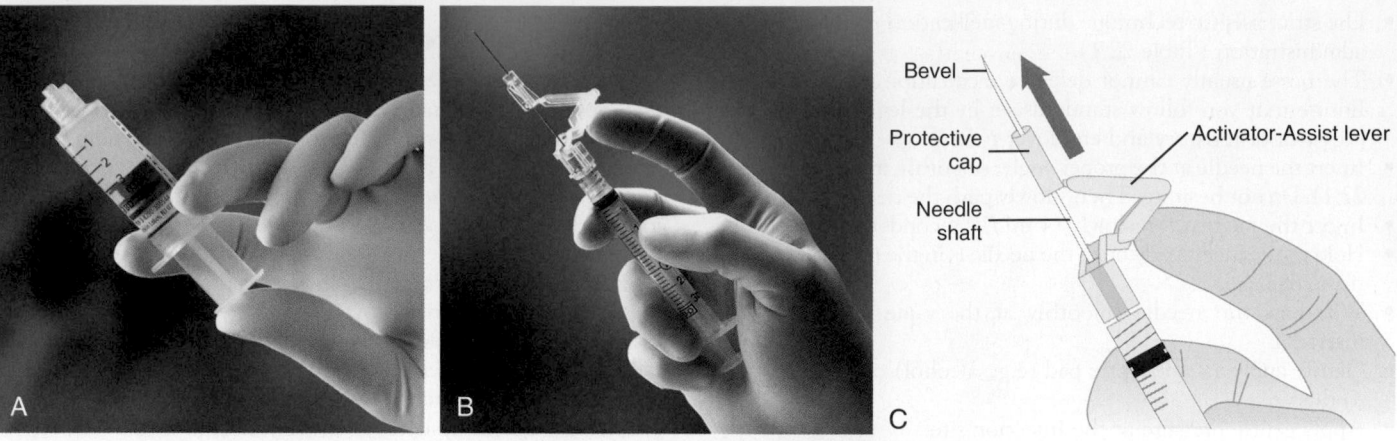

FIG 22.2 A, Needleless system. **B,** Safety needle system. **C,** Detail of safety needle system. (**A** *and* **B** *Courtesy and © Becton, Dickinson and Company.*)

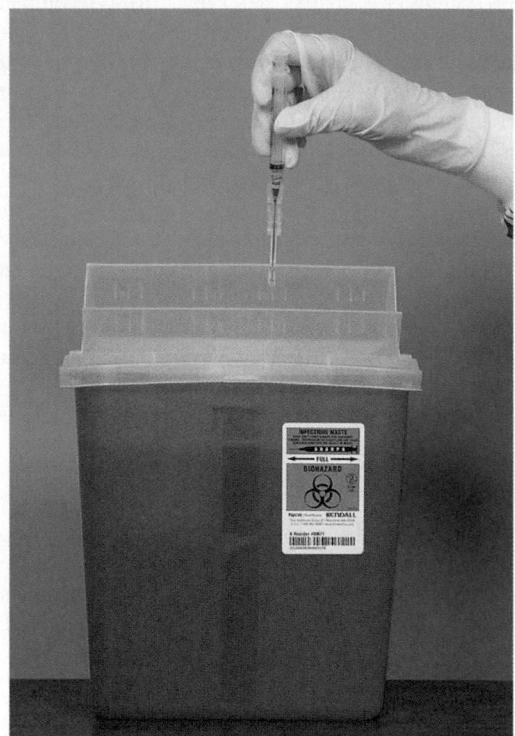

FIG 22.3 Sharps disposal using only one hand.

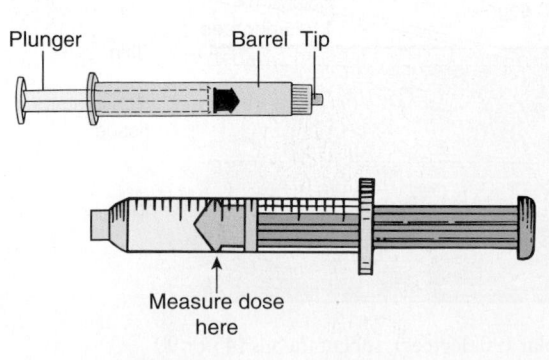

FIG 22.4 Parts of a syringe.

BOX 22.1

Recommendations for the Prevention of Needle-Stick Injuries

- Avoid using needles when effective needleless systems or sharps with engineered sharps injury protection (SESIP) safety devices are available.
- Do not recap any needle after medication administration.
- Plan safe handling and disposal of needles before beginning a procedure.
- Immediately dispose of needles, needleless systems, and SESIP into puncture-proof and leak-proof sharps disposal containers.
- Establish a surveillance program that tracks the rate and type of injuries, causative factors, and areas where improvement is needed.
- Maintain privacy and confidentiality of employees who have had sharps injuries.
- Attend education offerings on bloodborne pathogens and follow recommendations for infection prevention, including receiving the hepatitis B vaccine.
- Participate in the selection and evaluation of SESIP devices with safety features within your facility whenever possible.

Data from Public Health Agency of Canada. (2016). *Routine practices and additional precautions for preventing the transmission of infection in healthcare settings.* Retrieved from https://www.canada.ca/content/dam/phac-aspc/documents/services/publications/diseases-conditions/routine-practices-precautions-healthcare-associated-infections/routine-practices-precautions-healthcare-associated-infections-2016-FINAL-eng.pdf.

syringes use needles or needleless devices that slip onto the tip. Luer-Lok syringes (Fig. 22.5, A) use standard needles or needleless devices that are twisted onto the tip and lock themselves in place. The Luer-Lok design prevents the accidental removal of a needle from the syringe and allows the syringe to be connected to a needleless connector on an IV line or subcutaneous butterfly, avoiding the use of a needle and thereby reducing the risk of needle-stick injury.

Syringes come in a variety of sizes, ranging in capacity from 0.5 to 60 mL (see Fig. 22.5). When selecting a syringe, choose the smallest syringe size possible to improve accuracy of medication preparation. In addition, avoid injecting a large volume of fluid into tissues. A 1- to 3-mL syringe is usually adequate for a subcutaneous or IM injection. Larger volumes create pain and discomfort for a patient. Syringes are most commonly marked in a scale of

tenths of a millilitre (see Fig. 22.5, A). Tuberculin (TB) syringes are used to prepare small amounts of medication for intradermal (ID) and subcutaneous injections because they are marked in a scale of hundredths of a millilitre (see Fig. 22.5, B). Use a larger syringe to administer some IV medications and irrigate drainage tubes. Before use, carefully examine the syringe to determine the measurement scale and ensure that you use the correct syringe for preparing the prescribed medication.

Insulin syringes (see Fig. 22.5, C–D) hold 0.3 mL to 1 mL, and low-dose insulin syringes (30 units per 0.3 mL or 50 units per 0.5 mL) hold 0.3 mL to 1 mL. Both come with preattached needles and are calibrated in units. Most insulin syringes are U-100s, designed for use with U-100–strength insulin. Each milliliter of solution contains 100 units of insulin.

Needles

Some needles come attached to syringes. Others come packaged individually to allow flexibility in selecting the right needle for a patient. Needles are disposable, and most are made of stainless steel. A needle has three parts: the hub, which fits onto the tip of a syringe; the shaft, which connects to the hub; and the bevel, or slanted tip (Fig. 22.6). The needle hub, shaft, and bevel must remain sterile at all times. To prevent contamination, use gentle force to place the needle onto the syringe with the cap intact (Fig. 22.7, A–B). Some needles come with filters for preparation of medications (e.g., withdrawing medication from a glass ampoule to avoid any glass particles; the filter is to be removed and discarded after the medication has been drawn up [Krevesky & Whittaker, 2015]).

The tip of a needle, or the bevel, is always slanted. The bevel creates a narrow slit when injected into tissue that quickly closes after the needle is removed to prevent leakage of medication, blood, or serum. Longer bevelled tips are sharper and narrower, which minimizes tissue discomfort during a subcutaneous or IM injection.

Most needles vary in length from 6.4 mm (1.4 inch) to 76 mm (3 inches) (Fig. 22.8). Choose the needle length according to the type of tissue into which the medication is to be injected. Current evidence suggests that needle length should also be based on the patient's gender and anthropometric data, such as weight, body mass index (BMI), and waist circumference (Larkin, Ashcroft, Hickey, et al., 2018). A child or slender adult generally requires a shorter needle. Females have greater subcutaneous fat thicknesses at the ventrogluteal site and, therefore, require longer needles to ensure muscle penetration (Larkin et al., 2018). Use longer needles (2.5 mm [1 inch] to 40 mm [1½ inches] for IM injections and a shorter needle (9 mm [3/8 inch] to 16 mm [5/8 inch]) for subcutaneous injections. As the needle gauge becomes smaller, the needle diameter becomes larger. The selection of a gauge depends on the viscosity of fluid to be injected or infused; the greater the viscosity, the larger the gauge.

Disposable Injection Units

Single-dose, prefilled, disposable syringes are available for some medications. You do not need to prepare medication doses, except perhaps to expel unneeded parts of medication or remove air. Before

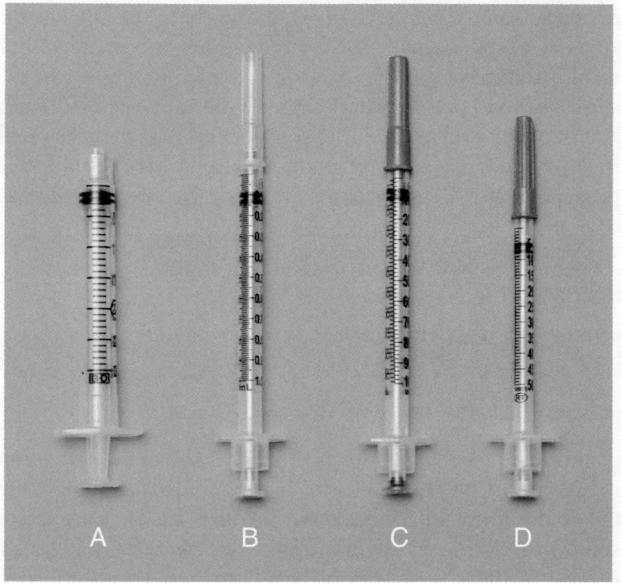

FIG 22.5 Examples of types of syringes. **A,** 3-mL syringe. **B,** Tuberculin syringe marked in 0.01 for doses of less than 1 mL. **C,** Insulin syringe marked in units (100). **D,** Insulin syringe marked in units (50).

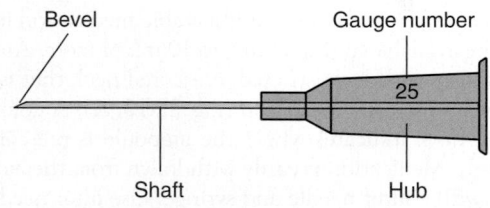

FIG 22.6 Parts of a needle.

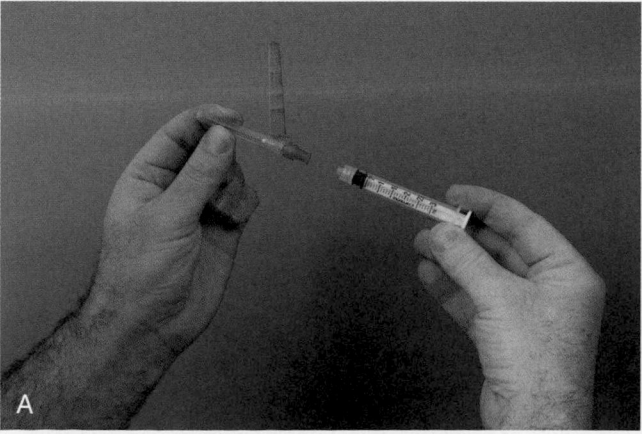

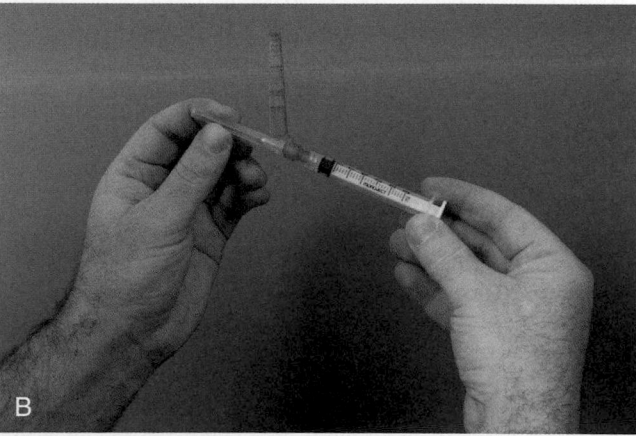

FIG 22.7 A, Capped needle placed on syringe tip. **B,** Needle secured.

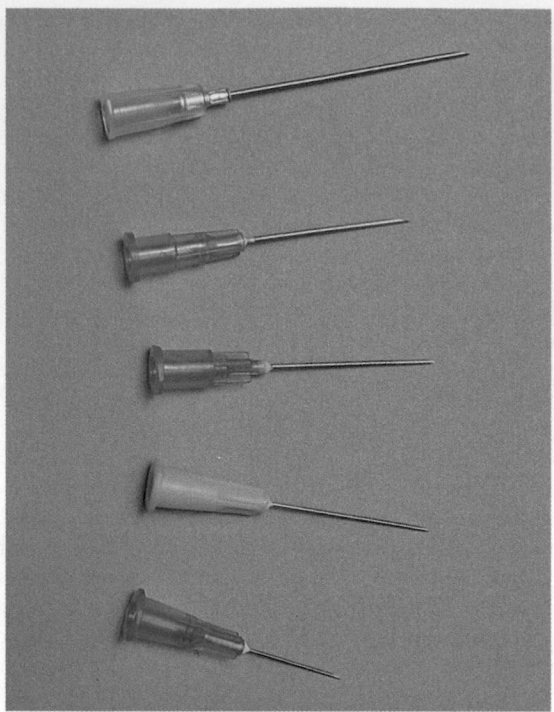

FIG 22.8 Needles: **Top to bottom:** 19 gauge, 38 mm length; 20 gauge, 25 mm length; 21 gauge, 25 mm length; 23 gauge, 25 mm length; and 25 gauge, 16 mm length. (*Astle, B. J., Duggleby, W., Potter, P. A., Perry, A. G., Stockert, P. A., & Hall, A. M. [Eds.]. (2019). Canadian Fundamentals of Nursing [6th ed., p. 776, Fig. 34-17]. Toronto: Elsevier Canada.*)

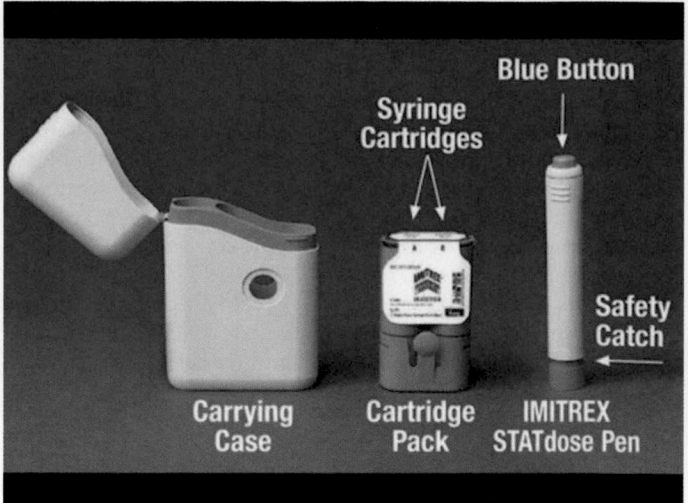

FIG 22.9 Prefilled syringe system: sumatriptan (Imitrex). (*From GlaxoSmithKline Canada*)

expelling air from a prefilled syringe, always check the manufacturer's recommendation, because the air bubble is *not* be removed prior to administration of some medications. It is important to check the medication and concentration carefully because prefilled syringes appear very similar. Prefilled unit-dose systems (e.g., Imitrex prefilled syringe system [Fig. 22.9]) include a reusable syringe holder and disposable, prefilled, sterile, cartridge units. This design reduces the risk for needle-stick injury.

◆ SKILL 22.1   Preparing Injections: Ampoules and Vials

NSO *Nursing Skills Online Administration of Parenteral Medications: Injections Module 7 / Lesson 2*

Ampoules contain single doses of injectable medication in a liquid form and are available in sizes from 1 to 10 mL or more. An ampoule is made of glass with a constricted, prescored neck that is snapped off to allow access to a medication (Fig. 22.10, A). A coloured ring around the neck indicates where the ampoule is prescored to be broken easily. Medication is easily withdrawn from the ampoule by aspirating with a filter needle and syringe. Use filter needles when preparing medication from a glass ampoule, to prevent glass particles from being drawn into the syringe (Alexander, Corrigan, Gorski, et al., 2014; Nicoll & Hesby, 2002). *Do not* use the filter needle to administer the medication because the filter has a one-way flow and once used to withdraw a medication and trap glass particles, it should not be "pushed" in the other direction during injection. In addition, filter needles have large, blunt ends that would be painful and cause tissue damage. Place an appropriate-size needle for injection on the syringe after withdrawing the medication.

A vial is a single- or multi-dose plastic or glass container with a rubber seal at the top (see Fig. 22.10, B). After you open a single-dose vial, discard it, regardless of the amount of medication used (Dolan, Meehan Arias, Felizardo, et al., 2016). A multi-dose vial contains several doses of a medication and thus can be used several times, although only for a single patient. When using a multi-dose vial, write the date the vial is opened on the vial label. Verify employer policy as to how long an opened multi-dose vial may be used. Properly discard a multi-dose vial when the allowed time for being open has expired.

A metal or plastic cap protects the rubber seal of the vial. Remove the cap when first preparing the vial for use. Vials may contain liquid or dry forms of medications; medications that are unstable in solution are packaged in dry form. Drugs that are time-sensitive injectable medication and must be administered within a specific time period to guarantee full drug effectiveness are often supplied in a powdered or dry form. When the drug is supplied in this form, the vial label specifies the solvent or diluent used to dissolve or reconstitute the medication and the amount needed to prepare a desired medication concentration. Normal saline and sterile water are the most common solutions.

Unlike an ampoule, a vial is a closed system. The user must inject air into the vial to permit easy withdrawal of the solution. Some medications, even when in a vial, may need to be drawn up with a filter needle because of the nature of the medication. Employer policies and package inserts from the manufacturer indicate drugs that should be prepared with a filter needle. Some vials have two chambers separated by a rubber stopper. One chamber contains the diluent solution; the other contains the dry medication. Before preparing the medication, push on the upper chamber to dislodge the rubber stopper and allow the powder and the diluent to mix.

Delegation and Collaboration

The skill of preparing injections from ampoules and vials cannot be delegated to unregulated care providers (UCPs).

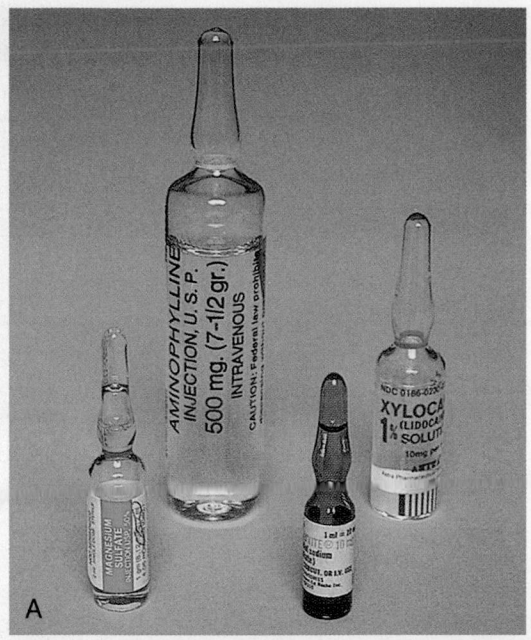

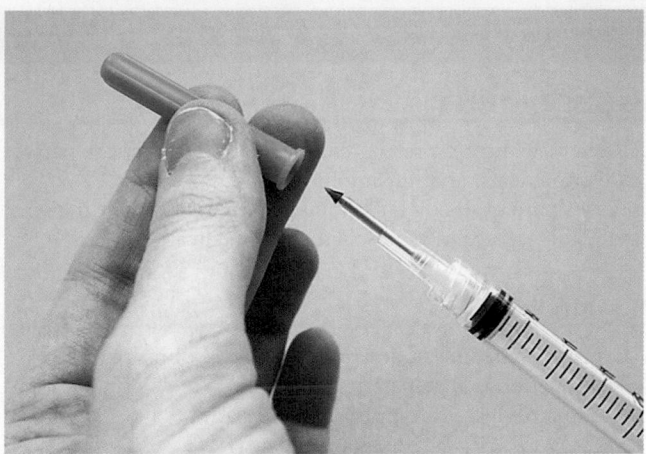

FIG 22.11 Syringe with needleless vial access adapter.

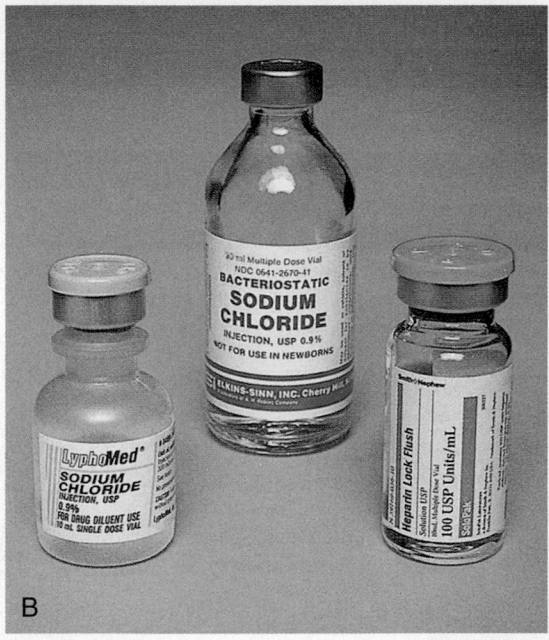

FIG 22.10 A, Medication in ampoules. **B,** Medication in vials.

Equipment
Medication in an Ampoule
- Syringe, needle, and filter needle
- Alcohol swab
- Small gauze pad or unopened alcohol swab

Medication in a Vial
- Syringe
- Two needles:
  - Needleless blunt-tip vial access cannula (Fig. 22.11) or needle (with safety sheath) for drawing up medication (if needed); filter needle if indicated
- Small gauze pad or alcohol swab
- Diluent (e.g., 0.9% sodium chloride or sterile water if indicated)

Medication in an Ampoule or Vial
- Medication administration record (MAR) or computer printout
- Sharps with engineered sharps injury protection (SESIP) safety needle for injection
- Medication in vial or ampoule
- Puncture-proof container for disposal of syringes, needles, and glass

STEP	RATIONALE

ASSESSMENT

1. Check accuracy and completeness of each MAR or computer printout with health care provider's prescription. Check patient's name, medication name and dosage, route of administration, and time of administration. Recopy or reprint any part of the MAR that is difficult to read.

The prescription sheet is the most reliable source and only legal record of medications that the patient is to receive. Computer order entry (COE) and barcode systems are technology recently introduced in many settings to reduce medication errors (Cochran, Barrett, & Horn, 2016; Lapkin, Levett-Jones, Chenoweth, et al., 2016).

2. Assess patient's medical and medication history.

Determines need for medication or possible contraindications for medication administration.

3. Assess patient's history of allergies. Know type of allergies and normal allergic response.

Do not prepare medication if there is a known patient allergy.

STEP	RATIONALE

ASSESSMENT

4. Review medication reference information for action, purpose, adverse effects, and nursing implications.

Allows you to administer drug properly and monitor patient's response.

5. Assess patient's body build, muscle size, and weight if giving subcutaneous or intramuscular (IM) medication.

Determines type and size of syringe and needle for injection.

PLANNING

1. Expected outcomes following completion of procedure:
- Proper dose is prepared.
- No air bubbles are in the syringe barrel.

Air bubbles displace medication. Elimination of air ensures accuracy of dose.

IMPLEMENTATION

1. Perform hand hygiene and prepare supplies.

Reduces transmission of microorganisms.

2. Prepare medications.

   a. If using a medication cart, move it outside patient's room.

Organization of equipment saves time and reduces occurrence of error.

   b. Unlock medication drawer or cart or log onto computerized medication dispensing system.

Medications are safeguarded when locked in the cabinet, cart, or computerized medication dispensing system.

   c. Follow employer's no-interruption zone (NIZ) policy. Prepare medications for one patient at a time. Keep all pages of MARs or computer printouts for one patient together or look at only one patient's electronic MAR at a time.

Preventing distractions reduces medication preparation errors. Use NIZ when possible (Lapkin et al., 2016; Tompkins McMahon, 2017).

   d. Select correct drug from stock supply or unit-dose drawer. Compare label of medication with MAR computer printout or computer screen.

Reading label and comparing it with transcribed prescription reduce errors. *This is the first check for accuracy.*

   e. Check expiration date on each medication, one at a time.

Expired medications are sometimes inactive, less effective, or harmful to patients.

   f. Calculate drug dose as necessary. Double-check calculation. Ask another nurse to check calculations if needed.

Double-checking reduces occurrence of error.

   g. If preparing a controlled substance, check record for previous drug count and compare with supply available.

Controlled substance laws require careful monitoring of dispensed narcotics.

   h. Do not leave drugs unattended.

The nurse is responsible for safekeeping of drugs.

3. Prepare ampoule. Compare medication label with MAR, computer screen, or computer printout.

This is the second check for accuracy.

   a. Tap top of ampoule lightly and quickly with finger until fluid moves from its neck (see illustration).

Dislodges any fluid that collects above neck of ampoule. All solution moves into lower chamber.

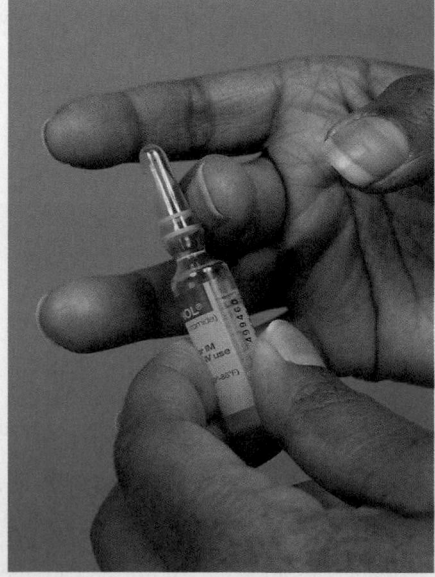

STEP 3a Tapping ampoule moves fluid down neck.

STEP	RATIONALE

IMPLEMENTATION

b. Cleanse the neck of the ampoule with antiseptic swab and allow it to dry. Place small gauze pad around neck of ampoule (see illustration).

Disinfects the neck of the ampoule and reduces risk of contamination (INS, 2016). Protects fingers from trauma as glass tip is broken off. Do not use opened alcohol swab to wrap around top of ampoule because alcohol may leak into ampoule.

c. Snap neck of ampoule quickly and firmly away from hands (see illustration).

Protects your fingers and face from shattering glass.

d. Draw up medication quickly, using filter needle long enough to reach bottom of ampoule to access medication.

System is open to airborne contaminants. Filter needles filter out any fragments of glass (Dolan et al., 2016).

e. Hold ampoule upside down or set it on flat surface. Insert filter needle into centre of ampoule opening. Do not allow needle tip or shaft to touch rim of ampoule.

Broken rim of ampoule is considered contaminated. When ampoule is inverted, solution dribbles out if needle tip or shaft touches rim of ampoule.

f. Aspirate medication into syringe by gently pulling back on plunger (see illustration).

Withdrawal of plunger creates negative pressure within syringe barrel, which pulls fluid into syringe.

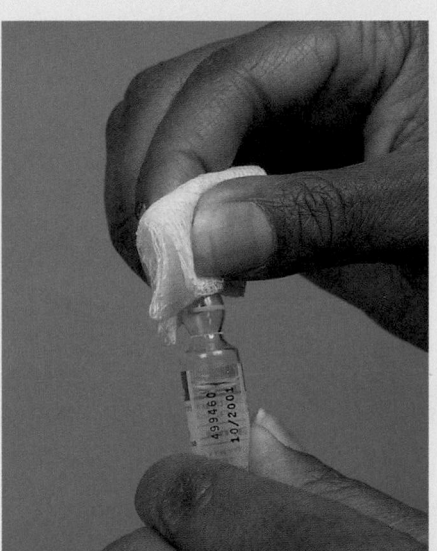

STEP 3b Gauze pad placed around neck of ampoule.

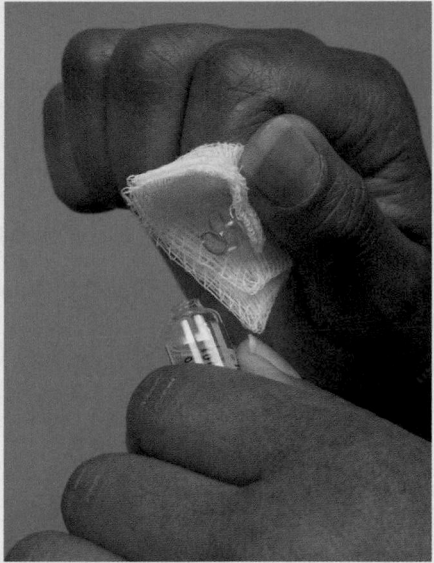

STEP 3c Neck snapped away from hands.

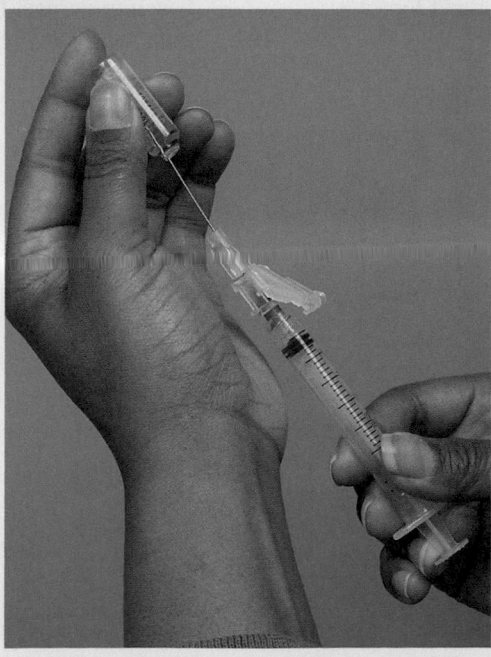

STEP 3f Medication aspirated with ampoule inverted.

STEP	RATIONALE

IMPLEMENTATION

g. Keep needle tip under surface of liquid. Tip ampoule to bring all fluid within reach of needle.

Prevents aspiration of air bubbles.

h. If you aspirate air bubbles, do not expel air into ampoule.

Air pressure forces fluid out of ampoule, and medication will be lost.

i. To expel excess air bubbles, remove needle from ampoule. Hold syringe vertically with needle pointing up. Tap side of syringe to cause bubbles to rise toward needle. Draw back slightly on plunger and push plunger upward to eject air. Do not eject fluid.

Withdrawing plunger too far removes it from barrel. Holding syringe vertically allows fluid to settle in bottom of barrel. Pulling back on plunger allows fluid within needle to enter barrel so fluid is not expelled. You then expel air at top of barrel and within needle.

j. If syringe contains excess fluid, use sink for disposal. Hold syringe vertically with needle tip up and slanted slightly toward sink. Slowly eject excess fluid into sink. Recheck fluid level in syringe by holding it vertically.

Safely disperses excess medication into sink. Position of needle allows you to expel medication without having it flow down needle shaft. Rechecking fluid level ensures proper dose.

k. Cover needle with its safety sheath or cap. Replace filter needle with regular SESIP needle.

Minimizes needle-sticks. Filter needles cannot be used for injection.

4. Prepare vial containing a solution.

a. Remove cap covering top of unused vial to expose sterile rubber seal. If a multi-dose vial has been used before, cap is already removed. Firmly and briskly wipe rubber seal with alcohol swab and allow it to dry.

Vial comes packaged with cap that cannot be replaced after seal removal. Not all drug manufacturers guarantee that rubber seals of unused vials are sterile. Swabbing with alcohol reduces transmission of microorganisms. Allowing alcohol to dry prevents alcohol from coating needle and mixing with medication.

b. Pick up syringe and remove needle cap or cap covering needleless access device. Pull back on plunger to draw amount of air into syringe equivalent to volume of medication to be aspirated from vial.

Injecting air into vial prevents buildup of negative pressure in vial when aspirating medication.

Clinical Decision Point *Some medications require use of a filter needle when preparing medications from vials. Check employer policy or medication reference. If you use a filter needle to aspirate medication, you need to change it to a regular SESIP needle of the appropriate size to administer medication (Dolan et al., 2016).*

c. With vial on flat surface, insert tip of needle or needleless device through centre of rubber seal (see illustration). Apply pressure to tip of needle during insertion.

Centre of seal is thinner and easier to penetrate. Using firm pressure prevents dislodging of rubber particles that could enter vial or needle.

d. Inject air into air space of vial, holding on to plunger. Hold plunger firmly; plunger is sometimes forced backward by air pressure within vial.

Injection of air creates vacuum needed to get medication to flow into syringe. Injecting into air space of vial prevents formation of bubbles and an inaccurate dose.

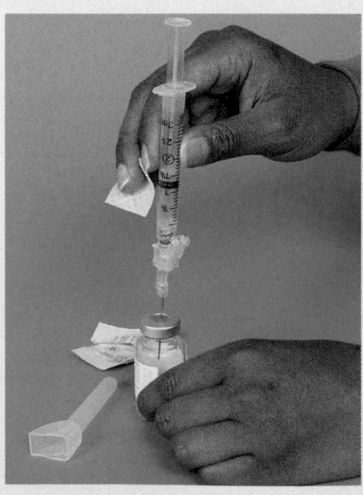

STEP 4c Insert safety needle through centre of vial diaphragm (with vial flat on table).

STEP	RATIONALE

IMPLEMENTATION

e. Invert vial while keeping firm hold on syringe and plunger. Hold vial between thumb and middle fingers of nondominant hand (see illustration). Grasp end of syringe barrel and plunger with thumb and forefinger of dominant hand to counteract pressure in vial.

Inverting vial allows fluid to settle in lower half of container. Position of hands prevents forceful movement of plunger and permits easy manipulation of syringe.

f. Keep tip of needle or needleless device below fluid level.

Prevents aspiration of air.

g. Allow air pressure from vial to fill syringe gradually with medication. If necessary, pull back slightly on plunger to obtain correct amount of medication.

Positive pressure within vial forces fluid into syringe.

h. When you obtain desired volume, position needle or needleless device into air space of vial; tap side of syringe barrel gently to dislodge any air bubbles (see illustration). Eject any air remaining at top of syringe into vial.

Forcefully striking barrel while needle is inserted in vial may bend needle. Accumulation of air displaces medication and causes dose errors.

i. Remove needle or needleless access device from vial by pulling back on barrel of syringe.

Pulling plunger rather than barrel causes plunger to separate from barrel, resulting in loss of medication.

j. Hold syringe at eye level at 90-degree angle to ensure correct volume and absence of air bubbles. Remove any remaining air by tapping barrel to dislodge any air bubbles. Draw back slightly on plunger; then push it upward to eject air. Do not eject fluid. Recheck volume of medication.

Holding syringe vertically allows fluid to settle in bottom of barrel. Tapping dislodges air to top of barrel. Pulling back on plunger allows fluid within needle to enter barrel so you do not expel fluid. You then expel air at top of barrel and within needle.

Clinical Decision Point *When preparing medication from a single-dose vial, do not assume that volume listed on the label is the total volume in vial. Some manufacturers provide a small amount of extra liquid, expecting loss during preparation. Be sure to draw up only desired volume.*

k. If you need to inject medication into patient's tissue, change needle with regular SESIP to appropriate gauge and length according to route of medication administration.

Inserting needle through rubber stopper dulls bevelled tip. The new needle is sharper and, because no fluid is along shaft, does not track medication through tissues. Filter needles cannot be used for injection.

l. Cover needle with its safety sheath or cap.

Minimizes needle-sticks.

m. For a multi-dose vial, make label that includes date of opening, concentration of drug per millilitre, and your initials.

Ensures that nurses will prepare future doses correctly. You discard some drugs within a certain time frame after mixing.

5. Prepare vial containing powder (reconstituting medications).

a. Remove cap covering vial of powdered medication and cap covering vial of manufacturer-recommended diluent. Firmly swab both rubber seals with alcohol swab and allow alcohol to dry.

Allowing alcohol to dry prevents it from coating needle and mixing with medication.

b. Draw up recommended volume of diluent into syringe following Steps 4b through 4j.

Prepares diluent for injection into vial containing powdered medication.

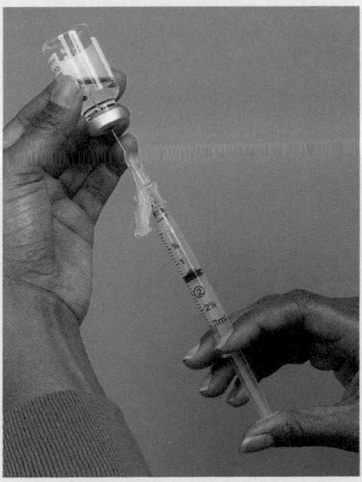

STEP 4e Withdraw fluid with vial inverted.

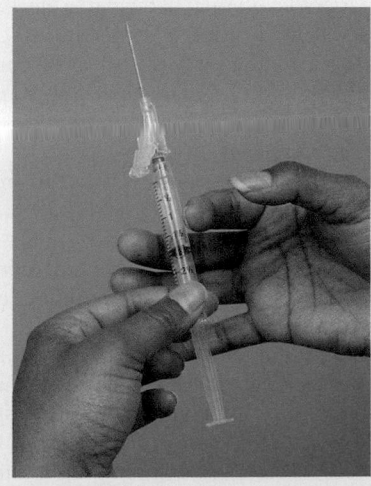

STEP 4h Hold syringe upright; tap barrel to dislodge air bubbles.

STEP	RATIONALE

IMPLEMENTATION

c. Insert tip of needle or needleless device through centre of rubber seal of vial of powdered medication. Inject diluent into vial. Remove needle.	Diluent begins to dissolve and reconstitute medication.
d. Mix medication thoroughly. Roll in palms. Do not shake.	Ensures proper dispersal of medication throughout solution and prevents formation of air bubbles.
e. Reconstituted medication in vial is ready to be drawn into new syringe. Read label carefully to determine dose after reconstitution.	Once you add diluent, concentration of medication (mg/mL) determines dose you give. Reading medication label carefully decreases medication errors.
f. Draw up reconstituted medication into syringe. Insert needleless device/needle into vial. Do not add air. Then follow Steps 4e through 4l.	Prepares medication for administration.

Clinical Decision Point *Some employers require that you verify the dose of certain medications (e.g., insulin and heparin) for accuracy with another nurse.*

6. Compare label of medication with MAR, computer screen, or computer printout and compare dose in syringe with desired dose before discarding the vial/ampoule.	*This is the third check for accuracy.*
7. Dispose of soiled supplies. Place broken ampoule and/or used vials and used needle or needleless device in puncture- and leak-proof container. Clean work area and perform hand hygiene.	Proper disposal of glass and needle prevents accidental injury to staff. Controls transmission of infection.

Unexpected Outcomes
1. Air bubbles remain in syringe (unless contraindicated by type of medication).
2. Incorrect dose is prepared.

Related Interventions
- Expel air from and add medication to it until you prepare correct dose.

- Discard prepared dose.
- Prepare correct new dose.

PROCEDURAL GUIDELINE 22.1 *Mixing Parenteral Medications in One Syringe*

Some medications need to be mixed from two vials or from a vial and an ampoule. Mixing compatible medications avoids the need to give a patient more than one injection. First, as the nurse you must check that the drugs are compatible and can be mixed in one syringe. Compatibility charts are in drug reference guides, posted within patient care units, or available electronically. If you are uncertain about medication compatibilities, consult a pharmacist. When mixing medications, you must correctly aspirate fluid from each type of container, especially a multi-dose vial, without contaminating the medication with the contents from another vial or ampoule.

When mixing medications from a vial and an ampoule, prepare medications from the vial first. Then withdraw medication from the ampoule using the same syringe and a filter needle. When mixing medications from two vials, do not contaminate one medication with another, ensure that the final dose is accurate, and maintain aseptic technique.

Give special consideration to the proper preparation of insulin, the hormone used to treat diabetes mellitus. Insulin is supplied in vials or cartridges for injection pens and is classified by onset, peak effect, and duration of action (Table 22.2). Often patients with diabetes mellitus receive a combination of different types of insulin to control their blood glucose levels. Before preparing

insulin, gently roll all cloudy insulin preparations (e.g., Humulin-N) between the palms of your hands to resuspend the insulin (Burchum & Rosenthal, 2016).

If more than one type of insulin is required to manage a patient's diabetes, you can mix them into one syringe if they are compatible. Always prepare the short- or rapid-acting insulin first to prevent it from being contaminated with the longer-acting insulin (Burchum & Rosenthal, 2016). In some settings insulin is not mixed. Box 22.2 lists recommendations for mixing insulins.

Delegation and Collaboration
The skill of mixing medications in one syringe cannot be delegated to an unregulated care provider (UCP). The nurse directs the UCP about:
- Potential adverse effects of medications and the need to immediately report their occurrence to the nurse.

Equipment
- Single- or multi-dose vials and ampoules containing medication
- Syringe
- Two needles:
  - Needleless blunt-tip vial access cannula or needle for drawing up medication
  - Filter needle if indicated

PROCEDURAL GUIDELINE 22.1 *Mixing Parenteral Medications in One Syringe—cont'd*

TABLE 22.2

Comparison of Insulin Preparations

Insulin Type* (Trade Name)	Onset	Peak Effect (Hours)	Duration of Action (Hours)
Bolus Insulins (Mealtime or Preprandial)			
Rapid-Acting (Clear)			
Insulin lispro (Humalog)	10–15 min	1–2	3–4.75
Insulin aspart (NovoRapid)	9–20 min	1–1.5	3–5
Insulin glulisine (Apidra)	10–15 min	1–1.5	3.5–5
Faster-acting insulin aspart (Fiasp)	4 min	0.5–1.5	3–5
Short-Acting (Clear)			
Regular insulin† (e.g., Humulin R, Novolin ge Toronto)	30 min	2–3	6.5
Basal Insulins			
Intermediate-Acting (Cloudy)			
Isophane insulin suspension (Novolin ge NPH, Humulin N)	1–3 h	5–8	Up to 18
Long-Acting (Clear)			
Insulin glargine (Lantus)‡	1–1.5 h	No peak identified	Up to 24
Insulin detemir (Levemir)‡	1–1.5 h	Peak unknown	16–24

Data from Lipsombe, L., Booth, G., Butalia, S., Dasgupta, K., Eurich, D., Goldenberg, R., … Simpson, S. (2018). Diabetes Canada 2018 clinical practice guidelines for the prevention and management of diabetes in Canada: Pharmacologic glycemic management of type 2 diabetes in adults. *Canadian Journal of Diabetes, 42*, S88–S103.
*All insulins are available in 100-unit strengths.
†This is the only insulin approved for intravenous or intramuscular use.
‡Cannot be mixed with other insulins.

BOX 22.2

Recommendations for Mixing Insulins

- Patients whose blood glucose levels are well controlled on a mixed-insulin dose need to maintain their individual routine when preparing and administering their insulin.
- Do not mix insulin with any other medications or diluents unless approved by prescriber.
- Never mix insulin glargine (Lantus) or insulin detemir (Levemir) with other types of insulin.
- Inject rapid-acting insulins mixed with NPH insulin within 15 minutes before a meal.
- Verify insulin doses with another nurse while you are preparing the injection.

- Sharp with engineered sharps injury protection (SESIP) needle for injection
- Alcohol swab
- Puncture-proof container for disposing of syringes, needles, and glass
- Medication administration record (MAR) or computer printout

Procedural Steps

1. Check accuracy and completeness of MAR or computer printout with health care provider's prescription. Check patient's name, medication name and dosage, route of administration, and time of administration. Recopy or reprint any part of MAR that is difficult to read.
2. Review pertinent information related to medication, including action, purpose, adverse effects, and nursing implications.
3. Assess patient body build, muscle size, gender, and weight if giving subcutaneous or intramuscular (IM) medication.

4. Consider compatibility of medications to be mixed and type of injection.
5. Check expiration date of medication printed on vial or ampoule.
6. Perform hand hygiene.
7. Prepare medication for one patient at a time following the 10 rights of medication administration (see Chapter 20). Select an ampoule or vial from the unit-dose drawer or automated dispensing system. Compare the label of each medication with the MAR or computer printout. In the case of insulin, ensure that correct type or types of insulin are prepared. *This is the first check for accuracy*.
8. Mixing medications from two vials (see illustration):
   a. Take syringe with needleless device or filter needle and aspirate volume of air equivalent to first medication dose (vial A).
   b. Calculate drug dose as necessary. Double-check calculation.
   c. Compare the medication label of both vials with MAR, computer screen, or computer printout. *This is the second check for accuracy.* Inject air into vial A, making sure that needle or needleless device does not touch solution (see illustration A).
   d. Holding on to plunger, withdraw needle or needleless device and syringe from vial A. Aspirate air equivalent to second medication dose (vial B) into syringe.
   e. Insert needle or needleless device into vial B, inject volume of air into vial B, and withdraw medication from vial B into syringe (see illustration B).
   f. Withdraw needle or needleless device and syringe from vial B. Ensure that proper volume has been obtained.
   g. Determine on syringe scale what the combined volume of medications should measure.

Continued

PROCEDURAL GUIDELINE 22.1 *Mixing Parenteral Medications in One Syringe—cont'd*

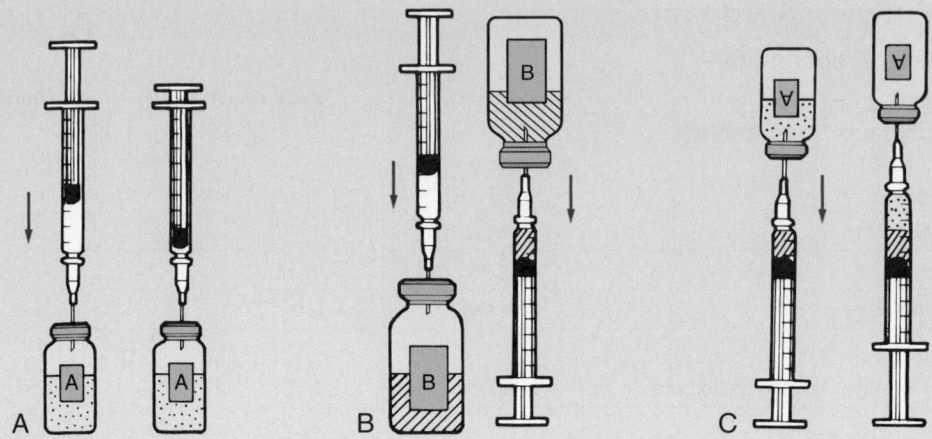

STEP 8 A, Inject air into vial A. **B,** Inject air into vial B and withdraw dose. **C,** Withdraw medication from vial A; medications are now mixed.

h. Insert needle or needleless device into vial A, being careful not to push plunger and expel medication within syringe into vial. Invert vial and carefully withdraw the desired amount of medication from vial A into syringe (see illustration C).

i. Withdraw needle or needleless device and expel any excess air from syringe. Check fluid level in syringe for proper dose. Medications are now mixed.

Clinical Decision Point *If too much medication is withdrawn from second vial, discard syringe and start over. Do not push medication back into either vial.*

j. Change needle or needleless device for appropriate-size needle if medication is being injected. Keep needle or needleless device capped until administration time.

9. Mixing insulin:

a. If patient takes insulin that is cloudy, roll bottle of insulin between hands to resuspend insulin preparation.

b. Wipe off tops of both insulin vials with alcohol swab.

c. Verify insulin dose against MAR.

Clinical Decision Point *If long-acting insulin glargine (Lantus) or detemir (Levemir) is prescribed, it should not be mixed with other insulin preparations.*

d. If mixing rapid- or short-acting insulin with intermediate- or long-acting insulin, take insulin syringe and aspirate volume of air equivalent to dose to be withdrawn from intermediate- or long-acting insulin first (see illustration). If two intermediate- or long-acting insulins are mixed, it makes no difference which vial is prepared first.

e. Insert needle and inject air into vial of intermediate- or long-acting insulin. Do not let tip of needle touch solution.

f. Remove syringe from vial of insulin without aspirating medication.

g. With the same syringe, inject air equal to the dose of rapid- or short-acting insulin into vial and withdraw correct dose into syringe (see illustration).

h. Remove syringe from rapid- or short-acting insulin and remove any air bubbles to ensure accurate dose.

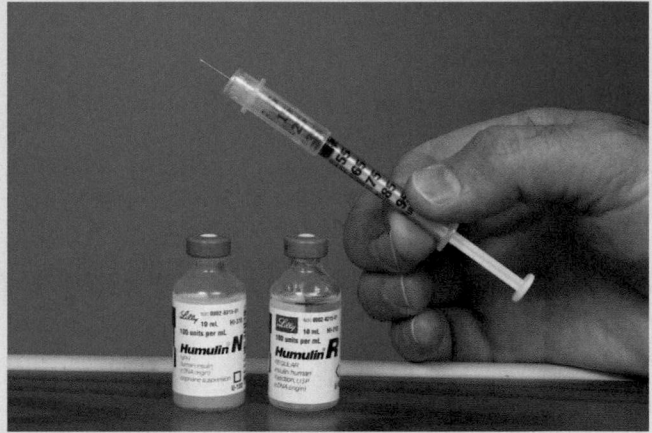

STEP 9d Aspirate air equivalent to dose to be withdrawn from intermediate insulin.

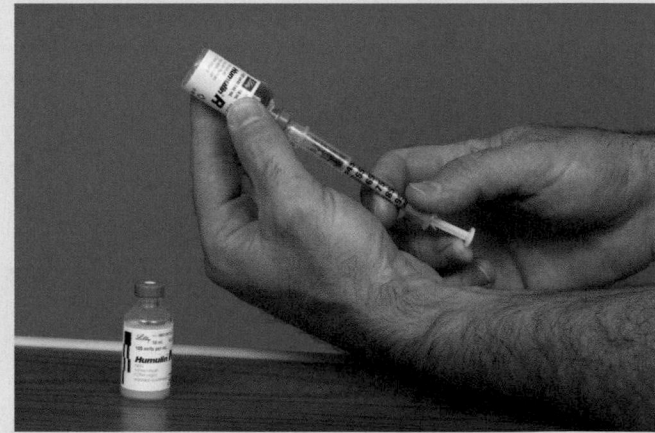

STEP 9g Withdraw short-acting insulin.

i. Verify short-acting insulin dosage with MAR and show insulin prepared in syringe to another nurse to verify that correct dosage of insulin was prepared. Determine which point on syringe scale the combined units of insulin should measure by adding the number of units of both insulins

PROCEDURAL GUIDELINE 22.1 *Mixing Parenteral Medications in One Syringe—cont'd*

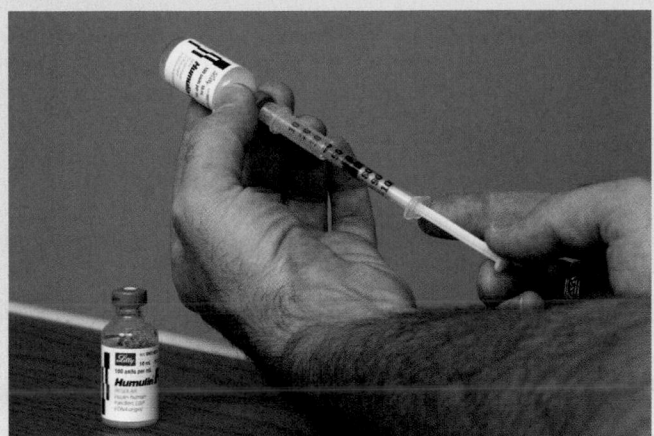

STEP 9k Withdraw intermediate insulin.

together (e.g., 4 units Regular + 10 units NPH = 14 units total). Verify combined dosage.

j. Place needle of syringe back into vial of intermediate- or long-acting insulin. Be careful not to push plunger and inject insulin in syringe into vial.

k. Invert vial and carefully withdraw desired amount of insulin into syringe (see illustration).

l. Withdraw needle and check fluid level in syringe. Verify with another nurse that correct total dose was prepared. Keep needle of prepared syringe sheathed or capped until ready to administer medication.

10. Mixing medications from a vial and an ampoule:
   a. Prepare medication from vial first, following Skill 22.1, Step 4.
   b. Determine on syringe scale what combined volume of medications should measure.

Clinical Decision Point *If needleless access device was used in preparing medication from vial, change needleless system to a filter needle to remove medication from ampoule.*

   c. Next, using the same syringe, prepare second medication from ampoule, following Step 3 in Skill 22.1.
   d. Withdraw filter needle from ampoule and verify fluid level in syringe. Change filter needle to appropriate SESIP needle. Keep device or needle sheathed or capped until administering medication.
   e. Check syringe carefully for total combined dose of medications.

11. Compare MAR, computer screen, or computer printout with prepared medication and labels on vials/ampoules. *This is the third check for accuracy.*

12. Dispose of soiled supplies. Place used ampoules and/or vials and needle or needleless device in puncture- and leak-proof container.

13. Clean work area and perform hand hygiene.

14. Check syringe again carefully for total combined dose of medications.

✦ SKILL 22.2   Administering Intradermal Injections

 Video Clip   **NSO**   *Nursing Skills Online Administration of Parenteral Medications: Injections Module 7 / Lesson 4*

Intradermal (ID) injections are used for skin testing (e.g., tuberculosis screening and allergy tests) or for treatment (e.g., immunotherapy for diagnosed allergies). Because these medications are potent, they are injected into the dermis, where blood supply is reduced, and drug absorption occurs slowly. A patient may have an anaphylactic reaction if the medications enter the circulation too rapidly. For patients with a history of multiple allergies, the health care provider may perform skin testing. Skin testing often requires you to visually inspect the test site; therefore, make sure that the ID sites are free of lesions and injuries and relatively hairless. The inner forearm and upper back are ideal locations.

Use a tuberculin (TB) or small syringe with a short (3.2 mm [1.8 inch] to 16 mm [5/8 inch]), fine-gauge (25 to 27) needle to administer an ID injection. The angle of insertion for an ID injection is 5 to 15 degrees (see Fig. 22.1). Inject only small amounts of medication (0.01 to 0.1 mL) intradermally. If a bleb does not appear or if the site bleeds after needle withdrawal, the medication may have entered subcutaneous tissues. In this situation skin test results will not be valid.

Delegation and Collaboration

The skill of administering ID injections cannot be delegated to an unregulated care provider (UCP). The nurse directs the UCP about:

- Potential medication adverse effects or allergic response signs and to report their occurrence to the nurse.
- Reporting any change in the patient's vital signs or condition to the nurse.

Equipment

- Syringe, 1 mL TB syringe with preattached 25- or 27-gauge needle, 3.2 mm (1/8 inch) to 16 mm (5/8 inch)
- Small gauze pad
- Alcohol swab
- Vial or ampoule of medication
- Clean gloves
- Medication administration record (MAR) or computer printout
- Puncture-proof container
- Anaphylaxis kit

STEP	RATIONALE

ASSESSMENT

1. Check accuracy and completeness of MAR or computer printout with health care provider's prescription. Check patient's name, medication name and dosage, route of administration, and time of administration. Recopy or reprint any part of MAR that is difficult to read.

The prescription sheet is the most reliable source and only legal record of medications that the patient is to receive. Computer order entry (COE) and barcode systems are technology recently introduced in many settings to reduce medication errors (Cochran et al., 2016; Lapkin et al., 2016).

2. Review medication reference information about expected reaction or anticipated effects when testing skin with specific allergen or when giving medication and appropriate time to read site.

Type of reaction depends on patient's ability to mount a cell-mediated immune response. Knowledge of expected and adverse reactions to skin testing helps you determine which symptoms to monitor for, how frequently, and when to reassess the patient.

3. Assess patient's history of allergies: known type of allergens and normal allergic reaction.

Do not administer any medication if there is known patient allergy. Medications are potent and can cause severe anaphylaxis.

4. Assess for contraindication to ID injections such as reduced local tissue perfusion. Assess for history of severe adverse reactions or necrosis from previous ID injection.

Decreased perfusion reduces absorption of medication. Prior history of severe reactions increases the risk for future severe reactions.

5. Assess patient's knowledge of purpose and response to skin testing.

Patients need to know when to return for follow-up reading of a skin test and when and how to report any reaction.

6. Check date of expiration.

Dose potency increases or decreases when outdated.

NURSING DIAGNOSES

- Anxiety
- Fear
- Insufficient knowledge regarding skin testing

Related factors are individualized on the basis of patient's condition or needs.

PLANNING

1. Expected outcomes following completion of procedure:
   - Patient experiences very mild burning sensation during injection but no discomfort after injection.
   - Small, light-coloured bleb approximately 6 mm (1/4 inch) in diameter forms at site and gradually disappears. Minimal bruising may be present.
   - Patient can identify signs of skin reaction and their significance.

Normal reaction to medication deposited in dermis.
Medication is in dermis and eventually absorbed. Bruising is result of minor bleeding from capillaries.
Demonstrates learning.

IMPLEMENTATION

1. Prepare medications for one patient at a time using aseptic technique and avoiding distractions (see Skill 22.1). Check label of medication carefully with MAR or computer printout three times (see Skill 22.1 or Procedural Guideline 22.1) when preparing medication.

Ensures that medication is sterile. Preventing distractions reduces medication preparation errors. Use no-interruption zone (NIZ) when possible (Lapkin et al., 2016; Tompkins McMahon, 2017).

Three checks for accuracy must occur when preparing medications:
1. Before removing the medication vial/container from the drawer.
2. When the prescribed amount of the medication is drawn up.
3. Before returning the vial to storage/drawer or disposing of an empty or single-use vial or ampoule.

2. Take medication(s) to patient at correct time (see employer policy). Apply 10 rights of medication administration.

Employer policies regarding timing of medications must consider the nature of the prescribed medication, specific clinical application, and patient needs (ISMP, 2011).

Clinical Decision Point *Before administering an ID injection, ensure an emergency anaphylaxis kit is on site and easily accessible (Mersey Care, 2017). Drugs given via the ID route are extremely potent and carry an increased risk of anaphylaxis.*

STEP	RATIONALE

IMPLEMENTATION

3. Close room curtain or door.

Provides privacy.

4. Identify patient using at least two person-specific identifiers (e.g., name and date of birth or name and medical record number) according to employer policy. Compare identifiers with information on patient's MAR or medical record.

Ensures correct patient. Complies with Accreditation Canada's standards and improves patient safety (Accreditation Canada, 2019).

5. Ask patient if they have any allergies.

Confirms patient's identity and allergy history.

6. Discuss purpose of each medication, action, and possible adverse effects. Allow patient to ask any questions. Tell them that the injection will cause slight burning or sting.

Patient has the right to be informed, and patient's understanding of each medication improves adherence to drug therapy. Helps minimize patient's anxiety.

7. Perform hand hygiene and apply clean gloves. Keep sheet or gown draped over body parts not requiring exposure.

Reduces transmission of infection.

8. Select appropriate site. Note lesions or discolorations of skin. If possible, select site three to four finger widths below antecubital space and one hand width above wrist. If you cannot use forearm, inspect upper back. If necessary, use sites appropriate for subcutaneous injections.

An ID injection site is free of discoloration, moles, scars, or hair so you can see results of skin test and interpret them correctly (Doyle & McCutcheon, 2015).

9. Help patient to comfortable position. Have them extend the elbow and support it and forearm on flat surface.

Stabilizes injection site for easy accessibility.

10. Clean site with antiseptic swab. Apply swab at centre of site and rotate outward in circular direction for about 5 cm (2 inches). *Option:* Use vapocoolant spray (e.g., ethyl chloride) before injection.

Mechanical action of swab removes secretions containing microorganisms.

Decreases pain at injection site.

11. Hold swab or gauze between third and fourth fingers of nondominant hand.

Gauze or swab remains readily accessible when withdrawing needle.

12. Remove needle cap from needle by pulling it straight off.

Preventing needle from touching sides of cap prevents contamination.

13. Hold syringe between thumb and forefinger of dominant hand with bevel of needle pointing up.

Smooth injection requires proper manipulation of syringe parts. With bevel up, you are less likely to deposit medication into tissues below dermis.

14. Administer injection.

   a. With nondominant hand, stretch skin over site with forefinger or thumb.

Needle pierces tight skin more easily.

   b. With needle almost against patient's skin, insert it slowly at 5- to 15-degree angle until resistance is felt. Advance needle through epidermis to approximately 3.2 mm (1/8 inch) below skin surface. You will see bulge of needle tip through skin (see illustration).

Ensures that needle tip is in dermis. You obtain inaccurate results if you do not inject needle at correct angle and depth (Doyle & McCutcheon, 2015).

   c. Inject medication slowly. Normally you feel resistance. If not, needle is too deep; remove and begin again.

Slow injection minimizes discomfort at site. Dermal layer is tight and does not expand easily when you inject solution.

Clinical Decision Point *It is not necessary to aspirate because dermis is relatively avascular.*

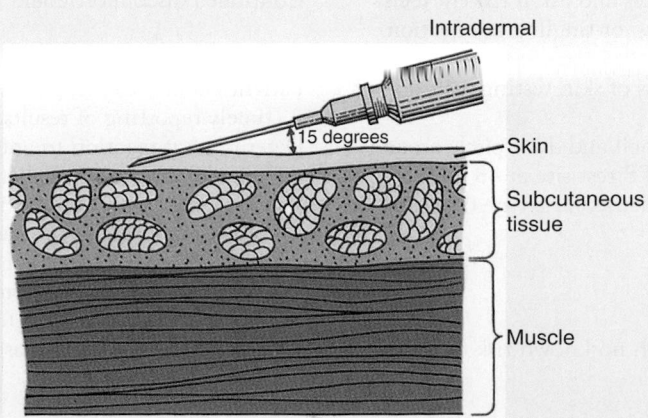

STEP 14b Intradermal needle tip inserted into dermis.

STEP	RATIONALE

IMPLEMENTATION

d. While injecting medication, note that small bleb (approximately 6.4 mm [1/4 inch]) resembling mosquito bite appears on skin surface (see illustration).

Bleb indicates that you deposited medication in dermis.

e. After withdrawing needle, apply alcohol swab or gauze gently over site.

Do not massage site. Apply bandage if needed.

15. Help patient to comfortable position.

Gives patient sense of well-being.

16. Discard uncapped needle or needle enclosed in safety shield and attached syringe in puncture- and leak-proof receptacle.

Prevents injury to patients and health care personnel. Recapping needles increases risk for a needle-stick injury (Elmi, Babaie, Malek, et al., 2018).

17. Remove gloves and perform hand hygiene.

Reduces transmission of microorganisms.

18. Stay with patient for several minutes and observe for any allergic reactions. If the patient received allergy immunotherapy, instruct the patient to stay for 30 minutes following the injection.

Dyspnea, wheezing, and circulatory collapse are signs of severe anaphylactic reaction and are likely to occur immediately after injection, or within 30 minutes of the injection.

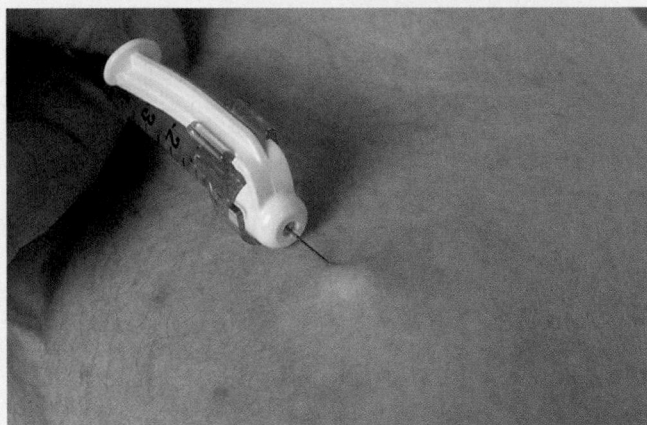

STEP 14d Injection creates small bleb.

EVALUATION

1. Return to room in 15 to 30 minutes and ask if patient feels any acute pain, burning, numbness, or tingling at injection site.

Continued discomfort could indicate injury to underlying tissues.

2. Ask patient to discuss implications of skin testing and signs of hypersensitivity.

Patient's ability to recognize signs of skin testing helps to ensure timely reporting of results.

3. Inspect bleb. *Option:* Use skin pencil and draw circle around perimeter of injection site. Read TB test site at 48 to 72 hours; look for induration (hard, dense, raised area) of skin around injection site of:

Determines if reaction to antigen occurs; indication positive for tuberculosis or tested allergens.

Site must be read at various intervals to determine test results. Pencil marks make site easy to find. You determine results of skin testing at various times, based on type of medication used or type of skin testing completed. Manufacturer directions determine when to read test results.

- 15 mm or more in patients with no known risk factors for tuberculosis.

Degree of reaction varies based on patient condition.

STEP	RATIONALE

EVALUATION

- 10 mm or more in patients who are recent immigrants; injection drug users; residents or employees of high-risk settings; patients with certain chronic illnesses; children less than 4 years of age; and infants, children, and adolescents exposed to high-risk adults.
- 5 mm or more in patients who are human immunodeficiency virus (HIV) positive, have fibrotic changes on chest X-ray film consistent with previous tuberculosis infection, have had organ transplants, or are immunosuppressed.

4. **Use Teach-Back:** "I want to be sure I explained to you the purpose of TB skin testing and what you might see after the test. Explain to me what the injection site might look like in 2 to 3 days." Develop a revised teaching plan if patient or caregiver is not able to teach back correctly.

Determines patient's and caregiver's level of understanding of instructional topic.

Unexpected Outcomes	Related Interventions
1. Patient complains of localized pain or continued burning at injection site, indicating potential injury to nerve or vessels.	• Assess injection site. • Notify patient's health care provider.
2. Raised, reddened, or hard zone (induration) forms around ID test site.	• Notify patient's health care provider. • Document sensitivity to injected allergen or positive test if tuberculin skin testing was completed.
3. Patient has adverse reaction with signs of urticaria, pruritus, wheezing, and dyspnea.	• Notify patient's health care provider. • Follow employer policy for appropriate response to drug reactions (e.g., administration of antihistamine such as diphenhydramine or epinephrine). • Add allergy information to patient's record.

Communication and Documentation

- Document drug, dose, route, site, time, and date on MAR in nurses' notes in electronic health record (EHR) or chart immediately after administration, not before. Correctly sign MAR according to employer policy.
- Document area of ID injection and appearance of skin in nurses' notes in EHR or chart.
- Document any undesirable or adverse effects from medication and report these to patient's health care provider.
- Document patient teaching, validation of understanding, and patient's response to medication in nurses' notes in EHR or chart.

Special Considerations
Teaching
- Instruct patient not to squeeze medication out of injection site.
- Teach patient that negative skin tests may not rule out allergies, especially when low concentrations of medication are used.

- Patient should wear medical identification band listing all allergies.
- Caution patient not to wash off pencil markings around injection site.
- Explain to patient how to observe for skin reactions.

Pediatric
- Children who are exposed to people with confirmed or suspected infectious tuberculosis should be tested for it immediately following exposure (Hockenberry & Wilson, 2015).
- Children with ongoing exposure to high-risk individuals (e.g., HIV-infected, homeless, incarcerated) should be tested for tuberculosis every 2 to 3 years (Hockenberry & Wilson, 2015).

Gerontological
- The skin of the older person is less elastic and must be held taut to ensure that ID injection is administered correctly.

✦ SKILL 22.3 Administering Subcutaneous Injections

 Video Clip **NSO** *Nursing Skills Online Administration of Parenteral Medications: Injections Module 7 / Lesson 3*

Subcutaneous injections involve depositing medication into the loose connective tissue underlying the dermis. Because subcutaneous tissue does not contain as many blood vessels as muscles, medications are absorbed more slowly than with intramuscular (IM) injections. Physical exercise or application of hot or cold compresses influences the rate of drug absorption by altering local blood flow to tissues. Any condition that impairs blood flow is a contraindication for subcutaneous injections.

Subcutaneous tissue contains pain receptors, so patients often experience discomfort with injection. The tissue is sensitive to

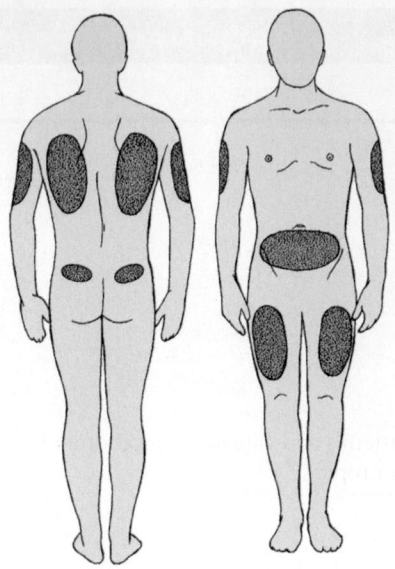

FIG 22.12 Common sites for subcutaneous injections.

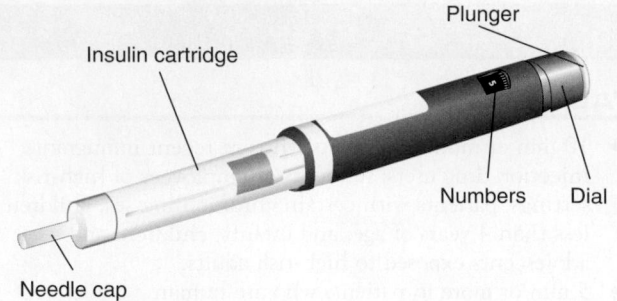

FIG 22.13 Insulin injection pen. *(From Lewis, S. L., et al. [2017]. Medical-surgical nursing: Assessment and management of clinical problems [10th ed.]. St. Louis: Mosby.)*

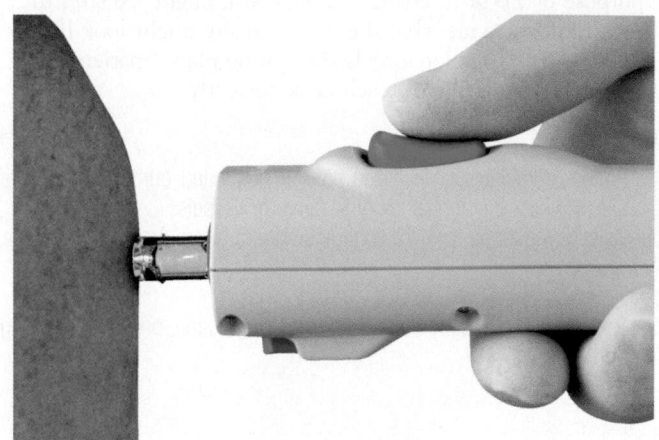

FIG 22.14 Jet injection system is held perpendicular to skin. *(Image courtesy Pharmajet. All rights reserved.)*

irritating solutions and large volumes of medications. Thus, only small volumes (0.5 to 1.5 mL) of water-soluble medications are administered subcutaneously to adults. In children, give smaller volumes—up to 0.5 mL (Hockenberry & Wilson, 2015). Examples of subcutaneous medications include epinephrine, insulin, allergy medications, opioids, and heparin.

The best subcutaneous injection sites include the outer aspect of the upper arms, the abdomen from below the costal margins to the iliac crests, and the anterior aspects of the thighs (Fig. 22.12). These areas are easily accessible and are large enough to allow rotating multiple injections within each anatomical location.

Choose an injection site that is free of skin lesions, bony prominences, and large underlying muscles or nerves. Site rotation prevents the formation of lipohypertrophy or lipoatrophy in the skin. A patient's body weight and adipose tissue are assessed when determining the depth of the subcutaneous layer. Choose the needle length and angle of insertion on the basis of a patient's weight and an estimation of the amount of subcutaneous tissue (Larkin et al., 2018). Gender should be considered, since females have more nonabdominal fat and total fat than males (Larkin et al., 2018). Nurses typically use a 25-gauge, 16 mm (5/8–inch) needle inserted at a 45-degree angle or a 13 mm (1/2–inch) needle inserted at a 90-degree angle to administer subcutaneous medications to a normal-size adult patient. Some children require only a 13 mm (1/2–inch) needle. If the patient is obese, pinch the tissue and use a needle long enough to insert through fatty tissue at the base of the skinfold. Thin patients often do not have sufficient tissue for subcutaneous injections; the upper abdomen is usually the best site in this case. To ensure that a subcutaneous medication reaches the subcutaneous tissue, follow this rule: If you can grasp 5 cm (2 inches) of tissue, insert the needle at a 90-degree angle; if you can grasp only 2.5 cm (1 inch) of tissue, insert the needle at a 45-degree angle.

Research on insulin administration shows that insulin needles that are 8 mm or longer often enter the muscles of men and people with a body mass index (BMI) of 25 kg/m^2 or less. Shorter 4- to 5-mm needles are associated with less pain, adequate control of blood sugars, and minimal leakage of medication (ISMP, 2017a; Spollett, Edelman, Mehner, et al., 2016). Thus, when administering insulin, needles of 4–8 mm are recommended (start with the shortest needle available). Administer at a 90-degree angle to reduce pain

and achieve adequate control of blood sugars with minimal adverse effects for people of all BMIs, including children (Diabetes Canada Clinical Practice Guidelines Expert Committee, 2018).

Several different devices are available for administration of subcutaneous injections. *Injection pens* allow patients to self-administer medications (e.g., epinephrine, insulin, or interferon) subcutaneously (Fig. 22.13). They offer a convenient delivery method using prefilled, disposable cartridges. The patient pinches the skin, inserts the needle, and injects a predetermined medication dose. Teaching is essential to ensure that patients use the correct injection technique and deliver the correct dose of medication. Teach patients the importance of priming the pen before use. Priming involves pointing the pen needle up in the air, dialing one or two units (see package directions) on the pen, and then pressing the plunger fully with the thumb, repeating until a drop appears. This clears the needle of air and ensures that a full dose is ready (Fit Forum, 2017). The disadvantages of this device include increased risk for needle-stick injury and user's lack of knowledge and skill in administration technique (Fit Forum, 2017). The *needleless jet injection system* administers subcutaneous medications without the use of needles. Needle-free injections use high pressure to penetrate the skin with the medication into the subcutaneous tissue (Fig. 22.14). Another option for subcutaneous injection is the *subcutaneous injection device* (e.g., insuflon) (Fig. 22.15), which is inserted into the subcutaneous tissue; the needle is then removed, leaving the cannula in the tissue to provide an avenue for administering medications for up to 3 days without having to puncture the skin with each injection. The

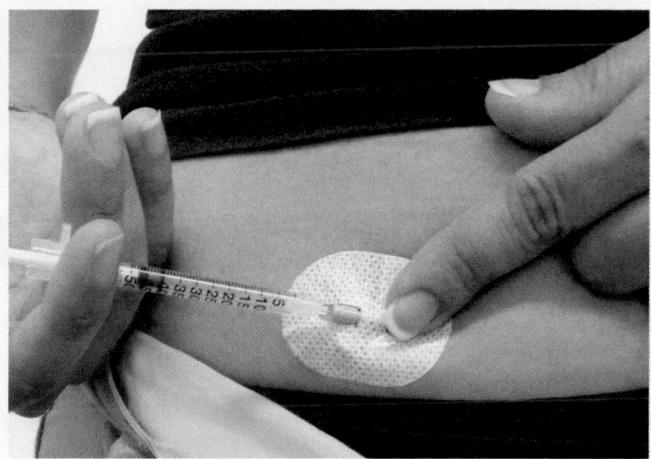

FIG 22.15 Subcutaneous device. *(Image courtesy IntraPump Infusion Systems. All rights reserved.)*

General Guidelines for Insulin Administration

- Store vials of insulin in the refrigerator, not the freezer. Keep vials currently being used at room temperature for up to 1 month. Do not inject cold insulin.
- Inspect vials before each use for changes in appearance (e.g., clumping, frosting, precipitation, change in clarity or colour), indicating lack of potency.
- Do not interchange insulin types unless approved by the patient's health care provider.
- Preferred injection sites include the abdomen, avoiding a 5-cm (2-inch) radius around the umbilicus and the outer aspect of the thighs.
- Have patient self-administer insulin whenever possible.
- Patients who take insulin need to self-monitor their blood glucose.
- Insulin syringes with needles attached and insulin pen needles should be used only once.
- All patients who take insulin should carry at least 15 g carbohydrate (e.g., glucose tablets—preferred choice, 15 mL table sugar dissolved in water, 175 mL juice or regular soft drink) in the event of a hypoglycemic reaction.

Adapted from Clinical Practice Guidelines Expert Committee (2018). Diabetes Canada 2018 Diabetes Canada 2018 clinical practice guidelines for the prevention and management of diabetes in Canada. *Canadian Journal of Diabetes, 42*(Suppl. 1), S1–S325. Retrieved from http://guidelines.diabetes.ca/docs/CPG-2018-full-EN.pdf.

subcutaneous butterfly is also an option frequently used for postoperative or palliative patients who are receiving frequent doses of analgesia or antiemetics subcutaneously. The subcutaneous butterfly reduces the frequency of puncturing the skin barrier and thereby contributes to patient comfort.

Special Considerations for Administration of Insulin

Most patients manage type 1 diabetes mellitus with insulin injections. Nurses need to be knowledgeable and vigilant when preparing insulin because it is considered a high-alert medication; medications are identified as high-alert when associated with the highest risk of injury when used in error (ISMP, 2017a). Anatomical injection site rotation is no longer necessary because newer human insulins carry a lower risk for skin hypertrophy. Patients choose one anatomical area (e.g., the abdomen) and systematically rotate sites within that region, which maintains consistent insulin absorption from day to day. Absorption rates of insulin vary, based on the injection site. Insulin is most quickly absorbed in the abdomen and most slowly in the thighs (Burchum & Rosenthal, 2016; Fit Forum, 2017).

The timing of insulin injections is critical. Health care providers plan insulin injection times based on blood glucose levels; when a patient will eat; and the onset, peak, and duration of the insulin to be administered. Knowing the peak action and duration of the insulin is essential when developing an effective diabetes management plan. Table 22.2 compares a variety of insulin preparations. Box 22.3 provides general guidelines for insulin administration.

Special Considerations for Administration of Heparin

Heparin therapy provides therapeutic anticoagulation to reduce the risk for thrombus formation by suppressing clot formation. Therefore, patients receiving heparin are at risk for bleeding, including bleeding gums, hematemesis, hematuria, or melena. Results from coagulation blood tests (e.g., activated partial thromboplastin time [aPTT] and partial thromboplastin time [PTT]) allow the nurse to monitor the desired therapeutic range for heparin therapy.

Before administering heparin, which is also identified as a high-alert medication, assess for pre-existing conditions that contraindicate its use, including cerebral or aortic aneurysm, cerebrovascular hemorrhage, severe hypertension, and blood dyscrasias. In addition, assess for conditions in which increased risk for hemorrhage is present: recent childbirth; severe diabetes and

renal disease; liver disease; severe trauma; and active ulcers or lesions of the gastrointestinal (GI), genitourinary (GU), or respiratory tract. Assess the patient's current medication regimen, including use of over-the-counter (OTC) and herbal medications (e.g., garlic, ginger, ginkgo, horse chestnut, or feverfew), for possible interaction with heparin. Other medications that interact with heparin include aspirin, nonsteroidal anti-inflammatory drugs (NSAIDs), cephalosporins, antithyroid agents, probenecid, and thrombolytics.

Low-molecular-weight heparins (LMWHs) (e.g., enoxaparin) are more effective than heparin in some patients. The anticoagulant effects are more predictable (Burchum & Rosenthal, 2016). LMWHs have a longer half-life and require less laboratory monitoring but are expensive. To minimize the pain and bruising associated with LMWH, it is given subcutaneously on the right or left side of the abdomen, at least 5 cm (2 inches) away from the umbilicus. Administer LMWH in its prefilled syringe with the attached needle and do not expel the air bubble in the syringe before giving the medication. There is some evidence to support a slower injection rate of 30 seconds to reduce bruising and pain (Athira & Rohini, 2016; Sanofi-Aventis Canada, 2018).

Delegation and Collaboration

The skill of administering subcutaneous injections cannot be delegated to an unregulated care provider (UCP). The nurse instructs the UCP about:

- Potential medication adverse effects and to immediately report their occurrence to the nurse.

Equipment

- Medication administration record (MAR) or computer printout
- Proper size syringe and sharps with engineered sharps injury protection (SESIP) needle:
  - Subcutaneous: syringe (1- to 3-mL) and needle (25- to 27-gauge, 3.2 mm [1/8 inch] to 16 mm [5/8 inch])
  - *Immunizations:* 23- to 25-gauge needle, 16 mm (5/8 inch) (Beirne, Hennessy, Cadogan, et al., 2015)

- Subcutaneous U-100 insulin: insulin syringe (1 mL) with preattached needle (30 to 32 gauge, 4–8 mm; start with shortest needle available)
- Subcutaneous U-500 insulin: Pen recommended but if not available, use 1 mL tuberculin (TB) syringe with needle (25- to 31-gauge, 6 mm preferred)

- Small gauze pad (*optional*)
- Alcohol swab
- Medication vial or ampoule
- Clean gloves
- Puncture-proof container

STEP	RATIONALE

ASSESSMENT

1. Check accuracy and completeness of each MAR or computer printout with health care provider's prescription. Check patient's name, medication name and dosage, route of administration, and time of administration. Recopy or reprint any part of MAR that is difficult to read.	The prescription sheet is the most reliable source and only legal record of medications that the patient is to receive. Computer order entry (COE) and barcode systems are technology recently introduced in many settings to reduce medication errors (Cochran et al., 2016; Lapkin et al., 2016).
2. Assess patient's medical and medication history.	Determines need for medication or possible contraindications for medication administration.
3. Assess patient's history of allergies: known type of allergies and normal allergic reaction.	Do not prepare medication if there is known patient allergy.
4. Review medication reference information for medication action, purpose, normal dose, adverse effects, time and peak of onset, and nursing implications.	Allows you to administer medication safely and monitor patient's response to therapy.
5. Check date of expiration for medication.	Dose potency increases or decreases when outdated.
6. Observe patient's previous verbal and nonverbal responses regarding injection.	Anticipating patient's anxiety allows you to use distraction to reduce pain awareness.
7. Assess for contraindication to subcutaneous injections, such as circulatory shock or reduced local tissue perfusion.	Reduced tissue perfusion interferes with drug absorption and distribution.
8. Assess patient's symptoms before initiating medication therapy.	Provides information to evaluate desired effect of medication.
9. Assess adequacy of patient's adipose tissue.	Adipose tissue influences methods for administering injections.
10. Assess relevant laboratory results (e.g., blood glucose, partial thromboplastin).	Provides baseline for measuring drug response.
11. Assess patient's knowledge of medication.	Poses implications for patient education.

NURSING DIAGNOSES

- Acute pain
- Anxiety

- Insufficient knowledge regarding medication administration or drug therapy

- Fear
- Reduced health maintenance

Related factors/Risk factors are individualized on the basis of patient's condition or needs.

PLANNING

1. Expected outcomes following completion of procedure:	
• Patient experiences no pain or mild burning at injection site.	Medications may cause minor tissue irritation.
• Patient achieves desired effect of medication with no signs of allergies or undesired effects.	Medication administered without patient injury.
• Patient explains purpose, dosage, and effects of medication.	Demonstrates learning.

IMPLEMENTATION

1. Perform hand hygiene and prepare medication using aseptic technique. Check label of medication carefully with MAR or computer printout three times (see Skill 22.1 or Procedural Guideline 22.1) when preparing medication.	Ensures that medication is sterile. **Three checks for accuracy** must occur when preparing medications: 1. Before removing the medication vial/container from the drawer. 2. When the prescribed amount of the medication is drawn up. 3. Before returning the vial to storage/drawer or disposing of an empty or single use vial or ampoule.

STEP	RATIONALE

IMPLEMENTATION

2. Take medication(s) to patient at correct time (see employer policy). During administration apply 10 rights of medication administration.

Hospitals must adopt medication administration policy and procedure for timing of medication administration that considers nature of the prescribed medication, specific clinical application, and patient needs (ISMP, 2011).

3. Close room curtain or door.

Provides privacy.

4. Identify patient using at least two person-specific identifiers (e.g., name and date of birth or name and medical record number) according to employer policy. Compare identifiers with information on patient's MAR or medical record.

Ensures correct patient.

5. Ask patient if they have allergies.

Confirms patient's allergy history.

6. Discuss purpose of each medication, action, and possible adverse effects. Allow patient to ask any questions. Tell patient that injection will cause slight burning or sting.

Patient has the right to be informed, and patient's understanding of each medication improves adherence to drug therapy. Helps minimize patient's anxiety.

7. Perform hand hygiene and apply clean gloves. Keep sheet or gown draped over body parts not requiring exposure.

Reduces transmission of infection. Respects dignity of patient while exposing injection area.

8. Select appropriate injection site. Inspect skin surface over sites for bruises, inflammation, or edema. Do not use an area that is bruised or has signs associated with infection.

Injection sites are free of abnormalities that interfere with drug absorption. Sites used repeatedly become hardened from lipohypertrophy (increased growth in fatty tissue).

Clinical Decision Point *Applying ice to the injection site for 1 minute before the injection may decrease the patient's perception of pain* (Hockenberry & Wilson, 2015).

9. Palpate sites and avoid those with masses or tenderness. Be sure that needle is correct size by grasping skinfold at site with thumb and forefinger. Measure fold from top to bottom. Make sure that needle is one-half length of fold.

You can mistakenly give subcutaneous injections in muscle, especially in abdomen and thigh sites. Appropriate size of needle ensures that you inject medication into subcutaneous tissue (Larkin et al., 2018).

  a. When administering insulin or heparin, use abdominal injection sites first, then posterior arms, and lastly, thigh injection site.

Risk for bruising is not affected by site.

  b. When administering LMWH subcutaneously, choose site on right or left side of abdomen, at least 5 cm (2 inches) away from umbilicus.

Injecting LMWH on side of abdomen helps decrease pain and bruising at injection site (Sanofi-Aventis Canada, 2018

  c. Rotate insulin site within an anatomical area (e.g., abdomen) and systematically rotate sites within that area.

Rotating injection sites within same anatomical site maintains consistency in day-to-day insulin absorption.

10. Help patient into comfortable position. Have them relax arm, leg, or abdomen, depending on site selection.

Relaxation of site minimizes discomfort.

11. Relocate site using anatomical landmarks.

Injection into correct anatomical site prevents injury to nerves, bone, and blood vessels.

12. Clean site with antiseptic swab. Apply swab at centre of site and rotate outward in circular direction for about 5 cm (2 inches) (see illustration).

Mechanical action of swab removes secretions containing microorganisms.

13. Hold swab or gauze between third and fourth fingers of nondominant hand.

Swab or gauze remains readily accessible for use when withdrawing needle after the injection.

14. Remove needle cap or protective sheath by pulling it straight off.

Preventing needle from touching sides of cap prevents contamination.

15. Hold syringe between thumb and forefinger of dominant hand; hold as dart (see illustration).

Quick, smooth injection requires proper manipulation of syringe parts.

16. Administer injection:

  a. For average-size patient, hold skin across injection site or pinch skin with nondominant hand.

Needle penetrates tight skin more easily than loose skin. Pinching elevates subcutaneous tissue and desensitizes area.

  b. Inject needle quickly and firmly at 45- to 90-degree angle (see illustration). Release skin if pinched. *Option:* When using injection pen or giving heparin, continue to pinch skin while injecting medicine.

Quick, firm insertion minimizes discomfort. (Injecting medication into compressed tissue irritates nerve). Correct angle prevents accidental injection into muscle.

  c. For obese patient pinch skin at site and inject needle at 90-degree angle below tissue fold.

Obese patients have fatty layer of tissue above subcutaneous layer.

STEP	RATIONALE

IMPLEMENTATION

d. After needle enters site, grasp lower end of syringe barrel with nondominant hand to stabilize it. Move dominant hand to end of plunger and slowly inject medication over several seconds (see illustration). When giving heparin, inject over 30 seconds (Sanofi Aventis Canada, 2018; Yi, Shuai, Tian, et al., 2016). Avoid moving syringe.

Movement of syringe may displace needle and cause discomfort. Slow injection of medication minimizes pain intensity and duration, and there is lower bruising at 48–72 hours postinjection (Yi et al., 2016).

Clinical Decision Point *Aspiration before injecting a subcutaneous medication, including heparin and insulin, is not necessary. Piercing a blood vessel in a subcutaneous injection is very rare (Lilley, Collins, & Snyder, 2017).*

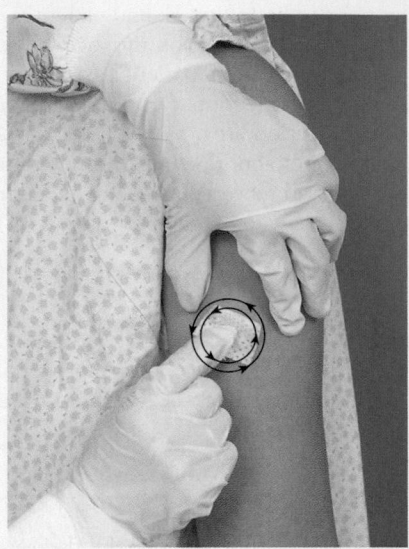

STEP 12 Subcutaneous site: Posterior aspect of upper arm. Clean site with circular motion.

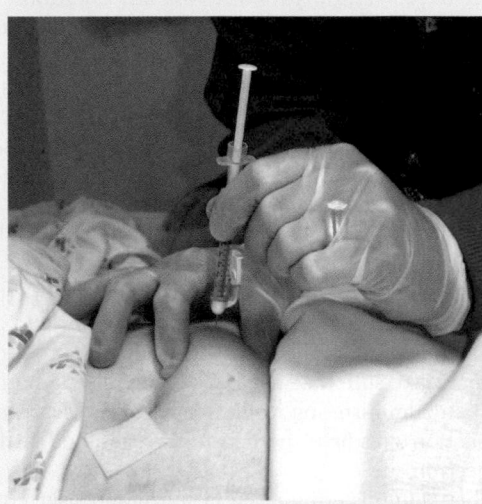

STEP 16b Subcutaneous injection. Angle and needle length depend on thickness of skinfold.

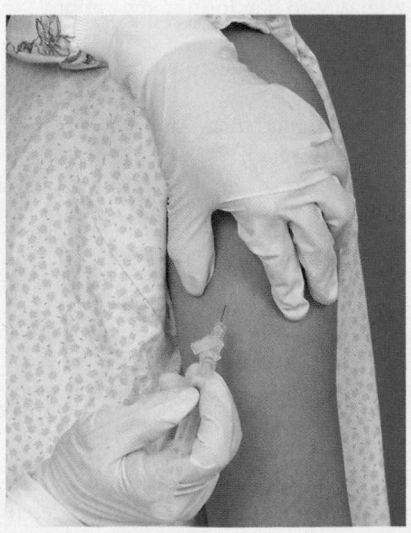

STEP 15 Subcutaneous injection in the posterior aspect of the upper arm. Hold syringe as if grasping a dart.

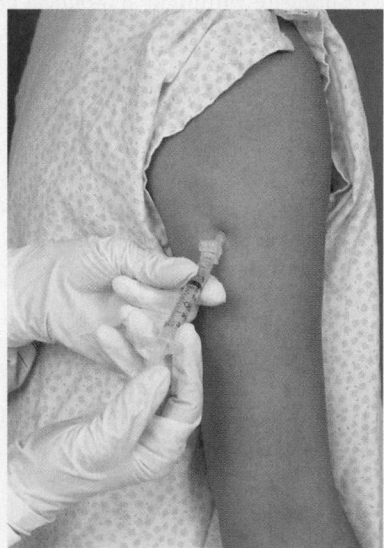

STEP 16d Inject medication slowly.

STEP	RATIONALE

IMPLEMENTATION

e. Withdraw needle quickly while placing antiseptic swab or gauze gently over site.

17. Apply gentle pressure to site. *Do not massage site.* (If heparin is given, hold alcohol swab or gauze to site for 30 to 60 seconds.)

18. Help patient to comfortable position.

19. Discard uncapped needle or needle enclosed in safety shield (see illustrations) and attached syringe into puncture- and leak-proof receptacle.

20. Remove gloves and perform hand hygiene.

21. Stay with patient for several minutes and observe for any allergic reactions.

Supporting tissues around injection site minimizes discomfort during needle withdrawal. Dry gauze may minimize patient discomfort associated with alcohol on nonintact skin.

Aids absorption. Massage can damage underlying tissue. Time interval prevents bleeding at site.

Gives patient sense of well-being.

Prevents injury to patients and health care personnel. Recapping needles increases risk for needle-stick injury (Elmi et al., 2018).

Reduces transmission of microorganisms.

Dyspnea, wheezing, and circulatory collapse are signs of severe anaphylactic reaction.

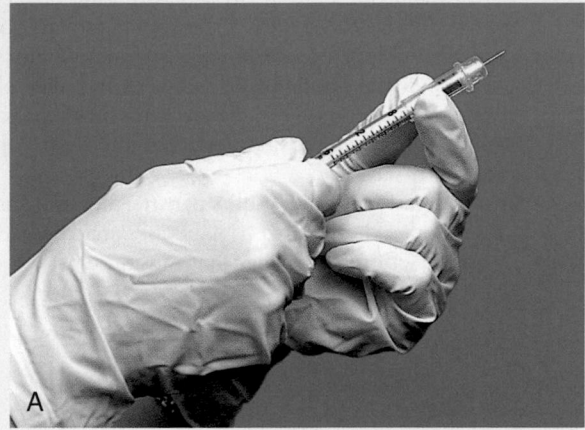 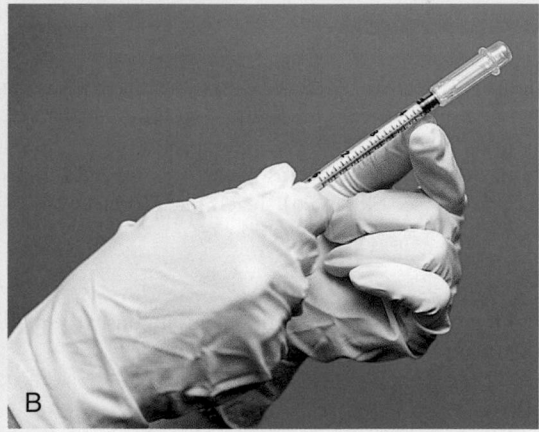

STEP 19 Needle with plastic guard to prevent needle-sticks. **A,** Position of guard before injection. **B,** After injection guard locks in place, covering needle.

EVALUATION

1. Return to room in 15 to 30 minutes and ask if patient feels any acute pain, burning, numbness, or tingling at injection site.

2. Inspect site, noting bruising or induration. Provide warm compress to site.

3. Observe patient's response to medication at times that correlate with onset, peak, and duration of medication. Review laboratory results as appropriate (e.g., blood glucose, partial thromboplastin).

4. Use Teach-Back: "I want to be sure I explained to you the reason for this subcutaneous injection. Tell me why you are receiving this injection." Develop a revised teaching plan if patient or caregiver is not able to teach back correctly.

Continued discomfort may indicate injury to underlying bones or nerves.

Bruising or induration indicates complication associated with injection.

Adverse effects of parenteral medications develop rapidly. Evaluate effect of medication on basis of onset, peak, and duration of action.

Determines patient's and caregiver's level of understanding of instructional topic.

STEP	RATIONALE

EVALUATION

Unexpected Outcomes

1. Patient experiences localized pain, numbness, tingling, or burning at injection site.
2. Patient displays adverse reaction with signs of urticaria, eczema, pruritus, wheezing, and dyspnea.

3. Hypertrophy of skin develops from repeated subcutaneous injection.

Related Interventions

- Assess injection site; may indicate potential injury to nerve or tissues.
- Notify patient's health care provider and do not reuse site.
- Monitor patient's vital signs.
- Follow employer policy for appropriate response to allergic reactions (e.g., administration of antihistamine such as diphenhydramine or epinephrine) and notify patient's health care provider immediately.
- Add allergy information to patient's record.
- Do not use site for future injections.
- Instruct patient not to use site for 6 months.

Communication and Documentation

- Immediately after administration, document medication, dose, route, site, time, and date given on MAR in nurses' notes in electronic health record (EHR) or chart. Correctly sign MAR according to employer policy.
- Document patient teaching, validation of understanding, and patient's response to medication in nurses' notes in EHR or chart.
- Document any undesirable or adverse effects from medication and report to patient's health care provider.

Special Considerations
Teaching

- Instruct patient to wear medical identification bracelet indicating important medical information, including bleeding tendencies, illnesses (e.g., diabetes mellitus), and allergies.
- Patients who require daily injections need to learn techniques of self-administration (see Skill 43.6). Teach injection techniques to a caregiver.

Pediatric

- Administer amounts up to 0.5 mL only subcutaneously to small children (Hockenberry & Wilson, 2015).

Gerontological

- Older persons have less elastic skin and reduced subcutaneous skinfold thickness. The upper abdominal site is the best site to use when the patient has little subcutaneous tissue.

Care in the Community

- Improper disposal of used needles and sharps in the home setting poses a health risk to the public and to waste management employees. Several options for safe sharps disposal at home exist, including allowing patients to transport their own sharps containers from home to collection sites (e.g., hospital or pharmacy); syringe exchange programs; or special devices that destroy the needle on the syringe, rendering it safe for disposal. If the patient cannot implement any of these options, have them dispose of needles and other sharps in a hard plastic or metal container with a tightly sealed lid (e.g., empty detergent bottle or coffee can). Pamphlets for safe home disposal of sharps are available from provincial public health services and most pharmacies, as are numerous online sites, such as https://www.pshsa.ca/products/safe-handling-disposal-of-sharps-medical-supplies-in-home-health-settings/.
- Instruct patients that insulin pen needles and insulin syringes should be used only once (Diabetes Canada, 2018).
- Teach injection techniques that minimize patient discomfort to patient and caregiver.

♦ SKILL 22.4   Administering Continuous Subcutaneous Medications

NSO *Nursing Skills Online Administration of Parenteral Medications: Intravenous Medications Module 7 / Lesson 3*

The continuous subcutaneous infusion (CSQI or CSCI) route of medication administration is used for selected medications (e.g., opioids, insulin) and for infusion of fluids for hydration or nutrition (Caccialanza, Constans, Cotogni, et al., 2018). The route is also effective with medications to stop preterm labour (e.g., terbutaline) and to treat pulmonary hypertension (e.g., treprostinil sodium). One factor that determines the infusion rate of CSQI is the rate of medication absorption. Most patients can absorb 1 to 2 mL/hour of medication, but the rate of absorption is more dependent on osmotic pressure than rate of administration (Alexander et al., 2014; Arthur, 2015). The procedure to initiate and discontinue CSQI therapy is similar, regardless of the type of medication being delivered. However, nursing assessment and interventions vary, depending on the type of medication administered.

With CSQI, patients are able to manage their illness and pain without the risks and expenses involved with intravenous (IV) medication administration (Caccialanza et al., 2018). The route is relatively easy for patients and families to learn and understand in the home setting. CSQI is often used for oncological and postoperative pain control in infants, children, and adults (Arthur, 2015). Box 22.4 summarizes benefits associated with the use of CSQI for pain management.

Patients with diabetes mellitus who use CSQI for management of blood glucose levels are carefully selected and receive intense diabetes self-management education from qualified diabetes educators and insulin pump trainers. The Medtronic MiniMed (Sheldon, 2019) integrates an insulin pump with real-time continuous glucose monitoring (Fig. 22.16). Adults and children living with diabetes

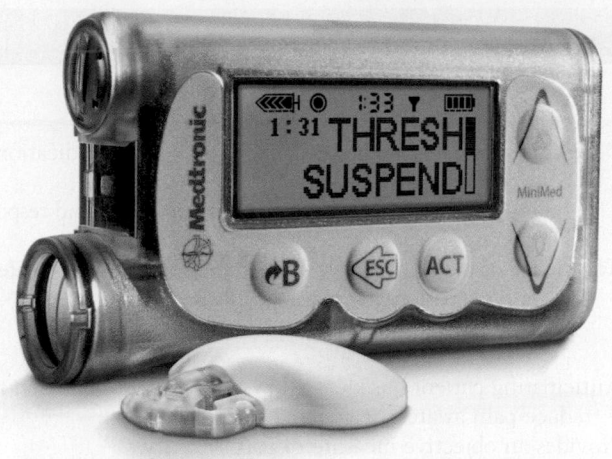

FIG 22.16 Mini-Med Paradigm REAL-Time Insulin CSQI pump and continuous glucose monitoring system. (*Courtesy Medtronic, Inc., Northridge, CA.*)

BOX 22.4

Pain Management Benefits With Use of Continuous Subcutaneous Infusion

- Benefits patients with poor venous access
- Provides pain relief to patients who are unable to tolerate oral pain medications
- Allows patients greater mobility
- Onset of action about 20 minutes
- Better pain control than intramuscular injections
- Lower rates of infection

Modified from Arthur, A. (2015). Innovations in subcutaneous infusions. *Journal of Infusion Nursing, 38*(3), 179; Bartz, L., et al. (2014). Subcutaneous administration of drugs in palliative care: Result of a systematic observational study. *Journal of Pain Symptom Management, 48*(4), 540.

---

mellitus who use insulin pumps require less insulin, have superior glycemic control, and better health-related quality of life (Pozzilli, Battelino, Danne, et al., 2016). Insulin pumps are becoming the treatment of choice for children living with type 1 diabetes. Age-appropriate education for the child and the entire family and, ideally, school personnel is essential and should include psychosocial support and nutritional information, including counting carbohydrates (Pozzilli et al., 2016).

A small-gauge (25- to 27-gauge) winged butterfly needle or special commercially prepared Teflon cannula is used to deliver medications. Although Teflon cannulas generally are more expensive, they are more comfortable for the patient, have lower rates of complications, and are associated with fewer needle-stick injuries. The choice of needle type is based on employer guidelines or patient preference.

Use the needle with the shortest length and the smallest gauge necessary to establish and maintain the infusion.

Use the same anatomical sites for subcutaneous injections and the upper chest. Site selection depends on a patient's activity level and the type of medication delivered. For example, pain medications given to ambulatory patients are best delivered in the upper chest, which allows a patient to move freely. Insulin is absorbed most consistently in the abdomen; thus, choose a site in the abdomen away from the waistline. Always avoid sites where the tubing of the pump could be disturbed. Rotate sites used for medication administration at least every 2 to 7 days or whenever complications such as leaking occur (Arthur, 2015; INS, 2016).

The CSQI route requires a computerized pump with safety features, including lockout intervals and warning alarms. Ideally, medication pumps are individualized on the basis of the medication being delivered and patient needs. Nurses also need to consider the availability and cost of the pump and supplies. When possible, patients should select the pump that fits their individual and home needs and is easiest to use.

Delegation and Collaboration

The skill of administering CSQI medications cannot be delegated to an unregulated care provider (UCP). The nurse instructs the UCP about:

- Potential medication adverse effects or reactions and to immediately report their occurrence to the nurse.
- Reporting complications (e.g., leaking, redness, discomfort) at the CSQI needle insertion site to the nurse.
- Obtaining any required vital signs and reporting them to the nurse.

Equipment
Initiation of CSQI

- Clean gloves
- Alcohol swab
- Antibacterial skin preparation such as chlorhexidine
- Small (25- to 27-gauge) winged catheter with attached tubing or CSQI-designed catheter (e.g., Sof-Set)
- Infusion pump
- Occlusive, transparent dressing
- Tape
- Medication in appropriate syringe or container
- Medication administration record (MAR) or computer printout

Discontinuing CSQI

- Clean gloves
- Small gauze dressing
- Tape or adhesive bandage
- Alcohol swab and chlorhexidine (*optional*)
- Puncture-proof container

STEP	RATIONALE

ASSESSMENT

1. Check accuracy and completeness of each MAR or computer printout with health care provider's prescription. Check patient's name, medication name and dosage, route of administration, and time of administration. Recopy or reprint any part of MAR that is difficult to read.

The prescription sheet is the most reliable source and only legal record of medications that the patient is to receive. Computer order entry (COE) and barcode systems are technology recently introduced in many settings to reduce medication errors (Cochran et al., 2016; Lapkin et al., 2016).

STEP	RATIONALE

ASSESSMENT

2. Assess patient's medical and medication history.

Determines need for medication or possible contraindications for medication administration.

3. Assess patient's history of allergies: known type of allergens and normal allergic reaction.

CSQI administration of medications may cause a rapid response. Allergic response is immediate.

4. Collect drug reference information necessary to administer drug safely, including action, purpose, adverse effects, normal dose, time of peak onset, how slowly to give medication, and nursing implications.

Knowledge of medication allows you to give medication safely and monitor patient's response to therapy.

5. Assess patient's previous verbal and nonverbal response to needle insertion.

Anticipating patient's anxiety allows you to use distraction to reduce pain awareness.

6. If an analgesic is being administered, assess patient's pain severity using an appropriate pain rating scale or tool.

Provides an objective measure of pain severity.

7. Assess for contraindications to CSQI (e.g., thrombocytopenia or reduced local tissue perfusion).

Any existing coagulation disorder contraindicates heparin infusion. Reduced tissue perfusion interferes with medication absorption and distribution.

8. Assess adequacy of patient's adipose tissue to determine appropriate infusion site.

Physiological changes of aging or patient illness influence amount of subcutaneous tissue, which affects choice of catheter insertion site.

9. Assess patient's knowledge regarding medication to be received and use of medication pump.

Provides background to determine need for patient education.

10. Assess patient's symptoms before initiating medication therapy. Determine severity of pain (if using analgesia) or measure blood glucose level (if using insulin).

Provides information to evaluate desired effects of CSQI medication.

NURSING DIAGNOSES

- Pain (acute, chronic)
- Anxiety
- Fear

- Insufficient knowledge regarding CSQI therapy
- Inadequate health maintenance

- Potential for infection
- Potential for injury

Related factors/Risk factors are individualized on the basis of patient's condition or needs.

PLANNING

1. Expected outcomes following completion of procedure:
   - Needle insertion site remains free from infection.

   Risk for infection at needle insertion site is potential complication of CSQI therapy.

   - Patient achieves desired effect of medication with no signs of adverse reactions.

   Medication is delivered safely with desired therapeutic effect achieved.

   - Patient explains purpose, dosage, and effects of medication and verbalizes understanding of CSQI therapy.

   Demonstrates learning.

IMPLEMENTATION

1. Review manufacturer directions for pump.

Ensures proper use of equipment.

2. Perform hand hygiene. Prepare medication using aseptic technique or if using a prefilled syringe, check dose on prefilled syringe. Connect syringe and prime tubing with medication, being careful not to lose any medication. Compare label of medication with MAR or computer printout three times.

Ensures that medication is sterile. Checking label of medication with transcribed prescription reduces occurrence of error.

Three checks for accuracy must occur when preparing medications:
1. Before removing the medication vial/container from the drawer.
2. When the prescribed amount of the medication is drawn up or when the prefilled syringe is connected to the tubing.
3. Before returning the vial to storage/drawer or disposing of an empty or single-use vial or ampoule. Or if using a prefilled syringe, once the syringe is placed in the pump, as in the next step.

STEP	RATIONALE

IMPLEMENTATION

3. Obtain and program medication administration pump. Place syringe in pump.

Ensures that medication dose administered is accurate.

4. Identify patient using at least two person-specific identifiers (e.g., name and date of birth or name and medical record number) according to employer policy. Compare identifiers with information on patient's MAR or medical record.

Ensures correct patient.

5. Ask patient if they have allergies.

Confirms patient's allergy history.

6. Discuss purpose of each medication, action, and possible adverse effects. Allow patient to ask any questions. Tell patient that needle insertion will cause slight burning or stinging.

Patient has right to be informed, and patient's understanding of each medication improves adherence to drug therapy.

7. Position patient supine, drape, and provide for privacy.

Respects patient's dignity.

8. Initiate CSQI:

   a. Be sure that patient is comfortable, sitting or lying down.

Eases pain associated with insertion of needle.

   b. Select appropriate injection site free of irritation and away from bony prominences and waistline. Most common sites used are subclavicular and abdomen.

Ensures proper medication absorption.

   c. Perform hand hygiene and apply clean gloves. Clean injection site with alcohol using circular motion, followed by antiseptic, using straight cleaning strokes. Allow both agents to dry.

Reduces risk for infection at insertion site.

   d. Hold needle in dominant hand and remove needle guard.

Prepares needle for insertion.

   e. Gently pinch or lift up skin with nondominant hand.

Ensures that needle will enter subcutaneous tissue.

   f. Gently and firmly insert needle at 45- to 90-degree angle (see illustration). Some shorter prepackaged needles (e.g., Sof-Set, Subcutaneous-Set) are inserted at a 90-degree angle. Refer to manufacturer directions.

Decreases pain related to insertion of needle.

   g. Release skinfold and apply tape over "wings" of needle.

Secures needle.

Clinical Decision Point *Some cannulas have a sharp needle covered with a plastic catheter. In this case, remove the needle and leave the plastic catheter in the skin.*

   h. Place occlusive, transparent dressing over insertion site (see illustration).

Protects site from infection and allows you to assess site during medication infusion.

   i. Attach tubing from needle to tubing from infusion pump and turn pump on.

Allows you to administer medication.

   j. Dispose of any sharps in appropriate leak- and puncture-proof container. Discard used supplies, remove gloves, and perform hand hygiene.

Prevents accidental needle-stick injuries and follow employer guidelines for disposal of sharps.

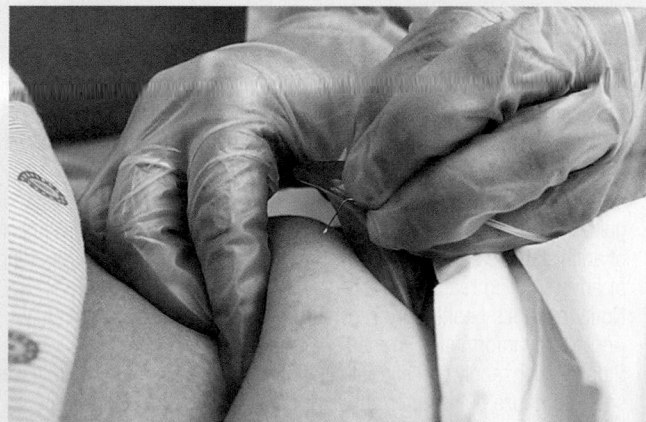

STEP 8f Insert butterfly needle into subcutaneous tissue of abdomen.

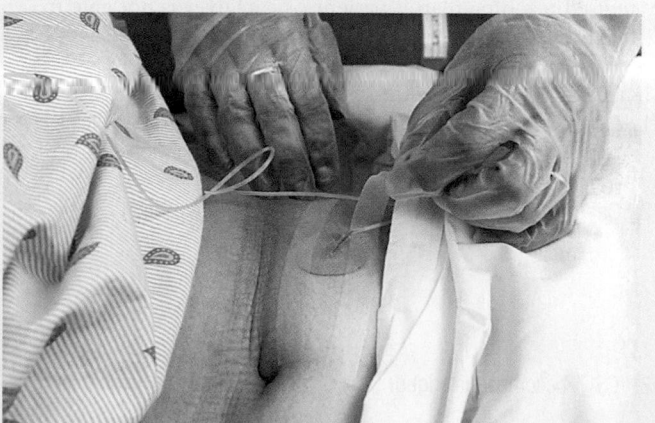

STEP 8h Place transparent dressing over insertion site.

STEP	RATIONALE

IMPLEMENTATION

k. Inspect site before leaving patient and instruct patient to inform you if site becomes red or begins to leak.

Initiate new site with new needle whenever erythema or leaking occurs. If site is free from complications, rotate needle every 2 to 7 days (Arthur, 2015; INS, 2016).

l. Stay with patient for several minutes and observe for any allergic reactions.

Dyspnea, wheezing, and circulatory collapse are signs of severe anaphylactic reaction.

9. Discontinue CSQI:

a. Verify prescription and establish alternative method for medication administration if applicable.

If medication will be required after discontinuing CSQI, a different medication and/or route is often necessary to continue to manage patient's illness or pain.

b. Stop infusion pump.

Prevents medication from spilling.

c. Perform hand hygiene and apply clean gloves.

Hand hygiene reduces risk of contamination of equipment. Gloves provide barrier in event of exposure to blood or body fluids (Infection Prevention & Control Canada [IPAC], 2017).

d. Remove dressing without dislodging or removing needle. Discard properly.

Exposes needle.

Clinical Decision Point *If site is infected, clean it with alcohol and antiseptic. Apply triple antibiotic cream to site if it is excoriated (abraded).*

e. Remove tape from wings of needle and pull needle out at same angle at which it was inserted.

Minimizes patient discomfort.

f. Apply gentle pressure at site until no fluid leaks out of skin.

Dressing adheres to site if skin remains dry.

g. Apply small sterile gauze dressing or adhesive bandage to site.

Prevents bacterial entry into puncture site.

10. Dispose of uncapped needles and syringes in puncture- and leak-proof container.

Prevents accidental needle-stick injuries and follows guidelines for disposal of sharps (CCOHS, 2019; PHAC 2013).

11. Remove and dispose of gloves and perform hand hygiene.

Reduces transmission of microorganisms.

EVALUATION

1. Evaluate patient's response to medication.

Determines effect of therapy. Decreased or absent response to medication may indicate that patient is not receiving medication into subcutaneous tissue (e.g., pump malfunction, medication leaking at site).

2. Assess site at least every 4 hours for redness, pain, drainage, or swelling.

Indicates infection at insertion site.

3. Use Teach-Back: "I want to be sure you understand your continuous infusion into your skin and the medication you are receiving. Tell me in your own words why you have a continuous infusion to receive your medication." Develop a revised teaching plan if patient or caregiver is not able to teach back correctly.

Determines patient's and caregiver's level of understanding of instructional topic.

Unexpected Outcomes

1. Patient indicates localized pain or burning at insertion site; or site appears red or swollen or is leaking, indicating potential infection or needle dislodgement.
2. Patient displays signs of allergic reaction to medication.

3. CSQI becomes dislodged.

Related Interventions

- Remove needle and place new needle in different site.
- Continue to monitor original site for signs of infection and notify health care provider if you suspect infection.
- Stop delivering medication immediately and follow employer policy or guidelines for appropriate response to allergic reaction (e.g., administration of antihistamine such as diphenhydramine or epinephrine) and reporting of adverse drug reactions.
- Notify patient's health care provider of adverse effects immediately.
- Add allergy information to medical record.
- Stop infusion, apply pressure at site until no fluid leaks out of skin, cover site with gauze dressing or adhesive bandage, and initiate new site.
- Assess patient to determine effects of not receiving medication (e.g., assess patient's pain level using age-appropriate pain scale, obtain blood glucose level).

Communication and Documentation

- After initiating CSQI, immediately chart medication, dose, route, site, time, date, and type of medication pump in nurses' notes in electronic health record (EHR) or chart. Use initials or signature.
- If medication is an opioid, follow employer policy to document waste.
- Document patient's response to medication and appearance of site every 4 hours or according to employer policy in nurses' notes in EHR or chart.
- Document patient teaching, validation of understanding, and patient's response to medication in nurse's notes in EHR or chart.
- Document any undesirable or adverse effects from medication and report these to patient's health care provider.

Special Considerations
Teaching

- Instruct patient to wear medical alert bracelet along with medical information, including disease (e.g., diabetes mellitus), allergies, and a contact phone number for the pump manufacturer for technical support.
- Instruct patients to carry backup batteries and extra medication if they are going to be away from home.
- Patients receiving insulin require intensive diabetes management education (Box 22.5).
- Never immerse pumps in water or expose them to X-ray films or magnetic resonance imaging.

Pediatric

- CSQI improves glycemic control in children and adolescents. There is a decreased rate of severe hypoglycemia, catheter-site infection, and weight gain (Hockenberry & Wilson, 2015).
- Insulin pumps offer more flexibility for adolescents, placing the responsibility of diabetes management with the child. Extensive child and family education is needed in using CSQI (Hockenberry & Wilson, 2015).
- Clean and change CSQI sites in children every 48 to 72 hours or at the first signs of inflammation (Hockenberry & Wilson, 2015).

Gerontological

- CSQI delivers isotonic IV solutions to dehydrated older persons; this is known as *hypodermoclysis therapy*. This method of providing

---

BOX 22.5

Education Topics for Patients Receiving Insulin With Continuous Subcutaneous Infusion

- Blood glucose monitoring
- Meal planning and food choices
- Incorporating exercise into daily routine
- How to program and use the insulin pump
- Illness guidelines and management
- Management of hypoglycemia
- Prevention and management of hyperglycemia
- Prevention of infection, especially at CSQI infusion site
- Problem-solving and decision-making skills when pump malfunctions
- Special considerations and precautions (e.g., what to do with pump when showering and sleeping)

Modified from Diabetes Canada Clinical Practice Guidelines Expert Committee. (2018). Diabetes Canada 2018 clinical practice guidelines for the prevention and management of diabetes in Canada. *Canadian Journal of Diabetes, 42*(Suppl. 1), S1–S325. Retrieved from http://guidelines.diabetes.ca/docs/CPG-2018-full-EN.pdf.

hydration avoids the need to transfer a patient from home or long-term care facility to an acute care hospital. A health care provider may prescribe use of hyaluronidase to facilitate dispersion and absorption of 1000 mL or more of hydration solutions (INS, 2016). Infuse fluids slowly (e.g., 30 mL/hour) during the first hour of therapy. If the patient remains comfortable, you can increase the rate of infusion. Usually infusion rates do not exceed 60 mL/hour. The rate and volume should not exceed those used for IV infusion (INS, 2016). Hypodermoclysis is an easy-to-use, safe, and cost-effective alternative to IV hydration for older persons (Caccialanza et al., 2018).

Care in the Community

- Patients in the home using CSQI need a responsible caregiver, if available. Educate the patient and caregiver about the desired effect of the medication, adverse effects of the medication, operation of the pump, how to evaluate the effectiveness of the medication, when and how to assess and rotate injection sites, and when to call a health care provider because of problems. Patients need to know where and how to obtain and dispose of all required supplies.
- Patients managing CSQI at home may use an antibacterial soap (e.g., Hibiclens) instead of alcohol and chlorhexidine to clean the insertion site.

◆ SKILL 22.5 Administering Intramuscular Injections

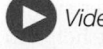 *Video Clip* **NSO** *Nursing Skills Online Administration of Parenteral Medications Module 7 / Lesson 5*

The intramuscular (IM) injection route deposits medication into deep muscle tissue, which has a rich blood supply, allowing medication to absorb faster than by the subcutaneous route. Any factor that interferes with local tissue blood flow affects the rate and extent of drug absorption. There is an increased risk for injecting drugs directly into blood vessels using the IM route. Therefore, whenever administering a medication by the IM route, first verify that the injection is justified (Nicoll & Hesby, 2002; WHO, 2018).

The viscosity of the medication, injection site, patient's weight, and amount of adipose tissue influence needle size selection. Determine needle gauge by the medication to be administered.

Some medications such as hepatitis B and tetanus, diphtheria, and pertussis (Tdap) immunizations are only given intramuscularly. Use a longer and heavier-gauge needle to pass through subcutaneous tissue and penetrate deep muscle tissue (see Fig. 22.1). A patient's body mass index (BMI), gender, and the amount of adipose tissue influence needle size selection. Because most facilities have needles that range in length from only 9.5 mm (3/8 inch) to 40 mm (1½ inches), investigate different medication routes, especially when IM injections are prescribed for patients who are obese.

The angle of insertion for an IM injection is 90 degrees. Muscle is less sensitive to irritating and viscous medications. A normal,

well-developed adult patient tolerates 2 to 5 mL of medication into a larger muscle without severe muscle discomfort (Nicoll & Hesby, 2002). However, larger volumes of medication (4 to 5 mL) are unlikely to be absorbed properly. Children, older persons, and thin patients tolerate only 2 mL of an IM injection. Do not give more than 1 mL to small children and older infants, and do not give more than 0.5 mL to smaller infants (Hockenberry & Wilson, 2015).

Rotate IM injection sites to decrease the risk for hypertrophy. Emaciated or atrophied muscles absorb medication poorly; thus, avoid their use when possible. The Z-track method, a technique for pulling the skin during an injection, is recommended for IM injections (Nicoll & Hesby, 2002). It prevents leakage of medication into subcutaneous tissues, seals medication in the muscle, and minimizes irritation. To use the Z-track method, apply the appropriate-size needle to the syringe and clean and select an IM site, preferably in a large, deep muscle such as the ventrogluteal. Pull the overlying skin and subcutaneous tissues approximately 2.5 to 3.5 cm (1 to 1½ inches) laterally to the side with the ulnar side of the nondominant hand. Hold the skin in this position until you have administered the injection (Fig. 22.17, A). Inject the needle deeply into the muscle. To reduce injection site discomfort, the Canadian Immunization Guide recommends that there is no longer any need to aspirate after the needle is injected when *administering vaccines* (PHAC, 2017). A recent summary of evidence (Paull, 2018) indicates that, historically, aspiration during IM injections has been based on expert opinion. Paull (2018) concludes that aspiration is largely unnecessary; it increases pain and should be avoided unless the medication could cause anaphylaxis or death if injected into a blood vessel (e.g., immunotherapy medication). Always follow employer policy for aspirating vaccines or other

medications during an IM injection and be alert to those medications that indicate aspiration must be done before an IM injection. Keep the needle inserted for 10 seconds to allow the medication to disperse evenly. Release the skin after withdrawing the needle. This leaves a zigzag path that seals the needle track wherever tissue planes slide across one another (see Fig. 22.17, B). The medication is sealed in the muscle tissue.

Injection Sites

When selecting an IM site, determine that the site is free of pain, infection, necrosis, bruising, and abrasions. Also consider the location of underlying bones, nerves, and blood vessels and the volume of medication to be administered. Because of the sciatic nerve location, the dorsogluteal muscle is not recommended as an injection site.

Ventrogluteal Site

The ventrogluteal muscle involves the gluteus medius; it is situated deep and away from major nerves and blood vessels. This site is the preferred and safest site for all adults, children, and infants, especially for medications that have larger volumes and are more viscous and irritating (Atay, Kurt, Akkaya, et al., 2017; Hockenberry & Wilson, 2015). Immunizations administered to infants and children are an exception, in which case the vastus lateralis is the preferred site (Hockenberry & Wilson, 2015). The ventrogluteal site is recommended for volumes greater than 2 mL (Hopkins & Arias, 2013; Nicoll & Hesby, 2002). Research shows that injuries such as fibrosis, nerve damage, abscess, tissue necrosis, muscle contraction, gangrene, and pain are associated with all the common IM sites *except* the ventrogluteal site (Hopkins & Arias, 2013).

To locate the ventrogluteal muscle, have the patient lie in either the supine or lateral position; place the heel of your hand over the greater trochanter of the patient's hip with the wrist almost perpendicular to the femur. Use your right hand for the left hip and the left hand for the right hip. Point the thumb toward the patient's groin; point the index finger to the anterior superior iliac spine; and extend the middle finger back along the iliac crest toward the buttock. The index finger, the middle finger, and the iliac crest form a V-shaped triangle. The injection site is the centre of the triangle (Fig. 22.18, A) To relax this muscle, the patient lies on their side or back, flexing the knee and hip (see Fig. 22.18, B).

Vastus Lateralis Muscle

The vastus lateralis muscle is another injection site used in adults and is the preferred site for administration of biologics (e.g., immunizations) to infants, toddlers, and children (Hockenberry & Wilson, 2015). The muscle is thick and well developed; it is located on the anterior lateral aspect of the thigh. It extends in an adult from a hand breadth above the knee to a hand breadth below the greater trochanter of the femur (Fig. 22.19, A). Use the middle third of the muscle for injection. The width of the muscle usually extends from the midline of the thigh to the midline of the outer side of the thigh. With young children or cachectic patients, it helps to grasp the body of the muscle during injection to be sure that the medication is deposited in muscle tissue. To help relax the muscle, ask the patient to lie flat with the knee slightly flexed and foot externally rotated or assume a sitting position (see Fig. 22.19, B).

Deltoid Muscle

Although the deltoid site is easily accessible, it is not well developed in many adults. There is potential for injury because the axillary, radial, brachial, and ulnar nerves and the brachial artery lie within the upper arm under the triceps and along the humerus. *Carefully assess the condition of the deltoid muscle; consult medication references*

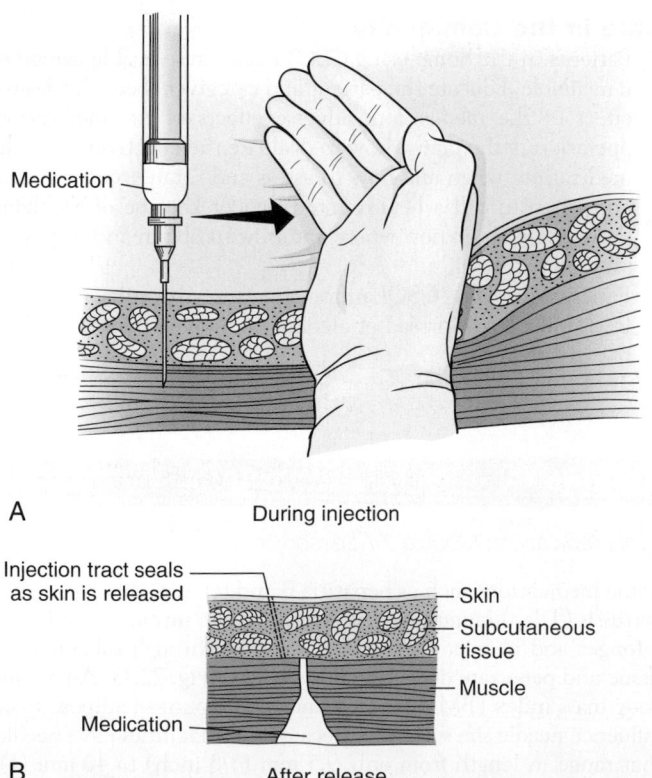

Medication

A   During injection

Injection tract seals
as skin is released

Skin

Subcutaneous
tissue

Muscle

Medication

B   After release

FIG 22.17 A, Pulling on overlying skin with dorsum of hand during IM injection moves tissue to prevent later tracking. **B,** Z-track left after injection prevents deposit of medication through sensitive tissue.

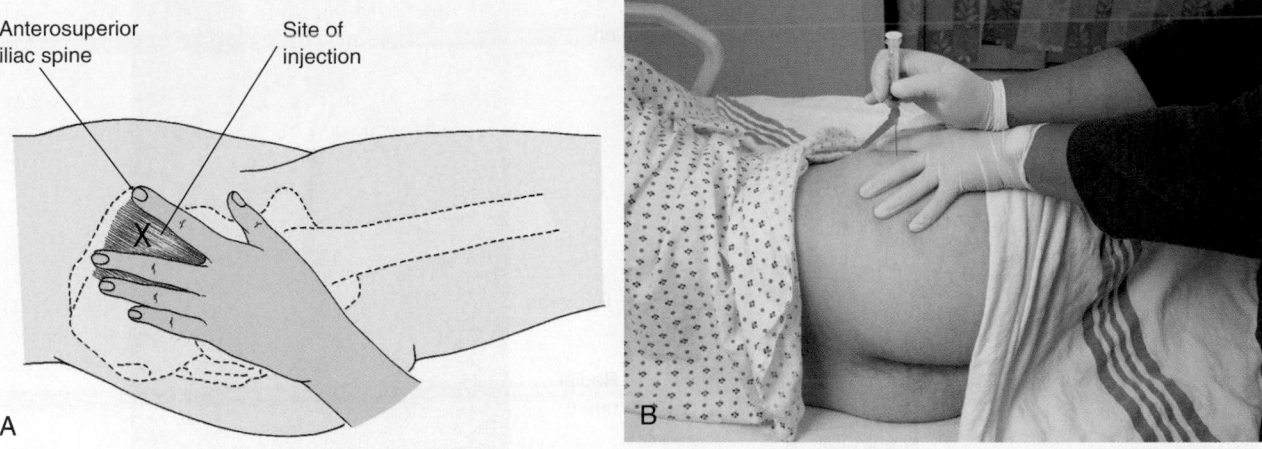

FIG 22.19 A, Anatomical view of ventrogluteal injection site. **B,** Injection at ventrogluteal site avoids major nerves and blood vessels.

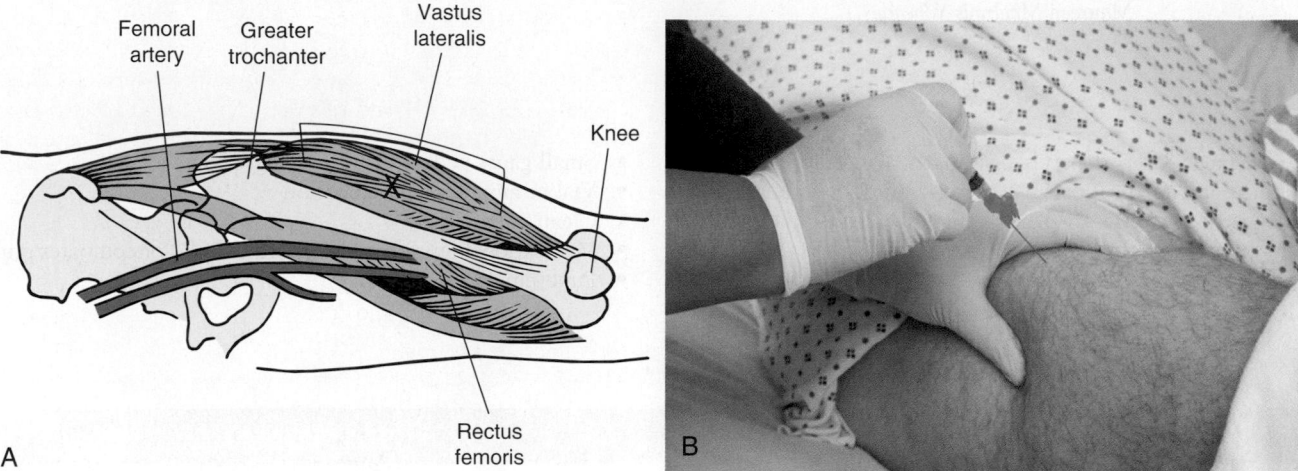

FIG 22.19 A, Landmarks for vastus lateralis site. **B,** Giving IM injection in vastus lateralis site.

for suitability of medication; and carefully locate the injection site using anatomical landmarks. Use this site for small medication volumes (2 mL or less) (Hopkins & Arias, 2013; Nicoll & Hesby, 2002); for administration of routine immunizations in toddlers, older children, and adults; or when other sites are inaccessible because of dressings or casts.

Locate the deltoid muscle by fully exposing the patient's upper arm and shoulder and asking them to relax the arm at the side or by supporting the patient's arm and flexing the elbow. Do not roll up any tight-fitting sleeve. Allow the patient to sit, stand, or lie down. Palpate the lower edge of the acromion process, which forms the base of a triangle in line with the midpoint of the lateral aspect of the upper arm. The injection site is in the centre of the triangle, about 3 to 5 cm (1.2 to 2 inches) below the acromion process (Fig. 22.20, A). Locate the apex of the triangle by placing four fingers across the deltoid muscle with the top finger along the acromion process. The injection site is three finger widths below the acromion process (see Fig. 22.20, B).

Delegation and Collaboration

The skill of administering IM injections cannot be delegated to an unregulated care provider (UCP). The nurse instructs the UCP about:

- Potential medication adverse effects and to immediately report their occurrence to the nurse.
- Reporting any change in the patient's condition to the nurse.

Equipment

- Proper-size syringe and sharps with engineered sharps injury protection (SESIP) needle:
  - *IM:* Syringe 2 to 3 mL for adult, 0.5 to 1 mL for infants and small children
  - Needle length corresponding to site of injection, age, gender, and size of patient. Refer to the following guidelines; length needed may vary outside of these guidelines for patients who are smaller or larger than average.

NEEDLE LENGTH FOR IMMUNIZATIONS (PHAC, 2017)

Site	Child	Adult
Anterolateral thigh (SUBCUT)	16 mm (⅝ inch)	16 mm (⅝–1 inch)
Anterolateral thigh (IM)	25–32 mm (1–1¼ inches)	25–40 mm (1–1½ inches)
Deltoid (IM)	16–25 mm (⅝–1 inch)	Gender- and weight-specific

SPECIFIC DELTOID NEEDLE LENGTH BASED ON GENDER AND WEIGHT

Gender—Male (>12 Years>	Gender—Female (>12 Years)	Needle Length
<60 kg	<60 kg	16–25 mm (⅝–1 inch)
60–118 kg	60–90 kg	25 mm (1 inch)
>118 kg	>90 kg	20 mm (1½ inches)

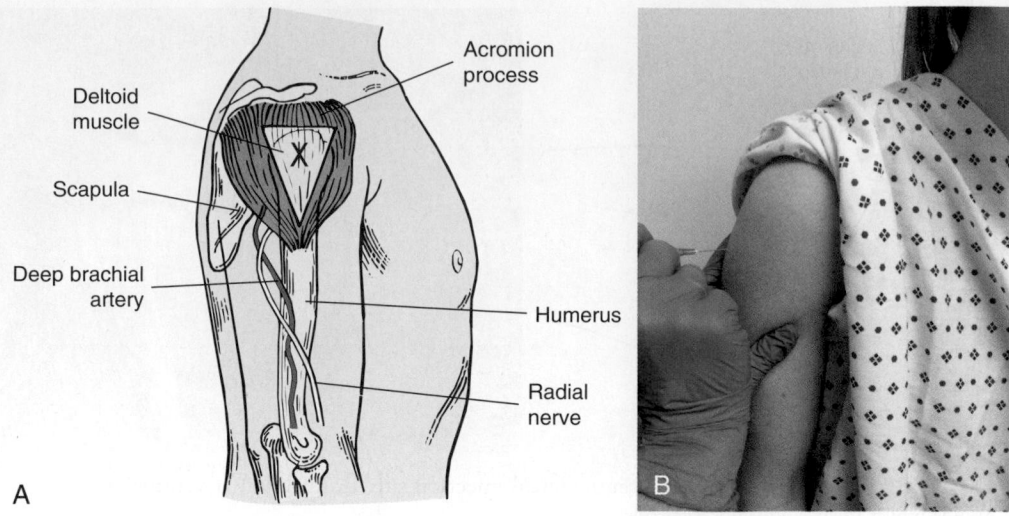

FIG 22.20 A, Landmarks for deltoid site. **B,** Giving IM injection in deltoid site. (*B, Courtesy of Maureen MacInnis-Wheatley.*)

- Needle gauge often depends on length of needle; administer biologics and medication in aqueous solution with a 20- to 25-gauge needle. Use 18- to 21-gauge needles for medications in oil-based solutions.
- Alcohol swab

- Small gauze pad
- Vial or ampoule of medication
- Clean gloves
- Medication administration record (MAR) or computer printout
- Puncture-proof container

STEP	RATIONALE

ASSESSMENT

1. Check accuracy and completeness of each MAR or computer printout with health care provider's prescription. Check patient's name, medication name and dosage, route of administration, and time of administration. Recopy or reprint any part of MAR that is difficult to read.	The prescription sheet is the most reliable source and only legal record of medications that the patient is to receive. Computer order entry (COE) and barcode systems are technology recently introduced in many settings to reduce medication errors (Cochran et al., 2016; Lapkin et al., 2016).
2. Assess patient's medical and medication history.	Determines need for medication or possible contraindications for medication administration.
3. Assess patient's history of allergies: known type of allergies and normal allergic reaction.	Do not prepare medication if there is a known patient allergy.
4. Review medication reference information for medication action, purpose, normal dose, adverse effects, time of peak onset, and nursing implications.	Allows you to administer medication safely and monitor patient's response to therapy.
5. Check date of expiration for medication.	Dose potency increases or decreases when outdated.
6. Observe patient's previous verbal and nonverbal responses to injection.	Anticipating patient's anxiety allows you to use distraction to reduce pain awareness.
7. Perform hand hygiene. Assess for contraindication to IM injections, such as muscle atrophy, reduced blood flow, or circulatory shock. Assess adequacy of adipose tissue.	Atrophied muscle absorbs medication poorly. Factors interfering with blood flow to muscles impair drug absorption.
8. Assess patient's symptoms before initiating medication therapy.	Provides information for you to evaluate desired effects of medication.

Clinical Decision Point *Because of the documented adverse effects of IM injections, other routes of medication injection are preferred. Consider contacting health care provider for alternative route of medication administration.*

9. Assess patient's knowledge regarding medication to be received.	Provides background to determine need for patient education.

STEP	RATIONALE

NURSING DIAGNOSES

- Acute pain
- Anxiety
- Fear

- Insufficient knowledge regarding medication administration or drug therapy

Related factors/Risk factors are individualized on the basis of patient's condition or needs.

PLANNING

1. Expected outcomes following completion of procedure:

   - Patient experiences no pain or mild burning at injection site.

     Medications may cause minor tissue irritation.

   - Patient achieves desired effect of medication with no signs of allergies or undesired effects.

     Medication administered without patient injury.

   - Patient explains purpose, dosage, and effects of medication.

     Demonstrates learning.

IMPLEMENTATION

1. Prepare medications for one patient at a time using aseptic technique. Keep all pages of MARs or computer printouts for one patient together or look at only one patient's electronic MAR at a time. Check label of medication carefully with MAR or computer printout three times (see Skill 22.1 and Procedural Guideline 22.1) when preparing medication.

   Ensures that medication is sterile. Preventing distractions reduces medication preparation errors. Use no-interruption zone (NIZ) when possible (Tomkins McMahon, 2017).

   Three checks for accuracy must occur when preparing medications:

   1. Before removing the medication vial/container from the drawer.
   2. When the prescribed amount of the medication is drawn up.
   3. Before returning the vial to storage/drawer or disposing of an empty or single use vial or ampoule.

2. Take medication(s) to patient at correct time (see employer policy). During administration apply 10 rights of medication administration.

   Hospital policies regarding timing of medications must consider the nature of the prescribed medication, specific clinical application, and patient needs.

3. Close room curtain or door.

   Provides privacy.

4. Identify patient using at least two person-specific identifiers (e.g., name and date of birth or name and medical record number) according to employer policy. Compare identifiers with information on patient's MAR or medical record.

   Ensures correct patient.

5. Ask patient if they have allergies.

   Confirms patient's allergy history.

6. Discuss purpose of each medication, action, and possible adverse effects. Allow patient to ask any questions. Tell patient that injection will cause a slight burning or sting.

   Patient has right to be informed, and patient's understanding of each medication improves adherence to drug therapy. Helps minimize patient's anxiety.

7. Perform hand hygiene and apply clean gloves. Keep sheet or gown draped over body parts not requiring exposure.

   Reduces transmission of infection. Respects patient's dignity while exposing injection site.

8. Select appropriate site. Note integrity and size of muscle. Palpate for tenderness or hardness. Avoid these areas. If patient receives frequent injections, rotate sites. Use ventrogluteal if possible.

   Ventrogluteal is preferred injection site for adults. It is also preferred site for children of all ages (Hockenberry & Wilson, 2015).

9. Help patient to comfortable position. Position patient depending on chosen site (e.g., sit, lie flat, on side, or prone).

   Reduces strain on muscle and minimizes injection discomfort.

Clinical Decision Point *Ensure that medical condition (e.g., circulatory shock, orthopedic surgery) does not contraindicate patient's position for injection.*

10. Relocate site using anatomical landmarks.

    Injection into correct anatomical site prevents injury to nerves, bone, and blood vessels.

11. Clean site with antiseptic swab. Apply swab at centre of site and rotate outward in circular direction for about 5 cm (2 inches).

    Mechanical action of swab removes secretions containing microorganisms.

12. Hold swab or gauze between third and fourth fingers of nondominant hand.

    Swab or gauze remains readily accessible for use when withdrawing needle after injection.

STEP	RATIONALE

IMPLEMENTATION

STEP	RATIONALE
13. Remove needle cap or sheath by pulling it straight off.	Preventing needle from touching sides of cap prevents contamination.
14. Hold syringe between thumb and forefinger of dominant hand; hold as dart, palm down.	Quick, smooth injection requires proper manipulation of syringe parts.
15. Administer injection:	
a. Position ulnar side of nondominant hand just below site and pull skin laterally approximately 2.5 to 3.5 cm (1 to 1½ inches). Hold position until medication is injected. With dominant hand inject needle quickly at 90-degree angle into muscle (see Fig. 22.17, A).	Z-track creates zigzag path through tissues that seals needle track to avoid leakage or tracking medication. A quick dartlike injection reduces discomfort. Use Z-track for all IM injections (Nicoll & Hesby, 2002; Ogston-Tuck, 2014).
b. *Option:* If patient's muscle mass is small, grasp body of muscle between thumb and forefingers.	Ensures that medication reaches muscle mass (Hockenberry & Wilson, 2015).
c. After needle pierces skin, still pulling on skin with nondominant hand, grasp lower end of syringe barrel with fingers of nondominant hand to stabilize it. Move dominant hand to end of plunger. Avoid moving syringe.	Smooth manipulation of syringe reduces discomfort from needle movement. Skin remains pulled until after medication is injected to ensure Z-track administration.
d. If aspiration is indicated by employer policy or manufacturer's medication directions, pull back on plunger 5 to 10 seconds. If no blood appears, inject medication slowly at rate of 10 sec/mL (Nicoll & Hesby, 2002).	Aspiration of blood into syringe indicates possible placement into a vein. Aspiration of blood into syringe indicates intravenous (IV) placement of needle. Slow injection rate reduces pain and tissue trauma and reduces chance of leakage of medication back through needle track (Hockenberry & Wilson, 2015; Nicoll & Hesby, 2002). The Canadian Immunization Guide (PHAC, 2017) no longer recommends aspiration when administering an immunization. The literature is inconsistent regarding recommendations of aspirating for other medications given IM. Some authors recommend no aspiration for all IMs (Sisson, 2015), while others suggest this recommendation is premature and that further research and evidence are needed (Thomas, Mraz, & Rajcan, 2016).

Clinical Decision Point *If blood appears in syringe, remove needle, dispose of medication and syringe properly, and prepare another dose of medication for injection to prevent injection of medication directly into the bloodstream.*

STEP	RATIONALE
e. Once medication is injected, wait 10 seconds, then smoothly and steadily withdraw needle, release skin, and apply gauze gently over site (see Fig. 22.17, B).	Allows time for medication to absorb into muscle before removing syringe. Dry gauze minimizes discomfort associated with alcohol on nonintact skin.
16. Apply gentle pressure to site. *Do not massage site.* Apply bandage if needed.	Massage damages underlying tissue.
17. Help patient to comfortable position.	Gives patient sense of well-being.
18. Discard uncapped needle or needle enclosed in safety shield and attached syringe into puncture- and leak-proof receptacle.	Prevents injury to patients and health care personnel. Recapping needles increases risk for needle-stick injury (Elmi et al., 2018).
19. Remove gloves and perform hand hygiene.	Reduces transmission of microorganisms.
20. Stay with patient for several minutes and observe for any allergic reactions.	Dyspnea, wheezing, and circulatory collapse are signs of severe anaphylactic reaction.

STEP	RATIONALE

EVALUATION

1. Return to room in 15 to 30 minutes and ask if patient feels any acute pain, burning, numbness, or tingling at injection site.

2. Inspect site; note any bruising or induration. Apply warm compress to site.

3. Observe patient's response to medication at times that correlate with onset, peak, and duration of medication.

4. **Use Teach-Back:** "I want to be sure I explained to you the purpose of this IM injection. Explain to me why you are receiving the injection and what you might expect to feel during the injection." Develop a revised teaching plan if patient or caregiver is not able to teach back correctly.

Continued discomfort may indicate injury to underlying bones or nerves.

Bruising or induration indicates complication associated with injection. Document findings and notify health care provider.

IM medications are absorbed rapidly. Adverse effects of parenteral medications develop rapidly.

Determines patient's and caregiver's level of understanding of instructional topic.

Unexpected Outcomes

1. Patient indicates localized pain or continued burning at injection site, indicating potential injury to nerve or vessels.

2. During injection blood is aspirated.

3. Patient displays adverse reaction with signs of urticaria, eczema, pruritus, wheezing, and dyspnea.

Related Interventions

- Assess injection site.
- Notify patient's health care provider.
- Immediately stop injection and remove needle.
- Prepare new syringe of medication for administration.
- Follow employer policy or guidelines for appropriate response to allergic reactions (e.g., administration of antihistamine such as diphenhydramine or epinephrine).
- Notify patient's health care provider immediately.
- Add allergy information to patient's record.

Communication and Documentation

- Immediately after administration, record medication, dose, route, site, time, and date given on MAR in nurses' notes in electronic health record (EHR) or chart. Correctly sign MAR according to employer policy.
- Document patient teaching, validation of understanding, and patient's response to medication in nurse's notes in EHR or chart.
- Document any undesirable or adverse effects from medication and report these to the health care provider.

Special Considerations
Teaching

- Patients who require regular injections (e.g., vitamin B$_{12}$) need to learn techniques of self-administration. Teach a family member or caregiver injection techniques and the importance of rotating sites to decrease the risk for hypertrophy.
- Instruct patient and caregiver to observe injection sites for complications and immediately report complications to the health care provider.
- Instruct patient and caregiver to observe for effectiveness of medication and adverse reactions and report ineffectiveness of medication and adverse reactions to the health care provider.
- Have patient perform several return demonstrations of medication preparation to validate that learning has taken place.

Pediatric

- Children can be very anxious or fearful of needles. Help with proper positioning and holding the child is sometimes necessary. Distraction such as blowing bubbles and pressure at the injection site before giving the injection can help alleviate anxiety (Hockenberry & Wilson, 2015).

Gerontological

- Older persons may have decreased muscle mass, which reduces drug absorption from IM injections. In addition, older persons may have loss of muscle tone and strength that impairs mobility, placing them at high risk for falls from guarding an injection site.

Care in the Community

- Self-administration of an IM injection is difficult, especially in the ventrogluteal site. Teach a caregiver to identify and administer injections in this site.
- Instruct adult patients who require frequent injections to apply EMLA cream to the injection site before administration.
- Instruct patients about the need for safe disposal of syringes and needles (see Skill 22.3, Care in the Community).
- See Skill 42.1 for information about modifying safety risks in the home.

✦ SKILL 22.6   Administering Medications by Intravenous Bolus

NSO *Nursing Skills Online Administration of Parenteral Medications: Intravenous Medications Module 8 / Lesson 3*

In the past, nurses often mixed medications into large volumes of intravenous (IV) fluids (500 to 1000 mL). However, today's safety standards and evidence-informed practice no longer support this practice on a routine basis (INS, 2016; ISMP, 2011). Many patient safety risks such as incorrect calculation, poor aseptic technique, incorrect labelling, pump programming errors, lack of medication knowledge, and mix-up with another medication occur when nurses have to prepare medications in IV containers on patient care units. There are a number of current best practices for preparation and administration of IV medication (Box 22.6).

An IV bolus is one method of medication administration that is becoming more common on patient care units. It introduces a concentrated dose of a medication directly into a vein by way of an existing IV access. An IV bolus or "push" usually requires small volumes of fluid, which is an advantage for patients who are at risk for fluid overload. Administering medications by IV bolus is common in emergencies when nurses need to deliver a fast-acting medication quickly. Because these medications act quickly, it is essential to monitor patients closely for adverse reactions. Employer policies identify specific medications that nurses can administer by IV push and other IV routes. These policies are based on the medication, compatibility and availability of staff, and type of monitoring equipment available. There are advantages and disadvantages to administering IV push medications (Box 22.7).

The IV bolus is a dangerous method for administering medications because it allows no time to correct errors. Administering an IV

push medication too quickly can cause death. Therefore, be very careful in calculating the correct amount of the medication to give and the rate of administration (see employer policy or manufacturer directions). Always ensure the reversal agent is on hand for the medication you are about to administer via IV push (ISMP, 2017b). In addition, a bolus may cause direct irritation to the lining of blood vessels; thus, always confirm placement of the IV catheter or needle. Never give an IV bolus if the insertion site appears edematous or reddened or if the IV fluids do not flow at the prescribed rate. Accidental injection of some medications into tissues surrounding a vein can cause pain, abscesses, and tissue necrosis.

Verify the rate of administration of IV push medication using employer policy or a medication reference manual. The Institute for Safe Medication Practices (ISMP, 2015) has identified the following strategies to reduce harm from rapid IV push medications:

- Use commercially available or pharmacy-prepared IV push medication whenever possible.
- Do NOT dilute IV push medications unless recommended by the manufacturer, employer policy, or reference literature.
- Administer at the rate recommended by the manufacturer, employer policy, or reference literature.
- Appropriately label syringes containing prepared medication.

Verify the rate of administration of IV push medication and compatibility using employer guidelines or a medication reference manual. Review the amount of medication that a patient will receive each minute, the recommended concentration, and rate of administration. For example, if a patient is to receive Lasix 20 mg IV push, calculate how many *millilitres per second* the dose should be administered to ensure that the drug is administered at a constant, controlled rate rather than the majority of the dose being rapidly administered randomly during the recommended push time. Reducing the volume (*to tenths of a millilitre*) and time (*to 10- to 15-second*

BOX 22.6

Best Practices for Administration of Intravenous Solutions and Medications

- Use standardized concentrations and dosages of medication.
- Use standardized procedures for prescribing, preparing, and administering intravenous (IV) medications.
- Administer solutions and medications prepared and dispensed from the pharmacy or commercially prepared when possible.
- Never prepare high-alert medications (e.g., heparin, dopamine, dobutamine, nitroglycerin, potassium, antibiotics, or magnesium) on a patient care unit.
- Use standardized infusion concentrations of "high-alert" medications.
- Limit the use of add-on devices to reduce risk of contamination and accidental disconnection.
- Standardize the storage of IV medications.
- Do not add medications to infusing containers of IV solutions.
- Use the mnemonic CATS PRRR to help remember safety checks for administering IV medications: *C*, compatibilities; *A*, allergies; *T*, tubing correct; *S*, site checked; *P*, pump safety checked; *R*, right rate; *R*, release clamps; *R*, return and reassess the patient.
- Use standardized label practices. Bold patient name, generic drug name, and patient-specific dose.
- Perform a medication reconciliation at each care transition (e.g., transfer, discharge) and when a new medication is prescribed.
- Correctly use technology such as intelligent-infusion devices, bar code–assisted medication administration, and electronic medication administration record.

Adapted from Infusion Nurses Society. (2016). Infusion therapy standards of practice. *Journal of Intravenous Nursing, 39*(1S); Institute for Safe Medication Practices (ISMP). (2010). *Guidelines for standard order sets*. Retrieved from http://www.ismp.org/tools/guidelines/StandardOrderSets.pdf; Institute for Safe Medication Practices (ISMP). (2019). *Principles of designing a medication label for IV piggyback medication for patient specific, inpatient use*. Retrieved from https://forms.ismp.org/Tools/guidelines/labelFormats/Piggyback.asp.

BOX 22.7

Advantages and Disadvantages of the Intravenous Push Method

Advantages

- Rapid onset of medication effects (useful in patients experiencing critical or emergent health problems).
- Medications can be prepared quickly and given over a shorter time than by intravenous (IV) piggyback.
- Doses of short-acting medications can be titrated on basis of a patient's needs and responses to the drug therapy. This is important for infants, children, and older patients.
- Method provides a more accurate dose of medication delivered because no medication is left in the IV line.

Disadvantages

- *Not all medications can be delivered by IV push.*
- Higher risk for infusion reactions; some are mild to severe because the medication action peaks quickly.
- When giving medication quickly (e.g., less than 1 minute), there is very little opportunity to stop the injection if an adverse reaction occurs.
- Risk for infiltration and phlebitis is increased, especially if a highly concentrated medication, a small peripheral vein, or a short venous access device is used.
- Hypersensitivity reaction can cause an immediate or delayed systemic reaction to a medication, requiring supportive measures.

blocks) allows accurate control of the push rate and avoids the most common error of pushing too fast. If the reference manual states the drug must be given over 1 minute, and the drug is supplied as 20 mg/2 mL, calculate as follows:

$$\frac{mL}{second\ (sec)} = \frac{2\ mL}{1} \times \frac{1}{60\ sec} = \frac{2\ mL}{60\ sec} = \frac{1\ mL}{30\ sec} = \frac{0.5\ mL}{15\ sec} = \frac{0.1\ mL}{3\ sec}$$

Understand the purpose of the medication and any potential adverse reactions related to the rate and route of administration. Some IV medications can only be given IV push safely when a patient is being monitored continuously for dysrhythmias, blood pressure changes, or other adverse effects. Therefore, you can push some medications only in specific areas within a health care facility (e.g., critical care unit). Confirm employer policy regarding requirements for special monitoring.

IV push medications are given through either an existing continuous IV infusion or an intermittent venous access (commonly called a *saline lock*). A saline lock is an IV catheter with a small "well" or chamber covered by a rubber cap. An IV catheter can be converted into a lock by inserting a special rubber-seal injection cap into the end of the catheter (see Chapter 29). Use of a lock saves time by eliminating constant monitoring of an IV line. It also offers better mobility, safety, and comfort for patients by eliminating the need for a continuous IV line. After you administer an IV bolus through an intermittent venous access, flush with a normal saline solution to keep it patent.

Delegation and Collaboration

The skill of administering medications by IV bolus cannot be delegated an unregulated care provider (UCP). The nurse instructs the UCP about:

- Potential medication actions and adverse effects of the medications and to immediately report their occurrence to the nurse.
- Reporting any patient complaints of moisture or discomfort around IV insertion site.
- Obtaining any required vital signs and reporting them to the nurse.

Equipment

- Watch with second hand
- Clean gloves
- Antiseptic swab
- Medication in vial or ampoule
- Proper-size syringes for medication and saline flush with needleless device or sharps with engineered sharps injury protection (SESIP) needle (21- to 25-gauge)
- Intravenous lock: Vial of normal saline flush solution (saline recommended [INS, 2016]) or prefilled normal saline flush; if employer continues to use heparin flush, the most common concentration is 10 units/mL; check employer policy
- Medication administration record (MAR) or computer printout
- Puncture-proof container

STEP	RATIONALE

ASSESSMENT

1. Check accuracy and completeness of each MAR or computer printout with health care provider's prescription. Check patient's name, medication name and dosage, route of administration, and time of administration. Recopy or reprint any part of MAR that is difficult to read.

2. Assess patient's medical and medication history.

3. **a.** Review medication reference information for medication action, purpose, adverse effects, normal dose, time of peak onset, how slowly to give medication, and nursing implications, such as need to dilute medication or administer it through a filter.

   b. Calculate the push rate in mL/second.

4. If you give medication through an existing IV line, determine compatibility of medication with IV fluids and any additives within IV solution.

5. Perform hand hygiene. Assess condition of IV needle insertion site for signs of infiltration or phlebitis.

6. Assess patency of patient's existing IV infusion line or saline lock (see Chapter 29).

7. Check patient's history of medication allergies: known allergens and normal allergic response.

8. Assess patient's symptoms before initiating medication therapy.

9. Assess patient's understanding of purpose of drug therapy.

The prescription sheet is the most reliable source and only legal record of medications that the patient is to receive. Computer order entry (COE) and barcode systems are technology recently introduced in many settings to reduce medication errors (Cochran et al., 2016; Lapkin et al., 2016).

Identifies need for medication.

Knowledge of medication allows you to give it safely and monitor patient's response to therapy.

IV medication is not always compatible with IV solution and/or additives, and a new site may need to be initiated.

Do not administer medication if site is edematous or inflamed.

For medication to reach venous circulation effectively, IV line must be patent, and fluids must infuse easily.

IV bolus delivers medication rapidly. Allergic response is immediate.

Provides information to evaluate desired effects of medication.

Provides background to determine need for patient education.

NURSING DIAGNOSES

- Acute pain
- Insufficient knowledge regarding medication administration or drug therapy

Related factors/Risk factors are individualized on the basis of patient's condition or needs.

STEP	RATIONALE

PLANNING

1. Expected outcomes following completion of procedure:
  - Patient experiences no medication adverse effects or allergic reactions.
  - IV site remains intact, without signs of swelling or inflammation or tenderness at site.
  - Patient explains purpose and side effects of medication.

Medication administered safely with desired therapeutic effect achieved.
Medication infuses without complications to IV site and surrounding tissues.
Demonstrates learning.

IMPLEMENTATION

1. Prepare medications for one patient at a time using aseptic technique. Keep all pages of MARs or computer printouts for one patient together or look at only one patient's electronic MAR at a time. Check label of medication carefully with MAR or computer printout three times (see Skill 22.1 and Procedural Guideline 22.1) when preparing medication.

Ensures that medication is sterile. Preventing distractions reduces medication preparation errors. Use no-interruption zone (NIZ) when possible (Tomkins McMachon, 2017).
Three checks for accuracy must occur when preparing medications:
1. Before removing the medication vial/container from the drawer.
2. When the prescribed amount of the medication is drawn up.
3. Before returning the vial to storage/drawer or disposing of an empty or single use vial or ampoule.

Clinical Decision Point *Current guidelines recommend that medications NOT be diluted unless specified by the manufacturer and peer-reviewed literature (INS, 2016; ISMP, 2015). Diluting medications when it is not required adds to the complexity of administering the drug and increases the risk for error (ISMP, 2015).*

2. Take medication(s) to patient at correct time (see employer policy). During administration apply 10 rights of medication administration.

Hospital policies regarding timing of medications must consider the nature of the prescribed medication, specific clinical application, and patient needs (ISMP, 2011).

3. Close room curtain or door.

Provides privacy.

4. Identify patient using at least two person-specific identifiers (e.g., name and date of birth or name and medical record number) according to employer policy. Compare identifiers with information on patient's MAR or medical record.

Ensures correct patient.

5. Ask patient if they have allergies.

Confirms patient's allergy history.

6. Discuss purpose of each medication, action, and possible adverse effects. Allow patient to ask any questions. Explain that you will give medication through existing IV line. Encourage patient to report symptoms of discomfort at IV site.

Keep patient informed of planned therapies, minimizing anxiety. Patients who verbalize pain at IV site help in detecting IV infiltrations early, lessening damage to surrounding tissues.

7. Perform hand hygiene and apply clean gloves.

Reduces transmission of infection.

8. IV push (existing IV line):
  a. Select injection port of IV tubing closest to patient. Use needleless injection port.

Needleless systems reduce the risk of needle-stick injury (INS, 2016).

Clinical Decision Point *Never administer IV medications through tubing that is infusing blood, blood products, or parenteral nutrition solutions.*

  b. Clean injection port with antiseptic swab, 0.5% chlorhexidine is preferred (INS, 2016). Allow to dry.

Prevents transfer of microorganisms during blunt cannula insertion.

  c. *Connect syringe to IV line:* Insert needleless tip of syringe containing drug through centre of port (see illustration).

Prevents introduction of microorganisms. Prevents damage to port diaphragm and possible leakage from site.

  d. Occlude IV line by pinching tubing just above injection port (see illustration). Pull back gently on plunger of syringe to aspirate for blood return.

Final check ensures that medication is being delivered into bloodstream.

Clinical Decision Point *In the case of smaller-gauge IV needles, blood return sometimes is not aspirated even if IV line is patent. If IV site does not show signs of infiltration and IV fluid is infusing without difficulty, give IV push.*

STEP	RATIONALE

IMPLEMENTATION

e. Keep the tubing above the injection port occluded and inject medication within the recommended amount of time. Use watch to time administrations (see illustration).

Ensures safe medication infusion. Rapid injection of IV drug can be fatal.

f. After injecting medication, withdraw syringe and recheck IV fluid infusion rate.

Injection of bolus may alter rate of fluid infusion. Rapid fluid infusion can cause circulatory fluid overload.

g. If IV medication is incompatible with IV fluids, stop IV fluids, clamp IV line, and flush with 10 mL of normal saline or sterile water (see employer policy). Then give IV bolus over appropriate amount of time and flush with another 10 mL of normal saline or sterile water at *same rate* as medication was administered.

Allows IV bolus to be administered without risks associated with IV incompatibilities. Ensure that employer guidelines permit flushing lines with incompatible medications. A new site may need to be initiated.

h. If IV line currently hanging is a medication, disconnect it and administer IV push medication as outlined in Step 9. Verify employer policy for stopping IV fluids or continuous IV medications. If unable to stop IV infusion, start new IV site (see Chapter 29) and administer medication using IV push (IV lock) method.

Avoids giving patient a sudden bolus of medication in existing IV line.

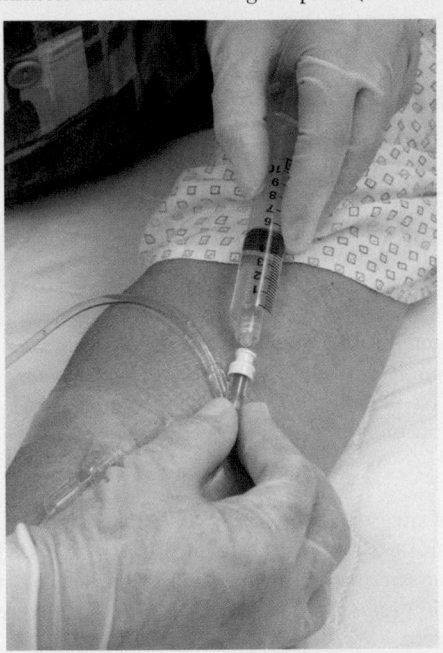

STEP 8c Connect syringe to IV line with needleless blunt cannula tip.

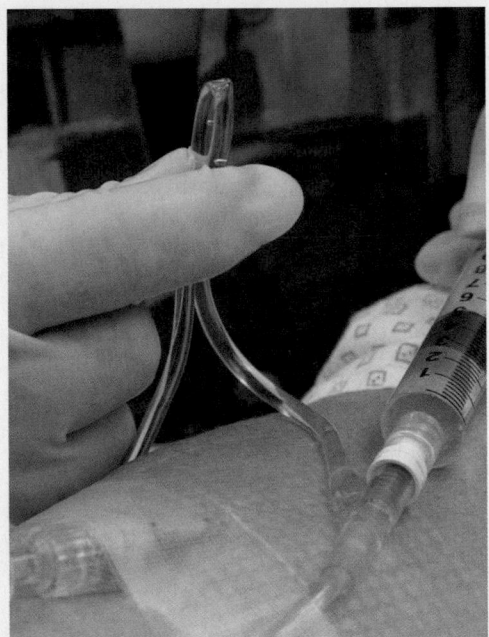

STEP 8d Occlude IV tubing above injection port.

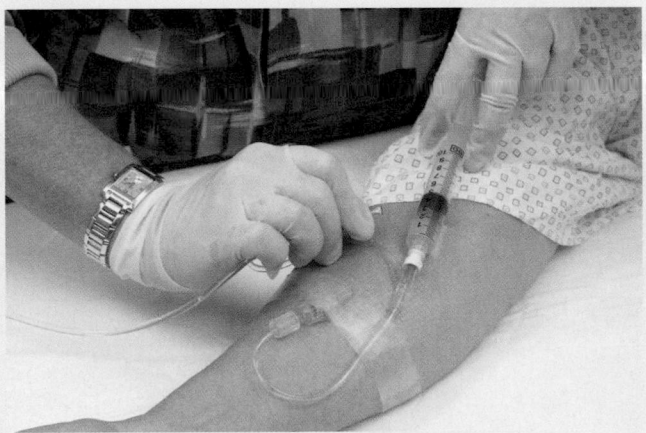

STEP 8e Use watch to time IV push medication.

STEP	RATIONALE

IMPLEMENTATION

9. IV push (saline lock):

a. Prepare flush solutions according to employer policy.

(1) *Saline flush method (preferred method):* Prepare two syringes filled with 2 to 3 mL of normal saline (0.9%) or use prefilled normal saline syringes if available. | Normal saline is effective in keeping IV locks patent and is compatible with wide range of medications. The S-A-S method is preferred:
S—Saline (to assess patency of site)
A—Administer medication
S—Saline (to clear medication from IV tubing) (INS, 2016).

(2) Heparin flush method (refer to employer policy).

b. Administer medication:

(1) Clean injection port with antiseptic swab; 0.5% chlorhexidine is preferred (INS, 2016). | Prevents transfer of microorganisms during needle insertion.

(2) Insert needleless tip of syringe with normal saline 0.9% through centre of injection port of IV lock (see illustrations).

(3) Pull back gently on syringe plunger and check for blood return. | Indicates if needle or catheter is in vein.

(4) Flush IV site with normal saline using a pulsatile technique (stop-start) to create turbulence (INS, 2016). | Clears needle and reservoir of blood. Flushing without difficulty indicates patent IV line.

Clinical Decision Point *Carefully observe the area of skin above the IV catheter. Note any puffiness or swelling as the IV site is flushed, which could indicate infiltration, requiring removal of catheter.*

(5) Remove saline-filled syringe.

(6) Clean injection port with antiseptic swab, 0.5% chlorhexidine is preferred (INS, 2016). | Prevents transmission of microorganisms.

(7) Insert needleless tip of syringe containing prepared medication through injection port of IV lock. | Allows administration of medication.

(8) Inject medication within recommended amount of time (calculate rate in mL per 10- or 15-second blocks). Use watch to time administration. | Many medication errors are associated with IV pushes being administered too quickly. Following guidelines for IV push rates promotes patient safety.

(9) After administering bolus, withdraw syringe.

(10) Clean injection port with antiseptic swab; 0.5% chlorhexidine is preferred (INS, 2016). | Prevents transmission of microorganisms.

(11) Flush injection port.

(a) Attach syringe with normal saline and inject flush at same rate that medication was delivered. | Flushing IV line with saline prevents occlusion of IV access device and ensures that all medication is delivered. Flushing IV site at same rate as medication ensures that any medication remaining within IV needle is delivered at the correct rate.

10. Dispose of SESIP covered needles and syringes in puncture- and leak-proof container. | Prevents accidental needle-stick injuries and follows guidelines for disposal of sharps (Dolan et al., 2016).

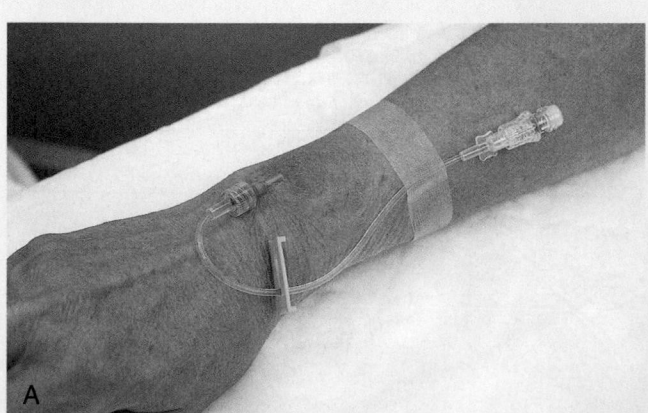
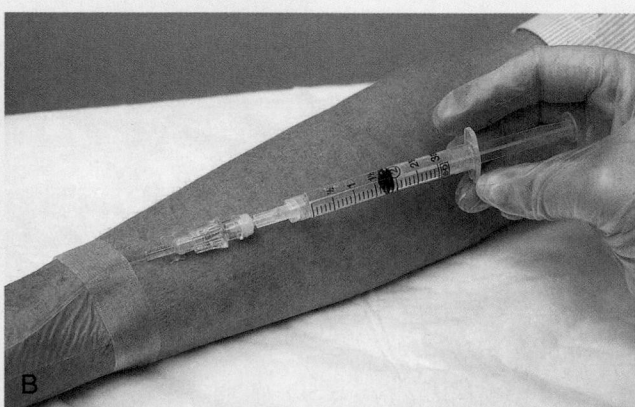

STEP 9b(2) A, IV catheter with saline lock adapter. **B,** Syringe inserted into injection port.

STEP	RATIONALE

IMPLEMENTATION

11. Stay with patient for several minutes and observe for any allergic reactions.

Dyspnea, wheezing, and circulatory collapse are signs of anaphylactic reaction.

12. Remove clean gloves and perform hand hygiene.

Reduces transmission of microorganisms.

EVALUATION

1. Observe patient closely for adverse reactions during administration and for several minutes thereafter.

IV medications act rapidly.

2. Observe IV site during injection for sudden swelling and for 48 hours after IV push.

Swelling indicates infiltration into tissues surrounding vein. Signs of infiltration may not occur for 48 hours.

3. Assess patient's status after giving medication to evaluate effectiveness of the medication.

Some IV bolus medications can cause rapid changes in patient's physiological status. Some medications require careful monitoring and assessment and possibly future laboratory testing (e.g., vasopressors and antiarrhythmics require blood pressure and heart rate monitoring, and heparin requires laboratory studies after administration to determine therapeutic levels).

4. Use Teach-Back: "I want to be sure I explained to you why you are receiving this IV medication. Can you explain to me what the medication is for and when to call the nurse?" Develop a revised teaching plan if patient or caregiver is not able to teach back correctly.

Determines patient's and caregiver's level of understanding of instructional topic.

Unexpected Outcomes

1. Patient develops adverse reaction to medication.

Related Interventions

- Stop delivering medication immediately and follow employer policy or guidelines for appropriate response to allergic reaction (e.g., administration of antihistamine such as diphenhydramine or epinephrine) and reporting of adverse drug reactions.
- Notify health care provider of adverse effects immediately.
- Add allergy information to patient's record.

2. IV medication is incompatible with IV fluids (e.g., IV fluid becomes cloudy in tubing) (see employer policy).

- Stop IV fluids and clamp IV line.
- Flush IV line with 10 mL of 0.9% sodium chloride or sterile water.
- Give IV bolus over appropriate amount of time.
- Flush with another 10 mL of 0.9% sodium chloride or sterile water at same rate as medication was administered.
- Restart IV fluids with new tubing at prescribed rate.
- If unable to stop IV infusion, start new IV site (see Chapter 29) and administer medication using IV push (IV lock) method.

3. IV site shows symptoms of infiltration or phlebitis (see Chapter 29).

- Stop IV infusion immediately or discontinue access device and restart in another site.
- Determine how much damage IV medication can produce in subcutaneous tissue.
- Provide IV extravasation care (e.g., injecting phentolamine around IV infiltration site) as indicated by employer policy, use a medication reference, and consult pharmacist to determine appropriate follow-up care.

Communication and Documentation

- Immediately document medication administration, including drug, dose, route, time instilled, and date and time administered on MAR in nurses' notes in electronic health record (EHR) or chart. Include initials or signature.
- Document patient teaching, validation of understanding, and patient's response to medication in nurse's notes in EHR or chart.
- Report any adverse reactions to patient's health care provider. Patient's response sometimes indicates need for additional medical therapy.

- Document patient's medication response in nurses' notes in EHR or chart.

Special Considerations
Teaching

- Teach patient and caregiver that effects of IV push medications occur rapidly. Explain reasons for giving medication slowly and teach signs of adverse effects.

Pediatric

- The therapeutic dosage of IV push medications for infants and children is often small and difficult to prepare accurately, even

with a tuberculin syringe. These medications need to be infused slowly and in small volumes because of the risk for fluid volume overload (Hockenberry & Wilson, 2015). Carefully follow employer policy when administering medications via IV bolus to pediatric patients.

Gerontological

- The renal and metabolic systems do not function as efficiently because of the aging process. Older persons may tolerate IV push medications if they are given over longer periods of time.

Care in the Community

- IV push medications are frequently given in the home. Use interprofessional collaboration (e.g., nurses, pharmacists, physicians) in the care of these patients. Patients and caregivers who are responsible for managing IV medications need to understand all aspects of administration safety. Adequate eyesight and manual dexterity are necessary to manipulate the syringe. Patients need to understand their venous access device, rate to give medications, and how to flush their access device. Patients need to store their medications safely and dispose of their IV supplies, and they should know whom to contact in case of an emergency.

◆ SKILL 22.7   Administering Intravenous Medications by Piggyback, Intermittent Infusion Sets, and Mini-Infusion Pumps

NSO *Nursing Skills Online Administration of Parenteral Medications: Intravenous Medications Module 8 / Lesson 2*

One method of administering intravenous (IV) medications uses small volumes (25 to 250 mL) of compatible IV fluids infused over a desired period of time. This method reduces the risk for rapid dose infusion and provides independence for patients. Patients must have an established IV line that is kept patent by either a continuous infusion or intermittent flushes of normal saline. Nurses can administer intermittent infusion of medication with any of the following methods.

- *Piggyback.* A piggyback is a small (25- to 250-mL) IV bag or bottle connected to a short tubing line that connects to the *upper* Y-port of a primary infusion line. The IV container that holds the medication is labelled following the IV piggyback medication format of the Institute for Safe Medication Practices (ISMP, 2019). The set is called a *piggyback* because the small bag or bottle is set *higher* than the primary infusion bag. In the piggyback setup, the main line does not infuse when a compatible piggybacked medication is infusing. The port of the primary IV line contains a back-check valve that automatically stops the flow of the primary infusion once the piggyback infusion flows. After the piggyback solution infuses and the solution within the tubing falls below the level of the primary infusion drip chamber, the back-check valve opens, and the primary infusion starts to flow again.
- *Volume-Control Administration.* Volume-control administration sets (e.g., Volutrol, Buretrol) are small (50- to 150-mL) containers that attach just below the primary infusion bag. The set is attached and filled in a manner similar to that used with a regular IV infusion. However, the priming of the set is different, depending on the type of filter (floating valve or membrane) within the set. Follow package directions for priming sets.
- *Mini-Infusion Pump.* The mini-infusion pump is battery operated and delivers medication in very small amounts of fluid (5 to 60 mL) within controlled infusion times using standard syringes (Fig. 22.21).

Needle Safety

Needleless injection systems are widely available and help to reduce needle-stick injuries by allowing direct connection with the IV line via a Luer lock port, a blunt-ended cannula, or shielded-needle device.

Delegation and Collaboration

The skill of administering IV medications by piggyback, intermittent infusion sets, and mini-infusion pumps cannot be delegated to an unregulated care provider (UCP). The nurse instructs the UCP about:

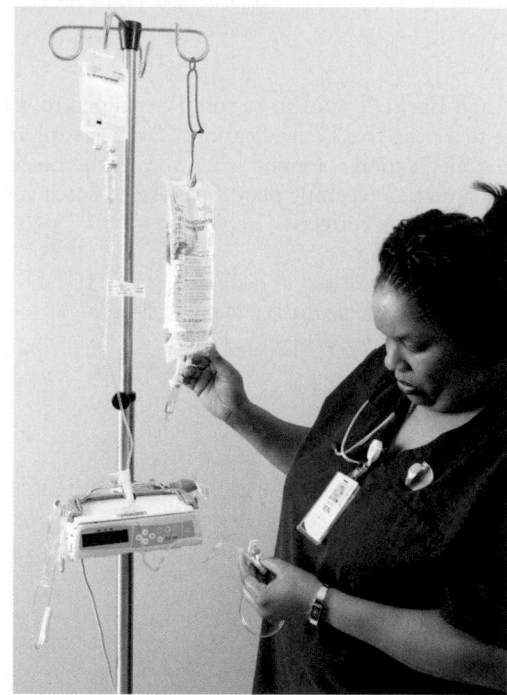

FIG 22.21 Mini-infusion pump.

- Potential medication actions and adverse effects and to immediately report their occurrence to the nurse.
- Reporting any patient indications of moisture or discomfort around IV insertion site.
- Reporting any change in patient's condition or vital signs to the nurse.

Equipment

- Adhesive tape (optional)
- Antiseptic swab—0.5% chlorhexidine preferred
- Clean gloves
- IV pole
- Medication administration record (MAR) or computer printout
- Puncture-proof container

Piggyback or Mini-Infusion Pump

- Medication prepared in 50- to 250-mL labelled infusion bag or syringe
- Prefilled syringe of normal saline flush solution (for saline lock only)
- Short microdrip, macrodrip, or mini-infusion IV tubing set with blunt-end (needleless) cannula attachment
- Needleless device
- Mini-infusion pump if indicated

Volume-Control Administration Set

- Volutrol or Buretrol
- Infusion tubing with needleless system attachment
- Syringe (1 to 20 mL)
- Vial or ampoule of prescribed medication

STEP	RATIONALE

ASSESSMENT

1. Check accuracy and completeness of each MAR or computer printout with health care provider's prescription. Check patient's name, medication name and dosage, route of administration, and time of administration. Recopy or reprint any part of MAR that is difficult to read.

The prescription sheet is the most reliable source and only legal record of medications that the patient is to receive. Computer order entry (COE) and barcode systems are technology recently introduced in many settings to reduce medication errors (Cochran et al., 2016; Lapkin et al., 2016).

2. Assess patient's medical and medication history.

Determines need for medication or possible contraindications for medication administration.

3. Assess patient's history of allergies: known type of allergens and normal allergic reaction.

IV administration of medication may cause rapid response. Allergic response is immediate.

4. Review medication reference information for medication action, purpose, normal dose, adverse effects, time and peak of onset, how slowly to give medication, and nursing implications (e.g., need to dilute medication, administer through filter).

Allows you to administer medication safely and monitor patient's response to therapy.

5. If you give medication through an existing IV line, determine compatibility of medication with IV fluids and any additional additives within IV solution.

IV medication is sometimes not compatible with IV solution and/or additives.

Clinical Decision Point *Never administer IV medications through tubing that is infusing blood, blood products, or parenteral nutrition solutions.*

6. Assess patency and placement of patient's existing IV infusion line or saline lock (see Chapter 29).

Do not administer medication if site is edematous or inflamed.

Clinical Decision Point *If patient's IV site is saline locked, clean the port with 0.5% chlorhexidine (INS, 2016) and assess the patency of the IV line by flushing it with 2 to 3 mL of sterile sodium chloride.*

7. Assess patient's symptoms before initiating medication therapy.

Provides information to evaluate desired effects of medication.

8. Assess patient's knowledge of medication.

Provides background to determine need for patient education.

NURSING DIAGNOSES

- Insufficient knowledge regarding medication administration or drug therapy
- Potential for imbalanced fluid volume
- Potential for ineffective health maintenance

Related factors/Risk factors are individualized on the basis of patient's condition or needs.

PLANNING

1. Expected outcomes following completion of procedure:
   - Patient experiences no adverse reactions.

   Medication was administered safely with desired therapeutic effect.

   - Medication infuses within desired time frame.

   IV line remains patent.

   - IV site remains intact without signs of swelling, inflammation, or symptoms of tenderness at site.

   Fluid infuses into vein, not tissues.

   - Patient explains medication purposes, action, side effects, and dosage.

   Demonstrates learning.

STEP	RATIONALE

IMPLEMENTATION

1. Prepare medications for one patient at a time using aseptic technique. Check label of medication carefully with MAR or computer printout three times (see Skill 22.1 and Procedural Guideline 22.1) when preparing medication.

Ensures that medication is sterile. Preventing distractions reduces medication preparation errors. Use no-interruption zone (NIZ) when possible (Tomkins McMahon, 2017).

Three checks for accuracy must occur when preparing medications:

1. Before removing the medication vial/container from the drawer.

2. When the prescribed amount of the medication is drawn up.

3. Before returning the vial to storage/drawer or disposing of an empty or single use vial or ampoule.

2. Take medication(s) to patient at correct time (see employer policy). During administration apply 10 rights of medication administration.

Hospital policies regarding timing of medications must consider the nature of the prescribed medication, specific clinical application, and patient needs (ISMP, 2011).

3. Close room curtain or door. Perform hand hygiene and apply clean gloves.

Provides privacy. Reduces infection transmission.

4. Identify patient using at least two person-specific identifiers (e.g., name and date of birth or name and medical record number) according to employer policy. Compare identifiers with information on patient's MAR or medical record.

Ensures correct patient.

5. Ask patient if they have allergies.

Confirms patient's allergy history.

6. Discuss purpose of each medication, action, and possible adverse effects. Allow patient to ask any questions. Explain that you will give medication through existing IV line. Encourage patient to report symptoms of discomfort at site.

Keep patient informed of planned therapies, minimizing anxiety. Patients who verbalize pain at IV site help in detecting IV infiltrations early, lessening damage to surrounding tissues.

7. Administer infusion.

a. Piggyback infusion:

(1) Connect infusion tubing to medication bag (see Chapter 29). Squeeze the drip chamber to fill it, and prime the tubing by opening regulator flow clamp. Once tubing is primed (all the air is removed by fluid), close clamp and cap end of tubing.

Filling infusion tubing with solution and freeing air bubbles prevent air embolus.

(2) Hang piggyback (see illustration) medication bag above level of primary fluid bag. (Use hook to lower main bag.)

Height of fluid bag affects rate of flow to patient.

(3) Connect tubing of piggyback infusion to appropriate connector on upper Y-port of primary infusion line:

Connection allows IV medication to enter main IV line.

(a) *Needleless system:* Wipe off needleless port of main IV line with 0.5% chlorhexidine swab, allow to dry, and insert cannula tip of piggyback infusion tubing (see illustrations).

Use needleless connections to prevent accidental needle-stick injuries (INS, 2016.).

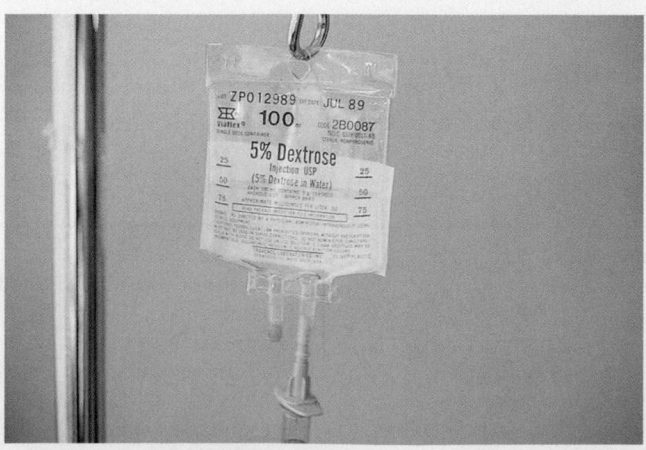

STEP 7a(2) Small-volume minibag for piggyback infusion.

STEP	RATIONALE

IMPLEMENTATION

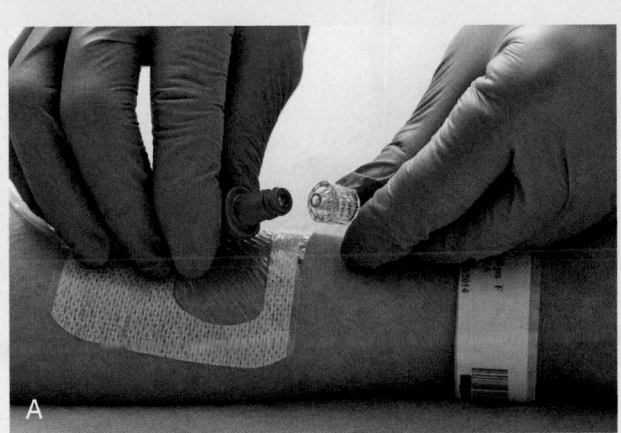 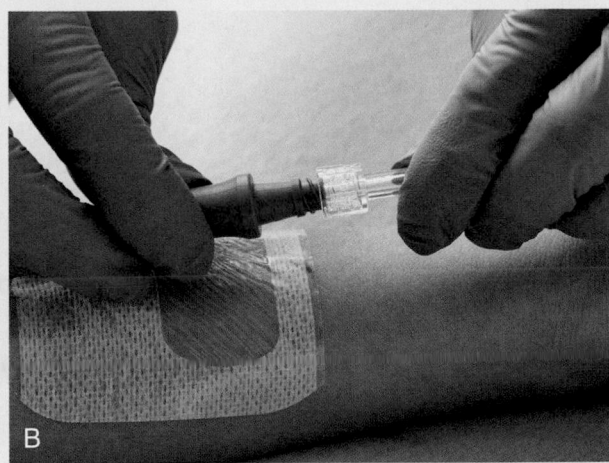

STEP 7a(3)(a) A, Needleless lock cannula system. **B,** Blunt-ended cannula inserts into port and locks.

(4) *Option:* Normal saline lock: Follow Steps 9a(1) through 9b(6) in Skill 22.6 to flush and prepare lock. Wipe off port with 0.5% chlorhexidine swab, let dry, and insert tip of piggyback infusion tubing via needleless access.

Flushing of lock ensures patency.

(5) Infusion times vary. Refer to medication reference or employer policy for recommended infusion time. If the medication is infusing by gravity, calculate the drip rate (gtt/min) and regulate the flow rate by adjusting the regulator clamp on the primary IV line (the regulator clamp on the piggyback line should be open all the way). If infusing by IV pump, calculate the rate (mL/hr) and set the pump.

Provides slow, safe, intermittent infusion of medication and maintains therapeutic blood levels.

(6) Once medication has infused:

(a) *Continuous infusion:* Check flow rate of primary infusion. Primary infusion automatically begins after piggyback solution is empty.

Back-check valve on piggyback prevents flow of primary infusion until medication infuses. Checking flow rate ensures proper administration of IV fluids.

(b) *Normal saline lock:* Disconnect tubing, clean port with 0.5% chlorhexidine, and flush IV line with 2 to 3 mL of sterile 0.9% sodium chloride. Maintain sterility of IV tubing between intermittent infusions.

(7) Regulate continuous main infusion line to prescribed rate.

Infusion of piggyback sometimes interferes with main line infusion rate.

(8) Leave IV piggyback and tubing in place for future drug administration (see employer policy) or discard in puncture- and leak-proof container.

Secondary line produces route for microorganisms to enter main line. Repeated changes in tubing increase risk for infection transmission. The INS (2016) recommends changing tubing every 96 hours.

b. Volume-control administration set (e.g., Volutrol):

(1) Fill Volutrol with desired amount of IV fluid (50 to 100 mL) by opening clamp between Volutrol and main IV bag (see illustration).

Small volume of fluid dilutes IV medication and reduces risk of fluid infusing too rapidly.

(2) Close clamp and check to be sure that clamp on air vent Volutrol chamber is open.

Prevents additional leakage of fluid into Volutrol. Air vent allows fluid in Volutrol to exit at regulated rate.

(3) Clean injection port on top of Volutrol with 0.5% chlorhexidine swab.

Prevents introduction of microorganisms during needle insertion.

STEP	RATIONALE

IMPLEMENTATION

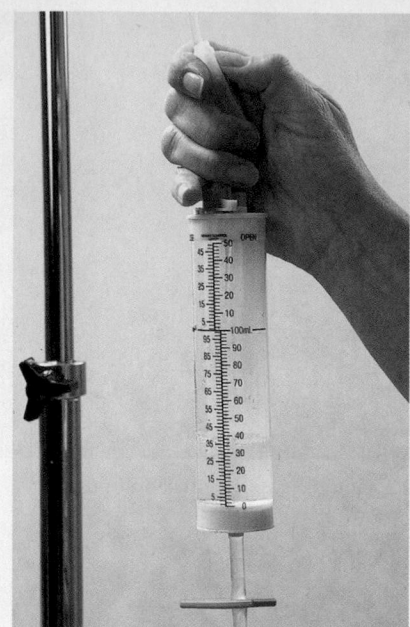

STEP 7b(1) Fill volume-control administration device.

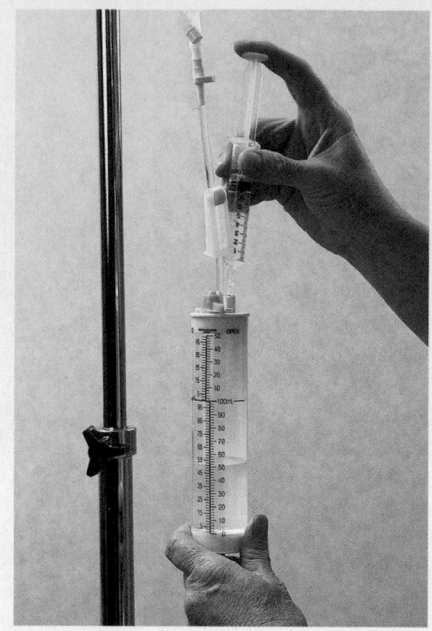

STEP 7b(4) Medication injected into device.

STEP	RATIONALE
(4) Remove needle cap or sheath and insert needleless syringe or syringe needle through port and inject medication (see illustration). Gently rotate Volutrol between hands.	Rotating mixes medication with solution to ensure equal distribution.
(5) Calculate the infusion rate and regulate the IV to allow medication to infuse in time recommended by employer policy, pharmacist, or medication reference manual.	For optimal therapeutic effect, medication should infuse in prescribed time interval.
(6) Label Volutrol with name of medication; dosage, total volume, including diluent; and time of administration following ISMP (2019) safe-medication label format.	Alerts nurses to medication being infused. Prevents other medications from being added to Volutrol.
(7) If patient is receiving continuous IV infusion, check infusion rate after Volutrol infusion is complete.	Ensures appropriate rate of administration.
(8) Dispose of uncapped needle or needle enclosed in safety shield and syringe in puncture- and leak-proof container. Discard supplies in appropriate container. Perform hand hygiene.	Prevents accidental needle-sticks. Reduces transmission of microorganisms.
c. Mini-infusion administration:	
(1) Connect prefilled syringe to mini-infusion tubing; remove end cap of tubing.	Special tubing designed to fit syringe delivers medication to main IV line.
(2) Carefully apply pressure to syringe plunger, allowing tubing to fill with medication.	Ensures that tubing is free of air bubbles to prevent air embolus.
(3) Place syringe into mini-infusion pump (follow product directions) and hang on IV pole. Be sure that syringe is secured (see illustration).	Secure placement is needed for proper infusion.
(4) Connect end of mini-infusion tubing to main IV line or saline lock:	Establishes route for IV medication to enter main IV line.
(a) *Existing IV line:* Wipe off needleless port on main IV line with 0.5% chlorhexidine swab, allow to dry, and insert tip of mini-infusion tubing through centre of port.	Needleless connections reduce risk for accidental needle-stick injuries.

STEP	RATIONALE

IMPLEMENTATION

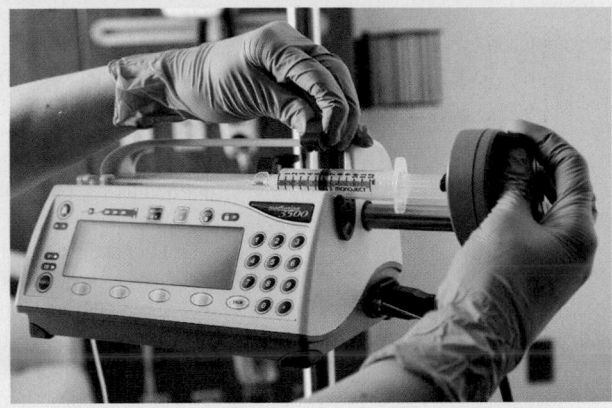

STEP 7c(3) Ensure that syringe is secure after placing it into mini-infusion pump.

<table>
<tr><td>

(b) *Normal saline lock:* Follow Steps 9a(1) through 9b(6) in Skill 22.6 to flush and prepare lock. Wipe off port with 0.5% chlorhexidine swab, allow to dry, and insert tip of mini-infusion tubing.

</td><td></td></tr>
<tr><td>

(5) Set pump to deliver medication within time recommended by employer policy, pharmacist, or medication reference manual. Press button on pump to begin infusion.

</td><td>

Pump automatically delivers medication at safe, constant rate based on volume in syringe.

</td></tr>
<tr><td>

(6) Once medication has infused:

(a) *Main IV infusion:* Check flow rate. Infusion automatically begins to flow once pump stops. Regulate infusion to desired rate as needed.

</td><td>

Maintains patent primary IV fluids.

</td></tr>
<tr><td>

(b) *Normal saline lock:* Disconnect tubing, clean port with 0.5% chlorhexidine, and flush IV line with 2 to 3 mL of sterile 0.9% sodium chloride. Maintain sterility of IV tubing between intermittent infusions.

</td><td></td></tr>
<tr><td>

8. Dispose of supplies in puncture- and leak-proof container.

</td><td>

Prevents accidental needle-sticks.

</td></tr>
<tr><td>

9. Remove gloves and perform hand hygiene.

</td><td>

Reduces transmission of microorganisms.

</td></tr>
<tr><td>

10. Stay with patient for several minutes and observe for any allergic reactions.

</td><td>

Dyspnea, wheezing, and circulatory collapse are signs of severe anaphylactic reaction.

</td></tr>
</table>

EVALUATION

1. Observe patient for signs or symptoms of adverse reaction.	IV medications act rapidly.
2. During infusion periodically check infusion rate and condition of IV site.	IV must remain patent for proper drug administration. Infiltration of IV site requires discontinuing infusion,
3. Ask patient to explain purpose and side effects of medication.	Evaluates patient's understanding of instruction.
4. Use Teach-Back: "I want to be sure I explained to you the reason for this IV medication. Can you explain to me why you are receiving the medication and what to report to the nurse?" Develop a revised teaching plan if patient or caregiver is not able to teach back correctly.	Determines patient's and caregiver's level of understanding of instructional topic.

STEP	RATIONALE

EVALUATION

Unexpected Outcomes
1. Patient develops adverse or allergic reaction to medication.

Related Interventions
- Stop medication infusion immediately.
- Follow employer policy for appropriate response to allergic reaction (e.g., administration of antihistamine such as diphenhydramine or epinephrine) and reporting of adverse medication reactions.
- Notify patient's health care provider of adverse effects immediately.
- Add allergy information to patient record per employer policy.

2. Medication does not infuse over established time frame.

- Determine reason (e.g., improper calculation of flow rate, poor positioning of IV needle at insertion site, infiltration).
- Take corrective action as indicated.

3. IV site shows signs of infiltration or phlebitis (see Chapter 29).

- Stop IV infusion and discontinue access device.
- Treat IV site as indicated by employer policy.
- Insert new IV catheter if therapy continues.
- For infiltration determine how harmful IV medication is to subcutaneous tissue. Provide IV extravasation care (e.g., injecting phentolamine around IV infiltration site) as indicated by employer policy or consult pharmacist to determine appropriate follow-up care.

Communication and Documentation

- Immediately document medication, dose, route, infusion rate, and date and time administered on MAR in nurses' notes in electronic health record (EHR) or chart. Include initials or signature.
- Document volume of fluid in medication bag or Volutrol on intake and output (I&O) form.
- Document patient teaching, validation of understanding, and patient's response to medication in nurse's notes in EHR or chart.
- Report any adverse reactions to patient's health care provider.

Special Considerations
Teaching

- Review all IV medications with patient and caregivers, including why patient is receiving the medication and potential adverse effects, including allergic responses.
- Teach patient and caregiver not to alter the prescribed rate of infusion without consulting the health care provider. IV medications need to be infused at a specified rate to achieve their desired effect and avoid adverse effects.
- Teach patient and caregiver to report any adverse effects immediately.

Pediatric

- Infants and young children are more vulnerable to alterations in fluid balance and do not adjust quickly to changes in it. Therefore, to assess fluid balance, monitor I&O carefully when infusing IV medications (Hockenberry & Wilson, 2015).

Gerontological

- Altered pharmacokinetics of medications and the effects of polypharmacy place older persons at risk for medication toxicity. Carefully monitor the response of older persons to IV medications (Touhy & Jett, 2018).
- Older persons are at risk for developing fluid volume overload and require careful assessment for signs of overload and heart failure.

Care in the Community

- Patients or caregivers who administer IV medications at home require education about the steps of medication administration. The patient or caregiver needs to perform several return demonstrations of IV medication administration before performing this skill independently. In addition, patients and caregivers need to know signs of IV medication administration complications such as phlebitis and infiltration and what to do for any problems.

✦ CLINICAL DEBRIEF

The nurse is developing a plan of care for an alert and oriented patient with thrombophlebitis of the left leg who received heparin 5000 units subcutaneously on admission to the unit and every 8 hours; this is the fourth day after admission. The heparin comes prepared from the pharmacy in a single-dose vial.

1. Which information does the nurse need to know about the medication and the vial before administration?

2. Which information does the nurse need to know about the patient before administration of the heparin?
3. Which aspects of the patient's care related to the administration of heparin can the nurse delegate to the unregulated care provider (UCP)?
4. The male patient weighs 100 kg (220 lb). The drug calculation has determined that 1 mL of heparin needs to be administered. Which size syringe and needle will be used to administer the injection?
5. The patient indicates soreness and tenderness at the heparin injection site. Using SBAR, show how you would communicate with the health care team about this patient.

✦ REVIEW QUESTIONS

1. Place the steps of administering an intradermal injection in the correct order.
   1. Inject medication slowly.
   2. Note the presence of a bleb.
   3. Advance needle through epidermis to 3 mm.
   4. Using nondominant hand, stretch skin over site with forefinger.
   5. Insert needle at a 5- to 15-degree angle into skin until resistance is felt.
   6. Clean site with antiseptic swab.

2. A patient with diabetes mellitus is receiving insulin using a continuous subcutaneous infusion pump. Place the steps of discontinuing the insulin pump in the correct order.
   1. Perform hand hygiene and apply clean gloves.
   2. Stop infusion pump.
   3. Remove dressing and discard properly.
   4. Apply gentle pressure to site until no fluid is leaking from skin.
   5. Verify prescription and establish an alternate route for medication if applicable.
   6. Apply small sterile gauze dressing to site.
   7. Remove tape from wings of needle and pull needle out.

3. The nurse is administering an intravenous (IV) push medication to a patient who has a compatible IV fluid running through IV tubing. Place the following steps in the appropriate order.
   1. Keep tubing pinched and inject medication within amount of time recommended by employer policy, pharmacist, or medication reference manual. Use watch to time administration.
   2. Select injection port of IV tubing closest to patient. Whenever possible, injection port should accept a needleless syringe. Use IV filter if required by medication reference or employer policy.
   3. After injecting medication, release tubing, withdraw syringe, and recheck fluid infusion rate.
   4. Connect syringe to port of IV line. Insert needleless tip or small-gauge needle of syringe containing prepared drug through centre of injection port.
   5. Clean injection port with antiseptic swab. Allow to dry.
   6. Occlude IV line by pinching tubing just above injection port. Pull back gently on syringe plunger to aspirate blood return.

ⓔ *Visit the Evolve site for a complete list of Clinical Debrief and Review Questions answers.*

REFERENCES

Accreditation Canada. (2019). *Required organizational practices handbook—Version 14.* Ottawa, ON: Author. Retrieved from http://www.wrha.mb.ca/quality/files/2019ROPHandbook.pdf

Alexander, M., Corrigan, A., Gorski, L., & Phillips, L. (2014). *Core curriculum for infusion nursing* (4th ed.). Philadelphia: Williams & Wilkins.

Arthur, A. (2015). Innovations in subcutaneous infusions. *Journal of Infusion Nursing,* 38(3), 179.

Atay, S., Kurt, F. Y., Akkaya, G., Karatag, G., Demir, S. I., & Calidag, U. (2017). Investigation of suitability of ventrogluteal site for intramuscular injections in children aged 36 months and under. *Journal for Specialists in Pediatric Nursing,* 22(4), e12187. doi:10.1111/jspn.12187

Athira, K., & Rohini, T. (2016). Effect of time duration in injecting subcutaneous low molecular weight heparin (LMWH) on pain and bruising among patients with myocardial infarction (MI). *International Journal of Nursing Education,* 8(4), 76–79. doi:10.5958/0974-9357.2016.00128.8

Beirne, P. V., Hennessy, S., Cadogan, S. L., Shiely, F., Fitzgerald, T., & MacLeod, F. (2015). Needle size for vaccination procedures in children and adolescents. *The Cochrane Database of Systematic Reviews,* (6), Art. No.: CD010720, doi:10.1002/14651858.CD010720.pub2

Burchum, J., & Rosenthal, L. (2016). *Lehne's pharmacology for nursing care* (9th ed.). St. Louis: Saunders.

Caccialanza, R., Constans, T., Cotogni, P., Zaloga, G. P., & Pontes-Arruda, A. (2018). Subcutaneous infusion of fluids for hydration or nutrition: A review. *Journal of Parenteral and Enteral Nutrition,* 42(2), 296–307. doi:10.1177/0148607116676593

Canadian Centre for Occupational Health and Safety (CCOHS). (2019). *Needlestick and sharps injury.* Retrieved from http://www.ccohs.ca/oshanswers/diseases/needlestick_injuries.html

Canadian Nurses Association (CNA). (2017). *Code of ethics for registered nurses.* Ottawa: Author. Retrieved from https://www.cna-aiic.ca/~/media/cna/page-content/pdf-en/code-of-ethics-2017-edition-secure-interactive.pdf?la=en

Cochran, G. L., Barrett, R. S., & Horn, S. D. (2016). Comparison of medication safety systems in critical access hospitals: Combined analysis of two studies. *American Journal of Health-System Pharmacy,* 73(15), 1167–1173. doi:10.2146/ajhp150760

Diabetes Canada Clinical Practice Guidelines Expert Committee. (2018). Diabetes Canada 2018 clinical practice guidelines for the prevention and management of diabetes in Canada. *Canadian Journal of Diabetes,* 42(Supp1), S1–S325. Retrieved from http://guidelines.diabetes.ca/docs/CPG-2018-full-EN.pdf

Dolan, S., Meehan Arias, K., Felizardo, G., et al. (2016). APIC position paper: Safe injection, infusion, and medication vial practices in health care. *American Journal of Infection Control,* 44(7), 750–757. doi:10.1016/j.ajic.2016.02.033

Doyle, G. R., & McCutcheon, J. A. (2015). *Clinical procedures for safer patient care.* Victoria, BC: BCcampus. Retrieved from https://opentextbc.ca/clinicalskills/

Elmi, S., Babaie, J., Malek, M., Motazedi, Z., & Shahsavari, K. (2018). Occupational exposures to needle stick injuries among health care staff: A review study. *Journal of Analytical Research in Clinical Medicine,* 6(1), 1–6. doi:10.15171/jarcm.201.001

FIT Forum for Injection Technique Canada. (2017). *Recommendations for best practice in injection technique* (3rd ed.). Retrieved from http://www.fit4diabetes.com/files/2314/8777/6632/FIT_Recommendations_3rd_Edition_2017.pdf

Giger, J. N. (2017). *Transcultural nursing: Assessment and intervention* (7th ed.). St. Louis: Mosby.

Greenway, K. (2014). Rituals in nursing: Intramuscular technique. *Journal of Clinical Nursing,* 23(23), 3583.

Hockenberry, M. J., & Wilson, D. (2015). *Wong's nursing care of infants and children* (10th ed.). St Louis: Mosby.

Hopkins, U., & Arias, C. (2013). Large-volume IM injections: A review of best practices. *Oncology Nurse Advisor,* 32. Retrieved from http://www.oncologynurseadvisor.com/chemotherapy/large-volume-im-injections-a-review-of-best-practices/article/281208/

Infection Prevention and Control Canada (IPAC). (2017). *IPAC Canada Practice Recommendations: Hand hygiene in health care settings.* Retrieved from https://ipac-canada.org/photos/custom/Members/pdf/17JulHand%20Hygiene%20Practice%20Recommendations_final.pdf

Infusion Nurses Society (INS). (2016). Infusion therapy standards of practice. *Journal of Intravenous Nursing,* 39(Suppl. 1), 1S.

Institute for Safe Medication Practices (ISMP). (2011). *Guidelines for timely administration of scheduled medications (acute).* Retrieved from http://www.ismp.org/Tools/guidelines/acutecare/tasm.pdf

Institute for Safe Medication Practices (ISMP). (2012). *Side tracks on the safety express. Interruptions lead to errors and unfinished. Wait, what was I doing?* Retrieved from http://www.ismp.org/newsletters/acutecare/showarticle.aspx?id=37

Institute for Safe Medication Practices (ISMP). (2015). *Safe practice guidelines for adult IV push medications.* Retrieved from https://www.ismp.org/sites/default/files/attachments/2017-11/ISMP97-Guidelines-071415-3.%20FINAL.pdf

Institute for Safe Medication Practices (ISMP). (2017a). *Guidelines for optimizing safe subcutaneous insulin use in adults.* Retrieved from http://www.ismp.org/Tools/guidelines/Insulin-Guideline.pdf

Institute for Safe Medication Practices (ISMP). (2017b). *2018–2019 Targeted medication safety best practices for hospitals.* Retrieved from https://www.ismp.org/sites/default/files/attachments/2017-12/TMSBP-for-Hospitalsv2.pdf

Institute for Safe Medication Practices (ISMP). (2019). *Principles of designing a medication label for IV piggyback medication for patient-specific, inpatient use.* Retrieved from https://forms.ismp.org/Tools/guidelines/labelFormats/Piggyback.asp

Krevesky, J., & Whittaker, C. (2015). *Information sheet: Filter needles.* Winnipeg, MB: Winnipeg Regional Health Authority. Retrieved from http://www.wrha.mb.ca/professionals/immunization/files/FilterNeedles.pdf

Lapkin, S., Levett-Jones, T., Chenoweth, L., & Johnson, M. (2016). The effectiveness of interventions designed to reduce medication administration errors: A synthesis of findings from systematic reviews. *Journal of Nursing Management,* 24, 845–858. doi:10.1111/jonm.12390

Larkin, T. A., Ashcroft, E., Hickey, B. A., & Elgellaie, A. (2018). Influence of gender, BMI and body shape on theoretical injection outcome at the ventrogluteal and dorsogluteal sites. *Journal of Clinical Nursing,* 27, e242–e250. doi:10.1111/jocn.13923

Lilley, L. L., Collins, S. R., & Snyder, J. S. (2017). *Pharmacology and the nursing process* (8th ed.). St. Louis: Mosby.

Mersey Care. (2017). *Clinical guideline for the administration of medication via an intradermal/subcutaneous/intramuscular injection*. Retrieved from https://www.merseycare.nhs.uk/media/4759/LCH-136%20Injection%20Policy.pdf

Nicoll, L., & Hesby, A. (2002). Intramuscular injection: An integrative research review and guideline for evidence-based practice. *Applied Nursing Research*, 16(2), 159.

Ogston-Tuck, S. (2014). Intramuscular injection technique: An evidence-based approach. *Nursing Standard*, 29(4), 55.

Paull, T. (2018). Evidence summary. Intramuscular injection: Aspiration. *The Joanna Briggs Institute EBP Database*, JBI10441.

Pozzilli, P., Battelino, T., Danne, T., Hovorka, R., Jarosz-Chobot, P., & Renard, E. (2016). Continuous subcutaneous insulin infusion in diabetes: Patient populations, safety, efficacy, and pharmacoeconomics. *Diabetes/Metabolism Research and Review*, 32(1), 21–39. doi:10.1002/dmrr.2653

Public Health Agency of Canada (PHAC). (2013). *Canadian needle stick surveillance network: Analysis of occupational exposures to blood, body fluids and blood borne pathogens (1 January 2008 to 30 June 2012), Final Program Report*. Ottawa: Centre for Communicable Diseases and Infection Control, Public Health Agency of Canada. Retrieved from http://publications.gc.ca/collections/collection_2014/aspc-phac/HP40-88-2013-eng.pdf

Public Health Agency of Canada (PHAC). (2017). *Canadian immunization guide: Guide: Part 1—Key Information*. Retrieved from https://www.canada.ca/en/public-health/services/publications/healthy-living/canadian-immunization-guide-part-1-key-immunization-information/page-8-vaccine-administration-practices.html#t3

Sanofi Aventis Canada. (2018). *Lovenox and Lovenox HP product monograph*. Retrieved from http://products.sanofi.ca/en/lovenox.pdf

Sheldon, A. (2019). *MiniMed Paradigm REAL-Time System fact sheet*. Retrieved from http://wwwp.medtronic.com/Newsroom/LinkedItemDetails.do?itemId=1101849348583&format=pdf&lang=de_CH

Sisson, H. (2015). Aspirating during the intramuscular injection procedure: A systematic literature review. *Journal of Clinical Nursing*, 24, 2368–2375. doi:10.1111/jocn.12824

Spollett, G., Edelman, S. V., Mehner, P., Walter, C., & Perfornis, A. (2016). Improvement of insulin injection technique: Examination of current issues and recommendations. *The Diabetes Educator*, 42(4), 379–394. doi:10.1177/0145721716648017

Tantisira, K., & Weiss, S. (2019). Overview of pharmacogenomics. *UpToDate*. Retrieved from http://www.uptodate.com/contents/overview-of-pharmacogenomics

Thomas, C., Mraz, M., & Rajcan, L. (2016). Blood aspiration during IM injection. *Clinical Nursing Research*, 25(5), 549–559. doi:10.1177/1054773815575074

Tompkins McMahon, J. (2017). Improving medication administration safety in the clinical environment. *Medsurg Nursing*, 26(6), 374–409.

Touhy, T. A., & Jett, K. F. (2018). *Ebersole and Hess' gerontological nursing & healthy aging* (5th ed.). St. Louis: Elsevier.

World Health Organization (WHO). (2018). *Tuberculosis*. Retrieved from http://www.who.int/mediacentre/factsheets/fs104/en/

Yi, L., Shuai, T., Tian, X., Zeng, Z., Ma, L., & Song, G. (2016). The effect of subcutaneous injection duration on patients receiving low-molecular-weight heparin: Evidence from a systematic review. *International Journal of Nursing Sciences*, 3(1), 79–88. doi:10.1016/j.ijnss.2016.02.008

23 | Oxygen Therapy

Written by **C.J. Wright-Boon, RN, MSN, and Noelle Ozog, RN, MScN(c)**

SKILLS AND PROCEDURES

OBJECTIVES

Mastery of content in this chapter will enable the nurse to:
- Discuss indications for oxygen therapy.
- Describe methods for administering oxygen therapy.
- Demonstrate applying an oxygen-delivery device.
- Demonstrate administering oxygen therapy to a patient with an artificial airway.
- Demonstrate obtaining peak expiratory flow rate (PEFR) measurements.

- Demonstrate proper use of incentive spirometry.
- Describe the use of noninvasive positive-pressure ventilation (NPPV) using continuous positive airway pressure (CPAP) or bi-level positive airway pressure (BiPAP).
- Demonstrate care of a patient receiving mechanical ventilation.

MEDIA RESOURCES

- evolve http://evolve.elsevier.com/Canada/Perry/clinicalskills/
- Review Questions
- Audio Glossary

- Case Studies
- ▶ Video Clips
- Clinical Debrief and Review Questions Answers

PURPOSE

Oxygen therapy is the administration of supplemental oxygen (O_2) to a patient to prevent or treat hypoxemia. Routes of administration include nasal cannula, face masks, noninvasive ventilation, and positive-pressure ventilators. Special care is required for each delivery device.

STANDARDS OF CARE

- Accreditation Canada, 2019—*Required Organizational Practices Handbook—Version 14* (http://www.wrha.mb.ca/quality/files/2019ROPHandbook.pdf)
- Canadian Patient Safety Institute (CPSI), 2012—*Prevent Ventilator Associated Pneumonia* (http://www.patientsafetyinstitute.ca/en/toolsResources/Documents/Interventions/Ventilator-Associated Pneumonia/VAP Getting Started Kit.pdf)
- Keenan, Sinuff, Burns, et al., 2011—*Clinical Practice Guidelines for the Use of Noninvasive Positive-Pressure Ventilation and Noninvasive Continuous Positive Airway Pressure in the Acute Care Setting* (http://www.cmaj.ca/content/cmaj/early/2011/02/14/cmaj.100071.full.pdf)

- O'Driscoll, Howard, Earis, et al., 2017—*BTS Guideline for Oxygen Use in Adults in Healthcare and Emergency Settings* (https://www.brit-thoracic.org.uk/document-library/clinical-information/oxygen/2017-emergency-oxygen-guideline/bts-guideline-for-oxygen-use-in-adults-in-healthcare-and-emergency-settings/)
- Rochwerg, Brochard, Elliott, et al., 2017—*European Respiratory Society (ERS)/American Thoracic Society (ATS) Clinical Practice Guidelines: Noninvasive Ventilation for Acute Respiratory Failure* (https://www.thoracic.org/statements/resources/cc/niv-guidelines.pdf)

PRINCIPLES FOR PRACTICE

- Oxygen therapy is used to treat hypoxia, a condition in which there is insufficient oxygen to meet the metabolic demands of the tissues and cells (Box 23.1).
- Hemoglobin is the carrier of respiratory gases, oxygen, and carbon dioxide (CO_2). It combines with a gas to carry it to and from the cells. Decreased hemoglobin levels reduce the amount of oxygen transported to the cells and CO_2 transported away from the cells.

Signs and Symptoms Associated With Acute Hypoxia

- Apprehension, anxiety, behavioural changes
- Decreased level of consciousness, confusion, drowsiness, altered concentration
- Increased pulse rate
- Increased rate and depth of respiration or irregular respiratory patterns
- Decreased lung sounds, adventitious lung sounds (e.g., crackles, wheezes)
- Elevated blood pressure evolving to decreased blood pressure
- Pulse oximetry (SpO_2) less than 90%, or less than 88% in a patient at risk of hypercapnia
- Dyspnea
- Use of accessory muscles of respiration, rib retractions
- Cardiac dysrhythmias
- Pallor, cyanosis
- Increased fatigue
- Dizziness

- Hemoglobin levels and acid–base status directly affect oxygenation. Acidemia increases the ability of hemoglobin to release oxygen to the tissues, whereas alkalemia decreases it.
- Pain and anxiety affect patient oxygenation. Nurses must assess patient's pain, pulse oximetry (SpO_2) values, level of consciousness, developmental level, and observed behaviours (Hockenberry & Wilson, 2015; Lewis, Bucher, Heitkemper, et al., 2019).
- Visual assessment of a patient for cyanosis is a difficult clinical skill; it should be assessed in conjunction with SpO_2, respiratory rate, and other vital signs (O'Driscoll, Howard, Earis, et al., 2017). Good lighting is essential for a proper assessment, regardless of skin tone or colour. Use the palmar surface of a patient's fingertips, a spot where it is easier to notice colour changes in any skin tone, to assess for cyanosis (Baranoski, Van Leeuwen, & Chen, 2017). Ask the patient and caregiver if they have noticed a colour change in the patient from the patient's baseline (Lewis et al., 2019).
- Nurses should treat oxygen therapy as a medication. It is important to continuously monitor the dosage or concentration of oxygen and routinely check prescription to verify that the patient is receiving the prescribed concentration. Follow the 10 rights of medication administration (see Chapter 20).
- Contraindications to oxygen therapies include conditions that increase the patient's risk for respiratory failure. In patients with congenital heart defects, oxygen affects blood flow through the heart and lungs. In patients with chronic pulmonary diseases, uncontrolled oxygen therapy increases the patient's risk for elevated CO_2 in the blood (hypercapnia [also called hypercarbia or CO_2 retention]). This hypercapnia is thought to be mainly due to an inhibition of pulmonary vasoconstriction, the body's mechanism of reducing perfusion to poorly ventilated alveoli, resulting in further mismatch between ventilation and perfusion (Cousins, Wark, & McDonald, 2016, pp. 1067–1068). These patients should receive oxygen sparingly.

PERSON-CENTRED CARE

- Explain to the patient and caregiver the oxygen setup and necessary safety precautions needed when oxygen is in use.
- Patients and visitors with limited English proficiency may need help with signs posted in the room.
- Safely accommodate valued practices when using oxygen. For example, some cultures light candles to honour holidays and may

Ventilator-Associated Pneumonia (VAP) Bundle and Additional Evidence-Informed Components of Care

1. Elevate the head of the bed to 45 degrees when possible; otherwise, attempt to maintain the head of the bed at more than 30 degrees.
2. Evaluate readiness for extubation daily.
3. Use endotracheal tubes with subglottic secretion drainage.
4. Conduct oral care and decontamination with chlorhexidine.
5. Initiate safe enteral nutrition within 24–48 hours of critical care unit admission.

Preventing VAP in Children:
1. Elevate the head of the bed.
2. Properly position oral or nasal gastric tubes.
3. Perform oral care.
4. Eliminate the routine use of instillation for suctioning.
   Additional evidence-informed components of care:
   - Hand hygiene
   - Practices that promote patient safety, mobility, and autonomy
   - Venous thromboembolism prophylaxis

From Canadian Patient Safety Institute (CPSI). (2012). *Prevent ventilator associated pneumonia*. Retrieved from http://www.patientsafetyinstitute.ca/en/toolsResources/Documents/Interventions/Ventilator-Associated Pneumonia/VAP Getting Started Kit.pdf.

accept the use of battery-operated candles while in the hospital. Another example is smudging, a ceremony that involves burning sweet grass, sage, cedar, or tobacco for spiritual purposes that is a part of some Indigenous cultures. Practise person-centred care and collaborate with the patient, caregivers, elders, and employer to determine how to accommodate cultural healing practices.

EVIDENCE-INFORMED PRACTICE

- Evidence is currently insufficient to recommend that high-flow nasal cannula (HFNC) is safer or more effective than other oxygen delivery systems (Corley, Rickard, Aitken, et al., 2017, p. 2).
- Early studies indicate that the use of ventilator-associated pneumonia (VAP) prevention bundles have decreased the rates of VAP (Chahoud, Semaan, & Almoosa, 2015). The Canadian Patient Safety Institute (CPSI, 2012) recommends a five-step "VAP bundle" (Box 23.2).
- VAP and ventilator-associated events (VAEs) are difficult to define (Waters & Muscedere, 2015). Throughout the literature, there is conflicting information related to the incidence of VAEs, proportions of VAEs classified as infection related, and ventilator use within and among location types (Magill, Li, Gross, et al., 2016).
- Adult patients who have received mechanical ventilation report experiencing:
  - Fear caused by dependence on the ventilator and loss of control of their life
  - Disconnection from reality
  - Impaired sense of body image
  - Development of adaptation patterns, including maintaining a strong belief and developing communication methods
  - Feeling concern and caring from others, including health care providers, who helped patients' sense of security (Tsay, Mu, Lin, et al., 2013).
- NPPV is an effective intervention in patients with chronic obstructive pulmonary disease (COPD) experiencing an acute episode of respiratory failure with hypercapnia (Shah, D'Cruz, & Murphy, 2018, p. S75).

- NPPV does not have a significant effect on exercise tolerance or lung function as part of routine care in chronic COPD but may improve outcomes for patients who remain hypercapnic after an acute episode or who have disordered sleep breathing (Shah et al., 2018).
- There is no evidence to support use of incentive spirometer (IS) alone to prevent pulmonary complications in patients who have undergone upper abdominal surgery (do Nascimento, Modolo, Andrade, et al., 2014; Tyson, Kendig, Mabedi, et al., 2015).

SAFETY GUIDELINES

- Know a patient's normal range of vital signs, including pulse oximetry (SpO$_2$).
- Be aware of environmental conditions. Patients with chronic respiratory diseases have difficulty maintaining optimal oxygen levels in polluted environments.
- If a patient is to receive long-term oxygen therapy, complete an environmental assessment to determine hazards in the home, such as the use of gas stoves or kerosene space heaters or the presence of smokers (see Chapter 42).
- Document a patient's smoking history. Smoking damages the mucociliary clearance mechanism of the lungs and paralyzes the ciliary action, resulting in a decreased ability to clear mucus from the airways. Chronic bronchitis is caused primarily by smoking and results in pooling of mucus in the airways, creating an environment for the development of infections. Long-term chronic bronchitis ultimately results in hypoxia.
- Know a patient's past and current hemoglobin and arterial blood gas (ABG) values.
- Oxygen is a medication. Increasing the oxygen litre flow rate for shortness of breath is similar to changing other medications.

BOX 23.3

Oxygen Safety Guidelines

- Remind patients that oxygen is a medication and is not adjusted without a health care provider prescription.
- In the home setting place an "Oxygen in Use" sign on the door of the residence.
- Keep oxygen delivery systems at least 3 metres (10 feet) from any heat source (Lacasse, Bernard, & Maltais, 2015).
- Oxygen supports combustion; however, it will not explode.
- No smoking is allowed on the premises.
- When using oxygen cylinders, secure them so they will not fall over.
- Determine that all electrical equipment in the room is functioning correctly and properly grounded (see Chapter 14). An electrical spark in the presence of oxygen will result in a serious fire.
- Avoid using items that create a spark (e.g., electric razor) with a nasal cannula in use; an electrical or mechanical toy in oxygen tent; or objects of synthetic fabrics that cause static electricity.
- Check the oxygen level of portable tanks before transporting a patient to ensure ample oxygen supply. Do not remove patient oxygen to allow the patient to use the washroom; use extension tubing or a wheeled portable oxygen cylinder as appropriate in the setting.

- Provide education to the patient and caregiver about long-term oxygen therapy, so they understand proper use of the equipment, and about safety measures (see Chapter 42) (Box 23.3).
- Have suction equipment available to help clear airway secretions, particularly in patients with artificial airways, such as an endotracheal tube or tracheostomy.
- Most employers require that a self-inflating resuscitation bag and appropriate-size mask be available in patient rooms, particularly for patients requiring mechanical ventilation.

✦ SKILL 23.1   Applying an Oxygen-Delivery Device

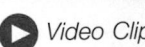 *Video Clip*

Various diseases (e.g., pneumonia, chronic obstructive pulmonary disease [COPD]) require the use of oxygen therapy. Pneumonia results in impaired gas exchange because of fluid and secretions in the lung, which decrease diffusion of oxygen from the lungs to the arterial blood supply. Some patients with COPD require long-term oxygen. These patients may require oxygen 24 hours a day; therefore, care is taken to plan administration around patient needs (Grindrod, 2015).

Oxygen-Delivery Devices

Oxygen therapy is inexpensive and widely available. Patients with decreased tissue oxygenation benefit from controlled oxygen administration. Long-term oxygen treatment can improve survival in COPD (Grindrod, 2015).

Selection of the oxygen delivery system is made on the basis of the level of oxygen support needed, the severity of the hypoxia, and the disease process. The patient's age, developmental level, health, level of orientation, presence of an artificial airway, the setting (acute or community), home environment, and support available after discharge all need to be considered.

Oxygen-delivery devices are categorized as high flow or low flow, depending on their ability to provide enough *flow* to match the patient's spontaneous minute volume. This is imperative for patient comfort and adequate oxygen delivery. High-flow devices provide

a higher flow of oxygen to meet the higher minute volume of patients in respiratory distress or failure. Both types of devices can deliver a range of inspired oxygen concentration (FiO$_2$) to patients. High-flow devices control the FiO$_2$ with less dependence on the patient's breathing pattern, and include Venturi masks (Fig. 23.1), large-volume nebulizer, blender masks, and the high-flow nasal cannula (Fig. 23.2). Low-flow devices include low-flow nasal cannula (Fig. 23.3), oxygen-conserving nasal cannula (Fig. 23.4), simple face masks (Fig. 23.5), partial rebreather masks, and nonrebreather masks (Fig. 23.6). Advantages and disadvantages of each are listed in Table 23.1.

An oxygen flowmeter regulates the flow rate in litres per minute (L/min). Fig. 23.7 shows a float ball oxygen flowmeter, set to 1 L/min. The flow rate is read from the middle of the ball (O'Driscoll et al., 2017). Oxygen cylinders include large H cylinders and smaller E cylinders (Fig. 23.8). Even smaller, easily transported cylinders are available for use in the home. Patients using long-term oxygen commonly use concentrators, some of which are portable.

Nasal Cannula

Several types of oxygen cannula are used to deliver oxygen to the patient (see Table 23.1). A low-flow nasal cannula is a simple, effective, and comfortable device for delivering oxygen to a patient (see Fig. 23.3). It enables a patient to breathe through the mouth or nose and

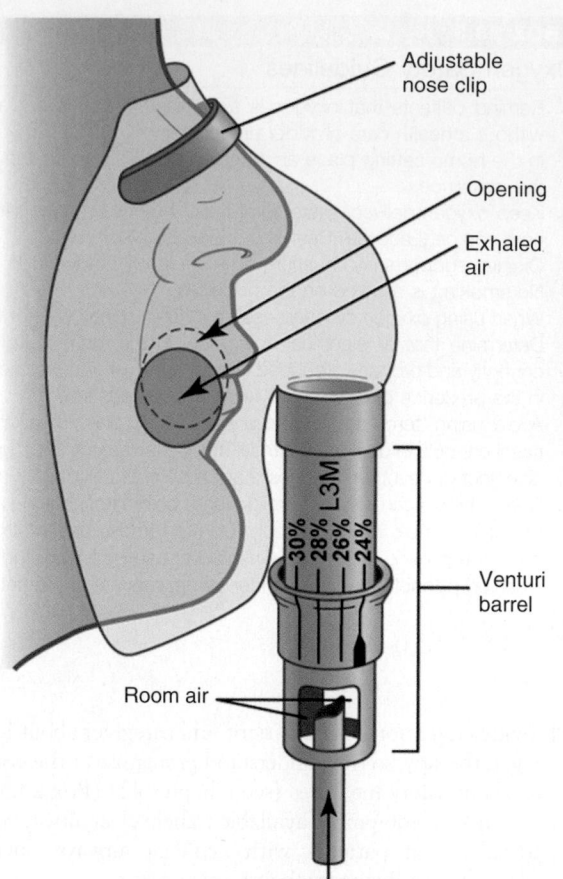

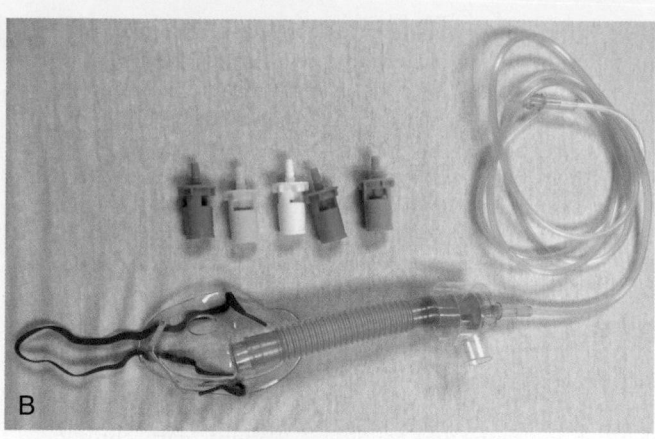

Copyright © 2014, 2011, 2007, 2004, 2000, 1996, 1992, 1987, 1983 by Mosby, an imprint of Elsevier Inc.

FIG 23.1 A, Venturi mask with one adjustable entrainment port. **B,** VentiMask with interchangeable ports. (*B, Courtesy Noelle Ozog.*)

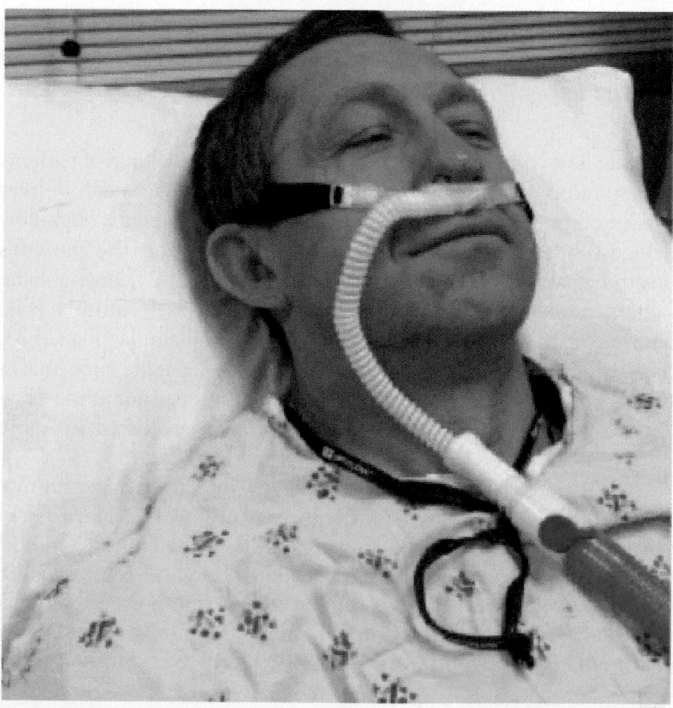

FIG 23.2 High-flow nasal cannula. (*Courtesy Fisher & Paykel Healthcare.*)

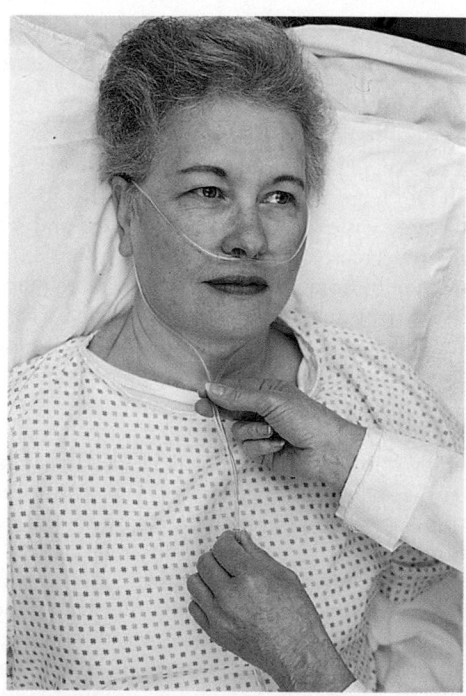

FIG 23.3 Low-flow nasal cannula adjusted for proper fit.

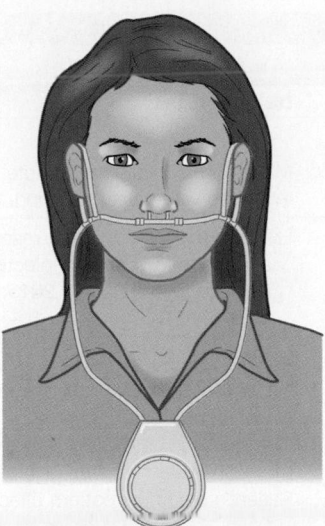

FIG 23.4 Oxygen-conserving cannula. *(From Lewis, S., et al. [2014]. Medical-surgical nursing: assessment and management of clinical problems [9th ed.]. St. Louis: Mosby.)*

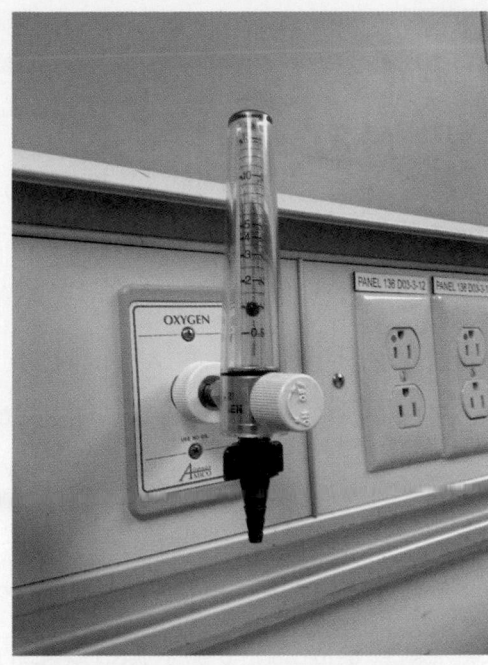

FIG 23.7 Oxygen flowmeter, set at 1 L/min. *(Courtesy Noelle Ozog.)*

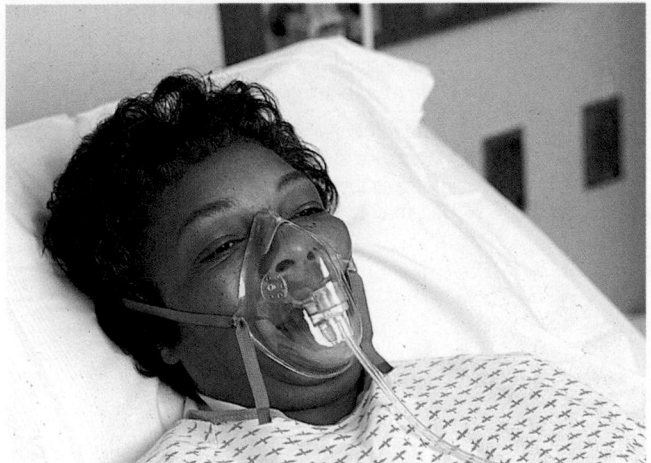

FIG 23.5 Simple face mask.

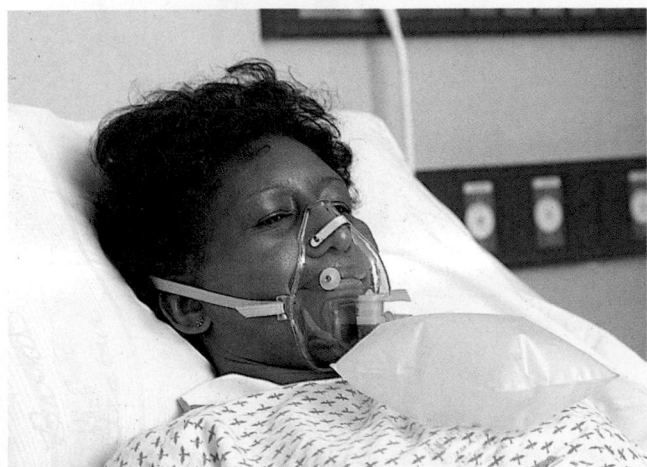

FIG 23.6 Plastic face mask with reservoir bag, being used as a non-rebreather (note one-way valve on exhalation port).

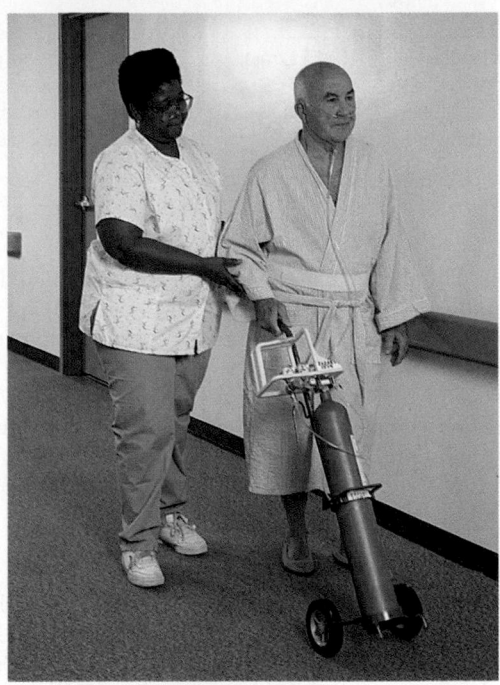

FIG 23.8 Smaller E tank for portability.

is available for all ages, for any length of use. The two prongs of the cannula (about 1.5 cm [½ inch] long) protrude from the centre of a disposable tube and are inserted into the nostrils. Oxygen is delivered via the cannula and does not require humidification at low flow rates (O'Driscoll et al., 2017). An oxygen-conserving cannula is indicated for patients who require higher oxygen concentrations than what can be provided via traditional nasal cannulae. The cannula possesses a built-in reservoir that allows for increasing oxygen concentration at a lower flow rate (see Fig. 23.4).

A high-flow nasal cannula (HFNC) has larger-diameter prongs than low-flow cannulae (Corley et al., 2017). The HFNC is connected to an air-oxygen blender that has an adjustable FiO_2

TABLE 23.1

Common Oxygen Delivery Systems

Delivery System	FiO₂ Delivered	Advantages	Disadvantages
High-Flow Delivery Devices			
Venturi mask (see Fig. 23.1)	24–50%	Provides specific amount of O₂ with humidity added Administers low, constant O₂	Mask and humidity may irritate skin Interferes with eating, drinking, and talking
High-flow nasal cannula (see Fig. 23.2)	Adjustable FiO₂ (21–100%) with a modifiable flow (up to 60 L/min)	Wide range of FiO₂; can be used on adults, children, and infants	FiO₂ dependent on patient respiratory pattern and input flow; risk for infection (Messika, Ben Ahmed, Gaudry, et al., 2015; Urden et al., 2016)
Low-Flow Delivery Devices			
Low-flow nasal cannula (see Fig. 23.3)	1–2 L/min: 24–28% 3–4 L/min: 32–36% 5–6 L/min: 40–44%	Safe Simple Easily tolerated Effective for low concentrations Does not impede eating or talking Inexpensive, disposable	Unable to use with nasal obstruction Drying of mucous membranes Can dislodge easily May cause skin irritation or breakdown Patient's breathing pattern affects exact FiO₂
Oxygen-conserving cannula (Oxymizer) (see Fig. 23.4)	8 L/min: up to 30–60%	Indicated for long-term O₂ Allows increased O₂ concentration at lower flow	More expensive than standard cannula
Simple face mask (see Fig. 23.5)	5–10 L/min: 40–60% (O'Driscoll et al., 2017)	Useful for short periods of time	Contraindicated for patients who retain CO₂ May induce feelings of claustrophobia Interferes with eating and drinking Increased risk for aspiration Patient's breathing pattern affects exact FiO₂
Partial rebreather Partial nonrebreather Full nonrebreather (see Fig. 23.6)	10–15 L/min; 60–80%	Useful for short periods of acute hypoxia Delivers increased FiO₂ Easily humidifies O₂ Does not dry mucous membranes	Hot and confining May cause skin irritation Interferes with eating, drinking, and talking Bag may twist and deflate

FiO₂, Fraction of inspired oxygen concentration.

(Fig. 23.9). This system can deliver a heated and humidified air/oxygen mixture at up to 60 L/min (Corley et al., 2017; Spoletini, Alobtaibi, Blasi, et al., 2015). It is used in patients prone to severe oxygen desaturation and is currently used in critical care settings. The HFNC has been used in the neonatal population. There is also increasing evidence to support its use in adults with acute respiratory failure (Gaunt, Spillman, Halub, et al., 2015; Roca & Masclans, 2015), though evidence is not conclusive to recommend it over other oxygenation devices (Corley et al., 2017).

Oxygen Masks

The simple face mask (see Fig. 23.5) is for short-term oxygen therapy. It fits loosely and delivers FiO₂ from 40 to 60% (O'Driscoll et al., 2017).

A face mask with a reservoir bag (including partial rebreathers, partial and full nonrebreather masks [see Fig. 23.6]) maintains a high-concentration oxygen supply in the reservoir bag. The nurse should frequently inspect the bag to make sure that it is fully inflated; if not, the patient may breathe in large amounts of exhaled carbon dioxide (Herren, Achermann, Hegi, et al., 2017). In partial rebreathers there is a two-way valve between the mask and the reservoir bag. In nonrebreathers it is a one-way valve that allows oxygen into the mask, but not exhaled CO₂ into the reservoir. Nonrebreathers also have one-way valves on either one (partial nonrebreathers) or both (full nonrebreathers) exhalation ports. (Herren et al., 2017, p. 2). A nonrebreather delivers 60 to 90% oxygen at an appropriate flow rate (O'Driscoll et al., 2017).

A Venturi mask is a cone-shaped high-flow device with entrainment ports at the base of the mask, which delivers a more precise concentration of oxygen. Some Venturi masks have one adjustable

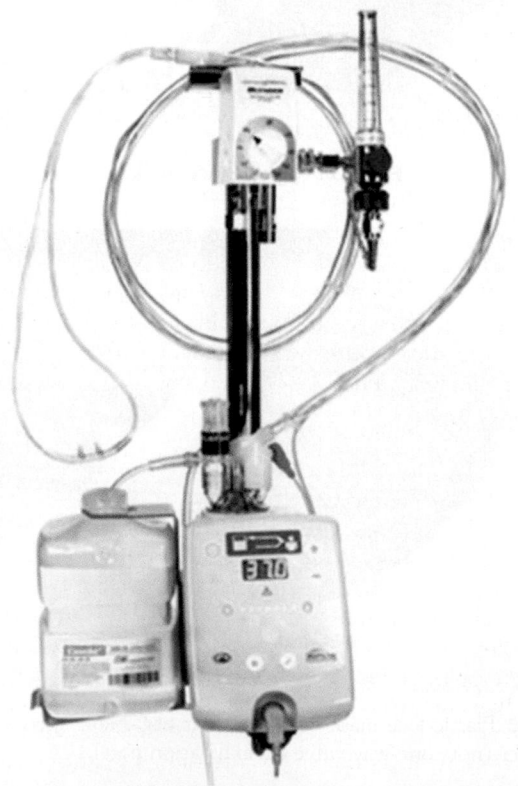

FIG 23.9 High-flow nasal cannula blender. (*Comfort Flo® Humidification System courtesy Teleflex Medical.*)

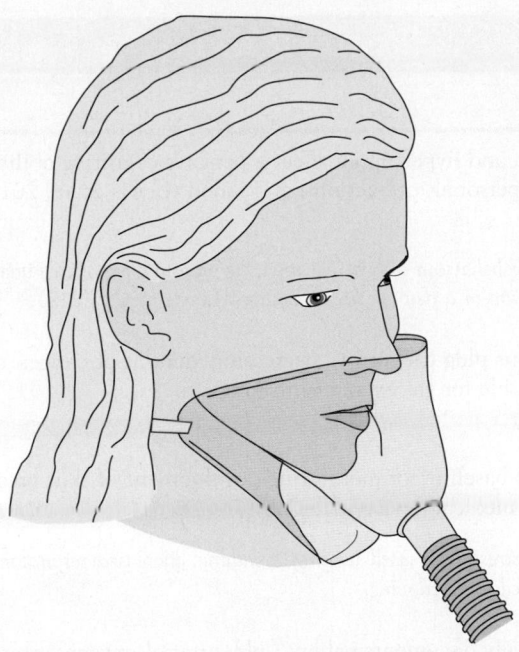

FIG 23.10 Face tent for oxygen delivery. *(From Hockenberry, M. J., & Wilson, D. [2015]. Wong's nursing care of infants and children [10th ed.]. St. Louis: Mosby.)*

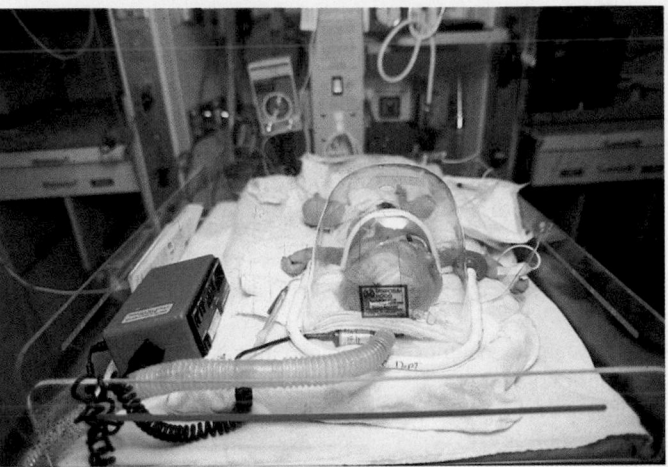

FIG 23.11 Oxygen tent.

entrainment port (see Fig. 23.1, A), whereas others have several interchangeable attachments (see Fig. 23.1, B). The FiO_2 delivered ranges from 24 to 50% and is based on the flow of the gas.

The face tent is a shield-like device that fits under a patient's chin and sweeps around the face (Fig. 23.10). It is used primarily for humidification and for oxygen only when a patient does not tolerate a tight-fitting mask. There is no way to estimate how much oxygen is delivered to the patient.

Oxygen tents (Fig. 23.11) are commonly used in the pediatric setting to provide high concentrations of humidified oxygen. This is particularly useful in the child with airway inflammation, croup, or other respiratory tract infections.

Delegation and Collaboration

The skill of applying a nasal cannula or oxygen mask can be delegated to an unregulated care provider (UCP), depending on the competence of the UCP to perform this skill in a particular situation and on employer policy. The nurse is responsible for assessing the patient's respiratory system, response to oxygen therapy, and setup of oxygen therapy, including adjustment of oxygen flow rate. The nurse directs the UCP by:

- Informing how to safely adjust the device (e.g., loosening the strap on the oxygen cannula or mask) and clarifying its correct placement and positioning.
- Instructing to inform the nurse immediately about any changes in vital signs; changes in pulse oximetry (SpO_2); changes in level of consciousness (LOC); skin irritation from the cannula, mask, or straps; or patient complaints of pain or breathlessness.
- Instructing personnel to provide extra skin care around the patient's ears and nose.
- Practising interprofessional collaboration, which is essential, especially in situations in which the patient suddenly needs a higher concentration of oxygen to maintain their SpO_2 within the target range or is having difficulty breathing despite normal SpO_2 levels.

Equipment

- Oxygen-delivery device as prescribed and as appropriate for current clinical condition of patient
- Oxygen tubing (consider extension tubing)
- Humidifier, indicated for high-flow and long-term oxygen use (O'Driscoll et al., 2017)
- Sterile water for humidifier, if indicated
- Face shield as needed for splash risk
- Clean gloves, if secretions are present
- Oxygen source
- Oxygen flowmeter
- Appropriate "Oxygen in Use" signs
- Pulse oximeter
- Stethoscope

STEP	RATIONALE

ASSESSMENT

1. Identify patient using at least two person-specific identifiers (e.g., name and date of birth or medical record number) according to employer policy.

2. Perform hand hygiene. Perform respiratory assessment, including symmetry of chest wall expansion, chest wall abnormalities (e.g., kyphosis), temporary conditions (e.g., pregnancy, trauma) affecting ventilation, respiratory rate and depth, sputum production, and lung sounds (see Chapter 8), and assess for signs and symptoms associated with hypoxia (see Box 23.1).

Ensures correct patient. Complies with Accreditation Canada's standards and improves patient safety (Accreditation Canada, 2019).

Reduces transmission of microorganisms. Changes in ventilation and gas exchange resulting in hypoxia require oxygen therapy.

STEP	RATIONALE

ASSESSMENT

3. Observe for behavioural changes (e.g., apprehension, anxiety, confusion, decreased ability to concentrate, decreased LOC, fatigue, and dizziness).

Hypoxia and hypercapnia affect a person's cognitive abilities, interpersonal interactions, and mood (Lewis et al., 2019).

Clinical Decision Point *Patients with sudden changes in their vital signs, LOC, or behaviour may be experiencing profound hypoxia. Patients who demonstrate subtle changes over time may have worsening of a chronic or existing condition or a new medical condition (Lewis et al., 2019).*

4. Assess airway patency and remove airway secretions by having patient cough and expectorate mucus or by suctioning (see Chapter 25). **NOTE:** Apply clean gloves if there is risk of mucus contact.

Secretions plug the airway, decreasing amount of oxygen that is available for gas exchange in lungs.

5. Inspect condition of skin around nose and ears.

Provides baseline for monitoring development of skin breakdown from medical device irritation.

Clinical Decision Point *Excessive amounts of secretions, signs of respiratory distress (increased work of breathing, increased respiratory rate), rhonchi on auscultation, excessive coughing, or decrease in patient SpO_2 can indicate need for suctioning.*

6. If available, note patient's most recent arterial blood gas (ABG) results or SpO_2 value. Remove and discard gloves if worn; perform hand hygiene.

Objectively documents patient's pH, arterial oxygen, arterial carbon dioxide, or arterial oxygen saturation.

7. Review patient's medical record for prescription for oxygen, noting delivery method, flow rate, duration of oxygen therapy, and parameters for titration of oxygen settings.

Ensures safe and accurate oxygen administration. Safe oxygen delivery includes the 10 rights of medication administration (see Chapter 20).

8. Assess patient's and caregiver's level of understanding about oxygen therapy.

Determines level of instruction required.

NURSING DIAGNOSES

- Reduced airway clearance
- Inadequate breathing pattern
- Reduced gas exchange
- Fatigue
- Anxiety
- Potential for impaired skin integrity
- Insufficient knowledge regarding purpose of oxygen therapy

Related factors/Risk factors are individualized on the basis of patient's condition or needs.

PLANNING

1. Expected outcomes following completion of procedure:
   - Patient's SpO_2 and/or ABGs return to or remain within normal limits or baseline levels.

Objective determinants of stable or improved oxygenation.

   - Patient's vital signs remain stable or return to baseline.

When there is no underlying cardiovascular disease, patients adapt to decreased oxygen levels by increasing pulse and blood pressure. This is a short-term adaptive response. Once signs of hypoxia are reduced or controlled, patient's vital signs usually return to normal.

   - Patient's work of breathing decreases.

Pulmonary conditions such as pneumonia or asthma cause varying degrees of airway narrowing. With improved oxygenation, patient's airways are open, and work of breathing decreases.

   - Patient experiences increased lung expansion.

Improved oxygenation helps to resolve collapsed and constricted airways, improves work of breathing, and thus improves lung expansion.

   - Patient's LOC returns to baseline.

Improvement in oxygenation relieves hypoxia and improves patient's mental status.

   - Patient verbalizes improved levels of comfort; and subjective sensations of anxiety, fatigue, and breathlessness decrease.

Increased oxygen levels in the blood reduce patient's anxiety, fatigue, and breathlessness.

   - Patient's ears, nares, and nasal mucosa remain intact.

Intact skin indicates no device-related pressure to underlying skin and mucous membrane (Pittman, Beeson, Kitterman, et al., 2015; Schallom, Cracchiolo, Falker, et al., 2015).

STEP	RATIONALE

PLANNING

2. Explain procedure to patient and caregiver.

Explanation decreases patient's anxiety and reduces oxygen consumption. Increases adherence to treatment and cooperation of patient and caregiver.

3. Gather equipment and supplies according to employer policy.

Provides organized implementation of the oxygen-delivery device.

IMPLEMENTATION

1. Perform hand hygiene and appropriate personal protective equipment (PPE). Apply face shield if there is risk of exposure to splashing mucus. Apply gloves if patient has oral or nasal secretions.

Reduces transmission of microorganisms.

2. Adjust bed to appropriate height and lower side rail on side nearest you. Check locks on bed wheel.

Minimizes caregiver's muscle strain and prevents injury. Prevents bed from moving.

3. Attach oxygen-delivery device (e.g., cannula, mask) to oxygen tubing and attach end of tubing to oxygen source adjusted to prescribed flow rate (see Fig. 23.7), with humidification if appropriate.

Humidity prevents drying of nasal and oral mucous membranes and airway secretions at high-flow rates or for long-term use (O'Driscoll et al., 2017).

4. Apply oxygen device:

   a. *Nasal cannula:* Place tips of the cannula into patient's nares. If tips are curved, they should point downward inside nostrils. Then loop cannula tubing up and over patient's ears. Adjust lanyard against patient's chin so cannula fits snugly but does not put pressure on patient nares and ears (see Fig. 23.3).

Tips of cannula direct flow of oxygen into patient's upper respiratory tract.

   b. *Masks:* Apply a mask by placing it over patient's mouth and nose. Then bring straps over patient's head and adjust to form a comfortable but tight seal (see Fig. 23.5).

A properly fitting device that does not create pressure on nares or ears is comfortable, and patient is more likely to keep it in place; reduces risk for skin breakdown (Schallom et al., 2015).

5. Maintain sufficient slack on oxygen tubing and secure to patient's clothes.

Allows patient to turn head without causing mask to shift position or dislodge nasal cannula.

6. Observe for proper function of oxygen-delivery device:

Ensures patency of delivery device and accuracy of prescribed oxygen flow rate (see Table 23.1).

   a. *Nasal cannula:* Cannula is positioned properly in nares; oxygen flows through tips.

Provides prescribed oxygen rate and reduces pressure on tips of nares.

   b. *Oxygen-conserving cannula (Oxymizer):* Fit as for nasal cannula. Reservoir is located under patient's nose or worn as a pendant.

Delivers higher flow of oxygen with nasal cannula. Delivers 2:1 ratio (e.g., 6 L/min nasal cannula is approximately equivalent to 3.5 L/min with Oxymizer device).

   c. *Simple face mask:* Select appropriate flow rate (see Fig. 23.5).

For short-term oxygen therapy.

   d. *Partial rebreather mask* (see Fig. 23.6): Mask seals tightly around mouth. Reservoir fills on exhalation and almost collapses on inspiration. Reservoir should not collapse completely.

For short-term therapy of 24 hours or less.

   e. *Nonrebreather mask:* Apply as regular mask. Can be combined with nasal cannula to provide higher inspired oxygen concentration (FiO_2). Reservoir should not collapse.

First choice for short-term high FiO_2 delivery. Valves on expiration ports permit exhalation but close during inhalation to prevent inhaling room air.

   f. *Venturi mask* (see Fig. 23.1): Apply as regular mask. Select appropriate flow rate (see Table 23.1).

Used when high-flow device is desired.

   g. *High-flow nasal cannula* (see Fig. 23.2): Fit as for nasal cannula.

Used when high oxygen delivery is required.

   h. *Face tent* (see Fig. 23.10): Apply tent under patient's chin and over mouth and nose. It will be loose, and a mist is always present.

Excellent source of humidification; however, FiO_2 cannot be controlled, so patients who require high FiO_2 cannot use this device.

7. Verify setting on flowmeter and oxygen source for proper setup and prescribed flow rate.

Ensures delivery of prescribed oxygen therapy in conjunction with specific cannula/mask.

STEP	RATIONALE

IMPLEMENTATION

8. Check cannula/mask every 8 hours or as employer policy indicates. If using humidification, keep container filled at all times.

Ensures patency of cannula and oxygen flow. Oxygen is a dry gas; when it is administered via high-flow systems for more than 24 hours, or if the patient reports dryness, add humidification (O'Driscoll et al., 2017)

9. Post "Oxygen in Use" signs on wall behind bed and at entrance to room.

Alerts visitors and care providers that oxygen is in use.

10. Properly dispose of gloves (if used) and perform hand hygiene.

Reduces transmission of microorganisms.

EVALUATION

1. Monitor patient's response to changes in oxygen flow rate with SpO$_2$. **NOTE:** Monitor ABGs when prescribed; however, obtaining ABG measurement is an invasive procedure and ABGs are not measured frequently.

Continual monitoring with SpO$_2$ is required for patients on oxygen therapy. Base changes in supplemental oxygen on individual patient's oxygen saturation levels.

2. Perform physical assessment, listening to lung sounds; palpating chest excursion; inspecting colour and condition of skin; and observing for decreased anxiety, improved LOC and cognitive abilities, decreased fatigue, and absence of dizziness. Measure vital signs.

Evaluates patient's response to supplemental oxygen. As patient's oxygen level improves, physical signs and symptoms improve.

3. Assess adequacy of oxygen flow each shift or per employer policy.

Ensures patency of oxygen delivery device.

4. Observe patient's external ears, bridge of nose, nares, and nasal mucous membranes for evidence of skin breakdown.

Oxygen therapy sometimes causes drying of nasal mucosa. The delivery device can cause skin breakdown where device comes in contact with face, neck, and ears (Schallom et al., 2015).

5. **Use Teach-Back:** "I want to be sure I explained how oxygen will help you. Explain to me why oxygen is beneficial for you to use right now." Develop a revised teaching plan if patient or caregiver is not able to teach back correctly.

Determines patient's and caregiver's level of understanding of instructional topic.

Unexpected Outcomes

1. Patient experiences skin irritation or breakdown (e.g., at ears, bridge of nose, nares, other pressure areas), sinus pain, or epistaxis.
2. Patient experiences continued hypoxia.

3. Patient experiences nasal and upper airway mucosa drying.

Related Interventions

- Provide appropriate skin care. Do not use petroleum-based gel around oxygen because it is flammable (Davidson, Banham, Elliott, et al., 2016).
- Notify health care provider.
- Obtain prescription for follow-up SpO$_2$ monitoring or ABG determinations.
- Consider measures to improve airway patency, including but not limited to coughing techniques and oropharyngeal or orotracheal suctioning.
- If oxygen flow rate is less than 5 L/min, humidification provides no difference in nose/throat dryness (Wen, Wang, Zhang, et al., 2017). At rates greater than 5 L/min, nasal mucous membranes dry, and pain in frontal sinuses may develop (Lewis et al., 2019).
- Assess patient's fluid status and increase fluids if appropriate.
- Provide frequent oral care.

Communication and Documentation

- Document the respiratory assessment findings, method of oxygen delivery, oxygen flow rate, patient's response to intervention, any adverse reactions or side effects.
- Document your evaluation of patient and caregiver learning.
- Communicate any unexpected outcome to health care provider or nurse in charge.

Special Considerations
Teaching

- If oxygen therapy continues after discharge, teach patient and caregiver the importance of and rationale for it, how to use the oxygen-delivery device, how to contact the supplier of medical equipment, and when to contact the health care provider (see Chapter 43).
- Discuss safety precautions for oxygen use (see Box 23.3) with patient and caregiver.
- Discuss signs of carbon dioxide retention (e.g., confusion, headache, decreased LOC, somnolence, carbon dioxide narcosis, respiratory arrest) that patient or caregiver needs to report to the health care provider.

Pediatric

- Some infants and small children are able to tolerate a nasal cannula. Secure the prongs of the cannula with transparent tape or strips of transparent dressing over the child's cheek.
- Sometimes infants receive oxygen therapy via an oxygen tent. Place the tent over the patient's head (see Fig. 23.10).
- Inspect toys placed in the tent for safety and suitability. Any source of sparks (e.g., from mechanical or electrical toys) is a potential fire hazard (Hockenberry & Wilson, 2015).
- Provide comfort and reassurance to the child. Make sure that they are able to see someone nearby. Children may still be held by their parents while receiving oxygen via nasal cannula or face mask (Hockenberry & Wilson, 2015).

Gerontological

- Because of the fragility of older persons' skin and mucous membranes, offer oral hygiene and skin care more frequently. Water-based gels such as Biotène are useful but also dry quickly and need more frequent application.

Care in the Community

Obtain appropriate referrals to determine if patient meets the standards for long-term oxygen therapy. Eligibility is assessed by measuring ABGs. Generally, criteria is a PaO_2 of 55 mm Hg or less when patient is clinically stable (Lacasse, Bernard, & Maltais, 2015). When patients have peripheral edema (cor pulmonale); hematocrit ≥55% (polycythemia); or right ventricular hypertrophy, pulmonary hypertension, or erythrocytosis, they are often eligible with a PaO_2 of 56 to 59 mm Hg (Lacasse et al., 2015). However, each province and territory has its own eligibility and reimbursement criteria for long-term oxygen use. Funding may be different for people whose health care is delivered through Veterans Affairs Canada (http://www.veterans.gc.ca/eng/services) or the Non-Insured Health Benefits Program (https://www.canada.ca/en/indigenous-services-canada/services/non-insured-health-benefits-first-nations-inuit.html).

- Oxygen tubing in the home setting is available in lengths of 15 m (50 feet).
- Provide information about a reliable oxygen-therapy equipment vendor within the community to determine if patient and caregiver are able to use a home-fill system with an oxygen concentrator, which provides patient with the opportunity to fill a portable canister as needed (Aguiar, Davidson, Carvalho, et al., 2015).
- Consider using oxygen-conserving devices (e.g., Oxymizer) that administer oxygen in a pulse-dosed flow during inhalation only. These reduce the use and cost of long-term oxygen therapy.

◆ SKILL 23.2   Administering Oxygen Therapy to a Patient With an Artificial Airway

Patients with an artificial airway require constant humidification to the airway (see Chapter 25). An artificial airway bypasses the normal filtering and humidification process of the nose and mouth. The two devices that supply humidified gas to an artificial airway are a T tube and a tracheostomy collar.

The T tube, also called a *Briggs adaptor*, is a T-shaped device with a 15-mm (¾-inch) connection that connects an oxygen source to an artificial airway such as an endotracheal (ET) tube or tracheostomy (Fig. 23.12). A tracheostomy mask is a curved device with an adjustable strap that fits around a patient's neck (Fig. 23.13).

Delegation and Collaboration

The skill of administering oxygen therapy to a patient with an artificial airway cannot be delegated to an unregulated care providers (UCP). The nurse instructs the UCP about:

- Patient-specific variations for application or adjustment of the T tube or tracheostomy collar (e.g., methods to avoid device-related pressure areas or pulling on the artificial airway, methods for handling accumulated secretions in devices).
- Immediately reporting to the nurse an increase in anxiety, changes in vital signs, and increase in airway secretions.
- Optimizing patient outcomes—the nurse uses interprofessional collaboration when caring for this patient. For example, the

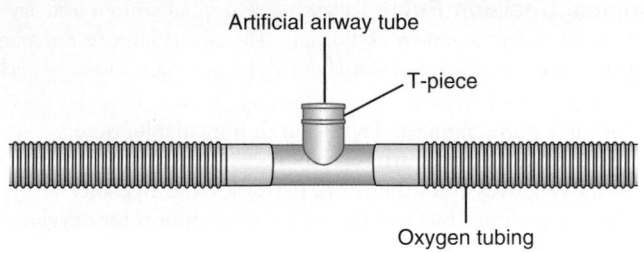

FIG 23.12 T tube.

nurse and respiratory therapist may work together to find the level of humidification and oxygenation that meets the oxygen needs of a patient.

Equipment

- T tube or tracheostomy collar
- Large-bore oxygen tubing
- Nebulizer
- Sterile water for nebulizer
- Oxygen or gas source
- Clean gloves

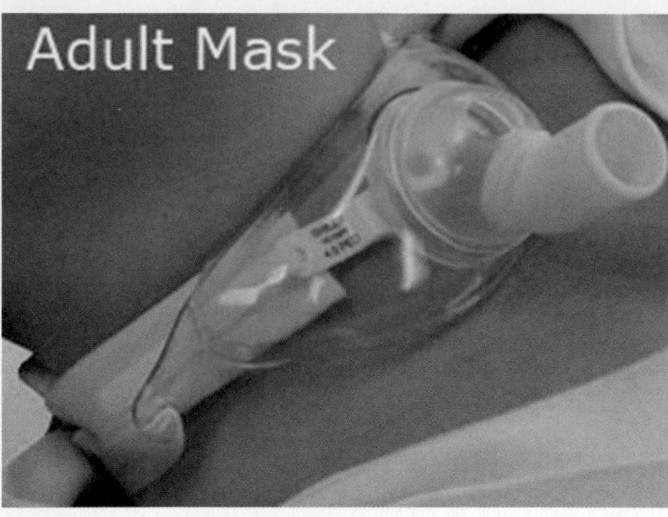

FIG 23.13 Tracheostomy mask. (*Courtesy Marcpac Company.*)

- Mask and/or barrier gown (refer to routine practices and additional precautions prescribed)
- Goggles (if splash risk)
- Flowmeter
- Yankauer or tonsillar tip suction catheter
- Connecting tubing (at least 1.8 m [6 feet])
- Suction machine or wall suction device
- Pulse oximeter
- Stethoscope

STEP	RATIONALE

ASSESSMENT

1. Identify patient using at least two person-specific identifiers (e.g., name and date of birth or medical record number) according to employer policy.

   Ensures correct patient. Complies with Accreditation Canada's standards and improves patient safety (Accreditation Canada, 2019).

2. Perform hand hygiene. Assess patient's respiratory status, including symmetry of chest wall expansion, respiratory rate and depth, sputum production, and lung sounds (see Chapter 8); assess for signs and symptoms associated with hypoxia (see Box 23.1). Assess condition of lips around endotracheal tube or of tracheal stoma. **NOTE:** Wear appropriate PPE.

   Changes in ventilation and gas exchange resulting in hypoxia require oxygen therapy. Provides baseline for monitoring of tissue breakdown from irritation of medical device. Reduces transmission of microorganisms.

3. Observe for patent airway and remove airway secretions by having patient cough and by suctioning (see Chapter 25).

   Secretions plug airway, decreasing amount of oxygen available for gas exchange in lung. Secretions also occlude T tube or tracheostomy collar, impeding oxygen delivery.

4. Observe for behavioural changes (e.g., apprehension, anxiety, confusion, decreased ability to concentrate, decreased LOC, fatigue, and dizziness).

   Hypoxia and hypercapnia affect a person's cognitive abilities, interpersonal interactions, and mood (Lewis et al., 2019).

Clinical Decision Point *Patients with artificial airways who develop sudden changes in their vital signs, LOC, or behaviour may be experiencing hypoxia secondary to airway obstruction. The airway must be determined to be patent before oxygen is administered. If patients continue with signs of hypoxia once obstruction is removed or ruled out, oxygen should be applied.*

5. Monitor pulse oximetry (SpO_2) and, if available, note patient's most recent arterial blood gas (ABG) results. Remove gloves and other PPE, perform hand hygiene.

   Objectively documents patient's pH, arterial oxygen, arterial carbon dioxide, or arterial oxygen saturation.

6. Review patient's medical record for prescription for oxygen, noting delivery method, flow rate, and duration of oxygen therapy.

   Ensures safe and accurate oxygen administration. Safe oxygen delivery includes the appropriate medication administration (see Chapter 20).

   Determines level of instruction or support needed.

NURSING DIAGNOSES

- Ineffective airway clearance
- Ineffective breathing pattern
- Impaired gas exchange
- Fatigue
- Anxiety
- Potential for impaired tissue integrity
- Deficient knowledge regarding purpose of therapy

Related factors/Risk factors are individualized on the basis of patient's condition or needs.

STEP	RATIONALE

PLANNING

1. Expected outcomes following completion of procedure:
   - Patient's signs of hypoxia are reduced or eliminated.
   - Patient's vital signs remain stable or return to baseline.

   Patient demonstrates improved oxygenation.

   When there is no underlying cardiovascular disease, patient adapts to decreased oxygen levels by increasing pulse and blood pressure. This is a short-term adaptive response. Once signs of hypoxia are reduced or controlled, patient's vital signs usually return to normal.

   - Patient's work of breathing decreases.

   With improved oxygenation, tissue oxygen demand is met, and work of breathing decreases.

   - Patient experiences increased lung expansion.

   Improved oxygenation helps to resolve collapsed and constricted airways, improve work of breathing, and thus improve lung expansion.

   - Patient's LOC returns to baseline.

   Improvement in oxygenation relieves hypoxia and improves patient's mental status.

   - ABG values or SpO_2 saturation returns to normal or baseline.

   Documents physiological response to oxygen therapy.

   - Tracheal stoma remains intact without irritation or peristomal skin breakdown.

   Tension on tracheal stoma from oxygen therapy equipment has potential to cause pressure on stoma and surrounding skin (Pittman et al., 2015).

2. Explain purpose of T tube or tracheostomy collar to patient and caregiver.

   Explanation decreases patient's anxiety and reduces oxygen consumption. Education increases adherence to treatment plan and cooperation of patient and caregiver.

IMPLEMENTATION

1. Gather equipment and supplies needed and complete necessary charges according to employer policy.

   Ensure that you have the necessary equipment to apply oxygen-delivery device appropriately.

2. Perform hand hygiene, apply clean gloves and goggles; consider use of barrier gown and mask.

   Reduces transmission of microorganisms by preventing contact with pulmonary secretions. Patients with excessive secretions or forceful productive coughs place caregiver at risk for splash contact.

3. Set up suction equipment at patient's bedside.

   Humidification increases airway secretions.

4. Attach T tube or tracheostomy mask to large-bore oxygen tubing and to humidified room air or oxygen source as indicated.

   Provides supplemental humidification to avoid drying of airway. This is necessary because of loss of oral and nasal passages that naturally humidify air.

5. If oxygen is prescribed, adjust flow rate to 10 L/min or as prescribed. Adjust nebulizer to proper oxygen concentration (FiO_2) setting. Attach T tube to artificial airway. Place tracheostomy collar over tracheostomy tube and adjust straps so it fits snugly.

   Flow rate ensures humidification; nebulizer regulates FiO_2.

6. Observe that T tube does not pull on artificial airway or cause pressure on adjacent skin and tissue. Observe for secretions within T tube or tracheostomy collar and suction as necessary (see Chapter 25).

   Pulling effect on tube increases patient's discomfort and causes pressure to side of patient's mouth or tracheal stoma, which increases risk for device-related pressure injuries (Pittman et al., 2015; Schallom et al., 2015).

7. Observe oxygen tubing frequently for accumulation of fluid caused by condensation. If fluid is present, drain tube away from patient, disconnect from collar or T tube, and discard fluid in proper receptacle.

   Fluid water is medium for bacterial growth. Draining contaminated water into proper receptacle prevents contamination of entire humidifying unit.

8. Remove PPE (gloves, goggles, mask, and/or gown); perform hand hygiene.

   Reduces transmission of microorganisms.

EVALUATION

1. Monitor patient's vital signs and SpO_2.

   Continuous monitoring of vital signs and SpO_2 allows for continual noninvasive, cost-effective trending of patient's vital signs and oxygen saturation.

2. Perform respiratory assessment and observe for any behavioural changes indicative of hypoxia.

   Monitors changes in patient's respiratory assessment and cognitive status in response to supplemental oxygen.

STEP	RATIONALE

EVALUATION

3. Observe position of oxygen-delivery device and condition of adjacent tissues to ensure that there is no pulling on artificial airway or pressure areas.

Pulling on artificial airway or pressure on adjacent tissues results in damage to oral cavity or stoma.

4. Use Teach-Back: "I want to be sure I explained how oxygen will help your mother. Explain to me why oxygen is attached to your mother's tracheostomy tube." Develop a revised teaching plan if patient or caregiver is not able to teach back correctly.

Determines patient's and caregiver's level of understanding of instructional topic.

Unexpected Outcomes

1. Patient experiences tracheal stoma or lip irritation; thick, tenacious secretions; pressure areas on neck or near stoma site.

2. Patient experiences continued hypoxia.

Related Interventions

- Implement measures to protect patient from medical device pressure injuries (MDPIs) (see Chapter 39).
- Increase frequency of suctioning and airway care (see Chapter 25).
- Determine if cause of continued hypoxia is oxygen-delivery device, plugging of airway, oxygen flow rate, or a new clinical problem.
- Notify health care provider of continued or worsening hypoxia.

Communication and Documentation

- Document the respiratory assessment findings; method of oxygen delivery, flow rate, condition of tracheal stoma or lips, patient's response; and any adverse reactions.
- Document your evaluation of patient and caregiver learning.
- Report any unexpected outcome to health care provider or nurse in charge.

Special Considerations
Teaching

- See teaching considerations for Skill 23.1.

Care in the Community

- Some patients who are at home have both a permanent tracheostomy and a T tube or a tracheostomy collar. The patient or caregiver needs to be physically able to perform tracheostomy care and suctioning techniques and must understand how to manage oxygen (see Chapters 25 and 43).
- In some jurisdictions, a community-based care provider can provide tracheostomy care and suctioning in the patient's home. These services may be expensive or of limited availability, so patient and caregiver teaching remain essential.

✦ SKILL 23.3 Using Incentive Spirometry

Incentive spirometry helps a patient deep breathe. It works by providing visual feedback that helps encourage the patient to take long, deep, slow breaths (Smetana, 2018). The use of an incentive spirometer (IS) alone is not recommended to prevent postoperative pulmonary complications. It should be used in combination with other pulmonary manoeuvres such as deep breathing and coughing (see Chapter 37), early mobilization of the patient, and directed coughing (do Nascimento et al., 2014; Smetana, 2018).

The two types of ISs are flow oriented and volume oriented. Flow-oriented ISs have one or more plastic chambers with freely movable coloured balls. The advantage of a flow-oriented IS is the slow, steady expansion of the lung. As a patient inhales slowly, the balls elevate to a premarked area (Fig. 23.14). A patient's goal is to keep the balls elevated for as long as possible to ensure maximal sustained inhalation. Even if a very slow inspiration does not elevate the balls, this pattern helps a patient improve lung expansion.

Volume-oriented devices use a bellows that a patient must raise to a predetermined volume by inhaling slowly (Fig. 23.15). The advantage of the volume-oriented IS is that a patient can achieve a known inspiratory volume and measure it with each breath.

Delegation and Collaboration

The skill of helping a patient to use incentive spirometry can be delegated to an unregulated care provider (UCP) depending on the

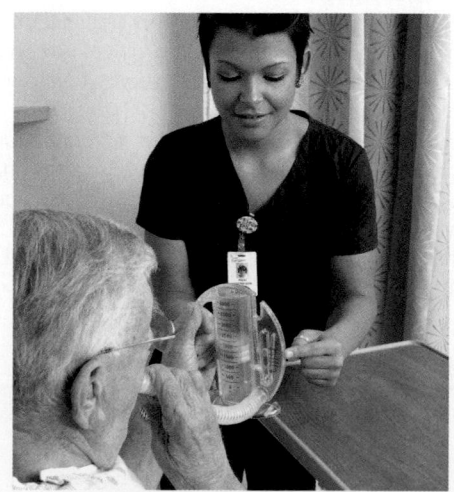

FIG 23.14 Flow-oriented incentive spirometer.

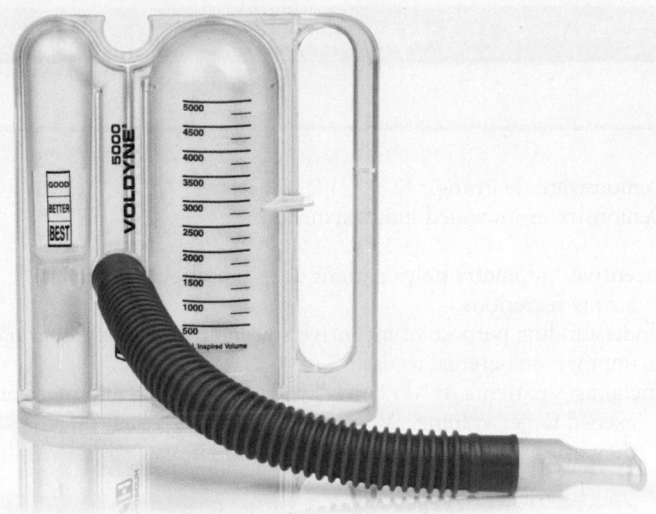

FIG 23.15 Volume-oriented incentive spirometer.

competence of the UCP to perform this skill in a particular situation and employer policy. The nurse is responsible for assessing and monitoring the patient, evaluating the patient response, educating the patient about the proper use of the IS, and evaluating that education. The nurse instructs the UCP by:

- Informing about the patient's target goal for incentive spirometry.
- Informing to immediately notify the nurse about any unexpected outcomes, such as chest pain, excessive sputum production, and fever.

Equipment

- Flow- or volume-oriented IS
- Stethoscope
- Pulse oximeter monitor

STEP	RATIONALE
ASSESSMENT	
1. Identify patient using at least two person-specific identifiers (e.g., name and date of birth or medical record number) according to employer policy.	Ensures correct patient. Complies with Accreditation Canada's Required Organizational Practices and improves patient safety (Accreditation Canada, 2019).
2. Review medical record to identify patients who will benefit from the use of an IS (e.g., existing pulmonary disease, obesity, debilitating chronic illness, heavy smokers, neuromuscular disease, or sickle cell disease with acute chest syndrome [Smetana, 2018]). In addition, identify patients able to combine IS with other airway clearance measures such as deep breathing and coughing (Tyson et al., 2015) or early mobilization.	Alerts health care personnel to patients at risk for respiratory complications during illness or after surgery.
3. Assess patient for confusion, cognitive impairment, ability to follow directions, age, developmental level, level of consciousness, and decreased necessary motor skills (Smetana, 2018).	Determines risks for difficulty performing incentive spirometry.

Clinical Decision Point *Patients who are unable to follow directions or who are not developmentally or physically able to perform the actions associated with this skill are not candidates for this intervention. This assessment helps the nurse determine whether to use the flow-oriented or volume-oriented IS.*

4. Perform hand hygiene. Assess patient's respiratory status, including symmetry of chest wall expansion, respiratory rate and depth, sputum production, and lung sounds (see Chapter 8). Also obtain a pulse oximeter reading.	Reduces transmission of microorganisms. Decreased chest wall movement, crackles or decreased lung sounds, increased respiratory rate, or increased sputum production can indicate a need for incentive spirometry to improve lung expansion.
5. Assess level of pain at rest and during activity (e.g., coughing) using appropriate pain rating scale (e.g., rate your pain on a 0-to-10 scale, with 0 being no pain and 10 being the worst pain ever).	Pain decreases effective incentive spirometry by restricting chest expansion.
6. Review interprofessional team recommendations and prescriptions for incentive spirometry.	Ensures appropriate incentive spirometry use.

NURSING DIAGNOSES

- Impaired breathing pattern
- Ineffective airway clearance
- Acute pain
- Impaired gas exchange

Related factors/Risk factors are individualized on the basis of patient's condition or needs.

STEP	RATIONALE

PLANNING

1. Expected outcomes following completion of procedure:
   - Patient demonstrates correct use of IS.
   - Patient achieves target volume and number of repetitions per hour.
   - Patient has improved breath sounds and increased pulse oximeter reading.
2. Explain procedure to patient and caregiver.

3. Indicate to patient where target volume is on IS. NOTE: If possible, demonstrate use of IS.

Demonstrates learning.
Demonstrates increased lung expansion.

Incentive spirometry helps patient deep breathe and manage airway secretions.
Understanding purpose of incentive spirometry and its proper use improves adherence to use.
Encourages patients to "do better" with each breath and meet or exceed target volume. When patients have a visual target, they can gauge their improvement.

IMPLEMENTATION

1. Gather equipment and supplies and complete necessary charges according to employer policy.
2. Perform hand hygiene.
3. Position patient in most erect position (e.g., high-Fowler's if tolerated) in bed or chair.
4. Instruct patient to hold IS upright, exhale normally and completely through mouth, and place lips tightly around mouthpiece (Fig. 23.16).

5. Instruct patient to take a slow, deep breath and maintain constant flow, like pulling through a straw. If flow-oriented IS is used, inhalation should raise the ball. If volume-oriented IS is used, inhalation should raise the piston. Remove mouthpiece at point of maximal inhalation; then have patient hold their breath for 3 seconds and exhale normally.

Ensures that you have the necessary equipment.

Reduces transmission of microorganisms.
Promotes optimal lung expansion during respiratory manoeuvre.
Allows for proper function of IS (Smetana, 2018). Showing patient how to correctly place mouthpiece is reliable technique for teaching psychomotor skill and enables patient to ask questions.
Maintains maximal inspiration; reduces risk for progressive collapse of individual alveoli.

Clinical Decision Point *Some patients are unable to hold their breath for 3 seconds. Encourage them to do their best and try to extend the duration of breath holding. Allow patients to rest between IS breaths to prevent hyperventilation and fatigue.*

6. Have patient repeat manoeuvre, encouraging them to reach prescribed goal.
7. Encourage patient to independently use IS at prescribed frequency. Frequently prescribed timing schedules of IS use are up to 30 deep breaths with 30- to 60-second rests between sets of 10 (Smetana, 2018).
8. Perform hand hygiene.

Ensures correct use of IS and patient's understanding of use.

Repeated use of IS improves lung expansion and promotes clearing of airways. Encouraging patients to perform independently gives them a sense of control over their care.
Reduces transmission of microorganisms.

EVALUATION

1. Observe patient's ability to use incentive spirometry by return demonstration.
2. Assess if patient is able to achieve target volume or frequency.
3. Auscultate chest during respiratory cycle and obtain pulse oximeter reading (Smetana, 2018).

4. **Use Teach-Back:** "I want to be sure I explained how and when to use the IS. Show me how to use your IS, and tell me how frequently you should use it." Develop a revised teaching plan if patient is not able to teach back correctly.

Determines patient's ability to perform breathing exercise correctly.
Measures adherence to therapy and lung expansion.
Documents lung expansion, identifies any abnormal lung sounds, and determines if airways are clear. Identifies improvement in pulse oximeter readings.
Determines patient's level of understanding of instructional topic.

STEP	RATIONALE

EVALUATION

Unexpected Outcomes	Related Interventions
1. Patient is unable to achieve incentive spirometry target volume.	• Encourage patient to attempt incentive spirometry more frequently, followed by rest periods. • Teach cough-control exercises. • Teach patient how to splint and protect incision sites during deep breathing (see Chapter 37). • Administer prescribed analgesic if acute pain is inhibiting use of IS.
2. Patient has decreased lung expansion and/or abnormal breath sounds or decreased pulse oximeter readings.	• Teach patient cough-control exercises. • Provide help with suctioning if patient cannot cough up secretions effectively.
3. Patient develops hyperventilation.	• Encourage longer rest periods between breaths.

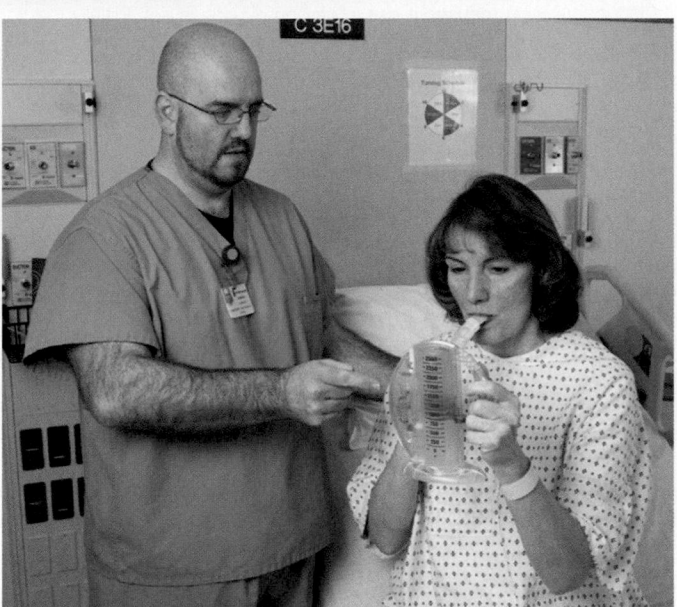

FIG 23.16 Proper placement of lips around incentive spirometer.

Communication and Documentation

- Document lung sounds, respiratory rate, and pulse oximeter readings before and after incentive spirometry; frequency of use; volumes achieved; and any adverse effects.
- Document your evaluation of patient learning.

Special Considerations
Teaching

- Teach patient to examine sputum for consistency, amount, and colour changes. Sputum should become clearer over time and decrease in volume.

Pediatric

- Incentive spirometry is not typically used in pediatrics except for school-age children; a pediatric patient needs the fine-motor skills and ability to follow instructions to use an IS effectively (Hockenberry & Wilson, 2015).
- Allowing a child to play with and try out the IS helps to decrease their anxiety and encourages participation in care.
- Use games or bubbles and pinwheels to encourage small children to take deep breaths. These activities help achieve the same goals as incentive spirometry in some children.

Gerontological

- Older persons with chronic illnesses or arthritis may have difficulty coordinating the use of the IS. They may require additional time to demonstrate the procedure (Touhy & Jett, 2018, p. 51).
- Weakened respiratory muscles and decreased elastic recoil properties of the lungs affect a patient's ability to cough and deep breathe. Therefore, it takes an older person longer to achieve the target volume (Touhy & Jett, 2018, pp. 30–31).
- Use volume-oriented IS: More muscle activity is required for an older person to achieve the same increase in chest wall volume using flow-oriented IS compared to volume-oriented IS (Lunardi, Porras, Barbosa, et al., 2014, pp. 423–424).

✦ SKILL 23.4   Care of a Patient Receiving Noninvasive Positive-Pressure Ventilation

Noninvasive positive-pressure ventilation (NIPPV or NPPV), or noninvasive ventilation (NIV), maintains positive airway pressure and improves alveolar ventilation in the spontaneously breathing patient without the need for an artificial airway. There are two types of NIPPV: continuous positive airway pressure (CPAP) and bi-level positive airway pressure (BiPAP). BiPAP and CPAP are usually applied via a mask covering the nose (Fig. 23.17) or both the mouth and nose, but those who require home CPAP may wear nasal prongs instead (Hill & Kramer, 2018; Pooboni & Markowitz, 2018).

NIPPV is increasingly used in care settings in the community, to treat a variety of conditions including obstructive sleep apnea (OSA), chronic obstructive pulmonary disease (COPD), and neuromuscular disorders. In the Canadian acute care setting, it is used in patients with acute respiratory failure due to cardiogenic pulmonary edema or COPD exacerbation (Digby, Keenan, Parker, et al., 2015; Keenan et al., 2011). NIPPV is only appropriate if these patients are cooperative, able to protect their own airway, and are not acutely deteriorating (Rochwerg et al., 2017).

The advantages of NIPPV over invasive ventilation include an increased ability to communicate with caregivers, better ability to cough and clear secretions, and allowance for eating and drinking. NIPPV can also decrease the risk of invasive ventilation complications such as pneumonia, and in some cases can decrease the

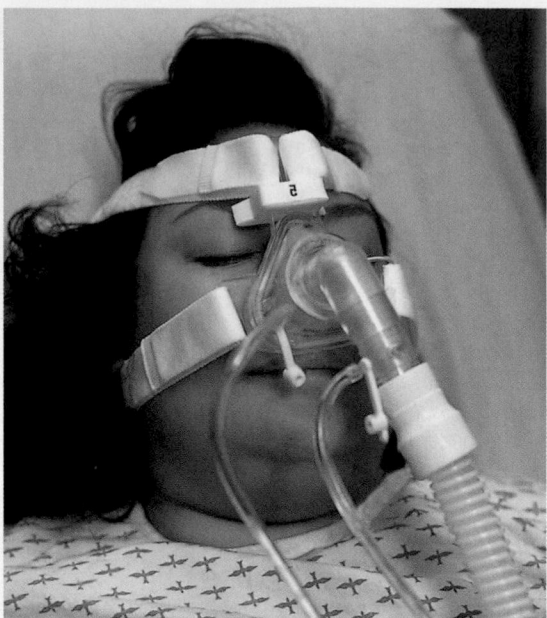

FIG 23.17 Nasal CPAP mask.

TABLE 23.2

Problems Associated With Continuous Positive Airway Pressure and Bi-Level Positive Airway Pressure

Problem	Cause
Discomfort	Mask that fits over patient's nose is tight fitting. Oxygen flow rate causes dry mucous membranes, which may cause eye irritation in full face masks.
Psychosocial	Relationship with sleep partner is difficult. There are possible sensations of claustrophobia.
Risks to skin integrity	Fit of mask causes pressure, and increased risk for skin breakdown. Patients may need to remove mask to relieve pressure.
Hypercapnia	Although CPAP improves alveolar function, which increases carbon dioxide clearance from the blood, it also causes air trapping. In some patients, this causes a rise in carbon dioxide levels. Initially the nurse needs to monitor patient's ABG levels.
Gastric distension	CPAP/BiPAP force more air into the stomach, which causes distension and discomfort.
Noise	Some patients find the older machines very noisy, interfering with sleep and leisure activities such as watching television or listening to music.

Data from Pooboni, S. K., & Markowitz, J. E. (2018). *Noninvasive ventilation procedures.* Retrieved from http://emedicine.medscape.com/article/1417959-overview.
ABG, Arterial blood gas; *BiPAP*, bi-level positive airway pressure; *CPAP*, continuous positive airway pressure.

need for sedation and the length of a patient's hospital stay (Rochwerg et al., 2017). There are also disadvantages to this type of ventilation (Table 23.2). The mask should be moulded against the patient's face and have a good seal to prevent air from leaking. This can cause feelings of claustrophobia and intolerance in patients, which can lead to issues with adherence to therapy. Wearing an overtight mask can also lead to skin breakdown, particularly on the bridge of the nose (Davidson et al., 2016).

Delegation and Collaboration

The skill of caring for a patient receiving noninvasive ventilation cannot be delegated to an unregulated care provider (UCP). However, the skills of patient positioning, therapeutic coughing, and CPAP/BiPAP mask application can be delegated to UCP, depending on the competence of the UCP to perform this skill in a particular situation and on employer policy. The nurse directs the UCP to immediately:
- Report to the nurse any changes in patient's vital signs; oxygen saturation; mental status; skin colour; or skin abrasions, bruising, or blistering around mask area.
- Report to the nurse any ventilator or CPAP/BiPAP machine alarms or patient monitor alarms.
- Report to the nurse any change in settings or patient comfort.
Interprofessional collaboration is essential when providing care for the patient. In some settings, the respiratory therapist may be responsible for managing the CPAP/BiPap machine, but the nurse retains primary responsibility for the patient. Nurses must communicate their assessment of the patient's respiratory status in response to NIPPV, as well as any concerns, to all team members to optimize patient care and safety.

Equipment

(**NOTE:** When device is used in the community setting, the equipment vendor provides the equipment.)
- Nasal mask/full face mask (with quick-release straps), or nasal pillows
- Oxygen source and tubing
- CPAP/BiPAP health care provider prescription
- Humidification source, if indicated
- BiPAP and/or CPAP ventilator
- Delivery tubing
- Pulse oximetry
- Clean gloves
- Personal protective equipment (PPE) as appropriate
- Stethoscope
- Suction equipment
- Self-inflating manual-resuscitation bag-valve-mask device

STEP	RATIONALE

ASSESSMENT

1. Identify patient using at least two person-specific identifiers (e.g., name and date of birth or medical record number) according to employer policy.

Ensures correct patient. Complies with Accreditation Canada's Required Organizational Practices and improves patient safety (Accreditation Canada, 2019).

STEP	RATIONALE

ASSESSMENT

2. Assess patient's respiratory status, including symmetry of chest wall expansion, respiratory rate and depth, oxygen saturation, sputum production, and lung sounds (see Chapter 8). When possible, ask patient about dyspnea and observe for signs and symptoms associated with hypoxia (see Box 23.1).

Decreased chest wall movement, crackles or decreased lung sounds, increased respiratory rate, increased sputum production, or signs of worsening hypoxia may make patient a candidate for NIPPV or changes in NIPPV settings.

3. Observe patient's skin over bridge of nose, around external ears, and back of head.

The mask can place pressure on skin and increase risk for skin breakdown (Schallom et al., 2015).

4. Observe patient's ability to clear and remove airway secretions by coughing.

Secretions plug the airway, decreasing amount of oxygen that is available for gas exchange in the lung.

5. Perform hand hygiene. Assess patient's vital signs and pulse oximetry; when available, note patient's most recent arterial blood gas (ABG) results.

Objectively documents patient's pH, arterial oxygen, arterial carbon dioxide, or arterial oxygen saturation. Identifies need for NIPPV.

6. Assess patient's level of consciousness, behaviours, and ability to maintain and protect airway.

Patients who cannot maintain their own airway or who are uncooperative are not candidates for NIPPV.

Clinical Decision Point *NIPPV is contraindicated in patients in cardiac or respiratory arrest, with facial deformities, hemodynamic instability, airway patency issues (including blood, emesis, secretions, or inability to protect airway), severe agitation, or impaired level of consciousness (DynaMed Plus., 2018). It may also be used in palliative and end-of-life care for dyspneic patients (Rochwerg et al., 2017).*

7. Review patient's medical record for prescription for CPAP/BiPAP and appropriate settings.

A health care provider prescription is necessary for this therapy.

8. Assess patient's and caregiver's understanding of purpose of CPAP and ongoing maintenance.

Determines level of instruction required.

NURSING DIAGNOSES

- Impaired gas exchange
- Reduced stamina
- Impaired comfort

- Sleep deprivation
- Deficient knowledge regarding purpose of CPAP

- Potential for aspiration
- Potential for impaired skin integrity

Related factors/Risk factors are individualized on the basis of patient's condition or needs.

PLANNING

1. Expected outcomes following completion of procedure:
   - Patient has increased lung expansion.

   Patient experiences improved gas exchange when lungs are expanded.

   - Patient maintains ABG levels and/or pulse oximetry (SpO_2) readings improve or remain normal.

   NIPPV delivered appropriately based on patient assessment data.

Clinical Decision Point *When first initiating CPAP/BiPAP, it is important to monitor gas exchange, especially in patients with COPD, cardiogenic pulmonary edema, or acute respiratory failure. You do this to observe for carbon dioxide retention. If patient has "do not resuscitate/allow natural death" directives, has a resuscitation care plan, or is receiving palliative care services, noninvasive ventilation may reduce breathlessness (Rochwerg et al., 2017), but careful consideration should be given to patient comfort and goals of care.*

   - Patient experiences reduction in feelings of dyspnea and work of breathing.

   In patients with acute conditions dyspnea usually improves.
   Patients with chronic pulmonary diseases may require nocturnal CPAP/BiPAP indefinitely to achieve long-term benefits.

   - Patient's vital signs and respiratory assessment parameters improve.

   Reduced pulse and respiratory rate, improved mental status, improved skin colour, and decreased use of accessory and abdominal muscles occur because patient's work of breathing decreases as level of oxygenation improves.

   - Patient's skin around bridge of nose, ears, and back of head remains clear without breakdown.

   Mask is applied properly and monitored for pressure occurrence.

   - Patient is able to describe how to use CPAP in the home setting.

   Demonstrates learning.

2. Explain to patient and caregiver the purpose and reasons for CPAP/BiPAP.

   Helps reduce sense of claustrophobia from mask. In addition, information reduces anxiety and increases cooperation and adherence to therapy.

STEP	RATIONALE

IMPLEMENTATION

1. Use interprofessional collaboration (e.g., respiratory therapist) to gather correct equipment and supplies and complete necessary charges according to employer policy.

   Ensures that you have necessary equipment to apply the NIPPV system.

2. Perform hand hygiene; apply clean gloves. Use appropriate PPE (goggles, mask, gown) if secretions are projectile or if patient is on additional precautions.

   Reduces transmission of microorganisms and exposure to pulmonary secretions.

3. Adjust bed to appropriate height and lower side rail on side nearest you. Check locks on bed wheels.

   Minimizes caregiver's muscle strain and prevents injury. Prevents bed from moving.

4. Determine correct mask size. Use masking chart to determine correct size (S, M, L, XL). **NOTE:** *It is imperative that mask have quick-release straps.*

   Mask should fit snugly over patient's nose (CPAP) or nose and/or mouth (BiPAP) to create a tight seal for delivering positive pressure. In case of emergency (e.g., vomiting, respiratory arrest), quick-release straps allow mask to be removed quickly. This system also allows patient to remove mask quickly as needed (Urden, Stacy, & Lough, 2016).

Clinical Decision Point *A patient receiving NIPPV via a full face mask should **never** be restrained. The patient must be able to remove the mask if they begin to vomit, need to remove excess secretions, or reposition a mask that has moved. A displaced mask can force the patient's jaw inward, which can obstruct the patient's airway (Urden et al., 2016).*

5. Connect CPAP/BiPAP device-delivery tubing to pressure generator.

   Ensures that patient is receiving proper NIPPV as prescribed.

6. Connect patient to pulse oximetry.

   It is important to continually monitor patient's level of oxygenation when initiating NIPPV.

7. Set CPAP/BiPAP initial settings per prescription.

   Interprofessional collaboration after initiation to determine initial patient response.

   a. *CPAP:* 5 to 15 cm H_2O is the typically prescribed pressure range (Pooboni & Markowitz, 2018).

   CPAP provides single positive pressure throughout breathing cycle, which helps to keep alveoli open at end-expiration.

   b. *BiPAP:* Inspiratory pressure is usually set at 10 to 12 cm H_2O initially and can be titrated up to 15–20 cm H_2O as patient condition dictates; expiratory pressure is usually set at 5–7 cm H_2O initially and can be titrated up as patient condition warrants (Pooboni & Markowitz, 2018).

   BiPAP supplies pressure at both inhalation and exhalation. The inhalation pressure is set according to health care provider's prescription and helps prevent airway closure. Expiratory pressure is set according to health care provider's prescription and keeps alveoli open at end-expiration (Davidson et al., 2016).

8. Select FiO_2 level as indicated and per prescription.

   Patients on NIPPV may also need supplemental oxygen to decrease signs and symptoms of hypoxia (Hill & Kramer, 2018).

9. If using humidification, ensure that humidification and heating appliances are connected and on.

   Humidification is not required but can be used if patient is experiencing dryness or thick secretions (Davidson et al., 2016).

10. Ensure that mask is fitted according to manufacturer instructions, no air leak is present, and there are no excessive pressure points.

   An ill-fitting mask leads to loss of pressure getting into airways, dyssynchrony with ventilator, and patient discomfort (Davidson et al., 2016). Pressure points around mask area can cause device-related pressure injuries (Schallom et al., 2015).

11. If patient is to use CPAP at home, have patient or caregiver demonstrate mask placement and adjustment of settings.

   Return demonstration indicates learning.

12. Dispose of supplies as appropriate, remove gloves and other PPE, and perform hand hygiene.

   Reduces transmission of microorganisms.

13. Continuous care of patient

   a. Ensure that all alarms are on and active and that ventilator circuit is intact and properly functioning.

   Ensures patient safety.

   b. Ensure that emergency resuscitation equipment is at bedside.

   Allows for quick resuscitation in case of worsening patient condition.

   c. Investigate any and all alarms that come with ventilator/CPAP machine and/or patient monitor.

   Alarms can alert the interprofessional team to problems with patient or with circuit that adversely affects patient status.

   d. Change patient's position every 2 hours or encourage patient to change position every 2 hours.

   Reduces incidence of atelectasis or pneumonia secondary to stasis of secretions.

STEP	RATIONALE
EVALUATION	
1. Observe for decreased anxiety, improved level of consciousness and cognitive abilities, decreased fatigue, and absence of dizziness.	Determines patient's response to NIPPV. As hypoxia and hypercapnia are reduced or corrected, patient's behavioural assessment parameters improve.
2. Measure vital signs, perform respiratory assessment and observe skin colour, and ask patient to describe sense of dyspnea.	Physical assessment parameters reveal oxygenation status.
3. Monitor pulse oximetry.	Documents patient's level of oxygenation. When first initiating NIPPV, it is important to obtain ABG levels in patients in whom abnormal gas exchange is suspected, after the first hour, and per employer protocol.
4. Observe skin integrity over bridge of patient's nose every 2 hours. Ask patient about level of comfort (Hill & Kramer, 2018).	Mask that is too tight causes skin breakdown, and frequent skin assessment is necessary (Pittman et al., 2015; Schallom et al., 2015).
5. If NIPPV is planned for use in home, observe and monitor patient's and caregiver's ability to manipulate CPAP or BiPAP machine/ventilator and face mask.	Determines patient's ability to perform self-care and adhere to CPAP/BiPAP plan. Success of noninvasive ventilation depends largely on patient acceptance and adherence (Gale, Jawad, Dave, et al., 2015).
6. Use Teach-Back: "I want to be sure I explained how NIPPV works and why you are receiving this therapy. Explain to me why this therapy is necessary." Develop a revised teaching plan if patient or caregiver is not able to teach back correctly.	Determines patient's and caregiver's level of understanding of instructional topic.

Unexpected Outcomes	Related Interventions
1. Patient experiences hypoxia, hypercapnia, or other signs of worsening respiratory function.	• Notify health care provider. • Reassess patient. • Determine correct settings and integrity of NIPPV.
2. Patient develops skin breakdown at mask sites or sites where mask straps are located, such as bridge of nose, nasal septum, or ears.	• Notify health care provider. • Place protective synthetic coverings on nasal bridge or areas of irritation or possible irritation to protect skin. • Fit mask appropriately to patient's face—it is tight enough to not cause air leak but loose enough to not cause skin breakdown. • Reassess patient (Davidson et al., 2016).
3. Patient states sense of smothering or claustrophobia.	• Explain system to patient again. • Demonstrate use of quick-release straps. • Have patient demonstrate use of quick-release straps. • Consider alternate mask style, if available.
4. Stomach distension secondary to positive-pressure air being forced into esophagus and trachea (Pooboni & Markowitz, 2018).	• Notify health care provider. • Be prepared for possible insertion of nasogastric tube (see Chapter 35).

Communication and Documentation

- Document respiratory assessment findings, CPAP/BiPAP settings, vital signs and pulse oximetry, patient response, patient teaching outcomes, and skin assessment.
- Document your evaluation of patient and caregiver learning.
- Communicate sudden changes in patient's behaviour or respiratory status and any decline in ABG levels or pulse oximetry values to charge nurse or health care provider.

Special Considerations

Teaching

- Teach patient and caregiver the prescribed hours to use the machine. If it is not in use for 24 hours/day, work with the patient and/or caregiver to identify the ideal time for use (e.g., bedtime, watching television).
- Teach patient and caregiver how to apply the mask, connect it to the machine, and add oxygen if prescribed.
- Instruct caregiver to bring the machine, along with a list of correct settings, to the hospital any time patient is admitted.

Care in the Community

- Using interprofessional collaboration, develop a teaching plan to ensure that the patient and caregiver have working knowledge of the system before discharge.
- When patients require home NIPPV, instruct in complete care of the CPAP/BiPAP system. Skills include assembling the system, cleaning it, and maintaining the equipment daily.
- Teach patient and caregiver what to do in case of respiratory distress or power failure.
- Notify appropriate power company so that in the event of a power outage the home is on priority for restoring power.
- Follow the safety precautions for oxygen use (see Box 23.3).

PROCEDURAL GUIDELINE 23.1 *Use of a Peak Flowmeter*

For patients who have measurable changes in the flow of their airways, such as patients with asthma or reactive airway disease, peak expiratory flow rate (PEFR) measurements are useful. The PEFR is the maximum flow that a patient forces out during one quick, forced expiration and is measured in litres per minute. These measurements are used as an objective indicator of a patient's current status or the effectiveness of treatment. Decreased PEFR may indicate the need for further interventions, such as increased doses of bronchodilators, anti-inflammatory medications, or even seeking emergency medical attention. Normal PEFR values vary according to a person's age, gender, and size.

Patients with asthma perform PEFR measures in the home to monitor the status of their airways. Asthma Canada (n.d.) recommends that patients measure their PEFR three times in succession, and then record the best reading. This can be done once or twice daily, before and after taking asthma medicines, and other times recommended by their health care provider.

Delegation and Collaboration

Initial assessment of the patient's condition is a nursing responsibility and cannot be delegated. The skills of follow-up PEFR measurements in a stable patient can be delegated to an unregulated care provider (UCP), depending on the competence of the UCP to perform this skill in a particular situation and on employer policy. The nurse instructs the UCP to:

- Report immediately to the nurse the patient's difficulty breathing or decrease in PEFR measurement.

Equipment

- Peak flowmeter (Fig. 23.18)
- Patient diary/action plan (if appropriate)

Procedural Steps

1. Review medical record for patient's baseline PEFR (if available).
2. Assess previous PEFR readings and the target set by patient's health care provider.
3. Help patient to stand or to high-Fowler's position or any other position that promotes optimum lung expansion.
4. Assess patient's baseline knowledge of when and how to use PEFR and correct response to results.
5. Slide clean mouthpiece into base of the numbered scale.
6. Instruct patient to take a deep breath through the nose and slowly blow out through the mouth. Have patient take a second deep breath.
7. Have patient place meter mouthpiece in the mouth and close lips, making a firm seal.
8. Have patient blow out as hard and fast as possible through the mouth only.
9. Monitor PEFR results and assess if patient is in expected range.
10. Inform patient of their individualized acceptable range and mark on meter.
11. If patient is to record PEFR at home, have them demonstrate how to record it accurately on chart using "traffic light" pattern.

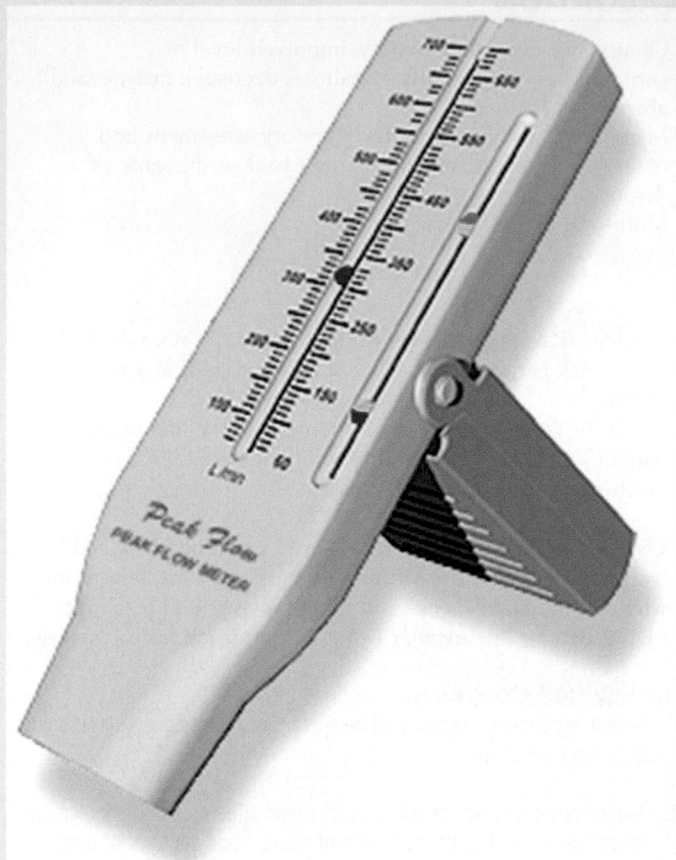

FIG 23.18 Peak flowmeter. (*Courtesy Philips Respironics.*)

A system of asthma zones—green, yellow, and red—is commonly used. Green indicates that the PEFR is 80 to 100% of patient's personal best value and means that they should continue with the currently prescribed treatment regimen. Yellow indicates that the PEFR is 60 to 80% of the personal best and that the person should add the prescribed quick-relief medication to the treatment regimen and continue with their daily long-term control medications. Red indicates that the PEFR is less than 60% of the patient's personal best and that the person should take the prescribed quick-relief medication and seek medical attention (The Lung Association, n.d.) (Fig. 23.19).

12. **Use Teach-Back:** "I want to make sure that I showed you how to correctly measure your PEFR. Show me how you would use this PEFR device." Develop a revised teaching plan if patient or caregiver is not able to teach back correctly.
13. Compare patient's PEFR with their personal best.
14. Record PEFR measurement before and after therapy and patient's ability and effort to perform PEFR in electronic health record (EHR) or chart.
15. Instruct patient to clean unit weekly following manufacturer instructions.

PROCEDURAL GUIDELINE 23.1 *Use of a Peak Flowmeter—cont'd*

Asthma Action Plan

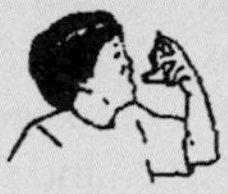

Name: _____

Doctor: _____ **Date:** _____

Phone for doctor or clinic: _____

Emergency contact phone and name: _____

You can use the colors of a traffic light to help learn about your asthma medicines.

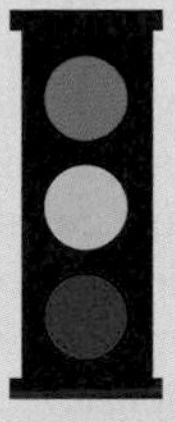

1. **Green** means **Go.**
   Use preventive medicine.
2. **Yellow** means **Caution.**
   Use quick-relief medicine.
3. **Red** means **Stop.**
   Get help from a doctor.

1. Green — Go

- Breathing is good
- No cough or wheeze
- Can work and play

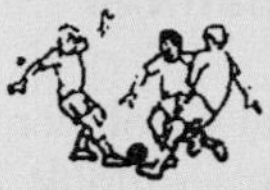

Peak flow number

_____ to _____

Personal best peak flow _____

Use preventive medicine.

Medicine	How much to take	When to take it

5 to 60 minutes before exercise, use this medicine:

_____

2. Yellow — Caution

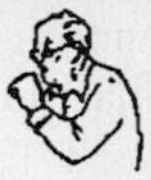

Cough 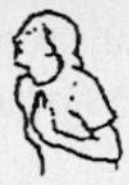 Wheeze 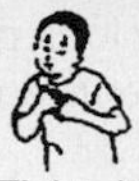 Tight chest

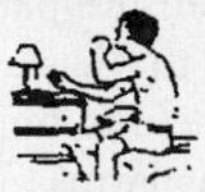

Wake up at night

Peak flow number _____ to _____

(50% to 80% of my best peak flow)

Take quick-relief medicine to keep an asthma attack from getting bad

Medicine	How much to take	When to take it
(short-acting beta$_2$ agonist)		

If symptoms return to Green Zone after 1 hour of taking above quick-relief medication, take _____ (medicine) and _____ (medicine).

If symptoms **do not** return to Green Zone after 1 hour of taking the quick-relief medication, take _____ (medicine) and add _____ (medicine).
(short-acting beta$_2$ agonist)   (oral steroid)

Call your doctor if symptoms do not improve within _____ hours after taking the oral steroid or if your symptoms are in the Red Zone.

3. Red — Stop — Danger

- Medicine is not helping
- Breathing is hard and fast
- Nose opens wide
- Can't walk
- Ribs show
- Can't talk well

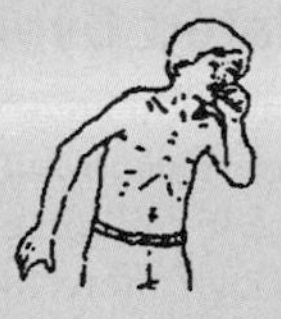

Peak flow number

_____ to _____

(50% or less of personal best)

Get help from a doctor now!
Take these medicines until you talk with the doctor.

Medicine	How much to take	When to take it
(short-acting beta$_2$ agonist)		
(oral steroid)		

Go to the emergency department immediately or call the ambulance if you cannot reach your doctor and you are still in the Red Zone after 15 minutes.

These signs signal **DANGER:**
- Difficulty walking or breathing
- Mental confusion
- Fingernails or lips are blue

Call the ambulance.

FIG 23.19 Asthma action plan. (*From Hockenberry, M. J., & Wilson, D. [2015]. Wong's nursing care of infants and children [10th ed.]. St. Louis: Mosby.*)

✦ SKILL 23.5   Care of a Patient on a Mechanical Ventilator

Mechanical ventilation is a life-saving therapy used for patients who have an inability to protect their airway or an illness that leads to respiratory failure. It can be used for a short period of time or as a long-term means of support for those who cannot support their own respiratory effort, such as those with neuromuscular disorders (Lewis et al., 2019). Patients receiving mechanical ventilation are most often in a critical care unit but may be seen in skilled nursing facilities or other community settings. The nurse must collaborate with the respiratory therapist when caring for patients receiving mechanical ventilation. At many institutions, the respiratory therapist is charged with caring for and monitoring the ventilator.

There are two types of mechanical ventilation: positive pressure and negative pressure. Positive-pressure ventilation is the usual method of ventilation that delivers a positive pressure to inflate the lungs (Fig. 23.20). An artificial airway such as an endotracheal (ET) tube or tracheostomy tube is necessary for positive-pressure mechanical ventilation (see Chapter 25). Multiple complications are associated with positive-pressure ventilation, including decreased cardiac output, aspiration, barotrauma, and ventilator-associated events (VAEs) such as ventilator-associated pneumonia (VAP) (see Chapter 25). Be alert for these side effects.

Negative-pressure ventilation is a noninvasive, negative-pressure ventilation technique that mimics normal physiological ventilation. It is used for the chronic management of patients with primary neuromuscular illnesses that interfere with normal respiratory muscle function, such as multiple sclerosis and muscular dystrophy. It generally is not used during acute illness. The patient is fitted with a poncho or shell that is connected to the ventilator. Air is removed from between the patient's chest wall and the interior wall of the poncho or shell, causing the negative pressure that allows the chest to pull outward, in turn causing the patient to inhale. Exhalation is passive. A patient using negative-pressure ventilation does not need an artificial airway (Lewis et al., 2019).

The skill described in this chapter focuses on positive-pressure mechanical ventilation frequently used in acute, subacute, and some selective community care settings.

Using the Mechanical Ventilator

Mechanical ventilation controls or helps a patient's respirations when they are unable to maintain adequate gas exchange because of respiratory or ventilatory failure. The ventilator takes over the physical work of moving air into and out of the lungs, but it does not replace or alter the physiological function of the lung. Mechanical ventilation maintains or improves ventilation, oxygenation, and breathing pattern. Patients with impaired ventilation have low oxygen level (hypoxemia), retained carbon dioxide (hypercapnia), and difficulty breathing.

Ventilator Settings

The mechanical ventilator has a number of settings to adjust the amount of oxygen delivered, the number of breaths per minute, the amount of tidal volume, the time for inspiration and expiration, and the pressure at which each breath is delivered. The goal of providing oxygenation is to maintain a PaO_2 of >60 mm Hg using an FiO_2 of 40% or less. Table 23.3 lists the ventilator parameters with which you need to become familiar to care for a patient on positive-pressure mechanical ventilation.

Modes of Positive-Pressure Mechanical Ventilation

There are many different modes of mechanical ventilation to support different conditions and physiological processes (Table 23.4).

It is important that patients remain on mechanical ventilation only as long as necessary because there is an increased mortality risk associated with positive-pressure ventilation. In addition, as the length of time needed for mechanical ventilation increases, there is an increased risk of failure to wean from the ventilator (Urden et al., 2016). Caring for a patient on mechanical ventilation and weaning from it require interprofessional collaboration.

Alarms

There are several alarms on the ventilator to ensure patient safety. Each ventilator is a little different; however, the basic alarms are similar. Alarms common to all ventilators include high-pressure, low-pressure, low-exhaled volume, and oxygen alarms (Table 23.5). Nurses need to know how to respond to the ventilator alarms and which nursing actions are required to preserve the patient's respiratory status. The two most frequent alarms are the high-pressure and low-pressure alarms. The high-pressure alarm is usually set at 10 to 20 cm greater than the peak inspiratory pressure (Lewis et al., 2019). When this alarm sounds, it indicates that the ventilator has met resistance to delivering the tidal volume and requires more pressure to inflate the lungs. The low-pressure alarm sounds when the ventilator has no resistance to inflating the lung. All ventilator alarms require immediate nursing intervention to prevent patient harm.

Ventilator-Associated Events

VAP, a type of VAE, has an estimated 5.8% mortality rate in patients receiving mechanical ventilation and costs the Canadian health care system an estimated $46 million each year (Muscedere, Martin, & Heyland, 2008), although more recent Canadian estimates are limited. The simplified way to identify VAP includes observing deterioration in the patient's respiratory status after a period of stability while on the ventilator, objective evidence of inflammation or infection, and laboratory evidence of respiratory infection. A patient can be considered for VAP only after they have received mechanical ventilation for more than 2 calendar days (Centers for Disease Control and Prevention [CDC], 2019).

In an attempt to decrease the incidence of VAEs, practice bundles have been developed and implemented at health care facilities across the country. The Canadian Patient Safety Institute's (2012)

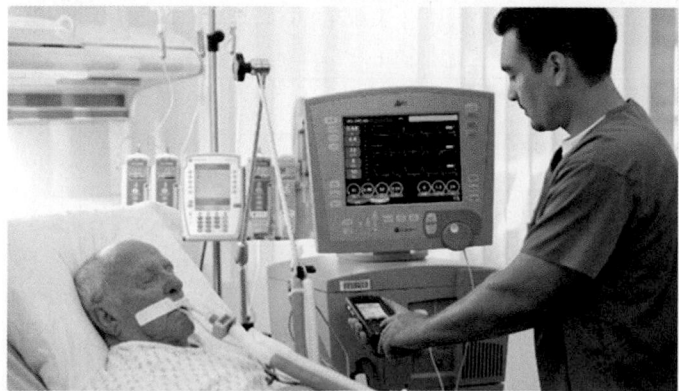

FIG 23.20 An intubated patient on a positive-pressure ventilator. (*Courtesy and © Becton, Dickinson and Company.*)

TABLE 23.3

Ventilator Parameters

Parameter	Definition	Ventilator Setting
Tidal volume (V_t)	Amount of air inspired and expired with each breath; can be set by ventilator or can measure patient's own spontaneous breaths	<10 mL/kg of patient body weight 4–6 mL/kg in patients with ARDS to avoid lung injury
Respiratory rate (R or RR)	Number of breaths delivered by ventilator per minute	Usually 10–20 breaths/min Usually adjusted with a set V_t to maintain specific $PaCO_2$, and depending on clinical goals (rest vs. weaning)
Fraction of inspired oxygen (FiO_2)	Amount of oxygen that patient receives	Ideally less than 50% to maintain PaO_2 >60 mm Hg and SpO_2 >90%
Positive end-expiratory pressure (PEEP)	Positive pressure applied at end-expiration of ventilator breaths to open alveoli and improve oxygenation	5 cm H_2O approximates physiological PEEP. May require higher levels (10–20 cm H_2O) in respiratory failure (e.g., refractory hypoxemia). If patient has a PEEP greater than 10 cm H_2O, the circuit should not be interrupted.
Sensitivity	Determines patient's inspiratory effort required to trigger the ventilator	A breath can be triggered by a change in either flow or pressure. Pressure trigger is usually 1–1 cm below baseline. Flow trigger is usually 1–3 L/min below baseline.
I:E ratio	Comparison of inspiratory (I) to expiratory (E) time	Example: Inspiration 0.5 seconds, expiration 1 second, then I : E = 1:2. Usually set at 1:2 to 1:3 because expiration is typically longer than inspiration. Can use inverse ratios for certain disease states such as ARDS in attempt to open alveoli.
Exhaled minute ventilation (V_E)	Measures exhaled minute ventilations in litres	Alarm set at 15% greater than patient's average V_E

Data from Urden, L., et al. (2016). *Priorities in critical care nursing* (7th ed.). St. Louis: Mosby; and Gallagher, J. (2017). Invasive mechanical ventilation (through an artificial airway). In D. L. Wiegand (Ed.), *AACN procedure manual for high acuity, progressive, and critical care* (7th ed., pp. 226–248). St. Louis: Elsevier.
ARDS, Acute respiratory distress syndrome; *PEEP,* positive end-expiratory pressure.

TABLE 23.4

Modes of Mechanical Ventilation

Mode	Ventilator Controls	Patient Controls	Indications	Nursing Considerations
Continuous positive airway pressure (CPAP)	Positive pressure during entire respiratory cycle.	Spontaneous breathing	Hypoxemic respiratory failure Weaning.	Helps open alveoli at end expiration, thereby improving oxygenation. Patients with COPD may tire after long hours of CPAP and require increased pressure support. Used in both invasive and noninvasive ventilation modes.
Pressure support ventilation (PSV)	Preset amount of positive pressure.	Patient determines rate and tidal volume	Augmenting a spontaneously breathing patient's inspiratory efforts.	Helps overcome resistance of airway and ventilator tubing. Reduces patient work of breathing and improves ventilator-patient synchrony.
Assist-control (AC) or continuous mandatory ventilation (CMV)	Backup control delivers preset number of breaths at set volume.	Initiation of breathing	*Volume-controlled CMV:* patients with weak respiratory muscles. *Pressure-controlled CMV:* patients with increased airway resistance or decreased lung compliance.	Watch for volutrauma in volume-controlled CMV. Watch for hypercapnia in pressure-controlled CMV. Sedation may be needed to control respiratory rate.
Synchronized intermittent mandatory ventilation (SIMV)	Set number of breaths at specified volume.	Some patients breathe spontaneously between SIMV breaths at volumes differing from those set.	Primary method of ventilation in many settings.	Requires frequent monitoring during weaning from mechanical ventilation. May increase patient's work of breathing.

Continued

TABLE 23.4

Modes of Mechanical Ventilation—cont'd

Mode	Ventilator Controls	Patient Controls	Indications	Nursing Considerations
Pressure-regulated volume-control ventilation (PRVCV or PRVC)	A preset tidal volume at the lowest possible airway pressure (pressure will not exceed preset maximum limit).		Patient with changing pulmonary mechanics and dynamics.	Variation of CMV combining the feature of both volume- and pressure-control settings. Potential complications are limited when compared with AC or pressure controlled–intermittent mandatory ventilation (PC-IMV) modes.
Airway pressure release ventilation (APRV)	Inspiratory and expiratory levels of CPAP are applied for predetermined periods of time.	Spontaneous breathing mode, spontaneous breathing can occur at both levels.	Recruits alveoli with decreased risk of high peak pressures, decreasing risk of barotrauma.	Patient should be monitored for hypercapnia.
High-Frequency				
High-frequency jet ventilation (HFJV)	Delivers gas rapidly under low pressure via special injector cannula. Delivers 100–600 cycles/min with lower-than-normal tidal volumes.		Uncommon in adults; more commonly used in neonates.	Patient on any mode of high-frequency ventilation requires continuous sedation and neuromuscular blocking agent administration. Requires intensive monitoring and care.
High-frequency oscillatory ventilation (HFOV)	Delivers 900–3000 cycles/min with very small tidal volumes. Airway pressure controlled.		Most common high-frequency type. Uncommon in adults; more commonly used in infants and children.	Maintains alveolar ventilation with low airway pressure; useful for treating esophageal or bronchopleural fistulas; helps avert barotraumas in high-risk patients if used early in treatment. Requires use of continuous sedation and neuromuscular blocking agent. Requires intensive monitoring and care.

Data from Urden, L., et al. (2016). *Priorities in critical care nursing* (7th ed.). St. Louis: Mosby.
COPD, Chronic obstructive pulmonary disease.

TABLE 23.5

Troubleshooting Mechanical Ventilation

Ventilator Alarm	Possible Causes	Nursing Interventions
Sudden increase in peak airway pressure (high-pressure alarm)	Coughing Airway plugging/excess secretions Changes in patient position Pneumothorax Incorrect ET tube position Kinked ventilator circuit Excessive water in ventilator circuit Patient biting tube Patient not in synchrony with ventilator Ventilator malfunction	Clear secretions by suctioning. Reposition patient. Assess breath sounds and chest wall movement. Verify placement of ET tube. Verify centimetre level of ET tube. Check circuit; unkink tubing. Drain ventilator tubing. Insert bite block. Sedate patient. Notify health care provider if interventions are not effective.
Gradual increase in peak airway pressure	Decreasing lung compliance Exacerbation of acute process	Evaluate breath sounds; suction. Check for reversible causes: airway plugging, bronchospasm. Notify health care provider if interventions are not effective.
Decrease in peak airway pressure (low-pressure alarm)	Patient disconnected from ventilator Leak in ventilator circuit ET tube displaced into pharynx Cuff not inflated properly Improved lung compliance Decrease in amount of secretions	Check for disconnection. Evaluate circuit connections; tighten loose connections. Assess cuff for appropriate pressure (see Skill 25.4).
Change in minute ventilation or tidal volume	Leak in ET cuff Patient stops spontaneously breathing Other conditions that trigger low- or high-pressure alarms	Check cuff seal (see Skill 25.4). Evaluate patient.
Increase in respiratory rate	Patient anxiety Increased metabolic demand Hypoxia	Reassure patient. Evaluate body temperature, heart rate, and rhythm. Monitor pulse oximetry.

TABLE 23.5

Troubleshooting Mechanical Ventilation—cont'd

Ventilator Alarm	Possible Causes	Nursing Interventions
Apnea	Respiratory arrest Oversedation Incidental extubation	Reverse/discontinue sedating medications. Provide breaths via self-inflating resuscitation bag. Prepare for reintubation if tube is dislodged and patient requires it.
Ventilator inoperative or low battery	Equipment malfunction Machine not plugged in	Plug in machine. Notify respiratory therapist. Provide breaths via self-inflating resuscitation bag if necessary.

Data from Urden, L., et al. (2016). *Priorities in critical care nursing* (7th ed.). St. Louis: Mosby; and Gallagher, J. (2017). Invasive mechanical ventilation (through an artificial airway). In D. L. Wiegand (Ed.), *AACN procedure manual for high acuity, progressive, and critical care* (7th ed., pp. 226–248). St. Louis: Elsevier.
ET, Endotracheal.

initiative, *Safer Healthcare Now!* has developed a widely used ventilator bundle (see Box 23.2).

Another care practice that is implemented for patients receiving mechanical ventilation is the ABCDE bundle. This bundle includes *a*wakening and *b*reathing coordination, *d*elirium monitoring and management, and early *e*xercise and mobility. Although this care bundle has not been used in practice for very long, there is some evidence of a decreased amount of time spent on the ventilator, decreased amount of delirium, and lower mortality when it is used (Lamb, 2015; Urden et al., 2016).

Other interventions exist, although they are not listed specifically within the care bundles being used to decrease the risk of VAEs. One of these interventions is to maintain continuous ET tube cuff pressure between 20 and 30 cm H_2O pressure to decrease the risk of microaspiration of oral secretions and gastric contents or tracheal ischemic lesions (Rouzé, Jaillette, Poissy, et al., 2017). Refer to Skill 25.4 for directions for this procedure. Other interventions include specially coated ET tubes, using ET tubes that allow for drainage of subglottic secretions (Rouzé et al., 2017; Urden et al., 2016), and turning and repositioning the patient every 2 hours.

Delegation and Collaboration

The skill of caring for a patient on a mechanical ventilator cannot be delegated to an unregulated care provider (UCP). The nurse directs the UCP to:
- Report immediately to the nurse any change in the patient's respiratory status, vital signs, or oxygen saturation and if patient indicates breathlessness.
- Inform the nurse immediately if any of the ventilator alarms sound.
- Help in daily care, such as bathing and repositioning the patient.

Interprofessional collaboration is essential in optimizing care and ensuring patient safety. In some settings, the respiratory therapist may be responsible for managing the ventilator, but the nurse retains primary responsibility for the patient. As well, in some settings the health care provider may prescribe the ventilator settings, whereas some employer policies will dictate the settings.

Using interprofessional collaboration, the nurse must continually communicate assessment findings of the patient's respiratory status in response to mechanical ventilation, and any concerns, to maintain patient safety and provide the best care possible.

Equipment

- Artificial airway
- Appropriate mechanical ventilator
- Heater and humidifier for circuit
- Oxygen source
- Pulse oximetry (SpO_2) probe and monitor
- Electrocardiogram (ECG) monitoring (if in a critical care unit or by institution policy)
- Capnography ($EtCO_2$) window and monitor (if available)
- Stethoscope
- 5- or 10-mL syringe
- Oral airway/bite block, as needed
- Manual self-inflating resuscitation bag (bag-valve-mask) with oxygen connecting tubing and flowmeter
- Appropriately sized resuscitation face mask
- Cuff pressure monitoring device
- Sedation monitoring scale (e.g., Richmond Agitation Sedation Scale) if patient is receiving sedation
- Clean gloves
- Appropriate personal protective equipment (PPE) (goggles, if splash risk; mask and gown if patient is on additional precautions)
- Suction equipment at bedside (in-line/individual catheters)
- Suction equipment for subglottic and oral suctioning
- Chlorhexidine solution (0.12%), oral swab, and toothbrush for oral care
- Method for patient communication (e.g., letter/picture board, common word lists)
- Ventilator flow sheet to document ventilator changes and settings (may be a paper flow sheet part of the electronic health record (EHR)

STEP	RATIONALE

ASSESSMENT

1. Identify patient using at least two person-specific identifiers (e.g., name and date of birth or account number, according to employer policy).

Ensures correct patient. Complies with Accreditation Canada's *Required Organizational Practices* and improves patient safety (Accreditation Canada, 2019).

STEP	RATIONALE

ASSESSMENT

2. Assess patient's level of consciousness (LOC) and ability to cooperate with mechanical ventilation and tolerate need for special positioning, such as head of bed (HOB) at 30 degrees.

Determines patient's ability to cooperate and understand aspects of care. Anxious and combative patients may require sedation to tolerate mechanical ventilation.

3. Assess patient's need for sedation (check employer policy).

Sedation is often used to improve patient tolerance of the ventilator (Davidson et al., 2016)

Clinical Decision Point *When patients on mechanical ventilation become excessively anxious or combative or try to override the ventilator, sedation is often used. Be aware that sedation is associated with increased length of time on the ventilator, increased risk of delirium, and increased mortality (Davidson et al., 2016). Follow employer policy for administering sedation agent and monitoring sedation levels.*

4. Perform hand hygiene. Assess patient's respiratory status, including symmetry of chest wall expansion, respiratory rate and depth, sputum production, and lung sounds (see Chapter 8), and assess for signs and symptoms associated with hypoxia (see Box 23.1).

Reduces transmission of microorganisms. Decreased chest wall movement; crackles, decreased, or absent lung sounds; increased respiratory rate; increased sputum production; or signs of worsening hypoxia indicate need for mechanical ventilation or changes in current ventilator settings to improve oxygenation and ventilation.

5. Assess patient's cardiovascular condition, including blood pressure, heart rate, regularity of heart rate, and quality of peripheral pulses (see Chapter 8).

Positive-pressure mechanical ventilation can increase patient's intrathoracic pressure. This can cause a decrease in cardiac output and cardiovascular function (Davidson et al., 2016).

6. Assess for signs and symptoms of inadvertent extubation (able to vocalize, low-pressure ventilator alarms, decreased or absent breath sounds, gastric distension, changes in ET tube depth according to markings, changes in $EtCO_2$ waveform and values, patient holding tube with hand).

Inadvertent extubation can lead to a decrease in patient oxygenation and cardiopulmonary status.

Clinical Decision Point *Sometimes patients tolerate inadvertent extubation. The nurse needs to carefully assess the patient and be prepared to apply a different type of oxygen-delivery device (nasal cannula, face mask, or noninvasive positive-pressure ventilation [NIPPV]) or to reintubate the patient (Hill & Kramer, 2018). The nurse may need to perform bag-valve-mask ventilation until a health care provider who can reintubate the patient arrives in the room.*

7. Check ventilator, $EtCO_2$ (if available), SpO_2, and ventilator and cardiac alarms at beginning of each shift and periodically throughout care and compare with health care provider prescription.

Verifies that ventilator settings are as prescribed. Ensures patient safety.

8. Apply clean gloves and verify placement of artificial airway through auscultation of lung sounds, verification of distal tip marking on ET tube and/or $EtCO_2$ value. Determine that tube is secure and stable (see Chapter 25).

Prevents migration of tube into right or left bronchus and accidental extubation.

Clinical Decision Point *When patients have periodic chest X-ray film examinations, verify placement of the artificial airway.*

a. Auscultate over trachea for presence of air leak. When air leak is present, you will hear movement of air over trachea. Assess and compare inhaled and exhaled tidal volumes as measured by ventilator.

Cuff of artificial airway needs to be inflated to create a seal for positive-pressure ventilation to occur.

b. Use cuff pressure monitoring device.

Cuff pressure of ET tube should be between 20 and 30 cm H_2O (Rouzé et al., 2017). Use 10-mL syringe to inflate or deflate cuff to achieve desired pressure.

Clinical Decision Point *ET tube cuff pressures need to be monitored carefully. Pressures that are too low lead to microaspiration of oral and subglottic secretions, which increase the patient's risk of developing VAP. If the cuff pressures are too high, the patient is at risk of developing tracheal mucosa damage (Rouzé et al., 2017). Hypopharyngeal suctioning should be performed before a cuff is deflated to decrease risk of aspiration of secretions (Hyzy, 2018).*

9. Ensure that suctioning system is functioning properly.

It is important to know that the emergency equipment is functioning before needing it (Schreiber, 2015).

10. Observe for patent airway and, if necessary, remove airway secretions by suctioning (see Chapter 25). Remove and dispose of gloves and perform hand hygiene.

Secretions plug airway, decreasing amount of oxygen that is available for gas exchange in lung. Secretions also occlude T tube or tracheostomy collar, impeding oxygen delivery to patient.

STEP	RATIONALE

ASSESSMENT

Clinical Decision Point *Routine suctioning of the patient should be avoided. Indications for suctioning include coarse crackles auscultated over trachea, the presence of a saw-tooth pattern in the pressure and flow curves on the ventilator, increased peak inspiratory pressures or decreased tidal volumes, decrease in patient's SpO_2, arterial blood gas (ABG) changes, visible secretions in the airway, inability of patient to cough effectively, or suspected aspiration (Sole, Bennett, & Ashworth, 2016).*

STEP	RATIONALE
11. Assess integrity of patient's oral mucous membrane and skin around tube stabilization device (Pittman et al., 2015).	Provides baseline to recognize signs of oral mucous membrane or skin breakdown.
12. If available, note patient's most recent ABG results or SpO_2. Determine if any factors have changed during mechanical ventilation.	Objectively documents patient's pH, arterial oxygen, arterial carbon dioxide, or arterial oxygen saturation.
13. Determine method for communication with patient. If possible, review previous communication techniques with patient and caregiver.	Patients with an artificial airway and mechanical ventilation cannot communicate verbally. Practise person-centred care and choose a communication tool based on patient preference, and reassess and document its effectiveness regularly (ten Hoorn, Elbers, Girbes, et al., 2016).
14. Review patient's medical record for prescription for mechanical ventilation, noting mode of ventilation, respiratory rate, oxygen setting, pressure support, positive end-expiratory pressures (PEEP), and tidal volume.	Mechanical ventilation and changes in ventilator settings require health care provider prescription. Knowing mode of ventilation should inform nurse on priority values to monitor.

NURSING DIAGNOSES

- Ineffective airway clearance
- Impaired spontaneous ventilation
- Ineffective breathing pattern
- Impaired gas exchange

- Dysfunctional ventilatory weaning response
- Impaired verbal communication

- Potential for infection
- Potential for impaired oral mucous membrane

Related factors/Risk factors are individualized on the basis of patient's condition or needs.

PLANNING

STEP	RATIONALE
1. Expected outcomes following completion of procedure:	
• Patient has improved lung expansion.	As patient's lungs and lung mechanics improve, lung expansion increases.
• Patient maintains or has improving partial pressures of oxygen (PaO_2) and carbon dioxide ($PaCO_2$), as well as pH levels and oxygen saturation within normal range or at patient baseline.	Verifies that ventilator settings are effective in improving or maintaining patient's level of oxygenation and ventilation.
• Patient's vital signs and respiratory assessment parameters improve.	Reduced pulse and respiratory rate, improved mental status, improved skin colour, and decreased use of accessory and abdominal muscles occur because patient's work of breathing decreases as level of oxygenation improves.
• Patient experiences reduction in feelings of dyspnea and work of breathing. **NOTE:** Dyspnea scales, such as the Medical Research Council Dyspnea Scale, are available to provide more objective data.	Indicates effectiveness of therapy.
• Patient uses communication board, paper and pencil, mobile device, or computer to state needs.	Appropriate communication system matches patient's abilities. Helps to express patient's needs and wishes (ten Hoorn et al., 2016).
2. Explain ventilator system to patient and caregiver and be sure to include purpose of and reasons for initiation of mechanical ventilation.	Reinforces need for ventilation to improve patient condition.
3. Position patient with HOB elevated 30 to 45 degrees (unless contraindicated).	Positioning patients with HOB elevated 30 to 45 degrees or higher is thought to reduce gastric reflux, thereby decreasing risk for aspiration and VAP (CPSI, 2016; Wang, Li, Yang, et al., 2016).

STEP	RATIONALE

IMPLEMENTATION

1. Perform hand hygiene; apply clean gloves. Apply PPE (mask, gown, and goggles if secretions are projectile or if patient is on additional precautions).	Reduces transmission of microorganisms and exposure to pulmonary secretions.
2. Attach mechanical ventilator to ET or tracheostomy tube if not already attached or connected to patient. Observe for proper functioning of mechanical ventilator.	Connects artificial airway to ventilator and ensures closed system, which enables ventilator to exert appropriate pressure or volume to meet patient's oxygen and ventilation demands.

Clinical Decision Point *The mechanical ventilator requires programming of accurate settings before attaching to the patient. This is most often the responsibility of the respiratory therapist as prescribed by the health care provider; it requires interprofessional collaborative and is a nursing responsibility.*

3. Verify that ET or tracheostomy tube is properly positioned during an inspiratory and expiratory cycle by listening to both lungs and assessing chest wall symmetry. Capnography can also be used to verify proper placement (Hyzy, 2018). When chest X-ray film is available, observe tube placement.	Properly placed artificial airway ensures that both lungs are ventilated equally. Improper airway placement leads to unilateral lung ventilation or inadequate oxygenation.
4. Observe patient for synchronization with mechanical ventilation and response to therapy.	Ensures that patient is comfortable using ventilator and has not experienced any adverse hemodynamic effects.
5. Monitor heart rate, blood pressure, respiratory rate, temperature, and cardiac rhythm routinely (see employer policy).	Implementation of mechanical ventilation results in decreased venous return and associated hemodynamic changes. The patient is also at increased risk for developing an infection (Waters & Muscedere, 2015); thus, temperature needs to be monitored.
6. Reassess and mark level of ET tube at lips or nares (see Chapter 25). Ensure that ET tube is secured.	Provides measure to compare with baseline for depth of tube placement. ET tube must be placed through vocal cords into trachea. Helps to ensure that tube is not too close to carina or in right main-stem bronchus. ET tube may be secured with use of tape or commercial tube holder.
7. Ensure that suction equipment is set up and functioning, including oral suctioning (see Chapter 25).	The nurse needs to provide airway care and suctioning of ET or tracheostomy tube as needed to prevent plugging of airway and reduce risk for infection.
8. Reposition patient regularly (minimum of every 2 hours), maintaining an HOB elevation of 30 to 45 degrees. In some instances, patient may even be placed in prone position. Monitor SpO$_2$ levels during and after positioning.	Elevated HOB positioning improves oxygenation and ventilation. It reduces stasis of secretions, which can lead to atelectasis or pneumonia. In addition, HOB elevation reduces risk for VAP (Wang et al., 2016). SpO$_2$ drops during position change and but should recover once patient is completely positioned. A sustained drop in SpO$_2$, indicates that patient is unable to tolerate that particular position at that time. Regular turning reduces risk of pressure injury development involving the skin.
	Some patients cannot safely have the HOB elevated. Prone positioning requires assistance of four or five staff members or a specialty bed, and may reduce VAP in patients with acute respiratory failure (Kallet, 2015). **NOTE:** A systematic review shows no clear evidence on the effectiveness of routine lateral repositioning or the effects of a single turn for critically ill patients (Hewitt, Bucknall, & Faraone, 2016).

Clinical Decision Point *Assess oral cavity for need for suctioning before repositioning. After repositioning, check cuff pressures and level of ET tube.*

9. Collaborate with health care provider frequently about status of patient, response to therapy, and ongoing monitoring.	Assesses oxygenation status and continued need for mechanical ventilation.
a. Monitor SpO$_2$ continuously.	Provides ability to continually assess oxygenation levels.

STEP	RATIONALE

IMPLEMENTATION

b. Monitor $EtCO_2$ continually (if available and indicated) and serial ABG levels to detect possible overventilation or inadequate alveolar ventilation.

Overventilation causes respiratory alkalosis from decreased carbon dioxide. Inadequate alveolar ventilation causes respiratory acidosis from increased carbon dioxide retention.

c. Obtain ABG levels with changes in patient's condition or ventilator changes per provider prescription.

Provides more accurate measure of oxygen saturation and PaO_2 and $PaCO_2$.

10. Perform hourly safety checks on patient and ventilator system:

a. Make sure that patient can reach call light.

Provides mechanism for patient to contact health care personnel.

b. Check security of all ventilator connections; make sure that alarms are all turned on, including both high- and low-pressure alarms and volume alarms.

Ensures continuous safe and proper functioning of ventilator system. Enables you to identify and correct problems in a timely manner.

c. Verify that all ventilator settings are correct and correspond to health care provider prescription.

Maintains integrity of system and ensures that all settings are consistent with health care provider prescription.

d. Check and refill humidifier as needed. Check corrugated tubing for condensation; drain away from patient but not into humidifier and appropriately discard liquid.

Ensures continuous humidification. Condensation that returns to humidifier can cause possible bacterial contamination. Condensation that drains into patient can cause pneumonia or severe coughing episode that can lead to increased patient distress (CPSI, 2012).

e. When present, observe temperature gauges on panel of mechanical ventilator, making sure that gas is delivered at correct temperature. Desired temperature of inspired gas is 35° to 37°C (95° to 98.6°F).

The temperature of inspired gas artificially alters patient's body temperature.

11. Perform mouth care at least every 12 hours (can be every 1–2 hours, depending on patent status) with chlorhexidine (CPSI, 2016) to brush teeth, gums, and tongue with soft toothbrush. Water-based moisturizer should be applied every 2–4 hours (see Chapter 18).

VAP is common, and it is associated with microaspiration of oropharyngeal secretions. Frequent mouth care reduces patient's risk for VAP. Oral care helps reduce risk for pneumonias (Hess, 2018).

12. Insert bite block if patient bites ET tube.

Prevents patient from occluding airway. Oral mucous membranes and tongue need to be monitored for any signs of breakdown.

13. Administer sedating drugs only as prescribed.

Sedating medications help to keep patient comfortable and breathe in synchrony with ventilator, but in excess, they can increase length of critical care stay (Davidson et al., 2016).

14. Perform daily interruption in sedation; assess readiness to extubate.

This step is supportive of the CPSI (2012) ventilator bundle. Sometimes patients need to be sedated to keep them comfortable or to increase synchrony with ventilator (Davidson et al., 2016). Providing daily interruptions of sedation allows assessment for weaning, delirium, and readiness to extubate (CPSI, 2012).

15. Administer medications (H_2 antagonists, sucralfate, or proton pump inhibitors [PPIs]) as prescribed for peptic ulcer disease (PUD) prophylaxis.

PUD prophylaxis is standard of care in most critical care settings to prevent stress ulcer formation.

Clinical Decision Point *There is some concern regarding the increased risk of developing a Clostridium difficile infection while adding these medications. This increased risk, thought to result from decreased gastric pH, leads to increased growth of bacteria in the gastrointestinal system (Wombwell, Chittum, & Leeser, 2017). Use interprofessional collaboration to determine the appropriate treatment regimen for the patient.*

16. Institute venous thromboembolism (VTE) prophylaxis as prescribed. This includes use of anticoagulants (if no contraindications such as bleeding are present) and sequential compression devices.

VTE prevention protocols reduce patient's risk (CPSI, 2012).

17. Perform nursing activities to prevent hazards of immobility (e.g., help patient change position, perform range-of-joint motion exercise, and encourage independence and early mobility as tolerated) (see Chapter 12).

Maintaining activity and promoting early mobility avoids complications associated with decreased mobility, such as pressure injuries, pneumonia, VTE, and activity intolerance. Patients receiving mechanical ventilation need help with activity but can ambulate.

STEP	RATIONALE

IMPLEMENTATION

18. Ensure that communication method is in place for patient. Practise person-centred care and use methods that the patient prefers (e.g., letter/picture boards, common word and phrase lists, writing utensil and paper, or a computer, tablet, or smartphone).	Patients report feeling frightened, anxious, and disconnected during their time of short-term mechanical ventilation (Tsay et al., 2013). Communication strategies help patient communicate their needs and feelings, which helps to decrease anxiety and fear (ten Hoorn et al., 2016).
19. Keep patient and caregiver informed about progress and plan for weaning from mechanical ventilator.	Apprehension and anxiety occur when patient and caregiver are not properly informed about progress, changes in care, or changes in ventilator setting.
20. Remove and dispose of PPE; perform hand hygiene.	Reduces transmission of microorganisms and exposure to pulmonary secretions.

EVALUATION

1. Monitor and evaluate patient's response to mechanical ventilation every 1 to 4 hours.
  a. *Neurological assessment:* LOC, orientation, sleepiness, changes in anxiety, sedation levels
  b. *Pulmonary assessment:* Lung sounds, airway clearance, work of breathing, breathing pattern, rate of respirations, SpO_2, $EtCO_2$
  c. *Cardiovascular assessment:* Vital signs, heart rhythm, heart sounds, lower-extremity edema, pulse quality
	Patients requiring mechanical ventilation have unstable physiological status. It is important to perform key focused evaluation measures frequently as patient's condition warrants.

2. Observe SpO_2 and $EtCO_2$ and monitor gas exchange.	Documents patient's level of oxygenation and ventilation.
3. Observe integrity of patient ventilator system.	Ensures adequate delivery of mechanical ventilation.

4. Observe and evaluate effectiveness of person-centred communication methods:
  a. Ask patient if needs and concerns are addressed.
  b. Observe for signs of frustration (e.g., patient shaking head in irritation, crying, withdrawal).
  c. Observe patient and caregiver and health care personnel use communication methods.
	Communication, or lack of it, increases patient's frustration, anxiety, and depression during mechanical ventilation and weaning process.

5. **Use Teach-Back:** "I want to be sure I explained how the ventilator works and why we are using it to treat your husband. Explain to me why mechanical ventilation is necessary." Develop a revised teaching plan if caregiver is not able to teach back correctly.	Determines patient's and caregiver's level of understanding of instructional topic.

Unexpected Outcomes	Related Interventions
1. Patient experiences a VAE such as VAP.	• Notify health care provider. • Remain with patient. • Conduct complete cardiac and pulmonary assessment. • Be prepared for initiation of antibiotic therapy.
2. Patient experiences no improvement in or worsening of respiratory status.	• Notify health care provider. • Reassess patient. • Assess integrity of ventilator system. • Expect ventilator change (increased PEEP levels, increase in respiratory rate or tidal volume). • Maintain patent airway by suctioning and inserting oral airway. • Provide oxygen.
3. Patient experiences self-extubation.	• Assess patient's respiratory status and level of oxygenation and ventilation. • Notify health care provider. • Patient may need sedation and/or use of restraints to prevent this complication from occurring in the future (see Chapter 14).

STEP	RATIONALE

EVALUATION

4. Patient experiences barotrauma such as tension pneumothorax (an emergency situation).	• Remain with patient, remove patient from ventilator, and ventilate with bag-valve-mask (see Chapter 28). • Notify health care provider. • Ask UCP to obtain chest tube insertion kit. • Ask additional personnel to obtain patient's vital signs.
5. Patient develops hemodynamic instability.	• Notify health care provider. • Stay with patient. • Be prepared to change ventilator settings or initiate intravenous inotropes or vasopressors.

Communication and Documentation

- Document the following: respiratory assessment findings, mode of mechanical ventilation, oxygen level, actual patient tidal volume, actual patient respiratory rate, peak inspiratory pressure, vital signs, size and level of the ET tube, ABG results (if performed as a point of care test), patient level of comfort, sedation level scores (if sedation is used), and degree of bed elevation.
- Document any nursing interventions that are performed, including oral care, repositioning, range-of-motion exercises, medications that were administered, and suctioning.
- Document your evaluation of patient and caregiver learning.
- Communicate sudden change in patient's respiratory status, ventilator-associated problems, or adverse reactions to nurse in charge or health care provider.

Special Considerations
Teaching

- Teach patient and caregiver about the rationale for mechanical ventilation and the alarms and what they mean.
- Teach patient and caregiver preferred alternative communication techniques to reduce frustration and fear.
- Teach patient about rationale for all interventions, including oral care and frequent repositioning.

Pediatric

- Increasing numbers of children are on home mechanical ventilation. For this reason, it is important to include the parent in the child's care as appropriate. Parents also need to be prepared that, when a readmission to a hospital occurs, because of the chronic nature of the illness the child may not be readmitted to a critical care unit but rather may remain on the general medical or surgical area (Hockenberry & Wilson, 2015).

- Once the child is stable on the mechanical ventilator, promote normal or near-normal activities as the child's condition warrants (e.g., promote play, resume school activities, and encourage mobility).

Gerontological

- Presence of comorbidities increase patient's risk for longer critical care, hospital stays.
- Older persons do not usually tolerate sedative or antianxiety medications prescribed. The prescribed dose is based on the patient's baseline kidney and liver functions (Touhy & Jett, 2018).

Care in the Community

- Planning for home ventilation is performed by an interprofessional team.
- Patients need to be assessed for acceptance of ventilator dependence and the ability to understand and demonstrate daily care of the artificial airway, ventilator, and ventilator circuit.
- Patients also need their home environment, personal/monetary resources, and availability of community care resources assessed. Insufficient funding, lack of available caregivers, and lack of transition support are the largest perceived barriers to Canadians receiving home ventilation (Rose, McKim, Katz, et al., 2015).
- Evaluate the following areas during each visit: environmental safety assessment, oxygen flow, alarm system, inspiratory pressure, high-pressure alarm, tidal volume setting, humidifier, respiratory rate, tubing, temperature, resuscitation bag, tracheostomy care, breath sounds, suctioning, and tubing changes.
- Teach patient and caregiver what to do in case of respiratory distress or power failure. Check to determine availability of emergency batteries and instruct caregiver in use of the bag-valve-mask (see Chapter 28).

✦ CLINICAL DEBRIEF

A 59-year-old man with a history of well-controlled chronic obstructive pulmonary disease (COPD) developed an upper respiratory tract infection 2 weeks ago and was treated with antibiotics. He completed his full course of antibiotics, but his symptoms continued. He has a 4-day history of fever greater than 39.4°C (102.8°F), fatigue, productive cough with yellow sputum, worsening dyspnea, and decreased activity tolerance. His health care provider does a complete examination, prescribes a chest X-ray, and obtains a sputum specimen. Preliminary chest X-ray results indicate right lower lobe pneumonia. He is admitted to a general medicine floor for treatment with intravenous (IV) antibiotics, supplemental oxygen at 2 L/min via nasal cannula, and pulmonary hygiene measures.

1. The nurse observes the patient and notices that he is fatigued, has difficulty speaking, and in general looks very uncomfortable. The nurse decides to do a focused assessment. Which system(s) will the nurse assess, and what information does the nurse expect to find?

2. The patient's condition continues to worsen, and the nurse pages the health care provider. The health care provider, who is in the room, tells the unregulated care provider (UCP) to place the patient on a simple face mask at 50% FiO_2 with a flow rate of 10 L/min and to encourage the patient to use an incentive spirometer. Why should the nurse question this prescription?

3. The patient is placed on a Venturi mask at 45% FiO_2, the first dose of IV antibiotic is administered, and the patient continues to be in distress. SpO_2 now is 85%, with a respiratory rate of 32 breaths/min, heart rate of 110 beats/min, BP 144/76, and temperature of 38.7°C (101.8°F). Crackles persist in the right lower lobe. In all other lobes lung sounds are clear but diminished. The patient is using accessory muscles to breathe, and cough is no longer productive. The patient states, "I can't breathe, I am going to die." The nurse recognizes that the health care provider needs to be notified. Using SBAR format, how should the nurse communicate the patient's status to the health care provider?

◆ REVIEW QUESTIONS

1. The nurse is caring for a patient receiving BiPAP ventilation via face mask for treatment of respiratory distress. Which interventions can usually be delegated to an unregulated care provider (UCP)? *(Select all that apply.)*
   a. Educating the patient and caregiver about the use of BiPAP
   b. Repositioning patient in bed or chair
   c. Titrating patient's FiO_2
   d. Adjusting mask if it becomes displaced
   e. Recording patient's SpO_2 level
   f. Assessing patient's respiratory status

2. The nurse is assessing a patient with no history of chronic lung disease who is experiencing respiratory distress. Which findings would best indicate the need for supplemental oxygen therapy? *(Select all that apply.)*
   a. Shortness of breath
   b. PaO_2 58 mm Hg
   c. SpO_2 89%
   d. Diminished breath sounds in all lobes
   e. Cyanosis of oral mucous membranes

3. The nurse is teaching the patient how to use the peak flowmeter. The nurse asks the patient to demonstrate the procedure. Place the steps of using a peak flowmeter in the correct order.
   a. Have patient take a deep breath and hold it.
   b. Place marker of meter at bottom of scale.
   c. Have patient place mouthpiece in the mouth.
   d. Have patient blow out as hard and fast as possible.
   e. Have patient stand up, if able.
   f. Record the value.

ⓔ *Visit the Evolve site for a complete list of Clinical Debrief and Review Questions answers.*

REFERENCES

Accreditation Canada. (2019). *Required organizational practices handbook—Version 14.* Retrieved from http://www.wrha.mb.ca/quality/files/2019ROPHandbook.pdf

Aguiar, C., Davidson, J., Carvalho, A. K., Iamonti, V. C., Cortopassi, F., & Jardim, J. R. (2015). Tubing length for long-term oxygen therapy. *Respiratory Care,* 60(2), 179–182. doi:10.4187/respcare.03454

Asthma Canada. (n.d.). *Peak flow meters.* Retrieved from https://www.asthma.ca/get-help/asthma-3/control/how-to-monitor/

Baranoski, G. V. G., Van Leeuwen, S. R., & Chen, T. F. (2017). On the detection of peripheral cyanosis in individuals with distinct levels of cutaneous pigmentation. In *2017 39th Annual International Conference of the IEEE Engineering in Medicine and Biology Society (EMBC)* (pp. 4260–4264). doi:10.1109/EMBC.2017.8037797

Canadian Patient Safety Institute (CPSI). (2012). *Prevent ventilator associated pneumonia.* Retrieved from http://www.patientsafetyinstitute.ca/en/toolsResources/Documents/Interventions/Ventilator-Associated Pneumonia/VAP Getting Started Kit.pdf

Canadian Patient Safety Institute (CPSI). (2016). *Ventilator-associated pneumonia (VAP).* Retrieved from http://www.patientsafetyinstitute.ca/en/Topic/Pages/Ventilator-Associated-Pneumonia-(VAP).aspx

Centers for Disease Control and Prevention (CDC). (2019). *Ventilator-associated event.* Retrieved from http://www.cdc.gov/nhsn/PDFs/pscManual/10-VAE_FINAL.pdf

Chahoud, J., Semaan, A., & Almoosa, K. F. (2015). Ventilator-associated events prevention, learning lessons from the past: A systematic review. *Heart and Lung: The Journal of Critical Care,* 44(3), 251–259. doi:10.1016/j.hrtlng.2015.01.010

Corley, A., Rickard, C. M., Aitken, L. M., et al. (2017). High-flow nasal cannulae for respiratory support in adult intensive care patients (Review). *The Cochrane Database of Systematic Reviews,* (5), CD010172, doi:10.1002/14651858.CD010172.pub2

Cousins, J. L., Wark, P. A. B., & McDonald, V. M. (2016). Acute oxygen therapy: A review of prescribing and delivery practices. *International Journal of COPD,* 11(1), 1067–1075. doi:10.2147/COPD.S103607

Davidson, A. C., Banham, S., Elliott, M., et al. (2016). BTS/ICS guideline for the ventilatory management of acute hypercapnic respiratory failure in adults. *Thorax,* 71(Suppl. 2), ii1–ii35. doi:10.1136/thoraxjnl-2015-208209

Digby, G. C., Keenan, S. P., Parker, C. M., et al. (2015). Noninvasive ventilation practice patterns for acute respiratory failure in Canadian tertiary care centres: A descriptive analysis. *Canadian Respiratory Journal: Journal of the Canadian Thoracic Society,* 22(6), 331–340. doi:10.1155/2015/971218

do Nascimento, P., Modolo, N. S., Andrade, S., Guimarães, M. M., Braz, L. G., & El Dib, R. (2014). Incentive spirometry for prevention of postoperative pulmonary complication in upper abdominal surgery. *Cochrane Database of Systemic Reviews,* (2), CD006058, doi:10.1002/14651858.CD006058.pub3

DynaMed Plus. (2018). *Noninvasive positive pressure ventilation (NPPV) in adults.* Ipswich, MA: EBSCO Information Services. Retrieved from http://www.dynamed.com/topics/dmp~AN~T483077/Noninvasive-positive-pressure-ventilation-NPPV-in-adults

Gale, N. K., Jawad, M., Dave, C., & Turner, A. M. (2015). Adapting to domiciliary non-invasive ventilation in chronic obstructive pulmonary disease: A qualitative interview study. *Palliative Medicine,* 29(3), 268–277. doi:10.1177/0269216314558327

Gaunt, K. A., Spillman, S. K., Halub, M. E., Jackson, J. A., Lamb, K. D., & Sahr, S. M. (2015). High-flow nasal cannula in mixed adult ICU. *Respiratory Care,* 60(10), 1383–1389. doi:10.4187/respcare.04016

Grindrod, K. (2015). Management of stable chronic obstructive pulmonary disease. *British Journal of Community Nursing,* 20(2), 58.

Herren, T., Achermann, E., Hegi, T., Reber, A., & Stäubli, M. (2017). Carbon dioxide narcosis due to inappropriate oxygen delivery: A case report. *Journal of Medical Case Reports,* 11(1), 4–7. doi:10.1186/s13256-017-1363-7

Hess, D. (2018). The ventilator circuit and ventilator-associated pneumonia. *UpToDate.* Retrieved from http://www.uptodate.com/contents/the-ventilator-circuit-and-ventilator-associated-pneumonia

Hewitt, N., Bucknall, T., & Faraone, N. M. (2016). Lateral positioning for critically ill adult patients. *Cochrane Database for Systematic Reviews,* (5), CD007205, doi:10.1002/14651858.CD007205.pub2. Retrieved from http://onlinelibrary.wiley.com/doi/10.1002/14651858.CD007205.pub2/abstract;jsessionid=9F9AF8BEE55142635440D69ECD18468B.f04t01. May 12, 2016.

Hill, N., & Kramer, N. (2018). Troubleshooting problems with noninvasive positive pressure ventilation. *UpToDate.* Retrieved from http://www.uptodate.com/contents/troubleshooting-problems-with-noninvasive-positive-pressure-ventilation

Hockenberry, M. J., & Wilson, D. (2015). *Wong's nursing care of infants and children* (10th ed.). St. Louis: Mosby.

Hyzy, R. (2018). Complications of the endotracheal tube following initial placement: Prevention and management in adult intensive care patients. *UpToDate.* Retrieved from http://www.uptodate.com/contents/endotracheal-tube-management-and-complications

Kallet, R. H. (2015). A comprehensive review of prone position in ARDS. *Respiratory Care,* 60(11), 1660–1687. doi:10.4187/respcare.04271

Keenan, S. P., Sinuff, T., Burns, K. E. A., Muscedere, J., Kutsogiannis, J., & Mehta, S.; Canadian Critical Care Trials Group/Canadian Critical Care Society Noninvasive Ventilation Guidelines Group. (2011). Clinical practice guidelines for the use of noninvasive positive-pressure ventilation and noninvasive continuous positive airway pressure in the acute care setting. *CMAJ : Canadian Medical Association Journal = Journal de l'Association Medicale Canadienne,* 183(3), E195–E214. doi:10.1503/cmaj.100071

Lacasse, Y., Bernard, S., & Maltais, F. (2015). Eligibility for home oxygen programs and funding across Canada. *Canadian Respiratory Journal,* 22(6), 324–330. doi:10.1155/2015/280604

Lamb, K. D. (2015). Year in review 2014: Mechanical ventilation. *Respiratory Care*, 60(4), 606.

Lewis, S., Bucher, L., Heitkemper, M. L., Harding, M. M., Barry, M. A., & Goldsworthy, S. (Eds.), (2019). *Medical-surgical nursing in Canada. Assessment and management of clinical problems* (4th ed.). Toronto, ON: Elsevier Canada.

Lunardi, A., Porras, D., Barbosa, R., et al. (2014). Effect of volume-oriented versus flow-oriented incentive spirometry on chest wall volumes, inspiratory muscle activity, and thoracoabdominal synchrony in the elderly. *Respiratory Care*, 59(3), 420–426. doi:10.4187/respcare.02665

Magill, S., Li, Q., Gross, C., Dudeck, M., Allen-Bridson, K., & Edwards, J. (2016). Incidence and characteristics of ventilator-associated events reported to the national healthcare safety network in 2014. *Critical Care Medicine*, 44(12), 2154–2162. doi:10.1097/CCM.0000000000001871

Messika, J., Ben Ahmed, K., Gaudry, S., et al. (2015). Use of high-flow nasal cannula oxygen therapy in subjects with ARDS: A 1-year observational study. *Respiratory Care*, 60(2), 162–169. doi:10.4187/respcare.03423

Muscedere, J. G., Martin, C. M., & Heyland, D. K. (2008). The impact of ventilator-associated pneumonia on the Canadian health care system. *Journal of Critical Care*, 23(1), 5–10. doi:10.1016/j.jcrc.2007.11.012

O'Driscoll, B. R., Howard, L. S., Earis, J., & Mak, V.; British Thoracic Society (BTS) Emergency Oxygen Guideline Group & BTS Emergency Oxygen Guideline Development Group. (2017). BTS guideline for oxygen use in adults in healthcare and emergency settings. *Thorax*, 72(Suppl. 1), ii1–ii90. doi:10.1136/thoraxjnl-2016-209729

Pittman, J., Beeson, T., Kitterman, J., Lancaster, S., & Shelly, A. (2015). Medical device related hospital-acquired pressure ulcers. *JWOCN: Journal of Wound, Ostomy and Continence Nursing*, 42(2), 151–154. doi:10.1097/WON.000000000000011

Pooboni, S. K., & Markowitz, J. E. (2018). *Noninvasive ventilation procedures.* Retrieved from http://emedicine.medscape.com/article/1417959-overview

Roca, O., & Masclans, J. (2015). High-flow nasal cannula oxygen therapy: Innovative strategies for traditional procedures. *Critical Care Medicine*, 43(3), 707.

Rochwerg, B., Brochard, L., Elliott, M. W., et al. (2017). Official ERS/ATS clinical practice guidelines: Noninvasive ventilation for acute respiratory failure. *European Respiratory Journal*, 50(2), 1602426. doi:10.1183/13993003.02426-2016

Rose, L., McKim, D. A., Katz, S. L., et al. (2015). Home mechanical ventilation in Canada: A national survey. *Respiratory Care*, 60(5), 695–704. doi:10.4187/respcare.03609

Rouzé, A., Jaillette, E., Poissy, J., Préau, S., & Nseir, S. (2017). Tracheal tube design and ventilator-associated pneumonia. *Respiratory Care*, 62(10), 1316–1323. doi:10.4187/respcare.05492

Schallom, M., Cracchiolo, L., Falker, A., et al. (2015). Pressure ulcer incidence in patients wearing nasal-oral versus full-face noninvasive ventilation masks. *American Journal of Critical Care*, 24(4), 349–356. doi:10.4037/ajcc2015386

Schreiber, M. (2015). Tracheostomy: Site care, suctioning, and readiness. *Medsurg Nursing*, 24(2), 121.

Shah, N. M., D'Cruz, R. F., & Murphy, P. B. (2018). Update: Non-invasive ventilation in chronic obstructive pulmonary disease. *Journal of Thoracic Disease*, 10(Suppl. 1), S71–S79. doi:10.21037/jtd.2017.10.44

Smetana, G. (2018). Strategies to reduce postoperative complications. *UpToDate.* Retrieved from http://www.uptodate.com/contents/strategies-to-reduce-postoperative-pulmonary-complications

Sole, M. L., Bennett, M., & Ashworth, S. (2016). Clinical indicators for endotracheal suctioning in adult patients receiving mechanical ventilation. *American Journal of Critical Care*, 24(4), 318–324. doi:10.4037/ajcc2015794

Spoletini, G., Alobtaibi, M., Blasi, F., & Hill, N. S. (2015). Heated humidified high-flow nasal oxygen in adults: Mechanism of action and clinical implications. *Chest*, 148(1), 253–261. doi:10.1378/chest.14-2871

ten Hoorn, S., Elbers, P. W., Girbes, A. R., & Tuinman, P. R. (2016). Communicating with conscious and mechanically ventilated critically ill patients: A systematic review. *Critical Care: The Official Journal of the Critical Care Forum*, 20(1), 1–14. doi:10.1186/s13054-016-1483-2

The Lung Association. (n.d.). My *asthma action plan*. Retrieved from https://www.lung.ca/sites/default/files/media/asthma_action_plan.pdf

Touhy, T., & Jett, K. (2018). *Ebersole & Hess' gerontological nursing & healthy aging* (5th ed.). St. Louis: Elsevier.

Tsay, S., Mu, P., Lin, S., Wang, K., & Chen, Y. (2013). The experiences of adult ventilator-dependent patients: A meta-synthesis review. *Nursing & Health Sciences*, 15(4), 525–533. doi:10.1111/nhs.12049

Tyson, A. F., Kendig, C. E., Mabedi, C., Cairns, B. A., & Charles, A. G. (2015). The effect of incentive spirometry on postoperative pulmonary function following laparotomy: A randomized clinical trial. *JAMA Surgery*, 150(3), 229–236. doi:10.1001/jamasurg.2014.1846

Urden, L. D., Stacy, K. M., & Lough, M. E. (2016). *Priorities in critical care nursing* (7th ed.). St. Louis: Mosby.

Wang, L., Li, X., Yang, Z., et al. (2016). Semi-recumbent position versus supine position for the prevention of ventilator-associated pneumonia in adults requiring mechanical ventilation (review). *The Cochrane Database of Systematic Reviews*, (1), CD009946, doi:10.1002/14651858.CD009946.pub2

Waters, B., & Muscedere, J. (2015). A 2015 update on ventilator-associated pneumonia: New insights on its prevention, diagnosis, and treatment. *Current Infectious Disease Reports*, 17(8), 1–9. doi:10.1007/s11908-015-0496-3

Wen, Z., Wang, W., Zhang, H., Wu, C., Ding, J., & Shen, M. (2017). Is humidified better than non-humidified low-flow oxygen therapy ? A systematic review and meta-analysis. *Journal of Advacned Nursing*, 73(11), 2522–2533. doi:10.1111/jan.13323

Wombwell, E., Chittum, M. E., & Leeser, K. R. (2017). Inpatient proton pump inhibitor administration and hospital-acquired *Clostridium difficile* infection: Evidence and possible mechanism. *American Journal of Medicine*, 131(3), 244–249. doi:10.1016/j.amjmed.2017.10.034

24 | Performing Chest Physiotherapy

Written by **Anne Griffin Perry, RN, MSN, EdD, FAAN, and Maureen Loft, NP-Adult, MScN, PhD**

OBJECTIVES

Mastery of content in this chapter will enable the nurse to:

- Assess for the need to perform chest physiotherapy (CPT) manoeuvres.
- Determine the need to modify or discontinue CPT manoeuvres.
- Explain how to prepare a patient and caregiver for the performance of each CPT manoeuvre.
- Perform the outlined CPT manoeuvres, including standard and modified versions.

- Describe the use of a positive expiratory pressure (PEP) device and high-frequency chest wall oscillation (HFCWO) vest airway clearance system.
- Describe expected and unexpected outcomes of each CPT manoeuvre.
- Describe discharge teaching and planning related to the use of each CPT manoeuvre in the home setting.

MEDIA RESOURCES

- e∨olve http://evolve.elsevier.com/Canada/Perry/clinicalskills/
- Review Questions

- Audio Glossary
- Clinical Debrief and Review Questions Answers

PURPOSE

Chest physiotherapy (CPT) is external chest wall manipulation, which includes one of a combination of or all of percussion, vibration, and postural drainage (PD) therapy to loosen and remove secretions from patients' airways (Strickland, Rubin, Haas, et al., 2015). CPT is usually followed by productive coughing or suctioning to remove secretions. The effectiveness of traditional CPT has been shown to be highly influenced by the patient population to which it is applied (Torres-Sanchez, Cruz-Ramirez, Cabrera-Martos, et al., 2017). Routine use of CPT does not improve mortality rates of adults with pneumonia (Yang, Yuping, Yin, et al., 2013), nor does it help children with pneumonia, bronchiolitis, or asthma, and it does not prevent atelectasis after extubation (Makic, Rauen, Jones, et al., 2015). However, CPT has shown benefits in patients with chronic obstructive pulmonary disease (COPD) (Torres-Sanchez et al., 2017) and is an essential therapy in patients with cystic fibrosis (CF). For these patients, the use of manual percussion and vibration, positive expiratory pressure (PEP), and high-frequency chest wall oscillation (HFCWO) device modalities is determined by patient preference and varies at different stages of the disease (Morrison & Milroy, 2018). An HFCWO system is a method for delivering CPT that uses high-frequency chest wall compressions created by bursts of air for external chest wall compression. A PEP device uses positive airway pressure to increase airway pressure and oscillations to loosen secretions, which helps a patient's ability to clear secretions. Each of these therapies is broadly classified as an airway clearance therapy (ACT) (Brown, White, & Tobin, 2017).

Careful patient assessment is a prerequisite for administering any ACTs. The auscultation of all the lung fields is essential to determine which regions would benefit from CPT. CPT manoeuvres move secretions into the large central airways; then these secretions are removed through coughing or suctioning. PD requires specific positioning of a patient so that the targeted lung segment is positioned in such a way that gravity helps in removing secretions. PEP and HFCWO devices are more commonly used by CF patients in the community but may also be used by patients with COPD or neuromuscular diseases.

STANDARDS OF CARE

- Accreditation Canada, 2019—*Required Organizational Practices Handbook—Version 14* (http://www.wrha.mb.ca/quality/files/2019 ROPHandbook.pdf)
- Strickland et al., 2015—*AARC Clinical Practice Guideline: Effectiveness of Nonpharmacological Airway Clearance Therapies in Hospitalized Patients* (https://www.aarc.org/wp-content/uploads/2014/08/pharm_cpg.pdf)

PRINCIPLES FOR PRACTICE

- Careful patient assessment is a prerequisite for administering any CPT and PD manoeuvre because the therapy is usually targeted to the affected areas and not all the lung fields (Strickland et al., 2015).
- The aim of CPT and PD is to remove secretions that accumulate in the airways of patients with CF.
- Surgical patients in the postoperative period and critically ill patients have excess secretions because of the effects of anaesthesia, ineffective coughing because of incision pain or muscle weakness, and reduced mobility (Ambrosino & Makhabah, 2014). Mucus plugs, atelectasis, and lobular collapse occur when secretions accumulate in the airways. Early mobility and ambulation are more successful in promoting airway clearance than routine CPT (Strickland et al., 2015; Yang et al., 2013).
- CPT and PD are often used in combination with other therapies, including antibiotics, bronchodilators, mucolytic agents, and inhaled and nebulized medications in CF patients (Strickland et al., 2015). These other therapies reduce mucus production and promote airway clearance. The goals of these therapies are (1) to clear the airways of excessive secretions to reduce the work of breathing and (2) to improve a patient's ability to cough up secretions (Morrison & Milroy, 2018).
- In the normal lung, the mucociliary transport system clears the airways of excessive mucus and inhaled particles. Airways normally remain clear, and mucus is constantly being cleared almost as fast as it is made. Normal mucus remains thin, white, and watery.
- In various disease states, mucus clearance slows down, or the cilia are overwhelmed by production of large quantities of mucus. The lungs no longer clear the mucus as fast as it is produced, allowing for bacterial colonization leading to infection. Altered ion clearance causes an overwhelming inflammatory response (Brown et al., 2017).

PERSON-CENTRED CARE

- When patients' physiological capacities are weakened, they are often anxious because of their illness or surgery, and they may be in pain. It is important to complete a pain assessment and administer prescribed analgesics 20 to 30 minutes before initiating any CPT manoeuvres. Premedication ensures that the patient is comfortable and as pain free as possible.
- Assess the patient's activity tolerance. Patients with cardiopulmonary disease, severe arthritis, and certain musculoskeletal diseases often have diminished activity tolerance and cannot tolerate a complete CPT session. Plan CPT during short periods interspersed with rest periods, at a time when the patient is rested, and not immediately after a meal.
- Encourage mobility and ambulation to reduce postoperative pulmonary complications and promote airway clearance (Strickland et al., 2015).
- The patient with chronic pulmonary illnesses such as CF poses different challenges. These patients must devote several hours of their day to activities to assist in airway clearance. It is important that CPT and other airway clearance techniques do not impact a patient's quality of life (QOL). To maintain this QOL try to integrate CPT and airway techniques into their routine, personal goals, and social activities (Wilson, 2018).
- CPT skills include a great deal of patient touching. Some cultures consider it offensive to touch in public. In addition, the skills of CPT sometimes involve a gentle percussion or vibration of a patient's rib cage. Patients and families from cultures where violence is an everyday occurrence need detailed information about the procedure so that they do not misunderstand the intent and objective of CPT. Always explain which type of touching is involved and what a patient may feel during the treatment. Provide an opportunity for the patient to temporarily stop and rest during the procedure (Giger, 2016).

EVIDENCE-INFORMED PRACTICE

- ACTs such as CPT and PD manoeuvres are effective only in selected patients, such as those with CF, bronchiectasis, other chronic pulmonary diseases, and some surgeries (Strickland et al., 2015). When disease processes alter the normal mechanisms of the body to clear the airway, therapies must be instituted to ensure that the airways remain free of secretions so the risk for pulmonary infection is reduced and the oxygen demands of the body are met. When secretions are stagnant, they obstruct airways, are conduits for bacterial colonization and infections, stimulate an inflammatory response, and contribute to airway and tissue damage (Mikesell, Kempainen, Laguna, et al., 2017).
- CPT is not recommended routinely as additional treatment for pneumonia in adults (Makic et al., 2015). Careful assessment of medical history for smoking, pulmonary infections, and other conditions may indicate the need for CPT in selected adults at risk for complicated pneumonia (Yang et al., 2013).
- ACT is not recommended as routine therapy in patients with COPD unless secretion retention is present (Strickland et al., 2015).
- In selected intubated patients in the critical care unit (CCU), early and routine CPT benefits patients and improves airway patency, secretion clearance, and oxygen delivery to the tissues. In addition, early CPT reduces some CCU complications, such as health care–acquired infections.
- High-frequency chest wall oscillators such as the vest airway clearance system (see Procedural Guideline 24.2) are effective in aiding sputum clearance for a variety of adult and pediatric lung diseases (Rimler, 2017).
- The use of a PEP device (see Procedure Guideline 24.1) improves patient satisfaction and adherence to airway clearance therapies (Rimler, 2017).

SAFETY GUIDELINES

- Assess the patient's normal range of vital signs. Conditions such as CF and complicated pneumonia requiring CPT can affect a patient's vital signs. The degree of change is related to the level of hypoxia, overall cardiopulmonary status, and tolerance of the procedure.
- Assess the patient's current medications. Some medications, particularly diuretics and antihypertensives, cause fluid and hemodynamic changes. These changes affect a patient's tolerance of the positional changes. Steroid medications, age, and malnutrition increase a patient's risk for pathological rib fractures and often contraindicate rib vibration.
- Review the patient's medical and surgical history. Certain conditions such as increased intracranial pressure, spinal cord injuries, abdominal aneurysm resection, bone metastases, or severe osteoporosis contraindicate the positional changes of postural drainage (Box 24.1). Thoracic trauma contraindicates percussion and vibration.
- Assess the patient's level of cognitive function. Alteration in mental status often makes it difficult or impossible for a patient

BOX 24.1

Contraindications for Postural Drainage

- Increased intracranial pressure
- Head and neck injury, until stabilized
- Active hemorrhage with hemodynamic instability
- Recent spinal surgery (e.g., laminectomy) or acute spinal injury
- Active hemoptysis
- Empyema
- Bronchopleural fistula
- Pulmonary edema associated with heart failure
- Large pleural effusions
- Pulmonary embolism
- Older, confused, or anxious patients who are unable to tolerate position change
- Rib fracture, with or without flail chest
- Surgical wound or healing tissue

Trendelenburg's position is contraindicated for the following:

- Uncontrolled hypertension
- Distended abdomen
- Esophageal surgery
- Recent gross hemoptysis
- Uncontrolled airway at risk for aspiration

Modified from White, G. (2013). *Basic clinical lab competencies for respiratory care: An integrated approach* (5th ed.). Clifton Park, NY: Cengage Learning.

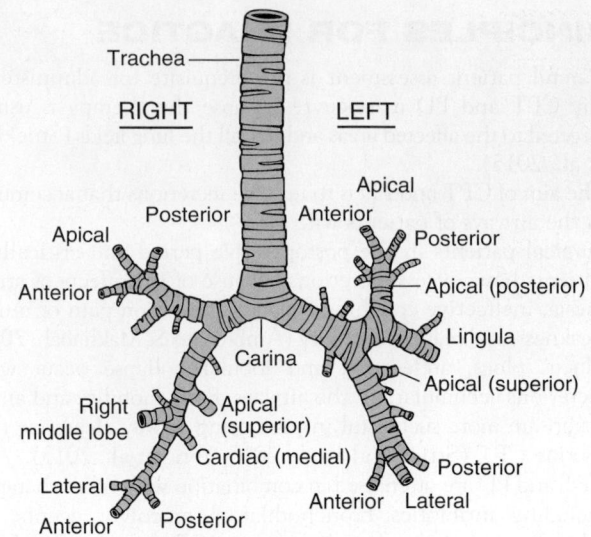

FIG 24.1 Tracheobronchial tree. (*Modified from Frownfelter, D. L., & Dean, E. [2006]. Principles and practice of cardiopulmonary therapy [43rd ed.]. St. Louis: Mosby.*)

to understand the procedure and participate in coughing and expectorating secretions.

- Have suction machine equipment available to help clear airway secretions (see Chapter 25).
- Patients who receive long-term steroid therapy are at risk for pathological fractures. Physical manoeuvres such as chest percussion and vibration may be contraindicated because of the risk for rib fractures. These patients benefit from individualized airway clearance measures such as use of a PEP device (dos Santos, Guimaraes, de Carhalho, et al., 2013; Strickland et al., 2015).

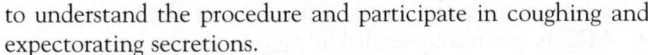

♦ SKILL 24.1   Performing Postural Drainage

Postural drainage (PD) is the use of positioning techniques to drain secretions from specific segments of the lungs and bronchi into the trachea (Fig. 24.1). Each position drains a specific corresponding section of the tracheobronchial tree from the upper, middle, or lower lung field into the trachea (Table 24.1). Additional coughing or airway suctioning helps remove secretions from the trachea.

Use physical assessment findings and a review of chest X-ray to determine which lung segments require PD. Patients needing PD usually have chronic conditions, which affect their activity tolerance. Knowing which lung segments require PD promotes patient cooperation, adherence to therapy, and prevention of excessive fatigue. In addition, use knowledge of a patient's condition and disease process and the extent of the pathological condition to individualize the PD therapy.

Delegation and Collaboration

The skill of PD can be delegated to an unregulated care provider (UCP). It is the nurse's responsibility to assess the patient, review laboratory and chest X-ray results, and determine that the patient is stable and able to tolerate the procedure. The nurse instructs the UCP to:

- Immediately report to the nurse changes in the patient's comfort level, changes in breathing pattern, and tolerance of the procedure.

- Use specific precautions related to the disease, mobility status, position restrictions, and treatment.

Equipment

- Stethoscope
- Pulse oximeter
- Trendelenburg's hospital bed or tilt table (more common in pediatric facilities)
- Water in pitcher and glass
- Tissues and paper bag
- Chair (for draining upper lobes)
- Extra pillows
- Clear graduated screw-top container for sputum collection (*optional*)
- Oral hygiene-care products
- Suction equipment (if patient is unable to cough and clear own secretions)
- Personal protective equipment (PPE) as required
- Patient education materials

TABLE 24.1

Positions and Procedures for Drainage, Percussion, and Vibration

Area and Procedure	Anatomical Area	Position of Patient

Left and Right Upper Lobe Anterior Apical Bronchi

Position patient in chair, or high-Fowler's, leaning back. Percuss and vibrate with heel of hands at shoulders and fingers over collarbones (clavicles) in front; do both sides at same time. Note body posture and arm position of nurse. Nurse's back is kept straight, and elbows and knees are slightly flexed.

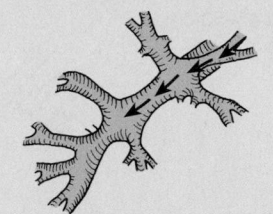 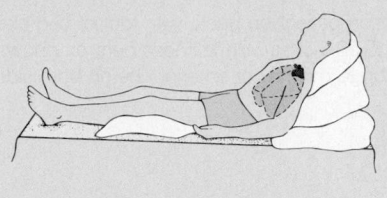

Anterior apical segments

Direction of mucus flow through upper lobe anterior apical bronchi.

Position hands for chest physiotherapy over left and right upper anterior apical bronchi.

Left and Right Upper Lobe Posterior Apical Bronchi

Position patient in chair, leaning forward on pillow or table. Percuss and vibrate with hands on either side of upper spine. Do both sides at same time.

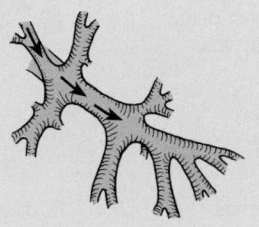 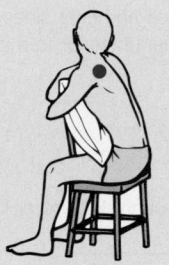

Posterior apical segments

Direction of mucus flow through upper lobe posterior apical bronchi.

Position hands for chest physiotherapy over left and right upper lobe posterior apical bronchi.

Left and Right Upper Lobe Anterior Bronchi

Position patient flat on back with small pillow under knees. Percuss and vibrate just below clavicle on either side of sternum.

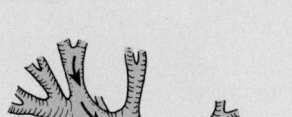 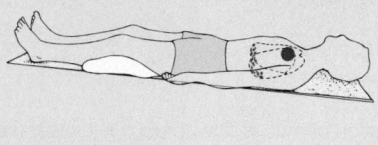

Anterior upper lobe segments

Direction of mucus flow through anterior upper bronchi.

Position hands for chest physiotherapy over right and left anterior upper lobe bronchi.

Left Upper Lobe Lingular Bronchus

Position patient on right side with arm overhead in Trendelenburg's position, with foot of bed raised 30 cm (12 inches), as tolerated.* Place pillow behind back, and roll patient one-quarter turn onto pillow. Percuss and vibrate lateral to left nipple below axilla.

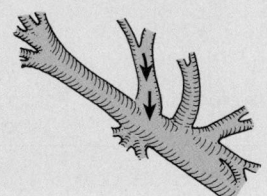 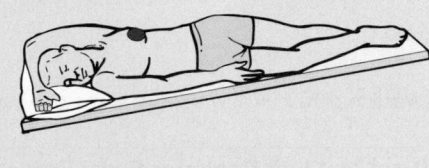

Left upper lobe lingular segment

Direction of mucus flow through left upper lobe lingular bronchus.

Position hands for chest physiotherapy over left upper lobe lingular bronchus.

Right Middle Lobe Bronchus

Position patient on left side or abdomen. Place pillow behind back, and roll patient one-quarter turn onto pillow. Percuss and vibrate to right nipple below axilla.

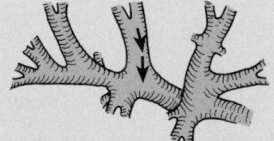 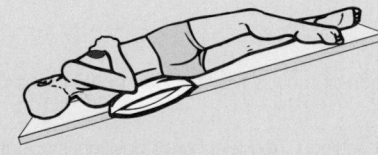

Right middle lobe segment

Direction of mucus flow through right middle lobe bronchus.

Position hands for chest physiotherapy over right middle lobe bronchus.

Continued

TABLE 24.1

Positions and Procedures for Drainage, Percussion, and Vibration—cont'd

Area and Procedure	Anatomical Area	Position of Patient
Left and Right Lower Lobe Anterior Bronchi Position patient on back, with foot of bed elevated 45–50 cm (18–20 inches). Have knees bent on pillow. Percuss and vibrate over lower anterior ribs on both sides. Direction of mucus flow through anterior lower lobe bronchi.	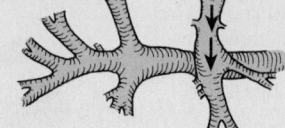	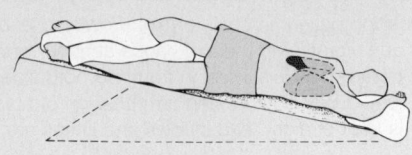 Anterior lower lobe segments Position hands for chest physiotherapy over left and right anterior lower lobe bronchi.
Right Lower Lobe Lateral Bronchus Position patient on abdomen in Trendelenburg's position with foot of bed raised 45–50 cm (18–20 inches), as tolerated. Percuss and vibrate on left and right sides of chest below shoulder blades (scapulae) posterior to midaxillary line. Direction of mucus flow through right lower lobe lateral bronchus.	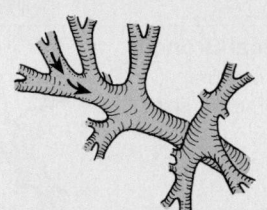	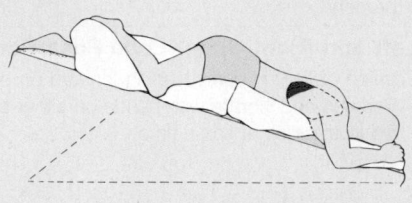 Right lower lateral lobe segment Position hands for chest physiotherapy over right lower lobe lateral bronchus.
Left Lower Lobe Lateral Bronchus Position patient on right side in Trendelenburg's position with foot of bed raised 45–50 cm (18–20 inches), as tolerated. Percuss and vibrate on left side of chest below scapulae posterior to midaxillary line. Direction of mucus flow through left lower lobe lateral bronchus.	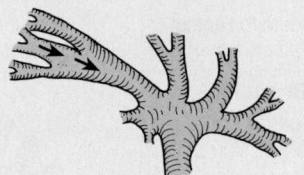	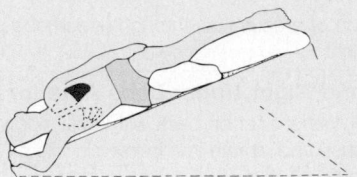 Left lower lobe lateral segment Position hands for chest physiotherapy over left lower lobe lateral bronchus.
Right and Left Lower Lobe Superior Bronchi Position patient flat on stomach with pillow under stomach. Percuss and vibrate below scapula on either side of spine. Direction of mucus flow through lower lobe superior bronchi.	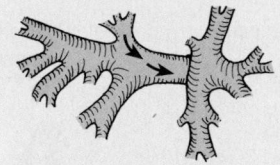	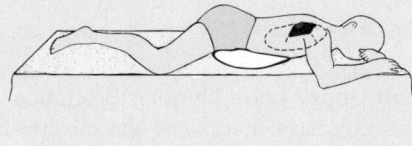 Lower lobe superior segments Position hands for chest physiotherapy over right and left lower lobe superior bronchi.
Right and Left Posterior Basal Bronchi Position patient on stomach in Trendelenburg's position with foot of bed raised 45–50 cm (18–20 inches), as tolerated. Percuss and vibrate over low posterior ribs on either side of spine. Direction of mucus flow through posterior basal bronchi.	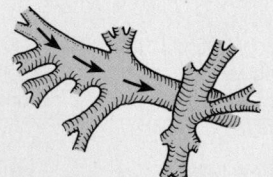	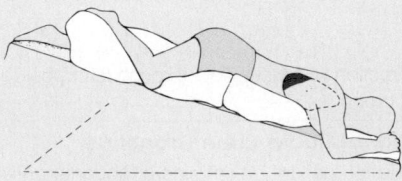 Posterior segments Position hands for chest physiotherapy over right and left posterior lower lobe bronchi.

*In adult settings, Trendelenburg's position is not used as frequently. Verify use with employer policy and health care provider's prescription.

STEP	RATIONALE

ASSESSMENT

1. Identify patient using at least two person-specific identifiers (e.g., name and date of birth or name and medical record number) according to employer policy.

Ensures correct patient. Complies with Accreditation Canada's standards and improves patient safety (Accreditation Canada, 2019).

2. Assess patient for history of decreased level of consciousness, decreased activity tolerance, and muscle weakness or chronic disease processes such as complicated pneumonia and chronic obstructive pulmonary disease (COPD) (see Box 24.1).

Conditions that pose risk for impaired airway clearance require PD.

Clinical Decision Point *If the use of Trendelenburg's position or other postures causes severe hypertension, severe hypoxemia, or severe shortness of breath, therapy is contraindicated (see Box 24.1). In addition, when patients have a risk for or a history of gastroesophageal reflux disease (GERD), which is regurgitation of stomach contents into the esophagus, the head-down positions should not be used.*

3. Review medical record and assess patient for signs and symptoms, including X-ray film changes consistent with atelectasis, lobar collapse pneumonia, or bronchiectasis; ineffective coughing; thick, sticky, tenacious, and discoloured secretions that are difficult to cough up.

Indicates need to perform postural drainage. X-ray and signs and symptoms indicate accumulation of pulmonary secretions and ineffective airway clearance. Chest physiotherapy (CPT) is an additional therapy to improve removal of airway secretions (Ambrosino & Makhabah, 2014).

4. Auscultate all lung fields for decreased breath sounds and adventitious lung sounds.

Findings identify specific lung segments needing drainage.

5. Obtain vital signs and pulse oximetry (SpO$_2$) before PD treatment.

Provides baseline to evaluate patient's response and tolerance to therapy.

6. Determine patient's and caregiver's understanding of and ability to perform home postural drainage.

Identifies potential areas for instruction for discharge planning. Home PD is essential for airway secretion management in patients with cystic fibrosis (CF) (Morrison & Milroy, 2018).

7. Use a 0-to-10 pain scale (0 being no pain, 10 being the worst pain ever) to determine patient's level of comfort.

Determines patient's level of pain and if preprocedure analgesia is needed.

NURSING DIAGNOSES

- Insufficient airway clearance
- Inadequate breathing pattern
- Reduced gas exchange
- Acute pain
- Insufficient knowledge regarding postural drainage and airway clearance

Related factors/Risk factors are individualized on the basis of patient's condition or needs.

PLANNING

1. Expected outcomes following completion of procedure:
   - Lung sounds improve or become clear to auscultation.
   - Sputum is more easily expectorated or suctioned out.

   Clearing of airways confirms effectiveness of procedure.
   PD manoeuvres loosen airway secretions, facilitating secretion removal.

   - Secretions appear more normal in colour and consistency.

   When infection is present, returning to normal secretion characteristics indicates resolving infection.

   - SpO$_2$ levels increase and dyspnea decreases.

   As secretions are removed, patient exchange of respiratory gases improves, and dyspnea gradually declines.

   - Chest X-ray shows improvements; lobar collapse and atelectasis are decreased or eliminated.

   PD drains secretions into major airways, facilitating removal during coughing and CPT. As a result, there is visual improvement on chest X-ray.

2. Prepare patient for procedure:
   a. If patient has an increased pain rating on assessment, administer analgesia 20 minutes before CPT manoeuvres.

   Pain control is essential for patient to actively participate in PD manoeuvres and cough forcefully to clear airways.

   b. Explain purpose and rationale for procedure. Explain positioning, sensations, how long it will take, and any discomforts or side effects.

   Helps promote cooperation. A well-prepared patient is usually more relaxed and comfortable, which is essential for effective drainage.

   c. Unless contraindicated, encourage high fluid intake (minimum of 1500 mL) daily. Maintain record of fluid intake and output.

   Fluids may thin secretions and make them easier to cough up. Patients need close monitoring and encouragement when first starting a high-fluid intake program.

STEP	RATIONALE

PLANNING

d. Plan treatments so they do not overlap with meals or tube feeding. Avoid PD 1 to 2 hours before or 1 to 2 hours after meals or bolus tube feedings. Stop all continuous gastric tube feedings for 30 to 45 minutes before PD. Check for residual feeding in patient's stomach; if greater than 100 mL, hold treatment.

Performing PD when patient's stomach is empty helps avoid gastric reflux or vomiting and aspiration of stomach contents.

e. Schedule treatments at appropriate times during day.

Scheduling of PD avoids conflict with other interventions and diagnostic testing.

Clinical Decision Point *If patient is receiving inhaled bronchodilator, nebulizers, or aerosol treatment, provide PD 20 minutes after such therapy. PD following bronchodilator therapy enhances patient oxygenation during procedure (Strickland et al., 2015).*

f. Have patient remove any tight or restrictive clothing.

Helps patient relax and promotes deep breathing.

IMPLEMENTATION

1. Close room door or pull curtains around patient's bed. Perform hand hygiene and apply clean gloves as indicated.

Maintains privacy. Reduces transmission of microorganisms.

2. Use findings from physical assessment and chest X-ray to select congested areas for draining. Consult with primary health care provider as needed.

Individualized treatment helps relieve specific areas of congestion identified during patient assessment.

3. Help patient to desired position to drain congested areas (see Table 24.1). Place pillows for support and comfort. Drape patient appropriately.

Proper patient positioning assists gravity in helping movement of secretions from peripheral airways to larger bronchi, where they can be cleared (Volsko, 2013).

4. Have patient maintain position for 10 to 15 minutes.

In adults draining each area takes time.

5. After 10 to 15 minutes of drainage in selected postures, perform chest percussion and vibration (see Procedural Guideline 24.2) over affected lung region. Table 24.1 shows all postures and hand placement for percussion and vibration.

Provides mechanical forces to help move airway secretions.

6. After 10 to 15 minutes of drainage in first posture, have patient sit up and cough. If indicated, save expectorated secretions in clear container. If patient cannot cough, suctioning is necessary (see Chapter 25).

Any secretions moved to central airways are removed by cough or suctioning before placing patient into next drainage position. Coughing is most effective when patient is sitting up and leaning forward.

Clinical Decision Point *Sometimes patients experience transient dyspnea and fatigue because of airway irritation and bronchospasm from the secretions. These patients often benefit from an oscillating or vibrating positive expiratory pressure device (see Procedural Guideline 24.1).*

7. Have patient rest briefly if necessary between positions. Note pulse oximeter readings.

Short rest periods between postures prevent fatigue and increase tolerance. SpO_2 values may fall slightly.

8. Have patient take sips of water.

Keeping mouth moist aids in expectoration of secretions.

9. Repeat Steps 3 to 8 until all affected areas selected are drained. Make sure that each treatment does not exceed 30 to 60 minutes.

Drainage is used only to drain areas involved and is based on individual assessment.

10. Offer to help patient with oral hygiene.

Promotes comfort and reduces foul-smelling breath.

11. Remove gloves and perform hand hygiene.

Reduces transmission of microorganisms.

EVALUATION

1. Auscultate lung fields.

Clearance of secretions usually relieves gurgling, early inspiratory crackles, and palpable crepitus.

2. Inspect character and amount of sputum.

Determines if more secretions are coughed up and if they are thinned adequately.

3. Review diagnostic reports, including sputum collections and cultures, chest X-rays, and arterial blood gas (ABG) levels.

Provides objective data on improvements in lung function.

4. Obtain vital signs, pulse oximetry.

Procedure can result in dysrhythmias and decreases in oxygen saturation, below 90%, in some patients.

STEP	RATIONALE

EVALUATION

5. Use Teach-Back: "I want to be sure I explained why you need to position yourself over the back of a chair with a pillow supporting your chest. Tell me why this position is important." Develop a revised teaching plan if patient or caregiver is not able to teach back correctly.

Determines patient's and caregiver's level of understanding of instructional topic.

Unexpected Outcomes	Related Interventions
1. Patient experiences severe dyspnea, bronchospasm, hypoxemia, or hypercarbia and/or is unable to tolerate treatment.	• Discontinue, modify, or shorten treatments. • Administer bronchodilator or nebulizer therapy 20 minutes before CPT. • Suction and ventilate with bag-valve-mask to improve patient oxygenation. Closely monitor ABG levels, oxygen saturation, and vital signs. • Initially increase treatments and encourage and teach coughing exercises. • Increase hydration (if medically appropriate). • Notify health care provider, because patient may need sputum culture, change in antibiotics, mucolytics, or a bronchoscopy to remove thick mucus plugs.
2. No improvement in chest assessment or chest X-ray examination results.	
3. Hemoptysis occurs; or patient develops acute hypotension, severe chest pain, vomiting, aspiration, and/or dysrhythmias.	• Stop therapy, place patient in high-Fowler's position, and obtain vital signs. • Call for help and notify health care provider. • Remain with patient; keep patient comfortable, calm, warm, and quiet. • If patient vomits or aspirates, suction airway and place them on their side. • Reapply patient's oxygen device if prescribed.

Communication and Documentation

• Document pretherapy and post-therapy assessment findings, SpO_2 readings, and chest X-ray results; frequency and duration of treatment; postures used and bronchial segments drained; cough effectiveness; need for suctioning; colour, amount, and consistency of sputum; hemoptysis or other unexpected outcomes; and patient's tolerance and reaction in the nurses' notes in electronic health record (EHR) or chart.
• Document your evaluation of patient and caregiver learning.

Special Considerations
Teaching

• Instruct patient and caregiver that the best times for treatments are (1) in the morning before breakfast, when patient can clear secretions that accumulate overnight; and (2) about 1 hour before bedtime, so lungs are clear before sleeping and patient has time after treatment to cough up any mobilized secretions. Frequency depends on need and patient's tolerance and varies from once daily to every 2 to 4 hours in an acute situation.
• Instruct caregiver how to recognize when patient's respiratory status requires breathing exercises or PD.

Pediatric

• In a child with CF, PD is a cornerstone therapy and is usually performed at least twice daily, on rising in the morning and in the evening (Hockenberry & Wilson, 2015).
• Many CF patients benefit from the use of the vest airway clearance system (see Procedural Guideline 24.2) (Hockenberry & Wilson, 2015; Morrison & Milroy, 2018).

• CPT is not beneficial in the treatment of bronchiolitis in children younger than 2 years of age (Roqué i Figuls, Giné-Garriga, Granados-Rugeles, et al., 2016).
• Children with pneumonia, bronchiolitis, and asthma have limited benefits with the administration of CPT (Makic et al., 2015).

Gerontological

• Take extra care and thoroughly assess patient when using PD in older persons. Certain medications such as antihypertensive and cardiac medications may increase the risk for dizziness when positions are changed rapidly (Salvo, 2018, p. 258). Therefore, change positions more slowly and closely assess for any changes in oxygen saturation or vital signs with position changes.
• Older persons with chronic cardiac and pulmonary conditions do not always tolerate a supine or side-lying position for PD. If a patient experiences a decrease in oxygen saturation (decreased SpO_2) or increased breathlessness in these positions, reposition them to a semi-Fowler's position and perform CPT.

Care in the Community

• Teach patient and caregiver how to assume PD positions at home. Some positions need modification to meet patient needs. For example, if the patient is very short of breath, place them in a supine, side-lying semi-Fowler's or side-lying Trendelenburg's position to drain lateral lower lobes.
• Obtain foam wedge or multiple pillows for correct positioning.
• If eligible, refer patient to a pulmonary rehabilitation program.

PROCEDURAL GUIDELINE 24.1 *Using a Positive Expiratory Pressure (PEP) Device*

A PEP device is a handheld airway clearance device (Fig. 24.2). The device has a control that can adjust the frequency of oscillations and resistance to expiratory flow. Positive expiratory pressure stabilizes airways and improves aeration of the distal lung areas. During exhalation, pressure from the airways is transmitted to the PEP device, which helps mucus dislodge from the airway walls and as a result prevents airway collapse, accelerates expiratory flow, and moves mucus toward the trachea (Strickland et al., 2015). Some patients living with cystic fibrosis (CF) may benefit more from this device than from standard chest physiotherapy (Volsko, 2013). However, CF patients must receive some type of routine airway clearance therapy daily.

Delegation and Collaboration

The skill of using a PEP device can be delegated to an unregulated care provider (UCP). The nurse is responsible for performing respiratory assessment, determining that the procedure is appropriate and that a patient can tolerate it, and evaluating a patient's response to it. Interprofessional collaboration is required when preparing to use a PEP device (e.g., respiratory therapist). When delegating to an UCP the nurse instructs the UCP to:

- Be alert for patient's tolerance of the procedure, such as comfort level and changes in breathing pattern, and to immediately report changes to the nurse.
- Use specific patient precautions, such as positioning restrictions related to disease or treatment.

Equipment

- Stethoscope
- Pulse oximeter
- Water and glass
- Chair
- Tissues and paper bag
- Clear graduated screw-top container
- Suction equipment (if patient is unable to cough and clear own secretions)
- PEP device (see Fig. 24.2)
- Personal protective equipment (PPE)
- Patient education materials

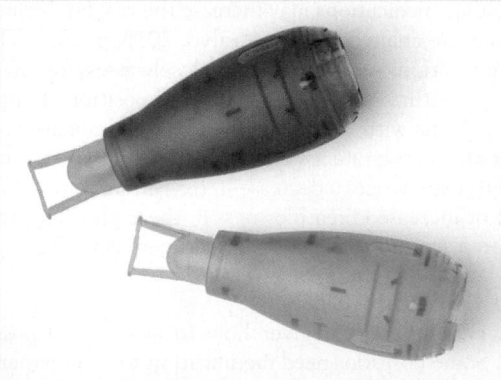

FIG 24.2 PEP device example—Acapella device. (*Used with permission from Smithsmedical.com.*)

Procedural Steps

1. Identify patient using at least two person-specific identifiers (e.g., name and date of birth or name and medical record number) according to employer policy (Accreditation Canada, 2019).
2. Verify the need for a health care provider's prescription per employer policy.
3. Perform respiratory assessment to determine lung segments requiring percussion and/or vibration (Volsko, 2013).
4. Assess patient's and caregiver's understanding of the device and procedure and explain and clarify procedure as needed.
5. Prepare prescribed PEP device as per manufacturer's recommendations

Clinical Decision Point *Verify that the correct device is used to match patient's expiratory flow rate. Refer to manufacturer's instructions and health care provider's prescription.*

   a. Initial setting: As prescribed by health care provider.
   b. As patient improves or is more proficient, adjust the proper resistance level upward as prescribed by health care provider.

Clinical Decision Point *Determine if aerosol medications therapy is prescribed. If so, attach a nebulizer to the end of the PEP valve if indicated.*

6. Instruct patient to:
   a. Sit comfortably.
   b. Take in a breath that is larger than normal but not to fill lungs completely. Instruct patient to inhale to about 75% of inspiratory capacity.
   c. Place mouthpiece into mouth, maintaining a tight seal.
   d. Hold breath for 2 to 3 seconds.
   e. Try not to cough and to exhale slowly for 3 to 4 seconds through the device while it vibrates.

Clinical Decision Point *If patient cannot maintain an exhalation for this length of time, adjust the PEP device as indicated by the manufacturer to allow the patient to exhale at a lower flow rate.*

   f. Repeat cycle for 5 to 10 breaths as tolerated.
   g. Remove mouthpiece and perform one or two forceful exhalations and "huff" coughs.
   h. Repeat Steps a to g, as required.
7. Auscultate lung fields.
8. Obtain vital signs, SpO_2.
9. Inspect colour, character, and amount of sputum.
10. Help patient with oral hygiene and cleaning of the PEP device.
11. **Use Teach-Back:** "I want to be sure that you can use this device safely. Show me how you use the PEP device during this airway treatment." Develop a revised teaching plan if patient or caregiver is not able to teach back correctly.
12. Review Unexpected Outcomes for Skill 24.1.
13. Document procedure and patient's tolerance. Document your evaluation of patient learning.

PROCEDURAL GUIDELINE 24.2 *Performing Percussion and Vibration*

During postural drainage a nurse, respiratory therapist, or trained caregiver sometimes uses physical manoeuvres such as percussion and vibration on the rib cage over lung tissue. The clinician uses techniques on specific parts of the rib cage over each affected lung region. Normally the mucociliary escalator and cough transport of the body can clear airway secretions effectively. However, when a patient's ability to clear the airways is reduced, the techniques of percussion and vibration are combined with postural drainage (see Skill 24.1).

Percussion is the manual external clapping of a patient's chest wall with cupped hands or with a mechanical device in a rhythmic fashion to loosen secretions from the bronchial walls. To apply vibration to a patient's external chest wall, place both hands (one over the other) over the areas to be vibrated. Then tense and contract the shoulder and arm muscles to create a vibration while the patient exhales to mobilize secretions (Strickland et al., 2015). Vibration augments the natural movement of the rib cage during exhalation and helps with secretion clearance. Never use the clavicles, breast tissue, sternum, spine, waist, or abdomen for percussion and vibration; only perform these manoeuvres over the ribs.

High-Frequency Chest Wall Oscillation

High-frequency chest wall oscillation (HFCWO) consists of an inflatable vest linked to an air-pulse generator. One HFCWO device is the vest airway clearance system, which helps to loosen and remove secretions from the airways (Fig. 24.3). HFCWO systems deliver high-frequency, small-volume expiratory pulses to a patient's external chest wall. This mechanical action helps to loosen and mobilize airway secretions (Wilson, 2018). It is beneficial for selected patients with neuromuscular diseases, cystic fibrosis (CF), and ineffective coughing and airway clearance. In addition, patients with sputum production of 25 to 30 mL/day also benefit from this device because HFCWO decreases the viscosity of mucus, making it easier to cough productively (Volsko, 2013).

Delegation and Collaboration

The skill of performing percussion and vibration can be delegated to an unregulated care provider (UCP) (refer to employer policy). The nurse is responsible for the respiratory assessment and review

of the patient's chest X-ray (in collaboration with a health care provider) to determine patient stability, which areas of the lungs are affected, and specific positions for the patient to assume. The nurse instructs the UCP about:

- Any patient precautions related to disease or treatment.
- Reporting to the nurse any problems the patient has with tolerance of the procedure, pain, or dyspnea, or changes in vital signs.

Equipment

- Stethoscope
- Hospital bed (tilt table placed in Trendelenburg's position, optional; check employer policy)
- Chair (for upper lobes)
- One to four pillows
- Water pitcher and glass
- Tissues and paper bag
- Clear graduated screw-top container
- Mechanical vibrator or percussor (*optional*)
- HFCWO device, such as the vest airway clearance system
- Single layer of clothing
- Personal protective equipment (PPE)
- Oral hygiene care: toothbrush, toothpaste, mouthwash, or chlorhexidine oral rinse if prescribed
- Suction equipment (*optional*)
- Stethoscope, pulse oximeter

Procedural Steps

1. Identify patient using at least two person-specific identifiers (e.g., name and date of birth or name and medical record number) according to employer policy (Accreditation Canada, 2019).
2. Assess patient and review medical record for signs, symptoms, and conditions that indicate need to perform percussion and vibration (see Skill 24.1, Assessment).
3. Perform respiratory assessment (including vital signs, pulse oximetry, inspection, and palpation) to assess breathing pattern, including muscles used for breathing, respiratory rate and depth, extent of excursion, chest wall movement, and oxygen saturation.
4. Auscultate lung sounds over lung segments drained during postural drainage (see Skill 24.1).

Clinical Decision Point *Percussion and vibration are contraindicated with rib fracture, fracture of other rib cage structures such as the clavicle or sternum, pain, severe dyspnea, and severe osteoporosis. Thin, weak patients with osteoporosis are most susceptible to injury and are taught other secretion-control manoeuvres (e.g., forceful coughing, humidification).*

5. Inspect and gently palpate rib cage over affected bronchial segment(s) for pain, tenderness, abnormal configuration, abnormal excursion or chest wall movement during breathing, and muscle tension. Percussion or vibration is contraindicated if one of these assessment findings is present, because the treatment has the potential to cause further injury and impair chest wall motion.
6. Determine patient's understanding and assess ability to cooperate with therapy, both in hospital and at home.
7. Explain procedure in detail: patient's positioning, sensations, how it will be done, how long it will take, use of vest (if applicable), and any discomforts or side effects.

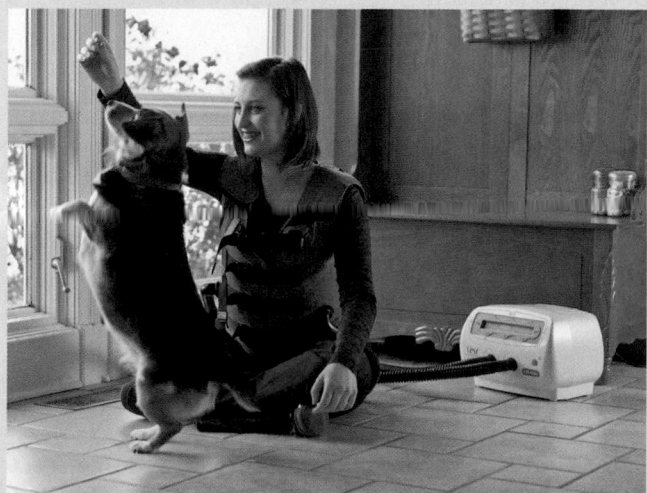

FIG 24.3 High-frequency chest wall oscillation vest for home use. (*Copyright © 2012 Hill-Rom Services, Inc. Reprinted with permission. All rights reserved.*)

Continued

PROCEDURAL GUIDELINE 24.2 *Performing Percussion and Vibration—cont'd*

8. Help patient relax and deep breathe during procedure. Have them practise exhaling slowly through pursed lips while relaxing chest wall muscles and blow out using abdominal muscles, not rib cage muscles.
9. Perform hand hygiene and apply clean gloves as appropriate.
10. Elevate bed to comfortable working height and stand close to bed with arms directly in front and knees slightly bent.
11. Use findings from physical assessment and chest X-ray to select congested areas of lung. Position patient in appropriate drainage position (see Table 24.1) and place pillows for support and comfort.
12. Perform percussion and vibration.
    a. *Percussion and vibration with hands:*
       (1) Perform percussion for 3 to 5 minutes in each position as tolerated. Begin on appropriate part of chest wall over draining area (see Table 24.1). Always ask if patient is experiencing any discomfort such as undue pressure or stinging of the skin.
       (2) Place hands side by side on chest wall over area to be drained. Cup hands with fingers and thumbs held tightly together. Make sure that entire outer part of hand makes contact with chest wall to avoid air leaks (see illustration).

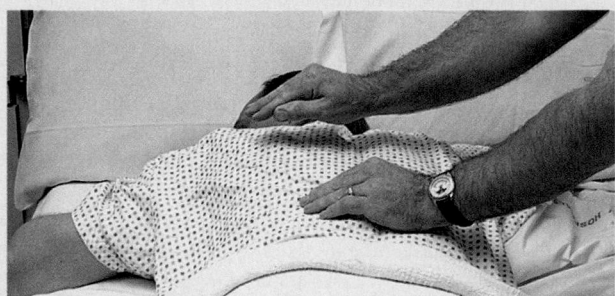

STEP 12a(2) Chest wall percussion, alternating hand clapping against patient's chest wall.

       (3) When clapping, most arm movement comes from the elbow and wrist joints. Clapping is often done for 5 minutes without stopping or for 2 to 3 minutes, alternating with vibration.
       (4) Alternately clap chest with cupped hands to create rhythmic popping sound resembling galloping horse. Perform clapping at moderate or fast speed, whichever is most comfortable and effective.
       (5) Perform chest wall vibration over each affected area (see Table 24.1). Perform vibrations in sets of three followed by coughing so any loosened secretions are expectorated.
          (a) Place flat part of hand over area and have patient take slow, deep breath through nose.
          (b) Gently resist chest wall as it rises during inhalation.
          (c) Have patient hold breath for 2 to 3 seconds and exhale through pursed lips, while contracting abdominal muscles and relaxing chest wall muscles. Chest wall relaxes and falls.
          (d) While patient is exhaling, gently push down and vibrate chest wall with flat part of hand (Volsko, 2013).

          (e) Repeat vibration three times and have patient cascade cough by taking a deep breath and doing a series of small coughs until end of breath. Instruct patient not to inhale between coughs. Vibrate chest wall as patient coughs. When applying pressure to ribs, always follow natural movement of the rib cage. Allow patient to sit up and cough as needed.

Clinical Decision Point *When a patient has excessive pulmonary secretions, which occur with CF, a mechanical vibrator instead of manual vibration is more effective in removing them.*

          (f) Monitor patient's tolerance of vibration and ability to relax chest wall and breathe properly as instructed.
          (g) Perform a total of three or four sets of three vibrations with vibration followed by coughing over each lung segment as tolerated. Strength and frequency of vibration will vary.
    b. *HFCWO device:*
       (1) Apply PPE.
       (2) Place vest on patient and assess for proper fit.
          (a) With vest deflated, adjust closures so it fits comfortably.
          (b) Vest should rest on shoulder and extend to top of hip bone.
       (3) Assess chest wall motion. Breathing should not be restricted when vest is deflated.
       (4) Connect tubing to the generator and ports of the vest. Turn on power.
       (5) Adjust pressure control as prescribed; usually pressure is between 5 and 6.
       (6) Adjust frequency; usually it is set between 10 and 15 Hz.
       (7) Administer any aerosol therapy as prescribed.
       (8) Depress and maintain pressure on the hand or foot control to initiate vest therapy.
       (9) After 5 to 10 minutes, release hand or foot control.
13. Instruct patient to cough or suction if they are unable to cough up mucus (see Chapter 25).
14. Continue with treatment, usually 15 to 30 minutes.
15. Help patient with oral hygiene.
16. Remove PPE and perform hand hygiene.
17. If long-term therapy is needed, teach patient and caregivers the procedure for home use for PEP or HFCWO devices. If they are not able to learn, use interprofessional collaboration to determine outpatient or community care follow-up requirements.
18. Auscultate lung fields.
19. Obtain vital signs, pulse oximetry.
20. Inspect colour, character, and amount of sputum.
21. **Use Teach-Back:** "We discussed the importance of using this vest to manage your respiratory secretions. Tell me why it is important to keep your airways clear of secretions." Develop a revised teaching plan if patient or caregiver is not able to teach back correctly.
22. Document procedure and patient's response. Document your evaluation of patient learning.

✦ CLINICAL DEBRIEF

A 29-year-old university student has a 22-year history of cystic fibrosis (CF). He is on the lung transplant list and adheres to his chest physiotherapy (CPT) and medication regimen. One week ago, he developed a cold, which continued to worsen, and his respiratory secretions were difficult to clear with his usual treatments. He was admitted to the hospital 3 days ago for complicated pneumonia, with a temperature of 40°C, pulse 100 beats/min, respiratory rate of 34 breaths/min, BP 130/80 mm/Hg, and 85% saturation (SaO_2) on 2 L/min of oxygen via nasal cannula. Chest X-ray showed bilateral lower lobe pneumonia and lobar collapse of his right middle lobe.

1. Based on the chest X-ray findings, what should the nurse expect to find on physical examination of the chest, and which additional signs and symptoms should the nurse expect to see?
2. Chest physiotherapy (CPT) was prescribed. Which positions should the nurse use for postural drainage (PD)?
3. After 24 hours of aggressive CPT and PD, a chest X-ray examination was repeated. It showed no improvement. Using SBAR, show how the nurse should communicate with the health care team about this patient.

✦ REVIEW QUESTIONS

1. The nurse is caring for a patient who is to have postural drainage three times a day. Which of the following are necessary to prepare the patient for postural drainage? *(Select all that apply.)*
   1. Encourage adequate fluid intake.
   2. Provide a light meal 30 minutes beforehand.
   3. Explain the procedure and positioning techniques.
   4. Review any chest X-rays and auscultate all lung fields.
   5. Coordinate treatments with other respiratory or medical therapies.
   6. Plan on performing chest physiotherapy (CPT) on all lung regions.
2. The nurse is implementing postural drainage (PD) on a patient. Place the following steps in correct order.
   1. Obtain vital signs and pulse oximetry.
   2. Position patient in proper position to drain selected lung segment.
   3. Maintain position for 10 to 15 minutes.
   4. Perform chest physiotherapy manoeuvres.
   5. Perform respiratory assessment.
   6. Provide a rest period between positions.
3. The nurse is caring for a patient who experiences severe dyspnea and hemoptysis during a session of percussion and vibration. After stopping the treatment, what is the priority nursing intervention?
   1. Notify the health care provider.
   2. Administer a bronchodilator to ease the dyspnea.
   3. Assess the patient.
   4. Elevate the head of the patient's bed.

ⓔ *Visit the Evolve site for a complete list of Clinical Debrief and Review Questions answers.*

REFERENCES

Accreditation Canada. (2019). *Required organizational practices handbook—Version 14.* Retrieved from http://www.wrha.mb.ca/quality/files/2019ROPHandbook.pdf

Ambrosino, N., & Makhabah, D. (2014). *Physiotherapy in the ICU.* Retrieved from http://www.rtmagazine.com/2014/07/physiotherapy-icu/

Brown, S., White, R., & Tobin, P. (2017). Keep them breathing: Cystic fibrosis pathophysiology, diagnosis, and treatment. *Journal of the American Academy of Physician Assistants, 30*(5), 23–27.

dos Santos, A. P., Guimaraes, R. C., de Carhalho, E. M., & Gastaldi, A. C. (2013). Mechanical behaviors of Flutter VRP1, Shaker, and Acapella devices. *Respiratory Care, 58*(2), 298–304. doi:10.4187/respcare.01685

Giger, J. N. (2016). *Transcultural nursing* (7th ed.). St. Louis: Mosby.

Hockenberry, M. J., & Wilson, D. (2015). *Wong's nursing care of infants and children* (10th ed.). St. Louis: Mosby.

Makic, M. B. F., Rauen, C., Jones, K., & Fisk, A. C. (2015). Continuing to challenge practice to be evidence based. *Critical Care Nurse, 35*(2), 39–50. doi:10.4037/ccn2015693

Mikesell, C., Kempainen, R., Laguna, T., et al. (2017). Objective measurement of adherence to out-patient airway clearance therapy by high-frequency chest wall compression in cystic fibrosis. *Respiratory Care, 62*(7), 920–927.

Morrison, L., & Milroy, S. (2018). Oscillating devices for airway clearance in people with cystic fibrosis. *Paediatric Respiratory Reviews, 25*, 30–32. doi:10.1016/j.prrv.2017.07.001

Rimler, R. (2017). *For CF patients, no one right device for airway clearance therapy.* RT, August 2017, 16–20. Retrieved from http://www.rtmagazine.com/2017/08/cf-patients-no-one-right-device-airway-clearance-therapy/

Roqué i Figuls, M., Giné-Garriga, M., Granados-Rugeles, C., Perrotta, C., & Vilaró, J. (2016). Chest physiotherapy for acute bronchiolitis in paediatric patients between 0 and 24 months old. *The Cochrane Database of Systematic Reviews,* (2), Art. No.: CD004873, doi:10.1002/14651858.CD004873.pub5

Salvo, S. (2018). *Mosby's pathology for massage therapists* (4th ed.). St. Louis, MO: Elsevier.

Strickland, S. L., Rubin, B., Haas, C., Volsko, T., Drescher, G., & O'Malley, C. (2015). AARC clinical practice guideline: Effectiveness of pharmacologic airway clearance therapies in hospitalized patients. *Respiratory Care, 60*(7), 1071–1077. doi:10.4187/respcare.04165

Torres-Sanchez, I., Cruz-Ramirez, R., Cabrera-Martos, I., Diaz-Pelegrina, A., & Valenza, M. C. (2017). Results of physiotherapy treatments in exacerbations of chronic obstructive pulmonary disease: A systematic review. *Physiotherapy Canada. Physiothérapie Canada, 69*(2), 122–132. doi:10.3138/ptc.2015-78

Volsko, T. A. (2013). Airway clearance therapy: Finding the evidence. *Respiratory Care, 58*(10), 1669.

Wilson, A. (2018). Oscillating devices for airway clearance in people with cystic fibrosis. *International Journal of Nursing Studies,* doi:10.1016/j.ijnurstu.2018.02.007. Online publication.

Yang, M., Yuping, Y., Yin, X., et al. (2013). Chest physiotherapy for pneumonia in adults. *The Cochrane Database of Systematic Reviews,* (2), CD006338, doi:10.1002/14651858.CD006338.pub2

25 | Airway Management

Written by **C.J. Wright-Boon, RN, MSN, and Jane Tyerman, RN, MScN, PhD**

SKILLS AND PROCEDURES

OBJECTIVES

Mastery of content in this chapter will enable the nurse to:
- Identify safety guidelines for managing a patient's airway.
- Discuss person-centred approaches to airway management.
- Describe the nursing interventions for airway management.
- Discuss the indications for airway suctioning.
- Discuss the indications for tracheostomy care.

- Correctly perform oropharyngeal, nasopharyngeal and nasotracheal, and tracheal suctioning; endotracheal care; and tracheostomy tube care.
- Correctly inflate a cuff on an endotracheal or tracheostomy tube.
- Change a tracheostomy tube or inner cannula.

MEDIA RESOURCES

- evolve http://evolve.elsevier.com/Canada/Perry/clinicalskills/
- Review Questions
- ▶ Video Clips

- Audio Glossary
- **NSO** Nursing Skills Online
- Clinical Debrief and Review Questions Answers
- Animations

PURPOSE

Airway management involves nursing interventions to maintain the patency of a patient's nose, mouth, upper airway, trachea, and lower airway of the respiratory system. The primary goal of airway management is to protect the airway, which will help promote and maintain adequate tissue oxygenation.

STANDARDS OF CARE

- Accreditation Canada, 2019 —*Required Organizational Practices Handbook—Version 14* (http://www.wrha.mb.ca/quality/files/2019ROPHandbook.pdf)
- American Association of Respiratory Care (AARC), 2004—* *AARC Clinical Practice Guidelines: Nasotracheal Suctioning—2004 Revision & Update* (https://www.aarc.org/wp-content/uploads/2014/08/09.04.1080.pdf)
- American Association of Respiratory Care (AARC), 2010— **AARC Clinical Practice Guidelines: Endotracheal Suctioning of

Mechanically Ventilated Patients with Artificial Airways 2010 (https://www.aarc.org/wp-content/uploads/2014/08/06.10.0758.pdf)
- American Association of Respiratory Care (AARC), 2011— **AARC Clinical Practice Guidelines: Capnography/Capnometry During Mechanical Ventilation: 2011* (https://www.aarc.org/wp-content/uploads/2014/08/04.11.0503.pdf)
- American Association of Respiratory Care (AARC), 2012— **AARC Clinical Practice Guidelines: Humidification During Invasive and Noninvasive Mechanical Ventilation: 2012* (https://www.aarc.org/wp-content/uploads/2014/08/12.05.0782.pdf)
- Canadian Patient Safety Institute (CPSI), 2009—*The Safety Competencies* (http://www.patientsafetyinstitute.ca/en/toolsResources/safetyCompetencies/Documents/Safety%20Competencies.pdf)
- Canadian Patient Safety Institute (CPSI), 2012—*Prevent Ventilator-Associated Pneumonia* (http://www.patientsafetyinstitute.ca/en/toolsResources/Documents/Interventions/Ventilator-Associated%20Pneumonia/VAP%20Getting%20Started%20Kit.pdf#search=canadian%20vap%20guidelines)
- Hellyer, Ewan, Wilson, et al., 2016—*The Intensive Care Society Recommended Bundle of Interventions for the Prevention of Ventilator-Associated Pneumonia* (https://journals.sagepub.com/doi/abs/10.1177/1751143716644461)

NOTE: AARC Clinical Practice Guidelines are used in Canada and are seminal publications.

- Institute for Healthcare Improvement (IHI), 2012—*How-To Guide: Prevent Ventilator-Associated Pneumonia* (http://www.ihi.org/resources/Pages/Tools/HowtoGuidePreventVAP.aspx)

PRINCIPLES FOR PRACTICE

- Various techniques for airway management are available to promote an open or patent airway, which has the potential to become blocked by mucus, a mechanical obstruction (i.e., soft tissue in upper airway), or a foreign body.
- Hydration, positioning, nutrition, chest physiotherapy techniques, deep breathing, coughing, humidity, incentive spirometry, and aerosol therapy are noninvasive techniques that are helpful in maintaining a patent airway.
- When patients are unable to protect their own airway or clear airway secretions with coughing, chest physiotherapy, or other noninvasive techniques, more invasive measures such as suctioning or inserting an artificial airway are needed.
- An artificial airway is a plastic or rubber device (such as a tracheostomy or endotracheal tube) that is inserted into the upper or lower respiratory tract to facilitate ventilation or the removal of secretions.
- Mechanical assistance may be needed to maintain airway patency.
- Indications for mechanical ventilation include (a) upper airway obstructions (e.g., secondary to burns, tumour, bleeding), (b) apnea, (c) high risk for aspiration, (d) inability to clear secretions, and (e) respiratory distress.

PERSON-CENTRED CARE

- Artificial airways alter patients' ability to communicate, possibly causing feelings of fear, frustration, anxiety, and vulnerability.
- Recommendations to improve communication for patients with an altered airway include developing alternate means of and establishing an environment that promotes effective communication among the patient, the caregivers, and the members of the interprofessional health care team (Baumgarten & Poulsen, 2015; ten Hoorn, Elbers, Girbes, et al., 2016).
- It is important to assess for anger and frustration when patients with artificial airways try to communicate and to consider the need for individualized and creative communication methods (Baumgarten, & Poulsen, 2015).
- Nurses need to thoroughly educate patients and their caregivers using plain language that is culturally sensitive and verify that they understand any procedures or tests.
- Collaboration with caregivers is essential when providing alternative means of communication for patients. Once communication is established, a patient and caregiver will have more trust in the care provided, which will promote cooperation and rapport.
- Use interprofessional collaboration when caring for patients who have English as their second language or do not speak English, to prevent misunderstanding of treatment options.
- Obtain professional translators or other communication aids so patients and caregivers understand the need for an artificial airway and the subsequent treatments.
- Assess the functional skills of the patient. Ensure that functioning hearing aids are in place and working so communication with a hearing-impaired patient is possible. Allow patients to wear their glasses and use communication devices such as picture or letter boards. Assess the patient's dominant hand and muscle strength if writing boards are to be used (Baumgarten, & Poulsen, 2015; ten Hoorn et al., 2016).

EVIDENCE-INFORMED PRACTICE

- There are significant concerns regarding the definition of ventilator-associated pneumonia (VAP) and ventilator-associated events (VAEs). As an interprofessional collaborative intervention, the Centers for Disease Control and Prevention (CDC, 2019) developed a lengthy algorithm for health care providers to use to accurately diagnose these complications.
  - The key points in the definition of VAE are "deterioration in respiratory status after a period of stability or improvement on the ventilator, evidence of infection or inflammation, and laboratory evidence of respiratory infection" (CDC, 2019, p. 10-4)
  - The patient must be mechanically ventilated for more than 2 calendar days to be eligible for VAE (CDC, 2019).
- VAP/VAE bundles are available to help guide nursing practice (see also Skill 23.5). Key interventions included in these bundles are the following:
  - Elevation of the head of bed (HOB) between 30 and 45 degrees
  - Daily interruption of sedation and daily assessment of a patient's readiness to extubate
  - Peptic ulcer disease prophylaxis
  - Deep venous thrombosis prophylaxis (unless contraindicated)
  - Daily oral care with chlorhexidine
  - Delirium monitoring and management
  - Early exercise and mobility
- Closed endotracheal suctioning techniques are preferred over open endotracheal suctioning techniques in patients who have undergone open heart surgery. Closed suctioning has fewer traumatic effects on mean arterial blood pressure and pulse oximetry than open suctioning (Kuriyama, Umakoshi, Fujinaga, et al., 2015).
- Closed-circuit suctioning has more advantages than disadvantages when compared with open-circuit suctioning, such as avoiding loss of positive end-expiratory pressure (PEEP), which decreases amount of hypoxemia, costs, and caregiver exposure to pulmonary secretions (Wiegand, 2017).
- New products are being developed to decrease the risk of biofilm formation on endotracheal tubes (ETs). Biofilm is associated with increased risks of developing VAP.
  - These new products include systems that scrape the inside of the ET to remove the secretions.
  - Silver-coated, gardine-coated, and gendine-coated ETs are also being investigated for their effectiveness in preventing biofilm formation (Tokmaji, Vermeulen, Muller, et al., 2015).
- Automated cuff pressure-control devices used to measure cuff pressures on artificial airways are not recommended because they interfere with the self-sealing characteristics of tracheal cuffs (Muir, Rodriguez, Galudes, et al., 2015).

SAFETY GUIDELINES

- Know a patient's baseline range of vital signs and oxygen saturation levels. Baseline physiological measures aid in identifying individual abnormalities and recognizing worsening of an illness.
- Know a patient's medical history. Smoking alters normal mucociliary clearance. Certain disorders such as chronic obstructive pulmonary disease (COPD), asthma, cystic fibrosis (CF), pneumonia, thoracic surgery, chest trauma, and abdominal surgery place patients at increased risk for an obstructed airway.
- Identify conditions that increase a patient's risk for aspiration of gastric contents into the lung, which can result in airway

obstruction. These include the presence of enteral feeding tubes or nasal and oral gastric tubes, a decreased level of consciousness, and a decreased swallowing ability.

- Use caution when suctioning patients with head injuries. The suction procedure causes an elevation in intracranial pressure (ICP) (Galbiati & Paola, 2015). Reduce this risk by presuctioning hyperventilation, which results in hypocarbia. This in turn induces vasoconstriction, thereby reducing the risk of elevated ICP.
- Determine if a patient has a history of nasal problems such as nasal trauma, nasal polyps, deviated nasal septum, or chronic sinusitis. Allergy problems may cause mucosal swelling that narrows nasal passages, which affects the ability to easily pass a suction catheter.
- Review a patient's respiratory assessments from the past 12 or 24 hours. These are relative baseline measurements that help in distinguishing between gradual and acute changes in a patient's status.
- Perform a systematic pulmonary assessment of upper and lower airways, including respiratory rate, respiratory pattern, accessory muscle use, breath sounds, ability to cough effectively, integrity of the rib cage, and the characteristics of sputum production.

- Identify and become familiar with the use of equipment available at the facility. Many types of artificial airways, suction catheters, and suction machines are available. Knowing how to operate the equipment before use helps lead to positive outcomes.
- Test all equipment before use. Have adequate supplies on hand at the bedside. Equipment must work properly to provide safe nursing care. Determine that the suction machine is generating adequate negative suction pressure and that suction catheters and appropriate equipment are available at the bedside.
- Know the adverse effects of medications and other therapies. Some medications, such as beta-adrenergic blockers, have the adverse effect of bronchospasm. An adverse effect of opioids and sedatives is respiratory depression. Similarly, too much oxygen reduces the drive to breathe in patients with chronic hypercapnia (elevated arterial carbon dioxide tension). Some position changes can affect a patient adversely. For example, in patients with impaired spinal cord innervations of the respiratory muscles, supine positions place the diaphragm at a mechanical disadvantage and increase the risk for aspiration.
- The instillation of normal saline when performing endotracheal suctioning is not a supported practice (Wiegand, 2017).

✦ SKILL 25.1   Performing Oropharyngeal Suctioning

▶ *Video Clip*   **NSO**   *Nursing Skills Online Airway Management Module 9 / Lesson 2*

Prior to initiating oropharyngeal suctioning, it is important that supplemental oxygen with appropriate delivery devices be readily available at the bedside. A Yankauer, or tonsillar tip, suction device is used for oropharyngeal suctioning (i.e., the removal of pharyngeal secretions through the mouth) (Fig. 25.1). A Yankauer suction catheter is made of rigid, minimally flexible plastic. The tip of this suction catheter usually has one large and several small openings through which the mucus enters with application of negative pressure. The Yankauer suction catheter is angled to facilitate removal of secretions through a patient's mouth. Oropharyngeal suctioning only removes secretions from the back of the throat. Perform oral suctioning when a patient is able to cough effectively but is unable to clear secretions, such as for patients with a neuromuscular injury who cannot manage their own oral secretions. Patients with artificial airways and impaired swallowing require use of the Yankauer suction device to provide oral hygiene.

Delegation and Collaboration

The skill of performing oropharyngeal suctioning may be delegated to an unregulated care provider (UCP), depending on employer policy. Do not delegate this skill for patients with oral or neck surgery in the immediate postoperative period. The nurse is responsible for assessing the patient's respiratory status. The nurse instructs the UCP about:

- Appropriate suction limits for oropharyngeal suctioning for a particular patient (e.g., the appropriate suction pressure, expected frequency of suctioning, and expected colour and volume of secretions).
- The risks of applying excessive or inadequate suction pressure.
- Avoiding mouth sutures, applying suction against sensitive tissues, and dislodging tubes in the patient's nose or mouth.
- Avoiding stimulation of the gag reflex.
- Immediately reporting to the nurse any change in vital signs, pulse oximetry (SpO_2), sputum (i.e., bloody), difficulty breathing, or discomfort during or after the procedure.

Equipment

- Yankauer or tonsillar tip suction catheter
- Clean gloves
- Towel, cloth, or disposable paper drape
- Personal protective equipment (PPE), as indicated
- Disposable cup or nonsterile basin
- Tap water or normal saline (about 100 mL)
- Suction machine or wall suction device with regulator
- Connecting tubing (1.8 metres [6 feet])
- Oral airway (if indicated)
- Washcloth (if indicated)
- Pulse oximeter, stethoscope
- Manual self-inflating resuscitation bag (bag-valve-mask) with oxygen-connecting tubing

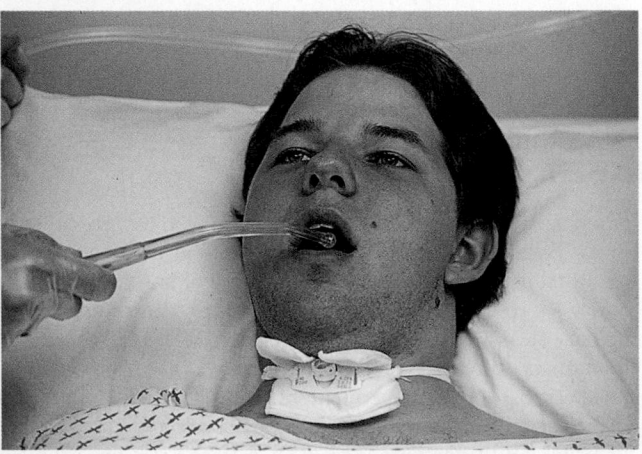

FIG 25.1 Oropharyngeal suctioning.

STEP	RATIONALE

ASSESSMENT

1. Identify patient using at least two person-specific identifiers (e.g., name and date of birth or name and medical record number) according to employer policy.

Ensures correct patient. Complies with Accreditation Canada's standards and improves patient safety (Accreditation Canada, 2019).

2. Identify risk factors for airway obstruction: impaired cough or gag reflex, weakened respiratory muscles, impaired swallowing, and decreased level of consciousness.

Risk factors prevent patient from protecting airway from aspiration or clearing secretions safely.

3. Assess for signs and symptoms of hypoxia: anxiety, change in level of consciousness, change in vital signs, decreased SpO_2, adventitious sounds (see also Box 23.1).

Suctioning of oropharyngeal airway is indicated with alterations in oxygenation associated with secretion accumulation.

4. Obtain patient's oxygen saturation level via SpO_2 (see Chapter 7). Keep pulse oximeter in place.

Provides an objective baseline measure of oxygen saturation and an early indication of changes in oxygenation status. Aids in assessment of patient during and after oropharyngeal suctioning.

5. Determine patient's ability to hold or manipulate catheter and their knowledge about use of suction catheter and procedure.

Encourages cooperation; minimizes risks and anxiety. Identifies teaching needs. Physical factors such as impaired mobility of upper extremities prevent patient from using catheter to help control oral secretions.

6. Assess for signs and symptoms of upper airway obstruction: gurgling on inspiration or expiration, restlessness, obvious excessive oral secretions, drooling, gastric secretions or vomitus in mouth, or coughing without clearing secretions from upper airway.

Secretions pool in the upper airway, which can cause total airway obstruction and hypoxia. The risk for aspiration of gastric contents and airway obstruction is increased in patients with vomiting; delayed gastric emptying; impairment in esophageal sphincter control, cough, swallowing, or gag reflex; or patients receiving enteral feedings.

7. Auscultate for presence of adventitious sounds (see Chapter 8 and Skill 25.2).

Determines if lower airway secretions are present and establishes baseline.

NURSING DIAGNOSES

- Reduced airway clearance
- Inadequate breathing pattern
- Reduced gas exchange
- Inadequate swallowing
- Insufficient knowledge regarding use of suction
- Potential for aspiration
- Potential for infection

Related factors/Risk factors are individualized on the basis of patient's condition or needs.

PLANNING

1. Expected outcomes following completion of procedure:
   - No gurgling sounds are heard in patient's pharynx on inspiration and expiration.

   Suctioning is effective. Secretions are removed from large upper airway.

   - Drooling is diminished or absent.

   Excessive drooling indicates that patient is unable to handle oral secretions.

   - Vomitus or gastric secretions are absent from mouth.

   Gastric secretions retained in oral cavity increase patient's risk for aspiration pneumonia.

   - SpO_2 improves or remains at patient's normal baseline.

   Removal of secretions helps to improve oxygen saturation level.

Clinical Decision Point *In patients living with chronic pulmonary disease, the SpO_2 value may remain the same after oropharyngeal suctioning. This baseline value may be lower than the typical normal values of greater than 95% (Grindrod, 2015).*

2. Perform hand hygiene. Gather equipment and supplies. Close room door or curtain.

Ensures well-organized procedure. Provides patient privacy as part of person-centred care.

3. Explain to patient how procedure helps clear airway secretions and relieves some breathing problems. Explain that coughing, gagging, or (less commonly) sneezing is normal and lasts only a few seconds. Encourage patient to cough out secretions and show how to splint painful areas during procedure. Have patient practice coughing, if able.

Gagging or coughing occurs when the posterior pharynx is suctioned or because of excess secretions. Coughing secretions out of lower airway or the posterior pharynx decreases the amount of suctioning required. Splinting reduces abdominal incision discomfort during coughing or gagging.

4. Position patient in semi-Fowler's or sitting position. Place towel, cloth, or paper drape across patient's neck and chest.

Promotes patient comfort and removal of airway secretions. Towel protects gown and bed linen from contamination by secretions.

STEP	RATIONALE

IMPLEMENTATION

1. Apply clean gloves and appropriate PPE (e.g., apply mask or face shield if splashing is likely; gown if transmission-based precautions are indicated).

Reduces transmission of microorganisms.

2. Fill cup or basin with approximately 100 mL of water or normal saline.

Helps to clean catheter after suctioning and assesses that equipment functions.

3. Connect one end of connecting tubing to suction machine and other to Yankauer suction catheter. Turn on suction machine; set vacuum regulator to appropriate setting (infants 80–100 mm Hg; children 100–120 mm Hg; adults 100–150 mm Hg) (AARC, 2004).

Prepares suction apparatus. Pressures should not exceed 150 mm Hg because elevated pressure settings increase risk for trauma to oral mucosa (AARC, 2004).

4. Check that suction machine is functioning properly, by placing tip of catheter in water or normal saline and suctioning small amount from cup or basin.

Ensures that equipment functions and lubricates catheter.

5. Remove patient's oxygen mask if present. Nasal cannula may remain in place. Keep oxygen mask near patient's face.

Allows access to mouth. Reduces chance of hypoxia.

Clinical Decision Point *Be prepared to quickly reapply supplemental oxygen if SpO₂ value falls below 90% or respiratory distress develops during or at the end of oropharyngeal suctioning. Be prepared to use the bag-valve-mask if patient has serious acute respiratory distress or decline in SpO₂.*

6. Insert catheter into mouth along gum line to pharynx. Move catheter around mouth until secretions have cleared. Encourage patient to cough. Replace oxygen mask.

Movement of catheter prevents suction tip from invaginating oral mucosal surfaces and causing trauma. Coughing moves secretions from lower airway into mouth and upper airway.

Clinical Decision Point *Be careful when using a Yankauer tip suction catheter with a patient who has had recent oral or head and neck surgery. Aggressive suctioning and excessive coughing should not be used or encouraged in patients who have undergone throat surgery, such as a tonsillectomy. These acts can aggravate the operative site, increasing the risk of infection or bleeding (Hockenberry & Wilson, 2015).*

7. Rinse catheter with water or normal saline in cup or basin until connecting tubing is cleared of secretions. Turn off suction. Place catheter in clean, dry area.

Rinses catheter and reduces probability of transmission of microorganisms. Clean suction tubing enhances delivery of set suction pressure.

8. Wash face if secretions are present on patient's skin.

Prevents skin breakdown.

9. Observe respiratory status. Repeat procedure if indicated. You may need to use a standard suction catheter to reach into the trachea if respiratory status is not improved (see Skill 25.2).

Directs nurse to continue, cease intervention, or choose another intervention.

10. Remove towel, cloth, or disposable drape and place in garbage or in laundry. Reposition patient; Sims' or side-lying position encourages drainage and should be used if patient has decreased level of consciousness.

Reduces transmission of microorganisms. Facilitates drainage of oral secretions.

11. Discard remainder of water or normal saline into appropriate receptacle. Rinse basin in warm, soapy water and dry with paper towels (check employer policy). Discard disposable cup into appropriate receptacle.

Reduces transmission of microorganisms and maintains medical asepsis. Moist environment encourages microorganism growth.

Clinical Decision Point *Keep catheter in non-airtight container such as brown paper or plastic bag attached to bedrail or in suction canister area. Do not store the catheter where it will come in contact with secretions or excretions, which promote bacterial growth.*

12. Remove PPE and dispose of in appropriate receptacle. Perform hand hygiene.

Reduces transmission of microorganisms to other patients and equipment.

13. Position patient and provide oral hygiene as needed.

Promotes patient's comfort.

STEP	RATIONALE

EVALUATION

1. Compare assessment findings before and after procedure.

2. Auscultate chest and airways for adventitious sounds.

3. Inspect mouth for any vomitus or remaining secretions.

4. Obtain and record postsuction SpO$_2$ value. Compare with presuction level.

5. **Use Teach-Back:** "I want to ensure that you understand why I need to suction your mouth. Can you tell me why I need to do this?" Develop a revised teaching plan if patient or caregiver is not able to teach back correctly.

Identifies physiological response to suction procedure.

Presence of lower airway adventitious sounds suggests need for lower airway suctioning.

A clear oral airway is necessary to prevent aspiration.

Provides objective measure of effectiveness of suction procedure (AARC, 2004).

Determines patient's and caregiver's level of understanding of instructional topic.

Unexpected Outcomes

1. Patient's respiratory distress increases.

2. Bloody secretions are suctioned.

Related Interventions

- Suction further or implement nasal or tracheal suctioning (Skill 25.2).
- Evaluate need for other means to protect airway (e.g., oral intubation, oral airway, positioning).
- Provide supplemental oxygen.
- Notify health care provider.
- Assess oral cavity for trauma or lesions.
- Reduce amount of suction pressure used.
- Observe catheter tip for nicks, which cause mucosal trauma.
- Increase frequency of oral hygiene.

Communication and Documentation

- Document the amount, consistency, colour, and odour of secretions; number of times suctioned; patient's response to suctioning; and presuction and postsuction cardiopulmonary assessment findings on flow sheet or nurses' notes in electronic health record (EHR) or chart.
- Document patient's and caregiver's understanding through teach-back of reasons for safe oral suctioning.
- Interprofessional collaboration should be prioritized by promptly notifying the health care provider of any unresolved outcomes, such as worsening respiratory distress.

Special Considerations
Teaching

- Instruct patient and caregiver not to allow catheter to fall to the floor. If this occurs, teach patient and caregiver how to clean or obtain a clean catheter (see Care in the Community).
- Provide information regarding signs and symptoms of worsening respiratory status.

Pediatric

- Airways of infants and children are smaller than those of an adult; even small amounts of mucus cause airway obstruction. Smaller suction catheters may need to be used (Hockenberry & Wilson, 2015).
- Bulb syringes may be used to suction the oral cavity in newborns and infants. To properly use a bulb syringe, compress the bulb before inserting into mouth to decrease the risk of forcing the secretions into lower airways. If the bulb syringe cannot remove the secretions, use appropriate-size mechanical suction equipment (Hockenberry & Wilson, 2015).
- Use lower suction pressures with infants and children than with adults (Hockenberry & Wilson, 2015).
- Position infants with breathing problems or excessive vomitus in side-lying position to decrease risk of aspiration (Hockenberry & Wilson, 2015).

- Suctioning, particularly for young infants, should be completed for only 5 seconds because of risk of deoxygenation. Allow 30 to 60 seconds for patient to reoxygenate (Hockenberry & Wilson, 2015).
- Complete oral suctioning first and then nasal suctioning, to decrease the risk of aspiration, particularly for newborn infants (Hockenberry & Wilson, 2015).

Gerontological

- Patients with dysphagia may benefit from oral suctioning before, during, and after meals.
- The oral mucosa in older persons is fragile (Touhy, Jett, Boscart, et al., 2019). Use a lower suction pressure if bleeding starts to occur.
- Older persons are prone to aspiration of oral secretions because of decreased cough and gag reflexes and increased incidence of dysphagia (Touhy et al., 2019).

Care in the Community

- Make sure that patient and caregiver know how to clean and disinfect or change the secretion collection container every 24 hours according to home care protocol. Many facilities seal and dispose of the entire disposable secretion collection canister as biohazardous material.
- Assess knowledge level of patient and caregiver to determine amount of instruction required and frequency of home health visits necessary to reach goals.
- Assess home for the presence of respiratory irritants, including cigarette smoke, dust, pollen, animal dander, mould, and chemicals.

Long-Term Care

- As many as 60% of patients who live in longterm care facilities have evidence of dysphagia, which makes them prone to aspiration. Ensure that dysphagia screens are performed for all patients and that properly functioning equipment is available (Touhy et al., 2019).

✦ SKILL 25.2 Airway Suctioning

NSO *Nursing Skills Online Airway Management Module 9 / Lessons 1, 2, and 3*

Suctioning is necessary when patients are unable to clear respiratory secretions. If the secretions are only in the nose and mouth, only the pharynx requires suctioning. However, in most instances both the pharynx and the trachea will be suctioned. Suction secretions from the pharynx as often as necessary using oropharyngeal suctioning (see Skill 25.1). Secretions that are not removed are more likely to be aspirated into the lungs, increasing the risk for infection, ventilator-associated pneumonia, and respiratory failure. Retained lower airway secretions require the use of tracheal suctioning to remove them. If frequent nasotracheal suctioning is indicated, consider application of a nasopharyngeal airway to prevent trauma.

Prior to initiating airway suctioning, it is important that supplemental oxygen with appropriate delivery devices be readily available at the bedside.

Tracheal airway suctioning is a sterile procedure. It extends into the lower airway and is indicated to remove respiratory secretions and maintain optimum ventilation and oxygenation in patients who are unable to remove these secretions independently. This skill can be performed in people with or without an artificial airway.

Tracheal suctioning has many complications, including hypoxemia, cardiac dysrhythmias, changes in blood pressure (either hypertensive or hypotensive), laryngeal or bronchospasm, pain, infection, or bradycardia. Bradycardia is associated with stimulation of the vagus nerve. Respiratory or cardiac arrest can even occur as a result of tracheal suctioning. Nasal trauma and bleeding can develop from a suction catheter being introduced through the nares (Urden, Stacy, & Lough, 2016).

Patient assessment, not routine suctioning, guides the frequency of airway suctioning (Urden et al., 2016). Patient assessment factors indicating the need for suctioning include oxygen saturation below 90%; visible secretions in the airway; patient's inability to produce an effective, productive cough; auscultation of coarse crackles over the trachea; and acute respiratory distress. If the patient has an artificial airway in place or is mechanically ventilated, other indications for suctioning include the presence of a saw-tooth pattern on the flow-volume loop on the ventilator monitor, increased peak inspiratory pressure or decreased tidal volumes noted on the ventilator monitor, abnormal capnography waveforms, or suspected aspiration (American Association of Critical Care Nurses [AACN], 2010; AARC, 2010; Sole, Bennett, & Ashworth, 2015; Timbrell & Jankowski, 2018; Wiegand, 2017).

Artificial Airway Suctioning

Endotracheal tubes (ETs) and tracheostomy tubes (TTs) are artificial airways inserted to maintain respiratory flow and prevent airway obstruction, provide a route for mechanical ventilation, permit easy access for secretion removal, and protect the airway from gross aspiration in patients with impaired cough or gag reflexes.

Endotracheal Tubes

NSO *Nursing Skills Online Airway Management Module 9 / Lesson 4*

ET intubation is a procedure performed by a health care provider or other specially trained personnel (e.g., certified registered nurse anaesthesiologist, respiratory therapist, or rescue personnel). An ET is inserted through the nares (nasotracheal tube) or most commonly through the mouth (oral ET) past the epiglottis and

vocal cords into the trachea (Fig. 25.2, A–B). Oral ETs are usually made of plastic or rubber. Adult (and some pediatric) sizes of ETs have a cuff moulded onto the tube. When the cuff is inflated, it seals the airway around the tube to prevent the aspiration of oral secretions or gastric contents into the lung and to obstruct the escape of air from mechanical ventilator breaths through the upper airway. Some newer ETs also contain a port that can be connected for continuous subglottal suctioning.

The length of time that an ET should remain in place is in dispute. Complications from long-term intubation include laryngeal and tracheal stenosis or a cricoid abscess (Urden et al., 2016). Sources differ on when a patient should be changed from an ET to a TT. The range of recommended length of time to be intubated is 7 to 10 days to as long as 21 days (Urden et al., 2016; Vargas, Sutherasan, Antonelli, et al., 2015). It is appropriate to consult with a health care provider if a patient begins to show signs of complications from the airways themselves, such as erosion of the oral mucosa. Known benefits of having a TT versus an ET include less need for deeper sedation, shorter ventilator weaning time (time it takes to

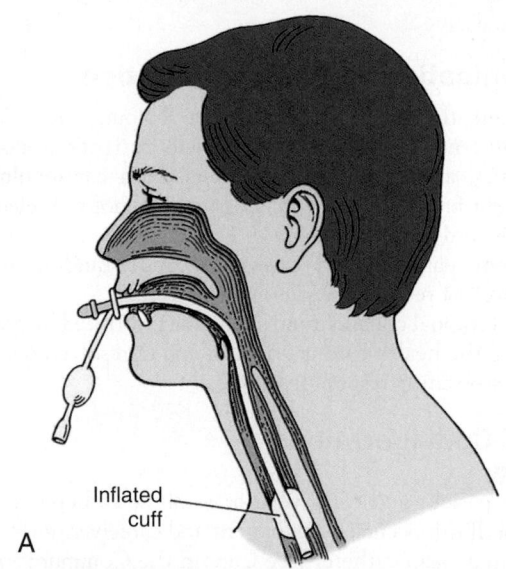

A

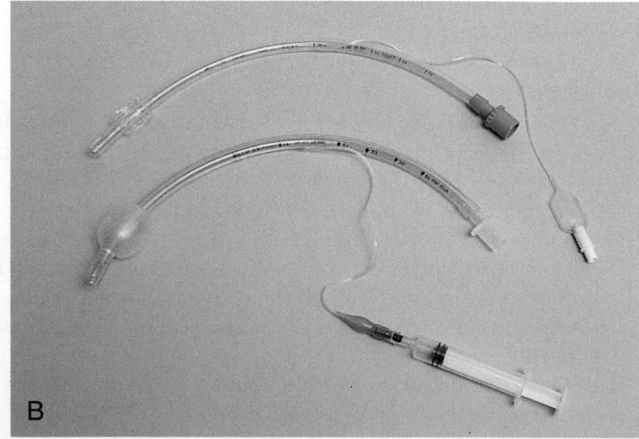

B

FIG 25.2 A, Endotracheal (ET) tube with inflated cuff. **B,** ET tubes with uninflated and inflated cuffs and syringe for inflation.

get a patient off a ventilator), and shorter critical care unit (CCU) and hospital stay (Hyde, Savage, Zarzaur, et al., 2015).

Tracheostomy Tubes

A TT can be temporary or permanent, depending on a patient's condition. It is inserted either surgically or percutaneously directly into the trachea through a small incision made in a patient's neck. Reasons for using a TT include the need for prolonged mechanical ventilation, upper airway obstruction secondary to trauma or tumour, and difficulties with airway clearance that occurs in conditions such as spinal cord injury or neuromuscular disease (Myatt, 2015; Urden et al., 2016). TTs are made of several different materials, including polyvinyl chloride or silicone-based plastics and stainless steel or metallic compounds. Metal TTs are thermal sensitive and must be protected from extreme heat and cold to prevent tissue injury in a patient. Most metal and plastic TTs contain an inner cannula that is withdrawn temporarily for cleaning airway-occluding mucus without removing the entire TT. The inner cannula can be cleaned and reused or may be a disposable plastic device (see Skill 25.4) (Myatt, 2015; Urden et al., 2016).

The use of closed-system suction catheters for suctioning artificial airways has increased in recent years. Use of a closed-system catheter (in-line) allows quicker lower airway suctioning without applying sterile gloves or a mask and does not interrupt ventilation and oxygenation in critically ill patients (see Procedural Guideline 25.1). With a closed-system method, the patient's artificial airway is not disconnected from the mechanical ventilator; therefore, there is no loss of positive end-expiratory pressure (PEEP) (Kuriyama et al., 2015). Other advantages of this system include a quicker, more efficient performance of the suctioning procedure. When comparing closed-versus-open suctioning, the incidence of ventilator-associated pneumonia (VAP) is unchanged (Elmansoury & Said, 2017). However, with a closed system there is decreased risk of infection for a health care provider from exposure to patient secretions (Urden et al., 2016). Recommended frequency for replacing closed-system suction catheters is every 24 to 48 hours, or according to employer policy.

Delegation and Collaboration

The skill of artificial airway suctioning of newly inserted artificial airways cannot be delegated to an unregulated care provider (UCP). The nurse instructs the UCP about:

- Any modifications of the skill, such as the need for supplemental oxygen or the use of a clean-versus-sterile suction technique.
- Appropriate suction limits for suctioning ETs and TTs and risks of applying excessive or inadequate suction pressure.
- Reporting any changes in the patient's respiratory status, level of consciousness, restlessness, secretion colour and amount, and unresolved coughing or gagging.
- Reporting any change in the patient's colour, vital signs, or indications of pain.

Equipment

- Stethoscope
- Pulse oximeter
- Portable or wall suction machine
- Connecting tubing (1.8 metres [6 feet])
- Bedside table
- Personal protective equipment (PPE) as indicated

Endotracheal or Tracheostomy Suctioning

- Appropriate-size suction catheter, usually 12–16 Fr (smallest diameter that will remove secretions effectively, preferably one that is no more than half the internal diameter of the artificial airway, to minimize decrease in PaO_2) (AACN, 2010; AARC, 2010)
- Two sterile gloves or one sterile and one clean glove
- Clean towel or paper drape
- Small Y-adapter (if catheter does not have a suction control port)
- Sterile basin or solution container
- Sterile normal saline solution or water, about 100 mL
- Pulse oximeter, stethoscope, and end-tidal carbon dioxide (CO_2) detector
- Manual self-inflating manual resuscitation bag-valve device with appropriate-size mask
- PEEP valve for resuscitation bag

STEP	RATIONALE

ASSESSMENT

1. Identify patient using at least two person-specific identifiers (e.g., name and date of birth or name and medical record number) according to employer policy.

   Ensures correct patient. Complies with Accreditation Canada's standards and improves patient safety (Accreditation Canada, 2019).

2. Perform hand hygiene and apply gloves if risk of exposing self to secretions. Assess for signs and symptoms of upper and lower airway obstruction requiring suctioning: abnormal respiratory rate, adventitious lung sounds, nasal secretions, gurgling, drooling, restlessness, gastric secretions or vomitus in mouth, and coughing without clearing airway secretions or improving adventitious lung sounds.

   Physical signs and symptoms result from secretions in upper and lower airways and decreased oxygen to the tissues. Presuction assessment provides baseline data for identifying need for suctioning and for measuring effectiveness of suction procedures.

3. Assess vital signs and signs and symptoms associated with hypoxia and hypercapnia: decreased pulse oximetry (SpO_2), increased pulse and blood pressure, apprehension, anxiety, lack of concentration, lethargy, decreased level of consciousness, confusion, dizziness, behavioural changes (e.g., irritability), irregular heart pulse, pallor, and cyanosis (a very late sign of hypoxia). Keep pulse oximeter on patient.

   Physical signs and symptoms resulting from decreased tissue oxygenation. Provides presuction baseline to measure patient tolerance of suctioning and effectiveness of suctioning on SpO_2 levels.

STEP	RATIONALE

ASSESSMENT

4. Assess for risk factors for upper and lower airway obstruction, including chronic obstructive pulmonary disease (COPD), impaired mobility, decreased level of consciousness, nasal feeding tube, decreased cough or gag reflex, and decreased swallowing ability.

Risk factors can impair patient's ability to clear secretions from airway, increase risk for retaining secretions, and necessitate nasopharyngeal or nasotracheal suctioning (Urden et al., 2016).

5. Identify patients with an increased risk for inadequate airway clearance (e.g., patients with decreased level of consciousness, neuromuscular or neurological impairment, or anatomical factors that influence upper or lower airway function, such as recent head or neck surgery, or neck tumours).

Changes in neurological status and neuromuscular impairment increase the likelihood that the patient is unable to clear respiratory secretions. Abnormal anatomy or head and neck surgery or trauma and tumours in and around the lower airway impair normal secretion clearance. Accumulating pulmonary secretions impede patient's ability to effectively clear airway through cough mechanism (Urden et al., 2016).

6. Assess for excessive amounts of secretions or secretions visible in the artificial airway, signs of respiratory distress (increased work of breathing, increased respiratory rate), presence of rhonchi on auscultation, excessive coughing, or decrease in patient pulse oximeter; if patient is on mechanical ventilation, also assess for increased peak inspiratory pressures, saw-tooth pattern on ventilator monitor, or changes in capnography waveform.

Suctioning should only be performed as patient condition indicates and not in a scheduled fashion, such as hourly (Lewis, Bucher, Heitkemper, et al., 2019; Myatt, 2015).

7. Assess patency of ET with capnography/end-tidal CO_2 detector.

ET may become displaced or blocked by secretions. CO_2 detector is pH sensitive and can be used to identify changes in CO_2 levels caused by retained secretions.

8. Assess factors that may affect volume and consistency of secretions.

Thickened or copious secretions increase risk for airway obstruction.

   a. Fluid balance

Fluid overload increases amount of secretions. Dehydration promotes thicker secretions.

   b. Lack of humidity

Environment influences secretion formation and gas exchange. Airway suctioning is needed when patient cannot clear secretions effectively.

   c. Infection (e.g., pneumonia)

Patients with respiratory infections are prone to increased secretions that are thicker and sometimes more difficult to expectorate.

9. For endotracheal suctioning assess patient's peak inspiratory pressure when on volume-controlled ventilation or tidal volume during pressure-controlled ventilation.

Increased peak inspiratory pressure or decreased tidal volume may indicate airway obstruction (Urden et al., 2016).

Clinical Decision Point *The patient's vital signs, pulse oximetry, end-tidal CO_2, and respiratory status will be assessed before and continuously throughout the procedure.*

10. Identify contraindications to nasotracheal suctioning (AARC, 2004): occluded nasal passages; nasal bleeding; epiglottis or croup; acute head, facial, or neck injury or surgery; coagulopathy or bleeding disorder; irritable airway; laryngospasm or bronchospasm; gastric surgery with high anastomosis; myocardial infarction.

These conditions are contraindicated because passage of a suction catheter through the nasal route causes trauma to existing facial trauma or surgery, increases nasal bleeding, or causes severe bleeding in presence of coagulopathy or bleeding disorders. In presence of epiglottis or croup, laryngospasm, or irritable airway, passage of a suction catheter through the nose causes intractable coughing, hypoxemia, and severe bronchospasm, necessitating emergency intubation or tracheostomy. Hypoxemia could worsen cardiac damage in myocardial infarction (AARC, 2004).

11. Review sputum microbiology data in laboratory report.

Certain bacteria are easier to transmit or require isolation because of virulence or antibiotic resistance.

12. Determine presence of apprehension, anxiety, decreased ability to concentrate, lethargy, decreased level of consciousness (especially acute), increased fatigue, dizziness, behavioural changes (especially irritability), pallor, cyanosis, dyspnea, or use of accessory muscles.

These are signs and symptoms of hypoxia and/or hypercapnia, which can indicate need for suction. These signs can also help in identifying patient's ability to cooperate with procedure.

13. Assess for patient's understanding of procedure and presence of any apprehension.

Reveals need for instruction or psychosocial support.

STEP	RATIONALE

NURSING DIAGNOSES

- Inadequate spontaneous ventilation
- Inadequate breathing pattern
- Inadequate gas exchange
- Inadequate swallowing

- Reduced airway clearance
- Anxiety
- Insufficient knowledge regarding suctioning

- Fatigue
- Reduced comfort
- Potential for aspiration
- Potential for infection

Related factors/Risk factors are individualized on the basis of patient's condition or needs.

PLANNING

1. Expected outcomes following completion of procedure:
- Upper and lower airways demonstrate absent or diminished gurgles, crackles, rhonchi, and wheezes on inspiration and expiration.

Absent or diminished adventitious sounds indicate that airways are cleared of secretions and are patent.

- Heart rate, blood pressure, respiratory rate, and effort are within normal range for patient.

When airway secretions are removed and oxygenation improves, patient's vital signs and respiratory assessment findings improve.

- Patient's SpO_2 is at or above baseline, whereas end-tidal CO_2 concentration, if being monitored, is at or below baseline.

Demonstrates improvement in gas exchange (Wiegand, 2017).

Clinical Decision Point *While normal end-tidal CO_2 ranges from 35 to 45 mm Hg, it is important to ensure that the patient's value is below the normal baseline. Persons with pulmonary diseases often have abnormal CO_2 values.*

- Patient's peak inspiratory pressure decreases back to baseline, and exhaled tidal volume increases back to baseline.

Demonstrates removal of secretions (Lium, Jin, Ma, et al., 2015; Wiegand, 2017).

2. Help patient to comfortable position, typically semi-Fowler's or high Fowler's.

Reduces stimulation of gag reflex, promotes patient comfort and secretion drainage, and prevents aspiration.

3. If not already present, place pulse oximeter on patient's finger. Take reading and leave oximeter in place.

Provides continuous SpO_2 value to determine patient's response to suctioning.

4. Explain to patient how procedure will help clear airway and relieve breathing difficulty. Explain that temporary coughing, sneezing, gagging, or shortness of breath is normal during procedure.

Encourages cooperation and minimizes risks, anxiety, and pain of procedure.

IMPLEMENTATION

1. Perform hand hygiene and apply appropriate PPE, as indicated.

Reduces transmission of microorganisms.

2. Adjust bed to appropriate height (if not already done) and lower side rail on side nearest you. Check locks on bed wheel.

Minimizes caregiver's muscle strain and prevents injury. Prevents bed from moving.

3. Connect one end of connecting tubing to suction device and place other end in convenient location near patient. Turn suction device on and set suction pressure to a level as low as possible and yet able to effectively clear secretions. This value is typically between 100 and 150 mm Hg in adults (between 60 and 100 mm Hg in neonates) (AACN, 2010; AARC, 2010). Occlude end of suction tubing to check pressure.

Ensures equipment function. Excessive negative pressure damages tracheal mucosa and induces greater hypoxia (Wiegand, 2017).

4. Prepare suction catheter for all types of open suctioning.
- **a.** Using aseptic technique, open suction kit or catheter package. If sterile drape is available, place it across patient's chest or on bedside table. Do not allow suction catheter to touch any nonsterile surfaces.

Prepares catheter, maintains asepsis, and reduces transmission of microorganisms. Provides sterile surface on which to lay catheter between passes.

STEP	RATIONALE

IMPLEMENTATION

b. Unwrap or open sterile basin and place on bedside table. Be careful not to touch inside of basin. Fill with about 100 mL sterile normal saline solution or water (see illustration).

Saline or water is used to clean tubing after each suction pass.

c. If performing nasotracheal suctioning, open packet of water-soluble lubricant and apply small amount to catheter.
NOTE: *Lubricant is not necessary for artificial airway suctioning.*

Water-soluble lubricant helps avoid lipid aspiration pneumonia. An excessive amount of lubricant occludes catheter.

5. Apply sterile gloves to each hand or nonsterile glove to nondominant hand and sterile glove to dominant hand.

Reduces transmission of microorganisms and maintains sterility of suction catheter.

6. Pick up suction catheter with dominant hand without touching nonsterile surfaces. Pick up connecting tubing with nondominant hand. Secure catheter to tubing (see illustration).

Maintains catheter sterility. Connects catheter to suction.

7. Place tip of catheter into sterile basin and suction small amount of normal saline solution from basin by occluding suction vent.

Ensures equipment function. Lubricates internal catheter and tubing.

8. Suction airway.

a. Nasopharyngeal and nasotracheal suctioning:

(1) Have patient take deep breaths, if able, or increase oxygen flow rate with delivery device through cannula or mask (if prescribed).

May help to decrease risks of hypoxemia.

(2) Lightly coat distal 5–8 cm (2–3 inches) of catheter with water-soluble lubricant.

Lubricates catheter for easier insertion.

(3) Remove oxygen-delivery device, if applicable, with nondominant hand.

Allows access to nares and catheter.

Clinical Decision Point *Be sure to insert the catheter during patient inhalation, especially if inserting it into the trachea, because the epiglottis is open. Do not insert during swallowing or the catheter will most likely enter the esophagus.* **Never apply suction during insertion.** *The patient should cough. If patient gags or becomes nauseated, the catheter is most likely in the esophagus and you need to remove it.*

(a) *Nasopharyngeal* (without applying suction): As patient takes a deep breath, insert catheter following natural course of naris; slightly slant catheter downward and advance to back of pharynx. Do not force through naris. In adults, insert catheter approximately 16 cm (6½ inches); in older children, 8–12 cm (3 to 5 inches); in infants and young children, 4–7.5 cm (1½–3 inches). The rule of thumb is to insert catheter the distance from tip of nose (or mouth) to angle of mandible.

Ensures that catheter tip reaches pharynx for suctioning.

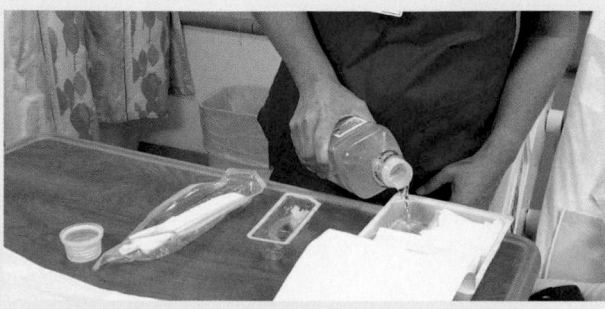

STEP 4b Pouring sterile saline into tray.

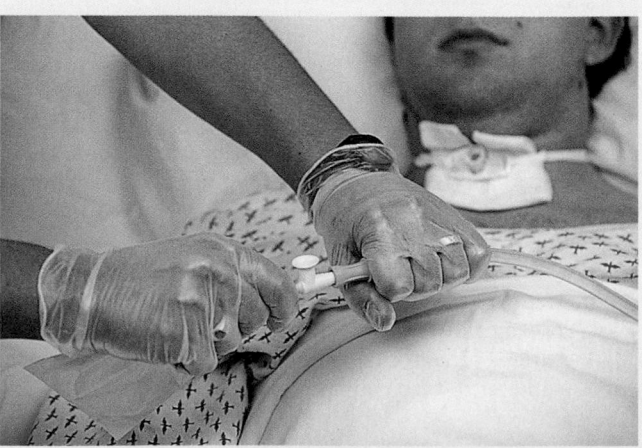

STEP 6 Attaching suction catheter to suction tubing.

STEP	RATIONALE

IMPLEMENTATION

Clinical Decision Point *If resistance is met during insertion, you may need to try the other naris. Do not force the catheter up the nares because this will cause mucosal damage.*

(i) Apply intermittent suction for no more than 10 seconds by placing and releasing nondominant thumb over catheter vent. Slowly withdraw catheter while rotating it back and forth between the thumb and forefinger.

Intermittent suction up to 10 seconds safely removes pharyngeal secretions. Suction time greater than 10 seconds increases risk for suction-induced hypoxemia (AACN, 2010; AARC, 2010; Wiegand, 2017).

(b) *Nasotracheal (without applying suction):* As patient takes a deep breath, advance catheter following natural course of naris. Advance catheter slightly slanted and downward to just above entrance into larynx and then trachea. While patient takes a deep breath, quickly insert catheter: for adults, insert approximately 15–20 cm (6–8 inches) into trachea (see illustration). Patient will begin to cough; then pull back catheter 1–2 cm (0.4–0.8 inches) before applying suction. **NOTE:** In older children, 15–20 cm (6–8 inches); in infants and young children, 8–14 cm (3–5½ inches).

Ensures that catheter tip reaches trachea for suctioning.

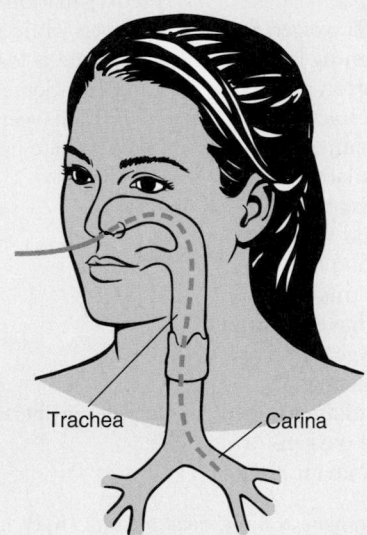

Trachea   Carina

STEP 8a(3)b Distance of insertion of nasotracheal catheter.

Clinical Decision Point *When using the nasal approach, perform tracheal suctioning before pharyngeal suctioning whenever possible. The mouth and pharynx contain more bacteria than the trachea. If copious oral secretions are present before beginning the procedure, suction mouth with oral suction device first.*

Clinical Decision Point *When there is difficulty in passing the catheter, ask patient to cough or say "ahh," or try to advance the catheter during inspiration. Both measures help to open the glottis to permit passage of the catheter into the trachea.*

(i) *Positioning option:* In some instances, turning patient's head helps you suction more effectively. If you feel resistance after insertion of the catheter, use caution; it has probably hit the carina. Pull catheter back 1–2 cm (0.4–0.8 inches) before applying suction (AARC, 2004).

Turning patient's head to side elevates bronchial passage on opposite side. Turning head to right helps with suctioning of left main-stem bronchus; turning head to left helps with suctioning right main-stem bronchus. Suctioning too deep may cause tracheal mucosa trauma.

STEP	RATIONALE

IMPLEMENTATION

(ii) Apply intermittent suction for no more than 10 seconds by placing and releasing nondominant thumb over catheter vent. Slowly withdraw catheter while rotating it back and forth between thumb and forefinger.

Suction time greater than 10 seconds increases risk for suction-induced hypoxemia (AACN, 2010; AARC, 2010; Wiegand, 2017). Suctioning too frequently or for a prolonged time can cause an increase in secretions. Intermittent suctioning and rotation of catheter prevents injury to tracheal mucosa. If catheter "grabs" mucosa, remove thumb to release suction.

Clinical Decision Point *Monitor patient's vital signs and oxygen saturation throughout suctioning process. Stop suctioning if there is a 20 beats/min change (increase or decrease) in pulse rate or if SpO_2 falls below 90% or deviates 5% from baseline.*

(4) Reapply oxygen-delivery device and encourage patient to take some deep breaths, if able.

Helps to decrease risk of hypoxia. Increases patient comfort.

(5) Rinse catheter and connecting tubing with normal saline or water until cleared.

Secretions that remain in suction catheter or connecting tubing decrease suctioning efficiency.

(6) Assess for need to repeat suctioning. Do not perform more than two passes with catheter. Allow patient to rest at least 1 minute (AACN, 2010; AARC, 2010). Ask patient to deep breathe and cough.

Observe for alterations in cardiopulmonary status. Suctioning induces hypoxemia, irregular pulse, laryngospasm, and bronchospasm (AACN, 2010; AARC, 2010). Hyperoxygenation is recommended before, during, and after open suctioning to reduce suction-induced hypoxemia (Galbiati & Paola, 2015).

b. Artificial airway:

(1) When patient has an artificial airway, hyperoxygenate the patient with 100% oxygen for at least 30 to 60 seconds before suctioning by (1) pressing suction hyperoxygenation button on ventilator OR (2) increasing baseline fraction of inspired oxygen (FiO_2) level on mechanical ventilator OR (3) disconnecting ventilator, attaching self-inflating resuscitation bag-valve device to tube with nondominant hand (or have assistant do this), and administering 5–6 breaths over 30 seconds (or have assistant do this). NOTE: Some mechanical ventilators have a button that, when pushed, delivers 100% oxygen for a few minutes and then resets to previous setting.

Preoxygenation decreases risk of decreased arterial oxygen levels while ventilation or oxygenation is interrupted, and volume is lost during suctioning (AACN, 2010; AARC, 2010). Some models of resuscitation bags do not deliver 100% oxygen; therefore, this is not the best way to oxygenate patient (Wiegand, 2017).

(2) If patient is receiving mechanical ventilation, open swivel adapter or, if necessary, remove oxygen- or humidity-delivery device with nondominant hand.

Exposes artificial airway.

Clinical Decision Point *Suctioning can cause elevations in intracranial pressure (ICP) in patients with head injuries. Reduce this risk by using presuction hyperoxygenation, which results in hypocarbia, which in turn induces vasoconstriction. Vasoconstriction reduces the potential for an increase in ICP (Urden et al., 2016).*

(3) Advise patient that you are about to begin suctioning. Without applying suction, gently but quickly insert catheter into artificial airway using dominant thumb and forefinger (it is best to try to time catheter insertion into artificial airway with inspiration) (see illustration). Advance catheter until you meet resistance or patient coughs; then pull back 1 cm (0.4 inch) (Wiegand, 2017).

Application of suction pressure while introducing catheter into trachea increases risk for damage to tracheal mucosa and increased hypoxia. Pulling back stimulates cough and removes catheter from mucosal wall so catheter is not resting against tracheal mucosa during suctioning. Shallow suctioning is recommended to prevent tracheal mucosa trauma (AACN, 2010; Wiegand, 2017).

Clinical Decision Point *If you are unable to insert the catheter past the end of the ET, the catheter is probably caught in the Murphy eye (i.e., side hole at the distal end of the ET that allows for collateral airflow in the event of tracheal main-stem intubation). If this happens, rotate the catheter to reposition it away from the Murphy eye or withdraw it slightly and reinsert with the next inhalation. Usually the catheter meets resistance at the carina. One indication that the catheter is at the carina is acute onset of coughing because the carina contains many cough receptors. Pull the catheter back 1 cm (0.4 inch).*

STEP	RATIONALE

IMPLEMENTATION

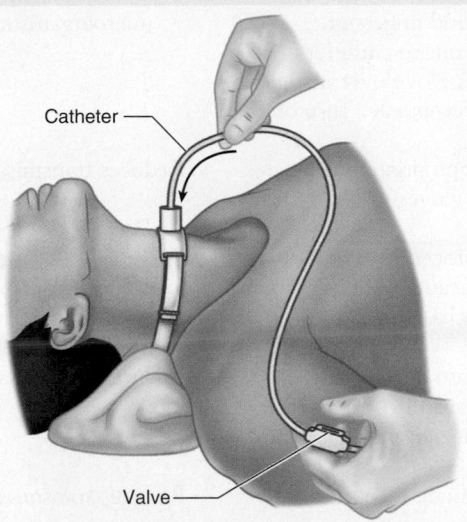

STEP 8b(3) Suctioning tracheostomy.

(4) Apply intermittent suction for 10 seconds (AACN, 2010; AARC, 2010; Wiegand, 2017). Apply intermittent suction by placing and releasing nondominant thumb over vent of catheter; slowly withdraw catheter while rotating it back and forth between dominant thumb and forefinger. Do not use suction for greater than 15 seconds. Encourage patient to cough. Watch for respiratory distress.

Suction time greater than 10 seconds increases risk for suction-induced hypoxemia (AACN, 2010; AARC, 2010; Wiegand, 2017). Intermittent suction and rotation of catheter prevent injury to tracheal mucosa. If catheter "grabs" mucosa, remove thumb to release suction.

Clinical Decision Point *If patient develops respiratory distress during the suctioning procedure, immediately withdraw catheter and supply additional oxygen and breaths as needed. In an emergency administer oxygen directly through the catheter. Disconnect suction and attach oxygen at prescribed flow rate through the catheter. If the patient does not tolerate the suctioning procedure, you may need to consider switching to closed (in-line) suctioning or allowing longer recovery times. Notify health care provider if patient develops significant cardiopulmonary compromise during suctioning (Urden et al., 2016; Wiegand, 2017).*

(5) If patient is receiving mechanical ventilation, close swivel adapter or replace oxygen-delivery device. Hyperoxygenate patient for 30–60 seconds.

Re-establishes artificial airway. Helps to decrease risks of hypoxia.

(6) Rinse catheter and connecting tubing with normal saline until clear. Use continuous suction.

Removes catheter secretions. Secretions left in tubing decrease suctioning efficiency and provide environment for microorganism growth.

(7) Assess patient's vital signs, cardiopulmonary status, and ventilator measures for secretion clearance. Repeat Steps (1) through (6) once or twice more to clear secretions. Allow adequate time (at least 1 full minute) between suction passes.

Suctioning can induce dysrhythmias, hypoxia, and bronchospasm and impair cerebral circulation or adversely affect hemodynamic stability (Wiegand, 2017).

Clinical Decision Point *The number of suction passes should be based on patient assessment and presence of secretions. If secretions persist after two passes, allow patient more time to rest and recover from these procedures (Wiegand, 2017).*

(8) When pharynx and trachea are sufficiently cleared of secretions, perform oropharyngeal suctioning (Skill 25.1) to clear mouth of secretions. Do not suction nose again after suctioning mouth.

Removes upper airway secretions. More microorganisms generally are present in mouth. Upper airway is considered "clean," and lower airway is considered "sterile." You can use the same catheter to suction from sterile to clean areas (e.g., tracheal suctioning to oropharyngeal suctioning) but not from clean to sterile areas.

STEP	RATIONALE

IMPLEMENTATION

9. When suctioning is complete, disconnect catheter from connecting tubing. Roll catheter around fingers of dominant hand. Pull glove off inside out so catheter remains coiled in glove. Pull off other glove over first glove in same way. Discard in appropriate receptacle. Turn off suction device.

Seals contaminants in gloves. Reduces transmission of microorganisms (Wiegand, 2017).

10. Remove towel, place in laundry or appropriate receptacle, and reposition patient. (Apply clean gloves to continue personal care.)

Reduces transmission of microorganisms. Promotes comfort.

11. If oxygen level was changed during procedure, readjust oxygen to original prescribed level because patient's blood oxygen level should have returned to baseline.

Prevents absorption atelectasis (i.e., tendency for airways to collapse if proximally obstructed by secretions). Prevents oxygen toxicity while allowing patient time to reoxygenate blood.

12. Discard remainder of normal saline into appropriate receptacle. If basin is disposable, discard into appropriate receptacle. If basin is reusable, rinse it out and place it in soiled utility room.

Reduces transmission of microorganisms.

13. Remove PPE and discard into appropriate receptacle. Perform hand hygiene.

Reduces transmission of microorganisms.

14. Place unopened suction kit on suction machine table or at head of bed.

Provides immediate access to suction catheter for next procedure.

15. Help patient to comfortable position and provide oral hygiene as needed.

EVALUATION

1. Compare patient's vital signs, cardiopulmonary assessments, and end-tidal CO_2 and SpO_2 values before and after suctioning. If patient is on ventilator, compare FiO_2 and tidal volumes and peak inspiratory pressures.

Identifies physiological effects of suction procedure to restore airway patency.

2. Ask patient if breathing is easier and if congestion is decreased.

Provides subjective confirmation that suctioning procedure has relieved airway.

3. Auscultate lungs and compare patient's respiratory assessment before and after suctioning.

Provides objective information about any change in lung sounds.

4. Observe character of airway secretions.

Provides data to document presence or absence of respiratory tract infection or thickened secretions.

5. Use Teach-Back: "I need to suction your father and I want to be sure that I explained the suctioning procedure and when I need to do it. Please tell me in your own words why I'm suctioning him." Develop a revised teaching plan if patient or caregiver is not able to teach back correctly.

Determines patient's and caregiver's level of understanding of instructional topic.

Unexpected Outcomes

1. Patient has decrease in overall cardiopulmonary status as evidenced by decreased SpO_2, increased end tidal CO_2, continued tachypnea, continued increased work of breathing, and cardiac dysrhythmias.

2. Bloody secretions are returned after suctioning.

Related Interventions

- Limit length of suctioning.
- Determine need for more frequent suctioning, possibly of shorter duration.
- Determine need for supplemental or increase in supplemental oxygen. Supply oxygen between suctioning passes.
- Notify health care provider.
- Determine amount of suction pressure used. It may need to be decreased.
- Ensure that suction is completed correctly using intermittent suction and catheter rotation. Do not apply suction until after catheter has been pulled back 1 cm (0.4 inches) to prevent applying suction while catheter is touching carina.
- Evaluate suctioning frequency.
- Provide more frequent oral hygiene.

STEP	RATIONALE

EVALUATION

3. Patient has paroxysms of coughing or bronchospasm.	• Administer supplemental oxygen. • Allow patient to rest between passes of suction catheter. • Consult with health care provider regarding need for inhaled bronchodilators or topical anaesthetics.
4. Inability to obtain secretions during suction procedure.	• Evaluate patient's fluid status and adequacy of humidification on oxygen-delivery device. • Assess for signs of infection. • Determine need for chest physiotherapy (see Chapter 24).

Communication and Documentation

- Document the amount, consistency, colour, and odour of secretions; size of catheter; route of suctioning; and patient's response to suctioning on flow sheet in nurses' notes in electronic health record (EHR) or chart.
- Document need for hyperoxygenation, type of hyperoxygenation, and percent of oxygenation used.
- Document patient's and caregiver's understanding through teach-back.
- Document patient's presuctioning and postsuctioning vital signs, cardiopulmonary status, and ventilation measures on flow sheet in nurses' notes in EHR or chart.
- Report patient's intolerance to procedure or unexpected physiological changes to health care provider.

Special Considerations

Teaching

- Instruct patient that coughing increases and that there will be some discomfort during the procedure.
- Explain why supplemental oxygen is given before and after suctioning if indicated.

Pediatric

- The size of the suction catheter should occlude less than 70% of the artificial airway in infants and less than 50% of the artificial airway in children (AACN, 2010; AARC, 2010).
- Hyperoxygenate with 100% oxygen in pediatric patients and 10% increase of baseline in neonates before suctioning (Hockenberry & Wilson, 2015).
- Perform ET suctioning only when clinically indicated in infants and neonates. Clinical signs are notable changes in respiratory rate and breath sounds, increased secretions, bradycardia, or restlessness (Hockenberry & Wilson, 2015).

- Thick secretions are more difficult to remove because of the small diameter of the suction catheter. Normal saline should not be instilled in the airway in an attempt to thin the secretions (AACN, 2010; AARC, 2010).
- Make sure that distance suctioned is not greater than 0.5 cm (0.2 inches) beyond the tip of the artificial airway. To determine distance, place catheter near a sample artificial airway (Hockenberry & Wilson, 2015).
- Infant airways have less cartilage and may collapse easily, especially in premature infants or those with reactive airways.
- Suctioning should not last beyond 5 seconds, and negative pressure should not exceed 100 mm Hg (Hockenberry & Wilson, 2015).

Gerontological

- Older persons lose some properties of elastic recoil and gas exchange.
- Capillaries of older persons are often fragile, predisposing patients to bleeding problems.
- Patients with coronary artery disease are at greater risk for cardiopulmonary compromise.

Care in the Community

- Most patients with airway clearance problems at home have a tracheostomy.
- Instruct patient and caregiver to clean and disinfect or change the secretion collection container every 24 hours according to employer policy.
- In the home setting, stress the importance of brief intervals of applying suction pressure. Instruct those performing suctioning to hold their breath during the application of negative suction pressure to help them remember to not suction too long.

PROCEDURAL GUIDELINE 25.1 *Closed (In-Line) Suction*

NSO *Nursing Skills Online Airway Management Module 9 / Lesson 4*

Closed suctioning (or in-line suctioning) is another method of suctioning an artificial airway. It involves the use of a multiuse suction catheter that is housed within a plastic sleeve and is attached to a patient's artificial airway (Fig. 25.3, A–B). This method of suctioning is associated with decreased risk of hypoxia and cardiovascular complications when compared to open suctioning. It is also the recommended method of suctioning for patients who cannot tolerate loss of positive end-expiratory pressure

(PEEP), such as those with severe respiratory disorders who require high amounts of PEEP or oxygen requirements (Wiegand, 2017).

Delegation and Collaboration

The skill of airway suction with a closed (in-line) suction catheter cannot be delegated to an unregulated care provider (UCP). In special situations, such as suctioning a well-established permanent tracheostomy, this procedure may be delegated to the UCP (refer

Continued

PROCEDURAL GUIDELINE 25.1 *Closed (In-Line) Suction—cont'd*

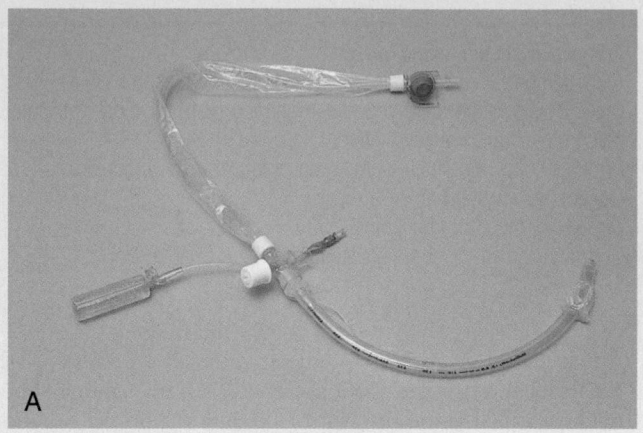

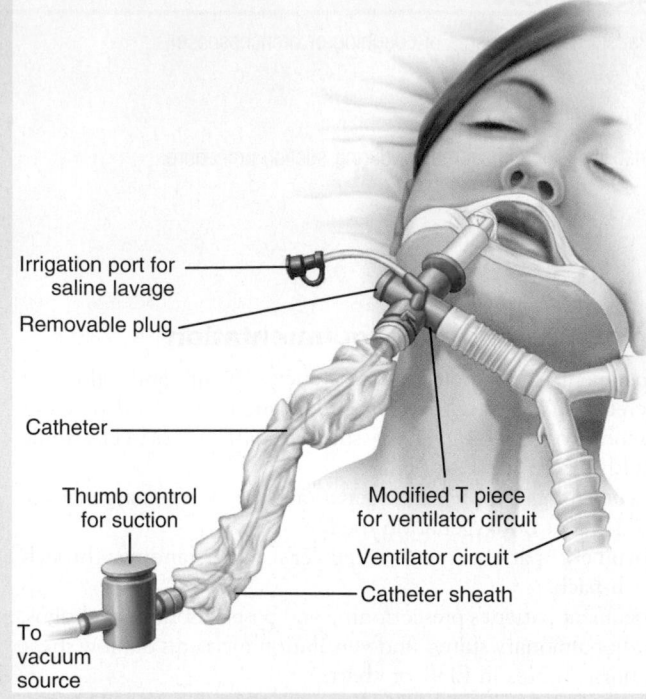

Irrigation port for saline lavage

Removable plug

Catheter

Thumb control for suction

To vacuum source

Modified T piece for ventilator circuit

Ventilator circuit

Catheter sheath

B

FIG 25.3 A, Closed-system suction catheter attached to endotracheal tube. **B,** Closed suction system attached to an endotracheal tube. (**B** *from Blanchard, B. [2011]. Thoracic surgery. In Rothrock, J. C., & McEwen, D. R. (Eds.), Alexander's care of the patient in surgery [14th ed.] St. Louis: Mosby.*)

to employer policy). The nurse is responsible for cardiopulmonary assessment and evaluation of the patient. The nurse often uses interprofessional collaboration (e.g., respiratory therapist) when assessing the patient and performing the suction procedure. The nurse instructs the UCP about:

- Any individualized aspects of patient care that pertain to suctioning (e.g., position, duration of suction, pressure settings).
- Expected quality, quantity, and colour of secretions, and informing the nurse immediately if there are changes.
- Patient's anticipated response to suction, and reporting immediately to the nurse changes in vital signs, indications of pain, shortness of breath, confusion, or increased restlessness.

Equipment

- Closed-system or in-line suction catheter
- Sterile saline solution lavage containers (5 to 10 mL)
- Suction machine/source with regulator
- Connecting tubing (1.8 metres [6 feet])
- Two clean gloves
- Oral suction kit/supplies for oropharyngeal suctioning
- Mask, goggles, or face shield; gown if isolation precautions indicate
- Oral mucus trap for specimen collection (if prescribed)
- Pulse oximeter and stethoscope
- Manual self-inflating resuscitation bag (bag-valve-mask) with appropriate-size mask, while not necessary for the procedure, is safe to have on hand.

Procedural Steps

1. Perform assessment as in Skill 25.2.
2. Perform hand hygiene. Gather equipment and supplies and close room door or curtain.

3. Identify patient using at least two person-specific identifiers (e.g., name and date of birth or name and medical record number) according to employer policy (Accreditation Canada, 2019).
4. Explain procedure to patient and the importance of coughing during the suctioning procedure. Even if patients cannot speak, they deserve to have information regarding the procedure.
5. Adjust the bed to an appropriate height and lower side rail on the side nearest you. Check locks on the bed.
6. Help patient assume a position of comfort for both patient and nurse, usually semi- or high-Fowler's position. Place towel across patient's chest.
7. Apply clean gloves and face shield and attach suction:
   a. In many facilities, a respiratory therapist attaches the catheter to the mechanical ventilator circuit. If the catheter is not already in place, open suction catheter package using aseptic technique and attach closed suction catheter to ventilator circuit by removing swivel adapter and placing closed suction catheter apparatus on endotracheal tube (ET) or tracheostomy tube (TT). Connect Y on mechanical ventilator circuit to closed suction catheter with flex tubing (see Fig. 25.3, A).
   b. Connect one end of connecting tubing to suction machine; connect other end to the end of a closed-system or in-line suction catheter. Turn suction device on, set vacuum regulator to appropriate negative pressure, and check pressure. Many closed-system suction catheters require slightly higher suction pressures (consult manufacturer guidelines).
8. Hyperoxygenate patient (usually 100% oxygen) by adjusting the fraction of inspired oxygen (FiO$_2$) setting on the ventilator or by using a temporary oxygen-enrichment program available on microprocessor ventilators according to employer policy. (Manual ventilation is not recommended.)

PROCEDURAL GUIDELINE 25.1 *Closed (In-Line) Suction—cont'd*

9. Unlock suction control mechanism if required by manufacturer. Open saline port and attach saline syringe or vial.
10. Pick up suction catheter enclosed in plastic sleeve with dominant hand.
11. Wait until patient inhales to insert catheter. Then insert catheter using a repeating manoeuvre of pushing catheter and sliding (or pulling) plastic sleeve back between thumb and forefinger until resistance is felt or patient coughs. Pull back 1 cm (0.4 inches) before applying suction to avoid tissue damage to tracheal carina.
12. Encourage patient to cough, and apply suction by squeezing on suction control mechanism while withdrawing catheter. **NOTE:** It is difficult to apply intermittent pulses of suction and nearly impossible to rotate the catheter compared to a standard catheter. Apply continuous suction for 10 seconds as you remove the suction catheter (AACN, 2010; AARC, 2010; Wiegand, 2017). Be sure to withdraw the catheter completely into the plastic sheath and past the tip of the airway so it does not obstruct airflow.
13. If specimen collection is prescribed, connect the long, soft end of the mucus specimen trap (Fig. 25.4) to the output for suction vacuum (b) and the suction catheter to collection port (d). Follow steps 11 and 12. Mucus will then be collected into the collection bottle (a). Label and send sample to laboratory immediately.

14. Reassess cardiopulmonary status, including pulse oximetry (SpO$_2$) and ventilator measures, to determine need for subsequent suctioning or complications. Repeat Steps 8 to 12 one more time to clear secretions if patient condition indicates. Allow adequate time (at least 1 full minute) between suction passes for ventilation and reoxygenation.
15. When airway is clear, withdraw catheter completely into sheath. Be sure that coloured indicator line on catheter is visible in the sheath. Attach sterile solution lavage container or sterile saline or water syringe to side port of suction catheter. Squeeze vial or push syringe while applying suction to rinse inner lumen of catheter. Use at least 5 to 10 mL of saline to rinse the catheter until it is clear of retained secretions, which can cause bacterial growth and increase the risk for infection (AARC, 2004). Lock suction mechanism if applicable and turn off suction.
16. Hyperoxygenate for at least 1 minute by following the same technique used to preoxygenate (Wiegand, 2017).
17. If patient requires oral or nasal suctioning, perform Skill 25.1 or 25.2 with separate standard suction catheter.
18. Place the Yankauer catheter on a clean, dry area for reuse with suction turned off or within patient's reach with suction on if patient is capable of suctioning their own mouth.
19. Reposition patient. Remove gloves, face shield, and other PPE; discard into appropriate receptacle; and perform hand hygiene.
20. Compare patient's vital signs and SpO$_2$ before and after suctioning.
21. Auscultate lung fields and compare with baseline.
22. Observe airway secretions.
23. Ask patient if breathing is easier and congestion is decreased.
24. **Use Teach-Back:** "I want to be sure I explained this suctioning procedure correctly. Please squeeze my hand if you understand these steps. Each time I suction you I will explain these steps again." Develop a revised teaching plan as indicated if patient is not squeezing hand in response.

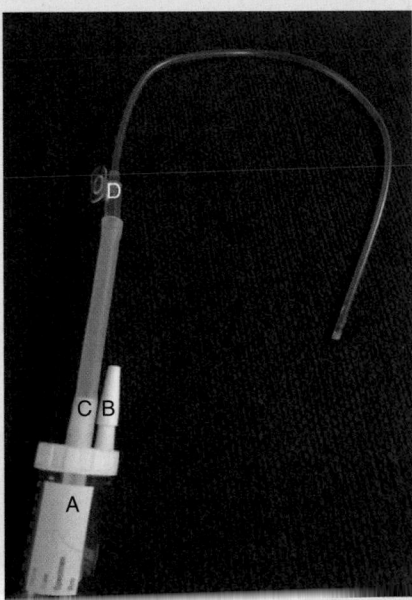

A - Collection bottle
B - Output for suction vacuum
C - Entry for secretions
D - Suction catheter

FIG 25.4 Arrangement of the device used in the collection of mucus. **a,** Collection bottle. **b,** Output for suction vacuum. **c,** Entry of secretions. **d,** Suction catheter. *(Courtesy of Jane Tyerman.)*

◆ SKILL 25.3   Performing Endotracheal Tube Care

NSO *Nursing Skills Online Airway Management Module 9 / Lesson 4*

Endotracheal tubes (ETs) are flexible, plastic tubes placed in the mouth or through the nose and advanced down into the trachea to establish short-term artificial airways to administer mechanical ventilation, relieve upper airway obstruction, protect against aspiration, and clear secretions (see Fig. 25.2). Routine care maintains correct position of the tube and good hygiene. Prior to performing endotracheal tube care, it is crucial that supplemental oxygen with appropriate delivery devices be readily available at the bedside.

After insertion of an ET, the cuff is inflated, and the tube is secured with tape or a commercially available device. A cuff on an ET prevents the escape of air between the tube and the walls of the trachea and reduces the risk of aspiration when a patient is receiving mechanical ventilation (Box 25.1). The amount of air or water inserted in a cuff is based on two factors (i.e., the size of the patient's trachea and the external diameter of the artificial airway). If the cuff pressures are too high, permanent damage to the tracheal mucosa occurs, leading to complications such as tracheomalacia; tracheoesophageal fistula; or erosion of the innominate artery, which is rare but almost always fatal (Karsli, Kayacan, Ince, et al., 2016). If the cuff pressure is too low, the mechanical ventilation will not be effective, and the patient has an increased risk of aspiration, which increases the risk of developing ventilator-associated pneumonia (VAP) (Myatt, 2015).

Preventing tube-related complications is a critical component of care and depends on securing the tube and inflating the cuff properly. In many facilities, these functions are the responsibility of respiratory therapists. However, the nurse is responsible for assessing the patient's respiratory status, ventilator settings and functioning, and integrity of the airway cuff.

Properly securing an ET prevents inadvertent extubation from coughing, gagging, or accidental pulling on the tube. Additional risks of movement of an artificial airway are tracheal stenosis (narrowing of windpipe); tracheomalacia (flaccidity of supporting tracheal cartilage); barotrauma (excess alveolar air during mechanical ventilation); erosion of the innominate artery; and tracheoesophageal fistula, particularly when the cuff is overinflated (Donatelli, Gupta, Santhosh, et al., 2015). In addition, the risk for device-related pressure injuries increases because of pressure from the artificial airway on adjacent tissues (e.g., lips, oral mucosa) (Pittman, Beeson, Kitterman, et al., 2015).

Once a tube is inserted, confirmation of placement is achieved using a chest X-ray film and a disposable end-tidal carbon dioxide (CO_2) detector (Fig. 25.5) (Wiegand, 2017). Capnography, the noninvasive measurement of the partial pressure of CO_2 in exhaled breath expressed as the CO_2 concentration over time, is used to continuously monitor CO_2 once the patient is placed on mechanical ventilation. It is recommended as a reliable way to validate the correct placement of an ET (AARC, 2011). The CO_2 monitor measures CO_2 directly from the airway, with the sensor located on the airway adapter at the hub of the ET.

After a tube is inserted and secured and the cuff is inflated, the nurse's chief concern is to maintain patency of the ET and prevent a ventilator-associated event (VAE). Please refer to Chapter 23 for more information regarding VAE. In patients who cannot clear their secretions, periodic suctioning of the artificial airway achieves airway patency.

Delegation and Collaboration

This skill of performing ET care cannot be delegated an unregulated care provider (UCP). The UCP may assist the nurse with ET care. Often the nurse uses interprofessional collaboration (e.g., respiratory therapist) in performing this care. The nurse directs the UCP to immediately:

- Report any signs of respiratory problems or increased airway secretions.
- Report if the ET appears to have moved or become obstructed or dislodged.
- Report changes in the patient's mood, level of consciousness, irritability, vital signs, decreased pulse oximetry value, or changes in end-tidal CO_2 values.

Equipment

- Towel
- ET and oropharyngeal suction equipment
- 1.3 cm (1/2 inch)– or 2.5 cm (1 inch)–wide adhesive or waterproof tape (do not use paper or silk tape) or commercial ET holder and mouth guard (follow manufacturer instructions for securing)
- Oral airway and bite block (bite block is optional and only used is patient is biting ET)

BOX 25.1

Indications for Cuff Inflation

Mechanical Ventilation
- Continuous positive airway pressure
- Positive end-expiratory pressure (PEEP)
- Inability to meet ventilatory requirements with cuff down
- Inability to meet oxygen requirements with cuff down

Risk of Aspirating Gastric Contents
- Feeding tube, especially large-bore, in stomach
- Gastroesophageal reflux disease
- Hiatal hernia
- During and after meals
- Impaired gastric emptying
- Decreased gag reflex
- Impaired swallowing

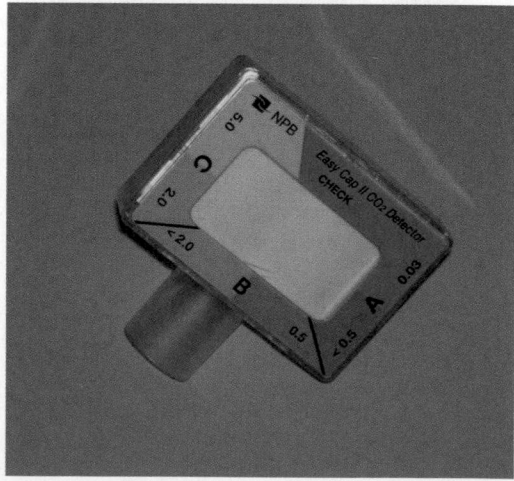

FIG 25.5 End-tidal CO_2 detector. (*Used by permission from Nellcor Puritan Bennett LLC, Boulder, CO, doing business as Covidien.*)

- Suction equipment
- Clean gloves
- Adhesive remover swab or acetone on cotton ball
- Oral hygiene supplies: pediatric toothbrush (or suction tooth-brush), toothette for edentulous patients
- Cleaning solution: 0.12 to 0.20% chlorhexidine mouthwash, rinse, or gel
- Face cleaner (e.g., wet washcloth, towel, soap, shaving supplies)
- Clean 5 cm × 5 cm (2 in × 2 in) gauze
- Tincture of benzoin, liquid adhesive, or skin preparation pads

- Tongue blade (optional)
- Mask, goggles, face shield (if indicated); gown if isolation procedures indicate
- Stethoscope
- Pulse oximeter, end-tidal CO_2 detector
- Another interprofessional team member (two people are needed to perform some of the steps)
- Communication device (letter or picture board, tablet, paper and pen)

STEP	RATIONALE

ASSESSMENT

1. Identify patient using at least two person-specific identifiers (e.g., name and date of birth or name and medical record number) according to employer policy.	Ensures correct patient. Complies with Accreditation Canada's standards and improves patient safety (Accreditation Canada, 2019).
2. Auscultate lungs and observe respiratory rate and depth.	Provides baseline measure of ventilation.
3. Perform hand hygiene and apply gloves. Observe condition of tissues surrounding ET for impaired skin integrity (e.g., blistering, abrasions, pressure injuries) on nares, lips, cheeks, or corner of mouth; excess nasal or oral secretions; patient moving tube with tongue, biting tube or tongue, and foul-smelling mouth.	Presence of ET impairs ability of patient to swallow oral secretions. Patient is at increased risk for developing pressure areas from impaired circulation as tube is pulled or pressed against mucosal tissues (Pittman et al., 2015).
4. Observe patency of airway: excess intratracheal or endotracheal secretions, diminished airflow, and sign and symptoms of airway obstruction.	Buildup of secretions in ET impairs oxygen delivery and subsequent tissue oxygenation.
5. Observe for signs and symptoms of gurgling on expiration, decreased exhaled tidal volume (mechanically ventilated patient), signs and symptoms of inadequate ventilation (rising end-tidal CO_2 concentration, patient–ventilator dyssynchrony, or dyspnea), spasmodic coughing, tense test balloon on tube, flaccid test balloon on tube, and ability to speak or vocalize.	Cuff underinflation increases risk for aspiration, allows secretions to enter the trachea, and permits vocalization. Cuff overinflation may cause ischemia or necrosis of tracheal tissue from obstruction of capillary bed, resulting in tracheomalacia or tracheoesophageal fistula (Myatt, 2015).
6. Observe for factors that increase risk for complications from ET: type and size of tube, movement of tube up and down trachea (in and out), duration of tube placement, presence of facial trauma, malnutrition, and neck or thoracic radiation.	Tube rotating from side to side can cause medical device–related pressure injuries. Tube can become dislodged from lower airway (incidental extubation), or it can enter right main-stem bronchus. Longer duration of intubation is associated with increased risk for lower airway complications such as VAE or VAP (Lewis, Dehne, Morbitzer, et al., 2018).
7. Assess for patient's ability to verbalize around ET or for presence of audible air leak.	Underinflated cuff allows passage of air through patient's vocal cords and increases patient's risk for aspiration (Rouze, De Jonckheere, Zerimech, et al., 2016).

Clinical Decision Point *When assessment indicates possible overinflation or underinflation of ET cuff, notify respiratory therapy and follow employer policy for correcting cuff pressures. Most sources agree that 20 cm H_2O is the lowest accepted pressure, but some sources recommend that the highest pressure to maintain the cuff is 25 cm H_2O (AACN, 2016; Myatt, 2015).*

8. Determine proper ET depth as noted by centimetres at lip or gum line. This line is marked on tube and recorded in patient's record at time of intubation and every shift.	Ensures that tube is at proper depth to adequately ventilate both lungs and that it is not too high, which causes vocal cord damage, or too low, which results in right main-stem intubation, in which only the right lung is ventilated.
9. Assess patient's knowledge of procedure.	Encourages cooperation, minimizes risks and anxiety. Identifies teaching needs.

NURSING DIAGNOSES

- Reduced airway clearance
- Insufficient breathing pattern
- Reduced gas exchange
- Fatigue

- Inadequate verbal communication
- Reduced skin integrity (or potential for)
- Potential for aspiration

- Potential for impaired oral mucous membrane
- Potential for infection

Related factors/Risk factors are individualized on the basis of patient's condition or needs.

STEP	RATIONALE

PLANNING

1. Expected outcomes following completion of procedure:
- ET remains in correct position in patient's trachea, evidenced by depth of tube being same as when started or as prescribed (same centimetre marking at gums or lips); bilateral breath sounds are equal; end-tidal CO_2 values remain at patient baseline.

Maintaining ET position promotes adequate ventilation of lungs. Complications of lower airway and vocal cord trauma are prevented.

- Patient's skin around mouth and oral mucous membranes remains intact without evidence of pressure or other injury from biting or from ET itself.

ET does not place undue pressure against corners of mouth, which could cause pressure area. Patient is not able to bite inner cheeks or tongue.

2. Perform hand hygiene. Gather equipment and supplies and arrange at bedside. Close room curtain or door.

Ensures that nurse has necessary equipment to implement all interventions that should be completed for patient. Ensures patient privacy.

3. Obtain assistance from available staff for this procedure.

Reduces risk for accidental extubation of ET.

4. Assist patient in assuming comfortable position for both patient and you. Elevate patient's head of bed at least 30 degrees, unless patient is at risk for pressure injury.

Provides access to site and facilitates completion of procedure. Prepares patient for oropharyngeal suctioning. Position may decrease risk of aspiration (Hellyer et al., 2016).

5. Explain procedure and patient's need to participate, including not biting or moving ET with tongue, trying not to cough when tape is off ET, keeping hands down, and not pulling on tubing.

Reduces anxiety, encourages cooperation, and reduces risk of accidental extubation.

IMPLEMENTATION

1. Perform hand hygiene. Apply clean gloves and mask, goggles, or face shield if indicated. Have assistant do so as well.

Reduces transmission of microorganisms.

2. Place clean towel across patient's chest.

Reduces soiling of bed clothes and linen.

3. Perform endotracheal or oropharyngeal suctioning if indicated (see Skills 25.1 and 25.2 and Procedural Guideline 25.1).

Removes secretions. Diminishes patient's need to cough during procedure.

4. Connect Yankauer suction catheter to suction source and have it ready to use. Ensure that suction source/machine for oral suctioning is on and functioning properly.

You need to have functioning equipment to perform oral care appropriately. Prepares suction apparatus.

5. Remove oral airway or bite block, if present, and place on towel.

Provides access to and complete observation of patient's oral cavity.

Clinical Decision Point *If patient is biting the tube, do not remove bite block until absolutely necessary. This prevents obstruction of the ET and occlusion of the airway.*

6. Brush teeth with soft toothbrush, using solution or toothpaste that helps to break down plaque buildup on teeth. Suction oropharyngeal secretions as necessary.

There may be need for a pediatric toothbrush, depending on size of patient's oral cavity. There are no definitive guidelines to support the frequency of oral brushing.

7. Use chlorhexidine solution and oral swabs to clean mouth. Suction oropharyngeal secretions as necessary. Apply mouth moisturizer to oral mucosa and lips after each cleaning.

This step should be completed every 2 to 4 hours (Wiegand, 2017). The swabs, solution, and moisturizer may come in a prepackaged kit from the manufacturer. The use of chlorhexidine mouthwash or gel is effective in reducing VAP (El-Rabbany, Zoghlol, Bhandari, et al., 2015).

Clinical Decision Point *It may be useful to have the assistant constantly suction the oral cavity during the procedure. This helps to prevent the pooling and aspiration of oral secretions. Use continuous subglottic suctioning if available at your place of employment (Wiegand, 2017).*

8. Prepare ET securement options:
  a. *Tape method:* Prepare tape by cutting a piece of tape long enough to go completely around patient's head from naris to naris plus 15 cm (6 inches). This is typically 30–60 cm (12–24 inches) in total length. Lay tape adhesive-side up on bedside table. Cut and lay 8–15 cm (3–6 inches) of second piece of tape, adhesive sides together, in centre of the long strip to prevent tape from sticking to hair. A smaller strip of tape should cover area between the ears around the back of the head.

Preparing tape ahead of time decreases amount of time one has to manually hold ET throughout procedure, therefore decreasing risk of tube dislodgement. Adhesive tape needs to encircle head below ears with sufficient tape left to wrap around tube.

STEP	RATIONALE

IMPLEMENTATION

b. *Commercially available ET holder:* Open package per manufacturer instructions. Set device aside with head guard in place. If using Velcro strips instead of cloth ties, ensure strips are in the open position.

Commercial devices are latex free, fast, convenient, and disposable.

Clinical Decision Point *It is a nursing decision whether to use tape or a commercially available ET holder. There are advantages and disadvantages to both (Smith & Pietrantonio, 2016).*

9. Remove old tape or device.
   a. *Tape:* While one person is holding and stabilizing ET, the other person removes tape from patient, using adhesive tape remover. The tape will also need to be removed from ET itself.

Provides access to skin under tape for assessment and hygiene. Adhesive tape remover ensures easier, less traumatic removal of the tape.

Clinical Decision Point *Clean ET tube with soap and water as needed. Do not apply adhesive tape remover to the ET itself. This action will make it nearly impossible for the new tape to appropriately stick to the ET, which increases risk of tube dislodgement.*

   b. *Commercially available device:* Remove Velcro strips from ET and remove ET holder from patient.

Velcro adhesive strips hold ET in place and provide marker to measure distance to patient's lips or gums. These devices all permit access to patient's mouth and lips for ease in oropharyngeal suctioning and oral hygiene.

Clinical Decision Point *Do not allow assistant to hold the tube away from the lips or nares. Doing so allows too much movement in the tube and increases the risk for tube movement and accidental extubation. Never let go of the ET because it could become dislodged.*

10. Remove excess secretions or adhesive from patient's face. Clean facial skin with mild soap and water and dry thoroughly. Apply tape adherence product such as tincture of benzoin to face.

Application of tape adherence product is necessary for new tape or device to stay on patient's face (Wiegand, 2017).

Clinical Decision Point *Do not remove oral airway or bite block if patient is actively biting. Wait until the new tape or commercial device is partially or completely secured to ET.*

11. Note level of ET by looking at mark or noting centimetre value on tube itself. Move oral ET to other side of mouth and ensure that tube marking at lip is unchanged. Perform oral care as needed on side where tube was initially positioned. Clean oral airway or bite block with warm, soapy water and rinse well. Reinsert as necessary.

Changing sides of ET removes pressure and decreases risk of breakdown at corners of mouth and oral mucosa (Pittman et al., 2015).

Clinical Decision Point *The patient may cough excessively when the tube is being moved. The person who is holding the tube in place should be prepared for this and take extra caution while holding it. In some instances, the ET may need to be secured with tape before the rest of the oral care is performed. In some cases, the patient may need to be administered a dose of an anti-anxiety or sedating medication.*

The cuff of the ET may need to be deflated before changing its position. If this step needs to be performed, deep oral suctioning should be completed before deflation of the cuff, and oral care should not be performed until the cuff is properly reinflated (Wiegand, 2017).

12. Secure tube (assistant continues to hold ET).
   a. Tape method:
      (1) Slip tape under patient's head and neck, adhesive side up. Take care not to twist tape or catch hair. Do not allow tape to stick to itself. It helps to gently stick end of tape to tongue blade, which serves as guide. Then slide tongue blade under patient's neck. Centre tape so double-faced tape extends around back of neck from ear to ear.

Positions tape to secure ET in proper position. Don't allow tape to go over earlobe.

STEP	RATIONALE

IMPLEMENTATION

(2) On one side of face, secure tape from ear to naris (nasal ET) or over lip to ET (oral ET). Tear remaining tape in half lengthwise, forming two pieces that are 1–1.5 cm (0.4–0.6 inch) wide. Secure bottom half of tape across upper lip (oral ET) or across top of nose (nasal ET) to opposite ear (see illustration A). Wrap top half of tape around tube and up from bottom (see illustration B). Tape should encircle tube at least two times for security.

Secures tape to face. Using top tape to wrap prevents downward drag on ET.

(3) Gently pull other side of tape firmly to pick up slack and secure to opposite side of face and ET same as first piece (see illustration). **NOTE:** ET is secured. Assistant can release hold. Check depth mark at lips or gum line.

Secures tape to face and tube. ET should be at same depth at lips or gum line. Check earlier assessment for verification of tube depth in centimetres.

b. Commercially available ET tube securement device:

Clinical Decision Point *This step will only need to be completed if the device is visibly soiled and cannot be cleaned or if it is no longer adhering to the face and keeping the ET secure.*

(1) Thread ET through opening designed to secure it. Be sure that pilot balloon is accessible.

Commercially available holders have a slit in front of holder designed to secure ET.

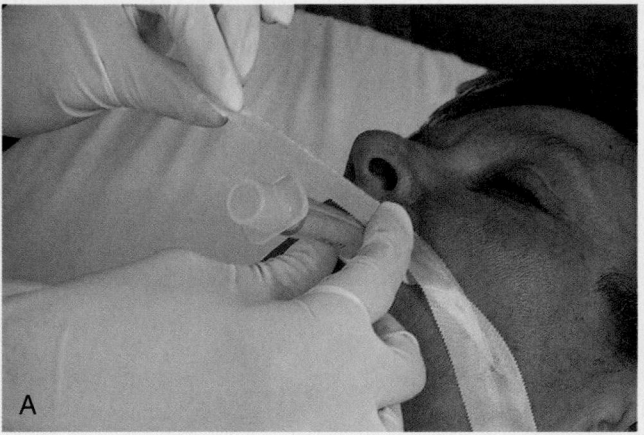 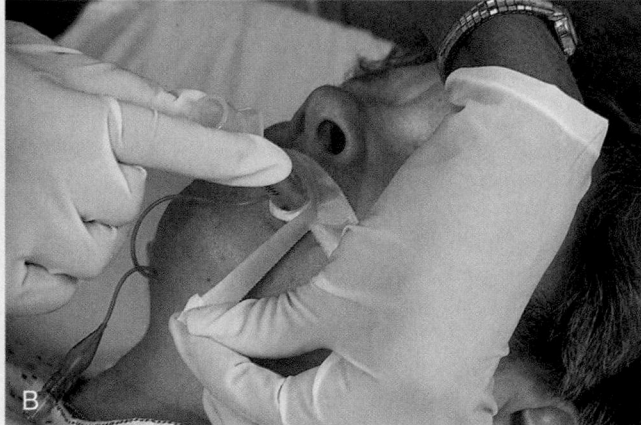

STEP 12a(2) **A,** Securing bottom half of tape across patient's upper lip. **B,** Securing top half of tape around tube.

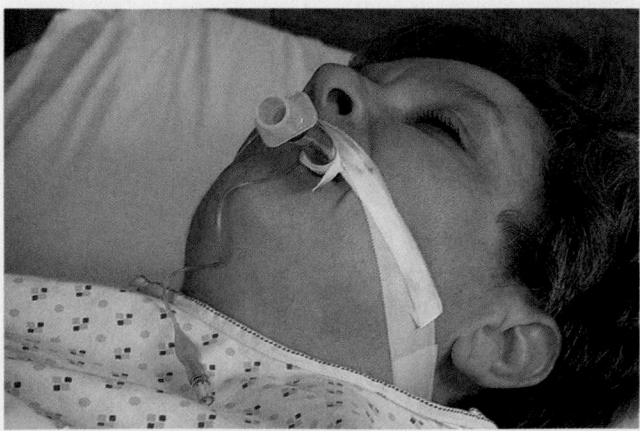

STEP 12a(3) Tape securing endotracheal tube.

STEP	RATIONALE

IMPLEMENTATION

(2) Place strips of ET holder under patient at occipital region of head.

(3) Verify that ET is at established depth, using lip or gum line marker as guide.

Ensures that ET remains at correct depth as determined during assessment.

(4) Attach Velcro strips at base of patient's head. Leave 1 cm (0.4 inch) slack in strips.

(5) Verify that tube is secure, it does not move forward from patient's mouth or backward down into patient's throat, and there are no pressure areas on oral mucosa or occipital region of head (see illustration).

Tube must be secure so it remains at correct depth. It can be secured without being tight and causing pressure.

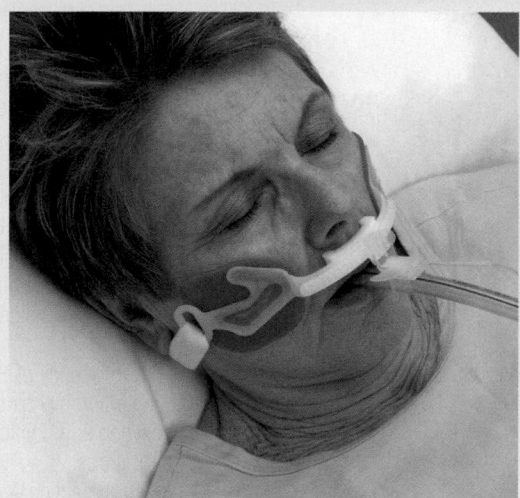

STEP 12b(5) Commercial endotracheal tube holder. (*Modified from Sills, J. R. [2000]. Entry-level respiratory therapist exam guide. St. Louis: Mosby.*)

13. For unconscious patient reinsert oral airway without pushing tongue into oropharynx and secure with tape.

Prevents patient from biting ET and allows access for oropharyngeal suctioning. An oral airway is not used in a conscious, cooperative patient because it causes excessive gagging and pressure areas to mouth and tongue.

14. Clean rest of face and neck with soapy washcloth, rinse, and dry. Shave male patient as necessary.

Moisture and beard growth prevent adhesive tape adherence.

Clinical Decision Point *When shaving patients, take great care to keep the cuff inflation port away from the razor. The razor can inadvertently cut or nick the tubing, causing air loss from the cuff and the possible need for reintubation.*

Clinical Decision Point *If a nasotracheal tube is in place, all of the preceding steps will be completed, except that the tube will not be moved, nor its position changed. It is out of the scope of nurse practice to move the ET from one naris to another and could cause great harm to the patient. For more information, see the Regulated Health Professions Act, 1991, available at https://www.ontario.ca/laws/statute/91r18*

15. Discard soiled items in appropriate receptacle. Remove towel and place in laundry.

Reduces transmission of microorganisms.

16. Reposition patient and ask them what else they need.

Promotes comfort; gives patients opportunity to communicate their needs.

17. Remove gloves and mask, goggles, or face shield or gown; discard in receptacle; and perform hand hygiene. (Assistant performs same steps.) Place clean items (e.g., tincture of benzoin, oral care solution, excess swabs) in a place of storage.

Reduces transmission of microorganisms. Ensures that contaminated gloves and hands do not touch clean items.

STEP	RATIONALE

EVALUATION

1. Compare respiratory assessments before and after ET care.

Identifies any physiological changes, including presence and quality of breath sounds after procedure.

2. Observe depth and position of ET according to health care provider recommendation.

Position of ET should not be altered.

3. Assess security of tape by *gently* tugging at tube.

Tape should remain attached to face. Patient may cough during tugging.

4. Assess skin around mouth and oral mucous membranes for intactness and pressure sores.

Tape should not tear skin. Pressure areas should be absent.

5. Compare end-tidal CO_2 values from before and after ET care.

Changes in end-tidal CO_2 can help identify displacement or dislodgement of ET.

6. Observe for excessive phonation, presence of gastric secretions in airway secretions, or tracheoesophageal fistula.

Occurs with inadequate or excessive cuff inflation.

Unexpected Outcomes	Related Interventions
1. Patient is extubated accidentally.	• Remain with patient while calling for help. • Ventilate with bag-valve-mask as needed. • Assess patient for airway patency, spontaneous breathing, and vital signs. • Prepare for reintubation.
2. ET moves in airway and becomes malpositioned.	• Call for help and repeat taping or securing procedure. Be prepared for chest X-ray film to confirm placement. • In very active patients without facial injury who are at risk for self-extubation, consider applying second piece of tape around back of head.
3. Patient has pressure injury in mouth or on lips and nares.	• Increase frequency of ET care. • Apply antimicrobial ointment per employer policy. • Align oxygen and humidity supply tubing so they do not pull ET, creating pressure sores. • Monitor for infection. If skin tear is present on cheeks or over nose or upper lip, apply protective barrier, such as stoma adhesive patch or hydrocolloid dressing, and apply tape to it.
4. Cuff leak develops.	• Verify position of tube, notify respiratory therapy, and follow employer policy.

Communication and Documentation

- Document respiratory assessments before and after care, patient's tolerance of procedure, prescribed and actual depth of ET, frequency of ET care, integrity of oral and nasal mucosa, pressure sore care (if performed), and frequency and extent of ET care on flow sheet in nurses' notes in electronic health record (EHR) or chart.
- Document repositioning of ET, side on which it is placed, and the securement technique used.
- Report unequal breath sounds, accidental extubation, cuff leak, or respiratory distress to the health care provider.

Special Considerations
Teaching
- Instruct patient and caregivers not to manipulate the ET, tape, or ET holder. If patient is complaining or appears uncomfortable, instruct caregiver to ask for the nurse.
- Instruct patient and caregiver to inform the nurse if the tube causes gagging. Repositioning of the tube, sedation, or both are options for reducing gagging.

Pediatric
- Neonatal and pediatric procedures for securing ETs and suctioning airways vary. Refer to employer policy for specific procedures (Hockenberry & Wilson, 2015).
- Infant skin is more prone to tearing when removing tape (Hockenberry & Wilson, 2015).
- Because of infants' delicate skin, you will not always use adhesive tape remover to remove the tape or skin preparation before securing the ET. ET holders are best used in this population as long as appropriate-size holders are available for the child.

Gerontological
- Older persons' skin is more prone to tearing when removing tape.
- Older persons with a tendency toward inadequate nutrition are more prone to complications (e.g., infection, breakdown of oral mucosa).

✦ SKILL 25.4 Performing Tracheostomy Care

▶ *Video Clip* **NSO** *Nursing Skills Online Airway Management Module 9 / Lesson 5*

A tracheostomy is a surgical or percutaneous creation of a stoma through the neck and into the trachea that allows for the insertion of an artificial airway called a *tracheostomy tube (TT)*. TTs are placed in patients who require long-term airway management because of airway obstruction, airway clearance needs, or long-term need for mechanical ventilation (Myatt, 2015). A TT offers advantages over long-term endotracheal tube (ET) placement such as decreased risk of laryngeal and tracheal injury, less sedation, shorter ventilator weaning time (the time it takes to get a patient off a ventilator) (Lim, 2015), and improved comfort for the patient. Some TTs even allow more patient freedom in the performance of activities of daily living such as feeding, speaking, and mobility.

TTs consist of several components (Fig. 25.6). The shaft is the main component of the TT and is what sits inside the trachea, keeping the airway open. Flanges rest against the patient's neck and prevent the TT from migrating into the trachea. The 15-mm connector is located on the shaft or the inner cannula and is where the ventilator tubing or resuscitation bag attaches to the TT. The obturator is placed inside the TT and used during the TT insertion process and is replaced with an inner cannula (if necessary) once inserted. The inner cannula is located inside the shaft of the TT and is a safety feature because it can be quickly removed and replaced if obstructed (Wiegand, 2017). TTs are curved and are commonly made of a synthetic material such as polyvinyl chloride (PVC), silicone, or polyurethane. The curved nature of the TT improves the ability of the tube to fit within the trachea (Wiegand, 2017). Metal tubes are rarely used because of their increased costs, their rigidity, and their lack of a cuff.

A TT is cuffed or uncuffed. A cuff on a TT serves the same purpose as the cuff on an ET. Cuffs are made of a balloonlike inflatable plastic typically inflated with air, although there are brands that are inflated with liquid such as water or saline. Uncuffed tubes allow patients the ability to clear the airway, but they provide no protection from aspiration. It is also more difficult to use positive-pressure ventilation in patients with these types of TTs (Myatt, 2015).

Some TTs allow a patient to speak. This ability to verbalize needs and wants provides psychological benefits to the patient. The openings in fenestrated tubes allow air to flow from the lungs over the vocal cords. However, these tubes must be used with caution; only patients who can swallow without aspiration should use them. There are speaking valves that can be used with TTs. The patient must have a cuffless TT in place or be able to tolerate the cuff being deflated without risk of respiratory distress or aspiration. Patients may not tolerate the speaking valves when first placed; therefore, they will need to be carefully monitored for signs of intolerance or respiratory distress.

Nurses also need to monitor for emergency events, such as tube obstruction or dislodgement. Box 25.2 provides a list of equipment that should be kept in the room or at the bedside of any patient who has a tracheostomy. Table 25.1 describes the signs of tracheal tube obstruction or dislodgement and the interventions that should be performed.

Delegation and Collaboration

The skill of performing tracheostomy care is not routinely delegated to an unregulated care provider (UCP). In some settings patients who have well-established TTs may have the care delegated to a UCP (refer to employer policy). The nurse is responsible for assessing a patient and evaluating for proper artificial airway care, often using interprofessional collaboration (e.g., respiratory therapist). The nurse

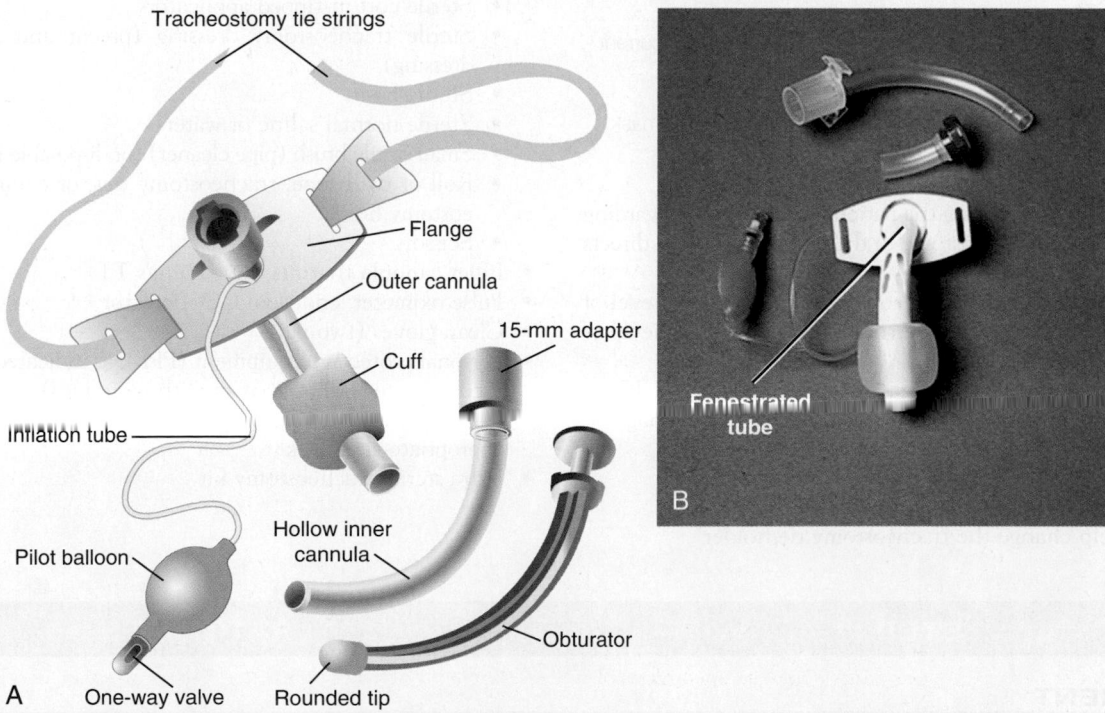

FIG 25.6 A, Parts of tracheostomy tube. **B,** Fenestrated tracheostomy tube with cuff, inner cannula, decannulation plug, and pilot balloon. (*From Lewis, S., et al. [2014]. Medical-surgical nursing: Assessment and management of clinical problems [9th ed.]. St. Louis: Mosby.*)

TABLE 25.1

Tracheostomy Emergencies

Emergency Type	Signs and Symptoms	Interventions

Tube dislodgement/ decannulation	• Inability to pass suction catheter past the length of the tube
	• Presence of subcutaneous emphysema near incision or stoma
	• Signs of respiratory distress
	• High-pressure alarm on ventilator
	• Flange of TT not flush with neck
	• Decreased SpO_2
	• Patient able to speak around the TT
		• Call for help
		• If stoma is less than 1 week old:
		  • Notify surgeon
		  • Bag-mask ventilation
		  • Prepare for intubation or surgical reinsertion of new TT
		• If stoma is well established: (typically greater than 1 week old)
		  • Replace with a new TT, inserting at a 90-degree angle into the trachea, then angling downward another 90 degrees

Tube obstruction	• Respiratory distress
	• Inability to pass suction catheter
	• Resistance felt when using the self-inflating resuscitation bag
		• Call for help
		• Remove and inspect the inner cannula (if one present); clean or replace with a new one
		• Mature site (>1 week)
		  • Replace the TT (if changing inner cannula did not relieve the obstruction)
		  • Patient may need more invasive intervention, such as bronchoscopy
		• Immature site (<1 week)
		  • Ensure TT is in correct position
		  • Prepare for more invasive intervention, such as oral endotracheal intubation, tracheostomy revision, or placement of a longer TT

Hemorrhage	• More than minimal bleeding at stoma site	• Notify health care provider • Provide oxygen, if not already in place

Data from Dawson, D. (2014). Essential principles: Tracheostomy care in the adult patient. *Nursing Critical Care, 19*(2), 63–72; Morris, L. L., et al. (2013). Tracheostomy care and complications in the intensive care unit. *Critical Care Nurse, 33*(5), 18.
TT, Tracheostomy tube.

BOX 25.2

Bedside Equipment for a Tracheostomy Patient

- Oxygen administration equipment with appropriate delivery devices
- Suction machine and equipment
- Suction tubing
- Suction catheters (Yankauer and tracheal)
- Sterile saline
- Additional tracheostomy tubes, one the same size as the current tube and another that is one size smaller
- Obturator
- Manual self-inflating resuscitation bag with appropriate-size mask
- 10-mL syringe
- Towel
- Artificial airway suction supplies (see Skill 25.2)
- Oropharyngeal suction supplies (see Skill 25.1)
- Sterile tracheostomy care kit, if available (be sure to collect supplies listed that are not available in kit), or two sterile 10 × 10–cm (4 × 4–inch) gauze pads
  - Sterile cotton-tipped applicators
  - Sterile tracheostomy dressing (precut and sewn surgical dressing)
  - Sterile basin
  - Sterile normal saline or water
  - Small sterile brush (pipe cleaner) (or disposable inner cannula)
  - Roll of twill tape, tracheostomy ties, or commercial tracheostomy holder
  - Scissors
- Inner cannula that fits the patient's TT
- Pulse oximeter, end-tidal CO_2 detector
- Clean gloves (two pair)
- Personal protective equipment (PPE), as indicated (e.g., goggles if concern regarding contact with secretions)
- Self-inflating manual resuscitation bag-valve device and appropriate-size mask
- Extra sterile tracheostomy kit

is also responsible for educating the patient and caregiver regarding care of an established tracheostomy in the home. The nurse directs the UCP to immediately:

- Report any changes in the patient's respiratory status, level of consciousness, confusion, restlessness or irritability, or level of comfort.
- Report any dislodgement or excessive movement of the TT.
- Report abnormal colour of the tracheal stoma and drainage.

Equipment

- Bedside table
- Person to help change the tracheostomy tie/holder

STEP	RATIONALE

ASSESSMENT

1. Identify patient using at least two person-specific identifiers (e.g., name and date of birth or name and medical record number) according to employer policy.	Ensures correct patient. Complies with Accreditation Canada's standards and improves patient safety (Accreditation Canada, 2019).

STEP	RATIONALE

ASSESSMENT

2. Perform hand hygiene and apply clean gloves. Observe for signs and symptoms of gurgling on expiration, decreased exhaled tidal volume (mechanically ventilated patient), signs and symptoms of inadequate ventilation (rising end-tidal CO_2 concentration, patient–ventilator dyssynchrony, or dyspnea), spasmodic coughing, tense test balloon on tube, flaccid test balloon on tube, and ability to speak or vocalize (see Box 25.1).

Reduces contact with infectious microorganisms. Cuff underinflation increases risk for aspiration and allows secretions to enter trachea and permits vocalization. Cuff overinflation may cause ischemia or necrosis of tracheal tissue from obstruction of capillary bed, resulting in tracheomalacia or tracheoesophageal fistula (Myatt, 2015).

3. Observe for excess peristomal secretions, excess intratracheal secretions, soiled or damp tracheostomy ties, soiled or damp tracheostomy dressing, diminished airflow through tracheostomy tube, or signs and symptoms of airway obstruction requiring suctioning (see Skill 25.2).

These signs indicate the need for tracheostomy care caused by presence of secretions at stoma site or within tracheostomy tube. Irritation of mucosa caused by tube itself can also cause increase in secretions (Wiegand, 2017).

4. Observe skin around tracheal stoma, under TT, and under tracheal ties for skin breakdown: blistering, erythema, drainage, or other discolouration.

Pressure areas related to TT increase patient's risk for medical device–related pressure injury (MDPI) formation (Pittman et al., 2015).

5. Assess patient's hydration status, humidity delivered to airway, status of any existing infection, patient's nutritional status, and ability to cough.

Determines factors that affect amount and consistency of secretions in tracheostomy and patient's ability to clear airway.

6. Assess patient's cardiopulmonary status, including pulse oximetry (SpO_2), end-tidal CO_2, vital signs, respiratory effort, lung sounds, and level of consciousness. Keep pulse oximeter in place.

Provides baseline for determining patient response to and tolerance of therapy.

7. Assess patient's or caregiver's understanding of and ability to perform tracheostomy care.

Allows you to identify potential need for instruction.

8. Check when tracheostomy care was last performed.

Tracheostomy care is provided at least every 4 to 8 hours and more often if indicated (e.g., increased airway or stoma secretions, infection [airway or stoma]) (Wiegand, 2017).

NURSING DIAGNOSES

- Inadequate airway clearance
- Inadequate breathing pattern
- Reduced gas exchange
- Insufficient knowledge regarding tracheostomy care
- Reduced comfort
- Reduced verbal communication
- Potential for aspiration
- Potential for infection

Related factors/Risk factors are individualized on the basis of patient's condition or needs.

PLANNING

1. Expected outcomes following completion of procedure:
   - Inner and outer cannulas of TT are free of secretions; ties are clean, secured snugly, and tied in double square knot.

   TT is patent and secure, optimizing amount of oxygen delivered to patient and limiting risk of infection from retained secretions.

   - Stoma site is pink; does not bleed; and is free of secretions, signs of infection, skin breakdown and pressure areas, and signs of granuloma formation.

   Indicates absence of infection at stoma site. Dry, intact tracheostomy stoma reduces risk for subsequent systemic infection.

   - No evidence of skin breakdown under tracheostomy ties or commercial tube holder.

   Patients with excessive secretions or diaphoresis are at risk for skin breakdown under TT stabilizer.

2. Have another nurse, UCP, or respiratory therapist help in this procedure (Wiegand, 2017).

   Prevents accidental extubation of TT.

3. Perform hand hygiene. Gather supplies and arrange at bedside. Close room door or curtain.

   Ensures a well-organized procedure. Demonstrates person-centred care by ensuring patient privacy.

4. Assist patient to comfortable position, raise head of bed to level of comfort.

5. Explain procedure and patient's participation.

   Encourages cooperation, minimizes risks, and reduces anxiety.

Clinical Decision Point *At some facilities, it is standard practice to have an extra TT that is the same size as the patient's current TT and a TT one size smaller at the bedside at all times in case there is an emergent need to replace the TT because of obstruction or dislodgement (Wiegand, 2017).*

STEP	RATIONALE

IMPLEMENTATION

1. Apply PPE as indicated.
2. Adjust bed to appropriate height and lower side rail on side nearest you. Check locks on bed wheel.
3. Preoxygenate patient for 30 seconds or ask patient to take five to six deep breaths. Then suction tracheostomy (see Skill 25.2). Before removing gloves, remove soiled tracheostomy dressing and discard in glove with coiled catheter.

Reduces transmission of microorganisms.
Minimizes caregiver's muscle strain and prevents injury. Prevents bed from moving.
Removes secretions to avoid occluding outer cannula while inner cannula is removed. Reduces need for patient to cough.

4. Perform hand hygiene. Prepare equipment on bedside table.

Prepares equipment and allows for smooth, organized completion of tracheostomy care.
Tracheostomy cares should be performed every 4 to 8 hours or per employer policy (Wiegand, 2017).

   a. Open sterile tracheostomy kit. Open two 10 × 10-cm (4 × 4–inch) gauze packages using aseptic technique and pour normal saline on one package. Leave second package dry. Open two cotton-tipped swab packages and pour normal saline on one package. Do not recap normal saline.
   b. Open sterile tracheostomy dressing package.
   c. Unwrap sterile basin and pour about 0.5–2 cm (0.2–0.8 inch) of normal saline into it.
   d. Open small sterile brush package and place aseptically into sterile basin.
   e. Prepare TT fixation device.
      (1) *If using twill tape:* Prepare length of twill tape long enough to go around patient's neck two times, about 60–75 cm (24–30 inches) for an adult. Cut ends on diagonal. Lay aside in dry area.

Cutting ends of tie on diagonal aids in inserting tie through eyelet.

      (2) *If using commercially available TT holder:* open package according to manufacturer directions.
   f. Open inner cannula package (if new one is to be inserted, such as with disposable inner cannulas or if patient does not tolerate being disconnected from oxygen source while cleaning reusable inner cannula).
5. Apply sterile gloves. Keep dominant hand sterile throughout procedure.

Reduces transmission of microorganisms.

6. Remove oxygen source if present.

Clinical Decision Point *It is important to stabilize the TT at all times during tracheostomy care to prevent injury, unnecessary discomfort, or accidental extubation. Have an assistant such as a UCP help during the procedure. Instruct the UCP to apply clean gloves.*

7. **Care of tracheostomy with reusable inner cannula:**
   a. While touching only outer aspect of tube, unlock and remove inner cannula with nondominant hand following line of tracheostomy. Drop inner cannula into normal saline basin.

Removes inner cannula for cleaning. Normal saline loosens secretions from inner cannula.

Clinical Decision Point *If the patient is receiving mechanical ventilation, you may want the person assisting you to hold the TT stable and remove the ventilator tube from the connection while you remove the inner cannula. This action helps to ensure that the TT itself is not removed accidentally if difficulties removing the ventilator from the TT or removing the inner cannula from the TT occur.*

   b. Place tracheostomy collar, T tube, or ventilator oxygen source over outer cannula. (**NOTE:** You may not be able to attach T tube and ventilator oxygen devices to all outer cannulas when inner cannula is removed.)

Maintains supply of oxygen to patient as needed.

Clinical Decision Point *If the patient is unable to tolerate being disconnected from the ventilator, replace the inner cannula with a clean new one and reattach the ventilator to the tracheostomy. Then proceed with cleaning the original inner cannula as described in the next steps and store it in a sterile container until the next inner cannula change (Wiegand, 2017).*

STEP	RATIONALE

IMPLEMENTATION

c. To prevent oxygen desaturation in affected patients, quickly pick up the inner cannula and use a small brush to remove secretions inside and outside the inner cannula (see illustration).

A tracheostomy brush provides mechanical force to remove thick or dried secretions.

d. Hold inner cannula over basin and rinse with sterile normal saline, using nondominant (clean) hand to pour normal saline.

Removes secretions and normal saline from inner cannula.

e. Remove oxygen source, replace inner cannula (see illustration), and secure "locking" mechanism. Reapply ventilator, tracheostomy collar, or T tube. Hyperoxygenate patient if needed.

Secures inner cannula and re-establishes oxygen supply.

8. Tracheostomy with disposable inner cannula:

a. Remove new cannula from manufacturer packaging.

Prepares you for change of inner cannula.

b. While touching only outer aspect of tube, withdraw inner cannula and replace with a new cannula. Lock it into position.

Provides clean, sterile inner cannula for patient.

Clinical Decision Point *If the patient is receiving mechanical ventilation, you may want the person assisting you to hold the TT stable and remove the ventilator tube from the connection while you remove the inner cannula. This action helps to ensure that the TT itself is not accidentally removed if difficulties removing the ventilator or the inner cannula from the TT occur.*

c. Dispose of contaminated cannula in appropriate receptacle and reconnect to ventilator or oxygen supply.

Prevents transmission of infection. Restores oxygen delivery.

9. Using normal saline-saturated cotton-tipped swabs and 10 × 10–cm (4 × 4–inch) gauze, clean exposed outer cannula surfaces and stoma under faceplate extending 5–10 cm (2–4 inches) in all directions from stoma (see illustration). Clean in circular motion from stoma site outward with dominant hand to handle sterile supplies. Do not go over previously cleaned area.

Aseptically removes secretions from stoma site. Moving in outward circle pulls mucus and other contaminants from stoma to periphery.

10. Using dry 10 × 10–cm (4 × 4–inch) gauze, pat lightly at skin and exposed outer cannula surfaces.

Dry surfaces prohibit formation of moist environment for microorganism growth and skin excoriation (Wiegand, 2017).

11. Secure tracheostomy.

Clinical Decision Point *Some facilities do not recommend changing the securement device for the first 72 hours after insertion of the TT because of risk of stoma closure if the tube were to become dislodged accidentally (Wiegand, 2017).*

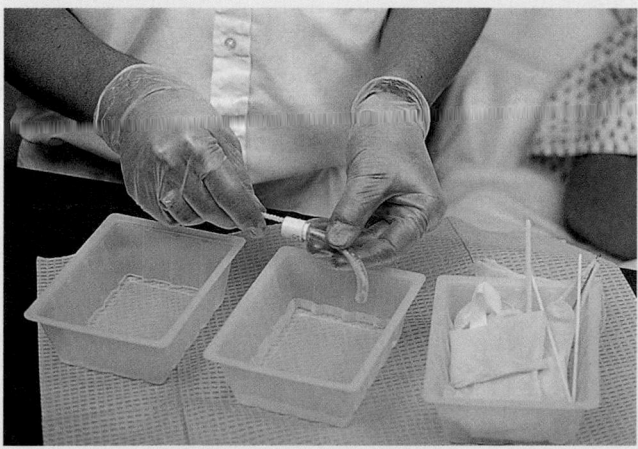

STEP 7c Cleaning tracheostomy inner cannula.

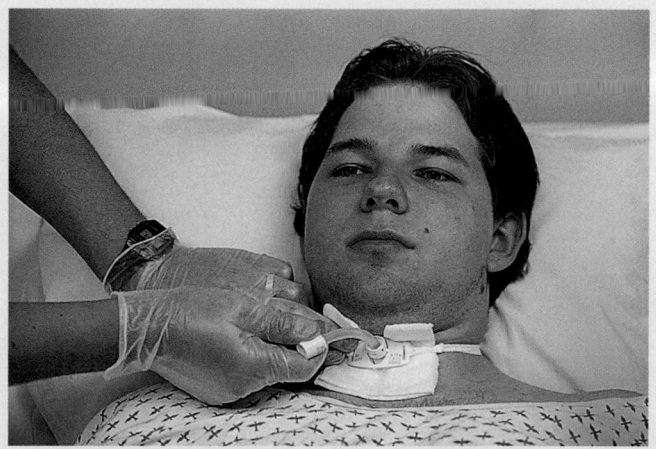

STEP 7e Reinserting inner cannula.

STEP	RATIONALE

IMPLEMENTATION

a. Tracheostomy tie method:

(1) Instruct assistant, if available, to apply clean gloves and securely hold TT in place. With assistant holding TT, cut old ties. Be sure to not cut pilot balloon of cuff.

Prevents transmission of infection. Secures TT to prevent incidental dislodgement. If pilot balloon is cut, there is no ability to inflate cuff (Wiegand, 2017).

Clinical Decision Point *Assistant must not release hold on the TT until new ties are firmly tied. If working without an assistant, do not cut old ties until new ties are in place and securely tied (Lewis et al., 2019). When ties are off, this is a good time to clean the back of the patient's neck and assess the patient's skin under the TT flange and under the ties or tube holder, making sure that skin is intact, free of pressure, and dry before applying securement device.*

(2) Take prepared twill tape, insert one end of tie through faceplate eyelet, and pull ends even (see illustration).

Diagonal cuts ensure ease of threading end of tie through holes of eyelet (Wiegand, 2017).

(3) Slide both ends of tie behind head and around neck to other eyelet and insert one tie through second eyelet.

(4) Pull snugly.

Secures TT.

(5) Tie ends securely in double square knot, allowing space for insertion of only one loose or two snug finger widths between tie and neck (see illustration).

One finger width of slack prevents ties from being too tight when tracheostomy dressing is in place and also prevents movement of tracheostomy tube into lower airway (Wiegand, 2017).

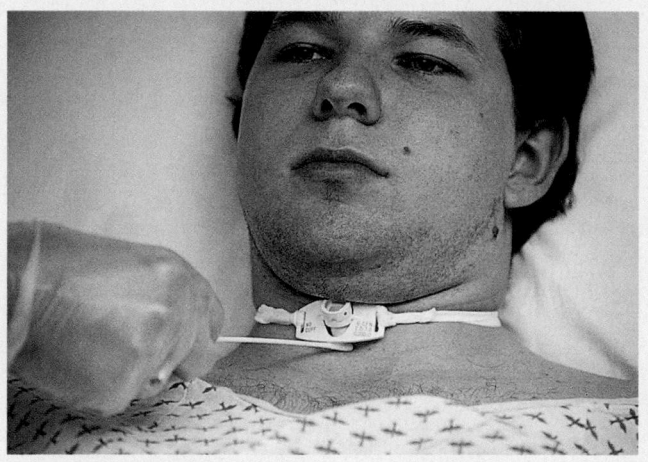

STEP 9 Cleaning around stoma.

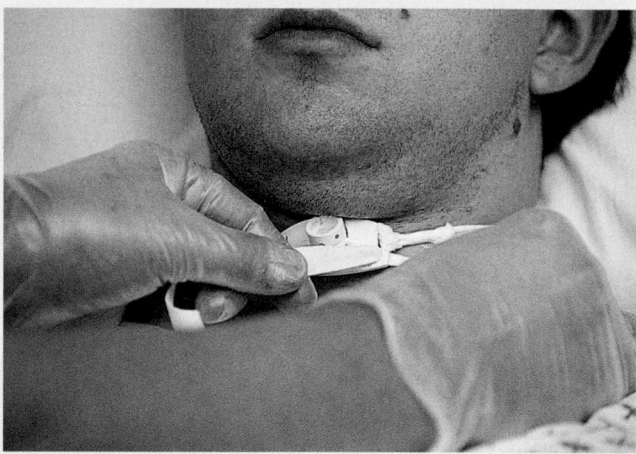

STEP 11a(2) Replacing tracheostomy ties. Do not remove old tracheostomy ties until new ones are secure.

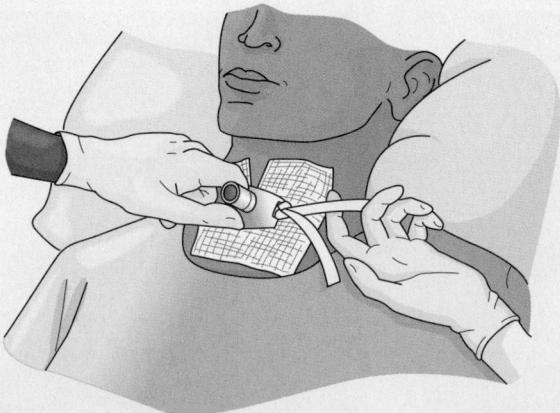

STEP 11a(5) Tracheostomy ties properly placed. (*From Sorrentino, S. A. [2013]. Mosby's textbook for nursing assistants [8th ed.]. St. Louis: Mosby.*)

STEP	RATIONALE

IMPLEMENTATION

(6) Insert new 10 × 10-cm (4 × 4-inch) tracheostomy dressing under clean ties and faceplate (see illustration).

Absorbs drainage. Dressing prevents pressure on clavicle heads (Wiegand, 2017).

b. Tracheostomy tube holder method:

(1) Instruct assistant, if available, to apply clean gloves and securely hold TT in place. When an assistant is not available, leave old TT holder in place until new device is secure.

Prevents incidental dislodgement of tube.
Ensures that tracheostomy stays in correct position.

(2) Align strap under patient's neck. Be sure that Velcro attachments are on either side of TT.

(3) Place narrow end of ties under and through faceplate eyelets. Pull ends even and secure with Velcro closures (see illustration).

Ensures proper securement of TT.

(4) Verify that there is space for only one loose or two snug finger widths to be inserted under neck strap.

Ensures proper securement of TT without securement device being too tight.

Clinical Decision Point *Never cut a gauze pad to fit around TT. The cut fibres from the gauze pad may shed fibres that could be inhaled by patient and lead to pulmonary damage or infection. Use a manufactured pad for this purpose (Wiegand, 2017).*

12. Perform oral care with toothbrush or oral swabs and chlorhexidine rinse.

Use of chlorhexidine may decrease patient risk of developing a ventilator-associated event (VAE) or ventilator-associated pneumonia (VAP) and promotes patient comfort.

13. Reposition patient comfortably, with head of bed elevated at least 30 degrees (unless at risk for pressure injury) and assess respiratory status.

Promotes comfort. Some patients require post-tracheostomy care suctioning.

14. Be sure that oxygen- or humidification-delivery sources are in place and set at correct levels.

Humidification provides moisture for airway, makes it easier to suction secretions, and decreases risk of mucus plugs (AARC, 2012; Wiegand, 2017).

15. Remove gloves and face shield and discard in appropriate receptacle. Perform hand hygiene.

Reduces transmission of microorganisms.

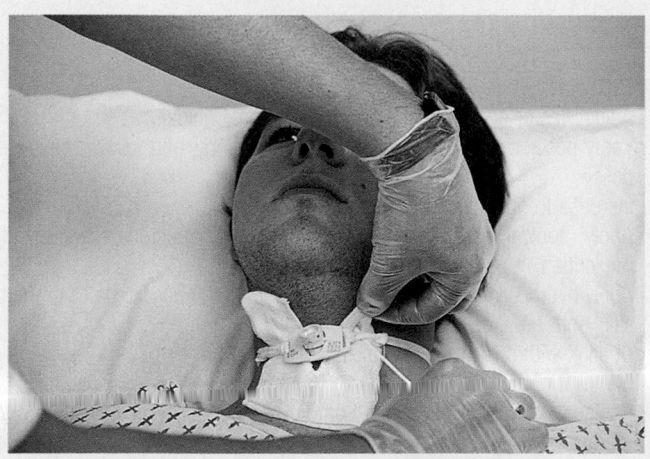

STEP 11a(6) Applying tracheostomy dressing.

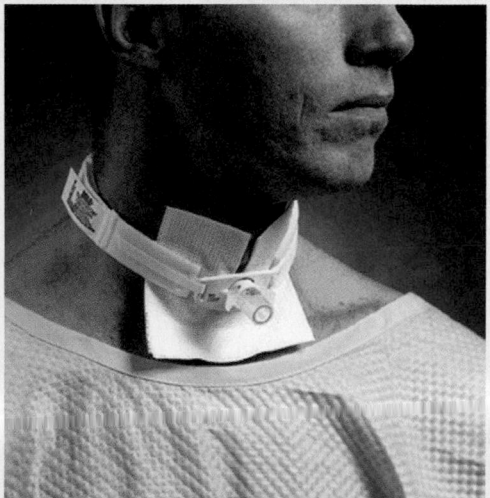

STEP 11b(3) Tracheostomy tube holder in place. *(Courtesy Dale Medical Products, Plainesville, MA.)*

STEP	**RATIONALE**

IMPLEMENTATION

16. Replace cap on reusable normal saline bottles. Store reusable liquids, date container, and store unused supplies in appropriate place.

Once opened, normal saline is considered free of bacteria for 24 hours.

EVALUATION

1. Compare assessments before and after tracheostomy care.

Determines effectiveness of tracheostomy care and patient's tolerance of procedure.

2. Assess fit of new tracheostomy ties and ask patient if tube feels comfortable. Palpate tube for pulsation for air under the skin.

Tracheostomy ties are uncomfortable and place patient at risk for tissue injury when they are too loose or too tight. A pulsating feeling in a TT can indicate early signs of innominate artery erosion. Air under skin suggests presence of subcutaneous emphysema.

3. Inspect inner and outer cannulas for secretions.

Presence of secretions on cannulas indicates need for more frequent tracheostomy care.

4. Assess stoma, surrounding skin, and skin under ties for inflammation, edema, bleeding, or discoloured secretions.

Broken skin places patient at risk for infection.
Stoma infection requires change in tracheostomy skin care plan.
Stomas located below second and third cartilage rings are at risk of causing innominate artery erosion (Wiegand, 2017).

5. Observe for excessive phonation, presence of gastric secretions in airway secretions, or tracheoesophageal fistula.

Occurs with inadequate or excessive cuff inflation.

6. Use Teach-Back: "I want to be sure I explained how to clean your tracheostomy tube and place new ties. Let's take time now and you can show me how to clean the tubing and place new ties." Develop a revised teaching plan if patient or caregiver is not able to teach back correctly.

Determines patient's and caregiver's level of understanding of instructional topic.

Unexpected Outcomes

1. Excessively loose or tight tracheostomy ties or tracheostomy holder.
2. Cuff leak develops.

3. Inflammation of tracheostomy stoma or pressure area around TT.

4. Accidental decannulation or dislodgement

5. Respiratory distress from mucus plugs in cannula.

Related Interventions

- Adjust ties or apply new ties or tracheostomy holder.
- Verify position of tube, notify respiratory therapy, and follow employer policy.
- Increase frequency of tracheostomy care.
- Apply topical antibacterial solution; apply bacterial barrier if prescribed.
- Apply hydrocolloid or transparent dressing just under stoma to protect skin from breakdown.
- Consult with skin care specialist.
- Call for help.
- Replace old TT with new tube. Some experienced nurses or respiratory therapists may be able to reinsert TT quickly.
- Same-size ET can be inserted in stoma in an emergency.
- Insert suction catheter to confirm that new tube is in trachea.
- Be prepared to manually ventilate patients in whom respiratory distress develops with self-inflating resuscitation bag until tracheostomy is replaced.
- Notify health care provider.
- Remove inner cannula if applicable for cleaning or suction cannula.
- Notify health care provider if TT requires replacement.

Communication and Documentation

- Document respiratory assessments before and after care; type and size of TT and inner cannula; frequency and extent of care, including inner cannula, dressing and securement device changes; type, colour, and amount of secretions; patient tolerance and understanding of procedure; and special care in event of unexpected outcomes in nurses' notes in electronic health record (EHR) or chart.
- Document condition of stoma and skin around stoma site and under dressing.
- Document any interventions that were performed to address patient complications.
- Document patient's and caregiver's understanding through teach-back.
- Report accidental decannulation or respiratory distress to the health care provider.

Special Considerations
Teaching

- Different types of TTs have different faceplates. Some are rigid; others are not. Instruct caregivers not to lift up rigid faceplates or they will dislodge the tube.
- Some commercial TT holders require removal of excess tie material to fit properly.
- If you anticipate long-term placement of tracheostomy, plan to teach patient and caregiver tracheostomy care.

- Patients with new tracheostomy frequently have bloody secretions for 2 or 3 days after tubing change (Wiegand, 2017).

Pediatric

- Children generally have shorter necks, making the stoma more difficult to clean.
- Pediatric TTs (smaller than size 4) do not contain an inner cannula.
- Nurses perform routine TT changes weekly after a tract has formed, generally 5 days (Hockenberry & Wilson, 2015).

Gerontological

- Some older persons may have more fragile skin and are more prone to skin breakdown from secretions or pressure (Touhy et al., 2019).
- Some older persons with impaired nutrition do not heal well.

Care in the Community

- Coordinate with patient, caregiver, and community care facility to ensure ability to secure appropriate supplies for use at home.
- Coordinate with community care services to ensure that home has appropriate electricity to support the equipment, particularly if patient is receiving mechanical ventilation or requires suctioning.
- See Skill 23.5, Care in the Community.

◆ CLINICAL DEBRIEF

A 65-year-old male experienced a severe stroke 2 days ago and at this time cannot communicate verbally. The interprofessional team is monitoring him for the ability to control his secretions and maintain an airway. The nurse walks into his room and notices cyanotic oral mucous membranes, pulse oximeter reading of 78%, and a large amount of oral secretions. The patient is gasping for air and tachypneic.

1. What should the nurse do first?
2. The nurse attempted to clear the patient's airway, but the patient continues to gasp for air; and the pulse oximeter improved only to 82%, even with the addition of 10 L oxygen via nonrebreather face mask. Rhonchi are noted on auscultation of breath sounds and trachea. The patient also continues to present with a large amount of oral secretions. The nurse recognizes that the health care provider needs to be notified. Using SBAR format, how should the nurse communicate the patient's status to the provider?
3. The patient was intubated; however, because of an inability to control secretions and maintain an airway, he was unable to be weaned off the ventilator. The decision was made to perform a tracheostomy. The nurse is teaching the patient's spouse about how the nurses will manage the tracheostomy tube. What should be included in the teaching plan, and why are these interventions performed?

◆ REVIEW QUESTIONS

1. The nurse is assessing a patient with an endotracheal tube (ET) and receiving positive-pressure mechanical ventilation. Which assessment findings should alert the nurse for the need to perform endotracheal suctioning? (Select all that apply.)
   1. Increased exhaled tidal volume above patient baseline
   2. Auscultation of rhonchi in the lungs

3. Elevated exhaled carbon dioxide levels
4. Decreased peak inspiratory pressures noted on the ventilator
5. Presence of yellow fluid within the ET
6. Patient speaking around the ET tube

2. A patient who is receiving mechanical ventilation via tracheostomy tube (TT) is preparing for discharge home. Which statements, made by the patient's primary caregiver, indicate an understanding of the care of this patient? (Select all that apply.)
   1. "We should suction the tracheostomy tube every 4 hours during the day."
   2. "We will need to rinse the nondisposable inner cannula with sterile saline to clean it."
   3. "We should make sure that the tracheostomy holder is tight against the skin."
   4. "We should check the pressure in the cuff at least three times a day."
   5. "We will need to clean the stoma site at least every 8 hours and more frequently if there are secretions or signs of infection."

3. Put the steps of tracheal suctioning in the correct order.
   1. Hyperoxygenate the patient.
   2. Assess for the need for suctioning.
   3. Perform oropharyngeal suctioning.
   4. Withdraw catheter while applying suction.
   5. Insert catheter into endotracheal or tracheostomy tube.

ⓔ Visit the Evolve site for a complete list of Clinical Debrief and Review Questions answers.

REFERENCES
Accreditation Canada. (2019). *Required organizational practices handbook—Version 14*. Retrieved from http://www.wrha.mb.ca/quality/files/2019ROPHandbook.pdf

American Association of Critical Care Nurses (AACN). (2010). *AACN practice alert: Oral care for patients at risk for ventilator-associated pneumonia.* Retrieved from https://www.aacn.org/docs/EventPlanning/WB0011/oral-care-patients-at-risk-vap-r44spvmp.pdf

American Association of Critical Care Nurses (AACN). (2016). *AACN practice alert: Prevention of aspiration.* Retrieved from http://www.aacn.org/wd/practice/content/practicealerts/aspiration-practice-alert.pcms?menu=practice

American Association of Respiratory Care (AARC). (2004). AARC clinical practice guideline: Nasotracheal suctioning—2004 revision & update. *Respiratory Care,* 49(9), 1080–1084. Retrieved from http://www.rcjournal.com/cpgs/pdf/09.04.1080.pdf

American Association of Respiratory Care (AARC). (2010). AARC clinical practice guidelines: Endotracheal suctioning of mechanically ventilated patients with artificial airways 2010. *Respiratory Care,* 55(6), 758–764.

American Association of Respiratory Care (AARC). (2011). AARC clinical practice guidelines: Capnography/capnometry during mechanical ventilation. *Respiratory Care,* 56(4), 503–509. doi:10.4187/respcare.01175

American Association of Respiratory Care (AARC). (2012). Humidification during invasive and noninvasive mechanical ventilation. *Respiratory Care,* 57(5), 782–788. doi:10.4187/respcare.01766

Baumgarten, M., & Poulsen, I. (2015). Patients' experiences of being mechanically ventilated in an ICU: A qualitative metasynthesis. *Scandinavian Journal of Caring Sciences,* 29(2), 205–214. doi:10.1111/scs.12177

Canadian Patient Safety Institute (CPSI). (2009). *The safety competencies.* Retrieved from http://www.patientsafetyinstitute.ca/en/toolsResources/safetyCompetencies/Documents/Safety%20Competencies.pdf

Canadian Patient Safety Institute (CPSI). (2012). *Prevent ventilator-associated pneumonia.* Retrieved from http://www.patientsafetyinstitute.ca/en/toolsResources/Documents/Interventions/Ventilator-Associated%20Pneumonia/VAP%20Getting%20Started%20Kit.pdf#search=canadian%20vap%20guidelines

Centers for Disease Control and Prevention (CDC). (2019). *Ventilator-associated event (VAE).* Retrieved from http://www.cdc.gov/nhsn/PDFs/pscManual/10-VAE_FINAL.pdf

Donatelli, J., Gupta, A., Santhosh, R., et al. (2015). To breathe or not to breathe: A review of artificial airway placement and related complications. *Emergency Radiology,* 22(2), 171–179. doi:10.1007/s10140-014-1271-8

Elmansoury, A., & Said, H. (2017). Closed suction system versus open suction. *Egyptian Journal of Chest Diseases and Tuberculosis,* 66(3), 509–515. doi:10.1016/j.ejcdt.2016.08.001

El-Rabbany, M., Zoghlol, N., Bhandari, M., & Azarpazhooh, A. (2015). Prophylactic oral health procedures to prevent hospital-acquired and ventilator-associated pneumonia: A systematic review. *International Journal of Nursing Studies,* 52(1), 452–462. doi:10.1016/j.ijnurstu.2014.07.010

Galbiati, G., & Paola, C. (2015). Effects of open and closed endotracheal suctioning on intracranial pressure and cerebral perfusion pressure in adult patients with severe brain injury: A literature review. *The Journal of Neuroscience Nursing: Journal of the American Association of Neuroscience Nurses,* 47(4), 239–246. doi:10.1097/JNN.0000000000000146

Grindrod, K. (2015). Management of stable chronic obstructive pulmonary disease. *British Journal of Community Nursing,* 20(2), 58–64. doi:10.12968/bjcn.2015.20.2.58

Hellyer, T. P., Ewan, V., Wilson, P., & Simpson, A. J. (2016). The Intensive Care Society recommended bundle of interventions for the prevention of ventilator-associated pneumonia. *Journal of the Intensive Care Society,* 17(3), 238–243. doi:10.1177/1751143716644461

Hockenberry, M. J., & Wilson, D. (2015). *Wong's nursing care of infants and children* (10th ed.). St. Louis: Mosby.

Hyde, G. A., Savage, S. A., Zarzaur, B. L., et al. (2015). Early tracheostomy in trauma patients saves time and money. *Injury,* 46(1), 110–114. doi:10.1016/j.injury.2014.08.049

Institute for Healthcare Improvement (IHI). (2012). *How-to guide: Prevent ventilator-associated pneumonia.* Retrieved from http://www.chpso.org/sites/main/files/file-attachments/ihi_howtoguidepreventvap.pdf

Karsli, B., Kayacan, N., Ince, U. K., & Mutlu, H. (2016). Tracheostomy and innominate artery bleeding: A later complication. *British Journal of Pharmaceutical Research,* 14(6), 1–5. doi:10.9734/BJPR/2016/31700

Kuriyama, A., Umakoshi, N., Fujinaga, J., & Takada, T. (2015). Impact of closed versus open tracheal suctioning systems for mechanically ventilated adults: A systematic review and meta-analysis. *Intensive Care Medicine,* 41(3), 402–411. doi:10.1007/s00134-014-3565-4

Lewis, S. L., Bucher, L., Heitkemper, M. L., et al. (Eds.). (2019). *Medical-surgical nursing in Canada: Assessment and management of clinical problems* (4th ed.). Toronto: Elsevier.

Lewis, T. D., Dehne, K. A., Morbitzer, K., Rhoney, D. H., Olm-Shipman, C., & Jordan, J. D. (2018). Influence of single-dose antibiotic prophylaxis for early-onset pneumonia in high-risk intubated patients. *Neurocritical Care,* 28(3), 362–369. doi:10.1007/s12028-017-0490-8

Lim, C. (2015). Effect of tracheostomy on weaning parameters in difficult-to-wean mechanically ventilated patients: A prospective observational study. *PloS One,* 10(9), 1–14. doi:10.1371/journal.pone.0138294

Lium, X., Jin, Y., Ma, T., Qu, B., & Liu, Z. (2015). Differential effects of endotracheal suctioning on gas exchanges in patients with acute respiratory failure under pressure-controlled and volume-controlled ventilation. *BioMed Research International,* 2015. doi:10.1155/2015/941081. Article ID: 941081.

Myatt, R. (2015). Nursing care of patients with a temporary tracheostomy. *Nursing Standard: Official Newspaper of the Royal College of Nursing,* 29(26), 42–49. doi:10.7748/ns.29.26.42.e9742

Nseir, S., Rodriguez, A., Saludes, P., et al. (2015). Efficiency of a mechanical device in controlling tracheal cuff pressure in intubated critically ill patients: A randomized controlled study. *Annals of Intensive Care,* 5(1), 12–19. doi:10.1186/s13613-015-0054-z

Pittman, J., Beeson, T., Kitterman, J., Lancaster, S., & Shelly, A. (2015). Medical device–related hospital-acquired pressure ulcers: Development of an evidence-based position statement. *Journal of Wound, Ostomy, and Continence Nursing: Official Publication of The Wound, Ostomy and Continence Nurses Society / WOCN,* 42(2), 151–154. doi:10.1097/WON.0000000000000113

Rouze, A., De Jonckheere, J., Zerimech, F., et al. (2016). Efficiency of an electronic device in controlling tracheal cuff pressure in critically ill patients: A randomized controlled crossover study. *Annals of Intensive Care,* 6(1), 930–938. doi:10.1186/s13613-016-0200-2

Smith, S. G., & Pietrantonio, T. (2016). Best method for securing an endotracheal tube. *Critical Care Nurse,* 36(2), 78–79. doi:10.4037/ccn2016214

Sole, M. L., Bennett, M., & Ashworth, S. (2015). Clinical indicators for endotracheal suctioning in adult patients receiving mechanical ventilation. *American Journal of Critical Care: An Official Publication, American Association of Critical-Care Nurses,* 24(2), 318–324. doi:10.4037/ajcc2015794

ten Hoorn, S., Elbers, P. W., Girbes, A. R., & Tuinman, P. R. (2016). Communicating with conscious and mechanically ventilated critically ill patients: A systematic review. *Critical Care: The Official Journal of the Critical Care Forum,* 20(1), 333–347. doi:10.1186/s13054-016-1483-2

Timbrell, D., & Jankowski, S. (2018). Management of an indication for tracheostomy in care of the critically ill patient. *Surgery,* 36(4), 187–195. doi:10.1016/j.mpsur.2018.01.006

Tokmaji, G., Vermeulen, H., Muller, M. C., Kwakman, P. H., Schultz, M. J., & Zaat, S. A. (2015). Silver-coated endotracheal tubes for prevention of ventilator-associated pneumonia in critically ill patients. *The Cochrane Database of Systematic Reviews,* 12(8), 1–42. doi:10.1002/14651858.CD009201.pub2

Touhy, T. A., Jett, K. F., Boscart, V., & McCleary, L. (2019). *Ebersole and Hess' gerontological nursing & healthy aging* (2nd Canadian ed.). Toronto: Elsevier Canada.

Urden, L., Stacy, K., & Lough, M. (2016). *Priorities in critical care nursing* (7th ed.). St. Louis: Mosby.

Vargas, M., Sutherasan, Y., Antonelli, M., et al. (2015). Tracheostomy procedures in the intensive care unit: An international survey. *Critical Care: The Official Journal of the Critical Care Forum,* 191(6), 637–645. doi:10.1186/s13054-015-1013-7

Wiegand, D. (2017). *AACN procedure manual for critical care* (7th ed.). St. Louis: Mosby.

26 | Cardiac Care

Written by **Giuliana Harvey, RN, MN; Heather MacLean, RN, MN; and Nelda K. Martin, RN, ANP-BC, CCNS**

OBJECTIVES

Mastery of content in this chapter will enable the nurse to:
- Identify the indications to perform a 12-lead electrocardiogram (ECG) and cardiac monitor application.
- Determine correct electrode placement to obtain an accurate ECG tracing.
- Describe measures to reduce false alarms.

MEDIA RESOURCES

- evolve http://evolve.elsevier.com/Canada/Perry/clinicalskills/
- Review Questions
- Audio Glossary
- **NSO** Nursing Skills Online
- Clinical Debrief and Review Questions Answers
- Animations

PURPOSE

The electrocardiogram (ECG) is the graphic representation of the electrical activities, or conduction system, of the heart used for diagnostic and treatment purposes. Accuracy of these waveforms depends on the correct placement and clean application of electrodes to the skin.

STANDARDS OF CARE

- Accreditation Canada, 2019—*Required Organizational Practices Handbook—Version 14* (http://www.wrha.mb.ca/quality/files/2019ROPHandbook.pdf)
- American Association of Critical Care Nurses (AACN), 2013—*AACN Practice Alert: Alarm Management* (http://ccn.aacnjournals.org/content/33/5/83.full.pdf+html)
- O'Gara, Kushner, Ascheim, et al., 2013—*2013 American College of Cardiology Foundation (ACCF)/American Heart Association (AHA), Guideline for the Management of ST-Elevation Myocardial Infarction* (http://circ.ahajournals.org/content/circulationaha/early/2012/12/17/CIR.0b013e3182742cf6.full.pdf)
- Sandau, Funk, Auerbach, et al., 2017—*Update to Practice Standards for Electrocardiographic Monitoring in Hospital Settings: A Scientific Statement from the American Heart Association* (http://circ.ahajournals.org/content/early/2017/10/03/CIR.0000000000000527)

PRINCIPLES FOR PRACTICE

- A 12-lead ECG provides a snapshot of the electrical activity of the heart from multiple views. It is a diagnostic tool to determine emergency treatment of patients with acute coronary syndrome or acute onset of potential life-threatening dysrhythmias. Accuracy and timeliness are the key principles of acquisition (O'Gara et al., 2013; Sandau et al., 2017).
- Cardiac monitoring provides continuous ECG observation of the acutely ill patient. Proper placement of the ECG electrodes is essential to ensure real-time detection of arrhythmias (Sandau et al., 2017) (Table 26.1).

PERSON-CENTRED CARE

- Placement of the electrodes requires exposure of a patient's chest. Measures to maintain the person's privacy and modesty are essential.
- Females require special consideration with the placement of electrodes as close to the chest wall as possible, avoiding the breast tissue.
- Patients and caregivers, especially those with a cultural need for modesty, may need detailed information about the procedure so they do not misunderstand the intent and objective of cardiac monitoring.
- Always explain which type of physical interaction is involved to avoid misinterpretation of interventions.

EVIDENCE-INFORMED PRACTICE

The clinical indications for the acquisition of continuous cardiac monitoring and 12-lead ECG have been well established over the last several years (Sandau et al., 2017). Patient selection for ECG monitoring is the first step toward establishing appropriate alarms and response expectations. Indications and contraindications for 12-lead ECG acquisitions follow.

TABLE 26.1

Common Basic Cardiac Rhythms

Rhythm Characteristics	Appearance	Clinical Considerations
Normal sinus rhythm (NSR): Regular rhythm, rate 60–100 beats/min, normal PQRST complex	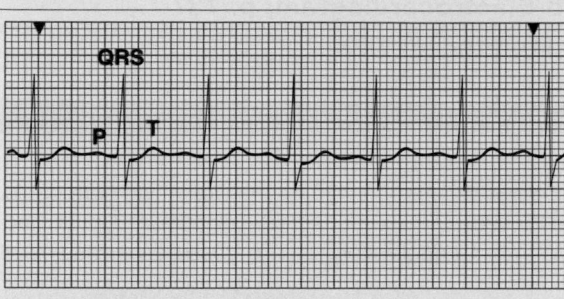 NSR	Normal heart rate and rhythm
Sinus tachycardia: Regular rhythm, rate greater than 100–180 beats/min, normal PQRS complex	Sinus tachycardia	Normal response to exercise, emotion, pain, fever, hyperthyroidism, and certain drugs
Atrial fibrillation: Abnormal and irregular rhythm; atrial rate 350–600 beats/min, ventricular rate <100 (controlled) and >100 (uncontrolled); abnormal P waves, f waves present, no PR interval, and normal QRS complex	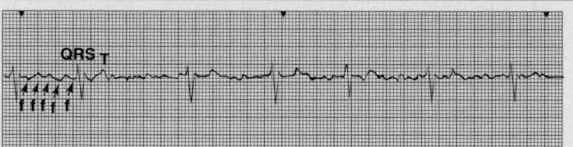 Coarse atrial fibrillation	Associated with mitral valve disease, coronary heart disease, and heart failure
Sinus bradycardia: Regular rhythm; rate less than 60 beats/min; normal P wave, PR interval, and QRS complex	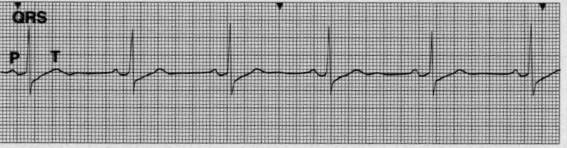 Sinus bradycardia	Associated with decreased cardiac output, dizziness, syncope, and chest pain
Ventricular tachycardia (V-Tach): Rhythm slightly irregular, rate 100–250 beats/min, P wave absent, PR interval absent, QRS complex wide and bizarre	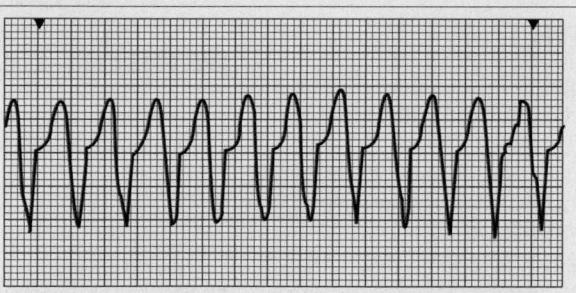 V-Tach	Often a forerunner of ventricular fibrillation; may cause pulselessness; if patient is unstable or pulseless, requires electrical defibrillation as soon as possible
Ventricular fibrillation: Rate 300–500; totally irregular, chaotic rhythm with no identifiable P wave, PR and QRS complex	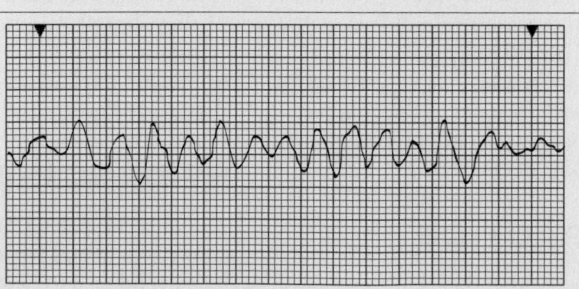 Coarse ventricular fibrillation	Lethal arrhythmia; patient pulseless and requires electrical defibrillation as soon as possible followed by immediate cardiopulmonary resuscitation (CPR)

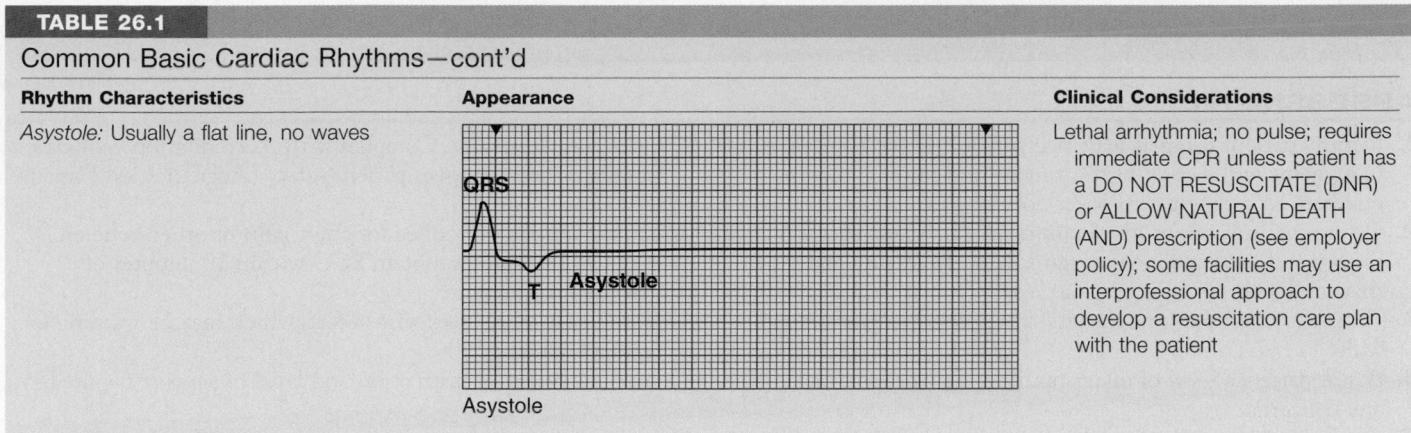

TABLE 26.1		
Common Basic Cardiac Rhythms—cont'd		
Rhythm Characteristics	**Appearance**	**Clinical Considerations**
Asystole: Usually a flat line, no waves	QRS T Asystole Asystole	Lethal arrhythmia; no pulse; requires immediate CPR unless patient has a DO NOT RESUSCITATE (DNR) or ALLOW NATURAL DEATH (AND) prescription (see employer policy); some facilities may use an interprofessional approach to develop a resuscitation care plan with the patient

Data and images from Wesley, K. (2017). *Huszar's ECG and 12-lead ECG interpretation* (5th ed.). St. Louis, MO: Elsevier.

Indications

- Suspected acute coronary syndrome, including myocardial infarction
- Evaluation of implanted defibrillators and pacemakers
- Disorders of the cardiac rhythm
- Evaluation of syncope
- Evaluation of metabolic disorders
- Effects and adverse effects of pharmacotherapy
- Evaluation of primary and secondary cardiomyopathic processes

Contraindications

- There are no absolute contraindications to performing an ECG other than patient refusal.
- Some patients may have allergies or, more commonly, sensitivities to the adhesive used to affix the leads. In these cases, hypoallergenic alternatives are available from various manufacturers.

SAFETY GUIDELINES

- Know the indications for a 12-lead ECG. Patients experiencing chest pain need to have their 12-lead ECG within 10 minutes of the assessment and onset of pain. Nonetheless, only 29% of women receive an ECG within 10 minutes, compared to 38% of men (Heart and Stroke Foundation of Canada, 2018). A 12-lead ECG will determine the next step in their treatment plan.
- Know a patient's current medications. Some medications, particularly beta blockers, and some calcium channel blockers and other antiarrhythmics can cause dysrhythmias.

✦ SKILL 26.1 Obtaining a 12-Lead Electrocardiogram

NSO *Nursing Skills Online Cardiac Care Module 10 / Lesson 2*

Electrical impulses of the heart are conducted to the surface of the body and are detected by electrodes placed on the skin of the limbs and torso. The electrodes carry these impulses to either a continuous monitor or a 12-lead electrocardiogram (ECG) machine. The appearance of the ECG pattern or waveform helps in diagnosing whether there are any abnormalities in the electrical conduction through the heart. The 12-lead ECG provides a snapshot of the waveforms from 12 different angles or views of the heart. One electrode is placed on each of the four extremities, and six electrodes are placed at specific sites on the chest for a total of 10 electrodes on the patient's skin. They are bipolar limb leads I, II, III; augmented limb leads aV_R, aV_L, aV_F; and precordial chest leads V_1 to V_6. The leads view a specific part of the surface of the heart and can help determine which part of the heart has sustained damage and the origin and flow of the impulse.

Delegation and Collaboration

The skill of obtaining a 12-lead ECG is restricted to health care providers who are specifically trained in this skill (see employer policy) and cannot be delegated to an unregulated care provider (UCP). The nurse directs the UCP to:

- Immediately report to the nurse changes in the patient's cardiac status, such as indications of chest pain.
- Immediately deliver the completed 12-lead ECG recording to a health care provider for interpretation.
- Use specific patient precautions related to disease, mobility status, or position restrictions.

Equipment

- 12-lead ECG machine
- 10 ECG leads with alligator clip, suction cup, or snap-on attachments
- 10 ECG electrodes (disposable, self-adhesive) or electrode paste
- Clean, dry towel or sponge wipes
- Hair clippers (optional depending on hair at electrode sites)

STEP	RATIONALE

ASSESSMENT

1. Identify patient using at least two person-specific identifiers (e.g., name and date of birth or name and medical record number) according to employer policy.	Ensures correct patient. Complies with Accreditation Canada's standards and improves patient safety (Accreditation Canada, 2019).
2. Determine indications for obtaining ECG. Assess patient's history and cardiopulmonary status (e.g., heart rate and rhythm, blood pressure, respirations).	If 12-lead ECG is prescribed for chest pain or other ischemic signs and symptoms, obtain ECG within 10 minutes of patient's pain report.
3. Assess for chest pain; rate acuity on appropriate pain rating scale.	Determines level of chest discomfort, which may be warning for cardiac ischemia.
4. Assess patient's level of understanding of procedure, including any concerns.	Determine extent of instruction and level of support required.
5. Assess patient's ability to follow directions and remain still in supine position if there are no patient-specific contraindications to this position (e.g., certain surgical procedures, continuous tube feedings).	Provides clear, accurate recording without artifact; however, patient's position may need to be altered based on patient health status (e.g., semi-Fowler's position).

NURSING DIAGNOSES

- Acute pain
- Anxiety
- Insufficient knowledge regarding purpose and steps of procedure
- Fear

Related factors/Risk factors are individualized on the basis of patient's condition or needs.

PLANNING

1. Expected outcomes following completion of procedure: • Patient tolerates procedure without anxiety or discomfort.	Appropriate preparation and education decrease anxiety.
• Clear, accurate recording of ECG waveform is obtained.	
2. Close room door or bedside curtains.	Provides privacy.

IMPLEMENTATION

1. Prepare patient for procedure: a. Remove or reposition patient's clothing to expose only patient's chest and arms. Keep abdomen and thighs covered.	Facilitates correct placement of cardiac leads and maintains patient's modesty. Improper lead placement produces artifact, which necessitates repeating test or interpretation errors.
b. Place patient in supine position with head of bed no higher than 30 degrees.	Electrodes must be placed on anterior chest for standard 12-lead ECG (Sandau et al., 2017).
c. Instruct patient to lie still without talking and do not cross legs.	Body movement or talking produces artifact, which may necessitate repeating the test.
2. Turn on machine; enter required demographic information.	Turning machine on first helps you identify electrode and lead issues on application.
3. Perform hand hygiene.	Reduces transmission of microorganisms.
4. Clean and prepare skin with soap and water for isolated electrode placement. Wipe area with a dry washcloth (Sandau et al., 2017). Clip excessive hair from electrode area.	The skin should be prepared before ECG electrodes are placed (Sandau et al., 2017). Proper skin preparation decreases skin impedance signal noise, thereby producing a clean, accurate recording. Do not use alcohol to clean area (Sandau et al., 2017). Clipping hair in the electrode area is preferred. Shaving leaves nicks that predispose the area for infection.

STEP	RATIONALE

IMPLEMENTATION

5. Apply electrodes in correct positions. If using leads with suction cups, apply electrode paste to areas before attaching leads.

    a. Chest (precordial) leads (Fig. 26.1)
    - V_1—Fourth intercostal space (ICS) at right sternal angle
    - V_2—Fourth ICS at left sternal border
    - V_3—Midway between V_2 and V_4
    - V_4—Fifth ICS at midclavicular line
    - V_5—Left anterior axillary line at level of V_4 horizontally
    - V_6—Left midaxillary line at level of V_4 horizontally

    b. Extremities: One lead on each extremity (Fig. 26.2); right wrist, left wrist, left ankle, right ankle.

6. Check 12-lead machine for messages to correct electrode or lead issues. If no messages occur, press button to obtain 12-lead ECG.

7. If you obtain ECG tracing without artifact, disconnect leads and wipe off excess electrode paste from patient's chest.

8. If STAT, immediately deliver ECG tracing (if not computerized) to appropriate health care provider for interpretation.

Proper placement of leads is very important for accurate interpretation of a 12-lead ECG. Ensure that the correct lead is in the correct location. If any leads are misplaced, the ECG reading will be inaccurate and can result in misdiagnosis and inappropriate treatment (Sandau et al., 2017).

Promotes comfort and hygiene.

If non-STAT 12-lead ECG, place this in patient's chart or designated area.

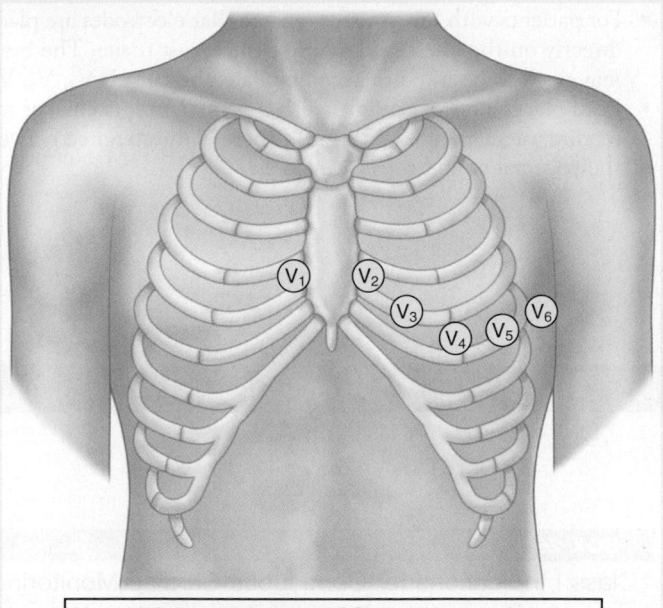

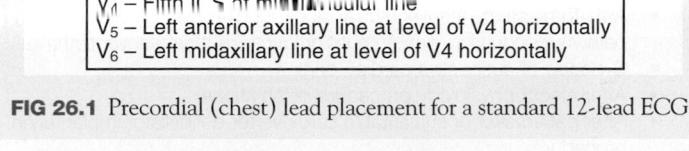

V₁ – 4th intercostal space (ICS) at right sternal angle
V₂ – 4th ICS at left sternal border
V₃ – Midway between V2 and V4
V₄ – Fifth ICS at midclavicular line
V₅ – Left anterior axillary line at level of V4 horizontally
V₆ – Left midaxillary line at level of V4 horizontally

FIG 26.1 Precordial (chest) lead placement for a standard 12-lead ECG.

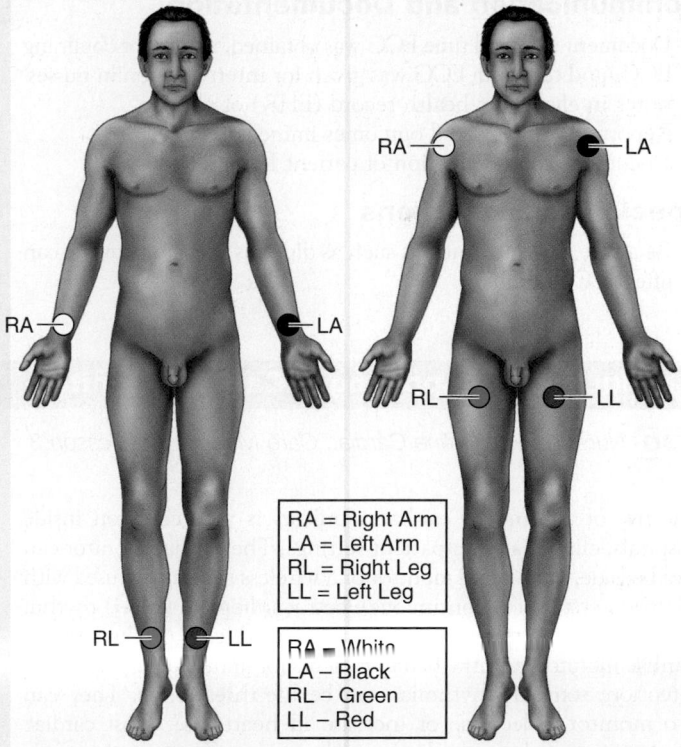

RA = Right Arm
LA = Left Arm
RL = Right Leg
LL = Left Leg

RA – White
LA – Black
RL – Green
LL – Red

FIG 26.2 Limb lead placement for a standard 12-lead ECG.

EVALUATION

1. Note and document if patient is experiencing any chest discomfort during procedure.

2. Discuss findings and results of 12-lead ECG with health care provider to determine next steps in patient's treatment plan.

Helps correlate ECG changes to symptoms of chest pain.

If myocardial infarction is identified, immediate steps will need to be taken to get patient to cardiac catheterization laboratory or consider use of thrombolytic medications.

STEP	RATIONALE

EVALUATION

3. Use Teach-Back: "I want to be sure I explained why you need this ECG. Why are you receiving an ECG?" Develop a revised teaching plan if patient is not able to explain rationale for procedure correctly.

Determines patient's level of understanding of instructional topic.

Unexpected Outcomes

1. ECG cannot be interpreted:
   - Absence of tracing on one or more leads
   - Presence of artifact in ECG tracings

Related Interventions

- Inspect electrodes for secure placement.
- Reposition any wires that move as a result of patient breathing or movement or vibrations in environment. Do not reposition electrodes if in correct position.
- Remind patient who is moving that lying still is necessary to obtain good tracing.
- If artifact looks like 60-cycle interference (very thick-lined waveform), unplug battery-operated equipment in room one item at a time to see if interference disappears. **NOTE:** 60-cycle interference is rare.
- Repeat tracing.

2. Patient has chest pain or anxiety.

- Continue to monitor patient.
- Reassess factors contributing to anxiety or distress.
- Follow specific prescriptions related to findings.
- Notify health care provider.

Communication and Documentation

- Document date and time ECG was obtained, reason for obtaining ECG, and to whom ECG was given for interpretation in nurses' notes in electronic health record (EHR) or chart.
- Report any unexpected outcomes immediately.
- Document your evaluation of patient learning.

- For patients with breast tissue, ensure that electrodes are placed directly on the chest wall and not the breast tissue. The breast may need to be lifted to accommodate chest leads V_4, V_5, V_6.
- Lead placement for patients with a permanent pacemaker may require an augmented position if there is interference between the pacemaker and intrinsic signals.

Special Considerations

- Be aware that medications such as digitalis and amiodarone can affect ECG results.

◆ SKILL 26.2 Applying a Cardiac Monitor

NSO *Nursing Skills Online Cardiac Care Module 10 / Lesson 3*

The use of continuous cardiac monitors is very common inside hospitals, clinics, and outpatient settings. The cardiac monitor can be a bedside, hard-wired monitor or a wireless transmitter used with telemetry systems. A continuous electrocardiogram (ECG) rhythm is obtained using three or five electrodes and leads on the patient. Cardiac monitors are attached to patients for immediate dysrhythmia detection; some dysrhythmias can be life-threatening. They can also monitor a decrease or increase in heart rate. Most cardiac monitor systems have dysrhythmia detection software and provide alarms when dysrhythmias appear or heart rate limits are exceeded.

It is important to monitor only patients with clinical indications for cardiac monitoring. This can significantly decrease the number of false alarms (AACN, 2013). There are certain patients, such as those with bundle branch blocks or ventricular pacing, who are more likely to initiate a higher number of false arrhythmia alarms. (Harris, Zegre-Hemsey, Schindler, et al., 2017). In 2017, the American Heart Association updated existing standards for ECG monitoring in hospitalized patients (Sandau et al., 2017) (Box 26.1) These standards are used in Canada.

BOX 26.1

Class I Indications for Continuous Cardiac Monitoring

- Chest pain/coronary artery disease (e.g., early phase acute coronary syndrome)
- Major cardiac interventions (e.g., cardiac surgery)
- Arrhythmias (e.g., atrioventricular block, long QT syndrome, accessory pathway conduction, symptomatic bradycardia, atrial tachyarrhythmias)
- Syncope of suspected cardiac origin
- After electrophysiology procedure or ablations
- After pacemaker or implantable cardioverter-defibrillator implantation procedure
- Temporary or transcutaneous pacing
- Noncardiac conditions (e.g., postconscious sedation)
- Medical conditions (e.g., moderate-to-severe imbalance of potassium or magnesium, drug overdose)

Data from Sandau, K., Funk, M., Auerbach, A., Barsness, G., Blum, K., Cvach, M., … Council on Cardiovascular Disease in the Young. (2017). Update to practice standards for electrocardiographic monitoring in hospital settings: A scientific statement from the American Heart Association. *Circulation, 136*(19), e1–e72.

Alarm fatigue occurs when a person is exposed to an excessive number of false alarms, leading to sensory overload (Sandau et al., 2017). This may cause the person to become desensitized to the alarms and potentially influence their response time (Sandau et al., 2017). Patient safety may be jeopardized if the alarms are silenced or ignored (Sendelbach, Wahl, Anthony, et al., 2015). The American Association of Critical Care Nurses (AACN, 2013) has provided strategies for alarm management to reduce alarm fatigue and enhance patient safety (Box 26.2). These strategies are applicable in the Canadian health care environment.

BOX 26.2

Expected Practice and Nursing Actions for the Reduction of Alarm Fatigue

- Provide proper skin preparation for ECG electrodes.
- Change ECG electrodes daily.
- Customize alarm parameters and levels of ECG monitors.
- Customize delay and threshold settings on oxygen saturation via pulse oximetry (SpO_2) monitors.
- Provide initial and ongoing education about devices with alarms.
- Establish interprofessional teams to address issues related to alarms, such as through development of policies and procedures.
- Monitor only patients with clinical indications for monitoring.

ECG, Electrocardiogram.
Adapted from American Association of Critical Care Nurses (AACN). (2013). *AACN practice alert: Alarm management.* Retrieved from http://ccn.aacnjournals. org/content/33/5/83.full.pdf+html.

Delegation and Collaboration

The skill of applying a cardiac monitor is restricted to health care providers who are specifically trained in ECG monitoring (see employer policy), and it cannot be performed by an unregulated care provider (UCP). The nurse directs the UCP to:

- Immediately report alarms or patient statements of pain or evidence of shortness of breath or hypotension.
- Ensure that the parameters for alarms and heart rate are set per health care provider prescription.

Equipment

- Bedside cardiac monitor or telemetry transmitter
- Three or five ECG electrodes (disposable, self-adhesive)
- Three or five ECG leads with snap-on attachments
- Clean, dry towel, washcloth, or gauze
- Hair clippers (optional, depending on hair at electrode sites)

STEP	RATIONALE

ASSESSMENT

1. Identify patient using at least two person-specific identifiers (e.g., name and date of birth or name and medical record number) according to employer policy.	Ensures correct patient. Complies with Accreditation Canada's standards and improves patient safety (Accreditation Canada, 2019).
2. Determine reason for continuous cardiac monitoring. Assess patient's history and cardiopulmonary status.	Knowing reason for monitoring allows for focused, improved response to an alarm.
3. Assess patient's level of understanding of procedure, including any concerns. Also assess for chest pain.	Determine extent of instruction and level of support required.
4. Check skin for excess oil or moisture. If present, wipe chest or limbs with clean, dry towel.	Provides clear, accurate recording without artifact.
5. Ensure patient's cellular phone is turned off.	Cellular phones can interfere with the ECG and cause artifacts (Mariappan, Raghavan, Aleem, et al., 2016).

NURSING DIAGNOSES

- Acute pain
- Anxiety
- Insufficient knowledge regarding purpose and steps of procedure
- Fear

Related factors/Risk factors are individualized on the basis of patient's condition or needs.

PLANNING

1. Expected outcomes following completion of procedure: • Patient tolerates procedure without anxiety or discomfort. • Clear, accurate ongoing recording of ECG rhythm is obtained.	Appropriate preparation decreases anxiety.
2. Close room door or bedside curtains.	Provides privacy.

STEP	RATIONALE

IMPLEMENTATION

1. Prepare patient for procedure:
   a. Remove or reposition patient's gown to expose only patient's chest. Keep abdomen and thighs covered.
   b. Place patient in supine position.
2. Perform hand hygiene.
3. Clean and prepare chest area with soap and water for electrode placement. Wipe area with a dry washcloth (Sandau et al., 2017). Clip excessive hair from electrode area rather than shaving.

4. Apply electrodes in correct positions for either a three- or five-electrode system (Fig. 26.3).
5. Attach monitor leads to electrodes. Colours of leads represent their polarity. White is negative. Black is positive. Red is ground or neutral. Two additional leads on five-lead system would include a green lead (positive or negative) and a brown lead (positive), which can be placed at V lead locations on precordial chest.
6. Check bedside monitor or telemetry station for any messages indicating electrode or lead issues. Troubleshoot as needed.
7. Check that the ECG rhythm can be visualized on bedside monitor, central station, or remote viewing station.

8. Change ECG electrodes daily or more often if electrode contact to skin is loose.
9. Customize alarm limits within 1 hour of assuming care of patient and on condition changes. Changes made should be in accordance with employer policies and health care provider prescription.

Facilitates correct placement of cardiac leads and maintains patient's modesty.
Electrodes must be placed on anterior chest.
Reduces transmission of microorganisms.
Proper skin preparation before ECG electrodes decreases skin impedance and signal noise, thus providing an accurate recording. Do not use alcohol to clean area, because it will dry the skin (Sandau et al., 2017). Clipping excessive hair rather than shaving reduces the risk for infection.
Proper placement of leads is very important for accurate dysrhythmia interpretation.
Colouring system (labelling) allows for consistent application of leads.

Monitoring system itself may detect bad electrode contact with skin or loose connection.
If staff is watching monitor remotely, communicate with them before you leave the room so you can correct any issues while on the phone with viewers. This call can also serve as notification that monitoring has started.
Changing ECG electrodes decreases the number of false alarms.
Customize alarms to individual patient needs in order to reduce false alarms and focus true alarms on reasons for monitoring (AACN, 2013).

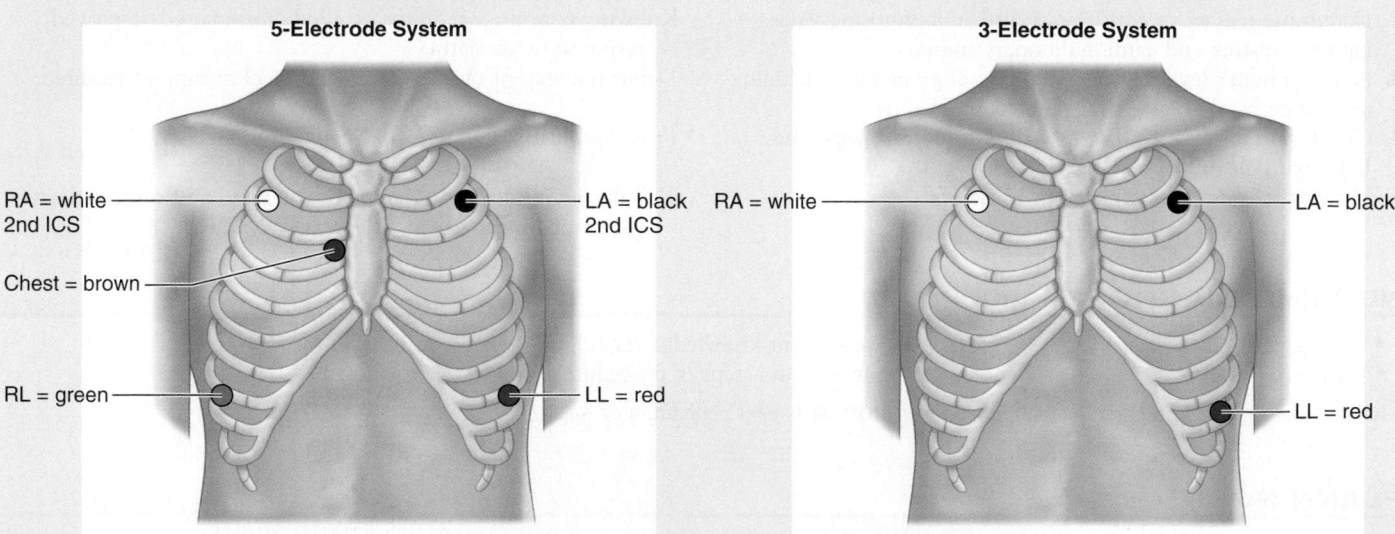

FIG 26.3 Cardiac monitor lead placement: three- or five-electrode systems. *ICS,* Intercostal space; *LA,* left arm; *LL,* left leg; *RA,* right arm; *RL,* right leg.

STEP	RATIONALE

EVALUATION

1. Although procedure is painless, it is important to note and document if patient experienced any distress.
2. Ensure that all appropriate alarms are ON.
3. **Use Teach-Back:** "I want to be sure I explained to you why you need this monitoring. Why is this monitoring important?" Develop a revised teaching plan if patient or caregiver is not able to explain rationale for procedure correctly.

Ensures accurate monitoring. Refer to employer policies.
Determines patient's and caregiver's level of understanding of instructional topic.

Unexpected Outcomes
1. Monitor tracing cannot be interpreted:
   - Absence of tracing on one or more leads
   - Presence of artifact in ECG tracings

Related Interventions
- Inspect electrodes for secure placement. Replace as needed and provide new skin preparation.
- Reposition any wires that move as a result of patient breathing or movement or vibrations in environment. Do not reposition electrodes if in correct position.
- If artifact looks like 60-cycle interference (very thick–lined waveform), unplug battery-operated equipment in room one item at a time to see if interference disappears. **NOTE:** 60-cycle interference is rare.

Communication and Documentation
- Review alarm trends and waveforms at least once a shift and on report of an alarm.
- Document at least one rhythm strip per shift (see employer policy), either on patient chart or electronic health record (EHR).
- Document your evaluation of patient and caregiver learning.
- Report and document any unexpected outcomes immediately to the health care provider.

Special Considerations
Pediatric
- In general, the mechanisms of dysrhythmias are the same in children as they are in adults; however, the appearance of the

dysrhythmias on the ECG may differ because of developmental issues such as heart size, baseline heart rate, sinus and arteriovenous (AV) node function, and autonomic innervation.
- Be aware that medications such as digitalis and antiarrhythmics can affect ECG rhythms.
- The position of the brown lead can be changed to mirror one of the precordial (chest) lead positions, V_1 to V_6. The standard placement is for V_1 at fourth intercostal space (ICS), right sternal border.

✦CLINICAL DEBRIEF

A 76-year-old female patient is postoperative day 2 following a partial colectomy. She has a history of a previous myocardial infarction (MI) with two stents; thus she is prescribed to be on continuous cardiac monitoring. The patient informs the nurse that she is experiencing chest pain, nausea, and shortness of breath. Vital signs are BP 100/50 mm Hg (previous BP 128/70), pulse 150 beats/min and regular (previous pulse 95), respiratory rate 28 breaths/min, pulse oximetry (SpO₂) 90% on room air, temperature 37.5°C (99.5°F). The patient's lungs have crackles in the bases bilaterally. The current telemetry rhythm is shown below. The nurse decides to call the health care provider.

Current telemetry rhythm:

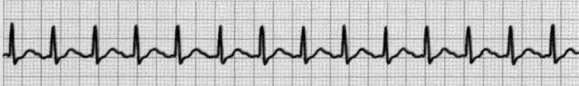

1. What does the nurse suspect is the primary physical concern for this patient? Based on the current patient findings (listed above), what

further assessments would be required before contacting the health care provider?
2. Based on the patient's signs and symptoms, which prescription should the nurse anticipate?
3. Using SBAR, how would the nurse communicate with the health care provider about this patient?

✦REVIEW QUESTIONS

1. The nurse has initiated cardiac monitoring via telemetry and notices artifact on the patient's electrocardiogram (ECG) rhythm. How should the nurse troubleshoot this artifact problem? *(Select all that apply.)*
   1. Move electrodes to different locations on the chest
   2. Wipe electrode skin areas with alcohol
   3. Prepare skin by washing with soap and water and drying with a washcloth
   4. Not change electrodes for 2 days
   5. Inspect electrodes for secure placement
   6. Assess if patient has a cellular phone on

2. What are the indications for a 12-lead electrocardiogram (ECG)? *(Select all that apply.)*

1. Suspected acute coronary syndromes, including myocardial infarction
2. Evaluation of implanted defibrillators and pacemakers
3. Disorders of the cardiac rhythm
4. Evaluation of shortness of breath
5. Evaluation of metabolic disorders
6. Effects and adverse effects of pharmacotherapy

3. When preparing a patient for a 12-lead electrocardiogram (ECG), it is necessary to apply six precordial chest leads. Match the lead with the correct anatomical position on the patient's chest.

1.	V_1	a.	Fifth intercostal space (ICS) at midclavicular line
2.	V_2	b.	Left midaxillary line at level of V_4 horizontally
3.	V_3	c.	Left anterior axillary line at level of V_4 horizontally
4.	V_4	d.	Fourth ICS at right sternal border
5.	V_5	e.	Midway between V_2 and V_4
6.	V_6	f.	Fourth ICS at left sternal border

ⓔ *Visit the Evolve site for a complete list of Clinical Debrief and Review Questions answers.*

REFERENCES

Accreditation Canada. (2019). *Required organizational practices handbook—Version 14.* Retrieved from http://www.wrha.mb.ca/quality/files/2019ROPHandbook.pdf

American Association of Critical Care Nurses (AACN). (2013). *AACN practice alert: Alarm management.* Retrieved from http://ccn.aacnjournals.org/content/33/5/83.full.pdf+html

Harris, P. R., Zegre-Hemsey, J. K., Schindler, D., Bai, Y., Pelter, M. M., & Hu, X. (2017). Patient characteristics associated with false arrhythmia alarms in intensive care. *Therapeutics and Clinical Risk Management, 13,* 499–513. doi:10.2147-TCRM.S126191

Heart and Stroke Foundation of Canada. (2018). *Ms. understood: Women's hearts are victim of a system that is ill-equipped to diagnose, treat and support them.* Retrieved from http://www.heartandstroke.ca/-/media/pdf-files/canada/2018-heart-month/hs_2018-heart-report_en.ashx

Mariappan, P., Raghavan, D., Aleem, S., & Zobaa, A. (2016). Effects of electromagnetic interference on the functional usage of medical equipment by 2G/3G/4G cellular phones: A review. *Journal of Advanced Research, 7*(5), 727–738. doi:10.1016/j.jare.2016.04.004

O'Gara, P. T., Kushner, F., Ascheim, D., et al. (2013). 2013 ACCF/AHA guideline for the management of ST-elevation myocardial infarction: A report of the American College of Cardiology Foundation/American Heart Association Task Force on Practice Guidelines. *Circulation, 127*(4), e362–e425. doi:10.1016/j.jacc.2012.11.019

Sandau, K., Funk, M., Auerbach, A., et al. Council on Cardiovascular Disease in the Young. (2017). Update to practice standards for electrocardiographic monitoring in hospital settings: A scientific statement from the American Heart Association. *Circulation, 136*(19), e1–e71. doi:10.1161-CIR.00000000000527

Sendelbach, S., Wahl, S., Anthony, A., & Shotts, P. (2015). Stop the noise: A quality improvement project to decrease electrocardiographic nuisance alarms. *Critical Care Nurse, 35*(4), 15–22. doi:10.4037/ccn2015858

27 | Closed Chest Drainage Systems

Written by **Ann Petlin, RN, MSN, CCNS, CCRN-CSC, ACNS-BC, PCCN, and Jane Tyerman, RN, MScN, PhD**

OBJECTIVES

Mastery of content in this chapter will enable the nurse to:
- Explain the physiology of normal respiration.
- List three common sites for chest tube placement.
- List three conditions requiring chest tube insertion.
- Describe closed chest drainage systems: water-seal and waterless systems.
- Describe principles and mechanisms of chest tube suction.
- Discuss measures to maintain patient safety during chest tube insertion, maintenance, and removal.
- Describe methods of troubleshooting chest tube systems.
- Discuss the nursing principles in caring for patients with chest tubes.
- Describe autotransfusion.

MEDIA RESOURCES

- **evolve** http://evolve.elsevier.com/Canada/Perry/clinicalskills/
- Review Questions
- Audio Glossary

- **NSO** Nursing Skills Online
- Clinical Debrief and Review Questions Answers

PURPOSE

The purpose of a closed chest drainage system, with or without suction, is to promote drainage of air and fluid from the pleural space. Lung re-expansion occurs as the fluid or air is removed and the patient's oxygenation improves (Lewis, Bucher, Heitkemper, et al., 2019; Wiegand, 2017). When air enters the pleural space, a pneumothorax occurs. When blood enters the pleural space, a hemothorax occurs. Pleural effusions occur when fluid enters the pleural space in response to infection, inflammation, or cancer.

STANDARDS OF CARE

- Accreditation Canada, 2019—*Required Organizational Practices Handbook—Version 14* (https://accreditation.ca/required-organizational-practices/)
- Atrium, 2015b—*Evidence-Based Care of Patients with Chest Tubes* (http://www.atriummed.com/EN/chest_drainage/Documents/NTI%202016.pdf)
- Waters, 2017—*Chest Tube Placement (Assist)* (In Wiegand, D. [Ed.], *AACN Procedure Manual for Critical Care* [7th ed.]. St. Louis: Elsevier.)

PRINCIPLES FOR PRACTICE

- The chest cavity is a closed structure bound by muscle, bone, connective tissue, vascular structures, and the diaphragm. This cavity has three distinct sections, each sealed from the others: one section for each lung and a third section for the mediastinum, which surrounds structures such as the heart, esophagus, trachea, and great vessels. The lungs are covered with a membrane called the *visceral pleura*. The interior chest wall is lined with a membrane called the *parietal pleura* (Fig. 27.1). The space between the visceral and parietal pleura is called the *pleural space* and is filled with approximately 7 to 20 mL of lubricating fluid to help the pleura slide during respiration (Kane, York, & Minton, 2013).
- Trauma, disease, or surgery can result in air, blood, pus, or lymph fluid leaking into the intrapleural space, creating a positive pressure that collapses lung tissue (Lewis et al., 2019). Small leaks (24% or less) are sometimes absorbed spontaneously and may not require a chest tube.
- A number of clinical conditions such as cancer, infection, pancreatitis, connective tissue disease, autoimmune diseases, asbestos exposure, certain medications, or collagen vascular diseases increase pleural fluid entry or decrease fluid exit from

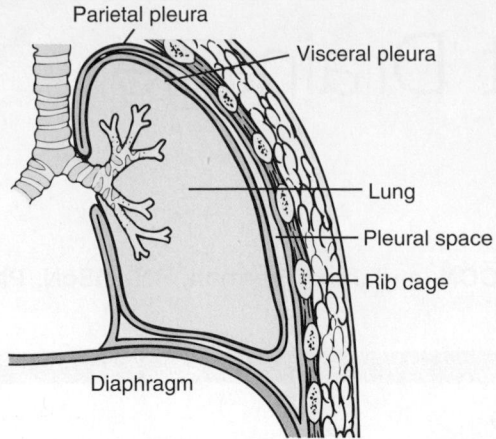

FIG 27.1 Partial structures of lungs.

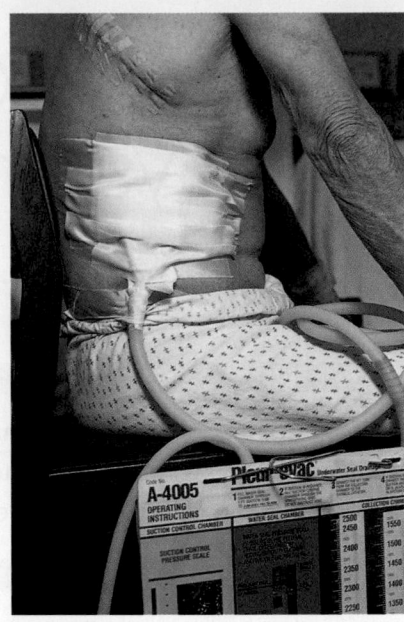

FIG 27.2 Pleural chest tube in place following thoracic surgery.

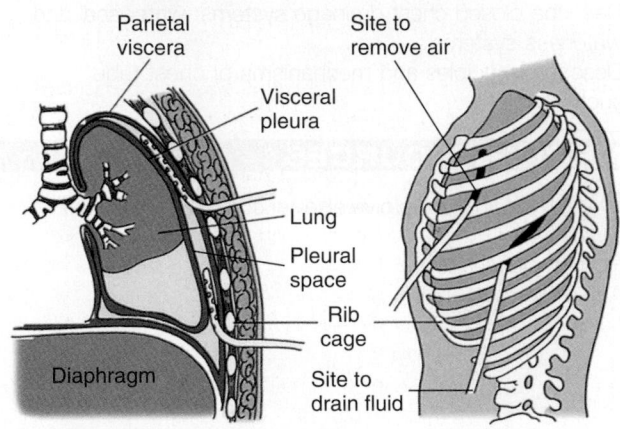

FIG 27.3 Diagram of sites for chest tube placement.

the lung. This is called a *pleural effusion;* when present, a patient usually needs a diagnostic thoracentesis and pleural fluid analysis to determine the cause of the exudate (see Chapter 10) (Bhatnagar & Maskell, 2015).

- A *pneumothorax* is collapse of the lung caused by a collection of air in the pleural space. The loss of negative intrapleural pressure causes the lung to collapse. A traumatic pneumothorax develops as a result of penetrating chest trauma such as a stabbing (open) or the chest striking the steering wheel in an automobile accident (closed). A spontaneous or primary pneumothorax sometimes occurs from the rupture of a small bleb (blister) on the surface of the lung or an invasive procedure, such as insertion of a subclavian intravenous (IV) line. Secondary pneumothorax occurs from an underlying disease, such as emphysema. A patient with a pneumothorax usually feels sharp chest pain that worsens on inspiration or coughing because atmospheric air irritates the parietal pleura.

- A tension pneumothorax, a life-threatening situation, occurs from rupture in the pleura when air accumulates in the pleural space more rapidly than it is removed. If left untreated, the lung on the affected side collapses, and the mediastinum shifts to the opposite (unaffected side), leading to tracheal deviation, reduced venous return, and subsequent decrease in cardiac output. Tracheal deviation is a late sign and may be absent in some cases (Welch & Saltarelli, 2018). Sudden chest pain, a fall in blood pressure, tachycardia, acute pleuritic pain, diaphoresis, dry cough, and cardiopulmonary arrest can occur.

- If emergent treatment is required, a needle decompression is achieved with a large-gauge needle (14 or 16 gauge) inserted into the second intercostal space, midclavicular line. A "hissing" sound is noted, followed by a rapid stabilization of the patient's vital signs and respiratory status (Wiegand, 2017).

- A *hemothorax* is collapse of the lung caused by an accumulation of blood and fluid in the pleural cavity between the chest wall and the lung, usually as a result of trauma. It produces a counterpressure and prevents the full expansion of the lung. A hemothorax is also caused by rupture of small blood vessels from inflammatory processes such as pneumonia or tuberculosis. In addition to pain and dyspnea, signs and symptoms of shock can develop if blood loss is severe (Mancini, Scalin, Serebrisky, & 2018).

- Chest tube insertion is the treatment for most types of effusions, pneumothorax, hemothorax, and postoperative chest surgery or trauma. A *chest tube* is a large catheter inserted through the thorax to remove fluid (effusions), blood (hemothorax), and/or air (pneumothorax).

- A pleural chest tube (Fig. 27.2) is inserted when air or fluid enters the pleural space, compromising oxygenation or ventilation.

- The location of the chest tube indicates the type of drainage expected. Apical (second or third intercostal space) and anterior chest tube placement promotes removal of air. Because air rises, these chest tubes are placed high, allowing evacuation of air from the intrapleural space and lung re-expansion (Fig. 27.3). The air is discharged into the atmosphere, and there is little or no drainage in the collection chamber.

- Chest tubes placed low (usually in the fifth or sixth intercostal space) and posterior or lateral drain fluid (see Fig. 27.3). Fluid in the intrapleural space is affected by gravity and localizes in the lower part of the lung cavity. Tubes placed in these positions drain blood and fluid. Fluid drainage is expected after open-chest surgery and with some chest trauma.

- A mediastinal chest tube is placed in the mediastinum, just below the sternum (Fig. 27.4), and is connected to a drainage system. This tube drains blood or fluid, preventing its accumulation

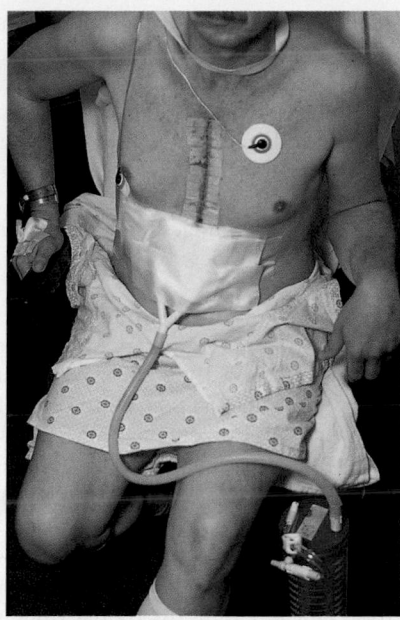

FIG 27.4 Mediastinal chest tube.

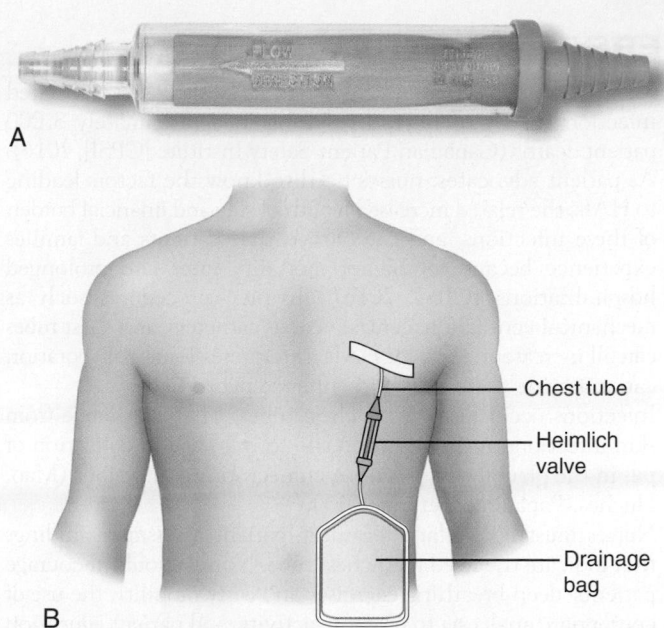

FIG 27.5 A, The Heimlich chest drain valve is a specially designed flutter valve that is used in place of a chest drainage unit for a small uncomplicated pneumothorax with little or no drainage and no need for suction. The valve allows for escape of air but prevents re-entry of air into the pleural space. **B,** Placement of valve between chest tube and drainage bag, which can be worn under clothing. (**A,** *Image courtesy Becton, Dickenson and Company, Franklin Lakes, New Jersey. All rights reserved.*)

around the heart. A mediastinal tube is commonly used after open-heart surgery.

- In emergent situations, a small pneumothorax catheter is inserted through the chest wall, and a rubber flutter one-way valve (e.g., a Heimlich valve) is attached to the catheter (Fig. 27.5, A–B). As a patient exhales, the positive pressure generated by the air leaving the chest enters the tubing, causing the valve to open so air is released. During inspiration the tube collapses on itself, preventing air from re-entering the chest. This type of valve is not used when patients need fluid drained, such as from a hemothorax or a pleural effusion (Lewis et al., 2019).

- Smaller "pigtail catheters" are also used and are less traumatic than the large-bore tubes. Ambulatory management with pigtail catheters is reasonable first-line treatment for spontaneous pneumothoraxes (Lewis et al., 2019).

- Mobile chest drains are devices that are lighter and self-contained; they allow patients to move with less restriction and cause less discomfort. These mobile systems rely on gravity or dry suction for drainage. They are ideal for home use for patients with persistent drainage or air leaks requiring prolonged use of a chest tube (Royer, Smith, Miller, et al., 2015).

- The disposable systems, such as an Atrium or Pleur-Evac chest drainage system, are one-piece moulded plastic units that provide for a single- or multiple-chamber closed drainage system (Fig. 27.6). A single-chamber system allows air from a pneumothorax to bubble out of the water seal and escape through the air outlet while preventing it from re-entering the intrapleural space. The drawback of a single-chamber system is that any chest drainage present collects in the same chamber that provides the water seal. If the single-chamber system fills with chest fluid, the water-seal level would rise, making it more difficult for the patient to expel any air. Thus, single-chamber systems are not recommended for the evacuation of fluid. An increased height of fluid in the water seal increases the resistance to drainage on expiration and eventually stops the drainage entirely.

- A two- or three-chamber system drains both a hemothorax and a pneumothorax effectively. The two-chamber system permits liquid to flow into the collection chamber, and air flows into

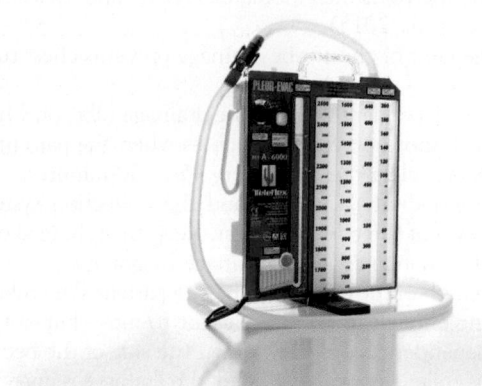

FIG 27.6 Disposable chest drainage systems. (*Multi-chamber Pleur-Evac image courtesy Teleflex Medical, Research Triangle Park, NC.*)

the water-seal chamber. A three-chamber system promotes the drainage of fluid and air with controlled suction. In both systems, the first chamber provides a compartment for fluid or blood drainage and a second compartment for either a water seal or a one-way valve. In the three-chamber system the third compartment is for suction control, which may or may not be used. The disposable units appear to be the system of choice because they are cost-effective and some facilitate autotransfusion; they are occasionally used in open-heart surgeries.

PERSON-CENTRED CARE

- More than 220,000 Canadians acquire a health care–associated infection (HAI) each year, resulting in approximately 8,000 patient deaths (Canadian Patient Safety Institute [CPSI], 2016). As patient advocates, nurses need to know the factors leading to HAIs, the related increased length of stay and financial burden of these infections, and the burden that patients and families experience because of higher mortality rates and prolonged hospitalizations (CPSI, 2016). Invasive procedures such as mechanical ventilation, central venous catheters, and chest tubes can all increase the risk for HAIs. Interprofessional collaboration can minimize these risks and enhance patient safety.
- Infections occur rarely with chest tubes. They can range from skin infections at the insertion site to *empyema* (a collection of pus in the pleural cavity) and even necrotizing infections (Mao, Hughes, Papadimos, et al., 2015).
- Nurses must be vigilant regarding patient assessment findings that indicate the need for a chest tube. Nurses should encourage patients' deep-breathing exercises and early mobility, the use of appropriate analgesia to promote activity, and patient education regarding these practices (Lewis et al., 2019).

EVIDENCE-INFORMED PRACTICE

- Small chest tubes often become blocked by blood clots and fibrin. Large-bore catheters (such as 28F) safely remove secretions (Zardo, Busk, & Kutschka, 2015).
- Milking and stripping a chest tube to clear the clots are controversial practices and when done on a routine basis can do more harm than good (Makic, Rauen, Jones, et al., 2015). Stripping causes a dangerous increase in intrathoracic pressure, which damages the lung tissue (Lewis, 2019; Wiegand, 2017). Chest drainage stripping or milking demonstrates no safety or efficacy benefits, slightly increases intrathoracic pressure, and risks tissue damage (Makic et al., 2015).
- Careful management of chest tube drainage prevents chest tube occlusion:
  - Avoid having dependent loops of the drainage tube; or, when these loops cannot be avoided (such as when the patient is sitting), lift and clear the tube every 15 to 30 minutes.
  - Keep the chest drainage tubing and the collection system below the level of the patient's chest. Keep the tubing above the collection system to allow drainage by gravity.
  - Tailor the length of the drainage tube to a patient. The tubing must be long enough to allow a patient to move but not so long that dependent loops hang down the side of the bed. If the tubing is coiled, looped, or clotted, the drainage is impeded and can result in a tension pneumothorax (Lewis et al., 2019).

SAFETY GUIDELINES

- Document patient's baseline vital signs, oxygen saturation, lung sounds, and respiratory status. Changes in vital signs or respiratory status often indicate a malfunction of a chest drainage system.
- Observe the water seal for intermittent bubbling or a rise and fall of fluid that is synchronous with respirations (Lewis et al., 2019). For example, in a spontaneously breathing patient the fluid level rises during inspiration and falls during expiration. When a patient is on a mechanical ventilator, the opposite occurs.
  - Constant bubbling in the water seal or a sudden, unexpected stoppage of water-seal activity is considered abnormal and requires immediate attention (Wiegand, 2017).

- Unexpected stoppage of chest tube activity may indicate a blockage or lung re-expansion. In these situations, immediate attention and correction are indicated. After 2 or 3 days, tidalling or bubbling on expiration is expected to stop, indicating that the lung has re-expanded (Wiegand, 2017).
- In a waterless system look for a rise and fall of fluid in the diagnostic air-leak indicator synchronous with respirations. Constant left-to-right bubbling (when facing the indicator) or violent rocking is considered abnormal and indicates an air leak.
- Note the expected amount of chest tube drainage and monitor drainage on a regular basis (e.g., every hour initially and then every 4 hours). At the end of the shift, make a mark to indicate the fluid level with the date and time on the side of the drainage collection chamber. Note the drainage amount as output.
  - A sudden decrease in the amount of chest tube drainage can indicate a possible clot or obstruction in the chest tube (Wiegand, 2017).
  - Notify a health care provider when there is a sudden increase of more than 250 mL of drainage over 1 hour, which can indicate fresh bleeding from the thorax (Mao et al., 2015).
  - Drainage from a pneumothorax is generally limited. Any fluid buildup is caused by chest tube insertion trauma. The chest tubes promote the removal of air from the intrapleural space.
- Know the expected colour of the drainage. Drainage from recent open-chest surgery initially is bright red and gradually becomes serous as the postoperative course continues. Blood-tinged fluid usually indicates malignancy, pulmonary infarction, or severe inflammation. Frank blood indicates a hemothorax. Pus indicates an empyema (Lewis et al., 2019).
- In the water-seal system observe for constant, gentle bubbling in the suction-control chamber when it is connected to suction. In the waterless system, a designated amount of suction is maintained by setting the suction source and dialling the prescribed suction level in the float ball column.
- Assess both types of systems for air leaks. If an air leak exists, determine whether it is in the patient (patient-centred air leak) or the chest tube system (system-centred air leak). To rule out an air leak as patient centred, assess the patient's respiratory status. Document and report any changes in lung sounds, pulse oximetry, respiratory rate, or mentation. Remember that continuous bubbling in the water-seal chamber with an absence of bubbles in the suction-control chamber indicates that there is a leak in the system (Wiegand, 2017). Ensure that all tubing connections are tight.
- Be sure that the drainage system is stable. Most chest drainage units have attached adjustable hangers that allow the device to hang on the side or end of the patient's bed. Many have a swing-out floor stand to reduce the chance of accidentally knocking over the chest drainage system if it is placed on the floor. Some manufacturers make a reusable drain caddy that allows the chest drainage system to be connected to an IV pole to facilitate patient movement and eliminate a chance of knocking over the system.
- Do not attempt to empty a chest tube drainage system.
- Chest tube drainage systems are replaced only when the collection chamber is full or if the system is contaminated.
- Never clamp a chest tube without a health care provider's prescription.
- Only clamp a chest tube if (1) changing the drainage system, (2) assessing for an air leak, (3) the chest tube becomes disconnected from the chest drainage system (short time only), or (4) removing chest tube.

✦ SKILL 27.1   Managing Closed Chest Drainage Systems

NSO Nursing Skills Online Closed Chest Drainage Systems Module 11 / Lessons 2 and 3

There are two types of commercial drainage systems: the water-seal and the waterless systems (Table 27.1). This procedure involves interprofessional collaboration, although the insertion of the chest tube is only performed by the health care provider. This skill reviews the nursing responsibilities and interventions related to safe management of chest tubes. Review the actions, roles, and responsibilities of the health care provider for chest tube placement (Table 27.2).

Water-Seal Systems

NSO Nursing Skills Online Closed Chest Drainage Systems Module 11 / Lessons 1 and 2

Two-Chamber Water-Seal System

On expiration, fluid or air is forced out of the intrapleural space. Suction pulls air or fluid through the chest tube into the drainage collection chamber. On entering the drainage collection chamber, this fluid or air displaces the air present in the chamber by pushing it through the water seal and out of the system into the atmosphere. The water-seal chamber is left open to air to drain. If the tubing is clamped, there is no mechanism for air to vent. To maintain the water-seal system, the chest tube system must remain upright. When it is tipped or overturned, the water seal is disrupted.

Three-Chamber Water-Seal System

If suction is used, the three-chamber water-seal system (Fig. 27.7) is set up with the suction-control chamber added. A prescribed amount of sterile fluid (e.g., 20 cm of water) is poured into the suction-control chamber, which is then attached to a suction source by tubing. The amount of sterile water added depends on manufacturer recommendations. The chamber is filled to the set volume for the prescribed amount of suction. It is the height of the water in the suction-control chamber that determines the amount of suction. Sterile water is added several times a day because of evaporation. As the fluid level decreases, the amount of suction also declines.

If the suction source delivers more negative pressure than the suction-control chamber water level allows, the extra air pulled into the chamber causes vigorous bubbling. If this occurs, lower the suction source setting to reduce noise and evaporation of the fluid. The absence of bubbling indicates that no suction is being

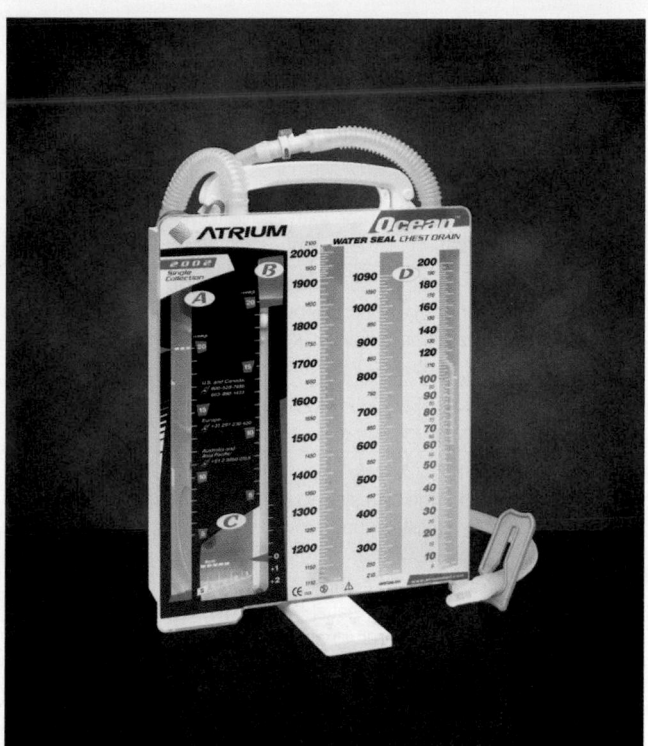

FIG 27.7 Disposable water-seal chest drainage system with suction. (*Used with permission, Atrium Medical Corp.*)

TABLE 27.1

Comparison of Chest Tube Drainage Systems

Drainage System Type	Function	Advantage	Disadvantage
Water-seal system (see Fig. 27.7)	Two-chamber system provides one-way valve for chest drainage. Water seal prevents re-entry of air into lung. Three-chamber system adds a chamber to aid evacuation of chest drainage.	Easy setup and use Cost effective	System must be kept upright to maintain seal Drainage chamber may fill up quickly if patient has large amount of drainage. Sterile water must be added several times a day to maintain suction and water seal because of evaporation.
Waterless system (see Fig. 27.8)	Also provides three chambers, but no water is required to establish a seal.	Seal is maintained by a one-way valve Accidental tipping of system does not compromise patient's condition More space provided for drainage	Water must be added to an air-leak indicator if patient requires evaluation of an air leak.
Dry suction system (see Fig. 27.9)	Also provides three chambers, but suction is controlled by an integrated valve.	Easy setup Quiet operation Can be used when higher levels of suction are required	Sterile water must be added to system to provide a water seal.

TABLE 27.2

Process for Insertion of Chest Tubes

Action	Purpose and Roles
Explain purpose, procedure, and possible complications to patient and ensure patient has signed the consent form.	The health care provider provides information and obtains informed consent.
Have pain medication available to administer before or immediately after chest tube insertion as appropriate according to patient's condition.	The nurse obtains the medication prescription prior to the procedure. Analgesia improves patient comfort throughout procedure and helps patient take appropriate deep breaths to promote lung expansion and drainage of fluid in pleural space.
Unless an emergent situation exists, perform "time-out" before initiating procedure (see Chapter 38).	This interprofessional collaborative protocol is performed immediately prior to a planned procedure as a universal patient safety initiative. During this procedure, the team confirms patient identity, surgical site, and planned procedure.
Perform hand hygiene. Clean chest wall with antiseptic.	All team members ensure aseptic technique is performed. Reduces transmission of microorganisms.
Apply mask and gloves.	All team members don appropriate personal protective equipment (PPE). Maintains surgical asepsis.
Drape area of chest tube insertion with sterile towels. Health care provider injects local anaesthetic and allows time for it to take effect.	Health care provider maintains surgical asepsis. Decreases pain during procedure.
Health care provider makes a small incision over the rib space where tube is to be inserted. Health care provider threads a clamped chest tube through the incision. Health care provider clamps chest tube until system is connected to water seal.	Inserts chest tube into intrapleural space. Clamping prevents entry of atmospheric air into chest and worsening of pneumothorax.
Health care provider sutures chest tube in place if suturing is policy or health care provider preference.	Secures chest tube in place.
Nurse covers chest tube insertion site with sterile 10 × 10–cm (4 × 4–inch) gauze and large dressing to form an occlusive dressing. Sterile petrolatum gauze is used around the tube.	Holds chest tube in place and occludes site around it. Helps stabilize chest tube and holds dressing tightly in place. Sterile petrolatum gauze helps prevent air leak.
Water-Seal System	
Remove connector cover from patient's end of chest drainage tubing with sterile technique. Secure drainage tubing to chest tube and drainage system.	Health care provider is responsible for making certain that system is set up properly, proper amount of water is in the water seal, dressing is secure, and chest tube is connected to drainage system securely.
Water-Seal Suction	
Connect system to suction or supervise a nurse connecting it to suction if suction is to be used.	Health care provider is responsible for determining and checking amount of fluid that is to be added to suction-control chamber and prescribing suction setting.
Waterless System	
Remove connector cover from patient's end of chest drainage tubing with sterile technique. Secure drainage tubing to chest tube and drainage system.	Health care provider is responsible for making certain that system is set up properly and chest tube is securely connected to drainage system.
Waterless Suction	
Turn on suction source. Set suction indicator (float ball or bellows) to prescribed setting.	Health care provider is responsible for prescribing suction level.
Health care provider or nurse adds sterile water or normal saline to diagnostic indicator on waterless system.	Allows quick assurance that system is functioning properly. Connects chest tube to drainage.
Health care provider or nurse unclamps chest tube.	Verifies correct chest tube placement.
Health care provider prescribes and assesses chest radiographic studies.	

exerted into the system. Raise the suction setting to restore gentle bubbling.

The middle chamber is the water seal. The water seal allows air to exit from the pleural space on exhalation and prevents it from entering the pleural cavity or mediastinum on inhalation. When the appropriate amount of sterile water is added, a 2-cm water seal is established. To maintain effective water seal, the chest drainage unit must remain upright; also, monitor the water level in the water-seal chamber to check for evaporation. Bubbling in the water-seal chamber indicates an air leak.

Waterless Systems

Two-Chamber Waterless System

The principles of the waterless system are similar to those of the water-seal system except that fluid is not required for setup. Because water is not used, accidentally tipping the system does not compromise the patient's condition.

The water seal is replaced by a one-way valve (Fig. 27.8) located near the top of the system. Most of the container serves as the drainage chamber. The suction chamber does not depend on water. Instead, it contains a float ball, which is set by a suction-control dial after the suction source is turned on. A diagnostic air-leak indicator is located on the face of the unit. It requires the addition of 15 mL of fluid for visualization. The function of the indicator is to identify one of the following:

1. The lung is expanding normally. This is indicated by a gentle tidalling of the fluid in the diagnostic indicator.
2. The lung is probably re-expanded if after 2 or 3 days the tidalling has stopped.
3. There is an air leak in the system if, when facing the system, the observer sees the fluid bubbling left to right. Locate and correct the source of the air leak.

Three-Chamber Waterless System

When suction is prescribed, attach the suction chamber port to the suction source by tubing, turn the suction on, and set the suction indicator (float ball or bellows) to the prescribed setting. If the suction indicator does not move to the prescribed level, increase the suction source setting until it does. The system is now functioning with suction.

There are usually two suction settings: one at either the suction-control chamber or the indicator setting and the other at the suction source. The settings are safety factors to reduce the

possibility that the intrapleural tissues receive too much suction, causing injury.

Dry Suction System

Dry suction-control systems provide many advantages (Fig. 27.9), including higher suction pressure levels if needed, easy setup, no

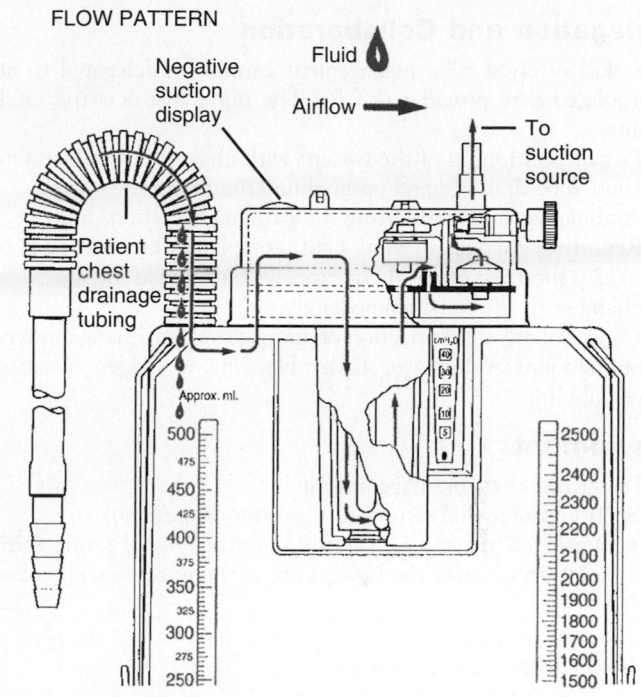

FIG 27.8 Disposable waterless chest drainage system with suction.

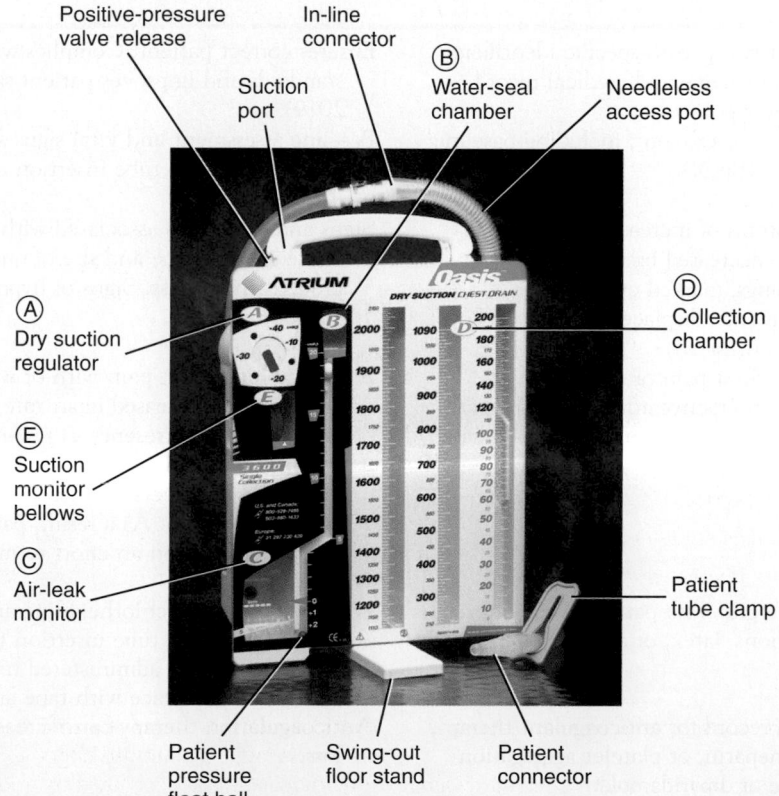

FIG 27.9 Dry suction chest drainage system. (*Used with permission, Atrium Medical Corp.*)

water in the suction-control chamber, and the absence of continuous bubbling, which provides for quiet operation. A self-compensating regulator controls the dry suction unit. A dial is set to the prescribed suction-control setting. These units are preset to −20 cm of water pressure, but they are adjustable from −10 to −40 cm. However, the dry suction-control systems require or have presealed sterile water to use in the water-seal chamber (Atrium, 2015a).

Delegation and Collaboration

The skill of chest tube management cannot be delegated to an unregulated care provider (UCP). The nurse instructs the UCP about:

- Proper positioning of the patient with chest tubes to facilitate chest tube drainage and optimal functioning of the system.
- Ambulating and transferring the patient with chest drainage.
- Reporting changes in vital signs, complaints of chest pain or sudden shortness of breath, or excessive bubbling in the water-seal chamber to the nurse immediately.
- Danger of any disconnection of drainage system, change in type and amount of drainage, sudden bleeding, or sudden cessation of bubbling.

Equipment

- Prescribed chest drainage system
- Suction source and setup (wall canister or portable)
  - *Water-seal system:* Add sterile water or normal saline (NS) solution to cover the lower 2 cm of the water-seal chamber.

Pour sterile water or NS into the suction-control chamber if suction is to be used (see manufacturer's directions)
- *Waterless system:* Add vial of 30- to 45-mL sterile sodium chloride or water (for diagnostic air-leak indicator), 20-mL syringe, 21-gauge needle, and antiseptic swab
- Dry suction system
- Clean gloves
- Sterile gauze sponges
- Local anaesthetic, if not an emergent procedure
- Chest tube tray (all items are sterile): knife handle (1), knife blade No. 10 or disposable safety scalpel No. 10, chest tube clamp, small sponge forceps, needle holder, size 3-0 silk sutures, tray liner (sterile field), curved 8-inch Kelly clamps (2), 10 × 10–cm (4 × 4–inch) sponges (10), suture scissors, hand towels (3), sterile gloves
- Dressings: Petrolatum or Xeroform gauze, split chest-tube dressings, several 10 × 10–cm (4 × 4–inch) gauze dressings, large gauze dressings (2), and 10-cm (4-inch) tape
- Head cover
- Face mask/face shield
- Sterile gloves
- Two rubber-tipped hemostats (shodded) for each chest tube
- 2.5-cm (1-inch) waterproof adhesive tape or plastic zip ties for securing connections
- Stethoscope, sphygmomanometer, and pulse oximeter

STEP	RATIONALE
ASSESSMENT	
1. Identify patient using at least two person-specific identifiers (e.g., name and date of birth or name and medical record number) according to employer policy.	Ensures correct patient. Complies with Accreditation Canada's standards and improves patient safety (Accreditation Canada, 2019).
2. Perform a complete respiratory assessment, including baseline vital signs and pulse oximetry (SpO_2).	Baseline assessment and vital signs are essential for any invasive procedure. Chest tube insertion often causes respiratory distress.
a. Assess for signs and symptoms of increased respiratory distress and hypoxia (e.g., decreased breath sounds over affected and unaffected lungs, marked cyanosis, asymmetrical chest movements, displaced trachea, shortness of breath, and confusion).	Signs and symptoms associated with respiratory distress are related to the type and size of pneumothorax, hemothorax, or pre-existing illness. Signs of hypoxia are related to inadequate oxygen to tissues.
b. Assess for sharp, stabbing chest pain or chest pain on inspiration, hypotension, and tachycardia. If possible, ask patient to rate level of comfort, using an appropriate pain rating scale.	Sharp stabbing chest pain with or without decreased blood pressure and increased heart rate may indicate tension pneumothorax. Presence of pneumothorax or hemothorax is painful, frequently causing sharp inspiratory pain. In addition, discomfort is associated with presence of a chest tube, not just with its insertion. As a result, patients tend to not cough or change position in an effort to minimize this pain (Wiegand, 2017).
3. Assess patient for known allergies. Ask patient if they have had a problem with medications, latex, or anything applied to the skin.	Povidone-iodine or chlorhexidine are antiseptic solutions used to clean skin before tube insertion (Porcel, 2018). Lidocaine is a local anaesthetic administered to reduce pain. The chest tube will be held in place with tape and sutures.
4. Review patient's medication record for anticoagulant therapy, including aspirin, warfarin, heparin, or platelet aggregation inhibitors such as ticlopidine or dipyridamole.	Anticoagulation therapy can increase procedure-related blood loss.
5. Review patient's hemoglobin and hematocrit levels.	Parameters reflect whether blood loss is occurring, which may affect oxygenation.

STEP	RATIONALE

ASSESSMENT

6. For patients who have chest tubes, observe:

    a. Chest tube dressing and site surrounding tube insertion.

Ensures that dressing is intact and occlusive seal remains without air or fluid leaks and that area surrounding insertion site is free of drainage or skin irritation.

    b. Tubing for kinks, dependent loops, or clots.

Maintains a patent, freely draining system, preventing fluid accumulation in chest cavity. When tubing is coiled, looped, or clotted, drainage is impeded, and there is an increased risk for tension pneumothorax or surgical emphysema (Lewis et al., 2019; Wiegand, 2017).

    c. Chest drainage system should remain upright and below level of tube insertion.

An upright drainage system facilitates drainage and maintains the water seal. To facilitate drainage and prevent backflow that would increase the risk for infection, the chest tube drainage system must be lower than the chest.

7. Determine patient's knowledge of procedure.

Encourages cooperation, minimizes risks and anxiety. Identifies teaching needs.

NURSING DIAGNOSES

- Reduced gas exchange
- Acute pain
- Anxiety
- Potential for infection

Related factors/Risk factors are individualized on the basis of patient's condition or needs.

PLANNING

1. Expected outcomes following completion of procedure:

- Patient is oriented and less anxious.

Hypoxia is relieved.

- Vital signs are stable.

Decreased hypoxia improves vital sign measures.

- Patient reports no chest pain.

Re-expansion of lung reduces chest pain.

- Breath sounds are auscultated in all lobes. Lung expansion is symmetrical, SpO$_2$ is stable or improved, and respirations are unlaboured.

Re-expansion of lung promotes normal respirations.

- Chest tube remains in place, and chest drainage system remains airtight.

Indicates correct placement and patency of chest tube drainage system.

- Gentle tidalling (fluctuations or rocking) is evident in water-seal or diagnostic indicator.

Indicates that system is functioning normally. Reflects changes in intrapleural pressure.

IMPLEMENTATION

1. Check employer policy and determine whether informed consent is needed. Complete "time-out" procedure.

Invasive medical procedures typically require informed consent. "Time-out" is completed to determine right patient, procedure, and location of insertion or incision site (Mayer, Sevdalis, Rout, et al., 2016).

2. Review health care provider's prescription for chest tube placement.

Insertion of chest tube requires health care provider prescription.

3. Perform hand hygiene.

4. Set up water-seal system (or dry system with suction); see manufacturer's guidelines.

    a. Obtain chest drainage system. Remove wrappers and prepare to set up two- or three-chamber system.

Maintains sterility of system for use under sterile operating room conditions.

    b. While maintaining sterility of drainage tubing, stand system upright and add sterile water or NS to appropriate compartments.

Reduces possibility of contamination.

        (1) *Two-chamber system (without suction):* Add sterile solution to water-seal chamber (second chamber), bringing fluid to required level as indicated.

Water-seal chamber acts as one-way valve so air cannot enter pleural space (Wiegand, 2017).

STEP	RATIONALE

IMPLEMENTATION

(2) *Three-chamber system (with suction):* Add sterile solution to water-seal chamber (second chamber). Add amount of sterile solution prescribed by health care provider to suction-control chamber (third chamber), usually 20 cm water pressure. Connect tubing from suction-control chamber to suction source. Tailor length of drainage tube to patient. **NOTE:** Suction-control chamber vent must not be occluded when using suction (see illustration).

Depth of fluid level dictates highest amount of negative pressure that can be present within system. For example, 20 cm of water is approximately 20 cm of water pressure. Any additional negative pressure applied to the system is vented into the atmosphere through the suction-control vent. This safety device prevents damage to pleural tissues from an unexpected surge of negative pressure from the suction source.

After chest tube is inserted, turn up the wall or portable suction device until water in suction-control bottle exhibits continuous, gentle bubbling.

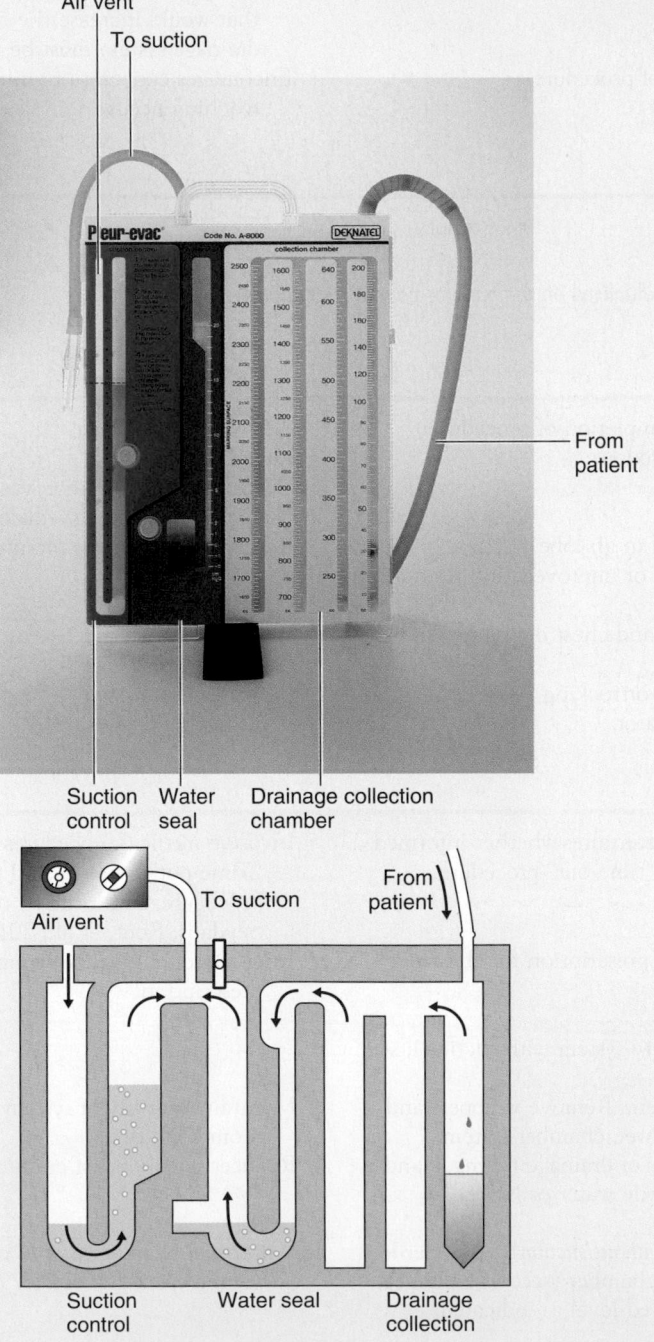

STEP 4b(2) Top, Pleur-Evac drainage system, a commercial three-chamber chest drainage device. **Bottom,** Schematic of drainage device.

STEP	RATIONALE

IMPLEMENTATION

Clinical Decision Point *When increasing suction, remember that increased bubbling does not result in more suction to the chest cavity, but only serves to evaporate the water more quickly.*

STEP	RATIONALE
(3) *Dry suction system:* Fill water-seal chamber with sterile solution. Adjust suction-control dial to prescribed level of suction; suction ranges from −10 to −40 cm of water pressure. Suction-control chamber vent is never occluded when suction is used. **NOTE:** On dry suction system, *DO NOT* obstruct positive-pressure relief valve. This allows air to escape.	Automatic control valve on dry suction-control device adjusts to changes in patient air leaks and fluctuation in suction source and vacuum to deliver prescribed amount of suction.
5. Set up waterless system (see manufacturer's guidelines).	
a. Remove sterile wrappers and prepare to set up.	Maintains sterility of system for use under sterile operating room conditions.
b. For two-chamber system (without suction), nothing is added or needs to be done to the system.	Waterless two-chamber system is ready for connecting to patient's chest tube after opening wrappers.
c. For three-chamber system (with suction), connect tubing from suction-control chamber to suction source.	Suction source provides additional negative pressure to system.
d. Instill 15 mL of sterile water or NS into diagnostic indicator injection port located on top of system.	Allows observation of rise and fall of water in diagnostic air leak window. Constant left-to-right bubbling or rocking is abnormal and indicates air leak. This is not necessary for mediastinal drainage because there is no tidalling. In an emergency, the system *does not* require water for setup.
6. Secure all tubing connections with tape in double-spiral fashion using 2.5-cm (1-inch) adhesive tape or zip ties (nylon cable) with a clamp (Wiegand, 2017). Check system for patency by:	Prevents atmospheric air from leaking into system and patient's intrapleural space. Provides chance to ensure airtight system before connection to patient.
a. Clamping drainage tubing that will connect to patient's chest tube.	
b. Connecting tubing from float ball chamber to suction source.	
c. Turning on suction to prescribed level.	
7. Turn off suction source and unclamp drainage tubing before connecting patient to system. Suction source is turned on again after patient is connected.	Having patient connected to suction when it is initiated could damage pleural tissues from a sudden increase in negative pressure. Tubing that is coiled or looped may become clotted and cause tension pneumothorax (Wiegand, 2017).
8. Administer premedication such as sedatives or analgesics as prescribed.	Reduces patient anxiety and pain during procedure.

Clinical Decision Point *During procedure, carefully monitor patient for changes in level of sedation.*

STEP	RATIONALE
9. Provide psychological support to patient.	
a. Reinforce preprocedure explanation.	Reduces patient anxiety and helps complete procedure efficiently.
b. Coach and support patient throughout procedure.	
10. Perform hand hygiene and apply clean gloves. Position patient in a supine position with the ipsilateral arm abducted, elbow flexed, and hand positioned above the head.	Reduces transmission of microorganisms. This position enhances accessibility to the insertion site (Wiegand, 2017).
11. Assist health care provider with chest tube insertion by providing needed equipment and local analgesic. Health care provider anaesthetizes skin over insertion site, makes small skin incision, inserts clamped tube, sutures it in place, and applies occlusive dressing.	Ensures smooth insertion.
12. Help health care provider attach drainage tube to chest tube; remove clamp. Turn on suction to prescribed level.	Connects drainage system and suction (if prescribed) to chest tube.

STEP	RATIONALE

IMPLEMENTATION

13. Tape or zip-tie all connections between chest tube and drainage tube. (**NOTE:** Chest tube is usually taped by health care provider at time of tube placement; check employer policy).	Secures chest tube to drainage system and reduces risk for air leak that causes breaks in airtight system (Wiegand, 2017).
14. Check systems for proper functioning. Health care provider prescribes chest radiography.	Verifies intrapleural placement of tube.
15. After tube placement, position patient: **a.** Use semi-Fowler's or high-Fowler's position to evacuate air (pneumothorax) (Wiegand, 2017). **b.** Use high-Fowler's position to drain fluid (hemothorax) (Wiegand, 2017).	Permits optimum drainage of fluid and/or air.
16. Check patency of air vents in system. **a.** Water-seal vent must have no occlusion. **b.** Suction-control chamber vent is not occluded when suction is used. **c.** Waterless systems have relief valves without caps.	Permits displaced air to pass into atmosphere. Provides safety factor of releasing excess negative pressure into atmosphere. Provides safety factor of releasing excess negative pressure.
17. Position excess tubing horizontally on mattress next to patient. Secure with clamp provided so it does not obstruct tubing.	Prevents excess tubing from hanging over edge of mattress in dependent loop. Drainage collected in loop can occlude drainage system, which predisposes patient to tension pneumothorax (Lewis et al., 2019).
18. Adjust tubing to hang in straight line from chest tube to drainage chamber.	Promotes drainage and prevents fluid or blood from accumulating in pleural cavity.
19. Place two rubber-tipped hemostats (for each chest tube) in easily accessible position (e.g., taped to top of patient's headboard). These should remain with patient when ambulating.	Chest tubes are double clamped under specific circumstances: (1) to assess for air leak (Table 27.3), (2) to empty or quickly change disposable systems, or (3) to assess if patient is ready to have tube removed.

Clinical Decision Point *In the event of a chest tube disconnection and risk of contamination, immediately re-establish the water-seal system and attach a new drainage system as soon as possible. Depending on employer policy, consider submerging the tube 2.5 to 5 cm (1 to 2 inches) below the surface of a 250-mL bottle of sterile water or NS until a new chest tube unit can be set up (Lewis et al., 2019).*

TABLE 27.3

Problem Solving With Chest Tubes

Assessment	Intervention
Air leak can occur at insertion site, at connection between tube and drainage device, or within drainage device itself. Determine when air leak occurs during respiratory cycle (e.g., inspiration or expiration). Continuous bubbling is noted in water-seal chamber that is attached to suction (Wiegand, 2017).	Check all connections between chest tube and drainage system to make sure they are tight. When in doubt, remove tape without disconnecting the tube to inspect connections. Inspect the chest drainage unit for cracks or breaks that can allow air into the system. Leaks are corrected when constant bubbling stops.
Assess for location of leak by squeezing the chest drainage tubing between your hands. If the bubbling stops, the air leak is inside patient's thorax or at chest insertion site.	Release the pressure on the drainage tube, reinforce chest dressing, and notify the health care provider immediately. Leaving the chest tube clamped can cause collapse of the lung, mediastinal shift, and eventual collapse of the other lung from buildup of air pressure within the pleural cavity.
If bubbling still continues, it indicates that the leak is in the drainage system.	Change the drainage system. Notify the health care provider, as a chest radiography may be required.
Assess for tension pneumothorax: • Severe respiratory distress • Low oxygen saturation • Chest pain • Absence of breath sounds on affected side • Tracheal shift to unaffected side • Hypotension and signs of shock • Tachycardia	Make sure that chest tubes are patent: Remove clamps, eliminate kinks, or eliminate occlusion. Notify health care provider immediately and prepare for another chest tube insertion. A one-way flutter (Heimlich) valve or large-gauge needle may be used for short-term emergency release of pressure in the intrapleural space. Have emergency equipment, oxygen, and code cart available because condition is life-threatening.
Water-seal tube is no longer submerged in sterile fluid because of evaporation.	Add sterile water to water-seal chamber until distal tip is 2 cm under surface level. Most chest drainage units are marked at the 2 cm level to indicate the fill line.

STEP	RATIONALE

IMPLEMENTATION

20. Dispose of sharps in proper container, dispose of used supplies, and perform hand hygiene.

Reduces transmission of microorganisms.

21. Care of patient after chest tube insertion:

   a. Perform hand hygiene and apply clean gloves. Assess vital signs, oxygen saturation; skin colour; breath sounds; rate, depth, and ease of respirations; and insertion site every 15 minutes for first 2 hours, and then at least every shift (see employer policy).

Provides immediate information about procedure-related complications such as respiratory distress and leakage.

   b. Monitor colour, consistency, and amount of chest tube drainage every 15 minutes for first 2 hours. Indicate level of drainage fluid, date, and time on write-on surface of chamber.

Provides baseline for continuous assessment of type and quantity of drainage. Ensures early detection of complications.

     (1) From mediastinal tube, expect less than 100 mL/hr immediately after surgery and no more than 500 mL in first 24 hours.

Sudden gush of drainage may result from coughing or changing patient's position (i.e., releasing pooled/collected blood rather than indicating active bleeding).

     (2) Report sudden fluctuations or changes in chest tube output (especially a sudden increase from previous drainage) or changes in colour (especially bright red blood, which could indicate hemorrhage) (Wiegand, 2017).

Acute bleeding indicates hemorrhage. Health care provider should be notified if there is more than 100 mL of bloody drainage in an hour, or according to health care provider prescription (Lewis et al., 2019; Wiegand, 2017).

     (3) Expect little or no output from anterior chest tube that is inserted for a pneumothorax.

   c. Observe chest dressing for drainage.

Drainage around tube may indicate blockage.

   d. Apply clean gloves. Palpate around tube for swelling and crepitus (subcutaneous emphysema) as noted by crackling.

Indicates presence of air trapping in subcutaneous tissues. Small amounts are commonly absorbed. Large amounts are potentially dangerous. Most occurrences of crepitus are minor (Mao et al., 2015).

Clinical Decision Point *Some patients may develop subcutaneous emphysema (i.e., a collection of air under the skin after chest tube placement), which can occur if tubing is blocked or kinked. When this occurs, a crepitus (a crackling sensation) is heard on auscultation.*

   e. Check tubing to ensure that it is free of kinks and dependent loops.

Promotes drainage.

   f. Observe for fluctuation of drainage in tubing and water-seal chamber during inspiration and expiration. Observe for clots or debris in tubing.

If fluctuation or tidalling stops, it means that either the lung is fully expanded or the system is obstructed (Wiegand, 2017). In a spontaneously breathing patient, fluid rises in water-seal or diagnostic indicator (waterless system) with inspiration and falls with expiration. The opposite occurs in a patient who is mechanically ventilated. This indicates that the system is functioning properly (Lewis et al., 2019; Wiegand, 2017).

   g. Keep drainage system upright and below level of patient's chest.

Promotes gravity drainage and prevents backflow of fluid and air into pleural space.

   h. Check for air leaks by monitoring bubbling in water-seal chamber: Intermittent bubbling is normal during expiration when air is being evacuated from pleural cavity, but continuous bubbling during both inspiration and expiration indicates leak in system.

Absence of bubbling may indicate that lung is fully expanded in patient with pneumothorax. Check all connections and locate sources of air leak as described in Table 27.3.

   i. Remove gloves and dispose of used soiled equipment in appropriate biohazard container. Perform hand hygiene.

Prevents accidents involving contaminated equipment.

EVALUATION

1. Evaluate patient for decreased respiratory distress and chest pain. Auscultate patient's lungs and observe chest expansion.

Determines status of lung expansion.

2. Monitor vital signs and SpO_2.

Determines if level of oxygenation has improved.

STEP	RATIONALE

EVALUATION

3. Reassess patient's level of comfort using an appropriate pain rating scale, comparing level with comfort before chest tube insertion.

Indicates need for analgesia. Patient with chest tube discomfort hesitates to take deep breaths and as a result is at risk for pneumonia and atelectasis.

4. Evaluate patient's ability to use deep-breathing exercises while maintaining comfort.

Indicates patient's ability to promote lung expansion and prevent complications.

5. Monitor continued functioning of system as indicated by reduction in amount of drainage, resolution of air leak, and complete re-expansion of the lung.

Detects early signs of system complications or indicates possible removal of chest tube.

6. **Use Teach-Back**: "I want to be sure I explained why you have a chest tube. Tell me the reason why you have it." Develop a revised teaching plan if patient or caregiver is not able to teach back correctly.

Determines patient's and caregiver's level of understanding of instructional topic.

Unexpected Outcomes

1. Patient develops respiratory distress. Chest pain, decrease in breath sounds over affected and unaffected lungs, marked cyanosis, asymmetrical chest movements, presence of subcutaneous emphysema around tube insertion site or neck, hypotension, tachycardia, and mediastinal shift are critical and indicate severe change in patient status, such as excessive blood loss or tension pneumothorax.

2. Air leak is unrelated to patient's respirations.

3. There is no chest tube drainage.

4. Chest tube is dislodged.

5. Substantial increase in bright red drainage is observed.

Related Interventions

- Notify health care provider immediately.
- Collect set of vital signs and SpO_2.
- Prepare for chest radiography.
- Provide oxygen as prescribed.

- See Table 27.3 for determining source of an air leak and for problem solving.
- Notify health care provider.
- Observe for kink in chest drainage system.
- Observe for possible clot in chest drainage system.
- Observe for mediastinal shift or respiratory distress (medical emergency).
- Notify health care provider.
- Immediately apply pressure over chest tube insertion site.
- Have assistant obtain sterile petroleum gauze dressing. Apply as patient exhales. Secure dressing with tight seal. Dressing with tape over three of four sides may allow for escape of air if there is residual pneumothorax.
- Notify health care provider.
- Obtain vital signs.
- Monitor drainage.
- Assess patient's cardiopulmonary status.
- Notify health care provider.

Communication and Documentation

- Document respiratory assessment, type of drainage device, amount of suction if used, amount of drainage in chamber, and presence or absence of air leak in nurses' notes in electronic health record (EHR) or chart. Document the integrity of the dressing and colour and type of drainage for comparison between shifts.
- Document patient teaching and validation of understanding on flow sheet or nurses' notes in EHR or chart.
- Document level of patient comfort and baseline vital signs, including oxygen saturation. For a postoperative patient, record vital signs and oxygen saturation every 15 minutes for at least 2 hours after surgery on flow sheet or nurses' notes in EHR or chart.
- Report any unexpected outcomes immediately to the nurse in charge or health care provider.

Special Considerations
Teaching

- Instruct patient and caregiver in proper functioning of chest tube and drainage system.
- Instruct patient to remain in bed if chest tube is attached to suction.
- Instruct patient to not lie on tubing or allow it to get kinked, to promote drainage.
- Instruct patient to immediately report any changes in chest comfort.
- Instruct patient to call immediately for help if the chest tube becomes dislodged.

Pediatric

- If possible, using pictures and special dolls, familiarize child and family with equipment before inserting chest drainage system (Hockenberry & Wilson, 2015).

- Chest tube drainage greater than 3 mL/kg/hr for more than 3 consecutive hours is excessive and may indicate postoperative hemorrhage. Notify the health care provider immediately (Hockenberry & Wilson, 2015).

Gerontological
- Fragility of the older person's skin requires special care and planning for management of chest tube dressing. Frequently assess surrounding skin for signs of skin breakdown.

Care in the Community
- Patients living with chronic conditions (e.g., uncomplicated pneumothorax, effusions, empyema) that require use of a long-term chest tube may be discharged with smaller mobile drains.
- Teach patient how to ambulate and remain active with a mobile chest tube drainage system.

- Instruct patient and caregiver about when to contact the health care provider regarding changes in the drainage system (e.g., chest pain, breathlessness, change in colour or amount of drainage, leakage on dressing around the chest tube).
- Provide patient and caregiver information specific to the type of drain; when possible, have patient demonstrate proper maintenance of the mobile drainage system. Most of these systems do not have a suction-control chamber and use a mechanical one-way valve instead of a water-seal chamber.
- Small-bore chest tubes and Heimlich valves should be used with caution in patients on mechanical ventilators owing to the potential for rapid accumulation of air and a tension pneumothorax (Lewis et al., 2019).

✦ SKILL 27.2   Assisting With Removal of Chest Tubes

NSO *Nursing Skills Online Closed Chest Drainage Systems Module 11/ Lesson 4*

Actual removal of a chest tube is most often the function of a physician or health care provider such as a physician's assistant or nurse practitioner (verify employer policy). Prepare a patient for chest tube removal by assessing the need for preremoval analgesia, obtaining the required medication prescriptions, and instructing the patient about the process and what will be requested of the patient. Instruct the patient to perform a Valsalva manoeuvre at either end inspiration or end expiration. The Valsalva manoeuvre is needed to provide positive pressure in the pleural cavity and prevent the patient from gasping when the tube is removed. If the patient is receiving ventilator support, remove the tube during peak inspiration (Wiegand, 2017). An occlusive dressing is applied immediately after tube removal to maintain a tight seal.

Delegation and Collaboration

The skill of assisting with removal of chest tubes cannot be delegated to an unregulated care provider (UCP). The nurse directs the UCP to:
- Immediately report to the nurse any patient sensations of shortness of breath, increased chest pain, dizziness, or increased anxiety.

- Report to the nurse any drainage on the dressing placed over the chest tube site.

Equipment
- Suture set
- Sterile scissors
- Sterile forceps
- Clean gloves
- Sterile gloves
- Face mask/face shield
- Prepared sterile dressing: petrolatum-impregnated gauze, 10 × 10–cm (4 × 4–inch) gauze dressings, and large dressings
- 10-cm (4-inch) adhesive tape or elastic bandage (Elastoplast) cut into strips
- Stethoscope, sphygmomanometer, pulse oximeter
- Disposable bed pad

STEP	RATIONALE

ASSESSMENT

1. Identify patient using at least two person-specific identifiers (e.g., name and date of birth or name and medical record number) according to employer policy.
2. Perform respiratory assessment and assess for lung re-expansion.
   a. Provide health care provider with results of chest radiography.
   b. Note trend in water-seal fluctuation over last 24 hours. Determine if bubbling is present.

Ensures correct patient. Complies with Accreditation Canada's standards and improves patient safety (Accreditation Canada, 2019).

Reveals position of lung tissue in chest cavity and whether sufficient lung re-expansion has occurred (Wiegand, 2017).
Pleura of expanded lung seals holes on internal tip of chest tube, halting fluctuation in water seal. Halt in fluctuation for 24 hours indicates that the lung is expanded. When bubbling is present, it usually indicates that the lung has not fully expanded (Wiegand, 2017).

STEP	RATIONALE

ASSESSMENT

c. Confirm that drainage has decreased to 50 to 200 mL in the prior 24 hours if the tube was placed for a hemothorax, empyema, or pleural effusion or less than 100 mL in 8 hours after cardiac surgery (Wiegand, 2017).

Pleural drainage was removed, allowing lung to re-expand.

d. Percuss lung for resonance (see Chapter 8).

Normal resonance occurs with re-expansion.

e. Auscultate lung sounds.

Normal breath sounds are heard bilaterally with re-expansion.

3. Assess patient's level of comfort using an appropriate pain rating scale and determine when the last analgesic medication was given.

Chest tube removal is often painful; additional analgesia or breathing exercises are often necessary (Lewis et al., 2019; Wiegand, 2017).

4. Determine patient's understanding of chest tube removal procedure.

Encourages cooperation and minimizes risks and anxiety. Identifies teaching needs.

5. Do not clamp chest tube before removal. Assess for changes in vital signs, oxygen saturation, chest pain, apprehension, and symptoms of tension pneumothorax.

Clamping chest tube before removal to assess patient's tolerance is no longer recommended because there is no benefit to the practice. If a chest tube that was continuing to bubble is clamped, tension pneumothorax may occur Mao et al., 2015; Wiegand, 2017).

NURSING DIAGNOSES

- Acute pain
- Anxiety
- Potential for impaired gas exchange

Related factors/Risk factors are individualized on the basis of patient's condition or needs.

PLANNING

1. Expected outcomes following completion of procedure:
- Lung re-expansion is maintained.
- Patient does not experience discomfort.
- Spontaneous healing of chest tube insertion site occurs after removal of tube without infection or other complications.

Source of air or fluid loss is sealed or has healed.
Pain management is achieved.
Large, nonporous occlusive dressing at puncture site promotes uncomplicated healing.

2. Explain procedure to patient.

Reduces anxiety and promotes patient cooperation.

IMPLEMENTATION

1. Administer prescribed medication for pain relief about 30 minutes before procedure.

Reduces discomfort and relaxes patient. Medication reaches peak effect at time of tube removal. Intravenous 4 mg morphine 20 minutes prior to tube removal, or 30 mg ketorolac 60 minutes before the procedure, produces substantial pain relief without excessive analgesia (Wiegand, 2017).

2. Perform "time-out" procedure with health care provider to verify patient identification, planned procedure, correct tube(s), and that chest tube is visible and patient position is correct.

The "time-out" step is intended to reliably identify patient as the individual for whom the procedure is intended and to match the procedure to the patient (Operating Room Nurses Association of Canada [ORNAC], 2017).

3. Perform hand hygiene and apply clean gloves and face shield if needed.

Reduces transmission of microorganisms.

4. Help patient to sitting position on edge of bed, or lying supine or on side without chest tubes. Place pad under chest tube site.

Health care provider prescribes patient's position to facilitate tube removal. Pad absorbs any drainage associated with tube removal.

5. Health care provider prepares an occlusive dressing of petrolatum-impregnated gauze on pressure dressing, sets it aside on sterile field, and applies sterile gloves.

Essential to prepare in advance for quick application to wound on tube withdrawal.

6. Support patient physically and emotionally while health care provider removes dressing and clips sutures.

Patients state that when they know the tube is being pulled, they can mentally prepare themselves for the procedure. Support from the health care team reduces anxiety and promotes cooperation.

STEP	RATIONALE

IMPLEMENTATION

7. Health care provider asks patient to exhale completely and hold it while bearing down (Valsalva manoeuvre).

Prevents accidental entrance of air into the pleural space (Wiegand, 2017).

8. Health care provider rapidly and smoothly pulls out chest tube and tightens and ties purse-string suture if present, after which patient is instructed to breathe normally.

This forms an airtight seal and prevents entry of air through the chest wound. Sutures decrease the possibility of air from entering the pleural space and aid in skin closure (Wiegand, 2017).

9. Health care provider applies sterile occlusive dressing over wound and firmly secures it in position with wide tape.

Keeps wound aseptic. Prevents entry of air into chest. Wound closure occurs spontaneously.

10. Health care provider inspects end of chest tube(s) before disposal to ensure entire removal.

If a portion of the tube is not fully removed, contact the health care provider immediately, because surgical removal may be required (Wiegand, 2017).

11. Help patient to upright position supported by pillows.

Restores patient's comfort. Patients report that proper positioning following chest tube removal helps to relieve procedure-related sensations of pain and pulling.

12. Remove used equipment from bedside. Dispose of in appropriate receptacle.

Helps prevent spread of microorganisms.

13. Remove gloves and perform hand hygiene.

Reduces transmission of microorganisms.

EVALUATION

1. Auscultate lung sounds.

Helps to confirm that lung remains expanded.

2. Palpate skin over area where tube was inserted for subcutaneous emphysema.

Subcutaneous emphysema results from entrance of air into the subcutaneous space. It is usually minor and resolves independent of interventions. If extensive, subcutaneous emphysema may be painful, preventing full lung expansion. Monitor area and document new or increased subcutaneous emphysema (Wiegand, 2017).

3. Evaluate for signs of respiratory distress immediately after tube removal and during first few hours after removal.

Provides for early notification of health care provider if adverse symptoms occur. Chest tubes may need reinsertion.

Critical Decision Point *If air is heard escaping from the chest tube site, reinforce the occlusive dressing and immediately notify the health care provider.*

4. Evaluate patient's vital signs, oxygen saturation, pulmonary status, and psychological status.

Detects early signs and symptoms of complications.

5. Review chest radiography, if prescribed.

Evidence does not support routine postremoval X-ray films in either adults or pediatric or neonatal patients (Johnson, Rylander, & Beres, 2017). If complications are noted, bedside ultrasound imaging or computed tomography (CT), which is better at identifying the chest cavity, may be prescribed.

6. Ask about patient's level of pain or comfort. Observe for nonverbal cues of pain and assess level of discomfort using an appropriate pain rating scale.

Indicates that wound did not close well. Determines patient's tolerance of procedure.

7. Check chest dressing for drainage and patency. When changing dressing, note wound for signs of healing.

Ensures occlusion and proper healing of chest wound.

Unexpected Outcomes

1. Dyspnea and laboured respirations noted after chest tube removal; potential recurrence of pneumothorax, hemothorax, or effusion.

2. Infection is noted at insertion site.

Related Interventions

- Notify health care provider.
- Obtain vital signs and oxygen saturation.
- Stay with patient.
- Prepare for possible chest tube reinsertion.
- Assess patient's vital signs for elevated temperature, tachypnea, and tachycardia. Assess wound for drainage, odour, erythema, or increased pain.

Communication and Documentation

- Document removal of tube, amount and appearance of drainage in the collection bottle, appearance of wound and dressing, and patient's response and understanding of the procedure on flow sheet or in nurses' notes in electronic health record (EHR) or chart.
- Document vital signs and respiratory assessment on flow sheet or nurses' notes in EHR or chart.
- Report unexpected outcomes to the nurse in charge or health care provider.

Special Considerations
Teaching

- Instruct patient and caregiver to immediately report signs of chest pain, shortness of breath, or sensations of chest discomfort.

Pediatric

- Pediatric patients usually require analgesia (e.g., morphine sulphate 0.1 mg/kg in combination with midazolam) before chest tube removal (Hockenberry & Wilson, 2015).
- EMLA (locally applied lidocaine/prilocaine anaesthetic patch) placed under the occlusive dressing at the chest tube insertion site 1 hour before tube removal reduces pain of the procedure. However, the child may still feel the "pulling" sensation (Hockenberry & Wilson, 2015).

◆ SKILL 27.3   Autotransfusion of Chest Tube Drainage

NSO *Nursing Skills Online Closed Chest Drainage Systems Module 11 / Lesson 5*

In autotransfusion blood lost from trauma, injury, or surgery is infused back into a patient's circulatory system. When reinfusion is linked with chest drainage, it is a relatively risk-free, inexpensive, and easy method of replacing blood. Benefits of autotransfusion include an immediate blood supply, no risk of transfusion reaction, and more oxygen supplied to vital organs (Wiegand, 2017). Patients must also have a patent intravenous (IV) line in place (see Chapter 29). Autotransfusion is contraindicated in patients with coagulation disorders, septicemia, cancer, and renal or hepatic insufficiency (Atrium, 2015a; Wiegand, 2017).

Delegation and Collaboration

The skill of autotransfusion of chest tube drainage cannot be delegated to an unregulated care provider (UCP). The nurse directs the UCP to immediately:

- Inform the nurse of changes in patient's vital signs or pulse oximetry (SpO$_2$) levels.
- Inform the nurse about increased or decreased drainage from chest tube.

Equipment

- Adult/pediatric single-use chest drainage and autotransfusion unit (Fig. 27.10)
- *Optional:* Continuous autotransfusion system (ATS) with a blood-compatible infusion pump (check employer policy)
- Microaggregate blood filter (40-micron filter, see manufacturer's instructions)

- Nonvented blood-compatible IV administration set
- Antiseptic swab
- Infusion pump (see manufacturer instructions)
- Replacement bag
- Personal protective equipment (PPE), as needed

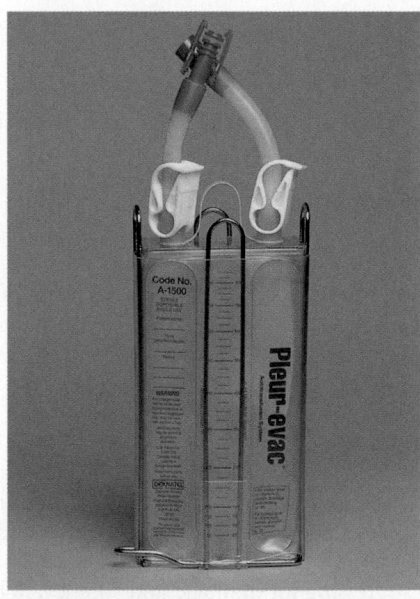

FIG 27.10 Example of autotransfusion unit.

STEP	RATIONALE

ASSESSMENT

1. Identify patient using at least two person-specific identifiers (e.g., name and date of birth or name and medical record number) according to employer policy. Compare identifiers with information on patient's medication administration record (MAR) or medical record.	Ensures correct patient. Complies with Accreditation Canada's standards and improves patient safety (Accreditation Canada, 2019).

STEP	RATIONALE

ASSESSMENT

2. See Assessment for Skill 27.1.
3. Determine presence of active bleeding (at least 50 to 100 mL/hr) through chest tube.

Indicates need for possible reinfusion of chest tube drainage.

Clinical Decision Point *Collected blood never remains in the chest drain or ATS blood bag for more than 6 hours before autotransfusion. Immediate use is preferred (Atrium, 2015a; Wiegand, 2017).*

4. Assess IV site (see Chapter 29); note size of IV catheter. An 18-gauge angiocatheter is preferred.
5. Obtain baseline laboratory data (e.g., hemoglobin and hematocrit).

Determines presence of adequate and patent IV site for administration of blood products.

Provides data to measure effectiveness of reinfusion of chest drainage on patient's circulating blood volume.

NURSING DIAGNOSES

- Reduced cardiac output
- Insufficient peripheral tissue perfusion
- Potential for infection

Related factors/Risk factors are individualized on the basis of patient's condition or needs.

PLANNING

1. Expected outcomes following completion of procedure:
   - Vital signs, hematocrit, and hemoglobin stabilize.

   - Drainage system functions correctly and lung re-expands in 48 to 72 hours.
   - IV line remains patent.

2. Explain procedure to patient.

Reinfusion reduces significant blood loss associated with closed chest drainage.

Negative pressure is re-established in intrapleural space.

Patent IV is necessary for reinfusion of cleansed mediastinal tube drainage.

Reduces anxiety and promotes patient cooperation.

IMPLEMENTATION

1. System setup:
   a. Set up ATS according to technique that maintains sterility of unit and following three steps printed on front of unit.
   b. Make certain that all connections are tight and all clamps are open.
   c. A 200-micron double-sided mesh filter is located in ATS bag to filter drainage.
   d. ATS collection bag has capacity of 1000 mL marked in increments of 25 mL and an area for marking times and amounts.

Contamination of unit provides ready source of infection to patient.

Tight connections ensure airtight system and open clamps allow chest drainage to enter ATS bag.

Filtering drainage removes extraneous materials and microemboli.

Dark red drainage is expected only during immediate postoperative period. This drainage turns serous over time.

Clinical Decision Point *Continuous ATS may be prescribed following cardiac surgery. This is a closed system with a specific infusion pump and IV circuit. This system requires specific education and is used in selected situations (Atrium, 2015a). Check employer policy.*

2. Perform hand hygiene and apply clean gloves.
3. Prepare chest drainage for reinfusion.
   a. Following manufacturer directions, open replacement bag, and close two white clamps.

   b. Use high-negativity relief valve to reduce excessive negativity.

Reduces transmission of microorganisms.

Contamination of unit provides ready source of contamination to patient. Closed clamps maintain closed system during replacement.

This eases removal of initial collection bag from metal support stand.

STEP	RATIONALE

IMPLEMENTATION

   c. *Bag transfer:*

     (1) Close clamp on chest drainage tubing.

     (2) Close clamps on top of initial ATS collection bag.

     (3) Connect chest drainage tube to new ATS bag.
     (4) Make certain that all connections are tight.
     (5) Open all clamps on chest drainage tube and replacement bag.

   d. Connect connectors on top of initial collection bag and remove bag by lifting it from side hook and then from foot hook.

   e. Secure replacement bag by connecting foot hook, replacing metal frame into side hook of chest drainage unit, and pushing down to secure frame onto hook.

   f. Place thumbs on top of metal frame and push up with fingers to slide bag out; remove replacement bag.

4. Reinfuse chest drainage.

   a. Use new microaggregate filter to reinfuse each autotransfusion bag.

   b. Access bag by inverting it, wiping off port with antiseptic swab, and spiking through port with microaggregate filter and twisting.

   c. With bag upside down, gently squeeze it to remove air and prime filter with blood.

   d. Hang bag on IV pole and continue to prime tubing until all air is gone. Clamp tubing, attach it to patient's IV access, and adjust clamp to deliver reinfusion at appropriate rate.

   e. If prescribed, anticoagulants (anticoagulant citrate dextrose solution-A or citrate phosphate dextrose solution, USP) are added to reinfusion through self-sealing port in autotransfusion connector.

   f. Monitor patient's vital signs and SpO_2 according to patient condition and employer policy. For some patients, this may be as frequently as every 15 minutes; for other patients it may be every hour.

5. Discontinue autotransfusion.

   a. Clamp chest drainage tube only briefly and only if prescribed by a health care provider and connect it directly to chest drainage unit with red and blue connectors.

   b. Open chest drainage tube clamp.

6. Discard used supplies and perform hand hygiene.

Rationale column:

Prevents air from entering chest cavity through tube and collapsing lung.
Maintains closed system for reinfusion, preventing contamination of blood.
Establishes new ATS.
Ensures airtight system.
Re-establishes ATS.

Maintains closed system within bag and removes it for use in autotransfusion.

Provides safe attachment of replacement bag to chest drainage unit.

Prevents infusion of microemboli and provides maximal filtration for each bag.
Connects autotransfusion bag to transfusion tubing.

Gentle pressure is used to prevent hemolysis.

Removes all air from transfusion tubing. Reinfusion is delivered by gravity, application of a blood cuff (not to exceed 150 mm Hg pressure), or blood-compatible IV pump (see Chapter 29).
Prevents clotting in autotransfusion. Reversing heparin with protamine to preoperative levels or collection of nonheparinized blood following emergency chest trauma may require a citrate anticoagulant (Atrium, 2015a).
Patients who require autotransfusion usually have complex physiological needs, and their vital signs change quite rapidly. Consistent, frequent monitoring allows for timely identification of changes and initiation of appropriate interventions to restore physiological stability.

Clamping chest tube for any length of time can cause tension pneumothorax (Lewis et al, 2019; Wiegand, 2017).

All drainage will be collected directly in drainage unit and discarded appropriately.
Reduces transmission of microorganisms.

EVALUATION

1. Monitor vital signs, hematocrit, and hemoglobin.
2. Monitor chest drainage system and patient's lung sounds.

3. Evaluate IV infusion site for infiltration and phlebitis.
4. **Use Teach Back:** "I want to be sure I explained why you needed this procedure. Tell me why this was important." Develop a revised teaching plan if patient or caregiver is not able to teach back correctly.

Rationale column:

Helps determine effects of treatment.
Helps determine proper functioning of system and its effectiveness.
Patent IV infusion site is maintained.
Determines patient's and caregiver's level of understanding of instructional topic.

STEP	RATIONALE

EVALUATION

Unexpected Outcomes

1. Chest tube is dislodged.

2. Patient has dyspnea, chest pain, and laboured respirations.

3. Patient has signs of infection, fever, and chills.

Related Interventions

- Immediately apply pressure over chest tube insertion site.
- Have assistant apply sterile petrolatum-impregnated occlusive dressing.
- Notify health care provider.
- Verify that chest tube is patent and draining.
- Obtain vital signs.
- Notify health care provider.
- Obtain wound cultures as prescribed.
- Obtain vital signs.

Communication and Documentation

- Document drainage and reinfusion with times and amounts of each; include patient's response to reinfusion in nurses' notes in electronic health record (EHR) or chart. Describe condition of IV infusion site.
- Document patient teaching and validation of understanding on flow sheet or in nurses' notes in EHR or chart.

Special Considerations
Teaching

- Prepare patient and caregiver for the procedure so they will understand when the patient's blood is reinfused. Patients and their caregivers may have had this instruction before surgery but need reinforcement.

✦ CLINICAL DEBRIEF

A patient is in the critical care unit following open-heart surgery. He has a right pleural and mediastinal chest tube to drainage. His last vital signs were blood pressure (BP) 110/64 mm Hg; pulse 86 beats/min; respirations on mechanical ventilator 16 breaths/min; SpO$_2$ 96%; temperature 37.2°C (99°F) axillary. The last hourly chest tube drainage was 75 mL from the pleural tube and 100 mL from the mediastinal tube.

1. Why is it important to check vital signs, check for air leaks, and note the amount of chest drainage every 15 to 30 minutes for at least 2 hours after the patient returns from surgery?
2. The patient is 12 hours postoperative and is no longer on mechanical ventilation. He is transferred from the bed to a chair. Immediately following this transfer, the nurse notes drainage of 50 mL of dark red fluid. What should the nurse do?
3. Using SBAR, how should the nurse document this episode with the patient's chest drainage as noted in Question 2?

✦ REVIEW QUESTIONS

1. Patients with chest tubes that remove bloody drainage from the chest cavity usually are at risk for respiratory problems. These patients have many care priorities. What are two important priorities related to management of the chest tube system?
   1. Monitoring chest tube drainage
   2. Promoting activity
   3. Promoting airway clearance
   4. Maintaining chest tube patency
   5. Observing dressing

2. The nurse is caring for a patient with a chest tube. Which activities can a nurse delegate to an unregulated care provider (UCP)? (Select all that apply.)
   1. Proper positioning of the patient to facilitate chest tube drainage
   2. Helping to remove a chest tube
   3. How to ambulate and transfer a patient with chest drainage
   4. Reporting any abnormal vital signs, complaints of chest pain or shortness of breath
   5. Reinfusion of chest tube drainage
   6. Reporting any change in the amount of drainage or sudden bleeding

3. Correctly organize the following steps to autoinfuse chest tube drainage.
   1. Hang the bag on an intravenous (IV) pole and continue to prime the tubing until all air is gone.
   2. Access the bag by inverting it and spiking it through the spike port with the microaggregate filter and twisting.
   0. Use a new microaggregate filter to reinfuse each autotransfusion bag.
   4. If prescribed, add anticoagulants to the reinfusion through the self-sealing port in the autotransfusion connector.
   5. With the bag upside down, gently squeeze it to remove the air and prime the filter with blood.
   6. Monitor patient's vital signs and SpO$_2$ according to patient condition and employer policy.

ⓔ *Visit the Evolve site for a complete list of Clinical Debrief and Review Questions answers.*

REFERENCES

Accreditation Canada. (2019). *Required organizational practices handbook—Version 14.* Retrieved from http://www.wrha.mb.ca/quality/files/2019ROPHandbook.pdf

Atrium. (2015a). *A personal guide to managing chest drainage: Dry suction water seal chest drainage.* Hudson, NH: Atrium Medical. Retrieved from http://www.atriummed.com/en/chest_drainage/Documents/Oasis-GreenHandbook-010139.pdf

Atrium. (2015b). *Evidence-based care of patients with chest tubes.* Hudson, NH: Atrium Medical. Retrieved from http://www.atriummed.com/EN/chest_drainage/Documents/NTI2015Evidence-BasedCareofPatientswithChestTubes.pdf

Bhatnagar, R., & Maskell, N. (2015). The modern diagnosis and management of pleural effusions. *British Medical Journal, 351,* h4520. doi:10.1136/bmj.h4520

Canadian Patient Safety Institute (CPSI). (2016). *Healthcare associated infections (HAI).* Retrieved from http://www.patientsafetyinstitute.ca/en/Topic/Pages/Healthcare-Associated-Infections-(HAI).aspx

Hockenberry, M. J., & Wilson, D. (2015). *Nursing care of infants and children* (10th ed.). St. Louis: Mosby.

Johnson, B., Rylander, M., & Beres, A. L. (2017). Do X-rays after chest tube removal change patient management? *Journal of Pediatric Surgery, 52*(5), 813–815. doi:10.1016/j.jpedsurg.2017.01.047

Kane, C., York, N. L., & Minton, L. A. (2013). Chest tubes in the critically ill patient. *Dimensions of Critical Care Nursing, 32*(3), 111–117. doi:10.1097/DCC.0b013e3182864721

Lewis, S. L., Bucher, L., Heitkemper, M. L., et al. (Eds.). (2019). *Medical-surgical nursing in Canada: Assessment and management of clinical problems* (4th ed.). Toronto, ON: Elsevier.

Makic, M. B., Rauen, C., Jones, K., & Fisk, A. C. (2015). Continuing to challenge practice to be evidence based. *Critical Care Nurse, 35*(2), 39–50. doi:10.4037/ccn2015693

Mancini, M., Scalin, T., & Serebrisky, D. (2018). *Hemothorax clinical presentation. Medscape.* Retrieved from https://emedicine.medscape.com/article/204791 6-clinical#b3

Mao, M., Hughes, R., Papadimos, T. J., & Stawicki, S. P. (2015). Complications of chest tubes: A focused clinical synopsis. *Current Opinion in Pulmonary Medicine, 21*(4), 376–386. doi:10.1097/MCP.0000000000000169

Mayer, E. K., Sevdalis, N., Rout, S., et al. (2016). Surgical checklist implementation project: The impact of variable WHO checklist compliance on risk-adjusted clinical outcomes after national implementation: A longitudinal study. *Annals of Surgery, 263*(1), 58–63. doi:10.1097/SLA.0000000000001185

Operating Room Nurses Association of Canada (ORNAC). (2017). *The ORNAC standards, guidelines, and position statements for perioperative registered nurses* (13th ed.). Kingston: Author.

Porcel, J. M. (2018). Chest tube drainage of the pleural space: A concise review for pulmonologists. *Tuberculosis and Respiratory Diseases, 81*(2), 106–115. doi:10.4046/trd.2017.0107

Royer, A. M., Smith, J. S., Miller, A., Spiva, M., Holcombe, J. M., & Headrick, J. R. (2015). Safety of outpatient chest tube management of air leaks after pulmonary resection. *The American Surgeon, 81*(8), 760–763.

Waters, J. (2017). Chest tube placement (assist). In D. Wiegand (Ed.), *AACN procedure manual for critical care* (7th ed.). St. Louis: Elsevier.

Welch, J. L., & Saltarelli, N. (2018). Tension pneumothorax: Lateral needle decompression. *Visual Journal of Emergency Medicine, 10,* 118–119. doi:10.1016/j.visj.2017.11.022

Wiegand, D. (2017). *AACN procedure manual for critical care* (7th ed.). St. Louis: Mosby.

Zardo, P., Busk, H., & Kutschka, I. (2015). Chest tube management: State of the art. *Current Opinion in Anaesthesiology, 28*(1), 45–49. doi:10.1097/ACO.0000000000000150

28 | Emergency Measures for Life Support

Written by **Nelda K. Martin, RN, ANP-BC, CCNS, and Danielle Byrne, RN, MN**

SKILLS AND PROCEDURES

OBJECTIVES

Mastery of content in this chapter will enable the nurse to:
- Discuss indications for basic airway adjunct insertion.
- State indications for cardiopulmonary resuscitation (CPR).
- Identify indications for use of an external defibrillator (automated or manual).
- Discuss the process of code management.

MEDIA RESOURCES

- evolve http://evolve.elsevier.com/Canada/Perry/clinicalskills/
- Review Questions
- Audio Glossary
- Clinical Debrief and Review Questions Answers

PURPOSE

This chapter addresses the basic aspects of cardiopulmonary resuscitation (CPR) skills and concepts of critical thinking applied during a cardiac arrest. Cardiopulmonary arrests are emergency situations that nurses must be prepared to handle at any time. Nurses are expected to follow current resuscitation guidelines in a systematic and organized manner. The goal is to provide resuscitation in a timely manner to restore cardiopulmonary function and avoid poor neurological outcomes. All nurses and nursing students are required to be certified and maintain certification in basic life support (BLS), which includes the use of an automatic external defibrillator (AED).

STANDARDS OF CARE

- American Heart Association (AHA), 2015/2018—*AHA Guidelines for CPR & ECC* (https://eccguidelines.heart.org/index.php/guidelines-highlights/)
- Heart and Stroke Foundation & American Heart Association (HSF & AHA), 2017—*Highlights of the 2015 American Heart Association Guidelines Update for CPR and ECC (Heart and Stroke Foundation of Canada Edition)* (https://www.heartandstroke.ca/-/media/pdf-files/canada/cpr-2017/ecc-highlights-of-2015-guidelines-update-for-cpr-ecclr.ashx)
- National Emergency Nurses Association (NENA), 2016—*Position Statement: Family/Primary Support Unit Presence During Bedside Invasive Procedures and Resuscitation* (http://nena.ca/w/wp-content/uploads/2014/11/FamilyPrimarySupport.pdf)

PRINCIPLES FOR PRACTICE

- In some cardiac arrests the cessation of circulating blood flow is caused by irregular heart rhythms known as *dysrhythmias*. The causes of dysrhythmias may include electrolyte disturbances, acute coronary syndrome, and certain prescribed or recreational medications. Lethal dysrhythmias include ventricular tachycardia (VT) and ventricular fibrillation (VF), which require a medically delivered electrical current for treatment (see Table 28.2).
- Early defibrillation (delivery of electrical current) may quickly return the heart to normal rhythm without further deterioration of a patient's status.
- Before most arrests, signs and symptoms of impending deterioration include tachycardia, hypotension, tachypnea, decreasing oxygen saturation below 90% despite provision of supplemental oxygen, and a decreasing urine output of less than 50 mL in 4 hours. These are reasons for activating a rapid response team (Agency for Healthcare Research and Quality [AHRQ], 2019).
- Know the employer's policy for activating the rapid response team. This can be composed of a critical care nurse, a physician or advanced practice nurse, and respiratory therapist, who are present in many hospitals (Tanguay & Bartel, 2017). This is an excellent example of interprofessional collaboration where a nurse can consult and discuss concerns with other team members for the betterment of patient care.
- Each employer has a specific code or signal to summon immediate assistance in the event of a cardiac and/or respiratory arrest; the arrest situation may be referred to as a "code" (e.g., "code blue," "code 7").

PERSON-CENTRED CARE

- When caring for people from diverse cultures and religions, nurses need to consider an individual's meaning and interpretation of life support and resuscitation. Although individuals may be part of a specific cultural or religious group, an individual may not follow all aspects of that culture or religion. Therefore, it is essential that nurses consider each person's interpretation and wishes to ensure the right of self-determination and implementation of culturally appropriate, person-centred nursing care.

- When necessary, use a professional language interpreter to explain the patient's health status to the patient and their caregiver. In addition, use cultural and religious support personnel to facilitate understanding of the events.

- Advance directives offer valuable information concerning a person's plan related to resuscitation status and decisions regarding resuscitation efforts. Although advance directives are often addressed before or during a person's hospitalization, nurses play an important role in advocating for and encouraging the person to discuss their wishes with the health care team.

- Follow employer's policy related to communicating and flagging a person's electronic health record or chart when a decision is made regarding do-not-resuscitate (DNR), do-not-attempt-resuscitation (DNaR), or allow-natural-death (AND) orders.

- Nurses need to be prepared for a large number of visitors who may remain at the bedside to provide support for the family or pray for the person. Nurses should collaborate with the family decision maker and leader to plan rotating visits at the bedside. Whenever a person requires resuscitation, a member of the interprofessional team (e.g., social worker, pastoral care worker) can support family presence at the bedside during the event.

EVIDENCE-INFORMED PRACTICE

The International Liaison Committee on Resuscitation (ILCOR) promotes, disseminates, and advocates for the international implementation of evidence-informed resuscitation for both initial care (BLS) and ongoing measures (advanced cardiac life support [ACLS]). The Heart and Stroke Foundation (HSF) is an active member of this consensus-building organization. The HSF, along with the American Heart Association (AHA), works collaboratively to develop North American guidelines (HSF & AHA, 2017). The 2015 AHA guidelines for in-hospital cardiac arrest chain of survival focus on the following aspects (Kleinman, Brennan, Goldberger, et al., 2015):

- Surveillance and prevention
- Recognition and activation of emergency medical response

- Immediate, high-quality CPR
- Rapid defibrillation with AED within 3–5 minutes of collapse
- Advanced life support and postarrest care

There is increased emphasis on high-quality CPR, ensuring chest compressions are of an adequate rate and depth while allowing the full chest to recoil between compressions. Interprofessional resuscitation teams need to work collaboratively to minimize interruptions of chest compressions and avoid excessive ventilation, with a goal of early defibrillation (if indicated) (Kleinman et al., 2015).

Family members might be at the bedside of the patient when a cardiac arrest occurs. Family presence during resuscitation (FPDR) should be considered an important part of person-centred care by the interprofessional resuscitation team. Through interprofessional collaboration a member of the team can be designated to help prepare the family for what they might see, hear, and smell prior to an event occurring. As well, this member can be there to support the family during the event (NENA, 2016). Development of policies and education for designated family members can support the safe and effective implementation of FPDR (Oczkowski, Mazzetti, Cupido, et al., 2015).

SAFETY GUIDELINES

- Know a patient's baseline vital signs, noting any irregularities in cardiac rhythm. Dysrhythmias can precipitate a cardiopulmonary arrest. Conditions that place a patient at risk for dysrhythmias include coronary artery disease, myocardial infarction, open-heart surgeries, acid–base imbalances, and toxicities.

- Know a patient's most recent serum electrolyte values. Electrolyte imbalances (e.g., potassium, magnesium, and calcium) can precipitate cardiopulmonary arrest.

- When a patient has been exposed to a chemical or drug, attempt to determine the type and amount of the substance involved. Certain chemicals (e.g., ethanol, tranquilizers, opiates) depress the respiratory centre, resulting in a respiratory arrest. Oversedation involving the use of patient-controlled analgesia (PCA) pumps or epidural administration can also contribute to respiratory depression. Overdoses of some medications can cause ventricular dysrhythmias and cardiopulmonary arrest.

- When electrical current is used during an emergency, good skin contact between the pad and patient's chest is essential to avoid the release of live electricity into the environment and to decrease the risk for skin burns (Link, Berkow, Kudenchuk, et al., 2015).

- Clear communication to all others in the room is essential at the time of defibrillation so that everyone is aware and does not touch the patient or the bed at the time of electrical current delivery.

✦ SKILL 28.1   **Inserting an Oropharyngeal Airway**

An *oropharyngeal airway (OPA)* is a semicircular, minimally flexible, curved piece of hard plastic (Fig. 28.1). When inserted, it extends from just outside the lips, over the tongue, and to the pharynx (Fig. 28.2). Oral airways allow nurses to suction through a central core or along the side of the airway and maintain airway patency in an unconscious patient. It is important to choose the correct size of an OPA based on a patient's age and the width and length of their mouth. Size is correct if, when the flange is held parallel to the

front teeth with the airway against the patient's cheek, the end of the curve reaches the angle of the jaw (Table 28.1).

Delegation and Collaboration

The skill of inserting an OPA cannot be delegated to an unregulated care provider (UCP). The nurse directs the UCP to:

- Immediately report to the nurse any signs of airway distress, vomiting, or change in level of consciousness.

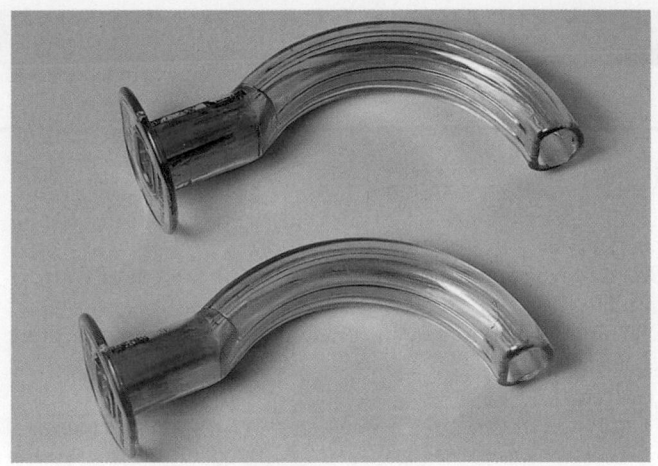

FIG 28.1 Oral airways.

TABLE 28.1

Oral Airway Guidelines for Size* by Age

Size	Age
30 mm or size 000	Premature neonates
45 mm or size 00	Newborn
55 mm or size 0	Newborn to 1 year
60 mm or size 1	1–2 years
70 mm or size 2	2–6 years
80 mm or size 3	6–18 years
90 mm or size 4	Adult medium
100 mm or size 5	Adult large
110 mm or size 6	Adult extra large

*Measure from the corner of the mouth to the angle of the jaw just below the ear for size estimation.

The nurse needs to use interprofessional collaboration (e.g., respiratory therapist) for safe OPA insertion.

Equipment

- Appropriate-size oral airway (see Table 28.1)
- Tongue blade
- Stethoscope
- Tissues or washcloths
- Clean gloves
- Face shield
- Gown if indicated
- Suction equipment if indicated
- Nonallergenic tape (*optional*)

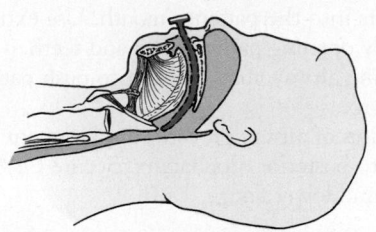

FIG 28.2 Placement of oral airway

STEP	RATIONALE

ASSESSMENT

1. Identify need to insert an OPA. Signs and symptoms include upper airway gurgling with breathing, absent cough or gag reflex, increased oral secretions, excessive drooling, grinding teeth, clenched teeth, biting endotracheal or gastric tubes, and laboured respirations.

These conditions place patient at risk for obstruction of the upper airway. Use OPAs only in unconscious patients. It may stimulate vomiting or laryngospasm if inserted in a semiconscious or conscious patient with a gag reflex.

2. Determine factors that may contribute to upper airway obstruction, such as age (children have a proportionally larger tongue) or presence of a nasal or oral airway and drainage tubes (swallowing is more difficult with tubes in place).

Allows you to accurately assess need for OPA placement. Patients at greater risk for upper airway obstruction are infants; children; and adults with upper airway congestion, loss of consciousness, seizure disorders, neuromuscular diseases, or increased oral secretions.

3. Ensure that patient does not have dentures in place before attempting an OPA insertion.

Oral airway insertion can dislodge dentures and cause worsening airway obstruction.

Clinical Decision Point *Never insert an OPA in a conscious patient with a gag reflex or a patient with recent oral or facial trauma, oral surgery, or loose teeth. Never force an airway into place.*

4. Assess caregiver's knowledge of procedure.

Identifies learning needs of caregiver. Patient will be unconscious.

NURSING DIAGNOSES

- Inadequate airway clearance
- Potential for aspiration

Related factors/Risk factors are individualized on the basis of patient's condition or needs.

STEP	RATIONALE

PLANNING

1. Expected outcomes following completion of procedure:
- Patient's respiratory status improves, as evidenced by respirations with normal rate, easier removal of secretions, and lack of gurgling noise in throat with respirations.
- Patient is not able to grind teeth or bite tubes.

- Patient's tongue does not obstruct airway.

2. Caregiver can verbalize understanding of need for oropharyngeal airway.

Airway is clear of secretions.

Oral airway prevents tooth contact with other teeth or with tubes.
Oral airway keeps tongue in correct position to maintain patent airway.
Teaching was successful.

IMPLEMENTATION

1. Position unconscious patient in semi-Fowler's position if possible.

2. Perform hand hygiene and apply clean gloves and face shield.

3. Whenever possible, use padded tongue blade to open patient's mouth; if necessary, use thumb and forefinger of nondominant hand to open jaws and teeth.

4. Insert OPA.

   a. Hold OPA with curved end up and insert distal end until airway reaches back of throat; then turn airway over 180 degrees and follow natural curve of tongue. *Option:* Hold airway sideways, insert halfway, and rotate 90 degrees while gliding it over natural curvature of the tongue. Make sure that outer flange is just outside the patient's lips.

Provides easy access to oral cavity.

Reduces transmission of microorganisms.

Provides access to oral cavity. To avoid a bite, do not insert your fingers into the patient's mouth. Use extreme caution if manually opening patient's jaw and teeth.
When inserting airway, take care not to push patient's tongue into pharynx.
Proper insertion of airway prevents displacement of patient's tongue into posterior oropharynx. Secure OPA with tape on upper and lower flange.

Clinical Decision Point *In a **pediatric patient**, **DO NOT** **rotate** the oral airway on insertion because the airway tip will damage the soft palate.*

5. Suction secretions as needed.
6. Reassess patient's respiratory status; auscultate lungs.
7. Clean patient's face with soft tissue or washcloth.
8. Discard tissue into appropriate receptacle, place washcloth in dirty or soiled linen bag, and remove gloves and face shield and discard in appropriate receptacle; perform hand hygiene.

9. Administer mouth care frequently.

Removes secretions; maintains patent airway.
Verifies respiratory status and patent airway.
Promotes hygiene.
Reduces transmission of microorganisms.

Increases patient comfort and removes debris. It also provides moisture to oral mucosal tissues.

Clinical Decision Point *Oral airways will need to be removed, cleaned or discarded, and replaced in patients with excessive oral secretions. Frequent suctioning of the oral cavity may be required. Oral airways are not a long-term solution. They can create pressure on underlying tissue and cause significant lip and tongue erosion, which can result in a medical device–related pressure injury (MDPI) (Norton, Parslow, Johnston, et al., 2018).*

EVALUATION

1. Observe patient's respiratory status and compare respiratory assessments before and after insertion of OPA.
2. Evaluate that airway is patent and that patient's tongue does not obstruct it.
3. Observe adjacent and underlying tissue for signs of redness, abrasion, or bruising.
4. Observe for patient pushing airway out with tongue or coughing.

Identifies patient's response to insertion of airway.

Ensures route for oxygen delivery to patient.

Identifies early signs of MDPI.

Patient's ability to clear own airway may have returned. Indicates reassessment of need for oral airway.

STEP	RATIONALE

EVALUATION

5. Use Teach-Back: "I want to be sure I explained why your loved one needs this oral airway. Tell me why it is important." Develop a revised teaching plan if caregiver is not able to teach back correctly.

Determines caregiver's level of understanding of instructional topic.

Unexpected Outcomes	Related Interventions
1. Patient continually coughs and gags when airway is inserted.	• Do not continue inserting airway if patient begins to gag. Stimulation of gag reflex can cause vomiting and aspiration. • Remove oral airway and position patient on side. • Reassess need for artificial airway prn.
2. Airway obstruction is not relieved.	• Obtain immediate assistance. • Reinsert airway or determine from health care provider if another form of airway is needed. • Assess for other causes of obstruction.
3. Patient pushes airway out of place or out of mouth.	• Reassess patient's need for OPA.
4. Unable to insert OPA; patient is combative or you are unable to open the patient's mouth.	• Get help. • Reassess patient's need for OPA. • Provide sedation as prescribed.

Communication and Documentation

• Document assessment findings indicating need for insertion and the patient's response while inserting the OPA; size of OPA; other interventions performed at the same time, especially positioning and suctioning; and patient's response to procedure, on flow sheet or in nurses' notes in an electronic health record (EHR) or chart.
• Document your evaluation of caregiver learning.

Special Considerations
Pediatric

• Oral airways are seldom used in treatment of airway obstruction in infants and children. Because the airway is narrow, OPAs are often more occlusive than beneficial (Hockenberry & Wilson, 2015).

◆ **SKILL 28.2** **Inserting a Nasopharyngeal Airway**

A *nasopharyngeal airway (NPA)* is a soft flexible rubber tube. The uncuffed tube is inserted nasally along the floor of the nasopharynx past the base of the tongue (Fig. 28.3). An NPA allows nurses to suction through a central core and maintain airway patency in conscious, semiconscious, or unconscious patients. It is important to choose the correct length by measuring from the tip of the patient's nose to the tragus of the ear (Fig. 28.4). The external diameter of the NPA should be slightly smaller than the patient's external nares opening but not be too large to blanch the nares on insertion.

Delegation and Collaboration

The skill of inserting an NPA cannot be delegated to an unregulated care provider (UCP). The nurse directs the UCP to:
• Immediately report to the nurse any signs of airway distress, vomiting, or change in level of consciousness.

Nurses need to use interprofessional collaboration (e.g., respiratory therapist) for safe NPA insertion.

Equipment

• Appropriate-size nasopharyngeal airway
• Stethoscope
• Water-soluble lubricant
• Tissues or washcloths
• Personal protective equipment (PPE) as required
• Suction equipment if indicated
• Nonallergenic tape (*optional*)

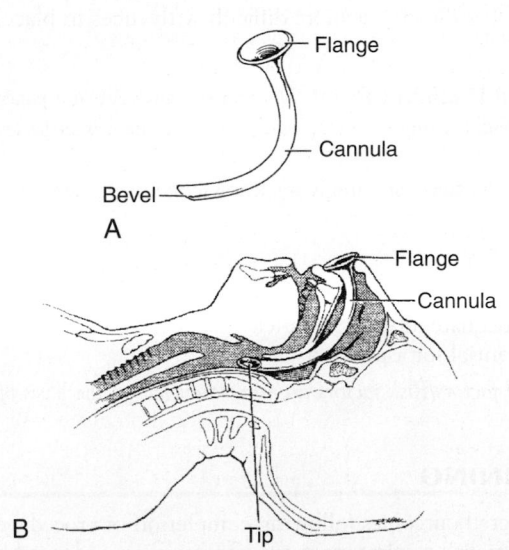

FIG 28.3 Nasopharyngeal airway. **A,** Airway parts. **B,** Proper placement. (*From Weigand, D. [2011]. AACN procedure manual for critical care [6th ed., Figure 10-1, p. 69]. Image is originally from Eubanks, D. H., & Bone, R. C. [1990]. Comprehensive respiratory care: A learning system. St. Louis: Mosby [p. 518].*)

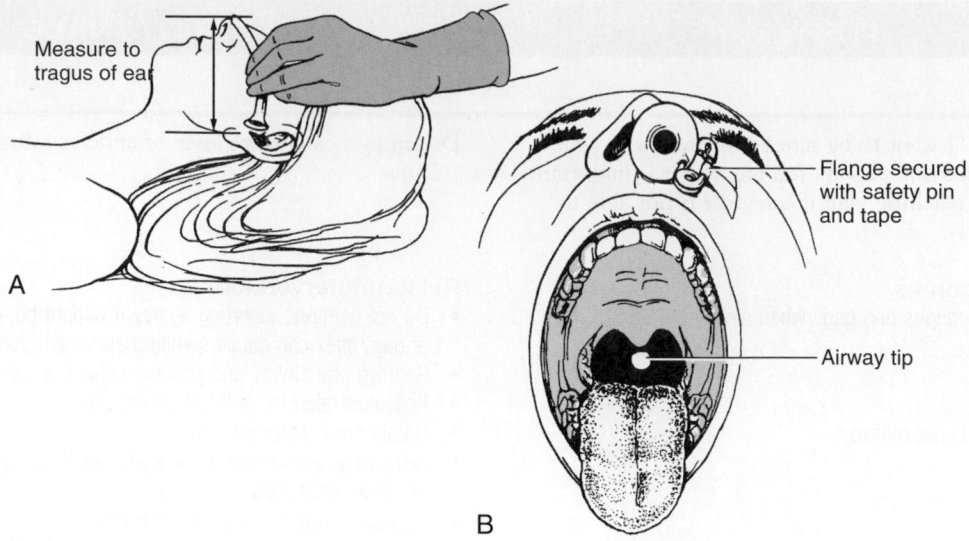

Measure to tragus of ear

Flange secured with safety pin and tape

Airway tip

A

B

FIG 28.4 A, Estimating nasopharyngeal airway size. **B,** Nasopharyngeal position after insertion. *(From Weigand, D. [2011]. AACN procedure manual for critical care [6th ed., Figure 10-2, p. 70]. Image is originally from Eubanks, D. H., & Bone, R. C. [1990]. Comprehensive respiratory care: A learning system. St. Louis: Mosby [p. 552].)*

STEP	RATIONALE

ASSESSMENT

1. Identify need to insert an NPA. Signs and symptoms include upper airway gurgling with breathing, increased oral secretions, and laboured respirations.

   These conditions place patient at risk for obstruction of the upper airway. Use an NPA on conscious, semiconscious, or unconscious patients. NPAs may stimulate vomiting or laryngospasm if measured incorrectly (i.e., they are too long).

2. Determine factors that may contribute to upper airway obstruction, such as age (children have a proportionally larger tongue) or presence of a nasal or oral airway and drainage tubes (swallowing is more difficult with tubes in place).

   Allows you to accurately assess need for NPA placement. Patients at greater risk for upper airway obstruction are infants; children; and adults with upper airway congestion, loss of consciousness, seizure disorders, neuromuscular disease, or increased oral secretions.

Clinical Decision Point *Never insert an NPA in a patient with obstructed nasal passages, prone to epistaxis, or with facial or head trauma when basilar skull fracture or cranial vault communication is suspected. Never force an airway into place.*

3. Assess patient or caregiver's knowledge of procedure.

   Identifies learning needs of patient and caregiver. Patient may be unconscious.

NURSING DIAGNOSES

- Inadequate airway clearance
- Potential for aspiration

Related factors/Risk factors are individualized on the basis of patient's condition or needs.

PLANNING

1. Expected outcomes following completion of procedure:
   - Patient's respiratory status improves, as evidenced by respirations with normal rate, easier removal of secretions, and lack of gurgling noise in throat with respirations.

     Airway is clear of secretions.

   - Patient's tongue does not obstruct airway.

     NPA keeps tongue in correct position to maintain patent airway.

2. Patient or caregiver can verbalize understanding of the need for an NPA.

   Teaching was successful.

STEP	RATIONALE

IMPLEMENTATION

1. Position patient in semi-Fowler's position if possible. — Provides easy access to oral cavity.
2. Perform hand hygiene and apply clean gloves and face shield. — Reduces transmission of microorganisms.
3. Insert NPA
   a. Generously lubricate the tip and outer tube with water-soluble lubricant. — When inserting an NPA, take care not to push the patient's tongue into the pharynx.
   b. With the bevel facing toward the septum, slide tube gently into the selected nostril with the dominant hand. Once the tip is beyond the septum, rotate the tube 180 degrees so curve faces downward. Advance until flange rests external to the nares. — Proper insertion of airway prevents displacement of patient's tongue into posterior oropharynx. Secure airway with tape on flange.
4. Suction secretions as needed. — Removes secretions; maintains patent airway.
5. Reassess patient's respiratory status; auscultate lungs. — Verifies respiratory status and patent airway.
6. Clean patient's face with soft tissue or washcloth. — Promotes hygiene.
7. Discard tissue into appropriate receptacle, place washcloth in dirty or soiled linen bag, and remove gloves and face shield and discard in appropriate receptacle; perform hand hygiene. — Reduces transmission of microorganisms.

Clinical Decision Point An NPA *will need to be removed, cleaned, or discarded, and replaced in patients with excessive secretions. They can create pressure on underlying tissue and pressure necrosis of the nasal ala, which can result in a medical device–related pressure injury (MDPI) (Norton et al., 2018).*

EVALUATION

1. Observe patient's respiratory status and compare respiratory assessments before and after insertion of airway. — Identifies patient's response to insertion of airway.
2. Evaluate that airway is patent. — Ensures route for oxygen delivery to patient.
3. Observe adjacent and underlying tissue for signs of redness, abrasion, or bruising. — Identifies early signs of MDPI.
4. Observe for patient pulling airway out. — Patient's ability to clear own airway may have returned. Indicates reassessment of need for airway.
5. **Use Teach-Back:** "I want to be sure I explained why your loved one needs this airway. Tell me why it is important." Develop a revised teaching plan if caregiver is not able to teach back correctly. — Determines caregiver's level of understanding of instructional topic.

Unexpected Outcomes	Related Interventions
1. Patient continually coughs and gags when airway is inserted.	• Do not continue inserting airway if patient begins to gag. Stimulation of gag reflex can cause vomiting and aspiration. • Remove airway and position patient on side. • Reassess need for artificial airway prn.
2. Airway obstruction not relieved.	• Obtain immediate assistance. • Reinsert airway or determine from health care provider if another form of airway is needed. • Assess for other causes of obstruction.
3. Patient pushes or pulls airway out of place.	• Reassess patient's need for NPA. • Get help.
4. Unable to insert airway; patient is combative, or you meet resistance when inserting airway.	• Reassess patient's need for NPA. • Provide sedation as prescribed.

Communication and Documentation

- Document assessment findings indicating need for insertion and those while inserting NPA; size of airway; other interventions performed at same time, especially positioning and suctioning; and patient's response to procedure, on flow sheet or in nurses' notes in an electronic health record (EHR) or chart.
- Document your evaluation of caregiver learning.

◆ SKILL 28.3   Code Management

All who respond to cardiopulmonary arrests should follow a simple, standardized, easy-to-remember approach. Initially a code is managed by the first responder performing the basic skills of cardiopulmonary resuscitation (CPR), which includes the primary survey and assessment of C (circulation/compressions), A (airway), B (breathing), and D (early defibrillation with an AED). The initial process also includes notification of the hospital interprofessional resuscitation team or code team. These interventions continue until the code team arrives. Most of the code team members have been trained in the advanced cardiac life support (ACLS) guidelines and the performance of the secondary survey and assessment: C (analysis of cardiac rhythm), A (airway intubation), B (confirmation of airway and ventilation), and D (differential diagnosis of the cause). Both surveys must be reassessed continually and managed as appropriate throughout the code situation.

The interprofessional code team usually includes a physician, critical care nurse, respiratory therapist, anaesthesiology personnel, and possibly radiology and laboratory technologists. A pastoral care representative or social worker is often available to be with the family.

The ability of a non-ACLS–certified nurse to initiate resuscitative efforts can prevent lethal dysrhythmias such as ventricular fibrillation (VF) from deteriorating to asystole (absence of cardiac electrical activity) and provide a chance for the heart to return to its normal rhythm. As soon as possible, the nurse needs to determine the patient's cardiac rhythm and, if appropriate, defibrillate the patient in VF or ventricular tachycardia (VT). Table 28.2 summarizes basic cardiac dysrhythmias. Early CPR and defibrillation delivered within the primary survey optimizes heart and brain function, leading to improved survivability. Equipment may be readily available at the bedside or in a designated area of the hospital unit. It is the nurse's responsibility to know how to use this equipment and to know its location and the contents of the resuscitation or crash cart.

Basic life support (BLS) certification with automatic external defibrillator (AED) training is a requirement of nurses and nursing students. Therefore, CPR will not be covered in detail within this chapter. Table 28.3 summarizes some points regarding CPR skills, including differences in adult, child, and infant techniques.

Delegation and Collaboration

The skill of code management cannot be delegated to unregulated care provider (UCP). However, a UCP who is certified in BLS techniques can perform the basic skills of CPR. Most UCPs are certified in BLS and can use an AED. Most facilities reserve the skill of manual defibrillation for licensed personnel who are ACLS certified or have received competency validation to perform manual defibrillation. All other skills in the code situation are directed by the code team leader and performed by nurses, respiratory therapists, and other health care providers.

Equipment

* Crash cart (Fig. 28.5)—Most adult carts have the following equipment:

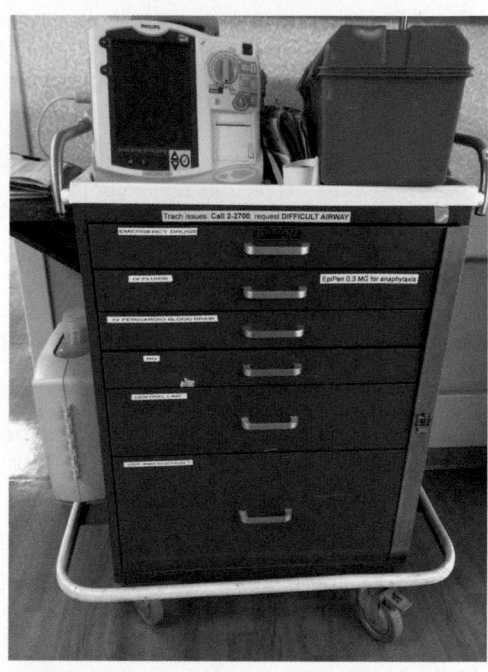

FIG 28.5 Emergency resuscitation cart.

TABLE 28.2

Common Cardiac Dysrhythmias*

Rhythm Characteristics and Etiology	Clinical Significance and Management
Sinus Tachycardia	
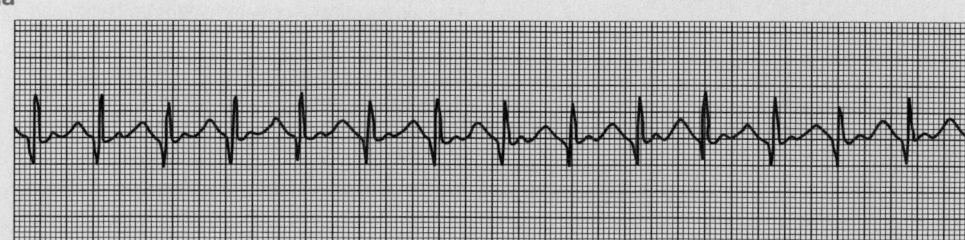	
Regular rhythm, rate 100–180 beats/min (higher in infants), normal P wave, normal QRS complex.	Some patients with heart disease are unable to increase their heart rate to meet increased oxygen demands.
Rate increase is often a normal response to exercise; emotion; or stressors such as pain, fever, pump failure, hyperthyroidism, and certain medications (e.g., caffeine, nitrates, epinephrine, nicotine).	Correct underlying factors; discontinue medications producing the adverse effect.

TABLE 28.2

Common Cardiac Dysrhythmias—cont'd

| **Rhythm Characteristics and Etiology** | **Clinical Significance and Management** |

Sinus Bradycardia

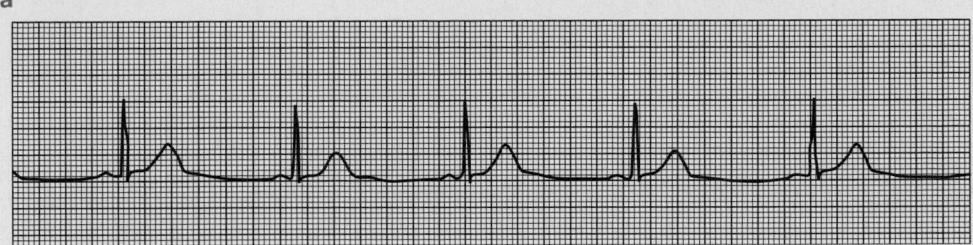

Regular rhythm, rate less than 60 beats/min, normal P wave, normal PR interval, normal QRS complex.	No clinical significance unless associated with signs and symptoms of reduced cardiac output such as dizziness or syncope or presence of chest pain.
Rate decrease is a normal response to sleep or in well-conditioned athlete; diminished blood flow to sinoatrial (SA) node, vagal stimulation, hypothyroidism, increased intracranial pressure, or medications (e.g., digoxin, propranolol, quinidine, procainamide) sometimes cause abnormal drops in rate.	Bradycardia with hypotension and decreased cardiac output is treated with atropine; pacemaker is sometimes necessary.

Atrial Fibrillation (A-fib)

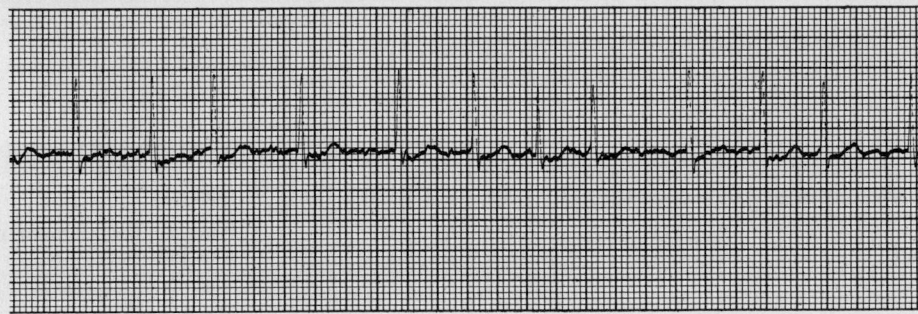

Chaotic, irregular atrial activity resulting in an irregular ventricular response. No identifiable P waves. Irregular ventricular response resulting in an irregular cardiac rate and rhythm. The conduction of the multiple atrial impulses across the atrioventricular (AV) node determines the rate. Caused by aging, calcification of the SA node, or changes in myocardial blood supply.	There is loss of the atrial kick (part of the cardiac output squeezed in the ventricles with a coordinated atrial contraction), pooling of blood in the atria, and development of microemboli. The patient often complains of fatigue, a fluttering in the chest, or shortness of breath if the ventricular response is rapid. Dysrhythmia occurs commonly in the aging and older person.

Ventricular Tachycardia

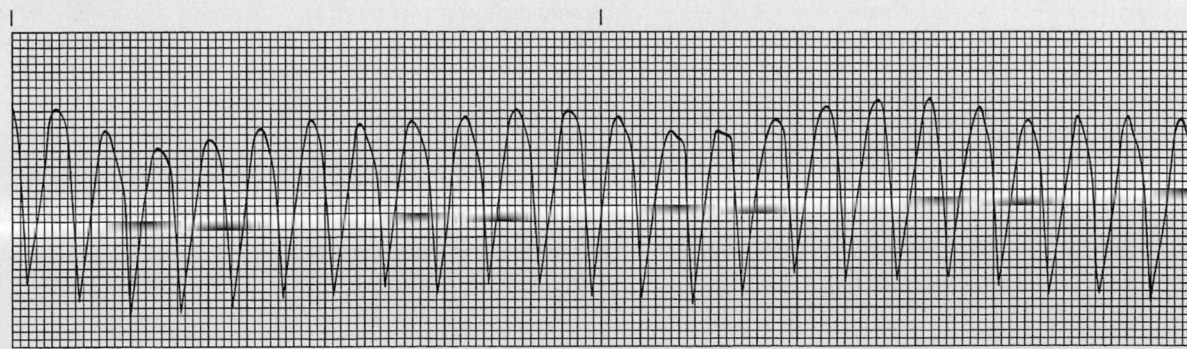

Rhythm slightly irregular, rate 100–200 beats/min, P wave absent, PR interval absent, QRS complex wide and bizarre, >0.12 second.	Results in decreased cardiac output caused by decreased ventricular filling time; often leads to severe hypotension and loss of pulse and consciousness.
Caused by changes in the normal pacemaker of the heart, such as decrease in blood flow, ischemia, or embolus.	Acute loss of pulse and respiration. Immediate chest compressions and defibrillation are required.

Continued

TABLE 28.2

Common Cardiac Dysrhythmias—cont'd

Rhythm Characteristics and Etiology   **Clinical Significance and Management**

Ventricular Fibrillation

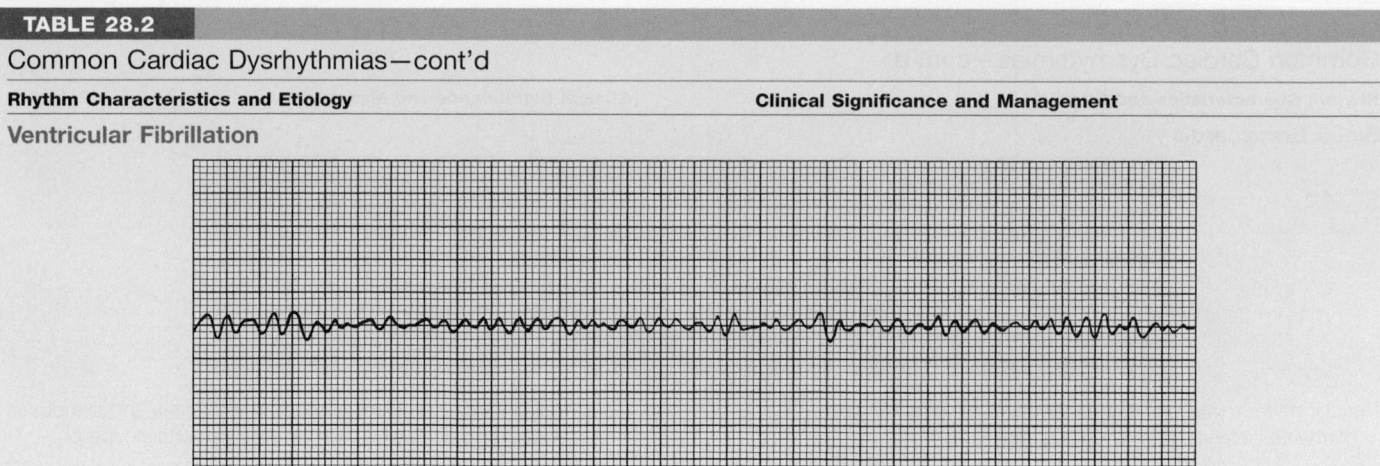

Uncoordinated electrical activity. No identifiable P, QRS, or T wave. Causes include sudden cardiac death, electrical shock, acute myocardial infarction, drowning, or trauma.

Acute loss of pulse and respiration. Immediate chest compressions and defibrillation are required. Availability of an automated external defibrillator (AED) is recommended in public and private places where large numbers of people gather or where people who are at high risk for heart attack live.

Modified from Kleinman, M. E., Brennan, E. E., Goldberger, Z. D., Swor, R. A., Terry, M., Bobrow, B. J., ... Rea, T. (2015). 2015 American Heart Association Guidelines for cardiopulmonary resuscitation and emergency cardiovascular care. Part 5: Adult basic life support and cardiopulmonary resuscitation quality. *Circulation, 132*(Suppl. 2), S414–S435.
*Refer to Table 26.1, Chapter 26, Cardiac Care, for common basic cardiac rhythms.

TABLE 28.3

Adult, Child, and Infant Cardiopulmonary Resuscitation Techniques (Health Care Providers)

Technique	Adult	Child (1–8 Years Old)	Infant (Under 1 Year); Does Not Include Newborns
Chest compressions: Push hard and fast to allow complete recoil	Begin compressions if no pulse Lower half of sternum, between nipples Heel of one hand, other hand on top 5–6 cm (2–2.4 inches) One to two rescuers: 100–120/min at a rate of 30 compressions to 2 breaths (30:2) Continue until AED is available and ready to analyze rhythm	Begin compressions if no pulse or pulse <60/min Lower half of sternum, between nipples Heel of one hand or as for adults At least ⅓ depth of chest One rescuer: 30 compressions, 2 breaths (30:2) Two rescuers: 15 compressions, 2 breaths (15:2)	Begin compressions if no pulse or pulse <60/min Just below nipple line (lower half of sternum) Two fingers, two thumbs (encircling hands) One rescuer: 30 compressions, 2 breaths (30:2) Two rescuers: 15 compressions, 2 breaths (15:2)
Defibrillation using AED	Use adult pads AED should be applied as soon as available, and shock as soon as advised Resume compressions immediately after shock	Use child pads whenever possible If none, use adult pads but do not overlap them Apply AED as soon as available, and shock as soon as advised	If there is a shockable rhythm, manual defibrillation is used.
Airway	Head tilt–chin lift (HCP: Suspected trauma, use jaw thrust)	Head tilt–chin lift (HCP: Suspected trauma, use jaw thrust)	Head tilt–chin lift (HCP: Suspected trauma, use jaw thrust)
HCP: Rescue breathing mouth-to-mask or bag-valve mask without chest compressions	10–12 breaths/min (approximately 1 breath every 5–6 seconds)	12–20 breaths/min (approximately 1 breath every 3 seconds)	12–20 breaths/min (approximately 1 breath every 3 seconds)
HCP: Rescue breaths for CPR with advanced airway (endotracheal tube/tracheotomy)	8–10 breaths/min (approximately 1 breath every 6–8 seconds)	8–10 breaths/min (approximately 1 breath every 6–8 seconds)	8–10 breaths/min (approximately 1 breath every 6–8 seconds)

Data from Kleinman, M. E., Brennan, E. E., Goldberger, Z. D., Swor, R. A., Terry, M., Bobrow, B. J., ... Rea, T. (2015). 2015 American Heart Association Guidelines for cardiopulmonary resuscitation and emergency cardiovascular care. Part 5: Adult basic life support and cardiopulmonary resuscitation quality. *Circulation, 132*(Suppl. 2), S414–S435; Atkins, D. L., et al. (2015). American Heart Association Guidelines for cardiopulmonary resuscitation and emergency cardiovascular care. Part 11: Pediatric basic life support and cardiopulmonary resuscitation quality. *Circulation, 132*(Suppl. 2), S519.
AED, Automated external defibrillator; *CPR,* cardiopulmonary resuscitation; *HCP,* health care provider.

- Clean and sterile gloves, gown, protective eyewear, masks, face shield
- Oxygen source
- Bag-valve mask device or resuscitation bag
- Oral and nasopharyngeal airways
- Laryngoscope, handle, and laryngoscope straight and curved blades
- Endotracheal (ET) tubes, various sizes (5 to 9 mm for adults; 0 to 4 mm for pediatrics)
- Carbon dioxide detector to confirm ET tube placement
- Tape or commercial ET tube holder
- Suction source and suction equipment if not with crash cart
- Backboard

- AED and/or manual defibrillator with AED/defibrillator pads
- Intravenous (IV) needles (sizes for adults and pediatrics)
- Central vascular access kit
- IV tubing and fluids (normal saline [NS] and 5% dextrose in water [D_5W])
- Syringes
- Laboratory specimen tubes
- Arterial blood gas kit
- Emergency medications
- ACLS guidelines or algorithms
  Follow employer's policy related to routine checks of emergency equipment functioning and supplies located on the crash cart.

STEP	RATIONALE

ASSESSMENT

1. Determine if patient is unconscious by gently shaking them and shouting, "Are you OK?" Assess patient unresponsiveness and call for help.

   Confirms that patient is unresponsive rather than intoxicated, sleeping, or hearing impaired. Substance misuse, hypoglycemia, toxicities, seizures, trauma, ketoacidosis, and shock also can cause unconsciousness.

2. Establish absence of respirations and lack of circulation within 10 seconds: no pulse, no respirations, no movement (Kleinman et al., 2015). Check carotid pulse on an adult or a child; use brachial or femoral pulse in an infant.

   Indicates need for emergency measures, including AED. Carotid pulse is the easiest to locate in adults and children. Femoral pulse may also be palpated in a child or an infant.

Clinical Decision Point *If an unresponsive person has adequate respirations and pulse, remain with the person until further help is present. Place the patient in a modified lateral recovery position (see illustration). Continue to assess for the presence of respirations and pulse because a recurrent arrest may develop.*

Determine if there is a resuscitation care plan on the patient's electronic health record (EHR) or chart, and proceed as per the employer's policy for do not resuscitate (DNR), do not attempt resuscitation (DNaR), or allow natural death (AND) prescriptions.

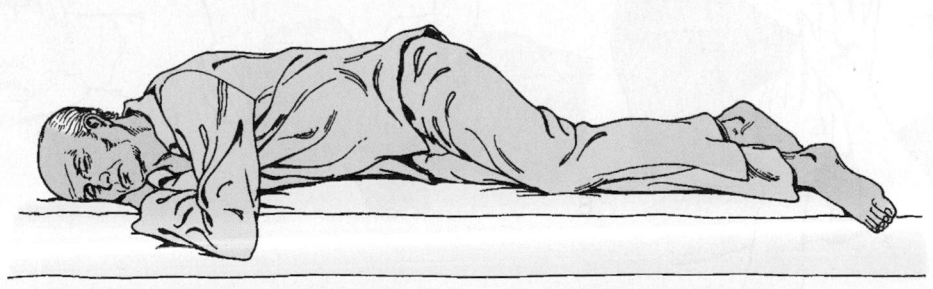

STEP 1 Modified recovery position.

NURSING DIAGNOSES

- Inadequate spontaneous ventilation
- Inadequate breathing pattern
- Reduced cardiac output
- Inadequate gas exchange

Related factors/Risk factors are individualized on the basis of patient's condition or needs.

STEP	RATIONALE

PLANNING

1. Immediately activate the code team or emergency medical services (EMS; 9-1-1). Tell coworkers to bring AED (if available) and crash cart to bedside.

Ensures timely application of defibrillation, CPR, and ACLS to the cardiac arrest patient.

2. Expected outcomes following completion of procedure:
- Patient regains pulse and respirations.
- Patient receives postresuscitation care.
- Patient is transported to critical care unit (CCU) for ongoing care.

CPR was successful.
Ongoing treatment and support are needed.
Resuscitation was successful.

IMPLEMENTATION

Primary Survey: C (Circulation/Compressions)

1. Place patient on hard surface such as floor, ground, or backboard. Patient must be flat. Logroll patient to flat, supine position using spine precautions if trauma is suspected.

External compression of heart is facilitated. Heart is compressed between sternum and spinal vertebrae, which must be on a hard and firm surface. Do *NOT* delay the start of CPR. Positioning patient on hard surface may take more than one or two rescuers. You may need to wait to safely move the patient. Place patient on backboard or position them as soon as appropriate help is present.

2. Start chest compressions and continue until AED is attached to patient and verbal prompt of device or code team advises you, "Do not touch the patient."

To minimize interruption time of chest compressions, continue CPR while AED pads are being applied and turned on.

   a. Assume correct hand position and compression ratio for patient (30:2 adult) (see Table 28.3; see illustrations).

Specific hand position, compression depth, and ratio are different for adults, children, and infants to avoid injury to the heart, lung, or liver (see Table 28.3).

Clinical Decision Point *Ensure that fingers are off the ribs and lowermost part of the xiphoid process. This minimizes the chance of rib fracture that could result in a punctured lung or liver laceration, which further compromises cardiopulmonary status. Continue chest compressions, ventilation, and AED use.*

Primary Survey: A (Airway)

3. Apply clean gloves and face shield.

Reduces transmission of microorganisms.

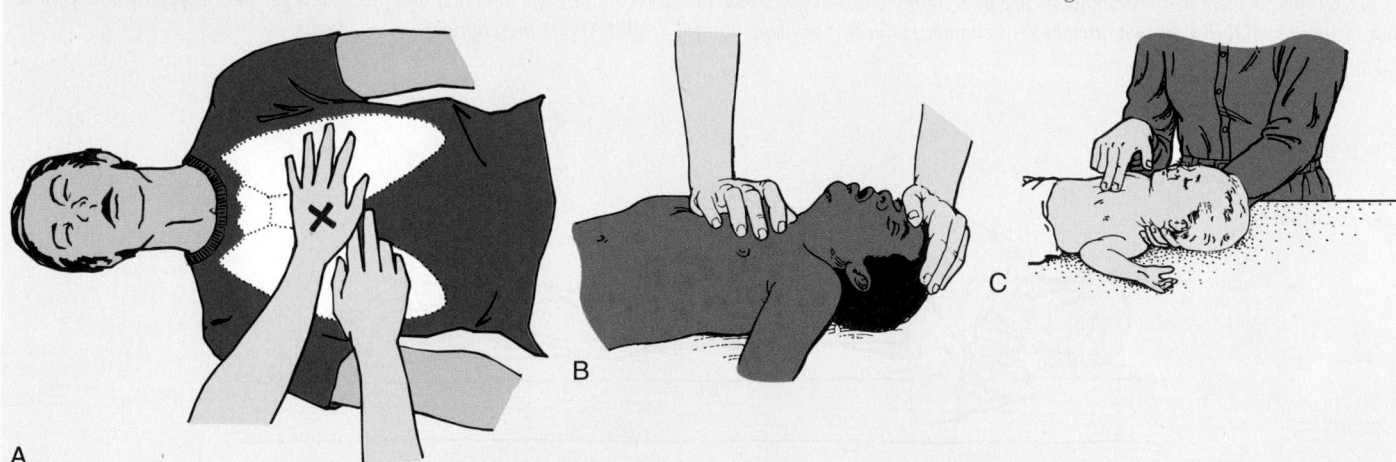

STEP 2a A, Proper hand position—adult. **B,** Proper hand position—child. **C,** Proper hand position—infant.

STEP	**RATIONALE**

IMPLEMENTATION

4. Open airway.

    a. Head tilt–chin lift (no trauma) (see illustration) *or*

    b. Jaw thrust (cervical trauma is suspected) (see illustration).

The tongue is the most common cause of a blocked airway in an unresponsive patient.

Suspect spinal cord injury in patients with trauma. Jaw-thrust manoeuvre prevents head extension and neck movement and further paralysis or spinal cord injury. Apply rigid cervical collar and immobilize patient as soon as possible to reduce cervical spine motion.

Primary Survey: *B* (Breathing)

5. Attempt to ventilate patient with slow breaths using one of the following methods:

    a. Mouth-to-mouth using barrier device.

    b. Mouth-to-mask using pocket mask (see illustration).

    c. Bag-valve mask device (see illustrations).

Slow breaths deliver air at low pressure to reduce risk of gastric distension.

Forms airtight seal to prevent air from escaping through nose.

Provides secure seal and permits use of supplemental oxygen.

Gives breaths with enough force to make chest rise.

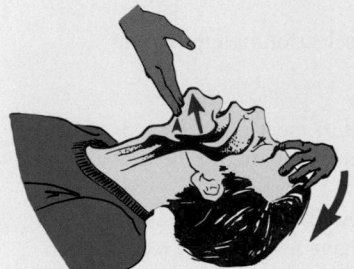

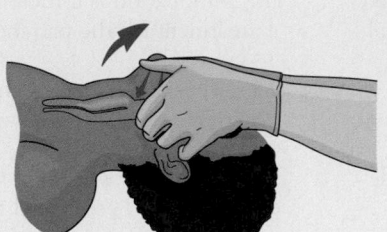

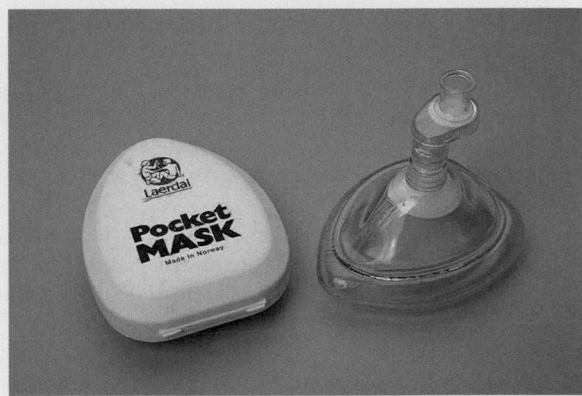

STEP 4a Head tilt–chin lift. *(From Sorrentino, S. [2008]. Mosby's textbook for nursing assistants [7th ed.]. St. Louis: Mosby.)*

STEP 4b Jaw thrust without head tilt.

STEP 5b Pocket mask.

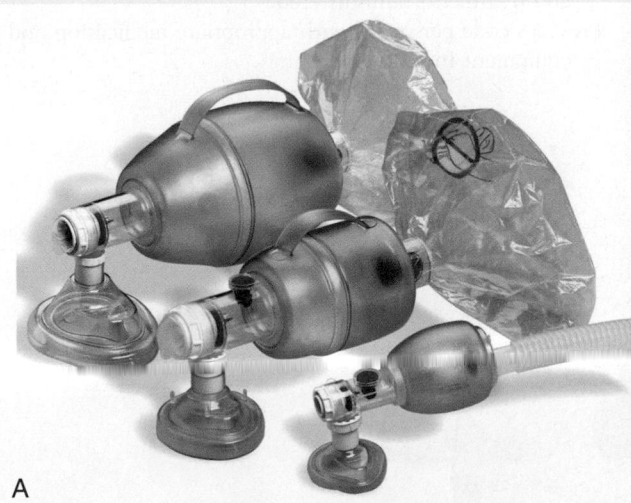

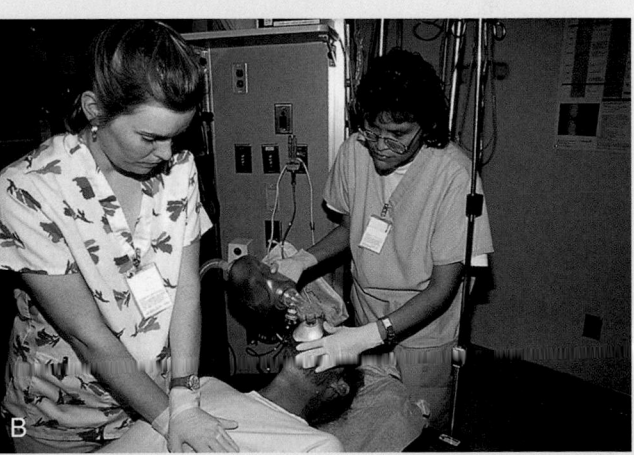

STEP 5c A, Bag-valve mask device. **B,** Two-rescuer breathing with bag-valve mask device. *(Courtesy Ambu USA.)*

STEP	RATIONALE

IMPLEMENTATION

6. If available, insert appropriate airway adjunct (see Skill 28.1 and Skill 28.2).

Maintains tongue on anterior floor of mouth and prevents obstruction of posterior airway by tongue.

7. Suction secretions if necessary or turn patient's head to one side unless trauma is suspected.

Suctioning prevents airway obstruction. Turning patient's head to one side allows gravity to drain any secretions, decreasing risk of aspiration.

Primary Survey: *D* (Defibrillation)

8. If pulse is absent and AED is available, apply AED or manual defibrillator "hands-off" pads immediately as appropriate (see illustration).

Most successful defibrillation rates occur when the AED is applied and used within 5 minutes following collapse. Survival rates decline when defibrillation is delayed. "Hands-off" pads are self-adhesive pads applied to the chest wall. You may need to clip chest hair to ensure good skin/pad contact or dry skin.

    a. After one shock, resume CPR for five cycles (30:2, adult compressions/breath ratio) and begin rhythm analysis and shock sequence again (see Table 28.3).

One shock followed by chest compressions for five cycles of 30:2 ratio (approximately 2 minutes) provides sufficient blood flow and perfusion before another set of shocks is delivered.

Secondary Survey: Implementation

1. Give code leader brief verbal report on events performed before code team's arrival (i.e., code, vital signs, medical diagnosis, and code intervention).

This information is critical in selection of appropriate treatment for the patient.

2. On arrival of sufficient personnel, delegate tasks as appropriate while core group continues with resuscitation efforts.

Delegation of duties is essential to meet critical needs of patient and their family in a timely matter.

    a. Help patient's roommate and visitors away from code scene. Assign pastoral care or other nurses to communicate with patient's family. Consider allowing family to witness resuscitation (see policy).

Family members who were allowed to witness resuscitation efforts have been found to have a significant reduction in posttraumatic stress and self-reports of a greater sense of resolution and fulfillment (American Association of Critical Care Nurses [AACN], 2016).

    b. Delegate someone to remove excess furniture or equipment from room.

Provides room for emergency equipment and responders.

    c. Have someone bring patient's chart to bedside or have access to patient's EHR.

Clarifies patient's medical condition, code status, and presence of any allergies.

    d. Assign nurse as recorder to record and document events of code.

Ensures accurate documentation of events of code, medications, and treatments administered.

    e. Assign another nurse to get medications and supplies from crash cart to hand off to code team members. The bedside nurse is involved in tasks such as medication administration, vital signs, and helping with procedures.

Provides code personnel with appropriate medication and equipment in a timely fashion.

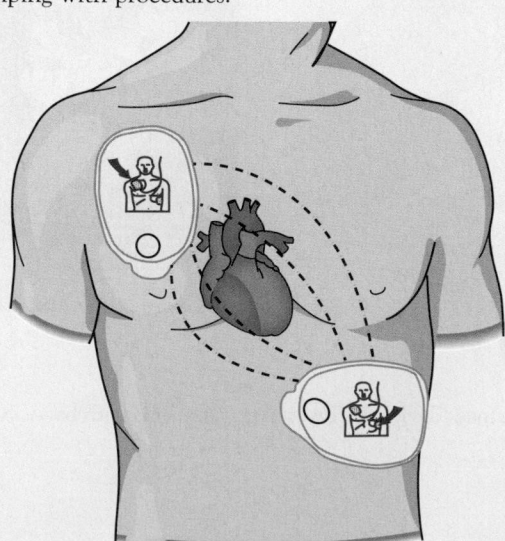

STEP 8 Paddle placement for defibrillation.

STEP	RATIONALE

IMPLEMENTATION

Secondary Survey: *C* (Analysis of Cardiac Rhythm and Defibrillation)

3. Turn on manual defibrillator. Attach manual defibrillator/monitor to patient using electrocardiogram (ECG) electrodes, quick-look paddles with gel pads, or "hands-off" defibrillation electrode to visualize cardiac rhythm (see illustration above in Step 8).

Cardiac rhythm monitor devices provide immediate rhythm display for analysis without disruption of rescue breathing and chest compression.

Good skin-to-paddle/pad contact ensures appropriate discharge of current and decreases chance of skin burns.

4. If cardiac rhythm is "shockable," continue CPR and help code team with manual defibrillation.

Manual defibrillation is performed by ACLS-certified personnel.

   a. Select proper energy level following the policy and equipment directions.

Energy is delivered in prescribed doses. Manual biphasic devices deliver shocks at a lower level (200 joules); monophasic waveforms use 360 joules.

   b. If using paddles with gel pads, place paddles on patient's chest wall.

   c. A warning must be called out before initiating charge (e.g., announce "Clear"). Verify that no one is in physical contact with patient, bed, or any item contacting patient during defibrillation.

Prevents accidental delivery of shock or injury to personnel.

   d. After one shock, resume CPR for five cycles (30:2, adult compressions/breath ratio) and begin rhythm analysis and shock sequence again (see Table 28.3).

One shock followed by chest compressions for five cycles of 30:2 ratio (approximately 2 minutes) provides sufficient blood flow and perfusion before another set of shocks is delivered.

5. Establish IV access (see Chapter 29) with large-bore IV needle (14- to 22-gauge) and begin infusion of 0.9% normal saline.

Provides a route for rapid drug administration and access for blood samples and fluid administration. Physiological saline is isotonic. Rapid fluid infusion facilitates dispersal of medication throughout cardiovascular system.

   a. If you cannot obtain peripheral IV access, the health care provider may pursue central venous or intraosseous (IO) access.

Administration of emergency medications is dependent on vascular or IO access.

6. Administer IV medications as prescribed. Some emergency medications are packaged as prefilled syringes for ease of use.

Medication used for treatment of VF and VT:
- Epinephrine: 1 mg every 3–5 minutes IV/IO
- Amiodarone: First dose—300 mg bolus IV/IO; second dose—150 mg bolus IV/IO.

Recorder needs to keep track of time intervals to prompt team for repeat doses when time has elapsed.

7. Help with procedures as needed.

Most equipment needed for special procedures during code is on the crash cart. Knowledge of crash cart contents is very helpful in the code to provide personnel with appropriate equipment.

8. Continue CPR until relieved (i.e., until patient regains spontaneous pulse and respiration, rescuer is exhausted and unable to perform CPR effectively, or health care provider prescribes discontinuation of CPR).

Interruptions in CPR are planned and organized. They usually occur during change of CPR personnel, defibrillation, and intubation. An interruption should not exceed 10 seconds (Kleinman et al., 2015).

Secondary Survey: *A* (Intubate Airway)

9. If respirations are absent, help code team with ET intubation.

Intubation provides a patent airway and facilitates pulmonary ventilation. A laryngeal mask airway or esophageal tracheal Combitube can also be used to provide advanced airway support.

   a. Have available laryngoscope handle, laryngoscope blades, curved and straight blades, ET tubes, stylet, suction, and tape or ET tube holder. Ensure that light source on laryngoscope is functional.

Light is necessary on laryngoscope to visualize vocal cords and intubate trachea. Batteries may need to be changed.

Secondary Survey: *B* (Confirmation of Airway and Ventilation)

10. Help in confirmation of ET tube placement or advanced airway support by auscultating lungs for bilateral breath sounds and monitoring the carbon dioxide (CO_2) detector to confirm correct airway placement.

Auscultation of lungs and monitoring of exhaled CO_2 or esophageal detector device further verify correct airway placement and adequacy of ventilation and gas exchange. (Link et al., 2015).

Chest X-ray film is usually obtained after patient has been stabilized to confirm placement of ET tube and central venous catheters.

STEP	RATIONALE

IMPLEMENTATION

11. Ventilate using bag device on intubation. **Avoid hyperventilation.**

Increased intrathoracic pressure caused by incomplete exhalation results in reduced cardiac output (Link et al., 2015).

Secondary Survey: *D* (Differential Diagnosis)
12. Obtain prescribed laboratory and diagnostic studies.

Aids in determination of cause of arrest.

EVALUATION

1. Reassess primary and secondary surveys throughout code event.

Keeps process organized and addresses immediate needs of patient.

2. Palpate carotid pulse at five cycles or 2 minutes of CPR.

Documents adequacy of external cardiac compressions.

3. Observe for spontaneous return of respirations or heart rate every 2 minutes.

Assessment of pulse, respiration, heart rate, and cardiac rhythm can occur after chest compressions and ventilation have been interrupted briefly every 2 minutes.

4. Ensure that interruptions in CPR are minimized.

Interruptions are associated with reduced coronary artery perfusion pressure and lower mean coronary perfusion pressure (Link et al., 2015).

5. Use Teach-Back: "I want to be sure I clearly explained what has happened to your loved one and why we performed cardiopulmonary resuscitation, known as CPR. In your own words, tell me why we had to perform CPR." Develop a revised teaching plan if caregiver is not able to teach back correctly.

Determines caregiver's level of understanding of instructional topic.

Unexpected Outcomes	Related Interventions
1. Patient develops skeletal injury such as fractured ribs or sternum or internal organ injury such as lacerated lung or liver as result of chest compressions.	• Obtain appropriate diagnostic tests to document injuries. • Assess patient's postarrest breathing for symmetry and pain. • Assess for intrathoracic or intra-abdominal bleeding (hematomas, increasing abdominal girth).
2. Patient's CPR is unsuccessful.	• Contact chaplain services, if appropriate. • Consult social worker. • Complete postmortem care on patient (see Chapter 17). • Notify coroner and organ and tissue donation organization in accordance with employer policy and provincial/territorial law. • Provide for privacy for patient's family to grieve and mourn loss of loved one.
3. Rescuer is unassisted, tires, and is unable to continue.	• Get help.

Communication and Documentation

• Immediately report arrest via the organization-wide communication system, indicating exact location of patient.
• Cardiopulmonary arrest requires precise documentation. Most employers use a form designed specifically for documenting patient arrests and subsequent care.
• Document in nurses' notes in an EHR or chart or on designated CPR worksheet: onset of arrest, time and number of AED shocks (you will not know the exact energy level used by the AED), time and energy level of manual defibrillations, medications given, procedures performed, cardiac rhythm, use of CPR, patient's response, and education and interventions provided to family.

Special Considerations
Teaching

• Patient and caregiver should keep emergency numbers taped to the phone or consider programming them into a speed dial function on both home and mobile phones. Stress the use of 9-1-1.

• If patient is at risk for cardiopulmonary arrest, encourage the family or caregiver to obtain BLS certification through a certified instructor.
• It is extremely helpful if the caregiver has a list of medications that the patient is presently taking and a description of purpose of medications.

Pediatric

• All people involved in administering CPR must understand different breathing/compression ratios, hand (fingers) placement, and depth of compression in children and infants compared with that in adults.
• Infants and children experience respiratory arrest much more frequently than full cardiopulmonary arrest.
• Quick reference, colour-coded guides are frequently used in pediatric codes to quickly determine appropriate drug doses and equipment sizes.
• Most AEDs are specifically designed for adult use only and are therefore not recommended for use with children younger than

8 years of age or weighing less than 25 kg (55 pounds) (Atkins, Berger, Duff, et al., 2015). Adult pads can be used if child pads are not available; place one pad on the front chest and the other on the back. Manual defibrillation performed by a health care provider using lower energy settings (2 to 4 joules/kg) is the most common method of pediatric defibrillation (Atkins et al., 2015).

Gerontological

- In older persons, compressions often result in rib or cartilage fractures.
- Remove loose-fitting dentures to avoid obstructing the airway. If dentures fit securely, leave them in to provide a tight seal when providing ventilations.

Care in the Community

- Cardiopulmonary arrest in the community setting requires activation of the emergency response system (call 9-1-1).
- In the community and in long-term care settings, patients may have implanted cardioverter defibrillators (ICDs), pacemakers, or both. For these patients, families need to know how to administer CPR and the specific capabilities of the patient's ICD or pacemaker. Placement of defibrillator or AED pads/paddles may need to be altered to avoid placement directly on top of an ICD or pacemaker generator. Remove medication patches from chest.
- Soft surfaces such as a mattress or car seat decrease efficiency of external cardiac compressions.
- AEDs are available for use in the community and home setting.

◆ CLINICAL DEBRIEF

You are the charge nurse for the night shift on a general medical floor. Your next patient is 85 years old and admitted with heart failure. On your rounds, you find your patient lying on the floor of the bathroom. You gently shake her and call her name. She is unresponsive. An automated external defibrillator (AED) is available down the hall.

1. What should you do first? Explain your choice.
   1. Apply the AED.
   2. Call for help.
   3. Check for a pulse.
   4. Open the airway and provide two breaths.
2. Your coworker arrives to the room with the AED. You've started chest compressions already. What is your next step? Explain your choice.
   1. Check for a pulse.
   2. Call for help.
   3. Tell your coworker to apply the AED.
   4. Continue with 8 to 10 breaths/min.
3. The code team has arrived to continue resuscitation attempts on the patient. Using an SBAR technique, how would you communicate to the arriving code team?

5. Assess for unresponsiveness, pulselessness, and breathlessness.
6. Announce "Clear."
7. Resume chest compressions.
8. Press the shock button.

ⓔ Visit the Evolve site for a complete list of Clinical Debrief and Review Questions answers.

REFERENCES

Agency for Healthcare Research and Quality (AHRQ). (2019). *Patient safety primer: Rapid response systems.* Retrieved from https://psnet.ahrq.gov/primers/primer/4/rapid-response-systems

American Association of Critical Care Nurses (AACN). (2016). Practice alert: Family presence during resuscitation and invasive procedures. *Critical Care Nurse, 36*(1), e11–e14. doi:10.4037/ccn2016980

American Heart Association (AHA). (2015/2018). *AHA guidelines for CPR & ECC.* Retrieved from https://eccguidelines.heart.org/index.php/guidelines-highlights/

Atkins, D. L., Berger, S., Duff, J. P., et al. (2015). Part 11: Pediatric basic life support and cardiopulmonary resuscitation quality: 2015 American Heart Association Guidelines update for cardiopulmonary resuscitation and emergency cardiovascular care. *Circulation, 132*(Suppl. 2), S519–S525. doi:10.1161/CIR.0000000000000265

Heart and Stroke Foundation & American Heart Association (HSF & AHA). (2017). *Highlights of the 2015 American Heart Association: Guidelines update for CPR and ECC. Heart and Stroke Foundation of Canada edition.* Retrieved from http://www.heartandstroke.ca/-/media/pdf-files/canada/cpr-2017/ecc-highlights-of-2015-guidelines-update-for-cpr-ecclr.ashx

Hockenberry, M. J., & Wilson, D. (2015). *Wong's nursing care of infants and children* (10th ed.). St. Louis: Mosby.

Kleinman, M. E., Brennan, E. E., Goldberger, Z. D., et al. (2015). 2015 American Heart Association Guidelines for cardiopulmonary resuscitation and emergency cardiovascular care. Part 5: Adult basic life support and cardiopulmonary resuscitation quality. *Circulation, 132*(Suppl. 2), S414–S435. doi:10.1161/CIR.0000000000000259

Link, M. S., Berkow, L. C., Kudenchuk, P. J., et al. (2015). Part 7: Adult advanced cardiovascular life support: 2015 American Heart Association guidelines update for cardiopulmonary resuscitation and emergency cardiovascular care. *Circulation, 132*(Suppl. 2), S444–S464. doi:10.1161/CIR.0000000000000261

National Emergency Nurses Association (NENA). (2016). *Position statement: Family primary support unit presence during bedside invasive procedures and resuscitation.* Chilliwack, BC: Author. Retrieved from http://nena.ca/w/wp-content/uploads/2014/11/FamilyPrimarySupport.pdf

Norton, L., Parslow, N., Johnston, D., et al. (2018). *Best practice recommendations for the prevention and management of pressure injuries.* Retrieved from http://www.woundscanada.ca/docman/public/health-care-professional/bpr-workshop/172-bpr-prevention-and-management-of-pressure-injuries-2/file

Oczkowski, S. J., Mazzetti, I., Cupido, C., & Fox-Robichaud, A. E. (2015). Family presence during resuscitation position paper for the Canadian Critical Care Society. *Canadian Respiratory Journal, 22*(4), 201–205. doi:10.1155/2015/532721

Tanguay, T., & Bartel, R. (2017). Implementation of a unique RRT model in a tertiary care center in Western Canada. *Canadian Journal of Critical Care Nursing, 28*(1), 34–37.

◆ REVIEW QUESTIONS

1. The nurse is performing CPR during a cardiac arrest. Which of the following techniques ensures the highest-quality chest compressions? *(Select all that apply.)*
   1. Minimizing interruption in chest compressions
   2. Avoiding full chest recoil
   3. Providing excessive ventilations
   4. Adequate depth and rate of compression
   5. Ensure the AED is in place
2. Place the following interventions in the correct sequence for beginning CPR.
   1. Check responsiveness.
   2. Begin 30 chest compressions.
   3. Provide two breaths.
   4. Attach the AED.
   5. Check for a pulse.
3. Review the following steps and place in correct order for using an external defibrillator (automatic or manual).
   1. Start chest compressions.
   2. Apply "hands-off" pads to the patient.
   3. Perform a visual check to ensure that no one is in contact with the patient.
   4. Turn on the power.

29 | Vascular Access and Infusion Therapy

Written by **Darlaine Jantzen, RN, MA, PhD; Adele deRosenroll, BSc; Selena Hebig, BSN, BScKin; and Carol Ann Liebold, RN, BSN, CRNI**

SKILLS AND PROCEDURES

OBJECTIVES

Mastery of content in this chapter will enable the nurse to:
- Discuss current evidence-informed practices for infusion therapy.
- Discuss common indications for intravenous (IV) therapy.
- Identify safety guidelines for IV fluid administration.
- Explain how to prepare a patient and caregiver for infusion therapy.
- Discuss complications of infusion therapy.
- Identify individualized person-centred care regarding infusion therapy, including cultural considerations and personal beliefs and values.
- Identify the educational needs of patients with vascular access devices (VADs) and those receiving infusion therapy.
- Explain techniques for preventing transmission of infection for a patient receiving infusion therapy.
- Demonstrate initiating infusion therapy, regulating IV flow rate, changing IV solutions, changing IV administration sets, changing peripheral vascular access device (PVAD) dressings, and discontinuing a PVAD.
- Identify common types of central vascular access devices (CVADs).
- Demonstrate assessment and maintenance of CVADs and discontinuation of a CVAD.

MEDIA RESOURCES

- evolve http://evolve.elsevier.com/Canada/Perry/clinicalskills/
- Review Questions
- Audio Glossary
- **NSO** Nursing Skills Online
- Clinical Debrief and Review Questions

PURPOSE

Vascular access is established when patients require infusion therapy or hemodynamic monitoring. Infusion therapy is used to correct or maintain fluid and electrolyte balance; administer continuous or intermittent medications, blood or blood products, and diagnostic agents and anaesthesia; and to correct or maintain nutritional status. Vascular access, one of the most common invasive procedures performed by health care providers worldwide, poses risks to patients; therefore, competence and dexterity are essential to safe patient care.

STANDARDS OF CARE

- Accreditation Canada, 2019—*Required Organizational Practices Handbook—Version 14.* (http://www.wrha.mb.ca/quality/files/2019 ROPHandbook.pdf)
- Canadian Vascular Access Association, 2013—*Occlusion Management Guideline for Central Venous Access* (http://cvaa.info/publications/occlusion-management-guideline-omg)
- Infusion Nurses Society (INS), 2016a—*Infusion Therapy Standards of Practice* (http://source.yiboshi.com/20170417/1492425631944540325.pdf)
- O'Grady, Alexander, Burns, et al., 2011—*Guidelines for the Prevention of Intravascular Catheter-Related Infections* (https://www.cdc.gov/infectioncontrol/guidelines/pdf/bsi/bsi-guidelines-H.pdf)
- Public Health Agency of Canada (PHAC), 2016—*Routine Practices and Additional Precautions for Preventing the Transmission of Infection in Healthcare Settings* (https://www.canada.ca/en/public-health/services/publications/diseases-conditions/routine-practices-precautions-healthcare-associated-infections.html)

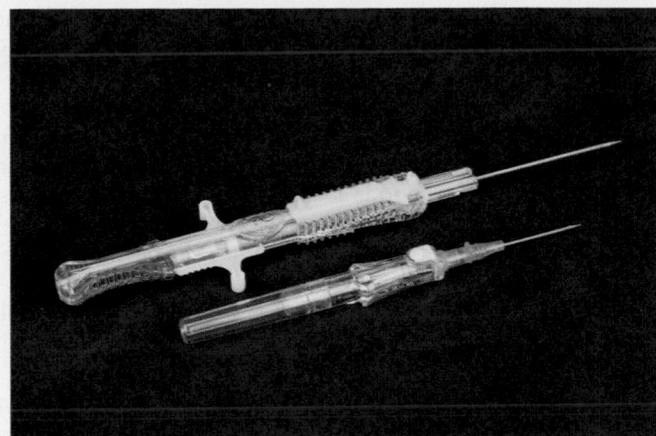

FIG 29.1 Peripheral venous access devices (PVADs): Midline (top) and short-peripheral (bottom). *(Courtesy Burl Jantzen.)*

PRINCIPLES FOR PRACTICE

- Evidence-informed practices guide the safe, efficient, high-quality care necessary to provide vascular access and infusion therapy.
- Successful vascular access depends on a thorough patient assessment, correct device and site selection, and catheter insertion technique.
- Indications and protocols for all aspects of vascular access and infusion therapy are established in practice guidelines and employer policies, informed by the best evidence, and carried out according to manufacturer directions for use (INS, 2016a).
- Assessments of a patient's anatomy and physiology of the circulatory system, fluid and electrolyte balance, disease pathophysiology, allergies, and response to illness are essential for safe infusion therapy.
- The 10 rights of medication administration for administrating parenteral solutions or medications are essential (see Chapters 20 and 22).
- Knowledge of the following is required to ensure safe infusion therapy: most appropriate vascular access device (VAD) required for the plan of care; medications or solutions to be infused; how to initiate and regulate the infusion; care and maintenance of the VAD and how to identity complications; use of infusion-related devices.

Intravenous (IV) Catheters

- To administer IV infusates and medications, a VAD is inserted into a vein. VADs can be peripherally (i.e., short-peripheral, midline [Fig. 29.1]) or centrally (i.e., tunnelled, nontunnelled, peripherally inserted central catheter [PICC], implanted port [intravenous access device, or IVAD]) located.
- When selecting the appropriate VAD, consider a patient's prescribed therapy, anticipated duration of treatment, and vascular characteristics, as well as the patient's age, comorbidities, history of infusion therapy, preference for VAD location, and resources available to care for the device (INS, 2016a).

Intravenous Solutions

- Many prepared IV solutions are available for use (Table 29.1).
- IV solutions fall into several categories: isotonic, hypotonic, and hypertonic. Isotonic solutions have the same osmolality as body fluids.
- Administer IV solutions as prescribed.

TABLE 29.1

Intravenous Solutions

Solution	Concentration	Other Names
Dextrose in Water Solutions		
Dextrose 5% in water*	Isotonic	D_5W
Dextrose 10% in water	Hypertonic	$D_{10}W$
Dextrose 50% in water	Hypertonic	$D_{50}W$
Saline Solutions		
0.45% sodium chloride (half NS)	Hypotonic	½ NS 0.45% NS
0.33% sodium chloride (one-third NS)	Hypotonic	⅓ NS
0.9% sodium chloride† (NS)	Isotonic	NS 0.9% NS 0.9% NaCl
3–5% sodium chloride	Hypertonic	3–5% NS 3–5% NaCl
Dextrose in Saline Solutions		
Dextrose 5% in 0.9% sodium chloride	Hypertonic	$D_5$0.9% NaCl $D_5$0.9% NS D_5 NS
Dextrose 5% in 0.45% sodium chloride	Hypertonic	$D_5$0.45% NaCl $D_5$0.45% NS D_5 ½ NS
Multiple Electrolyte Solutions		
Lactated Ringer's‡	Isotonic	LR
Dextrose 5% in lactated Ringer's	Hypertonic	D_5LR

LR, Lactated Ringer's; *NaCl,* sodium chloride; *NS,* Normal saline.
*Dextrose is quickly metabolized, leaving free water to be distributed evenly in all fluid compartments.
†Although it is isotonic because the total concentration of electrolytes equals plasma concentration, it contains 154 mmol of both sodium and chloride, which is a higher concentration of these electrolytes than is found in the plasma, which can cause fluid volume excess.
‡Contains sodium, potassium, calcium, chloride, and lactate.

- Isotonic solutions can cause increased risk for fluid overload in patients with renal or cardiac disease; hypotonic solutions can exacerbate a hypotensive state; and hypertonic solutions are irritating to the vein and can cause increased risk of heart failure and pulmonary edema.
- Short-peripheral catheters are not recommended for continuous vesicant therapy, parenteral nutrition, or infusates with an osmolarity greater than 900 mOsm/L (INS, 2016a). Solutions or medications with low or high pH (<5 or >9) may also contribute to infusion-related complications (e.g., phlebitis). To prevent these complications, a central venous access device (CVAD) is recommended. (INS, 2016a).
- Premixed solutions contain medications or electrolytes added by the manufacturer. These solutions have increased stability and allow for selecting the correct medication and diluents.
- Commercially prepared solutions are recommended for use, to reduce risks of infection and reconstitutions errors.
- A patient's specific fluid and electrolyte imbalance and serum electrolyte values guide selection of the appropriate IV fluid (Jantzen & Felver, 2018).

PERSON-CENTRED CARE

- Communication, comfort, and education are essential components of person-centred care.
- Person-centred nursing practice should be implemented: Engage patients in the decision-making process and collaborate on the plan of care. This includes soliciting and responding to patient preferences regarding their active involvement and the involvement of their caregivers.
- Preparing the patient prior to initiation of VAD or infusion therapy reduces their anxiety. Become familiar with the patient's past experience and current concerns and expectations. Speak directly to patients and answer questions as honestly as possible.
- Provide privacy throughout the procedure—during assessment, initiation of the VAD, and patient education.
- Patient education should be clear and concise and adapted for individual abilities and learning needs (Foster, Idossa, Lih-Wen, et al., 2016).
- When preparing for insertion, use techniques that minimize discomfort. Place patients in a comfortable position. Consider using local anaesthetic drugs (see employer policy) based on patient condition, needs, risks, benefits, and anticipated discomfort of the procedure (INS, 2016a).
- Effective education for patients and caregivers includes assessment of their learning needs, capabilities, and preferences. This includes attending to patients' cultural and linguistic needs and recognizing diversity.
- Consider the environment and context for treatment and education. Minimize distractions and interruptions during education, with initiation of VAD, and while initiating therapy.
- Patient teaching should also include information regarding care of the VAD, infection prevention, and potential VAD complications and the signs and symptoms to report (INS, 2016a).
- Infusion therapy skills that require hands-on care may present challenges for certain cultures; therefore, begin by explaining what kind of touching is required and ask permission before proceeding.
- Pain is an individual experience. Perception and expressions of pain vary with individuals and may be informed by cultural or personal beliefs and values and past experience.

EVIDENCE-INFORMED PRACTICE

Nurses must incorporate evidence-informed practice and clinical expertise when providing vascular access and infusion therapy (INS, 2016a).

- Nurses should critically evaluate and implement improvements to patient care based on current research and expert knowledge. Clinical quality indicators may include surveillance and analysis of infection rates (e.g., catheter-related bloodstream infections [CRBSI]) and infection prevention practices.
- Quality improvement engagement involves surveillance and analysis of infection rates, infection-prevention practices, and infusion-related patient quality indicators, such as occurrence of central line–associated bloodstream infection (CLABSI) and number of attempts at VAD insertion. Implementation of quality indicators and benchmarks develops a culture of accountability (INS, 2016a).
- For intermittent therapy, a short-peripheral IV (peripheral vascular access device [PVAD]) or midline device can be locked with preservative-free 0.9% sodium chloride (normal saline [NS]) in adults (INS, 2016a). Commercially available prefilled syringes

are used to reduce the risk of CRBSI. Use a minimum volume equal to twice the internal volume of the catheter system (INS, 2016a).
- To lock a central venous access device (CVAD) a number of solutions can be used, including sodium chloride or heparin solutions. Currently, there is insufficient evidence to recommend heparin or sodium chloride locking solutions for all CVADs. Heparin is derived from animal products (e.g., porcine, bovine) and may be in conflict with some patients' religious beliefs (INS, 2016a).
- Alternative locking solutions, such as sodium citrate, ethanol, taurolidine, or tetrasodium EDTA, may be considered for certain populations.
- Remove VADs for unresolved complication and when no longer necessary for the plan of care (INS, 2016a).
- Disinfection caps that contain a sponge saturated with 70% alcohol placed on the end of the needle-free connector between intermittent infusions provide active disinfection of the needle-free connector and thus do not require disinfection prior to the first access after removal. These caps have been shown to reduce intraluminal contamination, peripheral catheter bloodstream infections, and CLABSI rates (Voor in 't holt, Helder, Vos, et al., 2017).
- Primary and secondary continuous administration sets used to administer solutions other than lipid, blood, or blood products should be changed no more often than every 96 hours or according to employer policy (INS, 2016a).

SAFETY GUIDELINES

- Conduct a complete history and physical, including vital signs, and review laboratory findings before initiating any solutions or medications. Consider prolonged environmental conditions that affect a patient's fluid status (e.g., exposure to hot, humid weather) and lead to fluid and electrolyte imbalances, particularly in the infant, older person, and chronically ill.
- Know the indications for prescribed therapy before initiating infusion therapy. Obtain and review the health care provider's prescription to ensure appropriateness of the prescribed solution or medication for the patient's age, health status, medical diagnosis, allergy status, and acuity, and the VAD type and tip location, dose, frequency, and route of administration (INS, 2016b).
- Assess all VADs for patency and functioning before initiating infusion therapy. Observe site for signs and symptoms of complications (see Tables 29.3 and 29.4). Using a 10-mL syringe, assess for patency by slowly aspirating the VAD for blood return and flush to test for resistance. Do not force if resistance is evident. Palpate the site and ask patient if they are experiencing any discomfort (INS, 2016a, 2016b).
- Reduce risk for administration set misconnections by tracing the path between infusion and patient, labelling administration sets near patient connection and solution container, routing tubings with different purposes in different directions, and informing the patient, caregivers, and unregulated care providers (UCPs) to seek help, if needed, with connecting or disconnecting devices or infusions.
- Maintain sterility of VAD administration set at all times, and discard device if contamination is suspected (Box 29.1).
- Know and implement guidelines in *Routine Practices and Additional Precautions for Preventing the Transmission of Infection in Healthcare Settings* (PHAC, 2016) related to occupational exposure to bloodborne pathogens (Box 29.2).

BOX 29.1

Infusion Nurses Society (INS) Standards to Decrease Intravascular Infection Related to Intravenous Therapy

- Perform hand hygiene before providing any assessment or care and maintenance of a vascular access device (VAD).
- Use of an aseptic non-touch technique (ANTT) and good standards of hand hygiene can reduce the risk of infection when using central vascular access devices (CVADs). Refer to clinical guidelines on ANTT for intravenous therapy and hand hygiene (ANTT, 2018).
- Use an approved antiseptic solution to cleanse the skin prior to VAD insertion and for care and maintenance of the site. Chlorhexidine gluconate (CHG) 2% with 70% isopropyl alcohol is preferred for use on adult patients and on children older than 2 months of age. This solution has an immediate action to reduce bacteria load on the skin, as well as persistent activity for up to 7 days. If an alternative antiseptic is required because of patient sensitivity, consider the use of povidone-iodine, 70% alcohol, or tincture of iodine.
- Use a vigorous friction scrub to clean the skin; a back-and-forth motion in two different directions is recommended. This method promotes binding of the CHG to the layer of skin and improves efficacy.
- Always allow antiseptic solutions to completely dry prior to insertion and before applying a dressing. CHG and alcohol solutions require a minimum of 30 seconds' dry time; CHG in an aqueous solution requires 3 minutes and povidone iodine, at least 1.5–2 minutes. Do not blot or fan solution or wipe it away to dry.
- Assess PVAD insertion site and surrounding tissue a minimum of every 4 hours for patients in the hospital and daily when in the community.

- CVADs should be assessed at least once per day in acute care patients and with every scheduled community care visit.
- Assess VAD site for signs and symptoms of complication. Visually inspect for redness, swelling, drainage, or leaking; palpate through an intact dressing for any pain, discomfort, or cording along the vein pathway.
- Ensure that the dressing is dry and occlusive. If dressing is loose, wet, or soiled, change it immediately. The site must be cleaned with appropriate antiseptic before a new sterile dressing is applied.
- Frequency of dressing change is based on the type of dressing used. Transparent semipermeable membrane (TSM) dressings must be changed every 5–7 days, gauze dressings are changed every 2 days.
- Change needle-free connectors using ANTT, a minimum of every 7 days if removed for any reason, if contamination is suspected, or if it cannot be flushed clear of blood.
- Use an alcohol swab or CHG and alcohol to scrub the hub of the needle-free connector before each access.
- Change administration sets, including add-on devices, according to type of infusion (intermittent or continuous) and with placement of a new VAD. Always change immediately if contamination is suspected.
- Always attach a sterile end cap to the male end of intermittent tubing when not in use.

Modified from Infusion Nurses Society. (2016). Infusion therapy standards of practice. *Journal of Intravenous Nursing, 39*(Suppl. 1), 1S; Aseptic Non Touch Technique (ANTT). (2018). *ANTT core clinical guidelines, 2018*. Retrieved from http://antt.org/ANTT_Site/core_guidelines.html.

BOX 29.2

Standards for Reducing Occupational Exposure to Bloodborne Pathogens

1. Wear gloves when performing procedures if there is a reasonable expectation of contact with blood or body fluids (e.g., peripheral vascular access device [PVAD] initiation, dressing changes, blood draws).
2. Use safety-engineered equipment according to instruction for use, to reduce the risks of needle-stick injury.
3. Always place medical sharps in a puncture-resistant, leakproof container identified for biohazard use immediately after their use. Do not overfill sharps container over observer-recommended fill line, close the container securely, and discard appropriately according to employer policy.

4. Do not bend, shear, recap, or remove contaminated needles before disposing in sharps container.
5. Follow employer and Public Health Agency of Canada (2016) standards for safe handling of all medical sharps and hazardous substances.
6. Report and document all exposure to potentially infectious material, including sharps injuries, according to employer procedure.
7. Facilities must have engineering and work practice controls to eliminate or minimize employee exposure.

Modified from Public Health Agency of Canada. (2016). *Routine practices and additional precautions for preventing the transmission of infection in healthcare settings.* Ottawa: Author. Retrieved from https://www.canada.ca/content/dam/phac-aspc/documents/services/publications/diseases-conditions/routine-practices-precautions-healthcare-associated-infections/routine-practices-precautions-healthcare-associated-infections-2016-FINAL-eng.pdf.

◆ SKILL 29.1 Insertion of a Short-Peripheral Intravenous Access Device

NSO *Nursing Skills Online Intravenous Fluid Therapy Module 12 / Lessons 1 and 2*

A vascular access device (VAD) provides access to the venous system to deliver solutions and medications or blood and blood products. Assessment and selection of the most appropriate VAD are essential for safe, effective delivery of infusates. Peripheral vascular access devices (PVADs) are available in a variety of types, with a selection of gauge size and length (see Fig. 29.1; Table 29.2). The most commonly used PVAD is an over-the-needle catheter. This type includes a metal stylet to pierce the skin and a flexible catheter that is threaded into the vein. PVADs can be used to deliver continuous and intermittent infusion therapy; however, they are not recommended for continuous vesicant infusates, or solutions or medications with an osmolarity of greater than 900 mOsm/L (INS 2016a).

Delegation and Collaboration

The skill of inserting a PVAD may be completed by other members of the health care team who have appropriate education and if the skill is within their governing body's scope of practice. Assessment and care of PVADs requires interprofessional collaboration to ensure effective communication and enhance patient safety. Always refer to employer policy.

The skill of inserting a PVAD cannot be performed by an unregulated care provider (UCP). However, it is important for UCPs to report to the nurse the following immediately:

- Signs and symptoms of complications (redness, swelling, leaking, bleeding, or drainage under the dressing, or patient expression of pain or discomfort)

TABLE 29.2

Recommendations for Short-Peripheral Catheter Selection

Catheter Size (Gauge)	Clinical Indication
14, 16, 18	Trauma, surgery, rapid blood transfusions, and rapid fluid replacement
20	Continuous or intermittent infusions in adults; administration of blood transfusions in adults
22	Continuous or intermittent infusions in adults, children, neonates, and older persons; administration of blood or blood product in adults, children, neonates, and older persons
24	Continuous or intermittent infusions in adults, children, neonates, and older persons; administration of blood or blood product in adults, children, neonates, and older persons

Modified from Infusion Nurses Society (INS). (2016). *Policy and procedures for infusion therapy* (5th ed.). Norwood, MA: Author.

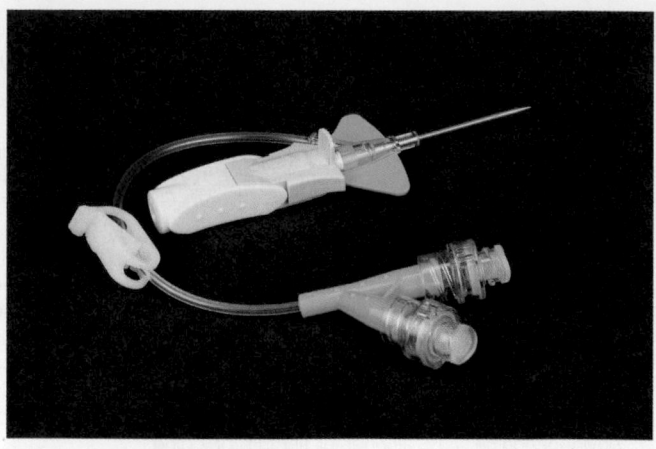

FIG 29.2 Short-peripheral IV catheter with integrated extension set and stabilization platform. (*Courtesy Burl Jantzen.*)

- A loose, wet, or soiled dressing
- Low volume in an intravenous (IV) solution bag
- Any electronic infusion device alarms

Equipment

- Use a commercially prepared IV start kit or collect the following:
  - Single-use tourniquet, selected PVAD, transparent semipermeable membrane (TSM) dressing with securement properties (preferred)
  - Antiseptic swab or wipe (chlorhexidine gluconate [CHG] and alcohol preferred; alternates include 2% CHG, povidone-iodine, or 70% alcohol)

- 5×5–cm (2×2–inch) gauze pads
- Tape
- Clean gloves (or sterile gloves if repalpation of the vein is required after skin antiseptics)
- 10-mL prefilled saline syringe
- Single-use hair clippers or scissors for hair removal, if indicated
- Skin barrier swab, for sensitive skin.
- Appropriate short-peripheral IV catheter with safety mechanism for venipuncture (Fig. 29.2)
- Short extension set with needle-free connector, if not using an integrated extension set. Vein visualization device, as needed
- Patient gown with snaps at shoulder seams, if available (makes removal during infusion therapy easier)
- Biomedical container for disposal of medical sharps

STEP	RATIONALE

ASSESSMENT

1. Confirm prescription for PVAD in patient's record.

A health care provider's prescription is required to initiate a VAD, except in the case of an emergency (INS, 2016a). A prescription for IV medications is sufficient for PVAD insertion. Verification that prescription is complete prevents medication errors.

2. Review patient allergies or skin sensitivities related to equipment required for insertion (e.g., latex, antiseptics, dressing adhesives, skin barrier solution).

Prevents unnecessary complications or discomfort. Equipment used during PVAD insertion may contain substances to which patient is allergic.

3. Review prescribed therapy, anticipated length of treatment, and patient characteristics to ensure the most appropriate VAD is selected. (e.g., PVAD or central venous access device [CVAD])

Infusions of continuous vesicants or solution with an osmolarity of greater than 900 mOsm/L are not recommended for PVADs.

Patient assessment must include age, history of vascular access, comorbidities, and patient preferences.

4. Consider most appropriate gauge of catheter required for infusion therapy or diagnostics.

Use the smallest gauge PVAD with the fewest number of lumens. This promotes vein preservation, reduces risks of phlebitis, and causes the least discomfort.

5. Assess patient's knowledge of procedure, reason for prescribed therapy, and arm placement preference.

Provides person-centred care by determining level of emotional support and instruction needed.

6. If administering IV fluid, assess for clinical factors or conditions that will respond to or be affected by administration of IV solutions (see Skill 29.2).

Provides baseline to determine effectiveness of prescribed therapy. A systems approach is recommended to assess for fluid and electrolyte imbalances (Jantzen & Felver, 2018).

STEP	RATIONALE

NURSING DIAGNOSES

- Anxiety
- Insufficient knowledge regarding infusion therapy

- Potential for pain related to vascular catheter insertion
- Potential for infection

- Potential for complications of vascular access
- Potential for electrolyte imbalance

Related factors/Risk factors are individualized on the basis of patient's condition or needs.

PLANNING

1. Expected outcomes following completion of procedure:
- PVAD selection is the most appropriate for prescribed therapy and vessel size.

- Patient's PVAD remains patent for delivery of infusion therapy and site is free of complications.
- Patient is able to explain purpose and risks related to PVAD placement and will be aware to report signs and symptoms of complications immediately.

2. Collect appropriate equipment.

Ensures patient safety, reinforces the importance of vein preservation, and improves patient's experience and satisfaction.

Ensures safe and effective delivery of required therapy; PVAD is without complications (INS, 2016a).

Demonstrates learning and conforms with informed consent (Foster et al., 2016). Ensures safe delivery of care with a person-centred approach (INS, 2016a).

Ensures patient safety and reduces anxiety when the insertion is done with dexterity and efficiency.

IMPLEMENTATION

1. Identify patient using at least two person-specific identifiers (e.g., name and date of birth or name and medical record number) according to employer policy. Compare identifiers with information on patient's medical record and armband.

2. Provide patient education about rationale for infusion, including solution and medications prescribed; procedure for initiating PVAD; and signs and symptoms of complications (e.g., redness, pain tenderness, swelling, bleeding, drainage, or leaking at insertion site). Include rationale for device selection (e.g., short-term therapy, comfort). Obtain informed consent.

3. Change patient's gown or clothing to allow for easy removal. A gown with snaps at the shoulder may be used, if available.

4. Ensure patient is sitting or lying in a comfortable position that provides adequate light and positioning for vein assessment and PVAD insertion.

5. Perform hand hygiene. Collect and organize equipment on clean, clutter-free bedside stand or over-bed table. Wipe surface with an antiseptic wipe prior to use.

6. Apply tourniquet on upper arm or at least 10 cm (4 in.) above intended insertion site. Do not apply too tightly. Assess patient level of comfort and confirm presence of pulse distal to the tourniquet.

Ensures correct patient. Complies with Accreditation Canada's standards and improves patient safety (Accreditation Canada, 2019).

Promotes person-centred care and patient safety.

Reduce risk of inadvertently dislodging VAD or administration set when changing.

Promotes comfort, relaxation, and vasodilation for the patient. Also enables good body mechanics to prevent injury and to increase opportunity for successful insertion.

Reduces transmission of infection and contamination of equipment (INS, 2016a). Easy access to equipment improves efficiency.

The tourniquet provides dilation of the vein for ease of visualization or palpation; it should impede venous flow while maintaining arterial circulation. Caution should be used with older persons or patients who have fragile skin. Apply over patient gown to prevent skin impairments or pulling of arm hair.

Consider use of a blood pressure cuff for patient comfort. Inflate to approximately 50 mmHg to apply appropriate amount of pressure.

STEP	RATIONALE

IMPLEMENTATION

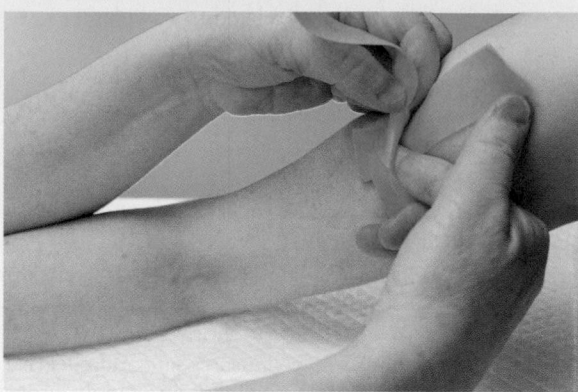

Step 6 Application of tourniquet (*Courtesy Patrick Coble.*)

7. Select the most appropriate vein and location through visual inspection and palpation (see illustration, Step 7A), using the following guidelines:
   - Veins should feel soft and bouncy and be adequate in size to accommodate the selected catheter gauge.
   - Use the most distal site above the wrist.
   - Do not use areas of flexion (e.g., antecubital fossa) unless required for less than 48 hours or in an emergency situation.
   - Avoid veins located in the hands unless for short-term use.
   - Do not use a site below a failed insertion attempt, unless completely healed.
   - Skin must be intact and free of signs of infection.
   - Ensure a minimum of 8 cm (3.2 in.) or three fingers above the wrist.
   - Do not use an arm that has a fistula or a graft for dialysis.
   - Avoid the use of veins in the upper extremity on the affected side of breast surgery with axillary node dissection or lymphedema, after radiation, or with arteriovenous (AV) fistulas or grafts, or in an affected extremity from a cerebrovascular accident (CVA) (INS, 2016a).
   - Consider use of heat (warm blanket or compress) to enhance vasodilation of the vein, to improve visualization and ability to palpate vein.

Use smallest-gauge peripheral catheter that will accommodate prescribed therapy and patient need (INS, 2016a).
   - Promotes insertion success and vein preservation and decreases risk of phlebitis.
   - Use of the hands can be very painful, limiting the patient's activities of daily living and ability to perform hand hygiene.
   - Areas of flexion cause patients discomfort and disrupt infusions. These patients have significantly higher risks of infiltration and of developing mechanical or bacterial phlebitis due to movement of the catheter and inability to maintain an occlusive dressing.
   - Venipuncture below a failed PVAD may lead to infiltration or extravasation of infusates.
   - Insertion attempt in an area of skin impairment increases risk of infection and patient discomfort.
   - Insertion sites at the wrist are associated with increased risks of nerve damage.
   - Using vein sites that may have impaired circulation or decreased sensation may increase risk of complications.
   - Use of heat promotes comfort, decreases anxiety, and prevents vasoconstriction.

Clinical Decision Point *Consider the use of vein visualization devices (Fig. 29.3) when no venous access is visible or easily palpated (if available in the facility). Options may include near-infrared light devices or ultrasound (requires additional education). Using vein visualization devices improves success of cannulation, decreases risks associated with traumatic or missed insertion attempts, and improves patient comfort.*

8. Remove tourniquet and prepare supplies.

9. Select appropriate-size catheter; open and prepare sterile packages using sterile aseptic technique (see Chapter 8) (see illustration).

If assessment of vein has taken longer than 1 minute, remove tourniquet to avoid vein fatigue and patient discomfort.
Use smallest-gauge peripheral catheter that will accommodate prescribed therapy and patient need (INS, 2016a). Do not remove backing from sterile dressing until ready to secure PVAD. Leave IV in the sterile packaging until ready to insert, to maintain aseptic technique.

Clinical Decision Point *Consider the required therapy and vein assessment to determine the most appropriate gauge of catheter and site selection.*

IMPLEMENTATION

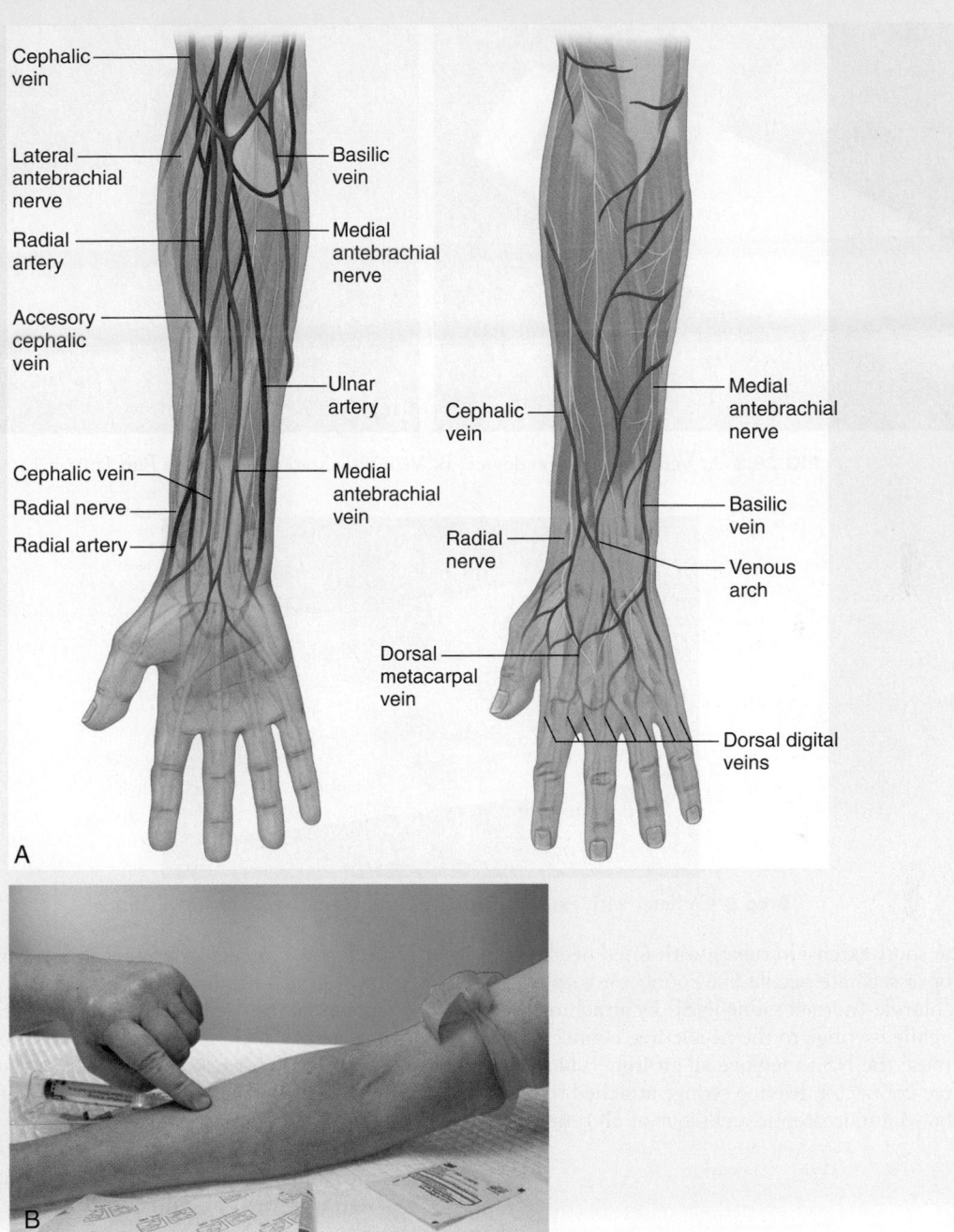

Step 7 A, Vein map. **B,** Palpate vein and select site. (*A, From Canadian Vascular Access Association. B, Courtesy Patrick Coble.*)

STEP	RATIONALE

IMPLEMENTATION

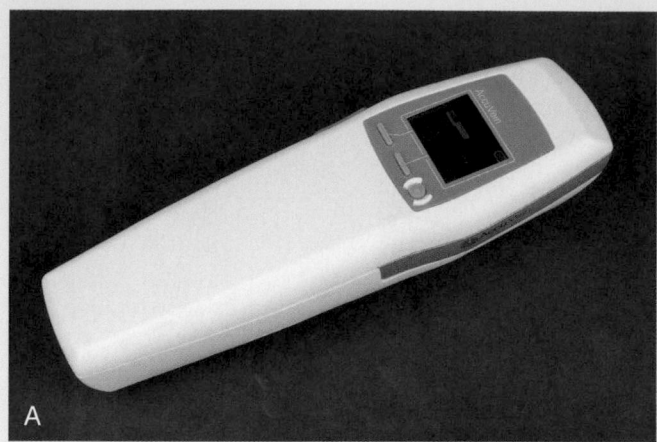
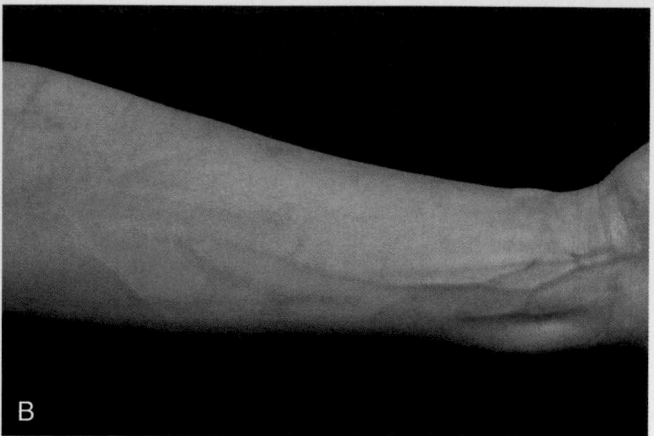

FIG 29.3 A, Vein visualization device. **B,** Vein visualization. *(Courtesy Burl Jantzen.)*

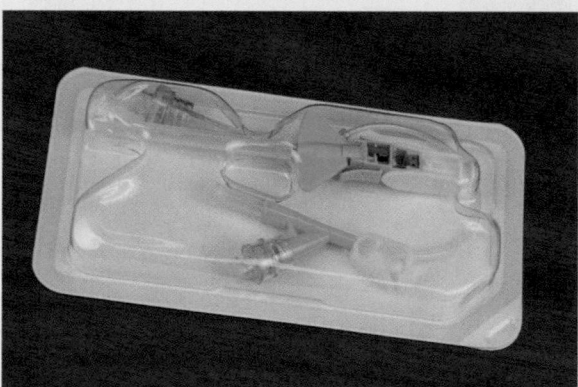

Step 9 Catheter with extension set sterile packaging. *(Courtesy Burl Jantzen.)*

10. Prime the short extension tubing with fused needle-free connector or separate needle-free connector with 0.9% sodium chloride (normal saline [NS]) by attaching the 10-mL prefilled syringe to the needle-free connector. Slowly infuse the NS to remove all air from tubing and needle-free connector, leaving syringe attached to the connector. Maintain aseptic technique at all times.

Needle-free connectors protect health care workers by providing a needle-free system, therefore eliminating potential for needle-stick injuries (INS, 2016a).

Integrated IV catheter and extensions provide a closed system, ensuring lower risk of blood exposure and less manipulation of the catheter hub, decreasing risks of mechanical and bacterial phlebitis.

Removing all air with NS or allowing blood to flow back in the integrated system prevents air from entering the patient's vein on PVAD insertion.

Clinical Decision Point *If an integrated IV extension set is not in use in the facility, short extension sets are recommended for use with PVAD for continuous and intermittent infusions. This reduces catheter manipulation and improves ease of IV administration set change, decreasing risks of contamination at catheter hub. All connections should be of a Luer-Lok type* (INS, 2016a).

11. Prepare insertion site. If hair removal is required, use surgical clipper or scissors to trim hair. If site is visibly soiled, clean with antiseptic soap and water prior to application of antiseptic solution.

Razors should not be used, as they cause micro-cuts in the skin that can lead to increased risks of infection (INS 2016a). Removal of hair is very important to obtain adequate skin antisepsis and maintain an occlusive dressing to prevent infection. Cleaning the skin prior to application of antiseptic solutions improves efficacy.

12. Perform hand hygiene before applying gloves.

Decreases potential risk of microbial contamination and cross-contamination (INS, 2016a).

STEP	RATIONALE

IMPLEMENTATION

Clinical Decision Point *Gloves are not necessary to locate the vein but must be applied for VAD insertion using a no-touch technique where the site is not palpated after skin antisepsis (INS, 2016a, 2016b).*

13. Reapply tourniquet using the same technique for vein assessment.	With more experienced inserters, assessment and insertion may be completed at the same application site of the tourniquet. Always be aware of the length of time the tourniquet is in place. It should not exceed 1 minute.
14. With your fingertip, palpate selected vein at intended insertion site by pressing downward. Note resilient, soft, bouncy feeling while releasing pressure.	Fingertip is more sensitive and better for assessing vein location and condition.

Clinical Decision Point *Vigorous friction, slapping, or hard tapping of a vein, especially in older persons, can cause venous constriction and bruising and hematoma (INS, 2016d).*

Clinical Decision Point *If vein palpation is necessary after performing skin antisepsis, use sterile gloves for palpation or perform skin antisepsis again, because touching a cleaned area introduces microorganisms from your finger to the site (INS, 2016a, 2016b).*

15. Clean insertion site with an antiseptic solution (see illustration) as follows: a) CHG and alcohol is preferred. Apply using a friction scrub in a back-and-forth motion for a minimum of 30 seconds. Solution must be allowed to completely air dry prior to PVAD insertion. b) Povidone iodine must remain on the skin for 1.5 to 2 minutes after application to completely dry and for adequate antisepsis. c) CHG without alcohol dry time is a minimum of 3 minutes for adequate antisepsis (INS, 2016b).	A combination of CHG and alcohol is preferred because it is a broad-spectrum biocide effective against Gram-positive and Gram-negative bacteria and fungi. It has a quicker kill rate than other antimicrobials and has been shown to inhibit growth for at least 48 hours. The addition of alcohol decreases drying time on the skin. All antiseptic solutions must be applied according to instructions for use to ensure adequate antisepsis to reduce risks of insertion-site and systemic infections. Mechanical friction enables penetration of the solution to the epidermal layers of skin. Antiseptics must be allowed to fully dry to assure efficacy. Do not wipe, blot, or fan the skin or blow on it to speed dry time (see Box 29.1).
16. Stabilize the vein with nondominant hand by placing fingers above and below intended insertion site, pulling skin taut.	Stabilization of the vein for needle insertion is key to preventing rolling of the vein. Stretching the skin taut decreases drag during insertion.
17. Perform venipuncture with bevel up, align catheter on top of intended insertion site at approximately a 10- to 15-degree angle, and puncture the skin and anterior vein wall (INS, 2016a). Observe for blood return in catheter (flashback) (see illustration). If patient experiences any paresthesia-like pain, including electrical shock, tingling, burning, or numbness, remove PVAD immediately to prevent potential nerve damage.	Ensure patient is aware of anticipating needle-stick and to remain as still as possible. Some manufactures require loosening of the catheter from the needle prior to insertion; follow specific instruction for use.

Clinical Decision Point *Use each VAD only once for each insertion attempt.*

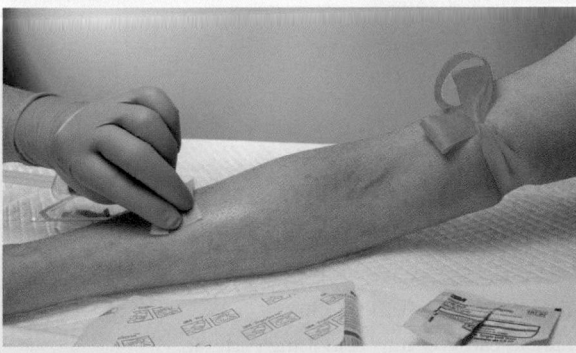

Step 15 Clean venipuncture site. (*Courtesy Patrick Coble.*)

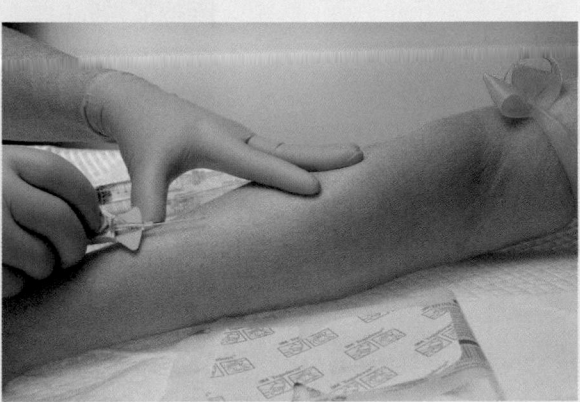

STEP 16 Stabilize vein. (*Courtesy Patrick Coble.*)

STEP	RATIONALE

IMPLEMENTATION

18. Once blood return is observed in the catheter or flashback chamber, lower the angle so it is parallel with the skin. Keeping skin taut, advance the needle slightly farther into the vein. Advance or thread catheter into the vein using the push-off tab and then release the tourniquet (see illustrations). If catheter does not thread, do not reinsert the needle into the catheter.

Lowering the angle after blood return decreases risk of puncturing the posterior vein wall.

Advancing with skin taut will ensure the catheter and needle tip are inside the vein wall.

Do not push using the catheter hub, as this contaminates the lumen. Using an integrated catheter/extension closed system eliminates this potential risk.

Reinsertion of the needle into the catheter can cause the catheter to shear off and embolize into the vein.

Advancing entire stylet into vein may penetrate wall of vein, resulting in hematoma.

Advancing catheter with your finger on the open hub causes contamination (INS, 2016a).

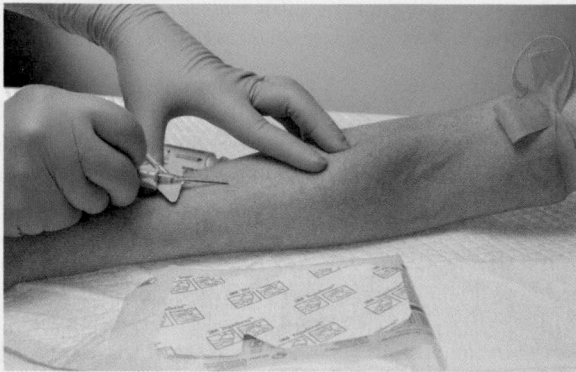

STEP 17 Perform venipuncture and observe for flashback. (*Courtesy Patrick Coble.*)

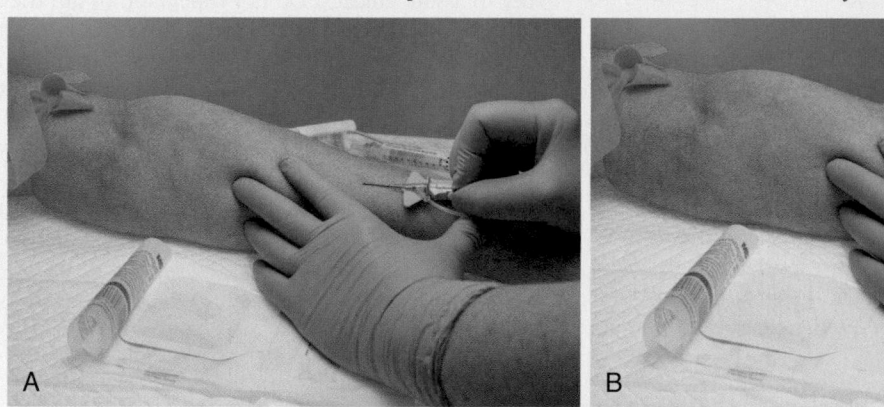

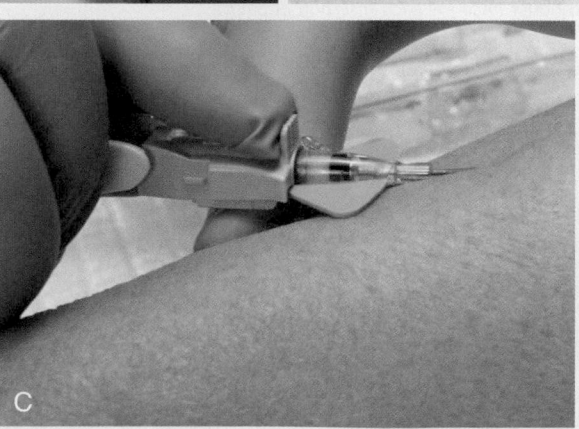

STEP 18 A, Lower catheter. **B,** Advance and thread. **C,** Thread catheter into vein using push tab. (*Courtesy Patrick Coble.*)

STEP	RATIONALE

IMPLEMENTATION

Clinical Decision Point *A single clinician should not make more than two attempts at initiating a PVAD, and total attempts should be limited to no more than four (INS, 2016a).*

19. **a)** Attach extension set or needle-free connector to catheter, depending on type of catheter used. If the PVAD has a blood-control mechanism (e.g., clamp on integrated extension or filter in hub), this will stop blood flow until add-on extension or needle-free connector is attached (see illustration). If PVAD does not have blood control, apply gentle but firm pressure above the insertion site to occlude blood flow, then attach add-on device. Avoid touching sterile connection ends.

  b) *Option:* Administration set can be attached directly to catheter hub in place of short extension tubing or needle-free connector.

Blood-control PVADs significantly decrease risk of blood exposure and enable attachment of add-on devices without risk of hub contamination.

Use aseptic technique when securing extension or needle-free connectors to catheter hub (see Box 29.2).

Prompt connection maintains patency of vein and reduces backflow of blood. Digital pressure minimizes blood loss and allows attachment of extension set or needle-free connector (INS, 2016b).

20. Apply sterile transparent securement dressing to cover and protect the insertion site (see illustration). Do not apply unsterile tape around the catheter, over the catheter hub, or under the sterile dressing.

Loop the extension tubing alongside the dressing and secure with a piece of tape for patient comfort and additional securement (see illustration). Do not obstruct the PVAD site.

Stretch netting may be used over the dressing to keep tubing from catching on clothing. Do not use rolled bandages.

Occlusive, dry dressings prevent mechanical and bacterial phlebitis and loss of access (see Box 29.1).

Dressing with securement properties or an addition of a stabilization device decreases risks of catheter dislodgement and movement.

Tape on top of TSM dressing prevents moisture from being carried away from skin. Removal of tape from TSM dressing can tear dressing and cause catheter dislodgement. Rolls of nonsterile tape can become contaminated with pathogenic bacteria and increased risk of PVAD contamination if applied under the sterile dressing.

Optional: A risk of medical adhesive-related skin injury (MARSI) is increased as a result of age, joint movement, and edema; therefore, a skin protectant prior to dressing application may be considered (INS 2016a). TSM dressing allows for visualization of the insertion site and surrounding area for assessment of complications.

If a gauze dressing is required because of patient sensitivities to the TSM dressing, assessment must be performed by palpation over the dressing, observing for any drainage and patient discomfort.

Rolled bandages can impair circulation or flow of infusion and obscure visualization for site assessment of complications.

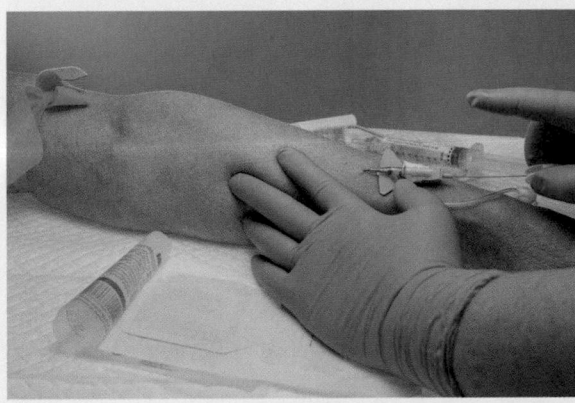

STEP 19 Engage safety mechanism. *(Courtesy Patrick Coble.)*

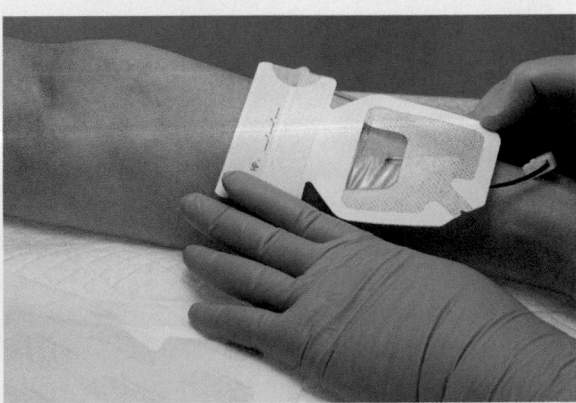

STEP 20 Apply dressing. *(Courtesy Patrick Coble.)*

STEP	RATIONALE

IMPLEMENTATION

21. Attach prefilled flush syringe of 0.9% sodium chloride to needle-free connector and flush using a push–pause technique to clear all visible blood from the extension set and needle-free connector. Leave a small amount of NS in the flush syringe to prevent syringe-induced blood reflux in the catheter (see illustration). If syringe was not previously attached to the extension set or needle-free connector when preparing supplies, scrub the connector and flush.	Clearing blood prevents risk of catheter occlusion and infection. If patient experiences discomfort or swelling, or leakage of fluid is observed during flushing, this indicates the catheter is no longer in the vein and must be removed immediately.
22. a) Remove flush syringe from needle-free connector, using the appropriate technique (see illustration A). **b)** Refer to Skill 29.2 if initiating infusion.	Needle-free connectors come in many types and styles; it is important to know if the connector has neutral, negative, or positive displacement properties to determine if a specific clamping sequence is required to prevent reflux of blood into the PVAD on removal of the syringe.

Clinical Decision Point *Needle-free connectors protect health care workers and decrease risk for needle-stick injuries. They have different internal mechanisms for fluid displacement and vary in the flush–clamp–disconnect sequence to prevent reflux of blood into the catheter on disconnection (INS, 2016a).*

The sequence depends on the type of internal mechanism:
- *Neutral displacement devices do not have a specified flush–clamp–disconnect sequence.*
- *For negative-pressure displacement devices, flush, clamp catheter, then disconnect syringe.*
- *For positive-pressure displacement, flush, disconnect syringe, then clamp catheter.*

23. Observe insertion site for swelling, with flush.	Swelling indicates catheter is no longer in the vein, which requires immediate catheter removal.
24. Label dressing according to employer policy (see illustration). Include date of insertion, and initials.	PVADs are changed on the basis of clinical assessment. It is important to know the insertion date to determine the length of time the PVAD has been in place and to alert the need for dressing change (see Box 29.1). Monitor for MARSI.
25. Dispose of any sharps in appropriate container, discard supplies, remove gloves, and perform hand hygiene.	Reduces transmission of microorganisms; prevents accidental needle-stick injuries (PHAC, 2016).
26. Review care and maintenance of PVAD and report any signs and symptoms of complications immediately to a health care provider.	Promotes patient engagement in care of PVAD.

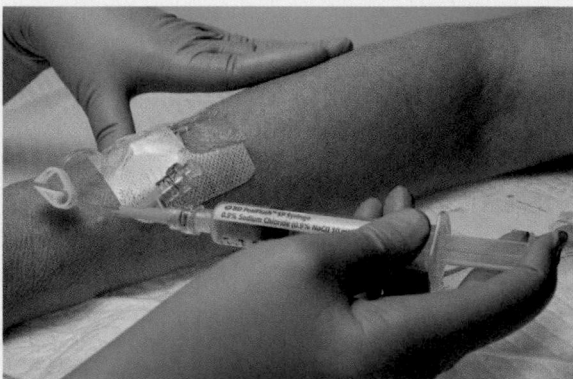

STEP 21 Flush PVAD. *(Courtesy Patrick Coble.)*

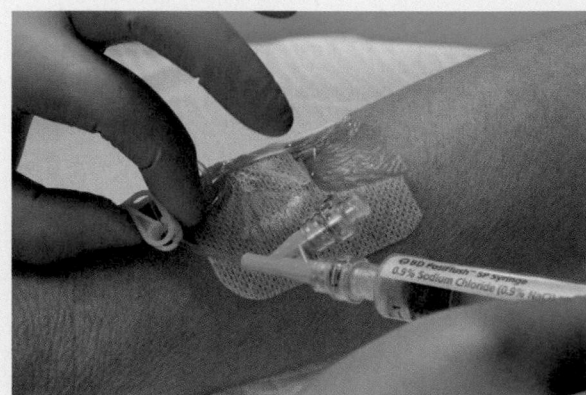

STEP 22 Close clamp. *(Courtesy Patrick Coble.)*

STEP	RATIONALE

IMPLEMENTATION

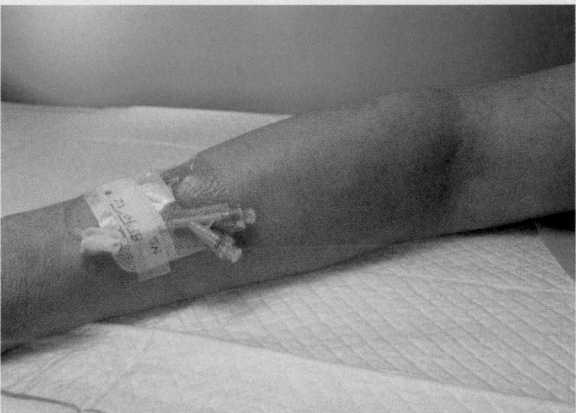

Step 24 Label dressing. *(Courtesy Patrick Coble.)*

EVALUATION

1. Assess PVAD for patency and complications, dressing, and patient-specific concerns, as per employer.
2. **Use Teach-Back:** "I want to make sure that I explained what you should watch for with your IV. Tell me the signs or symptoms that you should tell me or the other nurses about." Develop a revised teaching plan if patient or caregiver is not able to teach back correctly.

Frequent assessment prevents long-term damage, and early recognition leads to prompt treatment.
Determines patient's and caregiver's level of understanding of instructional topic.

Unexpected Outcomes

1. Catheter occlusion can occur from a bent catheter, positional catheter (catheter resting against catheter wall), kink or knot in infusion tubing, clot formation, or precipitate formation from administration of incompatible medications or solutions.
2. MARSI

3. Phlebitis (i.e., vein inflammation): pain, redness, warmth, swelling, induration, or presence of palpable cord along course of vein (INS, 2016a). Rate of infusion may be altered.

4. Catheter-related infection can present as redness, swelling around or above IV site, pain, purulent drainage at insertion site, and body temperature elevation (INS, 2016a).

5. Hematoma is bleeding under skin caused by trauma to vessel wall. It can occur during short-peripheral IV insertion if needle punctures either adjacent vessels or posterior vein wall or can be seen with multiple venipuncture attempts.

6. Nerve injuries during short-peripheral IV insertion can occur. Be alert for patient indications of paresthesias, including shocklike pain, tingling or pins and needles, burning, or numbness on insertion.

Related Interventions

- Determine cause and consider catheter removal.
- Positional catheters can be repositioned to improve IV flow.
- Remove occluded IV catheter. Occluded catheters should not be flushed because an embolus can result from dislodging a clot.
- Monitor site for signs of injury and change dressing, using a different type of dressing, if indicated.
- Consider infusate; confirm need for vascular access.
- Determine cause (e.g., chemical, mechanical, bacterial):
  - *Chemical phlebitis:* Apply warm compress, elevate limb, consider slowing infusion rate, and determine if catheter removal is necessary (INS, 2016a).
  - *Mechanical phlebitis:* Stabilize catheter, apply heat, elevate limb, continue to monitor, consider catheter removal if signs and symptoms persist (INS, 2016a).
  - *Bacterial phlebitis:* Remove IV catheter (INS, 2016a).
- Document phlebitis using a standardized scale, including nursing interventions per employer policy (Tables 29.3 and 29.4).
- Notify health care provider. Obtain prescription to culture drainage (INS, 2016a).
- Remove IV catheter and culture purulent drainage from around IV site (see Chapter 9) (INS, 2016a).
- Remove IV catheter immediately and apply pressure and dry, sterile dressing.
- Monitor for additional bleeding.
- Elevate extremity and monitor for circulatory, neurological, or motor dysfunction (INS, 2016b).
- Notify health care provider of any signs and symptoms of nerve injury (INS, 2016b).
- Immediately stop VAD insertion and remove device if patient indicates symptoms of paresthesias (INS, 2016a).
- Continue to monitor neurovascular status (INS, 2016b).

TABLE 29.3

Phlebitis Scale

Grade	Clinical Criteria
0	No symptoms
1	Erythema at access site with or without pain
2	Pain at access site with erythema and/or edema
3	Pain at access site with erythema and/or edema Streak formation Palpable venous cord
4	Pain at access site with erythema and/or edema Streak formation Palpable venous cord >2.5 cm (1 inch) in length Purulent drainage

Modified from Infusion Nurses Society (INS). (2016). *Policy and procedures for infusion therapy* (5th ed.). Norwood, MA: Author.

TABLE 29.4

Visual Infusion Phlebitis Scale

Score	Observation
0	IV site appears healthy
1	One of the following signs is evident: Slight pain near IV site *or* slight redness near IV site
2	Two of the following signs are evident: • Pain at IV site • Erythema • Swelling
3	All of the following signs are evident: • Pain along the path of cannula • Induration
4	All of the following signs are evident and extensive: • Pain along the path of cannula • Erythema • Induration • Palpable venous cord
5	All of the following signs are evident and extensive: • Pain along the path of cannula • Erythema • Induration • Palpable venous cord • Pyrexia

IV, Intravenous.
Modified from Infusion Nurses Society (INS). (2016). *Policy and procedures for infusion therapy* (5th ed.). Norwood, MA: Author.

Communication and Documentation

- Document PVAD insertion or unsuccessful attempts in the patient's EHR or chart (see employer policy). Include the following information:
  - Time and date
  - Location of PVAD insertion (e.g., cephalic vein on dorsal surface of right lower arm)
  - Gauge, length, and type of PVAD (e.g., 22 g × 2.5 cm [1.0 in.], brand name)
  - Number of attempts
  - Functionality of PVAD (i.e., flushes without resistance, no signs of complications)
  - Local anaesthetic, if used
  - Use of visualization technology, if used

- Patient response to procedure
- Patient education
- Document ongoing assessment a minimum of two times per shift and according to employer policy: flow rate; method of infusion (gravity or electronic infusion device [EID]); size, type, length, and brand of catheter; time infusion started; and patient's response to insertion. Use an infusion therapy flow sheet when available.
- If using an EID, document type and rate of infusion and device identification number.
- Document patient's status, IV fluid, amount infused, and integrity and patency of system according to employer policy.
- Document education provided to patient and caregiver. Include the following information: level of understanding, ability to follow instructions, awareness of reporting of signs and symptoms of complications.
- Provide a status report at change of shift, including:
  - Site assessment (e.g., no signs and symptoms of complication, dressing dry and occlusive)
  - Location and gauge of catheter
  - Patient's response
- Report to oncoming nursing staff the type of fluid, flow rate, status of VAD, amount of fluid remaining in present solution, expected time to hang subsequent IV container, and patient condition.
- Report to health care provider any signs and symptoms of IV-related complications.
- Document signs and symptoms of IV-related complications, including interventions and patient response to treatments.

Special Considerations
Teaching
- Educate patient to report any signs or symptoms of complications (e.g., redness, pain, tenderness, swelling, bleeding, drainage, or loose of soiled dressing), if flow rate slows or stops, or if patient sees blood in the IV administration set or on the dressing.

Pediatric
- Consider performing venipuncture in a neutral space to allow the child's room to be a safe place (INS, 2016c, p. 50).
- In addition to the usual venipuncture sites, other site selections may include the four scalp veins used in infants and toddlers and, if child is not walking, the dorsum of the foot.
- Needle selection is based on vein assessment and potential use. A typical gauge for PVAD is 26- to 24-gauge for neonates, 24- to 22-gauge for children.
- Use local anaesthetic and distraction strategies to minimize distress associated with venipuncture (INS, 2016c).
- Apply latex-free tubing or use a blood pressure cuff inflated to just below diastolic blood pressure.
- Allow older children to select IV site so they believe that they have some control over their treatment; this may increase their cooperation (INS, 2016c, p. 50).
- To increase success rate and improve safety for PVAD insertion, have assistance available to support and position the child. Use therapeutic holding, usually in a sitting position, to provide close contact and decrease movement that may result in unsuccessful initiation or dislodgement (Perry, Hockenberry, Lowdermilk, et al., 2017).
- Consider the use of securement devices to aid in preventing dislodging PVAD during daily activities and play.
- Choose age-appropriate activities compatible with maintenance of the IV infusion to support normal growth and development.

Gerontological

- Older persons may have fragile veins and skin. They have less subcutaneous support tissue, and their skin is thinning (INS, 2016d). Consider use of a barrier film before dressing application, to protect fragile skin.
- Avoid sites that are easily moved or bumped (e.g., the hand) and areas that may affect mobility and independence.
- Use a commercial protective device to protect the site and reduce manipulation.
- Appropriate gauge selection is a key factor in successful insertion and maintaining access (e.g., 22- or 24-gauge catheter). Smaller-gauge catheters are less traumatizing to the vein and will allow better blood flow, increasing hemodilution of infusates.
- If possible, avoid using the back of the older person's hand or the dominant arm for venipuncture because use of these sites interferes with their independence.

Care in the Community

- Ensure that a patient is able and willing to self-administer infusion therapy or that there is a reliable caregiver to provide infusion therapy care at home.

- Ensure that all sharps and equipment contaminated by blood are disposed of appropriately, based on community standards. Some suppliers provide sharps containers for needle disposal. Teach patient and caregiver appropriate sharps disposal.
- Instruct patient and caregiver about procedures of infusion therapy, including hand hygiene and aseptic technique while handling and proper disposal of syringes and other supplies. Observe patient and caregiver performing tasks.
- Provide patient with a contact number to access provider for 24-hour assistance in settings where this is available, in regard to therapy and equipment.
- Teach patient about activity restrictions (e.g., avoiding strenuous exercise of the arm with the IV line, protecting site while bathing or showering).
- Teach patient about complications and provide information and strategies for managing problems, including when to access a health care provider.

◆ SKILL 29.2   Initiating and Regulating Intravenous Infusions

NSO *Nursing Skills Online Maintenance of Intravenous Fluid Therapy Module 13 / Lesson 2*

Accurate infusion rates in intravenous (IV) therapy are essential in the safe delivery of solutions and medications (see Chapter 22). Appropriate regulation of infusion rates reduces complications (e.g., phlebitis, infiltration, fluid overload, or clotting of the vascular access device [VAD]) associated with infusion therapy (INS, 2016b). Infusion rates can be affected by changes in patient position, flexion of the IV site extremity, occlusion of the VAD, venospasm, venous trauma, or manipulation of the VAD. A patient achieves therapeutic outcomes and fewer complications when an IV system and flow rates are assessed systematically (INS, 2016b).

There are a variety of methods for regulating infusion rates. Electronic infusion devices (EIDs) maintain correct flow rates and catheter patency and prevent an unexpected bolus of IV infusion for patient safety (INS, 2016a). Many EIDs provide a record of the volume of fluid infused over a period of time. An EID delivers a measured amount of fluid over a period of time (e.g., 100 mL/hr) using positive pressure. An electronic sensor signals an alarm if the pressure in the system changes and the desired flow rate alters. The use of an EID does not absolve a nurse from checking to ensure that the pump is functioning and infusing at the prescribed rate, however (INS, 2016a). Hourly assessment is recommended to detect infiltration, extravasation, or phlebitis, regardless of the method for regulating infusion rates.

Manual flow-control devices include flow regulators (i.e., dial or barrel-shaped) and mechanical infusion devices without a power source (i.e., elastomeric devices, piston-driven pumps). These may be used when flow rate is not critical (Royal College of Nursing [RCN], 2016). They are not recommended for use in infants and children because accuracy cannot be guaranteed (INS, 2016c).

Flow regulators such as volume-control devices deliver small volumes with the aid of gravity. Patient and mechanical factors (e.g., height of the IV container, IV administration set size, or fluid viscosity) affect an IV gravity controller. One example of a volume-control device is a calibrated chamber placed between the IV container and the insertion spike and drip chamber of an administration set (see Chapter 22). A small volume of IV solution is placed in the chamber and regulated for administration. The advantage of this system is that, if the rate of the IV infusion is inadvertently increased, only a limited amount of solution will infuse. With either type of device, consistent monitoring is necessary to verify the accurate infusion of the IV solution and detect and prevent complications.

The capabilities of EIDs have increased over the years, allowing for enhanced patient safety. Multifunctional EIDs or "smart pumps" have an embedded computer system with a drug library and are associated with reduced risk for infusion-related medication errors. The built-in software is programmed from health care pharmacy databases with unit-specific profiles. The pump has an audible and visual alert when its setting does not match the preselected dose or volume limits, helping to prevent infusion errors. The use of a "smart pump" with the potential reduction in serious medication errors and improved patient outcomes is becoming the standard of care across all settings. Nurses should follow their employer policy and the manufacturer recommendations for selection and use of EIDs, alarm settings, pump controls, and features. Nurses need to practice diligence in assessing and monitoring patients because use of any EID or controller is not without risk of malfunction, placing a patient at risk for harm or injury.

Patients in alternative care settings (e.g., long-term care) can receive infusion therapy with ambulatory pumps, which promote independence and improved quality of life. Most pumps weigh less than 2.7 kg (6 lb) and range from palm size to fitting in a backpack. Programming capabilities range from rate adjustments, remote-site adjustments, and therapy-specific settings.

Delegation and Collaboration

The skill of regulating IV infusions cannot be delegated to an unregulated care provider (UCP). The licensed practical nurse (LPN)/registered practical nurse (RPN) scope of practice varies by province/territory and health authority. The skill of initiating and

regulating IV infusions may be delegated to other health care team members—always check employer policy. Caring for patients with IV infusions requires interprofessional collaboration for effective communication and patient safety. The nurse instructs the UCP to immediately report the following:

- When the IV solution bag is low and will require a new bag.
- When electronic infusion device is alarming.
- When the patient indicates any discomfort related to infusion, such as pain, burning, bleeding, or swelling at the VAD site.

Equipment

Supplies for initiation of infusion therapy:
- Prescribed IV solution or medication
- 70% alcohol or 2% chlorhexidine gluconate (CHG)/alcohol swabs

- IV administration set (IV tubing), either macrodrip or microdrip, depending on prescribed rate; if using EID, administration set must be compatible with the electronic device
- 0.2-micron filter, if recommended for type of infusion
- EID and IV pole
- Watch with second hand to calculate drip rate
- Calculator, paper, and pencil
- Tape
- Label
- Biomedical sharps container
- Stethoscope
- Patient gown with shoulder snaps for easy removal with continuous infusion therapy

STEP	RATIONALE

ASSESSMENT

1. Review accuracy and completeness of health care provider's prescription for patient name and correct solution: type, volume, additives, infusion rate, and duration of infusion therapy. Follow the 10 rights of medication administration (see Chapter 20).	Ensures delivery of correct IV solution and prescribed volume over prescribed time.
2. Perform hand hygiene.	Reduces transmission of microorganisms.
3. Assess for clinical factors and conditions that will be affected by infusion therapy, including laboratory values, clinical markers of volume, allergies, and behaviour and cognition.	Knowledge of infusion therapy modalities (e.g., peripheral vascular access device [PVAD], central vascular access device [CVAD], solution, medication, volume) is necessary to identify key assessments and treatment evaluation.
a. Body weight	Changes in body weight can be an indication of fluid loss or gain.
b. *Clinical markers of vascular volume:*	
(1) Urine output (decreased, dark yellow)	Kidneys respond to extracellular volume (ECV) deficit by reducing urine production and concentrating urine. Kidney disease can also cause oliguria.
(2) Vital signs: blood pressure, respirations, pulse, temperature	Changes in blood pressure may be associated with fluid volume status (fluid volume deficit [FVD]) seen in postural hypotension.
	Respirations can be altered in presence of acid–base imbalances.
	Temperature elevations increase need for fluid requirements (temperature of 38.3°C [101°F] to 39.4°C [103°F] require at least 500 mL of fluid replacement within a 24-hr period) (Weinstein & Hagle, 2014).
(3) Distended neck veins (Normally veins are full when person is supine and flat when person is upright.)	Indicator of fluid volume status: flat or collapsing with inhalation when supine with ECV deficit; full when upright or semi-upright with ECV excess.
(4) Auscultation of lungs	Crackles or rhonchi in dependent parts of lung may signal fluid buildup caused by ECV excess.
(5) Capillary refill	Indirect measure of tissue perfusion (sluggish with ECV deficit).
c. *Clinical markers of interstitial volume:*	
(1) Skin turgor (Pinch skin over sternum or inside of forearm.)	Failure of skin to return to normal position after several seconds indicates FVD.
(2) Dependent edema (pitting or nonpitting) (see Chapter 8).	Edema is not usually apparent until 2–4 kg (4.4–8.8 lbs) of fluid is retained. A weight gain of 1 kg (2.2 lbs) is equivalent to the retention of 1 L of body water (Phillips & Gorski, 2014).
(3) Oral mucous membrane between cheek and gum (see Chapter 8).	More reliable indicator than dry lips or skin. Dry between cheek and gums indicates ECV deficit.
d. Thirst	Occurs with hypernatremia and severe ECV deficit. Not a reliable indicator for older persons (Phillips & Gorski, 2014).

STEP	RATIONALE

ASSESSMENT

e. *Behaviour and level of consciousness:*

    (1) Restlessness and mild confusion

    (2) Decreased level of consciousness (lethargy, confusion, coma)

Occurs with FVD or acid–base imbalance

Occurs with severe ECV deficit.

May occur with osmolality, fluid and electrolyte, and acid–base imbalances.

4. Apply clean gloves; inspect and gently palpate skin around and above IV site over dressing. Ask patient how IV site feels. Assess VAD for patency and signs and symptoms of IV-related complications (e.g., infiltration, occlusion of VAD, phlebitis, infection, patient indication of pain, or leaking under dressing). Dispose of gloves; perform hand hygiene.

Identifies complications that compromise integrity of VAD and may necessitate replacement of VAD. Reduces transmission of infection.

5. Assess IV system for patency from IV container to insertion site.

Ensures delivery of prescribed volume over prescribed time.

6. Identify patient risk for fluid and electrolyte imbalance given type of IV solution (e.g., neonate, history of cardiac or renal disease).

Helps prioritize assessments. Volume control needs to be strict. Guides choice of infusion device.

7. Assess patient's knowledge of how positioning of IV site affects flow rate.

Fosters patient participation in maintaining most effective position of arm with IV equipment.

NURSING DIAGNOSES

- Insufficient fluid volume
- Excessive fluid volume
- Insufficient knowledge regarding infusion therapy
- Potential for infection

Related factors/Risk factors are individualized on the basis of patient's condition or needs.

PLANNING

1. Expected outcomes following completion of procedure:

- Fluid and electrolyte balance returns to, or remains within, normal range.
- Patient's VAD remains patent, and site is free from signs and symptoms of IV-related complications.
- Patient is able to explain how positioning of IV site affects rate and describe complications related to inaccurate flow rate.

Proper solution is infused at proper rate and monitored, resolving fluid and electrolyte imbalance (Jantzen & Felver, 2018).

Ensures that patient receives prescribed infusion therapy and that VAD is without complications (INS, 2016a).

Demonstrates learning (INS, 2016a).

2. Have paper and pencil or calculator to calculate flow rate.

Use mathematical calculations to obtain correct rate. Refer to medication math resources (or Evolve Calculations Tutorial) for assistance with calculations.

3. Prepare patient and caregiver by explaining procedure, its purpose, and what is expected of patient.

Decreases anxiety and promotes cooperation and adherence to therapy.

4. Check prescription to see how long each litre of fluid should infuse. If hourly rate (mL/hr) is not provided in prescription, calculate it by dividing volume by hours. For example:

Basis of calculation to ensure infusion of solution over prescribed hourly rate.

$$\text{mL/hr} = \frac{\text{Total infusion (mL)}}{\text{Hours of infusion}}$$
$$1000 \text{ mL/8 hr} = 125 \text{ mL/hr}$$

or if 3 L is prescribed for 24 hours:

$$3000 \text{ mL/24 hr} = 125 \text{ mL/hr}$$

Clinical Decision Point *It is common for health care providers to write an abbreviated IV prescription such as "D$_5$W with 20 mEq KCl 125 mL/hr continuous." This prescription implies that the IV should be maintained at this rate until a prescription has been written for the IV to be discontinued or changed to another prescription.*

STEP	RATIONALE

PLANNING

5. If "keep vein open" (KVO) or "to keep vein open" (TKVO) rate is prescribed, check employer policy regarding specific flow rate for this prescription.

Prevents catheter clotting, thus preserving venous access while infusing a minimal amount of fluid. A prescription for KVO (TKVO) rate must specify an infusion rate as required by the 10 rights of medication administration. Rates may vary from 0.5 mL/hr to 30 mL/hr based on type of VAD, patient-specific therapy, and method of infusion (gravity or EID).

6. Use hourly rate to program EID or, if gravity-flow infusion, use to calculate minute flow rate (gtt/mL).

EID automatically delivers correct minute flow rate. Gravity infusion requires calculation of gtt/mL.

7. Know calibration (drop factor), in drops per millilitre (gtt/mL), of infusion set used by employer:

   a. Microdrip: 60 gtt/mL. Used to deliver rates less than 100 mL/hr.

Microdrip tubing universally delivers 60 gtt/mL. Used when small or very precise volumes are to be infused.

   b. Macrodrip: 10 to 15 gtt/mL (depending on manufacturer). Used to deliver rates greater than 100 mL/hr.

There are different commercial parenteral administration sets for macrodrip tubing. Used when large volumes or fast rates are necessary. Know drip factor for tubing being used.

8. Select one of the following formulas to calculate minute flow rate (drops per minute) based on drop factor of infusion set:

Once you determine hourly rate, these formulas compute the correct flow rate.

   a. $mL/h/60\ min = mL/min$

$$Drop\ factor \times mL/min = Drops/min$$

   or

   b. $mL/h \times Drop\ factor/60\ min = Drops/min$

Calculate minute flow rate for a bag 1000 mL with 20 mEq KCl at 125 mL/hr.

Microdrip:

$$125\ mL/hr \times 60\ gtt/mL = 7500\ gtt/hr$$

$$7500\ gtt \div 60\ min = 125\ gtt/min$$

When using microdrip, millilitres per hour (mL/hr) always equals drops per minute (gtt/min).

Macrodrip:

$$125\ mL/hr \times 15\ gtt/mL = 1875\ gtt/hr$$

$$1875\ gtt \div 60\ min = 31 - 32\ gtt/min$$

Multiply volume by drop factor and divide product by time (in minutes).

IMPLEMENTATION

1. Identify patient using at least two person-specific identifiers (e.g., name and date of birth or name and medical record number) according to employer policy. Compare identifiers with information on patient's medication administration record (MAR) or medical record.

Ensures correct patient. Complies with Accreditation Canada's standards and improves patient safety (Accreditation Canada, 2019).

2. Perform hand hygiene.

Decreases potential risk of microbial contamination and cross-contamination (INS, 2016a).

3. Prepare IV administration set and solution for continuous or intermittent infusion just prior to administration.

Reviewing label for accuracy reduces risk for medication errors (INS, 2016a).

   a) Confirm IV solution using the 10 rights of medication administration (see Chapters 20 and 22). Verify that label information is accurate by reviewing name of medication or solution, dosage and concentration, beyond-use and expiration dates, and sterility state.

Medications cannot be added to an infusing bag.

   b) Check solution for colour and clarity. Check bag for leaks.

Sterility may be compromised if any of the following are observed:
- Leaking of the container or bag
- Discoloration of solution
- Precipitate is visible
- Solution is beyond use date or expiration has passed

Do not use if contamination is suspected.

STEP	RATIONALE

IMPLEMENTATION

c) Open administration set, maintaining sterility. **NOTE:** EIDs sometimes have a dedicated administration set; follow manufacturer's instructions.

Prevent touch contamination, which allows microorganisms to enter infusion equipment and bloodstream.

d) Place roller clamp about 2 cm to 5 cm below drip chamber and move roller clamp to "off" or "closed" position.

Close proximity of roller clamp to drip chamber allows more accurate regulation of flow rate. Moving clamp to "off" prevents accidental spillage of IV solution during priming.

e) Remove protective cap over spike port on infusion container or bag.

f) Remove protective cover from spike of administration set using aseptic technique. Insert spike into port of IV bag using a twisting motion (see illustration). If solution container is a glass bottle, clean rubber stopper on glass-bottled solution with antiseptic swab and insert spike into rubber stopper of IV bottle. Bottles require vented tubing. If sterility of spike is compromised, discard IV administration set and open a new set.

Provides access for insertion of IV administration set spike into solution using sterile technique.

g) Compress drip chamber and release, allowing it to fill one-third to one-half full.

Creates suction effect; fluid enters drip chamber to prevent air from entering tubing.

h) Purge air from tubing by slowly opening the roller clamp (see illustration). This will allow the IV solution to flow from the drip chamber to fill the tubing. If the administration set has in-line access ports, invert the port as the solution fills the tubing; this will ensure complete removal of air. When solution reaches the distal end of the tubing, close clamp. Label administration set with time and date, according to employer policy.

Priming ensures that IV administration set is clear of air and filled with IV solution before connecting to VAD. Slowly filling tubing decreases turbulence and chance of bubble formation.

Closing clamp prevents loss of solution.

Labelling IV administration set identifies when administration set needs to be changed.

i) Confirm by visual inspection that tubing is clear of air and air bubbles. To remove small air bubbles, firmly tap tubing where they are located.

Large air bubbles may act as emboli (Myers, 2017).

Optional: If using optional long extension tubing, remove protective cover and attach it to distal end of IV administration set, maintaining sterility. Then prime long extension tubing. Insert tubing into EID or hang solution and administration set to gravity.

Priming removes air from long extension tubing so it does not enter patient's vascular system.

Facilitates starting infusion as soon as IV site is ready.

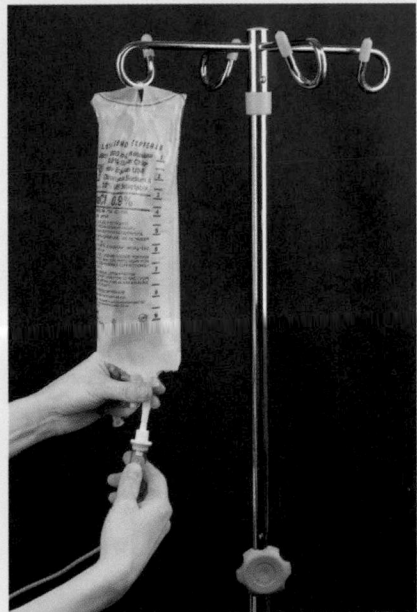

Step 3f Prepare infusate container and administration set. (*Courtesy Burl Jantzen.*)

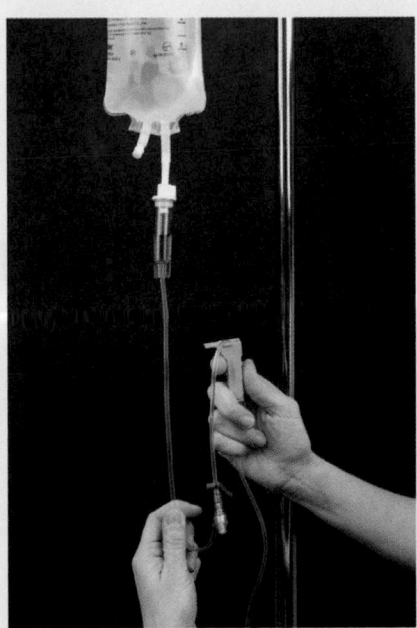

Step 3h Purge air from administration set using roller clamp. (*Courtesy Burl Jantzen.*)

STEP	RATIONALE

IMPLEMENTATION

4. To begin primary infusion, swab needle-free connector with alcohol swab or employer-approved antiseptic swab and attach Luer-Lok end of administration set to needle-free connector (see illustration).

Initiates flow of fluid through IV catheter, preventing clotting of VAD.

5. a) Regulate gravity infusion.
   - Ensure that IV container is at least 76.2 cm (30 in) above IV site for adults and increase height for viscous fluids (INS, 2016b).

Pressure caused by gravity is necessary to overcome venous pressure and resistance from tubing and catheter.

Clinical Decision Point *An anti–free flow safeguard (preventing bolus infusion in the event of machine malfunction or when tubing is removed from machine) is an important element of an EID and is required. Always check and follow manufacturer's recommendations for specific device features.*

   - Slowly open roller clamp on tubing until you can see drops in the drip chamber. Hold watch with a second hand at the same level as the drip chamber and count drip rate for 1 minute. Adjust roller clamp to increase or decrease rate of infusion.

Regulates flow to prescribed rate.

   b) Regulate using EID (see illustration) according to manufacturer's instructions.

6. Monitor infusion rate and IV site for complications at least hourly. Use watch to verify rate of infusion, even when using EID. Assess IV system from container to VAD insertion site when alarm signals.

Many factors influence drip rate; frequent monitoring ensures IV fluid administration, as prescribed.

Flow controllers and pumps do not replace frequent, accurate nursing evaluation.

EIDs can continue to infuse IV solutions after a complication has developed (INS, 2016a).

Alarm indicates a situation that requires attention. Empty solution container, tubing kinks, closed clamp, infiltration, clotted catheter, air in tubing, or low battery can trigger an EID alarm.

7. Attach labels to IV administration set, medication tubing, and solutions, based on employer policy.

Provides reference to determine next time for container change, especially with KVO rate that contains a specific infusion rate as prescribed by health care provider.

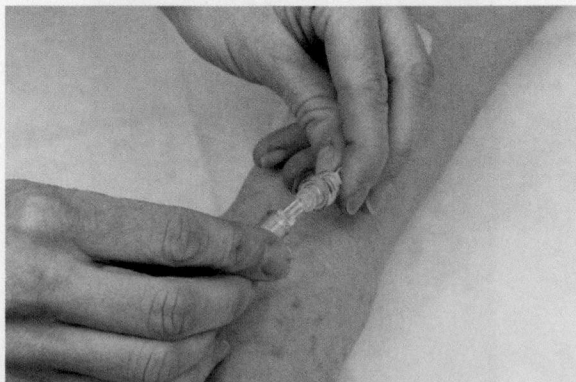

STEP 4 Attach administration set to scrubbed needle-free connector. (*Courtesy Patrick Coble.*)

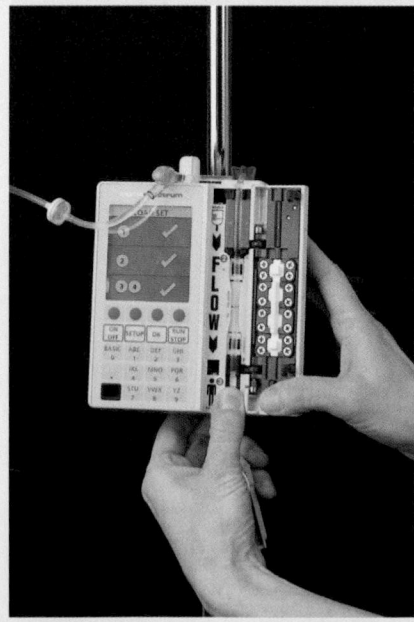

STEP 5b Insert administration set into EID. (*Courtesy Patrick Coble.*)

STEP	RATIONALE

IMPLEMENTATION

8. Teach patient purpose of EID if infusion therapy is delivered by EID, purpose of alarms, to avoid raising hand or arm that affects flow rate, and to avoid touching control clamp.

Information enables patient to protect IV site and informs them about rationale for not altering control rate.

9. Remove and dispose of any used supplies; perform hand hygiene.

Prevents transmission of infection.

EVALUATION

1. Observe patient every 1 to 2 hours (see employer policy), noting volume of IV fluid infused and rate of infusion.

Ensures delivery of prescribed volume over prescribed time and decreases risk for fluid and electrolyte imbalance.

2. Evaluate patient's response to therapy (e.g., laboratory values, input and output [I&O], weights, vital signs, postprocedure assessments).

Provides ongoing evaluation of patient's fluid status, including monitoring for fluid volume excess (FVE) or fluid volume deficit (FVD). Early recognition of complications leads to prompt treatment.

3. Evaluate patient at established intervals per employer policy for signs and symptoms of IV-related complications.

Prevents complications that compromise integrity of VAD or cause inaccurate IV solution flow rate.

4. **Use Teach-Back:** "I want to be sure that I explained the importance of your IV fluids running at the correct rate. Tell me what you think may cause the pump's alarm to go off and what you would do." Develop a revised teaching plan if patient or caregiver is not able to teach back correctly.

Determines patient's and caregiver's level of understanding of instructional topic.

Unexpected Outcomes

1. Solution does not infuse at prescribed rate.
   a. Sudden infusion of large volume of solution occurs; patient develops dyspnea, crackles in lung, dependent edema (edema in legs), and increased urine output, indicating FVE.

   b. IV solution runs slower than prescribed.

2. IV patency is lost subsequent to IV solution container running empty.

Related Interventions

- Slow infusion rate: KVO rates must have specific rate prescribed by health care provider.
- Notify health care provider immediately.
- Place patient in high-Fowler's position.
- Anticipate new IV prescriptions.
- Anticipate administration of oxygen per prescription.
- Administer diuretics if prescribed.
- Check for positional change that affects rate, height of IV container, kinking of tubing, or obstruction.
- Check VAD site for complications.
- Consult health care provider for new prescription to provide necessary fluid volume.
- Discontinue present IV infusion and restart new short-peripheral catheter in new site.

Communication and Documentation

- Document IV solution, rate of infusion in drops per minute (gtt/min) for infusions via gravity or milliliters per hour (mL/h).
- Document integrity and patency of system including VAD.
- Document use of any EID or control device and identification number on that device, if required by employer policy.
- Document patient response (e.g., laboratory values, I&O, weights, vital signs, postprocedure assessments) to therapy and unexpected outcomes (e.g., signs and symptoms of FVE, FVD, or IV-related complications).
- Document patient's and caregiver's level of understanding following instruction, in nurses' notes in electronic health record (EHR) or chart.
- At change of shift or when leaving on break, report rate of and volume left in infusion to nurse in charge or next nurse assigned to care for patient.

Special Considerations
Teaching

- Instruct patient to notify nurse if any signs or symptoms of IV complications are noted (e.g., redness, pain, tenderness, swelling, bleeding, drainage, or leakage from under dressing).
- Patient using an EID should know the significance of alarms and when to notify nursing staff.
- Teach patient about factors affecting flow rate, how to protect IV site, and about importance of not altering rate control.

Pediatric

- Do not use containers exceeding 150 mL in children younger than 2 years of age, exceeding 250 mL in children younger than 5 years of age, or exceeding 500 mL in children younger than 10 years of age. Always use tamper-resistant volume-controlled EIDs to ensure accurate fluid delivery (INS, 2016c).

Gerontological

- Use an EID and microdrip tubing to administer IV solutions to older persons. Monitor vital signs, electrolyte levels, blood urea nitrogen (BUN), creatinine, urine output, and body weight (INS, 2016d).

Care in the Community

- Ensure that patient is able and willing to operate an EID and administer infusion therapy. If patient is unable to provide self-care, be sure that a reliable caregiver is available in the home.

- Discuss proper EID function with patient. Consider use of an ambulatory-type device. Observe patient operating infusion EID and administering infusion therapy.
- Teach patient and caregiver what EID alarms mean, methods to troubleshoot them, and how to disconnect the IV administration set from the EID pump in the event of a pump failure.
- Ensure that patient's electrical outlets are properly grounded.
- Provide patient with a contact phone number to access 24 hours a day for addressing problems, if resources are available in the patient's setting.

✦ SKILL 29.3   Changing Intravenous Solution Containers

NSO *Nursing Skills Online Maintenance of Intravenous Fluid Therapy Module 13 / Lesson 3*

Patients receiving intravenous (IV) therapy periodically require changes of IV solutions. IV containers include plastic bags and glass bottles. The nurse changes a container when there is a prescription for a new solution or when it becomes time to add a sequential container. As patients respond to therapy, a new solution may be prescribed. The maximum hang time for routine replacement of IV containers is established by employer policy (INS, 2016a). Maximum hang time is based on assumptions that strict aseptic technique has been followed throughout and that the system remains closed. Stability of the solution or medication being infused determines hang time as well. Organizational skills are necessary to manage changing IV containers or solutions in a manner that decreases the risk of infusion-related complications such as an infusion container becoming empty or clotting of a vascular access device (VAD).

Delegation and Collaboration

The skill of changing IV solutions may be delegated to other health care team members if they have had appropriate education, the

skill is within their governing body scope of practice, and it is approved by employer policy. Caring for patients with IV infusions requires interprofessional collaboration for effective communication and patient safety.

The skill of changing IV solutions cannot be delegated to an unregulated care provider (UCP). The nurse instructs the UCP to report the following to the nurse immediately:

- When an IV container is near completion.
- Any cloudiness or precipitate in the IV solution.
- Alarm sounding on electronic infusion device (EID).
- Any patient indications of discomfort related to infusion, such as pain, burning, bleeding, or swelling.

Equipment

- Clean gloves
- IV solution as prescribed by health care provider
- Label

STEP	RATIONALE

ASSESSMENT

1. Review accuracy and completeness of health care provider's prescription in patient's medical record for patient name and correct solution: type, volume, additives, rate, and duration of infusion therapy. Follow the 10 rights of drug administration (see Chapter 20).	Ensures delivery of correct IV solution and prescribed volume over prescribed time (INS, 2016a).
2. Note date and time when IV administration set and solution were last changed.	Ensures correct timing of tubing changes.
3. Determine patient understanding of need for continued infusion therapy.	Indicates need for any patient education.
4. Perform hand hygiene and apply clean gloves; inspect and gently palpate skin around and above VAD site over dressing. Assess VAD for patency and signs and symptoms of IV-related complications (e.g., infiltration, occlusion of VAD, phlebitis, infection, patient indication of pain, or leakage under dressing). Discard gloves.	Identifies complications that compromise integrity of VAD and necessitate replacement of VAD.
5. Check infusion system from solution container down to VAD insertion site for integrity, including but not limited to discoloration, cloudiness, leakage, expiration date. Determine compatibility of all IV solutions and additives by consulting approved online database, drug reference, or pharmacist.	If there has been a break in integrity of solution container, a new bag is needed (INS, 2016a). May indicate need for IV administration set change. Incompatibilities cause physical, chemical, and therapeutic changes with adverse patient outcomes (see Chapter 8).
6. Check pertinent laboratory data.	Compare data with baseline to determine ongoing response to IV solution administration.

STEP	RATIONALE

NURSING DIAGNOSES

- Insufficient fluid volume
- Insufficient knowledge regarding IV infusion
- Potential for infection

Related factors/Risk factors are individualized on the basis of patient's condition or needs.

PLANNING

STEP	RATIONALE
1. Expected outcomes following completion of procedure:	
• IV solution is correct.	Patient receives solution prescribed for treatment of diagnosis.
• Fluid and electrolyte levels return to normal.	IV solution helps to maintain fluid and electrolyte levels.
• Patient's VAD remains patent, and site is free from signs and symptoms of IV-related complications.	Ensures access for delivery of prescribed infusion therapy (INS, 2016a).
• Patient and caregiver can explain purpose of IV solution change.	Demonstrates learning (INS, 2016a).
2. Perform hand hygiene. Collect equipment. Have next solution prepared at least 1 hour before needed. If solution is prepared in pharmacy, ensure that it has been delivered to patient care unit. Allow solution to warm to room temperature if it has been refrigerated. Check that solution is correct and properly labelled. Check solution expiration date. Ensure that any light sensitivity restrictions are followed.	Reduces transmission of infection and contamination of equipment (INS, 2016a). Proper handling of solutions prevents IV-related complications such as occlusion. Checking that solution is correct prevents medication error.
3. Prepare patient and caregiver by explaining procedure, its purpose, and what is expected of patient.	Promotes person-centred care and decreases anxiety.

IMPLEMENTATION

STEP	RATIONALE
1. Identify patient using at least two person-specific identifiers (e.g., name and date of birth or name and medical record number) according to employer policy. Compare identifiers with information on patient's medication administration record (MAR) or medical record.	Ensures correct patient. Complies with Accreditation Canada's standards and improves patient safety (Accreditation Canada, 2019).
2. Change solution when prescription changes or when a small amount, about 50 mL, remains.	Prevents waste of solution. Employer policy will specify maximum hang time for IV solution containers.
3. Perform hand hygiene.	Reduces transmission of microorganisms.
4. Prepare new solution for changing. If using plastic bag, hang on IV pole and remove protective cover from IV administration set port. If using glass bottle, remove metal cap and metal and rubber disks.	Permits quick, smooth, organized change from old to new container.
5. Close roller clamp on existing solution to stop flow rate. Remove IV administration set from EID if necessary to prevent contamination of the new solution port or tubing spike (if used). Then remove old IV solution container from IV pole. Invert solution container.	Prevents solution remaining in drip chamber from emptying while changing solutions. Prevents solution in bag from spilling.
6. Quickly remove spike from old solution container and, without touching tip, insert spike into new container.	Reduces risk for solution in drip chamber becoming empty and maintains sterility.

Clinical Decision Point *If spike becomes contaminated by touching an unsterile object, discard and open a new administration set.*

STEP	RATIONALE
7. Hang new container of solution on IV pole.	Gravity helps with delivery of fluid into drip chamber.
8. Check for air in IV administration set. If air bubbles have formed, remove them by closing roller clamp, stretching tubing downward, and tapping tubing with finger (bubbles rise in fluid to drip chamber).	Reduces risk of air entering tubing. Use of an air-eliminating filter also reduces risk.
9. Make sure that drip chamber is one-third to one-half full. If drip chamber is too full, level can be decreased by removing bag from IV pole, pinching off IV administration set below drip chamber, inverting container, squeezing drip chamber, releasing and turning solution container upright, and releasing pinch on tubing.	Reduces risk for air entering IV administration set. If chamber is completely filled, you cannot observe or regulate drip rate.

STEP	RATIONALE

IMPLEMENTATION

11. If infusing with gravity, place time label on side of container and label with time hung, time of completion, and appropriate hourly intervals. If using plastic bags, mark only on label and not container.

Provides visual comparison of volume infused compared with prescribed rate of infusion.

12. Where relevant, instruct patient on purpose of new IV solution, additives, flow rate, potential adverse effects, how to avoid occluding tubing, and what to report.

Information educates patient about purpose of continued infusion therapy, what to report, and how to protect VAD patency.

EVALUATION

1. Observe patient every 1 to 2 hours or at established intervals per employer policy for function, intactness, and patency of IV system; correct infusion rate; and type and amount of IV solution infused.

Ensures delivery of prescribed volume over prescribed time and decreases risk for fluid and electrolyte imbalance.

2. Evaluate patient to determine response to therapy (e.g., laboratory values, input and output [I&O], weights, vital signs, postprocedure assessments).

Provides ongoing evaluation of patient's fluid status.

3. Monitor patient for signs of fluid volume excess (FVE), fluid volume deficit (FVD), or signs and symptoms of electrolyte imbalances.

Early recognition of complications leads to prompt treatment.

4. Evaluate patient at established intervals per employer policy for signs and symptoms of IV-related complications.

Prevents complications that compromise integrity of VAD or cause inaccurate IV solution flow rate.

5. **Use Teach-Back:** "We talked about the importance of your IV solutions running continuously. I want to be sure I explained this clearly. Tell me in your own words what you should do if you notice that the IV is not dripping." Develop a revised teaching plan if patient or caregiver is not able to teach back correctly.

Determines patient's and caregiver's level of understanding of instructional topic.

Unexpected Outcomes	Related Interventions
1. Flow rate is incorrect; patient receives too little or too much solution.	• Notify health care provider if patient's anticipated infusion is 100 to 200 mL less than or greater than anticipated (per employer policy).
	• Evaluate patient for signs and symptoms of adverse effects of infusion (e.g., FVD or FVE).
	• Determine and correct cause of incorrect flow rate (e.g., change in position, tubing kink, loss of IV patency or intactness).
	• Use EID when accurate flow rate is critical.
2. Fluid and/or electrolyte imbalances	• Notify health care provider.
	• Anticipate prescriptions for changes in IV solution or additives.

Communication and Documentation

• Document in nurse's notes or on appropriate flow sheet in electronic health record (EHR) or chart the IV solution, rate of infusion, and integrity and patency of system.
• Document IV solution, rate of infusion in drops per minute (gtt/min) for infusions via gravity or millilitres per hour (mL/hr).
• Document integrity and patency of system including VAD according to employer policy.
• Document use of any EID or control device and identification number on that device, if required by employer policy.
• Document patient response (e.g., laboratory values, I&O, weights, vital signs, postprocedure assessments) to therapy and unexpected outcomes (e.g., signs and symptoms of FVE, FVD, or IV-related complications).
• Document patient's and caregiver's level of understanding following instruction in nurses' notes in EHR or chart.

• At change of shift or when leaving on break, report rate of and volume left in infusion to nurse in charge or next nurse assigned to care for patient.

Special Considerations
Teaching

• Inform patient of new solution, additives, and potential adverse effects, including those to report to the nurse.
• Instruct patient to notify nurse or UCP if flow rate slows or IV container is empty.

Care in the Community

• Ensure that patient and caregiver are willing and able to perform an IV solution change.
• Teach patient and caregiver how to perform an IV solution change. Observe them performing procedure.

✦ SKILL 29.4 Changing Administration Sets (Infusion Tubing)

NSO *Nursing Skills Online Maintenance of Intravenous Fluid Therapy Module 13 / Lesson 3*

Maintaining the integrity of the intravenous (IV) system through the conscientious use of infection-prevention principles is critical to positive patient outcomes. To prevent entry of bacteria into the bloodstream, sterility must be maintained during tubing and solution changes. In addition to the main tubing, patients may have add-on devices (e.g., filters, extension sets), which connect to the primary administration set. Secondary administration sets may be used as a method to administer medications in conjunction with the primary infusion (e.g., antibiotics). Luer-Lok connections are recommended to prevent accidental tubing disconnection (INS, 2016a). Administration sets are replaced whenever a vascular access site change occurs (INS, 2016a) or if the IV solution or tubing becomes damaged. Factors that determine administration set change include suspected contamination, type of solution infusing, and frequency of the infusion. Follow employer policy for specific requirements (Table 29.5).

Administration sets used for parenteral nutrition (see Chapter 33) and blood or blood products (see Chapter 30) have specific criteria with which nurses need to be familiar (see employer policy). Whenever possible, schedule IV administration set changes when it is time to hang a new IV container (see Skill 29.3).

Delegation and Collaboration

The skill of changing IV administration sets may be delegated to other health care team members if they have had appropriate education, the skill is within their governing body scope of practice, and it is approved by employer policy.

The skill of changing IV administration sets cannot be delegated to an unregulated care provider (UCP). The nurse instructs the UCP to report the following to the nurse immediately:
- Any leakage from or around the IV administration set.
- If tubing has become contaminated (lying on the floor).

Equipment

- Clean gloves
- Antiseptic swabs (CHG solution preferred, povidone-iodine, or 70% alcohol)
- Label
- Microdrip or macrodrip administration set of IV administration set as appropriate
- Add-on device as necessary (e.g., filters, extension set, needle-free connector)
- Tubing label
- 10-mL syringe with preservative-free 0.9% sodium chloride for intermittent infusion therapy

---

TABLE 29.5

Intravenous Administration Set Changes

Primary and Secondary Continuous Infusions	Primary Intermittent Infusions	Use of Add-on Devices
• Change no more frequently than every 96 hours for solutions *other* than lipid, blood, or blood products. • In addition to routine changes, change the administration set whenever the short-peripheral IV site is changed or a new CVAD is placed. • If the secondary set is removed from the primary set, the secondary set is now an intermittent set and should be changed every 24 hours.	• Should be changed every 24 hours because of increased risk of infection with repeated disconnecting and reconnecting of administration set. • Aseptically attach a new, sterile covering device to the Luer end of the administration set after each intermittent use. *Avoid* attaching the exposed end of the administration set to the port on the same set (e.g., looping).	• Should be minimized because each is a potential source of contamination and disconnection. • Use of administration sets with devices as part of the set is preferred. • Aseptically change with insertion of new VAD or with each administration set replacement. • Change if the integrity of the product is compromised or suspected of being compromised.

CVAD, Central vascular access device; *IV,* intravenous; *VAD,* vascular access device.
Modified from Infusion Nurses Society (INS). (2016b). *Policy and procedures for infusion therapy* (5th ed.). Norwood, MA: Author.

STEP	RATIONALE

ASSESSMENT

1. Note date and time when IV administration set was last changed (see Table 29.5 for recommendations on administration set changes).	Decreases risk of infection.
2. Perform hand hygiene. Assess IV administration set for puncture, contamination, or occlusion that requires immediate change.	Compromised tubing results in fluid leakage and bacterial contamination.
3. Determine patient understanding of need for continued infusion therapy.	Reinforces need for further instruction.

STEP	RATIONALE

NURSING DIAGNOSES

- Insufficient knowledge regarding infusion therapy
- Potential for infection

Related factors/Risk factors are individualized on the basis of patient's condition or needs.

PLANNING

1. Expected outcomes following completion of procedure:
   - Patient experiences no leakage of solution from or around IV administration set.
   - Patient's IV administration set is patent, and patient receives prescribed infusion therapy as prescribed.
   - Patient's VAD remains patent, and site is free from signs and symptoms of IV-related complications.
   - Patient and caregiver can explain purpose of tubing change and how patient can avoid occluding tubing.
2. Prepare patient by explaining procedure, its purpose, and what is expected of them.
3. Coordinate IV administration set changes with solution changes when possible.
4. Collect equipment.

Intact system decreases risk for microbial contamination.

Brief interruption of IV infusion does not result in occlusion of vascular access device (VAD).
Adherence to administration set changes decreases risk of complications.
Demonstrates learning.

Decreases anxiety, promotes cooperation, and prevents sudden movement of extremity, which could dislodge IV catheter.
Decreases number of times system is open.

Provides easy access to equipment for efficient procedure.

IMPLEMENTATION

1. Identify patient using at least two person-specific identifiers according to employer policy. Compare identifiers with information on patient's medication administration record (MAR) or medical record.
2. Perform hand hygiene. Open new infusion set and connect add-on pieces (e.g., filters, extension tubing) using aseptic technique. Keep protective coverings over infusion spike and distal adapter. Place roller clamp about 2–2.5 cm (1–2 inches) below drip chamber and move roller clamp to "off" position. Secure all connections.
3. Apply clean gloves. If patient's IV cannula hub is not visible, remove IV dressing (see Skill 29.5).
4. Prepare IV administration set with new IV container. See Skill 29.2, Step 2.
5. To prepare IV administration set (tubing) with existing continuous IV infusion bag:
   a. Move roller clamp on new IV administration set to "off" position.
   b. Slow rate of infusion through old tubing to keep vein open (KVO) rate using EID or roller clamp.
   c. Compress and fill drip chamber of old tubing.

   d. Invert container and remove old tubing by pulling out the spike. Hold previously used spike to retain pressure of gravity, while keeping the new spike sterile and upright.
   e. Insert spike of new infusion tubing into solution container. Hang solution bag on IV pole, compress drip chamber on new tubing, and release, allowing it to fill one-third to one-half full.
   f. Prime air out of IV administration set by filling with IV solution as per Skill 29.2. Return roller clamp to "off" position after priming tubing (filled with IV solution). Replace protective cover on end of IV administration set. Place end of adapter near patient's IV site.

Ensures correct patient. Complies with Accreditation Canada's standards and improves patient safety (Accreditation Canada, 2019).

Close proximity of roller clamp to drip chamber allows more accurate regulation of flow rate. Securing connections reduces risk later of air emboli and infection. Protective covers reduce entrance of microorganisms. All connections should be of Luer-Lok type (INS, 2016a).

Cannula hub must be visible to provide smooth transition when removing old tubing and inserting new tubing.
When possible, coordinate IV administration set changes with solution changes.
For when solution change is not required

Prevents fluid spillage.

Prevents occlusion of VAD.

Ensures that drip chamber remains full until new tubing is changed.
Solution in drip chamber will continue to run and maintain catheter patency.

Permits drip chamber to fill and promotes rapid, smooth flow of solution through tubing.

Priming ensures that IV administration set is clear of air before connection with VAD and filled with IV solution. Closing clamp prevents accidental loss of fluid.
Maintains sterility. Equipment is positioned for quick connection of new tubing.

STEP	RATIONALE
IMPLEMENTATION	
g. Stop EID or turn roller clamp on old tubing to "off" position.	Prevents fluid spillage.
6. Re-establish infusion.	
a. Gently disconnect old tubing from extension tubing (or from IV catheter hub) and quickly insert Luer-Lok end of new tubing or saline lock into extension tubing connection or IV catheter hub.	Allows smooth transition from old to new tubing, minimizing time that system is open.
b. For continuous infusion, open roller clamp on new administration set and regulate drip rate using roller clamp or insert tubing into EID, program according to prescribed rate, and initiate infusion.	Ensures catheter patency and prevents occlusion.
c. Attach piece of tape or preprinted label with date and time of IV administration set change onto tubing below drip chamber.	Provides reference to determine next time for tubing change.
d. Form loop of tubing and secure it to patient's arm with strip of tape.	Avoids accidental pulling against site and stabilizes catheter.
7. Remove spike and discard in sharps container. Discard old administration set. If necessary, apply new dressing (see Skill 29.5). Remove and dispose of gloves. Perform hand hygiene.	Reduces transmission of microorganisms.

EVALUATION

1. Observe patient every 1 to 2 hours or at established intervals per employer policy for function, intactness, and patency of IV system and leaking at connection sites.	Ensures that IV system is functioning appropriately and minimizes risk of infection caused by breach in system integrity.
2. Evaluate patient at established intervals per employer policy for signs and symptoms of IV-related complications.	Prevents complications that compromise integrity of VAD or cause inaccurate IV solution flow rate.

Unexpected Outcomes	**Related Interventions**
1. IV solution infuses more slowly than prescribed.	• Check for positional change that affects rate, height of IV container, kinking of tubing, or obstruction.
	• Check for patency by opening roller clamp.
	• Check VAD site for complications.
	• Consult health care provider for new prescription to provide necessary fluid volume.

Communication and Documentation

- Document tubing change, type of solution, volume, and rate of infusion in nurses' notes in electronic health record (EHR) or chart. Use a special infusion therapy flow sheet for parenteral solutions per employer policy.
- Document in nurses' notes in EHR or chart what IV problems the patient and caregiver know to report.

Special Considerations
Teaching

- Instruct patient to notify nurse if fluid leaks from or around IV site or tubing or if tubing separates from catheter.

Care in the Community

- Ensure that patient is able and willing to perform IV administration set change and maintain access site or that there is a reliable person at home to provide this infusion therapy care.
- Instruct patient or caregiver in procedure for performing a sterile tubing change. Observe them performing procedure.

◆ SKILL 29.5   Changing a Short-Peripheral Venous Access Device Dressing

NSO *Nursing Skills Online Maintenance of Intravenous Fluid Therapy Module 13 / Lesson 4*

Vascular access device (VAD) insertion and maintenance requires strict adherence to infection-prevention measures to prevent complications (i.e., catheter-related bloodstream infection [CRBSI],

phlebitis, loss of access). Transparent semipermeable membrane (TSM) dressing changes should be performed every 5 to 7 days, and gauze dressings every 2 days or when loose, wet, visibly soiled,

or integrity is compromised (INS, 2016a). If a gauze dressing is underneath a TSM, it should be changed every 2 days (INS, 2016a). Gauze dressing is no longer advised, except when required for patient care. Stabilization of short-peripheral catheters decreases the risk of catheter-related complications (mechanical and bacterial phlebitis) and premature loss of access caused by catheter movement. Preferred options for stabilization include a securement TSM dressing with border or a TSM film dressing with an additional engineered stabilization device (ESD). Use of sterile tape or surgical strips should be avoided because they are not an effective substitute for securement dressings or engineered stabilization devices (INS, 2016a, p. S73).

Delegation and Collaboration

The skill of changing a peripheral vascular access device (PVAD) dressing may be delegated to other health care professionals if they have had appropriate education, the skill is within their governing body scope of practice, and it is approved by employer policy.

Assessment and care of PVADs require effective communication and a collaborative team approach.

The skill of changing a PVAD dressing cannot be delegated to an unregulated care provider (UCP). The nurse instructs the UCP to report the following immediately:

- Report to the nurse if the dressing is visibly soiled, loose, or wet and if the patient indicates moistness or loosening of the PVAD dressing.
- Protect the PVAD dressing during hygiene and activities of daily living (ADLs).

Equipment

- Antiseptic swabs (CHG with alcohol solution preferred, povidone-iodine, or 70% alcohol)
- Sterile TSM dressing (with border preferred), or TSM dressing and added ESD
- Clean gloves

STEP	RATIONALE

ASSESSMENT

1. Determine when dressing was last changed. Dressing should be labelled to include date and time applied and insertion date.

Indicates when dressing change is required.

2. Perform hand hygiene and apply clean gloves. Observe present dressing for integrity and moisture. If moisture is present, determine source (site leakage or external source).

If the dressing integrity is compromised there is increased risk of infection or PVAD dislodgement.

3. Prior to removing dressing, assess the insertion site visually by gently palpating the skin around and above PVAD. Assess PVAD for signs and symptoms of PVAD- or infusion-related complications (e.g., infiltration, phlebitis, infection, patient indication of pain, or leakage under dressing). Remove dressing and discard gloves.

Identifies complications that compromise integrity of PVAD and may necessitate its replacement.

4. Assess patient's understanding of need for continued infusion therapy.

Promotes person-centred care.

NURSING DIAGNOSES

- Pain or discomfort
- Insufficient knowledge regarding infusion therapy
- Potential for infection
- Potential for loss of venous access

Related factors/Risk factors are individualized on the basis of patient's condition or needs.

PLANNING

1. Expected outcomes following completion of procedure:
   - Patient's PVAD remains patent, and site is free from signs and symptoms of infusion-related complications.

Proper care maintains IV site.

   - Patient and caregiver can explain procedure and purpose of PVAD dressing change.

Demonstrates learning.

2. Explain procedure and purpose to patient and caregiver. Explain that patient will need to hold affected extremity still. Explain how long procedure will take.

Decreases anxiety, encourages cooperation, and promotes active participation in person-centred care.

3. Collect equipment and organize on clean, clutter-free bedside stand or over-bed table. Apply clean gloves.

STEP	RATIONALE

IMPLEMENTATION

1. Identify patient using at least two person-specific identifiers (e.g., name and date of birth or name and medical record number) according to employer policy. Compare identifiers with information on patient's medication administration record (MAR) or medical record.

Ensures correct patient. Complies with Accreditation Canada's standards and improves patient safety (Accreditation Canada, 2019).

2. Perform hand hygiene.

Reduces transmission of infection and contamination of equipment.

3. Assess PVAD insertion site for signs and symptoms of infusion-related complications. If complication exists, determine if PVAD requires removal.

Presence of the following complication are indications for PVAD removal: redness, swelling, leakage, drainage, pain or discomfort.

4. Remove existing dressing. **NOTE:** ESDs must also be changed at the same time as the TSM dressing.

Technique minimizes discomfort and injury to skin during removal.

Use alcohol swab on TSM dressing next to patient's skin to loosen dressing.

Removing stabilization device allows for appropriate skin antisepsis before applying new stabilization device and dressing.

   a. *For TSM dressing:* Stabilize catheter with nondominant hand (see illustration). Remove dressing by pulling dressing away from the skin from proximal edge toward insertion site (INS, 2016a). Repeat on all sides until dressing has been removed.

Stabilization of the catheter is key to preventing loss of access.

Removing dressing parallel to the skin in slow motion helps prevent medical adhesive-related skin injury (MARSI).

Clinical Decision Point *Stabilize catheter throughout process while maintaining asepsis. If patient is restless or uncooperative, it is helpful to have another staff member help with the procedure.*

5. Perform skin antisepsis to insertion site with CHG/alcohol swab using friction in back-and-forth motion for at least 30 seconds, allow to dry completely (minimum of 30 seconds). Alternative antiseptic solutions may be used for patient sensitivities (alcohol, povidone-iodine, CHG). Always allow antiseptic solution to dry completely.

Reduces incidence of catheter-related infections (INS, 2016a). Allow any skin antiseptic agent time to fully dry for complete antisepsis and to prevent MARSI (INS, 2016a).

6. *Optional:* Apply skin protectant to areas where an adhesive will attach to skin. Avoid area directly around insertion site. Allow to dry.

Apply skin barrier solution to help protect skin integrity, prevent irritation from adhesive, and promote adhesion of dressing.

7. Apply sterile dressing over site (procedures differ; follow employer policy, and manufacturer's guidelines).

   a. *TSM dressing:* Apply TSM dressing as directed in Skill 29.1, Step 20.

Protects catheter insertion site and minimizes risk for infection. TSM dressing enables visualization of insertion site and surrounding area for assessment of complications (INS, 2016a).

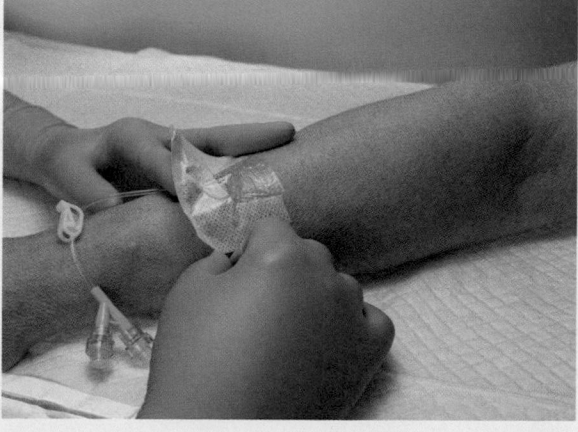

STEP 4a Remove TSM dressing. (*Courtesy Patrick Coble.*)

STEP	RATIONALE

IMPLEMENTATION

b. *Sterile gauze dressing:* Apply sterile gauze. This is not recommended; sterile gauze should only be used if patient does not tolerate TSM.

Use of sterile tape is not an effective stabilization device and is not recommended; however, if required, use only sterile tape under sterile dressing to prevent site contamination.

Gauze dressing obscures observation of insertion site and is changed every 2 days (INS, 2016a).

8. Remove and discard gloves and used equipment. Perform hand hygiene.

Prevents transmission of microorganisms.

9. Retape administration set tubing or extension set.

Prevents accidental dislodgement of PVAD. Provides safety and comfort for patient.

10. Label dressing per employer policy. Information on label includes date of dressing change and initials.

Communicates type of device and time interval for dressing change and site rotation.

11. Perform hand hygiene.

Reduces transmission of microorganisms.

EVALUATION

1. Evaluate function and patency of PVAD after dressing change by doing the following:

a) Swab the needle-free connector, then flush with a 10-mL prefilled syringe of 0.9% sodium chloride, assess the site for signs and symptoms of complications and ask patient if experiencing any discomfort.

b) Observe flow rate for continuous infusion, check for alarms if using an EID. Assess site for signs and symptoms of complications and ask patient if experiencing any discomfort.

Validates that the PVAD is patent and functioning correctly. Manipulation of catheter and tubing may cause PVAD dislodgement.

2. Assess patient and insertion site at established intervals per employer policy for signs and symptoms of PVAD- and infusion-related complications.

PVAD assessment for adult patients is required minimally every 4 hours, and every 1 to 2 hours for critically ill or sedated patients and for patients who have cognitive impairment (INS, 2016a). Outpatients must be provided with education to perform daily assessments and to report finding complications to a health care provider.

Assessment is critical to detect early signs of infection, infiltration, or extravasation or inaccurate infusion of solutions or medications.

3. Use Teach-Back: "I want to be sure that I explained reasons for why we change the IV dressing. Tell me in your own words the problems that you would report that would require us to change the dressing." Develop a revised teaching plan if patient or caregiver is not able to teach back correctly.

Determines if additional education is required to promote and support patient safety regarding IV dressing care and maintenance.

Unexpected Outcomes

1. PVAD is removed or dislodged accidentally.

2. Infusion of solutions or medications is not infusing at prescribed rate.

Related Interventions

- Restart new one in other extremity or above previous insertion site if continued therapy is required.
- Check PVAD and administration set tubing for bending, kinking, or dislodgement.
- Check if infusion is dependent on patient's arm position.
- Check and adjust height of infusion container.
- Ensure that there are no signs and symptoms of infiltration or extravasation at insertion site or surrounding PVAD location.

Communication and Documentation

- Document in patients' chart or in electronic health record (EHR) the time and date the PVAD dressing was changed, reason for change, type of dressing material used, patency of system, description of PVAD site, and patient tolerance.

Special Considerations
Pediatric

- More frequent assessment of the PVAD site and infusion therapy is required for neonatal and pediatric patients (at minimum, hourly) (INS, 2016a, p. s82).
- Pediatric patients are not always able to understand explanations fully. Presence of a parent or security toy during the procedure helps to decrease fear and increase patient cooperation. Performing the procedure on patient's toy or doll first may help with understanding and cooperation.
- Help from a second health care provider or parent is often required to keep patient still and protect PVAD dislodgement.
- Use CHG with care in premature infants and those under 2 months of age because of the risks of skin irritation and chemical burns (INS, 2016a).
- Dried povidone-iodine should be removed with sodium chloride or sterile water for neonates with compromised skin integrity (INS, 2016b).

Gerontological

- Many older persons have fragile skin; prevent skin tears by minimizing the use of tape or an ESD directly on the skin. Use a skin barrier solution prior to dressing application to decrease risks associated with MARSI.
- Site assessment by palpation is very important for detecting fluid infiltration. Visual assessment alone may not be adequate to detect accumulating fluid in the tissue because older persons tend to have decreased elasticity of skin and loose skinfolds. Patients may not experience discomfort before there is a large amount of fluid infiltration, owing to their decreased tactile sensations.

Care in the Community

- Educate patient and caregiver about the signs and symptoms of PVAD- and infusion-related complications.
- Acknowledge to patient and caregiver that dressing-change procedures in the community setting may be different from those in health care facilities and provide them with a rationale and reassurance.
- Observe patient and caregiver preforming hand hygiene.
- Ensure that patient is aware of the need to protect PVAD site during bathing or showering and understands that the site cannot be submerged in water. Instruct patient to cover the site with an occlusive plastic wrap or bag to keep the dressing dry and intact.
- Teach patient and caregiver what to do if dressing becomes compromised. If PVAD falls out or becomes dislodged, instruct them to apply gauze with enough pressure to stop any bleeding and to notify the health care provider.

PROCEDURAL GUIDELINE 29.1 *Removing a Short-Peripheral Venous Access Device*

NSO *Nursing Skills Online Intravenous Fluid Therapy Module 12 / Lesson 4*

A peripheral venous access device (PVAD) is removed when prescribed by the health care provider when the prescribed therapy is completed or is no longer needed for the plan of care, or if clinically indicated because of a complication (e.g., phlebitis, infiltration, or catheter occlusion). The technique for removing a PVAD follows infection-prevention guidelines to minimize the chance of the patient acquiring an infection.

Delegation and Collaboration

The skill of removing a PVAD may be delegated to other health care professionals if they have had appropriate education, the skill is within their governing body scope of practice, and it is approved by employer policy. Assessment and care of PVADs require interprofessional collaboration for effective communication and patient safety.

The skill of removing a PVAD cannot be carried out by an unregulated care provider (UCP). The nurse instructs the UCP to report the following to the nurse immediately:

- Any bleeding at the site after the catheter has been removed.
- Any indications of pain by the patient or observation of redness at the site.

Equipment

- Clean gloves
- Sterile 5 × 5–cm (2 × 2–inch) or 10 × 10–cm (4 × 4–inch) gauze sponge or small adhesive dressing
- Tape

Procedural Steps

1. Key assessments prior to removal of PVAD include identifying if the patient is on any anticoagulant or antiplatelet therapy or has a disorder that causes slow clotting.
2. Review accuracy and completeness of health care provider's prescription for discontinuation of PVAD, if required.
3. Perform hand hygiene and collect equipment.
4. Identify patient using at least two person-specific identifiers (e.g., name and date of birth or name and medical record number) according to employer policy. Compare identifiers with information on patient's medication administration record (MAR) or medical record.
5. Apply clean gloves. Palpate catheter site through intact dressing.
6. Assess patient's understanding of the reason for PVAD removal.
7. Explain procedure to patient before removing the catheter.
8. Turn administration set roller clamp to "off" position or turn electronic infusion device (EID) off and roller clamp to "off" position.
9. Carefully remove PVAD dressing and engineered stabilization device, if present, as per Skill 29.5, Step 4.
10. Stabilize PVAD hub with finger of nondominant hand.

Clinical Decision Point *Never use scissors to remove the tape or dressing because you may accidentally cut the catheter.*

Continued

PROCEDURAL GUIDELINE 29.1 *Removing a Short-Peripheral Venous Access Device—cont'd*

11. Place clean, sterile gauze above insertion site and, using dominant hand, withdraw catheter using a slow, steady motion and keeping the hub parallel to skin (see illustration).

Clinical Decision Point *Do not raise or lift catheter before it is completely out of the vein, to avoid trauma or hematoma formation.*

12. Apply pressure to site for a minimum of 30 seconds until bleeding has stopped. If patient has increased clotting time, maintain pressure until hemostasis occurs.
13. Inspect catheter for intactness after removal; note tip integrity and length.
14. Observe intravenous (IV) site for evidence of any complications such as redness, pain, tenderness, swelling, bleeding, or

drainage. Monitor for 24 to 48 hours after removal for postinfusion phlebitis.
15. Apply clean, folded gauze dressing over insertion site and secure with tape or a small adhesive dressing.
16. Discard used supplies, remove gloves, and perform hand hygiene.
17. Document procedure in patient's medical record in electronic health record (EHR) or chart.
18. Ensure patient understanding of why PVAD was removed and that dressing should remain in place for a minimum of 24 hours. Ensure that patient knows to report any signs and symptoms of complication at insertion site to health care provider.

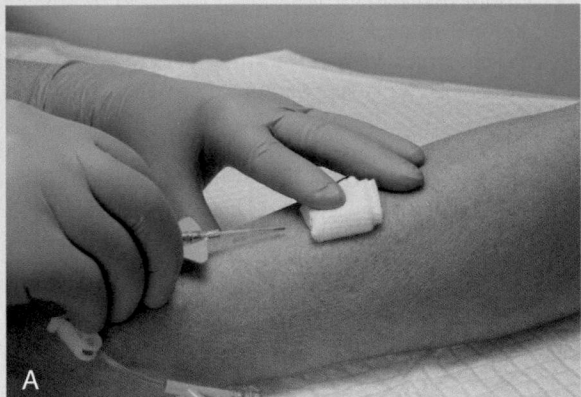
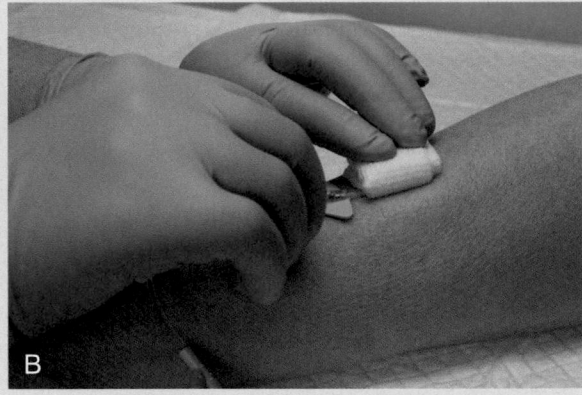

Step 11 PVAD removal. **A,** Apply pressure to site. **B,** Cover site and remove catheter. *(Courtesy Patrick Coble.)*

◆ SKILL 29.6 Caring for Patients With Central Vascular Access Devices

The selection of the most appropriate vascular access devices (VADs) for infusion therapy must be based on patient assessments, which may include intended length of treatment (greater than 7 days); type of infusion; patient characteristics such as age, vascular history, and comorbidities; and the care environment. Selecting the most appropriate device is critical to patient clinical outcomes, safety, and patient satisfaction.

Central vascular access device (CVAD) selection requires critical thinking and assessment, with interprofessional collaboration. The following are evidence-informed indications for use:
- Continuous vesicant therapy
- Solutions with an osmolarity greater than 900 mOsm/L
- History of poor peripheral access
- Clinical instability
- Complex care with multiple infusion needs, total parenteral nutrition (TPN), and for long-term infusion therapy

A CVAD differs from a peripheral VAD (PVAD) or midline in terms of where the tip of the catheter is located. PVADs and midlines terminate in peripheral veins; CVADs terminate in a centrally located vein. The ideal CVAD tip location for upper-body catheter insertion is in the superior vena cava at the cavoatrial junction. Catheters placed in the lower body terminate in the inferior vena cava above the level of the diaphragm (INS, 2016a). CVADs placed

in the femoral region are not recommended in adults (RCN, 2016, p. 36).

CVADs are categorized as nontunnelled, tunnelled, implanted (IVAD), and peripherally inserted (PICC) (Fig. 29.4). A tunnelled catheter is shown in Fig. 29.5. They may be designed for power injection and are made of different materials (e.g., polyurethane, silicone, or may be coated with antimicrobial or antithrombotic properties). Nurses must be able to identify each type of catheter and have knowledge of and education about appropriate access, use, care, and maintenance of the device.

CVADs can be nonvalved (clamps present) or have a valve either distally or proximally located. Distally located valves are referred to as Groshong catheters and have a rounded catheter tip (see Fig. 29.4, *B*). The valve is distally located on the side of the catheter and is pressure activated with infusion or aspiration. When the catheter is not in use, the valve remains closed. The valve helps prevent reflux of blood into the catheter, reducing risks of occlusion, and also prevents air embolism or blood loss if the needle-free connector is removed. Proximal valves are located close to the catheter hub and provide the same benefits (e.g., PASV or Solo). Valved catheters are locked with 0.9 % sodium chloride when not in use, to prevent occlusion and maintain patency.

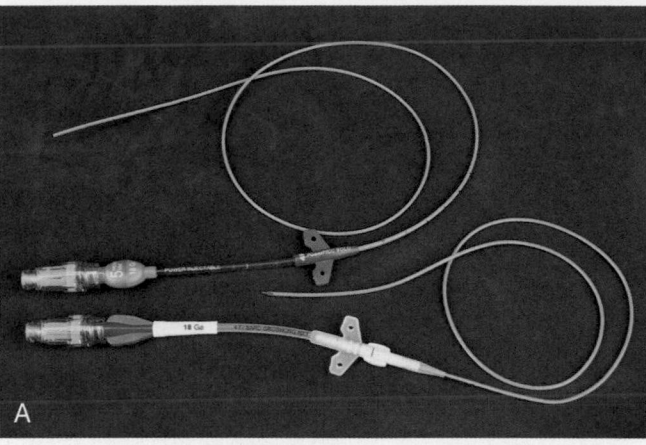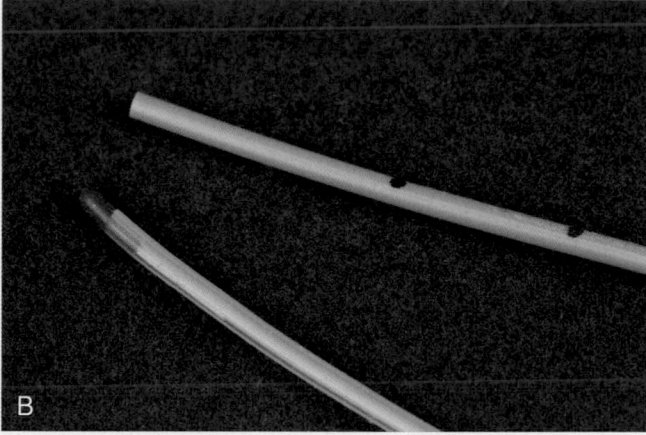

FIG 29.4 A, Peripherally inserted central catheters (PICCs). **B,** PICC tips. (*Courtesy Burl Jantzen.*)

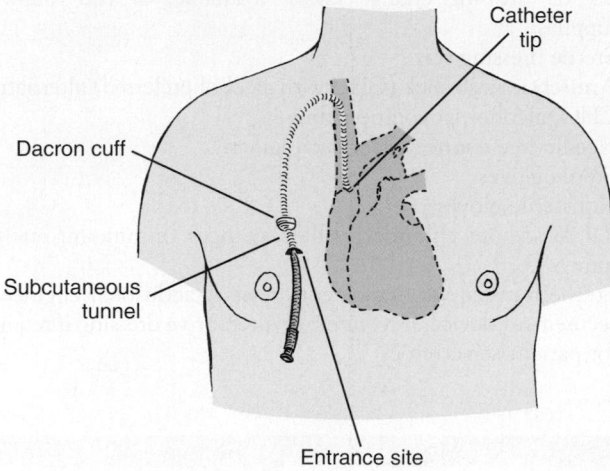

FIG 29.5 Tunnelled catheter is in place, threaded into superior vena cava.

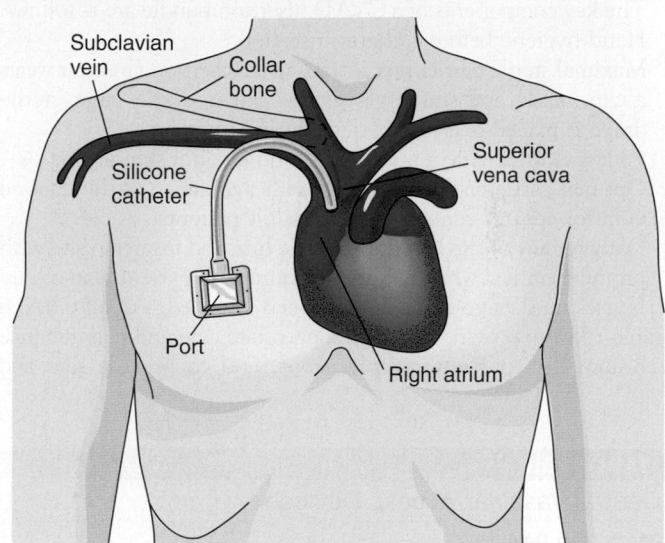

FIG 29.6 Implanted port and catheter.

Nonvalved CVADs, similar to a straw, are open and thus require clamps on the external segments to remain closed when the catheter is not in use, to prevent reflux of blood into the catheter tip and to prevent risk of air embolism or blood loss if the needle-free connector or administration set is removed. There is insufficient clinical evidence to recommend locking with heparin lock solution. Randomized controlled trials have shown equivalent outcomes with heparin lock and normal saline (INS, 2016a).

CVADs have single or multiple lumens. The choice of the number of lumens depends on the patient's condition and prescribed therapy. Evidence-informed practice recommends selecting the smallest gauge and the fewest number of lumens suitable for the patient's prescribed therapy. Patients who require numerous infusions and blood samplings may have a device placed with more than one lumen, allowing simultaneous administration of solutions and medications. In addition, multiple lumens allow for administration of incompatible solutions or medications at the same time. Access to each lumen is via the needle-free connector attached to the catheter hub.

An implanted vascular access device (IVAD) has a reservoir (port body) placed in a pocket under the skin with catheter tip placement at the cavoatrial junction (Fig. 29.6). IVADs have no external lumen or hub. They are accessed using a noncoring needle of the appropriate gauge and length. The noncoring needle is inserted using sterile technique at a 90-degree angle through the skin and into the port septum until it hits the back of the port body (Fig. 29.7).

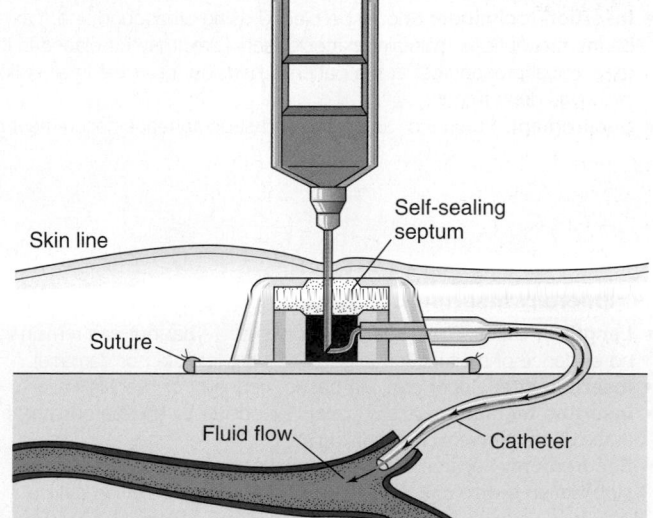

FIG 29.7 Cross-section of implanted port showing access of port with noncoring needle.

IVADs may be valved or nonvalved. To maintain patency when not required for infusion therapy, they require a monthly flushing with 0.9 % sodium chloride. Alternative locking solutions may be indicated according to patient condition, employer policy, and manufacturer's instruction for use.

Complications associated with CVADs can include local or systemic infection. A local infection can develop around the catheter insertion site or in the pocket of the implanted reservoir. A more serious infection of the bloodstream may be caused by contamination of the catheter from the skin of the patient's or health care provider's hands, contaminated solutions, or poor infection-prevention practices during insertion, care, and maintenance (INS, 2016b). Central line–associated blood stream infections (CLABSI) are very serious; therefore, bundling of prevention activities (e.g., CVAD insertion bundle) is recommended, as this has been shown to decrease this preventable complication (Canadian Patient Safety Institute [CPSI], 2016).

The key components of a CVAD insertion bundle are as follows:
- Hand hygiene before catheter insertion
- Maximal sterile barrier precautions with insertion (Inserter wears a cap, mask, and sterile gloves and gown, and a large, sterile drape is placed over the patient during insertion.)
- Chlorhexidine gluconate (CHG) and alcohol skin antisepsis
- Optimal catheter site selection, with avoidance of the femoral vein for central venous access in adult patients
- Daily review of the condition of the line and insertion site with prompt removal when no longer required for patient plan of care
Nurses must have evidence-informed knowledge of all CVADs (Table 29.6) to provide the most appropriate care and maintenance techniques, to prevent complications, and to provide safe and effective infusion therapy. Nurses need to use interprofessional collaboration when caring for patients with a CVAD to optimize patient safety.

Delegation and Collaboration

The skill of managing a CVAD cannot be delegated to an unregulated care provider (UCP). The nurse instructs the UCP to:
- Report the following to the nurse immediately: bleeding or swelling around CVAD insertion site; patient's shortness of breath; loosened or soiled dressing; patient developing a fever or indicating pain at the site; or catheter becoming dislodged.
- Inform the nurse if the electronic infusion device (EID) alarm signals or if fluid level in the container is low or empty.
- Assist with positioning patient during insertion and care.

Equipment
Site Care and Dressing Change
- CVAD dressing change kit, if available, or the following supplies:
- Sterile dressing tray
- Antiseptic swab stick (CHG with alcohol preferred) alternatives CHG, alcohol, povodine-iodine
- Needle-free connector for each lumen
- Sterile gloves
- Nonsterile gloves
- 0.9 % sodium chloride prefilled syringes (minimum, one per lumen)
- Sterile transparent securement dressing, additional engineered securement device, if required, or alternative dressing if required for patient sensitivities

---

TABLE 29.6

Central Vascular Access Devices

Short-Term Devices	Long-Term Devices
Nontunnelled Percutaneous	**External Tunnelled (Hickman, Broviac, Groshong)**
• **Length of dwell:** Days to several weeks	• **Length of dwell:** Recommended for long-term use, may remain in situ for many years if there are no unresolved issues with breakage, occlusion, or infections
• **Insertion sites:** Subclavian, external/internal jugular, and femoral veins	• **Insertion site:** Chest region through subclavian or jugular vein
• **Insertion technique:** Should be placed using ultrasound and maximum barrier precautions maintaining sterile technique, may be placed in the OR for surgical procedures, at the patient's bedside, or at the interventional radiology department	• **Insertion technique:** Surgically inserted in the OR, or in interventional radiology; tunnelling of proximal end subcutaneously from insertion site and exiting through skin at an exit site
• **Securement:** Sutures or an engineered subcutaneous securement device	• **Securement:** In place by a Dacron cuff coated in antimicrobial solution; in approximately 2–3 weeks scar tissue forms around cuff, fixing catheter in place. Sutures are present for the first 10 days to 2 weeks after insertion until secured by the Dacron cuff.
Peripherally Inserted Central Catheters (PICCs) (see Fig. 29.4)	**Implanted Venous Ports**
• **Length of dwell:** Recommended for up to 1 year but can remain in situ if no evidence of malfunction (e.g., occlusion, infection or damage)	• **Length of dwell:** Recommended for long-term use, may remain in situ for many years if there are no unresolved issues with breakage, occlusion, or infections
• **Insertion site:** Upper arm, via basilic, cephalic, or brachial veins	• **Insertion sites:** Subclavian or jugular vein is accessed with reservoir located in the chest, abdomen, or inner aspect of forearm
• **Insertion technique:** At the patient's bedside by an appropriately trained nurse or by interventional radiologist	• **Insertion technique:** Surgically inserted in the OR, or in interventional radiology; catheter is placed via subclavian or jugular vein and attached to reservoir located within a surgically created subcutaneous pocket (see Fig. 29.5)
• **Securement:** Securement dressing, adhesive-based engineered stabilization device, subcutaneous engineered stabilization device	• **Securement:** Reservoir is sutured in place within surgically created pocket. It is accessed using a noncoring needle through the skin (see Fig. 29.7).

OR, Operating room.

- Skin barrier swab (for sensitive skin)
- Alcohol swabs, minimum two per lumen

Blood Sampling
- Clean gloves
- Antiseptic swabs (CHG solution, povidone-iodine, or 70% alcohol)
- 5-mL Luer-Lok syringes
- 10-mL Luer-Lok syringes
- Vacuum system or blood transfer device (see employer policy)
- Blood tubes, including waste tubes, labels
- Needle-free connector injection cap
- Syringe (5 mL or 10 mL; see employer policy) for discarded blood
- 10-mL syringe with 5 to 10 mL preservative-free 0.9% sodium chloride (normal saline [NS])
- 10-mL syringe with heparin flush solution
- Sterile cap to maintain sterility of distal end of IV administration set

Changing the Needle-Free Connector
- Clean gloves
- Antiseptic swabs (CHG solution, povidone-iodine, or 70% alcohol)
- Needle-free injection cap(s)
- 10-mL syringe with 10 mL preservative-free 0.9% sodium chloride (NS)
- 10-mL syringe with heparin flush solution

Discontinuation of a Nontunnelled Catheter
- Personal protective equipment (PPE) as indicated (goggles, gown, mask, and clean gloves)
- CVAD dressing change kit, which includes sterile gloves, mask, antiseptic swabs for skin disinfection, TSM dressing, 10 × 10-cm (4 × 4-in) gauze pads, tape measure, sterile tape, label
- Petroleum-based ointment or petroleum-based gauze, sterile
- Suture removal kit (if sutures are in place)
- Stethoscope

STEP	RATIONALE

ASSESSMENT

1. Review accuracy and completeness of health care provider's prescription for insertion of CVAD for size and type. Assess treatment schedule: times for administration of IV solutions, medications, and blood sampling. Follow the 10 rights of medication administration (see Chapters 20 and 22). Confirm that informed consent has been obtained and witnessed by health care provider who will perform procedure.

Identifies patient's need for vascular access, evaluates response to therapy, and determines education needs. Insertion of central catheter requires informed consent (INS, 2016a).

2. Perform hand hygiene. Assess patient's hydration status: skin turgor, dryness of mouth, skin texture, and fluid intake and output.

Reduces transmission of infection. Provides baseline. In addition, dehydration makes insertion of CVAD more difficult.

3. Assess patient for any surgical procedures of upper chest or anatomical irregularities of proposed insertion site.

Previous surgical procedures or central vascular catheterizations indicate that you should not use a particular site. Spinal deformities and contractions make positioning difficult.

4. Assess CVAD placement site for skin integrity (open lesions) and signs of infection (i.e., redness, pain, tenderness, swelling, bleeding, or drainage). Apply gloves if drainage is present.

Compromised skin integrity contraindicates catheter insertion and can lead to secondary complications.

5. Assess patient for allergy to iodine, lidocaine, latex, or CHG.

Medications, solutions used during catheter insertion, and use of gloves and tape can cause serious allergic reactions.

6. Assess type of CVAD intended for placement. Review manufacturer's directions concerning catheter and maintenance.

Care and management depend on type and size of catheter or port, number of lumens, and purpose of therapy.

7. Assess for proper function of existing CVAD before therapy: integrity of catheter, ability to flush or infuse solution, and ability to aspirate blood. Remove and discard gloves (if worn). Perform hand hygiene.

Blood return should be obtained and patency confirmed before infusion of solutions or medications (INS, 2016a).

8. Assess if any catheter lumens require flushing or if CVAD site needs dressing change by referring to medical record, nurses' notes, employer policy, and manufacturer-recommended guidelines for use.

Provides guidelines for maintaining catheter patency and preventing infection.

NURSING DIAGNOSES

- Insufficient fluid volume
- Excessive fluid volume
- Insufficient knowledge regarding care of CVAD
- Reduced skin integrity
- Potential for infection
- Potential for injury

Related factors/Risk factors are individualized on the basis of patient's condition or needs.

STEP	RATIONALE

PLANNING

1. Expected outcomes following completion of procedure:
- Insertion occurs without complication.

- Optimal catheter tip placement is appropriate at or near the cavoatrial junction as confirmed by X-ray or fluoroscopy during insertion.
- Postinsertion CVAD will remain free of signs and symptoms of complications (redness, swelling, bleeding, or discomfort at insertion site), and suture or stabilization device will remain intact to prevent catheter migration.
- Solutions and medications infuse as prescribed.
- Patient's CVAD will have ongoing assessment and care and maintenance according to employer policies procedures and guidelines.

- Blood draws for diagnostics will be obtained following employer policy to prevent erroneous lab results and catheter occlusion.
- Patient and caregiver are able to explain purpose of CVAD and benefits to patient and caregiver. Patient will be still during procedure. Patient and caregiver are able to explain IV line therapy, care, and maintenance.

2. Explain procedure and purpose to patient and caregiver. Explain to patient that they must not move during procedure. Offer opportunity at this time for patient to use toilet, and offer pain medication (if needed).

3. Perform hand hygiene. Collect and organize equipment on clean, clutter-free bedside stand or over-bed table.

Rationale column:

Placement of nontunnelled CVAD carries risks such as pneumothorax, hematoma, air embolism, thrombosis, and infection.

Appropriate tip placement decreases risk of thrombotic complications or arrhythmias. Confirmation of tip location is required before use of CVAD (INS, 2016a).

Catheter is patent, properly placed, and without evidence of complications.

Catheter remains patent.

Care and maintenance of CVAD includes assessment, site care, dressing changes, needle-free connector, changes, and flushing. Aseptic technique must be maintained for all procedures (INS, 2016b).

Catheter remains patent after blood draws.

Demonstrates that patient and caregiver have understanding of and competency in caring for CVAD.

Decreases anxiety, promotes cooperation, and prevents sudden movement during sterile procedure.

Reduces transmission of infection and contamination of equipment (INS, 2016a).

IMPLEMENTATION

1. Identify patient using at least two person-specific identifiers (e.g., name and date of birth or name and medical record number) according to employer policy. Compare identifiers with information on medication administration record (MAR) or medical record.

Rationale: Ensures correct patient. Complies with Accreditation Canada's standards and improves patient safety (Accreditation Canada, 2019).

2. Assist with catheter insertion: nontunnelled device

Rationale: Ultrasound-guided venous access is recommended when the internal jugular vein is going to be used and equipment and clinical expertise are available. Ultrasound is also used to place PICCs using the brachial or basilic vein in children and adults (Heffner & Androes, 2018; Sabado & Pittiruti, 2018).

a. Health care provider, with help from nurse, positions patient in Trendelenburg's or supine position for placement in vessels above heart, unless contraindicated.

Rationale: Opens angle between clavicle and first rib; dilates veins to facilitate eventual catheter insertion.

Clinical Decision Point *Trendelenburg's position is contraindicated in patients with head injuries, increased intracranial pressure, certain respiratory conditions, and spinal cord injuries.*

(1) Nurse places rolled towel or bath blanket between patient's shoulder blades, rotating them slightly to 10-degree angle. Turn patient's head away from intended insertion site.

Rationale: Patient position of head down, below heart promotes maximum filling and distention with increase in diameter of subclavicular vein (Phillips & Gorski, 2014); a 10-degree tilt effectively achieves increase in diameter of vein.

b. Perform hand hygiene using antiseptic soap for 60 seconds.

Rationale: Handwashing technique removes transient and resident bacteria from skin.

STEP	RATIONALE

IMPLEMENTATION

c. If necessary, use scissors or electric clippers to remove any hair around insertion site. Explain rationale to patient.

Transient microorganisms reside in body hair. Shaving can cause increased risk for infection (INS, 2016a).

d. Health care provider and nurse apply cap, mask, eyewear, surgical gown, and powder-free sterile gloves.

Maximum barrier precautions are needed when inserting central vascular catheter (INS, 2016a).

e. Health care provider opens central vascular access kit. They may have nurse add needed sterile equipment to kit for use during insertion (see Chapter 10).

Maintains sterile field.

f. Site preparation:

Reduces incidence of catheter-related infections (PHAC, 2016).

(1) Perform skin antisepsis with CHG solution using friction in back-and-forth motion for 30 seconds and allow to dry completely.

Allow any skin antiseptic agent to fully dry for complete antisepsis (INS, 2016a).

g. After cleaning site, health care provider and nurse remove gloves. Health care provider changes into second pair of sterile gloves, and nurse performs hand hygiene. (Check employer policy, because some facilities require strict precautions.)

Gloves become contaminated from surface bacteria picked up in solution. Nurse functions as nonsterile circulator whose primary function is to ensure sterility of insertion field.

h. Health care provider uses large sterile drape and sterile towels to create sterile field. Health care provider finds anatomical landmarks and places sterile fenestrated drape appropriately over proposed insertion site.

Provides sterile work space for catheter insertion (INS, 2016a).

i. Health care provider arranges equipment in kit in preparation for catheter insertion.

Ensures smooth, orderly procedure.

j. Nurse sets up IV bag, primes and fills tubing, and covers end of tubing with sterile cap (see Skill 29.2).

IV administration set is ready to be connected to IV catheter.

k. Nurse scrubs top of 1% lidocaine bottle with antiseptic swab, allowing to dry completely, and holds bottle upside down if not in insertion kit. *Optional:* Topical local anaesthetic agents can be applied before insertion with health care provider's prescription.

Removes surface bacteria; enables health care provider to withdraw lidocaine while maintaining asepsis. Lidocaine has potential for creating allergic reaction and tissue damage.

l. Health care provider injects needle into bottle and withdraws approximately 3 to 4 mL lidocaine and injects needle into site for internal jugular puncture and anaesthetizes venipuncture site, waiting 1 to 2 minutes for effect to take place.

Minimizes discomfort that patient feels during venipuncture. Site has been documented to be safer for bedside insertion and ability to use ultrasound-guided insertion (Heffner & Androes, 2018; Sabado & Pittiruti, 2018).

Clinical Decision Point *Just before the time of catheter insertion, ask patient to hold their breath and strain. This is a Valsalva manoeuvre, the preferred method, which increases central venous pressure to prevent entry of air into the catheter. Breath holding and humming may be used in patients unable to perform the Valsalva manoeuvre. If the patient is unable to perform manoeuvres, compress patient's abdomen gently.*

m. Health care provider inserts IV catheter into internal jugular vein via ultrasound-guided access or using knowledge of vein anatomy. Usually this is done by locating the vein with a large-bore cannula, removing needle from cannula, threading wire into cannula and vein, removing cannula over wire, and threading central vein catheter over wire to appropriate location (Seldinger technique) (Heffner & Androes, 2018).

A large vein is selected because it will be less irritated by hypertonic solutions or medications.

n. Health care provider determines patency of line by withdrawing blood with 5-mL syringe, flushing with 0.9% sodium chloride, and placing needle-free connectors on hub of each lumen. *Option:* VAD may be flushed with heparin, based on type of catheter and employer policy.

Determines patency of device. Use of heparin, flush volume, and concentration vary by employer and type of catheter. Valved catheters are flushed with 0.9% sodium chloride only and do not require heparin.

o. Health care provider applies catheter securement device (e.g., engineered stabilization device, sutures, sterile tape, or surgical Steri-Strips) to secure central vascular catheter in place. Cover with TSM dressing.

Suturing catheter to skin at insertion site increases risk for infection. Catheter securement devices are noninvasive and preferred for preventing catheter dislodgement (INS, 2016a).

STEP	RATIONALE

IMPLEMENTATION

p. Health care provider removes sterile drapes and completes procedure. External catheter length is measured.

Measurement allows for comparison if dislodgement of CVAD is suspected (INS, 2016a).

q. Nurse initiates and regulates IV infusion to prescribed rate and connects to electronic infusion pump after receiving confirmation of tip location using electrocardiogram (ECG) reading. Although ECG technology is the gold standard for determining tip placement, a chest X-ray, transesophageal echocardiography, or fluoroscopy may be used.

Maintains patency of VAD. Confirmation of tip placement prevents complications.

3. Insertion site care and dressing change

a. Position patient in comfortable position with head slightly elevated. Have patient's arm extended for PICC or midline device.

Provides access to patient.

b. Prepare dressing materials.
TSM dressing: Change at least every 5–7 days.
Gauze dressing: Change at least every 2 days.
Gauze under TSM: Change at least every 2 days.

TSM dressings are preferred because they allow visualization of insertion site.

c. Perform hand hygiene and apply mask. Instruct patient to turn head away from site during dressing change or provide mask for patient.

Reduces transfer of microorganisms; prevents spread of airborne microorganisms over CVAD insertion site.

d. Apply clean gloves. Remove old TSM dressing by stabilizing catheter with nondominant hand. Remove dressing by pulling up one corner and gently pulling straight out and parallel to skin. Repeat on all sides until dressing has been removed.

Prevents unintentional catheter dislodgement and medical adhesive-related skin injuries (MARSI).

e. Remove catheter stabilization device, if present. Use alcohol to remove adhesive stabilization devices.

Enables visualization of insertion site and allows for appropriate skin antisepsis (INS, 2016a). Use of alcohol minimizes risk for MARSI (INS, 2016a).

Clinical Decision Point *If sutures are used for initial catheter stabilization and become loosened or are no longer intact, alternative stabilization measures should be used. Use of an engineered stabilization device is recommended because sutures are associated with increased risk of infection (INS, 2016a).*

f. Assess catheter, insertion site, and surrounding skin for signs and symptoms of complications (e.g., drainage). Measure the external segment of CVAD and compare to length at insertion. For PICC, measure upper-arm circumference 10 cm (4 in.) above antecubital fossa and compare with measurement on insertion.

Detection of complications for early intervention is critical. Comparison of measurements facilitates early recognition of dislodgement or migration. Increasing arm circumference could indicate thrombosis (INS, 2016a).

g. Remove and discard clean gloves; perform hand hygiene. Using sterile technique, open CVAD dressing kit and other supplies.

Sterile technique is required to apply new dressing.

h. Perform skin antisepsis with CHG/alcohol or alternate antiseptic. Apply solution using friction in back-and-forth motion for a minimum of 30 seconds and allow to air dry completely.

Allow any skin antiseptic agent to dry fully for complete antisepsis (INS, 2016a). Do not fan or wipe skin.

i. Apply skin barrier solution and allow to dry completely.

Protects irritated or fragile skin from dressing and stabilization device, if used, and minimizes risk for MARSI.

j. Apply sterile securement dressing or engineered stabilization device with TSM dressing. CHG-impregnated dressings are recommended for nontunnelled CVADs.

Use of engineered stabilization devices that enable visual inspection of insertion site can reduce risk for VAD complications (e.g., phlebitis, infection, migration) and unintentional loss of access (INS, 2016a). Use with caution in patients with fragile skin or complicated skin pathologies or in newborns and infants (INS, 2016a).

k. Apply label to dressing with date, initials, and external segment measurement.

Indicates when next dressing change is due and if catheter dislodgement or migration has occurred.

STEP	RATIONALE

IMPLEMENTATION

l. Dispose of soiled supplies. Remove gloves and perform hand hygiene.

Reduces transmission of microorganisms.

4. Blood sampling

a. Perform hand hygiene and apply clean gloves.

Reduces transmission of microorganisms.
Prevents transfer of body fluids.

b. Turn off all infusions for at least 1 to 5 minutes before drawing blood. **NOTE:** If you cannot stop infusion, draw blood from the peripheral vein.

Prevents dilution of sample, which may cause erroneous diagnostic results and misdiagnosis.

c. Draw blood through most appropriate lumen or as indicated by manufacturer's instructions.

Multi-lumen catheters may have different lumen sizes. The largest is usually the most suitable for blood draws.

d. Use syringe or vacuum tube method.

Check employer policy and manufacturer's instructions.

　　(1) Remove administration set or the needle-free connector. Apply sterile cap to male end of tubing.

Maintains sterility of end of IV administration set. Drawing from needle-free connector minimizes risk of blood exposure.

　　(2) Scrub catheter hub with antiseptic swab for at least 15 seconds and allow to dry completely.

Reduces risk of infection.

　　(3) Attach empty 10-mL syringe to needle-free connector, open clamp if required, and flush with 10 mL, then withdraw 5 to 6 mL of blood for discard sample.

Discard sample reduces risk of drug concentrations or diluted specimen. Drawing specimens for international normalized ratio (INR) studies from heparinized lines is not recommended (INS, 2016b).

　　(4) Clamp catheter (if necessary); remove syringe with blood and discard in appropriate biohazard container.

Valved catheters do not require clamping. Nonvalved catheters require clamping to prevent reflux of blood into catheter.

　　(5) Scrub catheter hub with another antiseptic swab and allow to dry completely.

Reduces risks of infection.
Refer to manufacturer's instruction for scrub time of needle-free connector (minimum 5 seconds).

　　(6) Attach a 10-mL sterile syringe and open clamp, if present. Draw required amount of blood for samples. If using transfer vacuum device method, attach device directly to needle-free connector and fill blood tube in correct order of draw (see illustration).

Syringe method may require more than one syringe if amount of blood exceeds 10 mL. Blood tubes must be filled in correct order to prevent errors in lab results.

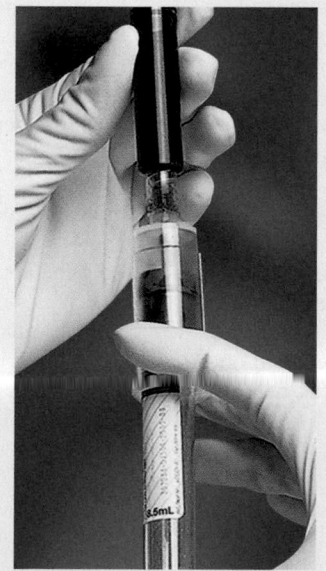

STEP 4d(6) Blood specimen transfer device. (*Courtesy © Becton Dickinson & Co.*)

STEP	RATIONALE

IMPLEMENTATION

(7) Attach a prefilled 10-mL 0.9% sodium chloride syringe to the needle-free connector and flush using a push–pause method. Note that the process may need to be repeated with a second flush syringe to completely clear blood from the needle-free connector and catheter.

Remove syringe using the appropriate flush–clamp–disconnect sequence based on the type of needle-free connector (e.g., neutral, negative, or positive displacement).

Nonvalved catheters require clamping to prevent reflux of blood into tip of catheter.

Flush with a minimum of volume twice the internal volume of the catheter to prevent thrombotic catheter occlusion.

Follow employer policy for flushing volumes and technique.

e. Instill catheter with heparin lock solution, if required, or reconnect administration set and resume infusion. Ensure that clamp is engaged (if applicable).

Prevents clot formation.

There is insufficient evidence to recommend heparin lock solution over NS. Alternative locking solutions may be considered for certain patient conditions.

Decreases risk of occlusion.

Clinical Decision Point *Always use a 10-mL syringe or syringe designed to generate lower injection pressure (i.e., 10-mL–diameter syringe barrel) on central lines in adults to minimize pressure during injection (INS, 2016a).*

f. Dispose of soiled equipment and used supplies. Remove gloves and perform hand hygiene.

Reduces transmission of microorganisms.

5. Changing needle-free connector:

a. Determine when needle-free connector is due for change, or if there are indications for change. Assess connector type and select.

Understanding of types of needle-free connector ensures appropriate flush–clamp–disconnect sequence based on type of device (e.g., positive, negative, or neutral displacement valves) (INS, 2016a). Needle-free connectors should be changed every 7 days, when removed for any reason, or if they cannot be flushed clear of blood. If contamination of needle-free connector is suspected, it should be changed, regardless of length of time in place. This decreases risk of occlusion and infection.

b. Perform hand hygiene and apply clean gloves.

c. Prepare new sterile, needle-free connector, attach connector to prefilled 0.9% sodium chloride syringe, and prime to remove air. Leave prefilled syringe in place. Repeat for number of lumen required.

Maintain sterility of connector while attaching to syringe to prevent risks of infection.

Priming with 0.9% sodium chloride prevents air from entering the circulatory system.

d. Close clamp on catheter if nonvalved, remove needle-free connector, maintaining aseptic technique, and discard.

Maintains sterility.

e. Scrub the catheter hub with an antiseptic swab and allow to air dry.

Ensures disinfection of catheter hub.

f. Attach new primed, sterile, needle-free connector to catheter hub. Open clamp, if present, and flush catheter using push–pause technique. Remove syringe using the appropriate flush–clamp–disconnect sequence based on the type of needle-free connector (e.g., neutral, negative, or positive displacement).

Using the appropriate flush–clamp–disconnect sequence decreases risk of catheter occlusion by preventing reflux of blood into the catheter tip.

If an alternative locking solution is required, scrub needle-free connector with antiseptic swab before attaching syringe, then instill.

g. Repeat process for each lumen.

6. Removing nontunnelled catheters:

a. Collaborate with interprofessional team to determine need for nontunnelled catheter. Confirm and review prescription for CVAD removal.

CVAD should be assessed daily and removed with unresolved complications (e.g., infection or occlusion) or when infusion therapy has been discontinued and venous access is no longer required for the plan of care.

Review employer policy to determine scope of practice and limitations associated with removal of CVAD.

b. Review patient allergies or skin sensitivity related to supplies (e.g., latex, antiseptic, dressings).

Prevents complications and discomfort.

c. Discontinue infusion of medications or solutions.

STEP	RATIONALE

IMPLEMENTATION

d. Position patient in a supine flat or Trendelenburg position unless contraindicated for patient care. Position patient for comfort and place moisture-proof pad appropriately.

Patient's position with exit site below level of the heart decreases risk of air embolus on catheter removal.
Maintains a clean environment.

e. Perform hand hygiene.

Decrease risk of transmission of microorganisms.

f. Prepare supplies using aseptic technique.

g. Apply appropriate PPE as indicated by employer policy (e.g., clean gloves and eye protection)

Decreases risks of bloodborne pathogen exposure to health care provider.

h. Gently remove CVAD dressing by stabilizing catheter and pulling dressing from proximal edge toward the insertion site. Remove adhesive or subcutaneous stabilization device, if present.

Prevents unintentional catheter dislodgement and MARSI.
Prevents skin tears. Allows inspection of CVAD insertion site before removal.

    (1) If adhesive stabilization device is present or CHG-impregnated dressing was used, apply moisture from alcohol swab or CHG/alcohol swab to lift device and remove it.

    (2) Assess site and surrounding skin for any signs and symptoms of complications (e.g., infection, drainage, skin irritation).

i. Perform skin antisepsis with CHG/alcohol or alternate antiseptic for patient sensitivities. Apply solution using friction in a back-and-forth motion for a minimum of 30 seconds. Allow to completely air dry.

Antiseptic agent must fully dry to complete antisepsis.
Site must air dry; do not fan or wipe antiseptic from skin.

j. Remove gloves and perform hand hygiene; Apply sterile gloves.

Decreases risk of transmission of microorganisms.

k. Remove sutures, if present for securement, maintaining aseptic technique.

Allows CVAD removal.

l. Fold sterile petroleum-based dressing and sterile gauze pad. Place at insertion site with petroleum dressing against skin and gauze on top; apply digital pressure.

Application of a petroleum-based dressing against the skin helps seal the skin to vein tract and decreases risk of air embolus.

m. Instruct patient to take a deep breath and perform Valsalva manoeuvre, or to hold breath as catheter is withdrawn.

The Valsalva manoeuvre creates increased intrathoracic pressure to decrease risk of air entering through the opening in the skin.
Gentle removal of catheter prevents it from being stretched and breaking. A damaged catheter may break off and leave a piece in the patient's arm.
Direct pressure reduces risk for bleeding and hematoma formation.

Clinical Decision Point *It is often necessary to apply pressure longer if the patient is receiving anticoagulation therapy or has prolonged clotting times.*

n. Slowly remove catheter while maintaining digital pressure. Instruct patient to breathe normally once digital pressure has been applied. Continue to hold until hemostasis occurs.
Do not pull against resistance; the catheter should be easily removed.
Apply petroleum-based ointment or gauze to exit site. Apply sterile occlusive dressing such as TSM dressing or sterile gauze to site. Change dressing every 24 hours until site is healed.

Slow removal helps prevent vasoconstriction and reduces risk of catheter breakage.
Direct pressure decreases risk of air embolus, bleeding, and hematoma formation.
Signs and symptoms of air embolus may include sudden onset of shortness of breath, coughing, chest pain, hypotension, altered level of consciousness, and tachyarrhythmias.

o. Apply TSM dressing over both petroleum-based gauze and sterile gauze pad at insertion site. Instruct patient to leave dressing in place for a minimum of 24 hours to ensure healing at site. Label dressing with date and initials.

Decreases risks of infection and protects site during healing process.
Identifies date of catheter removal.

STEP	RATIONALE

IMPLEMENTATION

p. Encourage patient to remain flat or reclining for 30 minutes postremoval (INS, 2016a).	Decreases risk of complications (e.g., air embolus, bleeding). If catheter tip is broken or compromised, place in container and label for possible follow-up and notify health care provider.
q. Inspect catheter according to knowledge of catheter type, purpose, and patient-specific factors (e.g. suspected breakage). Discard it in an appropriate biohazard container.	Catheter cultures should not be obtained routinely (INS, 2016a).
r. Dispose of soiled supplies; remove gloves and personal protective equipment. Perform hand hygiene.	Decreases risk of transmission of microorganisms.

EVALUATION

1. Consult chest X-ray or fluoroscopy report for confirmation of tip location prior to initiation of infusion therapy, or when clinical signs and symptoms indicate potential tip malposition. The ECG method of tip confirmation may be used during insertion process. It is considered the gold standard for tip location confirmation (e.g., PICCs).

   Radiology reviews chest X-ray to confirm tip location.
   An ECG is done in real time during insertion. It allows for greater accuracy of placement at the cavoatrial junction, enables immediate use of the catheter, decreases patient exposure to radiation, and is cost effective.

2. Daily assessment is required to determine need for CVAD.

   Prompt removal of all VADs is recommended when they are no longer required, to decrease risks associated with central line–associated bloodstream infection (CLABSI) (Garrett, 2015; INS, 2016a, p. S91).

3. Evaluate for immediate postinsertion complications:

   Complications after insertion can include pneumothorax, cardiac arrhythmias, and nerve injury (INS, 2016a, pp. S102, S106). Prompt identification can allow for treatment, repositioning of catheter, or removal, if necessary.

   a. Auscultate breath sounds and evaluate for shortness of breath, chest pain, and absent breath sounds.

   Signs and symptoms of pneumothorax develop if CVAD pierces intrathoracic space.

   b. Monitor vital signs, including heart rate and rhythm.

   Evaluates for signs of cardiac arrhythmias.

   c. Monitor patient indications of pain, numbness, tingling, or weakness.

   These are signs of nerve injury from catheter insertion.

4. Assess patient to determine response to infusion therapy (e.g., laboratory values, input and output [I&O], weights, vital signs, postprocedure assessments).

   Infusion therapy solutions and medications maintain or restore fluid and electrolyte balance. Early recognition of complications leads to prompt treatment.

5. Assess patient at established intervals for signs and symptoms of CVAD and infusion therapy-related complications (Table 29.7) according to employer policy.

   Complications may include site or systemic infection, inaccurate infusion rates, infiltration, extravasation, and occlusion. Frequently scheduled observation and assessment allow for early detection and treatment of potential complications.

6. Inspect administration set and needle-free connectors to ensure that connections are secure.

   Prevents accidental dislodgement of tubing and connectors, which may cause blood loss or entrance of air or microbes into the bloodstream.

7. **Use Teach-Back:** Educate patient and caregiver about plan of care. This may include expected outcomes of treatment, expected duration of therapy, care and maintenance of CVAD, risks associated with CVAD and infusion therapy, and aseptic technique. For long-term use, ask patient or caregiver to discuss steps in care and perform procedure (e.g., catheter site cleaning or dressing change). Instruct patient regarding when to report signs and symptoms of complications. "I want to be sure you understand when you need to report signs and symptoms of complications. Can you tell me when you should contact a health care provider?" Develop a revised teaching plan if patient or caregiver is not able to teach back correctly.

   Determines patient's and caregiver's level of understanding of instructional topic.
   Promotes safe, person-centred care.

STEP	RATIONALE

EVALUATION

Unexpected Outcomes	Related Interventions
1. For catheter complications, see Table 29.7.	• See Table 29.7.
2. Patient or caregiver is unable to explain or perform CVAD care.	• Indicates need for community care referral or additional instruction.

TABLE 29.7

Complications of Vascular Access Devices

Complication	Assessment	Prevention	Intervention
Catheter damage, breakage	Observe for holes or tears in catheter every shift. Observe insertion site when flushing for leaking of fluid.	When clamps are present move position every shift on the external segment to prevent kinks and catheter damage. Use needle-free connectors and administration sets. Use only 10-mL or larger-barrel syringe for flushing purposes. Small-barrel syringes exert more pressure. (They may be used when giving small volumes of medication at required infusion rate.) Do not flush against resistance. Do not use scissors near VADs.	Apply clamp between patient and catheter damage or break. Determine if catheter can be repaired or needs to be removed. Use repair kits that are specific to the catheter type and follow manufacturer's instructions. Collaborate with the interprofessional team, reassess the need for continued vascular access and replacement of device. Pressure-rated (power) catheters cannot be repaired and should be removed as soon as possible.
Occlusions such as: • Thrombotic • Medication precipitates • Mechanical, malposition • Pinch-off syndrome	Assess insertion site and sutures. Assess catheter external segment for kinks that may be causing occlusion. Check for blood return and presence of resistance when flushing with normal saline (e.g., sluggish or absent blood return). Assess for patient discomfort or edema at insertion site and surrounding area (neck, shoulder, upper arm). Pinch-off syndrome is compression of the catheter between the clavicle and the first rib. This causes a mechanical occlusion and potential fracture of the catheter. IVADs: Assess if correct placement of noncoring needle has been maintained.	Follow appropriate flushing and locking technique according to employer policy. Use a push–pause technique when flushing. Ensure that stabilization dressing or device is secure. Always flush VAD pre– and post– medication administration to prevent mixing of incompatible medications. Observer for signs of catheter malfunction, investigate cause, and notify health care provider to obtain prescription to resolve or remove VAD. If VAD malfunction is suspected, stop all infusion therapy and notify health care provider.	Reposition patient, ask patient to take a deep breath and cough, or raise patient's arm. Change in position may correct suspected occlusion. Perform dressing change if catheter is kinked at insertion site. In collaboration with the interprofessional team, instill thrombolytic, promptly when indicated. Obtain venogram or chest X-ray if prescribed. Collaborate with the interprofessional team to reassess the need for continued vascular access and replacement or removal of device.
Infection and sepsis: insertion site, tunnelled pathway, IVAD reservoir pocket, CRBSI	Assess VAD insertion site for signs and symptoms of infection (redness, drainage, edema, or tenderness). Assess for signs of systemic infection (e.g., increased temperature). Monitor laboratory findings.	Use aseptic technique for all aspects of insertion and maintenance of VAD. Always scrub the needle-free connector with an antiseptic swab before each access. Ensure that dressing is dry and intact at all times, and change it if compromised. Adhere to asepsis technique with dressing changes.	When infection of CVAD is suspected, obtain blood culture samples from the catheter and direct venipuncture. Follow employer policy for collection of samples. Remove CVAD if required as prescribed.

Continued

TABLE 29.7

Complications of Vascular Access Devices—cont'd

Complication	Assessment	Prevention	Intervention
Dislodgement or migration	Measure length of external segment every shift and compare with measurement at time of insertion. Observe insertion site for leakage or swelling. Assess for catheter patency. Ask patient to report loud swishing sound during flushing (reflects migration of catheter tip in the jugular vein). Assess for tachycardia or patient indication of heart flutter or irregular pulse. Palpate catheter skin junction and tunnel for coiling (catheter can feel cordlike underneath the skin).	Maintain a dry, occlusive securement dressing at all times. Use additional stabilization and securement devices as required. Educate patient on activities of daily living and care and maintenance of CVAD to prevent unintended dislodgement. Use additional catheter stabilization device as required. Avoid pulling on CVAD.	If external measurement has exceeded that recommended in employer policy, follow steps to reassess catheter tip location (chest X-ray). If assessment confirms catheter migration inward, catheter should be pulled back to external length at time of insertion when tip location was confirmed. If tip location is no longer acceptable for type and length of treatment, remove CVAD as prescribed. Reassess need for VAD. Replace as required for plan of care, and consider alternative stabilization and securement to prevent future loss of access.
Loss of skin integrity (e.g., hematoma, redness, blisters, erosion at catheter insertion site, cuff, or IVAD reservoir extrusion).	Assess insertion site daily through TSM and at time of dressing change for changes in skin integrity or drainage. Ask patient to report any signs or symptoms promptly (redness, itching, pain, blisters). Assess for drainage at catheter skin junction. Assess for redness. Assess for edema and contusions. Note if tunnelled catheter is exposed. (Dacron cuff is visible.)	Maintain nutritional status. Avoid unnecessary pressure to area surrounding the insertion site. Avoid trauma to skin while removing dressing. Always remove it slowly, keeping it parallel to the skin. Do not stretch TSM dressing when applying it. Always allow antiseptic solutions to dry before applying dressings. If possible, rotate site of noncoring needle when changed. Consider alternative antiseptic products with patient sensitivities. Consider use of skin-barrier products to prevent MARSI. Instruct patient to report signs and symptoms of infection.	Consider use of an alternative dressing or antiseptic. Perform a patch test in an alternate location to confirm patient sensitivities. Improve nutritional intake. Report extrusion of cuff or IVAD reservoir to health care provider.
Infiltration, extravasation	Assess for erythema, edema, local swelling at the insertion site, malposition of the catheter tip location, patient shortness of breath, lack of blood return, pain during infusion therapy (e.g., burning, stinging).	Perform ongoing assessment of insertion at regular intervals. Discontinue infusion immediately when infiltration is suspected. Instruct patient to report signs and symptoms of complications immediately (e.g., leaking, swelling, discomfort).	Administer antidote, when applicable, according to employer policy. Remove VAD as soon as possible. Elevate limb, if applicable, and apply warm or cold compresses appropriate for the solution or medication that has infiltrated. Mark area of infiltration and continue to assess for changes in skin integrity. Grade severity of infiltration according to recognized scale.
Pneumothorax, hemothorax, air emboli, hydrothorax	Observe for signs of subcutaneous emphysema by palpating skin around insertion site (e.g., crackling, crinkling paper sensation). Assess for patient discomfort, dyspnea, apnea, hypoxia, tachycardia, hypotension, nausea, or confusion.	Always engage clamps on external segment of catheter (if present) when removing needle-free connector or opening the catheter system. Valved CVADs do not require a clamp because the valve remains closed, unless aspirating or flushing. Purge all flush syringes and administration sets of air before connecting to VAD.	Administer oxygen as required. Report adverse signs and symptoms to health care provider immediately. If air emboli are suspected, place patient on left side with head down. Remove catheter as prescribed. Help with insertion of chest tubes as prescribed.

CLABSI, Central line–associated bloodstream infection; *CVAD,* central vascular access device; *IV,* intravenous; *IVAD,* implanted vascular access device; *MARSI,* medical adhesive-related skin injury; *PICC,* peripherally inserted central catheter; *TSM,* transparent semipermeable membrane; *VAD,* vascular access device.

Communication and Documentation

- Immediately notify health care provider of signs and symptoms of any complications.
- Document catheter site care in nurses' notes in electronic health record (EHR) or chart, including catheter location; size of catheter; number of lumens; condition of catheter insertion site or port site, including skin integrity, external catheter length, mid-arm circumference for PICC; condition and type of securement device; date and time of dressing change; change of needle-free connectors; flushes used; patency of catheter, including presence or absence of blood return; and patient's tolerance of the procedure.
- Document in EHR or chart the patient's and caregiver's ability to explain instructions.
- Document in nurses' notes in EHR or patient chart catheter removal: patient position, appearance of site, length of catheter removed, integrity of catheter after removal, dressing applied, patient's tolerance of procedure, presence or absence of bleeding from site every 15 minutes for 1 hour, and any problems with removal.
- Document in nurses' notes in EHR the blood draw: date, time, sample drawn, waste volume, and flushes used.
- Document in nurses' notes in EHR the unexpected outcomes and CVAD complications, health care provider notification, interventions, and patient response to treatment.

Special Considerations
Teaching

- Instruct patient to report discomfort around the site; discomfort in arms, shoulders, or side of the neck; or any shortness of breath.
- Discuss and provide written emergency measures and telephone numbers of health care personnel to be used in case of catheter damage, dislodgement, swelling, redness, or leakage at insertion site; occlusion of catheter; patient temperature above 38°C (100.4°F) (see employer policy); and shivering chills.
- Provide written instructions for dressing changes, inspection of insertion site, flushing, and tubing changes.
- Arrange for instruction and return demonstration of skills by patient or caregiver.
- Have patient or caregiver maintain a list of caregivers and telephone numbers (e.g., health care provider, nurse, social worker, pharmacist, dietitian).

Pediatric

- Central vein catheters that are of a smaller diameter and shorter length are available for children and infants.
- Take care to secure infant catheters in a manner that does not allow them to twist. Small-diameter catheters are fragile, and twisting them causes them to tear.
- The amount and dosage of flush solution (heparin/sodium chloride) vary with age, size, and catheter diameter and length.
- Record volume of blood draws on I&O record.

Gerontological

- Some older persons have difficulty lying flat in bed, and a modification of the totally supine position during CVAD insertion is often necessary.
- PICC insertion may provide an alternative route of administration and reduce the risk of complications associated with subclavian or jugular insertion.

Care in the Community

- Initiate early referral for discharge planning to social services, counsellor, or community care coordinator for assessment of resources.
- Provide patient with written list of providers for supplies and equipment.
- Provide patient with Kelly clamp *without* teeth (bulldog clamp) that can be used in the event of catheter rupture to prevent air embolism and instruct patient in its use.
- Instruct patient or caregiver in flushing technique, site care, and dressing change and observe them performing procedures.
- Instruct patient and caregiver in adaptations of hospital procedures that they can make at home (e.g., good hand hygiene instead of sterile gloves).
- Provide education to patient and caregiver about how to recognize signs and symptoms of IV-related complications, actions to take, how to report them, and methods for preservation of CVADs.
- Assess home environment and determine suitable area for dressing changes, avoiding areas where contaminants are potential hazards.
- Provide appropriate information about home disposal of soiled dressings and equipment (see Chapter 43).

◆ CLINICAL DEBRIEF

An 88 year old female with a history of heart failure and gastric cancer was admitted to the hospital 24 hours ago for dehydration with mild confusion, decreased urine output, postural hypotension, and poor oral intake after receiving chemotherapy. She has been receiving D₅LR at 100 mL/hr by gravity through a peripheral vascular access device (PVAD) infusion since admission. Today her daughter tells the nurse that her mother is having difficulty breathing and is asking for another pillow for her bed.

1. On the basis of her daughter's information, which clinical markers should the nurse assess, and which additional signs and symptoms would the nurse expect to find?

2. At morning rounds the health care team sees the patient and writes changes to the intravenous (IV) solution prescriptions. In addition, a prescription is received to administer furosemide 10 mg slow IV push daily for 3 days. Based on the patient's signs and symptoms, which prescriptions can the nurse anticipate? How would the nurse calculate the minute flow rate of an infusion set with a drop factor of 15 gtt/mL, and how would the nurse ensure an accurate flow rate?

3. The following morning the patient indicates tenderness at her PVAD site. However, she no longer has dyspnea or other signs of fluid volume excess. Her past 24-hour intake was 1 600 mL, and her output was 1 700 mL. Serum electrolyte levels drawn this morning were within normal limits. She reported that she put some tape on her IV dressing last night because it was falling off. There is marked swelling around the IV site with purulent drainage. Her temperature is 38.2°C (100.8°F). Using SBAR, show how you would communicate with the health care team about this patient.

✦ REVIEW QUESTIONS

1. A patient has a tunnelled central vascular access device (CVAD) placed, and the nurse will be performing catheter care and maintenance to include insertion site assessment, dressing change, needle-free connector change, and flushing with normal saline. Place the following steps in the correct order:

1. Attach needle-free connector to the catheter hub, flush with 0.9% sodium chloride, remove gloves, perform hand hygiene.
2. Apply new stabilization device, transparent semipermeable membrane (TSM) dressing, label dressing.
3. Perform hand hygiene, apply appropriate personal protective equipment (PPE), remove old dressing.
4. Perform skin antisepsis with chlorhexidine gluconate (CHG)/alcohol solution and allow to dry completely.
5. Remove needle-free connector, scrub exposed catheter hub with antiseptic swab, let dry completely.
6. Remove and discard clean gloves, perform hand hygiene, apply sterile gloves.

2. Which of the following steps are necessary when inserting a PVAD? *(Select all that apply.)*

1. Apply tourniquet to arm 10 to 15 cm (4 to 6 inches) above the intended insertion site.
2. Clean skin using an antiseptic agent (e.g., CHG/alcohol) and allow to dry thoroughly.
3. Stabilize the vein by placing the thumb proximal to the insertion site, stretching the skin in the direction of insertion.
4. Use the smallest-gauge, shortest-length catheter suitable for the plan of care and vein size.
5. Observe for blood in the catheter, lower catheter angle parallel to skin, and advance catheter off the needle into the vein.
6. Release the tourniquet once the catheter has been secured and the dressing has been applied.

ⓔ *Visit the Evolve site for a complete list of Clinical Debrief and Review Questions answers.*

REFERENCES

Accreditation Canada. (2019). *Required organizational practices handbook—Version 14*. Ottawa, ON: Author. Retrieved from http://www.wrha.mb.ca/quality/files/2019ROPHandbook.pdf

Aseptic Non Touch Technique (ANTT). (2018). *ANTT core clinical guidelines, 2017*. Retrieved from http://antt.org/ANTT_Site/core_guidelines.html

Canadian Patient Safety Institute (CPSI) (2016). *Central line infections*. Retrieved from http://www.patientsafetyinstitute.ca/en/Topic/Pages/Central-Line-Infections-(CLI).aspx

Canadian Vascular Access Association. (2013). *Occlusion management guideline for central venous access*. Retrieved from http://cvaa.info/publications/occlusion-management-guideline-omg

Foster, J., Idossa, L., Lih-Wen, M., & Murphy, E. (2016). Applying health literacy principles: Strategies and tools to develop easy-to-read patient education resources. *Clinical Journal of Oncology Nursing, 20*(4), 433–436. doi:10.1188/16.CJON.433-436

Garrett, J. H. (2015). Correlation between prevention of central line-associated bloodstream infections and health care reform. *Journal of the Association for Vascular Access, 20*(1), 20–21. doi:10.1016/j.java.2015.01.003

Heffner, A. C., & Androes, M. P. (2018). Overview of central venous access. *UpToDate*. Retrieved from http://www.uptodate.com/contents/overview-of-central-venous-access?source=search_result&search=central+line&selectedTitle=1%7E150

Infusion Nurses Society (INS). (2016a). Infusion therapy standards of practice. *Journal of Intravenous Nursing, 39*(1S). Retrieved from http://source.yiboshi.com/20170417/1492425631944540325.pdf

Infusion Nurses Society (INS). (2016b). *Policies and procedures for infusion therapy* (5th ed.). Norwood, MA: Author.

Infusion Nurses Society (INS). (2016c). *Policies and procedures for infusion therapy: Neonate to adolescent* (2nd ed.). Norwood, MA: Author.

Infusion Nurses Society (INS). (2016d). *Policies and procedures for infusion therapy of the older adult* (3rd ed.). Norwood, MA: Author.

Jantzen, D., & Felver, L. (2018). Fluid, electrolyte, and acid-base balances. In P. Potter, A. G. Perry, B. Astle, & W. Duggleby (Eds.), *Canadian fundamentals of nursing* (6th ed.). Toronto, ON: Elsevier Canada.

Myers, G. J. (2017). Air in intravenous lines: A need to review old opinions. *Perfusion, 32*(6), 432–435. doi:10.1177/0267659117706834

O'Grady, N. P., Alexander, M., Burns, L. A., et al. (2011). *Guidelines for the prevention of intravascular catheter-related infections*. Atlanta, GA: Centers for Disease Control and Prevention. Retrieved from https://www.cdc.gov/infectioncontrol/guidelines/pdf/bsi/bsi-guidelines-H.pdf

Perry, S., Hockenberry, M., Lowdermilk, D. L., Wilson, D., Keenan-Lindsay, L., & Sams, C. S. (2017). *Maternal-child nursing care in Canada* (2nd ed.). Toronto, ON: Elsevier Canada.

Phillips, L. D., & Gorski, L. (2014). *Manual of IV therapeutics: Evidence-based practice for infusion therapy* (6th ed.). Philadelphia: F.A. Davis.

Public Health Agency of Canada (PHAC). (2016). *Routine practices and additional precautions for preventing the transmission of infection in healthcare settings*. Ottawa, ON: Centre for Communicable Disease and Infection Control. Retrieved from https://www.canada.ca/content/dam/phac-aspc/documents/services/publications/diseases-conditions/routine-practices-precautions-healthcare-associated-infections/routine-practices-precautions-healthcare-associated-infections-2016-FINAL-eng.pdf

Royal College of Nursing (RCN). (2016). *Standards for infusion therapy* (4th ed.). London: Author.

Sabado, J. J., & Pittiruti, M. (2018). Principles of ultrasound-guided venous access. *UpToDate*. Retrieved from http://www.uptodate.com/contents/principles-of-ultrasound-guided-venous-access

Voor in 't holt, A. F., Helder, O. K., Vos, M. C., et al. (2017). Antiseptic barrier cap effective in reducing central line-associated bloodstream infections: A systematic review and meta-analysis. *International Journal of Nursing Studies, 69*, 34–40. doi:10.1016/j.ijnurstu.2017.01.007

Weinstein, S., & Hagle, M. (2014). *Plumer's principles and practice of infusion therapy*. Philadelphia: Lippincott, Williams & Wilkins.

30 | Blood Therapy

Written by **Christina Hurlock-Chorostecki, NP, MScN, PhD; and Carol Ann Liebold, RN, CRNI**

SKILLS AND PROCEDURES

Skill 30.1 **Initiating Blood Therapy, p. 836**

Skill 30.2 **Monitoring for Adverse Transfusion Reactions, p. 844**

OBJECTIVES

Mastery of content in this chapter will enable the nurse to:
- Discuss indications for blood therapy.
- Demonstrate the following skills on selected patients: initiating blood therapy and monitoring for adverse transfusion reactions.

- Describe various transfusion reactions.
- Explain techniques for managing symptoms of adverse transfusion reactions.

MEDIA RESOURCES

- **evolve** http://evolve.elsevier.com/Canada/Perry/clinicalskills/
- Review Questions
- ▶ Video Clips

- Audio Glossary
- **NSO** Nursing Skills Online
- Clinical Debrief and Review Questions Answers
- Animations

PURPOSE

The transfusion of blood and blood components restores and maintains quality of life for patients with hematological disorders, cancer, injury, or surgical intervention. To ensure patient safety, a competent nurse must know the complexities of the ABO and Rh system, the numerous components of blood that can be transfused, and the serious negative outcomes that can occur.

STANDARDS OF CARE

- Accreditation Canada, 2019—*Required Organizational Practices Handbook, Version 14* (http://www.wrha.mb.ca/quality/files/2019ROPHandbook.pdf)
- Canadian Blood Services (CBS), 2017–2019—*Clinical Guide to Transfusion* (https://professionaleducation.blood.ca/en/transfusion/clinical-guide-transfusion)
- Canadian Patient Safety Institute (CPSI), 2017—*Hospital Harm Improvement Resource. Infusion, Transfusion and Injection Complications.* (https://www.patientsafetyinstitute.ca/en/toolsResources/Hospital-Harm-Measure/Documents/Resource-Library/HHIR%20Infusion%20Transfusion%20and%20Injectibles.pdf)
- Canadian Society for Transfusion Medicine (CSTM), 2017a—*CSTM Standards for Hospital Transfusion Services, Version 4* (http://www.transfusion.ca/Home)
- Government of Canada, 2016—*Guidance Document: Blood Regulations* (https://www.canada.ca/en/health-canada/services/drugs-health-products/biologics-radiopharmaceuticals-genetic-therapies/applications-submissions/guidance-documents/blood-regulations/guidance-document-blood-regulations-1.html)
- National Advisory Committee on Blood and Blood Products, 2014—*NAC Companion Document to Red Blood Cell Transfusion: A Clinical Practice Guideline from the AABB* (https://www.nacblood.ca/resources/guidelines/Companion-Document-May-28-2014.pdf)
- Public Health Agency of Canada (PHAC), 2016—*Transfusion Transmitted Injuries Surveillance System (TTISS): 2009–2013 Summary Results.* (http://publications.gc.ca/collections/collection_2016/aspc-phac/HP40-168-2016-eng.pdf)

PRINCIPLES FOR PRACTICE

- Blood product transfusion therapy is the intravenous (IV) administration of red blood cells (Fig. 30.1), blood components (Fig. 30.2), or a plasma protein product (Fig. 30.3) for therapeutic purposes (De Biasio & Rymer, 2017). Transfusions are used to treat hemorrhage, treat symptomatic anemia, and improve oxygen delivery to tissues.
- The most common method of blood transfusion is *allogeneic* blood (blood donated from someone else).
- *Autologous transfusion* or *autotransfusion* is a method in which a patient's own blood is collected and reinfused for intravascular volume replacement (Pambrun, 2017). Preoperative autologous donation (PAD) has been an option for patients concerned with transfusion-related reactions or transmission of disease since the

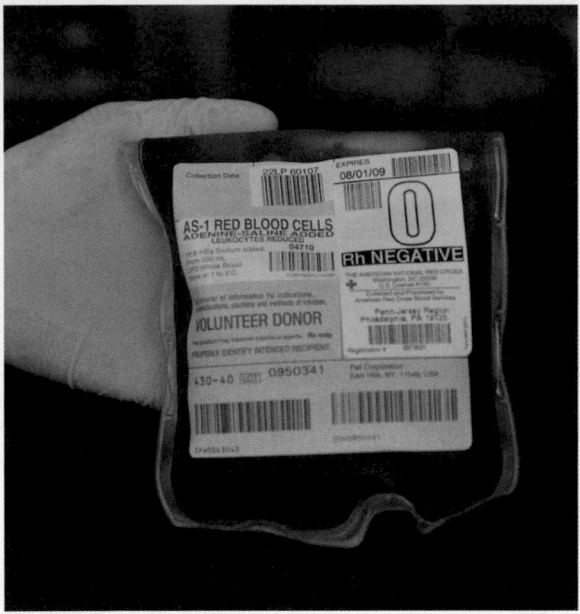

FIG 30.1 Unit of blood. (*Image courtesy of American Red Cross.*)

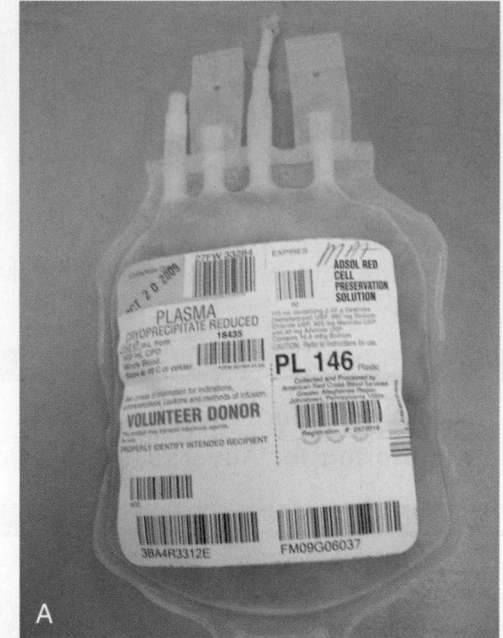

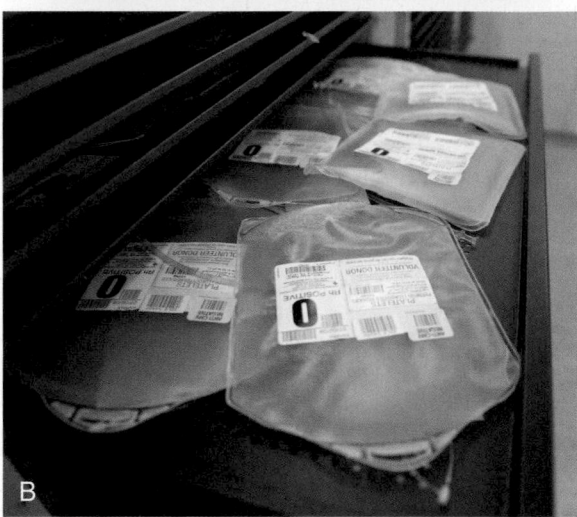

FIG 30.2 Bag of apheresis platelets (*A*) and pooled platelets (*B*). (*Images courtesy American Red Cross.*)

late 1990s. The use of PAD has significantly decreased in Canada because the rate of infection from allogenic blood is very low (Pambrun, 2017). Preoperative autologous donation may be beneficial for patients undergoing vascular and cardiothoracic surgeries where blood loss may be substantial. In the PAD process, patients can donate a maximum of 4 units of their own blood drawn one week apart. The last donation must occur more than 72 hours before surgery. The donated blood is stored in the same manner as allogenic blood for up to 42 days (Pambrun, 2017).

- To decrease transfusion-related adverse events, blood and its components are treated and stored in controlled environments. Blood is a living tissue; once obtained via the donor, it must remain healthy before transfusion. Various anticoagulants and preservatives are used internationally to maintain the shelf life of donated blood. In Canada, saline-adenine-glucose-mannitol (SAGM) is the preservative that is used, and citrate-phosphate-dextrose (CPD) is the anticoagulant used (Clarke, 2017; Lau, 2017).

- Caution is required when infusing multiple units of blood or a unit of blood nearing its expiration. When blood is stored, red blood cells are destroyed continually, which releases potassium (K) from the cells into the plasma. Often a laboratory test of a patient's K level is prescribed before administering a unit of blood.

- As a nurse, your role during a blood transfusion is to use the principles of interprofessional collaboration to carry out the health care provider's prescription by clearly and respectfully communicating with the blood bank personnel and the prescribing health care provider; safely administering the blood or blood products; assessing a patient before, during, and after the transfusion; and promptly identifying and reporting any transfusion reactions.

ABO System

There are three blood-typing systems: ABO, Rh, and human leukocyte antigen (HLA). These systems ensure a close match between transfused products and a recipient's blood. The ABO system uses the presence or absence of specific antigens on the surface of red blood cells to identify blood groups. When the type A antigen is present, the blood group is type A. When the type B

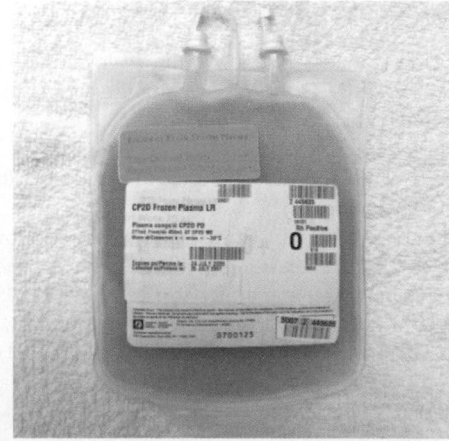

FIG 30.3 Bag of plasma. (*Image courtesy of Queens University School of Medicine. © qscalpel, photo by Adam Szulewski.*)}

TABLE 30.1

ABO Compatibilities for Transfusion Therapy

Component	Compatibilities	
Whole blood	Give type-specific blood only	
Packed red cells (stored, washed, or frozen/washed)	**Donor**	**Recipient**
	O	O, A, B, AB
	A	A, AB
	B	B, AB
	AB	AB
Fresh-frozen plasma	**Donor**	**Recipient**
	O	O
	A	A, O
	B	B, O
	AB	AB, B, A, O
Platelets	RBC: ABO and Rh compatible preferred	
	Donor	**Recipient**
	O	O, A, B, AB
	A	A, AB
	B	B, AB
	AB	AB

Data from Alexander, M., Corrigan, A. M., Gorski, L. A., et al. (2014). *Core curriculum for infusion nursing* (4th ed.). Philadelphia: Lippincott.

antigen is present, the blood group is type B. When both A and B antigens are present, the blood group is type AB, and when neither A nor B antigens are present, the blood group is type O (Lane, 2017) (Table 30.1).

Antibodies that react against the A and B antigens are naturally present in the plasma of people whose red blood cells do not carry the antigen. These antibodies (agglutinins) react against the foreign antigens (*agglutinogens*). Incompatible red blood cells agglutinate (clump together) and result in a life-threatening hemolytic transfusion reaction. People with type A blood have anti-B antibodies; people with type B blood have anti-A antibodies. People with type AB blood have neither antibody and can receive all blood types. People with type O blood have both A and B antibodies and can receive only type O blood (Lane, 2017). The most common transfusion reaction, acute hemolytic transfusion reaction (AHTR), results from ABO incompatibility, transfusing blood that is not compatible with the patient's ABO blood type.

Rh System

The Rh factor is considered when matching blood components for transfusion. The Rh factor is another antigen in red blood cell membranes. Although nearly 50 types of Rh antigen may be present on the surface of red blood cells, the type D antigen is widely prevalent and is most likely to elicit an immune response. It is the presence or absence of the D antigen that determines a person's Rh type. A person with the D antigen is Rh positive, and a person without the D antigen is Rh negative (Lane, 2017; Potter, Perry, Stockert, et al., 2019, p. 1064). Unlike the ABO antigens, naturally occurring antibodies to the Rh(D) antigen do not occur. A person with Rh-negative blood must first be exposed to Rh-positive blood before any Rh antibodies are formed. A person with Rh-negative blood who is exposed Rh-positive blood will develop enough antibodies to cause a severe transfusion reaction with repeated exposure (Lane, 2017). Generally, a person with Rh-negative blood receives Rh-negative blood, whereas a person with Rh-positive blood

can receive Rh-positive or Rh-negative blood (Potter et al., 2019, p. 1065).

An Rh-negative mother previously exposed to Rh antigen can transfer Rh antibodies across the placenta to an Rh-positive fetus. This can result in severe fetal hemolysis (i.e., the breakdown of red blood cells, with resultant anemia and jaundice) and is often fatal to the infant. To prevent current or future fetal hemolysis, Rh(D) immunoglobulin (e.g., WinRho) is given by intramuscular injection to the mother at 28 weeks' gestation and again within 72 hours of birth. WinRho significantly reduces alloimmunization by suppressing the immune response and antibody formation by the Rh-negative person who has been in contact with Rh-positive red blood cells (Clarke & Hannon, 2018). Since WinRho is made from human blood, there is a risk of pathogen transmission. To reduce the risk of future fetal hemolysis, it is recommended that in urgent situations females under the age of 45 receive O-negative red blood cells (Lane, 2017).

Acute Transfusion Reactions

- Clinical manifestations range from mild to severe and usually develop in the initial 15 minutes of the transfusion.
- Severe hemolytic reaction is rare (Lewis, Bucher, Heitkemper, et al., 2019).
- Acute transfusion reactions include the following:
  - Acute hemolytic reaction
  - Febrile nonhemolytic reaction (most common)
  - Mild allergic reaction
  - Anaphylactic and severe allergic reaction
  - Circulatory overload reaction
  - Sepsis reaction
  - Transfusion-related acute lung injury (TRALI) reaction

PERSON-CENTRED CARE

- Care is person centred when it is holistic, collaborative, and responsive (Sidani, Collins, Harbman, et al., 2015).
  - **Holistic care:** When administering blood products, the nurse needs to consider a patient's values and cultural and religious beliefs about blood therapy. It is important to seek to understand the patient's health values and goals. A person's perception of their disease or health condition affects how receptive they are to receiving blood. Blood transfusion is often equated to severity of illness.
  - **Collaborative care:** The nurse needs to facilitate the patient's engagement in treatment decisions. Provide accurate and unbiased information on risks and benefits of the transfusion and allay patient anxieties when possible.
  - **Responsive care:** The nurse needs to respect individuality. Provide the patient an opportunity to ask questions, address their concerns, and be consistent with the person's needs and preferences. An example of individuality is respecting the Jehovah's Witnesses religion prohibition of blood transfusions.
- When possible, it is helpful to consult a religious leader when caring for patients in need of blood therapy. Be familiar with employer policies and procedures to follow when patients choose an informed refusal. Immediately inform the prescribing health care provider of the patient's decision.
- By law, parents have the primary obligation to care for and make decisions about their minor children. However, the legal principle of *parens patriae* empowers the courts to act in the role of a parent for the protection of a child (Department of Justice, 2017). The nurse's role is to advocate for the patient and family.

- Patient safety is a priority—specifically the prevention of transfusion-related complications. Transfusion-related adverse reactions increased from 465 in 2009 to 874 in 2013, corresponding to an overall 5-year increase of 88% (PHAC, 2016). To ensure safe patient outcomes, the Transfusion Medicine Laboratory (TML), Canada Vigilance Program, and Transmitted Injuries Surveillance System (TTISS) (Québec Hemovigilance System in Quebec) monitor reported adverse reactions related to blood and blood product transfusions in Canada. All adverse reactions to a transfusion should be reported to TML for investigation. TTISS monitors more severe reactions, while Canadian Blood Services/Héma-Québec (CBS/HQ) investigates product-quality concerns.

INTERPROFESSIONAL COLLABORATION

In general, working collaboratively with all health care providers improves clinical outcomes and enhances workplace satisfaction. To engage well in interprofessional collaboration related to blood transfusion, the nurse must consider six essential elements: interdependence, partnership or collaboration, collective problem-solving, professional relationships, communication, and shared decision-making (Hurlock-Chorostecki et al., 2015). Interprofessional collaboration includes understanding the role of the transfusion laboratory personnel with respect to safe distribution of blood products, time required for compatibility testing, and monitoring of transfusion complications. Clear and respectful communication between the nurse and the prescriber of the blood products allows for timely and safe patient care. With interprofessional collaboration, all members of the health care team are comfortable asking questions, responding to concerns, and ensuring that patient needs are responded to in a consistent manner (Hurlock-Chorostecki, van Soeren, MacMillan, et al., 2015).

EVIDENCE-INFORMED PRACTICE

Compliance with standards and policies and ongoing education are essential to maintain patient safety and reduce potential errors. Safety and risk management are key factors in transfusion therapy. Transfusion-associated circulatory overload (TACO) is the leading cause of transfusion-related death in Canada (Government of Canada, 2016). A human error most often involves misidentification of the patient or of the unit of blood or mislabelling of the pretransfusion blood sample. Advances in technology have helped to decrease transfusion-related errors:

- Electronic bar-code technology helps prevent errors in the identification process between a patient and the compatible blood unit.
- International standard for labelling of blood components (ISBT 128) provides unique numbering of blood components (Fig. 30.4).
- Radiofrequency identification (RFID) is used to standardize and document key steps in the blood collection and confirm the recipient–blood unit matching at a patient's bedside.
- Advanced technological laboratory screening procedures help to ensure safe transfusions regarding bloodborne pathogens.
- Better assessment of blood and plasma cell integrity is available to avoid loss of blood component function.
- Blood alternative therapies with pharmacological developments such as colloids, crystalloids, erythropoietin, antifibrinolytics, and hematinics reduce the risks associated with transfusing human blood.

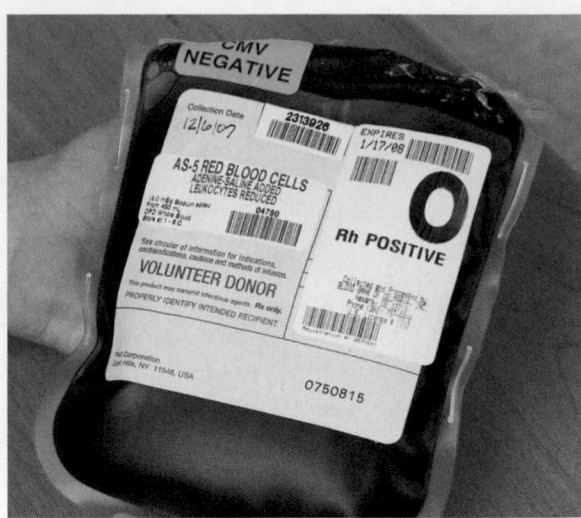

FIG 30.4 Red blood cells (unit of blood with a label). (*Image courtesy American Red Cross.*)

- Choosing Wisely, an Internet site and mobile app, provides rapid access to evidence-informed transfusion recommendations (Canadian Society for Transfusion Medicine, 2017b).

SAFETY GUIDELINES

- Administration of blood and blood components requires meticulous attention to detail (e.g., preparation, administration, and monitoring) to prevent life-threatening transfusion reactions (Table 30.2) and is usually administered via an electronic infusion device.
- Accurate labelling of the pretransfusion sample is important. The nurse needs to follow the employer policy for blood draws and clearly label blood tubes when with the patient.
- Appropriate pretransfusion blood work ensures safety and provides better red blood cell management in the blood bank. Crossmatch is prescribed to determine compatibility of red blood cells to the patient's blood when the patient requires a transfusion. When a patient is not likely to require blood products the Type-and-Screen is prescribed to determine a patient's ABO and Rh type and perform an antibody screen. This test allows a quick crossmatch should blood be required (Lane, 2017).
- Restrictive transfusion thresholds limit use of blood products until the hemoglobin level is 70 g/L (80 g/L in certain situations), thus reducing unnecessary transfusions (Canadian Society for Transfusion Medicine, 2017b).
- Multiple checks of the blood unit for correct labelling and verification of the correct patient are intended to reduce errors. The nurse follows the 10 rights of medication administration (Potter et al., 2019, p. 746) during a transfusion: the right medication, dose, patient, route, time, documentation, reason, patient education, and evaluation, and the patient's right to refuse the transfusion.
- The nurse reviews employer policy and procedures regarding administration of blood or blood products.
- Two nurses must verify the right blood unit and right patient immediately before administration.
- The patient must be wearing an ID armband.

Despite precautions, transfusion therapy carries risks. Infectious diseases such as viruses, bacteria, and parasites can be transmitted

TABLE 30.2

Transfusion Reaction Chart

IMMEDIATE ACTIONS!
1. STOP the transfusion.
2. Maintain intravenous (IV) access.
3. Check vital signs.
4. Recheck patient ID band and product label.
5. Notify health care provider.
6. Notify transfusion laboratory.

Signs and Symptoms		Usual Timing	Possible Etiology	Recommended Investigations	Suggested Treatment and Actions
Fever (at least 38°C and an increase of at least 1°C from baseline) **and/or** shaking chills/rigors	38°C to 38.9°C but **NO** other symptoms	During or up to 4 hours post-transfusion	Febrile nonhemolytic transfusion reaction	No testing required	• Antipyretic • With health care provider approval, transfusion may be resumed cautiously if product still viable.
	Less than 39°C but with other symptoms (e.g., rigors, hypotension) **or** 39°C or more	Usually within first 15 minutes but may be later	Febrile nonhemolytic transfusion reaction Bacterial contamination Acute hemolytic transfusion reaction	If hemolysis suspected (e.g., red urine or plasma)	**Do not restart transfusion.** • Antipyretic • Consider meperidine (Demerol) for significant rigors. • If bacterial contamination suspected, antibiotics should be started immediately. • Monitor for hypotension, renal failure, and DIC. • Return blood product to transfusion laboratory. • For additional assistance, contact the health care provider who wrote the prescription.
Urticaria (hives) Itching **or** rash	Less than two-thirds body but **NO** other symptoms	During or up to 4 hours post-transfusion	Minor allergic	No testing required	• Antihistamine • With health care provider approval, transfusion may be resumed cautiously if product is still available.
	Two-thirds body or more but **NO** other symptoms	Usually early in transfusion	Minor allergic (extensive)	No testing required	**Do not restart transfusion.** • Antihistamine • May require steroid
	Accompanied by other symptoms (e.g., dyspnea hypotension)	Usually early in transfusion	Anaphylactoid reaction/ anaphylaxis		**Do not restart transfusion.** • Epinephrine • Washed/plasma-depleted blood products pending investigation • Return blood products to transfusion laboratory. • For additional assistance, contact the health care provider who wrote the prescription.
Dyspnea **or** decrease in SpO$_2$% to 90% or less (and change of at least 5% from baseline)	Typically with hypertension	Within several hours of transfusion	Transfusion-associated circulatory overload (TACO)	If sepsis suspected	**Do not restart transfusion.** • Diuretics, oxygen, high Fowler's position • Return blood products to transfusion laboratory. • For additional assistance, contact the health care provider who wrote the prescription.
	Typically with hypotension	Within 6 hours of transfusion	Transfusion-related acute lung injury (TRALI)	If sepsis suspected	**Do not restart transfusion.** • Assess chest X-ray for bilateral pulmonary infiltrates. • If TRALI, the patient may require vasopressors and respiratory support.
		Usually within first 15 minutes but may be later	Bacterial contamination Acute hemolytic transfusion reaction Anaphylaxis	If sepsis suspected	• If bacterial contamination is suspected, antibiotics should be started immediately. • Monitor for hypotension, renal failure, and DIC. • If anaphylaxis is suspected, give epinephrine. • Return blood products to transfusion laboratory. • For additional assistance, contact the health care provider who wrote the prescription.

DIC, Disseminated intravascular coagulation.

From Ontario Transfusion Transmitted Injuries Surveillance System. (2018). Retrieved from https://ttiss.mcmaster.ca/?page_id=506. Originally published in *Bloody Easy Blood Administration Nurse* online course: http://transfusion Ontario.org/en/documents/?cat=bloody-bloody.

through blood transfusion. The risk is small owing to effective preventative strategies such as viral inactivation procedures and leukocyte reduction (MacDonald, O'Brien, & Delage, 2017). The majority of noninfectious risks are immune related and are the most common complications. Delayed hemolytic transfusion reaction (DHTR), transfusion-associated graft-versus-host disease (TA-GVHD), and post-transfusion purpura (PTP) may also occur.

Nonimmune reactions can be life-threatening (e.g., hemoglobinuria, hyperkalemia, hypocalcemia, hypothermia, or iron overload). Ensuring compatibility of the patient and donor is essential. Human-related errors (e.g., improper labelling, inadequate hand-off between nurses and the person transporting blood, or the method used to complete a blood requisition) that may lead to the administration of incompatible transfusions can occur in every step of the process.

✦ SKILL 30.1   Initiating Blood Therapy

 Video Clip **NSO** *Nursing Skills Online Blood Therapy Module 15 / Lesson 2*

Blood is administered for different clinical indications (Table 30.3). A patient's medical condition determines which blood component is indicated. A health care provider's prescription is required for the administration of a blood product. The nurse is responsible for understanding which blood components are appropriate in various situations. In addition, the nurse must ensure that an informed consent has been obtained and a blood sample has been collected and sent to the laboratory within 72 hours for typing and compatibility screening.

Blood is stored in a refrigerated environment. The refrigeration unit is regulated by the blood bank; blood is never stored in refrigerators on the hospital unit. The blood transfusion must be started soon after it is received. If it cannot be started, contact the blood bank. Blood that has been out of refrigeration for more than 60 minutes must be discarded (De Biasio & Rymer, 2017). In emergency situations, rapid transfusion of cold blood may lead to dysrhythmias and reduction of a patient's core temperature. A blood-warmer machine may be used for large transfusions of greater than 50 mL/kg/hr or patients with cold agglutinins (Fig. 30.5). Special tubing is required. Never heat blood products in a microwave or with hot water because it may destroy blood cells and result in hemolysis and severe reactions (Gehrie, Chandler, & Snyder, 2016).

Delegation and Collaboration

The skill of initiating transfusion therapy cannot be delegated to an unregulated care provider (UCP). The skill of initiating transfusion therapy by a registered practical nurse (RPN) or licensed practical nurse (LPN) varies by province and territory. After the transfusion has been started and the patient is stable, assistance with monitoring of a patient by a UCP does not relieve a registered nurse (RN) of the responsibility to continue to assess the patient during the transfusion. The nurse instructs the UCP about:

- What to observe, such as patient indication of shortness of breath, hives, or chills, and reporting this information to the nurse.

Equipment

- Y-type blood administration set with a 170- to 260-micron in-line filter (**NOTE:** Depending on the blood product, special tubing and filter are necessary.)
- Prescribed blood product
- 250-mL bag 0.9% sodium chloride (normal saline [NS]) for intravenous (IV) use
- 5- to 10-mL prefilled syringe with preservative-free 0.9% sodium chloride (NS)
- Antiseptic swabs (chlorhexidine solution preferred, povidone-iodine, or 70% alcohol)

- Clean gloves
- Tape
- Vital signs equipment: thermometer, blood pressure cuff, stethoscope, and pulse oximeter
- Signed transfusion consent form as required by employer policy. (Some employers may require consent for blood products on admission, while others require a separate consent.)

Optional Equipment

- Rapid infusion pump
- Electronic infusion device (Verify that the pump can be used to deliver blood and blood products.)
- Blood warmer (used mainly when large-volume or rapid transfusion is needed)
- Pressure bag
- Cardiac monitor for emergencies

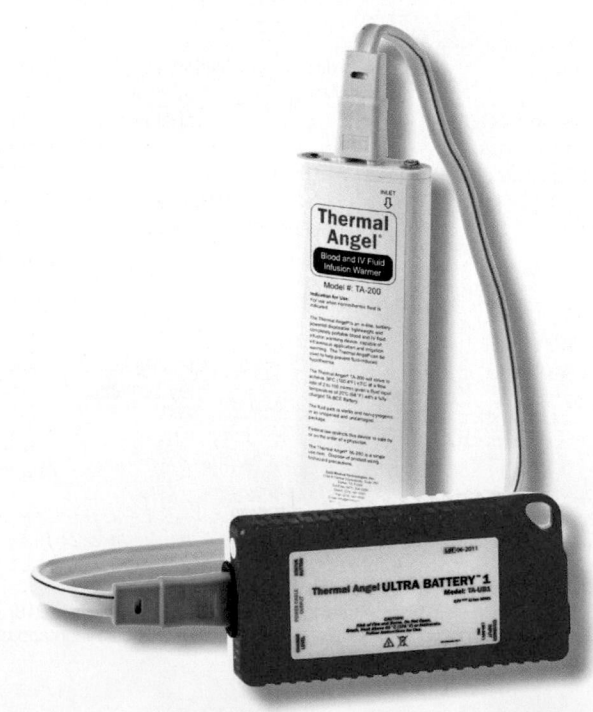

FIG 30.5 Blood-warming system. (*Used with permission of Estill Medical Technologies, Inc. All rights reserved.*)

TABLE 30.3

Blood and Blood Component Products

Blood Products	Major Uses	Storage and Expiration	Administration
Red blood cells (RBC)	Bleeding or anemic nonbleeding patients with signs and symptoms of impaired tissue oxygen delivery: • Tachycardia • Shortness of breath • Dizziness	2–6° C in approved refrigerator only Up to 42 days	• Blood tubing required • Initiate transfusion slowly for first 15 minutes, unless massive blood loss • Transfuse over no more than 4 hours • Typically, over 1½–2 hours, with slower rates for patients at risk for circulatory overload
Plasma	• Liver disease coagulopathy • Massive transfusion • Plasma exchange procedures for thrombotic thrombocytopenic purpura/ hemolytic uremic syndrome (TTP/HUS)	Frozen 1 year Once thawed, expires after 5 days stored at 1–6°C	• Blood tubing required • Initiate transfusion slowly for first 15 minutes unless massive blood loss • Transfuse over no more than 4 hours • Typically, over 30 minutes–2 hours
Platelets	Control or prevent bleeding in patients with: • Low platelet counts (thrombocytopenia) • Congenital platelet dysfunction • Platelets not functioning because of medications (ASA, clopidogrel) • Platelet dysfunction following cardiopulmonary bypass	20–24°C on an agitator to prevent clumping 5 days	• Blood tubing required • Initiate transfusion slowly for first 15 minutes unless massive blood loss • Transfuse over no more than 4 hours • Typically, over 60 minutes
Cryoprecipitate	To replace: • Fibrinogen in patients actively bleeding who have a low fibrinogen level • Specific coagulation factors when the specific factor concentrates are not available	Frozen 1 year Once thawed, expires after 4 hours; stored at 20–24°C	• Blood tubing required • Transfuse as rapidly as tolerated

Albumin (5% and 25%)	• Ascites patients undergoing large-volume paracentesis greater than 5 L
	• Spontaneous bacterial peritonitis (SBP)
	• Hepatorenal syndrome
	• Plasma exchange procedures
		Room temperature lower than 30°C
		Expires as indicated on packaging
			• Standard vented IV set—no blood tubing or filtering required
			• Bottles must be vented
			• Begin infusion slowly, then as tolerated
			• Maximum rate:
			  • Albumin 5%—300 mL/hr
			  • Albumin 25%—120 mL/hr

Intravenous immune globulin (IVIG)	• Replacement of immunoglobulins • Control of some infections and autoimmune diseases	Storage variable by brand Expires as indicated on packaging	• Standard vented IV set—no blood tubing or filtering required • Bottles must be vented • Infusion pump required • Begin infusion slowly, then as tolerated, maximum rate as indicated on package • Frequent vital sign monitoring
Prothrombin complex concentrate (Octaplex)	Reversal of warfarin or vitamin K deficiency in bleeding patients and those requiring emergency surgery	2–25°C Expires as indicated on packaging Use immediately once reconstituted	• Standard IV set—no blood tubing or filtering required • Infuse over 15–30 minutes • May be given slow IV push (usually by a physician) • Dosage based on weight and INR value—usually 2–4 vials • Effect is immediate and lasts 6–12 hours • For complete reversal, vitamin K10 mg IV must also be given

INR, International normalized ratio; *IV*, intravenous.

Data from Lima, A. (2010). *Bloody easy blood administration: A handbook for health professionals* (pp. 28–29, Appendix 1 and 2). Toronto, ON: Ontario Regional Blood Coordinating Network. Retrieved from http://www.transfusionontario.org/media/HOPE-EN-BloodAdminHdbk-Sprds.pdf; Callum, J., Pinkerton, P., Lima, A., Lin, Y., Karkouti, K., Leiberman, L., ... Webert, K. (2016). *Bloody easy 4. Blood transfusions, blood alternatives, and transfusion reactions* (4th ed.). Toronto: Ontario Regional Blood Coordinating Network. Retrieved from http://policyandorders.cw.bc.ca/resource-gallery/Documents/Transfusion%20Medicine/Bloody%20Easy%204. pdf

STEP	RATIONALE

ASSESSMENT

1. Identify patient using at least two person-specific identifiers (e.g., name and birthday or name and medical record number) according to employer policy.

Ensures correct patient. Complies with Accreditation Canada's standards and improves patient safety (Accreditation Canada, 2019).

2. Verify health care provider's prescription for specific blood or blood product with appropriate date, time to begin transfusion, special instructions (i.e., irradiated, leukocyte depleted), duration, and any pretransfusion or post-transfusion medications to administer.

A health care provider's prescription must be present before transfusing a blood product. Verifying the prescription helps to ensure that the appropriate blood component will be administered (De Biasio & Rymer, 2017). Premedications such as an antihistamine or antipyretic may be prescribed, especially if patient demonstrated previous transfusion sensitivity.

2. Obtain patient's transfusion history and note known allergies and previous transfusion reactions. Verify that type and crossmatch have been completed within 72 hours of transfusion.

Identifies patient's prior response(s) to transfusion of blood components. If patient has experienced a reaction in the past, anticipate a similar reaction and be prepared to rapidly intervene.

3. Verify that IV cannula is patent and without complications such as infiltration or phlebitis.

Patent IV ensures that transfusion will be infused within established time guidelines.

   a. Administer blood or blood components to an adult through a 16- to 22-gauge short-peripheral catheter and a 16- to 18-gauge when rapid infusion is required (Callum, Pinkerton, lima, et al., 2016).

The gauge of the IV cannula should be appropriate for accommodating the infusion of blood or blood components (De Biasio & Rymer, 2017). Large-gauge cannulas promote rapid flow of blood components. Rapid transfusion through a cannula that is too small can cause hemolysis of red blood cells (Callum et al., 2016).

   b. Transfuse a neonate, pediatric, or older adult patient with a 22- to 25-gauge device (Callum et al., 2016).

Use of smaller cannula gauges, such as 25-gauge, often requires a blood bank to divide the unit so that each half can be infused within the allotted time or with pressure-assisted devices.

   c. An appropriate-gauge central vascular access device (CVAD) may also be used.

Use of CVAD for administration of blood depends on catheter gauge and manufacturer recommendations for use. CVADs with multiple lumens allow medications to be administered through a different lumen while blood is infusing (De Biasio & Rymer, 2017).

4. Assess laboratory values such as hemoglobin, hematocrit, coagulation values, platelet count, and potassium.

Provides baseline for later evaluation of patient response to transfusion (INS, 2016; Potter at al., 2019, p. 1066).

5. Check that patient has completed and signed transfusion consent properly and is wearing an ID armband before retrieving blood.

Informed consent is required before transfusion. The consent form should include risks, benefits, and treatment alternatives; right to accept or refuse transfusion; and opportunity to ask questions. Administration of albumin does not require informed consent. ID armband ensures proper patient identification.

6. Know indications or reasons for transfusion (e.g., packed red blood cells [PRBCs] for patient with low hematocrit level from gastrointestinal bleeding or surgery blood loss).

Allows nurse to anticipate patient's response to therapy.

7. Obtain and record pretransfusion baseline vital signs (temperature, pulse, respirations, and blood pressure). If patient is febrile (temperature greater than 37.8°C [100°F]), notify health care provider before initiating transfusion.

Change from baseline vital signs during infusion alerts nurse to potential transfusion reaction or adverse effect of therapy (Lewis et al., 2019).

8. Assess patient's need for IV fluids or medications while transfusion is infusing.

If IV medications need to be administered during transfusion, second IV site is necessary. No other infusions are to be administered through same IV site as blood transfusion. Administer blood or blood components only with 0.9% sodium chloride (NS) (Callum et al., 2016).

9. Assess patient's understanding of procedure and rationale.

Alleviates some of the anxiety patient may have.

NURSING DIAGNOSES

- Decreased cardiac output
- Excessive fluid volume
- Inadequate fluid volume
- Inadequate peripheral tissue perfusion
- Potential for infection
- Reduced stamina
- Insufficient knowledge regarding transfusion

Related factors/Risk factors are individualized on the basis of patient's condition or needs.

STEP	RATIONALE

PLANNING

1. Expected outcomes following completion of the procedure:

- Patient verbalizes understanding of rationale for therapy.

  Indicates patient's understanding and ability to make informed decision for consent.

- Patient experiences improved activity tolerance.

  Oxygenation is improved.

- Mucous membranes are pink, and patient has brisk capillary refill.

  Tissue perfusion is improved.

- Patient's cardiac output returns to baseline.

  Intravascular volume is restored.

- Patient's systolic blood pressure improves, and urine output is 0.5 to 1 mL/kg/hr.

  Parameters reflect optimal fluid status and adequate renal blood flow.

- Patient's laboratory values improve in targeted areas (e.g., hemoglobin, hematocrit, coagulation values, platelet count).

  Indicates that patient responds appropriately to blood or blood component infusion.

IMPLEMENTATION

1. Preadministration protocol:

a. Obtain blood component from blood bank following employer protocol (see illustration). Check the unit of blood and patient documentation with lab personnel.

Timely acquisition ensures that the product is safe to administer. Employer protocol usually encompasses safeguards to ensure quality control throughout transfusion process.

b. Check blood bag for any signs of contamination (i.e., clumping or clots, gas bubbles, purplish colour) and presence of leaks.

Blood should not be infused if integrity is compromised. Air bubbles, clumping, clots, and discoloration can be an indication of bacterial contamination or inadequate anticoagulation of stored component and are contraindications for transfusion of that product (De Biasio & Rymer, 2017).

Blood serves as medium for bacterial growth.

c. Verbally compare and correctly verify patient, blood product, and type with another person considered qualified by your employer (e.g., RN or LPN) before initiating transfusion. The following verification process must be used:

Strict adherence to verification procedures before administration of blood or blood components reduces risk for administering wrong blood to patient. Approximately half of all transfusion reactions are related to the wrong patient receiving properly labelled blood (CPSI, 2017).

(1) Identify patient using at least two person-specific identifiers (e.g., name and date of birth or name and medical record number) according to employer policy. Compare identifiers with information on patient's medication administration record (MAR) or medical record.

Ensures correct patient. Complies with Accreditation Canada's standards and improves patient safety (Accreditation Canada, 2019).

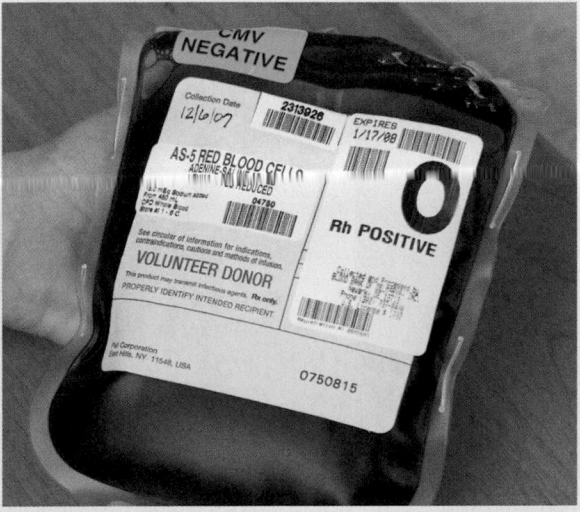

STEP 1a Unit of blood with label. (*Courtesy American Red Cross.*)

STEP	RATIONALE

IMPLEMENTATION

STEP	RATIONALE
(2) Transfusion record number and patient's identification number match.	Prevents accidental administration of wrong component.

Clinical Decision Point *If you notice a discrepancy during the verification procedure, do not administer the product. Notify the blood bank and appropriate personnel as indicated by employer policy. The product should be returned to the blood bank until the discrepancy is resolved (De Biasio & Rymer, 2017; INS, 2016).*

STEP	RATIONALE
(3) Patient's name is correct on all documents. Check patient identification number and date of birth on identification band and patient record.	
(4) Check unit number on blood bag with blood bank form to ensure that they are the same.	
(5) Blood type matches on transfusion record and blood bag. Verify that component received from blood bank is the same component that health care provider prescribed (e.g., packed red cells, platelets) (see illustration).	Ensures that patient receives correct therapy. Misidentification and improper labelling result in transfusing wrong ABO group (De Biasio & Rymer, 2017).
(6) Check that patient's blood type and Rh type are compatible with donor blood type and Rh type (e.g., Patient A+: Donor A+ or 0+).	Verifies accurate donor blood type and compatibility.
(7) Check expiration date and time on unit of blood.	Never use expired blood, because efficacy of cell components deteriorates and bacterial contamination may occur (Clarke, 2017).
(8) Just before initiating transfusion, check patient identification information with blood unit label information (see illustration). Do not administer blood to patient without identification bracelet or blood identification bracelet (see employer policy).	Serves as last point of patient and blood confirmation (De Biasio & Rymer, 2017).
(9) Both individuals verify patient and unit identification record process as directed by employer policy.	Documentation is legal medical record.
d. Review purpose of transfusion and ask patient to report any changes that they may feel during the transfusion.	Signs and symptoms of transfusion reactions include chills, low back pain, shortness of breath, rash, hives, or itching (Lewis et al., 2019). Prompt notification aids in early intervention.
e. Have patient void, or apply clean gloves and empty urine drainage collection container.	If transfusion reaction occurs, urine specimen containing urine produced after initiation of transfusion will be sent to laboratory (Callum et al., 2016).

Clinical Decision Point *Blood transfusion should be initiated within 30 minutes from the time of release from the blood bank. If this cannot be completed because of factors such as an elevated temperature, immediately return the blood to the blood bank and retrieve it when you can administer it (Lewis et al., 2019). It is important that the blood bag not be spiked until you ensure that no factors exist preventing transfusion.*

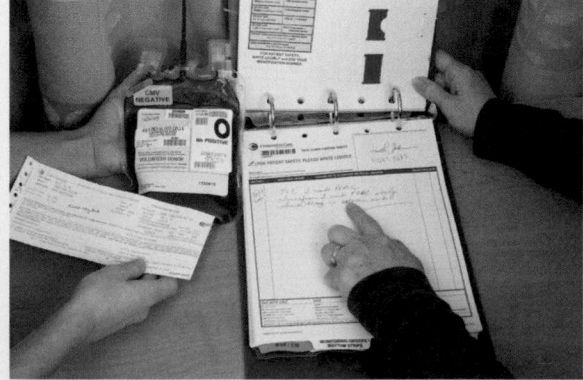

STEP 1c(5) Two clinicians verifying blood type with health care provider prescription.

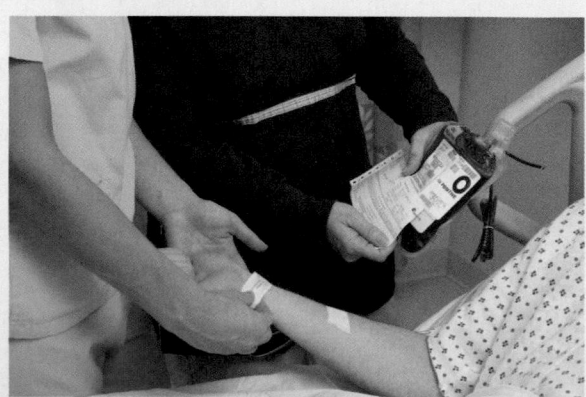

STEP 1c(8) Two clinicians verifying identification of patient and blood product.

STEP	RATIONALE

IMPLEMENTATION

2. Administration:

  a. Perform hand hygiene. Apply clean gloves. Reinspect blood product for signs of leakage or unusual appearance.

Using routine practices reduces risk for transmission of microorganisms. Provides ongoing verification of blood product.

  b. Open Y-tubing blood administration set for single unit. Use multi-set if multiple units are to be transfused.

Y-tubing facilitates maintenance of IV line access with NS in case patient will need more than 1 unit of blood.

  c. Set all clamp(s) to "off" position.

Setting clamps to "off" position prevents accidental spillage and waste of product.

  d. Use aseptic technique and spike bag of 0.9% sodium chloride (NS) IV bag with one of the Y-tubing spikes. Hang bag on IV pole and prime tubing. Open upper clamp on NS side of tubing and squeeze drip chamber until fluid covers filter and one-third to one-half of drip chamber (see illustration).

Primes tubing with fluid to eliminate air in Y-tubing. Closing clamp prevents spillage and waste of fluid.

  e. Maintain clamp on blood product side of Y-tubing in "off" position. Open common tubing clamp to finish priming tubing to distal end of tubing connector. Close tubing clamp when tubing is filled with saline. All three tubing clamps should be closed. Maintain protective sterile cap on tubing connector.

This will completely prime tubing with saline, and IV line is ready to be connected to patient's vascular access device (VAD).

  f. Prepare blood component for administration. Gently invert bag two or three times, turning back and forth. Remove protective covering from access port. Spike blood component unit with other Y-connection. Close NS clamp above filter, open clamp above filter to blood unit, and prime tubing with blood. Blood will flow into drip chamber (see illustration). Tap filter chamber to ensure that residual air is removed.

Gentle agitation suspends red blood cells in anticoagulant. A protective barrier drape may be used to catch any potential blood spillage. Tubing is primed with blood unit and ready for transfusion into patient.

Clinical Decision Point *NS is compatible with blood products, unlike solutions that contain dextrose, which cause coagulation of blood. Only use 0.9% sodium chloride (NS) to administer blood. No other solutions are to be administered with blood (piggybacked) (Callum et al., 2016; De Biasio & Rymer, 2017).*

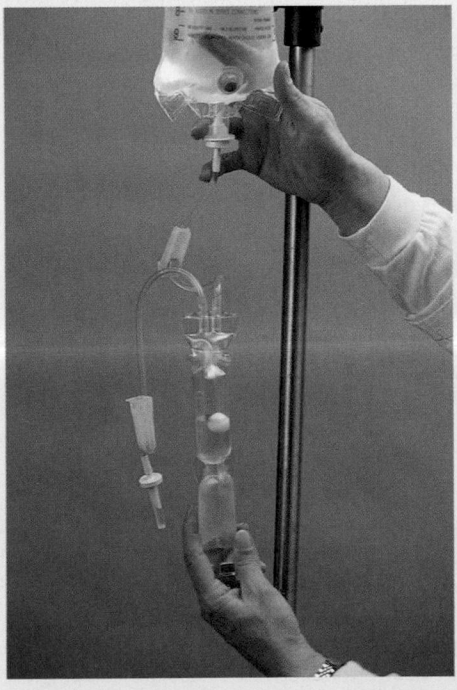

STEP 2d Blood administration set primed with normal saline.

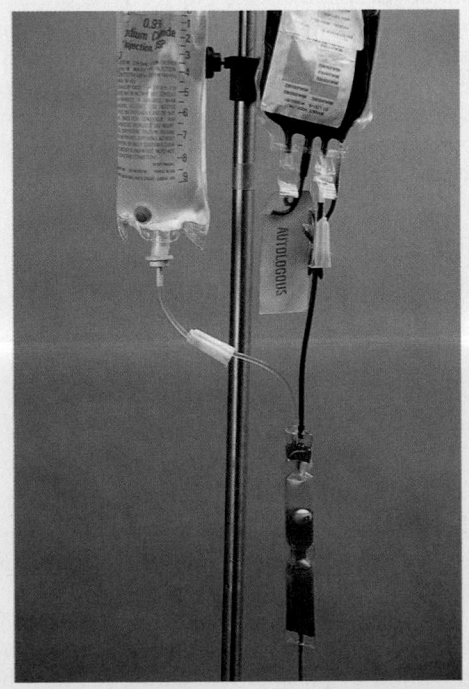

STEP 2f Unit of blood connected to Y-tubing setup.

STEP	RATIONALE

IMPLEMENTATION

g. Maintaining asepsis, attach primed tubing to patient's VAD by first cleansing the catheter hub with an antiseptic swab. Then quickly connect NS-primed blood administration tubing directly to patient's VAD.

> Reduces transmission of microorganisms from catheter hub. This initiates infusion of blood product into patient's vein.

h. Open common tubing clamp and regulate blood infusion to allow only 2 mL/min to infuse in initial 15 minutes. Remain with patient during first 15 minutes of transfusion. Initial flow rate during this time should be 1–2 mL/min or 10–20 gtt/min (drop factor: 10 gtt/mL).

> Many transfusion reactions occur within the first 15 minutes of transfusion. Infusing a small amount of blood component initially minimizes volume of blood to which patient is exposed, thereby minimizing severity of reaction (Lewis et al., 2019).

Clinical Decision Point *If signs of a transfusion reaction occur,* **immediately stop the transfusion,** *start 0.9% sodium chloride (NS) with a new primed tubing attached directly to the VAD hub, and notify the health care provider immediately (see Skill 30.2). Do not discard the blood product or tubing because they need to be returned to the blood bank. Do not infuse saline through existing tubing because it will cause blood in tubing to enter patient.*

i. Monitor patient's vital signs within 15 minutes of initiating transfusion, at prescribed intervals according to employer policy, at completion of transfusion, and post-transfusion (Lewis et al., 2019).

> Frequently monitoring patient helps to quickly alert you to transfusion reaction (De Biasio & Rymer, 2017).

j. If there is no transfusion reaction, regulate rate of transfusion according to health care provider's prescription based on drop factor for blood administration tubing (see Chapter 29).

> Maintaining prescribed rate of flow decreases risk for fluid volume excess while restoring vascular volume. Drop factor for most blood tubing is 10 gtt/mL.

Clinical Decision Point *Do not let a unit of blood hang for more than 4 hours because of danger of bacterial growth. When a longer transfusion time is indicated clinically, the unit may be divided by the blood bank, and the part not being transfused can be properly refrigerated (refer to employer policy). Administration sets should be changed at the completion of each unit or every 4 hours to reduce bacterial contamination (INS, 2016). Blood should only be stored in a refrigerator specific for blood or blood products to maintain appropriate temperature controls (Lewis et al., 2019).*

Clinical Decision Point *Medications and solutions should not be infused into the same IV line with a blood component because of the possibility of incompatibility unless the drug or solution has been approved by Health Canada for use with blood administration. Maintain a separate IV access if patient requires IV solutions or medications (De Biasio & Rymer, 2017). Always check employer policy.*

k. After blood has infused, clear IV line with 0.9% sodium chloride (NS) and discard blood bag according to employer policy. When consecutive units are prescribed, ensure line patency with 0.9% sodium chloride (NS) at keep vein open (KVO) rate as prescribed by health care provider and retrieve subsequent unit for administration.

> Infusing IV NS allows remainder of blood in IV tubing to infuse and keeps IV line patent for supportive measures in case of transfusion reaction (Lewis et al., 2019). KVO rate must specify infusion rate as required by rights of medication administration.

l. Appropriately dispose of all supplies. Remove gloves and perform hand hygiene.

> Routine practices during transfusion reduce transmission of microorganisms.

EVALUATION

1. Observe IV site and status of infusion each time vital signs are taken.

> Detects presence of IV-related complications (e.g., infiltration, occlusion, phlebitis) and verifies continuous and safe infusion of blood product.

2. Observe for any signs of transfusion reactions such as chills, flushing, itching, dyspnea, or rash during and for 6 hours after transfusion (De Biasio & Rymer, 2017).

> Compares presenting signs and symptoms to baseline assessment of patient before transfusion. These are early signs of transfusion reaction or late transfusion reaction (see Table 30.2).

STEP	RATIONALE

EVALUATION

3. Observe patient and assess laboratory values to determine response to administration of blood component.

Aids in determining whether goals of therapy have been reached or if further blood component therapy will be required. Laboratory results may not reflect transfusion reaction for several hours.

4. Use Teach-Back: "I want to be sure that I explained the reason for your blood transfusion? How can this transfusion help you?" Develop a revised teaching plan if patient or caregiver is not able to teach back correctly.

Determines patient's and caregiver's level of understanding of instructional topic.

Unexpected Outcomes	Related Interventions
1. Patient displays signs and symptoms of transfusion reaction such as chills, flushing, itching, dyspnea, or rash.	• Stop transfusion immediately. • Disconnect blood tubing at VAD hub and cap distal end with sterile connector to maintain sterile system. • Connect new NS solution and primed tubing directly to VAD hub to prevent any subsequent blood from infusing into patient from tubing. • Keep vein open with slow infusion of NS at 1–2 mL/min to ensure venous patency and maintain venous access for medication or to resume transfusion. • Notify health care provider. • See Table 30.2 for interventions.
2. Patient develops infiltration or phlebitis at venipuncture site.	• Transfusion should be stopped at first sign of infiltration, and IV line removed (see Procedural Guideline 29.1). • Insert new VAD in area above previous location or opposite arm. • Restart product if remainder can be infused within 4 hours of initiation of transfusion. • Institute nursing measures to reduce discomfort at infiltrated or phlebotic area.
3. Fluid volume overload occurs, and/or patient exhibits difficulty breathing or has crackles on auscultation of lungs.	• Slow or stop transfusion, elevate head of bed, and inform health care provider of physical findings. • Administer diuretics, morphine, and/or oxygen as prescribed by health care provider. • Continue frequent assessments and closely monitor vital signs and intake and output.

Communication and Documentation

- Before transfusion, document pretransfusion medications, vital signs, location and condition of IV site, and patient education in nurses' notes in electronic health record (EHR) or chart.
- Document the type and volume of blood component; blood unit, donor, and recipient identification; compatibility; and expiration date according to employer policy, along with patient's response to therapy. Document on the transfusion record in nurses' notes in EHR or chart, medication administration record, flow sheet, and/or intake and output sheet, depending on employer policy.
- Document volume of NS and blood component infused.
- Document amount of blood received and patient's response to therapy.
- Document vital signs before, shortly after initiation, during, and after transfusion.
- Document your evaluation of patient and caregiver learning.

- Report signs and symptoms of a transfusion reaction immediately to the health care provider and blood bank. Document in the patient record.
- Report to health care provider any intra-transfusion or post-transfusion deterioration in cardiac, pulmonary, or renal status. Document in the patient record.

Special Considerations
Teaching

- Educate patient and caregiver regarding rationale for transfusion and anticipated amount of time for completion of transfusion.
- Discuss with patient and caregiver the rationale for patient monitoring throughout the transfusion.
- Instruct patient and caregiver to notify the nurse if patient experiences itching, swelling, dizziness, dyspnea, low back pain, or chest pain because these may indicate a transfusion reaction.
- Instruct patient to inform the nurse if redness, pain, tenderness, swelling, bleeding, drainage, or leakage from under the dressing occurs at the IV site.

Pediatric

- Transfuse pediatric patients slowly (1 mL/kg/hr up to 50 mL/hr) for the first 15 minutes. Then increase the rate to 5 mL/kg/hr up to 150 mL/hr. The nurse should stay with the child during this time frame (Callum et al., 2016).
- Smaller portions of blood, from an assigned red blood cell unit, are commonly used for pediatric patients (Lau, 2017).
- A 22- or 24-gauge cannula can be used to infuse PRBCs in small veins that do not need rapid flow rates (Callum et al., 2016).
- Transfusion is not usually required in pediatric patients, unless the hemoglobin is less than 70 g/L. Neonates under 28 days old may require transfusion sooner (Callum et al., 2016).

Gerontological

- Some older persons have decreased cardiac function, thus requiring a slower infusion time. Half units may be obtained if a patient is unable to tolerate the volume in a whole unit of blood or blood component.
- In older persons at risk for circulatory overload, regulate flow rate at 1 mL/kg/hr.

Care in the Community

- Patients who have had prior transfusion reactions, acute angina, or heart failure are not good candidates for home transfusion.
- Nursing personnel must be present during the entire transfusion process and for 30 to 60 minutes after transfusion.
- Blood and blood products must be transported in a container with appropriate coolant. Verify and record the temperature at time of delivery.
- Initiate the transfusion as soon as possible after component is obtained from the blood bank.
- When blood sample is obtained for blood typing and cross-matching, attach identification band to patient with full name and identification number used by laboratory. This provides clear identification of patient when blood component transfusion is initiated.
- Instruct patient and caregiver in signs and symptoms of a delayed hemolytic transfusion reaction (i.e., unexplained fever, decrease in hemoglobin and hematocrit levels 2 to 14 days after transfusion) so they can report them and receive treatment, if necessary.
- Return the container, empty bags, and tubing to the community care employer after completion of the transfusion.

◆ SKILL 30.2   Monitoring for Adverse Transfusion Reactions

NSO *Nursing Skills Online Blood Therapy Module 15 / Lesson 3*

Adverse transfusion reactions may occur any time during a transfusion of blood products and up to 6 hours after a transfusion. Life-threatening reactions usually occur within the first 15 minutes of transfusion. The nurse must remain with the patient during this time to monitor physiological responses.

Several types of adverse reactions may result from a blood transfusion (see Table 30.2). A *hemolytic reaction* is a systemic response to the administration of a blood product that is incompatible with that of the recipient. The product contains allergens to which the recipient is sensitive or allergic, or it is contaminated with pathogens. Some patients who have a history of frequent transfusion may receive premedication with diphenhydramine to combat acquired sensitivities.

Before a transfusion each blood unit undergoes extensive serological testing to reduce the risk for patients acquiring a bloodborne disease. Symptoms that indicate an adverse reaction range from fever, chills, and skin rash to hypotension and cardiac arrest. Some patients also experience a delayed transfusion reaction, which sometimes does not occur for days or weeks after the transfusion (Lewis et al., 2019). Other possible adverse outcomes that result from transfusion therapy include transmission of diseases, circulatory overload reaction, sepsis reaction, and transfusion-related acute lung injury (TRALI) (Lewis et al., 2019). Facilities must report reactions and fatalities that occur as the result of a transfusion reaction to the Canada Vigilance Program, Canadian Blood Services or Héma-Québec, and Transfusion Transmitted Injuries Surveillance System (TTISS).

Delegation and Collaboration

The skill of administering and monitoring blood transfusions cannot be delegated to an unregulated care provider (UCP). The skill of administering and monitoring blood transfusion by a registered practical nurse (RPN) or licensed practical nurse (LPN) varies by provincial and territorial standards of practice as well as employer policy.

After the transfusion has been started and the patient is stable, a UCP can monitor a patient in collaboration with a nurse. This does not relieve a registered nurse (RN) of the responsibility to continue to assess the patient during the transfusion. The nurse instructs the UCP about:

- The signs and symptoms of a transfusion reaction that the patient may exhibit and to immediately report these to the nurse.

STEP	RATIONALE

ASSESSMENT

1. Identify patient using at least two person-specific identifiers (e.g., name and date of birth or name and medical record number) according to employer policy.	Ensures correct patient. Complies with Accreditation Canada standards and improves patient safety (Accreditation Canada, 2019).
2. With initiation of a transfusion, observe patient for fever with or without chills.	Fever indicates onset of acute hemolytic reaction, febrile nonhemolytic reaction, or bacterial sepsis.
3. Assess patient for tachycardia band/or tachypnea and dyspnea.	Indicates acute hemolytic reaction or circulatory overload. In case of circulatory overload, cough may accompany these symptoms.

STEP	RATIONALE

ASSESSMENT

4. Observe patient for drop in blood pressure.

Hypotension indicates infectious disease transmission, an acute hemolytic reaction, and anaphylaxis.

5. Observe patient for hives or skin rash, including assessment of trunk and back.

These are early indications of an allergic reaction, anaphylaxis, or graft-versus-host disease, which occurs after transfusion.

6. Observe patient for flushing.

This is an early indication of acute hemolytic reaction or febrile nonhemolytic reaction. Sometimes localized flushing presents with an allergic reaction.

7. Observe patient for gastrointestinal symptoms.

Nausea and vomiting are present in acute hemolytic transfusion reactions, anaphylactic reactions, or infectious disease transmission.

8. Observe patient for wheezing, chest pain, and possible cardiac arrest.

These are all indications of anaphylactic reaction.

9. Be alert to patient complaints of headache or muscle pain in presence of fever.

Both indicate febrile nonhemolytic reaction.

10. Monitor patient for disseminated intravascular coagulation (DIC), renal failure, anemia, and hemoglobinemia/hemoglobinuria by reviewing laboratory test results (complete blood count [CBC] with differential, hemoglobin [Hgb], hematocrit [Hct]).

All are late signs of an acute hemolytic reaction.

11. Auscultate patient's lungs before and during transfusion and monitor central venous pressure (CVP), if possible.

Crackles in base of lungs and rising CVP are indications of circulatory overload.

12. Observe patient for jaundice and increased liver enzyme levels, indicating liver damage; and decreased red blood cells (RBCs), white blood cells (WBCs), and platelets, indicating bone marrow suppression.

These indicate graft-versus-host disease and would occur following transfusion.

13. In patients receiving massive transfusions, observe for mild hypothermia, cardiac dysrhythmias, hypotension, hypocalcemia, and hemochromatosis (iron overload).

Cold blood products affect the cardiac conduction system, resulting in ventricular dysrhythmias. Other cardiac dysrhythmias, hypotension, and tingling indicate hypocalcemia, which occurs when citrate (used as a preservative for some blood products) combines with patient's calcium. Iron overload may occur after 10 transfusions (see Table 30.2). It usually occurs in patients who require chronic transfusions.

NURSING DIAGNOSES

- Inadequate gas exchange
- Excessive fluid volume
- Reduced cardiac output
- Hyperthermia
- Acute pain
- Potential for infection
- Anxiety
- Hypothermia

Related factors/Risk factors are individualized on the basis of patient's condition or needs.

PLANNING

1. Expected outcomes following completion of procedure:
   - Patient's cardiac parameters (heart rate, blood pressure, CVP) return to baseline.

   Intravascular volume is restored, reaction reversed.

   - Patient maintains core body temperature of 36° to 37.2°C (97° to 99°F).

   Helps to confirm absence of transfusion reaction, infection, and sepsis.

   - Patient has urine output of 0.5 to 1 mL/kg/hr.

   Reflects optimal fluid status.

   - Patient maintains oxygen saturation greater than 95%.

   Improved tissue perfusion.

   - Patient is comfortable.

   Absence of transfusion reaction. Appropriate nursing measures keep patient at ease.

2. Patient can explain signs and symptoms of a transfusion reaction.

   Calms anxiety and helps patient and caregiver anticipate nurse's actions.

STEP	RATIONALE

IMPLEMENTATION

1. If you suspect transfusion reaction:

  a. Immediately stop transfusion.

Severity of reaction is related to the amount of blood component infused and cause of the reaction. It is critical to prevent any more blood from infusing into patient.

  b. Remove blood component and tubing containing blood product. Replace them with new bag of 0.9% sodium chloride (normal saline [NS]) and tubing (see Chapter 29). Connect tubing directly to hub of vascular access device (VAD).

Prevents additional blood in tubing from being infused.

    Exception: If patient symptoms suggest mild allergic reaction, stop transfusion, administer antihistamine, and restart or discontinue transfusion per health care provider's prescription.

  c. Maintain patent VAD using 0.9% sodium chloride (NS) at rate prescribed by health care provider.

NS keeps IV patent and provides route for emergency medications and fluids.

  d. Obtain vital signs. Remain with patient for continuous monitoring and assessment. Do not leave patient alone.

Vital signs are objective measures of patient's condition, which can deteriorate rapidly.

  e. Notify health care provider.

Transfusion reactions require immediate medical intervention. Follow protocol for emergency interventions for anaphylactic reactions.

  f. Notify blood bank.

Blood bank has procedure to follow when notified of transfusion reaction.

  g. Obtain blood samples (if needed) from extremity opposite extremity receiving transfusion. Check employer policy regarding number and type of tubes to be used.

Typically, one tube of blood will be cross-matched to pretransfusion sample to ensure that correct blood was given to recipient. Blood will be checked for antibodies to determine type of reaction. Second sample will be checked for free hemoglobin in serum, indicating hemolysis, and bilirubin level should be obtained.

  h. Return remainder of blood component and attached blood tubing to blood bank according to employer policy.

Sample of this blood will be cross-matched to patient's pretransfusion and post-transfusion samples to determine if error in cross-matching occurred.

  i. Monitor patient's vital signs every 15 minutes or per employer policy.

Maintains ongoing assessment of patient's cardiopulmonary status and response to treatment.

  j. Administer prescribed medications according to type and severity of transfusion reaction.

Follow employer protocol or health care provider's prescription.

    (1) Epinephrine

Stimulates sympathetic nervous system to relieve respiratory distress and combat vasodilation in anaphylaxis.

    (2) Antihistamine

Diminishes some aspects of allergic response by blocking histamine receptors.

    (3) Antibiotics

Administered when bacterial contamination or sepsis is suspected.

    (4) Antipyretics/analgesics

Administered to relieve fever and discomfort in acute hemolytic reactions, febrile nonhemolytic reactions, graft-versus-host disease, and bacterial sepsis.

    (5) Diuretics/morphine

Treats circulatory overload by reducing intravascular volume (diuresis) and decreasing vascular tone (opioid effect).

    (6) Corticosteroids

Stabilizes cell membranes, decreasing histamine release. Administered in severe allergic reactions.

    (7) Intravenous (IV) fluids

Rapid administration of IV fluids counteracts some symptoms of anaphylactic shock.

  k. In event of cardiac arrest, initiate cardiopulmonary resuscitation (see Chapter 28).

Anaphylaxis can quickly lead to cardiopulmonary arrest. Prompt resuscitation may prevent further complications.

  l. Obtain first voided urine sample and send to laboratory. You may need to insert Foley catheter to obtain urine (see Chapter 34).

Hemoglobinuria occurs with acute hemolytic reactions. Degree of damage to kidneys is influenced by pH of urine and rate of urinary excretion. Attempts will be made to initiate diuresis and alkalinize urine. If kidney damage is severe, dialysis may be required.

STEP	RATIONALE

EVALUATION

1. Continue monitoring patient for signs and symptoms of transfusion reactions.

2. **Use Teach-Back:** "I want to be sure that I explained the reactions that can occur when you are getting a blood transfusion. What signs and symptoms would you report?" Develop a revised teaching plan if patient or caregiver is not able to teach back correctly.

Continued monitoring of patient's cardiopulmonary status and physiological response will indicate if reaction has been reversed.

Determines patient's and caregiver's level of understanding of instructional topic.

Unexpected Outcomes
1. Patient's physiological status worsens.

Related Interventions
- Appropriate interventions depend on type of transfusion reaction. Table 30.2 provides general guidelines.

Communication and Documentation

- Document the exact time the transfusion reaction was first noted, all vital signs and other physiological assessments, treatments instituted, and patient response in nurses' notes in electronic health record (EHR) or chart. Complete transfusion reaction report (according to employer policy).
- Document your evaluation of patient and caregiver learning.
- Immediately report presence of transfusion reaction and patient's physical assessment findings to health care provider.

Special Considerations
Teaching
- Teach patient and caregiver signs and symptoms of transfusion reactions and steps to take if they occur.

Pediatric
- Irradiated red blood cells and platelets are preferable in children under 6 years of age because of their immature immune systems

and to avoid graft-versus-host disease. Irradiation should occur immediately before use, since irradiation damage to the red blood cell membrane increases potassium loss, risking hyperkalemia in pediatric patients (Lau, 2017).

Gerontological
- Administer blood components cautiously to older persons, considering both the rate and amount of infusion, because they are at risk for developing circulatory overload.

Care in the Community
- Certain adverse outcomes (development of hepatitis) or transfusion reactions (delayed hemolysis) occur days to weeks after the patient has received transfusion and may become evident in the home setting.
- It is important that patients and caregivers are aware of signs and symptoms of adverse occurrences and of steps to take should they occur.

◆CLINICAL DEBRIEF

A 72-year-old man is admitted for a hip replacement and has donated 1 unit of autologous blood if he needs transfusion therapy after surgery. Three weeks earlier his surgery had been postponed because he had a case of pneumonia that required treatment with antibiotics. While he was awaiting hip surgery, he developed bleeding hemorrhoids, which were surgically repaired yesterday. Today he tells the nurse that he is very tired, and he passed a great deal of blood with several bowel movements during the night and earlier this morning. His colouring is pale, and his skin is cool to the touch. His blood pressure has dropped since admission, from 130/80 mm Hg to 100/66 mm Hg. His health care provider told him that he may need a blood transfusion. He had blood drawn this morning, and his hemoglobin has dropped from 100 g/L to 90 g/L. The patient states that he is very concerned about being transfused, and he thinks that the blood he donated will not be good since it was over a month ago.

1. Based on his concerns, which items would be assessed in preparation for a blood transfusion?
2. After the nurse obtains the unit of packed red blood cells (PRBCs) from the blood bank, the patient is taken to the operating room (OR) for a procedure to stop the rectal bleeding, which will last 1 to 2 hours before starting the blood transfusion. Which actions would the nurse take while waiting for him to return?
3. The patient has had no bleeding since his return to the unit from the OR and the nurse begins the blood transfusion as prescribed. About 30 minutes after initiating the first unit of PRBCs, he reports that he is itchy all over his body and presents with a rash and hives. His temperature is 37°C, pulse 112, respiration 24, and BP 126/80. Using SBAR, show how the nurse would communicate with the health care team about this patient.

✦ REVIEW QUESTIONS

1. Which of the following steps are necessary for initiating a transfusion of packed red blood cells (PRBCs)? *(Select all that apply.)*
 1. Infuse blood component with 5% dextrose (D_5W).
 2. Follow employer policy to verify correct patient and blood product.
 3. Check appearance of blood for leaks, bubbles, clots, or purplish colour.
 4. Infuse blood component over 4–6 hours to prevent fluid volume overload.
 5. Obtain vital signs before infusion, after 5 to 15 minutes of initiating infusion, and at its completion.
 6. Clear IV line with 0.9% saline after transfusion.

2. A patient is experiencing an acute hemolytic transfusion reaction while receiving packed red blood cells (PRBCs). Place the following steps in the correct order:
 1. Obtain vital signs and remain with the patient.
 2. Stop the infusion.
 3. Obtain blood and urine samples.
 4. Replace the blood component and tubing with a new bag of 0.9% sodium chloride (normal saline [NS]) and new tubing.
 5. Notify the blood bank.
 6. Notify the health care provider.

3. Which of the following items must be verified to ensure that the correct blood component is transfused to the correct patient? *(Select all that apply.)*
 1. Verbally compare and correctly identify the patient's identity using two patient identifiers.
 2. Verify that the transfusion record number matches the patient's identification number.
 3. Check that the expiration date is not passed.
 4. Confirm that the blood collection date is within 72 hours of the transfusion.
 5. Have two qualified individuals perform verifications before initiation of transfusion.
 6. Verify that the blood component and type to be infused match the patient's.

ⓔ *Visit the Evolve site for a complete list of Clinical Debrief and Review Questions answers.*

REFERENCES

Accreditation Canada. (2019). *Required organizational practices handbook—Version 14.* Ottawa, ON: Author. Retrieved from http://www.wrha.mb.ca/quality/files/2019ROPHandbook.pdf

Callum, J., Pinkerton, P., Lima, A., et al. (2016). *Bloody easy 4. Blood transfusions, blood alternatives, and transfusion reactions* (4th ed.). Toronto: Ontario Regional Blood Coordinating Network. Retrieved from http://policyandorders.cw.bc.ca/resource-gallery/Documents/Transfusion%20Medicine/Bloody%20Easy%204.pdf

Canadian Blood Services (CBS). (2017–2019). *Clinical guide to transfusion.* Retrieved from https://professionaleducation.blood.ca/en/transfusion/clinical-guide-transfusion

Canadian Patient Safety Institute (CPSI). (2017). *Hospital harm improvement resource. Infusion, transfusion and injection complications.* Retrieved from https://www.patientsafetyinstitute.ca/en/toolsResources/Hospital-Harm-Measure/Documents/Resource-Library/HHIR%20Infusion%20Transfusion%20and%20Injectibles.pdf

Canadian Society for Transfusion Medicine. (2017a). *Standards for hospital transfusion services* (Version 4). Retrieved from http://www.transfusion.ca/Resources/Standards

Canadian Society for Transfusion Medicine. (2017b). *Ten things physicians and patients should question.* Retrieved from https://choosingwiselycanada.org/transfusion-medicine/

Clarke, G. (2017). Blood components. In G. Clarke & S. Chargé (Eds.), *Clinical guide to transfusion.* Retrieved from https://professionaleducation.blood.ca/en/transfusion/clinical-guide-transfusion

Clarke, G., & Hannon, J. (2018). Hemolytic disease of the fetus and newborn and perinatal immune thrombocytopenia. In G. Clarke & S. Chargé (Eds.), *Clinical guide to transfusion.* Retrieved from https://professionaleducation.blood.ca/en/transfusion/clinical-guide-transfusion

De Biasio, L., & Rymer, T. (2017). Blood administration. In G. Clarke & S. Chargé (Eds.), *Clinical guide to transfusion.* Retrieved from https://professionaleducation.blood.ca/en/transfusion/clinical-guide-transfusion

Department of Justice. (2017). *Legal representation of children in Canada: Parens patriae jurisdiction.* Retrieved from http://www.justice.gc.ca/eng/rp-pr/other-autre/lrc-rje/p3.html

Gehrie, E., Chandler, J., & Snyder, E. (2016). Clinical and technical aspects of blood administration. In T. Simon, J. McCullough, E. Snyder, B. Solheim, & R. Strauss (Eds.), *Rossi's principles of transfusion medicine* (5th ed., pp. 23–29). Hoboken, NJ: Wiley-Blackwell.

Government of Canada. (2016). *Guidance document: Blood regulations.* Retrieved from https://www.canada.ca/en/health-canada/services/drugs-health-products/biologics-radiopharmaceuticals-genetic-therapies/applications-submissions/guidance-documents/blood-regulations/guidance-document-blood-regulations-1.html

Hurlock-Chorostecki, C., van Soeren, M., MacMillan, K., et al. (2015). A survey of interprofessional activity of acute and long-term care employed nurse practitioners. *Journal of the American Association of Nurse Practitioners, 27,* 507–513. doi:10.1002/2327-6924.12213

Infusion Nurses Society (INS). (2016). Infusion therapy standards of practice. *Journal of Intravenous Nursing, 39*(Suppl. 1), S1–S161. Retrieved from http://source.yiboshi.com/20170417/1492425631944540325.pdf

Lane, D. (2017). Pre-transfusion testing. In G. Clarke & S. Chargé (Eds.), *Clinical guide to transfusion.* Retrieved from https://professionaleducation.blood.ca/en/transfusion/clinical-guide-transfusion

Lau, W. (2017). Neonatal and pediatric transfusion. In G. Clarke & S. Chargé (Eds.), *Clinical guide to transfusion.* Retrieved from https://professionaleducation.blood.ca/en/transfusion/clinical-guide-transfusion

Lewis, S., Bucher, L., Heitkemper, M. L., Harding, M. M., Barry, M. A., & Goldsworthy, S. (Eds.). (2019). *Medical–surgical nursing in Canada. Assessment and management of clinical problems* (4th ed.). Toronto, ON: Elsevier Canada.

MacDonald, N., O'Brien, S., & Delage, G. (2017). Transfusion and risk of infection in Canada: Update 2012. *Paediatric Child Health, 17*(10), e102–e111. doi:10.1093/pch/17.10.e102

National Advisory Committee on Blood and Blood Products. (2014). *NAC companion document to red blood cell transfusion: A clinical practice guideline from the AABB.* Retrieved from https://www.nacblood.ca/resources/guidelines/Companion-Document-May-28-2014.pdf

Pambrun, C. (2017). Preoperative autologous donation. In G. Clarke & S. Chargé (Eds.), *Clinical guide to transfusion.* Retrieved from https://professionaleducation.blood.ca/en/transfusion/clinical-guide-transfusion

Potter, P. A., Perry, A. G., Stockert, P. A., Hall, A. M., Astle, B. J., & Duggleby, W. (Eds.). (2019). *Canadian fundamentals of nursing* (6th ed.). Toronto, ON: Elsevier Canada.

Public Health Agency of Canada (PHAC). (2016). *Transfusion transmitted injuries surveillance system (TTISS): 2009–2013 summary results.* Centre for Communicable Diseases and Infection Control. Ottawa, ON: Author. Retrieved from http://publications.gc.ca/collections/collection_2016/aspc-phac/HP40-168-2016-eng.pdf

Sidani, S., Collins, L., Harbman, P., et al. (2015). A description of nurse practitioners' self-report implementation of patient-centered care. *European Journal for Person Centered Healthcare, 3*(1), 11–18.

31 | Oral Nutrition

Written by **Kathryn Weaver, RN, MN, PhD; and Hope V. Bussenius, DNP, APRN, FNP-BC**

SKILLS AND PROCEDURES

Skill 31.1 **Performing a Nutritional Screening and Physical Examination, p. 853**

Skill 31.2 **Assisting an Adult Patient With Oral Nutrition, p. 859**

Skill 31.3 **Aspiration Precautions, p. 864**

OBJECTIVES

Mastery of content in this chapter will enable the nurse to:
- Perform an accurate nutritional screening.
- Identify the need for and collaborate with a dietitian when needed for a patient's nutritional assessment.
- Assess a patient's ability to swallow.
- Identify risk factors for aspiration.
- Evaluate a patient's tolerance of oral nutrition.
- Identify appropriate techniques to use to prevent a patient from aspirating.
- Demonstrate how to properly feed a patient who cannot self-feed.

MEDIA RESOURCES

- evolve http://evolve.elsevier.com/Canada/Perry/clinicalskills/
- Review Questions
- ▶ Video Clips
- Audio Glossary
- Clinical Debrief and Review Questions Answers

PURPOSE

Nutrition is a basic component of health that affects a patient's rate of recovery from short-term and chronic illness, surgery, and injury. Malnutrition develops as a result of deficiency in dietary intake, increased requirements associated with disease, complications of an underlying illness such as poor absorption, and excessive nutrient losses, or a combination of these factors (Bruins, Bird, Aebischer, et al., 2018). Malnutrition is a major concern for older persons and for patients with limited financial resources. Approximately one-third of community-dwelling Canadians aged 65 or older are at nutritional risk, with females more so than males, and those aged 75 or older at higher risk (Ramage-Morin, Gilmour, & Rotermann, 2017). Malnutrition is also highly prevalent for patients in acute hospital settings (Keller, McCullough, Davidson, et al., 2015b). As well, more than 50% of residents dwelling in long-term care homes in four Canadian provinces were found to consume inadequate amounts of folate, certain vitamins, calcium, magnesium, and zinc, with more than 90% consuming amounts below established dietary reference intakes for vitamins and magnesium (Keller, Lengyel, Carrier, et al., 2018). Amid limited staff resources, assisting patients with their meals competes with other duties, including bathing, toileting, and documenting (Lowndes, Armstrong, & Daly, 2015).

Every organ system is affected by malnutrition. Complications include alterations in muscle, cardiorespiratory and gastrointestinal function, immune function, wound healing, and psychosocial effects. As a nurse, you will provide nutritional screening and use interprofessional collaboration (e.g., dietitian, nutritionist, health care provider) to determine the best approaches for supporting patients' nutritional health.

STANDARDS OF CARE

- Accreditation Canada, 2019—*Required Organizational Practices Handbook—Version 14* (http://www.wrha.mb.ca/quality/files/2019ROPHandbook.pdf)
- Alberta Health Services, 2018—*Nutrition Guideline Seniors Health Overview (65 Years and Older)* (https://www.albertahealthservices.ca/assets/info/nutrition/if-nfs-ng-seniors-health-overview.pdf)
- Health Canada, 2015b—*Regulations Amending the Food and Drug Regulations—Nutrition Labelling, Other Labelling Provisions and Food Colours* (http://www.gazette.gc.ca/rp-pr/p1/2015/2015-06-13/html/reg1-eng.html)
- Health Canada, 2019a—*Canada's Dietary Guidelines for Health Professionals and Policy Makers* (https://food-guide.canada.ca/en/guidelines/)

- Health Canada, 2019b—*Food and Nutrition* (https://www.canada.ca/en/health-canada/services/food-nutrition.html)
- Health Canada, 2019c—*Health Canada's Healthy Eating Strategy* (https://www.canada.ca/en/services/health/campaigns/vision-healthy-canada/healthy-eating.html)
- Public Health Agency of Canada, 2014—*Canadian Best Practices Portal: Canadian Health Indicators* (http://cbpp-pcpe.phac-aspc.gc.ca/resources/health-indicators/canadian-health-indicators/)

PRINCIPLES FOR PRACTICE

- The Integrated Nutrition Pathway for Acute Care (INPAC) is a care pathway developed by the Canadian Malnutrition Task Force (Keller, Allard, Vesnaver, et al., 2015) that is undergoing uptake into practice. The INPAC requires routine identification of malnutrition with screening of patients in health care settings (Keller, Allard, Vesnaver, et al., 2015). For hospitalized patients, nutritional screening is completed during patient admission to a hospital (Keller, McCullough, Davidson, 2015a). When a nutritional screening is performed, one aim is to identify common risk factors for nutritional problems (Box 31.1).

BOX 31.1

Risk Factors for Potential Nutritional Problems

- Clear- or full-liquid diets for more than 3 days with inappropriate or insufficient nutrient supplementation
- Intravenous feeding (dextrose and saline or saline) or NPO (nothing by mouth) for more than 3 days without nutrient supplementation
- Low intake (<50%) of prescribed diet or tube feedings
- Weight 20% above or 10% below a healthy body weight (accounting for edema)
- Pregnancy weight gain deviating from the normal pattern of gaining 0.45 kg/week during the last 20 weeks of pregnancy; higher-than-normal maternal weight gain is associated with pre-eclampsia (high blood pressure and organ system damage during pregnancy), low birth weight, and perinatal death.
- Diagnoses that increase nutritional needs or decrease nutrient intake: cancer, malabsorption, diarrhea, hyperthyroidism, excessive inflammation, postoperative status, hemorrhage, infected or draining wounds, burns, infection, major trauma
- Chronic use of drugs, especially alcohol, which affects nutritional intake
- Alterations in chewing, swallowing, appetite, taste, and smell
- Body temperature consistently higher that 37°C (98.6°F) for more than 2 days, because fever increases both energy and micronutrient requirements
- Hematocrit: less than 43% in men, less than 37% in women; hemoglobin less than 140 g/L in men, less than 120 g/L in women can signal anemia, which may compromise tissue oxygen delivery (Mozos, 2015)
- Absolute decrease in lymphocyte count (<1 500 cells/mm³) is a predictor of nutritional risk and surgical complications (Rocha & Fortes, 2015)
- Elevated (>5 mmol/L) or decreased (<1.5 mmol/L) total plasma cholesterol, as this is associated with cardiovascular disease risk
- Serum albumin less than 30 g/L in patients without renal or liver disease, generalized dermatitis, or overhydration, as this is a predictor of nutritional risk and surgical complications (Rocha & Fortes, 2015)
- Remaining NPO

Modified from Grodner, M., Escott-Stump, S., & Dorner, S. (2015). *Foundations and clinical applications of nutrition: A nursing approach* (6th ed.). St. Louis: Elsevier Health Sciences.

- Nutrition assessment should be completed within 24 hours of screening (Keller, McCullough, Davidson, 2015a). Food intake, weight history, functional status, and body composition are assessed; the assessment takes approximately 10 minutes.
- Recommendations for nutritional care are based on the assessment. If the patient is at risk of malnutrition, optimal oral intake is provided and monitored. Barriers to food intake are assessed and body weight is measured at minimum once per week. Patients who are assessed as being at severe risk of malnutrition may be seen by a dietitian for specialized dietary treatment (Keller, McCullough, Davidson, 2015a).
- Food intake, and not change in body weight, is the primary mechanism for determining a change in nutrition care (Keller, McCullough, Davidson, 2015a).
- If a patient is malnourished at admission or during hospitalization, nutrition is flagged in the discharge summary note (completed by the dietitian, health care provider, or nurse). Education is provided to the patient and caregiver. Transfer of care recommendations include dietitian referral if nutrition rehabilitation is ongoing (Keller, McCullough, Davidson, 2015a).
- Nothing by mouth (NPO) status should be monitored daily. Being NPO for 3 days may necessitate a comprehensive nutritional assessment (Keller, McCullough, Davidson, 2015a).
- Patients who are malnourished have an increased length of hospital stay and may experience more complications (e.g., infection rates, mortality) during their period of hospitalization than patients who are in a well-nourished state (Bruins et al., 2018).
- As a nurse, you are responsible for assisting patients who are on an oral diet to successfully eat an adequate amount of food at a safe and comfortable pace.
- *Canada's Official Food Rules* was published in 1942 to maximize energy levels during wartime rations and poverty. Since then, worldwide food shortages, an increasing understanding of the health effects of overeating, and the most current evidence related to nutrition, physical activity, and health have been reflected in subsequent versions of the food guide. The intent is to promote health; reduce the risk of chronic diseases; and provide the basis for federal, provincial, and territorial food and nutrition policy and education initiatives. The newest food guide, *Canada's Dietary Guidelines* (Health Canada, 2019a) is based on three main guidelines: nutritious foods are the foundation of healthy eating (vegetables, fruits, whole grains, plant-based protein, unsaturated fats, and water); processed or prepared foods and beverages that contribute to excess sodium, free sugars, or saturated fat undermine healthy eating; and food skills are needed to navigate the current complex food environment and support healthy eating.
- Food insecurity occurs whenever the availability of nutritionally adequate and safe food or the ability to acquire food in socially accepted ways is inadequate. Food insecurity is more prevalent in households with children; those led by female lone parents; those with social assistance, worker's compensation, or employment insurance as the main source of income; where the highest level of education is less than secondary graduation; in urban areas; and in residences that are rented rather than owned. Food insecurity is higher in off-reserve Indigenous and recent immigrant households and in Nova Scotia, New Brunswick, and all the territories (Health Canada, 2017).

PERSON-CENTRED CARE

- An understanding of patients' values, beliefs, and attitudes about food and how these values affect food purchase, preparation,

and intake enables nurses to help patients make healthy food choices.

- Most Canadians need to improve some aspect of their diet. Nurses should use interprofessional collaboration (e.g., dietitian) in considering social factors that influence a person's diet: knowledge and attitudes about food and health, skills in being able to feed oneself and properly store and prepare food, social support, access to and use of food assistance programs, and the economic price system affecting a patient (Dietitians of Canada, 2014). Interprofessional collaboration has positive effects on patient health outcomes by increasing patient access to nutrition education, self-management training, and nutritional support.

- Individuals follow special patterns of food intake that are based on religion, cultural background, ethics, health beliefs, or concern about the environment. Such special diets (e.g., vegetarian, ovolactovegetarian) do not necessarily provide more or less nutritional benefit than diets based on the *Eat Well Plate* or other nutritional guidelines (Health Canada, 2019d).

- Some cultures believe in a hot-and-cold theory of health and illness based on the ancient Taoist concept of an essential life force, or qi, present in all objects and aspects of life. For a balanced diet, the yin (cold, dark, and passive) and the yang (heat, light, and active) are combined in the forms of food to create harmony within the body (Turchiaro, 2017). Foods are classified as hot or cold on the basis of their effect on metabolism after consumption, independent of the temperature at which they are served. Hotness in the body occurs after eating substances such as barbecued foods, red meat, fatty meat, and low-fibre foods such as soft drinks, coffee, honey, and milk, whereas coldness in the body follows consumption of foods such as vegetables, fruit, and grains. Foods affect the autonomic nervous and endocrine systems as well as the activity of the digestive enzymes. Substances that enhance activity of the whole system of the body are considered hot-natured, and those which reduce activity of the system are called cold-natured. Cold foods provide low energy and help balance hot foods. Hot foods provide greater energy for activity, are higher in calories, and are used to treat pallor and weakness. Different foods, in accordance with their temperature properties, are believed to directly influence health. For example, in an individual living with rheumatism, warming foods such as garlic can help alleviate pain. Also, in traditional Chinese medicine (TCM), most respiratory diseases (e.g., asthma) are perceived to be cold illnesses triggered by exposure to cold elements and require hot food treatment to restore the original balance (Ahmed, Salim, Steed, et al., 2017). Recently, a higher incidence of breast cancer was found among women who frequently consume hot foods (Zheng, Chen, Xie, et al., 2017). Use of TCM-based food classification could help people improve their dietary patterns—for example, by eating more cold foods and reducing consumption of high-risk hot foods to prevent breast cancer. This is consistent with the etiology and pathogenesis of breast cancer in Western medicine.

- Canada's Dietary Guidelines were developed by Health Canada (2019d) (Fig. 31.1) as a visual aid to suggest that Canadians fill half of their plate with vegetables and fruits at every meal.

EVIDENCE-INFORMED PRACTICE

Safe nutritional support of hospitalized adult patients living with obesity is an important priority of care. Following an extensive review of the literature, the Association of Parenteral and Enteral Nutrition (ASPEN) released clinical guidelines for the nutritional support of hospitalized adult patients with obesity (Choban, Dickerson, Malone, et al., 2013).

- Critically ill patients with obesity experience more complications than patients with optimal body mass index (BMI). These complications include an increase in mortality, longer critical care unit and hospital length of stay, greater need for mechanical ventilation, and higher incidence of infections and surgical complications.

- A nutritional support plan is recommended within 48 hours of admission to a critical care unit.

- A nutritional assessment is generally completed on patient admission to acute care facilities and additional nutritional screening within 24 hours, as indicated (Keller, McCullough, Davidson, 2015a).

Because weight is a sensitive issue for many patients, the Canadian Obesity Network (2011) has provided a toolkit with five steps to help health care team members better manage their patients' weight and related health issues. The 5As of obesity management include the following:

- **Ask** for permission to discuss weight and explore readiness.
- **Assess** obesity-related risks and "root causes" of obesity.
- **Advise** on health risks and treatment options.
- **Agree** on health outcomes and behavioural goals.
- **Assist** in accessing appropriate resources and providers.

Using the 5As, health care practitioners can discuss relevant epidemiology and causes of obesity with patients who experience obesity or are at risk. These patients can be counselled on complications of obesity and on the risk, benefits, and options available for management of obesity, including behavioural, pharmacological, and bariatric surgery management options.

Regarding older persons in long-term care homes, Dietitians of Canada (2013) has established best practices for nutrition, food service, and dining to improve residents' oral intake. Strategies include the following:

- Ensure that residents are given sufficient time to consume meals at a safe and comfortable pace.
- Help patients with any sensory aids such as hearing aids, glasses, and dentures before their food is served.
- Assign regular tables to team members so they become familiar with the residents and their personal needs, therapeutic diets, fluid consistencies, and dining preferences.
- Ensure that one team member, competent to handle risks such as choking and other response protocols, is assigned to be present at all times while residents are in the dining room.
- Provide nutritious snacks and beverages at times suitable to individual needs to provide person-centred care.

SAFETY GUIDELINES

- Improper handling, preparation, and storage practices may result in cases of foodborne illness (Health Canada, 2014a). Children younger than 5, pregnant women, adults over 65, and people with weak immune systems are more likely to become ill from contaminated food (Health Canada, 2015a). There are four principles for patients to follow in the home: cook to the right temperature, wash hands and surfaces (cutting boards, utensils, countertops) often, refrigerate promptly (summer—1 hour, winter—2 hours), and separate raw meats from other foods to prevent contamination (Box 31.2).

- Identify patients at risk for dysphagia (Hines, Kynoch, & Munday, 2016) and use interprofessional collaboration (e.g., speech-language pathologist) to minimize complications such as aspiration pneumonia (Herbert, Lindsay, McIntyre, et al.,

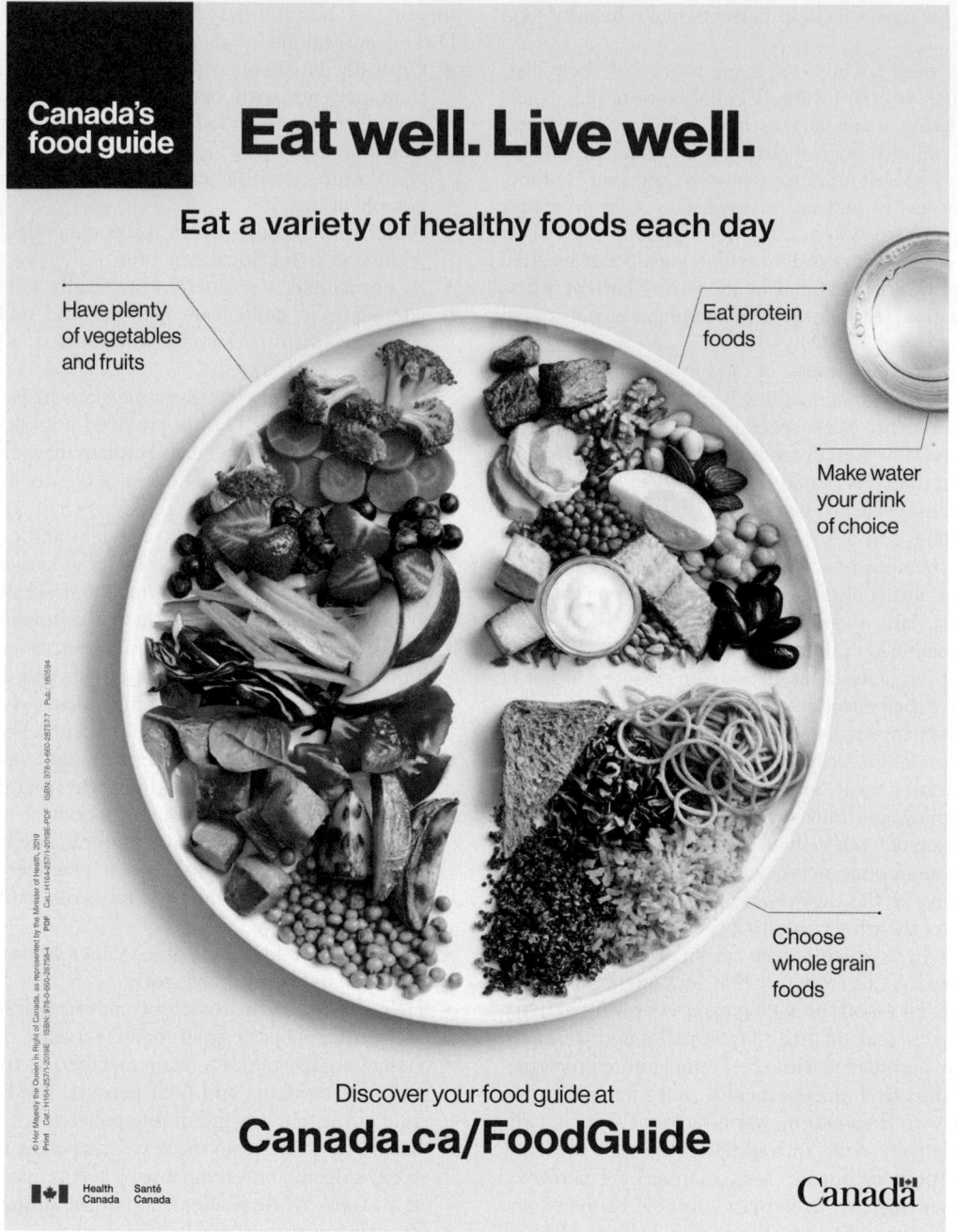

FIG 31.1 Canada's Dietary Guidelines. (© *Her Majesty the Queen in Right of Canada, as represented by the Minister of Health, 2019.*)

BOX 31.2

Food Safety Tips

- Wash hands, food-preparation surfaces, and utensils with warm, soapy water before touching food.
- For safe internal cooking temperatures for meat, poultry, fish, and eggs consult Health Canada's website (https://www.canada.ca/en/health-canada/services/general-food-safety-tips/safe-internal-cooking-temperatures.html).
- Wash all fresh fruits and vegetables thoroughly.
- Do not eat raw meats or drink unpasteurized milk or juices.
- Do not use food past the expiration date on a package.
- Keep foods refrigerated at 4.4°C (40°F) within 2 hours of cooking (1 hour in warmer temperatures).

- Place leftover foods in the refrigerator after cooking.
- Thaw frozen foods in the refrigerator.
- Discard food that you suspect is spoiled. Indicate date that food was first refrigerated.
- Sanitize countertops, cutting boards, and utensils after preparing food using a kitchen sanitizer (as directed) or a bleach solution (5 mL bleach to 750 mL of water). Rinse all items carefully with water.
- Clean the inside of the refrigerator, microwave, and other surfaces that come into contact with food regularly with bleach or soap.

Modified from Health Canada. (2014). *Food safety and you.* Retrieved from https://www.canada.ca/en/health-canada/services/general-food-safety-tips/food-safety-you.html.

2016). The role of speech-language pathologists is to evaluate the patient's ability to swallow and make recommendations to other interprofessional team members (Mittal, Mishra, & Nilakantan, 2015).

- Ensure that patients receive the correct therapeutic diet. Common dietary errors include wrong diet, meals meant for other patients, allergy conflicts, and meals delivered to a patient when NPO (Ross & Wallace, 2017).

- Assess a patient's level of consciousness before attempting any oral feeding. Hold oral nutrition if the patient's status has changed such that it may alter their ability to eat (e.g., decrease in level of consciousness) and consult with the health care provider.

✦ SKILL 31.1   Performing a Nutritional Screening and Physical Examination

Nurses screen for patients' actual and potential nutritional alterations by focusing on the effects of an illness, disease, or lifestyle on a patient's nutritional status, such as recent weight loss and decreased oral intake. *Nutrition risk screening* refers to use of a rapid and simple set of usually two or three questions that have been validated to predict if a patient is malnourished or at risk for malnutrition, which help determine if a detailed nutritional assessment is indicated (Steel & Wile, 2018). Nutrition screening tools most frequently used in Canadian care settings are shown in Box 31.3.

Part of nutritional screening is application of physical examination findings (including height and weight). A nurse conducts a complete or focused physical examination at the time of a patient's admission to a health care facility. The extent of an examination is determined by patient condition. During an examination, the nurse needs to recognize the physical signs that indicate a nutritional alteration (Table 31.1) and review laboratory results that further support a patient's nutritional status. The most commonly studied blood biomarker for malnutrition is albumin, followed by hemoglobin, total cholesterol, total lymphocyte counts, prealbumin, C-reactive protein, total protein, transferrin, creatinine, triglycerides, white blood cells, blood urea nitrogen, % hematocrit, iron, and estimated glomerular filtration rate (Zhang, Pereira, Luo, et al., 2017). Vitamin B_{12} and folate levels confirm a nutritional anemia diagnosis (Castellanos-Sinco, Ramos-Peñafiel, Santoyo-Sanchez, et al., 2015).

TABLE 31.1

Physical Signs of Nutritional Status Alteration

Body Area	Indicators of Malnutrition
General appearance	Listless, apathetic, cachectic
Posture	Sagging shoulders, sunken chest, humped back
Hair	Stringy, dull, brittle, dry, thin and sparse, depigmented, easily plucked
Face and neck	Greasy, discoloured, scaly, swollen, dark skin over cheeks and under eyes, lumpiness or flakiness of skin around nose and mouth
Skin	Rough, dry, scaly, pale, pigmented, irritated; bruises and petechiae
Lips	Dry, scaly, swollen, redness and swelling (cheilosis), angular lesions at corner of mouth or fissures or scars
Mouth, oral mucous membranes	Swollen, deep red or magenta mucous membranes, oral lesions
Gums	Spongy, bleed easily, marginal redness, inflamed, receding
Tongue	Swollen, scarlet and raw, magenta colour, beefy (glossitis), hyperemic and hypertrophic or atrophic papillae
Teeth	Missing, broken teeth
Eyes	Conjunctiva pale, redness of conjunctiva, dryness or infection, redness and fissuring of eyelid corners (angular palpebritis), Bitot's spots (dry-appearing patches on the conjunctiva)
Neck (glands)	Thyroid or lymph nodes enlarged
Nails	Spoon-shaped (koilonychias), brittle, ridged
Legs and feet	Edema, tender calf, tingling, weakness, lesions
Muscles	Flaccid, poor tone, undeveloped, tender, impaired ability to walk
Nerve conduction and mental status	Inattentive, irritable, confused, burning and tingling of hands and feet, loss of position and vibratory sense

BOX 31.3

Nutritional Screening Tools

- The Malnutrition Screening Tool (MST) (available at https://static.abbottnutrition.com/cms-prod/abbottnutrition-2016.com/img/Malnutrition%20Screening%20Tool_FINAL_tcm1226-57900.pdf) is a three-question tool used to assess recent weight and appetite loss, validated for use with general medical, surgical, and oncology patients. Designed for use by non–nutrition-trained staff, the MST uses a scoring system to identify patients at high nutrition risk, which can then provide a basis for dietetic referrals and intervention.

- The Mini Nutritional Assessment (MNA) (available at https://www.nestle.com/asset-library/documents/library/events/2010-malnutrition-in-older-people/mna_mini_english.pdf) was developed for patients at least 65 years of age. With its short six-question format, the MNA is easy to implement and has been validated in hospitals, long-term care facilities, and community care settings.

- The Canadian Nutrition Screening Tool (CNST) (available at http://nutritioncareincanada.ca/sites/default/uploads/files/CNST.pdf) consists of two questions developed by the Canadian Task Force on Malnutrition and tested for reliability in Canadian hospitals. Following a positive screening using the CNST, the Subjective Global Assessment (SGA) (available at http://subjectiveglobalassessment.com/) is used to assess nutritional status and help prioritize cases.

- The SGA requires completion of a questionnaire, which includes data on weight change, dietary intake change, gastrointestinal symptoms, changes in functional capacity in relation to malnutrition, and assessment of fat and muscle stores and the presence of edema and ascites. This tool allows for malnutrition diagnosis and classifies patients as follows: A—well nourished; B—mildly/moderately malnourished; or C—severely malnourished.

Adapted from Steel, C., & Wile, H. (2018). Nutrition screening practices across care settings: Results of a Canadian survey. *Canadian Journal of Clinical Nutrition,* 6(1), 7–19. doi:10.14206/canad.j.clin.nutr.2018.01.02

Modified from Nix, S. (2013). *Williams' basic nutrition and diet therapy* (14th ed.). St. Louis: Mosby.

The nurse also collects a patient history at the time of admission. Dietary information from the history provides helpful information that will enable the nurse to identify the adequacy of a patient's current diet, appetite changes, type of assistance needed to eat, and food preferences. Findings from a nutritional screening determine if there is a need for interprofessional collaboration (e.g., dietitian) to complete a more in-depth assessment of a patient's nutritional status. In addition, assessment findings can lead to a health care provider referral for a speech-language pathologist (SLP) if the patient has swallowing difficulties (Herbert et al., 2016).

Dietitians are considered to be the best-qualified provider to assess, design, and implement patients' nutritional treatment plans in collaboration with the health care team (Calloway, 2018). Dietitians use a problem-solving method, the nutrition care process, to think critically and make decisions regarding nutrition therapy (Hammond, Myers, & Trostler, 2014). The nutrition care process has four interrelated steps that are similar to those in the nursing process: nutrition assessment, nutrition diagnosis, nutrition intervention, and nutrition monitoring and evaluation (Hammond et al., 2014). The dietitian first comprehensively assesses a patient's nutritional status, including medical, social, nutritional, and medication history; physical examination; anthropometric measurements; and laboratory data. The goal of the assessment is to develop a nutritional plan of care that effectively addresses a patient's nutritional problems. The dietitian then makes a nutritional diagnosis describing alterations in a patient's nutritional status that the dietitian can treat independently or as part of the health care team (Swan, Vivanti, Hakel-Smith, et al., 2017). The nutritional intervention is a purposely planned activity intended to resolve nutrition diagnoses. Nutrition monitoring and evaluation are used to identify patient progress, including patient understanding of and adherence to treatment.

Delegation and Collaboration

The skill of performing and interpreting a nutritional screening and physical examination cannot be delegated to an unregulated care provider (UCP). However, measurement of a patient's height and weight can be delegated. The nurse directs the UCP to:
- Measure the patient's weight after voiding, at the same time of day and when wearing the same clothing.
- Use the internal bed scale according to employer policy (if applicable).
- Report inability to measure height if the patient is nonambulatory.
- Ensure that measurements take place in a private location to protect the patient's dignity.

Equipment
- Scale (beam, electronic, bed with scale, wheelchair or chair)
- Nutritional screening form (data sheet and pen or computerized assessment form)
- Tongue blade, clean gloves, pen light for physical examination

STEP	RATIONALE

ASSESSMENT

1. Identify patient using at least two person-specific identifiers (e.g., name and date of birth or name and medical record number) according to employer policy.

   Ensures correct patient. Complies with Accreditation Canada's standards and improves patient safety (Accreditation Canada, 2019).

2. Ask patient to report usual body weight (UBW), noting recent changes in weight. Ask if weight loss was intentional or unintentional.

   In adults, weight is usually stable. A weight loss of more than 5% within 1 month is an indicator for further assessment, especially in an adult older than 65 years (Table 31.2).

3. Perform hand hygiene. Measure actual body weight (ABW).

   Weight underreporting characterizes women who are overweight or practice restrained eating (Polivy, Herman, Trottier, et al., 2014).

   a. Have patient void. Be sure patient is wearing underwear or hospital gown. Weigh patient either barefoot or with same shoes. Weigh at same time of day.

   Improves accuracy of ABW for comparison over time.

   b. Make sure that any scale used has been calibrated. If ambulatory, help patient stand still on scale with weight evenly distributed on both feet.

   Accurate measurement requires regularly calibrated and maintained scales. Standing still with equal weight distribution helps in obtaining accurate weight (Grodner, Escott-Stump, & Dorner, 2015).

   c. If patient is unable to stand, use wheelchair or bed scale.

   Decreases risk of falling.

   d. Record weight to nearest 0.1 kg (0.25 lb).

   Provides precise measurement of weight.

4. Measure actual height.

   On average, when asked, people report being slightly taller than they are (Weir, 2017).

   a. Assist patient to standing position; if taking height with beam scale, have patient stand erect with weight equally distributed on both feet.

   Ensures accurate height (Grodner et al., 2015).

   b. Instruct patient to let arms hang free at sides with palms facing thighs.

   Prevents movement of shoulders, which will result in inaccurate measurement.

   c. Have patient look straight ahead, take a deep breath, and hold position while you bring horizontal bar firmly on top of head. Measure to nearest 0.1 cm (0.04 inch). Make sure your eyes are level with bar to read measurement.

   Steady position ensures accurate measurement. Provides precise measurement of height.

STEP	RATIONALE

ASSESSMENT

5. Calculate ideal body weight (IBW).

    a. Calculate via standard height and weight chart. IBW range for normal is 10% above and 10% below IBW.

    b. Use the following formulas:

      Male: 48.1 kg (106 lb) for first 152 cm (5 feet); add 2.7 kg (6 lb) per additional 2.5 cm (1 in).

      Female: 45.4 kg (100 lbs) for first 152 cm (5 feet); add 2.25 kg (5 lbs) per additional 2.5 cm (inch).

Use IBW to compare with patient's actual weight to determine if patient is at risk for nutritional alteration.

6. Calculate BMI (see illustration):

$$BMI = \frac{Actual\ Body\ Weight\ (kg)^2}{Height\ (m)^2}$$

$$BMI = \frac{Actual\ Body\ Weight\ (kg)^2}{Height\ (m)^2}$$

    a. Divide weight in kilograms by the square of height in meters (m²).

    b. Optional formula for BMI: weight (lbs)/ [height (in)]² × 703

Body mass index (BMI) is a measure of body fat based on adult height and weight that is widely used to assess health risk associated with under- and overweight. Use the following link for an automatic calculation:

https://www.diabetes.ca/diabetes-and-you/healthy-living-resources/weight-management/body-mass-index-bmi-calculator

Computes BMI kg/m² (Table 31.3).

TABLE 31.2

Weight Change as an Indicator of Nutritional Status

Weight Loss (% Body Weight)	Time Period	Nutritional Status
1–2	1 week	Moderate weight loss
Greater than 2	1 week	Severe weight loss
5	1 month	Moderate weight loss
Greater than 5	1 month	Severe weight loss

Adapted from Grodner, M., Escott-Stump, S., & Dorner, S. (2015). *Foundations and clinical applications of nutrition: A nursing approach* (6th ed.). St. Louis: Elsevier.

TABLE 31.3

Classification of Body Mass Index (BMI) in Adults

Degree of Adiposity	BMI
Underweight	Less than 18.5 kg/m²
Normal weight	18.5–24.9 kg/m²
Overweight	25–29.9 kg/m²
Obesity (class I)	30–34.9 kg/m²
Obesity (class II)	35–39.9 kg/m²
Extreme obesity (class III)	Greater than or equal to 40 kg/m²

From Health Canada. (2018). *Body mass index (BMI) nomogram.* Retrieved from https://www.canada.ca/en/health-canada/services/food-nutrition/healthy-eating/healthy-weights/canadian-guidelines-body-weight-classification-adults/body-mass-index-nomogram.html.

BMI Table (Metric)																			
	Underweight			Normal						Overweight					Obese				
BMI	16	17	18	19	20	21	22	23	24	25	26	27	28	29	30	31	32	33	34	35
Height (cm)	Body Weight (Kg)																		
145	34	36	38	40	42	44	46	48	50	53	55	57	59	61	63	65	67	69	71	74
150	36	38	41	43	45	47	50	52	54	56	59	61	63	65	68	70	72	74	77	79
155	38	41	43	46	48	50	53	56	58	60	62	65	67	70	72	74	77	79	82	84
160	41	44	46	49	51	54	56	59	61	64	67	69	72	74	77	79	82	84	87	90
165	44	46	49	52	54	57	60	63	65	68	71	74	76	79	82	84	87	90	93	95
170	46	49	52	55	58	61	64	66	69	72	75	78	81	84	87	90	92	95	98	101
175	49	52	55	58	61	64	67	70	74	77	80	83	86	89	92	95	98	101	104	107
180	52	55	58	62	65	68	71	75	78	81	84	87	91	94	97	100	104	107	110	113
185	55	58	62	65	68	72	75	79	82	86	89	92	96	99	103	106	110	113	116	120
190	58	61	65	69	72	76	79	83	87	90	94	97	101	105	108	112	116	119	123	126
195	61	65	68	72	76	80	84	87	91	95	99	103	106	110	114	118	122	125	129	133
200	64	68	72	76	80	84	88	92	96	100	104	108	112	116	120	124	128	132	136	140

STEP 6 Body mass index for BMI 35 and under. *(Retrieved from http://bmisite.net/bmi-chart.php.)*

STEP	RATIONALE

ASSESSMENT

7. Obtain dietary information as you complete nursing history (see Chapter 8):

   a. Assess patient's diet history, including current diet, food choices and preferences, appetite, food allergies (include on patient ID band), and food intolerances. **NOTE:** In outpatient settings have patient bring 7-day food diary report in electronic or paper format.

   Assesses factors affecting diet adequacy and appetite (Lentjes, McTaggart, Mulligan, et al., 2014). Web-based dietary records are more convenient for patients, produce statistically similar results, and have substantial logistic and cost advantages to clinicians (Benedik, Koroušić, Simčič, et al., 2014).

   b. Assess for any cultural and religious preferences and restrictions in diet. Ask patient if caregiver believes certain foods influence health changes to determine level of shared decision-making and areas for ongoing education.

   Knowing patient preferences demonstrates person-centred care and will improve ability to plan diet that patient will accept. As a resource, the Food and Agriculture Organization (FAO) of the United Nations provides advice on food, food groups, and dietary patterns for different cultures (FAO, 2019).

   c. Determine medications and other dietary or herbal supplements that patient is taking (over-the-counter and prescribed). Be aware of common drug–drug and drug–nutrient interactions (use interprofessional collaboration [e.g., pharmacist] as required).

   Certain medications inhibit or increase action of other medications. Some nutrients interact with medications. For example, vitamin K–rich foods (green leafy vegetables) interfere with action of warfarin (anticoagulant). Medications such as mineral oil laxatives impair nutrient use.

8. Perform physical assessment (see Chapter 8) (see Table 31.1), noting any physical changes reflecting nutritional deficiencies, patient's level of consciousness, responsiveness, and ability to swallow.

   The most obvious signs of malnutrition on physical examination are apparent in the skin, mouth, muscles, and central nervous system. Difficulty swallowing predisposes patient to aspiration when eating.

9. Review results of relevant laboratory tests (e.g., albumin, complete blood count [CBC]).

   Laboratory results can provide clues about nutritional status (refer to Box 31.1).

10. During first meal, determine patient's ability to set up food on plate, manipulate eating utensils, and self-feed.

   Difficulty in self-feeding creates a significant risk for malnutrition (Nyberg, Olsson, Pajalic, et al., 2015).

11. Complete a nutritional screening tool if required by employer (see Box 31.3).

   Valid tools include key elements for detecting patient's nutritional risk.

12. Explain to patient how you intend to apply nutritional assessment information in patient care.

   Allows time for patient to ask questions about assessment and improve understanding.

NURSING DIAGNOSES

- Reduced ability to swallow
- Inadequate nutrition
- Insufficient knowledge regarding
- nutritional needs/recommendations
- Obesity
- Overweight
- Potential for weight gain

Related factors/Risk factors are individualized on the basis of patient's condition or needs.

IMPLEMENTATION

1. Provide patient help with feeding based on assessment findings (see Skill 31.2).

   Level of assistance required depends on patient's motor skills, ability to attend, and ability to swallow and chew normally.

2. Institute aspiration precautions (see Skill 31.3) if needed.

   Precautions lessen chance of patient aspirating food or liquid into tracheobronchial tree.

EVALUATION

1. Review history and physical findings. Note abnormal findings or areas of concern.

   Permits prompt identification of risk for malnutrition and need for nutritional interventions.

2. Compare patient's BMI with recommended BMI for height/weight.

   Determines nutritional risk factors and health-related conditions.

3. Compare normal laboratory test levels with patient's levels.

   When considered with other nutritional parameters, abnormal values can indicate malnutrition (Grodner et al., 2015; Zhang et al., 2017).

4. Compute any score on nutritional screening tool.

   Valid tools use a scoring system to identify patients at high nutrition risk.

STEP	RATIONALE

EVALUATION

5. Use Teach-Back: "I want to be sure I explained why we need to do a nutritional screening for you. Tell me what the screening tells us. How will we use that information?" Develop a revised teaching plan if patient or caregiver is not able to teach back correctly.

Determines patient's and caregiver's level of understanding of instructional topic.

Unexpected Outcomes

1. Patient is overweight if BMI is 25–29 kg/m^2 in an adult. Patient is obese if BMI is greater than 29 kg/m^2.

2. Patient is underweight, taking in insufficient food.

3. Nutritional screening tool score reflects high nutrition risk.

Related Interventions

- Ensure patient is receiving correct caloric diet.
- Check that patient is being weighed on same scale, with same type of clothing and shoes, and at same time of day.
- Use interprofessional collaboration to conduct a nutritional assessment and calculate patient's caloric and protein intake and route of nutrition (enteral versus parenteral) (see Chapters 32 and 33).
- Consult with dietitian to determine needed calorie and protein intake and proper route of nutrition.
- Implement measures to improve patient's appetite: food appearance, room comfort, providing comfort measures before meal.
- Practice person-centred care and include patient and caregiver in meal plan development.
- Refer patient to dietitian.

Communication and Documentation

- Document assessment results and your evaluation of patient and caregiver learning on nurses' notes, flow sheet, and nutritional screening form in electronic health record (EHR) or chart.
- Notify health care provider of abnormal findings.
- Make referral to the dietitian as indicated.

Special Considerations
Teaching

- To increase the awareness of healthy nutrition, educate patient and caregiver about a case-specific nutritional diet.
- Provide patient and caregiver resources to promote healthy eating (e.g., *Eat Well Plate*, *My Food Guide* mobile app) (Health Canada 2019d) (Box 31.4). Technology nutrition applications and websites promote patient engagement with diet plan.

Cultural

- The eating community and the meal are the basic foundation of all societies. Food gives structure to daily life and ritualistically marks life-stage passages (e.g., eating cake at a wedding).
- Biological and geographic conditions, as well as cultural norms, determine changes in the food eaten within a certain community. Westerners' rejection of eating raw fish until recent years is one example of this: Westerners are more exposed to Japanese cuisine and thus eat more raw fish (Nordström, Coff, Jönsson, et al., 2013).
- Food creates bonds between people, and communities may exist whereby food differentiates "us" from "them." Inviting a friend for lunch is an example of the social role of food.
- Food also represents power. A person who does not have enough to eat is powerless, whereas a person who may control another person's food intake holds certain power over them.
- Food is an important part of gender relations. The traditional female role of feeding the family has been a factor in the exclusion

of women from public power; however, there is a dimension of power in the act of cooking and determining what other members of the family should eat. The person who controls food intake not only affects bodily functions and health but may also imprint values and virtues, especially on children.

- Culture and society shape a person's diet. "Unfortunately, as a society where cheap is good and fast is better, we've welcomed super-sized, low-cost fast food that has paved the way for a massive increase in the rate of obesity" (Group, 2016).
- There is a negative association between income and obesity. The cost of healthy food, such as fresh fruits and vegetables, has been found to be higher than that of less nutritious, energy-dense food (Kern, Auchincloss, Stehr, et al., 2018).
- Indigenous diets comprised of traditional foods were high in animal protein, nutrient-rich, and low in fat or high in marine sources of fat. Not only are traditional foods valued from cultural, spiritual, and health perspectives, but the activities involved in their acquisition and distribution allow for the practice of cultural values, such as sharing and cooperation. The energy spent in obtaining traditional foods is significant given the physical demands of hunting, fishing, trapping, growing, and gathering (Earle, 2011). *Traditional food* is the preferred term for First Nations and Métis peoples, and *country food* is the preferred term for Inuit people (Health Canada, 2019a).
- There is convincing evidence that the omega-3 fatty acids DHA and EHA found in fish and fish oils decrease the risk of cardio-vascular disease. Traditional diets, rich in sources of omega-3 fatty acids, beneficially affect the profile of fats consumed such that greater amounts of DHA and EHA are obtained, and a smaller percentage of the total fat in the diet is from saturated fats.
- Traditional Indigenous foods tend to be lower in carbohydrates, including simple sugars, which are significant in conditions such as obesity and diabetes mellitus. As well, good sources of vitamin

BOX 31.4

Building a Healthy Eating Style

Following Health Canada's (2019d) *Eat Well Plate* guidelines will result in a healthier eating style:

- When selecting food and beverages, focus on variety, amount, and nutrition. Include all food groups: fruits and vegetables, grain products, meat and alternatives, milk and alternatives, and oils and fats. Also include water intake.
- Eat the right amount for you based on your age, gender, height, weight, and physical activity level.
- A healthier eating style will help you avoid overweight and obesity and reduce your risk of diseases such as heart disease, diabetes mellitus, and cancer.
- Choose an eating style low in saturated fat, sodium, and added sugars.
- Read nutrition fact labels and ingredient lists carefully for the amounts of saturated fat, sodium, and added sugars when choosing your food and beverages.
- Eating foods with less sodium can reduce your risk of high blood pressure.
- Start with making a few small changes to create a healthier eating style. Think of each change as a personal "win" on your path to living healthier.
- Make half your plate fruits and vegetables.
- Focus on whole fruits, which are more nutritious than drinking juice.
- Vary your vegetables. Dark green and orange vegetables are packed with nutrients.
- Eat a variety of whole grains.
- Choose skim, 1%, or 2% milk or unsweetened fortified soy beverage.
- Choose meat alternatives such as split peas, chickpeas, kidney beans, black beans, lentils, or tofu. Eat heart-healthy fish such as char, herring, mackerel, salmon, sardines, and trout because these fish are high in omega-3 fats.
- Make calorie-free water your drink of choice.
- Create settings where healthy choices are available and affordable to you and others in your community.
- Professionals, policymakers, partners, industry, families, and individuals can help others make healthy eating a part of their lives.

See more at http://www.healthycanadians.gc.ca/eating-nutrition/healthy-eating-saine-alimentation/tips-conseils/interactive-tools-outils-interactifs/eat-well-bien-manger-eng.php.

C have been documented in the largely animal-based diets of Inuit peoples. Traditional wild plants contribute essential micronutrients to diets worldwide. For example, rose hips, consumed by many First Nations people in a variety of medicinal and food preparations, are high in vitamin C and demonstrate antibacterial and antioxidant properties.

- Given the benefits associated with traditional diets, a return to traditional dietary practices seems advisable. However, there are challenges in doing this. Many Indigenous communities face unique food security challenges related to consumption of traditional food. One-third of Indigenous households located off-reserve are food insecure owing to low income (Dietitians of Canada, 2016). Moreover, the willingness to consume country foods is affected by concerns over contaminants (e.g., cadmium, mercury, PCBs, and pesticides).
- Current dietary surveys among Indigenous groups, including First Nations peoples, reveal that often diets do not meet dietary recommendations for saturated fat, fibre, sodium, fruits, and vegetables. Poor dietary patterns also occur among Indigenous children, who consume snack foods frequently and consume less than the recommended servings of milk, fruits, and vegetables. Risk of specific dietary deficiencies have been identified in some Indigenous populations, including low intakes of zinc, calcium, and vitamin D among Cree schoolchildren, and low intakes of magnesium, folate, and vitamins A, C, and E among the women of 47 Yukon First Nation, Dene, Métis, and Inuit communities in the Canadian Arctic (Earle, 2011). Despite challenges such as food insecurity and biocontamination, traditional foods remain important for chronic-disease prevention; their use can be successfully promoted in Indigenous communities.
- In 2010, a national food guide was created to reflect the values, traditions, and food choices of First Nations, Inuit, and Métis peoples. This food guide includes both traditional (country) foods and store-bought foods that are generally available, affordable, and accessible across Canada and provides unique images and content.

Pregnant Female

Health Canada's (2019e) key recommendations for pregnant women include the following:

- Following *Canada's Dietary Guidelines* to eat the amount and type of food appropriate for a pregnant female
- Having at least two Food Guide servings of 150 g of cooked fish each week, as fish contains omega-3 fats and other important nutrients for pregnancy
- Limiting the amount of fresh or frozen tuna, shark, swordfish, escolar, marlin, and deep-sea perch because of mercury levels—to consume no more than 150 g per month
- Taking a multivitamin containing 0.4 mg of folic acid and 16–20 mg of iron every day
- Following food safety advice (see Box 31.2)
- Eating at least one dark-green and one orange vegetable each day
- Choosing vegetables and fruit prepared with little or no added fat, sugar, or salt
- Having vegetables and fruit more often than juice
- Making at least half of the daily grain products whole grain and choosing grain products that are lower in fat, sugar, or salt
- Drinking skim, 1%, or 2% milk each day
- Selecting lower fat alternatives
- Having meat alternatives such as beans, lentils, and tofu often
- Selecting lean meat and alternatives prepared with little or no added fat or salt
- Satisfying thirst with water as the beverage of choice
- Limiting foods and beverages high in calories, fat, sugar, or salt
- Being active regularly as part of a healthy pregnancy

Gerontological

- Nutrition, a major determinant of successful aging, promotes health and functionality. Food is critical to physical and physiological well-being and contributes to social, cultural, and psychological quality of life (Health Canada, 2017; Wren, 2015).

Pediatric

- Anthropometric data include measurement of length, weight, and head circumference in children. These measurements should be compared with standard growth charts to determine percentiles. The most commonly used growth charts in Canada are from the World Health Organization (WHO) and Centers for Disease Control and Prevention (CDC) (Lawrence, Cummings, Chanoine,

et al., 2015). These charts include BMI for age and weight for stature percentiles. WHO growth charts (www.whogrowthcharts.ca) have fewer percentile lines between the 3rd and 97th percentile; CDC charts (https://www.cdc.gov/growthcharts/cdc_charts.htm) include a wider range of percentile lines, enabling more precise description.

Care in the Community

- Instruct patient and caregiver about strategies for safe handling, preparation, and storage of food.
- Use interprofessional collaboration (e.g., occupational therapist) to assess the home environment to determine if the patient or caregiver can prepare a meal safely (see Chapter 42).

✦ SKILL 31.2   Assisting an Adult Patient With Oral Nutrition

Some patients are unable to feed themselves adequately because of the severity of their illness, which may cause musculoskeletal weakness, fatigue, or pain. For example, a patient who loses fine-motor skills will have difficulty getting food from the plate into the mouth. Helping adults with feeding requires time, patience, knowledge of a patient's limitations and nutritional needs, and understanding of a patient's preferences for foods and how to eat a meal. The nurse can improve a patient's nutritional intake by helping with feedings directly or teaching caregivers how to do so safely. To maintain a patient's dignity during feeding, encourage them to make decisions about food choices, times for eating, and correct use of assistive devices (when needed).

Hospitalized patients receive various therapeutic oral diets that require a health care provider's prescription. A therapeutic diet treats many illness and disease states (Table 31.4). Refer to employer dietary manual or consult a dietitian for specific information about therapeutic diets. There are two ways to modify a regular diet: quantitatively or qualitatively (Grodner et al., 2015). *Quantitative modifications* include number or size of meals served or amounts of specific nutrients, such as six small feedings or kcalorie diets. *Qualitative modifications* involve consistency, texture, or nutrients such as clear- or full-liquid diets. The nurse can supplement any diet with oral nutrition supplements. A prescription for a calorie count requires the nurse to record the percentage of each food a patient eats next to the food choice directly on the meal menu. The dietitian calculates caloric intake and determines the need for nutrition supplements or dietary change. For example, liquid supplements with or between meals significantly increase protein

---

TABLE 31.4

Progressive and Therapeutic Diets

Diet	Description
Clear-liquid	Foods that are clear and liquid at room or body temperature (e.g., water, apple or cranberry juice, gelatin, popsicles), leave little residue, and are easily absorbed; commonly prescribed for short-term use (24 to 48 hours) after surgery, before diagnostic tests, and after episodes of diarrhea and vomiting
Full-liquid	Includes foods on clear-liquid diet plus addition of smooth-textured dairy products (e.g., milk and ice cream), strained soups and custard, refined cooked cereals, vegetable juice, and pureed vegetables; commonly prescribed before or after surgery for patients who are acutely ill from infection or cannot chew or tolerate solid foods. Verify that patients can tolerate lactose before providing dairy products.
Pureed	Includes foods on full-liquid diet plus easily swallowed foods that do not require chewing (e.g., scrambled eggs, pureed meats, vegetables, fruits, mashed potatoes). Prescribed for patients with head and neck abnormalities or who have had oral surgery. Can be modified for low sodium or fat
Mechanical or dental-soft	Comprises all previous diets plus addition of ground or finely diced meats, flaked fish, cottage cheese, cheese, rice, potatoes, pancakes, light breads, cooked vegetables, cooked or canned fruit, bananas, and peanut butter; avoid tough meats, nuts, bacon, and fruits with tough skins or membranes; prescribed for patients who have chewing problems or mild GI problems; used as a transition diet from liquids to regular
Soft/low-residue/ low fibre	Addition of low-fibre, easily digested foods such as pastas, moist tender meats, and canned cooked fruits and vegetables; includes easy-to-chew and simply cooked foods; does not permit fatty, rich, and fried foods
High-fibre	Addition of fresh uncooked fruits, steamed vegetables, bran, oatmeal, and dried fruits; includes indigestible carbohydrates to relieve constipation, increase GI motility, and increase stool weight
Regular or diet as tolerated	No restrictions; permits patient preferences

Sample Therapeutic Diets

Diet	Description
Restricted fluids	Required in severe heart or kidney failure
Sodium-restricted	Low levels of sodium: may include a 4-g (no added salt), 2-g (moderate), 1-g (strict), or 500-mg (very strict) diet; often prescribed for patients with heart failure, renal failure, cirrhosis, or hypertension
Fat-modified	Cholesterol intake limited to less than 300 mg daily, and fat intake 30 to 35%; reduces fatty foods for hypercholesterolemia, malabsorption disorders, and diarrhea
Diabetic	Provides patients with an essential diet treatment for diabetes mellitus; recommended by Diabetes Canada; allows patients to select set amount of food from basic food groups

GI, Gastrointestinal.
Adapted from Grodner, M., Escott-Stump, S., & Dorner, S. (2015). *Foundations and clinical applications of nutrition: A nursing approach* (6th ed.). St. Louis: Mosby.

and calorie intake but do not replace scheduled meals (Gaddey & Holder, 2014).

Altered dentition, improperly fitted dentures, oral lesions or infections, or diseases causing impaired digestion may limit the types and consistencies of foods tolerated. Hemiplegia, a fractured arm, quadriplegia, debilitating illness, or generalized weakness limits self-feeding ability. The presence of intravenous (IV) catheters or tubing, dressings, and bandages also limits mobility needed for self-feeding. Use interprofessional collaboration (e.g., occupational therapist) to assess a patient's ability to self-feed and recommend adaptive equipment and supplies for self-feeding. Practise person-centred care when feeding an adult—use compassion, understanding, and common sense to provide a socially meaningful mealtime experience.

Delegation and Collaboration

The skill of assisting a patient with oral nutrition can be delegated to an unregulated care provider (UCP). However, the nurse is responsible for determining if a patient can receive oral nutrition, including swallowing ability and dietary restrictions. The nurse educates the UCP by:

- Explaining any specific swallowing strategies or techniques unique to the patient.
- Reviewing when to stop feeding and report immediately to the nurse incidences of coughing, gagging, pocketing of food in the mouth, or difficulty swallowing.
- Cautioning not to rush the patient during eating.

Equipment

- Stethoscope
- Washcloths and towels
- Tongue blade
- Adaptive utensils as needed for self-feeding
- Straw
- Oral hygiene supplies; *option:* solution for stomatitis care
- Clean gloves

STEP	RATIONALE

ASSESSMENT

1. Identify patient using at least two person-specific identifiers (e.g., name and date of birth or name and medical record number) according to employer policy.

Ensures correct patient. Complies with Accreditation Canada's standards and improves patient safety (Accreditation Canada, 2019).

2. Review prescribed diet for type of diet and supplements.

Helps to ensure that patient will receive proper diet.

3. Assess presence and condition of teeth. (Apply clean gloves if there is risk of exposure to saliva.) Determine if dentures are poorly fitted. Assess severity of mouth discomfort using an appropriate pain rating scale.

Absence of teeth and ill-fitting dentures inhibit normal chewing and influence preparation of food for safe swallowing (Laguna Cruañes & Chen, 2016) (see Skill 31.3). Pain can reduce appetite and ability to chew or swallow. These factors increase risk for dysphagia.

4. Have patient speak and swallow. Watch for laryngeal movement. Ask patient to say "Ah" while using tongue blade and penlight. Check for midline uvula and symmetrical rise of uvula and soft palate. Use tongue blade to elicit gag reflex (see Chapter 8).

Patients with chronic neurological disease may experience cranial nerve damage (Koch, Ferrazzi, Busatto, et al., 2017), specifically impaired swallowing (cranial nerve IX) or loss of gag reflex, hoarseness, and nasal voice (cranial nerve X).

5. Determine to what extent patient can self-feed. Assess physical motor skills (e.g., ability to grasp utensils, hold cup, and move utensil to mouth). Assess level of consciousness or ability to attend to feeding, visual acuity, and peripheral vision.

Patients with any level of independence should be encouraged to feed themselves. Understanding the patient's physical and cognitive limitations alerts you to the type of help the patient needs. Visual impairments make it difficult to see food and utensils (Nyberg et al., 2015).

6. Assess patient's appetite, recent food and fluid intake, cultural and religious preferences for participating in mealtime, and food likes and dislikes.

Determines type of foods and size of meals that can potentially improve oral intake.

7. Assess for presence of generalized fatigue, pain, or shortness of breath.

Symptoms affect appetite and ability to participate in feeding. Patients eat better when rested.

8. Assess nausea and recent bowel pattern. Is patient passing flatus? Auscultate for bowel sounds.

Determines baseline assessment of gastrointestinal function.

9. Assess need for elimination, hand hygiene, and oral care (including dentures) before feeding.

Reduces interruptions and improves patient's appetite.

10. Review nursing history (see Skill 31.1) for patient's most recent weight and laboratory values.

Provides ongoing monitoring of patient's nutritional status.

NURSING DIAGNOSIS

- Inadequate swallowing
- Acute pain
- Reduced feeding ability
- Reduced stamina
- Potential for insufficient fluid volume
- Potential for aspiration
- Potential for weight loss

Related factors/Risk factors are individualized on the basis of patient's condition or needs.

STEP	**RATIONALE**

PLANNING

1. Expected outcomes following completion of procedure:

- Patient's weight is maintained or trends toward desired level.

  Nutritional intake meets daily needs.

- Patient's nutrition-related laboratory values trend toward normal.

  Biochemical markers along with nutritional assessment may indicate nutritional status.

- Patient demonstrates increased ability to self-feed or open items on tray as appropriate.

  Indicates increased strength, improved mental status, and increased well-being.

- Patient coughs with no indication of respiratory compromise.

  Ineffective cough and respiratory compromise may indicate dysphagia and aspiration.

- Normal vital signs and skin colour while eating.

  Indicates tolerance to complete meal.

- Patient is able to describe foods allowed within prescribed diet.

  Demonstrates learning.

2. After assessment, allow patient to rest 30 minutes before mealtime.

Short rest improves patient's energy level and ability to participate in feeding.

3. Administer prescribed analgesic 30 minutes before meal if patient has discomfort.

Analgesic reaches peak level during meal, improving patient's ability to self-feed.

4. Explain to patient how you could set up and help with meal. Allow time for questions.

Minimizes anxiety and engages patient in mealtime.

IMPLEMENTATION

1. Prepare patient's room for mealtime.

  a. Perform hand hygiene. Clear over-bed table and arrange any needed supplies.

Reduces transmission of microorganisms and prepares room for food tray.

  b. Help patient to comfortable sitting position in chair or place bed in high-Fowler's position. If patient is unable to sit, turn patient on side with head of bed (HOB) elevated and chin tucked in position (see illustration).

Upright position facilitates swallowing, reducing aspiration risk.

Conditions such as pressure injury, traction, or spinal surgery prevent positioning with head elevated.

Chin-tuck position has been known to reduce risk of aspiration by narrowing the airway entrance (Leigh, Oh, Seo, et al., 2015) (see Skill 31.3).

2. Prepare patient for meal.

  a. Help patient with elimination needs and to perform hand hygiene.

Increases patient's comfort, enjoyment of meal, and nutritional intake.

  b. Apply clean gloves and offer oral hygiene. If patient has dentures, remove and rinse thoroughly and reinsert. Remove gloves and perform hand hygiene.

Moist, clean oral mucosa and teeth improve taste and appetite.

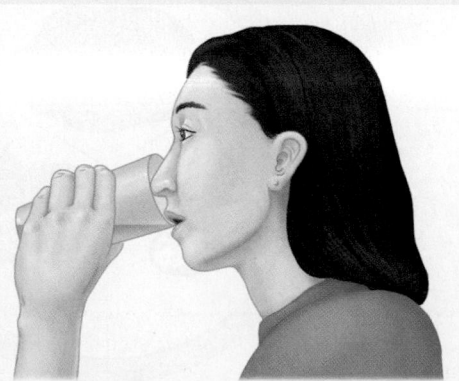 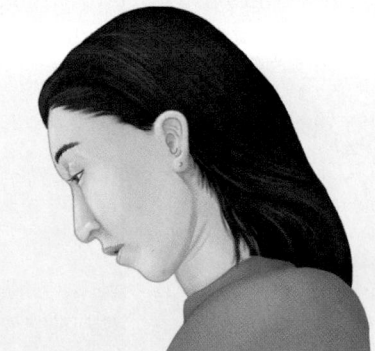

A   B

STEP 1b Chin-tuck position.

STEP	RATIONALE

IMPLEMENTATION

c. Patients with oral mucositis (inflammation of mucous membranes) benefit from rinsing with solutions such as saline, saline-sodium bicarbonate mouthwash, sodium bicarbonate solution, or topical anesthetics or using mucosal coating agents (Maria, Eliopoulos, & Muanza, 2017). Use interprofessional collaboration to determine best therapy.

Pain of stomatitis causes patients to avoid eating.

d. Help patient put on eyeglasses or insert contact lenses, if used (see Chapter 19).

Enhances patient's ability to self-feed and makes meal more visually appealing.

3. Check environment for distractions. Reduce noise level if possible. *Option:* If patient enjoys music, play a selection of their choice or soothing, low-volume music.

Pleasant environment enhances mealtime experience. Music intervention may reduce agitation in persons with dementia (Pedersen, Anderson, Lugo, et al., 2017).

4. Obtain special assistive devices as needed and instruct on use. For example:

Devices improve ability to grasp, pick up foods with utensils, and drink liquids.

- Two-handled cup with spout in lid makes it easier to handle cup and drink. Avoids spills. Cup's wide base prevents it from tipping over.
- Plate with plate guard (see illustration) and nonskid bottom helps person with limited flexibility of hands or poor motor coordination or who uses only one hand.
- Knife, fork, and spoon with large handles or attached splints help with limited hand function or a weak grip.

5. Assess meal tray for completeness and correct diet. Instruct patient about diet, rationale for diet, food options, and dysphagia risks.

Prevents intake of incomplete or incorrect diet. Instruction is more meaningful when applied during real-time activity.

6. Help set up meal tray if patient is unable to do so: open packages, cut up food, apply seasonings or condiments, place napkin.

Allows patient more independence and control. Small pieces are easier to chew and minimize risk for aspiration.

7. Watch patient successfully swallow first bites of food and drink. If patient is able to eat independently, stop here. Return after 15 or 20 minutes or stay nearby for communication and additional teaching.

Makes patient as self-sufficient as possible.

Clinical Decision Point *If patient is at risk for aspiration, stay at their side during feeding.*

8. Help patient who cannot eat independently.
a. Assume comfortable position.

Prevents you from rushing patient through meal.

b. If patient is visually impaired, identify food location on plate as if it were a clock (e.g., vegetables at 3 o'clock, meat at 12 o'clock) (see illustration).

Helps patient locate food items and to feed self if given adequate information about food placement on tray.

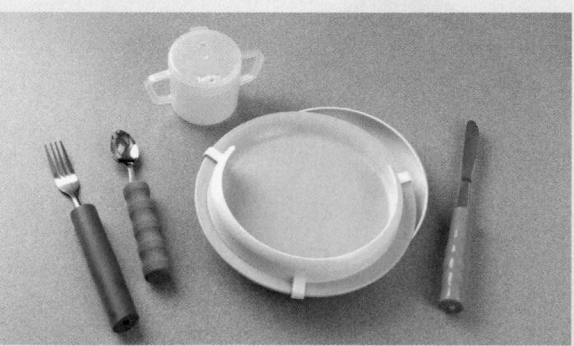

STEP 4 Mealtime adaptive equipment. *Clockwise from upper left:* Two-handled cup with lid, plate with plate guard, utensils with splints, and utensils with enlarged handles.

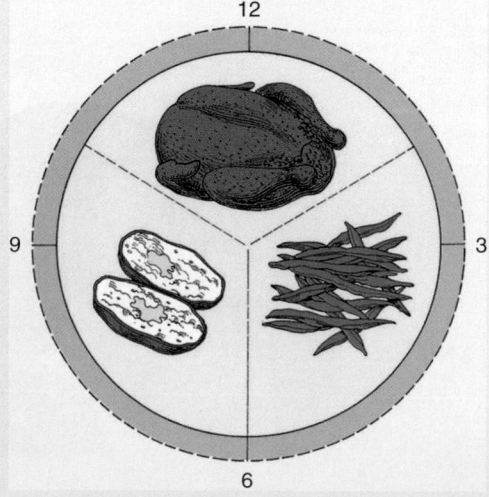

STEP 8b Clock setup to prepare food on a plate for the visually impaired patient.

STEP	RATIONALE

IMPLEMENTATION

c. Ask in which order patient would like to eat and cut food into bite-size pieces.

Gives patient more independence and control. Small bites reduce risk of aspiration (see Skill 31.3).

d. Provide fluids as requested. Discourage patient from drinking all fluids at beginning of meal.

Promotes swallowing. Prevents patient from filling up on fluids.

e. Pace feeding to avoid patient fatigue. Interact with patient, verbally encouraging self-feeding attempts.

Social interaction may improve appetite.

f. Use meal as opportunity to communicate with and educate patient about nutrition topics and discharge plan.

Offers extended time for teaching.

g. Have patient use chin-tuck position and place food in stronger side of the mouth.

Facilitates chewing and swallowing. Chin-tuck position may help to reduce aspiration risk (see Skill 31.3).

9. Use appropriate feeding techniques for patients with special needs:

Decreased saliva production impairs swallowing. Aspiration results from decreased or absent gag reflex.

a. *Older person:* Feed small amounts at a time, observing biting, chewing, ability to manipulate tongue to form bolus of food, swallowing, and fatigue. Ensure patient has swallowed food. Offer variety of foods and frequent rest periods.

Clinical Decision Point *If you suspect that patient is aspirating, stop feeding immediately and suction the airway (see Skill 31.3).*

b. *Patients living with neurological impairments:* Feed small amounts at a time, observing ability to chew, manipulate tongue to form bolus, and swallow. Have patient open mouth and check for food left inside cheeks (pocketing). Give small amount of thin liquid between bites.

Some patients with limited tongue strength and control are unable to move food to back of mouth for swallowing. Checking for "pocketed" food prevents aspiration (Remig & Weeden, 2016).

c. *Patients living with cancer:* Check for food aversions before and during meal. Monitor for fatigue.

Strong, abnormal sense of taste and smell and fatigue are adverse effects of chemotherapy.

10. Help patient with hand hygiene and mouth care after meal is completed. (Apply gloves as needed.)

Maintains comfort.

11. Help patient to resting position, leave head elevated at least 45 degrees for 30–60 minutes after meal.

Reduces risk of aspiration from regurgitation.

12. Remove and discard gloves and perform hand hygiene.

Reduces transmission of microorganisms.

EVALUATION

1. Monitor body weight at least weekly.

Determines ongoing nutritional status.

2. Monitor laboratory values as indicated.

Biochemical markers may help to identify changes in nutritional status.

3. Monitor intake and output (I&O) (see Chapter 8). Complete intake measurement (e.g., observed intake, calorie count).

4. Observe patient's ability to self-feed, including ability to feed self certain items and part or all of meal.

Informs what help patient needs with feeding.

5. Observe patient for choking, coughing, gagging, or food left in mouth during eating.

Indicates dysphagia and possible aspiration.

6. **Use Teach-Back:** "We discussed ways you can help feed your spouse that make it easier for him to swallow. Tell me two ways to help feed him and why it is important." Develop revised teaching plan if caregiver is not able to teach back correctly.

Determines caregiver's understanding of instructional topic.

STEP	**RATIONALE**
Unexpected Outcomes	**Related Interventions**
1. Patient is unable to eat entire meal or refuses to eat.	• Determine if patient has other food preferences and cultural or religious restrictions.
	• Assess factors to determine what is affecting patient's ability to eat.
	• Determine if patient's ability or desire to eat is better at other times of the day.
	• Determine if patient is in pain, nauseated, or constipated. Implement appropriate interventions (e.g., administering analgesic, antiemetic, or cathartic; providing food or liquid at a temperature patient prefers; offering small, frequent meals).
	• Provide more frequent oral care.
	• If inability to eat meal continues, use interprofessional collaboration to develop strategies to assist patient in meeting nutritional requirements.
2. Patient chokes on food.	• Stop feeding immediately; place on side with head forward and pointing down; suction mouth and airway.
	• Contact health care provider if choking occurs repeatedly.
	• Use interprofessional collaboration as required (e.g., SLP, dietitian) (see Skill 31.3).

Communication and Documentation

- Document in nurses' notes in electronic health record (EHR) or chart the patient's type of diet, amount of feeding assistance needed, tolerance of diet, and percentage of meal eaten (e.g., 25% of food consumed at breakfast).
- If evaluating I&O, document fluid intake on appropriate form (see Chapter 8).
- If patient is receiving oral nutritional supplements to fill or replace meals (e.g., Ensure, Boost), document the amount taken and patient's tolerance.
- Document any swallowing difficulties, food dislikes, or refusal to eat and report to health care provider and dietitian.
- Document your evaluation of caregiver learning.

Special Considerations
Teaching

- See Special Considerations, Teaching, Skill 31.1.

Pediatric

- Human breast milk is the most desirable complete diet for infants during the first 6 months. Infants who are breastfed or bottle-fed do not require additional fluids, especially water or juice, during the first 4 months of life. Excessive intake of water causes water intoxication, failure to thrive, and hyponatremia.

- Babies who are breastfed should receive daily vitamin D supplement of 10 micrograms (mcg) or 400 international units (IU) (Health Canada, 2014b).
- Typically, infants do not consume solid foods until 6 months of age. They should start with foods that contain iron and offer them a few times each day to support their growth and development (Health Canada, 2014b). Iron-fortified infant cereal is usually the first solid food to offer. Iron-rich foods include meats such as beef, lamb, game, poultry, and fish. Meat alternatives include eggs, tofu, and legumes such as beans and lentils.
- Solid foods should not be mixed in a bottle; they should be fed with a soft spoon (Hockenberry & Wilson, 2015).

Gerontological

- Some older persons have diminished appetite because of a decline in taste, smell, and number of taste buds (Ogawa, Annear, Ikebe, et al., 2017).
- Interactions between nutrients and medications affect taste of foods or metabolism, absorption, digestion, or excretion of drugs.

Care in the Community

- Assess financial resources of patient and caregiver to determine their ability to purchase nutritionally complete foods for patient.
- Help patient and caregiver identify ways to make meals in the home pleasant and enjoyable experiences.

◆ SKILL 31.3   Aspiration Precautions

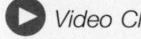 *Video Clip*

Aspiration is the entry of oropharyngeal secretions or gastric contents into the larynx and lower respiratory tract (Metheny, 2016). It often occurs from secretions in the oral pharynx or reflux of gastric content entering the throat and going down the trachea. Patients at risk for aspiration include those with *dysphagia* (difficulty swallowing). The ability to swallow effectively and safely is necessary for safe transport of food and fluid through the mouth, pharynx,

and esophagus to the stomach. It requires coordination of cranial nerves and the muscles of the tongue, pharynx, larynx, and jaw. Alteration or delay in the swallowing process causes dysphagia.

Some conditions that increase the risk for dysphagia include severity of illness (e.g., sepsis, acute stroke, head and neck cancer, head trauma, dementia, and Parkinson's disease), dehydration, and medical interventions (e.g., sedation, mechanical ventilation,

nasotracheal suctioning, and lying flat) compromising the gag reflex (Manabe, Teramoto, Tamiya, et al., 2015). Structural obstructions and medication adverse effects can also cause difficulty swallowing (Krishnan & Pandolfino, 2018) (Box 31.5). Factors found to best predict risk of aspiration are impaired or decreased gag reflex, dysphagia, and impaired physical mobility (Oliveira, Costa, Morais, et al., 2015). Symptoms of dysphagia vary, depending on the swallowing alteration. The nurse should suspect dysphagia if a patient has difficult or painful chewing or swallowing, frequent drooling, loss of food from the mouth during eating, pocketing food in the cheek, and spitting pieces of food out. In addition, a patient might experience choking or coughing when swallowing, a gurgling or wet-sounding voice quality, hoarseness, recurrent chest infection or unexplained temperature spikes, frequent throat-clearing, and having the sensation of food getting stuck in the throat after multiple attempts to swallow (Malhi, 2016).

Inability to coordinate the complex, sequential swallowing mechanism slows eating, results in food being left in the mouth, and may lead to aspiration (Scelza, Catiuscia, Lopes, et al., 2015). Aspiration pneumonia can be a fatal complication of dysphagia, especially in older persons. However, aspiration pneumonia will develop only if the material aspirated is pathogenic to the lungs and the patient's natural resistance to the material is compromised (Ebihara, Sekiya, Miyagi, et al., 2016; Zhao, Liu, & Huai-chen, 2015). *Tachypnea* (respirations above 26/min) is an early sign of aspiration (Zhao et al., 2015). Other signs include cough; *dyspnea* (difficult breathing); decreased breath sounds; and abnormal breath sounds such as wheezing, rales, and rhonchi (see Chapter 8).

Silent or *asymptomatic aspiration* refers to passage of food or liquid into the trachea and lungs without producing a protective cough or other signs consistent with aspiration (Ebihara et al., 2016). Lack of outward signs such as coughing reduces awareness by the patient, caregiver, and health team members that aspiration is occurring. This can result in longer periods of ingestion of food and liquid into the lungs and places the patient at higher risk for developing pneumonia (Shindo, Kikutani, Yoshida, et al., 2016). The subtle signs associated with silent aspiration are easy to miss and include lack of speech, decreased alertness, wet quality to voice, drooling, difficulty controlling secretions, and absence of gag reflex.

Dysphagia Evaluation

As a nurse, you are in a key position to identify your patients' swallowing difficulties and use interprofessional collaboration as required. Conduct your initial nutritional screening (see Skill 31.1) to determine the potential for both aspiration and safe oral intake. When you detect risk factors, use interprofessional collaboration (e.g., speech-language pathologist [SLP]) for dysphagia screening (Box 31.6). Dysphagia screening is a minimally invasive procedure that documents the likelihood that dysphagia is present, the need for further swallowing assessment, and the safety of patient intake. The single most important measure to prevent aspiration is to place the patient on NPO (nothing by mouth) until a dysphagia evaluation by an SLP is performed; then a safe diet can resume. A functional oral assessment by an SLP includes acceptance of liquid and food, bolus formation, lip seal, mastication, dentition, salivation, pocketing, tongue mobility, mandibular movements, propulsion of bolus along palatal vault, and impulsivity (Mittal et al., 2015). If the SLP finds serious abnormalities, the gold standard for dysphagia diagnosis is videofluoroscopy.

BOX 31.5

Causes of Dysphagia

Neurogenic
- Stroke
- Cerebral palsy
- Guillain-Barré syndrome
- Multiple sclerosis
- Amyotrophic lateral sclerosis (Lou Gehrig's disease)
- Diabetic neuropathy
- Parkinson's disease

Myogenic
- Myasthenia gravis
- Aging
- Muscular dystrophy
- Polymyositis

Obstructive
- Benign peptic stricture
- Lower esophageal ring
- Candidiasis
- Head and neck cancer
- Inflammatory masses
- Trauma or surgical resection
- Anterior mediastinal masses
- Cervical spondylosis

Other
- Gastrointestinal or esophageal resection
- Rheumatological disorders
- Connective tissue disorders
- Vagotomy

BOX 31.6

Criteria for Dysphagia Referral

Before Referral:
If the answer is yes to either of the following two questions, referral at this time is **not appropriate.**
- Is patient unconscious or drowsy?
- Is patient unable to sit in an upright position for a reasonable length of time?

Also Consider the Next Two Questions Before Making a Referral:
- Is the patient near the end of life?
- Does the patient have an esophageal problem that requires surgical intervention?

When Observing a Patient or Giving Mouth Care, Look for the Following:
- Open mouth (weak lip closure)
- Drooling liquids or solids
- Facial or tongue weakness
- Difficulty moving or swallowing secretions in the mouth
- Slurred, indistinct speech
- Hoarseness
- Poor posture or head control
- Weak involuntary cough
- Delayed cough (up to 2 minutes after swallow)
- General frailty, confusion, or dementia
- No spontaneous swallowing movements

If any of the above is present, the patient may have swallowing problems and need referral to a speech-language pathologist.

Dysphagia Management

Dysphagia management includes qualitative dietary modification by altering the consistency of food and liquids and is most effective when implemented using an interprofessional approach recommended by the SLP (Mittal et al., 2015). The SLP's treatment recommendations may include texture modifications for food and liquids (Mittal et al., 2015; Steele, Alsanei, Ayanikalath, et al., 2015). The dietitian ensures these recommendations are balanced with the nutritional and caloric needs of patients. The nurse assists patients with their mealtime feeding. Thus, interprofessional collaboration (e.g., SLP, dietitian) ensures appropriate food choices and consistency of liquids are individualized and based on which phase of swallowing is dysfunctional.

In 2018, Dietitians of Canada supported the *International Dysphagia Diet Standardisation Initiative* (IDDSI) to standardize terminology and descriptors for texture of foods and liquids that would meet the needs of individuals with dysphagia across all ages and care settings. The diet comprises eight levels: thin, slightly thick, mildly thick, liquidized/moderately thick, pureed/extremely thick, minced and moist, soft and bite-sized, and regular (Table 31.5). There is also a category of transitional foods that change from one texture into another when moisture is applied or temperature changed—for example, ice chips, ice cream, and certain wafers (IDDSI, 2017).

Thickened liquids are commonly prescribed to prevent aspiration pneumonia (Steele et al., 2015). A thickening agent alters flavour and texture qualities. Patients often dislike the taste and thickness, which increase nonadherence (Loret, 2015). It is important to

TABLE 31.5

International Dysphagia Diet Levels

Level	Description/Indications
0: Thin	Flows fast like water; can drink through any nipple, cup, or straw; requires functional ability to safely manage liquids of any type
1: Slightly thick	Thicker than water; requires more effort to drink than thin liquids; reduces speed of flow
2: Mildly thick	Sippable; pours quickly from a spoon, but slower than thin drinks; effort required to drink through standard-bore (5.3-mm) straw; suitable if tongue control is slightly reduced
3: Liquidized/Moderately thick	Smooth texture with no lumps; can be drunk from a cup; some effort required to drink through a standard or wide-bore (6.9-mm) straw; allows more time for oral control if pain on swallowing; needs some tongue propulsion effort
4: Pureed/Extremely thick	Cannot be drunk from a cup or sucked through a straw; does not require chewing; can be layered or moulded; suitable if pain on chewing or swallowing, or missing teeth, poorly fitting dentures.
5: Minced & moist	Can be scooped, shaped, and eaten with a spoon or fork; biting is not required; contains small lumps easy to squash with tongue. Suitable if pain or fatigue on chewing, missing teeth, poorly fitting dentures; tongue force needed to move bolus.
6: Soft & bite-sized	Can be eaten with a spoon, fork, or chopsticks; chewing required before swallowing; bite-sized pieces no larger than 8 mm (child) or 15 mm (adult). Suitable if pain or fatigue as above; tongue force and control needed to move food for chewing and move bolus for swallowing.
7: Regular	Normal, everyday foods that are developmentally and age appropriate; includes seeds, bones, and mixed consistencies. Requires ability to bite and chew for long enough to form a swallow-ready bolus and to remove bone or gristle from the mouth that cannot be swallowed safely

Modified from International Dysphagia Diet Standardisation Initiative (IDDSI). (2017). *Complete IDDSI framework: Detailed definitions.* Retrieved from http://iddsi.org/Documents/IDDSIFramework-CompleteFramework.pdf.

remember that the desired thickness of a liquid depends on a patient's swallowing deficit. Always read the label directions when modifying liquids to prepare the desired thickness correctly.

Consequences of Dysphagia

Physiological consequences of dysphagia include decreased appetite, weight loss, dehydration, malnutrition, and pneumonia (Wirth, Dziewas, Beck, et al., 2016). A patient's normal nutritional intake is altered when they are unable to consume oral nutrition or must make diet modifications to swallow without risk of aspiration. Malnutrition may occur secondary to insufficient protein, calorie, and micronutrient intake (Meiner, 2015). Losing the ability to eat and drink safely may affect quality of life. Emotional responses include altered body image, embarrassment, social isolation, and depression; a patient may feel as though they are a burden to caregivers.

Delegation and Collaboration

The skill of following aspiration precautions while feeding a patient can be delegated to an unregulated care provider (UCP). However, the nurse is responsible for the ongoing assessment of a patient's risk for aspiration and determination of positioning and any special feeding techniques. The nurse directs the UCP to:

- Position patient upright (45 to 90 degrees preferred) or according to medical restrictions during and after feeding.
- Use aspiration precautions while feeding patients who need help and explain feeding techniques that are successful for specific patients.
- Immediately report to the nurse any onset of coughing, gagging, "wet" voice, or pocketing of food.

Equipment

- Chair or bed that allows patient to sit upright
- Thickening agents as prescribed (rice, cereal, yogurt, gelatin, commercial thickener)
- Tongue blade
- Penlight
- Oral hygiene supplies (see Chapter 18)
- Suction equipment (see Chapter 25)
- Clean gloves
- *Option:* Pulse oximeter

STEP	RATIONALE

ASSESSMENT

1. Review results of nutritional screening in medical record (see Skill 31.1).	Reveals risk patterns (e.g., patients with dysphagia often alter their eating patterns or choose foods that provide inadequate nutrition).
2. Identify patient using at least two person-specific identifiers (e.g., name and date of birth or name and medical record number) according to employer policy.	Ensures correct patient. Complies with Accreditation Canada's standards and improves patient safety (Accreditation Canada, 2019).
3. Ask patient or caregiver if patient has difficulties chewing or swallowing various food textures.	Patients are likely to aspirate certain foods more than others.
4. Assess for conditions that cause dysphagia and present risk for aspiration (see Box 31.5). Also assess signs and symptoms of dysphagia (e.g., drooling, hoarseness, food pocketing). Use dysphagia screening tool if available.	Patients with neurological or neuromuscular disease and those with trauma to or surgery of oral cavity or throat are at risk.
5. Assess alertness, orientation, and ability to follow simple commands (e.g., open your mouth; stick out your tongue).	Disorientation and inability to follow commands present higher risk for dysphagia.
6. Assess patient's oral cavity, level of dental hygiene, missing teeth, or poorly fitting dentures. (Apply clean gloves if needed.)	Decayed teeth, plaque, and periodontal disease can cause growth of bacteria in the mouth, which can be aspirated (Cagnani, Barros, Sousa, et al., 2016).
7. Observe patient during mealtime for signs of dysphagia such as coughing, dyspnea, or drooling. Observe patient's attempt to feed self; note type of food consistencies and liquids able to swallow. Note during and at end of meal if patient tires.	Detects abnormal eating patterns such as frequent clearing of throat or prolonged eating time. Chewing and sitting up for feeding bring on fatigue (Meiner, 2015).
8. *Option:* Obtain baseline assessment oxygen saturation.	Research findings differ as to whether oximetry can reliably detect aspiration (Lancaster, 2015; Marian, Schröder, Muhle, et al., 2017).
9. Indicate on patient's electronic medical record, chart, or Kardex that dysphagia/aspiration risk is present. *Option:* Some facilities use different-coloured meal trays to signify patients at risk for aspiration.	Identifying patient as dysphagic reduces risk of improperly prepared oral nutrition without supervision.

NURSING DIAGNOSES

- Reduced ability to swallow
- Potential for aspiration

Related factors/Risk factors are individualized on the basis of patient's condition or needs.

STEP	RATIONALE

PLANNING

1. Expected outcomes following completion of procedure:
   - Patient does not exhibit signs or symptoms of aspiration.
   - Patient maintains stable weight.
2. Provide patient 30 minutes of rest.
3. Explain why you are observing patient while they eat.

4. Explain to patient and caregiver what you are going to do and why.

Interventions for preventing aspiration are successful.
Patient maintains adequate oral nutrition.
Fatigue increases risk of aspiration.
Indicators associated with aspiration require further swallowing evaluation such as fluoroscopic examination.
Increases patient cooperation and prepares caregiver to help.

IMPLEMENTATION

1. Perform hand hygiene and have patient or caregiver (if helping with feeding) perform hand hygiene.
2. Apply clean gloves. Provide oral hygiene, including brushing tongue, before meal.
3. Position patient upright (90 degrees) in chair or elevate height of bed (HOB) to a 45– to 90–degree angle or highest position allowed by medical condition during meal.

4. *Option:* Apply pulse oximeter to patient's finger; monitor during feeding.
5. Using penlight and tongue blade, gently inspect mouth for pockets of food.

6. Add thickener to thin liquids to create desired consistency according to prescription. Encourage patient to feed self.
7. Have patient assume chin-tuck position. Remind patient to not tilt head backward when eating or drinking.

8. If patient unable to feed self, place ½ to 1 teaspoon of food on unaffected side of mouth, allowing utensil to touch mouth or tongue.
9. Provide verbal coaching: remind patient to chew and think about swallowing.
   "Open your mouth.
   Feel the food in your mouth.
   Chew and taste the food.
   Raise your tongue to the roof of your mouth.
   Think about swallowing.
   Close your mouth and swallow.
   Swallow again.
   Cough to clear your airway."
10. Avoid mixing food of different textures in same mouthful. Alternate liquids and bites of food. Refer to dietitian for next meal if patient has difficulty with particular consistency.
11. Monitor swallowing and observe for throat clearing, coughing, choking, gagging, and drooling of food; suction airway as needed (see Chapter 25).
12. Minimize distractions, do not talk, and do not rush patient. Allow time for adequate chewing and swallowing. Provide rest period as needed during meal.

Educates about and prevents transmission of microorganisms.
Risk for aspiration pneumonia has been associated with poor oral hygiene (Cagnani et al., 2016).
Position facilitates safe swallowing and enhances esophageal motility (Alghadir, Zafar, Al-Eisa, et al., 2017). Side-lying position with chin-tuck is an option if patient cannot have head elevated.
Pulse oximetry may diagnose aspiration in dysphagic stroke patients (Marian et al., 2017).
Pockets of food found inside cheeks occur when patient has difficulty moving food from mouth into pharynx; may lead to aspiration (Luk, Chan, Hui, et al., 2017). Patient is usually unaware of pocketing, particularly persons living with dementia who lose ability to recognize objects and know when and how to chew or swallow (Cohen, Roffe, Beavan, et al., 2016).
Thin liquids are difficult to control in mouth and pharynx and are more easily aspirated (Steele et al., 2015).
Chin-tuck position is usually effective; however, severe cases of dysphagia may require a more aggressive approach, including enteral feeding (Saconato, Chiari, Lederman, et al., 2016). Hyperextension of neck makes it easier for food to enter airway.
Small bites help patient swallow (Grodner et al., 2015). Provides tactile cue to food; avoids pocketing of food on weaker side.
Verbal cueing keeps patient focused on normal swallowing. Positive reinforcement enhances patient's confidence in ability to swallow. Double- or repeat-swallowing helps clear any remaining food from unprotected airway (Mittal et al., 2015).

Single textures are easier to swallow than multiple textures. Alternating solids with liquids removes food residue in mouth and facilitates better transfer to the esophagus (Canham, 2016).
These indications suggest dysphagia and risk for aspiration (Malhi, 2016).

Environmental distractions during mealtime increase risk for aspiration (Desai, 2017). Avoiding fatigue reduces aspiration risk.

STEP	RATIONALE

IMPLEMENTATION

13. Use sauces, condiments, and gravies to facilitate cohesive food bolus formation.

Cohesive food bolus helps prevent pocketing, or small food particles from entering the airway (Steele et al., 2015).

14. Ask patient to remain sitting upright for at least 30 to 60 minutes after meal.

Remaining upright reduces chance of aspiration by allowing food particles remaining in pharynx to clear.

15. Provide thorough oral hygiene after meal (see Chapter 18).

Reduces plaque and secretions containing bacteria that can cause pneumonia, especially in patients with decreased immunity (Cagnani et al., 2016).

16. Remove gloves if worn. Perform hand hygiene.

Reduces spread of microorganisms.

EVALUATION

1. Throughout meal, cautiously observe patient's ability to swallow food and fluids of various textures and thickness without choking.

Identifies effort with swallowing and absence of signs related to aspiration. Sensitivity to how patients might feel being watched while eating or drinking enhances trust (Guthrie & Stansfield, 2017).

2. Monitor pulse oximetry readings for high-risk patients during eating.

Deteriorating oxygen saturation levels indicate aspiration.

3. Monitor patient's intake and output (I&O), calorie count, and food intake.

Helps detect malnutrition and dehydration.

4. Weigh patient daily or weekly.

Determines if weight is stable and reflects nutritional status.

5. Observe patient's oral cavity after meal.

Determines presence of food pockets after meal that could be aspirated.

6. Use Teach-Back: "We talked about why your husband is at risk to aspirate his food. Tell me the things to observe for that will tell you if he is having trouble swallowing. What should you do if these things happen during a meal?" Develop a revised teaching plan if caregiver is not able to teach back correctly.

Determines caregiver's level of understanding of instructional topic.

Unexpected Outcomes

1. Patient coughs, gags, indicates food "stuck in throat," and has wet quality to voice when eating.

2. Patient experiences weight loss over next several days or weeks.

Related Interventions

- Stop feeding immediately and place patient on NPO.
- Notify health care provider and suction as needed.
- Use interprofessional collaboration (e.g., SLP) for swallowing exercises and techniques to improve swallowing.
- Discuss findings with interprofessional team (e.g., health care provider, dietitian, SLP). Determine if nutritional supplementation or increasing frequency or quality of foods is needed.

Communication and Documentation

- Document in nurses' notes in electronic health record (EHR) or chart the assessment findings, patient's tolerance of liquid and food textures, amount of help required, position during meal, absence or presence of symptoms of dysphagia during feeding fluid intake, and amount eaten.
- Report any coughing, gagging, choking, or other swallowing difficulties to health care provider.

- Communicate that patient has dysphagia during hand-off communication at change of shift.
- Document your evaluation of caregiver learning.

Special Considerations
Pediatric

- Long-term effects for a child diagnosed with pediatric dysphagia include aspiration pneumonia, malnutrition,

dehydration, and increased risk of mortality and infectious complications. The consequences may be particularly severe because children have rapidly developing physiological systems and experience delayed development of oral-motor skills, food and fluid aversion, and altered bonding opportunities with parents (Dodrill & Gosa, 2015; Dziewas, Baiijens, Schindler, et al., 2017).

- The primary goals of feeding and swallowing interventions for children are to safely support adequate nutrition and hydration, determine the optimum feeding methods or technique to maximize swallowing safety and feeding efficiency, collaborate with the caregiver to incorporate dietary preferences, strive to develop age-appropriate eating skills, minimize the risk of pulmonary complications, and maximize quality of life (Dodrill & Gosa, 2015).

Gerontological

- Patients living with dementia are at high risk for eating and feeding difficulties and inadequate food and fluid intake. Depending on the severity of their cognitive impairment, they may forget to eat, forget they have eaten, fail to recognize food, or eat things that are not food.

- Eating difficulties are likely to worsen in a care facility because people living with dementia often become more confused in an unfamiliar place. Different mealtime routines and foods add to the problem.
- Patients living with dementia may not be able tell anyone they are hungry or need help eating or more time to chew and swallow.
- Minimize the use of sedatives and hypnotics, which impair the cough reflex and swallowing (Touhy, Boscart, & McCleary, 2019).

Care in the Community

- Educate patient and caregiver about aspiration precautions and techniques most effective for the patient to prevent development of pneumonia.
- Educate caregiver that older persons with pneumonia often express fewer symptoms than younger adults; therefore, aspiration pneumonia is underdiagnosed. Delirium may be the only manifestation of pneumonia in older persons.
- Dysphagia in the community setting is best managed with an interprofessional person-centred approach that includes the patient, caregiver, health care provider, nurse, occupational therapist, dietitian, and SLP (Department of Veterans Affairs, 2017).

✦ CLINICAL DEBRIEF

A 73-year-old patient with Alzheimer's disease is receiving medication that leaves him with a dry mouth. Results of a nutritional screening indicate difficulty swallowing. Symptoms include frequent coughing during a meal. The patient's respiratory rate is 18 breaths/min, heart rate 90 beats/min. The speech-language pathologist recommended a dysphagia mechanically altered diet with liquids thickened to the mildly thick level. The patient currently weighs 62.6 kg (138 lb) and is 177.8 cm (5'10") tall. His daughter visits frequently at the assisted-living facility. Although he can feed himself, she usually feeds him during scheduled mealtimes in the busy dining room. She frequently gives him sips of her coffee and bites of his favorite oatmeal cookies. The daughter encourages him to bend his head backward to make sure that he drinks all of the liquid in a cup or glass.

1. Determine the patient's body mass index (BMI) and rate his nutritional status.
2. Identify three ways you should teach the daughter to help him swallow and decrease his aspiration risk. Include rationales for your actions.
3. The patient is in the dining area where a UCP is feeding him. The UCP gives the patient some moist ground meat and then cooked fruit. The nurse walks up to the patient's table and notices the patient coughing and beginning to gag. The nurse instructs the UCP to stop feeding. The patient has a respiratory rate of 30 breaths/min and shows effort needed to breathe. Document a nursing note for this situation.

✦ REVIEW QUESTIONS

1. The nurse may delegate the following care to the UCP. (Select all that apply.)
   1. Nutritional screening
   2. Aspiration precautions
   3. Feeding a patient
   4. Interpreting pulse oximetry readings
   5. Measuring a patient's weight

2. A patient is unable to eat more than 25% of any meal because of pain and nausea. Which of the following interventions are most important for the nurse to perform? (Select all that apply.)
   1. Encourage the patient to eat small amounts several times during the day.
   2. Ask the patient which foods and beverages cause the least amount of nausea.
   3. Record a chronology of what the patient has been eating for the past 2 days.
   4. Provide an analgesic 30 minutes before a meal.

3. A nurse is examining a patient just admitted to an acute care facility in the hospital.
   List three assessment findings of the skin that would indicate a possible nutritional problem:
   1. _____
   2. _____
   3. _____

ⓔ *Visit the Evolve site for a complete list of Clinical Debrief and Review Questions answers.*

REFERENCES

Accreditation Canada. (2019). *Required organizational practices handbook—Version 14.* Ottawa, ON: Author. Retrieved from http://www.wrha.mb.ca/quality/files/2019ROPHandbook.pdf

Ahmed, S., Salim, H., Steed, L., & Pinnock, H. (2017). Blue inhalers: Blowing hot and cold. *NPJ Primary Care Respiratory Medicine, 27*(1), 6. doi:10.1038/s41533-016-0008-4

Alberta Health Services. (2018). *Nutrition guideline seniors health overview (65 years and older.* Retrieved from https://www.albertahealthservices.ca/assets/info/nutrition/if-nfs-ng-seniors-health-overview.pdf

Alghadir, A. H., Zafar, H., Al-Eisa, E. S., & Iqbal, Z. A. (2017). Effect of posture on swallowing. *African Health Sciences, 17*(1), 133–137. doi:10.4314/ahs.v17i1.17

Benedik, E., Koroušić, S., Simčič, M., et al. (2014). Comparison of paper- and web-based dietary records: A pilot study. *Annals of Nutrition & Metabolism, 64*(2), 156–166. doi:10.1159/000363336

Bruins, M. J., Bird, J., Aebischer, C., & Eggersdorfer, M. (2018). Considerations for secondary prevention of nutritional deficiencies in high-risk groups in high-income countries. *Nutrients*, 10(1), 1–15. doi:10.3390/nu10010047

Cagnani, A., Barros, A., Sousa, L., et al. (2016). Periodontal disease as a risk factor for aspiration pneumonia: A systematic review. *Journal of Biosciences*, 32(3), 813–821. doi:10.14393/BJ-v32n3a2016-33210

Calloway, S. D. (2018). *The CMS and Joint Commission dietary standards 2018: What hospitals need to know*. Retrieved from http://www.kyha.com/docs/Presentations/DietaryStandards.pdf

Canadian Obesity Network. (2011). *5As of obesity management*. Retrieved from https://obesitycanada.ca/resources/5as/

Canham, M. (2016). Looking into oropharyngeal dysphagia in older adults. *Nursing*, 46(6), 36–42. Retrieved from https://nursing.ceconnection.com/ovidfiles/00152193-201606000-00009.pdf

Castellanos-Sinco, H. B., Ramos-Peñafiel, C. O., Santoyo-Sanchez, A., et al. (2015). Megaloblastic anaemia: Folic acid and vitamin B_{12} metabolism. *Revista Médica Del Hospital General De México*, 78(3), 135–143. doi:10.1016/j.hgmx.2015.07.001

Choban, P., Dickerson, R., Malone, A., Worthington, P., & Compher, C. (2013). ASPEN Clinical guidelines: Nutrition support of hospitalized adult patients with obesity. *JPEN. Journal of Parenteral and Enteral Nutrition*, 37(6), 714–744. doi:10.1177/0148607113499374

Cohen, D. L., Roffe, C., Beavan, J., et al. (2016). Poststroke dysphagia: A review and design considerations for future trials. *International Journal of Stroke: Official Journal of the International Stroke Society*, 11(4), 399–411. Retrieved from http://clok.uclan.ac.uk/19750/

Department of Veterans Affairs. (2017). *Directive 1171. Management of patients with swallowing (oropharyngeal dysphagia) and feeding disorders*. Retrieved from https://www.va.gov/vhapublications/ViewPublication.asp?pub_ID=5387

Desai, R. V. (2017). *Caregiver's guide to dysphagia in dementia*. National Foundation of Swallowing Disorders. Retrieved from http://swallowingdisorderfoundation.com/caregivers-guide-dysphagia-dementia/

Dietitians of Canada. (2013). *Best practices for nutrition, food service and dining in long term care homes*. Retrieved from https://www.dietitians.ca/Downloads/Public/2013-Best-Practices-for-Nutrition,-Food-Service-an.aspx

Dietitians of Canada. (2014). *An inter-professional approach to malnutrition in hospitalized adults: Dietitians leading the way*. Retrieved from https://www.dietitians.ca/Downloads/Public/Interprofessional-Approach-to-Malnutrition-in-Hosp.aspx

Dietitians of Canada. (2016). *Aboriginal nutrition*. Retrieved from https://www.dietitians.ca/Dietitians-Views/Specific-Populations/Aboriginal-Nutrition.aspx

Dodrill, P., & Gosa, M. M. (2015). Pediatric dysphagia: Physiology, assessment, and management. *Annals of Nutrition & Metabolism*, 66(Suppl. 5), 24–31. Retrieved from https://www.karger.com/Article/FullText/381372#

Dziewas, R., Baiijens, L., Schindler, A., Verin, E., Michou, E., & Clave, P. (2017). European Society for Swallowing Disorders FEES accreditation program for neurogenic and geriatric oropharyngeal dysphagia. *Dysphagia*, 32(6), 725–733. doi:10.1007/s00455-017-9828-9

Earle, L. (2011). *Traditional aboriginal diets and health*. National Collaborating Centre for Aboriginal Health. Retrieved from https://www.ccnsa-nccah.ca/docs/emerging/FS-TraditionalDietsHealth-Earle-EN.pdf

Ebihara, S., Sekiya, H., Miyagi, M., Ebihara, T., & Okazaki, T. (2016). Dysphagia, dystussia and aspiration pneumonia in elderly people. *Journal of Thoracic Disease*, 8(3), 632–639. doi:10.21037/jtd.2016.02.60

Food and Agriculture Organization of the United Nations (FAO). (2019). *Food-based dietary guidelines*. Retrieved from http://www.fao.org/nutrition/education/food-dietary-guidelines/home/en/

Gaddey, H. L., & Holder, K. (2014). Unintentional weight loss in older adults. *American Family Physician*, 89(9), 718.

Grodner, M., Escott-Stump, S., & Dorner, S. (2015). *Foundations and clinical applications of nutrition: A nursing approach* (6th ed.). St. Louis: Elsevier Health Sciences.

Group, E. (2016). *How culture and society influence healthy eating*. Global Healing Center. Retrieved from https://www.globalhealingcenter.com/natural-health/how-culture-and-society-influence-healthy-eating/

Guthrie, S., & Stansfield, J. (2017). Teatime threats. Choking incidents at the evening meal. *Journal of Applied Research in Intellectual Disabilities*, 30(1), 47–60. doi:10.1111/jar.12218

Hammond, M. I., Myers, E., & Trostler, N. (2014). Nutrition care process and model: An academic and practice odyssey. *Journal of the Academy of Nutrition and Dietetics*, 114(12), 1879–1891. doi:10.1016/j.jand.2014.07.032

Health Canada. (2014a). *Food safety and you*. Retrieved from https://www.canada.ca/en/health-canada/services/general-food-safety-tips/food-safety-you.html

Health Canada. (2014b). *Infant nutrition*. Retrieved from https://www.canada.ca/en/health-canada/services/infant-care/infant-nutrition.html

Health Canada. (2015a). *Food safety for vulnerable populations*. Retrieved from https://www.canada.ca/en/health-canada/services/food-safety-vulnerable-populations/food-safety-vulnerable-populations.html

Health Canada. (2015b). *Regulations amending the Food and Drug Regulations—Nutrition labelling, other labelling provisions and food colours*. Retrieved from http://www.gazette.gc.ca/rp-pr/p1/2015/2015-06-13/html/reg1-eng.html

Health Canada. (2017). *Household food insecurity in Canada statistics and graphics (2011 to 2012)*. Retrieved from https://www.canada.ca/en/health-canada/services/nutrition-science-research/food-security/household-food-security-statistics-2011-2012.html

Health Canada. (2019a). *Canada's dietary guidelines for health professionals and policy makers*. Retrieved from https://food-guide.canada.ca/static/assets/pdf/CDG-EN-2018.pdf

Health Canada. (2019b). *Food and nutrition*. Retrieved from https://www.canada.ca/en/health-canada/services/food-nutrition.html

Health Canada. (2019c). *Health Canada's healthy eating strategy*. Retrieved from https://www.canada.ca/en/services/health/campaigns/vision-healthy-canada/healthy-eating.html

Health Canada. (2019d). *Make healthy meals with the Eat Well Plate*. Retrieved from http://www.healthycanadians.gc.ca/eating-nutrition/healthy-eating-saine-alimentation/tips-conseils/interactive-tools-outils-interactifs/eat-well-bien-manger-eng.php

Health Canada. (2019e). *Prenatal nutrition*. Retrieved from https://www.canada.ca/en/health-canada/services/food-nutrition/healthy-eating/prenatal-nutrition.html

Herbert, D., Lindsay, M., McIntyre, A., et al. (2016). Canadian stroke best practice recommendations: Stroke rehabilitation practice guidelines, update 2015. *International Journal of Stroke: Official Journal of the International Stroke Society*, 11(4), 459–484. doi:10.1177/1747493016643553

Hines, S., Kynoch, K., & Munday, J. (2016). Nursing interventions for identifying and managing acute dysphagia are effective for improving patient outcomes: A systematic review update. *The Journal of Neuroscience Nursing*, 48(4), 215–223. doi:10.1097/JNN.0000000000000200

Hockenberry, M. J., & Wilson, D. (2015). *Wong's nursing care of infants and children* (10th ed.). St. Louis: Mosby.

International Dysphagia Diet Standardisation Initiative (IDDSI). (2017). *Complete IDDSI framework: Detailed definitions*. Retrieved from http://iddsi.org/Documents/IDDSIFramework-CompleteFramework.pdf

Keller, H., Allard, J., Vesnaver, E., et al. (2015). Barriers to food intake in acute care hospitals: A report of the Canadian Malnutrition Task Force. *Journal of Human Nutrition and Dietetics*, 28(6), 546–557. doi:10.1111/jhn.12314

Keller, H., Lengyel, C., Carrier, N., et al. (2018). Prevalence of inadequate micronutrient intakes of Canadian long-term care residents. *The British Journal of Nutrition*, 1–10, doi:10.1017/S0007114518000107

Keller, H., McCullough, J., Davidson, B., et al. (2015a). *The integrated nutrition pathway for acute care (INPAC)*. Retrieved from http://nutritioncareincanada.ca/sites/default/uploads/files/INPAC.pdf

Keller, H. H., McCullough, J., Davidson, B., et al. (2015b). The integrated nutrition pathway for acute care (INPAC): Building consensus with a modified Delphi. *Nutrition Journal*, 14, 63. doi:10.1186/s12937-015-0051-y

Kern, D. M., Auchincloss, A. H., Stehr, M. F., et al. (2018). Neighborhood price of healthier food relative to unhealthy food and its association with type 2 diabetes and insulin resistance: The multi-ethnic study of atherosclerosis. *Preventive Medicine*, 106, 122–129. doi:10.1016/j.ypmed.2017.10.029

Koch, I., Ferrazzi, A., Busatto, C., et al. (2017). Cranial nerve examination for neurogenic dysphagia patients. *Otolaryngology*, 7(4), 1–6. doi:10.4172/2161-119X.1000319

Krishnan, K., & Pandolfino, J. E. (2018). Dysphagia and esophageal obstruction. In R. D. Kellerman & E. T. Bope (Eds.), *Conn's current therapy 2018* (pp. 199–204). Philadelphia: Elsevier.

Laguna Cruañes, L., & Chen, J. (2016). The eating capability: Constituents and assessments. *Food Quality and Preference*, 48(B), 345–358. doi:10.1016/j.foodqual.2015.03.008

Langmore, J. (2015). Dysphagia: Its causes, assessment and management. *British Journal of Community Nursing*, S28–S32.

Lawrence, S., Cummings, E., Chanoine, J., et al. (2015). Use of growth charts in Canada: A National Canadian Paediatric Surveillance Program survey. *Paediatrics & Child Health*, 20(4), 185–188.

Leigh, J.-H., Oh, B.-M., Seo, H. G., et al. (2015). Influence of the chin-down and chin-tuck maneuver on the swallowing kinematics of healthy adults. *Dysphagia*, 30(1), 89–98. doi:10.1007/s00455-014-9580-3

Lentjes, M. H., McTaggart, A., Mulligan, A. A., et al. (2014). Dietary intake measurement using 7 d diet diaries in British men and women in the European Prospective Investigation into Cancer–Norfolk study: A focus on methodological issues. *The British Journal of Nutrition*, 111(3), 516–526. doi:10.1017/S0007114513002754

Loret, C. (2015). Using sensory properties of food to trigger swallowing: A review. *Critical Reviews in Food Science and Nutrition*, 55(1), 140–145. doi:10.1080/10408398.2011.649810

Lowndes, R., Armstrong, P., & Daly, T. (2015). The meaning of 'dining': The social organization of food in long-term care. *Food Studies*, 4(1), 19–34.

Luk, J. K., Chan, F. H., Hui, E., & Tse, C. Y. (2017). The feeding paradox in advanced dementia: A local perspective. *Hong Kong Medical Journal*, 23(3), 306–310. doi:10.12809/hkmj166110

Malhi, H. (2016). Dysphagia: Warning signs and management. *British Journal of Nursing*, 25(10), 546–549.

Manabe, T., Teramoto, S., Tamiya, N., Okochi, J., & Hizawa, N. (2015). Risk factors for aspiration pneumonia in older adults. *PLoS ONE*, 10(10), e0140060. doi:10.1371/journal.pone.0140060

Maria, O. M., Eliopoulos, N., & Muanza, T. (2017). Radiation-induced oral mucositis. *Frontiers in Oncology*, 7, 89. doi:10.3389/fonc.2017.00089

Marian, T., Schröder, J., Muhle, P., et al. (2017). Measurement of oxygen desaturation is not useful for the detection of aspiration in dysphagic stroke patients. *Cerebrovascular Diseases Extra*, 7(1), 44–50.

Meiner, S. (2015). *Gerontologic nursing* (5th ed.). St. Louis: Mosby.

Metheny, N. A. (2016). Prevention of aspiration in adults. *Critical Care Nurse*, 36(1), e20–e24. doi:10.4037/ccn2016831

Mittal, R., Mishra, A. K., & Nilakantan, A. (2015). Therapeutic interventions by speech language pathologist in managing adult dysphagia: An evidence-based review. *Journal of Laryngology and Voice*, 5(1), 11–16. doi:10.4103/2230-9748.172105

Mozos, I. (2015). Mechanisms linking red blood cell disorders and cardiovascular diseases. *BioMed Research International*, 2015, 682054. doi:10.1155/2015/682054

Nordström, K., Coff, C., Jönsson, H., Nordenfelt, L., & Görman, U. (2013). Food and health: Individual, cultural, or scientific matters. *Genes & Nutrition*, 8(4), 357–363. doi:10.1007/s12263-013-0336-8

Nyberg, M., Olsson, V., Pajalic, Z., et al. (2015). Eating difficulties, nutrition, meal preferences and experiences among elderly—A literature overview from a Scandinavian context. *Journal of Food Research*, 4(1), 22–37. Retrieved from https://www.diva-portal.org/smash/get/diva2:771925/FULLTEXT01.pdf

Ogawa, T., Annear, M. J., Ikebe, K., & Maeda, Y. (2017). Taste-related sensations in old age. *Journal of Oral Rehabilitation*, 44(8), 626–635. doi:10.1111/joor.12502

Oliveira, A. R., Costa, A., Morais, H., Cavalcante, T., Lopes, M., & Araujo, T. (2015). Clinical factors predicting risk for aspiration and respiratory aspiration among patients with stroke. *Revista Latino-Americana de Enfermagem*, 23(2), 216–224. doi:10.1590/0104-1169.0197.2545

Pedersen, S. K. A., Anderson, P., Lugo, R., Andreassen, M., & Sutterlin, S. (2017). Effects of music on agitation in dementia: A meta-analysis. *Frontiers in Psychology*, 8, 742. doi:10.3389/fpsyg.2017.00742

Polivy, J., Herman, C. P., Trottier, K., & Sidhu, R. (2014). Who are you trying to fool: Does weight underreporting by dieters reflect self-protection or self-presentation? *Health Psychology Review*, 8(3), 319–338. doi:10.1080/17437199.2013.775630

Public Health Agency of Canada. (2014). *Canadian best practices portal: Canadian health indicators*. Retrieved from http://cbpp-pcpe.phac-aspc.gc.ca/resources/health-indicators/canadian-health-indicators/

Ramage-Morin, P. L., Gilmour, H., & Rotermann, M. (2017). Nutritional risk, hospitalization and mortality among community-dwelling Canadians aged 65 or older. *Health Reports*, 28(9), 17–27. Retrieved from https://www.statcan.gc.ca/pub/82-003-x/2017009/article/54856-eng.htm

Remig, V., & Weeden, A. (2016). Medical nutrition therapy for neurologic disorders. In L. K. Mahan & J. L. Raymond (Eds.), *Krause's food nutrition and the nutrition care process* (14th ed.). Philadelphia: Saunders.

Rocha, N. P., & Fortes, R. C. (2015). Total lymphocyte count and serum albumin as predictors of nutritional risk in surgical patients. *Brazilian Archives of Digestive Surgery*, 28(3), 193–196. doi:10.1590/S0102-67202015000300012

Ross, J., & Wallace, S. C. (2017). Safety risks in food services can be underestimated. *Healthcare Risk Management*, 39(3), 1–3. Retrieved from https://www.ahcmedia.com/articles/140212-safety-risks-in-food-services-can-be-underestimated

Saconato, M., Chiari, B., Lederman, H., & Goncalves, M. (2016). Effectiveness of chin-tuck maneuver to facilitate swallowing in neurologic dysphagia. *International Archives of Otorhinolaryngology*, 20(1), 13–17. doi:10.1055/s-0035-1564721

Scelza, L., Catiuscia, S. S. G., Lopes, A. J., & Lopes de Melo, P. (2015). Dysphagia in chronic obstructive pulmonary disease. In R. Speyer & H. Bogaardt (Eds.), *Seminars in dysphagia* (pp. 201–227). London: InTECH Open Ltd. Retrieved from https://cdn.intechopen.com/pdfs/48440.pdf

Shindo, H., Kikutani, T., Yoshida, M., Yajima, Y., & Tamura, F. (2016). Signs for identifying risk factors for aspiration pneumonia in elderly people needing nursing care. *Medical Research Archives*, 4(7), 1–14. Retrieved from https://journals.ke-i.org/index.php/mra/article/view/754

Steel, C., & Wile, H. (2018). Nutrition screening practices across care settings: Results of a Canadian survey. *The Canadian Journal of Clinical Nutrition*, 6(1), 7–19. doi:10.14206/canad.j.clin.nutr.2018.01.02

Steele, C. M., Alsanei, W. A., Ayanikalath, S., et al. (2015). The influence of food texture and liquid consistency modification on swallowing physiology and function: A systematic review. *Dysphagia*, 30(1), 2–26. doi:10.1007/s00455-014-9578-x

Swan, W. I., Vivanti, A., Hakel-Smith, N., et al. (2017). Nutrition care process and model update: Toward realizing people-centered care and outcomes management. *Journal of the Academy of Nutrition and Dietetics*, 117(12), 2003–2014. doi:10.1016/j.jand.2017.07.015

Touhy, T. A., Boscart, V., & McCleary, L. (2019). Nutritional needs. In T. A. Touhy, K. Jett, V. Boscart, & L. McCleary (Eds.), *Ebersole and Hess' gerontological nursing and healthy aging in Canada* (2nd Canadian ed., pp. 106–132). Toronto: Elsevier Canada.

Turchiaro, A. (2017). The energetics of food and nutrition according to traditional Chinese medicine. 5th European Nutrition and Dietetics Conference. College of Traditional Chinese Medicine Practitioners and Acupuncturists of Ontario, Canada. *Journal of Nutrition and Food Sciences*, doi:10.4172/2155-9600.C1.021

Weir, D. (2017). Biomarkers. In D. L. Vannette & J. A. Krosnick (Eds.), *The Palgrave handbook of survey research* (pp. 573–586). Cham, Switzerland: Palgrave Macmillan/Springer International.

Wirth, R., Dziewas, R., Beck, A., et al. (2016). Oropharyngeal dysphagia in older persons—From pathophysiology to adequate intervention: A review and summary of an international expert meeting. *Clinical Interventions in Aging*, 11, 189–208. doi:10.2147/CIA.S97481

Wren, A. (2015). *Nutrition & fall prevention*. Retrieved from https://physiotherapy.ca/nutrition-fall-prevention-spring-2015

Zhang, Z., Pereira, S., Luo, M., & Matheson, E. M. (2017). Evaluation of blood biomarkers associated with risk of malnutrition in older adults: A systematic review and meta-analysis. *Nutrients*, 9(8), E829. doi:10.3390/nu9080829

Zhao, J., Liu, Y., & Huai-Chen, L. (2015). Aspiration-related acute respiratory distress syndrome in acute stroke patients. *PLoS ONE*, 10(3), e0118682. doi:10.1371/journal.pone.0118682

Zheng, X., Chen, J., Xie, T., et al. (2017). Relationship between Chinese medicine dietary patterns and the incidence of breast cancer in Chinese women in Hong Kong: A retrospective cross-sectional survey. *Chinese Medicine*, 12, 17. doi:10.1186/s13020-017-0138-9

32 | Enteral Nutrition

Written by **Amy Spencer, MSN, RN-BC; April Ambalina, RN; and Alia Lagace, RN**

OBJECTIVES

Mastery of content in this chapter will enable the nurse to:
- Assess patients who are to have enteral tubes inserted.
- Assess patients who are to receive enteral tube feedings.
- Demonstrate the ability to insert a small-bore feeding tube correctly.
- Discuss the rationale for methods to determine nasogastric or nasoenteric feeding tube placement.

- Discuss the reasons for risks of pulmonary complications during the insertion and maintenance of a feeding tube.
- Demonstrate the appropriate technique for irrigating a feeding tube.
- Demonstrate three appropriate techniques for administering enteral formulas.
- Evaluate a patient's tolerance of enteral feeding.

MEDIA RESOURCES

- evolve http://evolve.elsevier.com/Canada/Perry/clinicalskills/
- Review Questions
- Audio Glossary

- **NSO** Nursing Skills Online
- Clinical Debrief and Review Questions Answers

PURPOSE

Enteral nutrition refers to the delivery of nutritional formulas through a tube that has been inserted into the gastrointestinal (GI) tract. Nasogastric (NG) feedings are delivered through a feeding tube introduced through the nose into the stomach. These gastric feedings can be either continuous, intermittent, or bolus and are delivered via gravity, syringe, or pump method, depending on the patient's needs and tolerance. Nasointestinal (NI) feedings are delivered through a feeding tube introduced through the nose into the small intestine. Intestinal (or small-bowel) feedings are continuous in nature and are therefore delivered via a pump (Winnipeg Regional Health Authority [WRHA, 2017a, p. 9]). Tubes are sometimes placed orally if a patient has trauma to the nose, cranial injury or surgery, or facial surgery. Candidates for tube feeding include patients who have adequate digestion and absorption but cannot ingest, chew, or swallow food safely or in adequate amounts.

STANDARDS OF CARE

- Accreditation Canada, 2019—*Required Organizational Practices Handbook—Version 14* (http://www.wrha.mb.ca/quality/files/2019ROPHandbook.pdf)
- Bankhead, Boullata, Brantley, et al.; Enteral Nutrition Practice Recommendations Task Force, 2009—*ASPEN Enteral Nutrition Practice Recommendations* (https://www.naspghan.org/files/documents/pdfs/training/curriculum-resources/nutrition/other-guidelines/Bankhead_Enteral_practice_recommendations.pdf)
- Canadian Patient Safety Institute (CPSI), 2009—*The Safety Competencies: Enhancing Patient Safety Across the Health Professions* (http://www.patientsafetyinstitute.ca/en/toolsResources/safetyCompetencies/Documents/Safety%20Competencies.pdf)
- Institute for Safe Medication Practices (ISMP) Canada, 2013—*Safety Bulletin: Some Liquid Medications May Be Unsuitable for Administration by Enteral Tube* (https://www.ismp-canada.org/

download/safetyBulletins/2013/ISMPCSB2013-05_LiquidMedicationsEnteralTube.pdf)
- Winnipeg Regional Health Authority (WRHA), 2017a—*Adult Enteral Nutrition Practice Guideline* (http://www.wrha.mb.ca/extranet/eipt/files/EIPT-34-005.pdf)

PRINCIPLES FOR PRACTICE

- The selection of an enteral feeding tube and placement method depends on the anticipated duration of feeding and other patient-related factors such as gastric emptying, GI anatomy, and risk for gastric reflux.
- Nasal tubes are associated with the development of sinusitis, otitis, vocal cord paralysis, and pressure injuries to the nose and sinuses.
- The reflux of tube-feeding formula into the oropharynx can lead to aspiration into the lung.
- It is recommended that the liquid form of medication be used for patients with feeding tubes. If a liquid form is not available, check with a pharmacist prior to crushing pills and tablets (WRHA, 2017a, p. 16).
- Radiographic film verification is recommended to confirm correct placement of any bedside inserted enteral tube before its initial use for feedings or medication administration (Bourgault, Heath, Hooper, et al., 2015).
- Marking and documenting the exit site of an enteral tube at the time of radiographic confirmation of correct placement will be helpful in subsequent monitoring of the location of the tube during its use for feedings (McCarthy & Martindale, 2015).

PERSON-CENTRED CARE

- The insertion and use of a feeding tube often raises emotional and psychological concerns. The patient and caregiver need reassurance and encouragement throughout the insertion procedure and once the tube feeding is in progress. If tube feeding is being considered by a patient's health care provider in the context of advanced illness, the Canadian Virtual Hospice website offers insightful information for health care providers, patients, and family members on navigating this controversial topic (see http://www.virtualhospice.ca/en_US/Utilities/Search.aspx?q=nutrition).
- Nursing interventions such as oral hygiene and care of the nasal passage or tube insertion site promote patient comfort during tube feeding and can reduce complications.
- Although tube feedings offer life-sustaining treatment, artificial nutrition can never replace the social and symbolic benefits of sharing meals. Social, religious, and cultural events involve food; patients requiring long-term tube feeding may feel a sense of loss regarding their ability to participate in life activities.
- Interprofessional collaboration among health care providers can help patients and caregivers use nutritional strategies to preserve or enhance quality of life. For example, a speech-language pathologist (SLP) can evaluate the ability of a patient to swallow safely.
- Encourage patients who require long-term tube feedings to use resources available to them, such as the Oley Foundation's website, or initiate a referral to their provincial/territorial home nutrition program, which can provide them with education, supplies, outreach, and networking (WRHA, 2017b).

- Patients with living wills or other forms of advance directives may refuse the use of artificial feeding via a feeding tube. An interprofessional approach to person-centred care that considers cultural, spiritual, and psychological dimensions of this issue should be considered, based on the patient's treatment goals.

EVIDENCE-INFORMED PRACTICE

Evidence-informed guidelines ensure correct technique for placing enteral feeding tubes, initiating and maintaining enteral nutrition, and reducing risks for feeding tube complications.

- Obtain radiographic confirmation of correct placement of any blindly inserted tube before its initial use for feeding or medication administration (Bourgault et al., 2015). The most common complication of blindly inserted feeding tubes is improper placement in the esophagus or pulmonary system (Bourgault et al., 2015).
- Feeding tubes are positioned into the small bowel to reduce the incidence of pulmonary aspiration of stomach contents. Research has not demonstrated this benefit consistently, but newer techniques for detecting aspiration provide some evidence that small-intestine feeding does reduce the incidence of pneumonia (Patel, Lemieux, McClace, et al., 2017).
- Gastric pH ≤ 5 likely indicates a gastric placement, and intestinal or respiratory pH is usually ≥ 7 (Fan, Tan, & Ang, 2017).
- Capnography and carbon dioxide (CO_2) detectors have been used to assess position of small-bore feeding tubes and can identify a tube placed in the airway by measuring CO_2 in expired air that directly reveals CO_2 being eliminated from the lungs. However, capnography does not verify proper position of the tube in the GI tract; therefore, final tube placement should be verified on radiographic film (Wallace & Gardner, 2015).
- Maintaining and monitoring tube location during enteral feeding and keeping the head-of-bed elevation at a minimum of 30–45 degrees effectively reduces aspiration and subsequent pneumonia (Saskatoon Health Region [SHR], 2017).
- Gastric residual volumes (GRVs) are measured routinely during tube feeding to identify risk for feeding intolerance. This technique involves withdrawing and measuring stomach contents at regular intervals during tube feeding. Feeding is stopped when GRVs exceed a specified level; however, studies have failed to demonstrate a consistent relationship between GRV and risk of pulmonary aspiration, regurgitation, or pneumonia (McCarthy & Martindale, 2015). Recommendations for stopping tube feeding for elevated GRVs range from 250 to 500 mL, but automatic cessation of feeding should not occur for GRV less than 500 mL in the absence of other signs of intolerance (McCarthy & Martindale, 2015; WRHA, 2017a).

SAFETY GUIDELINES

- Be aware of factors that increase a patient's risk for complications related to feeding tube insertion: altered level of consciousness, abnormal clotting, or impaired gag or cough reflex.
- Know the purpose of the feeding and the intended location of the tip of the feeding tube.
- Take precautions to prevent microbial contamination of enteral formulas.
- Be aware of safety measures to prevent pulmonary aspiration of gastric contents and accidental tube displacement by patients.

- Consult with a pharmacist regarding a patient's medications and their route of delivery to determine if administration via feeding tube is appropriate.
- Use an ENFit connector for all enteral nutrition sets, syringes, and feeding tubes to improve patient safety. The ENFit connector is not compatible with Luer-Lok connections or any other small-bore medical connectors and thus prevents misadministration of an enteral feeding or medication by the wrong route (ISMP, 2015; Kozeniecki & Fritzshall, 2015).

- A medical device–related pressure injury is a localized injury to the skin or underlying tissue that forms as a result of sustained pressure from a device. Choose the correct size of medical device(s) to fit the individual, cushion and protect the skin with dressings in high-risk areas (e.g., nasal bridge), and remove or move the device daily to assess skin (National Pressure Ulcer Advisory Panel [NPUAP], 2013).

| ✦ **SKILL 32.1** | **Inserting and Removing a Small-Bore Nasogastric or Nasoenteric Feeding Tube** |

NSO *Nursing Skills Online Enteral Nutrition Module 16 / Lessons 1 and 2*

Throughout this chapter nasally placed feeding tubes (8 to 12 French [Fr]) are referred to as *nasogastric (NG) tubes*; but some types of NG tubes, which are larger and more rigid, are used for gastric decompression instead of feeding (see Chapter 35). Small-bowel *nasointestinal (NI) tubes* such as nasojejunal (NJ) are also used for enteral tube feedings, and these are advanced into the jejunum of the small intestine by way of the nose. Feeding tubes are soft and flexible; many use a removable guidewire or stylet to provide stiffness during tube insertion. Although these wires facilitate placement of a tube, they also add to the risk of pulmonary or esophageal injury during insertion. Nurses can also pass feeding tubes through the mouth (oral gastric tube), especially in critical care when the patient is also intubated or when contraindications to nasal placement such as a basilar skull fracture or facial trauma exist.

Placement of a feeding tube requires a health care provider's prescription. All candidates for NG or NI tube placement require an assessment of their coagulation status. Anticoagulation and bleeding disorders pose a risk for epistaxis during nasal tube placement; the health care provider may prescribe platelet transfusion or other corrective measures before tube insertion.

Delegation and Collaboration

The skill of feeding tube insertion cannot be delegated to an unregulated care provider (UCP). However, UCPs may help with patient positioning and comfort measures during tube insertion.

Equipment
Insertion
- Small-bore NG or nasoenteric tube with or without stylet (select the smallest diameter possible to enhance patient comfort) (Fig. 32.1)
- 60-mL ENFit syringe
- Stethoscope, pulse oximeter, capnography (*optional*)
- Hypoallergenic tape, semipermeable (transparent) dressing, or tube fixation device
- Skin barrier protectant

- pH indicator strip (scale 1.0 to 11.0)
- Cup of water and straw or ice chips (for patients able to swallow)
- Water-soluble lubricant
- Emesis basin
- Towel or disposable pad
- Facial tissues
- Tape measure
- Clean gloves
- Suction equipment in case of aspiration
- Penlight to check placement in nasopharynx
- Tongue blade
- Oral hygiene supplies

Removal
- Disposable pad
- Tissues
- Clean gloves
- Disposable plastic bag
- Towel
- 60-mL ENFit syringe

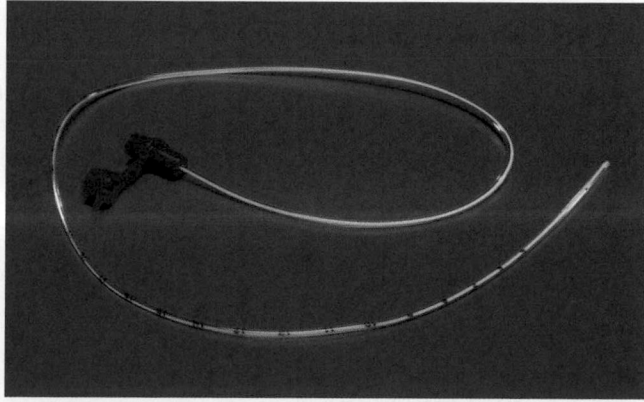

FIG 32.1 Small-bore feeding tube. (*Courtesy Kendall Brands, Mansfield, MA.*)

STEP	RATIONALE

ASSESSMENT

1. Verify health care provider's prescription for type of tube and enteric feeding schedule. Also check prescription to determine if health care provider wants prokinetic medications (e.g., metoclopramide) given before tube placement.

Health care provider's prescription is needed to insert feeding tube. Prokinetic medications given before tube placement may help advance tube into intestine.

2. Identify patient using at least two person-specific identifiers (e.g., full name, date of birth, personal identification number), according to employer policy.

Ensures correct patient. Complies with Accreditation Canada's standards and improves patient safety (Accreditation Canada, 2019).

3. Assess patient's knowledge of procedure.

Encourages cooperation, reduces anxiety, and minimizes risks. Identifies teaching needs.

4. Perform hand hygiene. Have patient close each nostril alternately and breathe. Examine each naris for patency and skin breakdown (apply clean gloves if drainage present).

Reduces transmission of microorganisms. Sometimes nares are obstructed or irritated, or septal defect is present. Place tube in most patent naris.

5. Review patient's medical history (e.g., for basilar skull fracture, nasal problems, nosebleeds, facial trauma, nasal-facial surgery, deviated septum, anticoagulant therapy, coagulopathy).

History of these problems may require you to consult with health care provider to change route of nutritional support. A risk of intracranial tube passage, causing neurological injury, exists for patients with basilar skull fractures and facial trauma.

Clinical Decision Point *If a patient is at risk for intracranial passage of the tube, avoid the nasal route. Oral placement or placement under medical supervision using fluoroscopic direct visualization is preferable. Insertion of a gastrostomy or jejunostomy tube is another alternative.*

6. Assess patient's height, weight, hydration status, electrolyte balance, and intake and output (I&O).

Provides baseline information to measure nutritional improvement after enteral feedings.

7. Assess patient's mental status (ability to cooperate with procedure, sedation), presence of cough and gag reflex, ability to swallow, critical illness, and presence of artificial airway.

Altered mental status or absence of gag or cough reflex increases risk of transbronchial placement (Caramia, 2018).

Clinical Decision Point *Recognize situations in which blind placement of a feeding tube poses an unacceptable risk for placement. Use of devices designed to detect pulmonary intubation such as CO_2 sensors or electromagnetic tracking devices enhances patient safety. While capnography has been found to be a valid verification tool, especially in mechanically ventilated patients, it is not commonly used on nursing units because of lack of availability, inadequate clinical research, and incompatible fitting onto an NG tube (Bennetzen, Håkonsen, Svenningsen, et al., 2015, p. 90).*

Alternatively, to avoid insertion complications from blind placement in high-risk situations, such as in critical care, clinicians trained in the use of visualization or imaging techniques should place tubes (Dharmalingam & Gunasekaran, 2016, p. 751; Mizzi, Cozzi, Beretta, et al., 2017, p. 49).

8. Perform physical assessment of abdomen (see Chapter 8). Remove and dispose of gloves (if worn). Perform hand hygiene.

Absent bowel sounds, abdominal pain, tenderness, or distension may indicate a medical problem contraindicating feedings.

NURSING DIAGNOSES

- Potential for aspiration
- Inadequate nutrition
- Reduced comfort

Related factors/Risk factors are individualized on the basis of patient's condition or needs.

PLANNING

1. Expected outcomes following completion of procedure:
   - Tube is successfully placed in stomach or small intestine.
   - Feeding tube remains patent.
   - Patient has no respiratory distress (e.g., increased respiratory rate, coughing, poor colour) or signs of discomfort or nasal trauma.

Proper position is essential before initiating feeding tube.
Proper irrigation clears tube of formula residue (Best, 2017).
Correctly placed tube causes no interference with airway.

2. Explain procedure to patient, including sensations (e.g., burning in nasal passages) that will be felt during insertion.

Increases patient's cooperation with intubation procedure and helps lessen anxiety.

3. Explain to patient how to communicate during intubation by raising index finger to indicate gagging or discomfort.

Patient must have a way of communicating to alleviate stress and enhance cooperation.

STEP	RATIONALE

IMPLEMENTATION

1. Perform hand hygiene. Prepare supplies at bedside.

Reduces transmission of microorganisms. Ensures organized procedure.

2. Stand on same side of bed as naris chosen for insertion and position patient upright in high-Fowler's position (unless contraindicated). If patient is comatose, raise head of bed as tolerated in semi-Fowler's position with head tipped forward, using a pillow chin to chest. If necessary, have a UCP help with positioning of confused or comatose patients. If patient is forced to lie supine, place in reverse Trendelenburg's position.

Allows for easier manipulation of tube.
Fowler's position reduces risk of aspiration and promotes effective swallowing. Forward head position helps with closure of airway and passage of tube into esophagus.

3. Apply pulse oximeter and measure vital signs.

Provides baseline for objective assessment of respiratory status during tube insertion.

   a. If patient has decrease in oxygen saturation, tube should not be inserted until you determine patient stability.

4. Place towel over patient's chest. Keep facial tissues within reach.

Prevents soiling of gown. Insertion of tube frequently produces tearing.

5. Determine length of tube to be inserted and mark location with indelible ink.

   a. Measure distance from tip of nose to earlobe to xiphoid process of sternum (see illustration). Mark this distance on tube with indelible ink.

Length approximates distance from nose to stomach. Tape is not to be used to mark distance as it can block the nares, be inhaled, collect mucus, and be difficult to remove once placement is confirmed.

   b. Measure distance from tip of nose to earlobe to mid-umbilicus for pediatric patient.

   c. Add 20 to 30 cm (8 to 12 inches) for NJ tubes.

Length approximates distance from nose to jejunum.

Clinical Decision Point *Tip of NG tube must reach the stomach to avoid the risk for pulmonary aspiration, which occurs when tubes terminate in the esophagus.*

6. Prepare NG or NJ tube for intubation.
   NOTE: Do not ice or freeze tubes.

Iced tube becomes stiff and inflexible, causing trauma to nasal mucosa.

   a. Obtain prescription for stylet tube and check employer policy for trained clinician to insert tube.

   b. If tube has guidewire or stylet, inject 10 mL of water from ENFit syringe into tube.

This aids in guidewire or stylet removal. Activates lubrication of tube for easier passage and ensures that tube is patent. ENFit devices will not be compatible with a Luer connection or any other type of small-bore medical connector, thus preventing misadministration of an enteral feeding (ISMP, 2015).

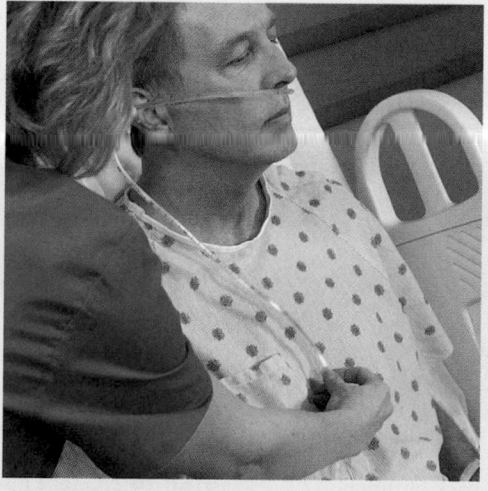

STEP 5a Measure to determine length of tube to insert.

STEP	RATIONALE

IMPLEMENTATION

c. If using stylet, make certain that it is positioned securely within tube. Inject 10 mL of water from ENFit syringe into tube.

Promotes smooth passage of tube into gastrointestinal (GI) tract. Improperly positioned stylet can cause tube to kink or injure patient. Ensures that tube is patent and aids in stylet removal. Once tube insertion is confirmed, have trained clinician remove stylet.

7. Prepare tube fixation materials. Cut hypoallergenic tape 10 cm (4 inches) long or prepare membrane dressing or other tube fixation device.

Used to secure tubing after insertion. Fixation devices allow tube to float free of nares, thus reducing pressure on nares, preventing device-related pressure injury.

8. Perform hand hygiene and apply clean gloves.

Reduces transmission of microorganisms.

9. *Option:* Dip tube with surface lubricant into glass of room-temperature water or apply water-soluble lubricant (see manufacturer directions).

Activates lubricant to facilitate passage of tube into naris and GI tract.

10. Provide alert patient a cup of water with straw (if able to swallow). If patient is unable to swallow, assist patient in tucking chin toward their chest.

Patient is asked to swallow water to facilitate tube passage. Closes off glottis and reduces risk for tube entering trachea.

11. Explain next steps to patient and gently insert tube through nostril to back of throat (posterior nasopharynx). This may cause the patient to gag. Aim back and down toward the ear (see illustration).

Natural contours facilitate passage of tube into GI tract.

12. Instruct patient to take deep breaths, relax, and flex head toward chest after tube has passed through nasopharynx.

Closes off glottis and reduces risk for tube entering trachea.

13. Encourage patient to swallow small sips of water. Advance tube as patient swallows.

Swallowing facilitates passage of tube past oropharynx. A distinct tug may be felt as the patient swallows, indicating that tube is following expected path.

14. Emphasize to patient the need to mouth breathe and swallow during insertion.

Helps facilitate passage of tube and alleviates patient's fears during procedure.

15. Do not advance tube during inspiration or coughing because it is more likely to enter the respiratory tract. Monitor oximetry and respiratory symptoms.

Can cause tube to inadvertently enter patient's airway, which will be reflected in changes in oxygen saturation and ability to speak.

16. Advance tube each time patient swallows until desired length has been reached (see illustration).

Reduces discomfort and trauma to patient. Helps facilitate tube passage.

Clinical Decision Point *Do not force the tube or push against resistance. If the patient starts to cough, experiences a drop in oxygen saturation, or shows other signs of respiratory distress, withdraw the tube into the posterior nasopharynx until normal breathing resumes.*

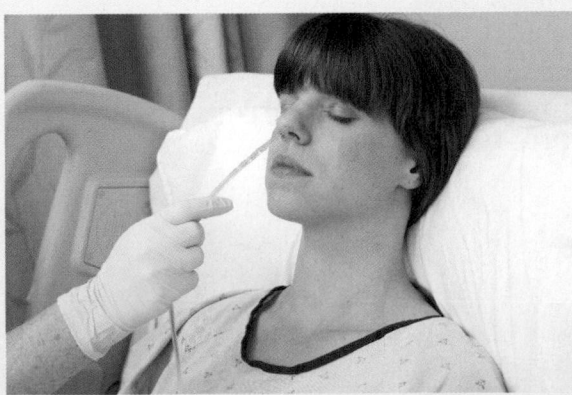

STEP 11 Insert tube through nostril to back of throat.

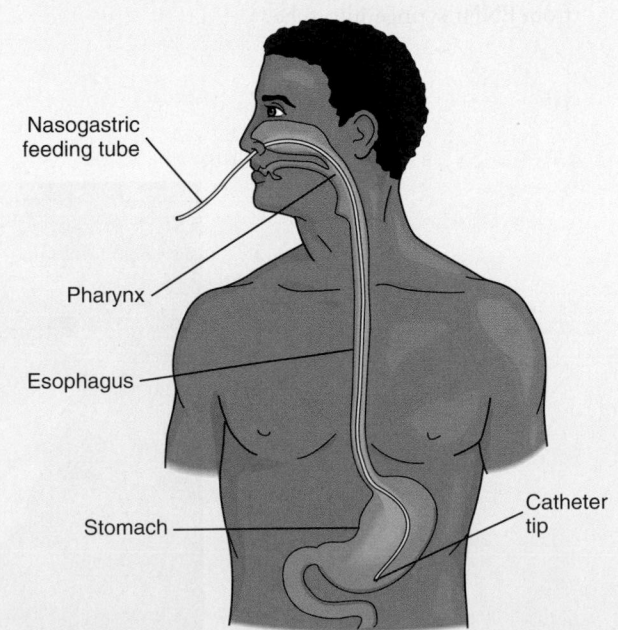

Nasogastric feeding tube

Pharynx

Esophagus

Stomach

Catheter tip

STEP 16 NG tube inserted through nasopharynx and esophagus into stomach.

STEP	RATIONALE

IMPLEMENTATION

17. Check for position of tube in back of throat using penlight and tongue blade.

Tube may be coiled, kinked, or entering trachea.

18. Temporarily anchor tube to nose with a small piece of tape.

Movement of tube stimulates gagging. Assesses general position before anchoring tube more securely.

19. Keep tube secure and check its placement by aspirating stomach contents to measure gastric pH (see Skill 32.2). Also measure amount, colour, and quality of return.

Proper tube position is essential before initiating feeding.

Clinical Decision Point *Insufflation of air into the tube while auscultating the abdomen is not a reliable means to determine the position of the feeding tube tip because air movement sounds can be heard when the NG tube is in the esophagus, stomach, or lung (Atalay, Aydin, Ertugrul, et al., 2016, p. 805).*

20. Carefully remove temporary tape and re-anchor tube to patient's nose, avoiding pressure on nares. Mark exit site on tube with indelible ink, measure and record external length of the tube (i.e., from naris to the end or tip of the NG tube). Select one of the following options for anchoring:

Marking and measuring the tube can alert nurses to possible displacement. A properly secured tube allows patient more mobility and prevents trauma to nasal mucosa.

Noting the external length helps determine possible tube dislodgement (Lord, 2018, p. 20).

a. Apply membrane dressing or tube fixation device:

Permits longer securement without need to change dressing.

  (1) *Membrane dressing:*

Allows membrane to adhere to skin.

    (a) Apply skin barrier or adhesive protectant ointment or spray to patient's cheek and area of tube to be secured.

    (b) Place tube against patient's cheek and secure tube with membrane dressing, out of patient's line of vision.

Eliminates application of tape around naris. Decreases risk for patient's inadvertent extubation.

  (2) *Tube fixation device:*

Secures tube and reduces friction on naris.

    (a) Apply wide end of patch to bridge of nose (see illustration).

    (b) Slip clamp around feeding tube as it exits naris (see illustration).

b. Apply tape:

Prevents pulling of tube. May require frequent change if tape becomes soiled.

  (1) Apply skin barrier or adhesive protectant ointment on tip of patient's nose and allow it to become "tacky."

Helps tape adhere better. Protects skin.

  (2) Remove gloves and tear a horizontal slit up the centre of the tape (see illustration).

  (3) Place intact end of tape over bridge of patient's nose. Wrap each strip around tube as it exits (see illustration).

Tube is free-floating in the naris with this taping method, resulting in movement of tube in pharynx. Securing tape to naris in this method reduces pressure on naris and risk for medical device–related pressure injury (Best, 2017).

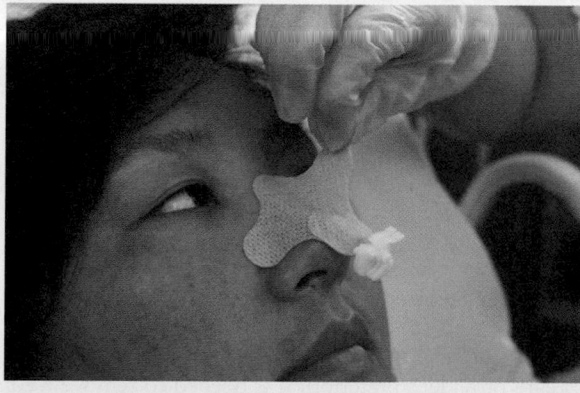

STEP 20a(2)(a) Apply tube fixation device to bridge of nose.

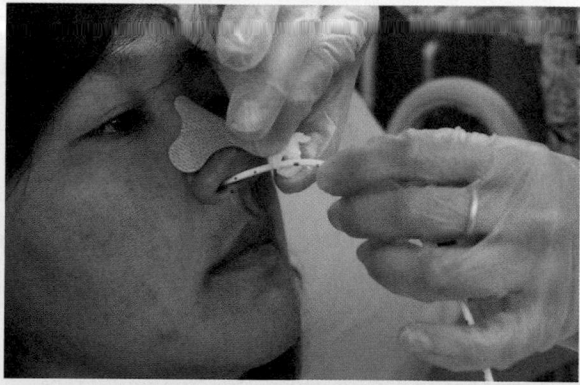

STEP 20a(2)(b) Slip clamp around feeding tube and gently close clamp around tube.

STEP	RATIONALE

IMPLEMENTATION

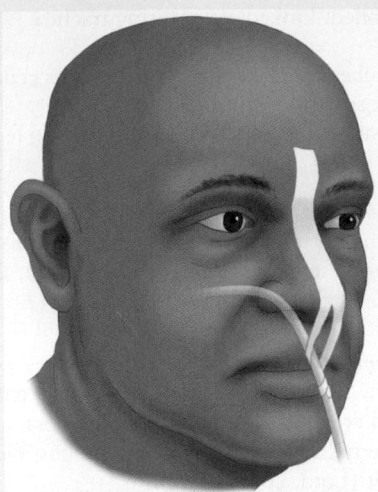

STEP 20b(2) Tear a horizontal slit up the centre of the tape.

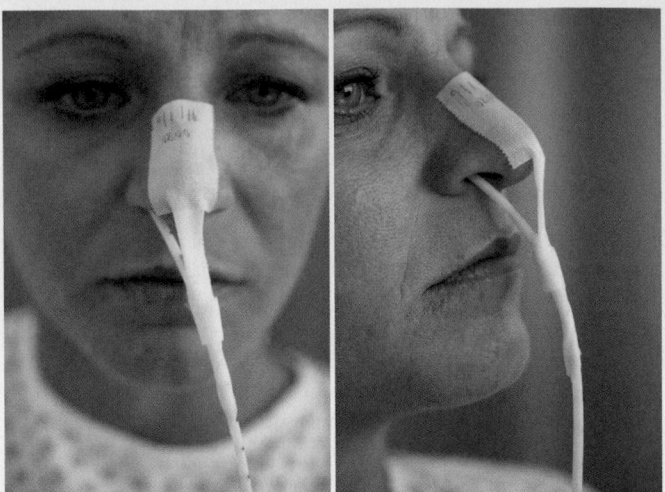

STEP 20b(3) A, Apply tape to anchor nasoenteral tube. **B,** Naris is free of pressure from tape and tube.

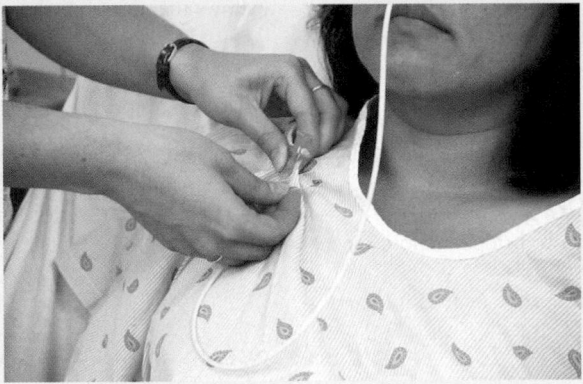

STEP 21 Fasten feeding tube to patient's gown.

STEP	RATIONALE
21. Fasten end of tube to patient's gown using clip (see illustration) Do not use safety pins to secure tube to gown.	Reduces traction on naris if tube moves. Safety pins can become unfastened and cause injury to patients.
22. Help patient to a comfortable position, maintain head of the bed elevated at least 30 degrees (preferably 45 degrees) unless contraindicated (SHR, 2017). For intestinal tube placement, place patient on right side, when possible, until radiographic confirmation of correct placement is made.	Promotes patient comfort while patient awaits radiographic (X-ray) confirmation of tube placement. Placing patient on right side promotes passage of NI tube into small intestine.
23. Remove gloves and perform hand hygiene.	Reduces transmission of microorganisms.

Clinical Decision Point *Leave stylet in place until correct position is verified by radiographic film. Never try to reinsert a partially or fully removed stylet while the feeding tube is in place. This can cause perforation of the tube and injure the patient.*

STEP	RATIONALE
24. Contact radiology to obtain radiographic film of chest or abdomen.	Radiographic film examination remains the gold standard of practice and is the most accurate method to determine feeding-tube placement (McFarland, 2017, pp. 201–202).
25. Perform hand hygiene. Apply clean gloves and administer oral hygiene (see Chapter 18). Clean tubing at nostril with dampened washcloth.	Promotes patient comfort and integrity of oral mucous membranes.
26. Remove gloves, dispose of equipment, and perform hand hygiene.	Reduces transmission of microorganisms.
27. **Tube removal:**	
a. Verify health care provider's prescription for tube removal.	Health care provider's prescription is needed to remove feeding tube.
b. Gather equipment.	Ensures organized procedure.

STEP	RATIONALE

IMPLEMENTATION

c. Explain procedure to patient.

Encourages cooperation, reduces anxiety, and minimizes risks. Identifies teaching needs.

d. Perform hand hygiene. Apply clean gloves.

Reduces transmission of microorganisms.

e. Position patient in high-Fowler's position unless contraindicated.

Reduces risk for pulmonary aspiration in event patient should vomit.

f. Place disposable pad or towel over patient's chest.

Prevents mucus and gastric secretions from soiling patient's clothing.

g. Disconnect tube from feeding administration set (if present) and instill 10 to 20 mL of air into the tube clamp or cap end.

Clears the tube and prevents formula from spilling from tube as it is removed.

h. Remove tape or tube fixation device from patient's nose. Unclip tube from patient's gown.

Allows tube to be removed easily.

i. Instruct patient to take a deep breath and hold it. Then as you kink the end of the tube securely, completely withdraw it by pulling it out steadily and smoothly onto the towel. Inspect intactness of tube (SHR, 2017), then dispose of it into appropriate receptacle.

Prevents inadvertent aspiration of gastric contents while tube is removed. Kinking prevents leakage of fluid from tube. Promotes patient comfort. Reduces transmission of microorganisms.

j. Offer tissues to patient to blow nose.

Clears nasal passages of remaining secretions.

k. Offer mouth care.

Promotes patient's comfort.

l. Remove and dispose of gloves; perform hand hygiene.

Reduces transmission of microorganisms.

EVALUATION

1. Observe patient's response to tube placement. Assess lung sounds; have patient speak; check vital signs; note any coughing, dyspnea, cyanosis, or decrease in oxygen saturation

Symptoms may indicate placement in the respiratory tract. Auscultation of crackles, wheezes, dyspnea, or fever may be a delayed response to aspiration.

2. Confirm radiographic film results with health care provider.

Verifies position of tube before initiating enteral feeding.

3. Remove stylet after radiographic film verification of correct placement. Review employer policy regarding requirement of trained clinician for insertion.

If placement needs adjustment, stylet is still in place.

4. Routinely check condition of nares, location of external exit site marking on tube, measurement of the external tube length, and colour and pH of fluid aspirated from tube.

Routine evaluation ensures no formation of medical device–related pressure injury and correct placement of tube.

Noting the external length helps in detecting possible tube dislodgement (Lord, 2018, p. 20).

5. After stylet removal, assess patient's level of comfort.

Provides for continued comfort of patient.

Use Teach-Back: "I want to make sure you know how to communicate with me during the tube insertion as it may be difficult for you to speak. Tell me how you will communicate with me during the tube insertion." Develop a revised teaching plan if patient is not able to teach back correctly.

Determines patient's level of understanding of instructional topic.

Unexpected Outcomes

1. Aspiration of stomach contents into respiratory tract (delayed response or small-volume aspiration) occurs, as evidenced by auscultation of crackles or wheezes, dyspnea, or fever.

2. Displacement of feeding tube to another site (e.g., from duodenum to stomach) possibly occurs when patient coughs or vomits.

Related Interventions

- Report change in patient condition to health care provider; if there has not been a recent chest radiographic film, suggest prescribing one.
- Position patient on side to protect airway.
- Suction nasotracheally and orotracheally.
- Prepare for possible initiation of antibiotics.
- Aspirate GI contents and measure pH.
- Remeasure external length and compare to records.
- Request a prescription for radiographic imaging to determine tube placement.
- If above verification methods confirm displacement of tube, discuss with health care provider the following options:
  a) Advancing current tube and reimaging to confirm, or
  b) Removing current displaced tube completely and reinserting new tube (see Skill 32-1).
- If there is question of aspiration, obtain chest radiographic film.

Communication and Documentation

- Document type and size of tube placed, external measurement of tube, patient's tolerance of procedure, condition of naris, and confirmation of tube position by radiographic film examination in nurses' notes in electronic health record (EHR) or chart.
- Document removal of tube, condition of naris, tube intactness, and patient's tolerance.
- Report any unexpected outcomes and the interventions performed.
- Document your evaluation of patient learning.

Special Considerations
Teaching

- Instruct patient or caregiver on the importance of frequent oral hygiene.
- Instruct patient or caregiver to report tension on feeding tube or displacement of tape or tube fixation device; instruct patient or caregiver to stabilize the tube and call for help.

Pediatric

- The distance from nose to ear to mid-umbilicus better predicts the insertion length for gastric tube placement in neonates and children than traditional nose-to-ear-to-xiphoid measurements (Hockenberry & Wilson, 2015).
- Radiographic film confirmation is the most accurate assessment of proper tube placement. The best bedside assessment of tube placement is to aspirate gastric contents for colour and pH (Hockenberry & Wilson, 2015). When inserting a feeding tube in an infant, the heart rate and blood pressure may change in response to vagal stimulation.

Care in the Community

- Assess patient's or caregiver's ability to maintain a tube for a feeding program.
- Assess the environmental safety (e.g., adequate space and electricity to operate and maintain needed equipment and supplies) and sanitation of the patient's home to determine potential for infection or injury.
- Teach patient or caregiver how to assess tube placement (see Skill 32.2).
- Teach caregiver correct method for securing a feeding tube and the routine care necessary to reduce pressure injuries.

◆ SKILL 32.2   Verifying Feeding Tube Placement

NSO *Nursing Skills Online Enteral Nutrition Module 16 / Lesson 3*

Nurses insert small-bore feeding tubes nasally for intermittent or continuous feeding. It is possible for the tip of a feeding tube to move or migrate into a different location (e.g., from the stomach into the intestine or esophagus, from the intestine into the stomach). Although all tubes should be marked to document the correct position, tube dislocation can sometimes occur without any external evidence that the tube has moved. The risk of aspiration of regurgitated gastric contents into the respiratory tract increases when the tip of the tube accidentally dislocates upward into the esophagus.

Following initial radiographic film verification of correct feeding tube position, the nurse must monitor the tube to ensure that the tube tip remains in the intended site. Based on a patient's clinical condition and employer policy, the nurse checks the feeding tube position at regular intervals (often every 4 to 6 hours) and before administering formula or medications through the tube. Radiographic verification is impractical every 4 to 6 hours and costly, but the reports of routine chest and abdominal films should be monitored for reference to the feeding tube location. No single bedside method of monitoring tube position during feeding is completely reliable; there are several techniques to use in combination to detect feeding tube dislocation:

- Monitor the external length of the tube and observe the appearance, volume, and pH of fluid aspirated through it. The colour of the fluid can help differentiate gastric from intestinal placement. Because most intestinal aspirates are stained by bile to a distinct yellow colour and most gastric aspirates are not, the difference in colour can often distinguish the sites (Fig. 32.2).

- Testing the pH of the aspirate at the bedside, auscultation, radiographic film, and colourimetric capnography are methods that have been suggested for verifying tube placement (Caramia, 2018). Results should be used in combination with other indicators with careful assessment of a patient in the clinical setting.
- Obtain repeat radiographic film confirmation if bedside methods create any doubt regarding the location of a tube.

Delegation and Collaboration

The verification of tube placement is the responsibility of the nurse and cannot be delegated to an unregulated care provider (UCP). The nurse directs the UCP to immediately inform the nurse if:

- Patient's respirations change or patient indicates shortness of breath, coughing, or choking.
- Patient vomits or the UCP notices vomitus in the patient's mouth during oral hygiene.
- Nasal skin irritation or excoriation is present.
- Change in the external length of the tube occurs.

Equipment

- 60-mL ENFit syringe
- Stethoscope
- Clean gloves
- pH indicator strip (scale of 1.0 to 11.0)
- Small medication cup
- Tape measure

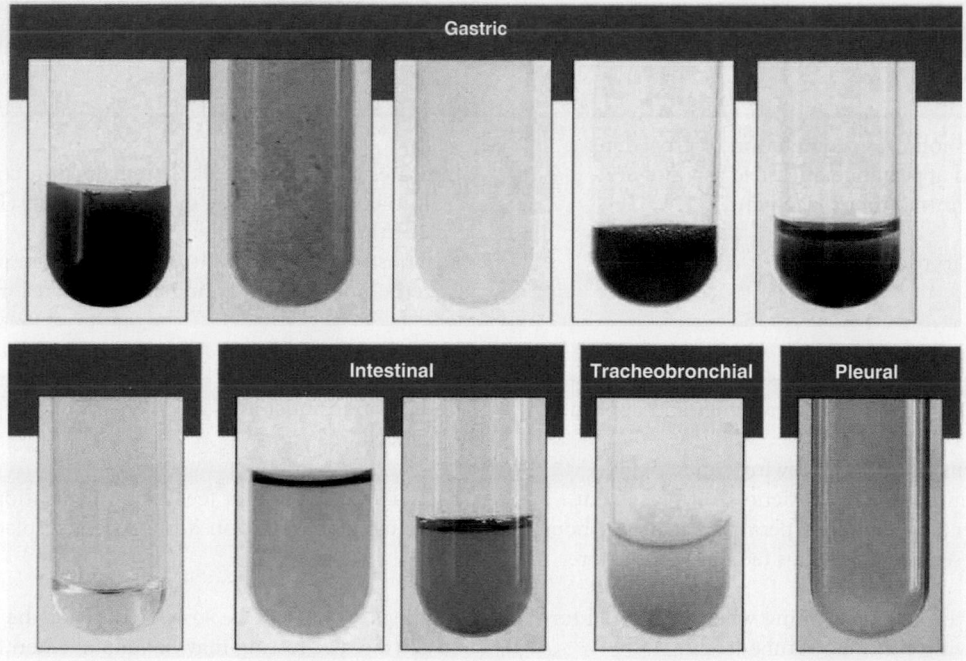

FIG 32.2 Typical colour of aspirates from stomach, intestine, and airway. (*Used with permission from Metheny, N.A., et al. [1998]. pH, color, and feeding tubes. RN, 61, 25.*)

STEP	RATIONALE

ASSESSMENT

1. Review employer policy for frequency and method of checking tube placement. **Do not insufflate air into tube to check placement.**

   Maintains quality of patient care. Listening for air instilled through the tube is unreliable (Atalay et al., 2016).

2. Identify patient using at least two person-specific identifiers (e.g., full name, date of birth, personal identification number) according to employer policy.

   Ensures correct patient. Complies with Accreditation Canada's standards and improves patient safety (Accreditation Canada, 2019).

3. Observe for signs and symptoms of respiratory distress during feeding: coughing, choking, or reduced oxygen saturation.

   Once tube has been correctly placed into the gastrointestinal (GI) tract, movement into the pulmonary system is unlikely. However, a tube that has been pulled back into the esophagus can lead to regurgitation and aspiration of formula.

4. Identify conditions that increase risk for spontaneous tube migration or dislocation: altered level of consciousness, agitation; retching, vomiting; nasotracheal suction.

   Feeding tubes may become dislocated by increases in intra-abdominal pressure or coughing, but most frequently they are displaced when the patient moves or pulls on the tube.

5. Observe and measure the external part of tube for movement of ink mark away from mouth or naris (see Skill 32.1).

   Increased external length of tube indicates that distal tip is no longer in correct position (Lord, 2018, p. 20).

6. Review patient's chart for prescriptions for continuous feeding. Review patient's medication record for a gastric acid inhibitor (e.g., ranitidine) or a proton pump inhibitor (e.g., omeprazole).

   The presence of enteral formula in aspirated secretions diminishes usefulness of pH measurements by buffering pH of the stomach. Similarly, H_2 receptor antagonists reduce acid content of secretions, also raising pH value (Bourgault et al., 2015).

7. Review patient's medical record for history of prior tube displacement.

   Patients are at increased risk for repeated tube displacement.

NURSING DIAGNOSES

- Inadequate gas exchange
- Potential for aspiration

Related factors/Risk factors are individualized on the basis of patient's condition or needs.

STEP	RATIONALE

PLANNING

1. Expected outcomes following completion of procedure:
   • Colour, pH, and appearance of gastric aspirate are consistent with initial tube placement.

   Indicates that tube has likely remained in correct location, initially confirmed by radiographic film (Bourgault et al., 2015).

2. Explain procedure to patient.

   Demonstrates person-centred care, because patient has the right to be informed regarding all procedures. Relieves anxiety.

IMPLEMENTATION

1. Prepare equipment, perform hand hygiene, and apply clean gloves.

   Reduces transmission of microorganisms. Organizes for procedure.

2. Verify tube placement at the following times:
   a. For intermittently tube-fed patients, test placement before each feeding (usually a period of at least 4 hours will have elapsed since previous feeding) and before medications.

   Each administration of feeding or medication can lead to pulmonary aspiration if the tube is displaced.

   b. Follow employer policy regarding when to test pH for patients receiving continuous tube feeding.

   Feedings should not be stopped only for the purpose of pH testing. pH testing may be helpful when feedings are interrupted for procedures or diagnostic studies (American Association of Critical Care Nurses [AACN], 2009; Bourgault et al., 2015). pH testing helps to determine the likelihood that the tube is in the desired location of the stomach (i.e., gastric secretions typically have a pH <5). However, tube feed formula alters the pH of gastric content; therefore, pH testing during continuous feeds may not be reliable (Lord, 2018, p. 19).

   c. Wait to aspirate gastric contents at least 1 hour after medication administration via tube.

   Premature withdrawal of contents will remove unabsorbed medication, reducing dose delivered to patient.

3. If tube feeding is infusing, turn off or place feeding on hold. Clamp or kink feeding tube and disconnect from feeding bag, or for intermittent feedings remove plug at end of tube. Draw up 30 mL of air into a 60-mL ENFit syringe. Flush tube with 30 mL of air before attempting to aspirate fluid. Repositioning patient from side to side is helpful. In some cases, more than one bolus of air is necessary.

   A burst of air helps to aspirate fluid more easily. Smaller syringes generate unnecessarily high pressures inside tube. A 60-mL syringe reduces pressure when flushing tube with air (SHR, 2017).

4. Draw back on syringe slowly and obtain 5 to 10 mL of gastric aspirate (see illustration). Observe appearance of aspirate (see Fig. 32.2). Aspirates from nasogastric (NG) tubes of continuously tube-fed patients often look like curdled enteral formula. Gastric aspirates from intermittently tube-fed patients typically are not bile stained (unless intestinal fluid has refluxed into stomach) (AACN, 2009).

   Drawing back quickly or using a smaller syringe may cause the tube to collapse.
   Quantity is sufficient for pH testing.
   Appearance of aspirate helps to assess position of the tube.

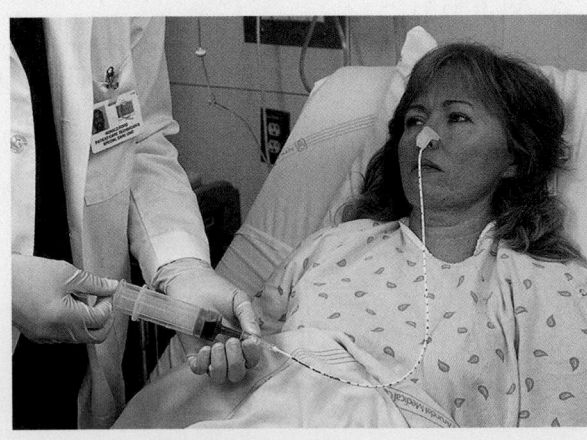

STEP 4 Obtain gastric aspirate.

STEP	RATIONALE

IMPLEMENTATION

5. Gently mix aspirate in syringe. Expel a few drops into a clean medicine cup. Measure pH of aspirated GI contents by dipping pH strip into fluid or applying a few drops of fluid to strip. Compare colour of strip with colour on chart (see illustration) provided by manufacturer.

Mixing ensures equal distribution of contents for testing. The most accurate readings of gastric pH levels are provided by pH paper covering a minimal range from 1.0 to 11.0.

   a. Gastric fluid from a patient who has fasted for at least 4 hours usually has a pH range of less than 5.0.

Using the pH value of 5.0 as the upper cut-off is the safest method for verification of tube location (Caramia, 2018).

   b. Fluid from a tube in the small intestine of a fasting patient usually has a pH ≥7 (Fan et al., 2017)

Intestinal contents are more basic than stomach contents. A pH ≥7 indicates intestinal or pulmonary placement (Fan et al., 2017).

6. If after repeated attempts it is not possible to aspirate fluid from a tube that was confirmed by radiographic and if (1) there are no risk factors for tube dislocation, (2) the tube has remained in the original taped position, and (3) the patient is not in respiratory distress, continue with irrigation (AACN, 2009; Bourgault et al., 2015).

Reports of routine chest or abdominal radiographic films can be used to monitor tube location. Repeat radiographic confirmation of tube position is indicated if external length of tube changes, tape holding the tube comes loose, or patient coughs forcefully or vomits (AACN, 2009; Bankhead et al., 2009).

7. Irrigate tube (see Skill 32.3).

Keeps tube patent.

8. Remove and dispose of gloves and supplies appropriately. Perform hand hygiene.

Reduces transmission of microorganisms.

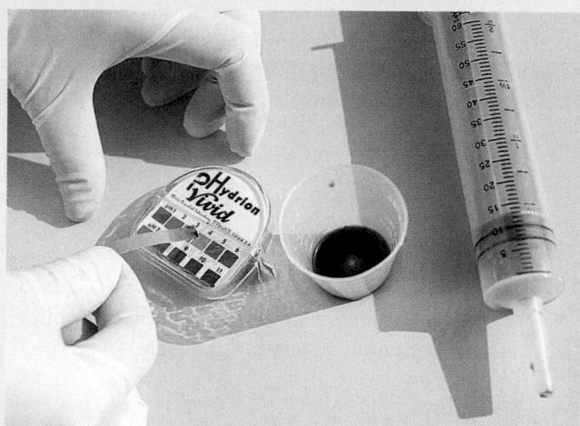 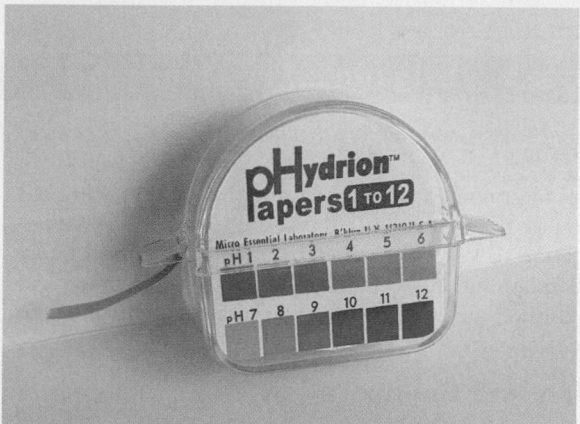

STEP 5 A, Compare colour on test strip with colour on pH chart. **B,** Test strips. (B, *Courtesy of Alia Lagace, University of Manitoba.*)

EVALUATION

1. Observe patient for respiratory distress: persistent gagging, coughing, drop in oxygen saturation, or changes in respiratory patterns (e.g., rate and depth).

Indicates that tube may be displaced in respiratory tract.

2. Verify that external length of tube, pH, and appearance of aspirate are consistent with initial tube placement.

Indicates that tip of tube is likely to be positioned in same place as it was following radiographic film confirmation.

3. **Use Teach-Back:** "I want to go over what I explained earlier. Tell me why it is important for me to test and assess your stomach contents colour and acidity before feedings." Develop a revised teaching plan if patient or caregiver is not able to teach back correctly.

Determines patient's and caregiver's level of understanding of instructional topic.

STEP	RATIONALE

Unexpected Outcomes

1. Red or brown colouring (coffee grounds appearance) of fluid aspirated from feeding tube indicates new or old blood, respectively, in GI tract.
2. Patient develops respiratory distress (e.g., dyspnea, decreased oxygen saturation, increased pulse rate) as a result of aspiration or tube displacement into lung.
3. Tube cannot be irrigated after testing.

Related Interventions

- If colour is not related to medications recently administered, notify health care provider.
- Stop any enteral feedings.
- Notify health care provider.
- Obtain chest radiographic film as prescribed.
- Reattempt to irrigate tube. Do not force fluid. If unsuccessful, notify health care provider.
- Prepare for unclogging procedure based on employer policy.

Communication and Documentation

- Document and report pH value and appearance of aspirate in nurses' notes in electronic health record (EHR) or chart.
- Document your evaluation of patient and caregiver learning.

Special Considerations
Teaching

- Have caregiver or patient demonstrate how to check tube placement while still in health care setting.
- Instruct patient to not pull or alter position of enteral tube.

Pediatric

- Decrease the amount of air insufflated according to patient's size (e.g., an infant may only need 1 mL of air; a small child, 5 mL) before withdrawal of gastric secretions.

Care in the Community

- See Special Considerations, Care in the Community, Skill 32.1.
- Instruct patient or caregiver not to proceed with feedings or medication administration via the tube if there is any doubt as to its correct placement.

◆ SKILL 32.3 Irrigating a Feeding Tube

NSO *Nursing Skills Online Enteral Nutrition Module 16 / Lesson 4*

Feeding tubes must remain patent to ensure that liquid nutritional formulas can pass through easily. All types of feeding tubes require routine irrigation to keep a tube patent. Inability to instill air or fluid suggests that a tube is occluded. Curdled enteral formula and improperly crushed medications are the most common causes of feeding tube occlusion.

Delegation and Collaboration

The skill of irrigating a feeding tube cannot be delegated to an unregulated care provider (UCP). The nurse directs the UCP to:

- Report when a tube feeding stops infusing.

Equipment

- 60-mL ENFit syringe
- Water (tap water or sterile [see employer policy], dated and initialed container at patient's bedside)
- Towel
- Clean gloves
- Stethoscope

STEP	RATIONALE

ASSESSMENT

1. Identify patient using at least two person-specific identifiers (e.g., full name, date of birth, personal identification number), according to employer policy.

2. Perform hand hygiene and apply clean gloves. Inspect volume, colour, and character of gastric aspirates (if obtainable) (see Skill 32.2). Remove and dispose of gloves and perform hand hygiene.

3. Note ease with which tube feeding infuses through tubing.

4. Monitor volume of continuous enteral formula administered during shift and compare with prescribed amount.

5. Refer to employer policy regarding routine irrigation parameters or health care provider's prescription for individual patient needs.

Ensures correct patient. Complies with Accreditation Canada's *Required Organizational Practices (ROP)* and ensures the correct patient receives the intended interventions (Accreditation Canada, 2019).

Determines correct tube placement.

Failure of formula to infuse as desired may indicate developing obstruction.

Indicates whether sufficient volume of feeding is infusing. Serves as baseline to determine tube patency.

Determines frequency of irrigations.

STEP	RATIONALE

NURSING DIAGNOSES

- Reduced fluid volume
- Excessive fluid volume
- Inadequate nutrition: less than body requirements

Related factors are individualized on the basis of patient's condition or needs.

PLANNING

STEP	RATIONALE
1. Expected outcomes following completion of procedure: • Feeding tube remains patent.	Irrigation fluid clears inner lumen of feeding tube of solids and secretions.
• Patient receives prescribed caloric intake.	Feeding infuses without interruption.
2. Explain procedure to patient; stress that you are not removing tube.	Decreases patient anxiety.
3. Position patient in high-Fowler's (if tolerated) or semi-Fowler's position.	Reduces reflux and risk for pulmonary aspiration during irrigation.

IMPLEMENTATION

STEP	RATIONALE
1. Perform hand hygiene, prepare equipment at patient's bedside, and apply clean gloves.	Reduces transmission of microorganisms. Ensures organized approach to irrigation.
2. Verify tube placement (see Skill 32.2) if fluid can be aspirated for pH testing and by verifying external tube length.	With tip of tube correctly placed in stomach or intestine, irrigation will not increase risk for pulmonary aspiration.
3. Irrigate routinely before, between, and after medication administration and before an intermittent feeding is administered.	Certain formulas have properties that predispose to tube clogging. Irrigation prevents mixing of medications in tube, which may cause clogging.
4. Draw up 30 mL of water in ENFit syringe. Patient should have individual bottle of solution.	This amount of solution will flush the length of the tube. Water is the most effective agent for preventing tube clogging.

Clinical Decision Point *Do not use carbonated beverages or fruit juices for flushing tubing.*

STEP	RATIONALE
5. Change irrigation container every 24 hours (according to employer policy).	Ensures clean equipment and solution. Sterile water is required for neonates and patients who are immune suppressed or critically ill (Bankhead et al., 2009; Hockenberry & Wilson, 2015). Tap water is appropriate in many clinical settings and home care if municipal water supply is safe (Bankhead et al., 2009).
6. Kink feeding tube while disconnecting it from administration tubing or while removing plug at end of tube.	Prevents leakage of gastric secretions.
7. Insert tip of ENFit syringe into end of feeding tube. Release kink and slowly instill irrigation solution.	Infusion of fluid clears tubing.
8. If unable to instill fluid, reposition patient on left side and try again.	Tip of tube may be against stomach wall. Changing patient's position may move tip away from stomach wall.
9. When water has been instilled, remove syringe. Reinstitute tube feeding or administer medication as prescribed. Flush each medication completely through tube.	Tubing is clear and patent. Ensures that full dose reaches stomach and medications do not mix with formula.
10. Remove and discard gloves; dispose of supplies in appropriate receptacle. Perform hand hygiene.	Reduces transmission of microorganisms.

EVALUATION

STEP	RATIONALE
1. Observe ease with which tube feeding instills through tubing.	Irrigated tube is patent, allowing for free flow of solution.
2. Monitor patient's caloric intake.	Total enteral nutrition infuses without difficulty.

STEP	RATIONALE

EVALUATION

3. **Use Teach-Back:** "I want to be sure that I explained why you need to flush your tube when you return home. Tell me why it is important to flush your tube." Develop a revised teaching plan if patient or caregiver is not able to teach back correctly.

Determines patient's and caregiver's level of understanding of instructional topic.

Unexpected Outcomes

1. Tube cannot be irrigated and remains obstructed.

2. Fluid and electrolyte imbalances occur. Insufficient irrigation can cause water deficiency; excessive irrigations can cause fluid volume excess.

Related Interventions

- Repeat irrigation; if unsuccessful, notify health care provider.
- There are several methods that can be prescribed to aid in unclogging an obstructed tube—for example, actuated devices, enzymatic mixtures, and warm water (Garrison, 2018, p. 149).
- Tube may need to be removed and a new tube placed.
- Notify health care provider of abnormal electrolyte levels or imbalanced intake and output.

Communication and Documentation

- Document time of irrigation and amount and type of fluid instilled, in nurses' notes in electronic health record (EHR) or chart.
- Report if tubing has become clogged.
- Document your evaluation of patient and caregiver learning.

Special Considerations
Pediatric

- Irrigation of a tube requires a smaller volume of solution in children: 1–2 mL for smaller tubes and 5–15 mL for larger tubes (Hockenberry & Wilson, 2015).

◆ **SKILL 32.4**   **Administering Enteral Nutrition: Nasoenteric, Gastrostomy, or Jejunostomy Tube**

NSO *Nursing Skills Online Enteral Nutrition Module 16 / Lesson 5*

Enteral nutrition, or tube feeding, is a method for providing nutrients to patients who are not able to meet their nutritional requirements orally. As a rule, candidates for enteral nutrition must have a sufficiently functional gastrointestinal (GI) tract to absorb nutrients. Examples of indications for enteral feeding include the following:

- Situations in which normal eating is unsafe because of high risk for aspiration: altered mental status, swallowing disorders, impaired gag reflex, dependence on mechanical ventilation, esophageal conditions (e.g., strictures or dysmotility), and delayed gastric emptying.
- Clinical conditions that interfere with normal ingestion or absorption of nutrients or create hypermetabolic states: surgical resection of oropharynx, proximal intestinal obstruction or fistula, pancreatitis, burns, and severe pressure injuries.
- Conditions in which disease- or treatment-related symptoms reduce oral intake: anorexia, nausea, pain, fatigue, shortness of breath, or depression.

Gastric feedings are the most common type of enteral nutrition, allowing tube-feeding formulas to enter the stomach and then pass gradually through the intestinal tract to ensure absorption. In contrast, small-bowel feeding occurs beyond the pyloric sphincter of the stomach, which reduces the risk for pulmonary aspiration (Lord, 2018, p. 20). General guidelines for timing of delivery of enteral tube feeds are categorized as continuous (typically 25–150 mL delivered continuously anywhere from 12 to 24 hours), intermittent (200–500 mL delivered over 30–90 minutes several times during the day), and bolus (50–100 mL delivered over less than 15 minutes several times a day). Feedings are also delivered by a predetermined method of either pump, gravity, or bolus. Pump feedings run through an enteral infusion pump that controls the rate. Pump feedings are used in situations where continuous feeding is prescribed and in cases of feeding via a small-bowel feeding tube. Gravity feeds are used for gastric feeds that are administered intermittently, where the tube feed formula bag is connected to the feeding tube port and the rate is controlled via a roller clamp along the tubing. Patients who receive gravity feeds have typically demonstrated tolerance of receiving their feed within 30 to 90 minutes. Bolus feeds, delivered by syringe method, are least common as they are instilled more quickly so present a higher risk for abdominal distension. The decision of what type and how much formula is typically determined by the dietitian, based on the patient's fluid, electrolyte, and caloric needs, in collaboration with the interprofessional team. The rule of thumb for initiating a new feed is start low and go slow. The rate and amount will often start low (e.g., 20 mL/hr) for the first 4 hours with instructions to increase the rate based on tolerance until desired amount is being delivered to the patient.

Aspiration of enteral nutrition is a serious complication and is a concern for all patients who receive enteral nutrition. Aspiration is the inhalation of oropharyngeal or gastric contents into the larynx and lower respiratory tract (Peterson, 2016, p. 37). Efforts should be made to prevent or minimize aspiration. AACN (2012) recommends several practices to minimize the risk of aspiration in tube-fed patients:

- Maintain head-of-bed elevation at an angle of 30 to 45 degrees unless contraindicated.
- For patients receiving tube feedings, assess tube placement and GI tolerance at 4-hour intervals.
- Avoid bolus feeding in patients deemed high risk for aspiration.

Delegation and Collaboration

The decision to delegate the skill of administration of nasoenteric tube feeding to an unregulated care provider (UCP) should be made

in accordance with employer policy. A nurse must first verify tube placement and patency. The nurse directs the UCP to:

- Elevate the head of bed to 30 to 45 degrees or sit the patient up in bed or a chair unless contraindicated.
- Not adjust the feeding rate; infuse the feeding as prescribed.
- Report any problems noted infusing the feeding or any discomfort voiced by the patient.
- Report any gagging, coughing, or choking.
- Provide frequent oral hygiene.

Equipment

- Disposable feeding bag, tubing, or ready-to-hang system
- 60-mL or larger ENFit syringe
- Stethoscope
- Enteral infusion pump for continuous feedings
- pH indicator strip (scale 1.0 to 11.0)
- Prescribed enteral formula
- Clean gloves
- ENFit connector

STEP	RATIONALE

ASSESSMENT

1. Identify patient using at least two person-specific identifiers (e.g., full name, date of birth, personal identification number) according to employer policy. | Ensures correct patient. Complies with Accreditation Canada *Required Organizational Practices (ROP)* and ensures the correct patient receives the intended interventions (Accreditation Canada, 2019). |

| 2. Assess patient's clinical status to determine potential need for tube feedings: decreased level of consciousness, nutritional deficits, head or neck surgery, facial trauma, or impaired swallowing. Use interprofessional collaboration to consult with nutrition support team and health care provider. | Identify candidates for enteral nutrition before they become nutritionally depleted. A health care provider's prescription is necessary for feedings. Some institutions in Canada have adopted prescription-writing privileges for registered dietitians. |

| 3. Assess patient for food allergies. | Prevents patient from developing allergic responses to feeding. |

| 4. Perform physical assessment of abdomen, including auscultation for bowel sounds, before feeding (see Chapter 8). | Objective measures for assessing tolerance include changes in bowel sounds, expanding girth, tenderness and firmness on palpation, increasing gastric residual volume (GRV), and vomiting (McCarthy & Martindale, 2015). Report findings to health care provider to determine if tube feeding can proceed safely (Bankhead et al., 2009). |

| 5. Obtain baseline weight and review serum electrolytes and blood glucose level. Assess patient for fluid volume excess or deficit, and metabolic abnormalities. | Enteral feedings should restore or maintain a patient's nutritional status. Measures provide objective data and baseline to determine selection of formula and measure effectiveness of feedings. |

| 6. Verify health care provider's prescription for type of formula, rate, route, and frequency. | Ensures that correct formula will be administered in appropriate volume. Enteral formulas are not interchangeable. |

NURSING DIAGNOSES

- Inadequate nutrition: less than body requirements
- Reduced swallowing
- Readiness for enhanced nutrition
- Potential for aspiration

Related factors/Risk factors are individualized on the basis of patient's condition or needs.

PLANNING

1. Expected outcomes following completion of procedure:
   - Patient achieves established target for body weight and fluid/electrolyte balance over time. | Indicates that patient's nutritional status is maintained or improved. |
   - Patient has no sign of respiratory distress. | Feeding tube does not enter airway, and patient does not aspirate feeding. |
   - Patient is free of abdominal cramping. | Feeding administered without abdominal distension. Demonstrates tolerance of tube feeding. |
2. Explain procedure to patient. | Decreases patient anxiety. |

IMPLEMENTATION

| 1. Perform hand hygiene. Apply clean gloves. | Reduces transmission of microorganisms and potential contamination of enteral formula. |

| 2. Verify correct formula and check expiration date; note integrity of container. | Ensures that correct therapy is administered and checks integrity of formula. |

STEP	RATIONALE

IMPLEMENTATION

3. Prepare formula for administration, following manufacturer guidelines.

   a. Have formula at room temperature.

   Cold formula causes gastric cramping and discomfort because liquid is not warmed by mouth and esophagus.

   b. Use aseptic technique to connect tubing to container as needed. Use proper ENFit connecter and avoid handling feeding system or touching can tops, container openings, spike, and spike port.

   Bag, connections, and tubing must be free of contamination to prevent bacterial growth (Lyman, 2017, p. 198).

   c. Shake formula container well. Clean top of canned formula with alcohol swab before opening it (Bankhead et al., 2009).

   Ensures integrity of formula; prevents transmission of microorganisms.

   d. For a closed system connect administration tubing to container. If using an open system, pour formula from Tetra Pak or can into administration bag (see illustration).

   Formulas are available in closed-system containers that contain a 24- to 48-hour supply of formula or in an open system, in which formula must be transferred from Tetra Paks or cans to a bag before administration.

4. Prime the tubing set by opening the roller clamp and allowing administration tubing to fill with formula. Clamp off tubing with roller clamp. Hang container on intravenous (IV) pole.

   Prevents introduction of air into stomach once feeding begins.

5. Place patient in high-Fowler's position or elevate head of bed at least 30 degrees (preferably 45 degrees). For a patient required to remain supine, place in reverse Trendelenburg's position, which raises head.

   Elevated head helps prevent pulmonary aspiration.

6. Verify tube placement (see Skill 32.2).

   Verifies if tip of tube is in stomach or intestine.

   a. *Nasoenteric tube:* Attach ENFit syringe and aspirate gastric contents. Observe appearance of aspirate and note pH. Measure external tube length and compare with patient record.

   Gastric fluid for patient who has fasted for at least 4 hours usually has pH of 1.0 to 4.0 (especially when patient is not receiving gastric acid inhibitor).

   b. *Gastrostomy tube:* Attach ENFit syringe and aspirate gastric contents. Observe appearance of aspirate and note pH.

   Continuous administration of tube feeding elevates pH (Simons & Abdallah, 2012). Noting the external length helps determine possible tube dislodgement (Lord, 2018, p. 20).

   c. *Jejunostomy tube:* Attach syringe and aspirate intestinal secretions. Observe appearance; if significant amounts are returned or resemble gastric secretions, check pH. Note the tube position by measuring external length or noting the outer measurement markings on the tube are consistent with the patient's medical record.

   Presence of intestinal fluid indicates that end of the tube is in the small intestine. If fluid tests acidic on pH test or looks like gastric fluid, tube may be displaced into the stomach.

   Noting the external length helps determine possible tube dislodgement (Lord, 2018, p. 20).

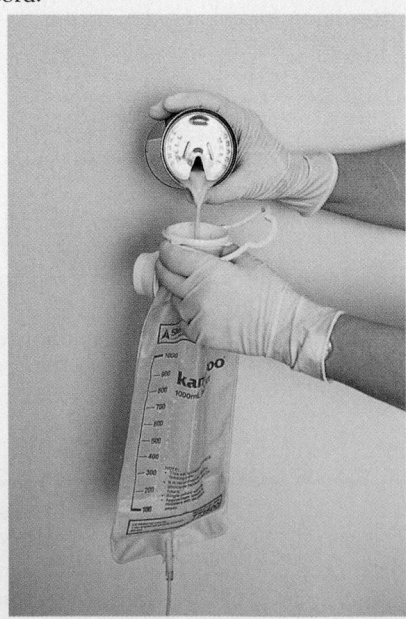

STEP 3d Pour formula into open feeding container.

STEP	RATIONALE

IMPLEMENTATION

7. Check GRV according to employer policy.

GRV determines if gastric emptying is delayed. Intestinal residual is usually very small. If intestinal feeding residual volume is greater than 10 mL, displacement of tube into stomach may have occurred.

  a. Draw up 10 to 30 mL air into ENFit syringe and connect to end of feeding tube. Inject air slowly into tube. Pull back slowly and aspirate total amount of gastric contents you can aspirate.

GRV may not be easy to obtain from small-bore feeding tube. A 60-mL syringe should be used to aspirate (Best, 2017).

  b. Return aspirated contents to stomach slowly unless volume exceeds 250 mL (see employer policy) (Patel et al., 2017).

Prevents loss of nutrients and electrolytes in discarded fluid. Some questions exist regarding safety of returning high volumes of fluid into stomach (Patel et al., 2017).

  c. GRVs in range of 200 to 500 mL should raise concern and lead to implementation of measures to reduce risk of aspiration. Automatic cessation of feeding shouldn't occur for GRV less than 500 mL in absence of other signs of intolerance (McCarthy et al., 2015; WRHA, 2017a, p. 12).

Elevated GRV should raise concern and lead to additional measures to reduce risk of aspiration (e.g., elevating the head of bed, regular oral hygiene care, use of prokinetic medications (Lord, 2018, p. 29; McCarthy & Martindale, 2015).

  d. Flush feeding tube with 30 mL water (see Skill 32.3).

Prevents clogging of tubing.

8. Intermittent feeding (administered at certain times during the day):

  a. Pinch proximal end of feeding tube and remove cap. Connect distal end of administration set tubing to ENFit device on feeding tube and release tubing.

Prevents leakage of gastric contents. Ensures that feeding will be administered into correct tubing (ISMP, 2015).

  b. Set rate by adjusting roller clamp on tubing (see illustration) or attach tubing to feeding pump. Allow bag to empty gradually over 30 to 45 minutes (length of time of a comfortable meal). Label bag with tube-feeding type, strength, and amount. Include date, time, and your initials.

Gradual emptying of tube feeding reduces risk for abdominal discomfort, vomiting, or diarrhea induced by bolus or too-rapid infusion of tube feedings. Labelling provides means to determine when to change administration set and confirms that patient is receiving the correct feeding.

Clinical Decision Point *Use pumps designated for tube feeding, not IV fluids.*

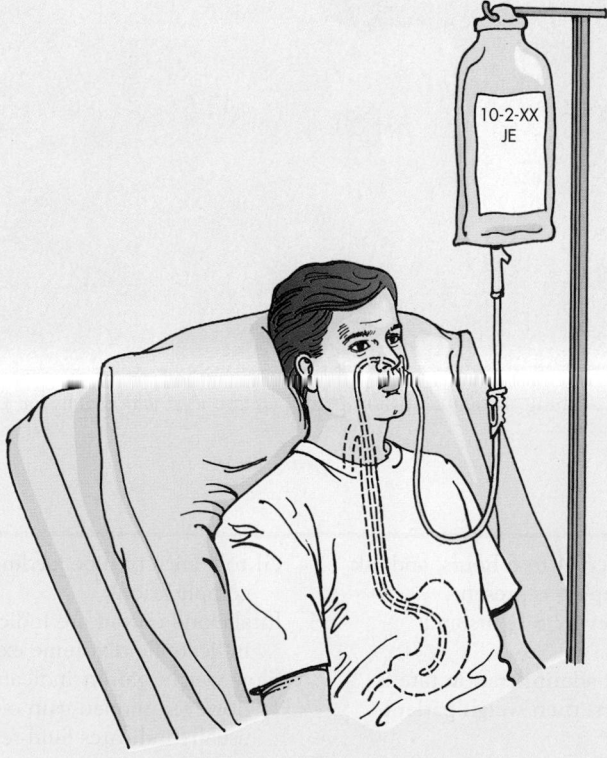

10-2-XX
JE

STEP 8b Administer intermittent feeding.

STEP	RATIONALE

IMPLEMENTATION

c. Immediately follow feeding with water (per health care provider's prescriptions and employer policy). Cover end of feeding tube with cap when not in use. Keep bag as clean as possible. Change administration set every 24 hours.

Prevents tube from clogging. Limits microbial contamination of system.

9. Continuous infusion method:

Method delivers prescribed hourly rate of feeding and reduces risk for abdominal discomfort.

a. Remove cap on tubing and connect distal end of administration set tubing to feeding tube using ENFit connector as in Step 8a.

Prevents leakage of gastric contents.

b. Thread tubing through feeding pump; set rate on pump and turn on (see illustration).

Delivers continuous feeding at steady rate and pressure. Feeding pump sounds alarm for increased resistance.

c. Advance rate of tube feeding (and concentration of feeding) gradually, as prescribed.

Tube feeding can usually begin with full-strength formula. Conservative initiation and advancement of enteral nutrition depend on factors such as patient's age, medical condition, nutritional status, and expected patient tolerance (Kozeniecki & Frtizshall, 2015).

Clinical Decision Point *Maximum hang time for formula is 12 hours in an open system; 24 to 48 hours in a closed, ready-to-hang system (if it remains closed). Refer to manufacturer guidelines and employer policy for specific guidelines on hang times (Malhi, 2017, pp. 11–12).*

10. After feeding, flush tubing with 30 mL water every 4 hours during continuous feeding (see employer policy) or before and after an intermittent feeding. Have dietitian prescribe total free-water requirement per day and obtain health care provider's prescription (see Skill 32.3).

Provides patient with source of water to help maintain fluid and electrolyte balance. Clears tubing of formula.

11. Rinse bag and tubing with warm water whenever feedings are interrupted.

Rinsing bag and tubing with warm water clears old tube feedings and reduces bacterial growth.

12. Dispose of supplies and perform hand hygiene.

Reduces transmission of microorganisms.

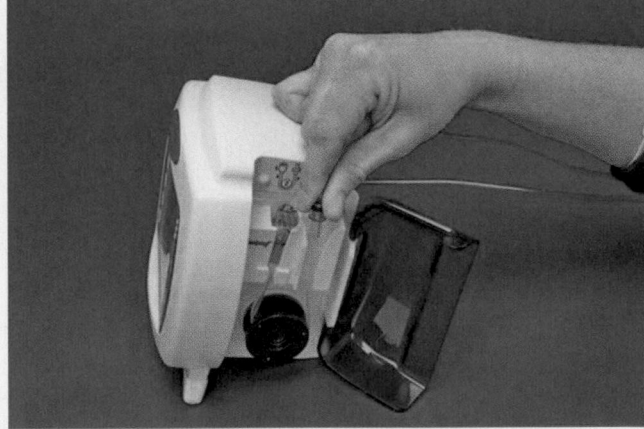

STEP 9b Connect tubing through infusion pump. (*Image used with permission Covidien. All rights reserved.*)

EVALUATION

1. Measure GRV per policy, usually every 4 to 6 hours, and ask patient if nausea or abdominal cramping is present.

GI tolerance of tube feedings must be monitored closely to avoid complications.

2. Monitor intake and output at least every 8 hours and calculate daily totals every 24 hours.

Intake and output are indications of fluid balance, which can indicate fluid volume excess or deficit.

3. Weigh patient daily until maximum administration rate is reached and maintained for 24 hours; then weigh patient three times per week.

Slow weight gain is indicator of improved nutritional status; however, sudden gain of more than 0.9 kg (2 lb) in 24 hours usually indicates fluid retention.

STEP	RATIONALE

EVALUATION

4. Monitor laboratory values as prescribed by health care provider.

Determines correct administration of formula rate and strength.

5. Observe patient's respiratory status.

Change in respiratory status may indicate aspiration of tube feeding into respiratory tract. Symptoms may include coughing, dyspnea, tachypnea, change in oxygen saturation, crackles, and hoarseness.

6. Examine abdomen and auscultate bowel sounds.

Evaluates status of gastric emptying and peristalsis.

7. For gastrostomy tubes, inspect site for signs of impaired skin integrity and symptoms of infection, injury, or tightness of tube (see Procedural Guideline 32.1).

Enteral tubes can cause pressure and excoriation at insertion site.

8. Observe nasoenteral tube insertion site at least daily (see employer policy). Note skin integrity and look for edema under device, excoriation, or presence of injury.

Allows for early detection of excoriation that can progress to a medical device–related pressure injury.

9. **Use Teach-Back:** "I want to be sure that I explained to you what you need to look for that means you're not tolerating your tube feeding. Tell me two signs you can look for that may mean you are not tolerating your tube feedings well." Develop a revised teaching plan if patient or caregiver is not able to teach back correctly.

Determines patient's or caregiver's level of understanding of instructional topic.

Unexpected Outcomes	Related Interventions
1. Feeding tube becomes clogged.	• Attempt to flush tube with warm water. • Special products are available for unclogging feeding tubes; do not use carbonated beverages and juices. • Hold feeding and notify health care provider. • Maintain patient in semi-Fowler's position. • Contact pharmacist to change medications to liquid form and flush before and after intermittent feedings and administering of medications (Kozeniecki & Fritzshall, 2015).
2. Patient develops large amount of diarrhea (more than three loose stools in 24 hours).	• Notify health care provider. • Use interprofessional collaboration (e.g., dietitian) to discuss need to change formula to prevent malabsorption. • Identify and treat underlying medical or surgical issues and infections (Kozeniecki & Fritzshall, 2015). • Provide perianal skin care after each stool. • Determine other causes of diarrhea (e.g., *Clostridium difficile* infection, contaminated tube feeding, medications containing sorbitol).
3. Patient develops nausea and vomiting.	• Administer antiemetic as prescribed. • Use prescribed medications to increase gastric motility. • Withhold tube feeding and notify health care provider. • Aspirate for residual.
4. Patient aspirates formula (auscultation of crackles or wheezes, dyspnea, or fever).	• Report change in condition to health care provider. • Position patient on side. • Suction nasotracheally or orotracheally.

Communication and Documentation

• Document amount and type of feeding, infusion rate, method of infusion, patient's response to tube feeding (e.g., GRV, cramping, bowel sounds, patency of tube, condition of skin at tube site) in nurses' notes in electronic health record (EHR) or chart.
• Document volume of formula and any additional water given on intake and output form.
• Report type of feeding, status of feeding tube, patient's tolerance, and adverse outcomes.
• Document your evaluation of patient and caregiver learning.

Special Considerations
Teaching

• Instruct patients and caregivers not to reconnect lines that have separated but to seek clinical assistance.
• Teach patient and caregiver that, if tolerated, patient should remain upright for 1 hour after feedings.
• Instruct patient or caregiver that patient may express feelings of fullness, increased gas, belching, or diarrhea.
• Teach patient or caregiver how to determine correct placement of feeding tube (see Skill 32.2).

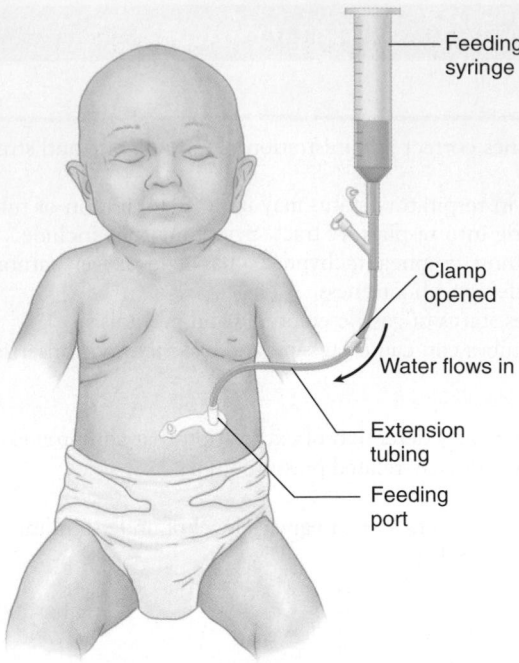

FIG 32.3 Infant being syringe fed.

Pediatric

- Preterm infants who are at risk for necrotizing enterocolitis frequently receive minimal enteral feeding (MEF) to limit stress on the GI tract. Use of breast milk for the MEF in premature infants reduces sepsis and necrotizing enterocolitis and improves patient outcomes (Cortez, Makker, Kraemer, et al., 2018).
- Infants who require MEF are sometimes fed using the syringe method while the parent or caregiver holds them to normalize the process and aid in bonding. The syringe can be held lower or higher to achieve the desired rate of instillation that the baby can tolerate (Fig. 32.3).

Gerontological

- Some older persons have decreased gastric emptying; therefore, formula remains in the stomach longer than for younger patients. GRV checks are especially important in patients with impaired cognition to decrease the risk for pulmonary aspiration.

Care in the Community

- See Special Considerations, Skill 32.1.
- Instruct patient or caregiver on technique for administering feedings in the home and proper storage and refrigeration of supplies.
- Instruct patient or caregiver about any symptoms or discomfort that may occur during enteral feedings. Reinforce instruction to contact health care provider if symptoms of discomfort occur.
- Teach patient or caregiver how to perform skin care around the gastrostomy or jejunostomy tube and signs and symptoms of infection at insertion site (see Procedural Guideline 32.1).

PROCEDURAL GUIDELINE 32.1 *Care of a Gastrostomy or Jejunostomy Tube*

Feeding tubes can be placed directly into the gastrointestinal (GI) tract through the abdominal wall in patients who cannot tolerate nasoenteric feeding tubes or require long-term (greater than 4–6 weeks) enteral nutrition. The stomach (gastrostomy tube) and jejunum (jejunostomy tube) are the most common sites for long-term feeding tubes. Long-term tubes require endoscopic, radiological, or surgical placement (Lord, 2018, p. 21). The insertion method used to place tubes may call for specific nursing interventions in the postinsertion period; but otherwise these tubes are used in a similar way to other feeding tubes. Feedings delivered via a gastrostomy tube are relatively safe to administer, provided the patient has normal gastric emptying. Gastrostomy tubes are often called G *tubes*; but they are also commonly referred to as *percutaneous endoscopic gastrostomy (PEG) tubes*, a term used to describe tubes placed endoscopically. Gastrostomy tubes range in size from 12 to 30 French (Fr) (Lord, 2018, p. 21) and exit through an incision/stoma in the upper left quadrant of the abdomen, where an internal bumper or balloon and an external bumper or disk hold the tube in place (Fig. 32.4).

Once the stoma tract is well formed, balloon gastrostomy tubes are replaced by specially trained nurses on the unit every 6 months (or as needed due to leaking, damage, or breakage of device).

Jejunostomy tubes are indicated when the risk of regurgitation and aspiration is especially high, as in cases of severely delayed gastric emptying or conditions such as pancreatitis that limit use of the stomach for feeding. They tend to be smaller in diameter at 5–16 Fr (Lord, 2018, p. 25). They can be placed directly into the small intestine in a surgical procedure or threaded through

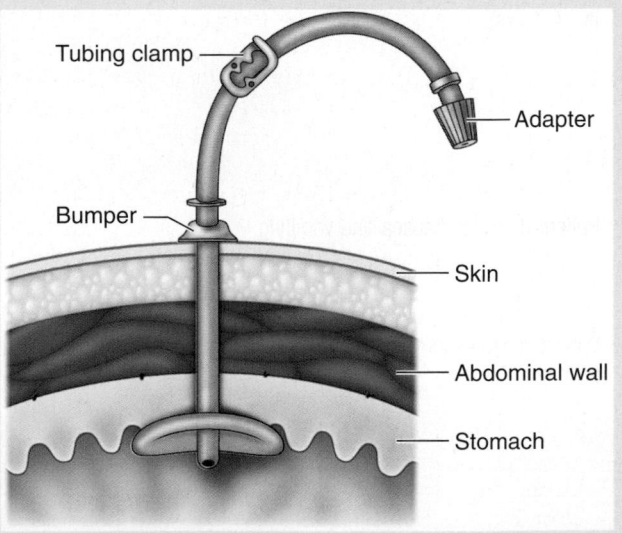

FIG 32.4 Placement of PEG tube into stomach.

the stomach into the jejunum under fluoroscopy. Some jejunal tubes inserted through this transgastric approach are dual-channel devices that have openings in both the stomach and the small-intestine part of the tube. These *combination tubes*, as they are called, allow simultaneous gastric decompression and intestinal feeding for patients with impaired gastric emptying or upper-GI cancers. Each lumen of a combination tube is clearly

PROCEDURAL GUIDELINE 32.1 *Care of a Gastrostomy or Jejunostomy Tube—cont'd*

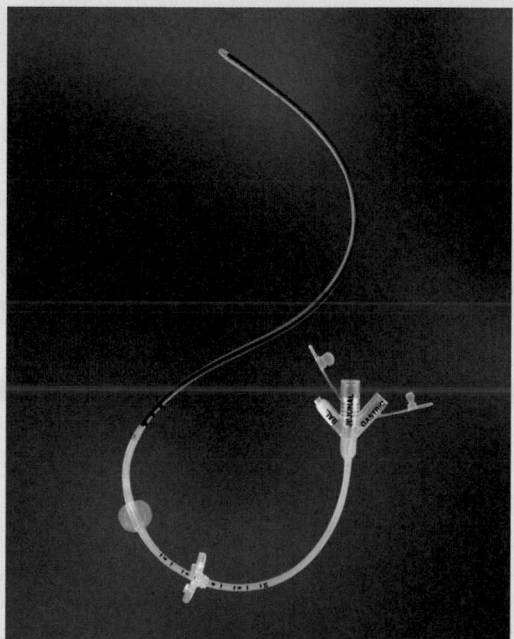

FIG 32.5 Dual lumen "combination tube" to allow jejunal feeding and gastric decompression. (*Image used with permission Kimberly-Clark Health Care. All rights reserved.*)

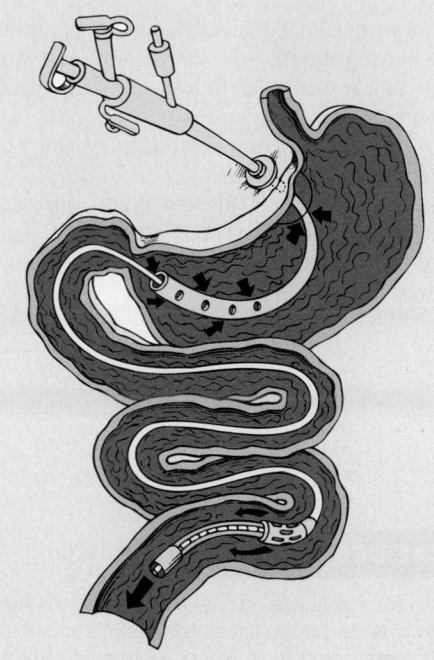

FIG 32.6 Endoscopic insertion of jejunostomy tube.

labeled to distinguish between the gastric and the jejunal ports (Fig. 32.5).

Sometimes a jejunostomy tube is placed through an existing PEG tube. The percutaneous endoscopic jejunostomy (PEJ) tube is passed through the PEG tube and advanced into the jejunum (Fig. 32.6). The PEJ tube occupies the lumen of the PEG tube; this tube-through-a-tube design does not allow drainage of the stomach during small-intestine feeding. In the case of both combination tubes and PEJ tubes, the nurse must know whether the intended site for formula delivery is gastric or jejunal to ensure safe and effective nutritional care.

For the first 48 to 72 hours after a new gastrostomy or jejunostomy tube is placed, the stoma tract is considered a surgical wound and is therefore to be cleaned using sterile technique. Postplacement (48–72 hours), with a noninfected stoma, clean technique of warm soap and water can be practised daily and the stoma may be left open to air.

For the first 4 weeks following stoma creation and tube insertion, the external bolster remains fairly tight against the abdomen and should generally not be adjusted. After 4 weeks, the external bolster on a gastrostomy/jejunostomy tube should be positioned approximately 0.5 to 1 cm (0.2 to 0.4 inches) from the patient's skin to prevent device-related pressure injury. Additionally, once the stoma site has healed and matured the tube should be gently rotated daily, 360 degrees, to prevent adhesion (WRHA, 2017a, p. 13).

Low-profile devices, sometimes referred to as *buttons*, are gastrostomy tubes that sit almost flush up against the patient's abdomen (Lord, 2018, p. 23). These types of devices are especially good for use in children or confused adults who may be inclined to pull on a longer tube (WRHA, 2017a, p. 8; Lord, 2018, p. 23).

Delegation and Collaboration

Care of a PEG or PEJ tube cannot be delegated to an unregulated care provider (UCP) (refer to employer policy). The nurse directs the UCP to:

- Inform the nurse of any patient indications of discomfort at the insertion site.
- Inform the nurse of any drainage on the insertion site dressing.

Equipment

- Normal saline, dated and initialed container at patient's bedside
- 10 × 10–cm (4 × 4–inch) gauze
- Prepared drain-gauze dressing
- Tape
- Clean gloves

Procedural Steps

1. Determine whether the exit site is left open to air or if a dressing is indicated. Check health care provider's prescription or verify employer policy.
2. Identify patient using at least two person-specific identifiers (e.g., name and date of birth or name and medical record number) according to employer policy.
3. Perform hand hygiene and apply clean gloves.
4. Remove old dressing. Fold dressing with drainage contained inside; remove gloves inside-out over dressing. Discard in appropriate container.
5. Assess exit site for evidence of tenderness, leakage, swelling, excoriation, infection, bleeding, or excessive movement (more than 6 mm [1/4 inch]) of the tube in or out of the stomach.
6. Clean skin around stoma site with warm water and mild soap or saline (according to employer policy) with 10 × 10–cm

Continued

PROCEDURAL GUIDELINE 32.1 *Care of a Gastrostomy or Jejunostomy Tube—cont'd*

(4 × 4–inch) gauze. (If drainage is present, apply clean gloves.) Clean, starting next to the stoma site, and work outward using circular strokes. Carefully clean under external bolster.

7. Rinse and dry site completely.
8. Apply a thin layer of protective skin barrier to exit site, if indicated (e.g., site excoriated).
9. If dressing is prescribed, place a drain-gauze dressing over external bar or disk. **NOTE:** Do not place dressing under external bar; this can cause gastric tissue erosion or internal abdominal wall pressure.

10. Secure dressing with tape.
11. Place date, time, and your initials on new dressing.
12. Remove gloves and dispose of supplies in appropriate receptacle. Perform hand hygiene.
13. Evaluate condition of site routinely (see employer policy).
14. Document in nurse's notes in electronic health record (EHR) or chart appearance of the exit site, drainage noted, and dressing application.
15. Report to health care provider any exit site complications.

✦ CLINICAL DEBRIEF

A 72-year-old male patient was admitted to the acute stroke unit following a cerebral hemorrhage. He has left-sided paralysis and is sometimes not responsive to verbal commands. He recognizes his family and at times has spoken a few words. The patient has been made NPO. The nutrition support team has recommended that he have a small-bore nasogastric feeding tube inserted for nutritional support. A continuous tube feeding of Isosource HN has been prescribed to run at 55 mL/hr.

1. The patient is now ready for his nasogastric tube insertion. Place the following steps in the correct order.
   1. Have patient swallow sips of water while advancing tube past nasopharynx.
   2. Perform hand hygiene.
   3. Tape or clip tube to gown to prevent pulling.
   4. Secure tube to nose.
   5. Measure to determine length of tube to be inserted.
   6. Apply pulse oximeter and measure vital signs.
   7. Obtain radiographic film to determine proper tube placement.
2. Before the patient's first feeding, the nurse aspirates a gastric residual volume of 150 mL. What is the correct nursing action? *(Select all that apply.)*
   1. Consult the dietitian.
   2. Stop the feeding immediately.
   3. Continue tube feeding as prescribed.
   4. Discard the fluid withdrawn through the tube.
   5. Continue to assess for feeding tolerance.
3. The patient has received feedings for about 12 hours. Four hours ago, the gastric residual volume (GRV) was 200 mL. The nurse is conducting rounds and finds the patient nauseated. Approximately 60 mL of vomitus is in the patient's emesis basin at the bedside. The nurse assesses the patient's abdomen to find it tender to touch and distended. Bowel sounds are decreased. The nurse aspirates 300 mL of gastric contents that have the appearance of formula. How does the nurse communicate this situation using SBAR?

✦ REVIEW QUESTIONS

1. Which of the following is the most reliable method of verifying the location of blindly inserted feeding tubes?
   1. pH testing of fluid withdrawn through the tube
   2. Auscultating over the epigastrium while instilling air through the tube

   3. Observing the colour and appearance of fluid aspirated through the tube
   4. Obtaining radiographic confirmation of tube placement
2. A nurse is preparing to set up enteral nutrition on a patient. What does the nurse need to use for patient safety?
   1. A Luer-Lok syringe
   2. A regular catheter tip syringe
   3. An ENFit connector
3. Which responsibilities can a nurse delegate to an unregulated care provider (UCP)? *(Select all that apply.)*
   1. Checking respirations or patient symptoms of shortness of breath, coughing, or choking
   2. Verifying tube placement
   3. Performing oral hygiene
   4. Inspecting skin around the insertion site for irritation or excoriation

ⓔ *Visit the Evolve site for a complete list of Clinical Debrief and Review Questions answers.*

REFERENCES

Accreditation Canada. (2019). *Required organizational practices handbook—Version 14.* Retrieved from http://www.wrha.mb.ca/extranet/eipt/files/EIPT-34-005.pdf

American Association of Critical Care Nurses (AACN). (2009). *Verification of feeding tube placement (blindly inserted).* Retrieved from https://seeiuc.org/wp-content/uploads/files/pdf/recursos/profesional/Colocacion_Sonda_de_Nutricion_AACN.pdf

American Association of Critical Care Nurses (AACN). (2012). Practice alerts 2012: Prevention of aspiration. *Critical Care Nurse, 32*(3), 71.

Atalay, Y. O., Aydin, R., Ertugrul, O., Gul, S. B., Polat, A. V., & Paksu, M. S. (2016). Does bedside sonography effectively identify nasogastric tube placements in pediatric critical care patients? *Nutrition in Clinical Practice, 31*(6), 805–809. doi:10.1177/0884533616639401

Bankhead, R., Boullata, J., Brantley, S., Corkins, M., & Guenter, P., ASPEN Board of Directors. (2009). ASPEN enteral nutrition practice recommendations. JPEN. *Journal of Parenteral and Enteral Nutrition, 33*(2), 122–167. doi:10.1177/0148607108330314

Bennetzen, L., Håkonsen, S., Svenningsen, H., & Larsen, P. (2015). Diagnostic accuracy of methods used to verify nasogastric tube position in mechanically ventilated adult patients: A systematic review. *JBI Database of Systematic Reviews and Implementation Reports, 13*(1), 188–223. doi:10.11124/jbisrir-2013-1179

Best, C. (2017). How to set up and administer an enteral feed via a nasogastric tube. *Nursing Standard, 31*(45), 42–47. doi:10.7748/ns.2017.e10509

Bourgault, A. M., Heath, J., Hooper, V., Sole, M. L., & Nesmith, E. G. (2015). Methods used by critical care nurses to verify feeding tube placement in clinical practice. *Critical Care Nurse, 35*(1), e1–e7. doi:10.4037/ccn2015984

Canadian Patient Safety Institute (CPSI). (2009). *The safety competencies: Enhancing patient safety across the health professions*. Retrieved from http://www.patientsafetyinstitute.ca/en/toolsResources/safetyCompetencies/Documents/Safety%20Competencies.pdf

Caramia, R. (2018). Commentary on "Intracranial placement of a nasogastric tube in non-trauma patient". *Journal of Intensive and Critical Care, 4*(1), 5. doi:10.21767/2471-8505.100108

Cortez, A., Makker, K., Kraemer, D., Neu, J., Sharma, R., & Hudak, M. (2018). Maternal milk feedings reduce sepsis, necrotizing enterocolitis and improve outcomes of premature infants. *Journal of Perinatology, 38*(1), 71–74. doi:10.1038/jp.2017.149

Dharmalingam, T., & Gunasekaran, V. (2016). Overcoming a difficult nasogastric tube insertion procedure with a video laryngoscope (C-Mac ®). *Indian Journal of Critical Care Medicine: Peer-Reviewed, Official Publication of Indian Society of Critical Care Medicine, 20*(12), 751–752.

Fan, E., Tan, S., & Ang, S. (2017). Nasogastric tube placement confirmation: Where we are and where we should be heading. *Proceedings of Singapore Healthcare, 26*(3), 189–195. doi:10.1177/2010105817705141

Garrison, C. M. (2018). Enteral feeding tube clogging: What are the causes and what are the answers? A bench top analysis. *Nutrition in Clinical Practice, 33*(1), 147–150. doi:10.1002/ncp.10009

Hockenberry, M. J., & Wilson, D. (2015). *Wong's nursing care of infants and children* (10th ed.). St. Louis: Elsevier.

Institute for Safe Medication Practices (ISMP). (2013). *Safety bulletin: Some liquid medications may be unsuitable for administration by enteral tube*. Retrieved from https://www.ismp-canada.org/download/safetyBulletins/2013/ISMPCSB2013-05_LiquidMedicationsEnteralTube.pdf

Institute for Safe Medication Practices (ISMP). (2015). *Safety Alert: ENFit enteral devices are on their way… Important safety considerations for hospitals*. Retrieved from https://www.ismp.org/newsletters/acutecare/showarticle.aspx?id=105

Kozeniecki, M., & Fritzshall, R. (2015). Enteral nutrition for adults in the hospital setting. *Nutrition in Clinical Practice, 30*(5), 634–651.

Lord, L. M. (2018). Enteral access devices: Types, function, care, and challenges. *Nutrition in Clinical Practice, 33*(1), 16–38. doi:10.1002/ncp.10019

Lyman, B. (2017). Enteral feeding set handling techniques: A comparison of bacterial growth, nursing time, labor, and material costs. *Nutrition in Clinical Practice, 32*(2), 193–200. doi:10.1177/0884533616680840

Malhi, H. (2017). Enteral tube feeding: Using good practice to prevent infection. *British Journal of Nursing: BJN, 26*(1), 8–12. doi:10.12968/bjon.2017.26.1.8

McCarthy, M. S., & Martindale, R. G. (2015). What's on the menu? Delivering evidence-based nutritional therapy. *Nursing, 45*(8), 36.

McFarland, A. (2017). A cost utility analysis of the clinical algorithm for nasogastric tube placement confirmation in adult hospital patients. *Journal of Advanced Nursing, 73*(1), 201–216. doi:10.1111/jan.13103

Mizzi, A., Cozzi, S., Beretta, L., Greco, M., & Braga, M. (2017). Real-time image-guided nasogastric feeding tube placement: A case series using Kangaroo with IRIS technology in an ICU. *Nutrition, 37*, 48–52. doi:10.1016/j.nut.2016.09.002

National Pressure Ulcer Advisory Panel (NPUAP). (2013). *Best practices for prevention of medical device–related pressure ulcers*. Retrieved from http://www.npuap.org/wp-content/uploads/2013/04/Medical-Device-Poster.pdf

Patel, J., Lemieux, M., McClace, S., Martindale, R., Hurt, R., & Heyland, D. (2017). Critical care nutrition support best practices: Key differences between Canadian and American guidelines. *Nutrition in Clinical Practice, 32*(5), 633–644. doi:10.1177/0884533617722165

Peterson, A. M. (2016). Aspiration pneumonia in the elderly tube fed patient—avoidable or unavoidable? Considerations for the LNC. *Journal of Legal Nurse Consulting, 27*(3), 36–40.

Saskatoon Health Region (SHR). (2017). *Policies and procedures: Enteral tube feedings*. Retrieved from https://www.saskatoonhealthregion.ca/about/NursingManual/1020.pdf

Simons, S. R., & Abdallah, L. M. (2012). Bedside assessment of enteral tube placement: Aligning practice with evidence. *The American Journal of Nursing, 112*(2), 40–46. doi:10.1097/01.NAJ.0000411178.07179.68

Wallace, S. C., & Gardner, L. A. (2015). Misplacements of enteral feeding tubes increase after hospitals switch brands. *The American Journal of Nursing, 115*(8), 44–46. doi:10.1097/01.NAJ.0000470401.28683.de

Winnipeg Regional Health Authority (WRHA). (2017a). *Adult enteral nutrition practice guideline*. Retrieved from http://www.wrha.mb.ca/extranet/eipt/files/EIPT-34-005.pdf

Winnipeg Regional Health Authority (WRHA). (2017b). *Manitoba home nutrition program—operational directive*. Retrieved from http://www.wrha.mb.ca/prog/nutrition/files/ManitobaHomeNutritionProgram-FINALapprovedAugust92017.pdf

33 | Parenteral Nutrition

Written by **Felicia Schaps, MSN-Ed, RN, CRNI, OCN, CNSC, IgCN, and Rachel Ollivier, RN, PhD(c)**

SKILLS AND PROCEDURES

OBJECTIVES

Mastery of content in this chapter will enable the nurse to:

- Describe the purpose and components of parenteral nutrition (PN).
- Identify patients who are candidates for PN.
- Discuss risks associated with PN.

- List the monitoring procedures used for patients receiving PN.
- Identify measures used to prevent complications of PN.
- Demonstrate appropriate nursing care and use of safe precautions when caring for a patient receiving PN.

MEDIA RESOURCES

- evolve http://evolve.elsevier.com/Canada/Perry/clinicalskills/
- Review Questions

- ▶ Video Clips
- Audio Glossary
- Clinical Debrief and Review Questions Answers

PURPOSE

Parenteral nutrition (PN) is a specialized form of nutritional support that is given intravenously by an infusion pump to patients who are unable to receive nutrients, such as food, by mouth or through the digestive system (Worthington, Balint, Bechtold, et al., 2017). For example, PN may be appropriate for patients recovering from bowel surgery, a bowel obstruction, or severe malnutrition (refer to Box 33.1 for a complete list of indications). PN may be referred to as total parenteral nutrition (TPN) or total nutrient admixture (TNA). In addition, PN meets long-term nutritional needs with infusions in the community if gastrointestinal (GI) issues are expected to be long term (months to years) (Box 33.1).

STANDARDS OF CARE

- Infusion Nurses Society (INS), 2016—*Infusion Therapy Standards of Practice* (http://source.yiboshi.com/20170417/1492425631944540325.pdf)
- Institute for Safe Medication Practices (ISMP), 2015—*Safe Practice Guidelines for Adult IV Push Medications* (https://www.ismp.org/guidelines/iv-push)
- O'Grady, Alexander, Dellinger, et al., 2002—*Guidelines for the Prevention of Intravascular Catheter-Related Infections* (https://www.cdc.gov/mmwr/preview/mmwrhtml/rr5110a1.htm)

PRINCIPLES FOR PRACTICE

- Peripheral parenteral nutrition (PPN) can be used for patients who are experiencing mild or moderate malnutrition for up to

weeks, as long as the formula has a final dextrose concentration of 5 to 10% and amino acid content of 3% (Alexander, Corrigan, Gorski, et al., 2014; Phillips, 2014).
- For patients with short-term GI dysfunction, the goal is to provide nutritional requirements while minimizing PN-related complications until patients can resume full oral diets or meet their needs with enteral tube feedings. PN is not intended for the purpose of meeting hydration or fluid needs (Guenter, Worthington, Ayers, et al., 2018).
- The type of catheter to use for administration of PN depends on patient factors and the expected length of PN therapy. The location of the catheter is defined on the basis of where the distal tip of the catheter lies. Concentrated PN solutions are diluted quickly when infused into a large-diameter central vein (Fig. 33.1).
- Patients who self-administer their PN solutions in the community will require a central catheter, which may be an implanted subcutaneous port, a peripherally inserted central catheter (PICC), or a tunnelled central access device (Fig. 33.2; see Chapter 29).
- Patients who require PN infusions do so for medical or surgical conditions that are often associated with GI losses (e.g., obstruction, diarrhea, fistula) and organ dysfunction; therefore, electrolyte monitoring is paramount. Thus, a typical laboratory panel relative to PN infusions would include a baseline assessment of electrolytes, serum proteins, complete blood count, triglyceride level, and liver function tests (Box 33.2).
- The components of the PN solution are amino acids, glucose, and lipids as energy sources, with the addition of electrolytes, minerals, trace elements, vitamins, and water. The addition of

BOX 33.1

Indications for Parenteral Nutrition

Nonfunctional GI Tract
- Small-bowel resection
- Small-bowel surgery or GI bleed
- Paralytic ileus
- Intestinal obstruction
- Trauma to abdomen, head, or neck
- Severe malabsorption
- Intolerant of slow rates of enteral tube feeding
- Chemotherapy, radiation therapy, bone marrow transplantation
- Severely catabolic patients when GI tract is not functioning for more than 7 days

Nonfunctional GI Tract
- Enterocutaneous fistula
- Inflammatory bowel disease
- Severe diarrhea
- Moderate-to-severe pancreatitis

Preoperative Parenteral Nutrition
- Preoperative bowel rest
- Severe malnutrition before surgery

GI, Gastrointestinal tract.

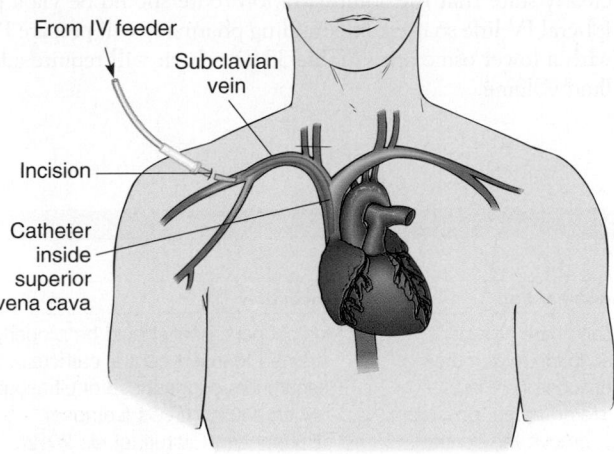

FIG 33.1 Placement of central venous catheter inserted into subclavian vein. *IV,* Intravenous. *(Courtesy Rolin Graphics.)*

BOX 33.2

Typical Monitoring and Laboratory Prescriptions for Patients With Parenteral Nutrition

Monitor
- Fluid intake, urine and gastrointestinal output every 8 hours
- Vital signs every 4 hours
- Body weight at least three times weekly

Initial and Repeated Weekly
- Complete metabolic panel with sodium (Na), potassium (K), chloride (Cl), carbon dioxide (CO_2), glucose, calcium (Ca), phosphate (PO_4), magnesium (Mg), triglycerides, transaminases, liver function
- Complete blood count (CBC) with hemoglobin, hematocrit, white blood count (WBC), red blood cells (RBCs), lymphocyte count
- Serum proteins, often including albumin, transferrin, C-reactive protein, and/or prealbumin

Daily Until Stable
- Electrolyte panel daily until stable, then weekly
- Glucose every 6 hours until within normal limits for 48 hours, then daily
- Glucose in preparation for cyclic parenteral nutrition (PN) in the community; monitor 2 hours after PN begins and 2 hours after PN ends; adjust insulin per prescriptions

Monthly or Biannually
- Trace elements such as zinc, copper, manganese, selenium (depending on underlying condition such as gastrointestinal issue or malabsorption) and for long-term community PN
- Selected vitamins for long-term community PN patients

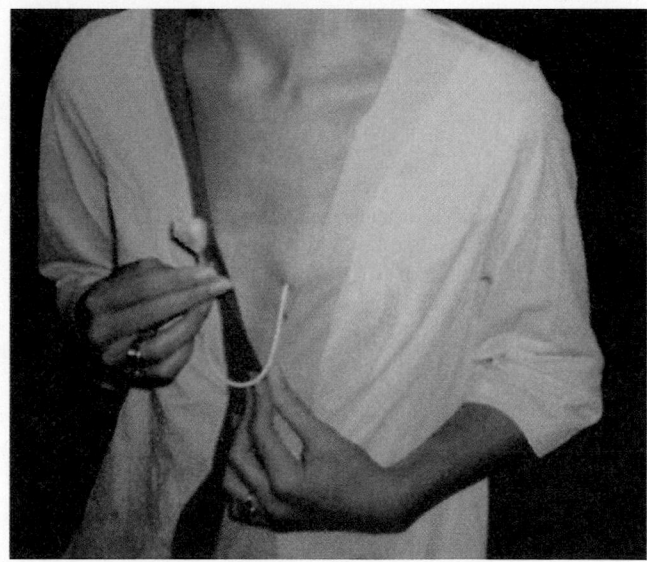

FIG 33.2 Tunnelled catheter used for home central parenteral nutrition. *(From Morgan, S. L., & Weinsier, R. L. [1998]. Fundamentals of clinical nutrition [2nd ed.]. St. Louis: Mosby.)*

lipid emulsion to the PN solution results in a preparation called a *3:1, 3-in-1,* or *TNA.*
- Because hyperglycemia has been linked to increased infection rates, monitoring blood glucose levels during a PN infusion is important. If possible, PN should not be interrupted for routine care or patient transport for diagnostic studies (Guenter et al., 2018, p. 298).
- When the goal is to prepare a patient for a cyclic infusion of PN in the community, it is very important to monitor glucose levels approximately 2 hours after an infusion begins (peak level) and 2 hours after it ends (trough level) to evaluate the need for adding regular human insulin to the infusion bag.
- Since a PN solution is typically provided in response to GI issues and to support nutritional needs, it is important to monitor data that describe patient progress (see Box 33.2). Measurement of intake and output is very important to document when a patient's GI function is changing and to provide information regarding the adequacy of fluid intake from the PN solution.

PERSON-CENTRED CARE

- Include the patient and caregiver in discussions and decisions, to promote person-centred care with patient autonomy, activities of daily living, individualized care planning, and socialization with friends and loved ones.
- Nurses collaborate with nutrition support teams and health care providers in administering PN and monitoring patients' response to PN therapy. Although practice patterns vary across employers, typically, dietitians or pharmacists provide advice on nutrition

support goals and write PN prescriptions in collaboration with other members of the health care team.

- PN may pose concerns for self-identified members of ethnic groups or people with philosophical, religious, or spiritual beliefs that include restriction of animal products. The components of PN are largely synthetic and do not contain pork. The lipid emulsion contains egg phospholipid, a product that may not be appropriate for vegan patients.
- It is important to be considerate of the sense of loss that a patient may experience when unable to consume food, which can be culturally tied for some patients.

EVIDENCE-INFORMED PRACTICE

When critically ill patients cannot tolerate enteral nutrition, PN provides an alternative route for nutritional delivery. PN has a decreased infection rate when it is initiated early rather than later in their care (Worthington et al., 2017). Key evidence-informed practice guidelines for management of critically ill patients in critical care units (CCUs) include the following (Taylor, McClave, Martindale, et al., 2016; Worthington et al., 2017):

- Enteral nutrition is preferred over PN for nutritional support (see Chapter 32).
- If the patient was healthy before this critical illness, with no evidence of protein calorie malnutrition, use of PN should be reserved and initiated only after the first 7 days of hospitalization (Worthington et al., 2017), when enteral nutrition is not available.

- PN should be initiated only if the duration of administration is anticipated to be greater than or equal to 7 days.
- In patients stabilized on PN, efforts should be made to reintroduce oral or enteral nutrition.
- PN should not be terminated until at least 50% of nutritional needs are being met by the oral or enteral route (Worthington et al., 2017).

SAFETY GUIDELINES

- Although the use of PN is an important technological advance that has allowed improved care for patients with GI issues, a number of complications are associated with the therapy. The most frequent complication is catheter-related bloodstream infection (CRBSI), a risk found in both hospitalized patients and those with PN in the community (Table 33.1). It is essential that appropriate care of the vascular access device, dressing, and site is instituted to minimize CRBSI, including avoiding blood draws and interruption of the infusions (INS, 2016; O'Grady, Alexander, Dellinger, et al., 2002) (see Chapter 29).
- Centrally administered PN (CPN) using concentrated dextrose solutions should not be infused into a peripheral intravenous (IV) or midline catheter because of the increased risk for phlebitis. If only peripheral lines are available, the prescriptions should clearly state that the administration route should be via a peripheral IV line so the compounding pharmacy will prepare PPN with a lower osmolarity (Table 33.2), which will require added fluid volume.

TABLE 33.1

Complications of Parenteral Nutrition

Problem	Cause	Symptoms	Immediate Action	Prevention
Pneumothorax	Tip of catheter enters pleural space during insertion, causing lung to collapse	Sudden chest pain, difficulty breathing, decreased breath sounds, cessation of normal chest movement on affected side, tachycardia	Per health care provider's prescription (e.g., nurse practitioner, certified registered nurse, physician) may remove the central catheter. Administer oxygen. Insert chest tube to remove air under water-seal drainage or dry one-way valve system.	Medical personnel should be properly trained to insert central catheters. Researchers suggest use of ultrasound when placing CVCs (Lamperti, Bodenham, Pittiruti, et al., 2012). Catheter should be secured properly to prevent migration and movement.
Air embolism	IV tubing disconnected; part of catheter system open or removed without being clamped	Sudden respiratory distress: decreased oxygen saturation levels, shortness of breath, coughing, chest pain, decreased blood pressure	Clamp catheter; position patient in left Trendelenburg's position; call health care provider; administer oxygen as needed (INS, 2016).	Make sure that all catheter connections are secure; clamp catheter when not in use. Never use a stopcock with a CVC. Unless contraindicated, instruct patient in Valsalva manoeuvre for tubing changes (INS, 2016).
Localized infection (exit site or tunnel)	Poor aseptic technique in removal of skin flora during site preparation and dressing care	*Exit site:* Erythema, tenderness, induration, or purulent drainage within 2 cm (0.8 inches) of skin at exit site. *Tunnel:* Same as above but extends beyond 2 cm from exit site	Call health care provider. *Exit:* Apply warm compress, provide daily care of site, give oral antibiotics. *Infection:* Collaborate with health care provider regarding removal of catheter (INS, 2016). *Tunnel:* Remove catheter.	Provide catheter site care using aseptic technique, visually inspect site (including cleaning site), applying new stabilization device, and applying sterile dressing (INS, 2016). Change transparent dressings at least every 5–7 days and gauze dressings every 48 hours (INS, 2016). Change dressing if damp, loosened, or soiled or when inspection of site is necessary (INS, 2016). Use chlorhexidine wipes to cleanse site (INS, 2016).

TABLE 33.1

Complications of Parenteral Nutrition—cont'd

Problem	Cause	Symptoms	Immediate Action	Prevention
Catheter-related sepsis or bacteremia	Catheter hub contamination; contamination of infusate; spread of bacteria through bloodstream from distant site	*Systemic:* Isolation of same microorganism from blood culture and catheter segment, with patient showing fever, chills, malaise, elevated white blood cell count	*Systemic:* Do not exceed hang time of 24 hours for PN that contains dextrose and amino acids either alone or with fat emulsion added as a 3-in-1 formulation (INS, 2016). Administer antibiotics intravenously; remove catheter per prescription.	Use full sterile-barrier precautions during catheter insertion and dressing change (INS, 2016). Do not disconnect tubing unnecessarily. Replace IV tubing and filter every 24 hours. In some selected situations it is necessary to change administration sets with each new PN container (INS, 2016).
Hyperglycemia	Possible blood-draw error, confirm with bedside glucose device; patient receiving too little insulin in PN solution; receiving steroids; new-onset infection	Excessive thirst, urination, blood glucose greater than 8.9 mmol/L, confusion	Call health care provider for prescription; may need to slow infusion rate.	Review medical history for blood drawn through central line with PN infusing (repeat peripheral blood draw or obtain reading using finger lancet device), glucose intolerance or diabetes, new infection, new medication such as steroids; keep rate as prescribed; never increase PN to "catch up." Maintain blood glucose in range prescribed by health care provider. Use aseptic technique and routine blood glucose monitoring.
Hypoglycemia	PN abruptly discontinued; too much insulin	Patient is shaky, dizzy, nervous, anxious, hungry; blood glucose level less than 4.4 mmol/L	Call health care provider; if PN discontinued abruptly, may need to restart D₁₀W at previous PN rate (check employer policy). Perform blood glucose monitoring; retest in 15 to 30 minutes.	Decrease PN, "tapering" gradually until discontinued; blood glucose monitoring is used to ensure adequate insulin.

CVC, central venous catheter; *IV*, intravenous; *IV*, intravenous; *PN*, parenteral nutrition.

TABLE 33.2

Comparison of Central Versus Peripheral Parenteral Nutrition Prescriptions

	Central Parenteral Nutrition	Peripheral Parenteral Nutrition
Osmolality	>600 mOsm/L	<900 mOsm/L (Worthington et al., 2017, p. 236)
Route of administration	Central venous catheter	Small peripheral vein
Usual daily caloric intake	20–35 calories/kg/day	5–10 calories/kg/day
Usual daily volume (mL)	1 000–2 000	2 000–3 000
Fat emulsion	Minor caloric source	Major caloric source

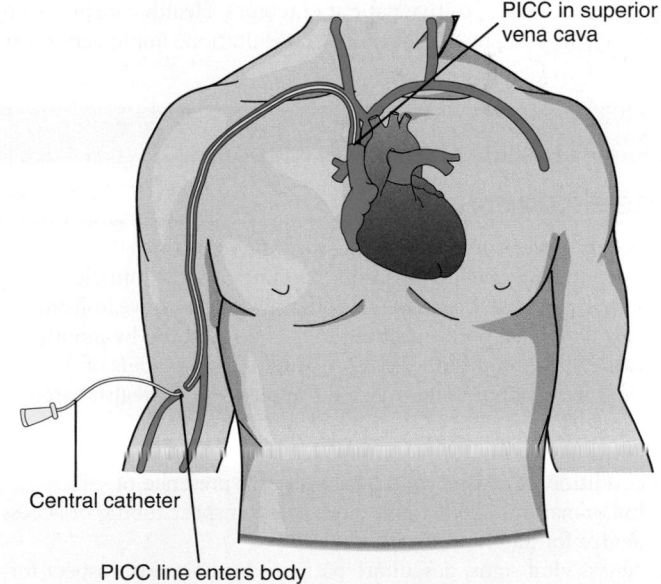

FIG 33.3 Peripherally inserted central catheter (PICC).

- PPN is used only for very short-term situations (maximum of 10–14 days) or when there is the need for very low caloric requirements (Worthington et al., 2017). It is difficult to meet total nutrient requirements with PPN because of the limitation of dextrose concentration peripherally and the inability to meet caloric goals without large volumes of solution.
- Many hospitals use PICCs, termed *PICC lines* (Fig. 33.3), which are typically placed by specially trained advanced vascular access teams or radiologists.
- Following central venous catheter insertion, PN should not be initiated until placement of a venous catheter tip is confirmed

by a radiograph or through the use of electrocardiographic (ECG) tip verification technology (INS, 2016).
- Appropriate aseptic technique is needed when handling the central line, dressings, tubing, and the needleless end cap PN port (see Skill 29.6).

- PN without lipids can be infused using tubing with a 0.20- or 0.22-micron filter, and lipid-containing emulsions (3-in-1) can be infused using a larger 1.2-micron filter (INS, 2016). A filter is necessary because it prevents particulate matter or large droplets of lipid from entering a patient, which could potentially result in a pulmonary embolism.
- In very malnourished patients, during a process termed *refeeding syndrome,* some electrolytes (e.g., potassium [K], magnesium [Mg] and phosphorus [P]) may shift intracellularly with glucose provided in the PN, potentially resulting in low serum levels with risk for arrhythmias and muscle weakness. Adequate electrolyte repletion should occur before the initiation of PN. There is an increased risk of pulmonary edema and heart failure when initiating feeding in malnourished patients at greater risk of refeeding syndrome.
- Since there is a risk of bloodstream infection in patients with catheters, regular monitoring of temperature and the catheter insertion site is important.

✦ SKILL 33.1   Administering Central Parenteral Nutrition

Administration of parenteral nutrition (PN) through a central line (CPN) requires the use of strict aseptic technique and application of critical thinking. Because of the composition of PN fluids, patients can experience metabolic and fluid balance changes quickly. In addition, the clinical condition of patients receiving CPN may be poor, especially when they have alterations in host defenses, severe underlying illnesses, and extremes of age. Nurses need to anticipate changes in a patient's condition that signal developing complications. Similarly, nurses need to use good judgment to maintain the intravenous (IV) system and ensure that it is functioning properly.

Delegation and Collaboration

The skill of administering PN to a hospitalized patient cannot be delegated to an unregulated care provider (UCP). The nurse directs the UCP to:
- Report when the pump sounds an alarm, or if the patient has shortness of breath or headaches, is feeling weakness or shaky, or has discomfort or bleeding at the IV site.
- Measure urinary output and weigh the patient per employer policy.

In addition, interprofessional collaboration is essential to improving and promoting positive patient outcomes. Health care providers involved in assessment, diagnosis, consultation, implementation, procedures, monitoring, and evaluation may include registered nurses, licensed (registered) practical nurses, nurse practitioners, dietitians, social workers, physicians, surgeons, and pharmacists, to name a few. These professions may comprise the nutritional support team.

Equipment

- Medication administration record (MAR) or computer printout
- PN solution (IV)
- Electronic infusion device (EID) with anti–free-flow control and alarms (INS, 2016)
- IV infusion tubing with Luer-Lok tip
- Appropriate IV filter (1.2-micron filter for 3-in-1 solutions or lipids containing a membrane that is particulate retentive and air eliminating; 0.20-micron filter for solutions that do not contain lipids) (INS, 2016).
- 5- to 10-mL syringe with sterile saline flush
- Bedside glucose monitoring kit
- Adhesive tape or tubing label
- Antimicrobial swab
- Clean gloves
- Stethoscope

STEP	RATIONALE

ASSESSMENT

1. Assess indications of and risks for protein/calorie malnutrition: weight loss from baseline or ideal, muscle atrophy or weakness, edema, lethargy, failure to wean from ventilatory support, chronic illness, and nothing by mouth (NPO) for more than 7 days. Confer with members of interprofessional team, such as the dietitian or health care provider.	These are clinical indications for PN. These baseline details provide a baseline from which change can be noted (Alexander et al., 2014).
2. Perform hand hygiene. Apply clean gloves as needed. Inspect condition of central vein access site for presence of inflammation, edema, and tenderness. Inspect tubing of access device for patency and kinking.	Reduces transmission of infection. Identifies early signs of infection, infiltration, or disruption in system integrity. Development of complication contraindicates infusion of fluids and indicates need to establish new IV site.
3. Assess vital signs, auscultate patient's lung sounds, inspect for edema of extremities, and measure patient's weight.	Provides baseline for monitoring patient's response to fluid infusion and nutrients. Crackles in lungs are early indication of fluid volume excess.
4. Assess medical record for levels of serum albumin, total protein, transferrin, prealbumin, and triglycerides and check blood glucose level by finger lancet. Remove gloves and perform hand hygiene.	Provides baseline for measuring patient's nutritional status. In addition, nutritional baseline identifies patient's unique requirements, and PN admixture is tailored to patient's specific needs (Alexander et al., 2014).
	Serum glucose determines patient's baseline, and tolerance of high levels of glucose in PN solution.
	Reduces transmission of microorganisms.

STEP	RATIONALE

ASSESSMENT

5. Assess patient's medical history for factors influenced by PN administration: electrolyte levels, and renal, cardiac, and hepatic function. Assess for history of allergies.

Some patients require that CPN therapy be adapted by composition or volume (requires health care provider prescription), based on medical history. PN includes constituents (e.g., medications) to which patient may be allergic.

6. Consult with primary health care provider or nurse practitioner, pharmacist, and dietitian on calculation of calorie, protein, and fluid requirements for patient. Physicians and dietitians often work together to form specific prescriptions, although it is essential that interprofessional collaboration is implemented in patient care.

Provides interdisciplinary plan for patient's nutritional support.

7. Verify prescription for nutrients, minerals, vitamins, trace elements, electrolytes, added medications, and infusion rate. Check for compatibility of added medications.

CPN is often prescribed daily in a hospital setting after review of laboratory values. In a community setting prescriptions may be obtained less frequently (e.g., weekly). Pharmacies that prepare parenteral solutions will check medication compatibility.

8. Assess patient's and caregiver's knowledge of PN, including any previous experience with community management.

Determines level and extent of instruction required.

NURSING DIAGNOSES

- Inadequate nutrition
- Insufficient fluid volume
- Excessive fluid volume
- Potential for unstable blood glucose level
- Potential for infection
- Insufficient knowledge regarding PN purpose and home management

Related factors/Risk factors are individualized on the basis of patient's condition or needs.

PLANNING

1. Expected outcomes following completion of procedure:
   - Patient's ideal weight gain is between 0.5 and 1.5 kg (1 to 3 lb) per week.

Weight is indicator of patient's nutritional status and determines fluid volume. Weight gain greater than 0.5 kg (1 lb) per day indicates fluid retention.

   - Blood glucose levels are maintained per health care provider's prescription for desired glucose range.

Glucose levels needed for specific populations differ on the basis of degree of illness, so a specific health care provider prescription is required (McClave, Taylor, Martindale, et al., 2016).

   - Central venous access device (CVAD) is patent, and site is free of pain, swelling, redness, purulent drainage, and inflammation.

Ensures that PN is infusing into vein rather than into surrounding tissues and that there are no signs of an access device infection.

   - Patient is afebrile.

Shows absence of systemic infection.

   - Patient and caregiver are able to discuss purpose and steps for care of PN.

Proper instruction informs patient and caregiver and prepares for community care if needed.

2. Explain purpose of PN to patient. Ensure that the patient and caregiver have the opportunity to ask questions or seek further information or clarification.

Promotes person-centred care through understanding of and involvement in their care plan and treatment.

3. If PN solution is refrigerated, remove from refrigeration 1 hour before infusion.

Ensures that solution will be administered at room temperature.

IMPLEMENTATION

1. Perform hand hygiene.

Reduces transmission of microorganisms.

2. Check label on PN bag with health care provider's prescription on MAR or computer printout and patient's name. Also check any additives and note solution expiration date. Steps 2–6 may require an independent double-check by another registered nurse, depending on employer policy.

Prevents medication error. ***This is the first check for accuracy.***

3. Inspect 2:1 PN solution for particulate matter; inspect 3:1 PN solution for separation of fat into layer.

Presence of particulate matter or fat emulsion separation requires that solution be discarded.

STEP	RATIONALE

IMPLEMENTATION

4. Before leaving medication room, check IV solution a second time using the 10 rights of medication administration (see Chapter 20), including route and rate of delivery. Check label of PN bag against MAR or computer printout.

This is the second check for accuracy.

5. Identify patient using at least two person-specific identifiers (e.g., name and date of birth, or name and medical record number) according to employer policy. Compare identifiers with information on patient's MAR or medical record.

Ensures correct patient. Complies with Accreditation Canada's standards and improves patient safety (Accreditation Canada, 2019).

6. Take PN solution to patient in advance of previous solution emptying. Compare names of solution and additives with MAR at bedside.

This is the third check for accuracy.

7. Apply clean gloves. Prepare IV tubing for PN solution:
   a. Attach appropriate filter to IV tubing.
   b. Prime tubing with PN solution, making sure that no air bubbles remain, and turn off flow with roller clamp (see Chapter 29). Some infusion pumps and IV tubing require that priming be done on the pump rather than by gravity.

Maintains sterility of solution. Air introduced into central circulation could result in air embolus, a fatal IV complication.

8. Wipe end port of CVAD with alcohol swab, allow to dry, then attach syringe of 0.9% normal saline (NS) solution to needleless port, aspirate for blood return, and flush saline per employer policy.

Scrubbing hub decreases amount of microorganisms (Alexander et al., 2014; INS, 2016). Determines patency of IV device before infusing PN.

9. Remove syringe. Trace tubing to the body before making the connection (Guenter et al., 2018, p. 299). Connect Luer-Lok end of PN IV tubing to end port of CVAD; for multi-lumen lines, label tubing used for PN.

Ensures that tubing is securely connected to IV line. A dedicated line should be used for multi-lumen devices. Labelling of high-risk catheters prevents connection with inappropriate tube or catheter.

10. Place IV tubing in EID. Open roller clamp. Set and regulate infusion rate as prescribed (see illustration). Depending on employer policy, infusion rate, as per the prescription, may need to be double-checked by another nurse.

PN infusion rates are prescribed to meet patient's metabolic and electrolyte needs. Maintaining rates prevents electrolyte imbalances.

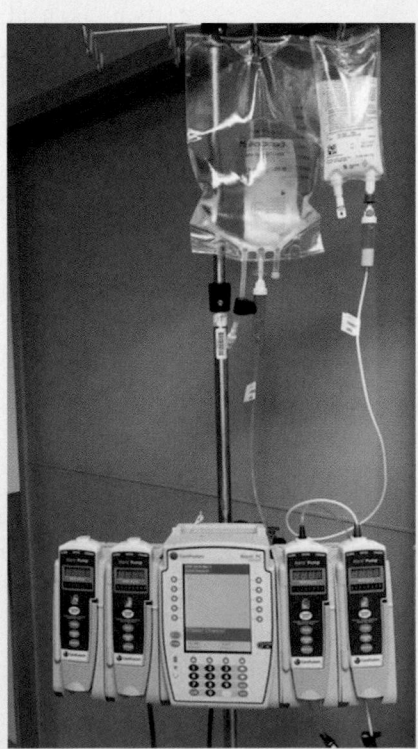

STEP 10 Parenteral nutrition solution infusing via infusion pump. *(Photo by Russell Flores, Vancouver General Hospital.)*

STEP	RATIONALE

IMPLEMENTATION

a. *Continuous infusion (optional):* Infusion rate is immediately set at prescribed rate and given over 24-hour period.

Ensures that blood glucose levels are maintained to prevent hypoglycemia or hyperglycemia (Alexander et al., 2014).

b. *Cycle infusion (optional):* Infusion rate is initiated at about 40 to 60 mL/hr, and the rate is gradually increased until patient's nutritional needs are met. Before completion of infusion, rate is decreased at about the same millilitre per hour until the CPN is completed. The infusion is usually given over a shorter time frame (12 to 18 hours).

Infusion rates are usually increased and decreased to prevent hypoglycemia or hyperglycemia, respectively (Alexander et al., 2014).

11. Infuse all IV medications or blood through alternative IV site or multi-lumen device. Do not obtain blood samples or central venous pressure readings through same lumen used for CPN.

Prevents drug incompatibility and IV device occlusion (Alexander et al., 2014).

12. Do not interrupt CPN infusion (e.g., during showers, transport to procedure, blood transfusion), and be sure that rate does not exceed prescribed rate (Guenter et al., 2018).

Prevents development of catheter-related bacteremia (INS, 2016).

13. PN containing dextrose and amino acids alone or with fat emulsion added as a 3:1 formulation should have a hang time not to exceed 24 hours. Fat emulsions alone should have a hang time not to exceed 12 hours.

Prevents bacterial infection and deterioration of emulsion (INS, 2016).

14. Change IV administration sets for PN every 24 hours and immediately on suspected contamination. Discard used supplies and perform hand hygiene.

Reduces transmission of infection.

EVALUATION

1. Monitor and document infusion rate according to employer policy. If infusion is not running on time, do not attempt to catch up; report this to the health care provider.

Too-rapid or too-slow infusion could result in metabolic disturbances such as hyperglycemia and fluid overload.

2. Monitor fluid intake and urine and gastrointestinal (GI) fluid output every 8 hours.

Prevents fluid imbalance from too-slow or too-rapid infusion.

3. Measure vital signs every 4 hours or as per employer policy.

Monitors for fluid overload response.

4. Obtain initial weight, and then weigh at least three times weekly.

Routine measurement of weights will reflect a gain/loss resulting either from caloric intake or fluid retention. Gradual weight gain, if weight gain is the goal, indicates adequate tolerance.

5. Evaluate for fluid retention; palpate skin of extremities; auscultate lung sounds.

Weight gain in excess of 0.5 kg (1 lb)/day, dependent edema, lung crackles, and intake greater than output per each 24-hour period indicate fluid retention.

6. Monitor patient's glucose levels every 6 hours or as prescribed and other laboratory parameters daily or as prescribed.

Maintenance of normal electrolyte levels, satisfactory fluid balance, acceptable serum glucose levels, and improvement in serum proteins indicate adequate tolerance of PN.

7. Inspect central venous access site for signs and symptoms of swelling, inflammation, drainage, redness, warmth, tenderness, or edema.

Determines IV patency and absence of infection, infiltration, or phlebitis.

8. Monitor for temperature, elevated white blood cell count, and malaise.

Signs of systemic infection.

9. **Use Teach-Back:** "I want to be sure that you know what to look out for. What signs and symptoms should you report to the nurse or doctor?" Develop a revised teaching plan if patient or caregiver is not able to teach back correctly, including the purpose for receiving PN.

Determines patient's or caregiver's level of understanding of instructional topic.

Unexpected Outcomes

1. Redness, swelling, and tenderness are visible around the central venous access site, indicating possible exit site infection.

Related Interventions

- Notify health care provider.
- Apply a warm compress and initiate daily site care as prescribed.
- Systemic antibiotic therapy may be started.

STEP	RATIONALE

EVALUATION

2. Patient develops fever, malaise, and chills, indicating systemic infection.	• Check exit site for signs of infection. • Notify health care provider and consult about need to obtain cultures of exit site or blood. • Systemic antibiotic therapy may be started.
3. Serum glucose level is greater than 8.3 mmol/L or target set by health care provider.	• Notify health care provider. • Indicates intolerance of glucose load in PN solution. • May indicate new-onset infection. • Verify that blood was not drawn with PN infusing or that proper procedures to interrupt PN and discard first blood draw were followed. • Possible need for addition of insulin to PN, modification of PN solution, or sliding-scale insulin coverage.

Communication and Documentation

- Document condition of CVAD, rate and type of infusion, catheter lumen used for infusion, intake and output (I&O), blood glucose levels, vital signs, and weights in nurses' notes in electronic health record (EHR) or chart.
- If signs of infection, occlusion, fluid retention, or infiltration occur, notify the health care provider.
- Document your evaluation of patient and caregiver learning.

Special Considerations
Teaching

- Instruct patient and caregiver in the purpose and goals of CPN. Keep them informed about daily care of the central line and progress with treatment.
- Inform patient of signs of central line infection to report to the nurse.

Pediatric

- Consider children's developmental needs when they are on long-term CPN. Perform regular assessments of development to determine child's progress. Implement interventions to encourage expected milestones (Hockenberry & Wilson, 2015).

Gerontological

- Some older persons have impaired ability to tolerate higher fluid volumes because of cardiac or renal impairment.

Care in the Community

- Patients requiring long-term CPN benefit from a referral to a community nutrition therapy team.
- Patients should have a home safety and physical, nutritional,

and psychological needs assessment conducted, if appropriate (INS, 2016).

- Patients receiving home CPN may have a peripherally inserted central catheter (PICC) line (see Fig. 33.3) or a tunnelled or implanted catheter (see Fig. 33.2) to reduce the possibility of infection. Patients or caregivers need to learn to perform catheter site care, dressing changes, techniques for connecting and disconnecting PN solutions, and infusion pump management.
- Some patients receive home CPN at night during sleep (cyclic TPN) to allow the freedom to leave home during the day. Some patients may also take an oral diet as tolerated, although their impaired GI function limits nutrient absorption. Encourage food and fluid intake for pleasure but monitor for diarrhea or increased output if eating to assess for dehydration.
- Teach patient and caregiver to monitor patient's temperature, weight, I&O, and serum glucose level and to recognize signs and symptoms of PN-related complications.
- Teach patient and caregiver about actions to take in case of emergency or unexpected outcomes, such as telephoning the health care provider or community infusion provider or going to the hospital, depending on the circumstances.
- If home CPN patients require insulin in their PN, they will need a home glucose monitoring device and instruction in its use.
- Patient teaching for community CPN administration will be given by community infusion staff after discharge or may be initiated in the hospital and continued in the community.

◆ SKILL 33.2 **Administering Peripheral Parenteral Nutrition with Lipid (Fat) Emulsion**

▶ *Video Clip*

The administration of peripheral parenteral nutrition (PPN) requires a lower dextrose content and is more appropriate for short-term use until central access can be achieved or the patient can be fed orally or enterally. Contraindications to the use of PPN include cardiac failure, severe liver disease, disorders of fat metabolism, uncontrolled diabetes mellitus, shock, and severe blood dyscrasias (Singh, 2018). This therapy is for short-term use, usually for 2 weeks or less. The PPN solution has lower concentrations of dextrose and

amino acids to reduce the osmolality (see Table 33.2) and decrease the risk for phlebitis. Adding lipid emulsion provides a source of calories with minimal impact on the osmolality. A lipid emulsion must be administered through vented intravenous (IV) tubing as a primary IV infusion or a piggyback.

This skill describes piggyback administration of PPN. Administration sets (including piggybacks) used for fat emulsions are changed every 24 hours and immediately on suspected contamination

(Alexander et al., 2014). The administration set must have a Luer-Lok design. Indications for PPN include the following:

- *Adequate peripheral access:* Despite its lower osmolality, PPN tends to cause phlebitis and often requires frequent changes in the access location. A midline catheter may be an alternative to the typical short-peripheral catheter.
- *Ability to tolerate larger volumes of fluid:* Because of the lower concentration of dextrose in PPN, a larger volume of fluid is required to obtain adequate calories. Some patients with impaired renal or cardiac function do not tolerate PPN.
- *Ability to tolerate lipid emulsions:* Lipid is the most calorically dense nutrient. A 1-L amount of 10% dextrose without lipid provides only 340 calories. A 250-mL amount of 20% lipid solution provides 500 calories.

Delegation and Collaboration

The skill of administering PPN for a hospitalized patient cannot be delegated to an unregulated care provider (UCP). The nurse directs the UCP to report to the nurse:

- Patient indication of burning, pain, or redness at peripheral IV site.
- Infusion pump alarms or a moist IV site dressing.
- Patient complaints of shortness of breath.

Equipment

- Medication administration record (MAR) or computer printout
- PPN solution
- Lipid emulsion in glass container or in a separate chamber, such as a prepared parental nutrition bag
- IV tubing for PPN with 0.20-micron filter for amino acid/dextrose solution
- IV tubing with a 1.2-micron filter for fat emulsion
- Bedside glucose monitoring kit
- Antimicrobial swab
- Electronic infusion pump with anti–free-flow control and alarms (INS, 2016)
- Clean gloves
- Stethoscope

STEP	RATIONALE

ASSESSMENT

1. Review medical record and assess patient for hypertriglyceridemia. Obtain prescriptions for serum triglyceride level before initiation of PPN and weekly.

Determines patient's ability to metabolize lipid.

2. Perform hand hygiene and apply clean gloves. Select or initiate appropriate functional IV site to administer PPN and lipid emulsion. Assess its patency and function (see Chapter 29).

PPN may cause phlebitis; therefore, appropriate vein selection is important.

3. Obtain blood glucose level with a finger lancet device.

Provides baseline to determine tolerance of glucose infusion.

4. Assess patient's fluid status by monitoring for edema in extremities, lung sounds, or fluid intake greater than fluid output.

Fluid intake given with PPN may cause fluid overload in older patients or those who have impaired renal or cardiac function.

5. Obtain patient's weight and vital signs. Remove gloves and perform hand hygiene.

Provides baseline information to determine effectiveness and tolerance of PPN solution. Reduces transmission of microorganisms.

6. Check health care provider's prescription against MAR for volume of fat emulsion, PPN solution, and administration time for fat emulsion. Then check name of solution on label with MAR.

The health care provider must prescribe fat emulsions and PPN. Fat emulsions may cause adverse symptoms if infused too rapidly as a separate infusion. Infusion time is normally at least 8 hours. Fat emulsions should hang no longer than 12 hours as a separate infusion from original container. *This is the first check for accuracy.*

7. Read label of fat emulsion solution.

Lipid emulsions are white and opaque; thus, be sure to avoid confusing enteral tube–feeding formula with parenteral lipids.

8. Assess patient's and caregiver's knowledge of PPN.

Determines level and extent of instruction required.

NURSING DIAGNOSES

- Inadequate nutrition
- Excessive fluid volume
- Potential for unstable blood glucose level
- Potential for infection

Related factors/Risk factors are individualized on the basis of patient's condition or needs.

PLANNING

1. Expected outcomes following completion of procedure:
   - Triglyceride level is less than 13.9 mmol/L in most patients.

Indicates adequate clearance of lipid.

STEP	RATIONALE

PLANNING

- Blood glucose levels are maintained per health care provider's prescription for desired glucose range.

- Venipuncture site is free of phlebitis, pain, swelling, redness, and inflammation.
- Patient does not show signs of systemic infection (e.g., elevated temperature).
- Patient does not show signs of allergy to lipids.

- Patient and caregiver are able to explain purpose of PPN and complications to watch for.

2. Explain purposes of PPN and fat emulsion.
3. Place patient in comfortable position for IV-line insertion or initiation of infusion. Explain associated procedures.
4. If PPN solution is refrigerated, remove from refrigeration 1 hour before infusion.

Glucose levels needed for specific populations differ, based on the degree of illness, so a specific health care provider prescription is needed (McClave et al., 2016).

Ensures proper administration and monitoring of PPN with lipids.

Temperature is indication of possible systemic infection related to PN.

Monitoring infusion requires observation for allergic response to infusion.

Proper instruction informs patient and caregiver.

Promotes understanding and allows for clarification or questions.

When patients are comfortable, they tolerate procedures more readily.

Solution should be removed from refrigeration before administration and should be administered at room temperature (Alexander et al., 2014).

IMPLEMENTATION

1. Perform hand hygiene.
2. Compare label of PPN bag and lipid emulsion bottle with MAR or computer printout; check for correct additives and solution expiration date. Also check patient's name. Steps 2–5 may require an independent double-check by another nurse, depending on employer policy.

3. Examine lipid solution for separation of emulsion into layers or fat globules or presence of froth.

4. Identify patient using at least two person-specific identifiers (e.g., name and date of birth or name and medical record number) according to employer policy. Compare identifiers with information on patient's MAR or medical record.

5. Compare identifiers with information on solution bag label and patient's MAR or medical record at the bedside.

6. Measure patient's vital signs.

7. Apply clean gloves. Prepare IV tubing for PPN solution; run solution through tubing to remove excess air. Turn roller clamp to "off" (clamped) position. Some infusion pumps and tubing require priming through the infusion pump. Add sterile capped needle or place sterile cap on end of tubing. Follow same procedure with separate infusion set for lipid infusion.

8. Wipe end port of peripheral IV infusion tubing with antimicrobial swab and allow to dry. Connect needleless connector at end of PPN tubing to end port of patient's functional peripheral IV line. Gently disconnect old PPN tubing from IV site and insert adapter of new PPN infusion tubing. Open roller clamp on new tubing. Allow solution to run to ensure that tubing is patent; regulate IV drip rate using electronic infusion pump.

9. Clean needleless peripheral line tubing injection cap with antimicrobial swab.

10. Attach fat emulsion infusion tubing to injection cap of IV line. Y-connector may be used if patient is receiving separate PPN and lipid infusions. Label tubing.

Reduces transmission of microorganisms.

Prevents medication error. *This is the second check for accuracy.*

Do not administer if these elements appear, as procedure may result in patient developing a fat embolism.

Ensures correct patient. Complies with Accreditation Canada's standards and improves patient safety (Accreditation Canada, 2019).

Ensures patient receives correct infusion. *This is the third check for accuracy.*

Provides baseline assessment. An immediate allergic reaction can develop once infusion begins.

To prevent air from entering vascular system, clear all tubing.

Prevents disruption of existing IV infusion and ensures patent infusion. Pump will deliver infusion at a prescribed rate.

Removes surface organisms at injection site and prevents organisms from entering blood system.

Fat emulsions cannot infuse through a 0.20-micron IV filter. Refer to employer policy; if larger 1.2-micron filter is used, lipids may be infused using a Y-connector (INS, 2016). Labelling high-risk catheters prevents connection with an inappropriate tube or catheter.

STEP	RATIONALE

IMPLEMENTATION

11. Open roller clamp completely on fat emulsion infusion and check infusion rate on pump. This step may require an independent double-check by another nurse, depending on employer policy.

Initial slow infusion allows you to observe for an allergic response.

12. Infuse lipids initially at 1 mL/min for adults and 0.1 mL/min for a child for the first 15 to 30 minutes; increase rate as prescribed.

Up to 2.5 g fat/kg per day may be infused, but current practice is generally to give less than 1 g fat/kg body weight per day in adults.

13. Begin PPN at prescribed rate. 20% of fats are infused over at least 8 hours. All lipids can hang for 12 hours as a separate infusion.

Rate of PPN administration does not need to be increased gradually. A lower concentration of dextrose allows most patients to tolerate a full administration rate without difficulty.

14. Remove and discard gloves and supplies and perform hand hygiene.

Reduces transmission of microorganisms.

EVALUATION

1. Monitor infusion rate routinely hourly or more frequently if necessary.

Too-rapid or too-slow infusion could result in metabolic disturbances such as hyperglycemia.

2. Measure vital signs and patient's general comfort level every 10 minutes for the first 30 minutes, then vital signs every 4 hours, or as per employer policy.

Monitors patient for lipid allergy.

3. Monitor patient's laboratory values (e.g., triglycerides, liver function tests) daily and perform blood glucose monitoring as prescribed. Measure serum lipids 4 hours after discontinuing infusion.

Provides objective data to measure response to therapy (e.g., ability of liver to metabolize lipids). Measurement of lipids too soon after infusion will yield incorrect blood values.

4. Monitor temperature every 4 hours and regularly inspect venipuncture site for signs of phlebitis or infiltration.

Onset of fever is a complication of intolerance of fat emulsion or sepsis. Determines integrity of IV system.

5. Evaluate patient's weight, intake and output (I&O), condition of peripheral extremities (for edema), and breath sounds.

Weight gain, I&O imbalance, peripheral edema, and crackles in lungs indicate fluid retention.

6. **Use Teach-Back:** "I want to be sure that I properly explained the reasons for your nutrition fluid. Why are you receiving this type of nutrition?" Develop a revised teaching plan if patient or caregiver is not able to teach back correctly.

Determines patient's or caregiver's level of understanding of instructional topic.

Unexpected Outcomes

1. There is intolerance of fat emulsion, as evidenced by increased triglyceride levels, increased temperature, chills, flushing, headache, nausea and vomiting, diaphoresis, muscle ache, chest and back pain, dyspnea, pressure over eyes, or vertigo.

2. See Unexpected Outcomes and Related Interventions for Skill 33.1.

Related Interventions

- Turn PPN infusion off.
- Inform health care provider.
- Prepare to treat anaphylactic reaction according to health care provider's prescriptions.
- Record lipid allergy in patient's medical record.

Communication and Documentation

- Document condition of IV site, type of solutions, rate and status of infusion, catheter lumen used for infusion, I&O, blood glucose levels, vital signs, weights, and other assessment findings in nurses' notes in electronic health record (EHR) or chart on the appropriate flow sheets.

- Document any adverse reactions in nurses' notes in EHR or chart.
- If signs of fat intolerance, infection, occlusion, fluid retention, or infiltration occur, notify the health care provider.
- Document your evaluation of patient and caregiver learning.

Special Considerations

Teaching

- PPN administration does not typically occur in the community unless the patient is in need of long-term nutritional support.

Pediatric

- See pediatric considerations for Skill 33.1, Administering Central Parenteral Nutrition

Gerontological

- Some older persons may have fragile peripheral veins or poor fluid tolerance because of cardiac or renal dysfunction, making PPN undesirable.

Care in the Community

- See care in the community considerations for Skill 33.1, Administering Central Parenteral Nutrition

◆ CLINICAL DEBRIEF

A 43-year-old patient is admitted to the hospital with a severe exacerbation of Crohn's disease. He has lost 4.5 kg (10 lb) over the last 3 weeks and has recurrent abdominal pain, cramping, and loose stools. He is unable to tolerate food orally and is becoming easily nauseated. He is to receive bowel rest and nutritional support with parenteral nutrition (PN) via central vascular access device (CVAD). The health care provider inserted a central line for 3:1 parenteral nutrition (PN) therapy.

1. Identify four physical parameters that can change quickly and should be part of the nurse's baseline assessment before initiating PN through a central line (CPN).
2. On the third day after central line insertion, the patient develops a fever and fatigue, preferring to stay in bed. What might the fever indicate, and what could be its source?
3. Two days after beginning CPN infusion, the patient experiences a 2-kg (5-lb) weight gain. He comments, "I'm gaining back some of the weight I lost." What should be the nurse's response? What should the nurse include in a nursing assessment?
4. The nurse takes the patient's vital signs: HR 100, RR 20 with bilateral rales, BP 130/86. The patient denies shortness of breath on exertion. Using SBAR, show how the nurse would communicate with the health care team about this patient.

◆ REVIEW QUESTIONS

1. A patient is being switched from a standard intravenous (IV) solution to peripheral parenteral nutrition (PPN). Which reason(s) should the nurse give the patient about why a large-diameter vein needs to be used for the infusion? *(Select all that apply.)*
   1. The fluid is very hyperosmolar.
   2. The fluid cannot flow through smaller veins.
   3. Peripheral veins become very irritated because of the content of the fluid.
   4. The patient will have the infusion for an extended amount of time, which will allow for the use of both hands without an IV line in them.
   5. Large veins allow the solution to infuse at an increased rate needed for PPN.
2. A patient with which of the following is a good candidate for short-term PPN? *(Select all that apply.)*
   1. Anastomotic leak
   2. Intestinal obstruction
   3. Severe mucositis
   4. Severe malnutrition before surgery
   5. Pneumonia
3. Place the three checks for accuracy before administering central parenteral nutrition (CPN) in the correct order.
   1. Before leaving the medication room, check intravenous (IV) solution a second time using the 10 rights of medication administration (see Chapter 20). Check label of PN bag against medication administration record (MAR) or computer printout.
   2. Identify patient using at least two person-specific identifiers (e.g., name and birthdate) according to employer policy. Compare contents of PN solution and additives on label of bag with information on patient's MAR or medical record at bedside.
   3. When preparing PN solution, check label on PN bag with health care provider's prescription on MAR or computer printout and patient's name.

ⓔ *Visit the Evolve site for a complete list of Clinical Debrief and Review Questions answers.*

REFERENCES

Accreditation Canada. (2019). *Required organizational practices handbook—Version 14*. Retrieved from http://www.wrha.mb.ca/quality/files/2019ROPHandbook.pdf

Alexander, M., Corrigan, A., Gorski, L. A., & Phillips, L. (Eds.). (2014). *Core curriculum for infusion nursing* (4th ed.). Philadelphia: Lippincott, Williams & Wilkins.

Guenter, P., Worthington, P., Ayers, P., Boullata, J. I., Gura, K. M., & Marshall, N., for the Parenteral Nutrition Safety Committee. (2018). Standardized competencies for parenteral nutrition administration: The ASPEN Model. *Nutrition in Clinical Practice*, 33(2), 295–304. doi:10.1002/ncp.10055

Hockenberry, M. J., & Wilson, D. (2015). *Wong's nursing care of infants and children* (10th ed.). St. Louis: Mosby.

Infusion Nurses Society (INS). (2016). Infusion therapy standards of practice. *Journal of Intravenous Nursing*, 39(Suppl. 1), S1.

Institute for Safe Medication Practices (ISMP). (2015). *Safe practice guidelines for adult IV push medications*. Retrieved from https://www.ismp.org/guidelines/iv-push

Lamperti, M., Bodenham, A. R., Pittiruti, M., et al. (2012). International evidence-based recommendations on ultrasound-guided vascular access. *Intensive Care Medicine*, 38(7), 1105–1117. doi:10.1007/s00134-012-2597-x

McClave, S. A., Taylor, B. E., Martindale, R. G., et al. American Society for Parenteral and Enteral Nutrition. (2016). Guidelines for the provision and assessment of nutrition support therapy in the adult critically ill patient. Society of Critical Care Medicine (SCCM) and American Society for Parenteral and Enteral Nutrition (A.S.P.E.N.). *JPEN. Journal of Parenteral and Enteral Nutrition*, 40(2), 159–211. doi:10.1177/0148607115621863

O'Grady, N. P., Alexander, M., Dellinger, E. P., et al. (2002). *Guidelines for the prevention of intravascular catheter-related infections*. Retrieved from https://www.cdc.gov/mmwr/preview/mmwrhtml/rr5110a1.htm

Phillips, L. (2014). *Manual of IV therapeutics: Evidence-based practice for infusion therapy* (6th ed.). Philadelphia: FA Davis.

Singh, A. (2018). Parental nutrition indications and complications. *Med Care Tips: Health and Medical Care*. Retrieved from http://medcaretips.com/parenteral-nutrition/

Taylor, B., McClave, S. A., Martindale, R. G., et al. American Society for Parenteral and Enteral Nutrition. (2016). Guidelines for the provision and assessment of nutrition support therapy in the adult critically ill patient. Society of Critical Care Medicine (SCCM) and American Society for Parenteral and Enteral Nutrition (A.S.P.E.N.). *Critical Care Medicine*, 44(2), 390–438. doi:10.1097/CCM.0000000000001525

Worthington, P., Balint, J., Bechtold, M., et al. (2017). When is parenteral nutrition appropriate? *JPEN. Journal of Parenteral and Enteral Nutrition*, 41(3), 324–377. doi:10.1177/0148607117695251

34 | Urinary Elimination and Catheterization

Written by **Wendy R. Ostendorf, RN, MS, EdD, CNE, and Shelley L. Cobbett, RN, GnT, MN, EdD**

SKILLS AND PROCEDURES

OBJECTIVES

Mastery of content in this chapter will enable the nurse to:
- Discuss nursing interventions that promote normal micturition when toilet access is compromised or after a catheter is removed.
- Discuss the relationship between fluid balance and urinary elimination.
- Describe how to use person-centred care principles when caring for patients with urinary elimination alterations.
- Describe ways to provide for patient safety when managing urinary elimination needs.

- Identify factors that increase risk for catheter-associated urinary tract infection (CAUTI).
- Perform the following skills: place and remove a urinal, insert a urinary catheter, care for an in-dwelling urinary catheter, measure postvoid residual (PVR) with catheterization and a bladder scan, irrigate a catheter, remove an in-dwelling catheter, apply a condom catheter, and care for a suprapubic catheter.

MEDIA RESOURCES

- evolve http://evolve.elsevier.com/Canada/Perry/clinicalskills/
- Review Questions
- ▶ Video Clips

- Case Studies
- Audio Glossary
- **NSO** Nursing Skills Online
- Clinical Debrief and Review Questions Answers

PURPOSE

A basic human function is urinary elimination, a function that can be compromised by a wide variety of illnesses and conditions. It is the role of a nurse to support bladder emptying as needed by helping the patient in toileting, which may include use of a commode, urinal, or bedpan. During acute illness, a patient may require urinary catheterization for close monitoring of urine output or to facilitate bladder emptying when bladder function is compromised. Some patients require long-term in-dwelling catheters, urethral or suprapubic, when the bladder fails to empty effectively. The nurse also implements measures to minimize risk for infection when bladder function is impaired or urinary drainage tubes are required.

STANDARDS OF CARE

- Canadian Nurse Continence Advisors, 2012—*Best Practice Guidelines: Promoting Continence Using Prompted Voiding* (http://www.cnca.ca/BPG.html)

- Canadian Patient Safety Institute (CPSI), 2016—*Hospital Harm Improvement Resource: Urinary Tract Infection* (http://www.patientsafetyinstitute.ca/en/toolsResources/Hospital-Harm-Measure/Improvement-Resources/pages/default.aspx)
- Registered Nurses' Association of Ontario (RNAO), 2011—*Nursing Best Practice Guideline: Promoting Continence Using Prompted Voiding* (http://www.cnca.ca/pdf/Promoting_Continence_Using_Prompted_Voiding.pdf)
- Wound Ostomy and Continence Nurses Society (WOCNS), 2016—*Care and Management of Patients with Urinary Catheters: A Clinical Resource Guide* (https://cdn.ymaws.com/www.wocn.org/resource/resmgr/publications/Care_&_Mgmt_Pts_w_Urinary_Ca.pdf)

PRINCIPLES FOR PRACTICE

- Adequate oral intake is essential for bladder health, especially if a patient has an in-dwelling urinary catheter. Some patients with

TABLE 34.1

Signs of Fluid Volume Deficit and Fluid Volume Excess

	Fluid Volume Deficit	Fluid Volume Excess
Eyes	Sunken eyes, dry conjunctivae, decreased or absence of tearing	Periorbital edema, blurred vision, papilledema
Mouth	Sticky, dry mucous membrane; dry, cracked lips; decreased saliva; increased viscosity of saliva; furrowed, shrunken tongue	Excessive salivation
Skin	Increased skin temperature; dry, scaly skin; poor turgor	Edema, anasarca
Cardiovascular	Increased pulse rate, weak pulse, hypotension, decreased pulse volume/ pressure, decreased capillary filling, increased hematocrit, flat neck veins	Bounding pulse rate, blood pressure normal with or without orthostatic changes, third heart sound (S_3), distended neck veins
Gastrointestinal	Sunken abdomen, vomiting, diarrhea, abdominal cramps	Vomiting, diarrhea, abdominal cramps
Renal	Oliguria or anuria, increased urine specific gravity (normal = 1.010 to 1.030)	Decreased urine specific gravity, diuresis (if kidneys are normal)

urinary problems limit fluid intake because of fear of incontinence or increased urinary frequency. The nurse must explain the importance of fluid intake in maintaining urinary health.

- The nurse must know the average output range for a patient. Adult urinary output averages 1 – 2 L in 24 hours; approximately 0.5 to 1.0 mL/kg/hr (Lewis, Bucher, Heitkemper, et al., 2019). An hourly output of less than 30 mL/hr for 2 consecutive hours shows the need for further assessment.
- It is important to know the signs of dehydration and fluid overload (Table 34.1). Start measurement of intake and output (I&O) when there is an actual or anticipated change in fluid balance.
- Excessive urination and extreme thirst can occur as a result of inadequate output of the pituitary hormone antidiuretic hormone (ADH) or the lack of normal response by the kidney to ADH. It is important to know that some patients (e.g., with brain tumour or brain surgery) often void very large amounts of urine (e.g., 20 L/day).
- The nurse must assess a patient's most recent serum electrolyte measurements. Abnormal values reflect alterations in fluid balance that can lead to deterioration in patients' health.
- Weigh a patient to determine fluid status. Ask them to empty their bladder. The patient must be weighed with the same scale, at the same time of day, and with comparable articles of clothing, including bed linen if bed weights are necessary.

PERSON-CENTRED CARE

- The personal level of touch required when helping patients with problems in urinary elimination requires you as a nurse to understand their values and preferences.

- Determine how patients feel about having to undergo procedures such as catheterization. Try to adapt procedures to minimize the invasive nature of catheterization and use a person-centred approach to maintain the patient's dignity and communicate respect.
- When caring for patients from diverse cultures, it is important to incorporate into the plan of care sensitivity and awareness of factors that may affect how you manage urinary elimination problems.
- Variations within a cultural group are common. Assess each patient and practise culturally sensitive care. Many cultures have specific beliefs and practices related to elimination, privacy, and gender-specific care. For example:
  - Some cultures emphasize female modesty and prohibit nonrelated males and females from touching; a same-gender caregiver needs to be provided.
  - Some cultures emphasize interdependence over independence; thus family presence at the bedside for important decision-making is common.
  - Privacy is important in many cultures; thus careful attention to draping is crucial.

EVIDENCE-INFORMED PRACTICE

- Major recommendations in evidence-informed guidelines to reduce catheter-related problems and infection include reducing inappropriate catheter use and removing catheters as soon as possible (CPSI, 2016; Fekete, 2018).
- Studies have shown that bacteriuria can occur within 4 days when open catheters are used and within approximately 30 days with closed systems. However, even with the closed drainage system, bacteriuria inevitably occurs over time, usually via breaks in the system (Centers for Disease Control and Prevention [CDC], 2009). Complications of long-term catheterization include chronic renal inflammation, chronic pyelonephritis, nephrolithiasis, cystolithiasis, and symptomatic urinary tract.
- Evidence-informed interventions for the prevention of CAUTI include the following:
  - Use aseptic catheter insertion with sterile equipment (Fekete, 2018).
  - Use only trained, dedicated personnel to insert and maintain urinary catheters (CPSI, 2016).
  - Use the smallest catheter possible.
  - Remove catheter as soon as possible (CPSI, 2016).
  - Secure in-dwelling catheters to prevent movement and pulling on the catheter.
  - Maintain a closed urinary drainage system.
  - Maintain an unobstructed flow of urine through the catheter, drainage tubing, and drainage bag.
  - Keep the urinary drainage bag below the level of the bladder at all times.
  - When emptying the urinary drainage bag, use a separate measuring receptacle for each patient. Do not let the drainage spigot touch the receptacle.
  - Perform routine perineal hygiene daily and after soiling.
  - Quality improvement and surveillance programs should be in place that alert providers that a catheter is in place; these include regular educational programming about catheter care.

SAFETY GUIDELINES

- Regularly assess and determine a patient's functional status, such as their ability to safely stand and transfer to a toilet or commode,

their ability to follow and understand directions, and their motivation to help in self-care activities such as using a toilet, commode, or urinal.

- Evaluate a patient's normal pattern of micturition. Patients taking diuretic medications should have a toilet, commode, or urinal close to their bed or chair. Respond to any request for toileting assistance in a prompt manner to lessen the chance of patients falling as they try to reach a toilet.
- Consider a patient's age when assessing voiding habits. Toilet training and enuresis are concerns for toddlers and preschoolers.

Frail older persons are at higher risk for incontinence because of multiple health care problems and associated physiological changes.

- Patients who need help with elimination should have a call bell within easy reach and an offer for help at regular intervals, especially in the morning after awakening, after meals, and before bedtime.
- Maintain aseptic technique when catheterizing a patient, to prevent CAUTI (CPSI, 2016; Fekete, 2018).

PROCEDURAL GUIDELINE 34.1 *Assisting With Use of a Urinal*

 Video Clip

A *urinal* is a container that collects and holds urine when access to a toilet is restricted. Patients who may need a urinal include those who have compromised mobility, severe dyspnea, or other illnesses that make walking to a bathroom impossible or excessively painful. In some instances, a male patient may be able to stand at the bedside and use a urinal. Most urinals are used by men, but there are specially designed urinals for women (Fig. 34.1). The female urinal has a larger opening at the top with a defined rim, which helps position the urinal closely against the genitalia. Usually a female will use a bedpan to void rather than a female urinal.

Delegation and Collaboration

The skill of assisting a patient with a urinal can be delegated to an unregulated care provider (UCP). The nurse directs the UCP to:

- Help the patient with special needs or adaptations, such holding a urinal for the patient.
- Provide personal hygiene as necessary after urination.
- Report immediately any changes in urine colour, clarity, and odour; development of incontinence (involuntary loss of urine); patient reports of dysuria, which could indicate an infection; and any changes in the frequency and amount of urine.

Equipment

- Urinal
- Clean gloves
- Graduated cylinder (used for measuring volume if on intake and output [I&O])
- Supplies for diagnostic urine tests and specimen collection (see Chapter 9).

- Wash basin, washcloths, towels, and soap
- Toilet tissue

Procedural Steps

1. Assess patient's normal urinary elimination habits, including any episodes of incontinence.
2. Determine how much help is needed to place and remove the urinal. (Ask the patient or observe previous use.)
3. Review health care provider prescriptions to determine if a urine specimen is to be collected.
4. Perform hand hygiene.
5. Explain procedure to patient.
6. Provide privacy by closing bedside curtain and room door.
7. Assess for a distended bladder by inspecting the lower one third of the abdomen or palpating gently above symphysis pubis.
8. Apply clean gloves.
9. Help patient into appropriate position: for a male patient—on side, back, sitting with head of bed elevated, or in standing position; for a female patient—lying supine. If needed, place an absorbent pad under patient's buttocks to protect bed linens from accidental spills.

Clinical Decision Point *Before having a patient stand to void, assess lower-extremity strength and mobility and assess blood pressure for orthostatic hypotension (Chapter 7), especially if there has been a period of prolonged bed rest.*

10. If possible, a male patient should hold urinal and position penis in urinal. If needed, help patient by positioning penis completely in urinal and holding urinal in place or by helping

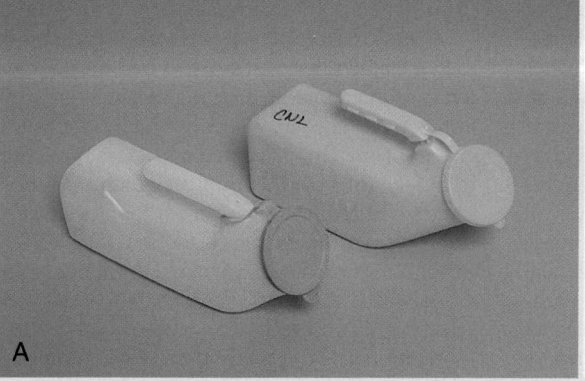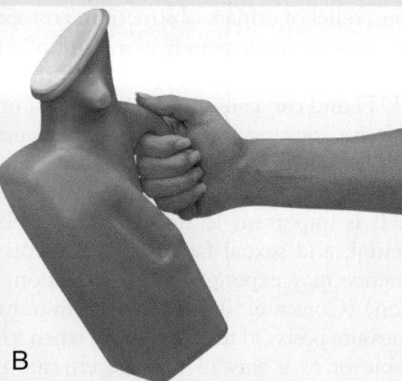

FIG 34.1 A, Male urinals. **B,** Female urinal. (**B** *Courtesy Briggs Medical Service Co.*)

Continued

PROCEDURAL GUIDELINE 34.1 *Assisting With Use of a Urinal—cont'd*

to hold the urinal. Ensure that the urinal is placed dependent of flow of urine.

11. Help a female patient by positioning her on a bedpan or, if using a female urinal, placing the urinal against the genitalia and stabilizing it to keep it in position and dependent of urine flow.

12. Cover patient with bed linens and place the call bell within reach. If possible, give patient further privacy by leaving the bedside after ensuring that they are in a safe and comfortable position. Remove gloves and perform hand hygiene.

13. After patient has finished voiding, apply gloves, remove urinal, and assess characteristics of urine for colour, clarity, odour, and amount. Help patient wash and dry penis or genitalia.

14. Measure urine and record output on I&O record, if needed (see Chapter 8).

15. Empty and clean urinal. Return urinal to patient for future use.

16. Help patient perform hand hygiene as needed.

17. Remove and dispose of gloves; perform hand hygiene.

◆ SKILL 34.1   Insertion of a Straight or an In-dwelling Urinary Catheter

NSO *Nursing Skills Online Urinary Catheterization Module 17 / Lessons 1 and 2*

Urinary catheterization is the placement of a tube through the urethra into the bladder to remove urine. This is an invasive procedure that requires a health care provider prescription and sterile technique (CPSI, 2016). Urinary catheterization may be short term (usually 2 weeks or less, but sources vary in terms of the exact time frame) or long term (more than 30 days) (WOCNS, 2016). Short-term catheterization is often used in patients who have acute urinary retention or have had urological and contiguous surgery and in critically ill patients requiring accurate measurement of urinary output. Examples of patients requiring long-term catheterization include those who have a bladder outlet obstruction that is not medically or surgically correctable and some patients with neurogenic bladder and retention.

Neurogenic bladder is a term used for bladder dysfunction due to neurological damage caused by internal or external trauma, disease, or injury (Gill, Vasavada, Firoozi, et al., 2018) and can be an indication for catheterization. Symptoms can include overflow or urge incontinence, frequency, urgency, incomplete bladder emptying, and urinary retention. Complications of neurogenic bladder may include continuous urine leakage causing reduced skin integrity, kidney damage, and urinary tract infection (UTI) (Shelat, 2019).

Conditions that require use of urinary catheters include the need to monitor urine output, relief of urinary obstruction, postoperative care, or a bladder that empties inadequately as a result of a neurological condition. Excessive accumulation of urine in the bladder increases the risk for UTI and can cause backward flow of urine up the ureters to the kidneys, causing kidney infection, damage, or both. *Urinary incontinence*, an involuntary leakage of urine, may require in-dwelling catheterization if the leaking urine interferes with wound healing. It is important to understand the physical, emotional, social, mental, and sexual factors that patients living with urinary incontinence may experience (e.g., isolation, sexual dysfunction, depression) (Corcos et al., 2017). Intermittent catheterization is used to measure postvoid residual (PVR) when a bladder scanner is not available or as a way to manage chronic urinary retention.

A patient with the diagnosis of overactive bladder (OAB) has urinary urgency, incontinence, frequency, and nocturia, with no UTI or obvious pathology (Corcos et al., 2017). Treatment of OAB includes behavioural therapies (e.g., bladder training and pelvic floor muscle therapy), lifestyle changes (e.g., fluid and caffeine restriction, weight loss), and patient education (Corcos, Przydacz, Campeau, et al., 2017). There are different strategies available for bladder training, all sharing a similar goal in restoring normal bladder function. Most bladder training programs include a voiding schedule, use of a diary or log to record voiding, and techniques for urgency control and suppression (Corcos et al., 2017).

The steps for inserting an in-dwelling and a single-use straight catheter are the same. The difference lies in the inflation of a balloon to keep the in-dwelling catheter in place and the presence of a closed drainage system. Urinary catheters are made with one to three lumens (Fig. 34.2). Single-lumen catheters (see Fig. 34.2, A) are used for intermittent catheterization (i.e., the insertion of a catheter for one-time bladder emptying). Double-lumen catheters, designed for in-dwelling catheters, provide one lumen for urinary drainage and a second lumen to inflate a balloon that keeps the catheter in place (see Fig. 34.2, B). Triple-lumen catheters (see Fig. 34.2, C) are used for continuous bladder irrigation or when it becomes necessary to instill medications into the bladder. One lumen drains the bladder, a second lumen is used to inflate the balloon, and a third lumen delivers irrigation fluid into the bladder.

A health care provider chooses a catheter on the basis of factors such as latex allergy, history of catheter encrustation, and susceptibility to infection. In-dwelling catheters are made of latex or silicone. Some have special coatings that reduce urethral irritation and encrustation. Silver-coated catheters have been used as a measure to reduce infection, but efficacy data have been inconsistent, with some studies reporting no benefit for prevention of catheter-associated urinary tract infection (CAUTI) (WOCNS, 2016). Straight or intermittent catheters are made of rubber (softer and more flexible) or polyvinyl chloride. Patients who self-catheterize have a large selection of catheters: some with special coatings that do not require lubrication and others that are self-contained systems consisting of a lubricated catheter and packaged with a connected drainage bag.

The size of a urinary catheter is based on the French (Fr) scale, which reflects the internal diameter of the catheter. Most adults

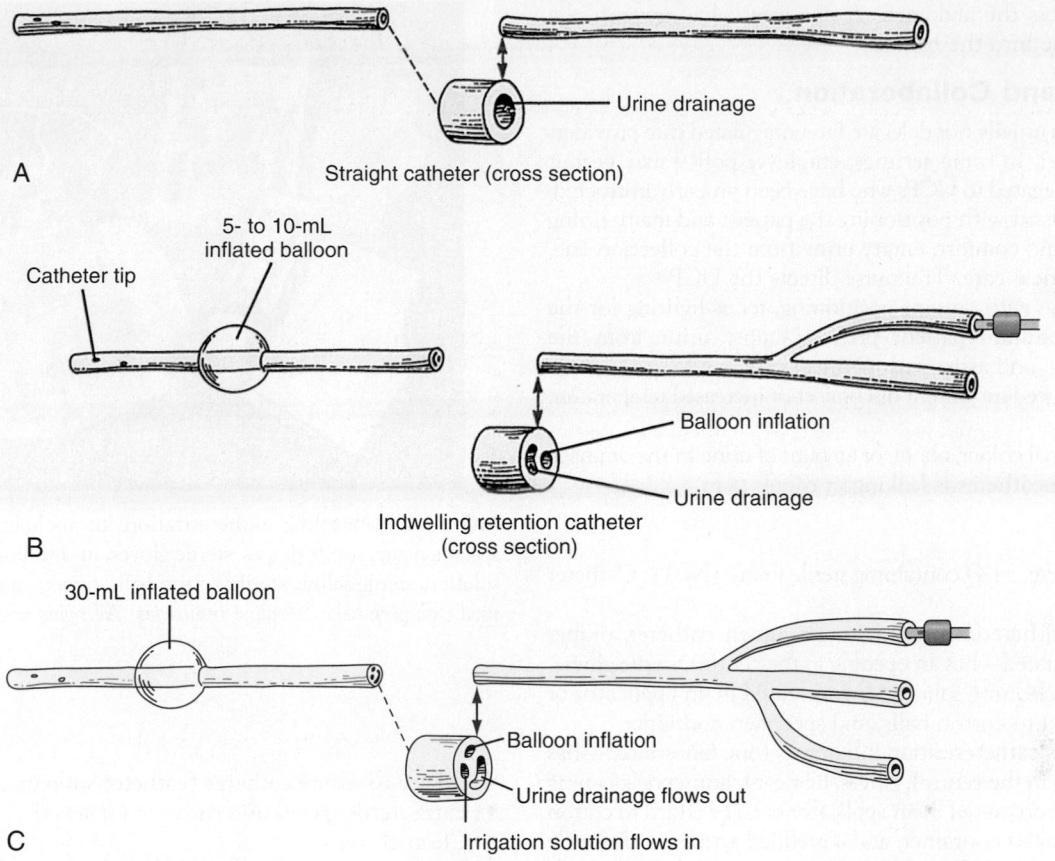

FIG 34.2 A, Single-lumen or straight catheter (cross section). **B,** Double-lumen or in-dwelling retention catheter (cross section). **C,** Triple-lumen catheter for continuous closed irrigation (cross section).

with an in-dwelling catheter should have a size 14 to 16 Fr to minimize trauma and risk for infection. Older persons or males with an enlarged prostate may need a smaller size (12 to 14 Fr). A coudé catheter is also available for men with an enlarged prostate with a urinary obstruction; it has a slightly bent tip designed to navigate past the obstruction. Larger-catheter diameters increase the risk for trauma to the bladder neck and urethra (Newman, Rovner, & Wein, 2017). However, larger sizes such as a 20 or 22 Fr are needed in special circumstances such as after urological surgery or in the presence of gross hematuria. Smaller sizes are needed, such as a 5 to 6 Fr for infants, and an 8 to 10 Fr for children.

In-dwelling catheters come in a variety of balloon sizes, from 3 mL for a child to 30 mL for continuous bladder irrigation (CBI). The size of the balloon is usually printed on the catheter port (Fig. 34.3). The recommended balloon size for an adult is a 5-mL balloon (filled with 10 mL). Long-term use of larger balloons (30 mL) has been associated with increased patient discomfort, irritation, and trauma; increased risk of catheter expulsion; and incomplete emptying of the bladder because of urine that pools below the level of the catheter drainage lumen (Newman et al., 2017).

For patients requiring long-term catheterization, catheter changes should be individualized, not changed at arbitrary times or specific intervals (CPSI, 2016). Catheters should be changed for leaking or blockage if disconnection of the system occurs, and before obtaining a sterile specimen for urine culture (CPSI, 2016). Long-term catheterization should be avoided because of its association with UTIs. Best practice involves removal of the catheter as soon as the patient can void (WOCNS, 2016).

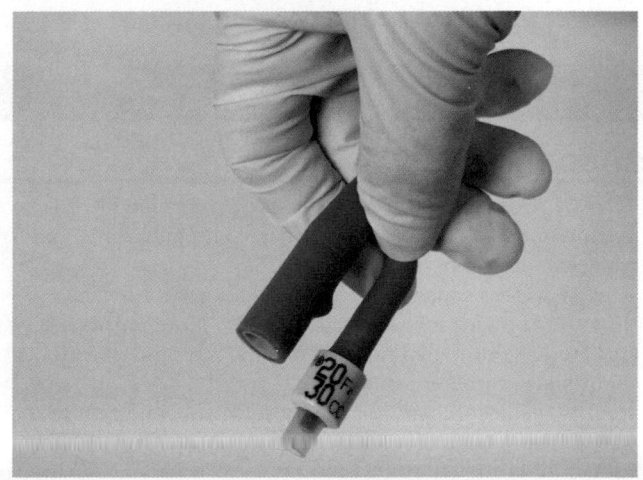

FIG 34.3 Size of catheter and balloon printed on catheter inflation valve.

An in-dwelling catheter is attached to a urinary drainage bag to collect the continuous flow of urine. The bag should always hang below the level of the bladder on the bedframe or a chair so urine drains down, out of the bladder. The bag should never touch the floor. When a patient ambulates, the bag is carried below the level of the patient's bladder. The only exception to this rule is when a catheter is attached to a specially designed drainage bag (belly bag)

that is worn across the abdomen. A one-way valve prevents the back flow of urine into the bladder.

Delegation and Collaboration

Catheterization is usually not delegated to unregulated care providers (UCPs). However, in some settings, employer policy may permit this skill to be delegated to UCPs who have been properly instructed. UCPs routinely assist with positioning the patient and maintaining patient privacy and comfort, empty urine from the collection bag, and provide perineal care. The nurse directs the UCP to:

- Help the nurse with patient positioning, focus lighting for the procedure, maintain patient privacy, empty urine from the collection bag, and assist with perineal care.
- Report postprocedure patient discomfort or increased temperature to the nurse.
- Report abnormal colour, odour, or amount of urine in the drainage bag and if the catheter is leaking or causes pain.

Equipment

- Catheter kit (Fig. 34.4) containing sterile items: (**NOTE:** Catheter kits vary.)
  - Straight catheterization kit: single-lumen catheter, drapes (one fenestrated—has an opening in the centre), sterile gloves, lubricant, cleaning solution incorporated in an applicator or to be added to cotton balls, and specimen container
  - In-dwelling catheterization kit: drapes (one fenestrated—has an opening in the centre), gloves, lubricant, antiseptic cleaning solution incorporated in an applicator or to be added to cotton balls, specimen container, and a prefilled syringe with sterile water (to inflate balloon). Some kits contain a catheter with an attached drainage bag; others contain only a catheter; others have no catheter.
- Sterile drainage tubing and bag (if not included in in-dwelling catheter insertion kit)

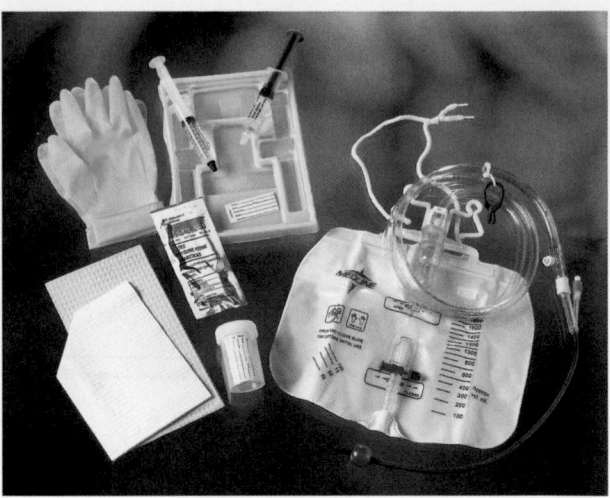

FIG 34.4 In-dwelling catheterization kit includes drainage device, specimen cup, sterile drapes, sterile gloves, in-dwelling catheter, cleaning solution, sterile saline, sterile cotton balls, forceps, and lubricant. (*Image used with permission Medline Industries. All rights reserved.*)

- Device to secure catheter (catheter strap or other device)
- Extra sterile gloves and catheter (*optional*)
- Clean gloves
- Basin with warm water, washcloth, towel, and soap for perineal care
- Flashlight or other additional light source
- Bath blanket, waterproof absorbent pad
- Measuring container for urine

STEP	RATIONALE

ASSESSMENT

1. Identify patient using at least two person-specific identifiers (e.g., name and date of birth, or name and medical record number), according to employer policy.

Ensures correct patient. Complies with Accreditation Canada's standards and improves patient safety (Accreditation Canada, 2019).

2. Review patient's medical record, including health care provider's prescription and nurses' notes. Note previous catheterization, including catheter size, response of patient, and time of catheterization.

Identifies purpose of inserting catheter (such as for measurement of PVR, preparation for surgery, or specimen collection) and potential difficulty with catheter insertion.

3. Review medical record for any pathological condition that may impair passage of catheter (e.g., enlarged prostate gland in men, urethral strictures).

Obstruction of urethra may prevent passage of catheter into bladder.

4. Perform hand hygiene. Ask patient about and check medical record for allergies.

Reduces transmission of microorganisms. Identifies allergy to antiseptic, tape, latex, and lubricant.

5. Assess patient's weight, level of consciousness, developmental level, ability to cooperate, and mobility.

Determines positioning for catheterization; indicates how much help is needed to properly position patient, ability of patient to cooperate during procedure, and level of explanation needed.

6. Assess patient's gender and age.

Determines catheter size.

7. Assess patient's knowledge of and prior experience with catheterization and feelings about procedure.

Reveals need for patient instruction, support, or both.

8. Assess for pain and bladder fullness. Palpate bladder over symphysis pubis or use bladder scanner (if available) (see Procedural Guideline 34.2).

Palpation of full bladder causes pain or urge to void, indicating full or overfull bladder.

STEP	RATIONALE

ASSESSMENT

9. Perform hand hygiene and apply clean gloves. Inspect perineal region, observing for perineal anatomical landmarks, erythema, drainage or discharge, and odour. Remove gloves and perform hand hygiene.

Assessment of female perineal landmarks improves accuracy and speed of catheter insertion.

NURSING DIAGNOSES

- Urinary retention
- Acute pain
- Reduced urinary elimination

- Anxiety
- Fear

- Insufficient knowledge regarding catheterization procedure
- Potential for infection

Related factors/Risk factors are individualized on the basis of patient's condition or needs.

PLANNING

1. Expected outcomes following completion of procedure:
   - Patient's bladder is not palpable.
   - Patient verbalizes absence of abdominal discomfort or bladder pressure or fullness.
   - Patient has urine output of at least 30 mL/hr as measured in urinary drainage bag.
   - Patient verbalizes purpose and expectations about procedure.

Bladder successfully emptied.
Catheterization and free flow of urine through catheter relieve bladder distension and discomfort.
Verifies presence of catheter in bladder, catheter patency, and adequate kidney function.
Reflects patient understanding of procedure.

2. Explain procedure to patient.
3. Arrange for extra personnel to help as necessary. Organize supplies at bedside.

Promotes cooperation.
Some patients are unable to assume positioning independently for procedure. Ensures more efficient procedure.

IMPLEMENTATION

1. Check patient's plan of care for size and type of catheter (if this is a reinsertion). Use smallest-size catheter possible.

Ensures that patient receives correct size and type of catheter. Larger catheter diameters increase risk for urethral trauma (Newman et al., 2017). A small catheter allows for adequate drainage of periurethral glands.

2. Perform hand hygiene.
3. Provide privacy by closing room door and bedside curtain.

Reduces transmission of microorganisms.
Promotes person-centred care and protects patient confidentiality.

4. Raise bed to appropriate working height. If side rails are in use, raise side rail on opposite side of bed and lower side rail on working side.
5. Place waterproof pad under patient.
6. Apply clean gloves. Clean perineal area with soap and water, rinse, and dry (see Chapter 18). Use gloves to examine patient and identify urinary meatus. Remove and discard gloves. Perform hand hygiene.

Promotes good body mechanics and patient safety.

Prevents soiling bed linen.
Hygiene before initiating aseptic catheter insertion removes secretions, urine, and feces that could contaminate sterile field and increase risk for CAUTI.

Clinical Decision Point *Obtain help to position and support weak, frail, obese, or confused patients.*

7. Position patient:
   a. **Female patient:**
      (1) Help to dorsal recumbent position (on back with knees flexed). Ask patient to relax thighs so you can rotate hips.
      (2) Alternate female position: Position side-lying (Sims') position with upper leg flexed at knee and hip. Support patient with pillows if necessary to maintain position.
   b. **Male patient:**
      (1) Position supine with legs extended and thighs slightly abducted.

Exposes perineum and allows hip joints to be externally rotated.

Alternate position is more comfortable if patient cannot abduct leg at hip joint (e.g., patient has arthritic joints or contractures).

Comfortable position for patient aids in visualization of penis.

STEP	RATIONALE

IMPLEMENTATION

8. Drape patient:

> Protects patient dignity by avoiding unnecessary exposure of body parts.

   a. Female patient:
   (1) Drape with bath blanket or use existing bed sheets; pull the bedspread up one side and the top sheet up the other side. Place blanket diamond fashion over patient, with one corner at patient's midsection, side corners over each thigh and abdomen, and last corner over perineum (see illustration).

   b. Male patient:
   (1) Drape patient by covering upper part of body with small sheet or towel; drape with separate sheet or bath blanket so only perineum is exposed (see illustration).

9. Position light to illuminate genitals or have assistant available to hold light source to visualize urinary meatus.

> Adequate visualization of urinary meatus helps with speed and accuracy of catheter insertion.

10. Open outer wrapping of catheterization kit. Place inner wrapped catheter kit tray on clean, accessible surface such as bedside. Patient size and positioning dictate exact placement.

> Provides easy access to supplies during catheter insertion.

11. Open inner sterile wrap covering tray containing catheterization supplies, using sterile technique (see Chapter 6). Fold back each flap of sterile covering one at a time, with last flap opened toward the nurse.

> Sterile wrap serves as sterile field.

   a. *In-dwelling catheterization open system:* Open separate package containing drainage bag, check to make sure that clamp on drainage port is closed, and place drainage bag and tubing in easily accessible location. Open outer package of sterile catheter, maintaining sterility of inner wrapper (see Chapter 6).

> Open drainage bag systems have separate sterile packaging for sterile catheter, drainage bag and tubing, and insertion kit.

   b. *In-dwelling catheterization closed system:* All supplies are in sterile tray and arranged in sequence of use.

> Closed drainage bag systems have catheter preattached to drainage tubing and bag.

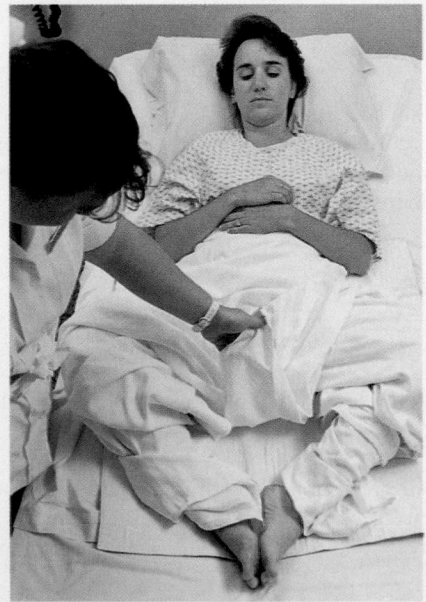

STEP 8a(1) Female patient draped and in dorsal recumbent position.

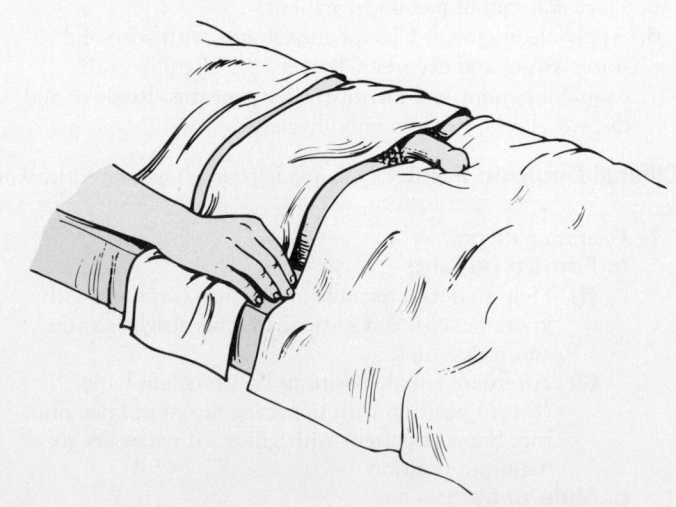

STEP 8b(1) Drape male patient with blankets.

STEP	RATIONALE

IMPLEMENTATION

c. *Straight catheterization:* All needed supplies are in sterile tray that contains supplies and can be used for urine collection.

12. Apply sterile gloves.

Maintains surgical asepsis.

13. *Option:* Apply sterile drape with ungloved hands when drape is packed as first item. Touch only edges of drape. Then apply sterile gloves.

Maintains surgical asepsis.

14. Drape perineum, keeping gloves and working surface of drape sterile.

Sterile drapes provide sterile field over which you will work during catheterization.

a. Drape female:

(1) Pick up square sterile drape touching only edges (2.5 cm [1 inch]).

(2) Allow drape to unfold without touching unsterile surfaces. Allow top edge of drape (2.5 to 5 cm [1 to 2 inches]) to form a cuff over both hands.

When creating cuff over sterile gloved hands, sterility of gloves and workspace is maintained.

(3) Place drape with shiny side down on bed between patient's thighs. Slip cuffed edge just under buttocks as you ask patient to lift hips. Take care not to touch contaminated surfaces with sterile gloves. If gloves are contaminated, remove and apply new pair.

(4) Pick up fenestrated sterile drape out of tray. Allow drape to unfold without touching unsterile surfaces. Allow top edge of drape to form a cuff over both hands. Apply drape over perineum so that opening is over exposed labia (see illustration).

Opening in drape creates sterile field around labia.

b. Drape male:

(1) Use of square drape is optional; you may apply fenestrated drape instead.

(2) Pick up edges of square drape and allow to unfold without touching unsterile surfaces. Place over thighs, with shiny side down, just below penis. Take care not to touch contaminated surfaces with sterile gloves.

(3) Place fenestrated drape with opening centred over penis (see illustration).

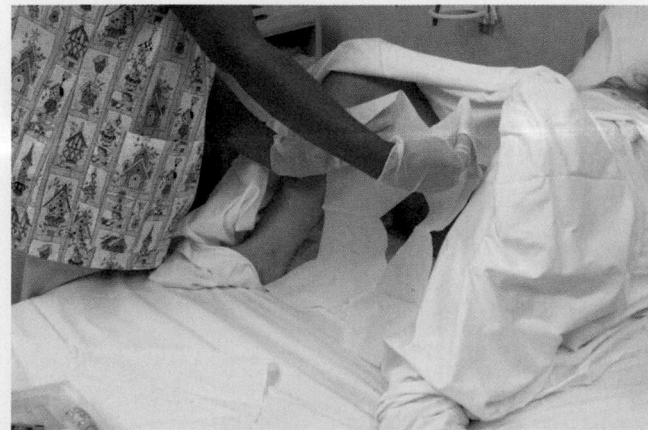

STEP 14a(4) Place sterile fenestrated drape (with opening in centre) over female's perineum.

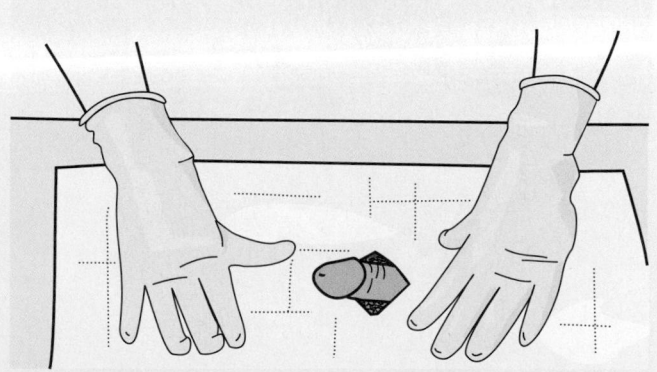

STEP 14b(3) Drape male with fenestrated drape.

STEP	RATIONALE

IMPLEMENTATION

15. Arrange remaining supplies on sterile field, maintaining sterility of gloves. Place sterile tray with cleaning solution (premoistened swab sticks or cotton balls, forceps, and solution), lubricant, sterile catheter, and prefilled syringe for inflating balloon (in-dwelling catheterization only) on sterile drape between the patient's legs.

Provides easy access to supplies during catheter insertion and helps to maintain aseptic technique. Appropriate placement is determined by size of patient and position during catheterization.

a. If kit contains sterile cotton balls, open package of sterile antiseptic solution and pour over cotton balls. Some kits contain package of premoistened swab sticks. Open end of package for easy access (see illustration and Fig. 34.4).

Use of sterile supplies and antiseptic solution reduces risk of CAUTI (CPSI, 2016).

b. Open sterile specimen container if specimen is to be obtained (see Chapter 9).

Makes container accessible to receive urine from catheter if specimen is needed.

c. For in-dwelling catheterization, open sterile wrapper of catheter and leave catheter on sterile field. If part of closed-system kit, remove tray with catheter and preattached drainage bag and place on sterile drape. Make sure that clamp on drainage port of bag is closed. If needed and if part of sterile tray, attach catheter to drainage tubing.

In-dwelling catheterization trays vary. Some have preattached catheters; others need to be attached but are part of the sterile tray; others do not have catheter or drainage system as part of tray.

d. Attach a prefilled water syringe into the balloon port on the catheter.

Preparation for inflating the balloon once the catheter is in place as the nondominant hand is used to stabilize the catheter while the dominant hand inflates the balloon with the syringe.

e. Open packet of lubricant and squeeze out on sterile field. Lubricate catheter tip by dipping it into water-soluble gel 2.5 to 5 cm (1 to 2 inches) for women and 12.5 to 17.5 cm (5 to 7 inches) for men (see illustration).

Lubrication minimizes trauma to urethra and discomfort during catheter insertion.
Male catheter needs enough lubricant to cover length of catheter inserted.

Clinical Decision Point *Pretesting a balloon on an in-dwelling catheter by injecting fluid from the prefilled sterile water syringe into the balloon port is no longer recommended. Testing the balloon may distort and stretch it and lead to damage, causing increased trauma on insertion.*

16. Clean urethral meatus:
    a. **Female patient:**
       (1) Separate labia with fingers of nondominant hand (now contaminated) to fully expose urethral meatus.

Optimal visualization of urethral meatus is possible.

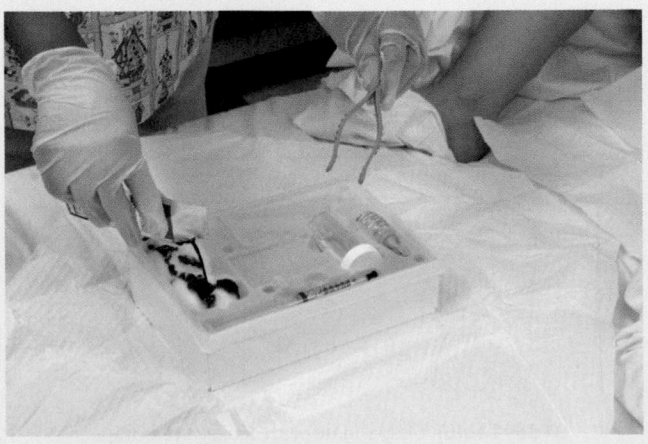

STEP 15a Sterile kit includes antiseptic swabs.

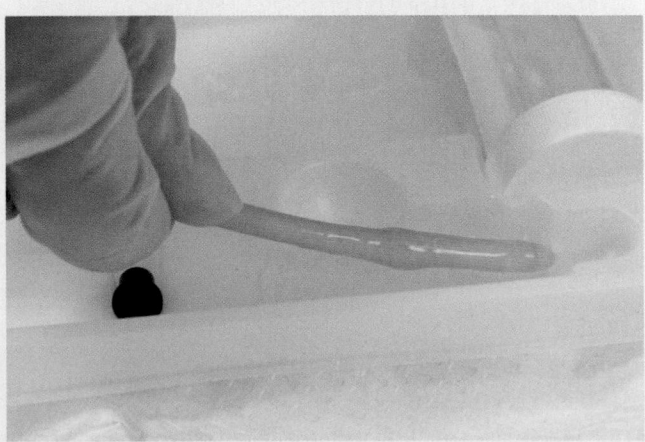

STEP 15e Lubricate catheter.

STEP	RATIONALE

IMPLEMENTATION

(2) Maintain position of nondominant hand throughout procedure.

(3) Holding forceps in dominant hand, pick up one moistened cotton ball or pick up one swab stick at a time. Clean labia and urinary meatus from clitoris toward anus. Use new cotton ball or swab for each area that you clean. Clean by wiping far labial fold, near labial fold, and directly over centre of urethral meatus (see illustration).

b. Male patient:

(1) With nondominant hand (now contaminated) retract foreskin (if uncircumcised) and gently grasp penis at shaft just below glans. Hold shaft of penis at right angle to body. This hand remains in this position for remainder of procedure.

(2) Using uncontaminated dominant hand, clean meatus with cotton balls or swab sticks, using circular strokes, cleaning from meatus toward glans in a spiral motion.

(3) Repeat cleaning three times using clean cotton ball or swab stick each time (see illustration).

17. Pick up and hold catheter 7.5 to 10 cm (3 to 4 inches) from catheter tip with catheter loosely coiled in palm of hand. If catheter is not attached to drainage bag, make sure to position urine tray so end of catheter can be placed there once insertion begins.

18. Insert catheter. Explain to patient that a feeling of burning, pinching, or pressure may be experienced as catheter is inserted into urethra. This sensation is normal and will go away quickly.

Closure of labia during cleaning means that area is contaminated and requires cleaning procedure to be repeated.
Front-to-back cleaning moves from area of least contamination toward highly contaminated area. Follows principles of medical asepsis (see Chapter 5). Dominant gloved hand remains sterile.

When grasping shaft of penis, avoid pressure on dorsal surface to prevent compression of urethra.
Losing grasp during cleaning means that area is contaminated and requires cleaning procedure to be repeated.

Circular cleaning pattern follows principles of medical asepsis (see Chapter 5).

Holding catheter near tip allows for its easier manipulation during insertion. Coiling catheter in palm prevents distal end from striking nonsterile surface.

Helps to minimize patient anxiety.

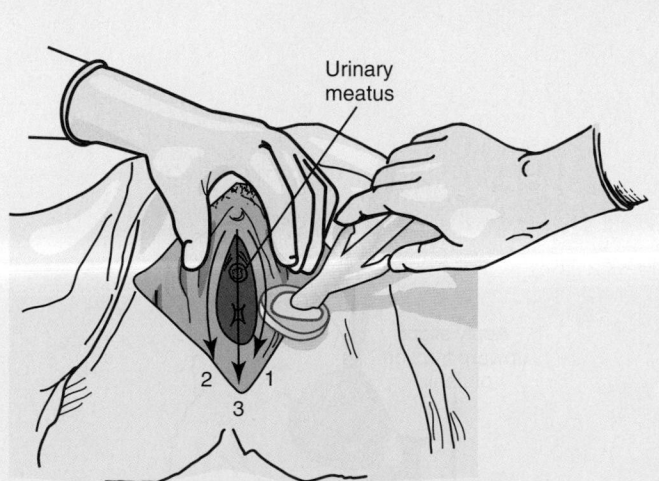

Urinary meatus

STEP 16a(3) Clean female perineum.

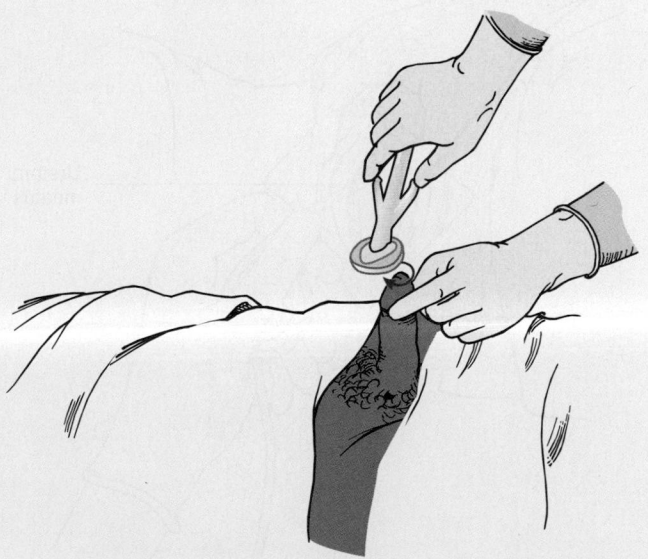

STEP 16b(3) Clean male urinary meatus.

STEP	RATIONALE

IMPLEMENTATION

a. Female patient:

(1) Ask patient to bear down gently, and slowly insert catheter through urethral meatus (see illustration).

Bearing down may help you visualize urinary meatus and promotes relaxation of external urinary sphincter, aiding in catheter insertion.

(2) Advance catheter a total of 5 to 7.5 cm (2 to 3 inches) or until urine flows out of catheter. When urine appears, advance catheter another 2.5 to 5 cm (1 to 2 inches). Do not use force to insert catheter.

Urine flow indicates that catheter tip is in the bladder or lower urethra.

(3) Release labia and hold catheter securely with nondominant hand.

Prevents accidental expulsion of catheter from the patient's bladder.

b. Male patient:

(1) Lift penis to position perpendicular (90 degrees) to patient's body and apply gentle upward traction (see illustration).

Straightens urethra to ease catheter insertion.

(2) Ask patient to bear down as if to void and slowly insert catheter through urethral meatus.

Relaxation of external sphincter aids in insertion of catheter.

(3) Advance catheter 17 to 22.5 cm (7 to 9 inches) or until urine flows out end of catheter.

Length of male urethra varies. Flow of urine indicates that tip of catheter is in the bladder or urethra but not necessarily that balloon part of in-dwelling catheter is in bladder.

(4) Stop advancing with straight catheter. When urine appears in in-dwelling catheter, advance it to bifurcation (inflation and deflation ports exposed) (see illustration).

Further advancement of catheter to bifurcation of drainage and balloon inflation port ensures that it is inserted sufficiently into the bladder (WOCNS, 2016).

(5) Lower penis and hold catheter securely in nondominant hand.

Prevents accidental expulsion of catheter from the patient's bladder.

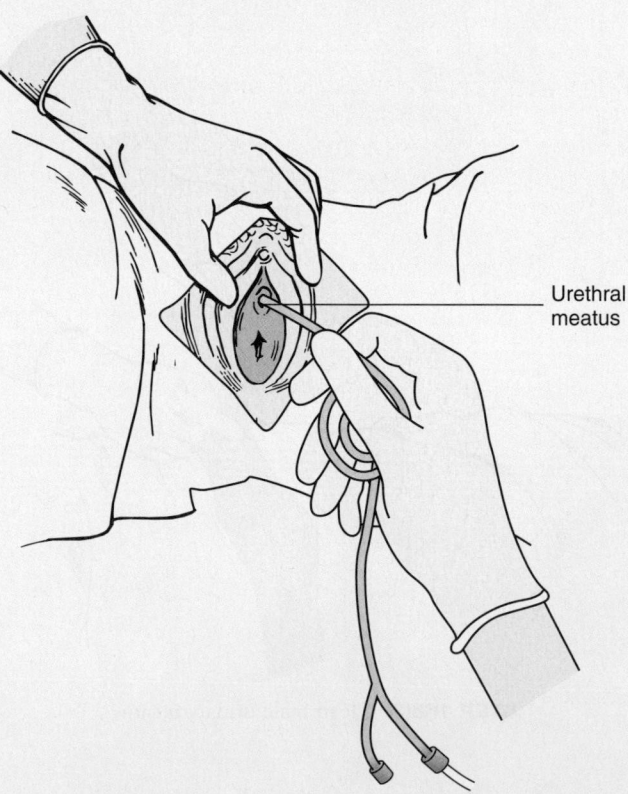

Urethral meatus

STEP 18a(1) Insert catheter into female urinary meatus.

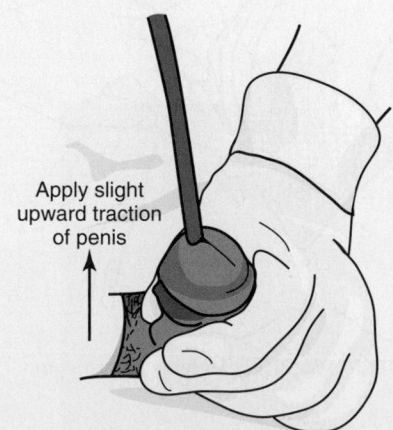

Apply slight upward traction of penis

STEP 18b(1) Insert catheter into male urinary meatus.

STEP	RATIONALE

IMPLEMENTATION

19. Allow bladder to empty fully unless employer policy restricts maximum volume of urine drained.

There is no definitive evidence regarding whether there is benefit in limiting maximal volume drained; however, draining too much volume at once can cause a large fluid shift in the patient (e.g., fluid volumes >1 L), resulting in dizziness and hypotension.

20. Collect urine specimen as needed (see Chapter 9). Fill specimen container to 20 to 30 mL by holding end of catheter over cup.

Sterile specimen for culture analysis can be obtained.

   a. Label and bag specimen according to employer policy. Label specimen in front of patient. Send to laboratory as soon as possible.

A fresh urine specimen ensures more accurate findings. Labelling ensures that diagnostic results will be connected to the correct patient.

21. Straight catheterization: When urine stops flowing, withdraw catheter slowly and smoothly until removed.

Minimizes trauma to urethra.

22. Inflate catheter balloon with amount of fluid designated by manufacturer.

Improper balloon inflation can result in an asymmetrical balloon, which may cause the catheter tip to bend, resulting in improper drainage, bladder spasms, or leakage (WOCNS, 2016).

   a. Continue to hold catheter with nondominant hand.

Holding on to catheter before inflating balloon prevents expulsion of catheter from urethra.

   b. With free dominant hand, pick up the prefilled syringe that is connected to the balloon port at end of catheter.

   c. Slowly inject total amount of solution (see illustration).

Full amount of solution needed to inflate balloon properly.

Clinical Decision Point *If the patient indicates sudden pain during inflation of a catheter balloon or when resistance is felt when inflating the balloon, stop inflation, allow the fluid from the balloon to flow back into the syringe, advance the catheter farther, and reinflate the balloon. The balloon may have been inflating in the urethra. If pain continues, remove the catheter and notify the health care provider.*

   d. After inflating catheter balloon, release catheter from nondominant hand. *Gently* pull catheter until resistance is felt. Then advance catheter slightly.

By moving catheter slightly back into bladder, pressure on bladder neck is avoided.

   e. Connect drainage tubing to catheter if it is not already preconnected.

23. Secure catheter with catheter strap or another securement device attached to the drainage bag tubing and the patient's leg. Leave enough slack to allow leg movement.

Securing catheter reduces risk of catheter migration, inflammation, necrosis, CAUTI, or accidental catheter removal (Yates, 2018). Leaving enough slack allows for leg movement and penile erection without causing urethral trauma.

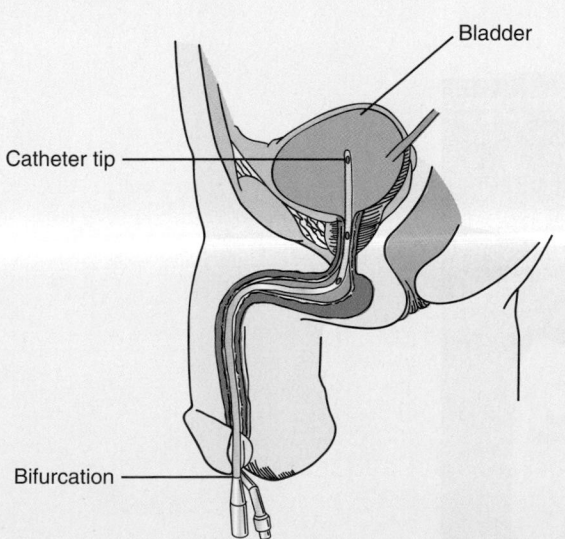

STEP 18b(4) Male anatomy with correct catheter insertion to bifurcation.

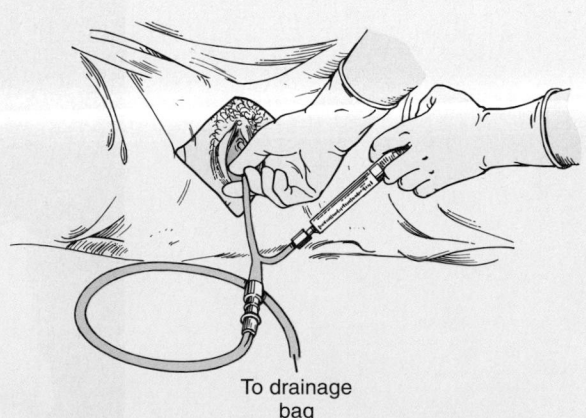

STEP 22c Inflate balloon (in-dwelling catheter).

STEP	RATIONALE

IMPLEMENTATION

a. Female patient:
(1) Secure catheter tubing to inner thigh, allowing enough slack to prevent tension (see illustration).

b. Male patient:
(1) Secure catheter tubing to upper thigh (see illustration) or lower abdomen (with penis directed toward chest). Allow slack in catheter so movement does not create tension on catheter.

Anchoring catheter reduces traction on urethra and minimizes urethral injury (Yates, 2018).

(2) If retracted, replace foreskin over glans penis.

Leaving foreskin retracted can cause discomfort and dangerous edema.

24. Clip drainage tubing to edge of mattress. Position drainage bag lower than bladder by attaching to bedframe. Do not attach to side rails of bed (see illustration).

Drainage bags that are below level of bladder ensure free flow of urine, thus decreasing risk for CAUTI (WOCNS, 2016). Bags attached to movable objects such as side rail increase risk for urethral trauma because of pulling or accidental dislodgement.

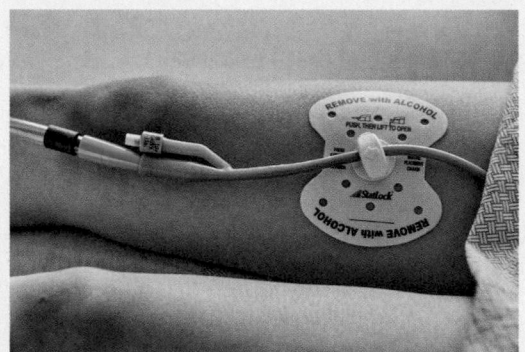

STEP 23a(1) Secure in-dwelling catheter on female with adhesive securement device.

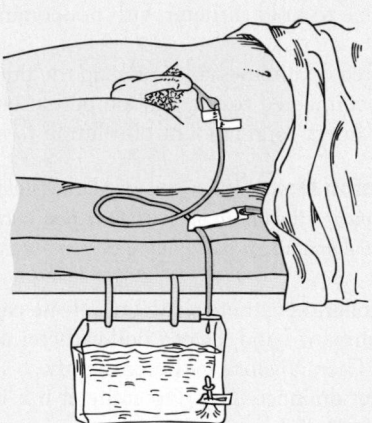

STEP 23b(1) Secure in-dwelling catheter on male with tape. (*From Sorrentino, S. A., Remmert, L. N., & Wilk, M. J. [2018]. Mosby's Canadian textbook for the support worker [4th ed., Fig. 31.11B]. Toronto: Elsevier.*)

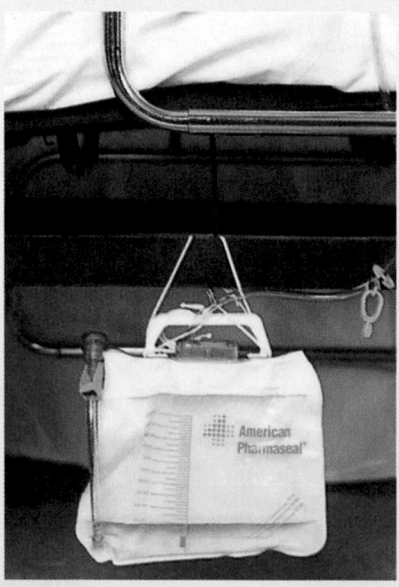

STEP 24 Drainage bag below level of bladder.

STEP	RATIONALE

IMPLEMENTATION

25. Check to ensure that there is no obstruction to urine flow. Coil excess tubing on bed and fasten to bottom sheet with clip or another securement device.

   Rationale: Obstruction to flow of urine increases risk for CAUTI (WOCNS, 2016).

26. Provide hygiene as needed. Help patient to comfortable position.

27. Dispose of supplies in appropriate receptacles.

28. Measure urine and record.

   Rationale: Provides baseline for urine output.

29. Remove gloves and perform hand hygiene.

   Rationale: Reduces transmission of infection.

EVALUATION

1. Palpate bladder for distension or use bladder scan (see Procedural Guideline 34.2) as per employer policy.

   Rationale: Determines if distension is relieved.

2. Ask patient to describe level of comfort.

   Rationale: Determines if patient's sensation of discomfort or fullness has been relieved.

3. *In-dwelling catheter:* Observe character and amount of urine in drainage system.

   Rationale: Determines if urine is flowing adequately.

4. *In-dwelling catheter:* Determine that there is no urine leaking from catheter or tubing connections.

   Rationale: Prevents injury to patient's skin and ensures closed sterile system.

5. **Use Teach-Back:** "I want to be sure I explained clearly about the tube in your bladder and some things you can do to ensure the urine flows out of the tube. Tell me what you can do to keep the urine flowing." Develop a revised teaching plan if patient is not able to teach back correctly.

   Rationale: Determines patient's level of understanding of instructional topic.

Unexpected Outcomes

1. Catheter goes into vagina.

2. Sterility is broken during catheterization by nurse or patient.

3. Patient indicates bladder discomfort, and catheter is patent as evidenced by adequate urine flow.

Related Interventions

- Leave catheter in vagina.
- Clean urinary meatus again. Using another catheter kit, reinsert sterile catheter into meatus (check employer policy). **NOTE:** If gloves become contaminated, start procedure again.
- Remove catheter in vagina after successful insertion of second catheter.
- Replace gloves if contaminated and start over.
- If patient touches sterile field but equipment and supplies remain sterile, avoid touching that part of sterile field.
- If equipment or supplies become contaminated, replace with sterile items or start over with new sterile kit.
- Check catheter to ensure that there is no traction on it.
- Notify health care provider. Patient may be experiencing bladder spasms or symptoms of UTI.
- Monitor catheter output for colour, clarity, odour, and amount.

Communication and Documentation

- Document and report the reason for catheterization, type and size of catheter inserted, amount of fluid used to inflate balloon, specimen collection (if applicable), characteristics and amount of urine, patient's response to procedure, and any education in nurses' notes in electronic health record (EHR) or chart.
- Document amount of urine on intake and output (I&O) flow sheet record in the EHR or chart.
- Report persistent catheter-related pain, inadequate urine output, and discomfort to health care provider.
- Document your evaluation of patient learning.

Special Considerations
Teaching

- Discuss with the patient routine care of the catheter and drainage system, which includes avoiding any kinking in the drainage tubing, keeping the drainage bag dependent, avoiding pulling on the catheter, and daily hygiene.
- Explain that adequate fluid intake helps prevent catheter blockage.

Pediatric

- When caring for an infant or a young child, explain procedures to parents. Describe procedure to a child at a level the child is able to understand (Hockenberry & Wilson, 2015).

- Children and adolescents will experience some discomfort during catheterization. Assistance and gentle holding may be necessary, especially with younger children. Most children prefer to have the parents remain with them during the procedure. Ask adolescents if they would like a parent to remain with them.
- Catheterization in infants and children may be made easier by use of an adequate amount of catheter lubricant containing 2% lidocaine (Hockenberry & Wilson, 2015).
- Teaching young children to blow into a straw or pinwheel can help to relax pelvic muscles during catheter insertion (Hockenberry & Wilson, 2015).

Gerontological

- The urethral meatus of an older female may be difficult to identify because of urogenital atrophy.
- Symptoms of a UTI in an older person may be difficult to recognize and may be indicated by cognitive changes, lethargy, anorexia, weakness, tachycardia, hypotension, and increased respiratory rate (WOCNS, 2016).
- Older persons have an increased risk for UTI related to increased prevalence of chronic disease such as diabetes mellitus and prostatic hypertrophy and a higher prevalence of incontinence.

- The presence of a urinary catheter and its drainage tubing and bag can interfere with the already compromised mobility of the older person.

Care in the Community

- Patients who are at home may use a leg bag during the day and switch to a larger-volume bag at night. If a patient changes from a large-volume bag to a leg bag, instruct them in the importance of hand hygiene and cleaning the connection ports with alcohol before changing bags.
- Teach patients and caregivers how to properly position the drainage bag; empty the urinary drainage bag; and observe urine colour, clarity, odour, and amount.
- Educate patients and caregivers about the signs of UTI and troubleshooting techniques for a leaking catheter.
- Arrange for home delivery of catheter supplies, always ensuring that there is at least one extra catheter, insertion kit, and drainage bag in the home.

◆ SKILL 34.2 Care and Removal of an In-dwelling Catheter

NSO *Nursing Skills Online Urinary Catheterization Module 17 / Lesson 5* *Video Clip*

Providing regular perineal hygiene, preventing catheter-related trauma, and removing in-dwelling catheters as soon as possible are important interventions to reduce risk of catheter-associated urinary tract infection (CAUTI) (CPSI, 2016; WOCNS, 2016). Prolonged in-dwelling catheterization is a major risk factor for CAUTI. When removing an in-dwelling catheter, it is important to ensure that the catheter balloon is fully deflated to minimize trauma to the urethra. Often clinicians clamp catheter tubing before removal in the belief that the practice allows the bladder to fill and obtain bladder tone. However, evidence is unclear that the practice of clamping a catheter before removal will improve bladder function after removal (WOCNS, 2016).

All patients should have their voiding monitored after catheter removal for at least 24 to 48 hours by using a voiding record or bladder diary. The nurse records the time and amount of each voiding, including any incontinence, in the patient record. A bladder scan is used (see Procedural Guideline 34.2) or ultrasound to monitor bladder functioning by measuring postvoid residual. Abdominal pain and distension, a sensation of incomplete emptying, incontinence, constant dribbling of urine, and voiding in very small amounts can indicate inadequate bladder emptying requiring intervention.

The risk of urinary tract infection (UTI) increases with the use of an in-dwelling catheter. Symptoms of infection can develop 2 or more days after catheter removal. Nurses need to inform patients of the risk for infection, prevention measures (e.g., perineal hygiene), and signs and symptoms that need to be reported to the primary care provider.

Delegation and Collaboration

The skill of performing routine catheter care can be delegated to an unregulated care provider (UCP). The skill of removing an in-dwelling catheter can be delegated to a UCP (see employer policy); however, the nurse must first assess a patient's status and verify the health care provider prescription. The nurse directs the UCP to:

- Report characteristics of the urine (colour, clarity, odour, and amount) before and after catheter removal.
- Report the condition of the patient's genital area (e.g., colour, rashes, open areas, odour, soiling from fecal incontinence, trauma to tissues around urinary meatus).
- If permitted by employer policy to remove catheter, check size of balloon and syringe needed to deflate balloon and report if balloon does not deflate and if there is bleeding after removal.
- Report time and amount of first voiding after catheter is removed.
- Report patient indications of fever, chills, burning, flank pain, back pain, and blood in the urine.
- Report patient indications of dysuria, hematuria, urgency, frequency, lower abdominal pain, change in mental status, and lethargy.

Equipment
Catheter Care

- Clean gloves
- Waterproof pad
- Bath blanket
- Soap, washcloth, towel, and basin filled with warm water. *Option:* chlorhexidine 2% cloth

Removing a Catheter

- 10-mL or larger syringe without needle (Information on balloon size [mL] is printed directly on balloon inflation valve [see Fig. 34.3].)
- Graduated cylinder to measure urine
- Toilet, bedside commode, urine "hat," urinal, or bedpan
- Bladder scanner (if indicated)

STEP	RATIONALE

ASSESSMENT

1. Identify patient using at least two person-specific identifiers (e.g., name and date of birth or name and medical record number), according to employer policy.

Ensures correct patient. Complies with Accreditation Canada's standards and improves patient safety (Accreditation Canada, 2019).

2. Perform hand hygiene.

Reduces transmission of microorganisms.

3. Assess need for catheter care:

   a. Observe urinary output and urine characteristics.

Reduces transmission of microorganisms. A sudden decrease in urine output may indicate occlusion of catheter. Cloudy, foul-smelling urine associated with other systemic symptoms may indicate CAUTI.

   b. Assess for history or presence of bowel incontinence.

The most common bacteria to cause CAUTI are *Escherichia coli*, a major colonizer of the bowel; thus fecal incontinence increases risk for CAUTI (WOCNS, 2016).

   c. Observe for any discharge, redness, bleeding, or presence of tissue trauma around urethral meatus (this may be deferred until catheter care).

Indicates inflammatory process, possible infection, or erosion of catheter through urethra.

   d. Assess patient's knowledge of catheter care.

Determines need for patient education related to catheter care.

4. Assess need for catheter removal:

   a. Review patient's medical record, including health care provider's prescription and nurses' notes. Note length of time catheter was in place.

Catheters in place for more than a few days cause higher risk for catheter encrustation and UTI.

   b. Assess patient's knowledge of and prior experience with catheter removal.

Reveals need for patient instruction and support.

   c. Assess urine colour, clarity, odour, and amount. Note any urethral discharge, irritation of genital region, or trauma to urinary meatus (this may be deferred until just before catheter removal).

May be indicator of inflammation or UTI and source of discomfort during catheter removal.

   d. Determine size of catheter inflation balloon by looking at balloon inflation valve.

Determines size of syringe needed to deflate balloon and amount of fluid expected in syringe after deflation.

NURSING DIAGNOSES

- Reduced urinary elimination
- Insufficient knowledge regarding catheter care
- Potential for infection

Related factors/Risk factors are individualized on the basis of patient's condition or needs.

PLANNING

1. Expected outcomes following catheter care:
- Genital area is free of secretions, fecal matter, and irritation.

Basic hygiene, especially after bowel movements, reduces risk for CAUTI (WOCNS, 2016).

- Patient verbalizes feeling of comfort.

Cleaning relieves local discomfort from irritation of catheter.

2. Expected outcomes after catheter removal:
- Patient voids at least 150 mL with each voiding no more than 6 to 8 hours after removal.

Indicates return of voluntary bladder function without urinary retention.

- Patient verbalizes feeling of complete bladder emptying and absence of discomfort.
- Patient identifies signs and symptoms of UTI.

Indicates patient learning.

3. Explain procedure to patient. Discuss signs and symptoms of UTI. If applicable, teach patient how to perform catheter hygiene.

Reduces anxiety and promotes cooperation.
Self-care supports patient's sense of autonomy.

IMPLEMENTATION

1. Close room door and bedside curtain.

Provides patient privacy.

2. Perform hand hygiene.

Reduces transmission of microorganisms.

3. Raise bed to appropriate working height. If side rails are raised, lower side rail on working side.

Promotes use of proper body mechanics.

STEP	RATIONALE

IMPLEMENTATION

4. Organize equipment for perineal care and/or removal of catheter.

Increases efficiency of procedure.

5. Position patient with waterproof pad under buttocks and cover with bath blanket, exposing only genital area and catheter (see Skill 34.1).

Demonstrates person-centred care and respect for patient dignity by only exposing genital area and catheter.

   a. Female is in dorsal recumbent position.

   b. Male is in supine position.

6. Apply clean gloves.

Reduces transmission of infection.

7. Remove catheter securement device while maintaining connection with drainage tubing.

Provides ability to easily clean around catheter and to remove it.

8. Catheter care:

   a. *Female:* Use nondominant hand to gently separate labia to fully expose urethral meatus and catheter. Maintain position of hand throughout procedure.

Provides full visualization of urethral meatus. Full separation of labia prevents contamination of meatus during cleaning.

   b. *Male:* Use nondominant hand to retract foreskin if not circumcised and hold penis at shaft just below glans. Maintain hand position throughout procedure.

Retraction of foreskin provides full visualization of urethral meatus.

Clinical Decision Point *Accidentally closing labia or dropping penis during cleaning requires procedure to be repeated.*

   c. Grasp catheter with two fingers to stabilize it.

Prevents unnecessary traction on catheter.
Pulling on catheter is a cause of discomfort for patient and can damage urethra and bladder neck.

   d. Assess urethral meatus and surrounding tissues for inflammation, swelling, discharge, or tissue trauma and ask patient if burning or discomfort is present.

Determines frequency and type of ongoing care required. Indicates possibility of CAUTI or catheter erosion through urethra.

   e. Provide perineal hygiene using mild soap and warm water (see Chapter 18). *Option:* Use chlorhexidine 2% cloth.

Antiseptic cleaners have not been proven conclusively to decrease risk for CAUTI. Chlorhexidine use has not been supported with sufficient evidence, and there have been rare cases of anaphylaxis due to use of chlorhexidine gel (WOCNS, 2016; Yates, 2015).

   f. Using clean washcloth, clean catheter.

      (1) Starting close to urinary meatus, clean catheter in circular motion along its length for about 10 cm (4 inches), moving away from body (see illustration). Remove all traces of soap. *For male patients:* Reduce or reposition foreskin after care.

Reduces presence of secretions or drainage on outside catheter surface.

   g. Reapply catheter securement device. Allow slack in catheter so movement does not create tension on it.

Securing in-dwelling catheter reduces risk of urethral trauma, urethral erosion, CAUTI, or accidental removal (CPSI, 2016; Yates, 2018).

9. Routinely check drainage tubing and bag.

   a. Catheter is secured to upper thigh (for women) or abdomen (for men).

Maintains unobstructed flow of urine out of bladder (CPSI, 2016; Yates, 2018).

   b. Tubing is coiled and secured onto bed linen.

   c. Tubing is not looped or positioned above level of bladder.

   d. Tubing is not kinked or clamped.

   e. Drainage bag is positioned below level of bladder with urine flowing freely into bag.

   f. Drainage bag is not overfull. Empty drainage bag when ½ full.

Overfull drainage bag creates tension and pulls on catheter, resulting in trauma to urethra and/or urinary meatus (Yates, 2018).

STEP	RATIONALE

IMPLEMENTATION

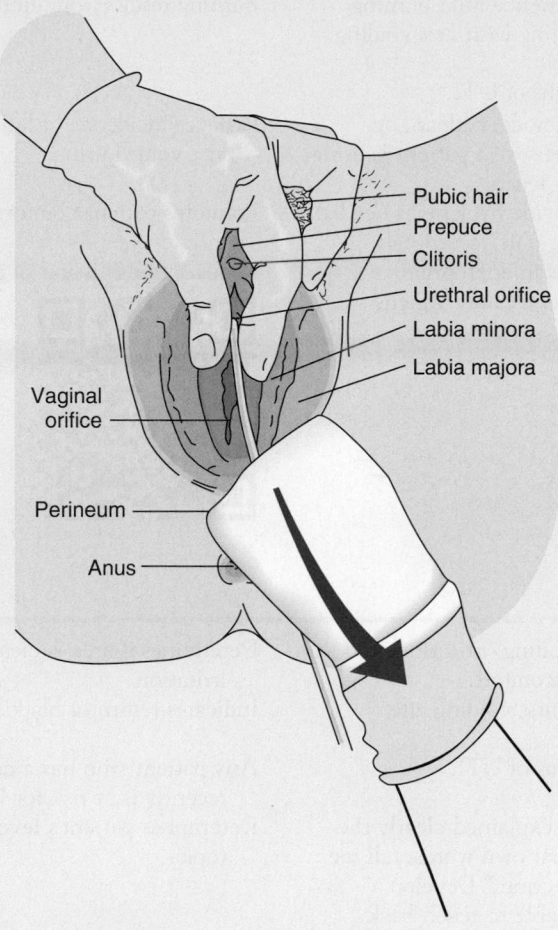

Pubic hair
Prepuce
Clitoris
Urethral orifice
Labia minora
Labia majora

Vaginal orifice

Perineum

Anus

STEP 8f(1) Clean catheter starting at meatus and moving downward while holding it securely.

10. Catheter removal:
(Follow Step 8, above, before catheter removal.)

   a. Move syringe plunger up and down to loosen and then pull it back to 0.5 mL. Insert hub of syringe into inflation valve (balloon port). Allow balloon fluid to drain into syringe by gravity. The syringe should fill. Make sure that the entire amount of fluid is removed by comparing removed amount to volume needed for inflation.

A partially inflated balloon can traumatize the urethral wall during removal. Passive drainage of catheter balloon prevents formation of ridges in balloon. These ridges can cause discomfort or trauma during removal.

   b. Pull catheter out smoothly and slowly. Examine it to ensure that it is whole. The catheter should slide out easily. Do not use force. If you note any resistance, repeat Step 10a to remove remaining water.

A nonwhole (not intact) catheter means that pieces of catheter may still be in the bladder. Notify health care provider immediately.

   c. Wrap contaminated catheter in waterproof pad. Unhook collection bag and drainage tubing from bed.

Promotes patient comfort and safety.

   d. Empty, measure, and record urine present in drainage bag (see Chapter 8).

Documents urinary output.

   e. Encourage patient to maintain or increase fluid intake (unless contraindicated).

Maintains normal urine output.

   f. Initiate voiding record or bladder diary. Instruct patient to tell you when the need to empty bladder occurs and that all urine needs to be measured. Make sure that patient understands how to use collection container.

Evaluates bladder function.

STEP	RATIONALE

IMPLEMENTATION

g. Explain that many patients experience mild burning, discomfort, or small-volume voiding with first voiding, which soon subsides.

Burning results from urethral irritation.

h. Instruct patient to report any signs of UTI.

i. Ensure easy access to toilet, commode, bedpan, or urinal. Place urine "hat" on toilet seat if patient is using toilet. Place call bell within easy reach.

Reduces incidence of falls during toileting. Urine hat collects first voided urine.

11. Reposition patient as necessary. Provide hygiene as needed. Lower level of bed and position side rails accordingly.

Promotes patient comfort and safety.

12. Dispose of all contaminated supplies in appropriate receptacle, remove gloves, and perform hand hygiene.

Reduces transmission of microorganisms.

EVALUATION

1. Inspect catheter and genital area for soiling, irritation, and skin breakdown. Ask patient about discomfort.

Determines if area is cleaned properly and if patient has any irritation.

2. Observe time and measure amount of first voiding after catheter removal.

Indicates return of bladder function after catheter removal.

3. Evaluate patient for signs and symptoms of UTI.

Any patient who has a catheter or has had a catheter removed recently is at risk for UTI.

4. Use Teach-Back: "I want to be sure I explained clearly the signs of a urinary tract infection. In your own words, tell me what signs indicate a urinary tract infection." Develop a revised teaching plan if patient is not able to teach back correctly.

Determines patient's level of understanding of instructional topic.

Unexpected Outcomes

1. Water from inflation balloon does not return into syringe.

2. Patient has cloudy urine, foul urine odour, fever, chills, dysuria, flank pain, back pain, hematuria, urgency, frequency, lower abdominal pain, change in mental status, and lethargy (Medline Plus, 2019).

3. Patient is unable to void after catheter removal, has sensation of not emptying, strains to void, or experiences small voiding amounts with increasing frequency.

Related Interventions

- Reposition patient; ensure that catheter is not pinched or kinked.
- Remove syringe. Attach new syringe and allow enough time for passive emptying.
- Attempt to empty balloon by gently pulling back on syringe plunger.
- If catheter balloon does not deflate, *do not* cut balloon inflation valve to drain water. Notify health care provider.
- Assess for bladder distension and tenderness.
- Monitor vital signs and urine output.
- Report findings to health care provider; signs and symptoms may indicate UTI.
- Consult with health care provider for prescription to remove catheter.
- Assess for bladder distension.
- Help to normal position for voiding and provide privacy.
- Perform bladder ultrasound or scan (see Procedural Guideline 34.2) to assess for excessive urine volume in bladder.
- If patient is unable to void within 6 to 8 hours of catheter removal or experiences abdominal pain, notify health care provider.

Communication and Documentation

- Document time for catheter care and appearance of urine; describe condition of meatus and catheter in nurses' notes in electronic health record (EHR) or chart.
- Document and report time of catheter removal; amount of water removed from balloon; condition of urethral meatus and catheter; the time, amount, and characteristics of first voided urine in nurses' notes in EHR or chart.
- Document teaching related to catheter care, catheter removal, and fluid intake in nurses' notes in EHR or chart.
- Report hematuria, fever, dysuria, inability or difficulty voiding, and any new incontinence after a catheter is removed to health care provider.
- For patient continuing to have a catheter in place, report signs of UTI to health care provider.

Special Considerations
Teaching

- Unless contraindicated, patients with a catheter should drink at least 2 L of fluid per day to promote continuous flushing of the bladder and prevent sediment from collecting in the catheter tubing.
- Instruct patient to hold collection bag below the level of the bladder when ambulating.
- Instruct patient not to disconnect the catheter from the collection tubing and bag.

Pediatric

- During catheter removal do not force catheter out of bladder if you meet resistance. When excessive tubing has been inserted in the bladder, there have been occurrences of knotting of the tube (Hockenberry & Wilson, 2015).

Gerontological

- Older persons may exhibit atypical signs and symptoms of CAUTI such as a change in mental status attributed to delirium. A change in mental status may include confusion, agitation, and lethargy.
- In contrast to UTI, asymptomatic bacteriuria (ASB) is more common in older persons than in younger adults. Nursing home residents often suffer from significant cognitive deficits, impairing their ability to communicate, and from chronic genitourinary symptoms (e.g., incontinence, urgency, and frequency), which make the diagnosis of symptomatic UTI in this group particularly challenging. Furthermore, when infected, nursing home residents are more likely to present with nonspecific symptoms of UTI, such as lack of appetite, confusion, and a decline in functional status; fever may be absent or diminished (WOCNS, 2016).

Care in the Community

- Assess the patient and caregiver for ability and motivation to participate in routine catheter care.

✦ SKILL 34.3 Performing Closed Urinary Catheter Irrigation

To maintain the patency of in-dwelling catheters, it is sometimes necessary to irrigate or flush a catheter with sterile solution. However, irrigation poses a risk of causing a urinary tract infection (UTI) and thus must be done maintaining a closed urinary drainage system. In some instances, the health care provider will determine that irrigations are needed to keep a catheter patent, such as after genitourinary surgery when there is a high risk for catheter occlusion from blood clots.

Closed catheter irrigation provides intermittent or continuous irrigation of a urinary catheter without disrupting the sterile connection between the catheter and the drainage system (Fig. 34.6). Continuous bladder irrigation (CBI) is an example of a continuous infusion of a sterile solution into the bladder, usually using a three-way irrigation closed system with a triple-lumen catheter. CBI is frequently used following genitourinary surgery to keep the bladder clear and free of blood clots or sediment.

Delegation and Collaboration

The skill of performing closed catheter irrigation cannot be delegated to an unregulated care provider (UCP). The nurse directs the UCP to:

- Report to the nurse if the patient indicates pain, discomfort, or leakage of fluid around the catheter.
- Monitor and document intake and output (I&O); report immediately any decrease in urine output.
- Report any change in the colour of the urine, especially the presence of blood clots.

Equipment

- Sterile irrigation solution at room temperature (as prescribed)
- Antiseptic swabs
- Clean gloves

PROCEDURAL GUIDELINE 34.2 *Bladder Scan and Catheterization to Determine Residual Urine*

A bladder scanner (Fig. 34.5) is a noninvasive device that creates an ultrasound image of the bladder for measuring the volume of urine in the bladder. The device makes calculations to report accurate urine volumes, especially lower volumes. A bladder scanner is used to assess bladder volume whenever inadequate bladder emptying is suspected, such as after the removal of in-dwelling urinary catheters, in the evaluation of new-onset incontinence, and after urological surgery. The most common use for the bladder scan is to measure postvoid residual (PVR) (i.e., the volume of urine in the bladder after a normal voiding). To obtain the most reliable reading, measure PVR within 5 to 15 minutes of voiding (Huether, McCance, El-Hussein, et al., 2018). A volume less than 50 mL is considered normal. Two or more PVR measurements greater than 100 mL require further investigation. If a bladder

Continued

PROCEDURAL GUIDELINE 34.2 *Bladder Scan and Catheterization to Determine Residual Urine—cont'd*

scanner is not available, obtain a PVR by measuring urine emptied from the bladder after a straight catheterization.

Delegation and Collaboration

The skill of measuring bladder volume by bladder scan can be delegated to an unregulated care provider (UCP). The nurse must first determine the timing and frequency of the bladder scan measurement and interpret the measurements obtained. The nurse also assesses the patient's ability to toilet before measuring PVR and the abdomen for distension if urinary retention is suspected. The nurse directs the UCP to:

* Follow manufacturer recommendations for use of the device.
* Measure PVR volumes within 5 to 15 minutes after helping the patient to void.
* Report and document bladder scan volumes.

Equipment

* Bladder scanner (follow manufacturer instructions for use)
* Ultrasound gel
* Cleaning agent for scanner head such as an alcohol pad
* Urethral catheterization tray with single-use catheter for straight/intermittent catheterization (see Skill 34.1).
* Paper towel or washcloth

Procedural Steps

1. Identify patient using at least two person-specific identifiers (e.g., name and date of birth or name and medical record number), according to employer policy (Accreditation Canada, 2019).
2. Assess intake and output (I&O) record to determine urine output trends and check the plan of care to verify correct timing of the bladder scan measurement.
3. Perform hand hygiene and apply clean gloves.
4. Provide privacy by closing the room door and bedside curtain.
5. Discuss procedure with the patient. If measurement is for PVR, ask patient to void and measure voided urine volume. Measurement should be within 5 to 15 minutes of voiding.
6. Measure PVR with the bladder scan.
   a. Help patient to a supine position with head slightly elevated. Raise bed to appropriate working height. If side rails are raised, lower side rail on working side.
   b. Expose patient's lower abdomen.
   c. Turn on scanner per manufacturer guidelines.
   d. Set gender designation per manufacturer guidelines. Women who have had a hysterectomy should be designated as male.
   e. Wipe scanner head with alcohol pad or other cleaner and allow to air dry.
   f. Palpate patient's symphysis pubis (pubic bone). Apply generous amount of ultrasound gel (or, if available, a bladder scan gel pad) to midline abdomen 2.5 to 4 cm (1 to 1.5 inches) above symphysis pubis.
   g. Place scanner head on gel, ensuring that scanner head is oriented per manufacturer guidelines.
   h. Apply light pressure, keep scanner head steady, and point it slightly downward toward bladder. Press and release the scan button (see illustration).
   i. Verify accurate aim (refer to manufacturer guidelines). Complete scan and print image (if needed).
7. Remove ultrasound gel from patient's abdomen with paper towel or moist cloth.
8. Remove ultrasound gel from scanner head and wipe with alcohol pad or other cleaner; allow to air-dry.
9. Help patient to comfortable position. Lower bed and replace side rails accordingly.
10. Remove gloves and perform hand hygiene.
11. Measure PVR after using straight/intermittent catheterization (see Skill 34.1). Compare results with prevoiding scan; urine volume should be less.
12. Review health care provider's prescription to determine how often to assess residual urine.
13. Review I&O record to determine urine output trends.

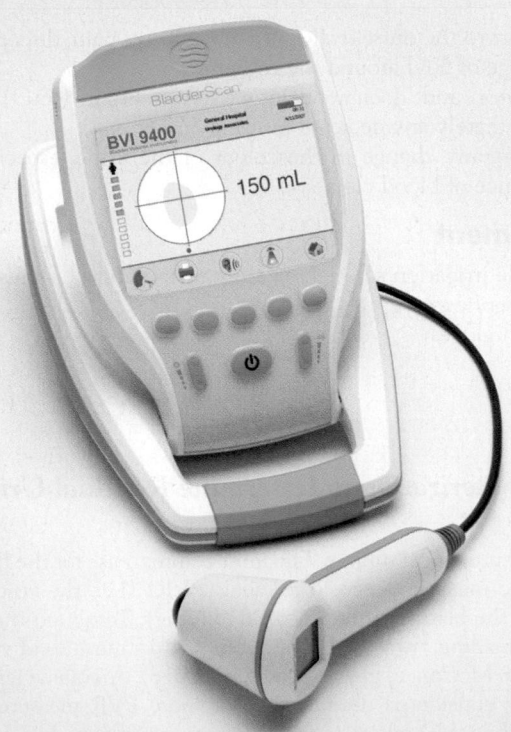

FIG 34.5 Bladder scanner with image.

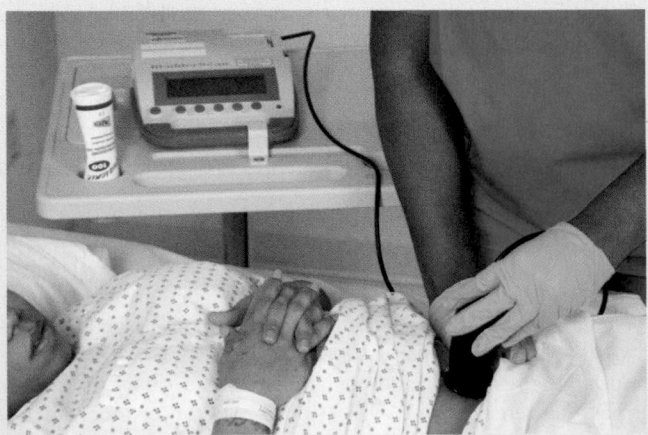

STEP 6h Placement of bladder scan head.

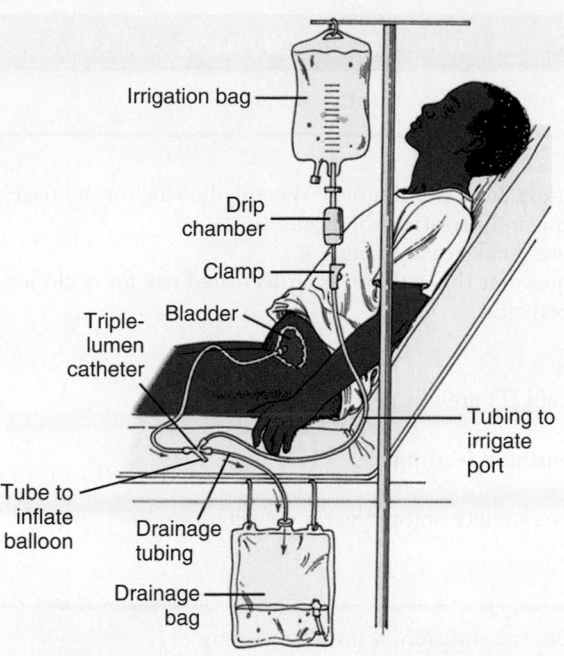

Irrigation bag

Drip chamber

Clamp

Bladder

Triple-lumen catheter

Tube to inflate balloon

Drainage tubing

Drainage bag

Tubing to irrigate port

FIG 34.6 Closed continuous bladder irrigation.

Closed Intermittent Irrigation
- Antiseptic swabs
- Sterile irrigation solution at room temperature as prescribed
- Sterile container
- Syringe to access system: Luer-Lok syringe for needleless access port (per manufacturer instructions)
- Screw clamp or rubber band (used to temporarily occlude catheter as irrigant is instilled)

Closed Continuous Irrigation
- Antiseptic swabs
- Sterile irrigation solution at room temperature as prescribed
- Irrigation tubing with clamp to regulate irrigation flow rate
- Y connector (optional) to connect irrigation tubing to double-lumen catheter
- Intravenous (IV) pole (closed continuous or intermittent)

STEP	RATIONALE
ASSESSMENT	
1. Identify patient using at least two person-specific identifiers (e.g., name and date of birth, or name and medical record number), according to employer policy.	Ensures correct patient. Complies with Accreditation Canada's standards and improves patient safety (Accreditation Canada, 2019).
2. Verify in medical record: **a.** Prescription for irrigation method (continuous or intermittent), type (sterile saline or medicated solution), and amount of irrigant.	A health care provider's prescription is required to initiate therapy. Frequency and volume of solution used for irrigation may be in the prescription or standardized as part of employer policy.
b. Type of catheter in place (see Fig. 34.2).	Single- and double-lumen catheters are used with open irrigation. Triple-lumen catheters are used for both intermittent and continuous closed irrigation.
3. Perform hand hygiene. Palpate bladder for distension and tenderness or use bladder scan (see Procedural Guidelines 34.2).	Reduces transmission of microorganisms. Bladder distension indicates that flow of urine may be blocked from draining.
4. Assess patient for abdominal pain or spasms, sensation of bladder fullness, or catheter bypassing (leaking).	May indicate overdistension of bladder caused by catheter blockage. Offers baseline to determine if therapy is successful.
5. Observe urine for colour, amount, clarity, and presence of mucus, clots, or sediment.	Indicates if patient is bleeding or sloughing tissue, which would require an increased irrigation rate or frequency of catheter irrigation.
6. Monitor I&O. If CBI is being used, the amount of fluid draining from the bladder should exceed the amount of fluid infused into the bladder.	If output does not exceed irrigant infused, catheter obstruction (i.e., blood clots, kinked tubing) should be suspected, irrigation stopped, and the prescriber notified (Lewis et al., 2019).
7. Assess patient's knowledge regarding purpose of performing catheter irrigation.	Reveals need for patient instruction and support.

NURSING DIAGNOSES

- Reduced urinary elimination
- Acute pain
- Insufficient knowledge regarding closed catheter irrigation
- Potential for infection

Related factors/Risk factors are individualized on the basis of patient's condition or needs.

STEP	RATIONALE

PLANNING

1. Expected outcomes following completion of this procedure:
- With CBI: Catheter fluid return is greater than volume of irrigating solution instilled.
- Patient reports relief of bladder pain or spasms.
- Urine output has decreased with an absence of blood clots and sediment. (**NOTE:** Urine will be bloody following bladder or urethral surgery, gradually becoming lighter and blood tinged in 2 to 3 days.)

- Absence of fever, lower abdominal pain, and cloudy or foul-smelling urine.
- Patient can explain purpose of the procedure and what to expect.

2. Explain procedure to patient.

Indicates patency of drainage system, allowing for drainage of urine and irrigating solution.
Indicates bladder emptying.
Indicates that the catheter is at decreased risk for occlusion with blood clots.

Signs of UTI are not present.

Demonstrates learning.

Reduces anxiety and promotes cooperation.

IMPLEMENTATION

1. Perform hand hygiene.

2. Provide privacy by closing room door and bedside curtain.

3. Raise bed to appropriate working height. If side rails are raised, lower side rail on working side.

4. Position patient supine and expose catheter junctions (catheter and drainage tubing).

5. Remove catheter securement device.

6. Organize supplies according to type of irrigation prescribed. Apply clean gloves.

7. Closed continuous irrigation:
   a. Close clamp on new irrigation tubing and hang bag of irrigating solution on IV pole. Insert (spike) tip of sterile irrigation tubing into designated port of irrigation solution bag using aseptic technique (see illustration).

Reduces transmission of microorganisms.
Demonstrates person-centred care by promoting patient comfort and self-esteem.
Promotes use of good body mechanics.
Position provides access to the catheter and promotes patient dignity as much as possible.
Position provides access to the catheter and promotes patient dignity as much as possible.
Eases access to catheter parts.
Ensures an efficient procedure.

Prevents air from entering tubing. Air can cause bladder spasms. Technique prevents transmission of microorganisms.

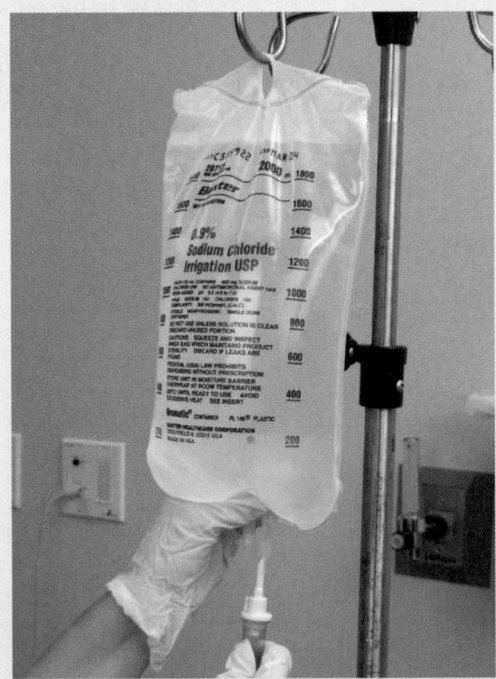

STEP 7a Spiking bag of sterile irrigation solution for continuous bladder irrigation.

STEP	RATIONALE

IMPLEMENTATION

b. Fill drip chamber half full by squeezing chamber. Remove cap at end of tubing, and then open clamp and allow solution to flow (prime) through tubing, keeping end of tubing sterile. Once fluid has completely filled tubing, close clamp and recap end of tubing.

Priming tubing with fluid prevents introduction of air into the bladder.

c. Using aseptic technique, remove cap and connect end of tubing securely to port for infusing irrigation fluid into double- or triple–lumen catheter.

Reduces transmission of microorganisms.

d. Adjust clamp on irrigation tubing to begin flow of solution into bladder. If set volume rate is prescribed, calculate drip rate and adjust rate at roller clamp. If urine is bright red or has clots, increase irrigation rate until drainage appears pink (according to prescribed rate or employer policy).

Continuous drainage is expected. It helps to prevent clotting in the presence of active bleeding in the bladder and flushes clots out of the bladder.

e. Observe for outflow of fluid into drainage bag. Empty catheter drainage bag as needed.

Discomfort, bladder distension, and possible injury can occur from overdistension of the bladder when bladder irrigant cannot adequately flow from the bladder. The bag will fill rapidly and may need to be emptied every 1 to 2 hours.

8. Closed intermittent irrigation:

Fluid is instilled through the catheter in a bolus, flushing system. Fluid drains out after irrigation is complete.

a. Pour prescribed sterile irrigation solution into sterile container.

b. Draw prescribed volume of irrigant (usually 30 to 50 mL) into sterile syringe using aseptic technique. Place sterile cap on tip of needleless syringe.

Ensures sterility of irrigating fluid.

c. Clamp catheter tubing below soft injection port with screw clamp (or fold catheter tubing onto itself and secure with rubber band).

Occluding catheter tubing below the point of injection allows irrigating solution to enter the catheter and flow into the bladder.

d. Using circular motion, clean catheter port (specimen port) with an antiseptic swab.

Reduces transmission of microorganisms.

e. Insert tip of needleless syringe using twisting motion into port.

Ensures that catheter tip enters lumen of catheter.

f. Inject solution using slow, even pressure.

Gentle instillation of solution minimizes trauma to bladder mucosa.

g. Remove syringe and clamp (or rubber band), allowing solution to drain into urinary drainage bag. (**NOTE:** Some medicated irrigants may need to dwell in the bladder for a prescribed period, requiring the catheter to be clamped temporarily before being allowed to drain.)

Allows drainage to flow out by gravity.
Medications must be instilled long enough to be absorbed by lining of bladder. Clamped drainage tubing and bag should not be left unattended.

9. Anchor catheter with a catheter securement device (see Skill 34.1).

Prevents trauma to urethral tissue caused by pulling catheter.

10. Help patient to a safe and comfortable position. Lower bed and place side rails accordingly.

Promotes patient comfort and safety.

11. Dispose of all contaminated supplies in an appropriate receptacle, remove gloves, and perform hand hygiene.

Reduces transmission of microorganisms.

EVALUATION

1. Measure actual urine output by subtracting total amount of irrigation fluid infused from total volume drained into basin.

Determines accurate urinary output.

2. Review I&O flow sheet to verify that hourly output into drainage bag is in appropriate proportion to irrigating solution entering bladder. Expect more output than fluid instilled, because of urine production.

Determines urinary output in relation to irrigation.

3. Inspect urine for blood clots and sediment and be sure that tubing is not kinked or occluded.

A decrease in blood clots means that the therapy is successful in maintaining catheter patency.
The system is patent.

STEP	RATIONALE

EVALUATION

4. Evaluate patient's comfort level.

5. Monitor for signs and symptoms of infection.
6. **Use Teach-Back:** "I want to be sure I explained clearly about the flushing of your catheter. Tell me in your own words the reason we are flushing your catheter." Develop a revised teaching plan if patient is not able to teach back correctly.

Indicates catheter patency by absence of symptoms of bladder distension.
Patients with in-dwelling catheters remain at risk for infection.
Determines patient's level of understanding of instructional topic.

Unexpected Outcomes	Related Interventions
1. Irrigating solution does not return (closed intermittent irrigation) or is not flowing at prescribed rate (CBI).	• Examine tubing for clots, sediment, and kinks. • Notify health care provider if irrigant does not flow freely from bladder, patient indicates pain, or bladder distension occurs.
2. Drainage output is less than the amount of irrigation solution infused.	• Examine drainage tubing for clots, sediment, or kinks. • Inspect urine for presence of or an increase in blood clots and sediment. • Evaluate patient for pain and distended bladder. • Notify health care provider.
3. Bright-red bleeding with the irrigation (CBI) infusion wide open.	• Assess for hypovolemic shock (vital signs, skin colour and moisture, anxiety level). • Leave irrigation infusion wide open and notify health care provider.
4. Patient experiences pain with irrigation.	• Examine drainage tubing for clots, sediment, or kinks. • Evaluate urine for presence of or increase in blood clots and sediment. • Evaluate for distended bladder. • Notify health care provider.

Communication and Documentation

- Document irrigation method, amount and type of irrigation solution, amount returned as drainage, characteristics of output, urine output, and patient tolerance of procedure in nurses' notes in the electronic health record (EHR) or chart.
- Report catheter occlusion, sudden bleeding, infection, or increased pain to the health care provider.
- Document I&O on the appropriate flow sheet.
- Document your evaluation of patient learning.

Special Considerations
Teaching
- Instruct patient and caregiver to observe urine daily for changes in colour, presence of mucus or blood, and odour.
- Inform patients that bleeding is common after many urological procedures and to expect bright red–tinged urine during the first

48 hours after surgery, followed by a change in urine ranging from pink-tinged to clear.
- Instruct patient to maintain adequate oral intake of at least 2 L/day (unless contraindicated).

Care in the Community
- Patients and caregivers can be taught to perform catheter irrigations with adequate support, demonstration and return demonstration, and written instructions.
- Teach patients and caregivers to observe regularly urine colour, clarity, odour, and amount.
- Arrange for home delivery and storage of catheter and irrigation supplies.
- Teach patients and caregivers signs of catheter obstruction or UTI.

♦ SKILL 34.4   Applying a Condom-Type External Catheter

NSO *Nursing Skills Online Urinary Catheterization Module 17 / Lesson 3*

The external urinary catheter, also called a *condom catheter* or *penile sheath*, is a soft, pliable condom-like sheath that fits over the penis, providing a safe and noninvasive way to contain urine. Most external catheters are made of soft silicone that reduces friction. The silicone is clear, allowing for easy visualization of skin under the catheter. Latex catheters are still available and used by some patients. It is important to verify that a patient does not have a latex allergy before applying this type of catheter.

Condom-type external catheters are held in place by an adhesive coating of the internal lining of the sheath, a double-sided self-adhesive strip, brush-on adhesive applied to the penile shaft, or, in rare cases, an external strap. The catheter may be attached to a small-volume (leg) drainage bag or a large-volume (bedside) urinary drainage bag, both of which need to be kept lower than the level of the bladder. The condom-type external catheter is suitable for incontinent patients who have complete and spontaneous

bladder emptying. The catheters come in a variety of styles and sizes. For the best fit and correct application, it is important to refer to manufacturer guidelines. Condom-type external catheters are associated with less risk for urinary tract infection (UTI) than in-dwelling catheters; thus they are an excellent option for the male with urinary incontinence. Other externally applied catheters are available for men who cannot be fitted for a condom-type external catheter. One type attaches to the glans penis by means of hydrocolloid strips that stay in place for multiple days and allows straight catheterization. Another option is a reusable condom-like device that is held in place by specially designed underwear.

Delegation and Collaboration

Assessment of the skin of a patient's penile shaft and determination of a latex allergy are done by a nurse before catheter application. The skill of applying a condom catheter can be delegated to an unregulated care provider (UCP), depending on employer policy. The nurse directs the UCP to:

- Follow manufacturer directions for applying the condom catheter and securing device.
- Monitor urine intake and output (I&O) and record them, if applicable.
- Immediately report any redness, swelling, or skin irritation or breakdown of the glans penis or penile shaft.

Equipment

- Condom catheter kit (condom sheath of appropriate size, securement device [internal adhesive or strap], skin preparation solution [per manufacturer directions])
- Urinary collection bag with drainage tubing or leg bag and straps
- Basin with warm water and soap
- Towels and washcloth(s)
- Bath blanket
- Clean gloves
- Scissors, hair guard, or paper towel

STEP	RATIONALE

ASSESSMENT

1. Identify patient using at least two person-specific identifiers (e.g., name and date of birth or name and medical record number), according to employer policy.

Ensures correct patient. Complies with Accreditation Canada's standards and improves patient safety (Accreditation Canada, 2019).

2. Review medical record and assess urinary pattern, ability to empty bladder effectively, and degree of urinary continence.

Incontinent patients are at risk for skin breakdown and thus are candidates for using a condom catheter.

3. Review medical record for history of allergy to rubber or latex. Check patient's allergy wristband.

Condoms are made of latex and can cause serious skin reaction.

4. Perform hand hygiene and apply clean gloves. Assess skin of penis for rashes, erythema, and open areas. (This may be deferred until just before catheter application.) Remove gloves and perform hand hygiene.

Reduces transmission of microorganisms. Provides baseline for comparing changes in condition of the skin after application of the condom catheter.

Clinical Decision Point *Apply condom catheters only when the skin on the penile surface is intact.*

5. Assess patient's mental status, knowledge of the purpose of using a condom-type catheter, and ability to apply the device. It may be appropriate to include the caregiver in this assessment.

Identifies patient learning needs and if self-application can be taught or if caregiver needs to be included in instruction.

6. Verify patient's size and type of condom catheter from plan of care or use manufacturer measuring guide to measure length and diameter of penis in flaccid state (apply gloves for measurement).

Identifies proper size of catheter needed. Penile shaft should be at least 2 cm (0.8 inch) in length to ensure successful application. If it is too small, the condom catheter may fall off and compress the urethra, stopping urine flow or causing local tissue trauma; if it is too big, the catheter may leak or fall off (Newman et al., 2017).

NURSING DIAGNOSES

- Urinary incontinence
- Insufficient knowledge regarding catheter application and care
- Potential for impaired skin integrity

Related factors/Risk factors are individualized on the basis of patient's condition or needs.

PLANNING

1. Expected outcomes following completion of procedure:
   - Patient's skin is free from urine wetness.
   - Glans and penile shaft are free of skin irritation or breakdown.
   - Patient explains purpose of procedure and what to expect.
2. Explain procedure to patient.

Catheter is applied correctly.
Catheter is secure and not too tight.

Helps to minimize anxiety and promotes cooperation.
Reduces anxiety and promotes cooperation.

STEP	RATIONALE

IMPLEMENTATION

1. Identify patient using at least two person-specific identifiers (e.g., name and date of birth, or name and medical record number), according to employer policy.

   Ensures correct patient. Complies with Accreditation Canada's standards and improves patient safety (Accreditation Canada, 2019).

2. Perform hand hygiene.

   Reduces transmission of microorganisms.

3. Provide privacy by closing room door and bedside curtain.

   Promotes patient comfort and self-esteem.

4. Raise bed to appropriate working height. Lower side rail on working side.

   Promotes use of good body mechanics.

5. Prepare urinary drainage collection bag and tubing (large-volume drainage bag or leg bag). Clamp off drainage bag port. Place nearby, ready to attach to condom after applied.

   Provides easy access to drainage equipment after applying condom catheter.

6. Help patient to a supine or sitting position. Place bath blanket over upper torso. Fold sheets so only penis is exposed.

   Respects patient dignity; draping prevents unnecessary exposure of body parts.

7. Apply clean gloves. Provide perineal care (see Chapter 18). Dry thoroughly before applying device. In an uncircumcised male, ensure that foreskin has been replaced to normal position before applying condom catheter. Do not apply barrier cream.

   Prevents skin breakdown from exposure to secretions. Removes any residual adhesives. Perineal care minimizes skin irritation and promotes adhesion of new external catheter. Barrier creams prevent sheath from adhering to penile shaft.

8. Clip hair at base of penis as necessary before application of condom sheath. Some manufacturers provide a hair guard that is placed over the penis before applying the device. Remove the hair guard after applying the catheter. An alternative to a hair guard is to tear a hole in a paper towel, place it over the penis, and remove it after application of device.

   Hair adheres to the condom and is pulled during condom removal or may get caught in adhesive as the external catheter is applied.

Clinical Decision Point *The pubic area should not be shaved because it may increase risk for skin irritation.*

9. Apply condom catheter. With nondominant hand, grasp penis along the shaft. With dominant hand, hold rolled condom sheath at tip of the penis with head of the penis in cone. Smoothly roll sheath onto the penis. Allow 2.5 to 5 cm (1 to 2 inches) of space between tip of the glans penis and end of the condom catheter (see illustration).

   Excessive wrinkles or creases in the external catheter sheath after application may mean that the patient needs a smaller size.

10. Apply appropriate securement device as indicated in manufacturer guidelines.

    The condom must be secured firmly so it is snug and stays on but not tight enough to cause constriction of blood flow. Application of gentle pressure ensures adherence of adhesive with penile skin.

    a. Self-adhesive condom catheters: After application, apply gentle pressure on the penile shaft for 10 to 15 seconds to secure catheter.

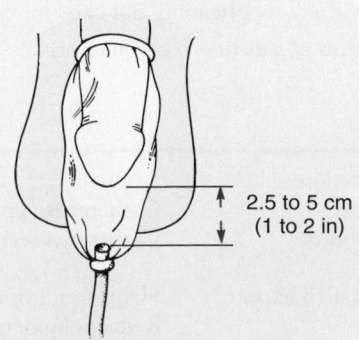

2.5 to 5 cm
(1 to 2 in)

STEP 9 Condom catheter.

STEP	RATIONALE

IMPLEMENTATION

b. Outer securing strip-type condom catheters: Spiral wrap penile shaft with strip of supplied elastic adhesive. Strip should not overlap itself. Elastic strip should be snug, not tight (see illustration).

Using the spiral wrap technique allows supplied elastic adhesive to expand so blood flow to penis is not compromised.

Clinical Decision Point *Never use regular adhesive tape to secure a condom catheter. Constriction from tape can reduce blood flow to tissues.*

11. Remove hair guard if used. Connect drainage tubing to end of the condom catheter. Be sure that condom is not twisted. If using a large drainage bag, secure tubing to thigh to prevent tension on the condom.

Allows urine to be collected and measured. Keeps patient dry. A twisted condom obstructs urine flow, causing urine pooling, skin irritation, and weakening and deterioration of adhesive, causing the catheter to come off.

12. Help patient to a safe, comfortable position. Lower bed and place side rails accordingly.

Promotes safety and comfort.

13. Dispose of contaminated supplies, remove gloves, and perform hand hygiene.

Reduces spread of microorganisms.

14. Remove and reapply daily after Steps 9 to 11 unless an extended-wear device is used. To remove condom, wash the penis with warm, soapy water and gently roll the sheath and adhesive off penile shaft.

Prevents trauma and irritation to penile sheath.

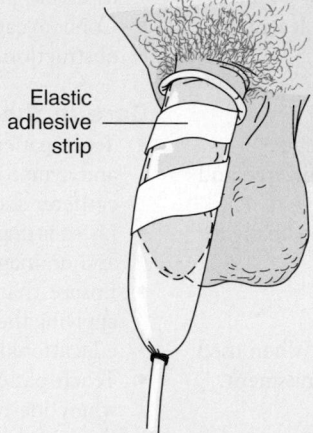

Elastic adhesive strip

STEP 10b Spiral application of adhesive strip.

EVALUATION

1. Observe urinary drainage.

A twisted condom prevents urine from draining into the collection bag.

2. Inspect penis with the condom catheter in place within 15 to 30 minutes after application. Assess for swelling and discoloration and ask patient if there is any discomfort.

Determines if condom is applied too tightly, impeding circulation to the penis.

3. Inspect skin on penile shaft for signs of breakdown or irritation at least daily, when performing hygiene, and before reapplying condom.

Changing the external catheter decreases the chance of infection.

4. **Use Teach-Back:** "I want to be sure I explained clearly use of your external condom catheter and some things you can do to prevent it from falling off. Tell me how you can help keep the catheter on without it slipping off." Develop a revised teaching plan if patient or caregiver is not able to teach back correctly.

Determines patient's and caregiver's level of understanding of instructional topic.

Unexpected Outcomes
1. Skin around penis is erythematous, ulcerated, or denuded.

Related Interventions
- Check for latex allergy or allergy to skin preparation or adhesive device.
- Remove condom and notify health care provider.
- Do not reapply until the penis and surrounding tissue are free from irritation.
- Ensure that the condom is not twisted and that urine flow is unobstructed after application.

STEP	**RATIONALE**

EVALUATION

2. Penile swelling or discoloration occurs.

- Remove external catheter.
- Notify health care provider.
- Reassess current condom size. See manufacturer size chart.

3. Condom catheter does not stay on.

- Ensure that catheter tubing is anchored and that patient understands to not pull or tug on the catheter.
- Reassess condom catheter size. Refer to manufacturer guidelines for sizing.
- Observe whether the condom catheter outlet is kinked and urine is pooling at the tip of the condom, bathing the penis in urine; reapply as necessary and avoid catheter obstruction.
- Assess need for another brand of external catheter (i.e., one that is self-adhesive).

Communication and Documentation

- Document condom application; condition of penis, skin, and scrotum; urinary output; and voiding pattern in nurses' notes in electronic health record (EHR) or chart.
- Report penile erythema, rashes, or skin breakdown.
- Document your evaluation of patient and caregiver learning.

Special Considerations
Teaching
- Teach patient about signs of skin breakdown or trauma.
- Teach patient to keep the condom and catheter kink free and positioned below the level of the bladder.
- Teach patient with a leg bag to assess leg straps periodically for tightness and loosen them as necessary.

Pediatric
- Use of condom catheters is uncommon in children. When used in adolescents, take precautions to minimize embarrassment.

Gerontological
- Evaluate patients with neuropathy carefully before applying a condom catheter. The patient may not feel the sensation of pressure from a condom device. Assess penile skin at more frequent intervals, at least twice daily.
- Condom catheters are not recommended in patients with prostatic obstruction.

Care in the Community
- Teach patient and caregiver appropriate assessments such as signs and symptoms of UTI, signs of skin irritation, or poor-fitting catheter sheath.
- Loose-fitting clothing may be needed to accommodate the catheter and drainage system.
- Ensure that patient and caregiver understand correct steps in applying the condom catheter. Manufacturers often supply patient educational materials.
- Teach patient and caregiver to empty drainage bag frequently when one-half full, to avoid unnecessary tension on the catheter that can lead to problems keeping the catheter intact.

✦ SKILL 34.5   Suprapubic Catheter Care

A *suprapubic catheter* is a urinary drainage tube inserted surgically into the bladder through the abdominal wall above the symphysis pubis (Fig. 34.7). The catheter may be sutured to the skin, secured with an adhesive material, or retained in the bladder with a fluid-filled balloon similar to an in-dwelling catheter.

Suprapubic catheters are placed when there is blockage of the urethra (e.g., enlarged prostate, urethral stricture, after urological surgery) and when a long-term urethral catheter causes irritation or discomfort or interferes with sexual functioning.

Delegation and Collaboration

The skill of caring for a newly established suprapubic catheter cannot be delegated to an unregulated care provider (UCP); however, care of an established suprapubic catheter may be delegated (refer to employer policy). The nurse directs the UCP to:
- Report the patient's discomfort (bladder fullness, abdominal pain, skin irritation) related to the suprapubic catheter.
- Empty the drainage bag and document urinary output on the intake and output (I&O) record.

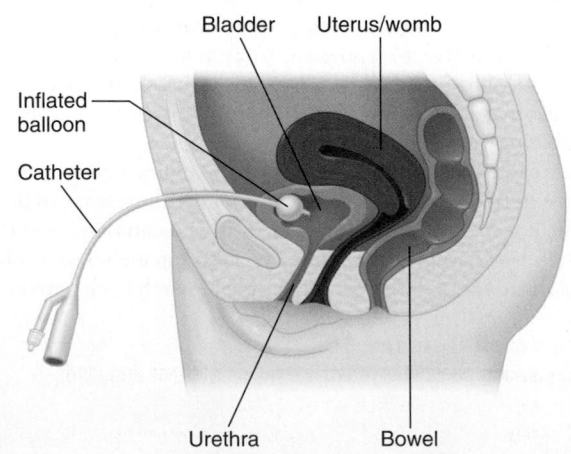

FIG 34.7 Suprapubic catheter.

- Report any change in the amount and character of the urine.
- Report any signs of redness, foul odour, or drainage around the catheter insertion site.

Equipment

- Clean gloves (sterile may be needed in some cases, see employer policy)

- Cleaning agent (sterile normal saline solution)
- Sterile cotton-tipped applicators
- Sterile surgical drainage gauze (split gauze)
- Sterile gauze dressing
- Washcloth, towel, soap, and water
- Tape
- Velcro tube holder or tube stabilizer (*optional*)

STEP	RATIONALE

ASSESSMENT

STEP	RATIONALE
1. Identify patient using at least two person-specific identifiers (e.g., name and date of birth, or name and medical record number), according to employer policy.	Ensures correct patient. Complies with Accreditation Canada's standards and improves patient safety (Accreditation Canada, 2019).
2. Assess urine in drainage bag for amount, clarity, colour, odour, and sediment.	Abnormal findings indicate potential complications such as urinary tract infection (UTI), decreased urinary output, and catheter occlusion.
3. Perform hand hygiene and apply clean gloves. Observe dressing for drainage and intactness.	Reduces transmission of infection. Drainage indicates a potential complication such as infection. Dressing may become nonocclusive because of tape choice or drainage.
4. Assess catheter insertion site (may be deferred until you clean site) for signs of inflammation (i.e., pain, erythema, edema, and drainage) and for growth of granulation tissue. Ask patient if there is any pain at the site; if so, assess for pain using an appropriate pain assessment tool. Remove gloves and perform hand hygiene.	If insertion is new, slight inflammation may be expected as part of normal wound healing but can also indicate infection. Hypergranulation tissue can develop at the insertion site as a reaction to the catheter. In some instances, intervention may be needed (WOCNS, 2016). Reduces transmission of microorganisms.
5. Assess for elevated temperature and chills.	Increased temperature may indicate UTI or skin site infection.
6. Assess patient's knowledge of purpose of catheter and its care.	Determines level of instruction and support required.
7. Check for allergies.	Patient may be sensitive to tape, latex, or antiseptic solution.

NURSING DIAGNOSES

- Reduced urinary elimination
- Acute pain
- Insufficient knowledge regarding catheter care
- Inadequate skin integrity
- Potential for infection

Related factors/Risk factors are individualized on the basis of patient's condition or needs.

PLANNING

STEP	RATIONALE
1. Expected outcomes following completion of procedure:	
• Patient indicates no pain or discomfort at insertion site and over bladder.	A patent catheter system keeps the bladder empty and the patient comfortable.
• Urine output is 30 mL or greater per hour.	Indicates that catheter is patent.
• Urine remains clear without foul odour, and patient is afebrile.	Indicates that patient is free of catheter-associated urinary tract infection (CAUTI).
• Catheter exit site is free of infection (i.e., erythema, edema, drainage, tenderness).	Indicates absence of infection and irritation of skin.
• Patient and caregiver can explain purpose of and methods for catheter care.	Evaluates learning.
2. Explain procedure to patient and caregiver.	Reduces anxiety and promotes cooperation. Patients with a suprapubic catheter frequently rely on caregivers for support.

IMPLEMENTATION

STEP	RATIONALE
1. Perform hand hygiene.	Reduces transmission of infection.
2. Provide privacy by closing room door and bedside curtain.	Displays person-centred care by promoting comfort and patient's self-esteem.
3. Raise bed to appropriate working height. If side rails are raised, lower side rail on working side.	Promotes use of good body mechanics.
4. Prepare supplies and open gauze packets in same manner as for applying dry dressing (see Chapter 40).	Keeps dressing sterile until application.

STEP	RATIONALE

IMPLEMENTATION

5. Apply clean gloves. Loosen tape and remove existing dressing. Note type and presence of drainage. Remove gloves and perform hand hygiene.

Provides baseline for condition of suprapubic wound. Reduces transmission of infection from dressing.

6. **Clean insertion site using sterile aseptic technique for newly established catheter:** This option is used less frequently; review employer policy or consider individual patient need. In some facilities, clean gloves are appropriate.
   a. Apply sterile gloves.

The catheter site is made surgically and thus is treated similarly to other incisions as designated by employer policy. Confirm if using either medical aseptic or sterile technique is recommended.

   b. Without creating tension, hold catheter up with nondominant hand while cleaning. Use sterile gauze moistened in saline and clean skin around insertion site in a circular motion, starting near the insertion site and continuing in outward widening circles for approximately 5 cm (2 inches) (see illustration).

Moves from area of least contamination to area of most contamination. Tension on the catheter may cause discomfort or damage to the wall of the bladder or cause catheter to slip out of place.

   c. With fresh, moistened gauze, gently clean base of catheter, moving up and away from site of insertion (proximal to distal).

Removes microorganisms that reside on any drainage that adheres to tubing.

   d. Once insertion site is dry, use a sterile gloved hand to apply drain dressing (split gauze) around the catheter (see illustration). Tape in place.

Collects drainage that develops around catheter insertion site.

7. **Clean long-term/established catheter:**
   a. Apply clean gloves.
   b. Without creating tension, hold catheter erect with nondominant hand while cleaning. Clean with soap and water in a circular motion, starting near catheter insertion site and continuing in outward widening circles for approximately 5 cm (2 inches).

Cleaning and drying suprapubic insertion site requires general hygienic measures; dressing is an option if drainage is not present.

   c. With a fresh washcloth or gauze, gently clean base of the catheter, moving up and away from site of insertion (proximal to distal).

Removes microorganisms that reside in any drainage that adheres to tubing.

   d. *Option:* Apply drain dressing (split gauze) around catheter and tape in place.

8. Secure catheter to lateral abdomen with tape or Velcro multipurpose tube holder.

Secures catheter and reduces risk of excessive tension on suture and catheter.

9. Coil excess tubing on bed. Keep drainage bag below level of bladder at all times.

Maintains free flow of urine, thus decreasing risk for CAUTI (CPSI, 2016; WOCNS, 2016).

10. Dispose of all contaminated supplies in an appropriate receptacle, remove gloves, and perform hand hygiene.

Reduces transmission of microorganisms.

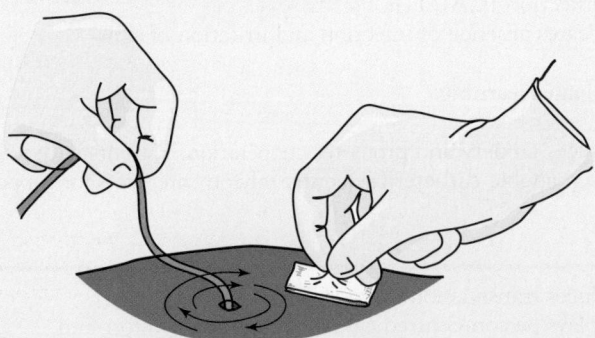

STEP 6b Clean around suprapubic catheter in a circular pattern.

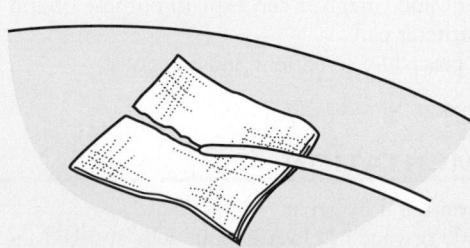

STEP 6d Split drain dressing for suprapubic catheter.

STEP	RATIONALE

EVALUATION

1. Ask patient to rate pain or discomfort from suprapubic catheter with an appropriate pain assessment tool.

Determines if bladder is draining and patient is free of infection.

2. Monitor for signs of infection (e.g., fever, elevated white blood count) and observe urine for clarity, sediment, unusual colour, or odour.

Suprapubic catheters increase risk for UTI.

3. Observe catheter insertion site for erythema, edema, discharge, and tenderness. Check dressing at a minimum of every 8 hours.

Indicators of an insertion site infection.

4. **Use Teach-Back:** "I want to be sure I explained clearly about the care of your suprapubic catheter. Tell me about some of the things you need to do to care for it at home." Develop a revised teaching plan if patient or caregiver is not able to teach back correctly.

Determines patient's and caregiver's level of understanding of instructional topic.

Unexpected Outcomes
1. Patient develops symptoms of UTI or catheter site infection.

Related Interventions
- Increase fluid intake to at least 2 L in 24 hours (unless contraindicated).
- Monitor vital signs, I&O; observe amount, colour, consistency of urine; assess site.
- Notify health care provider.

2. Suprapubic catheter becomes dislodged.

- Cover site with sterile dressing.
- Notify health care provider. If this is a newly established catheter, it will need to be reinserted immediately.

3. Skin surrounding catheter exit site becomes red or irritated or develops open areas.

- Notify health care provider.
- Change dressing (if used) more frequently to keep site dry.
- Consult with wound care nurse.

Communication and Documentation

- Document and report character of urine and type of dressing change, including assessments of insertion site and patient's comfort level with the catheter and dressing change in nurses' notes in electronic health record (EHR) or chart.
- Document urine output on the I&O flow sheet. When there is both a suprapubic and urethral catheter, document outputs from each catheter separately.
- Document your evaluation of patient and caregiver learning.
- Report any signs of UTI or insertion site infection to the health care provider.

Special Considerations
Teaching
- If not contraindicated, encourage patients to consume a minimum of 2 L of fluids daily.

- Teach patient to keep the drainage bag lower than the bladder and to keep tubing free of kinks.

Care in the Community
- Teach patient and caregiver how to clean and apply a dressing (if applicable) using clean technique.
- Caution patient and caregiver about avoiding the use of powders or creams around the catheter unless specifically instructed to do so.
- Teach patient and caregiver how to properly position the drainage bag; empty the urinary drainage bag; and observe urine colour, clarity, odour, and amount.
- Arrange for home delivery of catheter supplies, always ensuring that there is at least one extra catheter and drainage bag in the home.
- Teach patient and caregiver signs of catheter obstruction, UTI, and wound infection.

◆ CLINICAL DEBRIEF

The nurse is caring for an 80-year-old Inuit woman with a history of a stroke, type 2 diabetes mellitus, urinary retention, urinary incontinence, and recurrent urinary tract infections (UTIs). The health care provider has prescribed measurement of postvoid residual (PVR) by either straight catheterization or bladder scan. There is also a prescription for an in-dwelling catheter if the PVR exceeds 400 mL. The patient's spouse will not allow anyone to insert a catheter except her family.

1. Which assessments would be pertinent for this patient?
2. Explain why an assessment of PVR is important for this patient.
3. When measuring PVR, should the nurse use the bladder scanner, or should a straight catheterization be performed? Give the rationale for your answer.
4. Explain the teaching that would be appropriate when assessing PVR urine.
5. Using SBAR, show how you would communicate with the health care team about this patient.

✦ REVIEW QUESTIONS

1. Place the following steps for insertion of an in-dwelling catheter in a female patient in appropriate order.
   1. Insert and advance catheter.
   2. Lubricate catheter.
   3. Inflate catheter balloon.
   4. Clean urethral meatus with antiseptic.
   5. Drape patient with the sterile square and fenestrated drapes.
   6. When urine appears, advance catheter another 2.5 to 5 cm (1 to 2 inches).
   7. Prepare sterile field and supplies.
   8. Gently pull catheter until resistance is felt.
   9. Attach drainage tubing.

2. The nurse is preparing to remove an in-dwelling urinary catheter. Which nursing interventions should the nurse implement? *(Select all that apply.)*
   1. Attaching a 3-mL syringe to the inflation port
   2. Allowing the balloon to drain into the syringe by gravity
   3. Initiating a voiding record/bladder diary
   4. Pulling catheter quickly
   5. Clamping the catheter before removal

3. Which nursing interventions are appropriate in the care of a patient with a newly inserted suprapubic catheter? *(Select all that apply.)*
   1. Using sterile technique, clean the skin close to the catheter with a circular motion.
   2. Wipe away any drainage on the catheter by wiping down the catheter toward the insertion site.
   3. Inspect the insertion site for erythema, edema, discharge, or tenderness.
   4. Secure the catheter to the abdomen with tape or a tube-holder device.
   5. Apply upward tension to the catheter when cleaning the site and tubing.

ⓔ *Visit the Evolve site for a complete list of Clinical Debrief and Review Questions answers.*

REFERENCES

Accreditation Canada. (2019). *Required organizational practices handbook—Version 14.* Retrieved from http://www.wrha.mb.ca/quality/files/2019ROPHandbook.pdf

Canadian Nurse Continence Advisors. (2012). *Best practice guidelines: Promoting continence using prompted voiding.* Retrieved from http://www.cnca.ca/BPG.html

Canadian Patient Safety Institute (CPSI). (2016). *Hospital harm improvement resource.* Retrieved from http://www.patientsafetyinstitute.ca/en/toolsResources/Hospital-Harm-Measure/Improvement-Resources/pages/default.aspx

Centers for Disease Control and Prevention (CDC). (2009). *Guideline for prevention of catheter-associated urinary tract infections.* Retrieved from https://www.cdc.gov/infectioncontrol/guidelines/cauti/background.html

Corcos, J., Przydacz, M., Campeau, L., et al. (2017). CUA guidelines on adult overactive bladder. *Canadian Urological Association journal = Journal de l'Association des urologues du Canada, 11*(5), E142–E173. doi:10.5489/cuaj.4586

Fekete, T. (2018). *Catheter-associated urinary tract infections in adults.* UpToDate. Retrieved from http://www.uptodate.com/contents/catheter-associated-urinary-tract-infection-in-adults

Gill, B., Vasavada, S., Firoozi, F., & Rackley, R. (2018). Neurogenic bladder. *Medscape.* Retrieved from https://emedicine.medscape.com/article/453539-overview?pa=l-ZI0vnFehDH2cAqpwK2koRgNTIN6l7eUzu393gVl%2B4sjOK%2ByQOgbH-Q2VrDS9fBhXd%2FsGPYa%2BToEoLjuhFnUEHw%3D%3D#a6. [Art. 453539]

Hockenberry, M. J., & Wilson, D. (2015). *Wong's nursing care of infants and children* (11th ed.). St. Louis: Mosby.

Huether, S. E., McCance, K., El-Hussein, M. T., Power-Kean, K., & Zettel, S. (2018). *Understanding pathophysiology* (1st Canadian ed.). Toronto, ON: Elsevier Canada.

Lewis, S. L., Bucher, L., Heitkemper, M., et al. (Eds.). (2019). *Medical-surgical nursing in Canada: Assessment and management of clinical problems* (4th Canadian ed.). Toronto, ON: Elsevier Canada.

Medline Plus. (2019). *Catheter-related UTI.* U.S. National Library of Medicine. Retrieved from https://medlineplus.gov/ency/article/000483.htm

Newman, D., Rovner, E., & Wein, A. (2017). *Clinical application of urological catheters, devices and products.* New York: Springer.

Registered Nurses' Association of Ontario (RNAO). (2011). *Nursing best practice guideline: Promoting continence using prompted voiding.* Retrieved from http://www.cnca.ca/pdf/Promoting_Continence_Using_Prompted_Voiding.pdf

Shelat, A. (2019). *Neurogenic bladder. MedlinePlus.* Retrieved from https://medlineplus.gov/ency/article/000754.htm

Wound Ostomy and Continence Nurses Society (WOCNS). (2016). *Care and management of patients with urinary catheters: A clinical resource guide.* Retrieved from https://cdn.ymaws.com/www.wocn.org/resource/resmgr/publications/Care_&_Mgmt_Pts_w_Urinary_Ca.pdf

Yates, A. (2015). Selecting gel types for urinary catheter insertion. *Nursing Times, 111*(26), 18–20.

Yates, A. (2018). Catheter securing and fixation devices: Their role in preventing complications. *The British Journal of Nursing, 27*(6), 290–294. doi:10.12968/bjon.2018.27.6.290

35 | Bowel Elimination and Gastric Intubation

Written by **Lori Klingman, MSN, RN; and Maureen Loft, NP-Adult, MScN, PhD**

SKILLS AND PROCEDURES

OBJECTIVES

Mastery of content in this chapter will enable the nurse to:
- Describe factors that promote and impede normal bowel elimination.
- Discuss methods to relieve constipation or impaction.
- Describe precautions to follow when administering an enema.

- Describe approaches for managing a patient's comfort during nasogastric tube insertion.
- Perform the following skills: helping a patient use a bedpan, digitally removing stool, administering an enema, and inserting and removing a nasogastric tube.

MEDIA RESOURCES

- **evolve** http://evolve.elsevier.com/Canada/Perry/clinicalskills/
- Review Questions
- ▶ Video Clips

- Case Studies
- Audio Glossary
- **NSO** Nursing Skills Online
- Clinical Debrief and Review Questions Answers

PURPOSE

Regular elimination of bowel waste products is essential for normal body functioning. Alterations of bowel elimination often indicate early signs, symptoms, or problems in the gastrointestinal (GI) system across the lifespan, particularly in older persons and children (Davignon, Sham, Lappen, et al., 2016; Ferrara & Saccomano, 2017). A patient's overall lifestyle patterns, food and fluid intake, medications, functional status, and chronic conditions influence bowel function. Foods may induce symptoms that have a range of effects on bowel elimination (Singh, Salem, Nanavati, et al., 2018). To manage a patient's bowel elimination problems, nurses need to understand factors that promote, impede, or alter normal bowel elimination.

Patients may require the nurse's help to meet bowel elimination needs (e.g., using a bedpan). If a patient is constipated, the nurse will likely administer enemas or digitally remove impacted stool. If severe diarrhea exists, a fecal management system (FMS) protects a patient's perianal skin and collects contaminated fecal waste (Singh, Salem, et al., 2018). When patients undergo abdominal surgery or experience an alteration in GI peristalsis, a nasogastric (NG) tube is inserted for gastric decompression (Fan, Tan, & Aug, 2017).

STANDARDS OF CARE

- Accreditation Canada, 2019—*Required Organizational Practices Handbook—Version 14* (http://www.wrha.mb.ca/quality/files/2019ROPHandbook.pdf)
- Emergency Nurses Association (ENA), 2015—*Clinical Practice Guideline, Gastric Tube Placement Verification* (https://www.ena.org/docs/default-source/resource-library/practice-resources/cpg/gastrictubecpg7b5530b71c1e49e8b155b6cca1870adc.pdf?sfvrsn=a0e9dd7a_12)
- Norton, Parslow, Johnston, et al.; Wounds Canada, 2018—*Best Practice Recommendations for the Prevention and Management of Pressure Injuries* (https://www.woundscanada.ca/docman/public/health-care-professional/bpr-workshop/172-bpr-prevention-and-management-of-pressure-injuries-2/file)
- Registered Nurses Association of Ontario (RNAO), 2011—*Nursing Best Practice Guideline: Prevention of Constipation in the Older Adult Population* (http://rnao.ca/sites/rnao-ca/files/Prevention_of_Constipation_in_the_Older_Adult_Population.pdf)
- Rowan-Legg & Canadian Paediatric Society (CPS), Community Paediatrics Committee, 2011 (reaffirmed 2018)—*Managing Functional Constipation in Children* (https://www.cps.ca/en/documents/position/functional-constipation)

PRINCIPLES FOR PRACTICE

- Chronic constipation is a functional GI disorder and a condition frequently encountered in clinical practice (Box 35.1). Approximately 30% of people experience constipation during their lifetime, with older persons being most affected (DeGiorgio, Ruggeri, Stanghellini, et al., 2015).
- Opioid-induced constipation occurs frequently in the palliative care population. Opioids stimulate mu-opioid receptors, which induce analgesia. However, activation of these receptors reduces gastric emptying; increases pyloric, anal, and biliary sphincter tone; reduces biliary track secretions; and increases water absorption from the bowel. All of these factors reduce delayed intestinal transit time, and constipation occurs (Prichard & Bharucha, 2015).
- Constipation is also a complication of acute stroke, and, because of motor or sensory impairments, these patients need structured bowel-retraining programs to achieve bowel health (Casaubon, Boulanger, Glasser, et al., 2016).
- Patients with severe diarrhea may often require an FMS to protect the perianal skin from breakdown, pressure injury formation, and fecal containment (Beeson, Elfrid, Pike, et al., 2017; Norton et al., 2018).
- Postoperative ileus and severe abdominal distension, with or without nausea or vomiting, is an indication of failure for the return of adequate bowel function. This causes patient discomfort, increases recovery time, and increases length of hospital stay. When a postoperative ileus occurs, often an NG tube may need to be inserted (Sanfilippo & Spoletini, 2015).

PERSON-CENTRED CARE

- Nurses need to show respect for a person's privacy, provide necessary comfort and hygiene measures, and attend to the patient's emotional needs when performing required skills.
- When caring for patients from various cultural and ethnic groups who have elimination issues, nurses need to modify nursing interventions to meet their patients' elimination needs and provide for culturally sensitive hygiene needs. For example, hand hygiene can be practised for hygienic reasons, for ritual reasons during religious ceremonies, and for symbolic reasons in specific everyday life situations (World Health Organization [WHO], 2009).
- It is important to determine a patient's normal pattern of bowel elimination and accommodate that pattern while they are in a health care setting. The amount of help needed can be established according to the time a patient normally has a bowel movement.
- Nurses should consider developmental changes that affect bowel functioning throughout the lifespan. For example, an older person who becomes less active and has decreased muscle tone and changes in eating patterns is at higher risk for experiencing constipation (Huether, McCance, El-Hussein, et al., 2018).

EVIDENCE-INFORMED PRACTICE

- Nurses assess constipation by obtaining a thorough patient history (e.g., diet, exercise, bowel pattern history, medications). Nurses also need to review medications to identify those associated with an increased risk for developing constipation (e.g., chronic laxative use). Daily dietary fibre intake should be between 25 and 30 grams per day (RNAO, 2011).
- Research studies continue to investigate methods of correctly verifying NG tube placement, which is crucial to avoid tube position complications. Radiographic verification of placement of tube immediately following insertion is the gold standard and provides a clear and measurable placement of the tube. Likewise, aspiration of gastric contents and pH measurement of 5 or less are used in subsequent verifications for tube placement (Fan et al., 2017).
- Pressure applied to the mucous membranes lining the GI tract can cause ischemia and medical device–related pressure injuries (MDRPIs) (Pittman, Beeson, Kitterman, et al., 2015). The resultant pressure injury generally conforms to the pattern or shape of the device.
  - NG and nasoenteral tubes can cause tissue necrosis, skin breakdown, and pressure on the intubated nares. NG tube fixation methods that remove pressure from the nares help to reduce the risk for MDRPI (Pittman et al., 2015; Wound Ostomy and Continence Nurses Society [WOCN], 2016).
  - In-dwelling FMSs are effective in protecting perianal skin from fecal enzyme irritation and subsequent breakdown. However, there is a risk for rectal mucosa necrosis and tearing secondary to the cuff, which is placed internally (Sammon, Montague, Frame, et al., 2015; Singh, Bhargava, Vasantha, et al., 2018).
- Methods to reduce MDRPI related to bowel elimination and gastric decompression include:
  - Conducting routine and ongoing assessment of nares and secondary pressure sites underlying medical devices and implement skin-care practices such a taping method to reduce the risk for MDRPI (National Pressure Ulcer Advisory Panel [NPUAP], 2016; Pittman et al., 2015; WOCN, 2016).
  - Frequently removing tape or the fixation device to inspect underlying skin and provide skin care (Pittman et al., 2015).
  - Placing thin foam or breathable dressings under medical devices (NPUAP, 2016).
  - Positioning NG drainage tubing in such a manner as to not cause secondary pressure on the nares from the weight of the drainage tubing itself (NPUAP, 2012).
  - Verifying that the patient is not lying on drainage tubing.
  - For patients who have an FMS, routinely assessing anal and

---

BOX 35.1

Common Causes of Constipation

- Irritable bowel syndrome: constipation predominant
- Diseases/conditions (e.g., Parkinson's disease, diabetes, colon cancer, dehydration, diabetes mellitus, hypercalcemia/hypokalemia, immobility, and stroke) (RNAO, 2011)
- Low-fibre diet that is high in animal fats (e.g., meats, dairy products, eggs), refined sugars (rich desserts), high-carbohydrate diet, and low fluid intake, all of which slow peristalsis (Ball et al., 2015)
- Medications: antihypertensives, anticonvulsants, antidepressants, antacids, iron supplements, opioid medications (Costilla & Foxx-Orenstein, 2014; Prichard & Bharucha, 2015)
- Laxative misuse (Burchum & Rosenthal, 2016)
- Older persons: slowed peristalsis, loss of abdominal muscle elasticity, reduced intestinal mucus secretion, often eating low-fibre foods (Ball et al., 2015)
- Neurological conditions that block nerve impulses to the colon (e.g., spinal cord injury, tumour) (Lewis, Bucher, Heitkemper, et al., 2019)
- Colonic action slowed by medications such as anticholinergics, antispasmodics, anticonvulsants, antidepressants, antihistamines, antihypertensives, antiparkinsonism drugs, bile acid sequestrants, diuretics, antacids, iron supplements, calcium supplements (Burchum & Rosenthal, 2016)

perianal areas for redness, blistering, edema, and breaks in skin integrity (Singh, Bhargava, et al., 2018).

SAFETY GUIDELINES

- Promote comfort when a patient uses a bedpan. Encourage the patient to use the bathroom when able.
- Answer the call light promptly to prevent a patient from attempting to get out of bed without help. This is a common factor related to patient falls.
- Patients with neurological sensory or motor deficits are prone to constipation. They should be placed on an individualized bowel training schedule (Casaubon et al., 2016)
- Autonomic dysreflexia occurs in people with spinal injuries at T6 or above, exhibiting as marked hypertension and headache

(Peate, 2016). Assess these patients for flushing, sweating, chills, nasal congestion, blurred vision, and headache (Peate, 2016).
- When digital removal of impacted fecal material is prescribed, obtain patient baseline vital signs and periodically monitor heart rate during the procedure. Observe the patient for signs of distress, pain, discomfort, bleeding, and collapse (Peate, 2016).
- Follow employer policy to verify correct placement of NG tubes, which includes radiographic verification after insertion and subsequent pH verification of pH of 5 or less (Fan et al., 2017).
- When a patient with an NG tube indicates nausea or vomits, assess both placement and patency of the tube. Reposition and irrigate the tube as needed.
- When handling fecal matter, always use personal protective equipment (PPE) based on routine practices and additional precautions as required.

✦ SKILL 35.1   Providing a Bedpan

Encouraging patients to use a toilet or commode best supports optimal bowel hygiene. For patients who are on bed rest or unable to ambulate, the use of a bedpan may be required. Two types of bedpans are available (Fig. 35.1). The regular and most commonly used bedpan has a curved, smooth upper end and a tapered lower end. The upper end (wide end) of the regular pan fits under a patient's buttocks toward the sacrum, with the lower end (tapered end) fitting just under the upper thighs toward the foot of the bed. A fracture pan, designed for patients with body or leg casts or those who are restricted from raising their hips (e.g., following total hip joint replacement), slips easily under a patient. The shallow upper end of the pan with a flat, wide rim fits under a patient's buttocks

toward the sacrum, with the deep, lower open end toward the foot of the bed.

Delegation and Collaboration

The skill of providing a bedpan can be delegated to an unregulated care provider (UCP); however, providing or removing a bedpan is more readily facilitated with two people. The nurse needs to use interprofessional collaboration to provide optimal patient care and education and to complete patient care in a timely manner. The nurse instructs the UCP to:
- Correctly position patients with mobility restrictions or those who have therapeutic equipment such as wound drains, intravenous (IV) catheters, or traction.
- Provide perineal and hand hygiene for the patient as necessary after using a bedpan.

Equipment
- PPE for transmission-based precautions (e.g., contact)
- Bedpan (regular or fracture) (see Fig. 35.1)
- Bedpan cover
- Toilet tissue
- Specimen container (if necessary); plastic bag clearly labelled with date, patient's name, and identification number
- Basin, washcloths, towels, and soap
- Waterproof, absorbent pads (if necessary)
- Clean drawsheet (if necessary)
- Stethoscope

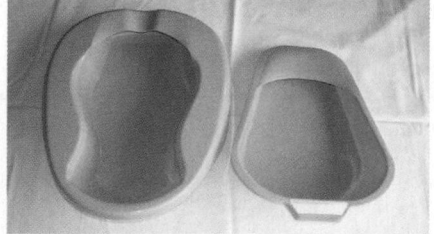

FIG 35.1 Types of bedpans. *Left*, Regular bedpan. *Right*, Fracture bedpan.

STEP	RATIONALE

ASSESSMENT

1. Assess patient's normal bowel elimination habits: routine pattern, character of stool, effect of certain foods or fluids and eating habits on bowel elimination, effect of stress and level of activity on normal bowel elimination patterns, current medications, and normal fluid intake.

   Managing a patient's elimination problems depends on thorough understanding of normal elimination and factors that create alterations. Peristalsis is strongest during the hour after the first meal of the day. Anticipate when to offer bedpan.

2. Perform hand hygiene. Auscultate abdomen for bowel sounds and palpate lower abdomen for distension.

   Normal bowel sounds occur irregularly at a rate of 5 to 35 per minute. Presence of feces in the colon, often mistaken for an abdominal mass, can be felt as a soft, rounded, boggy mass in the cecum and ascending, descending, or sigmoid colon (Ball, Dains, Flynn, et al., 2015).

STEP	RATIONALE

ASSESSMENT

3. Assess patient to determine level of mobility, including ability to sit upright and lift hips or turn.	Determines if patient can help in positioning on bedpan or if help is needed. Determines whether to use regular or fracture bedpan. Older persons, patients living with obesity, patients who have had hip or knee surgery or spinal injury, and debilitated patients often require assistance of two or more nurses to help them onto or off a bedpan.
4. Assess patient's level of comfort. Ask about presence of rectal or abdominal pain, presence of hemorrhoids, or irritation of skin surrounding anus.	Pain limits a patient's ability to help with positioning. Rectal or abdominal pain reduces a patient's ability to bear down during defecation.
5. Apply clean gloves. Inspect condition of perianal and perineal skin. Remove gloves and perform hand hygiene.	Repeated diarrhea can cause perineal and perianal skin irritation and skin breakdown (Sammon et al., 2015).
6. Determine need for stool specimen. This may have been prescribed by the health care provider, or the assessment findings may indicate that a sample is required (e.g., patient is oozing stool, foul odour).	Provides opportunity to obtain specimen container before placing patient on bedpan.

NURSING DIAGNOSES

- Acute pain
- Bowel incontinence
- Diarrhea
- Chronic pain
- Reduced physical mobility
- Chronic functional constipation
- Reduced self-toileting abilities
- Potential for constipation

Related factors/Risk factors are individualized on the basis of patient's condition or needs.

PLANNING

1. Expected outcomes following completion of procedure:	
• Perianal skin is clean and intact.	Hygiene technique after defecation keeps perianal skin clear of fecal secretions.
• Patient eliminates without pain or discomfort.	Patient is positioned comfortably on bedpan.
2. Explain procedure to patient, including self-help tips (e.g., how to use a trapeze, how to move hips).	Promotes independence, reduces anxiety, and helps patient to assist during procedure.
3. Obtain help from additional nursing personnel as warranted.	Adequate personnel resources minimize muscle strain for you and patient. Reduces patient's discomfort.

IMPLEMENTATION

1. Perform hand hygiene.	Reduces transmission of microorganisms.

Clinical Decision Point *Use a fracture pan if the patient had a total hip replacement. An abduction pillow may be placed between the legs when turning, to decrease the risk of possible dislocation of the new joint (refer to employer policy).*

2. Provide privacy by closing curtains around bed or door of room.	Demonstrates person-centred care by reducing embarrassment and promotes bowel elimination.
3. Raise side rail on opposite side of bed.	Protects patient from falling out of bed. Patient can grasp side rail to move about in bed and onto bedpan.
4. Raise bed horizontally according to your height.	Promotes use of good body mechanics and minimizes muscle strain for you and patient.
5. Have patient assume supine position.	Position eases eventual pan placement.

Clinical Decision Point *Observe for the presence of drains, dressings, IV fluids, and traction. These devices make it difficult for a patient to help with positioning, and as the nurse you will likely need more personnel to help place the patient on a bedpan.*

6. Place patient on bedpan:	
a. *For patients who can help themselves:*	
(1) Apply clean gloves. Raise head of patient's bed 30 to 60 degrees.	Prevents hyperextension of back and provides support to upper torso when patient raises hips. Sitting position promotes defecation.

STEP	RATIONALE

IMPLEMENTATION

(2) Remove upper bed linens so they are out of the way but do not expose patient.

Prevents embarrassment to patient; maintains persons' dignity and demonstrates respect as part of person-centred care.

(3) Have patient flex knees and lift hips upward.

If legs, upper torso, and arms are supporting body weight, little effort should be required of the patient.

(4) Place your hand that is closest to the patient's head palm up under the patient's sacrum to help lift. Ask patient to bend knees and raise hips. As patient raises hips, use the other hand to slip the bedpan under them (see illustrations). Be sure that open rim of the bedpan is facing toward foot of the bed. Do not force pan under patient's hips. (*Optional:* Have patient use overhead trapeze frame to raise hips.)

Positions bedpan high under buttocks so feces enters pan. Incorrect placement of bedpan causes discomfort for patient and spillage of contents. If legs, upper torso, and arms are supporting body weight, little effort should be required of patient. Forcing bedpan under patient increases risk of friction injury to underlying skin and tissues.

(5) *Optional:* If using a fracture pan, slip it under patient as hips are raised (see illustration). Be sure that deep, open, lower end of bedpan is facing toward foot of the bed.

Patient requires less manoeuvring and does not have to lift hips.

b. *For patients who are immobile or have mobility restrictions on bedpan:*

(1) Apply clean gloves. Lower head of bed flat or raise head slightly (if tolerated by medical condition).

Helps patient who cannot lift hips, must remain flat, or medically is not permitted to lift hips to roll onto bedpan.

(2) Remove top linens as necessary to turn patient while minimizing exposure.

Prevents embarrassment to patient; demonstrates respect for patient's sense of dignity.

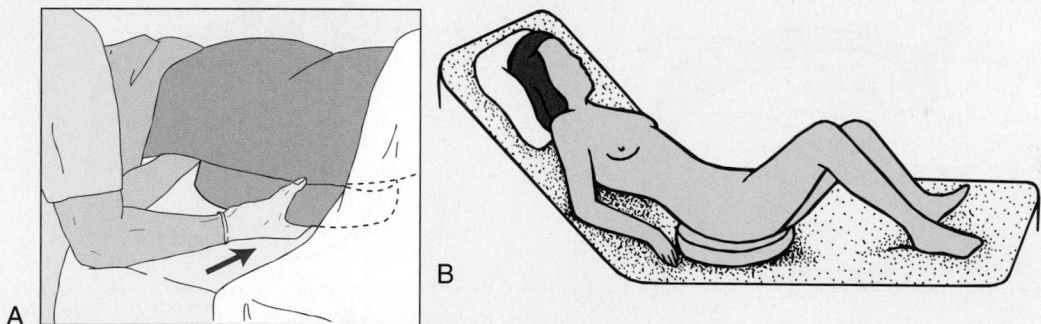

STEP 6a(4) A, Placing bedpan under patient's hips. **B,** Correct positioning for placing mobile patient on bedpan.

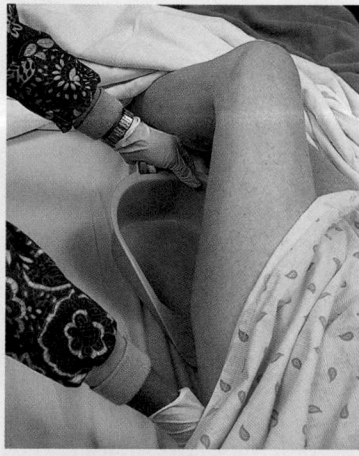

STEP 6a(5) Patient lifts hips as fracture pan is positioned.

STEP	RATIONALE

IMPLEMENTATION

(3) Help patient roll onto side with their back toward you. Place bedpan firmly against patient's buttocks and down into mattress. Be sure that open rim of bedpan is facing toward foot of the bed (see illustrations).

Incorrect placement causes discomfort to patient and spillage of contents.

Clinical Decision Point *If the patient has had total hip replacement, use a fracture pan; an abduction pillow may be used between the patient's legs while they are positioning themselves onto the fracture pan.*

(4) Keep one hand against bedpan; place the other around far hip of patient. Ask patient to roll back onto the bedpan, flat in bed. Do not force pan under patient.

Using minimal exertion, this places patient squarely on the pan. Avoid forcing the bedpan under patient, to decrease risk for friction injury to underlying skin and tissues.

(5) Raise patient's head 30 degrees or to a comfortable level (unless contraindicated).

Patient assumes sitting position unless condition necessitates maintaining a flat position.

(6) Have patient bend knees (unless contraindicated).

Relieves stress on back.

7. Maintain patient's comfort, privacy, and safety. Cover patient for warmth. Place a small pillow or rolled towel under lumbar curve of their back. Leave room but stay close by.

Provides added comfort. Pain reduces or eliminates urge to defecate, which will result in bowel elimination problems.

8. Have call bell and toilet tissue within reach for patient.

Promotes safety by preventing patient from reaching over edge of bed for objects out of reach.

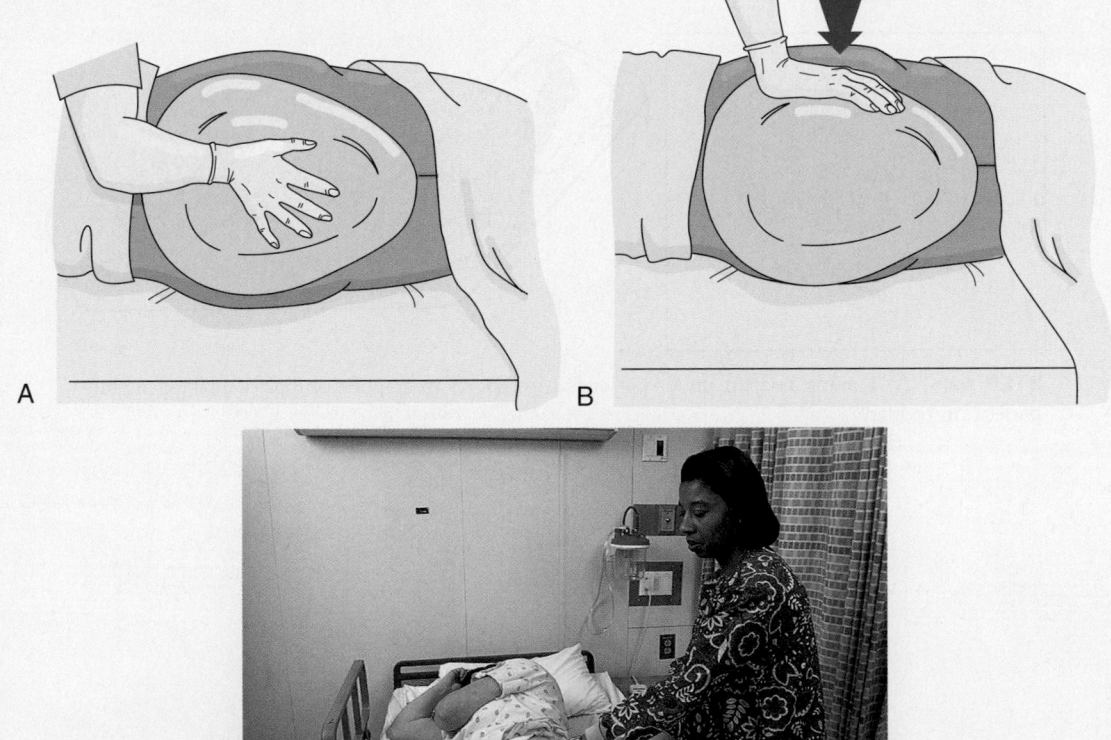

STEP 6b(3) A, Position patient on one side and place bedpan firmly against buttocks. **B,** Push down on bedpan and toward patient. **C,** Nurse places bedpan in position. (**A** *and* **B** *from Sorrentino, S. A. [2009]. Mosby's textbook for nursing assistants [7th ed.]. St. Louis: Mosby.*)

STEP	RATIONALE

IMPLEMENTATION

9. Ensure that bed is in lowest position, and raise upper side rails.

Promotes patient safety and enables patient to reposition pan as needed.

10. Remove PPE and perform hand hygiene if performing other tasks in the room while patient uses the bedpan.

Reduces transmission of microorganisms.

11. Allow patient to be alone but monitor status and respond promptly once patient signals they are finished using the bedpan.

Reassures patient. Removing the bedpan in a timely manner prevents pressure injuries.

12. Perform hand hygiene and reapply PPE if PPE was removed to perform other activities in the room (e.g., tidy bedside, chart).

Reduces transmission of microorganisms.

13. Remove bedpan:

   a. It is optimal to have assistance of a team member to assist with removal of the bedpan. If working alone, place the bedpan on the floor on a protective barrier.

Working with a team member allows one to immediately empty bedpan contents while the nurse finishes cleaning the patient. Provides area to place bedpan and contents on floor after removal from patient to prevent accidental spilling of full bedpan on bed surface.

   b. Maintain privacy; determine if patient is able to wipe own perineal area. If you clean perineal area, apply PPE and use several layers of toilet tissue or disposable washcloths. For female patients clean from mons pubis toward rectal area.

Maintains respect for privacy. Cleans from clean to dirty area of perineum.

   c. Deposit contaminated tissue in bedpan if no specimen or intake and output (I&O) is needed. Remove PPE and perform hand hygiene.

Toilet tissue contaminates specimen and affects accurate output measurement.

   d. For mobile patients:

     Apply PPE. Ask patient to flex knees, placing body weight on lower legs, feet, and upper torso; lift buttocks up from bedpan. At the same time place hand farthest from patient on side of the bedpan to support it (prevent spillage) and place the other hand (closest to patient) under their sacrum to help lift. Have patient lift, and remove bedpan. Place bedpan on draped bedside chair and cover it.

Avoids pulling or forcing pan from under hips; this action can pull skin and cause tissue injury.

   e. For immobile patients:

     Apply PPE. Lower head of bed. Help patient roll onto side away from you and off the bedpan. Hold bedpan flat and steady while patient is rolling off; otherwise spillage will occur. Place bedpan on draped bedside chair and cover it.

Reduces spread of microorganisms. Reduces spread of offensive odours.

14. Allow patient to perform hand hygiene. Change soiled linens, remove and dispose of PPE, and return patient to a comfortable position.

Reduces chance of skin breakdown when bedridden patient lies on dry, wrinkle-free linens.

15. Place bed in its lowest position. Ensure that call bell, phone, drinking water, and desired personal items (e.g., books) are within easy access.

Promotes comfort and reduces risk for injury to patient. Patients often fall when reaching for items.

16. *Option:* Obtain stool specimen as prescribed (see Skill 9.2). Wear PPE when emptying contents of bedpan into toilet or in special receptacle in utility room. Use spray faucet attached to most facility toilets to rinse bedpan thoroughly. Use disinfectant if required by employer; store pan. Remove PPE.

If bedpan becomes very soiled, replace it with a clean one.

17. Perform hand hygiene.

Reduces transmission of microorganisms.

EVALUATION

1. Assess characteristics of stool. Note colour, odour, consistency, frequency, amount, shape (see Fig. 35.2), and constituents. Assess characteristics of urine if patient voided in bedpan.

Helps to identify significant changes or findings.

STEP	RATIONALE

EVALUATION

2. Evaluate patient's ability to use bedpan.
3. Inspect patient's perianal area and surrounding skin while removing bedpan.
4. **Use Teach-Back:** "I want to make sure you're comfortable getting off and on the bedpan by using the trapeze to pull your body off the bed. Show me how you will use the trapeze." Develop a revised teaching plan if patient is not able to teach back correctly.

Provides continual assessment of patient's self-toileting ability.
Liquid stool predisposes patients to skin breakdown (Sammon et al., 2015).
Determines patient's level of understanding of instructional topic.

Unexpected Outcomes	Related Interventions
1. Patient is unable to successfully use bedpan.	• If patient's mobility allows, obtain prescription for use of bedside commode.
2. Patient is incontinent of stool. Avoid use of adult briefs for bedridden patient.	• Establish a regular schedule of offering a bedpan. Adult briefs mask toileting needs and may potentiate skin breakdown called *incontinence-associated dermatitis (IAD)* (Sammon et al., 2015).
	• Discuss with staff the need to answer the patient's request for toileting help promptly and to use a toileting schedule.
3. Patient develops irritation and breakdown of skin around perianal area.	• Administer perianal skin care using moisture barrier.
	• Reassess perianal skin with each bowel movement and each position change.

Communication and Documentation

- Document the type of help needed and if the patient tolerates getting on and off the bedpan, the character and amount of stool, and urine output (if patient also voids) on flow sheet or in nurses' notes in electronic health record (EHR) or chart.
- Document your evaluation of patient learning.
- Complete laboratory requisition if you collected a stool or urine specimen and send it to the laboratory. Document the type of specimen sent.

Special Considerations
Pediatric

- Constipation in early childhood results from environmental changes such as being hospitalized and reluctance to use a bedpan. Toilet-trained children often regress during hospitalization (Hockenberry & Wilson, 2015).
- Repeated withholding of stool leads to stretching or dilating of the rectum and decreases the sensation or "urge" to defecate (Hockenberry & Wilson, 2015).

- In children over the age of 4 years, encopresis (involuntary discharge of feces) is often the result of chronic constipation (Borowitz, 2017).

Gerontological

- Older persons have some loss of sphincter control and often require a quick response when requesting a bedpan (Ball et al., 2015).
- The use of continence aids such as pads or briefs is more common in older persons. Timely continence care and assessment of skin integrity are critical to prevent skin impairment (Francis, 2018).
- The incidence of constipation is greater because there is impaired rectal sensation to defecate. As a result, the older person does not perceive the need to defecate.
- With increased age, transit time through the bowel increases, causing a normal lengthening of the time between bowel movements (Ball et al., 2015).

◆ SKILL 35.2   Removing Fecal Impaction Digitally

Fecal impaction is the inability to pass a collection of hard stool. This condition occurs in all age groups. Physically and mentally incapacitated individuals and institutionalized older persons are at greatest risk. Patients with acute stroke and spinal cord injuries are also at greater risk for fecal impaction (RNAO, 2011).

Functional constipation is defined as including two or more of the following factors for at least 3 months: (1) straining with defecation at least one fourth of the time, (2) lumpy or hard stools (or both) one fourth of the time (Fig. 35.2), (3) sensation of anorectal blockage at least one fourth of the time, (4) loose stools rarely present without the use of laxatives, or (5) three or fewer bowel movements in a week (Wald, 2015).

Symptoms of fecal impaction include constipation, rectal discomfort, anorexia, nausea, vomiting, abdominal pain, abdominal bloating, diarrhea (leaking around the impacted stool), and urinary frequency (Ness, 2013). Prevention is the key to managing fecal impaction. With newer bowel management techniques such as transanal irrigation, digital removal of fecal material is not needed (Ness, 2013). However, once impaction occurs, digital removal of stool is the only alternative.

Delegation and Collaboration

The skill of removing a fecal impaction digitally cannot be delegated to an unregulated care provider (UCP). The nurse instructs the UCP to:

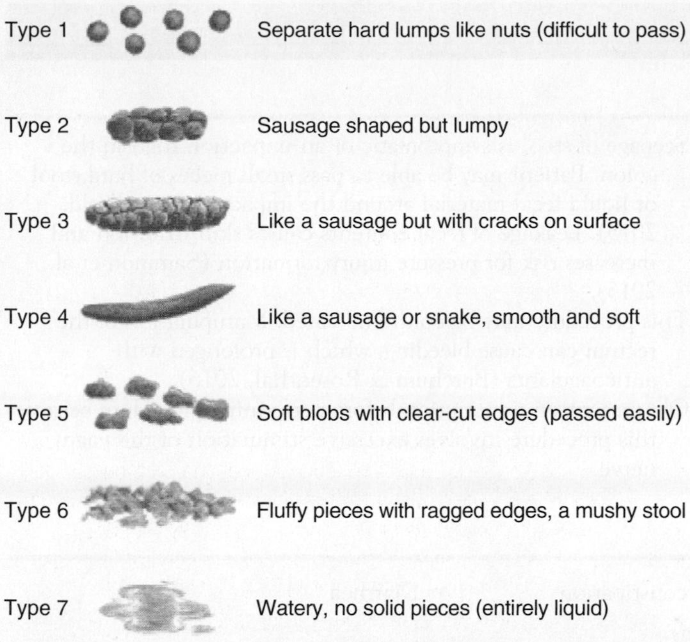

Type 1   Separate hard lumps like nuts (difficult to pass)

Type 2   Sausage shaped but lumpy

Type 3   Like a sausage but with cracks on surface

Type 4   Like a sausage or snake, smooth and soft

Type 5   Soft blobs with clear-cut edges (passed easily)

Type 6   Fluffy pieces with ragged edges, a mushy stool

Type 7   Watery, no solid pieces (entirely liquid)

FIG 35.2 Bristol Stool Form Scale. *(From O'Donnell, L.J., Virjee, J., & Heaton, K. W. [1990]. Detection of pseudodiarrhoea by simple clinical assessment of intestinal transit rate. British Medical Journal, 300(6722), 439. ©1990. Reprinted with permission of the BMJ Publishing Group.)*

- Help the nurse position the patient for the procedure.
- Monitor heart rate as the nurse removes impaction.
- Observe the stool for colour, consistency, rectal bleeding, or bloody mucus and report this immediately to the nurse.
- Provide perineal care following each bowel movement.

Equipment

- Personal protective equipment (PPE)
- Water-soluble local anaesthetic lubricant (**NOTE:** Some employers require use of water-soluble lubricant without anaesthetic.)
- Waterproof, absorbent pads
- Bedpan
- Bedpan cover (optional)
- Bath blanket
- Basin, washcloths, towels, and soap
- Vital sign equipment
- Stethoscope

STEP	RATIONALE

ASSESSMENT

STEP	RATIONALE
1. Identify patient using at least two person-specific identifiers (e.g., name and date of birth or name and medical record number), according to employer policy.	Ensures correct patient. Complies with Accreditation Canada's standards and improves patient safety (Accreditation Canada, 2019).
2. Ask patient about normal and current bowel elimination pattern, including frequency and characteristics of stool; use of laxatives, enemas, and other medications; level of exercise; urge to defecate but inability to do so; feelings of incomplete emptying; and sensations of bloating, cramping, and excessive gas.	Information provides data in determining contributing factors and preventive measures. Large fecal mass causes rectal distension and increases perception of urge to evacuate rectum (DeGiorgio et al., 2015).
3. Inspect patient's abdomen for distension.	Observation identifies distended or asymmetrical areas, which are then investigated on auscultation or palpation. Distension can contribute to, or be a result of, constipation.
4. Auscultate all four quadrants for presence of bowel sounds.	Hypoactive bowel sounds may result from partial obstruction of the gastrointestinal (GI) tract (Ball et al., 2015).
5. Palpate patient's abdomen for distension, discomfort, or masses.	Symptoms are related to accumulation of stool in intestinal tract. A palpable mass may be felt with severe constipation (Ball et al., 2015).
6. Measure patient's current vital signs, including pain level using a validated pain assessment score.	Provides baseline measurement. The sacral branch of the vagus nerve is stimulated during digital stimulation; this stimulation results in reflex slowing of heart rate (Ball et al., 2015).

Clinical Decision Point *Because of the potential to stimulate the sacral branch of the vagus nerve, patients with a history of dysrhythmias or heart disease have a greater risk for changes in heart rhythm. Monitor patient's pulse before and during the procedure. This procedure is often contraindicated in cardiac patients; if in doubt, verify with the health care provider.*

STEP	RATIONALE
7. If patient has a spinal cord injury (SCI), review their routine for digital removal of stool, and if this is part of the patient's routine bowel care, it is essential not to interrupt the routine (Peate, 2016).	The level of SCI and severity of injury affect the pattern of constipation. Injuries to cervicothoracic vertebrae increase the frequency of constipation. Patients with SCI are at risk for autonomic dysreflexia before and after the procedure, which may cause a sudden elevated blood pressure (BP). In these patients, digital removal of stool is a routine intervention for bowel health and should not be interrupted (Peate, 2016).

STEP	RATIONALE

ASSESSMENT

8. Perform hand hygiene and apply clean gloves. Observe consistency of stool (see Fig. 35.2), seepage of liquid stool, or continued passage of small amounts of hard stool. Observe anal area for signs of irritation or hemorrhoids. Remove gloves and perform hand hygiene.

Seepage of stool is symptomatic of an impaction high in the colon. Patient may be able to pass small pieces of hard stool or liquid fecal material around the impacted mass (Wald, 2015). Leakage of fecal contents causes skin irritation and increases risk for pressure injury formation (Sammon et al., 2015).

9. Determine if patient is receiving anticoagulant therapy or has a past history of rectal surgery.

This procedure may be contraindicated. Manipulation of the rectum can cause bleeding, which is prolonged with anticoagulants (Burchum & Rosenthal, 2016).

10. Check patient's record for health care provider's prescription for digital removal of impaction and use of anaesthetic lubricant.

Obtain written prescription before performing procedure because this procedure involves excessive stimulation of the vagus nerve.

NURSING DIAGNOSES

- Acute pain
- Chronic functional constipation
- Diarrhea

Related factors are individualized on the basis of patient's condition or needs.

PLANNING

1. Expected outcomes following completion of procedure:
  - Impacted stool is removed successfully.
  - Patient is free of abdominal or rectal discomfort.

  - Vital signs remain within patient's baseline.

Indicates that rectum is clear of stool.
Fecal impaction causes direct pain to rectum and indirect abdominal discomfort through abdominal distension (Ness, 2013).
Indicates absence of vagal stimulation.

2. Explain procedure to patient.

Information reduces anxiety and encourages patient participation in therapeutic elimination protocol.

3. Perform hand hygiene. Arrange supplies at bedside.

Ensures access to supplies during procedure.

IMPLEMENTATION

1. Obtain help to change patient's position if necessary. Raise bed horizontally to a comfortable working height.

Promotes patient safety and use of good body mechanics.

2. Pull curtains around bed or close door to room.

Maintains patient's sense of privacy and prevents unnecessary exposure of body parts.

3. Lower side rail on patient's right side. Keeping far side rail raised, help patient to a left side-lying position with the knees flexed and back.

Promotes patient safety. Provides access to rectum. The left side-lying position promotes rectal sphincter relaxation, mimics the squatting position to aid in defecation (RNAO, 2011), and promotes an anatomical approach for insertion of the index finger.

4. Drape patient's trunk and lower extremities with a bath blanket and place a waterproof pad under the patient's buttocks.

Maintains patient's sense of privacy and prevents unnecessary exposure of body parts.

5. Perform hand hygiene, apply clean gloves, and place bedpan next to patient.

6. Lubricate gloved index finger and middle finger of dominant hand with anaesthetic lubricant.

Prevents transmission of microorganisms. Reduces discomfort and permits smooth insertion of finger into anus and rectum.

7. Instruct patient to take slow, deep breaths during the procedure. Gradually and gently insert gloved index finger and feel anus relax around finger. Insert middle finger.

Slow, deep breaths help to relax the patient. Gradual insertion of the index finger helps to dilate the anal sphincter.

8. Gradually advance fingers slowly along rectal wall toward umbilicus.

Guiding finger toward rectal wall follows the natural direction of the colon, allowing for access to impacted stool high in the rectum.

9. Gently loosen fecal mass by moving fingers in scissors motion to fragment fecal mass. Work fingers into hardened mass.

Loosening and penetrating mass allows for removal of stool in small pieces, resulting in less discomfort to patient.

STEP	RATIONALE

IMPLEMENTATION

10. Work stool downward toward end of rectum. Remove small sections of feces and discard into bedpan.	Prevents need to force finger up into rectum and minimizes trauma to mucosa.
11. Observe patient's response and periodically assess heart rate and look for signs of fatigue.	Vagal stimulation slows the heart rate and causes dysrhythmias. This procedure often exhausts a patient.

Clinical Decision Point *Stop the procedure if the heart rate drops or rhythm changes from the patient's baseline or if the patient has dyspnea or indicates palpitations.*

12. Continue to clear rectum of feces and allow patient to rest at intervals.	Rest improves patient's tolerance of procedure, allowing heart rate to return to normal.
13. After removal of impaction, perform perineal hygiene (see Procedural Guideline 18.1).	Promotes patient's sense of comfort and cleanliness.
14. Remove bedpan and inspect feces for colour and consistency. Dispose of feces in toilet.	Reduces transmission of microorganisms.
15. If needed, help patient to toilet or clean and store bedpan. (Procedure may be followed by enema or cathartic.)	Removal of impaction stimulates defecation reflex.
16. Remove PPE. Remove gloves by turning them inside out and discarding in a proper receptacle. Perform hand hygiene.	Reduces transmission of microorganisms.

EVALUATION

1. Apply clean gloves, perform rectal examination for stool, and observe anal and perianal area for irritation or skin breakdown following the disimpaction. Remove and dispose of gloves; perform hand hygiene.	Determines if rectum is clear. Fecal material, especially diarrhea, causes irritation to perianal tissues (Sammon et al., 2015).
2. Reassess vital signs and compare to baseline value. Continue to monitor patient for 1 hour for bradycardia.	Determines extent of vagal stimulation.
3. Auscultate bowel sounds.	Determines presence of peristaltic activity.
4. Palpate abdomen to determine if it is soft and nontender.	Discomfort is relieved.
5. **Use Teach-Back:** "I want to make sure you include the high-fibre foods and fluids that we recommended for your diet to help prevent constipation. Tell me which foods you will add to your diet." Develop a revised teaching plan if patient or caregiver is not able to teach back correctly.	Determines patient's and caregiver's level of understanding of instructional topic.

Unexpected Outcomes	Related Interventions
1. Patient experiences trauma to rectal mucosa as evidenced by rectal bleeding.	• Assess anal and perianal region for source of bleeding. • Stop procedure if bleeding is excessive and notify health care provider.
2. Patient experiences bradycardia (heart rate <60 per minute), decrease in blood pressure, and decrease in level of consciousness as a result of vagus nerve stimulation.	• Stop procedure and measure vital signs. • Notify health care provider and remain with patient.
3. Patient has seepage of liquid stool after procedure is complete.	• Assess patient for continuing impaction. • Notify health care provider for possible rectal suppository (see Chapter 20) or enema. • Increase patient's fluid intake and dietary fibre.

Communication and Documentation

- Document patient's tolerance of procedure, amount and consistency of stool removed, vital signs, and adverse effects on flow sheet or in nurses' notes in electronic health record (EHR) or chart.
- Document patient's and caregiver's understanding through teach-back about the types of high-fibre foods to reduce the frequency of constipation.
- Report any changes in vital signs and adverse effects to the health care provider.

Special Considerations
Pediatric

- Do not digitally remove stool in a pediatric patient because of the risk for anal fissures and pain that trigger stool withholding (Hockenberry & Wilson, 2015).
- Dietary changes including increased fluid intake and increased fibre intake with whole vegetables and fruits instead of juice; bran cereal; dried fruits; lentils; and beans can help alleviate constipation in children (Dietitians of Canada, 2018; Rowan-Legg et al., 2018).

Gerontological

- Many older persons are especially prone to dysrhythmias and other problems related to vagal stimulation; monitor heart rate and rhythm closely (Ball et al., 2015).
- For older persons, instituting a diet adequate in dietary fibre adds bulk, weight, and form to the stool and improves defecation

(DeGiorgio et al., 2015). The recommended daily fibre intake is 25 to 30 grams daily (RNAO, 2011).

- Laxative use for chronic constipation in older persons must be individualized to the patient's cardiac and renal comorbidities, drug interactions, and adverse effects (DeGiorgio et al., 2015).

✦ SKILL 35.3   Administering an Enema

NSO *Nursing Skills Online Bowel Elimination/Ostomy Care Module 18 / Lesson 2* 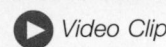 *Video Clip*

An *enema* is the instillation of a solution into the rectum and sigmoid colon to promote defecation by stimulating peristalsis. Typically, enemas treat constipation or empty the bowel before diagnostic procedures or certain types of abdominal surgery. The volume or type of fluid that breaks up the fecal mass stretches the rectal wall and initiates the defecation reflex. Table 35.1 summarizes common types of enemas.

Cleansing enemas promote complete evacuation of feces from the colon. They act by stimulating peristalsis through infusion of large volumes of solution. Oil-retention enemas act by lubricating the rectum and colon, allowing feces to absorb oil and become softer and easier to pass.

Medicated enemas contain pharmacological therapeutic agents. Some are prescribed to reduce dangerously high serum potassium levels (e.g., sodium polystyrene sulfonate enema) or to reduce bacteria in the colon before bowel surgery (e.g., neomycin enema).

Delegation and Collaboration

The skill of administering an enema can be delegated to an unregulated care provider (UCP). **NOTE:** If a medicated enema is prescribed, then it cannot be delegated to a UCP. The nurse instructs the UCP to:

- Properly position patients who have mobility restrictions or therapeutic equipment such as drains, intravenous (IV) catheters, or traction.
- Inform the nurse immediately about patient's new abdominal pain (*exception*: a patient reports cramping) or rectal bleeding.

- Inform the nurse immediately of the presence of blood in the stool or around the rectal area or any change in vital signs.

Equipment

- Personal protective equipment (PPE)
- Water-soluble lubricant
- Waterproof, absorbent pads
- Toilet tissue
- Bedpan, bedside commode, or access to toilet
- Bath blanket
- Basin, washcloths, towel, and soap
- Stethoscope

Enema Bag Administration

- Enema container with tubing and clamp (Fig. 35.3)
- IV pole
- Appropriate-size rectal tube (adult: 22 to 30 Fr; child: 12 to 18 Fr)
- Correct volume of warmed (tepid) solution (adult: 750–1000 mL; adolescent: 500–700 mL). For pediatric patients, the weight of the child usually determines the volume for the enema; for example, with a phosphate enema, calculate 6 mL/kg (up to 135 mL) for total volume; enemas are not recommended for children under 2 years of age (Rowan et al., 2018).

Prepackaged Enema

- Prepackaged enema container with lubricated rectal tip (Fig. 35.4)

TABLE 35.1

Types of Enemas

Type of Enema	Description and Implications
Tap-water (hypotonic) enema	Do not repeat after first installation because water toxicity or circulatory overload can develop.
Physiological normal saline	Safest enema to administer. Infants and children can tolerate only this type because of their predisposition to fluid imbalance.
Hypertonic solution (e.g., commercially prepared Fleet enema)	Useful for patients who cannot tolerate large volumes of fluid.
Harris flush enema	A return-flow enema that helps to expel intestinal gas. Administer a small amount (100–200 mL) of enema solution into the patient's rectum and colon. Lower the enema container to allow the total volume of solution to flow back. The repeated back-and-forth administration and return of the fluid reduces flatus and promotes return of peristalsis.
Soapsuds enema (SSE)	Pure castile soap added to either tap water or normal saline. Use only pure castile soap. The recommended ratio of pure soap to solution is 5 mL (1 teaspoon) to 1000 mL (1 quart) warm water or saline. Add soap to the enema bag after water is in place to reduce excessive suds.
Oil-retention enema	Oil-based solution. The colon absorbs a small volume, which softens stool for easier evacuation.
Carminative solution	Relieves gaseous distension. Example: MGW solution, which contains 30 mL of magnesium, 60 mL of glycerin, and 90 mL of water.

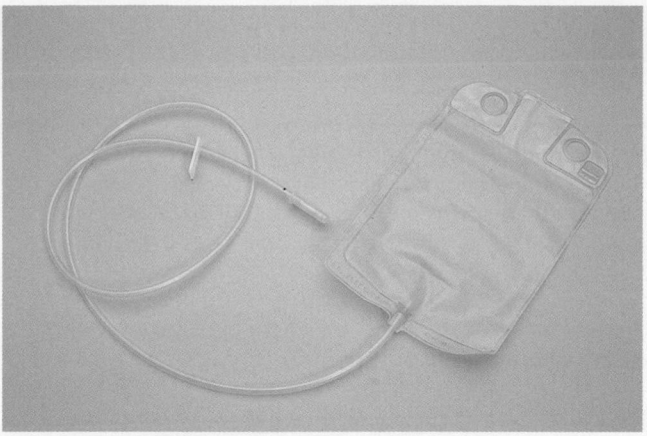

FIG 35.3 Enema bag with tubing.

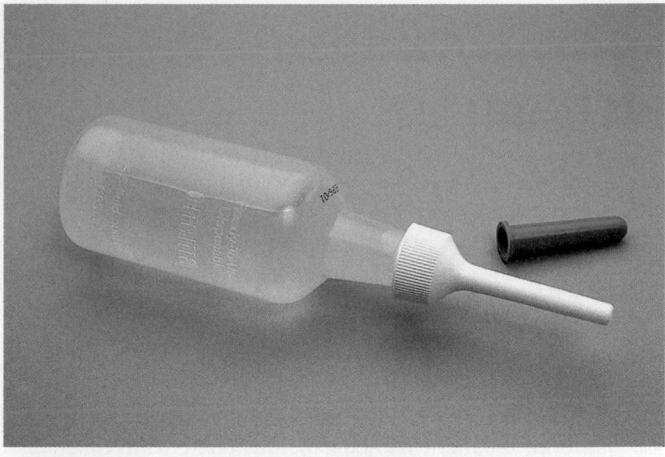

FIG 35.4 Prepackaged enema container with rectal tip and cap.

STEP	RATIONALE

ASSESSMENT

1. Identify patient using at least two person-specific identifiers (e.g., name and date of birth or name and medical record number), according to employer policy.

Ensures correct patient. Complies with Accreditation Canada's standards and improves patient safety (Accreditation Canada, 2019).

2. Review health care provider's prescription for an enema and clarify reason for administration.

A prescription by a health care provider is usually required for a hospitalized patient. The prescription states which type of enema the patient will receive.

3. Assess last bowel movement, normal versus most recent bowel pattern, presence of hemorrhoids, and presence of abdominal pain or cramping.

Determines need for enema and type of enema used. Also establishes baseline for bowel function. Hemorrhoids may obscure rectal opening and cause discomfort or bleeding during evacuation.

4. Assess patient's mobility and their ability to turn and position on their side.

Determines if assistance is needed for positioning patient.

5. Inspect abdomen for presence of distension and auscultate for bowel sounds.

Establishes baseline for determining effectiveness of enema.

6. Assess patient for allergy to any active ingredients of Fleet enema.

Reduces risk for allergic reaction.

7. Determine patient's level of understanding of purpose of the enema.

Allows for planning appropriate teaching measures.

Clinical Decision Point *"Enemas until clear" prescription means that enemas are repeated until the patient passes fluid that is clear of fecal matter. The fluid the patient passes may also be tinted and have small flecks of fecal matter. Check employer policy, but usually the patient should receive only three consecutive enemas to avoid disruption of fluid and electrolyte balance. It is essential to observe contents of solution passed.*

NURSING DIAGNOSES

- Acute pain
- Constipation
- Chronic functional constipation
- Potential for constipation

Related factors/Risk factors are individualized on the basis of patient's condition or needs.

PLANNING

1. Expected outcomes following completion of procedure:
   - Stool is evacuated.
   - Enema return is clear.
   - Abdomen is flat, nontender, with no distension.
2. Perform hand hygiene. Arrange supplies at bedside.

Solution clears rectum and lower colon of stool.
Indicates that all solid fecal material in colon has passed.
Gas and feces are expelled.
Ensures access to supplies during procedure.

STEP	RATIONALE

IMPLEMENTATION

1. If the enema is medicated, the skill is usually not delegated to a UCP (see employer policy). Check accuracy and completeness of each medication administration record (MAR) with the health care provider's written prescription. Check patient's name, type of enema, and time for administration. Compare MAR with label of enema solution.

The prescription is the most reliable source and only legal record of drugs or procedure that a patient is to receive. Ensures that patient receives correct enema.

2. Provide privacy by closing curtains around bed or closing door.

Reduces embarrassment for patient.

3. Place bedpan or bedside commode in easily accessible position. If patient will be expelling contents in toilet, ensure that toilet is available and place patient's nonskid slippers and bathrobe in an easily accessible position.

A bedpan is used if the patient is unable to get out of bed. Nonskid slippers help prevent a patient who may be rushing to the bathroom from falling. An extra gown provides modesty for patient.

4. Perform hand hygiene.

Reduces transmission of microorganisms.

5. With side rail raised on patient's right side and bed raised to an appropriate working height, help patient turn to a left side-lying (Sims') position with the right knee flexed. Encourage patient to remain in this position until the procedure is complete. Place a child in the dorsal recumbent position.

Allows enema solution to flow downward by gravity along the natural curve of the sigmoid colon and rectum, thus improving retention of solution.

Clinical Decision Point *Patients with poor sphincter control require placement of a bedpan under the buttocks. Administering an enema with the patient sitting on the toilet is unsafe because curved rectal tubing can abrade the rectal wall.*

6. Apply clean gloves and place waterproof pad, absorbent side up, under hips and buttocks. Cover patient with a bath blanket, exposing only the rectal area, clearly visualizing the anus.

Pad prevents soiling of linen. Blanket provides warmth, reduces exposure of body parts, and allows patient to feel more relaxed and comfortable.

7. Separate buttocks and examine perianal region for abnormalities, including hemorrhoids, anal fissure, and rectal prolapse.

Findings influence approach for inserting enema tip. Prolapse contraindicates enema.

8. Administer enema.

   a. **Administer prepackaged disposable enema:**

   (1) Remove plastic cap from tip of container. Tip may already be lubricated. Apply more water-soluble lubricant as needed.

   Lubrication provides for smooth insertion of rectal tube without causing rectal irritation or trauma. With presence of hemorrhoids, extra lubricant provides added comfort.

   (2) Gently separate buttocks and locate anus. Instruct patient to relax by breathing out slowly through the mouth.

   Breathing out promotes relaxation of external rectal sphincter.

   (3) Expel any air from enema container.

   Introducing air into the colon causes further distension and discomfort.

   (4) Insert lubricated tip of container gently into anal canal toward umbilicus (see illustration).
   Adult & Adolescent: 7.5–10 cm (3–4 inches)
   Child: 5–7.5 cm (2–3 inches)
   Infant: 2.5–3.75 cm (1–1½ inches)

   Gentle insertion prevents trauma to rectal mucosa.

Clinical Decision Point *If pain occurs or you feel resistance at any time during the procedure, stop and discuss this with the health care provider. Do not force insertion.*

   (5) Roll plastic bottle from bottom to tip until all of solution has entered rectum and colon. Instruct patient to retain solution until the urge to defecate occurs, usually 2 to 5 minutes.

   Prevents instillation of air into the colon and ensures that all content enters the rectum. Hypertonic solutions require only small volumes to stimulate defecation.

STEP	**RATIONALE**

IMPLEMENTATION

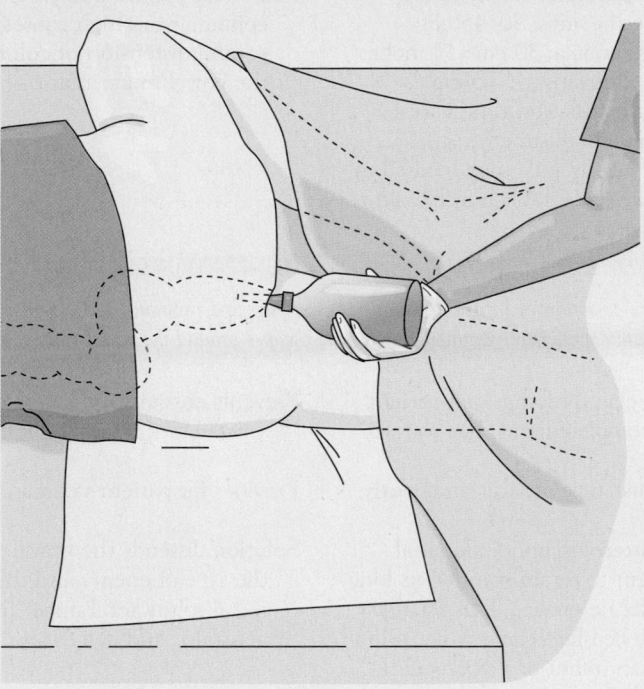

STEP 8a(4) With patient in left lateral Sims' position, insert tip of commercial enema into rectum. *(From Sorrentino, S. A. [2009]. Mosby's textbook for nursing assistants [7th ed.]. St Louis: Mosby.)*

b. Administer enema in standard enema bag:

(1) Add warmed prescribed type of solution and amount to enema bag. Warm tap water as it flows from faucet. Place saline container in a basin of warm water before adding saline to the enema bag. Check temperature of solution by pouring a small amount of solution over the inner wrist.	Hot water burns intestinal mucosa. Cold water causes abdominal cramping and is difficult to retain.
(2) If soapsuds enema (SSE) is prescribed, add castile soap after water.	Reduces suds in enema bag.
(3) Raise container, release clamp, and allow solution to flow long enough to fill tubing.	Removes air from tubing.
(4) Reclamp tubing.	Prevents further loss of solution.
(5) Lubricate 6–8 cm (2½ –3 inches) of tip of rectal tube with lubricant.	Allows smooth insertion of rectal tube without risk for irritation or trauma to mucosa.
(6) Gently separate buttocks and locate anus. Instruct patient to relax, by breathing out slowly through the mouth. Touch patient's skin next to the anus with tip of the rectal tube.	Patient's breathing out and feeling skin being touched with tube promotes relaxation of external anal sphincter.
(7) Insert tip of rectal tube slowly by pointing it in the direction of the patient's umbilicus. Length of insertion varies (see Step 8a[4]).	Careful insertion prevents trauma to rectal mucosa from accidental lodging of tube against the rectal wall. Insertion beyond the proper limit can cause bowel perforation.

Clinical Decision Point *If the tube does not pass easily, do not force it. Consider allowing a small amount of fluid to infuse and then try to reinsert the tube slowly. The instillation of fluid relaxes the sphincter and provides additional lubrication. If impaction is present, remove it (see Skill 35.2) before administering the enema.*

(8) Hold tubing in the rectum constantly until the end of fluid instillation.	Prevents expulsion of rectal tube during bowel contractions.
(9) Open regulating clamp and allow solution to enter slowly, with container at patient's hip level.	Rapid infusion stimulates evacuation of tubing and can cause cramping.

STEP	RATIONALE

IMPLEMENTATION

(10) Raise height of enema container slowly to an appropriate level above the anus: 30–45 cm (12–18 inches) for high enema; 30 cm (12 inches) for regular enema (see illustration); 7.5 cm (3 inches) for low enema. Instillation time varies with volume of solution administered (e.g., 1 L may take 10 minutes). An IV pole may be used to hold an enema bag once you establish a slow flow of fluid (see illustration).

Allows for continuous, slow instillation of solution. Raising the container too high causes rapid instillation and possible painful distension of colon. High pressure causes rupture of the bowel in an infant.

Clinical Decision Point *Temporary cessation of infusion minimizes cramping and promotes the ability to retain solution. Lower the container or clamp tubing if the patient indicates they are experiencing cramping or if fluid escapes around the rectal tube.*

(11) Instill all solution and clamp tubing. Tell patient that the procedure is completed and that you will remove the tubing.

Prevents entrance of air into rectum. Patients may misinterpret sensation of removing tube as loss of control.

9. Place layers of toilet tissue around tube at anus and gently withdraw rectal tube and tip.

Provides for patient's comfort and cleanliness.

10. Explain to patient that some distension and abdominal cramping are normal. Ask patient to retain solution as long as possible until the urge to defecate occurs. This usually takes a few minutes. Stay at the bedside. Have patient lie quietly in bed, if possible. (For an infant or a young child, gently hold buttocks together for few minutes.)

Solution distends the bowel. Length of retention varies with the type of enema and the patient's ability to contract the rectal sphincter. Longer retention promotes stimulation of peristalsis and defecation.

11. Discard enema container or disposable bag and tubing in a proper receptacle. Remove PPE and perform hand hygiene.

Reduces transmission and growth of microorganisms.

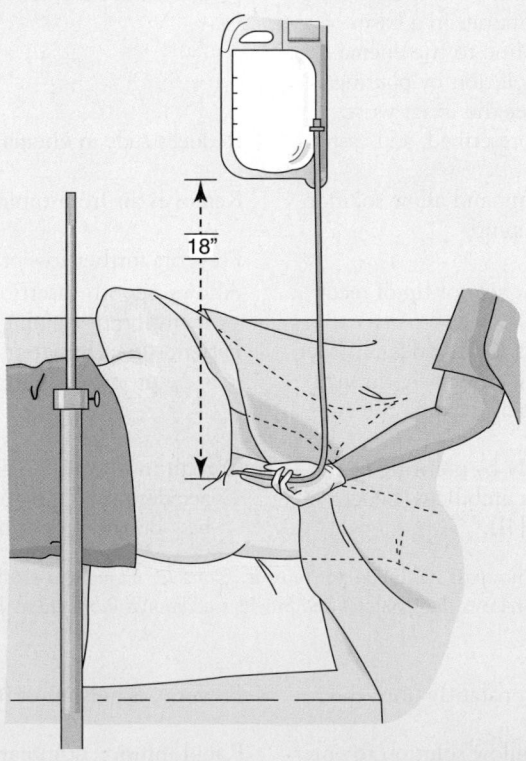

STEP 8b(10) IV pole is positioned so bottom of enema bag is 45 cm (18 inches) above anus. (*From Sorrentino, S. A. [2009]. Mosby's textbook for nursing assistants [7th ed.]. St. Louis: Mosby.*)

STEP	RATIONALE

IMPLEMENTATION

12. Help patient to the bathroom or commode, if possible. If using a bedpan, apply clean gloves and help patient to as near a normal position for evacuation as possible (see Skill 35.1).

Normal squatting position promotes defecation.

13. Observe character of stool and solution (caution patient against flushing toilet before inspection).

Determines if enema was effective.

14. Help patient as needed to wash anal area with warm soap and water (use gloves for perineal care).

Fecal contents irritate the skin. Hygiene promotes patient's comfort.

15. Remove and discard gloves and perform hand hygiene.

Reduces transmission of micro-organisms.

EVALUATION

1. Inspect colour, consistency, and amount of stool; odour; and fluid passed.

Determines if stool is evacuated or fluid is retained. Note abnormalities such as presence of blood or mucus.

2. Assess for abdominal distension.

Determines if distension is relieved.

3. **Use Teach-Back:** "I want to be sure I explained clearly how to position yourself in bed if you need to give yourself an enema. Tell me how you would position yourself." Develop a revised teaching plan if the patient is not able to teach back correctly.

Determines patient's level of understanding of instructional topic.

Unexpected Outcomes

1. Severe abdominal cramping, bleeding, or sudden abdominal pain develops and is unrelieved by temporarily stopping or slowing flow of solution.

2. Patient is unable to hold enema solution.

Related Interventions
- Stop enema.
- Notify health care provider.
- Obtain vital signs.
- If this occurs during installation, slow the rate of infusion.

Communication and Documentation

- Document the type and volume of enema given, time of administration, characteristics of results, and patient's tolerance of the procedure on flow sheet or in nurses' notes in electronic health record (EHR) or chart.
- Document patient's understanding through teach-back for self-administration of a prepackaged enema in nurses' notes in EHR or chart.
- Report the failure of patient to defecate and any adverse effects to the health care provider.

Special Considerations
Pediatric

- The use of oral stool softeners is the initial recommended treatment of constipation in children (Jordan-Ely, 2015).
- Children and infants usually do not receive free water and soap enemas because of the serious adverse effects of fluid shifts. Use

of sodium phosphate enemas should be limited to avoid hyperphosphatemia (Bernal, Dole, & Thame, 2018), and these are not recommended for children under 2 years of age (Rowan et al., 2018).

Gerontological

- Caution is warranted when administering enemas prescribed for older persons. Some older persons become tired, are at risk for fluid and electrolyte imbalances, and experience changes in vital signs (Roque & Bouras, 2015).
- Some older persons may have difficulty retaining the fluid. The nurse may gently hold the buttocks together to help with retention of fluid (DeGiorgio et al., 2015).

Care in the Community

- Assess patient's and caregiver's ability and motivation to administer enema and provide instruction as needed.

PROCEDURAL GUIDELINE 35.1 *Applying a Fecal Management System*

A fecal management system (FMS) protects the perineum from exposure to fecal enzymes and prevents feces from spreading to wounds (Beeson et al., 2017). In addition, the FMS is useful for patients with severe fecal incontinence, such as those with *Clostridium difficile*–associated diarrhea. FMS systems are latex-free, in-dwelling rectal catheters with a low-pressure balloon to hold the catheter in place in the rectum and soft, flexible drainage tubing attached to a containment device. These systems have an irrigation port to maintain patency of the catheter and promote fecal drainage. Risks associated with use of this in-dwelling device include rectal necrosis, loss of rectal tone, pressure injury, or fistula formation (Singh, Bhargava, et al., 2018). Nurses must use interprofessional collaboration to discuss options for patients; certain situations contraindicate the use of a FMS (Box 35.2).

Delegation and Collaboration
The skill of applying a topical (external) fecal containment device cannot be delegated to an unregulated care provider (UCP). The UCP can assist the nurse by helping to position a patient during device application. The nurse instructs the UCP to:
- Report to the nurse any instances of leakage or change in appearance of skin around the device noted during routine care.
- Report to the nurse immediately any increase in patient's rectal pain or sensation of pressure or rectal bleeding.

Equipment
- FMS, also called fecal containment device (FCD) kit (Fig. 35.5).
- Personal protective equipment (PPE)
- Protective bed pad
- Bath basin

Procedural Steps
1. Identify patient using at least two person-specific identifiers (e.g., name and date of birth or name and medical record number) according to employer policy (Accreditation Canada, 2019).
2. Review medical record for contraindications for use of an FMS (see Box 35.2).

3. Assess for frequency and amount of diarrhea over the last 24–48 hours.
4. Assess patient for allergy to silicone. Note that these devices are latex free.
5. Perform hand hygiene and apply PPE. Perform perineal hygiene, and observe patient's anal region for swelling, hemorrhoids, redness, irritation, or drainage. Presence of these findings may contraindicate placement of the device or may indicate need for other interventions to the perianal skin.
6. Change gloves and perform digital rectal examination to ensure that there is no rectal impaction. Remove and discard gloves.
7. Perform hand hygiene and apply new clean gloves.
8. Apply the FMS.
   a. Prepare system by connecting the collection bag to catheter tube assembly.
   b. Deflate cuff, usually done with 60-mL syringe supplied in the kit.
   c. Fill 60-mL syringe with manufacturer's recommended quantity of tap water and attach syringe to inflation port. *DO NOT* inflate at this time. Inflation port is colour coded.
   d. Position patient in left knee–chest position. This position helps to maximize sphincter relaxation.
   e. Place protective bed pad under patient's dependent hip.
   f. Fold cuff according to manufacturer directions and lubricate cuff. Note that a folded cuff should be the size of your index finger.
   g. Generously lubricate anal sphincter.
   h. Gently separate patient's buttocks (UCP can assist), exposing perianal area for entire procedure. Make sure that the perianal area is clean and dry. It may be necessary to perform perineal hygiene again.
   i. Insert cuff using your index finger as a guide. Once the cuff is in the rectal vault, it will open to its original shape.
      (1) Inflate cuff with manufacturer's recommended quantity of water by slowly depressing the syringe plunger; the cuff will inflate. Use the pilot balloon as a guide: If the balloon indicates overinflation or underinflation, withdraw all fluid from the cuff, reposition it in the rectal vault, and reinflate it.

BOX 35.2

Contraindications for Use of Fecal Management Systems

- Suspected or confirmed anal pathology
- Pediatric population
- Existing poor anal sphincter
- Anorectal stricture or stenosis
- Anorectal surgery
- Colorectal surgery in the preceding 12 months
- Severe hemorrhoids
- Rectal tumour
- Fecal impaction
- Allergy or sensitivity to silicone
- Inflammatory processes of the rectum: Crohn's disease, radiation proctitis
- Anticoagulated patients

From Whiteley, I., & Sinclair, G. (2014). Faecal management systems for disabling incontinence or wounds: Literature review. *British Journal of Nursing, 23*(16), 881.

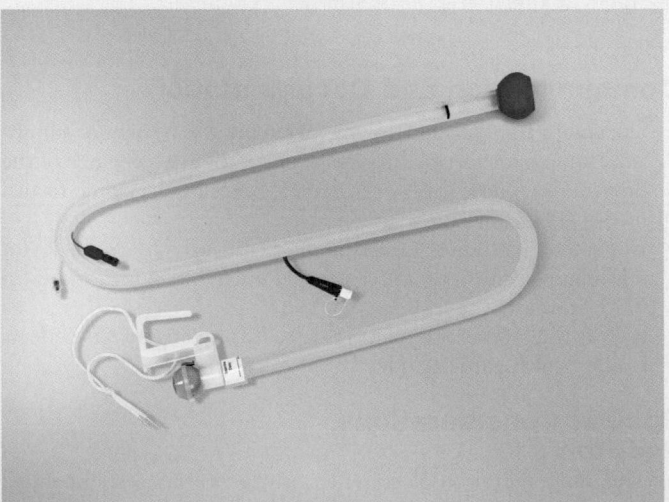

FIG 35.5 DIGNICARE® stool management system. (*Copyright © 2016 C.R. Bard, Inc. Used with permission.*)

PROCEDURAL GUIDELINE 35.1 *Applying a Fecal Management System—cont'd*

    (2) Remove syringe from injection port and gently pull on the catheter to ensure that cuff seats against the rectal floor.

  j. Note position of indicator line in relation to patient's anus. Changes in indicator line position may indicate need for the cuff to be repositioned. Remove gloves and perform hand hygiene.

9. Irrigate cuff as needed: Fill syringe with 45 mL of tap water and attach to clear irrigation port. Observe flow, but if leakage occurs, the cuff may need repositioning (see manufacturer instructions).

Clinical Decision Point *If the catheter tubing is obstructed with fecal contents, irrigate the catheter. Attach a filled syringe to the FLUSH port and irrigate. Ensure that the flush port remains parallel to the catheter to prevent kinking.*

10. If stool sampling is needed, use sample port (see Fig. 35.5). Apply clean gloves, open sample port, and either tilt or milk the catheter tubing to collect a sample or insert a slip-tip catheter to withdraw fecal material. Close sample port when finished. Remove gloves and perform hand hygiene.

11. Replace collection bag as needed. Perform hand hygiene and apply clean gloves.
  a. Disconnect drainage tubing from the collection bag.
  b. If necessary, attach bag plug into the collection bag hub.
  c. Connect new bag to tubing.
  d. Dispose of fecal contents per employer policy. Remove PPE and perform hand hygiene.

12. Removal of FMS. Perform hand hygiene and apply PPE.
  a. Attached depressed syringe 60 mL to cuff infusion port and slowly withdraw all water.
  b. Once cuff is deflated, grasp the catheter as close to the patient as possible and slowly slide it out of the anus.
  c. Dispose of FMS according to employer policy, remove PPE, and perform hand hygiene.

13. Position patient in a comfortable position and perform any hygiene needed.

14. Monitor patient for diarrhea and record amounts on intake and output (I&O) record every shift.

15. Record application of device and appearance of skin in nurses' notes in electronic health record (EHR) or chart.

✦ SKILL 35.4   Insertion, Maintenance, and Removal of a Nasogastric Tube for Gastric Decompression

There are times following major surgery or with conditions affecting the gastrointestinal (GI) tract when normal peristalsis is altered temporarily. Because peristalsis is slowed or absent, a patient cannot eat or drink fluids without causing abdominal distension. The temporary insertion of a nasogastric (NG) tube into the stomach serves to decompress the stomach, keeping it empty until normal peristalsis returns.

An NG tube is a hollow, pliable tube inserted through a patient's nasopharynx into the stomach. It allows for the removal of gastric secretions and the introduction of solutions into the stomach. Sometimes an NG tube is used for enteral feedings, but a softer, small-bore feeding tube is preferred for feeding purposes (see Chapter 32). The Levin and Salem sump tubes are the most common ones

used for stomach decompression. The Levin tube is a single-lumen tube with holes near the tip (Fig. 35.6). It is connected to a drainage bag or an intermittent suction device to drain stomach secretions.

The Salem sump tube is preferable for stomach decompression. The tube has two lumens: one for removal of gastric contents and one to provide an air vent, which prevents suctioning of gastric mucosa into eyelets at the distal tip of a tube. A blue "pigtail" is the air vent that connects with the second lumen (Fig. 35.7). When the main lumen of the sump tube is connected to suction, the air vent permits free, continuous drainage of secretions. ***Never clamp off the air vent, connect to suction, or use for irrigation.***

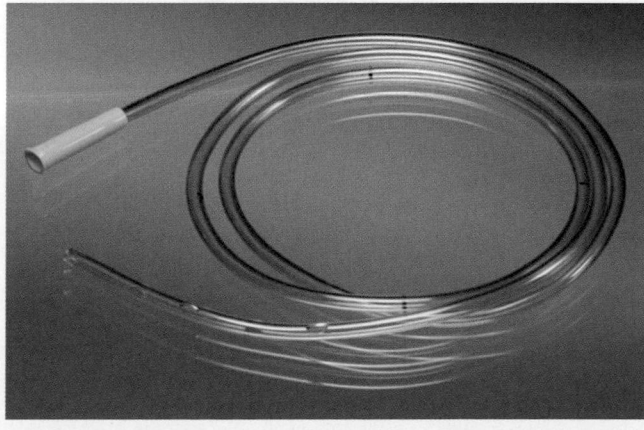

FIG 35.6 Levin tube. (*Courtesy Bard Medical, Covington, GA.*)

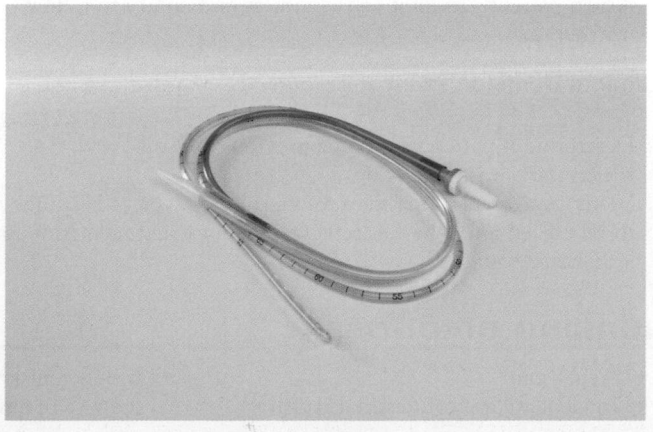

FIG 35.7 Salem sump tube. (*Courtesy Covidien, Mansfield, MA.*)

Insertion of an NG tube is uncomfortable; patients experience a burning sensation as the tube passes through the sensitive nasal mucosa. Following tube insertion, it is important to keep the patient comfortable and to observe skin around their nares because the tube is a constant irritation to mucosa and has the potential to cause a medical device–related pressure injury (MDRPI). Prevention of MDRPI is critical. The nurse needs to routinely assess the condition of the nares and mucosa for inflammation, blistering, and excoriation (Pittman et al., 2015).

Delegation and Collaboration

The skill of inserting and maintaining an NG tube cannot be delegated to an unregulated care provider (UCP). The nurse instructs the UCP to:

- Measure and record the drainage from an NG tube.
- Provide oral and nasal hygiene measures.
- Perform selected comfort measures, such as positioning or offering ice chips if allowed.
- Anchor the tube to the patient's gown during routine care to prevent accidental displacement.
- Immediately report to the nurse any signs of redness or irritation to the nares.

Equipment

- 14- or 16-Fr NG tube (Smaller-lumen catheters are not used for decompression in adults because they must be able to remove thick secretions.) (*Option:* A dual-purpose tube, one that is used for both gastric decompression and enteral feedings, may be prescribed for selected patients.)
- Water-soluble lubricant
- pH test strips (measure gastric aspirate acidity); use paper with a range of at least 1.0–11.0 or higher
- Tongue blade
- Flashlight
- Emesis basin
- Bulb or catheter-tipped syringe
- 2.5-cm (1-inch) wide hypoallergenic tape or commercial fixation device
- Safety pin and rubber band
- Clamp, drainage bag, or suction machine with pressure gauge if wall suction is to be used
- Towel
- Glass of water with straw
- Facial tissues
- Normal saline
- Tincture of benzoin (*optional*)
- Suction equipment
- Stethoscope
- Personal protective equipment (PPE)

STEP	RATIONALE

ASSESSMENT

1. Identify patient using at least two person-specific identifiers (e.g., name and date of birth or name and medical record number), according to employer policy.	Ensures correct patient. Complies with Accreditation Canada's standards and improves patient safety (Accreditation Canada, 2019).
2. Perform hand hygiene (apply appropriate PPE). Inspect condition of patient's nares and nasal and oral cavity.	Documents if skin on nares is intact or irritated before NG tube insertion. Determines need for special nursing hygiene measures after tube placement.
3. Ask if patient has a history of nasal surgery or congestion and allergies, and note if a deviated nasal septum is present.	Alerts nurse to potential obstruction. Insert tube into *uninvolved* nasal passage. Procedure may be contraindicated if surgery is recent.
4. Auscultate for bowel sounds. Palpate patient's abdomen for distension, pain, and rigidity. Remove and discard gloves if applied, and perform hand hygiene.	In the presence of diminished or absent bowel sounds, auscultate abdomen at least 1 minute in each quadrant (Ball et al., 2015). Documents baseline for any abdominal distension, GI ileus, and general GI function, which later serves as comparison once the tube is inserted.
5. Assess patient's level of consciousness and ability to follow instructions.	Determines patient's ability to help in the procedure.

Clinical Decision Point *If the patient is confused, disoriented, or unable to follow commands, get help from another staff member to insert the tube.*

6. Determine if patient has had a previous NG tube and, if so, which naris was used.	Patient's previous experience complements any explanations and prepares patient for NG tube placement.
7. Verify health care provider prescription for type of NG tube to be placed and whether tube is to be attached to suction or a drainage bag.	Requires prescription from health care provider. Adequate decompression depends on NG suction.

NURSING DIAGNOSES

- Acute pain
- Inadequate gastrointestinal motility
- Insufficient knowledge regarding purpose of gastric decompression
- Inadequate oral mucous membrane
- Potential for impaired skin integrity

Related factors/Risk factors are individualized on the basis of patient's condition or needs.

STEP	RATIONALE

PLANNING

1. Expected outcomes following completion of procedure:

- Abdomen is soft, nontender, and without distension.

    Correctly positioned NG tube remains patent, drains gastric secretions, and relieves gastric distension.

- Nares and nasal mucosa remain intact, clear, and without abrasions or excoriation.

    Ensures absence of irritation or pressure injury formation from NG tube.

- Patient's level of comfort improves or remains the same.

    A correctly inserted NG tube prevents abdominal discomfort from progressing.

2. Inform patient that the procedure may make them gag and that there will be a burning sensation in the nasopharynx as the tube is passed. Develop a hand signal with the patient.

Increases patient's cooperation and ability to anticipate nurse's action. If patient is unable to tolerate the procedure, use of a hand signal will alert the nurse.

3. Perform hand hygiene and arrange supplies at bedside.

Ensures access to supplies during procedure.

IMPLEMENTATION

1. Position patient upright in high-Fowler's position unless contraindicated. If patient is comatose, raise head of the bed as tolerated in a semi-Fowler's position with the head tipped forward, chin to chest.

Promotes patient's ability to swallow during procedure. Good body mechanics prevent injury to you or patient.

2. Place a bath towel over the patient's chest; give facial tissues to patient. Allow them to blow their nose, if necessary. Place an emesis basin within reach.

Prevents soiling of patient's gown. Tube insertion through nasal passages may cause tearing and coughing with increased salivation.

3. Pull curtain around bed or close room door.

Provides privacy and preserves dignity as part of person-centred care.

4. Wash bridge of nose with soap and water or alcohol swab. Dry thoroughly.

Removes oils from nose to allow fixation devices to adhere completely.

5. Stand on patient's right side if right-handed, on left side if left-handed. Lower side rail.

Allows easiest manipulation of tubing.

6. Instruct patient to relax and breathe normally while you are occluding one naris. Then repeat this action for the other naris. Select the nostril with greater airflow.

The tube passes more easily through the naris that is more patent.

7. Measure distance from tip of patient's nose to earlobe to xiphoid process of sternum (see illustration).

This length approximates the distance from nose to stomach. The NEX (nose-earlobe-xiphoid) method is commonly used in clinical settings with adult patients.

8. Mark length that will be inserted with indelible ink.

Indicates length of tube you will insert.

9. Prepare tube fixation materials. Cut hypoallergenic tape 10 cm (4 inches) long or prepare membrane dressing or another tube fixation device (see Step 24a[2]).

Fixation devices allow the tube to float free of the nares, thus reducing pressure on the nares and preventing MDRPI (Pittman et al., 2015).

10. Perform hand hygiene and apply clean gloves.

Reduces transmission of infection.

11. Apply pulse oximetry/capnography device and measure vital signs. Monitor oximetry/capnography during insertion.

Provides objective assessment of respiratory status before and during tube insertion.

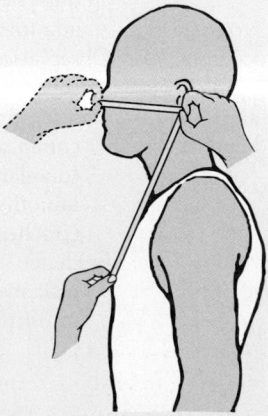

STEP 7 Determine length of tube to be inserted.

STEP	RATIONALE

IMPLEMENTATION

12. *Option:* Dip tube with surface lubricant into a glass of room-temperature water or lubricate 7.5–10 cm (3–4 inches) end of tube with water-soluble lubricant (see manufacturer directions).	Water activates lubricant, minimizes friction against nasal mucosa, and aids in insertion of the tube. Water-soluble lubricant is less toxic than oil-base lubricant if aspirated.
13. Hand an alert patient a cup of water if they are able to hold the cup and swallow, unless contraindicated. Check employer policy related to use of a straw when drinking. If the patient is unconscious do not use water, watch for patient coughing. Explain that you are about to insert the tube.	Swallowing water facilitates tube passage. The use of a straw may cause the patient to swallow additional air and worsen gastric distention. Coughing may indicate that the tube is inadvertently entering the lungs. Explanation decreases patient anxiety and increases patient cooperation.
14. Explain the next steps. Insert the tube gently and slowly through the naris to back of the throat (posterior nasopharynx). Aim back and down toward the patient's ear.	Natural contour facilitates passage of tube into GI tract and reduces gagging.
15. Have patient relax and flex head toward their chest after tube is passed through the nasopharynx.	Closes off glottis and reduces risk of tube entering the trachea.
16. Insert tube using swallow or no-swallow technique.	
a. Encourage patient to swallow by having them take small sips of water when possible. Advance tube as the patient swallows, rotate tube gently 180 degrees while inserting. Advance tube each time the patient swallows until you reach the desired length.	Swallowing facilitates passage of tube past the oropharynx. A tug may be felt as the patient swallows, indicating that tube is following the desired path.
b. If using the no-swallow technique, ask patient to take a deep breath and hold it when tube reaches the pharynx (Fan, Liu, & Gui, 2016). Once tube is inserted 15 to 20 cm, have the patient perform abdominal breathing.	In a recent randomized controlled trial, researchers found that a no-swallow technique of NG tube insertion decreased patient discomfort; increased success rate at first intubation; and reduced nausea, tearing, mucosal injury, and changes in vital signs (Fan et al., 2016).
17. Do not advance the tube during inspiration or coughing because it will likely enter the respiratory tract. Monitor oximetry/capnography.	When tube inadvertently enters the airway, changes in oxygen saturation or end-tidal carbon dioxide (CO_2) (capnography) occur.

Clinical Decision Point *Do not force NG tube. If the patient starts to cough or has a drop in oxygen saturation or increased CO_2, withdraw the tube into the posterior nasopharynx until normal breathing resumes.*

18. Using a penlight and tongue blade, check to be sure that tube is not positioned in the back of the throat.	Tube could become coiled or kinked or enter the trachea.
19. Temporarily anchor tube to the nose with a small piece of tape.	Securing the tube prevents movement of tube and subsequent gagging. Allows for verification of tube placement.
20. Verify tube placement. Check employer policy for recommended methods of checking tube placement.	
a. Follow prescription for bedside X-ray and notify radiology for examination of chest and abdomen.	Radiography is the gold standard for verification of initial placement of the tube (Lortie & Charbonney, 2016). This must be done before any medication or liquid is administered (Fan et al., 2017).
b. While waiting for radiography, follow these procedures: Attach a bulb or catheter-tipped syringe to the end of tube. Aspirate gently back on the syringe to obtain gastric contents, observing amount, colour, and quality of return (see illustration).	Observation of gastric contents is useful to determine initial tube placement. Gastric contents are usually green but are sometimes off-white, tan, bloody, or brown in colour. Other common aspirate colours include yellow or bile stained (duodenal placement), watery, pale yellow (esophagus), or tan/off-white and aspirate is of mucous consistency (tracheohronchial) (Lord, 2018).
c. Use pH test paper to measure aspirate for pH with colour-coded pH paper. Be sure that paper range of pH is at least from 1.0 to 11.0 (see illustration).	Evidence supports pH testing to be used as an indicator for placement: values of ≤5 likely indicate a gastric placement; intestinal or respiratory pH is usually ≥7 (Fan et al., 2017).

STEP	RATIONALE

IMPLEMENTATION

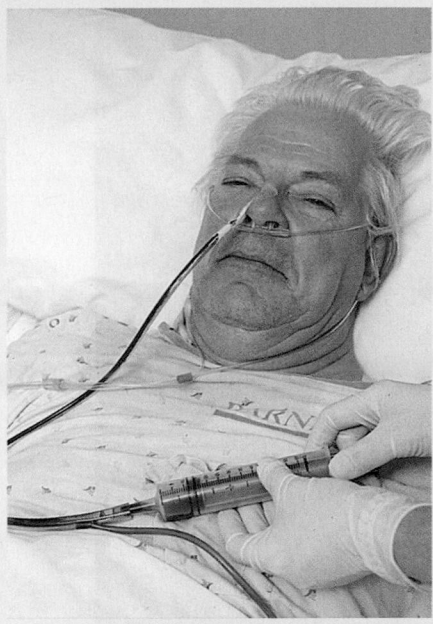

STEP 20b Aspiration of gastric contents.

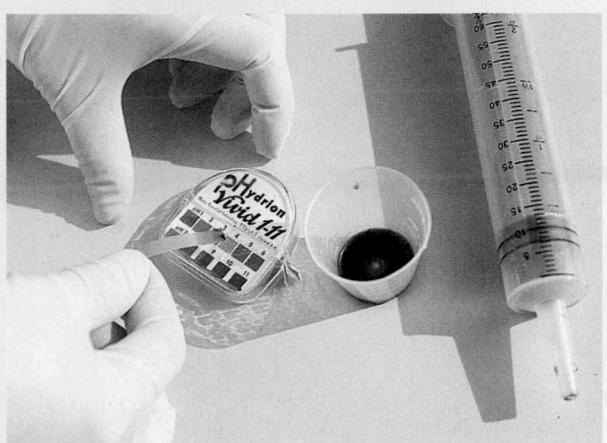

STEP 20c Checking pH of gastric aspirate.

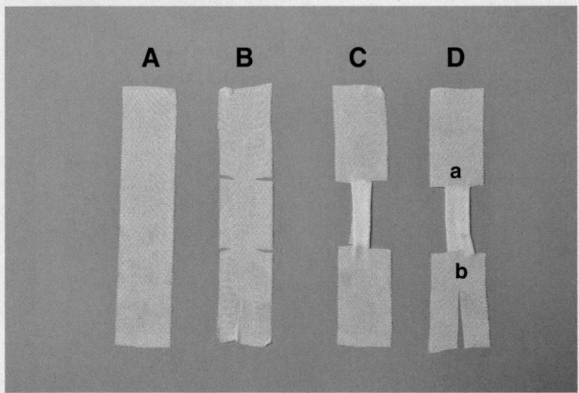

STEP 21a(2) Taping method. **A,** Start with a piece of tape. **B,** Make two slits on both sides of the tape. **C,** Fold the middle section inward. **D,** Tear a new slit in bottom of the tape. Top part (a) should attach to patient's nose; bottom part (b) should be wrapped around the tube.

21. Anchor tube with a fixation device, avoiding pressure on the nares. Select one of the following fixation methods.

   a. Apply tape.

   (1) Apply tincture of benzoin or other skin adhesive on bridge of patient's nose and allow it to become "tacky."

   (2) Tear small horizontal slits at $\frac{1}{3}$ and $\frac{2}{3}$ length of tape without splitting tape (see illustration). Fold middle sections toward one another to form a closed strip.

   (3) Print date and time on tape and place top end of tape over bridge of patient's nose.

   (4) Wrap bottom end of tape around tube as it exits the nose (see illustration).

Proper anchoring and marking of the tube helps prevent migration of tube and pressure injury formation.

Helps tape adhere better. Protects underlying skin.

The strip holds tubing to lessen rubbing against the soft palate and naris.

STEP	RATIONALE

IMPLEMENTATION

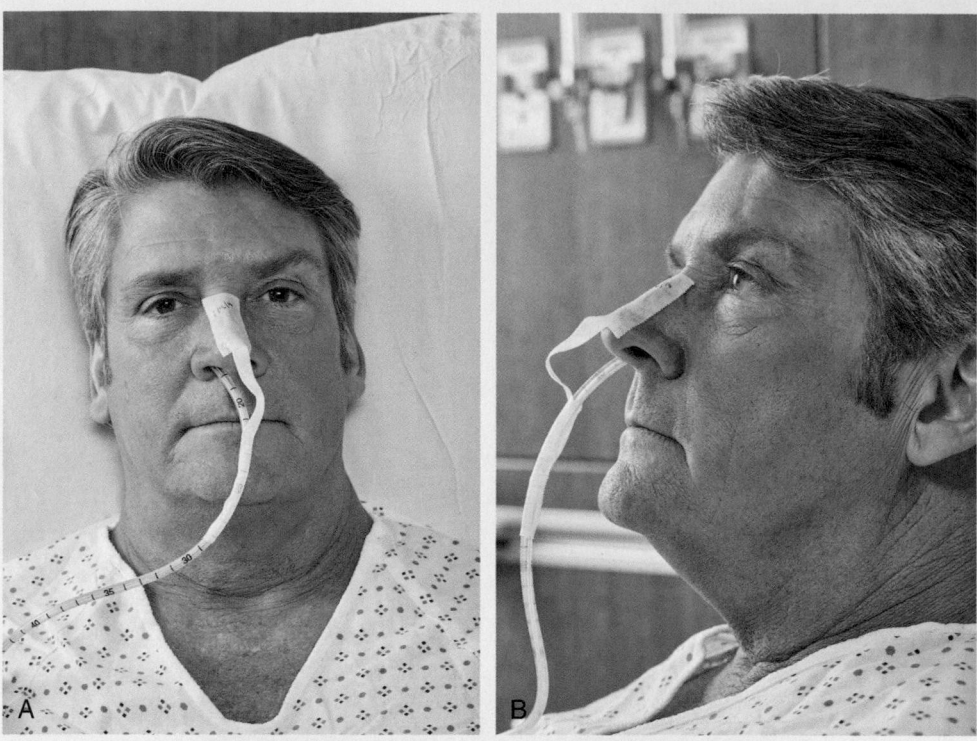

STEP 21a(4) A, Tape applied to anchor nasogastric tube. **B,** Nares are free of pressure from tape and tube.

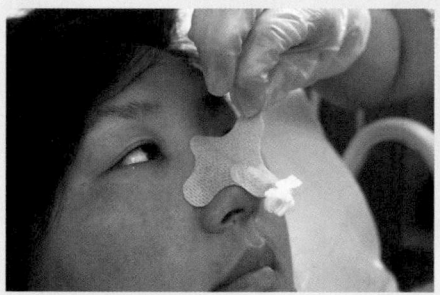 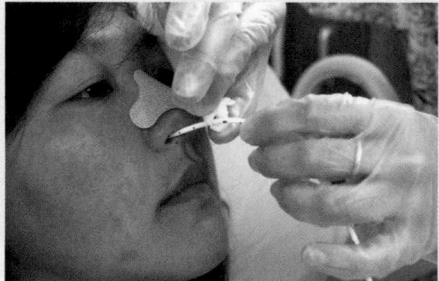 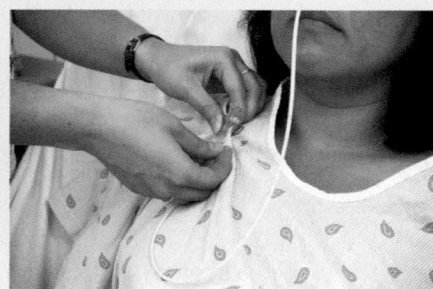

STEP 21b(1) Apply patch to bridge of nose. **STEP 21b(2)** Slip connector around NG tube. **STEP 22** Fasten NG tube to patient gown.

b. Apply tube fixation device using shaped adhesive patch (see manufacturer directions).	Secures tube and reduces friction on nares.
(1) Apply wide end of patch to bridge of nose (see illustration).	
(2) Slip connector around tube as it exits the nose (see illustration).	
22. Fasten end of nasogastric tube to patient's gown with a piece of tape (see illustration). Do not use safety pins to fasten tube to gown.	Anchors tubing to prevent pulling on nose.
23. Keep head of bed elevated at least 30 degrees (preferably 45 degrees) unless contraindicated or patient in semi-sitting position if upright (Best, 2016).	Reduces risk for aspiration of stomach contents.

Clinical Decision Point *If inserting a Salem sump tube, keep the pigtail of the tube above the level of the stomach. This prevents a siphoning action that clogs the tube.*

24. Assist radiology as needed in obtaining prescribed X-ray of the chest and abdomen.	Radiography is the gold standard for NG tube verification (Fan et al., 2017).

STEP	RATIONALE

IMPLEMENTATION

STEP	RATIONALE
25. Remove gloves, perform hand hygiene, and help patient to a comfortable position.	Reduces transmission of microorganisms.
26. Once placement is confirmed, measure amount of tube that is external and mark exit of tube at nares with indelible marker as guide for any tube displacement. Record this information in nurses' notes in electronic health record (EHR) or chart.	The mark alerts nurses and other health care providers to possible tube displacement, which will require confirmation of tube placement.

Clinical Decision Point *Never reposition an NG tube of a gastric surgical patient, as positioning can rupture the suture line.*

STEP	RATIONALE
27. Attach NG tube to suction as prescribed.	Suction setting is usually prescribed low intermittent, which decreases gastric irritation from NG tube.

Clinical Decision Point *If the lumen of the tube is narrow and secretions are thick, the NG tube will not drain as desired. Irrigate the tube (see Step 30). Use interprofessional collaboration to discuss need for a higher suction setting if unable to irrigate the tube because of thick secretions.*

STEP	RATIONALE
28. **NG tube irrigation:**	
a. Perform hand hygiene and apply clean gloves.	Reduces transmission of microorganisms.
b. Check for tube placement in stomach by disconnecting NG tube, connecting irrigating syringe, and aspirating contents (see Step 22b). Temporarily clamp NG tube or reconnect it to the connecting tube and remove syringe.	Prevents accidental entrance of irrigating solution into lungs.
c. Empty syringe of aspirate and use it to draw up 30 mL of normal saline.	Use of saline minimizes loss of electrolytes from stomach fluids.
d. Disconnect NG from connecting tubing and lay end of connection tubing on towel.	Reduces soiling of patient's gown and bed linen.
e. Insert tip of irrigating syringe into end of NG tube. Remove clamp. Hold syringe with tip pointed at the floor and inject saline slowly and evenly. Do not force solution.	Position of the syringe prevents introduction of air into vent tubing, which causes gastric distension. Solution introduced under pressure causes gastric trauma.

Clinical Decision Point *Do not introduce saline through blue pigtail air vent of the Salem sump tube.*

STEP	RATIONALE
f. If resistance occurs, check for kinks in tubing. Turn patient onto their left side. Repeated resistance should be reported to the health care provider.	The tip of the tube may lie against the stomach lining. Repositioning patient on their left side may dislodge the tube away from the stomach lining. Buildup of secretions causes distension.
g. After instilling saline, immediately aspirate or pull back slowly on the syringe to withdraw fluid. If the amount aspirated is greater than the amount instilled, record difference as output. If the amount aspirated is less than the amount instilled, record difference as intake.	Irrigation clears tubing so the stomach should remain empty. Measure and document amount of irrigant fluid inserted in the tube as intake.
h. Use a bulb syringe to place 10 mL of air into blue pigtail.	Ensures patency of air vent.
i. Reconnect NG tube to drainage or suction. (Repeat irrigation if solution does not return.)	Re-establishes drainage collection; may repeat irrigation or repositioning of tube until NG tube drains properly.
29. **Removal of NG tube:**	
a. Verify prescription to remove NG tube.	A health care provider prescription is required for this procedure.
b. Auscultate abdomen for presence of bowel sounds.	Verifies return of peristalsis.
c. Explain procedure to patient and reassure them that removal is less distressing than insertion.	Minimizes anxiety and increases cooperation. Tube passes out smoothly.
d. Perform hand hygiene and apply clean gloves.	Reduces transmission of microorganisms.
e. Turn off suction and disconnect NG tube from drainage bag or suction. With irrigating syringe, insert 20 mL of air into lumen of NG tube. Remove tape or fixation device from bridge of nose and patient's gown.	Have tube free of connections before removal. Clears gastric fluids from tube to prevent aspiration of contents or soiling of clothing and bedding.
f. Hand patient facial tissue; place a clean towel across their chest. Instruct patient to take and hold breath as tube is removed.	Some patients wish to blow their nose after the tube is removed. The towel keeps the gown from getting soiled. Temporary airway obstruction occurs during tube removal.

STEP	RATIONALE

IMPLEMENTATION

g. Clamp or kink tubing securely and pull tube out steadily and smoothly into towel held in the other hand while patient holds their breath.

Clamping prevents tube contents from draining into the oropharynx. Reduces trauma to mucosa and minimizes patient's discomfort. Towel covers tube, which is an unpleasant sight. Holding breath helps to prevent aspiration.

h. Inspect intactness of tube.

i. Measure amount of drainage and note character of content. Dispose of tube and drainage equipment into proper container.

Provides accurate measure of fluid output. Reduces transfer of microorganisms.

j. Clean nares and provide mouth care.

Promotes comfort.

k. Position patient comfortably and explain procedure for drinking fluids if not contraindicated. Instruct patient to notify you if nausea occurs.

Sometimes patients are not allowed anything by mouth (NPO) for up to 24 hours. When fluids are allowed, prescriptions usually begin with a small amount of ice chips each hour and increase as the patient is able to tolerate more.

30. For all procedures, clean equipment and return to their proper place. Place soiled linen in utility room or proper receptacle.

Proper disposal of equipment prevents spread of microorganisms and ensures proper exchange procedures.

31. Remove and discard gloves and perform hand hygiene.

Reduces transmission of microorganisms.

EVALUATION

1. Observe amount and character of contents draining from NG tube. Ask if patient feels nauseated.

Determines if tube is decompressing stomach of contents.

2. Auscultate for presence of bowel sounds. Turn off suction while auscultating.

Sound of the suction apparatus is sometimes misinterpreted as bowel sounds.

3. Palpate patient's abdomen periodically. Note any distension, pain, or rigidity.

Determines success of abdominal decompression and return of peristalsis.

4. Inspect condition of nares and nose.

Evaluates onset of skin and tissue irritation.

5. Observe position of tubing.

Prevents tension applied to nasal structures.

6. Explain that it is normal if patient has a sore throat or irritation in the pharynx.

Result of tube irritation.

7. Use Teach-Back: "I need to be sure I explained why you need the NG tube and the importance of letting me know if you are nauseated. Tell me why it is important for me to know if you feel nauseated." Develop a revised teaching plan if patient or caregiver is not able to teach back correctly.

Determines patient's and caregiver's level of understanding of instructional topic.

Unexpected Outcomes

1. Patient indicates nausea, or patient's abdomen is distended and painful.

2. Patient develops irritation or erosion of skin around naris.

3. Patient develops signs and symptoms of pulmonary aspiration: fever, shortness of breath, or pulmonary congestion.

Related Interventions

- Assess patency of tube. The NG tube may be occluded or no longer in the stomach.
- Irrigate tube.
- Verify that suction is on as prescribed.
- Notify health care provider if distension is unrelieved.
- Provide frequent skin care to area.
- Use taping method designed to reduce MDRPI (see taping methods Step 23a and 23b).
- Consider switching tube to the other naris.
- Perform complete respiratory assessment.
- Notify health care provider.
- Obtain chest X-ray examination as prescribed.

Communication and Documentation

- Document length, size, and type of gastric tube inserted and in which naris it was inserted. In addition, record patient's tolerance of procedure, confirmation of tube placement, location of distal tip of tube, character of gastric contents, pH value, results of radiography, whether the tube is clamped or connected to a drainage bag or to suction, and amount of suction supplied, on flow sheet or in nurses' notes in EHR or chart.
- Document patient's and caregiver's understanding through teach-back of what to report to the nurse and purpose of the NG tube in nurses' notes in EHR or chart.
- Document difference between amount of normal saline instilled and amount of gastric aspirate removed on intake and output (I&O) sheet. Record the amount and character of contents draining from the NG tube, every shift.
- Document removal of the tube "intact," patient's tolerance of procedure, and final amount and character of drainage.

Special Considerations
Gerontological

- Check for ill-fitting dentures and remove them for the patient's safety and comfort during the insertion.
- Oral and nasal mucosal drying is sometimes present. Adequately lubricate the tube for insertion.

◆ CLINICAL DEBRIEF

A 66-year-old man with a history of severe osteoarthritis is hospitalized following a total right knee replacement performed 2 days ago. At present he is allowed touch-down weight bearing on his right leg. His last bowel movement was the day before surgery; thus, he has gone 3 days without a bowel movement. Since surgery he received opioid pain medication through his intravenous (IV) line and began taking oral pain medication last night. His abdomen is nontender and slightly distended, with active bowel sounds in all four quadrants. He attempted a bowel movement with a great deal of straining and expelled small, hard, brown stool. The nurse has talked to the health care provider and obtained a prescription for a prepackaged enema.

1. The nurse has explained the enema procedure to the patient and has prepared the supplies. The nurse needs to provide a bedpan or commode for him to expel fecal material after the enema. Provide the rationale for the type of bedpan he should use or whether a commode can be used.
2. What is the expected outcome of the prepackaged enema? Which, if any, instructions will the nurse give to the unregulated care provider (UCP)?
3. Two days later the patient has the same symptoms as before receiving the enema. He has still not had a bowel movement. This time he has liquid stool seeping from the rectum. Using SBAR, show how the nurse would communicate with the health care team about this patient.

◆ REVIEW QUESTIONS

1. The nurse is caring for a patient who needs to use a bedpan. Which of the following comfort measures should the nurse use for proper positioning and general comfort? *(Select all that apply.)*
   1. Keep the head of the bed flat.
   2. Place toilet tissue within reach.
   3. Stay with patient while they are using the bedpan.
   4. Place a small pillow under the lumbar curve in the back.
   5. Place the head of the bed at a 45-degree angle.
2. The nurse has several activities to perform. Which can be delegated to the UCP? *(Select all that apply.)*
   1. Administering a tap-water enema
   2. Removing a fecal impaction
   3. Placing a patient on a bedpan
   4. Inserting a nasogastric (NG) tube
   5. Providing oral care for a patient with an NG tube

3. A patient is to have a nasogastric (NG) tube inserted. Place the following steps in the correct order.
   1. Measure distance to insert tube from tip of nose, to earlobe, and to xiphoid process.
   2. Verify the prescription for the NG tube.
   3. Tape tube to the nose.
   4. Perform hand hygiene and apply personal protective equipment.
   5. Identify patient using at least two identifiers.
   6. Pass the tube along the floor of nasal passage, then just past the nasopharynx.
   7. Instruct the patient to flex their head forward and swallow while the tube is advanced.

ⓔ *Visit the Evolve site for a complete list of Clinical Debrief and Review Questions answers.*

REFERENCES

Accreditation Canada. (2019). *Required organizational practices handbook—Version 14.* Retrieved from http://www.wrha.mb.ca/quality/files/2019ROPHandbook.pdf

Ball, J., Dains, J., Flynn, J., Solomon, B., & Stewart, R. (2015). *Seidel's guide to physical examination* (8th ed.). St. Louis: Mosby.

Beeson, T., Elfrid, B., Pike, C., & Pittman, J. (2017). Do intra-anal bowel management devices reduce incontinence-associated dermatitis and/or pressure injuries? *Journal of Wound Ostomy Continence Nursing,* 44(6), 583–588. doi:10.1097/WON.0000000000000381

Bernal, C., Dole, M., & Thame, K. (2018). The role of bowel management in children with bladder and bowel dysfunction. *Current Bladder Dysfunction Report.* doi:10.1007/s11884-018-0458-3

Best, C. (2016). How to insert a nasogastric tube and check gastric position at the bedside. *Nursing Standard,* 30(38), 36–40. doi:10.7748/ns.30.38.36.s43

Borowitz, S. (2017). Encopresis. *Medscape. Pediatrics: General medicine.* Retrieved from https://emedicine.medscape.com/article/928795-overview#a3

Burchum, J., & Rosenthal, L. (2016). *Lehne's pharmacology for nursing care* (9th ed.). St. Louis: Saunders.

Casaubon, L., Boulanger, J., Glasser, E., et al. (2016). Canadian stroke best practice recommendations: Acute inpatient stroke care guidelines, update 2015. *International Journal of Stroke: Official Journal of the International Stroke Society,* 11(2), 239–252. doi:10.1177/1747493015622461

Costilla, V. C., & Foxx-Orenstein, A. E. (2014). Constipation: Understanding mechanisms and management. *Clinics in Geriatric Medicine,* 30(1), 107–115. doi:10.1016/j.cger.2013.10.001

Davignon, A., Sham, R., Lappen, D., Martinussen, D., D'Angelo, M., & Aleong, R. (2016). Implementation and evaluation of a natural bowel care protocol in long-term care. *Perspectives—Gerontological Nursing Association,* 38(4), 7–15.

DeGiorgio, R., Ruggeri, E., Stanghellini, V., Eusebi, L., Bazzole, F., & Chiarioni, G. (2015). Chronic constipation in the elderly: A primer for the gastroenterologist. *BMC Gastroenterology,* 15, 130. doi:10.1186/s12876-015-0366-3

Dietitians of Canada. (2018). *Constipation in children.* Retrieved from http://www.unlockfood.ca/en/Articles/Childrens-Nutrition/Health-Conditions/Constipation-in-Children.aspx

Emergency Nurses Association (ENA). (2015). *Clinical practice guideline: Gastric tube placement verification.* Retrieved from https://www.ena.org/docs/default-source/resource-library/practice-resources/cpg/gastrictubecpg7b5530b71c1e49e8b155b6cca1870adc.pdf?sfvrsn=a8e9dd7a_8

Fan, E., Tan, S., & Aug, S. (2017). Nasogastric tube placement confirmation: Where we are and where we should be heading. *Proceedings of Singapore Healthcare,* 26(3), 189–195. doi:10.1177/2010105817705141

Fan, L., Lui, Q., & Gui, L. (2016). Efficacy of nonswallow nasogastric tube intubation: A randomized controlled trial. *Journal of Clinical Nursing,* 25(21–22), 3326–3332.

Ferrara, L., & Saccomano, S. J. (2017). Constipation in children: Diagnosis, treatment, and prevention. *The Nurse Practitioner,* 42(7), 30–34. doi:10.1111/jpc.12939

Francis, K. (2018). Damage control: Differentiating incontinence-associated dermatitis from pressure injury. *Nursing,* 48(6), 18–25. doi:10.1097/01.NURSE.0000532739.93967.20

Hockenberry, M. J., & Wilson, D. (2015). *Wong's nursing care of infants and children* (10th ed.). St. Louis: Mosby.

Huether, S., McCance, K., El-Hussein, M., Power-Kean, K., & Zettel, S. (2018). *Understanding pathophysiology* (1st Canadian ed.). Toronto: Elsevier.

Jordan-Ely, J. (2015). Disimpaction of children with severe constipation in 3-4 days in a suburban clinic using polyethylene glycol with electrolytes and sodium picosulphate. *Journal of Paediatrics and Child Health,* 51(12), 1195–1198.

Lewis, S. L., Bucher, L., Heitkemper, M., et al. (2019). *Medical-surgical nursing in Canada: Assessment and management of clinical problems* (4th Canadian ed.). Toronto, ON: Elsevier Canada.

Lord, L. (2018). Enteral access devices: Types, function, care, and challenges. *NCP. Nutrition in Clinical Practice,* 33(1), 16–38. doi:10.1002/ncp.10019

Lortie, M., & Charbonney, E. (2016). Confirming placement of nasogastric feeding tube. *CMAJ: Canadian Medical Association Journal = Journal de l'Association Medicale Canadienne,* 188(5), E96. doi:10.1503/cmaj.150609

National Pressure Ulcer Advisory Panel (NPUAP). (2012). *Mucosal pressure ulcers: An NPUAP position statement.* Retrieved from http://www.npuap.org/wp-content/uploads/2012/03/Mucosal_Pressure_Ulcer_Position_Statement_final.pdf

National Pressure Ulcer Advisory Panel (NPUAP). (2016). *Pressure injury prevention points.* Retrieved from http://www.npuap.org/wp-content/uploads/2016/04/Pressure-Injury-Prevention-Points-2016.pdf

Ness, W. (2013). Digital removal of faeces. *Nursing Times,* 109(17–18), 18–20.

Norton, L., Parslow, N., Johnston, D., et al. (2018). *Best practice recommendations for the prevention and management of pressure injuries.* Wound Care Canada. Retrieved from https://www.woundscanada.ca/docman/public/health-care-professional/bpr-workshop/172-bpr-prevention-and-management-of-pressure-injuries-2/file

Peate, I. (2016). How to perform digital removal of faeces. *Nursing Standard,* 30(40), 36–39.

Pittman, J., Beeson, T., Kitterman, J., Lancaster, S., & Shelly, A. (2015). Medical device–related hospital-acquired pressure ulcers. *Journal of Wound Ostomy & Continence Nursing,* 42(2), 151–154. doi:10.1097/WON.0000000000000113

Prichard, D., & Bharucha, A. (2015). Management of opioid-induced constipation for people in palliative care. *International Journal of Palliative Nursing,* 21(6), 272, 274–280. doi:10.12968/ijpn.2015.21.6.272

Registered Nurses' Association of Ontario (RNAO). (2011). *Nursing best practice guideline: Prevention of constipation in the older adult population.* Toronto, ON: Author. Retrieved from http://rnao.ca/sites/rnao-ca/files/Constipation_supplement_2011.pdf

Roque, M., & Bouras, E. (2015). Epidemiology and management of chronic constipation in elderly patients. *Clinical Interventions in Aging,* 10, 919–930. doi:10.2147/CIA.S54304

Rowan-Legg, A., Canadian Paediatric Society (CPS), Community Paediatrics Committee. (2011; Reaffirmed 2018). *Managing functional constipation in children.* Retrieved from https://www.cps.ca/en/documents/position/functional-constipation

Sammon, M. A., Montague, M., Frame, F., et al. (2015). Randomized controlled study of the effects of 2 fecal management systems on incidence of anal erosion. *Journal of Wound Ostomy & Continence Nursing,* 42(3), 279–286. doi:10.1097/WON.0000000000000128

Sanfilippo, F., & Spoletini, G. (2015). Perspectives on the importance of postoperative ileus. *Current Medical Research and Opinion,* 31(4), 675–676. doi:10.1185/03007995.2015.1027184

Singh, R., Salem, A., Nanavati, J., & Mullin, G. (2018). The role of diet in the treatment of irritable bowel syndrome: A systematic review. *Gastroenterology Clinics of North America,* 47(1), 107–137. doi:10.1016/j.gtc.2017.10.003

Singh, S., Bhargava, B., Vasantha, P., et al. (2018). Clinical evaluation of a novel intrarectal device for management of fecal incontinence in bedridden patients. *Journal of Wound Ostomy Continence Nursing,* 45(2), 156–162. doi:10.1097/WON.00000000000004

Wald, A. (2015). Constipation: Pathophysiology and management. *Current Opinion in Gastroenterology,* 31(1), 45–49. doi:10.1097/MOG.0000000000000137

World Health Organization (WHO). (2009). *WHO guidelines on hand hygiene in health care: First global patient safety challenge: Clean care is safer care.* Geneva: World Health Organization Press.

Wound Ostomy and Continence Nurses Society (WOCN). (2016). *Guideline for prevention and management of pressure ulcers (injuries)* (2nd ed.). Mount Laurel, NJ: Author.

36 | Ostomy Care

Written by **Jane Fellows, MSN, CWOCN; and Shelley L. Cobbett, RN, GnT, MN, EdD**

SKILLS AND PROCEDURES

Skill 36.1 **Pouching a Colostomy or an Ileostomy, p. 975**

Skill 36.2 **Pouching a Urostomy, p. 980**

Skill 36.3 **Catheterizing a Urinary Diversion, p. 984**

OBJECTIVES

Mastery of content in this chapter will enable the nurse to:
- Identify the types of fecal and urinary diversions.
- Explain the differences in consistency of effluent based on the type of ostomy.
- Pouch a fecal or a urinary diversion.
- Describe methods used to maintain integrity of the peristomal skin.
- Catheterize a urinary diversion.

MEDIA RESOURCES

- **evolve** http://evolve.elsevier.com/Canada/Perry/clinicalskills/
- Review Questions
- ▶ Video Clips
- Audio Glossary
- **NSO** Nursing Skills Online
- Clinical Debrief and Review Questions Answers

PURPOSE

With certain diseases or conditions a surgically created opening in the abdominal wall, called a *stoma*, is necessary to allow for the passage of urine or fecal matter. It is essential that a pouch be placed over a stoma correctly so the output from the stoma is contained, the skin around the stoma is protected, and a patient is free from odour or leakage.

STANDARDS OF CARE

- Nurses Specialized in Wound, Ostomy and Continence Canada (NSWOCC) & Canadian Association of Enterostomal Therapy (CAET), 2009—*Clinical Best Practice Guidelines, Ostomy Care and Management* (http://nswoc.ca/?s=best+practice+guidelines)
- Ostomy Canada Society, 2017—*Ostomy 101* (http://community.ostomycanada.ca/information/ostomy-101/)
- Registered Nurses Association of Ontario (RNAO), 2009—*Best Practice Guidelines: Ostomy Care and Management* (http://rnao.ca/sites/rnao-ca/files/Ostomy_Care__Management.pdf)

PRINCIPLES FOR PRACTICE

- An *ostomy*, such as a colostomy or ileostomy, is an artificial opening in an organ of the body, created during an operation. For example, a stoma in the large intestine or colon is called a *colostomy* (Fig. 36.1), which is usually placed in the descending colon and results in a stool similar to that normally passed through the rectum.

- A stoma placed in the transverse or ascending colon is an *ileostomy*, which drains fecal effluent that is watery to thick and contains some digestive enzymes (Fig. 36.2).
- The character of the output of a bowel stoma (called *effluent*) is influenced by a patient's medications and hydration status and the foods eaten. Diet and fluid therapy are important therapies in managing ostomy effluent.
- If removal of the urinary bladder is necessary, the ureters are inserted into a section of the ileum or small intestine, then an ileal conduit or a *urostomy* is created (Fig. 36.3) from which urine exits the body through the stoma.
- A patient with a colostomy, ileostomy, or ileal conduit has no sensation or control over the time or frequency of the output and must wear a pouch to collect effluent.
- There are surgical procedures that create continent internal fecal or urinary pouches, eliminating the need to wear an external pouch. An *ileal pouch* is an internal reservoir formed from a segment of the ileum that is then connected to the anal canal above the anal sphincter (Fig. 36.4, A–B). A *continent urinary reservoir* (Fig. 36.5) is a reservoir created from the intestine. A small stoma on the abdominal wall allows access via a catheter inserted to empty urine from the pouch. These surgeries are less common than the urostomy.

PERSON-CENTRED CARE

- A person with a newly created stoma for the elimination of urine or fecal matter from the body needs to be taught how to

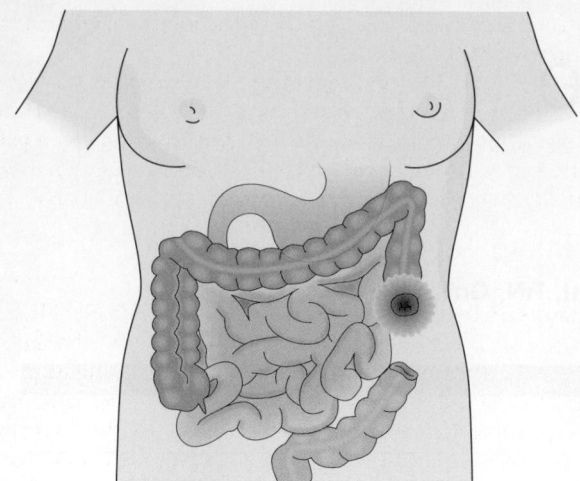

FIG 36.1 Sigmoid colostomy.

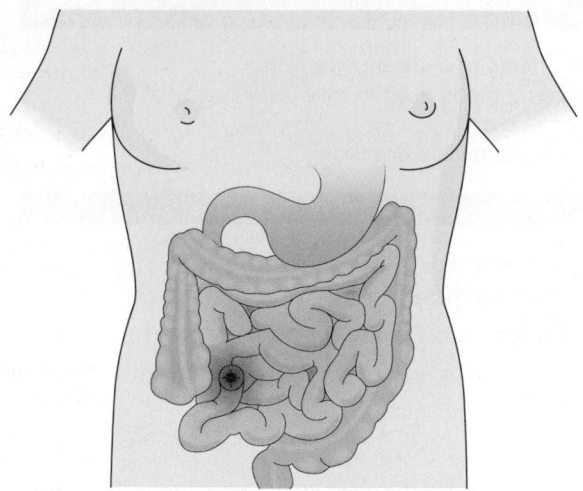

FIG 36.2 Ileostomy.

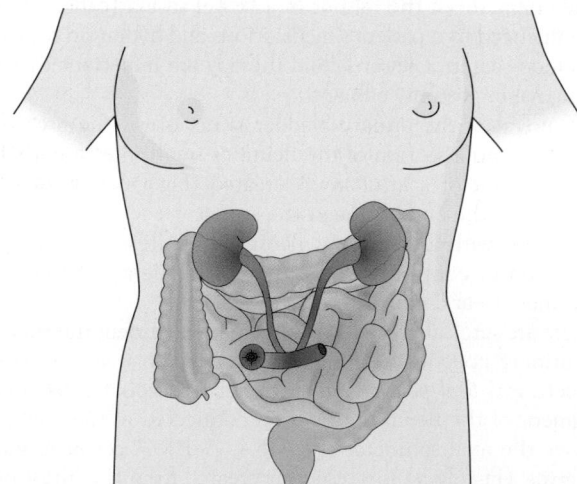

FIG 36.3 Urostomy (ileal conduit).

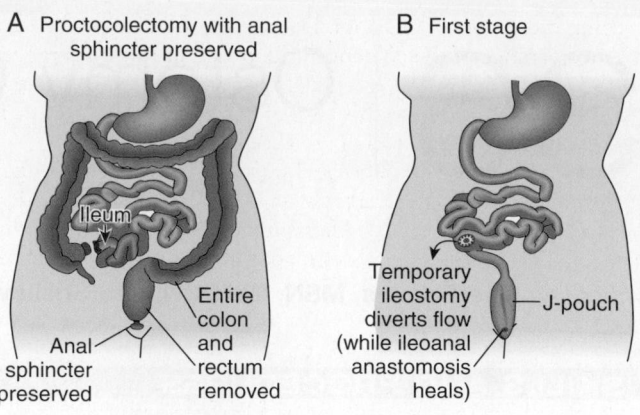

A Proctocolectomy with anal sphincter preserved

Ileum

Anal sphincter preserved

Entire colon and rectum removed

B First stage

Temporary ileostomy diverts flow (while ileoanal anastomosis heals)

J-pouch

FIG 36.4 Ileal pouch anal anastomosis.

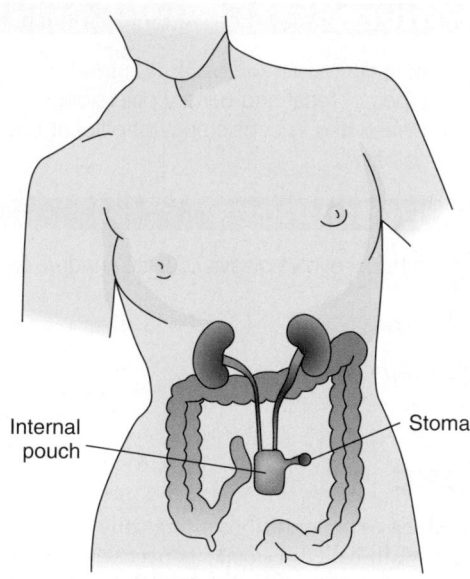

Internal pouch

Stoma

FIG 36.5 Continent urinary diversion.

care for the ostomy to regain autonomy in self-care for basic elimination. If a patient was not self-managing elimination before surgery, a caregiver may need to be taught to provide this care.

- With any ostomy requiring a pouching system, a secure seal to prevent leakage of the effluent and protect the skin around the stoma (peristomal skin) is vital to avoid peristomal skin problems (Colwell, McNichol, & Boarini, 2017).
- A reliable and effective pouching system is a very important factor in facilitating a patient's emotional adjustment to an ostomy (Carmel, Colwell, & Goldberg, 2016).
- In addition to the stress of illness and surgical recovery, patients with ostomies face fear of social rejection, concern about sexual function and intimacy, and the need for help with personal care (Carmel et al., 2016).
- Having an ostomy can have a significant impact on a patient's quality of life, with a range of physical, psychological, or social restrictions. Some patients also face significant change in their perceived body image, their lifestyle, and intimate relationships (Jayarajah & Samarasekera, 2017). Always practise person-centred care with these patients and encourage them to express their feelings about their ostomy.
- In communicating with a patient during ostomy care, it is important to be sensitive and avoid conveying anything that the patient may interpret as disrespect or disgust. Practise person-centred care, prepare adequately for the procedure, arrange interprofessional collaboration when necessary, and maintain a

calm, professional demeanor. Do not act offended by the odour or appearance of the effluent in the pouch or the appearance of the stoma. A negative reaction from caregivers only reinforces a patient's feelings that this alteration in bodily function makes them personally and socially unacceptable.

- When patients come to a hospital with an ostomy, encourage them to be able to resume self-care as soon as possible. Respect a patient's routine of care even if it differs from usual care in the facility. Offer educational materials to support the patient's development of ostomy self-care (Culha, Kosgeroglu, & Bolluk, 2016).

EVIDENCE-INFORMED PRACTICE

Evidence-informed guidelines exist for proper stoma measurement and the role of an ostomy nurse in caring for patients with a stoma.

- Before ostomy surgery, a health care provider or ostomy care nurse should see the patient to mark a stoma site. Assessing the patient's abdomen while they are lying, sitting, and standing allows the nurse and patient to find an optimal stoma location that will make it easy for the patient to see the stoma and apply a pouch with a reliable seal (Salvadena, Hendren, McKenna, et al., 2015a, b).
- The Canadian Society of Intestinal Research (CSIR) (2018) recommends that the site be marked on the abdomen away from abdominal scars, creases, skinfolds, or the belt line. Studies show that preoperative stoma site marking is crucial for improving patients' postoperative quality of life, promoting their

independence, and reducing the rates of postoperative complications (CSIR, 2018).

- Having the support and care of an ostomy nurse leads to better adjustment to an ostomy and improved health-related quality of life (Riemenschneider, 2015). Whenever possible, a patient with a new ostomy should be referred to an ostomy nurse who has advanced, specialized education in this type of care.

SAFETY GUIDELINES

- Change ostomy pouches when they are $\frac{1}{3} - \frac{1}{2}$ full to avoid leakage, which can lead to chemical or enzymatic injury to the skin.
- Know the signs of a healthy stoma and surrounding skin:
  - *Colour/moisture:* Stoma should be red or pink and moist. Report a grey, purple, black, or very dry stoma to the charge nurse or health care provider, as this finding indicates that the stoma is not healthy.
  - *Size:* In the 4–6 weeks after surgery, the stoma will likely decrease in size. Measure the stoma with each pouch change and adjust the size of the opening cut in the wafer.
  - *Peristomal skin:* It normally is intact with some reddening after the adhesive wafer is removed. Presence of blisters, a rash, or excoriated skin is abnormal.
- Wear personal protective equipment (PPE) as required (e.g., gloves during pouch and stoma care) to reduce exposure to and transmission of infectious microorganisms.

✦ SKILL 36.1   Pouching a Colostomy or an Ileostomy

▶ *Video Clip*   **NSO**   *Nursing Skills Online Bowel Elimination/Ostomy Care Module 18 / Lessons 1, 3, and 4*

Immediately after a fecal surgical diversion, it is necessary to place a pouch over a newly created stoma to contain effluent when the stoma begins to function. The pouch will keep a patient clean and dry, protect the skin from drainage, and provide a barrier against odour. A cut-to-fit, transparent pouching system is preferred because it will protect the peristomal skin, allow the stoma to be visualized, and accommodate changes in stoma size as swelling decreases after surgery.

Nurses need to recognize the difference between a budded stoma (Fig. 36.6) and a flush or retracted stoma (Fig. 36.7). In the immediate postoperative period, the stoma may be edematous and the abdomen distended. These symptoms will resolve over a 4- to 6-week period after surgery, but during this time it will be necessary to revise the pouching system to meet the changing size of the stoma and the changes in body contours (Carmel et al., 2016).

There are many types of pouching systems. All have a protective layer that adheres to the skin, called a *skin barrier*, and a pouch. A one-piece pouching system (Fig. 36.8) has the two parts integrated together. A two-piece system (Fig. 36.9) has a separate skin barrier and pouch. The flush or retracted stoma may require a convex wafer (Fig. 36.10) for successful placement of a pouch. This type of skin barrier provides gentle pressure on the peristomal skin to push the stoma through the opening in the wafer. The pouch is applied to the skin barrier by attaching it to a flange (a plastic ring) on the barrier. The nurse must use the skin barrier with a flange that fits the corresponding size pouch from the same manufacturer to avoid leakage between the skin barrier and the pouch. Some pouching systems have precut openings in the barrier for the stoma, whereas others need to be custom cut to size for a patient's stoma measurement. It is important

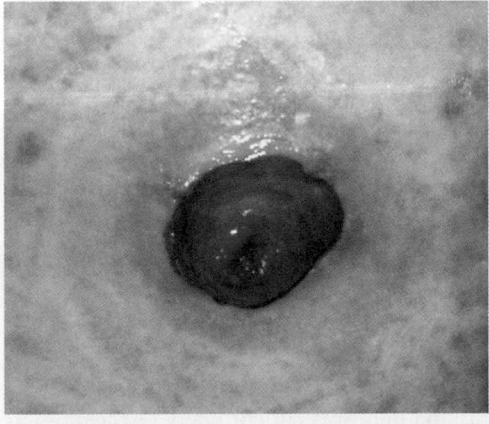

FIG 36.6 Budded stoma. (*Courtesy Jane Fellows.*)

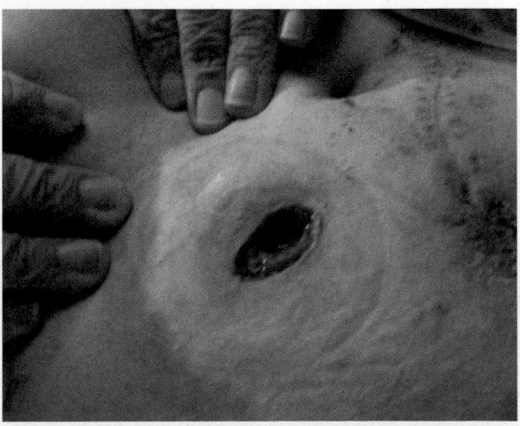

FIG 36.7 Retracted stoma. (*Courtesy Jane Fellows.*)

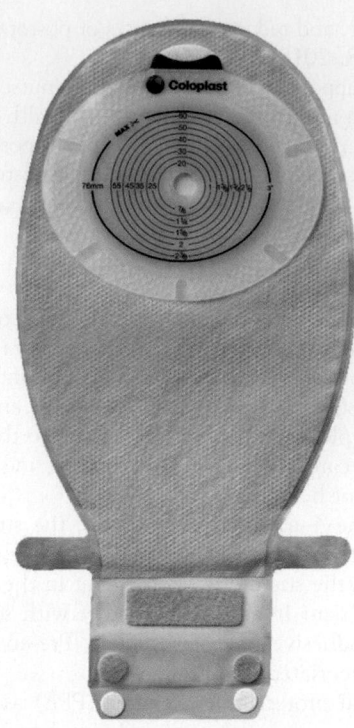

FIG 36.8 One-piece pouch with Velcro closure. *(Courtesy Coloplast, Minneapolis, MN.)*

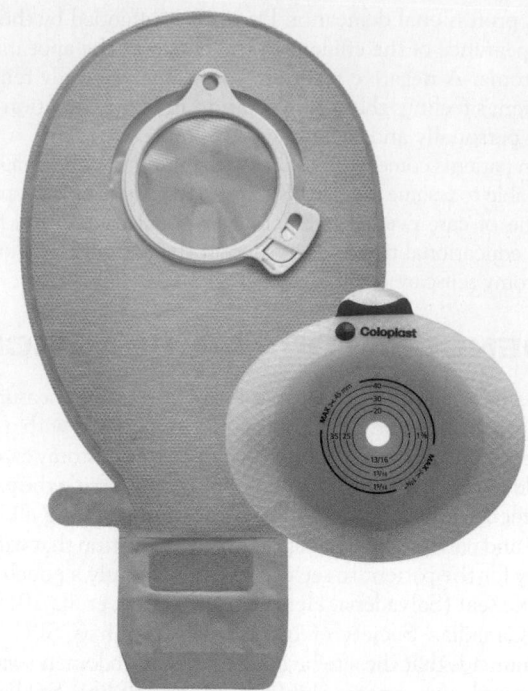

FIG 36.9 Two-piece pouching system with separate skin barrier and attachable pouch. *(Courtesy Coloplast, Minneapolis, MN.)*

to understand how to use each of these different pouching systems before applying them on patients (Carmel et al., 2016). The websites for the companies that make ostomy supplies have both patient and health care provider instructions that are helpful in understanding how to use the pouching systems (e.g., https://www.coloplast.ca; https://www.convatec.ca/; http://www.hollister.ca/en-ca/).

Delegation and Collaboration

The skill of pouching a new ostomy should not be delegated to an unregulated care provider (UCP). In some facilities care of an established ostomy (4–6 weeks or more after surgery) can be delegated to UCPs. The nurse directs the UCP about:

- The expected amount, colour, and consistency of drainage from an ostomy.
- The expected appearance of the stoma.
- Special equipment needed to complete a particular patient's pouching.
- The changes in a patient's stoma and surrounding skin integrity that should be reported.

Equipment

- Skin barrier/pouch—clear, drainable one-piece or two-piece, cut-to-fit or precut size
- Pouch closure device such as a clip, if needed
- Ostomy measuring guide
- Adhesive remover *(optional)*

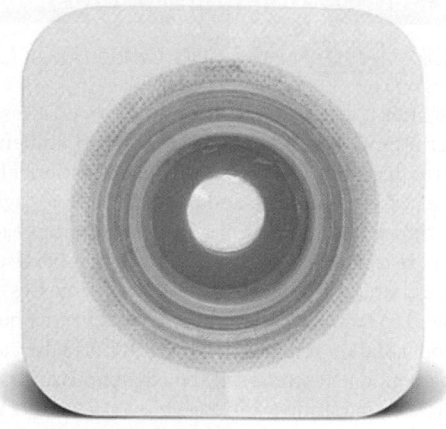

FIG 36.10 Convex skin barrier wafer. *(Used with permission Convatec, Inc. All rights reserved.)*

- Clean gloves
- Washcloth
- Towel or disposable waterproof barrier
- Basin with warm tap water
- Scissors
- Waterproof bag for disposal of pouch
- Personal protective equipment (PPE) (gown or goggles are optional if there is any risk of splashing when emptying pouch)

STEP	RATIONALE

ASSESSMENT

1. Identify patient using at least two person-specific identifiers (e.g., name and date of birth or name and medical record number), according to employer policy.	Ensures correct patient. Complies with Accreditation Canada's standards and improves patient safety (Accreditation Canada, 2019).

STEP	RATIONALE

ASSESSMENT

2. Perform hand hygiene and apply clean gloves.

Reduces transmission of microorganisms.

3. Observe existing skin barrier and pouch for leakage and length of time in place. Pouch should be changed every 3 to 7 days, not daily (Carmel et al., 2016). If an opaque pouch is being used, remove it to fully observe stoma. Dispose of this kind of pouch in a proper receptacle.

Assesses effectiveness of pouching system and detects potential for problems. To minimize skin irritation, avoid unnecessary changing of the entire pouching system. When the pouch leaks, skin damage from effluent causes more skin trauma than early removal of the wafer.

Clinical Decision Point *Repeated leakage may indicate the need for a different type of pouch or addition of products such as stoma putty. If the pouch is leaking, change it. Taping or patching it to contain effluent leaves the skin exposed to chemical or enzymatic irritation.*

4. Observe amount of effluent in pouch and empty it if it is more than ⅓–½ full by opening the pouch and draining it into a container for measurement of output. Note consistency of effluent and record intake and output (I&O).

Weight of the pouch may disrupt the seal of adhesive on the skin. Monitor fluid balance and bowel function after surgery. Normal colostomy effluent is soft or formed stool, whereas normal ileostomy effluent is liquid.

5. Observe stoma for type, location, colour, swelling, presence of sutures, trauma, and healing or irritation of peristomal skin.

Stoma characteristics influence selection of an appropriate pouching system. Convexity in the skin barrier is often necessary with a flush or retracted stoma.

6. Observe placement of stoma in relation to abdominal contours and presence of scars or incisions. Remove and dispose of gloves; perform hand hygiene.

Determines if current pouching system is effective or if a new selection is needed. Abdominal contours, scars, or incisions affect the type of system and adhesion to the skin surface. Reduces transmission of microorganisms.

7. Explore patient's attitudes, perceptions, knowledge, and acceptance of stoma; discuss interest in learning self-care. Identify others who will be helping patient after leaving hospital.

Determines patient's willingness to learn. Facilitates teaching plan and timing of care to coincide with availability of caregivers.

NURSING DIAGNOSES

- Reduced skin integrity
- Insufficient knowledge regarding pouching of an ostomy
- Alteration in body image
- Willingness for enhanced knowledge
- Potential for impaired skin integrity

Related factors/Risk factors are individualized on the basis of patient's condition or needs.

PLANNING

1. Expected outcomes following completion of procedure:
- Stoma is red and moist; peristomal skin is intact and free of irritation; sutures are intact.

Normal findings in patient with postoperative ostomy that is healing.

- Stoma drains a moderate amount of liquid or soft stool, and flatus is in pouch, which can be seen with bulging of pouch. (Flatus may not be observable if the pouch has a gas filter.)

Stoma is functioning normally. A snug seal around the stoma has been attained. Flatus indicates return of peristalsis after surgery.

- Patient and/or caregiver observe stoma and steps of procedure.

Reveals acceptance of alteration in body image and interest in self-care.

- Patient asks questions about the procedure and attempts to help with pouch change.

Indicates readiness to learn and begin self-care.

2. Explain procedure to patient; encourage patient's interaction and questions.

Lessens patient's anxiety and promotes person-centred care.

3. Assemble equipment and close room curtains or door.

Optimizes use of time; provides privacy.

IMPLEMENTATION

1. Have patient assume semi-reclining or supine position (same position assumed during assessment and pouching). (**NOTE:** Some patients with established ostomies prefer to stand.) If possible, provide patient with a mirror for observation.

When patient is semi-reclining, there are fewer skinfolds, which allows for ease of application of pouching system.

2. Perform hand hygiene and apply clean gloves.

Reduces transmission of microorganisms.

3. Place towel or disposable waterproof barrier under patient and across patient's lower abdomen.

Protects bed linen; maintains patient's dignity.

STEP	RATIONALE

IMPLEMENTATION

4. If not done during assessment, remove the used pouch and skin barrier gently by pushing skin away from barrier. Use adhesive remover to facilitate removal of skin barrier. Empty pouch and dispose of it in an appropriate receptacle. Measure output if needed. **NOTE:** There may be no output at the time of first pouch change.

Reduces skin trauma. Improper removal of pouch and barrier can cause peristomal skin irritation or breakdown.

5. Clean peristomal skin gently with warm tap water using a washcloth; do not scrub the skin. If you touch the stoma, minor bleeding is normal. Pat skin dry. Have washcloth handy for additional cleaning if there is output from the stoma while preparing the pouch.

Soap leaves residue on skin, which may irritate the skin. The pouch does not adhere to wet skin.
Ileostomies have frequent output, especially after eating.

6. Measure stoma (see illustration). Expect size of stoma to change in the first 4–6 weeks after surgery.

Allows for proper fit of pouch that will protect peristomal skin.

7. Trace pattern of stoma measurement on pouch backing or skin barrier (see illustration).

Prepares for cutting opening in pouch.

8. Cut opening on backing or skin barrier wafer (see illustration). If using mouldable or shape to fit barrier, use your fingers to mould shape to fit stoma.

Customizes pouch to provide appropriate fit over stoma.

9. Remove protective backing from adhesive backing or wafer (see illustration).

Prepares skin barrier for placement.

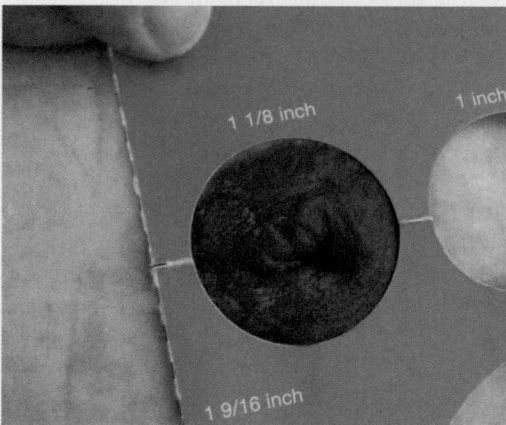

STEP 6 Measure stoma. (*Courtesy Coloplast, Minneapolis, MN.*)

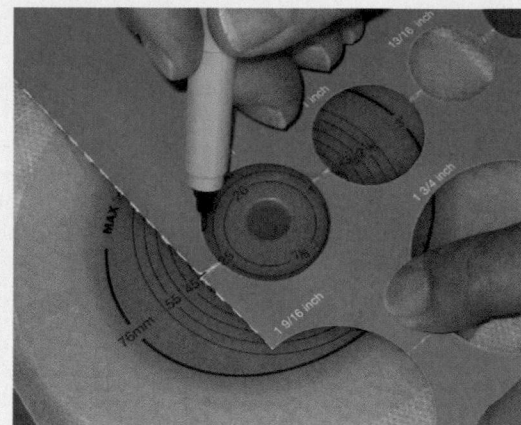

STEP 7 Trace measurement on skin barrier. (*Courtesy Coloplast, Minneapolis, MN.*)

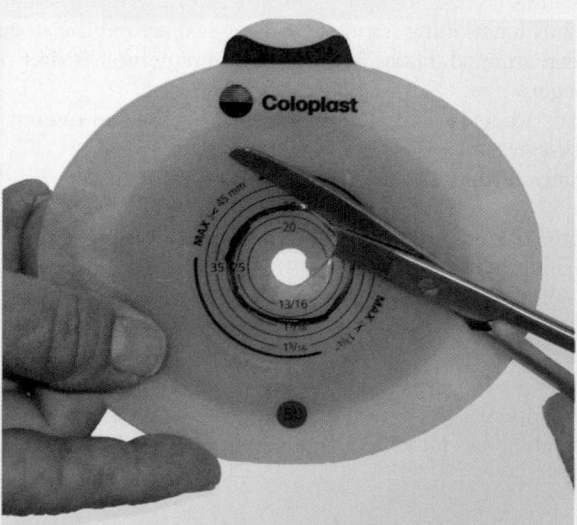

STEP 8 Cut opening in wafer. (*Courtesy Coloplast, Minneapolis, MN.*)

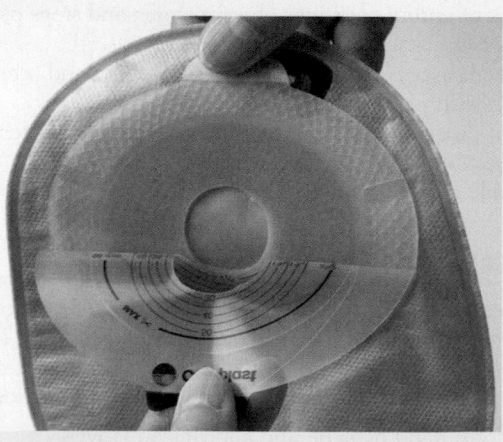

STEP 9 Remove protective backing. (*Courtesy Coloplast, Minneapolis, MN.*)

STEP	RATIONALE

IMPLEMENTATION

10. Apply pouch over stoma (see illustration). Press firmly into place around stoma and outside edges. Have patient hold their hand over the pouch to apply heat to secure seal.

Pouch adhesives are heat and pressure sensitive and hold more securely at body temperature.

11. Close end of pouch with clip or integrated closure. Remove drape from patient. Help patient to assume a comfortable position.

Ensures that pouch is secure. Contains effluent.

12. Remove and dispose of gloves and other PPE. Perform hand hygiene.

Reduces transmission of microorganisms.

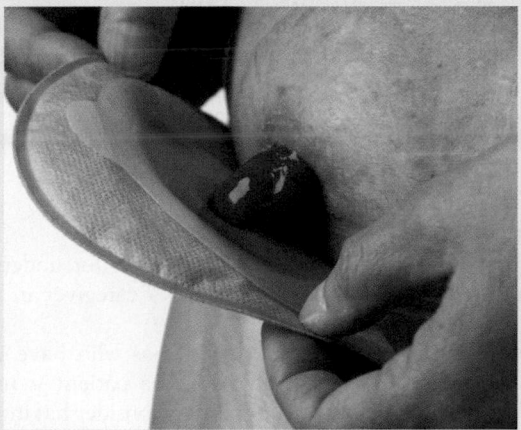

STEP 10 Apply pouch over stoma. (*Courtesy Coloplast, Minneapolis, MN.*)

EVALUATION

1. Observe condition of skin barrier and adherence of pouch to abdominal surface.

Determines presence of leaks.

2. Observe appearance of stoma, peristomal skin, abdominal contours, suture line, and presence of any flatus during pouch change.

Determines condition of stoma and peristomal skin and progress of wound healing.

3. Note if there is presence of any flatus during pouch change

Determines if peristalsis is returning.

4. Observe patient's and caregiver's willingness to view stoma and ask questions about procedure.

Determines level of adjustment to and understanding of stoma care and pouch application. Allows planning for future education needs and progress toward acceptance of altered body image.

5. **Use Teach-Back:** "I want to be sure you understand what is involved in changing your ostomy pouch. Tell me how often you should empty your pouch and things you can do to stop the skin around your stoma from becoming sore." Develop a revised teaching plan if patient or caregiver is not able to teach back correctly.

Determines patient's and caregiver's level of understanding of instructional topic.

Unexpected Outcomes

1. Skin around stoma is irritated, blistered, or bleeding or a rash is noted. This may be caused by undermining of pouch seal by fecal contents, causing irritant dermatitis, or by adhesive removal causing skin stripping or fungal or other skin eruption.

2. Necrotic stoma is manifested by purple or black colour, dry instead of moist texture, failure to bleed when washed gently, or tissue sloughing.

3. Patient refuses to view stoma or participate in care.

Related Interventions

- Remove pouch more carefully.
- Change pouch more frequently or use a different type of pouching system.
- Avoid use of acetone-based products.
- Arrange for interprofessional collaboration, including an ostomy care nurse.
- Report to nurse in charge or health care provider.
- Document appearance.

- Obtain referral for ostomy care nurse.
- Allow patient to express feelings.
- Encourage caregiver support.

Communication and Documentation

- Document type of pouch and skin barrier applied; time of procedure; amount and appearance of effluent in the pouch; location, size, and appearance of stoma; and condition of peristomal skin in the electronic health record (EHR) or chart.
- Document patient's and caregiver's level of participation, teaching that was done, and response to teaching.
- Report any of the following to the health care provider: abnormal appearance of stoma, suture line, peristomal skin, or character of output.

Special Considerations
Teaching

- Teach changing of a pouch whenever doing a pouch change, even if the patient does not appear interested. Do not insist that the patient look at the stoma; allow time for adjustment.
- Include the caregiver in teaching to facilitate the patient's readiness to learn.
- Some patients accept a stoma with minimal emotional difficulty; some may never completely adjust to it. Practise person-centred care—individualize care according to the patient's situation and circumstances (Riemenschneider, 2015).
- Give the patient plain-language teaching materials that clearly state each step for a pouch change. Audio, video, and online instructions are also available. Consider using materials that have illustrations for each step. For patients who do not speak English, provide a professional interpreter.
- Give patients a list of equipment and the name, address, phone number, and website of the supplier.

Pediatric

- Pediatric stoma surgery is usually done because the neonate has necrotizing enterocolitis (NEC), Hirschsprung's disease, or a congenital disorder (Soldes, 2016). The stomas frequently are temporary, with closure of the ostomy occurring when the surgical repair has healed and the neonate is medically ready for surgery. Children and adolescents may have ostomy surgery for conditions such as Gardner syndrome, typhlitis, inflammatory bowel disease, and trauma (Minkes, McHard, Mazziotti, et al., 2017).

- To prevent parastomal hernias, stomas should be brought through the rectus abdominis in older children and adolescents (Minkes et al., 2017).
- The most common complications with pediatric stomas are skin irritation and infection (e.g., candida infection, dermatitis). It is important to teach caregivers appropriate wound care (Minkes et al., 2017).
- The skin of a preterm infant is not fully developed and is more absorbent than that of a full-term infant. Avoid use of skin sealants and adhesive removers on these infants (RNAO, 2009).
- Select pediatric pouches designed especially for neonates, infants, and children. The pouches are smaller and have a more skin-sensitive adhesive on the barrier.
- Adolescents requiring an ostomy benefit from presurgical contact with other adolescents who have an ostomy. Practise person-centred care by facilitating conversations with adolescent patients about their care issues and concerns, as well as about their life in general (e.g., school, family, and spirituality) (Mohr & Hamilton, 2016).

Gerontological

- Evaluate an older person's cognitive status for understanding ostomy self-care instructions. Include a caregiver in the care plan (if appropriate).
- Adapt care approaches for older persons who have impaired manual dexterity or limited vision. If a patient is unable to custom-cut the size of the skin barrier, consider having barriers precut by an ostomy equipment supplier or using a precut pouching system.
- Costs of ostomy supplies and reimbursement are an issue for patients on a fixed income if not covered by insurance.

Care in the Community

- Evaluate home toileting facilities and patients' ability to empty the pouch directly into a toilet.
- A patient may shower without covering a pouch. A patient may take the pouch off in the shower to clean the peristomal skin if they wish to do so and if cleared by health care provider.
- Patients should avoid storing pouches in extremely hot or cold locations. Temperature affects barrier and adhesive materials.

◆ SKILL 36.2 Pouching a Urostomy

Because urine flows continuously from an incontinent urinary diversion, placement of a pouch is more challenging than with a fecal diversion. In the immediate postoperative period, urinary stents extend out from a stoma (Fig. 36.11). A surgeon places the stents to prevent stenosis of the ureters at the site where the ureters are attached to the conduit. The stents will be removed during the hospital stay or at the first postoperative visit with the surgeon.

The stoma is normally red and moist. It is made from part of the intestinal tract, usually the ileum. A normal stoma protrudes above the skin. An ileal conduit is usually located in the right lower quadrant of a patient's abdomen. While the patient is in bed, the pouch may be connected to a bedside drainage bag to decrease the need for frequent emptying. When the patient goes home, a bedside drainage bag may be used at night to avoid having to get up to empty the pouch. Each type of urostomy pouch comes with a connector for the bedside drainage bag (Fig. 36.12). Incorrect pouch placement, large volumes of urine in the pouch, or a urinary pouch without an antireflux valve promotes reflux of urine back into the

urostomy and ureters, causing the risk of infection. The risk of reflux is reduced by attaching a urinary pouch to straight drainage when high urinary output is expected. A patient must understand the importance of draining the pouch frequently and using clean technique during stomal and skin care. If the pouch does not contain an integrated gas (flatus) filter, the patient needs to be taught how to release built-up gas from the pouch.

Delegation and Collaboration

The skill of pouching a new incontinent urinary diversion cannot be delegated an unregulated care provider (UCP). In some facilities care of an established urostomy (4–6 weeks or more after surgery) can be delegated to UCPs. The nurse directs the UCP about:

- Expected appearance of the stoma.
- Expected amount and character of the output and when to report changes.
- Change in the patient's stoma and surrounding skin integrity that should be reported.

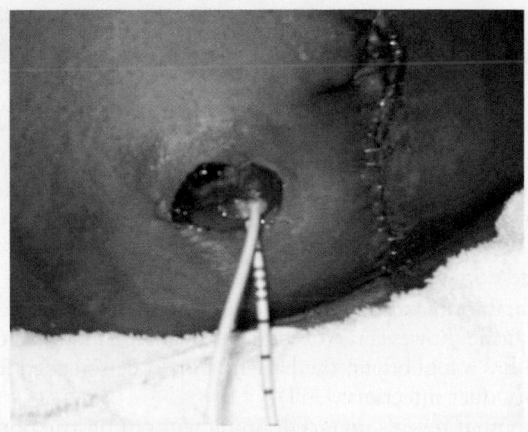

FIG 36.11 Urostomy stoma with stents in place. (*Courtesy Jane Fellows.*)

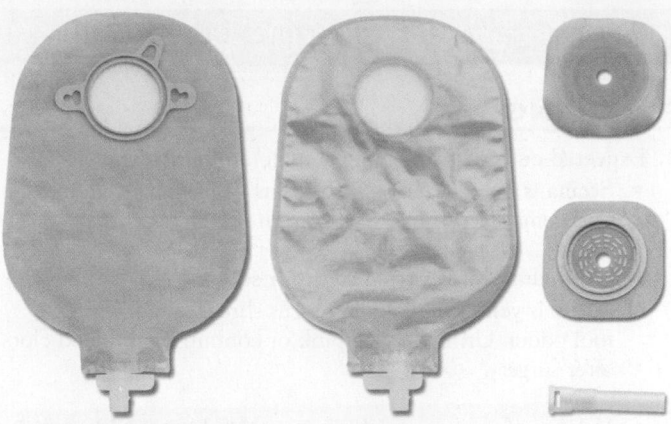

FIG 36.12 Urostomy pouching system with adapter to connect pouch to bedside drainage bag. (*Courtesy Hollister Inc, Libertyville, IL.*)

- Special equipment for a particular patient that is needed to complete the procedure.

Equipment

- Urinary pouch (with antireflux flap) and skin barrier; clear, drainable one- or two-piece, cut-to-fit or precut size
- Appropriate adapter for connection to bedside drainage bag
- Measuring guide
- Bedside urinary drainage bag
- Clean gloves
- Washcloth

- Towel or disposable waterproof barrier
- Basin with warm tap water
- Scissors
- Adhesive remover
- Absorbent wick made from gauze rolled tightly in the shape of a tampon
- Waterproof bag for disposal of pouch
- Mirror for patient to observe ostomy
- Personal protective equipment (PPE) as required (e.g., gown and goggles if there is any risk of splashing when emptying pouch)

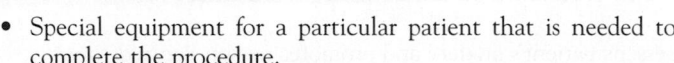

STEP	RATIONALE

ASSESSMENT

1. Identify patient using at least two person-specific identifiers (e.g., name and date of birth or name and medical record number), according to employer policy.

Ensures correct patient. Complies with Accreditation Canada's standards and improves patient safety (Accreditation Canada, 2019).

2. Perform hand hygiene and apply clean gloves.

Reduces transmission of microorganisms.

3. Observe existing skin barrier and pouch for leakage and length of time in place. Pouch should be changed every 3 to 7 days, not daily (Carmel et al., 2016). If urine is leaking under the wafer, change the pouch.

Assesses effectiveness of pouching system and allows for early detection of potential problems. To minimize skin irritation, avoid changing the entire pouching system unnecessarily. Repeated leakage may indicate need for a different type of pouch to provide a reliable seal.

4. Observe characteristics of urine in pouch or bedside drainage bag. Empty pouch if it is more than one-third to one-half full by opening valve and draining it into a container for measurement.

There may be blood or large amounts of mucus in urine after surgery, but this should resolve in the first 1–2 weeks after surgery. Weight of pouch can disrupt seal. Urine from ileal conduit will contain mucus because of flow through intestinal segment.

5. Observe stoma for colour, swelling, presence of sutures, trauma, and healing of peristomal skin. Assess type of stoma. Remove and dispose of gloves.

Consider stoma characteristics in selecting appropriate pouching system. Convexity in skin barrier is often necessary with a flush or retracted stoma.

6. Explore patient's perceptions, acceptance, and knowledge of stoma and interest in learning self-care. Identify others who will be helping patient after leaving hospital.

Facilitates teaching plan and timing of care to coincide with availability of caregivers.

NURSING DIAGNOSES

- Reduced skin integrity
- Insufficient knowledge regarding care of urostomy
- Alteration in body image
- Willingness for enhanced knowledge
- Potential for impaired skin integrity

Related factors/Risk factors are individualized on the basis of patient's condition or needs.

STEP	RATIONALE

PLANNING

1. Expected outcomes following completion of procedure:

- Stoma is red and moist with stents protruding from it. Peristomal skin is free of irritation and intact. Sutures are intact.

These are normal findings for postoperative urinary diversion.

- Urine drains freely from stents or stoma.

These are normal findings after surgery.

- Urine is yellow with some mucus shreds and is without foul odour. Urine may be pink or contain small blood clots after surgery.

It is normal for most individuals to have some mucus shreds in their urine; however, if the number of shreds increases or the urine has a foul odour, the patient should be screened for a urinary tract infection (UTI).

- Volume of output is within acceptable limits (≥30 mL/hr).

Normal output reveals ureters draining without obstruction.

- Patient and caregiver observe stoma and procedural steps.

Shows adjustment to change in body image and a willingness to learn self-care.

- Patient asks questions about procedure and may help with pouch change.

Indicates readiness to learn and begin self-care.

2. Explain procedure to patient; encourage their interaction and questions.

Lessens patient's anxiety and promotes person-centred care.

3. Assemble equipment and close room curtains or door.

Optimizes use of time; provides privacy.

IMPLEMENTATION

1. Position patient in semi-reclining or supine position. If possible, provide patient with a mirror for observation.

When patient is semi-reclining, there are fewer skin wrinkles, which allows for ease of pouch application.

2. Perform hand hygiene and apply clean gloves.

Reduces transmission of microorganisms.

3. Place towel or disposable waterproof barrier under patient and across patient's lower abdomen.

Protects bed linen; maintains patient's dignity.

4. If not done during assessment, remove the used pouch and skin barrier gently by pushing skin away from the barrier. If stents are present, pull pouch gently around them and lay towel underneath. Empty pouch and measure output. Dispose of pouch in an appropriate receptacle.

Reduces risk for trauma to skin and for dislodging stents. Keeps urine from leaking onto skin. Urine output provides information about renal status and whether volume is within acceptable limits (≥30 mL/hr).

5. Place rolled gauze at stoma opening. Maintain gauze at stoma opening continuously during pouch measurement and change.

Using wick at stoma opening prevents peristomal skin from becoming wet with urine during pouch change.

6. While keeping rolled gauze in contact with stoma, clean peristomal skin gently with warm tap water and washcloth; do not scrub skin. If you touch the stoma, minor bleeding is normal. Pat skin dry.

Avoid using soap. It leaves residue on the skin, which can irritate it. The pouch does not adhere to wet skin.

7. Measure stoma (see illustration, Skill 36.1, Step 6). Expect size of stoma to change during the first 4 to 6 weeks after surgery.

Allows for proper fit of pouch that will protect peristomal skin.

8. Trace pattern on pouch backing or skin barrier (see illustration, Skill 36.1, Step 7).

Prepares for cutting opening in pouch.

9. Cut opening in pouch (see illustration, Skill 36.1, Step 8). If using mouldable or shape to fit barrier, use your fingers to mould shape to fit stoma.

Customizes pouch to provide appropriate fit over stoma.

10. Remove protective backing from adhesive backing or wafer surface (see illustration, Skill 36.1, Step 9). Remove rolled gauze from stoma.

Prepares pouch for application to skin.

11. Apply pouch (see illustration Skill 36.1, Step 10). Press adhesive barrier firmly into place around stoma and outside edges. Have patient hold their hand over the pouch 1 to 2 minutes to secure seal.

Pouch adhesives are heat and pressure sensitive and will hold more securely at body temperature.

12. Use adapter provided with pouches to connect pouch to the bedside urinary bag. Keep tubing below level of the bag.

Allows patient to rest without having to empty pouch frequently. Tubing position allows for collection and measurement of urine and prevents backflow of urine into stoma.

STEP	RATIONALE

IMPLEMENTATION

13. Remove drape from patient. Help patient to assume a comfortable position. Remove and dispose of gloves and other disposables; perform hand hygiene.

Reduces transmission of microorganisms.

EVALUATION

1. Observe appearance of stoma, peristomal skin, and suture line during pouch change.

Determines condition of stoma and peristomal skin and progress of wound healing.

2. Evaluate character and volume of urinary drainage.

Determines if stoma and/or stents are patent. Character of urine reveals degree of concentration and whether there is possible UTI.

3. Observe patient's and caregiver's willingness to view stoma and ask questions about procedure.

Determines level of adjustment to and understanding of stoma care and pouch application.

4. Use Teach-Back: "I want to be sure you understand what is involved in changing your ostomy pouch. Let's review what we discussed. Tell me how often you should empty your pouch and how often you should change it." Develop a revised teaching plan if patient or caregiver is not able to teach back correctly.

Determines patient's and caregiver's level of understanding of instructional topic.

Unexpected Outcomes

1. Skin around stoma is irritated, blistered, or bleeding; or maceration is noted as result of chronic exposure to urine.

2. No urine output for several hours, or output is less than 30 mL/hr. Urine has foul odour.

3. Patient and caregiver are unable to observe stoma, ask questions, or participate in care.

Related Interventions

- Check stoma size and opening in skin barrier.
- Resize skin barrier opening, if necessary.
- Remove pouch more carefully.
- Consult ostomy care nurse.
- Increase fluid intake (if allowed).
- Notify health care provider.
- Obtain urine specimen for culture and sensitivity if prescribed.
- Consult ostomy care nurse.
- Allow patient to express feelings.
- Encourage caregiver support.

Communication and Documentation

- Document type of pouch, time of change, condition and appearance of stoma and stents and peristomal skin, and character of urine in the electronic health record (EHR) or chart.
- Document urinary output on I&O form.
- Document patient's and caregiver's reaction to stoma and level of participation.
- Document your evaluation of patient and caregiver learning.
- Report abnormalities in stoma or peristomal skin and absence of urinary output to nurse in charge or health care provider.

Special Considerations
Teaching

- Follow teaching considerations in Skill 36.1.
- Teach patients the significance and importance of drinking about 2 L (2 quarts) of fluid daily to decrease risk for developing UTI (Carmel et al., 2016). Explain that some mucus in the urine is expected but that patients should report any blood in their urine, excessively cloudy urine, chills, fever (38.3°C [101°F] or higher), or back (flank) pain to their health care provider.

Pediatric

- In neonates, urinary diversions are less common than fecal ostomies.
- Select pediatric pouches designed especially for neonates, infants, and children; these pouches are smaller and have a more skin-sensitive adhesive on the barrier.

Gerontological

- Follow gerontological considerations in Skill 36.1.
- Older persons have decreased thirst and may not normally consume adequate fluids. Explain the importance of fluid intake to promote healthy renal function and decrease risk for developing UTI.

Care in the Community

- Follow care-in-the-community considerations in Skill 36.1.
- Instruct patient that the pouch can be connected to straight drainage at night. Make sure that the patient understands that the adapter will be needed to connect the pouch to the bedside drainage bag (see Fig. 36.12).

✦ SKILL 36.3 Catheterizing a Urinary Diversion

Catheterization of a urinary diversion is the only method to obtain an accurate culture and sensitivity specimen to screen a patient for infection. Check employer policy to identify the appropriate health care team member to collect this specimen. When it is necessary to obtain a urine specimen from a urinary diversion, the best method is to insert a sterile catheter into the stoma. Obtaining a specimen of urine in a pouch does not provide an accurate finding because of the likely risk of contamination by microorganisms growing in the stagnant urine. With the use of strict aseptic technique, catheterization is relatively safe and easy. If a patient uses a two-piece system, remove the pouch from the skin barrier and replace it after catheterization without disturbing the skin barrier. If a patient uses a one-piece system, remove the pouch to obtain the specimen and replace it with a new pouch after the procedure. To prevent trauma to the tissues, one needs to understand how the stoma and implanted ureters are constructed for a patient (see Fig. 36.3).

Delegation and Collaboration

The skill of catheterizing a urinary diversion cannot be delegated an unregulated care provider (UCP). The nurse directs the UCP to:

- Inform the nurse if the patient has peristomal or flank pain (sign of kidney infection).
- Inform the nurse if there is a change in colour, odour, or amount of urine or if there is blood in the urine.

Equipment

- Urinary catheterization supplies (contained in prepackaged sterile catheter kit or gathered separately):
- 14- to 16-Fr sterile catheter
- Water-soluble lubricant
- Antiseptic swabs (e.g., povidone-iodine or chlorhexidine)
- Sterile gloves
- Sterile specimen container
- Absorbent gauze wick
- Bed protection barrier
- Towels
- Urinary pouch, if needed
- Clean gloves

STEP	RATIONALE
ASSESSMENT	
1. Identify patient using at least two person-specific identifiers (e.g., name and date of birth or name and medical record number), according to employer policy.	Ensures correct patient. Complies with Accreditation Canada's standards and improves patient safety (Accreditation Canada, 2019).
2. Obtain health care provider's prescription for catheterization.	This invasive procedure requires a health care provider's prescription.
3. Observe for signs and symptoms of urinary tract infection (UTI): elevated temperature, chills, foul-smelling urine, and elevated white blood cell (WBC) count.	Determines need to perform catheterization to obtain sterile specimen from urinary diversion. Having a urinary diversion poses a risk for reflux of urine back to the kidneys, resulting in infection.
4. Assess patient's understanding of need for the procedure and how it is done.	Determines willingness to cooperate and reduces patient's anxiety.

NURSING DIAGNOSES

- Insufficient knowledge regarding catheterization procedure
- Potential for infection
- Potential for injury: urinary tract

Related factors/Risk factors are individualized on the basis of patient's condition or needs.

PLANNING

1. Expected outcomes following completion of procedure:	
• Urine specimen is not contaminated with bacteria during procedure.	Urine is obtained correctly. Laboratory results are accurate.
• Patient describes risks for infection and techniques to prevent infection.	Demonstrates patient's learning.
2. Assemble equipment and close room curtain or door.	Optimizes use of time and provides privacy.
3. Explain procedure to patient, including sensations that will be felt. If possible, obtain specimen when the patient is due to change the pouch if using a one-piece system.	Lessens anxiety and promotes patient's cooperation. Cleaning the stoma and surrounding skin may cause a cool sensation. Insertion of the catheter may cause a sensation of mild pressure, or it may not be felt at all. Changing the pouch too frequently could result in skin trauma.

STEP	RATIONALE

IMPLEMENTATION

1. If possible, position patient sitting, and drape towel across their lower abdomen.

   Gravity facilitates flow of urine. Maintains patient's dignity. Towel absorbs urine.

2. Perform hand hygiene and apply clean gloves.

   Reduces transmission of microorganisms.

3. Remove pouch. If patient uses a two-piece system, remove the pouch but leave barrier attached to the skin.

   Allows access to stoma.

4. Remove gloves and perform hand hygiene.

   Avoids contamination.

5. Open sterile catheterization set according to instructions or open needed equipment and place on sterile barrier using aseptic technique (see Chapter 5). If not using a catheterization kit, place gauze pad on sterile field and squeeze a small amount of lubricant onto the gauze. Apply sterile gloves.

   Prepares sterile work field.

6. If needed, have patient hold absorbent gauze wick on the stoma while you prepare catheterization supplies.

   Prevents leakage of urine on peristomal skin, linens, and clothing.

7. Clean surface of stoma with antiseptic swabs using a circular motion from centre outward. Use a new swab each time; repeat process twice. Allow chlorhexidine antiseptic to dry or wipe off excess antiseptic with dry sterile gauze or cotton ball.

   Removes surface bacteria. Chlorhexidine must dry to achieve antibacterial effect.

Clinical Decision Point *If the patient has stents in place, use an antiseptic swab to clean the ends of the stents and place the stents in the sterile cup. Allow urine to drip into the cup until you obtain an adequate amount for a specimen. Then go directly to Step 13.*

8. Remove lid from sterile specimen container.

   Sterile container collects a small volume of urine.

9. Lubricate tip of catheter with water-soluble lubricant, keeping catheter sterile.

   Facilitates passage of catheter through the stoma.

10. With your dominant hand, gently insert catheter tip into the stoma. Do not force the catheter; redirect course as needed. Place distal end of the catheter into the specimen container. Have patient cough; massage their abdomen near the stoma or turn patient on their side.

    Use care to avoid trauma to conduit. Movement and coughing may facilitate flow of urine from conduit.

11. Hold container below level of the stoma. If needed, wait several minutes to get an adequate amount of urine.

    Culture and sensitivity studies only require 3 to 5 mL of urine (check employer policy).

12. Withdraw catheter slowly; place an absorbent pad over the stoma.

    Keeps skin dry.

13. Apply lid to specimen container.

    Prevents accidental spillage.

14. Reapply a new pouch or reattach pouch if patient uses a two-piece system (see Skill 36.2).

    The pouch is necessary to contain urine.

15. Dispose of used pouch and equipment properly.

    Avoids unpleasant odour in room.

16. Remove gloves; perform hand hygiene. Label specimen in presence of the patient, place it in a biohazard bag, and send it to the laboratory at once.

    Ensures that laboratory results are assigned to correct patient. Labelling ensures acceptance and processing of specimen by laboratory. Urine that sits for long periods at room temperature will adversely affect laboratory results.

EVALUATION

1. Compare results of culture and sensitivity with expected findings. Mucus is a normal finding if patient has an ileal conduit.

   Determines presence of infection. If contamination appears likely, a second specimen will be needed.

2. **Use Teach-Back:** "I want to be sure you understand the reason we needed to collect the urine. Tell me in your own words why we did this procedure to get urine from your stoma. What are the signs of a urinary tract infection when you have a urostomy?" Develop a revised teaching plan if patient or caregiver is not able to teach back correctly.

   Determines patient's and caregiver's level of understanding of instructional topic.

Unexpected Outcomes

1. Unable to obtain urine specimen.

2. Skin or stoma reveals complications.

Related Interventions

- Reposition patient.
- If there is still no urine, push fluids and try again later.
- Inform health care provider if unable to obtain specimen on second attempt.
- Notify health care provider.
- Consult with ostomy care nurse about pouching system or skin barrier to use.

Communication and Documentation

- Document time the specimen was collected; patient's tolerance of the procedure; and appearance of urine, skin, and stoma, in the electronic record (EHR) or chart.
- Document your evaluation of patient and caregiver learning.
- Report results of laboratory test to the nurse in charge or health care provider.

Special Considerations
Teaching

- Explain common symptoms of UTI: flank pain, dark or bloody urine, foul-smelling urine, fever (38.3°C [101°F] or higher), confusion.
- Encourage patient to notify a health care provider if symptoms of infection develop.
- Reinforce the importance of fluid intake of 2 L/day, or as tolerated.

◆CLINICAL DEBRIEF

A nurse is assigned to care for a 28-year-old fashion designer with a 10-year history of ulcerative colitis with an increase in bleeding, pain, and frequent episodes of diarrhea. Her health care provider has tried to control her symptoms with medications, but this approach has been unsuccessful in the last year. She has been admitted to the hospital for a colectomy with ileal pouch anal anastomosis and J-pouch construction (see Fig. 36.4). She will have a temporary ileostomy. An ostomy nurse has been consulted for stoma site marking and preoperative education.

1. Why is the consultation necessary?
2. When the patient returns from surgery, the nurse assesses her abdomen and finds that it is firm and distended. She has several sites on her abdomen where the laparoscopes were inserted; each has been closed with two staples, and no dressings are present on these sites. An ostomy pouch is placed on the right side of her abdomen. The stoma is visible through this pouch; it is red and round and protrudes above the abdomen. No output is present in the pouch. Using SBAR, show how the nurse communicates her assessment with the other health care providers.
3. On the first postoperative day the patient asks how often the pouch should be emptied and how frequently it will have to be changed. What should the nurse tell her?

◆ REVIEW QUESTIONS

1. The nurse has inserted a catheter into a patient's urinary stoma, but only a few drops of urine have drained. Which actions should the nurse perform to try to obtain an adequate sample? *(Select all that apply.)*
   1. Remove the catheter and obtain urine from the pouch.
   2. Gently insert the catheter further into the stoma.
   3. Massage the patient's abdomen.
   4. Have the patient turn on their side.
   5. Attempt to intubate the stoma with a larger-size catheter.

2. The nurse is caring for a recent postoperative patient with an ileostomy and notes a raw, weeping area of the skin around the stoma. Which actions are most appropriate in this situation? *(Select all that apply.)*
   1. Cleaning the area with alcohol to help dry the raw skin
   2. Consulting an ostomy care nurse
   3. Reviewing the pouch change procedure with the patient
   4. Having the patient continue their usual skin care regimen of cleaning gently with water and placing the pouch over the raw, moist skin
   5. Recommending that the patient measure the stoma again and cut a new pattern because the stoma may have changed size since surgery

3. Place the steps for an ostomy pouch change in the correct order.
   1. Close the end of the pouch.
   2. Measure the stoma.
   3. Cut the hole in the wafer.
   4. Press the pouch into place over the stoma.
   5. Remove the old pouch.
   6. Trace the correct measurement onto the back of the wafer.
   7. Observe the stoma and the skin around it.
   8. Clean and dry the peristomal skin.

ⓔ *Visit the Evolve site for a complete list of Clinical Debrief and Review Questions answers.*

REFERENCES

Accreditation Canada. (2019). *Required organizational practices handbook—Version 14*. Ottawa: Author. Retrieved from http://www.wrha.mb.ca/quality/files/2019ROPHandbook.pdf

Canadian Society of Intestinal Research (CSIR). (2018). *Stoma site selection*. Retrieved from https://www.badgut.org/information-centre/ostomies/stoma-site-selection/

Carmel, J. E., Colwell, J., & Goldberg, M. (Eds.), (2016). *Wound, ostomy, continence nurses society core curriculum: Ostomy management*. Philadelphia: Wolters Kluwer.

Colwell, J., McNichol, L., & Boarini, J. (2017). North America wound, ostomy, and continence and enterostomal therapy nurses current ostomy practice related to peristomal skin issues. *Journal of Wound, Ostomy, and Continence Nursing, 44*(3), 257–261. doi:10.1097/WON.0000000000000324

Culha, I., Kosgeroglu, N., & Bolluk, O. (2016). Effectiveness of self-care education on patients with stomas. *IOSR Journal of Nursing and Health Science*, 5(2), 70–76. doi:10.9790/1959-05217076

Jayarajah, U., & Samarasekera, D. (2017). A cross-sectional study of quality of life in a cohort of enteral ostomy patients presenting to a tertiary care hospital in a developing country in South Asia. *BMC Research Notes*, 10, 75. doi:10.1186/s13104-017-2406-2

Minkes, R., McHard, K., Mazziotti, M., et al. (2017). *Stomas of the small and large intestine in children—Treatment and management*. MedScape, Pediatrics: Surgery. Retrieved from https://emedicine.medscape.com/article/939455-treatment#d15

Mohr, L., & Hamilton, R. (2016). Adolescent perspectives following ostomy surgery: A grounded theory study. *Journal of Wound, Ostomy, and Continence Nursing*, 43(5), 494–498. doi:10.1097/WON.0000000000000257

Nurses Specialized in Wound, Ostomy and Continence Canada (NSWOCC) & Canadian Association of Enterostomal Therapy (CAET). (2009). *Clinical best practice guidelines, ostomy care and management*. Retrieved from http://nswoc.ca/?s=best+practice+guidelines

Ostomy Canada Society. (2017). *Ostomy 101*. Retrieved from http://community.ostomycanada.ca/information/ostomy-101/

Riemenschneider, K. (2015). Uncertainty and adaptation among adults living with incontinent ostomies. *Journal of Wound, Ostomy, and Continence Nursing*, 42(4), 361–367. doi:10.1097/WON

Registered Nurses Association of Ontario (RNAO). (2009). *Clinical best practice guidelines: Ostomy care and management*. Retrieved from http://rnao.ca/sites/rnao-ca/files/Ostomy_Care__Management.pdf

Salvadena, G., Hendren, S., McKenna, L., et al. (2015a). WOCN Society and ASCRS position statement on preoperative stoma site marking for patients undergoing colostomy or ileostomy surgery. *Journal of Wound, Ostomy, and Continence Nursing*, 42(3), 249–252. doi:10.1097/WON.0000000000000119

Salvadena, G., Hendren, S., McKenna, L., et al. (2015b). WOCN Society and AUA position statement on preoperative stoma site marking for patients undergoing urostomy surgery. *Journal of Wound, Ostomy, and Continence Nursing*, 42(3), 253–256. doi:10.1097/WON.0000000000000118

Soldes, O. (2016). Ileostomy and colostomy. In P. Mattei, P. Nichol, I. M. Rollins, & C. Murator (Eds.), *Fundamentals of pediatric surgery* (pp. 479–485). New York: Springer.

37 | Preoperative and Postoperative Care

Written by **Diane Rudolphi, MS, RN, and Nicole Lewis-Power, RN, MN, PhD(c)**

SKILLS AND PROCEDURES

OBJECTIVES

Mastery of content in this chapter will enable the nurse to:
- Explain how to integrate person-centred care into preoperative and postoperative care.
- Describe the physical preparations needed for a patient facing surgery.
- Identify risk factors that have a potential for affecting a patient's clinical outcomes postoperatively.
- Discuss cultural differences that might affect the implementation of preoperative and postoperative procedures.

- Describe the benefits of structured preoperative teaching.
- Explain the rationale for each of the postoperative exercises.
- Successfully teach a patient to perform postoperative exercises.
- Discuss the differences in nursing assessment during the immediate postoperative period and the convalescent phase of recovery.
- Conduct an assessment of a preoperative and a postoperative patient.

MEDIA RESOURCES

- evolve http://evolve.elsevier.com/Canada/Perry/clinicalskills/
- Audio Glossary
- Checklists
- Case Studies

- Review Questions
- ▶ Video Clips
- Clinical Debrief and Review Questions Answers

PURPOSE

Surgical care of patients is in a continuous state of technological advancement. As a result, patients have shortened lengths of stay because of less invasive surgery and less time spent in a hospital. During the preoperative phase, the nursing role focuses on physical, psychological, sociocultural, and spiritual preparation while also validating existing information, reinforcing patient education, and providing nursing care to prepare the patient and family for the surgical experience (American Society of PeriAnaesthesia Nurses [ASPAN], 2015). During the postoperative phase, when a patient returns from the operating room (OR), the nurse initially is responsible for completing a thorough assessment of the patient's physical and mental status while also providing continuous monitoring of their condition and ongoing education during the recovery process.

STANDARDS OF CARE

- Accreditation Canada, 2019—*Required Organizational Practices Handbook—Version 14* (http://www.wrha.mb.ca/quality/files/2019ROPHandbook.pdf)

- National Association of PeriAnaesthesia Nurses of Canada (NAPANc), 2018—*Standards for Practice*, 4th edition (http://napanc.ca/index.php/standards)
- Operating Room Nurses Association of Canada, 2017—*Standards, Guidelines and Position Statements for Perioperative Registered Nurses*, 13th edition (https://www.ornac.ca/en/standards)

PRINCIPLES FOR PRACTICE

- A variety of diagnostic tests are coordinated before surgery to ensure that the surgeon and anaesthesia care providers have the information needed to determine a patient's risks during surgery and the postoperative period.
- The National Association of PeriAnaesthesia Nurses of Canada (NAPANc, 2018) identifies patient assessment, data collection, and management as critical in all phases of the perianaesthesia environment, and has provided specific guidelines for care of the pediatric and older person population.
- The speed of a patient's recovery depends on how effectively the nurse anticipates potential complications, initiates necessary

supportive and preventive therapies, and actively involves the patient and caregiver in the recovery process.

- Preoperative and postoperative patient education improves outcomes after surgery. The shift in how surgical services are now provided poses special challenges to meeting patients' educational needs within a reduced time frame. Because most patients undergo surgery in an ambulatory setting and thus avoid a hospital stay, it is essential that they receive adequate information to ensure that they or their caregivers can manage postoperative care activities in the home setting.
- NAPANc (2018) advocates that the registered nurse (RN) take part in in the preanaesthesia phase in order to anticipate patient outcomes from surgery and anaesthesia and that the nurse use critical thinking and clinical judgement to interpret and analyze preoperative data and assessments. This analysis enables recognition of the need for further testing, interprofessional collaboration, or additional interventions to prevent intraoperative and postoperative complications.

PERSON-CENTRED CARE

- Engaging and involving patients and caregivers in patient care results in safer and more patient-centred care (Spruce, 2015).
- To provide culturally competent care to a surgical patient, the nurse should begin by assessing the family to determine not only who should be involved but also who legally is responsible for making decisions and giving consent for surgery.
- To better understand the culture and needs of the patient, the nurse may be required to request very specific information from the patient, family, or religious leader.
- When providing preoperative teaching, include caregivers. The use of professional interpreters for patients who do not speak English is necessary to provide competent informed patient care.
- Before surgery, it is important to accommodate a patient's religious and cultural needs and adapt the patient's care to encompass their practices and beliefs whenever possible. Identify cultural and religious beliefs and practices that may affect patients' and caregivers' reactions to the surgical experience, such as diet, pain, blood transfusions, and disposal of body parts, including hair.
- Both before and after surgery assess patient preferences for pain medication. Many patients believe that pain medication leads to addiction and will attempt to endure the pain without medication. Cultures that value males being in control of their emotions may prevent members from verbalizing pain.
- Persons of some religions or cultures may request to wear articles such as jewellery, medallions, or undergarments. To accommodate these needs and deliver person-centred care, nurses may need to allow such articles (e.g., medals, underclothing) to be worn until just before surgery. If articles are removed, the nurse must ensure that they are returned promptly after surgery.

EVIDENCE-INFORMED PRACTICE

Approximately 8 000 people in Canada die from health care–associated infections (HAIs) annually. Approximately 220 000 will get infected. The estimated cost for treatment of these infections was estimated at $129 million in 2010 (Canadian Patient Safety Institute [CPSI], 2016a). Surgical site infection (SSI) is the most common HAI among surgical patients, with 77% of patient deaths reported to be related to infection (CPSI, 2016b).

The following evidence-informed guidelines have been identified to reduce SSIs (CPSI, 2016b):

- Adequate perioperative antimicrobial coverage
- Appropriate hair removal
- Maintenance of perioperative glucose control
- Perioperative normothermia

There are also strict guidelines for use of antibiotics (Diaz & Newman, 2015). The goal of prophylactic antibiotic therapy is to select the most effective antibiotics for maximum coverage and administer them when they are most beneficial to protect patients from infection with as little risk as possible:

- Overall, it is recommended that prophylactic antibiotics be given as close to the time of incision as possible (within 60 minutes) and not be given for longer than 24 hours after surgery.
- Vancomycin and fluoroquinolones (i.e., ciprofloxacin, levofloxacin) may be given up to 2 hours before incision because of their longer infusion times. Antibiotic use after incision closure does not reduce infection rates, and when the antibiotics are continued, infections are more likely to be caused by a resistant organism (Centers for Disease Control and Prevention [CDC], 2016).
- Prophylactic antibiotics should be discontinued within 24 hours after the end of surgery in most cases.

SAFETY GUIDELINES

- Know the type and nature of any previous surgery. Anatomical and physiological alterations affect a patient's risk for operative problems.
- Identify the factors and conditions that increase a patient's risks during surgery. Preoperative preparation and postoperative care depend on knowledge of these risk factors.
- Know the rationale for and extent of impending surgery. Each type of surgical procedure requires a different type of nursing care and allows nurses to anticipate potential complications correctly.
- Ensure that the patient has signed the informed consent. A nurse may witness a patient's signature, but in most facilities this practice is discouraged, as it is the health care provider's (e.g., surgeon) responsibility to ensure informed consent has been obtained. Should the patient or family not be fully informed about the surgical procedure, it is the nurse's responsibility to advocate for the patient and inform the health care provider of this lack of knowledge. Informed consent is required by law to help protect patients' rights, their autonomy, and their privacy. The surgeon should give the patient information about the extent and type of surgery; alternative therapies; and usual risks, benefits, and consequences of not having surgery. See employer policy regarding consent (Table 37.1).
- Complete the preoperative checklist according to employer policy.
- Administer pain-relief therapies according to a patient's perioperative needs. Pain can slow a surgical patient's recovery.
- Restrict patient activity after administration of preoperative and postoperative sedatives to minimize the risk for patient falls.

TABLE 37.1

Information Needed for Informed Consent

Parameters	Examples
Name of procedure/surgery	Abdominal hysterectomy under general anaesthesia
Description of procedure/surgery	Removal of uterus only through an incision in the abdominal wall at the top of the pubic hairline; done while unconscious
Person performing procedure/surgery	Dr. Rachel Jones, assisted by Dr. William Smith
Benefits of procedure/surgery	To remove uterus with fibroids and stop excessive bleeding Abdominal route necessary because of anticipated adhesions from prior abdominal surgery
Potential risks and adverse effects of procedure/surgery	Risk of hemorrhage and infection from surgery; risk of excessive sedation and allergic reaction to medications used with general anaesthesia; accidental damage to bladder, intestines, and/or nerves controlling these organs
Approximate length of time for procedure/surgery	About 1 hour; 1 to 2 hours in postanaesthesia care unit (PACU)
Approximate length of time needed for recovery	3 to 4 days on surgical unit; 4 to 6 weeks before resuming physically stressful work
Alternative treatments	Removal of uterus vaginally; radiation to shrink fibroids
Consequences of refusing treatment	Continuation of pain and vaginal bleeding, risk for developing anemia; after menopause, fibroids should regress

---

✦ SKILL 37.1   **Preoperative Assessment**

A thorough preoperative nursing assessment of a patient's physiological and psychological condition allows a nurse to identify patient risks and plan for care during and after surgery. The assessment documents baseline data for future comparisons to determine the effect of instruction and whether complications have developed during the perioperative period. Many health care facilities have a designated department devoted to completing thorough preoperative screening and testing. Laboratory tests, electrocardiograms (ECGs), chest X-ray films, and other tests are often obtained 1 to 2 weeks in advance of the scheduled surgical procedure. Perioperative staff performs a thorough assessment and reviews the test results to identify any potential abnormalities that may need further evaluation and treatment before surgery.

The nurse assesses patients again 1 to 2 hours before the scheduled time of surgery to ensure that there are no changes in their physical condition. Advanced planning allows time for nurses to follow up on any unexpected outcomes. Before beginning this assessment, the nurse needs to establish a trusting relationship with the patient. It is not unusual for the patient to remember and report at this time facts that were not previously told to the surgeon. The nurse should provide the patient privacy and a location free of interruption to encourage open communication. The nurse initiates a preprocedure checklist, beginning with the decision to perform a procedure, maintained with ongoing data collection and assessment, and verified immediately before moving the patient to the procedure room (Accreditation Canada, 2019). Typically, the surgeon, anaesthetist, or nurse completes an assessment, and the patient signs a consent form after receiving an explanation of the procedure from the surgeon. Current test results and notices of any special considerations during the procedure such as a need for blood products or special equipment should be available.

Delegation and Collaboration

The skill of preoperative assessment cannot be delegated to an unregulated care provider (UCP). The nurse instructs the UCP to:
• Obtain vital signs and weight and height measurements.

Equipment

• Stethoscope
• Blood pressure monitoring equipment
• Pulse oximetry
• Thermometer
• Watch or clock with a second hand
• Method to measure height and weight
• Access to laboratory, ECG, X-ray films, and other diagnostic equipment as needed
• Preprocedure checklist
• Preoperative assessment form

STEP	RATIONALE

ASSESSMENT

1. Identify patient using at least two person-specific identifiers (e.g., name and date of birth or name and medical record number), according to employer policy.

Ensures correct patient. Complies with Accreditation Canada's standards and improves patient safety (Accreditation Canada, 2019).

2. Perform hand hygiene. Prepare equipment and room for assessment.

Reduces transmission of infection. Makes assessment more efficient.

STEP	RATIONALE

ASSESSMENT

3. Determine if patient has any communication impairment (e.g., blindness, hearing loss), can read and understand English, and is mentally competent. For example, give patient an informational brochure and have them explain part of the contents. Obtain a professional interpreter if needed.

The patient may not fully comprehend a diagnosis, understand proposed treatment, or effectively consider alternatives that are presented without effective communication. Relying on a family member as an interpreter cannot guarantee the accuracy of explanations.

4. Assess patient's understanding of the intended surgery and anaesthesia. Ask patient to offer a description rather than asking a simple yes-or-no question (e.g., "Tell me in your own words what your surgery will involve"). Ask about the patient's and caregiver's expectations of surgery and care. Include questions concerning fears, cultural practices, and religious beliefs, if applicable.

Patients may have misconceptions and incomplete knowledge. Asking about fears, cultural practices, and religious beliefs enables you to anticipate priorities of the patient and caregiver and adapt your plan so you can give appropriate instruction and support.

5. Ask if patient has an advance care plan (see Chapter 17).

Advance care plans protect patient's rights by communicating patient's treatment preferences if patient is unable to communicate.

6. Collect nursing history and identify surgical risk factors:

Allows for anticipation of possible complications and planning for interventions to reduce patient risks.

Clinical Decision Point *If patient is having emergency surgery, focus on assessment of primary body system affected.*

a. Condition requiring surgery.

Allows you to anticipate postoperative needs and possible complications.

b. Chronic illnesses and associated risks (e.g., hypertension—bleeding, and stroke; postoperative respiratory depression and arrest; asthma—impaired ventilation; hiatal hernia—aspiration; diabetes mellitus—impaired wound healing; methicillin-resistant *Staphylococcus aureus*—impaired wound healing and sepsis).

Some chronic conditions increase the risk of complications from surgery and anaesthesia.

c. Determine if patient has obstructive sleep apnea (OSA). Many facilities use the STOP-Bang assessment tool (http://www.stopbang.ca/):
STOP*
  • Do you SNORE loudly (louder than talking or loud enough to be heard through closed doors)?
  • Do you often feel TIRED, fatigued, or sleepy during the daytime?
  • Has anyone OBSERVED you stop breathing during your sleep?
  • Do you have or are you being treated for high blood PRESSURE?
BANG
  • BMI more than 35 kg/m^2
  • AGE over 50 years old
  • NECK circumference >16 inches (40 cm)
  • GENDER: Male
  *Any question answered *Yes* is a risk factor.

In the surgical population, a STOP-Bang score of 5–8 identifies patients with high probability of moderate/severe OSA. The STOP-Bang score helps the health care team to stratify patients for unrecognized OSA, practice perioperative precautions, or triage patients for diagnosis and treatment (Chung, Abdullah, & Liao, 2016).

Patients with OSA will require special anaesthesia precautions. Patients with OSA are often sensitive to sedative medications, especially if the OSA is untreated. Even minimal sedation can cause airway obstruction and ventilatory arrest, thus requiring close monitoring postoperatively (Chung et al., 2016).

d. Last menstrual period (for female patients in childbearing years).

Anaesthetic drugs and other medications could injure the fetus.

e. Previous hospitalizations.

Determines if patient is familiar with hospital procedures.

f. Full medication history, including prescription, over-the-counter (OTC), medicinal marijuana and herbal remedies, and date and time of last doses.

Patient may not report OTC medications and herbal remedies unless specifically asked. All may interact with anaesthetic drugs or other medications given during surgery. Patient may be instructed to take any routine blood pressure, cardiac, or seizure medications. Changes in dosages of oral diabetic drugs or insulin may be prescribed.

g. Previous experience with surgery and anaesthesia; have patient clarify if any undesirable outcomes occurred.

Information helps to prevent recurrent problems with planned surgery.

STEP	RATIONALE

ASSESSMENT

h. Family history of complications from surgery or anaesthesia.	Family history of reactions to anaesthetic drugs may indicate familial condition such as malignant hyperthermia, which is life-threatening.
i. Allergies to medications, food, or tape, including specific questions about natural rubber latex. Ask patients if they have had any problem with medication or anything placed on their skin.	Allergies to medications or latex can be life-threatening. Prevention of latex allergy in sensitized patients requires specific precautions. Often patients with latex allergies are scheduled as the first case of the day. In addition, many patients do not understand that rubber and latex are the same. Using both words helps obtain accurate information.
j. Physical impairment (e.g., paralysis, reduced range of motion of extremity).	Physical impairments may cause limited mobility and situations that could lead to problems with positioning and risk for pressure injury formation. Communicate this information to the operating room (OR) nurse because these patients may need special positioning or OR bed surfaces.
k. Prostheses and implants (e.g., implantable medication-delivery pump, dentures, hearing aid, pacemaker, internal defibrillator, hip prosthesis).	These devices are often removed prior to surgery (see employer policy) because they could become damaged or malfunction from electrical equipment used during surgery. Report this information to the OR nurse.
l. Smoking, alcohol, and drug use.	Preoperative alcohol consumption is associated with an increased risk of general postoperative morbidity, general infections, wound complications, pulmonary complications, prolonged stay at the hospital, and admission to a critical care unit (Rotevatn, Boggild, Olesen, et al., 2017). Preoperative use of illicit drugs can lead to pulmonary complications, poor pain control, and withdrawal symptoms. Smoking can lead to cardiopulmonary complications.
m. Occupation.	Anticipates how postoperative restrictions will affect the patient's return to work.
7. Obtain patient's weight, height, and vital signs (see Chapters 7 and 8).	Height and weight are used to calculate drug dosages. Vital signs provide a baseline for postoperative comparison.

Clinical Decision Point *Many patients with OSA are morbidly obese, placing them at increased risk for aspiration of acidic gastric fluid at the time of induction of anaesthesia. For this reason, many of these patients receive medications to suppress gastric acid production, neutralize the acid, or stimulate emptying of the stomach. Use interprofessional collaboration (e.g., health care provider) to discuss possible prescription for acid-suppressing medication.*

8. Assess patient's respiratory status, including auscultation of lungs, adventitious sounds, character and rate of respirations, oxygen saturation, ability to breathe lying flat, use of oxygen or continuous positive airway pressure (CPAP) at home, and chest X-ray film report.	Poor respiratory condition can affect the patient's response to general anaesthesia. Use of CPAP may indicate that the patient has OSA, a condition that poses risks after surgery.
9. Auscultate heart sounds and evaluate patient's circulatory status, including apical pulse, ECG report, and peripheral pulses (see Chapter 8).	Screens for possible cardiac problems that may contraindicate surgery. Circulation may be a factor in positioning patient on the OR table.
10. Assess for patient's risk for postoperative thrombus formation (e.g., older persons, immobilized patients, patients with personal or family history of blood clots, use of birth control pills, hormones). Ask patient about any leg pain. Observe calves for swelling, warmth, and redness; observe calves for symmetry; and palpate pedal pulses.	Circulation slows after general anaesthesia, increasing tendency for blood clot formation. Immobilization during surgical procedure promotes venous stasis. Manipulation and positioning can cause accidental trauma to leg veins.

Clinical Decision Point *Homans' sign is not always present when a deep vein thrombosis (DVT) exists (Schick & Windle, 2016). If you suspect a thrombus, notify the surgeon and refrain from manipulating the extremity any further. Surgery will usually need to be postponed. Antiembolism stockings or a venous flexus foot pump (Fig. 37.1) may be prescribed for patients at risk for thrombus formation (see Chapter 12).*

11. Complete a gastrointestinal assessment; identify time of patient's last intake of food or drink (see Chapter 8).	With patient under general anaesthesia, the esophageal sphincter relaxes, and the stomach contents can be aspirated.
12. Complete neurological assessment; determine patient's neurological status, including level of consciousness (LOC), cognitive function, and sensation, and note neurological deficits (see Chapter 8).	Patient's neurological status affects attentiveness to instruction. Offers important baseline for postoperative evaluation.

STEP	RATIONALE

ASSESSMENT

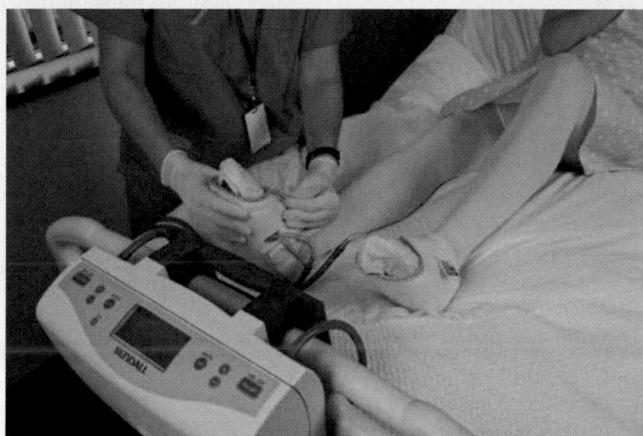

FIG 37.1 Venous plexus foot pump with bedside controls. (*Courtesy Tyco Healthcare Group LP.*)

13. Assess patient's musculoskeletal system, including range of motion (ROM) of joints (see Chapter 8). / If ROM is limited, extra care is needed to prevent injury related to positioning in surgery.

14. Examine patient's skin; identify any breaks in skin integrity and determine level of hydration (see Chapter 8). Pay particular attention to area of body on which patient will be positioned. / If skin is thin, broken, or bruised, extra padding is needed in surgery. Hydration may affect skin integrity.

15. Assess patient's emotional status, including level of anxiety, coping ability, and caregiver support. Assess potential for abuse from a partner or family member. / If patient has a high level of anxiety or fear, use interprofessional collaboration (e.g., social worker, pastoral care, advanced practice nurse) as required. Any suspected or reported abuse requires follow-up, according to provincial/territorial regulations.

16. Review results of laboratory tests, including complete blood count, electrolytes, urinalysis, and other diagnostic tests. / Laboratory work provides an assessment of major body systems.

NURSING DIAGNOSES

- Inadequate knowledge regarding preoperative plan of care
- Potential for perioperative positioning injury
- Potential for impaired skin integrity
- Potential for infection

Related factors/Risk factors are individualized on the basis of patient's condition or needs.

PLANNING

1. Expected outcomes following completion of procedure:
   - Patient provides appropriate preoperative information required to establish plan of care. / Identifies patient's knowledge of preoperative plan of care.
   - Patient remains alert and appropriately responsive to assessment questions. / Identifies patient readiness to learn.
   - Patient does not incur any injury during preoperative preparation in OR. / Precautions taken because of assessment findings prevent positional and skin injury.

IMPLEMENTATION

1. Communicate to preoperative team risk factors that have the potential for making the patient vulnerable to complications intraoperatively. / Limitations in mobility and sensation should affect how patient is positioned for surgery. Presence of OSA and any cardiopulmonary abnormalities can influence anaesthesia approach.

Clinical Decision Point *Even though the surgeon and anaesthesia provider will conduct a separate assessment, your findings may reveal surgical risk factors not identified previously.*

STEP	RATIONALE

IMPLEMENTATION

2. Based on the patient's cognitive status, experience, and nature of planned surgery, present preoperative instruction to patient and caregiver (see Skill 37.2).	Assessment findings influence the approach to instructions and topics to discuss.

EVALUATION

1. Determine if patient information is complete so plan of care can be established. Validate unclear information with patient and caregiver.	Provides preoperative baseline of assessment data.
2. Evaluate patient's ability to cooperate (e.g., makes eye contact, answers appropriately).	Establishes patient's ability to participate in assessment.
3. Use Teach-Back: "I want to be sure I explained what you need to know about your intended surgery and anaesthesia. Tell me why you are having surgery and when your surgery is scheduled." Develop a revised teaching plan if patient is not able to teach back correctly.	Determines patient's level of understanding of instructional topic.

Unexpected Outcomes
1. Patient does not understand what surgery will be performed.
2. Patient reports allergy to latex.

Related Interventions
- Notify surgeon.
- Remove all supplies containing latex from patient's room.
- Post latex precautions sign on door or stretcher.
- Notify surgeon, anaesthesia provider, and OR nurse.

Communication and Documentation

- Document findings on the preoperative part of the nurses' detailed preoperative notes or other designated employer form in electronic health record (EHR) or chart.
- Report abnormal laboratory values or other concerns to the health care provider (surgeon or anaesthesiologist).
- Document your evaluation of patient and caregiver learning.

Special Considerations
Pediatric

- Involve the parent or guardian in the preoperative preparation to decrease the child's anxiety.

- Consider a child's developmental level when performing preoperative assessment and preoperative preparation (e.g., use stories, films, books, tours, toys, and games) (Perry, Hockenberry, Lowermilk, et al., 2017).
- Encourage parent or guardian to accompany the child to the surgery holding area.

Gerontological

- Age-related changes may result in diminished short-term memory. Additional assessment and teaching may be necessary.
- An older person may have some limitation in ROM. If this limitation is significant, notify the OR nurse so the surgical position can be modified.

✦ SKILL 37.2   Preoperative Teaching

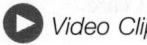 *Video Clip*

With shortened hospital lengths of stay and growth in ambulatory surgical procedures, there is a greater demand for patient preparation and support. Patient education must go beyond simply providing information because patients and families must be prepared to assume more preoperative and postoperative responsibilities. Preoperative patient teaching involves helping a patient understand and prepare mentally for the surgical experience. Effective education focuses on each patient's individual needs and leads to patients feeling empowered because they have sufficient knowledge that meets their needs, expectations, or preferences.

In the past, patients received preoperative teaching the day or evening before surgery, when patients are most anxious. Health care cost reduction practices now have most patients entering the hospital or ambulatory care centre the morning of surgery. Preoperative teaching is not effective at this time because of patient anxiety and stress related to surgical preparation (Wongkietkachorn, Wongkietkachorn, & Rhunsiri, 2018). Many health care facilities now provide outpatient education programs to prepare patients and their caregivers for a specific surgery. For example, patients who require a total knee replacement go to preoperative preparation classes with other patients requiring the same surgery. Effective preoperative teaching increases patient satisfaction, promotes psychological well-being, and may decrease complications leading to an increased length of hospital stay (Lewis, Bucher, Heitkemper, et al., 2019). As a nurse, plan your teaching based on the preoperative assessment. Make every attempt to ensure the patient's privacy.

Select the best learning method for the patient. In many settings video, written, and online materials are available to help you. Whenever possible, have the caregivers responsible for the patient's care after surgery present during teaching. Later the caregivers serve as coaches and help the patient perform postoperative exercises. Plan to have the patient demonstrate expected postoperative skills to allow for practice and facilitate understanding.

Patients and their families are often anxious about impending surgery, which hinders learning. Speak in a clear, slow voice to reduce the patient's anxiety and promote understanding. You may need extra time for teaching and reinforcement to ensure patient understanding. After surgery, high anxiety can lead to negative psychological and physiological outcomes. Preoperative information about expected perioperative sensations decreases the distress associated with surgery. By teaching and setting expectations before surgery (pain level, average length of surgery), the patient and the nurse can make a significant contribution to success in the postoperative recovery phase.

Delegation and Collaboration

The skills of preoperative teaching cannot be delegated to an unregulated care provider (UCP). The UCP can reinforce and help patients perform postoperative exercises. The nurse instructs the UCP about:

- Any precautions or safety issues unique to the patient (e.g., fall precautions, mobility limitations, bleeding precautions, weight-bearing issues, dietary concerns).
- Informing the nurse of any identified concerns (e.g., patient is unable to perform the exercises correctly).

Equipment

- Stretcher or bed
- Pillow
- Incentive spirometer
- Preoperative education flow sheet
- Positive expiratory pressure (PEP) device
- Stethoscope

STEP	RATIONALE
ASSESSMENT	
1. Identify patient using at least two person-specific identifiers (e.g., name and date of birth or name and medical record number), according to employer policy.	Ensures correct patient. Complies with Accreditation Canada's standards and improves patient safety (Accreditation Canada, 2019).
2. Ask about patient's previous experiences with surgery and anaesthesia.	This allows you to individualize teaching and address specific patient concerns.
3. Determine if patient and caregiver understand surgery.	This information determines if correction of misunderstanding is necessary.
4. Identify patient's cognitive level, language, and culture. If patient does not speak English, have a professional interpreter present to assist you.	These factors may alter the patient's ability to understand the meaning of the surgery and can affect the postoperative healing course if there are mixed messages or misunderstanding.
5. Assess patient's risk for postoperative respiratory complications (see Skill 37.1). Check nursing history for patient's height and age.	General anaesthesia predisposes a patient to respiratory problems (see Chapters 23 and 25). The presence of underlying respiratory conditions or patient's inability to perform postoperative respiratory exercises increases the patient's risk for pulmonary complications. Height and age are used to set incentive spirometer parameters.
6. Assess patient's anxiety related to surgery.	If anxiety is still high, directs you to provide additional emotional support. Indicates patient's readiness to learn.
7. Assess caregiver's willingness to learn and support patient following surgery.	Caregiver's presence after surgery can be a potential motivating factor for patient recovery. In addition, the caregiver can coach the patient through postoperative exercise and observe for any postoperative problems.
8. Assess patient's medical prescriptions.	Preoperative and postoperative prescriptions often require adaptations in the way patient performs exercises.

NURSING DIAGNOSES

- Anxiety
- Inadequate knowledge regarding postoperative exercises

Related factors/Risk factors are individualized on the basis of patient's condition or needs.

PLANNING

1. Expected outcomes following completion of procedure:	
• Patient demonstrates culturally appropriate eye contact, asks and answers questions appropriately.	Identifies patient's readiness to learn.

STEP	RATIONALE

PLANNING

- Patient correctly performs splinting, turning and sitting, breathing exercises, and leg exercises.
- Family identifies location of waiting room and time frame when they can expect status on their family member.
- Caregivers verbalize ability to help prepare patient at home before surgery.
- Caregivers provide emotional support for patient before surgery.

Patient will be prepared to participate in postoperative exercises following surgery.

Family anxiety may be reduced with preoperative expectations clearly provided.

Caregivers can assist patient with necessary preparations before surgery at home.

Both patient and caregiver have support for surgery.

IMPLEMENTATION

1. Perform hand hygiene. Inform patient and caregiver of date, time, and location of surgery; anticipated length of surgery; additional time in postanaesthesia recovery area; and where to wait.

   Reduces transmission of infection. Accurate information helps reduce stress associated with surgery.

2. Answer questions that patient and caregiver ask.

   Responding to patient and caregiver questions helps to decrease their anxiety and demonstrates your concern for them.

3. Instruct patient about preoperative bowel or skin preparations, as needed. Check medical prescriptions and employer policy regarding number of preoperative showers and drug to be used for each shower (2% chlorhexidine gluconate is used most often). Following each preoperative shower, instruct patient to rinse the skin thoroughly and dry with a fresh, clean, dry towel. Patient should don clean clothing.

   Proper skin preparation is a critical element in preventing surgical site infections (SSIs). Rinsing skin removes residual antiseptic preparation that may cause skin irritation. After use, towels contain microorganisms that can grow in the presence of moisture. Using fresh towel after each shower and donning clean clothing minimizes risk of reintroducing microorganisms to clean skin (Association of periOperative Registered Nurses [AORN], 2015).

4. Instruct patient about extent and purpose of food and fluid restrictions for period specified before surgery (e.g., no clear liquids at least 2 hours before surgery, no light meal [e.g., toast and a clear liquid] 6 hours or more before surgery, no meat or fried foods 8 hours before surgery, unless otherwise specified by surgeon or anaesthesiologist) (College of Physicians and Surgeons of British Columbia, 2017).

   During general anaesthesia muscles relax; and gastric contents can reflux into esophagus, leading to aspiration. Anaesthetic eliminates patient's ability to gag.

5. Describe perioperative routines (e.g., time-out, site marking, intravenous [IV] therapy, urinary catheterization, enema, hair clipping or removal, laboratory tests, transport to operating room [OR]).

   Allows patient to anticipate and recognize routine procedures, reducing anxiety.

6. Describe planned effect of preoperative medications.

   Provides information about what to expect, decreasing patient anxiety.

7. Review which routine medications patient needs to discontinue before surgery.

   Some medications are discontinued before surgery to minimize effects that can cause surgical risks. For example, anticoagulants may increase bleeding and are usually discontinued several days before surgery. Insulin dosages are usually adjusted because of reduced intake of food before surgery.

8. Describe perioperative sensations (e.g., blood pressure cuff tightening, electrocardiogram [ECG] leads, cool room, and beep of monitor).

   Misconceptions and concerns about anaesthesia have been ranked high among preoperative patients.

9. Describe pain-control methods to be used after surgery. Many patients have a patient-controlled analgesia (PCA) pump (see Chapter 16).

   Patients are fearful of postoperative pain. Explaining pain-management techniques reduces this fear. Establishes what pain is acceptable; patients will know they will not be pain-free, but their pain will be managed.

10. Describe what patient will experience after surgery (e.g., where patient will be on awakening, frequent vital signs, catheters, drains, tubes, alternating pressure from sequential compression device, postoperative exercises).

    Provides concrete description of what patient can expect after surgery so patient is prepared.

STEP	RATIONALE

IMPLEMENTATION

11. Teach turning:

  a. Instruct patient on turning and sitting up (especially suited for abdominal and thoracic surgery):

    (1) Turn onto right side: Have patient assume supine position and move to side of bed (in this case, left side) if permitted by surgery. Instruct patient to move by bending knees and pressing heels against mattress to raise and move buttocks (see illustration). The top side rails on both sides of the bed should be in up position.

      Promotes circulation and ventilation.

      Positioning begins on side of bed so turning to the other side does not cause patient to roll toward edge of bed. Buttocks lifting prevents shearing force against sheets. If patient's bed has a turn-assist feature, use it to help position them.

    (2) Have patient splint incision with right hand, or with right hand with pillow over incisional area; patient should keep right leg straight and flex their left knee up (see illustration); grab right side rail with their left hand, pull toward right, and roll onto their right side. Reverse process to turn to left side.

      Supports incision and decreases discomfort while turning.

    (3) Instruct patient to turn every 2 hours from side to side while awake. Often patient requires assistance with turning after surgery. If patient is unable to turn, assist or turn patient every 2 hours unless contraindicated by operative procedure.

      Reduces risk of vascular, pulmonary, and pressure injury complications.

Clinical Decision Point *Some patients, such as those who have had back surgery or vascular repair, are restricted from flexing their legs after surgery. Some patients are restricted from turning or may need help for positioning (see Chapter 11).*

    (4) Have patient sit up on right side of bed. Elevate head of bed and have patient turn onto their right side. While lying on right side, patient pushes on mattress with left arm and swings feet over edge of bed with nurse's help. For patient to sit up on left side of bed, reverse this process.

      Sitting position lowers diaphragm to permit fuller lung expansion.

Clinical Decision Point *Caution patient to always ask for assistance, particularly the first time sitting up on the side of the bed, to reduce risk of a fall.*

12. Teach coughing and deep breathing: If the patient has an abdominal or thoracic incision, teach patient to place a pillow over the incision area and their hands over the pillow, to splint the incision.

    Patient may be unable or reluctant to deep breathe because of weakness or pain, resulting in secretions remaining in base of the lungs. Collection of secretions increases risk of pulmonary atelectasis and pneumonia. Deep breathing and coughing exercises place a strain and stress on the suture line, causing discomfort. Splinting provides a firm support and reduces incisional pulling and pain.

  a. Help patient to high-Fowler's position in bed with their knees flexed, or have patient sit on side of bed or chair in an upright position.

    Sitting position facilitates diaphragmatic expansion.

  b. Instruct patient to place palms of their hands across from one another lightly along lower border of rib cage or upper abdomen (see illustration).

    This allows patient to feel the rise and fall of their abdomen during deep breathing.

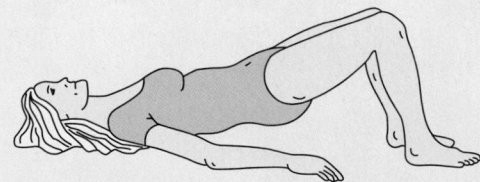

STEP 11a(1) Buttocks lift for moving to side of bed.

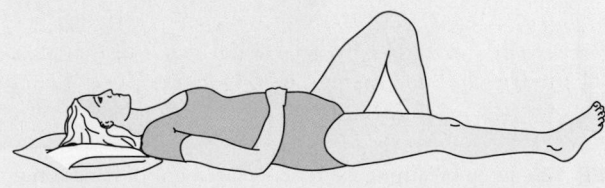

STEP 11a(2) Leg position when turning to right.

STEP	RATIONALE

IMPLEMENTATION

c. Have patient take slow, deep breaths, inhaling through the nose. Explain that patient will feel normal downward movement of the diaphragm during inspiration. Demonstrate as needed.

Helps to prevent hyperventilation or panting. Slow, deep breathing allows for more complete lung expansion.

d. Have patient avoid using chest and shoulder muscles while inhaling.

Increases unnecessary energy expenditure and does not promote full lung expansion.

e. Have patient take slow, deep breath; hold for count of 3 seconds; and slowly exhale through the mouth as if blowing out a candle (pursed lips).

Resistance during exhalation helps to prevent alveolar collapse.

f. Have patient repeat breathing exercise three to five times.

Repetition reinforces learning.

g. Have patient take two slow, deep breaths, inhaling through the nose and exhaling through pursed lips.

Deep breaths expand lungs fully so air moves behind mucus to facilitate coughing.

h. Have patient inhale deeply a third time and hold breath to count of 3. Have patient cough fully for two to three consecutive coughs without inhaling between coughs.

Deep breathing moves up secretions in the respiratory tract to stimulate cough reflex without voluntary effort on the part of the patient (Lewis et al., 2019).

i. Caution patient against just clearing throat.

Clearing the throat does not remove mucus from deeper airways.

j. Have patient practice several times. Instruct patient to perform turning, coughing, and deep breathing every 2 hours. Have caregiver coach patient to exercise.

Ensures mastery of technique. Frequent pulmonary exercises and movement decrease risk of postoperative pneumonia (Lewis et al., 2019).

13. Teach use of an incentive spirometer (see also Skill 23.3):

Provides visual aid of respiratory effort. Encourages deep breathing to loosen secretions in lung bases.

a. Position patient in sitting position in chair or in reclining position with head of bed elevated at least 45 degrees in bed.

Facilitates diaphragm lowering and lung expansion.

b. Either set or indicate to patient on the incentive spirometer device scale the volume level to be reached with each breath (targeted tidal volume). Use manufacturer directions to set volume.

Establishes goal of volume level necessary for adequate lung expansion. Manufacturers determine target on basis of patient height and age.

c. Explain to patient how to place mouthpiece of incentive spirometer so lips completely cover the mouthpiece (see illustration). Have patient demonstrate until position is correct.

Validates patient's understanding of instructions, evaluates psychomotor skills, and lets patient ask questions.

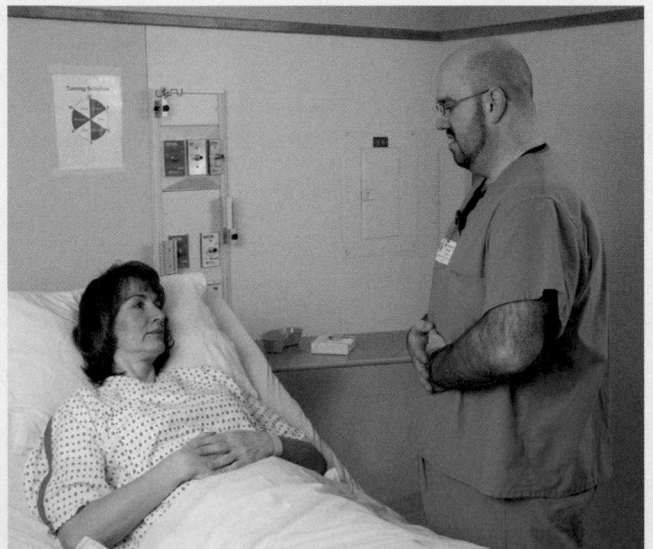

STEP 12b Deep-breathing exercise—placement of hands on upper abdomen during inhalation.

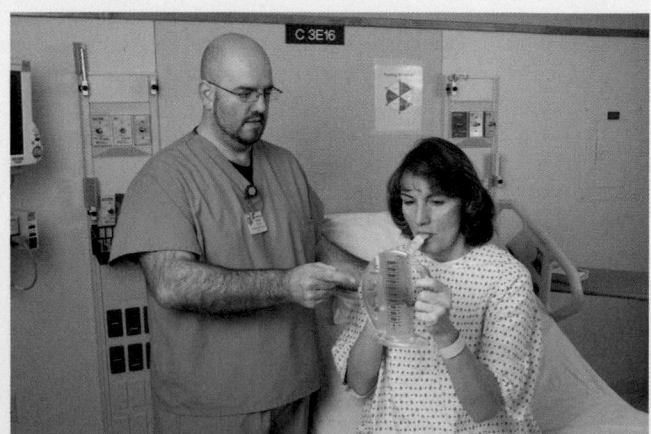

STEP 13c Patient demonstrates incentive spirometry.

STEP	RATIONALE

IMPLEMENTATION

d. Instruct patient to exhale completely, then position mouthpiece so lips completely cover it, and inhale slowly, maintaining constant flow through unit until reaching goal volume (see illustration).

Promotes complete inflation of lungs and minimizes atelectasis.

e. Once maximum inspiration is reached, have patient hold breath for 2 to 3 seconds and then exhale slowly.

Promotes alveolar inflation.

f. Instruct patient to breathe normally for a short period between each of the 10 breaths taken on incentive spirometer. Have patient repeat this every hour while awake.

Prevents hyperventilation and fatigue.

14. Teach PEP therapy and "huff" coughing:

a. Set PEP device for setting prescribed.

Higher settings require more effort.

b. Instruct patient to assume a semi-Fowler's or high-Fowler's position in bed or to sit in a chair, and place nose clip on patient's nose (see illustration).

Promotes optimum lung expansion and expectoration of mucus.

c. Have patient place lips around the mouthpiece. Instruct patient to take a full breath and exhale two or three times longer than inhalation. Repeat pattern for 10 to 20 breaths.

Ensures that patient does all breathing through the mouth. Ensures that patient uses device properly.

d. Remove device from mouth and have patient take a slow, deep breath and hold it for 3 seconds.

Promotes lung expansion before coughing.

e. Instruct patient to exhale in quick, short, forced "huffs." Repeat exercise every 2 hours while patient is awake.

"Huff" coughing, or forced expiratory technique, promotes bronchial hygiene by increasing expectoration of secretions.

15. Teach controlled coughing:

Deep breaths expand lungs fully so air moves behind mucus and facilitates effective coughing.

a. Explain importance of maintaining an upright position.

Position facilitates diaphragm excursion and enhances thorax and abdominal expansion.

b. Demonstrate coughing. Have patient take two slow, deep breaths, inhaling through the nose and exhaling through (pursed lips) mouth.

Consecutive coughs help remove mucus more effectively and completely than one forceful cough.

c. Have patient inhale deeply a third time and hold breath to count of 3. Patient should cough fully for two to three consecutive coughs without inhaling between coughs (see illustration). (Tell patient to push all air out of lungs.)

Clearing the throat does not remove mucus from deeper airways. A dull, forceful cough is most effective in removing mucus.

d. Caution patient against just clearing throat instead of coughing deeply.

Clearing throat does not remove mucus from deeper airways.

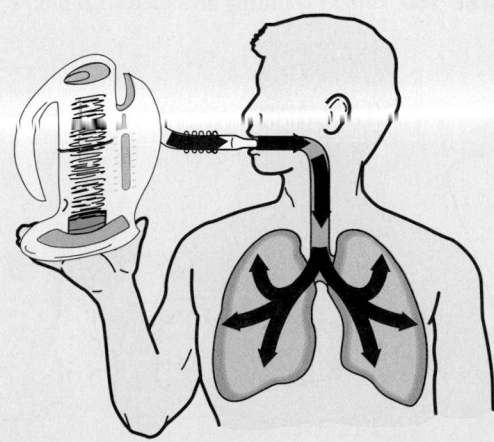

STEP 13d Diagram of use of incentive spirometer.

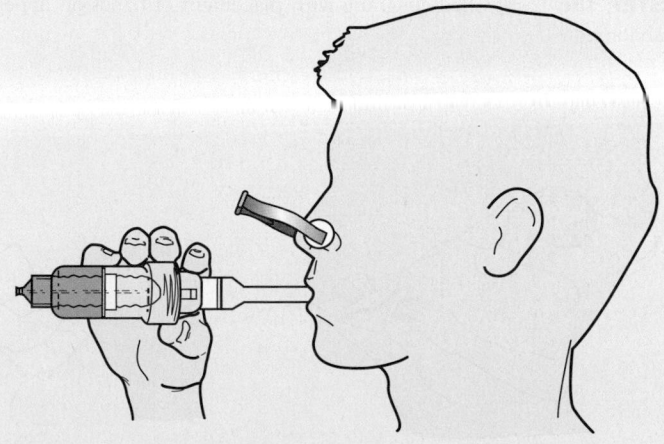

STEP 14b Diagram of use of positive expiratory pressure device.

STEP	RATIONALE

IMPLEMENTATION

e. If surgical incision is either thoracic or abdominal, teach patient to place either hands or pillow over incisional area and place hands over pillow to splint the incision (see illustration). During breathing and coughing exercises, patient should press gently against incisional area for splinting and support.

Surgical incision cuts through muscles, tissues, and nerve endings. Deep-breathing and coughing exercises place additional stress on the suture line and cause discomfort. Splinting the incision with hands or a pillow provides firm support and reduces incisional pulling and pain.

f. Patient continues to practice coughing exercises, splinting imaginary incision (see illustration). Instruct patient to cough two to three times every 2 hours while awake.

Deep coughing with splinting effectively expectorates mucus with minimal discomfort.

g. Instruct patient to examine sputum for consistency, odour, amount, and colour changes and notify a nurse if any changes are noted.

Sputum consistency, odour, amount, and colour changes indicate presence of a pulmonary complication such as pneumonia.

16. Teach leg exercises:

a. Instruct patient in leg exercises and encourage that they be performed every 1 to 2 hours while patient is awake: ankle rotation, dorsiflexion and plantar flexion, leg extension and flexion, and straight-leg raises.

Leg exercises facilitate venous return from lower extremities and reduce risk of circulatory complications such as venous thrombus.

b. Position patient supine.

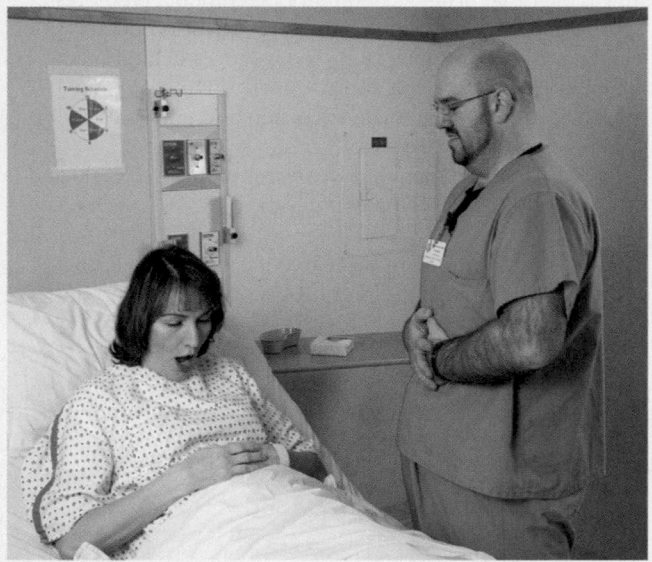

STEP 15c Controlled coughing with placement of hands on upper abdomen.

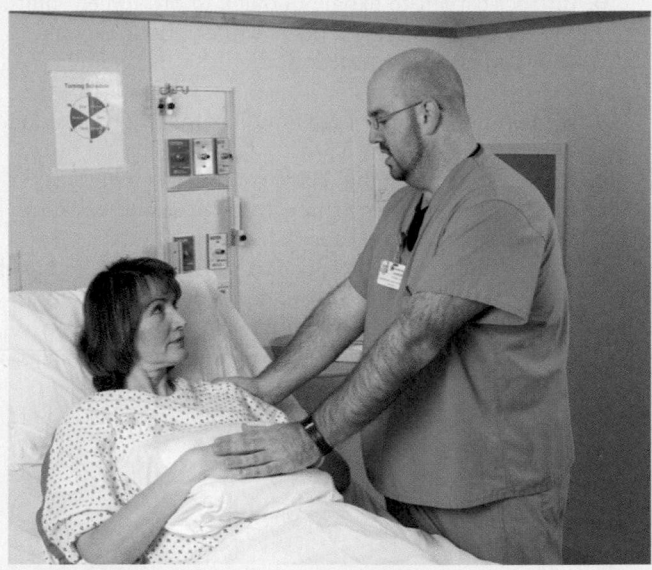

STEP 15e Patient splinting abdomen with pillow.

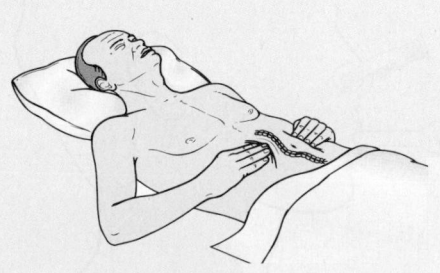
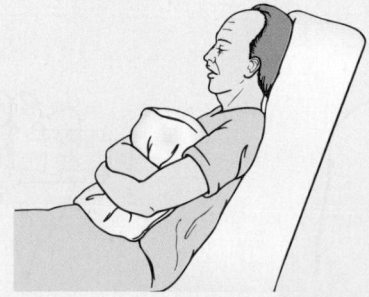
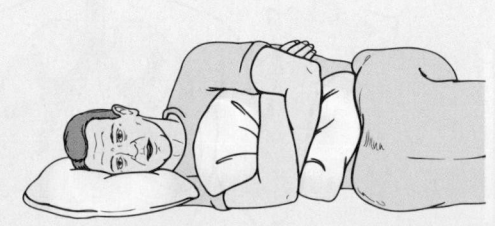

STEP 15f Techniques for splinting incisions.

STEP	RATIONALE

IMPLEMENTATION

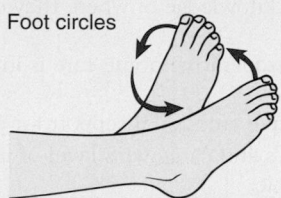

Foot circles

STEP 16c Foot circles. *(From Lewis, S., et al. [2019]. Medical-surgical nursing: assessment and management of clinical problems [4th Canadian ed.]. Toronto: Elsevier.)*

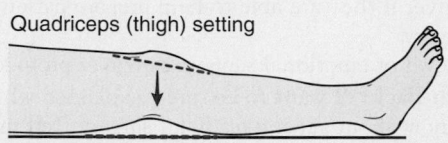

Quadriceps (thigh) setting

STEP 16e Quadriceps (thigh) setting. *(From Lewis, S., et al. [2019]. Medical-surgical nursing: assessment and management of clinical problems [4th Canadian ed.]. Toronto: Elsevier.)*

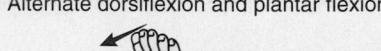
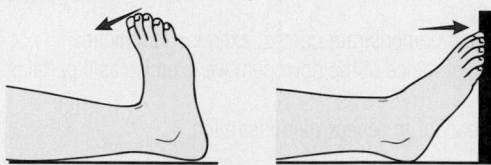

Alternate dorsiflexion and plantar flexion

STEP 16d Alternate dorsiflexion and plantar flexion. *(From Lewis, S., et al. [2019]. Medical-surgical nursing: assessment and management of clinical problems [4th Canadian ed.]. Toronto: Elsevier.)*

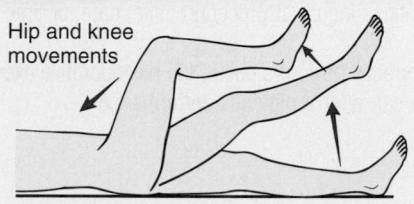

Hip and knee movements

STEP 16f Hip and knee movements. *(From Lewis, S., et al. [2019]. Medical-surgical nursing: assessment and management of clinical problems [4th Canadian ed.]. Toronto: Elsevier.)*

STEP	RATIONALE
c. Instruct patient to rotate each ankle in a complete circle and draw imaginary circles with the big toe five times (see illustration).	Promotes joint mobility and venous return.
d. Have patient alternate dorsiflexion and plantar flexion and instruct patient to feel calf muscles tighten and relax. Repeat five times (see illustration).	Helps maintain joint mobility and promote venous return to prevent thrombus formation.
e. Have patient perform quadriceps setting by tightening thigh and bringing knee down toward mattress and relaxing. Repeat five times (see illustration).	Quadriceps-setting exercises contract muscles of upper legs, maintain knee mobility, and improve venous return to the heart.
f. Instruct patient to alternate raising legs straight up from bed surface. Leg should be kept straight. Repeat five times (see illustration).	Causes quadriceps muscle contraction and relaxation, which help promote venous return (Lewis et al., 2019).
17. Have patient continue to practice exercises before surgery at least every 2 hours while awake. Teach patient to coordinate turning and leg exercises with diaphragmatic breathing and use of incentive spirometer.	Leg exercises stimulate circulation, which prevents venous stasis to help prevent formation of deep vein thrombosis (DVT) (Lewis et al., 2019).
18. Verify that patient's expectations of surgery are realistic. Correct expectations as needed.	Can prevent postoperative anxiety or anger.
19. Reinforce therapeutic coping strategies. If ineffective, encourage alternatives.	Therapeutic coping strategies promote postoperative adherence and recovery.

EVALUATION

1. Observe patient demonstrating splinting, turning and sitting, deep breathing, use of incentive spirometer, PEP therapy, and leg exercises.	Validates patient's ability to perform postoperative exercises and use devices.

STEP	RATIONALE

EVALUATION

2. Ask family to identify location of waiting room and validate if correct.

3. Ask caregiver if they are able to help prepare patient at home before surgery.

4. Observe level of emotional support caregiver provides patient.

5. **Use Teach-Back:** "I want to be sure I explained what you need to know about getting ready for surgery. Tell me which medications you should not take before surgery?" Develop a revised teaching plan if patient or caregiver is not able to teach back correctly.

Establishes family's knowledge of where they can wait for patient information.

Establishes that postoperative home care is in place for patient on discharge.

Identifies preoperative emotional support for patient.

Determines patient's and caregiver's level of understanding of instructional topic.

Unexpected Outcomes	Related Interventions
1. Patient identifies incorrect procedure, site, date, or time of surgery.	• Provide correct information verbally and in writing for patient and caregiver.
2. Patient incorrectly performs one of the postoperative exercises. Anxiety and fatigue can alter a patient's performance.	• Explain and demonstrate correct exercise technique. • Explain importance of the postoperative exercise as it pertains to patient recovery. • Instruct patient to repeat demonstration.

Communication and Documentation

• Document all preoperative patient and caregiver teaching in the nurses' notes in the electronic health record (EHR) or chart and their response to teaching.

Special Considerations
Teaching

• Nurses are responsible for ensuring that patient education material is clear, concise, in plain language, person-centred, and based on the patients' needs and abilities. In addition, the nurse must evaluate the effectiveness of the teaching (Box 37.1) (Schick & Windle, 2016).

Pediatric

• Use an age-appropriate level of communication and provide simple explanations using familiar terms.

• The use of pictures, models, equipment, and play rather than verbal explanations increases learning in preschool and school-age children.

• Teaching coughing, deep breathing, and leg exercises is not usually necessary for young children. The normal responses of crying and moving extremities will maintain lung expansion and peripheral circulation.

• Adolescents need to receive the same preoperative instructions and teaching as adults to support their developmental level.

Gerontological

• Physiological changes that occur with aging may require admission to hospital before surgery for additional diagnostic tests and stabilization of the condition (Table 37.2).

• Age-related changes in the central nervous system may diminish short-term memory. Additional time and reinforcement may be necessary for older persons to learn and comprehend information (van de Pol, Flit, Lagro, et al., 2017). The greater the number of different exposures to new material, the higher the probability that the material will be learned.

• Reinforce teaching with verbal explanations, audiovisual resources, pamphlets, and demonstrations. Consider sight and hearing deficits when providing both written and verbal instructions (van de Pol et al., 2017).

Care in the Community

• Review coughing, deep breathing, abdominal splinting, relaxation, leg exercises, and ambulation before patient admission and after discharge.

BOX 37.1

The Joint Commission Patient and Family Education Standards

Education provided is appropriate to the patient's needs. The assessment of learning needs addresses cultural and religious beliefs, emotional barriers, the desire to learn, physical or cognitive limitations, and barriers to communication as appropriate. When called for by the age of the patient and the length of stay, the hospital assesses and provides for the patient's education needs. Patients are educated about the following:

• The plan for care, treatment, and services (e.g., postoperative monitoring)

• Basic health practices and safety (e.g., out of bed [OOB] only with help)

• The safe and effective use of medication (e.g., the patient is the only one allowed to self-administer patient-controlled analgesia [PCA])

• Nutrition interventions, modified diets, or oral health (e.g., progression of diet after surgery)

• Safe and effective use of medical equipment or supplies when provided by the hospital (e.g., incentive spirometer)

• Pain—Understanding pain, the risk for pain, the importance of effective pain management, the pain-assessment process, and methods for pain management (e.g., reporting pain, frequency of medications, nonpharmacological pain-relief techniques)

• Habilitation or rehabilitation techniques to help the patient reach the maximum independence possible (e.g., early ambulation).

Modified from The Joint Commission (TJC). (2011). *Accreditation manual for hospitals.* Chicago: Author; and Schick, L., & Windle, P. (2016). *PeriAnaesthesia nursing core curriculum: Preprocedure, phase I and phase II PACU nursing* (3rd ed.). St. Louis: Saunders.

TABLE 37.2

Physiological Factors That Place Older Persons at Risk for Surgery

Alterations	Surgery Risks	Nursing Implications
Cardiovascular		
Degenerative change in myocardium and valves	Reduced cardiac reserve	Assess baseline vital signs.
Rigidity of arterial walls and reduction in sympathetic and parasympathetic innervation to the heart	Predisposes patient to postoperative hemorrhage and rise in systolic and diastolic blood pressure	Maintain adequate fluid balance to minimize stress to heart. Ensure that blood pressure is adequate to meet circulatory demands.
Increase in calcium and cholesterol deposits within small arteries; arterial walls thickened	Predisposes patient to clot formation in lower extremities	Teach patient techniques for performing leg exercises and proper turning. Apply bilateral antiembolism stockings, sequential compression devices (SCDs) (see Chapter 12).
Integumentary		
Decreased subcutaneous tissue and increased fragility of skin	Prone to pressure injuries and skin tears	Assess skin every 4 hours; pad all bony prominences during surgery. Turn or reposition (see Chapter 39).
Pulmonary		
Rib cage stiffens and enlarges	Reduced vital capacity	Teach patient proper technique for coughing and deep-breathing exercises and use of incentive spirometer.
Reduced diaphragm excursion	Greater residual capacity or volume of air left in lung after normal breath increases, reducing amount of new air brought into lungs with each inspiration	Encourage deep breathing. Use incentive spirometer to enhance exhalation.
Lung tissue is less distensible; alveoli enlarged	Reduced blood oxygenation	Assess oxygen saturation via oximetry (SpO_2).
Renal		
Reduced blood flow to kidneys	Blood loss that causes decrease in circulation to the kidney	Monitor urinary output and laboratory data (i.e., blood urea nitrogen [BUN], creatinine).
Reduced glomerular filtration rate and excretory times	Limits ability to remove medications or toxic substances	Assess for adverse effects of medications.
Reduced bladder capacity	Increase in voiding frequency; larger amount of urine stays in the bladder after voiding Sensation of need to void may not occur until bladder is filled	Instruct patient to notify nurse immediately when sensation of bladder fullness develops. Keep call light or bedpan within easy reach.
Neurological		
Sensory losses, including reduced tactile sense, increased pain tolerance	Patient is less able to respond to early warning signs of surgical complications	Inspect bony prominences for signs of pressure.
Decreased reaction time	Patient becomes confused easily after anaesthesia	Orient patient to surrounding environment. Observe for nonverbal signs of pain. Maintain a safe environment. Institute fall precautions.
Metabolic		
Lower basal metabolic rate	Reduced total oxygen consumption and nutritional needs	Ensure adequate nutritional intake once diet is resumed.
Reduced number of red blood cells and hemoglobin levels	Reduces ability to carry adequate oxygen to tissues	Administer necessary blood products. Assess for adequacy of oxygenation, fatigue, and infection.
Change in total amounts of body potassium and water volume	Greater risk for fluid or electrolyte imbalance	Monitor electrolyte levels.

✦ SKILL 37.3   Physical Preparation for Surgery

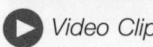 Video Clip

Preparing a patient for surgery involves activities and procedures that help to decrease anxiety, ensure patient safety, and decrease the risk for perioperative complications. The type of surgery determines the preparation required before surgery (e.g., low-residue and clear-liquid diets, enemas, cathartics, and oral antibiotics for patients who undergo bowel surgery). Smoking cessation should be encouraged, and patients should be offered nicotine substitutes. Nicotine delays wound healing, increases the risk of infection, and increases the risk for venous thromboembolism (VTE) (Rothrock, 2015). Patients whose blood work indicates a low hemoglobin level and/or abnormal electrolyte levels or coagulopathies often require inpatient therapy before surgery.

Because many patients are admitted on the day of surgery, much of the preoperative preparation is often the responsibility of the patient or the primary caregiver. Therefore it is important that a preadmission nurse or nurse in the surgeon's practice provide adequate instructions. Patient teaching should include any food and fluid restrictions; which medications, if any, are permitted on the morning of surgery; and the need for surgical site preparation the evening before surgery (see Skill 37.2). It is also important to include action that a patient will need to take if they omit any of these procedures by mistake. Written instructions are a useful adjunct to teaching because a patient and caregiver can refer to them for any points that are unclear or forgotten. Videos and pamphlets are also useful adjuncts in preparing patients and their families.

The revised Joint Commission Standards (2016) incorporated in the National Patient Safety Goals (NPSGs) implemented the Universal Protocol for Preventing Wrong Site, Wrong Procedure, Wrong Person surgery (The Joint Commission, 2016). This protocol was implemented as an added safety measure to ensure that the correct person, procedure, and surgical site are verified at the time of scheduling the procedure, on admission or entry into the facility, and each time the responsibility for care of the patient is transferred to another caregiver. A final verification check involving the entire surgical team occurs immediately before the start of the procedure. If the case involves laterality (right versus left), multiple structures (e.g., fingers, toes, lesions), or multiple levels (e.g., spine), the final verification should include a site marking by the person performing the procedure. The site markings need to be visible after the patient has been prepared and draped. Patients should be involved in this process when they are awake and aware. Immediately before starting the procedure a "time-out" is called. The entire operative team, using active communication, verifies correct patient identity, correct side and site, agreement on the procedure to be done, correct patient position, and availability of correct implants and any special equipment or special requirements. This final verification process should be documented.

Delegation and Collaboration

The skill of coordinating the patient's preparation for surgery cannot be delegated to an unregulated care provider (UCP). Depending on employer policy, the UCP may administer an enema; obtain vital signs in stable patients; apply antiembolism stockings; and help patients remove clothing, jewellery, and prostheses. The nurse instructs the UCP about:

- Using basic infection control practices and proper precautions when preparing a patient for surgery.
- Observing and using precautions if the patient has an intravenous (IV) catheter or other invasive devices in place.

Equipment

NOTE: Equipment varies by procedure prescribed.
- Vital sign equipment: stethoscope, blood pressure (BP) cuff, thermometer, pulse oximeter
- Oxygen equipment
- Suction equipment as prescribed
- Hospital gown
- IV solution and administration set (see Chapter 29)
- Skin-cleaning solution
- Compression (antiembolism) stockings (see Chapter 12)
- Intermittent compression devices (ICD)
- Venous foot pump
- Urinary catheterization kit (see Chapter 34)
- Preoperative checklist
- Medications (e.g., sedative)
- Clean gloves

STEP	RATIONALE

ASSESSMENT

STEP	RATIONALE
1. Identify patient using at least two person-specific identifiers (e.g., name and date of birth or name and medical record number), according to employer policy.	Ensures correct patient. Complies with Accreditation Canada's standards and improves patient safety (Accreditation Canada, 2019).
2. Complete preoperative assessment (see Skill 37.1).	Provides all baseline assessment data for surgical team.
3. Assess and record patient's heart rate, BP, respiratory rate, oxygen saturation, and temperature.	Provides baseline for patient's preoperative status.
4. If patient is same-day admission or an ambulatory patient, validate that admission preparations were completed as prescribed. Specific preparations to review, include NPO status, administration of medications, skin preparation, and bowel preparation, if applicable.	Failure to complete preparation could lead to perioperative or postoperative complications and may necessitate postponement or cancellation of surgery.
5. Ask if patient has advance care plan. If so, place it in their medical record.	Document conveys patient's wishes if life support measures are necessary.

STEP	RATIONALE

NURSING DIAGNOSES

- Inadequate knowledge regarding the surgical experience
- Fear
- Anxiety
- Acute pain

- Reduced oral mucous membrane
- Reduced physical mobility
- Potential for impaired skin integrity
- Potential for delayed surgical recovery
- Potential for infection

- Potential for perioperative-positioning injury
- Potential for disturbed body image

Related factors/Risk factors are individualized on the basis of patient's condition or needs.

PLANNING

1. Expected outcomes following completion of procedure:

- Patient can state which surgical procedure is being performed and risks and benefits of surgery.

Identifies preparation for informed consent.

- Patient states that anxiety is decreased.

Decreased anxiety increases participation.

IMPLEMENTATION

1. Perform hand hygiene. Help patient put on hospital gown and remove personal items. Patients are often anxious before surgery. Before any procedure, decrease their anxiety by explaining how equipment or preparation will feel (e.g., cold, tight) before touching patient.

Reduces transmission of infection. Allows patient to orient to surroundings and understand presurgical procedures.

2. Instruct patient to remove makeup, nail polish, hairpins, and jewellery.

Hair appliances and jewelry anywhere on the body may become dislodged and cause injury during positioning and intubation. Rings decrease circulation in fingers. Makeup, nail polish, and false nails impede assessment of skin and oxygenation. In addition, acrylic nails harbour pathogenic organisms (Rothrock, 2015).

3. Ensure that money and valuables have been locked up or given to a caregiver.

Patient may not return to the same location after surgery. Prevents valuables from being misplaced or lost.

4. Ensure that patient has followed appropriate fluid and food restrictions per surgeon or anaesthesiologist prescription (see Skill 37.2).

Extent and type of restriction vary by employer policy and health care provider. Under general anaesthesia, sphincters in the stomach relax, and contents can reflux into esophagus and trachea.

5. Verify presence of allergies and ensure that allergy/sensitivity band or other safety armbands are present.

Alerts surgeons and health care team to potential allergies and risk of falls.

6. Verify that patient has followed instructions about omission or ingestion of medications as instructed.

Missed or inaccurate dosage could precipitate complications.

7. Verify that bowel preparation (e.g., laxative, cathartic, enema) has been completed by patient or caregiver at home, if prescribed.

Proper bowel evacuation is needed for surgery to be performed.

Clinical Decision Point *In some situations, additional enemas and/or cathartics are prescribed. Emptying the bowel is necessary for bowel surgery and to decrease the risk of postoperative ileus. Enemas are used when surgery is near the lower intestine.*

8. Ensure that medical history and physical examination results are in the patient's record.

Ensures that pertinent laboratory and diagnostic test results are available and that all preoperative preparations are completed (Canadian Medical Protective Association, 2018).

9. Verify that surgical consent, anaesthesia consent, and consent for blood transfusion are complete. The name of procedure; name of surgeon(s); date; name of person authorized to obtain surgical consent; signature of surgeon (or authorized person) obtaining consent, anaesthesia provider delivering anaesthesia, and witness to the patient signature; and patient's signature all should be present.

Ensures patient's agreement to undergo intended procedure. In most settings the surgeon obtains consent, and the nurse verifies that it is complete and consistent with the patient's understanding (refer to employer policy).

10. Ensure that necessary laboratory work, electrocardiogram (ECG), and chest X-ray film studies are completed and results are on chart.

Diagnostic test results may indicate a medical problem and provide data for postoperative comparison.

STEP	RATIONALE

IMPLEMENTATION

11. Verify that blood type and cross-match are completed if prescribed by surgeon and that blood transfusions are available as needed.

In many cases surgery cannot begin without availability of blood units.

12. Instruct patient to void.

Prevents risk of bladder distension or rupture during surgery.

13. Initiate IV therapy; refer to employer policy or surgeon's prescriptions (see Chapter 29).

An IV line provides access for fluids and medications to be administered to patient when in the operating room (OR).

14. Administer preoperative medications as prescribed (e.g., preoperative antibiotics, prophylactic medications).

Preoperative medications are used for various reasons and should be administered as prescribed for maximum effectiveness.

15. Apply compression stockings, if prescribed (see Chapter 12).

Compression stockings promote circulation during periods of immobilization, reducing risk of embolism.

16. Apply intermittent compression devices (ICDs) if prescribed. **NOTE:** ICDs may or may not be used in combination with compression stockings. Verify prescription.

ICDs push blood from superficial veins into deep veins, decreasing venous stasis.

Clinical Decision Point *ICDs do not provide effective deep vein thrombosis (DVT) prophylaxis if the device is not applied correctly or if the patient does not wear the device continuously except during bathing, skin assessment, and ambulation. ICDs are not to be worn when a patient has an active DVT because of risk of pulmonary embolism.*

17. Perform hand hygiene. Apply clean gloves. Clean and prepare surgical site if prescribed.

Cleaning with antimicrobial soap decreases bacterial flora on skin.

18. Perform hand hygiene. Insert urinary catheter if prescribed (see Chapter 34). **NOTE:** There are times when a urinary catheter is placed in the OR.

Maintains bladder decompression and provides for monitoring output during surgery.

19. Allow patient to wear eyeglasses or a hearing aid as long as possible before surgery so the patient is able to sign consents and read materials. Remove contact lenses, eyeglasses, hairpieces, and dentures just before surgery (see checklist completed before surgery noting that all items are removed before proceeding to OR).

These aids facilitate patient cooperation by ensuring that the patient has clear vision and maximal auditory perception throughout the preoperative phase.

20. Place cap over patient's head and hair.

The cap contains hair and minimizes OR contamination during surgery. Plastic or reflective caps reduce heat loss during surgery.

21. Place patient on bed rest with call light within reach and inform them not to get out of bed without help. Allow family members to remain at the bedside until patient is transferred to surgical area. Maintain a quiet and relaxing environment.

There is an increased chance of injury when patient tries to ambulate to void when sedated and unattended.

22. Help patient onto stretcher for transport to the OR.

Some ambulatory surgery patients walk to the OR.

EVALUATION

1. Have patient describe surgical procedure and its benefits and risks.

Confirms level of knowledge needed to sign informed consent.

2. Have patient repeat preoperative instructions.

Provides evidence that patient understands instructions.

STEP	RATIONALE

EVALUATION

3. Monitor patient for signs and symptoms of anxiety and ask how patient and family are feeling.	Increased heart rate and blood pressure, dilated pupils, dry mouth, increased sweating, and muscle rigidity or shaking are responses to stress and anxiety. Asking patient about feelings gives them permission to express concerns, which can be further explored.
4. **Use Teach-Back:** "I want to be sure you understand what will happen after your surgery. Tell me what you expect to happen once you get to the recovery room." Develop a revised teaching plan if patient is not able to teach back correctly.	Determines patient's level of understanding of instructional topic.

Unexpected Outcomes	Related Interventions
1. Patient is unable to give consent, and family member is unavailable.	• In emergencies, obtain telephone consent from next of kin. Two people must witness oral consent (see employer policy). • Document explanation of situation and fact that oral consent was obtained and witnessed. • At earliest opportunity, person giving oral consent must sign written consent. A signed telegram or signed fax may also be considered oral consent. Follow employer policy.
2. Patient did not remain NPO, which may place them at risk for aspiration and may indicate that they did not understand instructions or forgot.	• Use interprofessional collaboration (e.g., surgeon, anaesthesiologist) to discuss food and fluid intake. Surgery may be postponed or cancelled.
3. Informed consent has not been signed and witnessed. Surgeon and anaesthesiologist did not provide information or ensure that consent forms were signed.	• Patient is not ready for surgery. Patient must sign consent before administration of preoperative medications or any medication that alters the central nervous system. Notify health care provider, surgeon, and anaesthesiologist.
4. Vital signs are above or below the patient's baseline or expected range.	• May indicate infection, pain, anxiety, or cardiovascular dysfunction. Notify surgeon and anaesthesiologist.
5. Patient did not void.	• Patient did not need to void or was unable to void. Assess for bladder distension.

Communication and Documentation

- Document preoperative physical preparation on preoperative checklist in the electronic health record (EHR) or chart.
- Document disposition of patient valuables and belongings (i.e., whether locked up according to employer policy or given to caregiver) in the EHR or chart.
- Report lack of signed and witnessed consent form or failure of patient to maintain NPO status and action taken.
- Document your evaluation of patient and caregiver learning.

Special Considerations
Pediatric
- Give the child as many choices related to procedures as possible.

- Keep parent–child separation to the minimum time possible. When a parent or guardian cannot be present, it is important to leave a favourite possession with the child.
- Allow the parent or guardian to accompany their child to the surgery holding area.

Gerontological
- Some older persons may have cognitive, sensory, or physical impairments and it may take an older person more time to dress for surgery and complete the needed physical preparation.

◆ SKILL 37.4	**Providing Immediate Anaesthesia Recovery in the Postanaesthesia Care Unit**

The first phase of postoperative care takes place during the immediate recovery period. This phase extends from the time the patient leaves the operating room (OR) to the time they are is stabilized in the postanaesthesia care unit (PACU), meets discharge criteria, and is transferred to the nursing unit.

The first 1 to 2 hours are the most critical period for assessing the aftereffects of anaesthesia, including airway clearance, cardiovascular complications, temperature control, and neurological function (Table 37.3). A patient's condition can change rapidly; assessments must be timely, knowledgeable, and accurate. Nurses

TABLE 37.3

Postanaesthesia Monitoring and Management of Complications

Condition	Interventions
Airway	
Mechanical obstruction: Decreased LOC and muscle relaxants, resulting in flaccid muscles and tongue blocking airway	Hyperextend neck; pull mandible forward; use nasal or oral airway; encourage deep breathing.
Retained thick secretions: Irritation from anaesthesia; anticholinergic medications; history of smoking	Suction; encourage coughing.
Laryngospasm: Stridor from excessive secretions or airway irritation	Encourage patient to relax and breathe through the mouth. If extreme, it may require positive-pressure ventilation with oxygen, a small dose of muscle relaxant (prescribed by anaesthesiologist), and intubation.
Laryngeal edema: Allergic reaction, irritation from ET tube, fluid overload	Administer humidified oxygen, antihistamines, steroids, sedatives; in some cases, perform reintubation.
Bronchospasm: Pre-existing asthma, anaesthetic irritation (expiratory wheeze)	Administer bronchodilators as prescribed.
Aspiration: Vomiting from hypotension, accumulated gastric secretions and delayed gastric emptying, pain, fear, position changes	Position patient on side; suction airway; administer antiemetic as prescribed.
Breathing: Hypoventilation/Hypoxemia	
CNS depression: Anaesthesia, analgesics, muscle relaxants (respiratory rate shallow)	Encourage patient to cough and deep breathe; use mechanical ventilator; administer narcotic antagonist and muscle-relaxant reversal medication.
Mechanical restriction: Obesity, pain, tight cast or dressings, abdominal distension	Reposition patient; give analgesic; loosen cast or dressings; implement measures to reduce gastric distension (e.g., NG intubation, NG suction).
Circulation	
Hypovolemia: Blood loss, dehydration	Administer IV fluids or blood replacement.
Hypotension: Anaesthesia/drug effects, vasodilation (possibly from spinal anaesthesia), narcotics	Elevate patient's legs; give oxygen, IV fluids, or blood replacement; administer vasopressors; monitor I&O, stimulation, hemoglobin, and hematocrit.
Cardiac failure: Pre-existing cardiac disease; circulatory overload; excessive/too-rapid fluid replacement	Provide digitalization and diuretics; monitor ECG.
Cardiac arrhythmias: Hypoxemia; MI; hypothermia; imbalance of potassium, calcium, magnesium	Provide IV fluid replacement; monitor ECG and urine output; identify and treat cause.
Hypertension: Pain, distended bladder, pre-existing hypertension, vasopressor medications	Compare with preoperative baseline; identify and determine cause.
Compartment syndrome: Pressure from edema causing enough compression to obstruct arterial and venous circulation resulting in ischemia, permanent numbness, loss of function; forearm and lower leg are most common sites	Obtain compartment pressures to diagnose, and elevate extremity no higher than heart level; remove or loosen bandage or cast to relieve compression; if left untreated, amputation may be required. Do not apply ice.

CNS, Central nervous system; *ECG,* electrocardiogram; *ET,* endotracheal; *I&O,* intake and output; *IV,* intravenous; *LOC,* level of consciousness; *MI,* myocardial infarction; *NG,* nasogastric.

need to be aware of the common complications and problems associated with the specific types of anaesthesia (Table 37.4). Quick judgement regarding the most appropriate interventions is essential. A patient is usually ready for discharge to the general unit when specific standardized criteria are met. The Aldrete score is one of several scoring systems for assessment (Table 37.5). It uses parameters of activity, respiration, circulation, consciousness, and oxygen saturation. A score of 8 or less indicates that additional monitoring is required. A score of 10 indicates full recovery of the patient.

Recovery from ambulatory surgery requires the same assessments. However, the depth of general anaesthesia may be less because the surgery is less involved and of shorter duration. Some patients have only intravenous (IV) conscious sedation, and intensive monitoring is required for a shorter time period. As soon as the patient is

stable and alert, the nurse needs to give instructions for home care to the patient and caregiver, including demonstrations and written instructions.

Delegation and Collaboration

The skill of initiating immediate anaesthesia recovery of a patient cannot be delegated to an unregulated care provider UCP. The UCP may provide basic comfort and hygiene measures. The nurse instructs the UCP by:

- Explaining any restrictions for how to provide comfort measures (e.g., repositioning, turning, applying warming blanket).
- Offering instruction in providing needed supplies.

NOTE: Other appropriate personnel may be allowed to do more in ambulatory surgery recovery, such as provide initial by-mouth (PO) liquids—always refer to employer policy.

TABLE 37.4

Focused Assessment of Patient Problems Related to Anaesthesia Type

Anaesthesia Type	Focused Assessment
General	Hypotension; changes in heart rate or rhythm; lowered body temperature; respiratory depression; emergence delirium in the form of shivering, trembling, confusion, or hallucinations
Spinal	Headache, hypotension, decreased cardiac output, cyanosis, difficulty breathing
Local	Skin rash; allergic reaction with edema of the face, lips, mouth, or throat; restlessness; bradycardia; hypotension; ischemic necrosis at injection site
Conscious sedation	Respiratory depression, bradycardia, hypotension, nausea and vomiting
Epidural	Cyanosis, breathing difficulties, decreased heart rate, irregular heart rate, pale skin colour, nausea and vomiting

Data from Lilley, L. L., Collins, S. R., & Snyder, J. S. (2014). *Pharmacology and the nursing process* (7th ed.). St. Louis: Mosby; and Rothrock, J. C. (2015). *Alexander's care of the patient in surgery* (15th ed.). St. Louis: Mosby.

TABLE 37.5

Aldrete Score for Postanaesthesia Monitoring

		Score
Respirations	Able to deep breathe and cough freely	2
	Dyspnea or limited breathing	1
	Apneic	0
O_2 Saturation	Able to maintain O_2 saturation >92% on room air	2
	Requires supplemental O_2 to maintain SpO_2 >90%	1
	O_2 saturation <90% even with supplemental O_2	0
Circulation	BP +/− 20% of preoperative level	2
	BP +/− 20–50% of preoperative level	1
	BP +/− >50% of preoperative level	0
Consciousness	Awake and oriented	2
	Wakens with stimulation	1
	Not responding	0
Movement	Moves four limbs on own	2
	Moves two limbs on own	1
	Moves no limbs on own	0

BP, Blood pressure; *O_2*, oxygen; *SpO_2*, pulse oximetry.
From College of Physicians and Surgeons of British Columbia. (2017). *Accreditation standards patient care: Post-anesthesia care (Appendix D)*. Retrieved from https://www.cpsbc.ca/files/pdf/NHMSFAP-AS-Post-Anesthesia-Care.pdf.

Equipment

- Equipment for physical assessment
- Various types and sizes of artificial airways
- Constant and intermittent suction
- Oxygen equipment such as mask, oxygen regulator and tubing, and positive-pressure delivery system
- Pulse oximeter
- End-tidal carbon dioxide (CO_2) monitor
- Blood pressure (BP) monitoring equipment
- Adjustable lighting
- Electrocardiogram (ECG) monitor
- Arterial blood gas supplies
- Bladder scanner

- Bedside portable ultrasound to assess pulses
- Thermoregulation equipment, including thermometers, blanket warmers, and cooling blankets
- IV supplies (if prescribed) (see Chapter 29)
- Adult and pediatric emergency cart with defibrillator
- Stock supplies (e.g., facial tissues, dressings, bedpans, urinals, emesis basins)
- Personal protective equipment
- Latex-free supplies and equipment

STEP	RATIONALE

ASSESSMENT

1. Identify patient using at least two person-specific identifiers (e.g., name and date of birth or name and medical record number), according to employer policy.

Ensures correct patient. Complies with Accreditation Canada's standards and improves patient safety (Accreditation Canada, 2019).

2. Receive hand-off report from circulating nurse and anaesthesia provider, including procedure performed, range of vital signs, any complications, estimated blood loss (EBL), other fluid loss, fluid replacement during surgery, type of anaesthesia, medications given, type of airway and size, extent of surgical wound, restrictions to movement of position during surgery, and any preoperative medical and nursing diagnoses.

Determines patient's general status and allows nurse to anticipate type of assessment needed, the need for special equipment, potential treatment measures, and nursing care interventions in PACU.

3. On patient's arrival in PACU, review surgeon's prescriptions.

Allows nurse to focus on priority interventions; assists nurse in organizing care.

4. Consider type of surgical procedure, restrictions to movement, and type of anaesthesia used.

Influences type of assessments necessary, type of complications for which to observe, and specific nursing interventions needed.

STEP	RATIONALE

ASSESSMENT

5. Perform hand hygiene. Perform thorough patient assessment, including vital signs; pulse oximetry; pain; assessment of body systems to include respiratory, cardiac, neurological, gastrointestinal (GI), genitourinary (GU), and metabolic; and fluid status. Assess patient's surgical site and drains, skin integrity, safety, and anxiety level.

Reduces transmission of infection. Provides baseline for ongoing postoperative evaluations. Identifies priority nursing interventions.

6. Take vital signs and monitor pulse oximetry during initial stabilization (ASPAN, 2015).

Monitors patient stability.

7. Discharge from phase I level of care is based on specific criteria, not a time limit. Criteria should address assessment of airway patency, oxygenation, hemodynamic stability, thermoregulation, neurological stability, intake and output (I&O), tube patency, dressings, pain and comfort management, and postanaesthesia scoring system if used. See employer policy for required frequency of assessment.

Discharge instructions are developed in consultation with anaesthesia department.

Clinical Decision Point *Be sure to turn patient on side (when possible) to observe underlying skin and accumulation of blood or serous drainage not visible otherwise.*

NURSING DIAGNOSES

- Inadequate airway clearance
- Inadequate breathing pattern
- Inadequate spontaneous ventilation
- Inadequate tissue perfusion
- Acute pain
- Inadequate gas exchange

- Inadequate swallowing
- Inadequate fluid volume
- Excessive fluid overload
- Inadequate thermoregulation
- Acute confusion
- Inadequate skin integrity

- Inadequate physical mobility
- Reduced verbal communication
- Inadequate protection
- Potential for aspiration
- Potential for urinary retention

Related factors/Risk factors are individualized on the basis of patient's condition or needs.

PLANNING

1. Expected outcomes following completion of procedure:
   - Patient's airway remains clear; respirations are deep, regular, and within normal limits by time of transfer. Oxygen saturation remains greater than 95%.

No occurrence of pulmonary changes except those expected from effects of anaesthetic or analgesic.

   - Patient's BP, pulse, and temperature remain within previous baseline or normal expected range by time of transfer.

No occurrence of cardiovascular, pulmonary, or thermoregulatory changes except those expected from effects of anaesthetic or analgesic.

   - Dressings are clean, dry, and intact by discharge from recovery.

Indicates wound stabilization without signs of bleeding or infection.

   - I&O is within expected parameters by discharge from recovery.

Adequate urinary elimination is maintained. Fluid intake (IV and/or PO) is adequately maintained.

   - Patient reports relief of discomfort after receiving analgesia or other pain-relief measures by time of transfer from immediate recovery area (usually 1 to 2 hours).

Pain-relief measures effectively alter patient's reception or perception of pain.

   - Patient's postoperative assessments are within expected normal postoperative parameters.

Patient is stable and may be prepared for the next phase of postoperative recovery.

2. Perform hand hygiene and prepare equipment for continued monitoring and care activities.

Reduces transmission of infection.

IMPLEMENTATION

1. While receiving hand-off report as patient enters PACU on stretcher or bed, immediately attach oxygen tubing to regulator, hang IV fluids, and check IV flow rates. Connect any drainage tubes to gravity drainage or continuous or intermittent suction as prescribed. Attach cardiac monitor. Ensure that in-dwelling catheter and bag are in drainage position and patent.

Maintaining oxygenation and circulation are two priorities. Inhaled oxygen improves the percentage of oxygen delivered to alveoli. IV fluids maintain circulatory volume and provide a route for emergency medications. Drainage tubes must remain patent and in proper position to allow fluid to drain.

STEP	RATIONALE

IMPLEMENTATION

2. Continue ongoing assessment of all vital signs every 5 to 15 minutes until patient stabilizes or more frequently if clinically indicated (see employer protocol). Compare findings with patient's baseline. Provide warm blankets as needed for patient comfort.

Vital signs reveal onset of postoperative complications from surgery or anaesthesia (e.g., respiratory depression, hypo- or hyperthermia, pulse irregularity, or hypotension). Acute blood loss may lead to hypovolemic shock with signs of reduced BP, elevated heart and respiratory rates, pale skin, and restlessness. General anaesthetic may affect the temperature-regulating centre, and a lower metabolic rate causes hypothermia. Malignant hyperthermia is a rare inherited condition that develops after receiving an anaesthetic and is a medical emergency (Rothrock 2015; Schick & Windle, 2016).

Clinical Decision Point *If the patient underwent a short procedure under procedural sedation, check employer policy for sedation recovery guidelines. The perianaesthesia registered nurse (RN) monitoring a patient who receives procedural sedation/analgesia should have no other responsibilities that compromise continuous patient monitoring. The nurse should monitor oxygenation until the patient is no longer at risk for hypoxemia. Ventilation and circulation are monitored at regular intervals until patients are suitable for discharge (NAPANc, 2018).*

3. Maintain patent airway after general anaesthesia.

  a. Position patient on their side with head facing down and neck slightly extended (see illustration). Never position a patient with hands over chest (reduces chest expansion).

Ensures appropriate oxygenation.

Extension prevents occlusion of airway at the pharynx. Downward position of head moves the tongue forward, and mucus or vomitus can drain out of the mouth, preventing aspiration.

Clinical Decision Point *Always stay with a sedated patient until respirations are well established. Patients with an artificial airway may gag and vomit, become restless, or stop breathing. Closely monitor patients with a history of obstructive sleep apnea.*

  b. Place a small folded towel or small pillow under the patient's head. If patient is restricted to a supine position, elevate head of bed approximately 10 to 15 degrees, extend patient's neck, and turn their head to the side. Have emesis basin available if patient becomes nauseated.

Supports head in extended position. Prevents aspiration if patient should vomit.

Clinical Decision Point *If the patient is not able to extend their neck, turn their head to the side, if possible; suction the oropharynx (see Chapter 25) frequently.*

  c. Encourage patient to cough and deep breathe on awakening and every 15 minutes.

  d. Suction artificial airway and oral cavity as secretions accumulate.

  e. Once gag reflex returns, have patient spit out oral airway (see illustration). Do not tape oral airway.

Promotes lung expansion and expectoration of mucous secretions.

Clears airway of secretions.

Indicates that patient can clear airway independently. If airway is taped, patient will gag and may obstruct the airway.

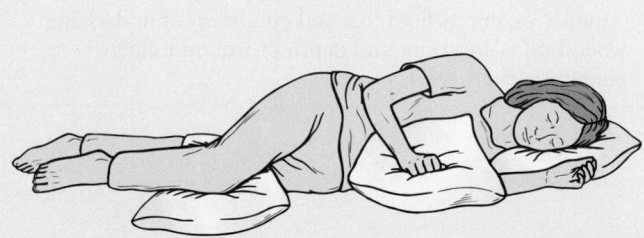

STEP 3a Position of patient during recovery from general anaesthesia.

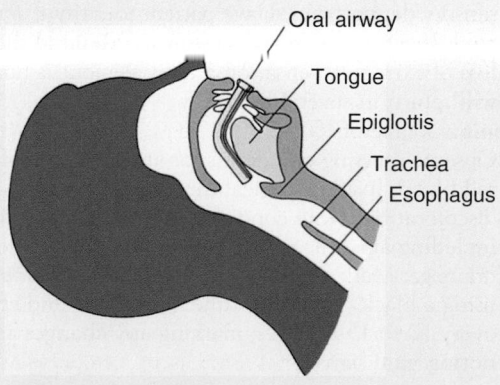

Oral airway
Tongue
Epiglottis
Trachea
Esophagus

STEP 3e Oral airway position before removal.

STEP	RATIONALE

IMPLEMENTATION

f. Avoid rapid position changes in patients who had spinal anaesthesia, which can cause changes in the patient's BP. Good body alignment is needed. Maintain IV infusion. Encourage fluid intake (only if patient can take fluids, such as with ambulatory surgery).	Rapid movements are avoided so as not to cause spinal headache from loss of cerebrospinal fluid. Increased IV or PO fluids help the body replace cerebrospinal fluid.

Clinical Decision Point *Because of the shorter half-life of medications used today, many patients have the oral airway removed before leaving the OR. PACU nurse must assess that respiratory effort is adequate; otherwise the airway may need to be replaced, and the patient may need a ventilator.*

4. Call patient by name in a normal tone of voice. If there is no response, attempt to arouse patient by touching or gently moving a body part. Explain that surgery is over and that the patient is in the recovery area.	Determines patient's level of consciousness and ability to follow commands.
5. Assess circulatory perfusion by inspecting colour of nail beds, mucous membranes, and skin. Palpate for skin temperature. Test for capillary refill (see Chapter 8).	Pink or normal colour of skin, nail beds, and mucous membranes and brisk (3 seconds or less) capillary refill indicate adequate perfusion. Warm extremities indicate adequate circulation.
6. Inspect colour of nail beds and skin. Palpate for skin temperature.	Indicators of peripheral tissue perfusion.
7. Assess closely for any behavioural or clinical changes reflecting potential cardiovascular and pulmonary complications of general anaesthesia (see Table 37.3). Monitor laboratory findings.	Postoperative patients who are sedated often become hypoxic.
8. If patient had general anaesthesia: As patient arouses, introduce yourself and orient them to surroundings.	
9. Monitor sensory, circulatory, pulmonary, and neurological responses after spinal or epidural anaesthesia.	Reflects return of spinal function.
a. Monitor for hypotension, bradycardia, and nausea and vomiting.	Blockage of the sympathetic nervous system results in vasodilation of major vessels and systemic hypotension.
b. Maintain adequate IV infusion.	Maintains BP by increasing fluid volume and fills temporarily expanded vascular space.
c. Keep patient supine or with head slightly elevated and maintain position.	Minimizes risk of postspinal anaesthesia headache from leakage of spinal fluid at injection site, with increased pressures caused by elevation of upper body. Headache is more common with spinal than epidural anaesthesia (Lewis et al., 2019).
d. Observe patients in PACU until they regain movement in extremities.	Patients fear permanent loss of function.
e. Assess respiratory status, level of spinal sensation, and mobility in lower extremities. Drowsiness will be apparent after IV sedation. Level of anaesthesia depends on location of sensation change. Have patient close eyes and use alcohol wipe to test sensation along sensory dermatomes. Have patient identify if warm or cold. *If patient had spinal anaesthesia:* Remind them that loss of extremity sensation and movement is normal and will return in several hours.	Spinal block is set within 20 minutes of onset. However, if level of anaesthesia moves above sixth thoracic vertebra (T6), respiratory muscles are affected. Patients often feel short of breath and may require mechanical ventilation if respiratory muscles are severely affected.
10. Monitor source of I&O.	
a. Observe dressing and drains for any evidence of bright red blood. Inspect surgical incision for swelling or discoloration. Note condition of surgical dressing, including amount, colour, odour, and consistency of drainage. Mark dressing with circle around drainage using a black pen. Place time of marking and check area every 10 to 15 minutes, marking any changes and noting vital signs.	Determines extent of fluid loss and condition of underlying wound. Size, location, and depth of wound influence amount of drainage.

STEP	RATIONALE

IMPLEMENTATION

b. Reinforce pressure dressing or change simple dressing if prescribed (see Chapter 40). Continue to monitor condition of incision, surrounding tissue, and amount and colour of any drainage if incision is exposed or covered with transparent dressing.

Pressure dressing should not be removed because it helps to maintain hemostasis (termination of bleeding) and absorb drainage. Changing dressings immediately after surgery can disrupt wound edges and aggravate drainage. The first dressing changes most often occur 24 hours after surgery and are usually done by the surgeon. Minor surgical wounds may not have dressings but simply skin closure; or wounds may be covered with a transparent dressing, which allows for observation of the incision and surrounding tissue (Rothrock, 2015).

c. Inform surgeon of unexpected bloody drainage and reinforce dressing as indicated. Apply direct pressure. Also look underneath patient for any pooling of bloody drainage. Monitor for decreased BP and increased pulse.

Progressive increase or changes in characteristics of drainage warrant a call to the surgeon because they could indicate hemorrhage (Lewis et al., 2019; Schick & Windle, 2016). Hemorrhage from a surgical wound is most likely within the first few hours, indicating inadequate hemostasis during surgery. As the dressing becomes saturated, blood often oozes down the patient's side and collects underneath them.

d. Inspect condition and contents of any drainage tubes and collecting devices. Note character and volume of drainage.

Determines patency of drainage tube and extent of wound drainage.

e. Observe amount, colour, and appearance of urine from in-dwelling Foley catheter (if present).

Urine output of less than 30 mL/hr is a sign of decreased renal perfusion or altered renal function.

f. If a nasogastric (NG) tube is present, assess drainage. If it is not draining, check placement and irrigate it if necessary with normal saline (see Chapter 35).

Maintains patency of tube to ensure gastric decompression. Expected drainage is dark or pale, yellow, or green and 100 to 200 mL/hr. Bloody drainage occurs after some surgeries.

g. Monitor and maintain IV fluid rates. Observe IV site for signs of infiltration (see Chapter 29).

Provides adequate hydration and circulatory function.

11. Promote comfort.

a. Provide mouth care by placing a moistened washcloth to the lips, swabbing oral mucosa with a dampened swab or soft toothbrush, or applying petrolatum to the lips.

The mouth is dry from NPO status and preoperative anticholinergics such as atropine.

b. Provide a warm blanket or active rewarming therapy to promote warmth and minimize shivering.

General anaesthesia impairs thermoregulation, the OR environment is cold, and exposure of body cavity results in internal heat loss. Shivering increases oxygen consumption, predisposes patient to arrhythmias and hypertension, impairs platelet function, alters drug metabolism, impairs wound healing, and increases hospitalization costs because of cumulative adverse outcomes (NAPANc, 2018).

c. Help with position changes and provide supportive pillows.

Improves ventilation and circulation.

12. Continue monitoring pain as the patient awakens and until transfer to the surgical unit or discharge, including quality, severity, and location (see Chapter 16). Do not assume that all postoperative pain is incisional pain.

Pain is often not directly related to the surgical procedure (e.g., chest pain [myocardial infarction or pulmonary embolism] or muscle pain [trauma from positioning]). Referred pain (in shoulder) often occurs after laparoscopy. Systematic assessment of pain helps patients achieve functional status

a. Provide pain medication as prescribed and when vital signs have stabilized.

Promotes patient comfort.

13. Explain patient's condition to patient and inform them of plans for transfer to nursing unit or discharge.

Decreases anxiety that can interfere with recovery process.

14. When patient's condition stabilizes, contact the anaesthesiologist to approve care transition (i.e., transfer to nursing unit or discharge to home).

The surgeon is responsible for authorizing transfer or discharge.

15. Before discharge to home from an ambulatory surgery unit, provide verbal and written instructions (Box 37.2).

Patients and home care providers must be aware of potential complications and follow-up care.

Clinical Decision Point *If the patient is to be discharged to home, ensure that the patient has someone to drive them home and observe them for signs and symptoms of complications. Review with the patient and driver reportable signs and symptoms and emergency care needed.*

STEP	RATIONALE

EVALUATION

1. Compare all vital sign assessment measurements with patient's baseline and expected normal levels.

Evaluates patient's respiratory, cardiovascular, and thermoregulatory status throughout recovery.

2. Inspect surgical wound and dressings for drainage. Be sure to assess for wound drainage under patient.

Provides data to measure progress of wound healing.

3. Measure I&O. Urine output should be at least 30 to 50 mL/hr.

Indicates onset of fluid imbalances.

4. Auscultate bowel sounds and ask if patient has passed flatus.

Allows you to evaluate return of peristalsis and diet tolerance.

5. Measure patient's perception of pain after implementing pain-relief measures such as positioning and use of analgesics.

Determines level of comfort achieved and effectiveness of pain-relief measures.

6. Complete system-specific physical assessments as appropriate according to patient's unique type of surgery (e.g., craniotomy—neurological assessment; neck surgery—airway status; vascular surgery—circulation and bleeding; orthopaedic surgery—neurovascular status and immobility or positioning).

Allows you to monitor course of recovery.

7. **Use Teach-Back:** "I want to be sure you know what to expect when you go home. Tell me the signs and symptoms to expect if you were to get an infection?" Develop a revised teaching plan if patient or caregiver is not able to teach back correctly.

Determines patient's and caregiver's level of understanding of instructional topic.

Unexpected Outcomes

1. Patient exhibits respiratory depression (pulse oximetry <95%, respiratory rate <10 breaths/min or shallow).

2. Patient exhibits signs of hypovolemia related to internal or incisional hemorrhage.

Related Interventions

- Promptly report to surgeon.
- Administer oxygen as prescribed by nasal cannula. Give patients with chronic obstructive pulmonary disease (COPD) 2 L/min or less of oxygen.
- Encourage deep breathing every 5 to 15 minutes.
- Position patient to promote chest expansion (on side or semi-Fowler's).
- Administer prescribed medications (e.g., epinephrine, muscle relaxant, narcotic reversal medication).
- Elevate patient's legs enough to maintain downward slope toward trunk of body. Do not lower head past flat position because this position increases respiratory effort and potentially decreases cerebral perfusion.
- Promptly report patient's present status to surgeon.
- Administer oxygen at 6 to 10 L/min by mask per prescription.
- Increase rate of IV fluid or administer blood products as prescribed.
- Monitor BP and pulse every 5 to 15 minutes.
- Apply pressure dressings as follows per prescription
- *Abdominal dressing:* Cover bleeding area with several thicknesses of gauze compresses and place tape 7 to 10 cm (3 to 4 inches) beyond width of dressing with firm, even pressure on both sides close to the bleeding source. Maintain pressure as you tape the entire dressing to maximize pressure at source of bleeding.
- *Dressing on extremity:* Apply rolled gauze, pressing gauze compress over bleeding site. Do not continue tape around entire extremity.
- *Dressing in neck region:* Cover with several thicknesses of gauze and place tape 7 to 10 cm (3 to 4 inches) beyond width of dressing. Apply with pressure but do not occlude carotid artery or airway. Assess every 5 to 15 minutes for carotid pulse and evidence of airway obstruction.
- Patient remains NPO because it is often necessary to return to surgery for control of bleeding.

BOX 37.2

Postanaesthesia and Ambulatory Surgery Discharge Criteria

Postanaesthesia Discharge Criteria

- Patient awake (or returns to baseline)
- Vital signs stable
- No excess bleeding or drainage
- No respiratory depression
- SaO$_2$ greater than 90%
- Pain controlled
- Report given

Ambulatory Surgery Discharge Criteria

- All postanaesthesia care unit (PACU) discharge criteria met
- No intravenous (IV) narcotics for last 30 minutes
- Minimal nausea and vomiting
- Pain controlled
- Voided (if appropriate to surgical procedure/prescriptions)
- Able to ambulate if age appropriate and not contraindicated
- Responsible adult present to accompany patient
- Discharge instructions given and understood

STEP	RATIONALE
3. Patient indicates severe incisional pain; analgesic dosage may be insufficient.	• Administer analgesics; reassess and provide analgesia before pain becomes severe. • Pain sometimes lowers BP; analgesia may restore vital signs to normal. Monitor vital signs carefully. • For patients with patient-controlled analgesia (PCA), be sure that patient is using device correctly. Teach caregiver not to manipulate PCA. • *Orthopaedic surgery:* The earliest symptom of compartment syndrome in an extremity is pain unrelieved by analgesics. Other symptoms include numbness, tingling, pallor, coolness, and absent peripheral pulses. The surgeon *must* be notified. Do not elevate extremity above level of the heart because this increases venous pressure. Application of ice is contraindicated because vasoconstriction will occur (Lewis et al., 2019).
4. Vital signs are above or below the patient's baseline or expected range.	• Alterations may result from anaesthetic effects. Ensure patient is fully awake. • Medicate for pain as indicated. • Notify health care provider.
5. I&O measurements are imbalanced.	• Possible fluid volume excess or deficit. Continue to monitor and notify health care provider.

Communication and Documentation

- Document in nurses' notes in electronic health record (EHR) or chart patient's arrival time at PACU; include vital signs and other physical parameters, level of consciousness (LOC), and pain severity. Also include condition of dressings and tubes, character of drainage, and all nursing measures initiated.
- Document vital signs and I&O on appropriate flow sheets.
- Report any abnormal assessment findings and signs of complications to the health care provider and/or surgeon.
- Document your evaluation of patient and caregiver learning.

Special Considerations
Teaching

- If patient had spinal or epidural anaesthetic, remind caregiver that loss of extremity movement is normal for several hours.
- Reinforce preoperative teaching regarding coughing, deep breathing, leg exercises, and information concerning ambulation and pain control.
- Patient teaching for ambulatory surgical patients includes the following:
  - Surgeon's office and surgery centre telephone number (or appropriate 24-hour emergency contact)
  - Follow-up appointment, date, time
  - Review of prescribed medications
  - Guidelines related to specific surgery
  - Dressing and wound care
  - Pain control
  - Activity restrictions
  - Guidelines related to possible effects of anaesthesia
  - Dietary restrictions
  - Activity restrictions
  - Signs and symptoms of complications

Pediatric

- Maintenance of body temperature in infants and children after surgery is a priority because of their immature temperature-control mechanisms.

- Infants and children normally have higher metabolic rates and differences in physiological makeup than adults, resulting in greater oxygen, fluid, and calorie needs.
- Vomiting is a major concern in young children because of increased risk for fluid and electrolyte imbalances and risk for aspiration. Vomiting is also more likely because surgery in children is often necessitated by accidental injuries without benefit of NPO status.
- Keep parent–child separation to a minimum. If the parent or guardian cannot be present, leave a favourite possession with the child.
- Refer to NAPANc (2018) Resource 6: PeriAnesthesia Care of the Pediatric Client.

Gerontological

- The ability of older persons to tolerate surgery depends on the extent of physiological changes that have occurred with aging, the presence of any chronic diseases, and the duration of the surgical procedure.
- When communicating with older persons, be aware of any auditory, visual, or cognitive impairment that may be present.
- Refer to NAPANc (2018): Appendix N: Alterations of Aging Clients and Effect of Anesthesia on Geriatric Response.

Care in the Community

- Teach ambulatory surgery patients and caregivers about any postoperative exercises, home modifications, or activity limitations.
- If the patient is discharged with dressing changes, suggest that the bedroom or bathroom is usually ideal for this procedure.
- Be informed as to which supports and services are available in the community where the patient lives, and provide the patient with a list of these services or where to obtain information on the services available.
- Assess need for a community health care referral. Check provincial/territorial regulations to see who is eligible to receive home care and what services community care nurses can provide in the patient's home.

✦ SKILL 37.5 Providing Early Postoperative and Convalescent-Phase Recovery

The second phase of recovery is the postoperative convalescent period. The American Society of PeriAnaesthesia Nurses (ASPAN) defines the phase II level of care as the period when the nursing roles focus on preparation for care in the home or an extended-care environment. This period extends from the time a patient is discharged from the postanaesthesia care unit (PACU) to the time they are discharged from the inpatient hospital. Outpatient surgical patients undergo convalescence at home. All patients who have undergone surgical procedures have similar postoperative needs. However, nursing care becomes very individualized and depends on the nature of a patient's surgery, pre-existing medical conditions, the onset of complications, and the speed of recovery. Not all surgical patients recover at the same rate. During the convalescent period, the nurse begins preparation for discharge and actively includes the patient and caregivers in the process. The nurse promotes the patient's independence, educates the patient and caregiver about any limitations imposed by surgery, and provides resources needed for the patient to assume an improved state of wellness.

Delegation and Collaboration

The skill of providing early postoperative and convalescent-phase recovery cannot be delegated to an unregulated care provider (UCP). The UCP may obtain vital signs (if the patient is stable), apply a nasal cannula or oxygen mask (but not adjust oxygen flow), and provide hygiene or repositioning for comfort. The nurse instructs the UCP by:

- Explaining how often to take vital signs.
- Reviewing specific safety concerns and what to observe and report back to the nurse.

- Explaining any precautions that affect how to provide basic hygiene and comfort measures.

Equipment

- Postoperative bed (recliner for day surgery recovery)
- Stethoscope, sphygmomanometer, thermometer
- Intravenous (IV) fluid poles and infusion pumps, as needed
- Emesis basin
- Washcloth and towel
- Waterproof pads
- Equipment for oral hygiene
- Pillows
- Facial tissue
- Oxygen equipment and bag-valve-masks and emergency cart with defibrillator available for adult and children
- Suction equipment (to suction airway)
- Dressing supplies
- Intermittent suction (to connect to nasogastric [NG] or wound drainage tubes)
- Orthopaedic appliances (if needed)
- Clean gloves
- Personal protective equipment (PPE) as indicated
- Malignant hyperthermia cart (Rothrock, 2015; Schick & Windle, 2016)
- Latex-free supplies and equipment
- Transport equipment, including wheelchair and cart

STEP	RATIONALE

ASSESSMENT

1. Obtain report from PACU nurse summarizing patient's current status.

2. Identify patient using at least two person-specific identifiers (e.g., name and date of birth or name and medical record number), according to employer policy.

3. On patient's arrival on nursing unit, collect a more detailed hand-off report from nurse accompanying patient.

4. Review patient's chart for information pertaining to type of surgery; complications; medications administered; preoperative medical risks; baseline vital signs, including PACU vitals; and patient's usual medications given or not given before surgery.

5. Review postoperative medical prescriptions.

6. Assess patient's and caregiver's knowledge and expectations of surgical recovery.

Allows you to prepare hospital room with necessary supplies and equipment for patient's special needs.

Ensures correct patient. Complies with Accreditation Canada's standards and improves patient safety (Accreditation Canada, 2019).

Detailed report helps nurse plan appropriate assessment and nursing care measures. Data provide baseline for detecting any change in patient's condition.

Nature of surgery, intraoperative complications, and presence of medical risks dictate complications for which to observe. Vital signs provide means for detecting postoperative changes. The list of patient's usual medications may necessitate a call to the surgeon for prescriptions concerning timing and dose of medications not given before surgery.

Offers additional guidelines for type of care to provide.

Patient will be better prepared to participate in care.

NURSING DIAGNOSES

- Reduced airway clearance
- Inadequate breathing pattern
- Reduced gas exchange
- Inadequate tissue perfusion
- Acute confusion
- Acute pain

- Dehydration
- Excessive fluid overload
- Inadequate knowledge regarding postoperative care
- Inadequate nutrition
- Inadequate physical mobility

- Reduced skin integrity
- Reduced verbal communication
- Inadequate protection
- Potential of aspiration
- Potential of urinary retention

Related factors/Risk factors are individualized on the basis of patient's condition or needs.

STEP	RATIONALE

PLANNING

1. Expected outcomes following completion of procedure:

- Patient's breath sounds remain clear bilaterally.

  No occurrence of pulmonary changes except those expected from effects of anaesthetic or analgesic.

- Patient's vital signs remain within normal limits consistent with preoperative baseline.

  No occurrence of cardiovascular, pulmonary, or thermoregulatory changes except those expected from effects of anaesthetic or analgesic.

- Incision wound edges are well approximated; no drainage is noted.

  Indicates wound healing without signs of bleeding or infection.

- Fluid balance is evident by intake and output (I&O) records.

  Adequate urinary elimination is maintained. Fluid intake (IV and/or by mouth [PO]) is adequately maintained.

- Patient describes pain as less than 4 on scale of 0 (no pain) to 10 (worst pain ever) while engaged in moderate activity by discharge.

  Pain-relief measures effectively alter patient's reception or perception of pain.

- Normal bowel sounds are present after bowel surgery or general anaesthesia within 48 to 72 hours after surgery.

  Indicates return of gastrointestinal (GI) function.

- Patient or caregiver describes signs that indicate complications that need to be reported, dietary modifications, and activity restrictions in the home. Identifies plans for follow-up visit and demonstrates incision care.

  Involves patient in plan of care and minimizes anxiety. As recovery progresses, the patient is able to make more choices regarding how procedures should be performed. The caregiver can serve as a coach or provide direct assistance and help the patient remember explanations given.

2. Perform hand hygiene and arrange equipment at bedside.

Reduces transmission of infection. Improves efficiency of care activity.

3. If patient is being transported by stretcher, prepare for transfer with bed in a high position (level with stretcher), with sheet folded to side and room for stretcher to be placed beside bed easily (see Chapter 11).

Arrangement of equipment facilitates safety and smooth transfer process.

IMPLEMENTATION

1. Early recovery initial postoperative care

a. Help transport staff, using slide board, to move patient from stretcher to bed (see Chapter 11). Identify patient using at least two person-specific identifiers (e.g., name and date of birth or name and medical record number), according to employer policy.

Ensures correct patient. Complies with Accreditation Canada's standards and improves patient safety (Accreditation Canada, 2019).

b. Attach any existing oxygen tubing, position IV fluids, verify IV flow-rate settings on infusion pump, and check drainage tubes (e.g., Foley catheter or wound drainage).

Maintains patency of IV and integrity of drainage tubing.

c. Maintain airway. If patient remains sleepy or lethargic, keep their head extended and support it in a side-lying position (see Chapter 25).

Minimizes chances of aspiration and obstruction of airway with tongue.

d. Conduct initial assessment of level of consciousness (LOC) and vital signs and compare findings with vital signs in recovery area and patient's baseline values. Continue monitoring as prescribed.

Patient's status may change during transfer. Movement of patient and their pain level influence stability of vital signs. Change in vital signs may reveal onset of postoperative complications.

e. Encourage patient coughing, deep breathing, and use of incentive spirometry and PEP device (see Skill 37.2) to prevent atelectasis.

Anaesthesia, medications, and intubation irritate airways, resulting in secretions and atelectasis. Coughing and use of devices expands chest, aerates lungs, and mobilizes secretions.

f. Assess GI system for return of bowel sounds.

Indicates return of GI function.

g. If NG tube is present, check placement and irrigate (see Chapter 35). Connect to a proper drainage device. Connect all other drainage tubes to an appropriate suction or collection device. Secure it to prevent tension on tubing.

Transfer and movement may dislodge tubes, which would interfere with drainage.

STEP	RATIONALE

IMPLEMENTATION

h. Assess patient's surgical dressing for appearance, presence, and character of drainage. Unless contraindicated by surgeon, outline drainage along edges with a pen and reassess in 1 hour for change. If no dressing is present, inspect condition of the wound (see Chapter 40).

The wound can hemorrhage quickly during the early postoperative period. Observations of wound and dressings provide data to measure progress of wound healing.

Clinical Decision Point *If unable to change dressing, mark area of drainage and label with time, date, and initials. Record frequency of reinforcement. Never use a felt-tip marker to mark the dressing because ink can bleed into gauze, contaminating the incision site.*

i. Palpate abdomen for bladder distension or use bladder ultrasound when available. If a Foley catheter is present, check placement. Ensure that it is draining freely and is properly secured. Patient may have continuous bladder irrigations or a suprapubic catheter (see Chapter 34).

Anaesthesia often contributes to urinary retention. Urinary stasis increases risk for urinary tract infection.

j. If no urinary drainage system is present, explain that voiding within 8 hours after surgery is expected. Male patients may void successfully if allowed to stand.

Anaesthetics and analgesics depress the sensation of bladder fullness. The patient may still have no sensations below the level of spinal or epidural anaesthetic.

k. Measure all sources of fluid I&O (including estimated blood loss during surgery).

Altered fluid and electrolyte balance is a potential complication of major surgery.

l. Describe purpose of equipment and frequent observations to patient and caregiver.

Unfamiliar sights (e.g., equipment, patient's appearance) often provoke anxiety.

m. Position patient for comfort, maintaining correct body alignment. Avoid tension on surgical wound site.

Reduces stress on suture line. Helps patient relax and promotes comfort.

n. Place call light within reach and raise side rails (one of two or three of four). Instruct patient to call for help to get out of bed.

Promotes patient's safety as effects of anaesthesia continue to diminish. Raising all side rails may be considered physical restraint.

o. Assess patient's level of pain on an age-appropriate pain scale. Check last time analgesic was given. Patient-controlled analgesia (PCA) may be used for pain control (see Chapter 16). Medicate patient as prescribed either around the clock or as needed (prn) as prescribed during the first 24 to 48 hours. Explain to the patient how you plan to assist with pain control; review prescriptions of what is prescribed and their frequency.

Determines level of discomfort. Adequate pain control is needed to enable patient to carry out breathing exercises, coughing, and ambulation.

2. Continued postoperative care

a. Assess vital signs at least every 4 hours or as prescribed.

Temperature greater than 38°C (100.4°F) in the first 48 hours may indicate atelectasis, the normal inflammatory response, or dehydration. A temperature greater than 37.8°C (100°F) on the third day or after often indicates wound infection, pneumonia, or phlebitis (Lewis et al., 2019). Altered blood pressure or pulse is associated with cardiovascular complications (see Table 37.3).

b. Closely monitor progress of wound healing, and change dressings as prescribed.

Wound infection occurs most often within 3 to 6 days after surgery. Wound dehiscence occurs most often 3 to 11 days after surgery (see Chapter 40).

c. Monitor drainage (see illustration A) and maintain wound drainage devices such as Jackson-Pratt, Hemovac, or Penrose drains. Jackson-Pratt and Hemovac drainage systems must be emptied when they are half full of drainage or air and recharged (compressed to discharge air) (see illustration B).

Wound drainage devices promote healing from inside to outside and relieve pressure on suture line. Compressing flexible closed container and then plugging drainage hole creates negative suction pressure.

d. Provide oral care at least every 2 hours as needed. If permitted, offer ice chips.

Medication such as an anticholinergic given before surgery makes the mouth dry. Oral care and ice chips promote comfort.

e. Encourage patient to turn, cough, deep breathe, and use incentive spirometer and PEP device at least every 2 hours (see Skill 37.2).

Promotes adequate ventilation and minimizes hypoventilation and atelectasis. This is especially necessary for patients with a history of smoking, pneumonia, or chronic obstructive pulmonary disease (COPD) or for patients who are confined to bed rest.

STEP	RATIONALE

IMPLEMENTATION

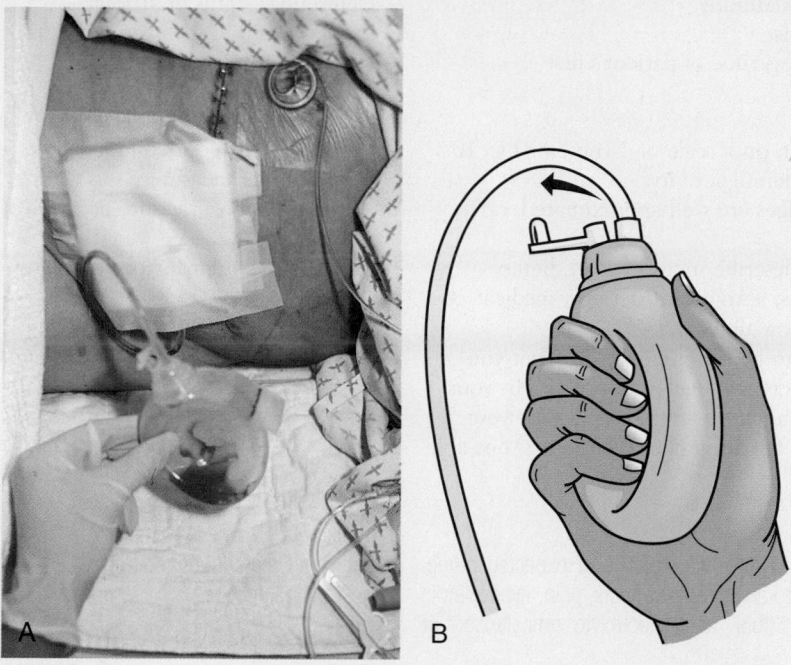

STEP 2c A, Note colour of drainage from device. **B,** Charging Jackson-Pratt drainage system.

f. Monitor function of sequential compression devices. If prescribed, apply elastic stockings to lower extremities (see Chapter 12). Explain to patient that compression device will inflate and deflate intermittently.

Stockings increase venous return (Elisha, Heiner, Nagelhout, et al., 2015). Explanation decreases anxiety and fosters cooperation.

g. Promote ambulation and activity as prescribed (see Chapter 12). Assess vital signs before and after activity to assess tolerance. Patients often are encouraged to be up in a chair the evening of surgery or the next morning and progress to walking in the room or hallway.

Ambulation is the most significant nursing intervention to prevent postoperative complications. Mobility promotes circulation, lung expansion, and peristalsis. Postural hypotension is caused by sudden position changes.

h. Progress patient's intake from clear liquids to regular diet as tolerated if nausea and vomiting do not occur.

Nausea and vomiting are associated with anaesthesia and surgery. IV fluids are usually discontinued when oral intake is tolerated. Some patients must be NPO for several days until flatus returns or bowel sounds are heard.

i. Include patient and caregiver in decision making; answer questions as they arise.

Promotes patient's sense of control and independence and improves self-esteem.

j. Provide an opportunity for patients who must adjust to change in body appearance or function to verbalize feelings.

Radical surgery, amputation, or inoperable cancer often results in anxiety and depression. Grief response to loss of a body organ is common and should be expected.

3. Convalescent phase

a. Assess patient's home environment for safety, cleanliness, and availability of community resources and help for patient. (**NOTE:** In many settings, this is done by a case manager and not a staff nurse. Use the information to revise any teaching you provide.)

Provides information about patient's need for home care. Verifies patient's and caregiver's level of knowledge and any additional teaching needs for discharge. Helps to promote uncomplicated discharge and patient's independence and participation in care.

b. Provide instruction on care activities that patient or caregiver will perform at home (e.g., dressing change, medication administration, exercises, IV therapy).

Enables patient to achieve self-care at home.

c. Keep patient and caregiver informed of progress made toward recovery. Explain time expected for discharge from hospital. Provide answers to individual patient questions or concerns.

Decreases anxiety and helps patient know what to anticipate participating in discharge planning.

STEP	RATIONALE

EVALUATION

1. Auscultate breath sounds bilaterally.	Determines status of airways.
2. Monitor trends in vital signs.	Provides data to measure progress of postoperative status.
3. Evaluate I&O records. Assess time of patient's first postoperative urination.	Indicates onset of urination.
4. Auscultate bowel sounds.	Allows you to evaluate return of peristalsis and diet tolerance.
5. Ask patient to describe pain on a scale of 0 (no pain) to 10 (worst pain ever) after moderate activity.	Determines level of comfort achieved and effectiveness of pain-relief measures.
6. Inspect incision (wound edges are well approximated, no drainage noted).	Provides data to measure progress of wound healing.
7. Have patient or caregiver describe incision care, dietary modifications or restrictions, activity restrictions, medication schedule, and plans for follow-up visit.	Identifies need for further teaching.
8. **Use Teach-Back:** "I want to be sure I explained what you need to know about your activity level after surgery. In your own words, tell me how you will be more active after your surgery." Develop a revised teaching plan if patient is not able to teach back correctly.	Determines patient's level of understanding of instructional topic.

Unexpected Outcomes	Related Interventions
1. Vital signs are above or below patient's baseline or expected range. Initially this could be related to anaesthesia effects, pain, hypovolemic shock, airway obstruction, fluid and electrolyte imbalance, or hypothermia.	• Identify contributing factors. • Notify surgeon.
2. Patient indicates severe incisional pain.	• Report to surgeon; discuss alternative analgesic option. • Try nonpharmacological pain control measures (see Chapter 16).

Communication and Documentation

- Document patient's arrival at the nursing unit, vital signs, assessment findings, and all nursing measures initiated in nurses' notes in electronic health record (EHR) or chart.
- Continue to document these factors every 4 hours or more frequently as patient's condition warrants.
- Document vital signs and I&O on appropriate flow sheet.
- Report any abnormal assessment findings and signs of complications to surgeon.
- Document your evaluation of patient and caregiver learning.

Special Considerations
Teaching

- Instruct patient and caregiver to identify signs and symptoms and appropriate actions to take for infection, respiratory, circulatory, or GI difficulties and wound disruptions.
- Provide important phone numbers to patient and caregiver for use in emergency and follow-up care on discharge.
- Teach patient about appropriate wound care, diet recommendations, and activity restrictions.

Pediatric

- Assessment of a child's perceptions of the surgical experience includes reinforcement of positive experiences and clarification of misconceptions. Drawing and storytelling are effective methods that allow children to share their thoughts and feelings (Perry et al., 2017).

- Use an appropriate pain assessment tools to determine the child's pain level.

Gerontological

- Older persons often experience a longer and more difficult postoperative recovery. Assess carefully for the development of postoperative complications.
- Assess for postoperative delirium and changes in mental status along with potential causes.
- Older persons may not request pain medication because they believe it should be tolerated as an expected effect of surgery (Lewis et al., 2019).

Care in the Community

- Teach the patient and caregiver about postoperative exercises, home modifications, activity limitations, wound dressing care, medications, and nutritional needs.
- If the patient is discharged with dressing changes, the bedroom or bathroom is usually ideal for the procedure. Have the patient and caregiver perform return demonstration of dressing change.
- Make referral to community health services if the patient and caregiver will have difficulty providing the expected level of care needed.
- Patients having surgery performed in ambulatory surgery centres must be accompanied by another person to allow for discharge after the procedure (see Box 37.2).

◆ CLINICAL DEBRIEF

The nurse is assigned to care for a 52-year-old female patient who is 152 cm (5 feet) tall and weighs 113.4 kg (250 lb). She is married with three adult children and is employed as an attorney. The nurse just received her from the postanaesthesia care unit (PACU) following an abdominal hysterectomy for fibroid tumours and a bladder neck suspension. Her previous medical history includes 30-year, 2-pack-per-day cigarette smoking and type 2 diabetes mellitus, and she has been on birth control pills for 20 years. She has an abdominal dressing that has a small amount of shadowing on it, is on oxygen at 2 L via nasal cannula, and has both a Foley catheter and a suprapubic catheter draining pink-tinged urine. She has an intravenous (IV) infusion of $D_5\frac{1}{2}$ normal saline (NS) infusing at 125 mL/hr and a morphine patient-controlled analgesia (PCA) device. She received cefazolin IV piggyback approximately 45 minutes before her incision was made and is to receive her second dose 8 hours later.

1. Which postoperative complications is this patient at risk for developing, and what are the nursing implications? Provide the rationale.

2. What postoperative teaching should she receive, and who should be included in the teaching?

3. On postoperative day 2 the patient appears anxious and has a pulse oxygenation of 82%. On assessment, her left lung sounds are diminished when compared to the right. She also indicates that her left leg is painful and swollen. Using SBAR, show how the nurse would communicate with the health care team about this patient.

◆ REVIEW QUESTIONS

1. Prevention of surgical site infections (SSIs) requires numerous actions by both the surgical team and the patient. Select the measures that are used to reduce SSIs. *(Select all that apply.)*
   1. Discharge patient from the hospital as soon as possible.
   2. Give prophylactic antibiotic therapy as close to the time of incision as possible.
   3. Shave excess hair with a razor just before the surgery begins.
   4. Control hyperglycemia in patients with and without diabetes.
   5. Give a shower or bath after the preoperative enema is evacuated.

2. There are numerous measures to prevent venous thromboembolism during the postoperative period. Which interventions are most appropriate before the surgery begins? *(Select all that apply.)*
   1. Performing an assessment for Homans' sign
   2. Ensuring that bilateral lower-extremity sequential compression devices are on and functioning
   3. Teaching patient coughing and breathing techniques
   4. Instructing patient how to ambulate after surgery
   5. Teaching patient how to do leg exercises

3. Which assignment would the nurse delegate to the unregulated care provider (UCP)? *(Select all that apply.)*
   1. Managing the postoperative care of the patient
   2. Initial assessments on arrival to the PACU
   3. Emptying the Foley catheter
   4. Caring for the patient requiring monitoring and providing comfort measures
   5. Assessing the intravenous (IV) site

ⓔ *Visit the Evolve site for a complete list of Clinical Debrief and Review Questions answers.*

REFERENCES

Accreditation Canada. (2019). *Required organizational practices handbook—Version 14.* Ottawa: Author. Retrieved from http://www.wrha.mb.ca/quality/files/2019ROPHandbook.pdf

American Society of PeriAnaesthesia Nurses (ASPAN). (2015). *2015–2017 perianaesthesia nursing standards, practice recommendations and interpretive statements.* Cherry Hill, NJ: Author.

Association of periOperative Registered Nurses (AORN). (2015). *Perioperative standards and recommended practices.* Denver, CO: AORN.

Canadian Medical Protective Association (CMPA). (2018). *Summary of key concepts and good practices.* Retrieved from https://www.cmpa-acpm.ca/serve/docs/ela/goodpracticesguide/pages/key_concepts/key_concepts-e.html?open=communication&to=documentation

Canadian Patient Safety Institute (CPSI). (2016a). *Healthcare associated infections (HAI).* Retrieved from http://www.patientsafetyinstitute.ca/en/Topic/Pages/Healthcare-Associated-Infections-(HAI).aspx

Canadian Patient Safety Institute (CPSI). (2016b). *Surgical site infection (SSI).* Retrieved from http://www.patientsafetyinstitute.ca/en/Topic/Pages/Surgical-Site-Infection-(SSI).aspx

Centers for Disease Control and Prevention (CDC). (2016). *Infection control standards for The Joint Commission, updated 2015.* Retrieved from www.cdc.gov/ncidod/dhqp/hai.html

Chung, F., Abdullah, H. R., & Liao, P. (2016). STOP-Bang questionnaire: A practical approach to screen for obstructive sleep apnea. *Chest,* 149(3), 631–638. doi:10.1378/chest.15-0903

College of Physicians and Surgeons of British Columbia. (2017). *Fasting guideline.* Retrieved from https://www.cpsbc.ca/files/pdf/NHMSFAP-Fasting.pdf

Diaz, V., & Newman, J. (2015). Surgical site infection and prevention guidelines: A primer for certified registered nurse anesthetists. *AANA Journal,* 83(1), 63–68.

Elisha, S., Heiner, J., Nagelhout, J., & Gabot, M. (2015). Venous thromboembolism: New concepts in perioperative management. *AANA Journal,* 83(3), 211–221.

Lewis, S. L., Bucher, L., Heitkemper, M., et al. (2019). *Medical-surgical nursing: Assessment and management of clinical problems* (4th Canadian ed.). Toronto: Elsevier.

National Association of PeriAnaesthesia Nurses of Canada (NAPANc). (2018). *Standards for practice* (4th ed.). New Brandon, MB: Author.

Operating Room Nurses Association of Canada (ORNAC). (2017). *The ORNAC standards, guidelines, and position statements for perioperative registered nurses* (13th ed.). Retrieved from https://www.ornac.ca/en/standards

Perry, S. E., Hockenberry, M. J., Lowermilk, D. L., & Wilson, D. (2017). *Maternal child nursing care in Canada* (2nd ed.). Toronto, ON: Elsevier.

Rotevatn, T., Boggild, H., Olesen, C., et al. (2017). Alcohol consumption and the risk of postoperative mortality and morbidity after primary hip or knee arthroplasty—A register-based cohort study. *PLoS ONE,* 12(3), e0173083. doi:10.1371/journal.pone.0173083

Rothrock, J. (2015). *Alexander's care of the patient in surgery* (15th ed.). St. Louis: Mosby.

Schick, L., & Windle, P. (2016). *PeriAnaesthesia nursing core curriculum: Preoperative, phase I and phase II PACU nursing* (3rd ed.). St. Louis: Saunders.

Spruce, L. (2015). Back to basics: Patient and family engagement. *AORN Journal,* 102(1), 34–37. doi:10.1016/j.aorn.2015.04.020

The Joint Commission. (2016). *National patient safety goals effective January 1, 2016.* Retrieved from https://www.jointcommission.org/assets/1/6/2016_NPSG_HAP.pdf

van de Pol, M., Flit, C., Lagro, J., Slaats, Y., Olde Rikkert, M., & Lagro-Janssen, L. (2017). Shared decision making with frail older patients: Proposed teaching framework and practice recommendations. *Gerontology & Geriatrics Education,* 38(4), 482–495. doi:10.1080/02701960.2016.1276014

Wongkietkachorn, A., Wongkietkachorn, N., & Rhunsiri, P. (2018). Preoperative needs-based education to reduce anxiety, increase satisfaction, and decrease time spent in day surgery: A randomized controlled trial. *World Journal of Surgery,* 42(3), 666–674. doi:10.1007/s00268-017-4207-0

38 | Intraoperative Care

Written by **Diane Rudolphi, MS, RN; Damilola Funke Iduye, RN, MN; and Steve Michael Iduye, RN, MHI**

OBJECTIVES

Mastery of content in this chapter will enable the nurse to:
- Describe the meaning of a sterile conscience.
- Describe the roles of a registered nurse in the operating room.
- Identify guidelines for use of sterile technique in the operating room.

- Perform surgical hand antisepsis correctly.
- Describe how to correctly don a sterile surgical gown.
- Apply sterile gloves using the closed technique.

MEDIA RESOURCES

- evolve http://evolve.elsevier.com/Canada/Perry/clinicalskills/
- Review Questions

- Audio Glossary
- Clinical Debrief and Review Questions Answers

PURPOSE

Nurses practising in the operating room (OR) support patients' surgical experiences from the preoperative phase throughout the intraoperative period and into the various postoperative phases (see Chapter 37). Working in collaboration with the health care team, perioperative nurses exercise critical thinking skills to provide individualized, holistic, and evidence-informed care to patients throughout their perioperative experience (Operating Room Nurses Association of Canada [ORNAC], 2017).

STANDARDS OF CARE

- Canadian Patient Safety Institute (CPSI), 2009—*Surgical Safety Checklist: Canada* (http://www.patientsafetyinstitute.ca/en/tools Resources/Pages/SurgicalSafety-Checklist-Resources.aspx)
- Canadian Patient Safety Institute (CPSI), 2016—*Surgical Care Safety* (http://www.patientsafetyinstitute.ca/en/Topic/Pages/Surgical-Care-Safety.aspx)
- Operating Room Nurses Association of Canada (ORNAC), 2017—*The ORNAC Standards, Guidelines, and Position Statements for Perioperative Registered Nurses* (https://www.ornac.ca/en/standards)
- World Health Organization (WHO), 2009—*Surgical Safety Checklist* (http://www.who.int/patientsafety/safesurgery/checklist/en/)
- World Health Organization (WHO), 2016—*Global Guidelines on the Prevention of Surgical Site Infection* (http://www.who.int/gpsc/ssi-prevention-guidelines/en/)

PRINCIPLES FOR PRACTICE

- The interprofessional surgical team includes the surgeon, physician's assistant (PA), registered nurse first assistant (RNFA) (Box 38.1), registered nurse anaesthesia assistant (RNAA) and/or physician anaesthesiologist, circulating nurse (RN), and scrub nurse/technician (RN, licensed practical nurse [LPN]/registered practical nurses [RPN]) (Box 38.2) or surgical technician. Interprofessional collaboration is an important element in the intraoperative environment to ensure patient safety. Nurses coordinate the OR personnel, monitor and advocate for the patient, maintain surgical standards of care, and communicate effectively with the other members of the team as appropriate. In the intraoperative phase, communication and teamwork are vital to ensuring patient safety and anticipated surgical outcome.
- The intraoperative phase begins when a patient enters the OR suite and ends with admission to the postanaesthesia care unit (PACU).
- A circulating nurse (Box 38.3) is an RN who both manages and collaborates closely with the interprofessional team while using the nursing process to guide the patient through the intraoperative phase (Rothrock, 2015). They are a "nonsterile" member of the surgical team who assumes responsibility and accountability for maintaining patient safety and continuity of quality care. This includes supervising the conduct of the scrub technician and delegating tasks to unregulated care providers (UCPs) as appropriate. The circulating nurse also assists the first assistant, scrub nurse/technician, and surgeon.

BOX 38.1

Role and Responsibilities of a Registered Nurse First Assistant

The role of the registered nurse first assistant (RNFA) is an expansion of the traditional perioperative nursing role, and areas of responsibility overlap. The roles of an RNFA include the following:

- Participating in "time-out" procedure with other surgical team members (safety measure taken to ensure correct patient; signed consent; correct procedure; correct site, side, and level; correct patient position; correct implants/equipment present; and provision of appropriate answers to any questions or concerns) (CPSI, 2009; ORNAC, 2017)
- Assisting with patient positioning, skin preparation, and draping
- Providing surgical exposure (assisting in retracting tissues and suctioning surgical field)
- Assessing the patient and monitoring hemostasis and blood loss
- Safe handling and/or cutting tissue
- Suturing and using surgical instruments and medical devices safely and correctly
- Performing wound closure
- Monitoring and protecting against contamination of the sterile field
- Applying human anatomical and physiological considerations in practice; recognizing structure, function, and location of tissues and organs; manipulating tissues accordingly to avoid injury
- Ensuring preoperative and postoperative patient management in collaboration with other health care providers
- Initiating intraoperative actions according to employer policy if surgeon becomes incapacitated
- Collaborating with the health care team to ensure optimal surgical outcome

From Association of periOperative Registered Nurses (AORN). (2015). *AORN standards and recommended practices for perioperative nursing—Position statement: AORN official statement on RN first assistants.* Denver, CO: The Association; Operating Room Nurses Association of Canada (ORNAC). (2017). *The ORNAC standards, guidelines, and position statements for perioperative registered nurses* (13th ed.). Kingston, ON: Author.

BOX 38.2

Role of the Scrub Nurse

- Helps circulating nurse prepare the OR and open supplies
- Performs surgical hand antisepsis and dons sterile gown and gloves
- Prepares sterile field with procedure-appropriate supplies and instruments, verifying that all are in working condition
- Participates in "time-out" procedure with other surgical team members (a safety measure taken to ensure correct patient; signed consent; correct procedure; correct site, side, and level; correct patient position; correct implants/equipment present; provision of appropriate answers to any questions or concerns) (CPSI, 2009; ORNAC, 2017)
- Performs sponge, sharps, and instrument counts with circulating nurse before incision is made, at the beginning of wound closure, and at the end of the surgical procedure to ensure that there is no retained foreign body in the patient (Rothrock, 2015)
- Labels all liquids and/or medications on the sterile field with a sterile marking pen when liquid or medication is out of the original container or package
- Gowns and gloves surgeons and assistants as they enter the OR
- Assists surgeons with sterile draping of patient
- Keeps sterile field orderly and monitors progress of procedure and any breaks in aseptic technique
- Passes sterile instruments and supplies to surgeons and assistants during surgery
- Handles surgical specimens per employer policy
- Constantly monitors location of all sponges and sharps in the sterile field

OR, Operating room.

BOX 38.3

Role of the Circulating Nurse

- Coordinates care of the patient undergoing surgery and collaborates with surgical team using evidence-informed practice and individualized approach for patient care
- Provides appropriate care during admission to the OR and preinduction, induction, intraoperative, and emergence phases
- Develops, modifies, and documents the individualized plan of care, or a clinical pathway to meet the specific needs of the patient
- Organizes and prepares OR before start of surgical procedure; checks to see that equipment works properly
- Gathers supplies for surgical procedure and opens sterile supplies for scrub nurse/technician
- Performs surgical counts and documents accurately sponges, sharps, and instruments with scrub nurse/technician before incision is made, at the beginning of wound closure, and at the end of surgical procedure
- Ensures that all liquids and/or medications on the sterile field are labeled with a sterile marking pen when liquid or medication is out of the original container or package
- Sends for patient at appropriate time
- Conducts preoperative patient assessment, including the following:
  - Explaining role and identifies patient
  - Reviewing medical record and verifies procedure and consents
  - Confirming that dentures and prostheses are removed
  - Confirming patient's allergies, nothing by mouth (NPO) status, laboratory values, ECG, X-ray film studies, skin condition, and circulatory and pulmonary status
- Safely transfers patient to operating table and positions patient according to surgeon preference and procedure type, and postoperatively, using safety precautions (e.g., safety belt, securing arms, padding bony prominences)
- Participates in "time-out" procedure with other surgical team members (safety measure taken to ensure correct patient; signed consent; correct procedure; correct site, side, and level; correct patient position; correct implants/equipment present; provision of appropriate answers to any questions or concerns) (CPSI, 2009; ORNAC, 2017)
- Applies conductive pad to patient if electrocautery used; may prepare patient's skin; may apply ECG electrodes
- Applies antiembolism stockings and sequential compression device per health care provider prescription
- Explains briefly to patient what the circulating nurse and the scrub nurse/technician are doing
- Assists surgical team by tying gowns and arranging equipment
- Assists anaesthesia personnel during induction and extubation
- Uses a surgical conscience to maintain and monitor integrity of the sterile field
- Strives to provide environmental conditions conducive to positive patient outcomes
- Continuously monitors procedure for any breaks in aseptic technique and anticipates needs of health care team; opens additional sterile supplies for scrub nurse/technician
- Continuously monitors patient throughout surgery
- Handles surgical specimens per employer policy
- Documents on perioperative nurses' notes
- Communicates to family and PACU personnel during surgical procedure

ECG, Electrocardiogram; *OR,* operating room; *PACU,* postanaesthesia care unit.

- It is essential that perioperative nurses develop a sterile conscience, that is, always knowing the location of a sterile field and what items are sterile and which are nonsterile. A sterile conscience requires knowledge of the principles of aseptic technique; self-discipline; good communication skills to identify, address, and correct any breaks in sterile technique; and the maturity to overcome personal preferences.

- While a patient is in the OR and the OR team is gowned and gloved, it is recommended that a surgical safety checklist or the World Health Organization (WHO) checklist be completed (WHO, 2009) (Fig. 38.1). The surgical safety checklist is a tool that is used to promote safety in any perioperative environment (CPSI, 2009; ORNAC, 2017). The WHO checklist identifies three phases of an operation, each corresponding to a specific period in the normal flow of work: before the induction of anaesthesia ("sign in"), before the incision of the skin ("time-out"), and before the patient leaves the operating room ("sign out") (WHO, 2009). In each phase, a checklist coordinator, usually the circulating nurse, must confirm that the surgery team has completed the listed tasks before it proceeds with the operation.

- The surgical safety checklist verifies the patient's identity, ascertains if the patient has any allergies, checks if the surgical site is marked and verifies the site marking, asks the patient if they have any questions, and ensures adherence to safety protocols (ORNAC, 2017; WHO, 2009). The surgical checklist consists of three parts: *briefing*, which is the period from the patient's transfer to the operating bed to the induction of anaesthesia; *time-out*, which is the time immediately prior to the incision; and *debriefing*, which is the period after the surgery is complete but before the patient's transfer to the PACU (ORNAC, 2017).

- Time-outs are standardized by each facility, initiated by a designated member of the team, and involve all the immediate members of the surgical/procedure team who will be participating in the procedure from start to finish. It is during the time-out that the team members agree, at a minimum, that the correct patient and site have been identified and the correct procedure is scheduled to be done. A designated member of the team must document the time-out according to employer policy before the procedure begins (ORNAC, 2017; Rothrock, 2015).

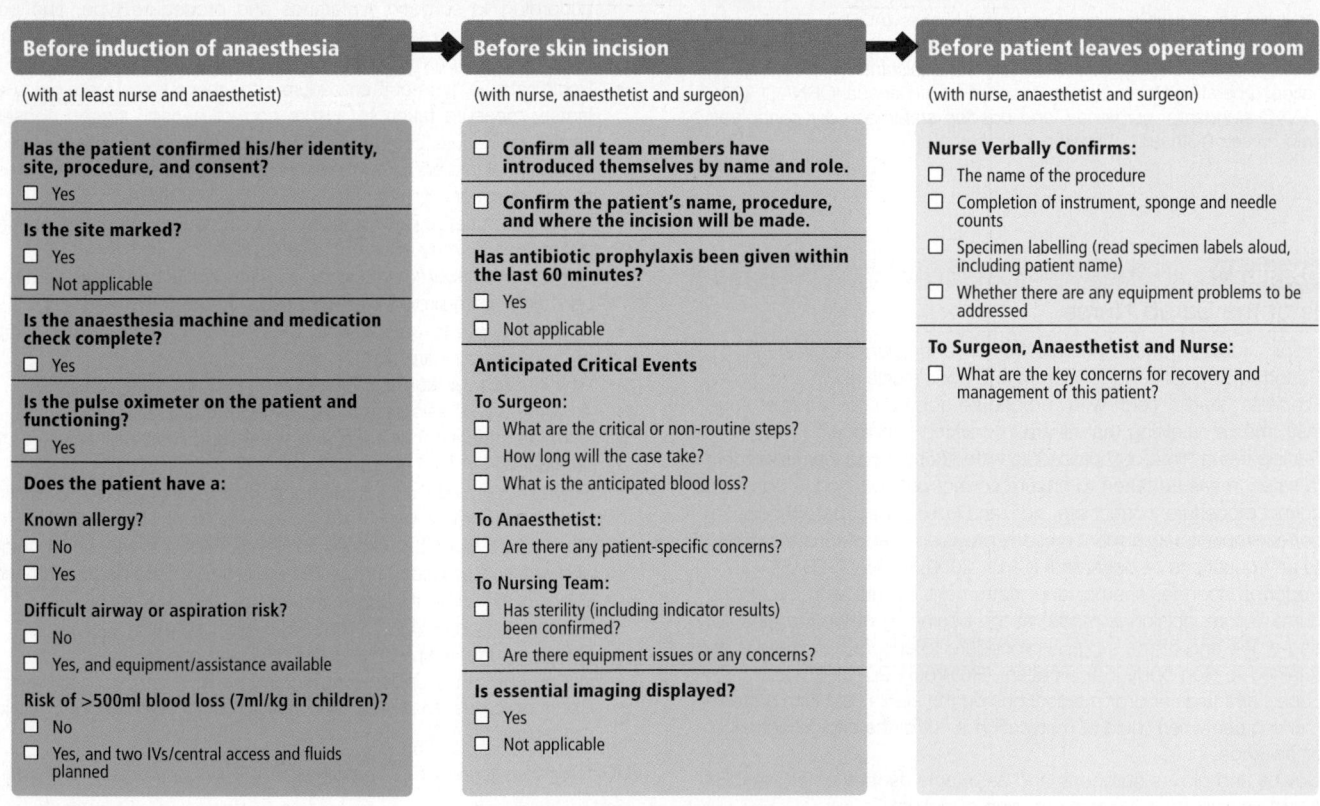

Surgical Safety Checklist

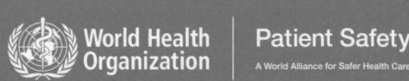 **World Health Organization** | **Patient Safety**
A World Alliance for Safer Health Care

Before induction of anaesthesia

(with at least nurse and anaesthetist)

Has the patient confirmed his/her identity, site, procedure, and consent?
- ☐ Yes

Is the site marked?
- ☐ Yes
- ☐ Not applicable

Is the anaesthesia machine and medication check complete?
- ☐ Yes

Is the pulse oximeter on the patient and functioning?
- ☐ Yes

Does the patient have a:

Known allergy?
- ☐ No
- ☐ Yes

Difficult airway or aspiration risk?
- ☐ No
- ☐ Yes, and equipment/assistance available

Risk of >500ml blood loss (7ml/kg in children)?
- ☐ No
- ☐ Yes, and two IVs/central access and fluids planned

Before skin incision

(with nurse, anaesthetist and surgeon)

- ☐ **Confirm all team members have introduced themselves by name and role.**
- ☐ **Confirm the patient's name, procedure, and where the incision will be made.**

Has antibiotic prophylaxis been given within the last 60 minutes?
- ☐ Yes
- ☐ Not applicable

Anticipated Critical Events

To Surgeon:
- ☐ What are the critical or non-routine steps?
- ☐ How long will the case take?
- ☐ What is the anticipated blood loss?

To Anaesthetist:
- ☐ Are there any patient-specific concerns?

To Nursing Team:
- ☐ Has sterility (including indicator results) been confirmed?
- ☐ Are there equipment issues or any concerns?

Is essential imaging displayed?
- ☐ Yes
- ☐ Not applicable

Before patient leaves operating room

(with nurse, anaesthetist and surgeon)

Nurse Verbally Confirms:
- ☐ The name of the procedure
- ☐ Completion of instrument, sponge and needle counts
- ☐ Specimen labelling (read specimen labels aloud, including patient name)
- ☐ Whether there are any equipment problems to be addressed

To Surgeon, Anaesthetist and Nurse:
- ☐ What are the key concerns for recovery and management of this patient?

This checklist is not intended to be comprehensive. Additions and modifications to fit local practice are encouraged.   Revised 1 / 2009   © WHO, 2009

FIG 38.1 The WHO surgical safety checklist. (*Used with permission, World Health Organization.*)

PERSON-CENTRED CARE

- The patient may be unsure of what to expect and have concerns regarding pain, disfigurement, and length of recovery. It is a nurse's responsibility to practise person-centred care and encourage questions.
- Care of the surgical patient requires specialized knowledge for the nurse who closely monitors a patient's intraoperative response to the experience.
- Patient needs vary on the basis of preoperative health, type of surgical procedure, and cultural and religious beliefs. Nurses need to obtain information regarding culture and religious preferences that may affect the patient's acceptance of education, blood administration, and surgical interventions.
- Information is communicated to the interprofessional team to ensure comprehensive intraoperative care.

EVIDENCE-INFORMED PRACTICE

- Decreased glove perforation results in decreased surgical site infection (SSI) and also protects the health care provider from exposure to contaminated blood and body fluids and subsequent infection (Mischke, Verbeek, Saarto, et al., 2014; ORNAC, 2017). Evidence-informed research offers the following gloving guidelines:
  - Double gloving is superior to single gloving.
  - Double gloving provides an additional barrier; there is a significant reduction in the perforation of the innermost layers when double gloving is used compared to single gloving (Makama, Okeme, Makama, et al., 2016; ORNAC, 2017; Rothrock, 2015).
  - In addition, double gloving and using the perforation indicator system (lighter pair of gloves worn over a darker pair) helps a health care provider better identify glove failure (Diaz & Newman, 2015).
- Current evidence-informed research links perioperative hypothermia with an increase in morbidity and mortality. Specifically, hypothermia can put patients at additional risk of SSI, cardiac arrhythmias, changes in medication metabolism, and increased incidence of surgical bleeding. Patients at risk for hypothermia include older persons, those with low body weight or metabolic disorders, those in a cold surgical environment or who receive cold infusions, and those undergoing open-cavity surgical procedures and general surgeries (Schick & Windle, 2016; Yang, Huang, Zhou, et al., 2015).
- Interventions effective in preventing hypothermia include forced-air warming. Commencement of active warming preoperatively and monitoring it throughout the intraoperative period is effective. Combined strategies, including preoperative commencement of warming and the use of warmed fluids plus forced-air warming during surgery, are also effective (Steelman, Chae, Duff, et al., 2018; Torossian, Bräuer, Höcker, et al., 2015).

OR personnel are responsible for adhering to specific infection-control practices based on individualized employer guidelines. Basic evidence-informed infection-control practices include the following:

- Hand hygiene should be performed (with specific attention given to areas between the thumb and first digit) when OR staff arrive at the health care facility, before and after patient contact, before and after donning gloves and other personal protective equipment, before and after eating, after contact with contaminated items, when items or hands are visibly soiled, and before leaving the health care facility (ORNAC, 2017; Rothrock, 2015).
- Hand scrub using alcohol-based hand-rub products should be approved by the employer's infection control department, and an established standardized protocol must be followed (ORNAC, 2017). The user must be made aware of and follow the manufacturer written instructions regarding storage, dispensing, technique, and amount of product required (ORNAC, 2017; Rothrock, 2015).
- OR personnel should use approved brushless, alcohol-based surgical hand-rub products (with added emollients) that limit damage to the user's skin, improve adherence to hand antisepsis protocols, simplify application technique, and reduce material waste (i.e., water, brushes, and packaging) (Rothrock, 2015).
- Fingernails should be clean, short, natural, and look healthy, and nail polish should not be worn. Avoid use of any nail enhancements (artificial nails, acrylics, extenders, and gels) (ORNAC, 2017).

SAFETY GUIDELINES

- Landers (2015) recommends an initiative to reduce intraoperative errors: using a time-out, decreasing distractions, nonpunitive error reporting, and increasing staff ratios and education.
- All items used within a sterile field must be sterile.
- Gowns used by scrub people must be sterile before donning. Once in place, gowns are sterile from the front chest and shoulders to table level and on the sleeves to 5 cm (2 inches) above the elbow.
- Persons who are sterile must keep their hands in view, above waist level and below neckline, to avoid contamination.
- When wearing a sterile gown, one should not fold the arms with hands tucked in the axillary region. This area is not considered sterile once the gown is donned. Perspiration can lead to strike-through, or contamination that occurs when moisture permeates a sterile barrier.
- Sterile-draped tables are sterile only at table level. Sides of the drape extending below table level are unsterile.
- All personnel moving around or within a sterile field must do so in a manner consistent with maintaining the sterility of that field. Scrubbed persons move from sterile areas to other sterile areas, contacting a sterile field only with sterile gowns and gloves. Unsterile health care team members always stay at least 30 cm (1 ft.) away from the sterile field while keeping it in constant view; they touch only unsterile areas.
- All sterile supplies and equipment are grouped around the sterile-draped patient.
- Unsterile people must avoid reaching over the sterile field.
- Scrubbed people remain close to the sterile field. When changing position, they need to turn face-to-face or back-to-back.
- Break-in aseptic technique should be monitored and corrected immediately.

✦ SKILL 38.1 Surgical Hand Antisepsis

In the operating room (OR) setting, surgical hand antisepsis must be achieved through effective surgical scrub or antiseptic hand rub (ORNAC, 2017; Rothrock, 2015). To reduce patient risk for acquiring postoperative infections, use of an antimicrobial preparation for hand antisepsis is an integral part of the presurgical scrubbing procedure for OR personnel. Although the skin cannot be sterilized, the number of microorganisms can be greatly reduced by chemical, physical, and mechanical means.

Through the use of an antimicrobial agent and sterile brushes or sponges, the surgical hand scrub removes debris and transient microorganisms from the nails, hands, and forearms; reduces the resident microbial count to a minimum; and inhibits rapid and rebound growth of microorganisms (ORNAC, 2017; Rothrock, 2015). Evidence suggests that completing a brushless hand-rub technique using approved hand-hygiene products, with or without water, is an alternative to the traditional hand scrub with a brush with the same microbial efficacy (Association of periOperative Registered Nurses [AORN], 2015). Both hand-antiseptic methods are currently used in OR settings.

AORN (2015) recommends a 3- to 5-minute hand and arm scrub with an approved antimicrobial agent for all surgical procedures. Surgical hand-scrub procedure for all staff using either the anatomical timed scrub or the counted-stroke method should be standardized (AORN, 2015; ORNAC, 2017) (follow employer policy). Some procedures, described as clean procedures (e.g., laryngoscopy and proctoscopy), require performing hand hygiene but are not necessarily surgical hand antisepsis.

Delegation and Collaboration

The skill of surgical hand antisepsis can be assigned to any member of the health care team. The registered nurse (RN) routinely observes surgical hand antisepsis for staff compliance.

Equipment

- Deep sink with foot or knee controls for dispensing water and soap
- Antimicrobial agent approved by employer (dispenser with foot controls)
- Surgical scrub brush with plastic nail file
- Paper face mask, cap or hood, surgical shoe covers
- Protective eyewear/face shield
- Sterile towel
- Sterile pack containing sterile gown

STEP	RATIONALE

ASSESSMENT

1. Determine type and length of time for hand hygiene (follow employer policy).

Guidelines vary regarding ideal time needed for surgical scrub.

2. Remove bracelets, rings, and watches.

Jewellery harbours and protects microorganisms. from removal. Jewellery interferes with hand hygiene and donning of personal protective equipment (ORNAC, 2017). Skin under rings has been shown to harbour more pathogens; therefore, rings should not be worn (AORN, 2015).

3. Inspect fingernails, which must be short, clean, natural, and healthy. Nail polish should not be worn. Never wear artificial nails, extenders or enhancers.

Long nails and chipped or old nail polish harbour microorganisms (ORNAC, 2017). Long fingernails can puncture gloves, causing contamination. Artificial nails interfere with hand hygiene and promote with the growth of *Staphylococcus aureus*, Gram-negative microorganisms, and fungus (ORNAC, 2017).

4. Inspect condition of cuticles, hands, and forearms for presence of abrasions, cuts, or open lesions.

Cuts, abrasions, exudative lesions, fresh tattoos, or hangnails tend to ooze serum, which may contain pathogens. Individuals with these conditions should not have patient contact until conditions heal (AORN, 2015).

NURSING DIAGNOSIS

- Potential for infection

Related factors/Risk factors are individualized on the basis of patient's condition or needs.

PLANNING

1. Expected outcomes following completion of procedure:
   - Patient does not develop signs of surgical site infection.

Indicates that microorganisms are not transferred to patient and sterile field.

STEP	RATIONALE

IMPLEMENTATION

STEP	RATIONALE
1. Don surgical shoe covers, cap or hood, face mask, and protective eyewear.	Protective eyewear prevents exposure to blood or body fluids splashing from sterile field, which causes risk for infection (e.g., human immunodeficiency virus [HIV], hepatitis B virus [HBV]).

Clinical Decision Point *Laser surgery requires special protective eyewear to prevent eye damage from stray laser energy.*

STEP	RATIONALE
2. Perform prescrub wash at beginning of work shift.	Prevents contamination of hands after scrub.
a. Turn water on using foot or knee control and adjust to comfortable temperature.	
b. Wet hands thoroughly with water. Follow manufacturer directions for application of soap.	
c. Rub hands, covering all surfaces with lather, including backs of hands, fingertips, inner webs, and palms, washing for at least 15 seconds.	A short prescrub wash/rinse at least 15 seconds at the beginning of the work shift removes gross debris and superficial microorganisms (AORN, 2015).
d. Rinse hands well. Dry hands thoroughly with disposable towel and discard towel.	Rinsing removes all soap and remaining debris.
3. Surgical hand scrub (with sponge):	
a. Turn on water using foot or knee control. Clean under nails of both hands with disposable nail pick or cleaner (see illustration). Rinse hands and forearms under running water.	Removes dirt and organic materials that harbour microorganisms.
b. Dispense antimicrobial scrub agent according to manufacturer instructions, often one to two full pumps (Provincial Infectious Diseases Advisory Committee [PIDAC], 2014). Apply agent to wet hands and forearms with soft, nonabrasive sponge.	Ensures removal of resident microorganisms on all surfaces of hands and arms (AORN, 2015).
c. Time a 2- to 5-minute scrub (follow manufacturer instructions). Visualize each finger, hand, and arm as having four sides (see illustrations). Wash all four sides effectively, keeping hand elevated, elbow down. Repeat for other hand, fingers, and arm.	Times vary by product. Scrubbing all surfaces ensures removal of resident microorganisms on hands and arms (AORN, 2015). The direction of the scrubbing procedure is from the hands to the elbows (PIDAC, 2014). Keeping hands elevated and elbows down prevents microorganisms from flowing back onto hands.
d. Avoid splashing surgical attire. Discard sponges in appropriate container.	
e. Rinse hands and arms, running water from fingertips to elbows in one continuous motion, holding hands higher than elbows and away from surgical site (see illustration).	Hands remain the cleanest part of the upper extremities.

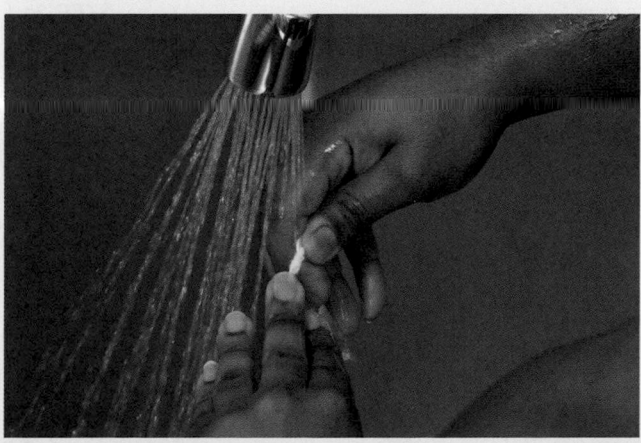

STEP 3a Clean under fingernails.

STEP	RATIONALE

IMPLEMENTATION

f. Turn off water using foot or knee controls, and back into the OR holding hands higher than elbows and away from surgical attire.

g. Approach sterile setup and grasp sterile towel, taking care not to drip water on sterile field (see illustration).

Water contaminates field.

h. Keeping hands and arms above the waist and outstretched, carefully grasp one end of sterile towel to dry one hand thoroughly, moving from fingers to elbow in rotating motion (see illustration).

Avoids sterile towel contacting unsterile scrub attire and transferring contamination to hands. Dries skin from cleanest (hands) to least clean (elbows).

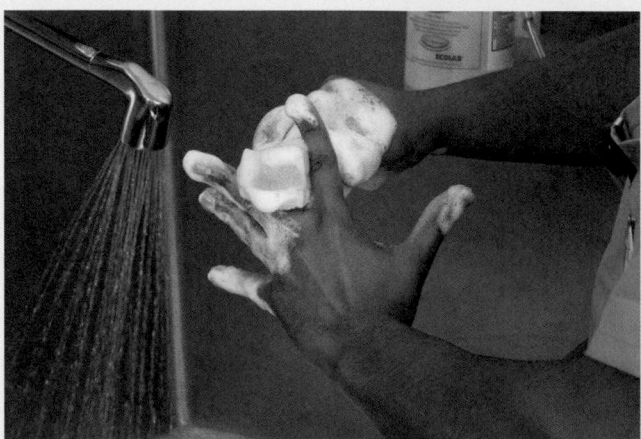 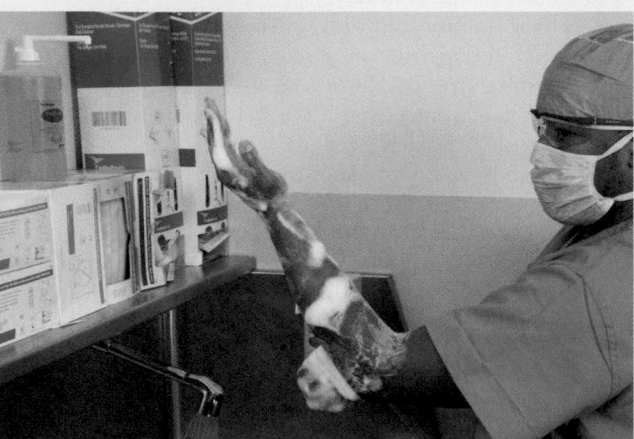

STEP 3c A, Scrub sides of fingers. **B,** Scrub forearms.

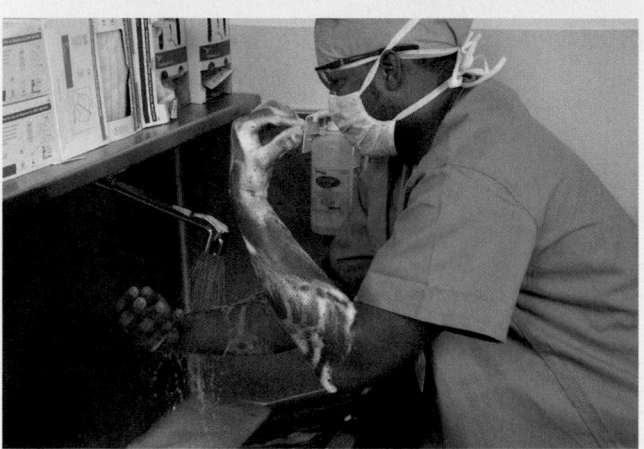 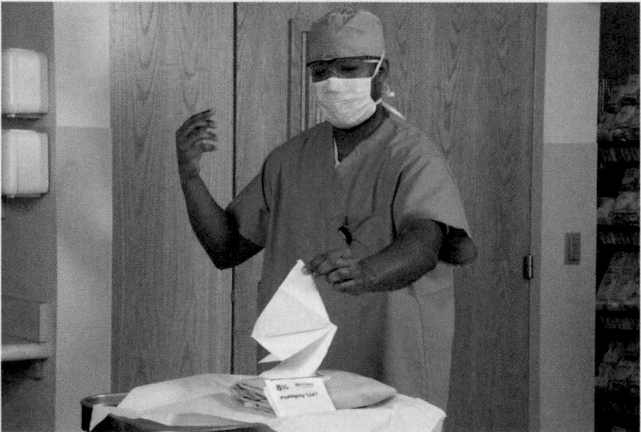

STEP 3e Rinse arms.   **STEP 3g** Grasp sterile towel.

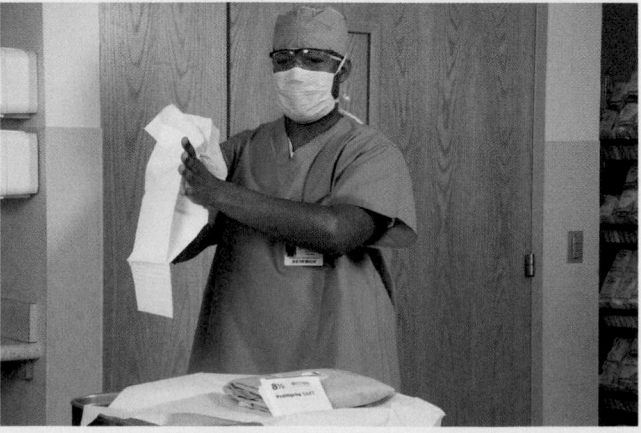

STEP 3h Dry hands thoroughly.

STEP	RATIONALE

IMPLEMENTATION

   i. Use opposite end of towel to dry other hand.

   j. Drop towel into linen hamper or into circulating nurse's hand.

4. Perform spongeless surgical hand scrub with alcohol-based hand-rub product:

   a. After prescrub wash (Step 2), turn on water using foot or knee control. Clean under nails of both hands with disposable nail pick or cleaner and rinse hands and forearms under running water. Dry hands thoroughly with paper towel. Turn off water.

   b. Dispense manufacturer-recommended amount of surgical hand antiseptic/scrub agent (see illustration). Apply agent to hands and forearms according to manufacturer's written instructions for application, recommended volume, and specified time.

   c. Repeat antimicrobial product application if indicated in manufacturer instructions.

   d. Rub thoroughly until completely dry (see illustration). Proceed to OR to don gloves.

Avoids transfer of microorganisms from elbow to opposite hand.

A broad-spectrum hand antiseptic agent has the ability to kill microorganisms when applied, promotes reduction in microorganism regrowth on all surfaces of hands and arms, and has a cumulative effect over time (ORNAC, 2017).

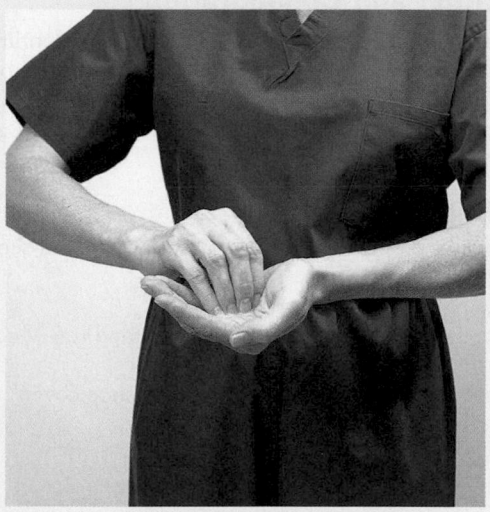

STEP 4b Dispense antimicrobial agent into hands. (*Photo Courtesy 3M Health Care.*)

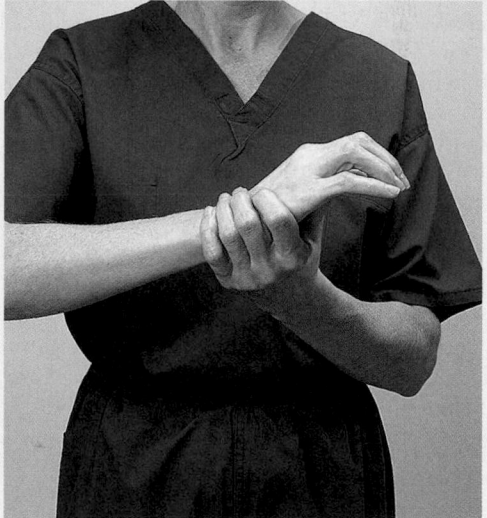

STEP 4d Rub thoroughly until completely dry. (*Photo Courtesy 3M Health Care.*)

EVALUATION

1. Monitor patient after surgery for signs of surgical site infection (usually occurs 2 to 3 days after surgery).

Signs of infection include redness, heat, swelling, pain, and purulent drainage.

Unexpected Outcomes

1. Redness, heat, swelling, pain, or purulent drainage may develop at surgical site, which often indicates wound infection.

Related Interventions

• Individualize interventions based on patient's situation (e.g., wound care, antibiotic therapy).

Communication and Documentation

• No documentation is required for surgical hand antisepsis.

• Document area and description of surgical site after surgery to provide baseline for monitoring wound.

BOX 38.4

Gloving and Gowning Guidelines

When to Change Surgical Sterile Gloves

- After each patient contact
- When a defect is noted
- Following suspected or actual contamination
- When perforation from a needle, suture, or other event occurs
- Immediately following use of methyl methacrylate
- If unintentional electric shock from the electrocautery device is received
- When gloves swell or become loose
- According to employer policy

Removal of Contaminated Gown and Gloves

- When a gown becomes contaminated, the scrubbed person steps away from the sterile field, the circulator dons protective gloves, unties the scrub nurse's gown, faces the scrub nurse, grasps the gown at the shoulders, and pulls it off while inverting the gown.
- The gloves are removed using a glove-to-glove and then skin-to-skin technique and are discarded immediately.
- The scrub nurse regowns and regloves self, using closed-glove technique (from another table) or gowns and gloves the other scrubbed personnel.

From Operating Room Nurses Association of Canada (ORNAC). (2017). *The ORNAC standards, guidelines, and position statements for perioperative registered nurses* (13th ed., pp. 149–152). Kingston, ON: Author.

✦ SKILL 38.2 Donning a Sterile Gown and Closed Gloving

Immediately following surgical hand antisepsis, surgical personnel apply a sterile gown and then apply sterile gloves. All members of the surgical team must prepare in this manner before entering the sterile field. Once applied, the surgical gown is considered sterile in the front from chest to waist or table level. The sleeves are considered sterile from 5 cm (2 inches) above the elbow to the level of the cuff (ORNAC, 2017). The neckline, shoulders, under the arms, sleeve cuffs, and the back of the gown are not considered sterile (ORNAC, 2017). Surgical gowns should cover all garments worn underneath. All sterile gowns that are free of tears, punctures, strain, and abrasion provide an effective barrier against microorganisms, particulates, and fluids passing between unsterile and sterile areas and prevent risk of contamination (ORNAC, 2017).

All members of the surgical team use the closed-glove method to apply gloves when entering the sterile field. If a glove becomes contaminated during the surgery, the circulating nurse, wearing protective unsterile gloves, grasps the outside of the glove and pulls it off inside out, leaving the stockinette cuff of the gown in place. Another sterile team member assists in regloving. The open method can be used when only one glove has been contaminated. In some

settings, the scrub nurse will wear two pairs of sterile gloves. If both of the scrub nurse/technician's gloves become contaminated, the gown is removed first, then the gloves are removed, and then the nurse regowns and regloves using the closed-glove method (Box 38.4).

Delegation and Collaboration

The registered nurse (RN) can assign the skills of donning a sterile gown and closed gloving to a surgical technologist or licensed practical nurse/registered practical nurse (LPN/RPN). The RN routinely observes sterile gown application and closed gloving for staff compliance.

Equipment

- Package of proper-size sterile gloves (latex-free if sensitivity or allergy is present)
- Sterile pack containing sterile gown
- Clean, flat, dry surface (table or Mayo stand) on which to open gown and gloves
- Paper face masks, cap or hood, surgical shoe covers
- Protective eyewear/face shield

STEP	RATIONALE

ASSESSMENT

1. Select proper size and type of sterile gloves. Select latex-free gloves if you know that the patient or any surgical personnel in room are latex sensitive.	Proper fit ensures ease of handling instruments and supplies. Prevents latex allergic response.

Clinical Decision Point *Know your employer's policy because double gloving may be recommended to reduce the risk for glove perforation during a surgical procedure (Makama et al., 2016; ORNAC, 2017).*

2. Select proper size and type of sterile surgical gown.	Ill-fitting gown impedes movement of extremities.

NURSING DIAGNOSIS

- Potential for infection

Related factors/Risk factors are individualized on the basis of patient's condition or needs.

STEP	RATIONALE

PLANNING

1. Expected outcomes following completion of procedure:
  • Patient does not develop signs of surgical site infection.

Nurse maintains aseptic technique and does not contaminate gown or gloves.

IMPLEMENTATION

1. Donning sterile gown:

a. Open sterile gown and glove package on clean, dry, flat surface. Scrub nurse (before scrubbing hands) or circulating nurse can do this for you, preferably on a small table separate from sterile field containing sterile instruments and supplies.

Provides sterile area for gloving.

b. Perform surgical hand antisepsis (see Skill 38.1). Dry hands thoroughly.

c. Pick up gown (folded inside out) from sterile package, grasping inside surface at collar.

Hands are not completely sterile. Inside surface of gown will contact surface of skin and thus is considered contaminated.

d. Lift folded gown directly upward and step back, away from table.

Prevents gown from touching unsterile object.

e. Locate neckband; with both hands grasp inside front of gown just below neckband.

Clean hands may touch inside of gown without contaminating outer surface.

f. Keeping gown at arm's length away from body, allow it to unfold with inside of gown toward body. Do not touch outside of gown or allow it to touch floor.

Outside of gown remains sterile.

g. With hands at shoulder level, slip both arms into armholes simultaneously (see illustration). Do not allow hands to move through cuff opening. Have circulating nurse pull gown over your shoulders by reaching inside the arm seams. Pull gown on, leaving sleeves covering hands.

Careful application prevents contamination. Gown covers hands to prepare for closed gloving.

h. Have circulating nurse tie gown at neck and waist (see illustration). If gown is wraparound style, do not touch sterile front flap until scrub nurse/technician has gloved (see Step 3b).

Secures gown without contaminating it.

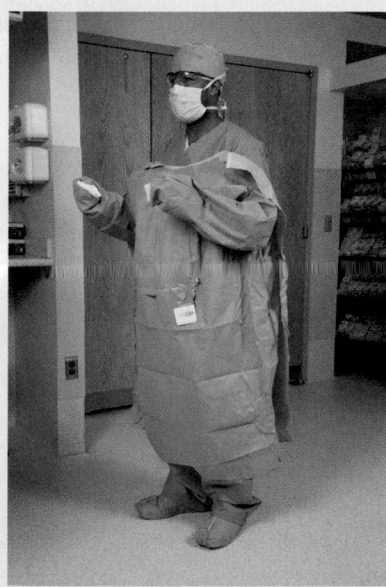

STEP 1g Place arms in sleeves.

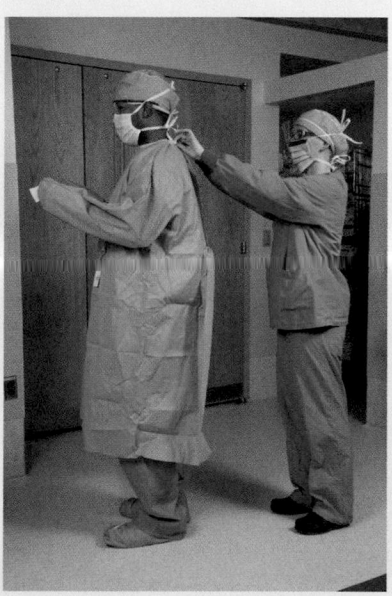

STEP 1h Circulating nurse ties scrub gown.

STEP	RATIONALE

IMPLEMENTATION

2. Applying gloves using closed-glove method:

a. With hands covered by gown cuffs and sleeves, open inner sterile glove package (see illustration).

Sterile gown cuff touches sterile glove surface.

b. Grasp folded cuff of glove for dominant hand with nondominant hand.

Sterile gown touches sterile glove.

c. Extend covered dominant hand and forearm forward with palm up and place palm of glove against palm of dominant hand. Glove fingers point toward elbow.

Positions glove for application over cuffed hand, keeping glove sterile.

d. While holding glove cuff through gown with dominant hand on which it was placed, grasp back of glove cuff with nondominant hand and turn glove cuff over end of dominant hand and gown cuff (see illustration).

Positions glove over gown for hand insertion.

e. Grasp top of glove and underlying gown sleeve with covered nondominant hand. Carefully extend fingers into glove, being sure that cuff of glove covers cuff of gown.

f. Glove nondominant hand in same manner with gloved dominant hand (see illustration A). Keep hand inside sleeve. Be sure that fingers are fully extended into both gloves (see illustration B).

Gloves remain sterile.

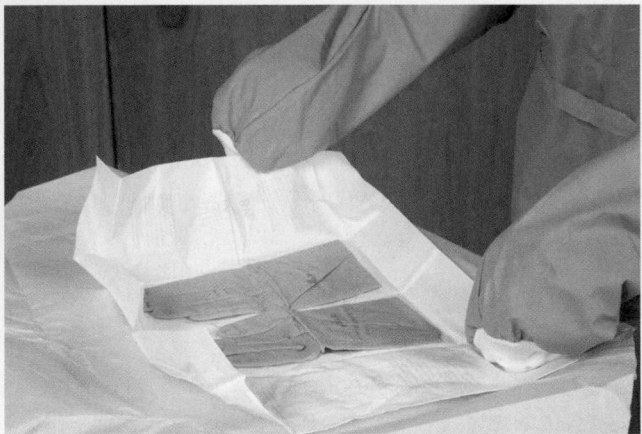

STEP 2a Scrub nurse opens glove package.

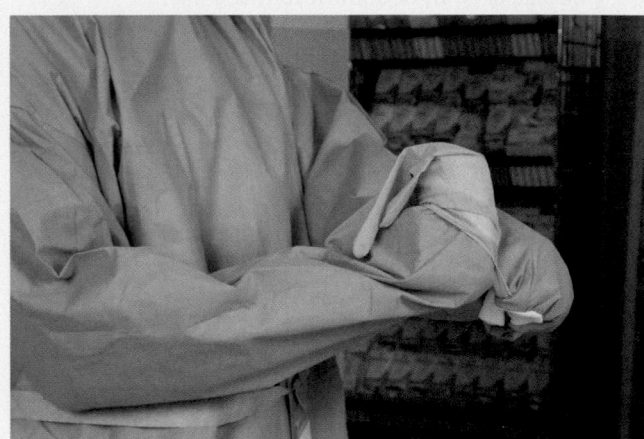

STEP 2d Glove applied as hands remain inside cuffs.

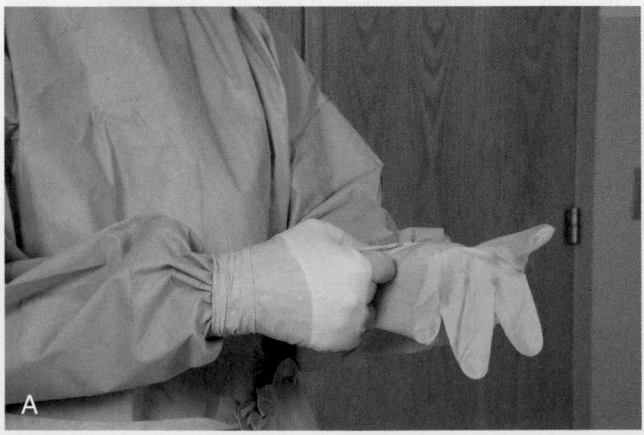

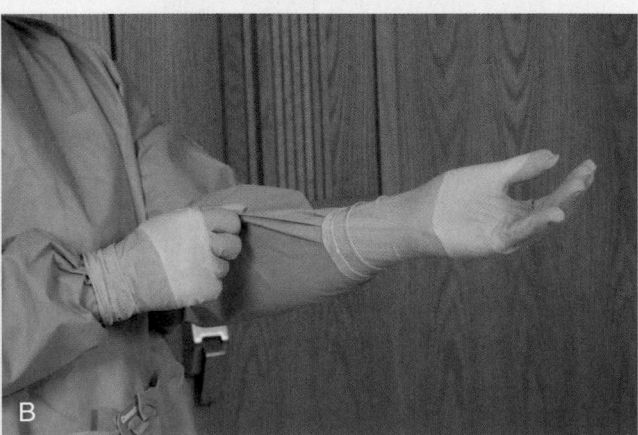

STEP 2f A, Second glove applied. **B,** Gloved fingers extended.

STEP	RATIONALE

IMPLEMENTATION

3. Donning wraparound gown:

a. Grasp sterile front flap/paper tab with gloved hands and untie.

Front of gown is sterile.

b. Pass sterile paper tab to a member of sterile surgical team or to nonsterile team member (e.g., circulating nurse) (see illustration). Keep gown tie in right hand. Circulating nurse stands still as scrub nurse/technician turns.

Nonsterile team member uses caution not to touch sterile tie when taking sterile paper tab while scrub nurse/technician turns.

c. Allowing margin of safety, turn to left one-half turn, covering back with extended gown flap. Retrieve sterile tie only from team member and secure both ties in place.

Manoeuvre covers entire body with gown.
Nonsterile team member pulls off paper tab and discards it.

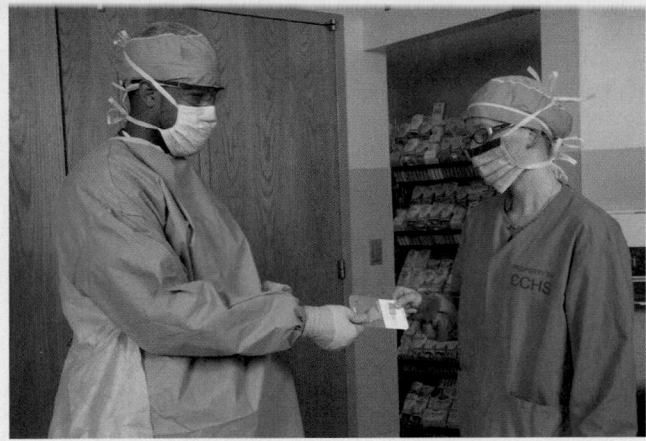

STEP 3b Paper tap on disposable gown is passed to circulating nurse.

EVALUATION

1. Monitor patient after surgery for signs of surgical site infection (usually occurs 2 to 3 days after surgery).

Signs of infection include redness, heat, swelling, pain, and purulent drainage.

Unexpected Outcomes
1. Redness, heat, swelling, pain, or purulent drainage develops at surgical site, which often indicates wound infection.

Related Interventions
- Individualize interventions based on patient's situation (e.g., wound care, antibiotic therapy).

Communication and Documentation

- No documentation is required for sterile gowning and gloving.
- Document area and description of surgical site after surgery to provide baseline for monitoring wound.

✦CLINICAL DEBRIEF

You are the circulating nurse in the general operating room, and your first case scheduled at 0730 is an 82-year-old female undergoing an exploratory laparotomy with lysis of adhesions. You are organized and have checked the supplies and equipment in the room. Anaesthesia and the surgeon are ready and available in the room while the scrub nurse is performing a surgical hand scrub. When the patient arrives, you introduce yourself and review the chart. The patient's chart states that she is 160 cm (5'1") tall and weighs 44 kg (96.8 lb). When you interview her and review her past medical history, she verifies the information in her chart, stating that she has hypothyroidism.

1. In thinking about risk factors, what are your main concerns?
2. What are the complications associated with hypothermia?
3. What should the circulating nurse be anticipating regarding intraoperative irrigations and infusions?
4. When you look closer at the patient's chart, you note that the "on call to OR antibiotic," cefazolin 1 g IV, that has been prescribed to infuse within 60 minutes of the time of the incision has not been administered and was never sent with the patient on transfer to the operating room. Using SBAR, note to whom you would address this issue, and show how you would communicate with the interprofessional team regarding this patient situation.

✦ REVIEW QUESTIONS

1. The nurse is performing a beginning-of-shift prescrub wash. Place the steps of the prescrub in the correct order.
   1. Wet hands and apply soap.
   2. Rinse well to remove all soap.
   3. Dry with disposable towel.
   4. Turn on water using foot or knee control.
   5. Rub hands covering all surfaces for at least 15 seconds.
2. Interprofessional collaboration is vital as part of the surgical team. What is included in the responsibilities of the circulating nurse? *(Select all that apply.)*
   1. Conducting perioperative assessments
   2. Reviewing medical records for accuracy and completeness
   3. Performing the surgical hand scrub and donning a sterile gown and gloves
   4. Participating in "time-out"
   5. Maintaining patient safety and continuity of care throughout the perioperative period
3. ORNAC (2017) recommends guidelines for changing damaged or contaminated gloves during a procedure. Which specific guidelines are included? *(Select all that apply.)*
   1. The glove should be changed at the moment the break is noted.
   2. The nonsterile member of the team should remove the contaminated gloves by touching only the gloves.
   3. The gown cuff should remain at the wrist level.
   4. One member of the sterile team should reglove the other.
   5. The nonsterile member of the team should reglove the other.

ⓔ *Visit the Evolve site for a complete list of Clinical Debrief and Review Questions answers.*

REFERENCES

Association of periOperative Registered Nurses (AORN). (2015). *Guidelines for perioperative practices*. Denver, CO: Author.

Canadian Patient Safety Institute (CPSI). (2009). *Surgical safety checklist. Why: Information, rationale, and FAQ, Version 1.0*. Ottawa: Author. Retrieved from http://www.patientsafetyinstitute.ca/en/toolsResources/Documents/Interventions/Surgical%20Safety%20Checklist/Information%20Rationale%20%20FAQ.pdf

Canadian Patient Safety Institute (CPSI). (2016). *Surgical care safety*. Retrieved from http://www.patientsafetyinstitute.ca/en/Topic/Pages/Surgical-Care-Safety.aspx

Diaz, V., & Newman, J. (2015). Surgical site infections and preventions guidelines: A primer for certified registered nurse anesthetists. *AANA Journal, 83*(1), 63–68.

Landers, R. (2015). Reducing surgical errors: Implementing a three-hinge approach to success. *AORN Journal, 101*(6), 657–665. doi:10.1016/j.aorn.2015.04.013

Makama, J. G., Okeme, I. M., Makama, E. J., & Ameh, E. A. (2016). Glove perforation rate in surgery: A randomized, controlled study to evaluate the efficacy of double gloving. *Surgical Infections, 17*(4), 436–442. doi:10.1089/sur.2015.165

Mischke, C., Verbeek, J., Saarto, A., Lavoie, M., Pahwa, M., & Ijaz, S. (2014). Gloves, extra gloves or special types of gloves for preventing percutaneous exposure injuries in healthcare personnel. *The Cochrane Database of Systematic Reviews, 2014*(3), CD009573, doi:10.1002/14651858.CD009573.pub2

Operating Room Nurses Association of Canada (ORNAC). (2017). *The ORNAC standards, guidelines, and position statements for perioperative registered nurses* (13th ed.). Kingston, ON: Author.

Provincial Infectious Diseases Advisory Committee (PIDAC). (2014). *Best practices for hand hygiene in all health care settings* (4th ed.). Toronto, ON: Queen's Printer for Ontario. Retrieved from http://www.publichealthontario.ca/en/eRepository/2010-12%20BP%20Hand%20Hygiene.pdf

Rothrock, J. (2015). *Alexander's care of the patient in surgery* (15th ed.). St. Louis: Mosby.

Schick, L., & Windle, P. (Eds.), (2016). *Perianesthesia nursing core curriculum*. St. Louis: Saunders.

Steelman, V. M., Chae, S., Duff, J., Anderson, M. J., & Zaidi, A. (2018). Warming of irrigation fluids for prevention of perioperative hypothermia during arthroscopy: A systematic review and meta-analysis. *Arthroscopy: The Journal of Arthroscopic and Related Surgery, 34*(3), 930–942, e2. doi:10.1016/j.arthro.2017.09.024

Torossian, A., Bräuer, A., Höcker, J., Bein, B., Wulf, H., & Horn, E. (2015). Preventing inadvertent perioperative hypothermia. *Deutsches Ärzteblatt International, 112*(10), 166–172. doi:10.3238/arztebl.2015.0166

World Health Organization (WHO). (2009). *Surgical safety checklist*. Retrieved from http://www.who.int/patientsafety/safesurgery/checklist/en/

World Health Organization (WHO). (2016). *Global guidelines for the prevention of surgical site infection*. Retrieved from http://www.who.int/gpsc/ssi-prevention-guidelines/en/

Yang, L., Huang, C., Zhou, Z., et al. (2015). Risk factors for hypothermia in patients under general anesthesia: Is there a drawback of laminar airflow operating rooms? A prospective cohort study. *International Journal of Surgery, 21*, 14–17. doi:10.1016/j.ijsu.2015.06.079

39 | Prevention and Care of Skin Breakdown

Written by **Rosemary Kohr, RN, MScN, PhD; and Janice C. Colwell, RN, MS, CWOCN, FAAN**

SKILLS AND PROCEDURES

OBJECTIVES

Mastery of content in this chapter will enable the nurse to:
- Discuss the response of the body during each stage of the wound-healing process.
- Differentiate between primary- and secondary-intention wound healing.
- Explain factors that promote or impair normal wound healing.
- Identify risk factors for development of skin breakdown (e.g., pressure injury).
- Describe guidelines for prevention of skin breakdown.
- Perform a skin assessment.
- Discuss the valid and reliable tools for assessing a patient's risk for pressure injuries.

- Identify outcome criteria for patients at risk for pressure injuries or impaired skin integrity.
- Discuss teaching needs of the patient and caregiver regarding prevention of and treatment for skin breakdown (particularly pressure injury).
- Perform a wound irrigation.
- Remove sutures or staples.
- Demonstrate care of a wound-drainage system.
- Discuss the purpose and use of negative-pressure wound therapy (NPWT) and wound vacuum treatment.

MEDIA RESOURCES

- evolve http://evolve.elsevier.com/Canada/Perry/clinicalskills/
- Case Studies
- Review Questions

- ▶ Video Clips
- NSO Nursing Skills Online
- Clinical Debrief and Review Questions Answers

PURPOSE

The skin is the body's largest organ. In its role as sensory protection, the skin defends the body in recognizing pain, touch and pressure, and temperature. The acidic pH of the skin creates an *acid mantle*, which further serves to protect the skin from external bacteria, viruses, or other potential contaminants. It also plays a major role in thermoregulation, metabolism, immunity, and fluid balance regulation (Bryant & Nix, 2016b). Intact skin is the first line of defense of the body against invasion by infectious microorganisms. If there is a break in the integrity of the skin, appropriate, evidence-informed wound care is necessary to promote wound closure and return to an intact skin layer (Orsted, Keast, Forest-Lalande, et al., 2018).

Care of a patient's skin is essential for both preventing and managing skin breakdown. Pressure injuries are of particular importance in health care settings because they are one type of skin breakdown that often can be prevented through implementation of evidence-informed practices such as pressure off-loading, management of incontinence, adequate nutritional intake, and consistent, regular repositioning schedules. In addition, frequent monitoring of the patient's skin can be done by educating the patient, caregiver, and unregulated care providers (UCPs) on wound assessment and prevention strategies (Orsted et al., 2018).

STANDARDS OF CARE

- Accreditation Canada, 2019—*Required Organizational Practices Handbook—Version 14* (http://www.wrha.mb.ca/quality/files/2019ROPHandbook.pdf)
- Canadian Patient Safety Institute (CPSI), 2016—*Pressure Ulcer: Resources* (http://www.patientsafetyinstitute.ca/en/toolsResources/Hospital-Harm-Measure/Improvement-Resources/HHI-Pressure-Ulcer/Pages/Resource-Library-Pressure-Ulcer-Resources.aspx)
- National Pressure Ulcer Advisory Panel (NPUAP), 2016—*National Pressure Ulcer Advisory Panel Announces a Change in Terminology from Pressure Ulcer to Pressure Injury and Updates the Stages of Pressure Injury* (http://www.npuap.org/national-pressure-ulcer-advisory-panel-npuap-announces-a-change-in-terminology-from-pressure-ulcer-to-pressure-injury-and-updates-the-stages-of-pressure-injury/)
- National Pressure Ulcer Advisory Panel (NPUAP), European Pressure Ulcer Advisory Panel (EPUAP), Pan Pacific Pressure Injury Alliance (PPPIA), & Haesler, 2014—*Prevention and Treatment of Pressure Ulcers: Quick Reference Guide* (http://www.epuap.org/wp-content/uploads/2016/10/quick-reference-guide-digital-npuap-epuap-pppia-jan2016.pdf)
- Orsted, Keast, Forest-Lalande, et al. (Wounds Canada), 2018—*Best Practice Recommendations for the Prevention and Management of Pressure Injuries* (https://www.woundscanada.ca/docman/public/health-care-professional/bpr-workshop/165-wc-bpr-prevention-and-management-of-wounds/file)
- Wound Ostomy and Continence Nurses (WOCN) Society, 2016—*Guideline for Prevention and Management of Pressure Ulcers (Injuries)* (https://www.wocn.org/)

PRINCIPLES FOR PRACTICE

- The skin is the largest external organ. It has two layers: the *epidermis* and the *dermis* (Fig. 39.1). The epidermis has five layers.
  - *Stratum corneum*, the outermost layer, consists of flattened dead keratinized cells. Stratum corneum prevents dehydration of underlying cells and is a physical barrier against entry of certain chemicals.
  - The next layers of the epidermis are the *stratum lucidum, stratum granulosum,* and *stratum spinosum.*
  - *Stratum germinativum*, the innermost layer, is sometimes called the *basal layer.* Important features of stratum germinativum are the epidermal protrusions, or "peaks and valleys," that point downward into the dermis. These provide resiliency and integrity to the skin structure. *Melanocytes*, the cells that give skin its colour, are also in this layer. As individuals age, this layer flattens out and decreases skin resiliency.

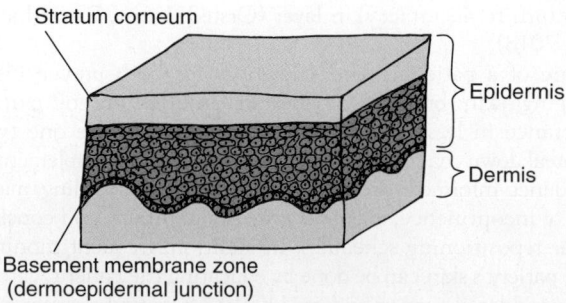

FIG 39.1 Diagram of layers of skin and subcutaneous tissue.

- The area that separates the epidermis from the dermis is called the *dermoepidermal junction* or the *basement membrane zone.*
- Beneath the epidermis is the dermis. Collagen (a tough fibrous protein layer), blood vessels, and nerves compose the dermal layer. Collagen comprises about 70% of the dermis and is essential in wound healing. The dermis restores the physical properties of the skin and its structural integrity. Restoration of both the epidermal and dermal layers is necessary to promote healing. Risk for local or systemic infection, impaired circulation, and breakdown of tissue directly impair the wound-healing ability of the skin layers (Doughty & Sparks-Defriese, 2016).
- Pressure injuries occur from unrelieved prolonged soft tissue compression, which interferes with the blood flow to the tissue; if this compression continues for a prolonged period of time, the tissue dies from lack of blood flow, or *tissue ischemia.* Ischemia develops when pressure on the skin is greater than vascular pressure inside the vessels, causing the vessels to collapse and decreasing tissue perfusion.
- The most common sites for development of pressure injuries are over bony prominences and can include the sacrum, coccyx, ischial tuberosities, greater trochanters, heels, scapulae, iliac crests, and lateral and medial malleoli (Pieper, 2016). Fig. 39.2 shows pressure points over bony prominences where pressure injuries can develop in sitting or lying positions.
- Wounds should be assessed on a scheduled basis. If the assessment indicates that the wound is not healing as expected, the plan of care needs to be changed to support wound healing.
- A thorough wound assessment includes the identification of the type of wound healing (e.g., primary, secondary, or tertiary intention) and the type of tissue and characteristics of the wound base, as well as the condition of the wound edges and periwound skin. All these parameters should be considered when determining treatment options. In the case of pressure injury, the assessment includes the stage of injury (NPUAP, 2016) and will be discussed later in this chapter.
- The healing process consists of *phases*, which for explanation purposes, are presented as distinct—but in real life, these phases overlap. In a full-thickness wound the phases are hemostasis, inflammation, proliferation, and remodelling or maturation (Box 39.1). Every wound or injury, no matter what type, follows the phases of wound healing. Chronic wounds are those wounds that stall at a particular point in the wound healing trajectory.
- During the proliferative stage, fibroblasts are at the site of injury. These fibroblasts increase synthesis of collagen, which forms the healing ridge that can be palpated under an intact healing incision by days 5 to 9 (Fig. 39.3) (Doughty & Sparks-Defriese, 2016).
- Wound healing occurs by primary, secondary, and tertiary intention (Fig. 39.4).
  - Healing by *primary intention* occurs when the edges of a clean surgical incision remain close together. The wound heals quickly, and tissue loss is minimal or absent (Doughty & Sparks-Defriese, 2016). The skin cells regenerate quickly, and capillary walls stretch across under the suture line to form a smooth surface as they join.
  - Wounds that are left open and allowed to heal by scar formation are classified as healing by *secondary intention* (Beitz, 2016). There are tissue loss and open wound edges. Granulation tissue gradually fills in the area of the defect (Fig. 39.5). This process is typical of severe laceration or massive surgical intervention with skin loss.
  - In *secondary intention*, there is a gap between the edges. Connective tissue develops, which supports new capillaries.

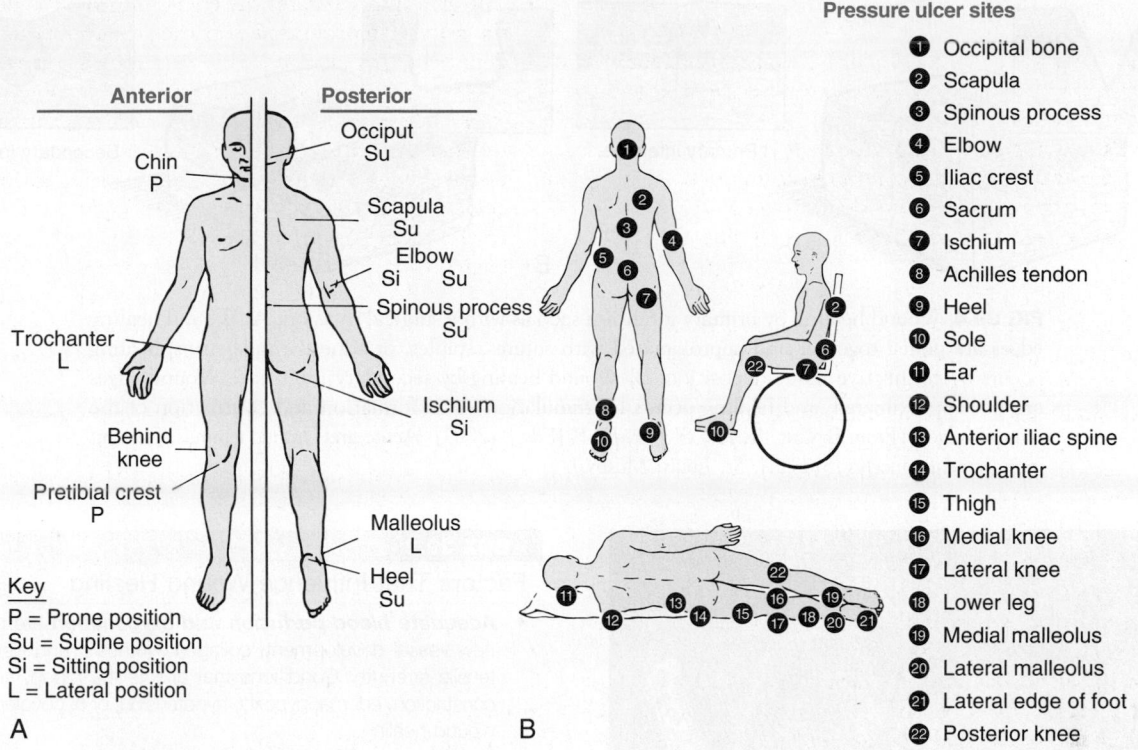

Pressure ulcer sites

1. Occipital bone
2. Scapula
3. Spinous process
4. Elbow
5. Iliac crest
6. Sacrum
7. Ischium
8. Achilles tendon
9. Heel
10. Sole
11. Ear
12. Shoulder
13. Anterior iliac spine
14. Trochanter
15. Thigh
16. Medial knee
17. Lateral knee
18. Lower leg
19. Medial malleolus
20. Lateral malleolus
21. Lateral edge of foot
22. Posterior knee

FIG 39.2 A, Bony prominences most frequently underlying pressure injuries. **B,** Pressure injury sites. *(From Trelease, C. C. [1988]. Developing standards for wound care. Ostomy & Wound Management, 26:50.)*

BOX 39.1

Phases of Wound Healing (Full-Thickness Wounds)

Hemostasis Phase

Immediately upon injury, blood vessels constrict; clotting factors activate coagulation pathways to stop bleeding. Clot formation seals the disrupted vessel(s) so blood loss is controlled and acts as a temporary bacterial barrier. Platelets release growth factors, which attract cells needed to begin the repair process.

Inflammatory Phase

Within the first few days, vasodilation occurs, allowing plasma and blood cells to leak into the wound, noted as edema, erythema, and exudate. Leukocytes (white blood cells) arrive in the wound to begin wound cleanup. Macrophages, a type of white blood cell, appear and begin to regulate the wound repair. The result of the inflammatory phase is a clean wound bed, ready to lay down epithelial cells to move into active healing, for a normal, noncomplicated wound.

Proliferative Phase

Now epithelialization (the construction of new epidermis) begins. At the same time new, pink granulation tissue is formed. New capillaries (angiogenesis) are created, restoring the delivery of essential oxygen and nutrients to the wound bed. Collagen is synthesized and begins to provide strength and structural integrity to the wound. Contraction, which occurs in open wounds, reduces the size of the wound and moves the wound toward closure.

Maturation (Remodelling) Phase

Collagen is remodelled to become stronger and provides tensile strength to the wound. The surface appearance in an uncomplicated wound will be that of a well-healed scar. This phase can last up to 2 years, and the tensile strength of the healed tissue is at most 80% of the original skin.

Data from Doughty, D. B., & Sparks-Defriese, B. (2016). Wound healing physiology. In R. A. Bryant & D. P. Nix (Eds.), *Acute and chronic wounds: Current management concepts* (5th ed.). St. Louis: Mosby.

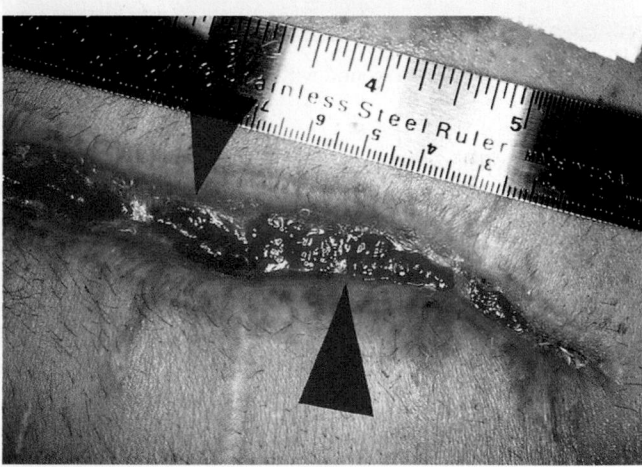

FIG 39.3 Surgical wound with epithelialization occurring: epithelial healing ridge apparent. *(From Bryant, R. A., & Nix, D. P. [Eds.]. [2007]. Acute and chronic wounds: Current management concepts [3rd ed.]. St. Louis: Mosby.)*

This form of healing results in the formation of scar tissue to close the wound. The slowness of this process places a patient at greater risk for infection because there is no epidermal barrier until later in the healing process.

- Healing by *tertiary intention* is sometimes called *delayed primary intention* or *closure*. It occurs when surgical wounds are not closed immediately but left open for 3 to 5 days to allow edema or infection to diminish. Then the wound edges are sutured or stapled closed (Doughty & Sparks-Defriese, 2016).

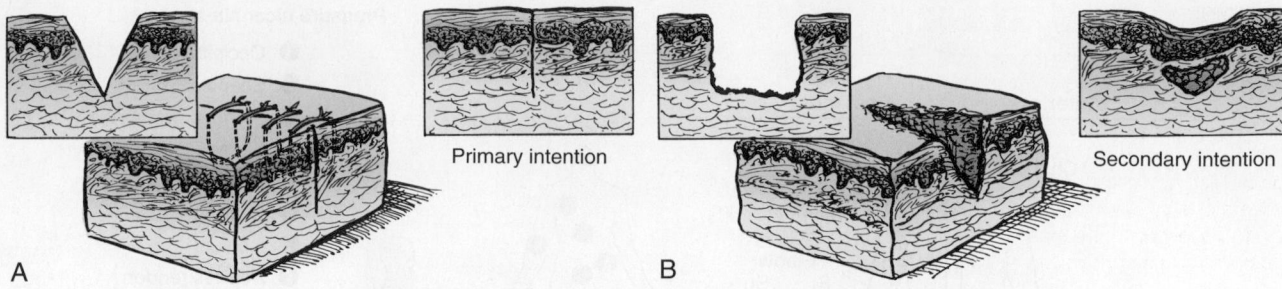

A   Primary intention

B   Secondary intention

FIG 39.4 Wound healing by primary intention such as with a surgical incision. **A,** Wound healing edges are pulled together and approximated with sutures, staples, or adhesive tape strips; healing occurs by connective tissue deposition. **B,** Wound healing by secondary intention. Wound edges are not approximated, and healing occurs by granulation tissue formation and contraction of the wound edges. *(From Bryant, R. A., & Nix, D. P. [Eds.]. [2007]. Acute and chronic wounds: Current management concepts [3rd ed.]. St. Louis: Mosby.)*

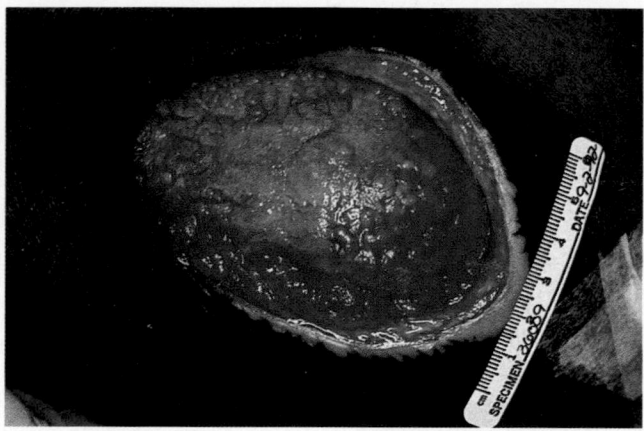

FIG 39.5 Open wound with granulation tissue.

- The percentage and type of tissue in the wound bed healing by secondary intention provide insight into the severity and duration of the wound, the extent to which it is progressing toward healing, and the effectiveness of current interventions (Nix, 2016). Viable tissue is normally red to pink in colour and moist in appearance. This type of tissue is called *granulation tissue* and indicates a wound moving toward healing. Black, brown, or tan tissue in the wound is slough or eschar and should be removed, or wound healing will be delayed.
- The location, severity, and extent of the injury and the tissue layer or layers involved all affect the wound-healing process (Doughty & Sparks-Defriese, 2016). In addition, there are underlying factors that prevent the ability of cells and tissues to regenerate, return to normal structure, or resume normal functioning (Box 39.2).
  - Partial-thickness wounds (loss of tissue limited to epidermis and possible partial loss of the dermis) heal by the process of regeneration.
  - Full-thickness wounds (total loss of skin layers and some deeper tissues) heal by scar formation.

Pressure Injury Versus Pressure Ulcer

The term *pressure injury* replaced *pressure ulcer* in the National Pressure Ulcer Advisory Panel (NPUAP) Pressure Injury Staging System as of April 2016 (Box 39.3). This update was the result of a consensus process to more accurately describe pressure injuries to both intact and ulcerated skin. In the previous staging system, stage

---

BOX 39.2

Factors That Influence Wound Healing

- ***Adequate blood perfusion and oxygenation*** are necessary for new vessel development, collagen synthesis, and development of tensile strength. Conditions that affects the blood, such as vasoconstriction, edema, hypoxia, hypotension, or hypovolemia, will affect wound healing.
- ***Nutrition and hydration*** are key factors to support collagen synthesis, tensile strength, and immune function. In a study conducted by Allard and colleagues (2016), it was determined that over 45% of patients admitted to acute care facilities were clinically malnourished on admission.
- ***Chronic moisture*** from fecal and urinary incontinence compromises the protective barrier of the skin and may macerate tissue, making skin more susceptible to breakdown. In addition, the alteration in pH (acid mantle) related to urine or feces can compromise the barrier effectiveness of the acid mantle (Elias, 2015).
- ***Pressure off-loading*** is a key element in skin breakdown, either through the unrelieved pressure from immobility or through friction or shear (NPUAP et al., 2014). Shear can damage the skin through dragging along a surface—for example, when "boosting" a person in bed, forgetting to support the heels, or when an individual with spinal cord injury is transferring from the bed to wheelchair without use of a support or slider device. Friction injury may result if a patient is agitated and frequently rubbing across a surface (Brienza, Antokal, Herbe, et al., 2015).
- ***Wound infection or increased bioburden*** in the wound bed will prolong the inflammatory response, and the microorganisms use nutrients and oxygen needed for wound repair.
- ***Advanced age*** can contribute to a diminished proliferation of cells critical to pressure injury repair.
- A patient with ***diabetes mellitus*** may have impaired wound healing because of abnormal and prolonged inflammation, reduced collagen synthesis, and impaired epithelial migration. Hyperglycemia is associated with compromised neutrophil function and impaired migration.
- ***Corticosteroid therapy or the use of other immunosuppressive agents*** such as chemotherapy increases the patient's susceptibility to infection.
- ***Medical devices*** can cause pressure injury or skin breakdown if the device is over a bony prominence or nonbony locations from a poorly positioned or ill-fitting device or incorrect device use. These types of skin injuries are called *medical device–related pressure injuries (MDRPIs)* and defined as injuries resulting from devices designed and applied for diagnostic or treatment purposes. The injury generally conforms to the shape of the device (WOCN, 2016).

From Doughty, D. B., & Sparks-Defriese, B. (2016). Wound healing physiology. In R. A. Bryant & D. P. Nix (Eds.), *Acute and chronic wounds: Current management concepts* (5th ed.). St. Louis: Mosby.

BOX 39.3

Staging of Pressure Injuries

Position

Stage 1 Pressure Injury: Nonblanchable erythema of intact skin

Intact skin with a localized area of nonblanchable erythema, which may appear differently in darkly pigmented skin. Presence of blanchable erythema or changes in sensation, temperature, or firmness may precede visual changes. Colour changes do not include purple or maroon discoloration; these may indicate deep tissue pressure injury.

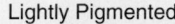

Lightly Pigmented

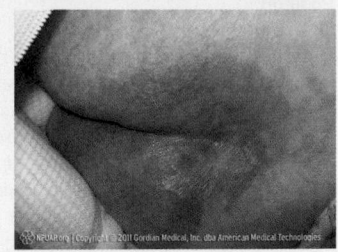

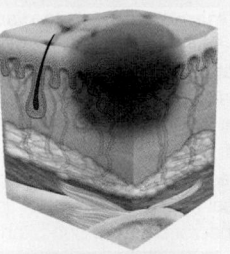

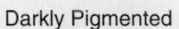

Darkly Pigmented

Stage 2 Pressure Injury: Partial-thickness skin loss with exposed dermis

Partial-thickness loss of skin with exposed dermis. The wound bed is viable, pink or red, and moist and may also present as an intact or ruptured serum-filled blister. Adipose (fat) and deeper tissues are not visible. Granulation tissue, slough, and eschar are not present. These injuries commonly result from adverse microclimate and shear in the skin over the pelvis and shear in the heel. This stage should not be used to describe moisture-associated skin damage (MASD), including incontinence-associated dermatitis (IAD), intertriginous dermatitis (ITD), medical adhesive–related skin injury (MARSI), or traumatic wounds (skin tears, burns, abrasions).

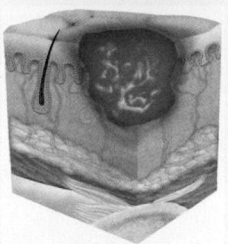

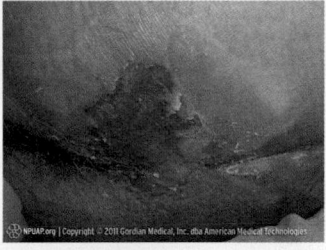

Stage 3 Pressure Injury: Full-thickness skin loss

Full-thickness loss of skin, in which adipose (fat) is visible in the injury and granulation tissue and epibole (rolled wound edges) are often present. Slough and/or eschar may be visible. The depth of tissue damage varies by anatomical location; areas of significant adiposity can develop deep wounds. Undermining and tunnelling may occur. Fascia, muscle, tendon, ligament, cartilage, and/or bone are not exposed. If slough or eschar obscures the extent of tissue loss, this is an *Unstageable Pressure Injury*.

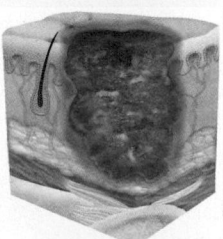

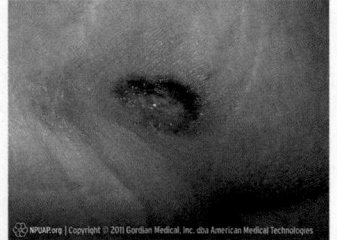

Stage 4 Pressure Injury: Full-thickness skin and tissue loss

Full-thickness skin and tissue loss with exposed or directly palpable fascia, muscle, tendon, ligament, cartilage, or bone in the injury. Slough and/or eschar may be visible. Epibole (rolled edges), undermining, and/or tunnelling often occur. Depth varies by anatomical location. If slough or eschar obscures the extent of tissue loss, this is an *Unstageable Pressure Injury*.

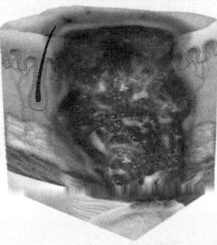

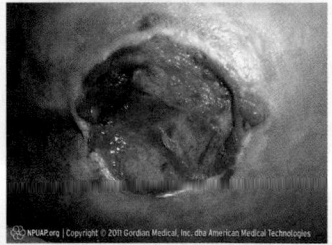

Continued

BOX 39.3

Staging of Pressure Injuries—cont'd

Position
Deep Tissue Pressure Injury:
Persistent nonblanchable deep red, maroon, or purple discoloration
Intact or nonintact skin with localized area of persistent nonblanchable deep red, maroon, or purple discoloration or epidermal separation revealing a dark wound bed or blood-filled blister. Pain and temperature change often precede skin colour changes. Discoloration may appear differently in darkly pigmented skin. This injury results from intense and/or prolonged pressure and shear forces at the bone–muscle interface. The wound may evolve rapidly to reveal the actual extent of tissue injury or may resolve without tissue loss. If necrotic tissue, subcutaneous tissue, granulation tissue, fascia, muscle, or other underlying structures are visible, this indicates a full-thickness pressure injury (unstageable, stage 3 or 4). Do not use *deep tissue pressure injury (DTPI)* to describe vascular, traumatic, neuropathic, or dermatological conditions.

Unstageable Pressure Injury:
Obscured full-thickness skin and tissue loss: Full-thickness skin and tissue loss in which the extent of tissue damage within the injury cannot be confirmed because it is obscured by slough or eschar. If slough or eschar is removed, a stage 3 or 4 pressure injury will be revealed. *Stable eschar* (i.e., dry, adherent, intact without erythema or fluctuance) on the heel or ischemic limb *should not be softened or removed.*

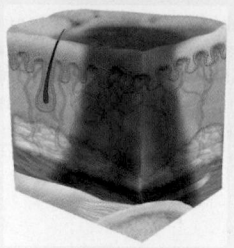
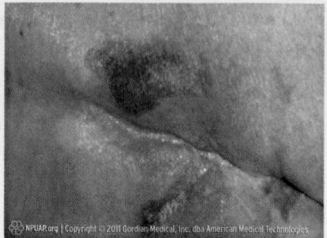

Dark Eschar

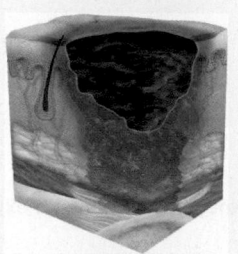
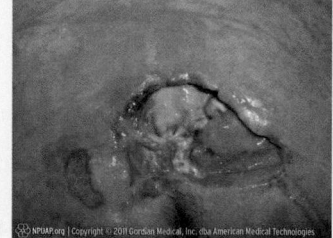

Slough Eschar

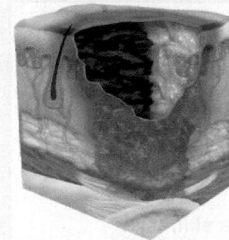

Used with permission of the National Pressure Ulcer Advisory Panel, (NPUAP), European Pressure Ulcer Advisory Panel (EPUAP), & Pan Pacific Pressure Injury Alliance (PPPIA). (2016). *Prevention and treatment of pressure ulcers: Quick reference guide.* Osborne Park, Western Australia: Cambridge Media.

1 and deep tissue injury described intact skin with underlying injury, whereas the other stages described open injuries. This description led to confusion because the definitions for each of the stages referred to the injuries as pressure *ulcer*, implying open wounds (NPUAP, 2016). This chapter will make some references to pressure ulcers because this was the terminology used when the cited literature was published; however, most of this text will use the evidence-informed term *pressure injury*.

PERSON-CENTRED CARE

- Actions that promote communication, being conscious of a patient's privacy (e.g., using drapes and sheets), and prompt removal of soiled dressings and bed linens are inherent aspects of care for every patient.
- Sensitivity toward cultural differences is essential. Paying attention to the patient's and family's cultural and religious needs will help to allay anxiety and miscommunication.
- In providing skin care, nurses need to recognize potentially sensitive issues, such as whether care needs to be provided by the same gender of health care personnel as that of the patient.

In some cultures, it may be inappropriate to expose body parts to a member of the opposite sex (Fearns, Heller-Murphy, Kelly, et al., 2017). Use of a professional translator may also be required, to ensure communication is clearly understood by the patient, caregiver, and health care provider. Unless unavoidable (e.g., emergency situation), family members or other staff members should not be used as translators.
- When changing dressings or assessing wounds, it is important to recognize that blood and secretions may have significance for some cultures (e.g., bed linens or gowns may be considered "dirty" and should be promptly changed; blood maybe seen as a life force, so the presence of it on dressings or sheets should first be explained and then removed as soon as possible).
- Some religious beliefs may prohibit dressings containing any animal-derived products (e.g., some dressings may contain animal-derived collagen) (Chong, Kok, Choke, et al., 2017).
- Encourage patients to talk about any traditional home remedies and practices that they may have used or might use. It is important to respectfully explain to the patient and caregiver when these practices need to be avoided if they could increase risk for infection or negatively affect wound healing.

EVIDENCE-INFORMED PRACTICE

- Risk assessment is a central component of clinical practice aimed at identifying individuals susceptible to skin breakdown, to target appropriate prevention and treatment interventions (NPUAP, EPUAP, PPPIA, et al., 2014; WOCN, 2016):
  - Ensure that a complete skin assessment is part of the risk assessment screening policy at all health care facilities (NPUAP et al., 2014; WOCN, 2016). Ongoing, regular skin assessment is necessary to detect early signs of skin breakdown, particularly pressure-related damage.
  - In individuals at risk for skin breakdown (see Factors, Box 39.2), a comprehensive skin assessment should be conducted as soon as possible, but within 8 hours of admission (or first visit in community setting). Ongoing assessment and evaluation should be part of the patient care plan, related to the level of risk, and prior to care transition or discharge from care (NPUAP et al., 2014; WOCN, 2016).
  - If risk is identified, relevant interventions need to be implemented immediately. For example, pressure relief strategies, including repositioning and use of pressure reduction surfaces, should be implemented. All interventions must be documented in relation to the identified risk.
- Skin integrity bundles that identify key areas of assessment, skin-care measures, repositioning, and pressure-reducing strategies are effective in reducing frequency and severity of pressure injuries in critically ill patients. Many facilities have implemented this approach, as these bundles provide health care providers with specific preventive and treatment measures for a select group of at-risk or high-risk patients (Coyer, Gardner, Duobrovsky, et al., 2015).
- There is some evidence of the effectiveness of silicon-foam dressings prophylactically applied in high-risk patients to prevent pressure injury development (Black, Clark, Dealey, et al., 2015; Byrne, Nichols, Sroczynski, et al., 2016). However, frequent repositioning, visual inspection of the area, and incontinence management are also essential.
- Routine assessment of skin under and around medical devices helps reduce the risk for pressure injury, aids in identifying early stages of skin breakdown, and prompts interventions (Black & Kalowes, 2016; Pittman, Beeson, Kitterman, et al., 2015).
- Nonviable tissue in a wound can delay wound healing and contribute to wound infection. *Debridement*, the removal of nonviable tissue from the wound, is an essential objective of topical therapy and a critical component of optimal wound management (Ramundo, 2016).
- Methods of debridement include enzymatic, mechanical, autolytic, and sharp. The type of debridement chosen depends on the condition of the wound, the goal of wound treatment, and the patient's overall condition (NPUAP et al., 2014; WOCN, 2016).
- Enzymatic debridement is the topical application of enzymes such as collagenase over the necrotic tissue. Collagenase digests the necrotic tissue by dissolving the collagen in the dead tissue (NPUAP et al., 2014). When collagenase is used on a wound, the necrotic tissue is covered with the collagenase, and a moisture-retentive dressing can be used to soften the tissue (Ramundo, 2016).
- World Health Organization (WHO) (2016) guidelines advocate the use of triclosan-coated sutures because there is moderate evidence to support their use for reducing the risk for surgical site infection or postoperative wound complications. It is important that the primary repair approximates the wound edges and the incision is adequately perfused.

SAFETY GUIDELINES

- Patients should be routinely assessed for risk of skin breakdown. This is particularly important for patients who have any underlying factors that would increase the risk of pressure injury. The Braden Risk Assessment Scale (Braden Scale) (Table 39.1) or the Norton Scale (WOCN, 2016) are valid and reliable tools that provide guidance for effective interventions to reduce the risk of skin breakdown. However, evidence is lacking to conclude that the use of risk assessment scales reduces the incidence of pressure injuries (WOCN, 2016). It is the combination of identified risk (based on a risk assessment tool), critical thinking, clinical judgement, and targeted interventions aimed at the specific risk factors that decreases potential pressure injury development.
- The standard risk assessment tools provide instructions for preventive interventions. These include documentation of the location of pressure points, and establishment of a repositioning routine and implementing it every 1–2 hours as patient condition allows, to ensure redistribution of pressure from the superficial capillaries and allow tissues to compensate for temporary ischemia. Nurses need to follow appropriate lifting and handling guidelines to avoid friction and shear (see Chapter 11).
- Patients at high risk for pressure injury should be placed on specialized beds, overlays, or mattresses (see Chapter 13), which redistribute pressure over the entire body surface to prevent excess pressure over bony prominences. By distributing pressure evenly over a patient's body surface, less pressure is applied to a concentrated area. Similar products to redistribute pressure (e.g., high-density foam, gel, or inflatable air cushion) should be provided for at-risk patients (e.g., those who sitting in a wheelchair or geriatric chair).
- Patients who are incontinent of stool or urine must be cleaned as soon as possible. Use gentle cleansing cloths and/or no-rinse perineal cleanser. Prolonged skin moisture from urinary and fecal incontinence creates alteration in skin pH as well as, in the case of fecal incontinence, fecal enzyme action on the skin—all significant risk factors for skin breakdown (Thayer, Rozenboom, & Baranoski, 2016). Areas subjected to repeated episodes of incontinence should be protected with a barrier ointment, cream, or paste, but these products must not interfere with the effectiveness of continence briefs (adult diapers). Avoid use of corn starch or baby powder (Yates, 2018). Fecal containment devices are available for difficult-to-manage fecal incontinence (see Chapter 35).
- Minimize friction and shear through use of lift sheets when repositioning patients, to reduce rubbing the skin against sheets. Ensure heels are not dragging when repositioning. Raise the head of the bed no more than 30 degrees (unless medically contraindicated) to prevent sliding and shear injury and to decrease pressure on the coccyx (WOCN, 2016).
- Adequate nutrition helps to prevent and treat pressure injuries (WOCN, 2016). A diet high in protein with enough calories, vitamins, and minerals helps maintain normal tissue status and promotes healing. With tissue injury, the body needs more energy (calories) for healing; nutrient deficiencies may result in impaired or delayed healing. Monitoring a patient's nutritional status is part of the nurse's total assessment (WOCN, 2016).
- Use interprofessional collaboration (e.g., wound care nurse, dietitian) to support optimal wound healing.
- Do not remove an initial surgical dressing for direct wound inspection until the health care provider writes a prescription for removal. If drainage has saturated the initial dressing or the patient is experiencing unanticipated or increased pain,

TABLE 39.1

Braden Scale for Predicting Pressure Injury Risk*

Sensory Perception

Ability to respond meaningfully to pressure-related discomfort	1. *Completely limited:* Unresponsive (does not moan, flinch, or grasp) to painful stimuli because of diminished level of consciousness or sedation *or* Limited ability to feel pain over most of the body	2. *Very limited:* Responds only to painful stimuli; cannot communicate discomfort except by moaning or restlessness *or* Has a sensory impairment that limits the ability to feel pain or discomfort over half of the body	3. *Slightly limited:* Responds to verbal commands but cannot always communicate discomfort or need to be turned *or* Has some sensory impairment, which limits ability to feel pain or discomfort in one or two extremities	4. *No impairment:* Responds to verbal commands; has no sensory deficit that would limit ability to feel or voice pain or discomfort

Moisture

	1. *Constantly moist:* Skin kept moist almost constantly by factors such as perspiration and urine; dampness detected every time patient is moved or turned	2. *Very moist:* Skin often but not always moist; linen must be changed at least once a shift	3. *Occasionally moist:* Skin occasionally moist, requiring extra linen change approximately once a day	4. *Rarely moist:* Skin usually dry; linen requires changing only at routine intervals

Activity

Degree of physical activity	1. *Bedfast:* Confined to bed	2. *Chairfast:* Ability to walk severely limited or nonexistent Cannot bear own weight and/or must be helped into chair or wheelchair	3. *Walks occasionally:* Walks occasionally during day but for very short distances with or without help; spends most of each shift in bed or chair	4. *Walks frequently:* Walks outside room at least twice a day and inside room at least once every 2 hours during waking hours

Mobility

Ability to change and control body position	1. *Completely immobile:* Does not make even slight changes in body or extremity position without help	2. *Very limited:* Makes occasional slight changes in body or extremity position but unable to make frequent or significant changes independently	3. *Slightly limited:* Makes frequent, although slight, changes in body or extremity position independently	4. *No limitations:* Makes major and frequent changes in position without help

Nutrition

Usual food intake pattern	1. *Very poor:* Never eats a complete meal Rarely eats more than one third of any food offered; eats two servings or less of protein (meat or dairy products) per day; takes fluids poorly; does not take a liquid dietary supplement *or* Is NPO and/or maintained on clear liquids or IV infusions for more than 5 days	2. *Probably inadequate:* Rarely eats a complete meal and generally eats only about half of any food offered Protein intake includes only three servings of meat or dairy products per day; occasionally takes a dietary supplement *or* Receives less than optimal amount of liquid diet or tube feeding	3. *Adequate:* Eats over half of most meals; eats a total of four servings of protein (meat, dairy products) each day; occasionally refuses a meal but usually takes a supplement when offered *or* Is on a tube-feeding or TPN regimen that probably meets most of nutritional needs	4. *Excellent:* Eats most of every meal; never refuses a meal; usually eats a total of four or more servings of meat and dairy products per day; occasionally eats between meals; does not require supplementation

Friction and Shear

	1. *Problem:* Requires moderate-to-maximum help to move; complete lifting without sliding against sheets is impossible Frequently slides down in bed or chair; repositioning with maximal help; spasticity, contractions, or agitation leads to almost constant friction	2. *Potential problem:* Moves feebly or requires minimal help; during a move skin probably slides to some extent against sheets, chair, restraints, or other devices; maintains relatively good position in chair or bed most of the time but occasionally slides down	3. *No apparent problem:* Moves in bed and chair independently and has sufficient muscle strength to sit up completely during move; maintains good position in bed or chair	

Adapted from Barbara Braden, PhD, RN, Creighton University School of Nursing, Omaha, NE.
IV, Intravenous; *NPO,* nothing by mouth; *TPN,* total parenteral nutrition.
*Score patient in each of the six subscales. Maximum score is 23, indicating little or no risk. A score of ≤18 indicates at risk; ≤9 indicates very high risk.

contact the health care provider for reassessment of the surgical site.

- If needed, provide analgesia 30 minutes before a dressing change.

- Healed skin from a prior injury or ulceration is weaker than skin that has never had an injury.

- Know a patient's nutritional status. Tissue repair and infection resistance are directly related to adequate nutrition, including proteins, carbohydrates, lipids, vitamins, and minerals. Patients who are malnourished are at increased risk for wound infections and wound infection–related sepsis (Stotts, 2016a). Recognize that culture and religion may prohibit certain foods and may also affect nutritional intake during designated religious holidays.

- Understand the risks of obesity. Inadequate vascularization decreases delivery of nutrients and cellular elements required for healing. The patient is at greater risk for wound infection and dehiscence or evisceration (Beitz, 2014).

- When a drain is present, clean the drain site using a circular stroke, starting with the area immediately next to the drain (Fig. 39.6). Using sterile gauze, clean immediately next to the drain and attempt to clean a little farther out from the drain.

- Identify factors that decrease oxygenation, such as decreased hemoglobin level, smoking, and underlying cardiopulmonary conditions. Adequate oxygenation at the tissue level is essential for white blood cell activity and phagocytosis, fibroblast proliferation and collagen synthesis, and re-epithelialization (Doughty & Sparks-Defriese, 2016). Tissue repair is negatively influenced by a hematocrit value below 33% and a hemoglobin value below 10 g/100 mL. Hemoglobin level and oxygen release to tissues are reduced in smokers.

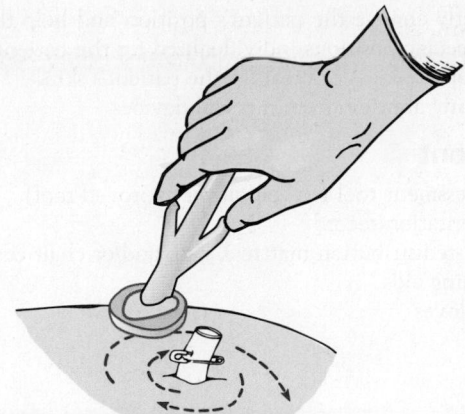

FIG 39.6 Cleaning drain site.

- Know the types of medications prescribed. Steroids reduce the inflammatory response and slow collagen synthesis. Cortisone depresses fibroblast activity and capillary growth. Chemotherapy depresses bone marrow production of white blood cells and impairs immune function.

- Identify the presence of chronic diseases or chronic trauma, such as diabetes mellitus or radiation. Decreased tissue perfusion and failure to release oxygen to tissues result from diabetes mellitus.

♦ SKILL 39.1 Risk Assessment, Skin Assessment, and Prevention Strategies: Pressure Injury

NSO *Nursing Skills Online Wound Care Module 19 / Lessons 1 and 4*

The goal in preventing the development of pressure injuries is early identification of an at-risk patient and the implementation of prevention strategies. The *Guidelines for Prevention and Management of Pressure Injuries* (WOCN, 2016) are a compilation of international research and expert reviews that include the following:

- Identify individuals at risk for developing pressure injuries and initiate an early prevention program.
- Implement appropriate strategies and plans to attain and maintain intact skin and prevent skin breakdown and complications.
- Promptly identify and manage complications.
- Involve patient and caregiver in patient's self-management of skin care and pressure injury.
- Implement cost-effective strategies and plans that prevent and treat pressure injuries.

The current recommendation is to perform a pressure injury risk assessment on patient admission to a health care facility and to repeat this on a regularly scheduled basis or when there is a significant change in a patient's condition (WOCN, 2016). For example, if a patient who was ambulatory on admission becomes confined to bed because of a surgical procedure, this person is potentially at higher risk for skin breakdown than when first admitted. When assessing patients, the nurse needs to use risk assessment tools such as the Braden Scale or the Norton Scale (WOCN, 2016).

The Braden Scale (see Table 39.1) has six subscale parameters: sensory perception, moisture, activity, mobility, nutrition, and risk

of friction and shear (Ayello & Braden, 2002; Braden & Bergstrom, 1989, 1994). Maximum score is 23, indicating little to no risk, and scores range from at risk to very high risk (Table 39.2). It is important to understand how to interpret the meaning of a patient's total score and, more importantly, the subscores. The higher the score, the lower the risk (see Table 39.1). Specific interventions related to the subscore results should be documented and implemented.

As a nurse, you need to inspect a patient's skin and bony prominences at least daily and in good light. Direct (artificial) lighting may be required in order to identify pressure-related skin changes on darker-skinned individuals. Remove medical devices or tape securing these devices, shoes, socks, antiembolic stockings and heel and elbow protectors for skin inspection (Black & Kalowes, 2016). Inspect all bony prominences, including back of head, shoulders, rib cage, elbows, hips, ischium, sacrum, coccyx, knees, ankles, and heels (see Fig. 39.2). Palpate any reddened or discoloured areas with a gloved finger to determine if the erythema blanches. Blanching is normal and expected. If you palpate an area that does not blanch (abnormal reactive hyperemia), this area is a site for potential skin breakdown.

Delegation and Collaboration

While the skill of pressure injury risk assessment cannot be delegated to an unregulated care provider (UCP), the nurse should instruct the UCP to:

- Frequently change the patient's position and help the patient to use specific positions individualized for the patient.
- Report any redness or break in the patient's skin.
- Report any abrasion from medical devices.

Equipment

- Risk assessment tool (use employer-approved tool)
- Documentation record
- Pressure-redistribution mattress, bed, and/or chair cushion
- Positioning aids
- Clean gloves

TABLE 39.2

Braden Risk Assessment Scale Score Interpretation

Classification	Risk Scores
At risk	15–18
Moderate risk	13–14
High risk	10–12
Very high risk	≤9

Data from British Columbia Provincial Nursing Skin and Wound Committee. (2014). *Braden scale for predicting pressure ulcer risk in adults & children/infants.* Retrieved from https://www.clwk.ca/buddydrive/file/guideline-braden-risk-assessment/

STEP	RATIONALE

ASSESSMENT

1. Identify patient using at least two person-specific identifiers (e.g., name and date of birth or name and medical record number), according to employer policy.

Ensures correct patient. Complies with Accreditation Canada standards and improves patient safety (Accreditation Canada, 2019).

2. Review medical record to assess patient's risk for pressure injury formation:

Determines need to administer preventive care and identifies specific factors that place patient at risk (NPUAP et al., 2014).

   a. Paralysis or immobilization caused by restrictive devices

Patient is unable to turn or reposition independently or relieve pressure.

   b. Presence of a medical device such as a nasogastric (NG) tube, oxygen equipment, artificial airways, drainage tubing, or mechanical devices (Doughty & McNichols, 2016).

Medical devices have the potential to exert pressure on a patient's nares or ears or on tissue adjacent to devices such as artificial airways and drainage tubes (Pittman et al., 2015).

    (1) If not medically contraindicated, remove medical device to observe and palpate skin and tissues under and around each medical device.

Pressure area assumes the same configuration as medical device (WOCN, 2016; Schallom, Cracchiolo, Falker, et al., 2015).

   c. Sensory loss (e.g., hemiplegia, spinal cord injury)

Patient is unable to feel discomfort from pressure and does not independently change position.

   d. Circulatory disorders (e.g., peripheral vascular diseases, vascular changes from diabetes mellitus, neuropathy)

Reduce perfusion of tissue layers in skin.

   e. Increased temperature

Increases metabolic demands of tissues.
Accompanying diaphoresis leaves skin moist.

   f. Anemia

Decreased hemoglobin level reduces oxygen-carrying capacity of blood and amount of oxygen available to tissues.

   g. Malnutrition

Inadequate nutrition leads to weight loss, muscle atrophy, and reduced tissue mass.
Nutrient deficiencies result in impaired or delayed healing (Stotts, 2016a).

   h. Fecal or urinary incontinence

Skin becomes exposed to a moist environment that contains bacteria. Excessive moisture macerates skin (Whitehead, Giampieri, Graham, et al., 2017).

   i. Heavy sedation and anaesthesia

Patient is not alert and does not turn or change position independently. Sedation alters sensory perception.

   j. Age

Neonates and very young children are at high risk for pressure injury, the head being the most common site (WOCN, 2016).
There is loss of dermal thickness in older persons, impairing the ability to distribute pressure (Pieper, 2016).

   k. Dehydration

Results in decreased skin elasticity and turgor.

   l. Edema

Edematous tissues are less tolerant of pressure, friction, and shear.

   m. Existing pressure injuries

Limit surfaces available for position changes, placing available tissues at increased risk.

   n. History of pressure injury

Tensile strength of skin from previously healed pressure injury is 80% or less; therefore, this area cannot tolerate pressure as much as undamaged skin (Doughty & Sparks-Defriese, 2016).

STEP	RATIONALE

ASSESSMENT

3. Use an employer-approved risk assessment tool such as the Braden Scale or Norton Scale. Perform risk assessment when patient enters the health care facility and repeat on a regularly scheduled basis or when there is significant change in patient's condition (WOCN, 2016).

Valid and reliable risk assessment tools help in evaluating a patient's risk for developing a pressure injury. Identifying risk factors that contribute to the potential for skin breakdown enables you to target specific interventions for decreasing risk for skin breakdown.

4. Obtain risk score (see Tables 39.1, 39.2, and 39.3) and evaluate its meaning based on patient's unique characteristics.

Risk cutoff score depends on the instrument used. Score involves identifying contributing risk factors and minimizing negative outcomes.

5. Perform hand hygiene. Assess condition of patient's skin over regions of pressure (see Fig. 39.2). Apply gloves as needed with open and draining wounds.

Body weight against bony prominences places underlying skin at risk for breakdown.

  a. Inspect skin for discoloration (see Box 39.2 for patients with darkly pigmented skin) and tissue consistency (firm or boggy) and palpate for abnormal sensations (Nix, 2016).

Indicates that tissue was under pressure; hyperemia is a normal physiological response to hypoxemia in tissues.

  b. Palpate discoloured area on skin and under and around medical devices. Release your fingertip and look for blanching.

If on palpation an area of redness blanches (lightens in colour), this indicates normal reactive hyperemia; tissue is not at risk for skin breakdown. Tissue that does not blanch when palpated indicates abnormal reactive hyperemia, an indication of possible ischemic injury.

  c. Inspect for pallor or mottling.

Persistent hypoxia in tissues that were under pressure is an abnormal physiological response.

  d. Inspect for absence of superficial skin layers.

Represents early pressure injury formation; usually a partial-thickness wound that may have resulted from friction, shear, or both.

  e. Inspect for changes in skin temperature, edema, and tissue consistency, especially individuals with darkly pigmented skin.

Localized heat, edema, and induration have been identified as warning signs for pressure injury development. Because it is not always possible to observe changes in skin colour on darkly pigmented skin, these additional signs should be considered in the assessment (NPUAP et al., 2014).

  f. Inspect for wound drainage.

Wound drainage increases risk for skin breakdown because it is caustic to skin and underlying tissues.

Tubing from drainage devices (e.g., Jackson-Pratt, Hemovac) causes pressure under the device and on adjacent skin (Black et al., 2015).

6. Assess skin and tissue around and beneath medical devices every nursing shift for additional areas of potential pressure injury resulting from medical devices (Black et al., 2015) (Table 39.4).

Patients at high risk have multiple sites for pressure necrosis from medical devices in areas other than bony prominences (Makic, 2015).

Pressure points around medical devices (e.g., oxygen cannula and masks, drainage tubing) can cause pressure injury to underlying tissue and become full-thickness pressure injuries (Black et al., 2015; Pittman et al., 2015; Schallom et al., 2015).

TABLE 39.3		
Pressure Injury Risk Assessment		
Level of Care	**Initial**	**Reassessment**
Acute care	Within 8 hours of admission (NPUAP et al., 2014)	• On a defined schedule (e.g., every 24 to 72 hours) • Whenever major change in patient's condition occurs
Critical care	On admission	• Every 24 hours (Tayyib & Coyer, 2016) (see employer policy)
Long-term care	On admission	• Weekly for first 4 weeks after admission • Routinely on quarterly basis • Whenever patient's condition changes or deteriorates
Community care	On admission	• As per employer policy

STEP	RATIONALE

ASSESSMENT

7. Observe patient for preferred positions when in bed or chair. Note and care for contractures; provide pressure relief with, for example, foam wedges.

Preferred positions result in weight of body being placed on certain body prominences.

Presence of contractures may result in pressure exerted in unexpected places.

8. Observe ability of patient to initiate and help with position changes.

Potential for friction and shear injuries increases when patient is dependent on others for position changes.

9. Assess patient's and caregiver's understanding of what a pressure injury is and the individual risks for patient to develop pressure injuries.

Gaps in understanding of the significance of pressure injury and thus its prevention may lead to exacerbation of skin breakdown.

NURSING DIAGNOSES

- Inadequate peripheral tissue perfusion
- Insufficient knowledge regarding pressure injury prevention
- Inadequate nutrition
- Reduced mobility
- Reduced skin integrity
- Potential for impaired skin integrity

Related factors/Risk factors are individualized on the basis of patient's condition or needs.

PLANNING

1. Expected outcomes following identification/assessment and intervention plan:
- Risk factors are identified.

Establishes approach to patient needs and baseline for future assessment.

- Patient experiences no change from baseline skin assessment.

Prevention interventions diminish occurrence or worsening of pressure injury.

- Skin is intact with no evidence of erythema or no signs of breakdown.

Prevention strategies reduce risk factors.

- Patient and caregiver are able to articulate and respond to patient's individual risk factors for pressure injury.

Demonstrates knowledge transfer.

2. Explain procedure(s) and purpose to patient and caregiver.

Relieves anxiety and provides opportunity for education.

IMPLEMENTATION

1. Implement prevention guidelines adapted from WOCN (2016) *Guideline for Prevention and Management of Pressure Ulcers.*

Reduces patient's risk for developing pressure injury.

2. Close room door or bedside curtain and perform hand hygiene.

Demonstrates person-centred care by maintaining patient privacy and reducing possibility of bacterial transmission.

3. If patient has open, draining wounds, wear sterile surgical gloves.

Use of routine practices and additional precautions prevents accidental exposure to body fluids.

4. Following initial assessment, continue to inspect skin at least once a day.

a. Observe patient's skin; pay particular attention to bony prominences and areas around and under medical devices and tubes. If you find a reddened area, gently press area with a gloved finger to check for blanching. If area does not blanch, ensure pressure off-loading; suspect tissue injury and recheck in 1 hour. Discoloration may vary from pink to deep red.

Routine skin inspection is fundamental to risk assessment and in selecting interventions to reduce risk of injury (WOCN, 2016). Persistent redness when lightly pigmented skin is pressed can indicate tissue injury. If the area of redness blanches (pales in colour), it indicates that the skin is likely not at risk for breakdown.

Clinical Decision Point *Do not massage reddened areas, because doing so may cause additional tissue trauma. Reddened areas indicate blood vessel damage, and massaging can further damage the vessel (Bryant & Nix, 2016a).*

b. If patient has darkly pigmented skin, look for colour changes that differ from their normal skin colour.

Darkly pigmented skin may not blanch. A change in colour may occur at the site of pressure; this change in colour *differs* from patient's usual skin colour (NPUAP et al., 2014) (see Box 39.2).

STEP	RATIONALE

IMPLEMENTATION

5. Each shift, check all treatment and assistive devices (e.g., catheters, feeding tubes, casts, braces) for potential pressure points (see Table 39.4).

Pressure from these devices increases risk on bony prominences and other areas.

    a. Verify that device is correctly sized, positioned, and secured.

Incorrect size, placement, and securing of medical device can cause excessive pressure and rubbing by device on underlying skin (Makic, 2015).

TABLE 39.4

Strategies to Prevent Medical and Immobilization Device–Related Pressure Injuries

Device	Pressure Areas	Prevention Strategies*
Nasogastric tubes	Nares Skin on nasal bridge	Secure tube using pressure-relieving techniques, which direct pressure from tube away from the nares (see Chapters 32 and 35). Reposition tube.
Endotracheal tubes	Lips Tongue	Remove securing device daily and inspect for pressure injury (Black & Kalowes, 2016). Rotate tube every shift or more often.
Nasotracheal tube	Nose/nasal bridge Nares	Remove securing device daily and inspect for pressure injury (Black & Kalowes, 2016). Reposition.
Tracheostomy tubes	Front of neck and stoma site Back of neck	Remove securing device daily. Increase stoma care. Apply pressure reduction dressing to back of neck.
Oxygen and cannula and tubing	Ears Nose	Apply pressure reduction dressing to external ear. Periodically remove cannula to relieve pressure and inspect for pressure injury (Schallom et al., 2015).
Noninvasive positive-pressure ventilation (NIPPV)/bilevel positive airway pressure (BiPAP)	Forehead Nose/nasal bridge	Pretreat bridge of nose with pressure reduction dressing before application of mask. If possible, remove mask for a few minutes.
Drainage tubing	Area immediately next to drainage tube Adjacent area during patient position changes	Apply appropriate dressing around drainage tube. Check tubing placement with each position change. Instruct patient not to lie on tubing (Pittman et al., 2015).
In-dwelling catheter	Thighs Female: urethra, labia Male: tip of penis	Provide meticulous perineal care. Anchor and secure catheter to reduce pressure.
Orthopaedic devices	All areas where device comes in contact with patient's skin and tissues	When possible and not contraindicated, inspect under the device.
Neck collar	Neck and occipital region Scalp	Remove hard collars as soon as possible and replace with softer collar (Black et al., 2015). Inspect scalp daily.
TED (thromboembolic deterrent) hose or stockings (*not the same as compression stockings*)	Calf Behind knee Heel Toes	Verify proper fit. Remove stockings for observation of pressure points. Are worn only by nonambulatory patients. *Compression stockings* must be fitted after circulation has been assessed (ankle-brachial pressure index or vascular flow studies), which should be documented in patient's history. Compression stockings are designed for ambulatory individuals and are generally applied on arising and removed at bedtime.
Immobilization devices	Wrists Ankles	Apply dressing between patient's skin and immobilizer (Black et al., 2015). Verify space between immobilizer and patient's skin. Ensure assistance from person (e.g., unregulated care provider) and remove restraints one at a time to inspect skin.

*In addition to routine inspection and cleansing of skin under and around medical device.

STEP	RATIONALE

IMPLEMENTATION

b. Consider shielding underlying skin with protective dressing (low-profile nonadherent [silicone] foam, hydrocolloid or dimenthecone barrier, applied as a wipe).

Silicone foam dressing provides moisture-vapour transfer to wick moisture away from body. Hydrocolloid is occlusive but can provide protection from friction and shear. Dimenthecone barrier wipes function as "second skin" barrier (Black et al., 2015; Makic, 2015).

Clinical Decision Point *Inspect skin around and beneath orthopaedic devices (e.g., cervical collar, braces, or cast). Note any abrasions or warmth in areas where devices can rub against the skin (Pittman et al., 2015; Schallom et al., 2015).*

6. Remove and dispose of gloves; perform hand hygiene.

Reduces transmission of microorganisms.

7. Review patient's pressure injury risk assessment score, paying attention to subscores.

Risk scores aid in identifying interventions to lessen or eliminate current risk factors.

8. If immobility, inactivity, or poor sensory perception is a risk factor(s) for patient, consider one of the following interventions:

Immobility and inactivity reduce a patient's ability or desire to independently change position. Poor sensory perception decreases a patient's ability to feel sensation or pressure discomfort.

a. Identify appropriate schedule to reposition patient (in consultation with patient). Plan regular assessment of skin condition to identify early signs of pressure damage. If skin changes occur, re-evaluate the plan.

Reduces duration and intensity of pressure. Some patients may require more frequent repositioning (NPUAP et al., 2014; WOCN, 2016).

b. When patient is in side-lying position in bed, use 30-degree lateral position (see illustration). Avoid using 90-degree lateral position.

Reduces contact of trochanter with support surface.

c. When needed, use pillow bridging (see illustration).

Use of pillows prevents direct contact between bony prominences.

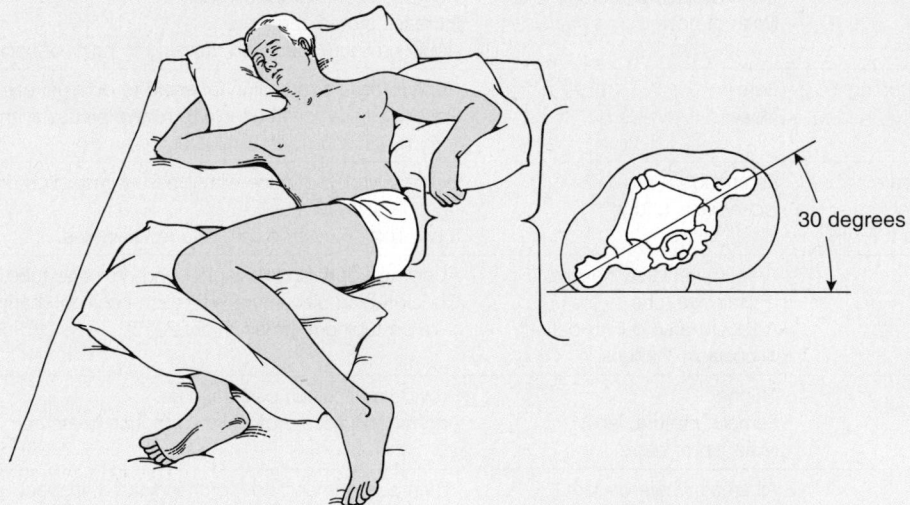

STEP 8b Thirty-degree lateral position with pillow placement.

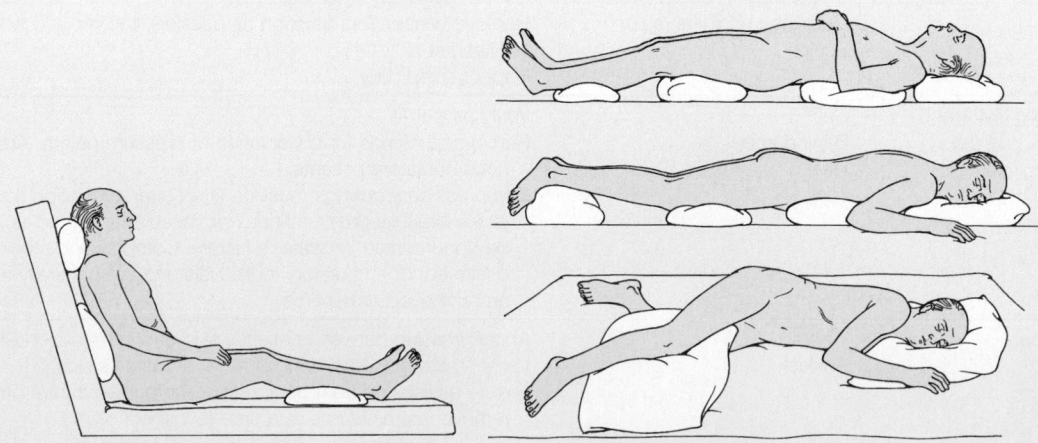

STEP 8c Pillow bridging.

STEP	RATIONALE

IMPLEMENTATION

d. In bed: Ensure pressure redistribution surface is in place for patient lying in bed. Make sure pressure on heels is reduced.

Reduces amount of pressure exerted on tissues.

e. In chair: Use pressure-redistribution device and shift points under pressure at least every hour (WOCN, 2016). Make sure heels are also provided with pressure off-loading.

Reduces amount of pressure on body areas (e.g., sacrum, ischium, heels).

9. If friction and shear are identified as risk factors, consider the following interventions:

Friction and shear damage tissue from the epidermis to below the dermis through repeated action.

a. Use safe patient handling guidelines to reposition patient (see Chapter 11). For example, use slide board or transfer sheets to move patient from bed to stretcher.

Proper repositioning of patient prevents creating shear from dragging patient along sheets. Slide board provides slippery surface to reduce friction. Use of "lift team," when appropriate, keeps patient's skin, including heels, off sheets.

b. Ensure that heels are free from surface of bed by using a pillow under calves to elevate heels or use a heel-suspension device; knees should be in 5- to 10-degree flexion (Bååth, Engström, Gunningberg, et al., 2016; WOCN, 2016).

"Floating" heels from bed surface offload the heel completely and redistribute weight of the leg along the calf without applying pressure on the Achilles tendon (Bååth et al., 2016).

c. Maintain head of bed at 30 degrees or lower or at the lowest degree of elevation consistent with patient's condition (do not lower head of bed if patient is at risk for aspiration (WOCN, 2016).

Decreases potential for patient to slide toward foot of bed and incur shear injury.

10. If patient receives *low score* on moisture subscale (e.g., Braden Scale), consider one of the following interventions:

Continual exposure of body fluids on patient's skin increases risk for skin breakdown and pressure injury development.

a. Apply clean gloves. Cleanse and pat skin dry after each incontinent episode (WOCN, 2016). Apply moisture barrier protectant (e.g., cream, ointment) to perineum and surrounding skin according to manufacturer's instructions.

Friction and shear are increased in the presence of moisture. Barrier protects skin from fecal or urinary incontinence. Some barrier products only require once/day application. Overuse leads to occlusion of skin.

b. If skin is denuded, use protective barrier cream or ointment (e.g., dimethicone or Vaseline) after each incontinent episode, depending on manufacturer's instructions (Lian, 2016).

Provides barrier between skin and stool or urine, allowing for healing.

Ensure barrier cream or ointment does not affect absorption of the continence brief.

c. If moisture source is from wound drainage, consider appropriate dressing. Ensure protective barrier to protect skin is in place. Use interprofessional collaboration to discuss collection device if indicated.

Avoids frequent exposure of wound drainage from skin, which can lead to maceration and skin breakdown.

11. If friction and shear are risk factors and patient is confined to a wheelchair:

Relief of pressure by changing from lying to sitting position is insufficient if sitting lasts a prolonged time. Patients should be encouraged to reposition; if pressure injury risk factors are present, provide pressure relief cushion (e.g., RoHo®, EHOB® or gel cushion) (WOCN, 2016).

a. Tilt patient's chair seat to prevent sliding forward; support arms, legs, and feet to maintain proper posture (NPUAP et al., 2014).

b. Limit amount of time patient spends in a chair without pressure relief (NPUAP et al., 2014).

c. For patients who can reposition themselves while sitting, encourage pressure relief every 15 minutes using chair push-ups, forward lean, or side-to-side movement (WOCN, 2016).

Assess ability of patient to comply. Continue to use pressure-reduction cushion for chair since most patients have difficulty managing repositioning on their own.

12. Educate patient and caregiver regarding pressure injury risk and prevention (WOCN, 2016).

Helps in adherence to interventions to reduce pressure injury risk.

13. Remove gloves and discard in appropriate receptacle. Perform hand hygiene.

Reduces transmission of microorganisms.

STEP	RATIONALE

EVALUATION

1. Observe patient's skin for areas at risk for tissue damage, noting change in colour, appearance, or texture (Table 39.5).

Enables you to evaluate success of prevention techniques.

2. Observe tolerance of patient for position change by measuring level of comfort on appropriate pain rating scale.

Position changes sometimes interfere with patient's sleep and rest pattern.

3. Compare subsequent risk assessment scores and skin assessments.

Provides ongoing comparison of patient's risk level to facilitate appropriateness of plan care.

4. Use Teach-Back: "I just to make sure you understand why your skin needs to be checked regularly. Can you tell me in your own words why we will be checking your skin on a regular basis?" Develop a revised teaching plan if patient or caregiver is not able to teach back correctly.

Determines patient's and caregiver's level of understanding of instructional topic.

Unexpected Outcomes

1. Skin becomes mottled, reddened, purplish, or bluish.

Related Interventions

- Notify health care provider; use interprofessional collaboration (e.g., wound care specialist, dietitian, physiotherapist [PT]) as necessary. Re-evaluate patient's circulation and oxygen saturation, immobility and position changes, and bed surface.

2. Areas under pressure develop persistent discoloration, induration, or temperature changes.

- Notify health care provider.
- Modify patient's positioning and turning schedule.
- Frequent reassessment of condition.

Communication and Documentation

- Document on flow sheet, in nurses' notes, and in electronic health record (EHR) any skin changes, patient's risk score and subscores, and skin assessment. Describe positions, turning intervals, pressure-redistribution devices, and other prevention measures. Note patient's response to the interventions.
- Document your evaluation of patient's and caregiver's understanding of the need for frequent skin and pressure injury assessment education.
- Report to health care provider the need for additional interprofessional collaboration for the high-risk patient and the time frame for consultation.

Special Considerations

Teaching

- Help patient and caregiver understand multiple factors involved in preventing and treating pressure injuries.
- Explain and demonstrate positioning options to achieve pressure redistribution.
- Explain the purpose and maintenance of pressure-redistribution devices (see Chapter 13).
- When teaching patients to change position for pressure redistribution, suggest using television programming and commercial intervals or a clock or phone with an alarm as reminders.

Pediatric

- Infants and young children in diapers are at risk for skin breakdown; also assess occiput area and ensure the child has a pressure-reduction pillow or mattress.

Gerontological

- Re-evaluate sitting posture and position because body weight and muscle tone change with age.
- In older persons, thinning skin leads to a decrease in padding protection over bony prominences, and the time for epidermal regeneration is diminished, leading to slower healing (Wysocki, 2016).
- When interpreting the Braden Scale score, consider a score of ≤18 as at risk for the older person (Ayello, 2012).

Care in the Community

- Identify community resources such as relatives, neighbours, or community (e.g., church) members who may be able to provide safe assistance (e.g., meals, transfer from bed or chair). Review available professional health care services and resources the patient and caregiver may wish to access (e.g., home care services).

TABLE 39.5

Wound Colour/Tissue

Black/brown wounds/eschar	Black or brown tissue is eschar, which represents full-thickness tissue destruction. Black is used to describe necrotic tissue or desiccated tissue such as tendon. It is also related to gangrenous lesions secondary to peripheral vascular disease.
Yellow wounds/ slough	Yellow tissue represents nonviable tissue and in some cases the presence of an infection. Sloughy tissue can be yellow, cream coloured, or grey slough, which is often accompanied by purulent drainage.
Red wounds/ granulation	Red tissue represents the presence of granulation tissue. The red colour is the result of an increasing amount of new blood vessels in the wound and is considered healthy.

- Closely monitor patients at home with the following risk factors: poor nutrition, dementia, wheelchair or bed dependence, incontinence, anemia, fracture, obesity, or skin drainage.
- Remind patient and caregiver that repositioning needs to occur while a patient is sitting in a chair. Consider shifting in position every 15 minutes. Small shifts such as moving or repositioning the legs redistributes pressure over bony prominences. Patients who sit for long periods in a wheelchair or a chair should have an appropriate and functional pressure-reduction cushion (WOCN, 2016). Ensure the wheelchair and the cushion are assessed for ongoing functionality.

PROCEDURAL GUIDELINE 39.1 *Performing a Wound Assessment*

▶ *Video Clip*　[**NSO**]　*Nursing Skills Online Wound Care Module 19 / Lesson 1*

Normal wound healing occurs in an organized fashion, and evaluation of wound status provides an ongoing assessment of wound healing and helps determine wound treatments. The frequency of wound assessment depends on the patient's overall condition, employer policy, the type of dressings used, and overall patient goals (Nix, 2016). Check employer policy for frequency of wound assessment and specific wound assessment tool.

Routine wound assessment, including documentation of wound measurement, provides valuable information regarding the status of the wound. For example, is wound healing progressing as expected, or is it delayed? Is there new drainage? Wound size may be affected by debridement. An expected finding is an increase in the size of the wound when necrotic tissue is removed. An increase in the amount and consistency of the drainage and new presence of odour may indicate a wound infection; and a wound culture may be necessary if systemic antibiotics are prescribed.

Assessment of the wound occurs before, during, and after the wound is cleaned and irrigated. The following parameters are included when performing a wound assessment:

- *Location:* Note the anatomical position of the wound.
- *Type of wound:* If known, identify the etiology of the wound (i.e., surgical, pressure, trauma).
- *Extent of tissue involvement:* A full-thickness wound involves both the dermis and epidermis. A partial-thickness wound involves only the epidermal layer. If it is a pressure injury, use the staging system of the NPUAP (2016) (see Box 39.3).
- *Type and percentage of tissue in wound base:* Describe the type of tissue (i.e., granulation, slough, eschar) and the approximate percentage of each type.
- *Wound size:* Follow employer policy to measure wound dimensions, which include width, length, and depth.
- *Wound exudate:* Describe the amount, colour, and consistency. Serous drainage is clear like plasma; sanguineous or bright red drainage indicates fresh bleeding; serosanguineous drainage is pink; and purulent drainage is thick and yellow, pale green, or white.
- *Presence of odour:* Note the presence or absence of odour, which may indicate infection.
- *Wound edge:* Determine if the wound edges are rolled, jagged, or smooth; pink (healing) or white (maceration) in colour.
- *Periwound area:* Assess the colour, temperature, and integrity of surrounding skin. Note any indication of reaction to dressing (e.g., redness from adhesive tape).
- *Pain:* Use a validated pain assessment scale to evaluate pain.

Delegation and Collaboration

The skill of wound assessment cannot be delegated to an unregulated health care provider (UCP). It is the nurse's responsibility to assess and document wound characteristics. The nurse directs the UCP to report the following to the nurse:

- Drainage from the wound that is present on sheets or as strike-through from the dressing.
- Presence of odour in the area of the wound.
- Patient indicating increasing pain at the wound site.
- Any dressing that is no longer adherent.

Equipment

- Personal protective equipment (PPE) (e.g., clean gloves, gown, and goggles if splash or spray risk exists)
- Employer tool to document assessment, including measuring guide
- Cotton-tipped applicator
- Dressing supplies, as prescribed
- Disposable waterproof biohazard bag

Procedural Steps

1. Identify patient using at least two person-specific identifiers (e.g., name and date of birth or name and medical record number) according to employer policy.
2. Examine patient record for the last wound assessment to use as a comparison for this wound assessment. Review record to determine etiology of the wound, interventions to treat the underlying cause, past dressing protocol, and wound characteristics from the last wound assessment.
3. Assess comfort level or pain on an appropriate pain rating scale and identify symptoms of anxiety. Offer pain medication prior to assessment, if indicated.
4. Perform hand hygiene. Close room door or bed curtains and position patient.
   a. Position patient comfortably to permit observation of wound in well-lit room.
   b. Expose only area of the wound and maintain patient privacy.
5. Explain procedure of wound assessment to patient and caregiver (if caregiver wishes to remain during the assessment to ensure patient permission).
6. Form a cuff on waterproof biohazard bag and place near bed.
7. Apply clean gloves and remove soiled dressings.
8. Examine dressings for quality of drainage (colour, consistency), presence or absence of odour, and quantity of drainage (note if dressings were saturated, slightly moist, or had no drainage). Discard dressings in waterproof biohazard bag. Discard gloves.
9. Perform hand hygiene and apply clean gloves.
10. Inspect wound and determine type of wound healing (e.g., primary or secondary intention).
11. Use employer-approved assessment tool and assess the following:
    a. Wound healing by primary intention (surgical wound):
       (1) Assess anatomical location of wound on body.
       (2) Note if incisional wound margins are approximated or closed together. The wound edges should be together with no gaps.

Continued

PROCEDURAL GUIDELINE 39.1 *Performing a Wound Assessment—cont'd*

(3) Observe for presence of drainage. A closed incision should not have any drainage.

(4) Look for evidence of infection (presence of erythema, odour, or wound drainage).

(5) Lightly palpate along incision to feel a healing ridge (see Fig. 39.3). The ridge will appear as an accumulation of new tissue presenting as firmness beneath the skin, extending to about 1 cm (½ inch) on each side of the wound between 5 and 9 days after the incision had been created. This is an expected positive sign (Doughty & Sparks-Defriese, 2016).

b. Wound healing by secondary intention (e.g., pressure injury or contaminated surgical or traumatic wound:

(1) Assess anatomical location of wound.

(2) Assess wound dimensions: Measure size of wound (including length, width, and depth). If using a ruler, use disposable centimetre measuring guide. Measure length by placing a ruler above wound at the point of greatest length (or head to foot). Measure width from side to side (Nix, 2016) (see illustration). Measure depth by inserting cotton-tipped applicator in area of greatest depth and placing a mark on applicator at skin level. Discard measuring guide and cotton-tipped applicator in a biohazard bag. If using an e-documentation system with automatic photo measurement, follow employer instructions for use.

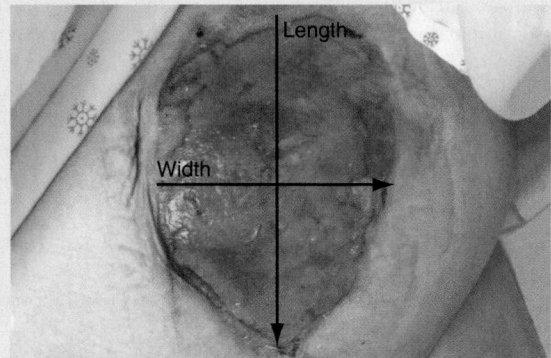

STEP 12b(2) Measuring wound length and width.

(3) Assess for *undermining* (i.e., the destruction of tissue under intact skin around the wound perimeter): Use cotton-tipped applicator to gently probe wound edges. Measure depth and note location using the face of a clock as a guide. The 12 o'clock position (top of wound) would be toward the head of the patient, and the 6 o'clock position would be the bottom of the wound toward the patient's feet. Document the number of centimetres that area extends from wound edge (e.g., underneath intact skin).

(4) Assess extent of tissue loss: If the wound is a pressure injury, determine the deepest viable tissue layer in the wound bed and determine its stage. If necrotic tissue does not allow visualization of the base of the wound,

the stage cannot be determined. If the wound is not a pressure injury, determine if there is partial-thickness loss (epidermis and part of the dermis) or full-thickness loss (loss of both the epidermis and the dermis). If it is a pressure injury, use the staging system of the NPUAP (2016) (see Box 39.3).

(5) Observe tissue type, including percentage of granulation, slough, and necrotic tissue.

(6) Note presence of exudate: amount, colour, consistency, and odour. Indicate amount of exudate by using part of dressing saturated (completely or partially saturated) or in terms of quantity (e.g., scant, moderate, or copious).

(7) Note if wound edges are rounded toward wound bed, macerated (white in colour), or jagged—any of these features may be an indication of delayed wound healing. Describe presence of epithelialization at wound edges (if present) because this indicates movement toward healing.

Clinical Decision Point *Compare the wound assessment to previous assessments and determine progress toward healing. If there is no movement toward healing or if you notice deterioration or increased drainage, consider a wound-care consultation. Lack of wound healing is often related to infection. Notify the health care provider and use interprofessional collaboration (wound care nurse) as indicated.*

12. Inspect the periwound skin, including colour, texture, and temperature, and describe skin integrity (e.g., open macerated areas, blistering). Periwound assessment provides clues about the effectiveness of wound treatment and possible wound deterioration (Nix, 2016).

13. Determine if previous dressing is still appropriate, based on wound characteristics. If it is, apply dressings as prescribed. If not, use interprofessional collaboration to discuss a change in treatment plan, or if the prescription states "according to best practice," decide which dressing is most appropriate and apply it. Use an indelible (waterproof) marker to write date on the new dressing.

14. Reassess patient's pain and level of comfort, including pain at wound site, using an appropriate pain rating scale after dressing is applied.

15. Discard biohazard bag, soiled supplies, and gloves per employer policy. Perform hand hygiene.

16. Document wound assessment findings and dressing details, including when the next dressing change should be completed. Confirm comparison of assessment with previous wound assessments to monitor wound healing (see Clinical Decision Point, above).

✦ SKILL 39.2   a Wound Irrigation

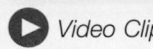 *Video Clip*

Wound irrigation is used to clean open surgical or chronic wounds such as pressure injuries. Typically, the irrigation of an open wound involves the use of clean gloves. Review the health care provider's prescription to determine if a sterile solution is required. Sterile solutions may be necessary with new traumatic wounds (Nelson, Crumbley, & Elster, 2016). Irrigation involves introducing the cleaning solution directly into the wound with a syringe, syringe and catheter, pulsed lavage device, or a handheld shower. A proper wound-cleaning solution is one that does not harm the tissue and uses an adequate force to agitate and wash away surface debris and devitalized tissue that contain bacteria (Table 39.6) (Jaszarowski & Murphree, 2016).

When using a syringe, the tip remains 2.5 cm (1 inch) above the wound. If a patient has a deep wound with a narrow opening, attach a soft catheter to the syringe to allow the fluid to enter the wound. Pulsed lavage delivers kinetic and mechanical energy and suction (a form of subatmospheric pressure). When pulsed lavage is used, normal saline may be delivered between 4 and 15 psi (pressurized irrigation) through a mechanical apparatus. Suction (subatmospheric pressure) may be used to aspirate wound debris and remove microorganisms. The use of mechanical energy through a pressurized spray also helps with the removal of wound debris. Ambulatory patients often benefit from the use of a handheld shower for wound cleaning, holding the shower spray approximately 30 cm (12 inches) from the wound.

Delegation and Collaboration

The skill of wound irrigation cannot be delegated to an unregulated health care providers (UCP) unless it is an established chronic wound and is permitted by employer policy. It is the nurse's responsibility to assess and document wound characteristics. If relevant, the nurse directs the UCP to:

- Notify the nurse when the wound is exposed so an assessment can be completed.
- Report to the nurse the patient's pain, presence of blood, and drainage.

Equipment

- Irrigant/cleaning solution (volume 1.5 to 2 times the estimated wound volume)
- Irrigation delivery system (as prescribed), depending on amount of pressure desired
- 35-mL syringe with a 19-gauge angiocatheter to facilitate optimum pressure for cleaning with minimal risk for tissue injury (Bryant & Nix, 2016c)
- Personal protective equipment (PPE) (e.g., clean gloves, gown, and goggles if splash or spray risk exists)
- Waterproof underpad if needed
- Dressing supplies (see Tables 39.3 and 40.1)
- Disposable waterproof biohazard bag
- Extra towels and padding (to use to protect bed)
- Wound assessment supplies (see Procedural Guideline 39.1)

TABLE 39.6

Wound-Cleaning Considerations

| | Mechanical Force | |
	High Pressure	Low Pressure
Wound base characteristics	Presence of necrotic tissue (eschar, fibrin slough), debris, or other particulate matter Significant bacterial burden Moderate/large amount of exudate	Presence of granulation tissue or new epithelial cells No/minimum serous or serosanguinous exudate
Clinical outcome(s)	Loosen, soften, and remove devitalized tissue from wound Separate eschar from fibrotic tissue/fibrotic tissue from granulating base	Prevent trauma to viable wound tissue Remove wound-care product residue
Solution	Normal saline or potable municipal tap water (warmed, if possible) Volume of solution depends on size of wound	Normal saline or potable municipal tap water (warmed, if possible) Volume of solution depends on size of wound
Delivery systems	35-mL syringe/19-gauge angiocatheter	Pouring saline directly from bottle Bulb syringe Piston syringe

Adapted from Spear, M. (2011). Wound cleansing: solutions and techniques. *Plastic Surgical Nursing, 31*(1), 29.

STEP	RATIONALE

ASSESSMENT

1. Identify patient using at least two person-specific identifiers (e.g., name and date of birth or name and medical record number), according to employer policy.

Ensures correct patient. Complies with Accreditation Canada's standards and improves patient safety (Accreditation Canada, 2019).

2. Review health care provider's prescription to ensure best practice for irrigation of open wound and type of solution to be used.

Open-wound irrigation requires a medical prescription, including type of solution(s) to use.

3. Assess patient's level of comfort, using an appropriate pain rating scale.

Provides baseline to determine tolerance of procedure.

4. Review patient's chart for signs and symptoms related to patient's open wound.

Provides ongoing data to indicate change in wound status (Nix, 2016).

  a. Extent of impairment of skin integrity, including size of wound

  b. Verify number of drains present (if any)

Awareness of drain position facilitates safe dressing removal and determines need for special dressings.

  c. Drainage, including amount, colour, consistency, and any odour noted

Ongoing data; drainage should decrease in healing wound. When drainage increases, it is often related to infection (Doughty & Sparks-Defriese, 2016).

  d. Wound tissue colour

Colour represents balance between necrotic and new scar tissue. Proper selection of wound-care products on the basis of wound colour facilitates removal of necrotic tissue and promotes new tissue growth (Nix, 2016).

  e. Culture reports and/or use of antimicrobial dressings.

An infected wound has an increase in bioburden and critical colonization of bacteria. Culture reports identify the type of bacteria and selection of appropriate systemic antibiotics. Wound cultures are relevant if systemic antibiotic treatment is required (Stotts, 2016b). Antimicrobial dressings may be used.

5. Assess patient for history of allergies to antiseptics, solutions, medications, tapes, or dressing material.

Known allergies suggest applying a sample of prescribed wound treatment as a skin test before flushing wound with a large volume of solution or selecting different tape or dressing material.

6. Assess patient's and caregiver's understanding of need for irrigation and signs of wound infection.

Determines extent of instruction required.

NURSING DIAGNOSES

- Acute pain
- Insufficient knowledge related to purpose of irrigation
- Reduced skin integrity
- Reduced tissue integrity
- Potential for infection
- Potential for injury

Related factors/Risk factors are individualized on the basis of patient's condition or needs.

PLANNING

1. Expected outcomes following completion of procedure:

- Patient states acceptable level of comfort and pain on a validated pain rating scale after wound irrigation.

Premedication, appropriately administered irrigation, application of clean dressing, and repositioning patient ensure comfort.

- Wound begins to demonstrate signs of healing; wound is free of excessive drainage, exudate, and inflammation.

Wound closure and healing progress in absence of debris and presence of protective dressing.

- Skin integrity is maintained; no redness, edema, or inflammation is noted in surrounding tissue.

No further skin and tissue damage has resulted from wound irrigation.

- Patient is able to describe signs of wound healing and infection.

Demonstrates learning.

2. Perform hand hygiene. Administer analgesic at least 30 minutes before starting wound irrigation procedure.

Promotes pain control and enables patient to move more easily and be positioned to facilitate wound irrigation (Krasner, 2016).

3. Explain procedure to patient and caregiver about procedure. Describe signs of healing and infection during irrigation.

Promotes cooperation and reduces anxiety.

STEP	RATIONALE

PLANNING

4. Gather appropriate supplies for wound irrigation and dressing.

Ensures an organized procedure.

5. Close room door or bed curtains, perform hand hygiene, and position patient.

Maintains privacy; frequent hand hygiene reduces amount of microorganisms.

   a. Position patient comfortably to permit gravitational flow of irrigating solution over wound and into collection receptacle (see illustration).

Directing solution from the top to bottom of a wound and from a clean to contaminated area prevents further infection. Position patient during planning stage, keeping in mind bed surfaces needed for later preparation of equipment.

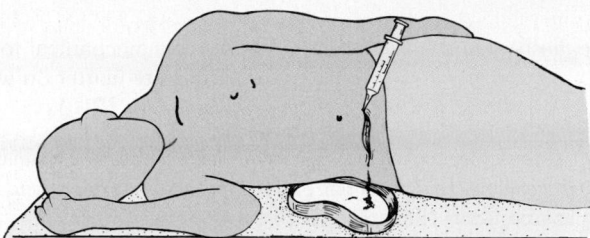

STEP 5a Patient position for wound irrigation.

   b. Position patient so wound is vertical to collection basin. Irrigant should be room temperature.

Room-temperature solution increases comfort and reduces vascular constriction response in tissues.

   c. Place padding or extra towel on bed under area where irrigation will take place.

Protects bedding from becoming wet.

IMPLEMENTATION

1. Perform hand hygiene.

While cleaning wound, use meticulous hand hygiene and proper infection-control procedures before and after removing soiled dressings to limit risk for health care–acquired infection (Jaszarowski & Murphree, 2016).

2. Form a cuff on waterproof biohazard bag and place near bed.

Cuffing helps to maintain a large opening, thereby enabling placement of contaminated dressings without touching bag itself.

3. Apply PPE (gown, mask, goggles as indicated); apply clean gloves and remove old dressing.

Reduces transmission of microorganisms. Protects nurse from splashes or sprays of blood and body fluids.

4. Discard old dressing and gloves in biohazard bag. Perform hand hygiene.

Reduces transmission of microorganisms.

5. Apply clean or sterile gloves (see employer policy). Perform wound assessment and examine recent charted assessment of patient's open wound (see Procedural Guideline 39.1).

Provides ongoing wound-healing data. Use sterile precautions when sterile gloves are needed.

6. Expose area near wound only.

Provides privacy and prevents chilling of patient.

7. Irrigate wound with wide opening:

   a. Fill a 35-mL syringe with warmed irrigation solution.

Irrigating a wound involves mechanical force, which helps with separation and removal of necrotic debris and surface bacteria (Jaszarowski & Murphree, 2016). Flushing a wound helps remove debris and facilitates healing by secondary intention. Warmed (body temperature) irrigant promotes wound healing.

   b. Attach 19-gauge angiocatheter.

Catheter lumen delivers ideal pressure for cleaning and removing debris (Ramundo, 2016). Mechanical debridement may include irrigation, which can be done through use of a 35-mL syringe with 19-gauge angiocatheter with irrigation pressures delivered between 4 and 15 psi (WOCN, 2016).

   c. Hold syringe tip 2.5 cm (1 inch) above upper end of wound and over area being cleaned.

Prevents syringe contamination. Careful placement of syringe prevents unsafe pressure of flowing solution.

   d. Using continuous pressure, flush wound; repeat Steps 7a to 7c until solution draining into basin is clear.

Flushing wound helps to remove debris; clear solution indicates removal of all debris.

STEP	RATIONALE

IMPLEMENTATION

8. Irrigate deep wound with very small opening:

    a. Attach soft catheter to filled irrigation syringe.

Catheter permits direct flow of irrigant into wound. Expect wound to take longer to empty when opening is small.

    b. Gently insert tip of catheter into opening about 1.3 cm (0.5 inch).

Prevents tip from touching fragile inner wall of wound.

Clinical Decision Point *Do not force the catheter into the wound because this will cause tissue damage. Ensure that irrigant solution will be flushed out of the wound; avoid irrigating when the wound base will not permit effective flushing out of solution.*

    c. Using slow, continuous pressure, flush wound.

Use of slow mechanical force of stream of solution loosens particulate matter on wound surface and promotes healing (Ramundo, 2016).

Clinical Decision Point *Pulsatile high-pressure lavage is often the irrigation of choice for necrotic wounds. Pressure settings should be set per provider prescription, usually between 4 and 15 psi, and should not be used on skin grafts, exposed blood vessels, muscle, tendon, or bone. Use with caution if the patient has a coagulation disorder or is taking anticoagulants (Ramundo, 2016).*

    d. While keeping catheter in place, pinch it off just below syringe.

Avoids contamination of sterile solution

    e. Remove and refill syringe. Reconnect to catheter and repeat until solution draining into basin is clear.

9. Clean wound with handheld shower:

    a. With patient seated comfortably in shower chair or standing if condition allows, adjust spray to gentle flow; make sure that water is warm.

Useful for patients able to shower with help or independently. May be accomplished at home.

    b. Shower for 5 to 10 minutes with shower head 30 cm (12 inches) from wound.

Ensures that wound is cleaned thoroughly.

10. When indicated (e.g., determining appropriate systemic antibiotic), obtain cultures (see Chapter 9) after cleaning with nonbacteriostatic saline.

WOCN (2016) recommends using quantitative bacterial cultures (tissue biopsy or swab cultures). The most common types of wound cultures are swab technique, aspirated wound fluid, or tissue biopsy (Stotts, 2016b).

Clinical Decision Point *Obtain a wound culture for systemic antibiotic use if presence of inflammation around the wound, purulent odour or drainage, or new drainage; when the patient is febrile and systemic infection is suspected; or when antimicrobial topical treatments are not effective.*

11. Dry wound edges with gauze; dry patient after shower.

Prevents maceration of surrounding tissue from excess moisture.

12. Remove and dispose of gloves. Perform hand hygiene. Apply clean or sterile gloves (see employer policy). Apply appropriate dressing and label with time, date, and nurse's initials.

Reduces transmission of microorganisms. Maintains protective barrier and healing environment for wound.

13. Remove mask, goggles, and gown.

Reduces transfer of microorganisms.

14. Dispose of equipment and soiled supplies; remove and dispose of gloves. Perform hand hygiene.

Reduces transmission of microorganisms.

15. Help patient to a comfortable position.

EVALUATION

1. Have patient rate level of comfort and pain using an appropriate pain rating scale.

Patient's pain should not increase as result of wound irrigation.

2. Monitor type of tissue in wound bed.

Identifies wound-healing progress and determines type of wound cleaning and dressing needed.

STEP	RATIONALE

EVALUATION

3. Inspect dressing periodically (see employer policy).

Determines patient's response to wound irrigation and need to modify plan of care.

4. Evaluate periwound skin integrity.

Determines if extension of wound has occurred or signs of infection are present (warm, red periwound skin).

5. Observe for presence of retained irrigant.

Retained irrigant is medium for bacterial growth and subsequent infection.

6. Use Teach-Back: "I want to be sure that I explained why your wound was cleaned (irrigated) today. Tell me why it is important to clean (irrigate) your wound." Develop a revised teaching plan if patient or caregiver is not able to teach back correctly.

Determines patient's and caregiver's level of understanding of instructional topic.

Unexpected Outcomes	Related Interventions
1. Bleeding or serosanguinous drainage appears.	• Review medications (e.g., anticoagulant therapy). • Notify health care provider of bleeding. • Flush wound during next irrigation using less pressure.
2. Increased pain or discomfort occurs.	• Decrease force of pressure during wound irrigation. • Assess patient for need for additional analgesia before wound care.
3. Suture line opening extends.	• Notify health care provider. • Re-evaluate amount of pressure to use for next wound irrigation.

Communication and Documentation

- Document wound assessment before and after irrigation; amount, colour, and odour of drainage on dressing removed; amount and type of solution used; irrigation device used; patient's tolerance of the procedure; and type of dressing applied after irrigation on flow sheet in nurses' notes in electronic health record (EHR) or chart.
- Document patient's and caregiver's understanding through teach-back of reasons for wound irrigations.
- Immediately report to the health care provider any evidence of fresh bleeding, sharp increase in pain, retention of irrigant, or signs of shock.

Special Considerations
Teaching

- Instruct patient and caregiver regarding wound-care technique, observe them doing a return demonstration, and provide written instructions.
- Explain the need for specialized supplies such as irrigating solutions and dressings and the need to maintain asepsis when performing care.
- Teach patient and caregiver signs of healing wound, improper wound healing, and wound infection.

Pediatric

- Some pediatric patients are very frightened. They might verbally and physically try to prevent the nurse from cleaning the wound. Having the child take active part in the procedure or working out their feelings about wound irrigation with play therapy on a doll with a wound helps the child to be more cooperative.
- Neonatal skin is immature and easily damaged from pressure and wound-care products. Check that products are approved for

use with this population. Remember that in neonates the skin readily absorbs products.

Gerontological

- Wound irrigations are traumatic, frightening, and painful to some older persons. Assess patient's cooperation before irrigating the wound. Be aware of patient's cognitive level of understanding when performing wound irrigation.

Care in the Community

- Assess patient's home environment to determine adequacy of resources for performing wound care; check especially for adequate lighting, safe (treated) water supply (municipal water that has standard government testing), and storage of supplies.
- Plan wound care in conjunction with patient's total rehabilitation goals. The objective of wound-care management in a subacute care setting is to return the patient to their home environment.
- Provide encouragement to address underlying factors (e.g., nutrition, continence management, pressure off loading), including education for patient and caregiver about wound-healing expectations of chronic wounds (Doughty & Sparks-Defriese, 2016).
- If ambulatory, patients will often be appropriate for wound-care management in an outpatient clinic. Be sure that the patient has directions to the clinic and knows where to park and where to obtain dressing supplies in advance (if necessary).
- Solutions to use for irrigation in the home include potable tap water, distilled water, cooled boiled water, and normal saline (WOCN, 2016). Normal saline can be made in the home: 8 teaspoons of salt in 3.5 litres of distilled water; keep it refrigerated for 1 month. The saline solution should be allowed to reach room temperature before use.

✦ SKILL 39.3   Removing Sutures and Staples

Nurses need to have the skills and equipment to remove sutures and staples. Generally, staple and suture removal is prescribed by the health care provider. The prescription will state whether staples or sutures be removed at one time or every other suture or staple is removed as the first phase, with the remainder removed in the second phase.

Sutures and staples generally are removed within 7 to 14 days after surgery if healing is adequate (Whitney, 2016). Retention sutures usually remain in place 14 to 21 days. Timing the removal of sutures and staples is important. They must remain in place long enough to ensure initial wound closure with enough strength to support internal tissues and organs. Sutures left in longer than 14 days generally leave suture marks (Whitney, 2016).

Sutures are threads of wire or other materials used to sew body tissues together. They come in different sizes and are absorbent or nonabsorbent. They are placed within tissue layers in deep wounds and superficially as the final means for wound closure. The choice of suture technique depends on the type and anatomical location of the wound, thickness of the skin, degree of tension, and desired cosmetic effect (Fig. 39.7) (Whitney, 2016). A patient's history of

wound healing, the site of the wound, tissues involved, and the purpose of the sutures determine the suture material selected. For example, a patient with repeated abdominal surgeries might require wire sutures for greater strength to promote wound closure.

Staples are stainless-steel wires, are quick to use, and provide strength. The location of the incision sometimes restricts their use because there must be adequate distance between the skin and structures that lie below the skin, including bone and vascular structures. They are used for skin closure of abdominal incisions and orthopaedic surgery when appearance of the incision is not critical. Removal requires a sterile staple extractor and aseptic technique.

If there is any sign of suture line separation during the removal process, the remaining sutures or staples are left in place, and a description is documented and reported to the health care provider. In some cases, these are removed several days to 1 week later. After sutures or staples are removed, the nurse applies Steri-Strips over the incision to provide support. The strips loosen over time (5 to 7 days) and can be removed when half of the strip is no longer attached to the skin.

Delegation and Collaboration

The skill of staple and suture removal cannot be delegated to an unregulated care provider (UCP). The nurse directs the UCP to report any of the following to the nurse:

- Drainage, bleeding, swelling at the incision site or an elevation in patient's temperature.
- Patient's indication of pain.
- Any dehiscence of the closed wound (following suture removal).

Equipment

- Disposable waterproof biohazard bag
- Sterile suture removal set (forceps and scissors) or sterile staple extractor
- Sterile antiseptic swabs
- Gauze pads
- Steri-Strips or butterfly adhesive strips
- Clean gloves (sterile gloves optional)

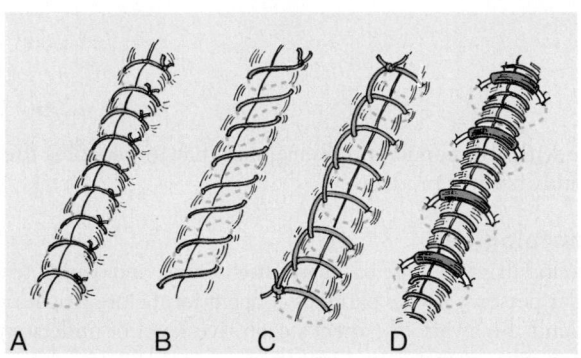

FIG 39.7 Types of sutures. **A,** Intermittent. **B** and **C,** Continuous. **D,** Blanket.

STEP	RATIONALE

ASSESSMENT

STEP	RATIONALE
1. Identify patient using at least two person-specific identifiers (e.g., name and date of birth or name and medical record number) according to employer policy.	Ensures correct patient. Complies with Accreditation Canada's standards and improves patient safety (Accreditation Canada, 2019).
2. Review patient's chart for the following information:	
a. Check health care provider's prescription.	Health care provider prescription is required for removal of sutures.
b. Review specific directions related to suture or staple removal.	Indicates specifically which sutures are to be removed (e.g., every other suture).
c. Determine history of conditions that may pose risk for impaired wound healing: advanced age, cardiovascular disease, diabetes, immunosuppression, radiation, obesity, smoking, poor nutrition, infection.	Pre-existing health disorders affect speed of healing and sometimes result in dehiscence.
3. Assess patient for history of allergies. Use latex-free gloves.	Determines if patient is sensitive to antiseptic, latex, or other supplies used (e.g., paper tape).

STEP	RATIONALE

ASSESSMENT

4. Assess patient's comfort level on an appropriate pain rating scale. Ensure comfort measures are in place prior to removal of sutures or staples (e.g., positioning, analgesia if prescribed).

Provides baseline of patient's comfort level to determine response to therapy.

5. Perform hand hygiene. Inspect incision for healing ridge and skin integrity of suture line for uniform closure of wound edges, normal colour, and absence of drainage and inflammation. Apply clean gloves, if necessary, to palpate wound. Remove and dispose of gloves after assessment.

Indicates adequate wound healing for support of internal structures without continued need for sutures or staples (Whitney, 2016).

6. Assess patient's or caregiver's knowledge of wound care and what observations the patient needs to make when doing their own wound care.

Determines extent of instruction required.

Clinical Decision Point *If wound edges are separated or signs of infection are present, the wound has not healed properly. Notify the health care provider because sutures or staples may need to remain in place or other wound care initiated.*

NURSING DIAGNOSES

- Acute pain
- Insufficient knowledge regarding incision care
- Reduced skin integrity
- Potential for infection

Related factors/Risk factors are individualized on the basis of patient's condition or needs.

PLANNING

1. Expected outcomes following completion of procedure:
- All suture material or staples are removed.
- Suture line is intact.
- Patient states acceptable level of comfort on an appropriate pain rating scale, following removal of sutures or staples.
- Patient or caregiver can describe wound care following suture removal.

Removes source of infection or irritation from retained sutures.
Wound is healing and does not require protective dressings.
Some patients require pain medication before suture or staple removal.

Demonstrates learning.

2. Explain to patient how you will remove staples and that suture removal is usually not a painful procedure, although patient may feel pulling or tugging of skin.

Gains patient cooperation and reduces anxiety.

3. Administer prescribed analgesic, if needed, at least 30 minutes before procedure.

Promotes patient comfort to help minimize movement during suture removal.

IMPLEMENTATION

1. Close curtains or room door.

Provides privacy.

Clinical Decision Point *For a patient who is highly anxious or who has an extensive wound, consider administering analgesic 30 minutes before suture removal, and assess patient comfort and pain level to ensure effectiveness of analgesic prior to suture or staple removal. Offer alternative comfort measures, such as squeezing a ball, distraction, or breathing techniques. Often talking through the procedure with the patient during suture removal is helpful to relieve anxiety.*

2. Position patient comfortably while exposing suture line. Ensure that direct lighting is on suture line.

Aids visibility and correct placement of forceps or extractor during removal process, ultimately reducing soft tissue injury.

3. Perform hand hygiene.

Reduces transmission of microorganisms.

4. Place cuffed waterproof disposal bag within easy reach.

Provides for easy disposal of contaminated dressings and prevents passing items over sterile work area.

5. Prepare materials needed for suture or staple removal:
- **a.** Open sterile suture removal kit or staple extractor kit.
- **b.** Open sterile antiseptic swabs and place on inside surface of kit.
- **c.** Obtain gloves (sterile gloves if policy indicates).

Ensures an organized procedure.

STEP	RATIONALE

IMPLEMENTATION

6. Apply clean gloves. Carefully remove dressing; discard dressing and gloves in prepared refuse disposal bag.

Reduces transmission of infection.

7. Inspect incision and suture line (see illustration).

Determines adequacy of wound healing.

8. Perform hand hygiene. Apply clean or sterile gloves as required by employer policy.

Reduces transmission of infection.

9. Clean sutures or staples and healed incision with antiseptic swabs. Start at sides next to incision and then wipe across suture line using a new antiseptic swab for each swipe.

Removes surface bacteria from incision and sutures or staples.

10. **Remove staples:**

   a. Place lower tips of staple extractor under the first staple. As you close handles, the upper tip of the extractor depresses the centre of the staple, causing both ends of the staple to be bent upward and simultaneously exit their insertion sites in the dermal layer (see illustration).

   Avoids excess pressure to suture line and secures smooth removal of each staple.

   b. Carefully control staple extractor.

   Avoids pressure on suture line and patient discomfort.

   c. As soon as both ends of staple are visible, move it away from the skin surface (see illustration) and continue until staple is over refuse bag.

   Prevents scratching tender skin surface with sharp pointed ends of staple, for comfort and infection control.

   d. Release handles of staple extractor, allowing staple to drop into refuse bag.

   Avoids contaminating sterile field with used staples.

   e. Repeat Steps 10a through 10d until all staples are removed.

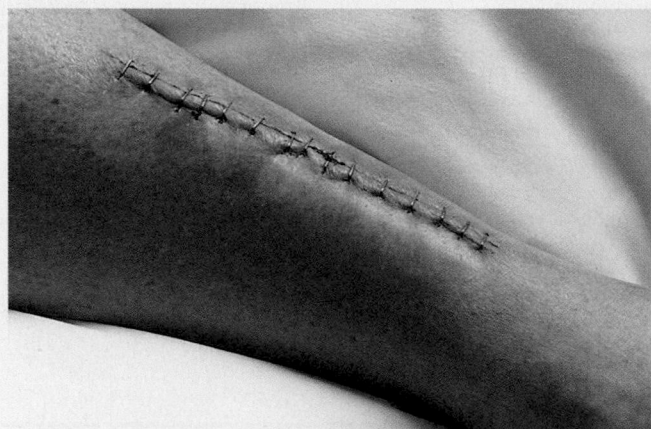

STEP 7 Suture line secured with staples.

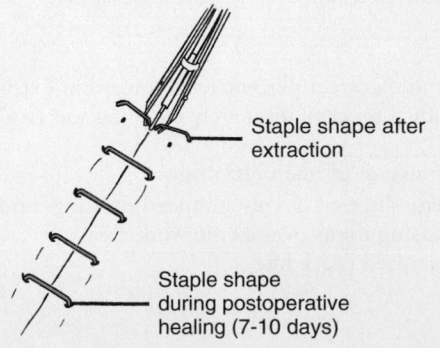

Staple shape after extraction

Staple shape during postoperative healing (7-10 days)

STEP 10a Staple extractor placed under staple.

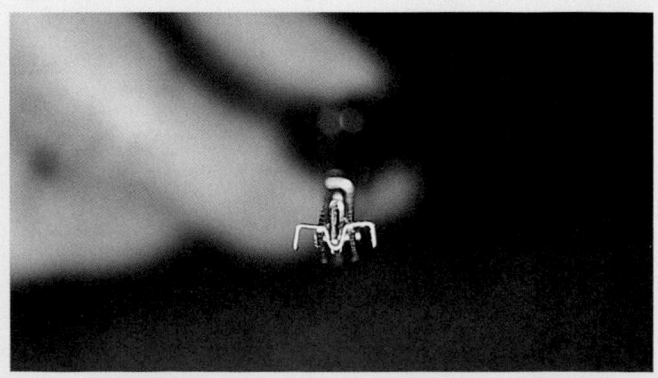

STEP 10c Metal staple removed by extractor.

STEP	**RATIONALE**

IMPLEMENTATION

11. Remove interrupted sutures:

    a. Place gauze a few centimetres from the suture line. Hold scissors in your dominant hand and forceps (clamp) in your nondominant hand.

Gauze serves as receptacle for removed sutures. Placement of scissors and forceps allows for efficient suture removal.

Clinical Decision Point *Placement of scissors and forceps is very important. Avoid pinching the skin around the wound when lifting up the suture. Likewise, avoid cutting the skin around the wound by accident when snipping the suture.*

    b. Grasp knot of suture with forceps and gently pull up knot while slipping tip of scissors under suture near skin (see illustration).

Releases suture.

    c. Snip suture as close to the skin as possible at end distal to knot.

Clinical Decision Point *Never snip both ends of the suture; there will be no way to remove the part of the suture situated below the surface.*

    d. Grasp knotted end with forceps and in one continuous smooth action pull suture through from the other side (see illustration). Place removed suture on gauze.

Smoothly removes suture without additional tension to suture line.

Clinical Decision Point *Never pull the exposed surface of any suture into tissue below the epidermis. The exposed surface of any suture is considered contaminated.*

    e. Repeat Steps 11a through 11d until you have removed every other suture.

    f. Observe healing level. Based on observations of wound response to suture removal and health care provider's original prescription, determine whether remaining sutures will be removed at this time. If so, repeat Steps 11a through 11d until you have removed all sutures.

Determines status of wound healing and if suture line will remain closed after all sutures are removed.

    g. If there is any doubt about wound healing, immediately stop suture removal and notify health care provider.

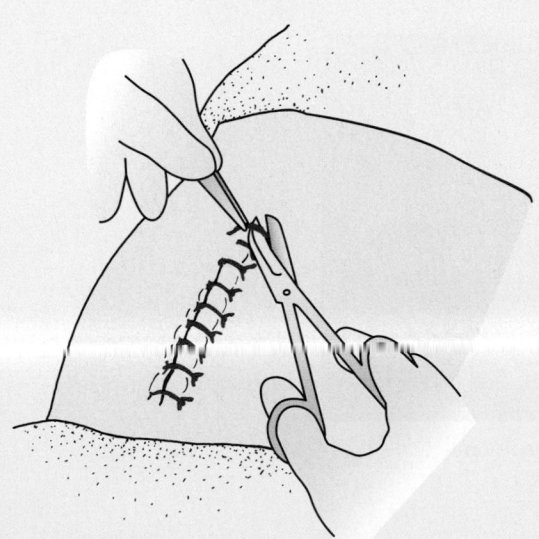

STEP 11b Removal of intermittent suture. Nurse cuts suture as close to the skin as possible, away from knot.

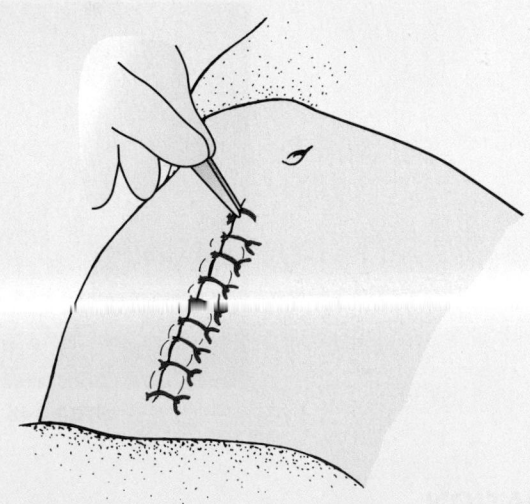

STEP 11d Nurse removes suture, never pulling contaminated stitch through tissues.

STEP	RATIONALE

IMPLEMENTATION

12. Remove continuous and blanket stitch sutures:

   a. Place sterile gauze a few centimetres from suture line. Grasp scissors in dominant hand and forceps in nondominant hand.

   b. Snip first suture close to skin surface at end distal to knot.

   c. Snip second suture on same side.

   d. Grasp knotted end and gently pull with continuous smooth action, removing suture from beneath skin. Place suture on gauze compress.

   e. Repeat Steps 12a to 12d in consecutive order until entire line is removed.

13. Inspect incision to make sure that all sutures are removed and identify any trouble areas. Gently wipe suture line with antiseptic swab to remove debris and clean incision.

14. Apply Steri-Strips if *any* separation greater than two stitches or two staples in width is apparent, to maintain contact between wound edges.

   a. Cut Steri-Strips to allow strips to extend 4 to 5 cm (1½ to 2 inches) on each side of incision.

   b. Remove from backing and apply across incision (see illustration).

   c. Instruct patient to take showers rather than soak in a bathtub, according to health care provider's preference.

15. Remove and discard gloves. Perform hand hygiene and apply a new pair of gloves. Apply light dressing or expose incision to air if no clothing will come in contact with suture line. Instruct patient about applying their own dressing, if needed, at home.

16. Discard all contaminated materials and remove and dispose of gloves.

17. Dispose of sharps (disposable staple extractor and/or scissors) in designated sharps disposal bin and perform hand hygiene.

Rationale column:

Gauze serves as receptacle for removed sutures. Placement of scissors and forceps allows for efficient suture removal.

Releases suture.

Releases interrupted sutures from knot.

Smoothly removes sutures without additional tension to suture line. Prevents pulling of contaminated part of suture through skin.

Reduces risk for further incision line separation.

Supports wound by distributing tension across wound and eliminates closure-technique scarring.

Steri-Strips are not removed and are allowed to fall off gradually.

Healing by primary intention eliminates need for dressing.

Reduces transmission of infection.

Provides a safe environment because instruments are sharp and contaminated. Reduces transmission of infection.

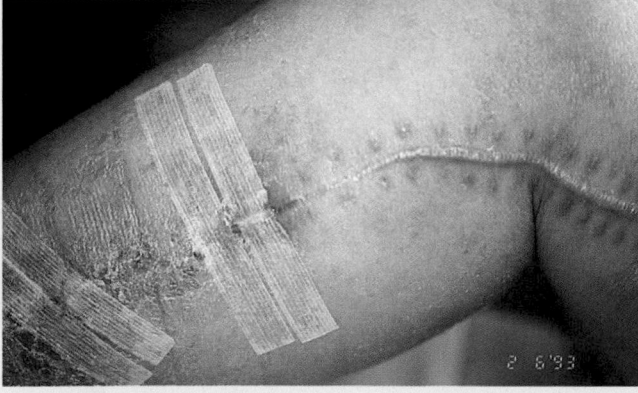

STEP 14b Steri-Strips over incision.

EVALUATION

1. Assess site where sutures or staples were removed; inspect condition of soft tissues, including skin. Look for any pieces of removed suture left behind.

     Ensures that sources of infection have been removed.

2. Determine if patient has pain along incision.

     Determines comfort level and can indicate if suture material remains in skin.

STEP	RATIONALE

EVALUATION

3. **Use Teach-Back:** "I want to be sure that I have told you about the signs of a wound or incision infection before you are discharged. Tell me what signs of infection you should watch for." Develop a revised teaching plan if patient or caregiver is not able to teach back correctly.

Determines patient's and caregiver's level of understanding of instructional topic.

Unexpected Outcomes
1. Retained suture is present.

2. Patient experiences wound separation or drainage secondary to healing problems.

Related Interventions
- Notify health care provider.
- Instruct patient to notify health care provider if signs of suture line infection develop following patient's discharge from facility.
- Leave remaining sutures or staples in place.
- Place Steri-Strip closures across suture line.
- Notify health care provider.

Communication and Documentation

- Document the time the sutures or staples were removed and the number of sutures or staples removed; cleaning of the suture line, appearance of the wound, level of healing of the wound, and type of dressing applied; and patient's response to suture or staple removal on flow sheet in nurses' notes in electronic health record (EHR) or chart.
- Document patient's and caregiver's understanding of why the sutures were removed.
- Immediately report to the health care provider any suture line separation, dehiscence, evisceration, bleeding, or purulent drainage.

Special Considerations
Teaching

- Teach patient to observe for any sign of separation of wound edges before removing remaining sutures or staples and inspect incision for continued healing.
- Reinforce instruction about resuming bathing and showering activities, avoiding abdominal strain during defecation, and getting adequate nutrition and ambulation.

- Teach patient not to put additional stress on suture line from such activities as lifting or bending. Patients who have had abdominal surgery or injury need to avoid heavy lifting for several weeks.
- Instruct patient that sometimes there is a small amount of drainage from wound immediately after suture removal.

Pediatric

- Help is sometimes necessary to keep infants from moving during the suture removal procedure.
- Topical anaesthetic solutions (e.g., lidocaine, EMLA) applied to intact skin may provide short-term (20 minutes) anaesthesia (Krasner, 2016).

Gerontological

- Some older persons need reassurance about suture or staple removal. Depending on their cognitive status, they may not understand the procedure.
- An older person's skin is often at higher risk for dehiscence after sutures or staples are removed.

✦ SKILL 39.4 Managing Wound Drainage Evacuation

NSO *Nursing Skills Online Wound Care Module 19 / Lesson 2*

If drainage accumulates in a wound bed, wound healing is delayed. Drainage is facilitated when the surgeon inserts either a closed- or an open-drain system, even if the amount of drainage is small. The drain is inserted directly through a small stab wound near the suture line into the area of the wound.

An open-drain system (e.g., a Penrose drain [Fig. 39.8]) is used to remove drainage from the wound and deposit it onto the skin surface. A sterile safety pin is inserted through this drain, outside the skin, to prevent the tubing from moving into the wound.

A closed-drain system such as the Jackson-Pratt (JP) drain (Fig. 39.9) or Hemovac drain relies on the presence of a vacuum to withdraw accumulated drainage from around the wound bed into the collection device. A JP drain collects fluid that is in the range of 100 to 200 mL/24 hr. A Hemovac or ConstaVac drainage system is used for larger amounts of drainage (500 mL/24 hr). The collection device is connected to a clear plastic drain with multiple perforations.

Drainage collects in a closed reservoir or a suction bladder. The closed system collects fluid but operates only if the tubing is patent and a vacuum exists. If the drainage device is half full, empty the chamber and measure the drainage. After measurement re-establish the vacuum and ensure that all drainage tubes are patent.

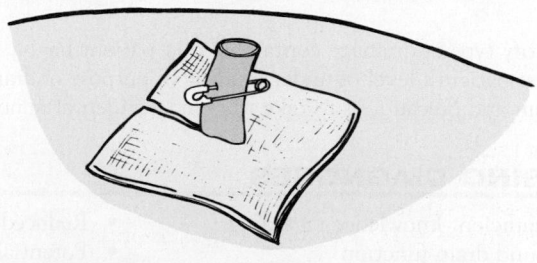

FIG 39.8 Penrose drain with drain-split gauze.

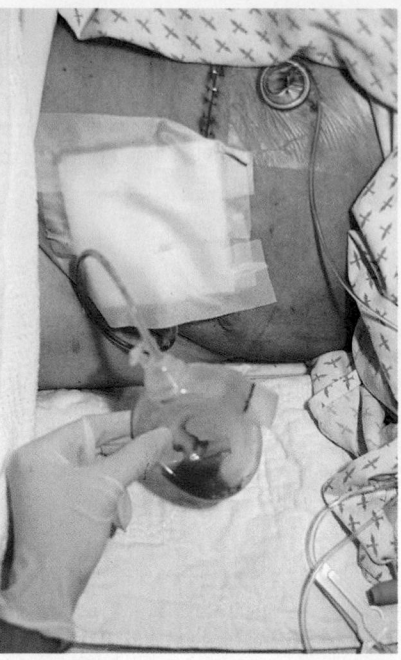

FIG 39.9 Jackson-Pratt wound drainage system.

Delegation and Collaboration

The assessment of wound drainage and maintenance of drains and the drainage system cannot be delegated to an unregulated care provider (UCP). However, the nurse may delegate emptying a closed drainage container or pouch, measuring the amount of drainage, and reporting the amount on the patient's intake and output (I&O) record to a UCP. The nurse instructs the UCP to:

- Report any increase in frequency of emptying the drain other than once a shift.
- Report any change in amount, colour, or odour of drainage.
- Review with the nurse the I&O procedure.

Equipment

- Graduated measuring cylinder or specimen container
- Antiseptic wipes
- Gauze sponges, including split gauze sponges for drain site
- Sterile gauze dressings as needed
- Clean gloves
- Safety pin(s)
- Protective equipment: goggles, mask, and gown if risk of spray from drain is present
- Disposable drape or barrier
- *Optional:* Normal saline for cleaning insertion site

STEP	RATIONALE

ASSESSMENT

1. Identify patient using at least two person-specific identifiers (e.g., name and date of birth or name and medical record number), according to employer policy.

   Ensures correct patient. Complies with Accreditation Canada's standards and improves patient safety (Accreditation Canada, 2019).

2. Review medical record to identify presence, location, and purpose of closed wound drain and drainage system as patient returns from surgery.

   Drainage tubing is usually placed near the wound through a small surgical incision.

3. Perform hand hygiene. Wear clean gloves if there is a risk of coming into contact with drainage or if indicated by employer policy. Assess drainage present on patient's dressing. Identify the number of wound drain tubes and what each one will be draining. Label each drain tube with a number or label.

   Assigning a labelling system to each drain helps with consistent documentation when the patient has multiple drainage tubes.

4. Inspect system to determine presence of one straight tube or Y-tube arrangement with two tube insertion sites.

   Allows nurse to plan skin care and identify quantity of sterile dressing supplies needed.

5. Inspect system to ensure proper functioning. A complete systematic inspection includes the insertion site, drainage moving through tubing in the direction of the reservoir, patency of drainage tubing, airtight connection sites, and presence of any leaks or kinks in the system. Remove and dispose of gloves. Perform hand hygiene.

   A properly functioning system maintains suction until the reservoir is filled or drainage is no longer being produced or accumulated. Tension on drainage tubing increases injury to skin and underlying muscle.

6. Determine if drain tube needs self-suction, wall suction, or no suction, according to health care provider's prescription.

   Some drain tubes, such as Hemovac, can be used with self-suction or wall suction.

Clinical Decision Point *Attach tape and a safety pin to drainage tubing and pin to the patient's gown so the suction device is below the level of the wound and does not pull on the insertion site.*

7. Identify type of drainage containers that patient has.

   Determines frequency for emptying drainage.

8. Assess patient's level of understanding of purpose of drainage system and precautions to take to avoid accidental removal.

   Determines extent of instruction required.

NURSING DIAGNOSES

- Insufficient knowledge regarding wound drain function
- Reduced skin integrity
- Potential for infection
- Potential for injury

Related factors/Risk factors are individualized on the basis of patient's condition or needs.

STEP	RATIONALE

PLANNING

1. Expected outcomes following completion of procedure:
   - Wound healing continues.
   - Vacuum is re-established.
   - Tubing is patent.
   - Patient describes precautions to avoid drain removal.
2. Explain procedure to patient.

Patient is comfortable, and wound drainage is collected.
Suction system is intact.
Fluid is draining away from wound area.
Demonstrates learning.
Promotes patient's cooperation and reduces anxiety.

IMPLEMENTATION

1. Close room door or bedside curtains.
2. Perform hand hygiene and apply clean gloves.
3. Place open specimen container or graduated container (for measuring output) on bed between you and the patient.
4. **Empty Hemovac or ConstaVac:**
   a. Maintain asepsis while opening the plug on port indicated for emptying drainage reservoir.
      (1) Tilt suction container in direction of the plug.
      (2) Slowly squeeze two flat surfaces together, tilting toward measuring container.
   b. Drain contents into measuring container (see illustration).
   c. Hold uncovered antiseptic swab in dominant hand. Place suction device on a flat surface with open outlet facing upward; continue pressing downward until bottom and top are in contact (see illustration).
   d. Holding surfaces together with one hand and using an antiseptic swab, quickly clean opening, plug with other hand, and immediately replace plug; secure suction device on patient's bed.
   e. Check device for re-establishment of vacuum, patency of drainage tubing, and absence of stress on tubing.

Provides privacy.
Reduces transmission of microorganisms.
Permits measuring and discarding of wound drainage.

Avoids entry of pathogens.
Vacuum will be broken, and the reservoir will pull air in until the chamber is fully expanded.
Drains fluid toward plug.
Prevents splashing of contaminated drainage. Squeezing empties reservoir of drainage.
Contents counted as fluid output (see Chapter 8).

Cleaning plug reduces transmission of microorganisms into drainage evacuation.

Compression of surface of Hemovac creates vacuum.

Facilitates wound drainage and prevents tension on drainage tubing.

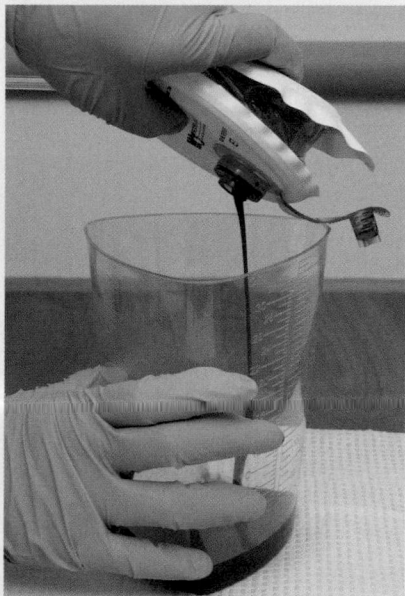

STEP 4b Hemovac contents drained into measuring container.

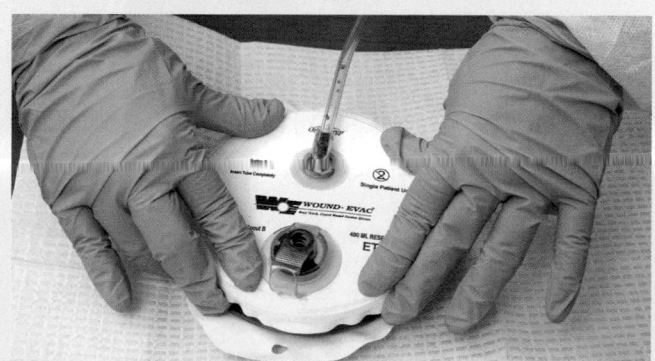

STEP 4c Hemovac compressed to create suction.

STEP	RATIONALE

IMPLEMENTATION

5. Empty Hemovac with wall suction:
   a. Turn off suction.
   b. Disconnect suction tubing from Hemovac port.
   c. Empty Hemovac as described in Step 4.
   d. Use an antiseptic swab to clean port opening and the end of suction tubing. Reconnect tubing to port.
   e. Set suction level as prescribed or on low if health care provider does not specify suction level.

6. Empty JP suction drain:
   a. Open port on top of bulb-shaped reservoir (see illustration).
   b. Tilt bulb in direction of port and drain toward opening. Empty drainage from device into measuring container (see illustration). Clean end of emptying port and plug with antiseptic wipe.
   c. Compress bulb over drainage container. While compressing bulb, replace plug immediately.

7. Place and secure drainage system below site with a safety pin on the patient's gown. Be sure that there is slack in tubing from reservoir to the wound.

8. Note characteristics of drainage in measuring container; measure volume and discard by flushing in commode.

9. Discard soiled supplies and remove and dispose of gloves. Perform hand hygiene.

10. Apply clean gloves. Proceed with dressing change (see Chapter 40) around drain site and inspection of skin if indicated. Split-drain sponge dressings are often used around drain tubes (see illustration) and taped in place.

11. Discard contaminated materials and remove gloves. Perform hand hygiene.

Empties drainage and re-establishes suction to wound bed.

Cleaning plug reduces transmission of microorganisms.

Re-establishes wound suction.

Breaks vacuum for drain.

Reduces transmission of microorganisms.

Re-establishes vacuum.

Pinning drainage tubing to patient's gown prevents tension or pulling on tubing and insertion site.

Contents count as fluid output.

Reduces transmission of microorganisms.

Prevents entrance of bacteria into surgical wound.

Reduces transmission of microorganisms.

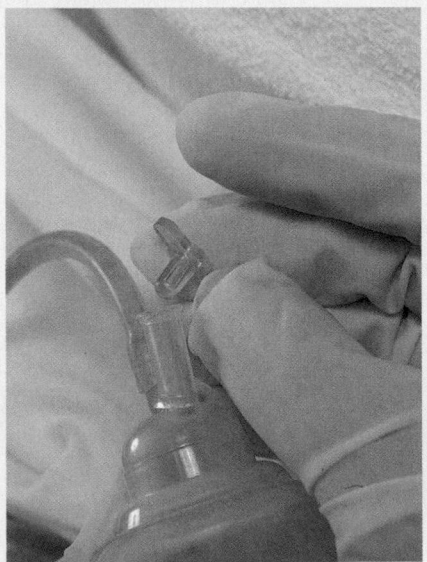

STEP 6a Opening port of Jackson-Pratt device.

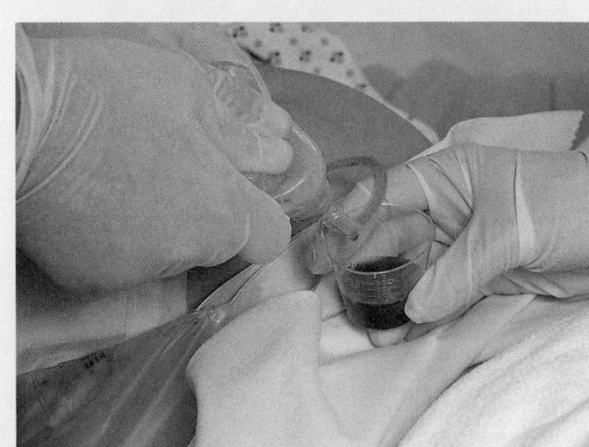

STEP 6b Emptying contents from Jackson-Pratt drainage device.

STEP	RATIONALE

IMPLEMENTATION

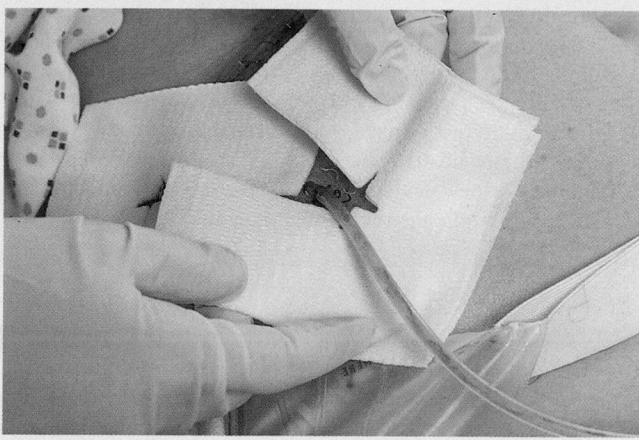

STEP 10 Applying split gauze dressing around Jackson-Pratt drain tube.

EVALUATION

1. Observe for drainage in suction device.	Indicates presence of vacuum, patency of tubing, and functioning of drainage suction device.

Clinical Decision Point *Inspect for clots or cellular debris. Clots or large collections of debris may block drainage flow. The Y-site in the drainage tubing is especially prone to clogging.*

2. Inspect wound for drainage or collection of drainage fluid under skin, causing seroma.	Drainage should not be significant under suture line. It may indicate inadequate functioning of drainage suction device.
3. Measure drainage from drainage system, and record on I&O form every 8 to 12 hours and as needed for large drainage volume.	Determines status of wound healing. Collect diagnostic specimen when there is unexpected purulence or a pungent odour, report findings to health care provider, and record in progress note.
4. Use Teach-Back: "I want to be sure I explained clearly why it is important for you not to pull on your drain. Tell me what can happen if you pull the drain out accidentally." Develop a revised teaching plan if patient or caregiver is not able to teach back correctly.	Determines patient's and caregiver's level of understanding of instructional topic.

Unexpected Outcomes	Related Interventions
1. Site where tube exits becomes infected.	• Notify health care provider about presence of signs of infection: purulent drainage, odour, reddened site, increased white blood cell count, and temperature elevation. • Use aseptic technique when changing dressings.
2. Bleeding appears in or around drainage collector.	• Determine amount of bleeding and notify health care provider if it is excessive. • Assess for tension on patient's drainage tubing. • Secure tubing to prevent pulling and pain.
3. Patient experiences pain.	• Assess patient's level of pain. • Medicate patient. • Stabilize drainage tubing to reduce tension and pulling against incision. • Notify health care provider if signs of wound infection are present.
4. Drainage suction device is not accumulating drainage.	• Assess drainage tubing for clots. • Assess drainage system for air leaks or kinks. • Notify health care provider.

Communication and Documentation

- Document emptying the drainage suction device; re-establishing vacuum in the suction device; amount, colour, and odour of drainage; dressing change to drain site; and appearance of drain insertion site on flow sheet in nurses' notes in electronic health record (EHR) or chart.
- Document amount of drainage on I&O record.
- Document your evaluation of patient and caregiver learning.
- Immediately report a sudden change in amount of drainage, either output or absence of drainage flow, to the health care provider. Also report pungent odour of drainage or new evidence of purulence, severe pain, or dislodgement of the drainage tube to the health care provider.

Special Considerations
Teaching

- Instruct patient about anticipated postoperative drainage, expected progress of wound healing and drainage volume, and estimated date of removal of drain as volume diminishes.

- Teach patient or caregiver how to empty and record amount of drainage. If patient is going home with a drainage device, ask the patient or caregiver to record the amount emptied and bring the recording to the next outpatient visit.

Pediatric

- Have parent or guardian help pediatric patients keep drainage tubes in place and not dislodge them.

Gerontological

- Be aware that older persons with large amounts of drainage will need additional fluid intake because they are more likely to become dehydrated.
- Take measures to prevent a confused patient from pulling out a drain collector.

Care in the Community

- Provide written instructions in drain care. Include the importance of measuring and documenting the amount of drainage. The patient should communicate the volume of drainage daily with the health care provider.

✦ SKILL 39.5   Negative-Pressure Wound Therapy

Negative-pressure wound therapy (NPWT) or wound vacuum is the application of a subatmospheric (negative) pressure to a wound through suction to facilitate healing and collect wound fluid (Netsch, Nix, & Haugen, 2016). There are a number of types of NPWT, from the large canister and vacuum that is attached to the bed and connected to a wall plug to small mini-NPWT products that provide the patient with complete mobility. When managing NPWT, the nurse needs to be familiar with how the product functions, and in some cases additional education is required before using the product (see employer policy).

The primary effects of negative pressure at the wound surface (Figs. 39.10 and 39.11) Netsch, 2016) are as follows:

- Removing wound exudates
- Maintaining a moist wound surface
- Reducing edema with improved perfusion
- Macrodeformation (traction on the sides of the wound), which promotes wound contraction
- Microdeformation and mechanical stretch on cells in the wound bed, which changes cell shape and activates intracellular processes to promote healing

Indications for NPWT include chronic, acute, traumatic, subacute, and dehisced wounds; partial-thickness burns; injuries (e.g., diabetic and pressure); flaps and grafts once nonviable tissue is removed; and select high-risk postoperative surgical incisions

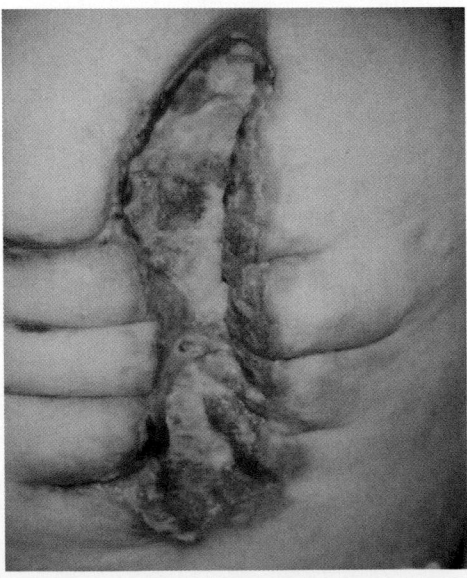

FIG 39.10 Dehisced wound before negative-pressure wound therapy. (*Courtesy KCI Licensing, San Antonio, TX*).

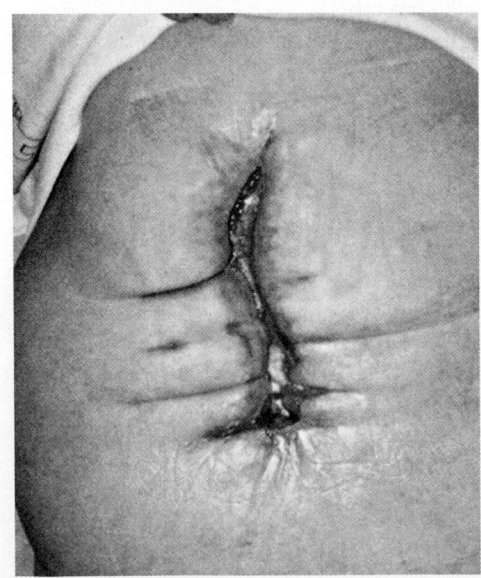

FIG 39.11 Dehisced wound after negative-pressure wound therapy. (*Courtesy KCI Licensing, San Antonio, TX*).

(e.g., orthopaedic, sternal). NPWT is also used in wounds with tunnels (i.e., a channel has formed that extends from any part of the wound through subcutaneous tissue or muscle), undermining, or sinus tracts as long as the wound filler can fill the dead space and is easily retrieved (Netsch et al., 2016). Research also supports use of an installation of wound-rinsing agents to facilitate healing in some chronic wounds (WOCN, 2016).

Contraindications to NPWT include necrotic tissue with eschar present; untreated osteomyelitis; nonenteric and unexplored fistulas; malignancy in the wound; exposed vasculature; and exposed nerves, anastomotic site, or organs. Safety precautions need to be considered for patients at high risk for bleeding or hemorrhage; patients taking anticoagulants; and patients requiring magnetic resonance imaging (MRI), hyperbaric chamber, or defibrillation (Netsch et al., 2016).

There are a number of different NPWT systems, some of which are gauze or foam based; some are designed for acute care settings or for outpatient care (Netsch, 2016).

NPWT can be delivered intermittently or continuously. Research and review of evidence show improved microvascular blood flow and granulation tissue formation with intermittent versus continuous therapy delivered at 125 mm Hg (WOCN, 2016). However, for patients with severe pain, lower levels of pressure (75–80 mm Hg)

can be used to reduce pain and discomfort without compromising effectiveness (EPUAP & NAPUAP, 2009; Netsch et al., 2016).

Delegation and Collaboration

The skill of NPWT cannot be delegated to an unregulated care provider (UCP). The nurse directs the UCP to:
- Use caution in positioning or turning the patient to avoid tubing displacement.
- Report to the nurse any change in dressing shape or integrity.
- Report to the nurse any change in the patient's temperature or comfort level.
- Report any wound fluid leakage around the edges of the adhesive drape.

Equipment

- The NPWT unit requires a health care provider's prescription. Vacuum-assisted closure (VAC) products are available in several different systems. The most appropriate approach when using a VAC system is to refer to the manufacturer's instructions. The following information is relevant to use of any type of VAC product.

STEP	RATIONALE

ASSESSMENT

1. Identify patient using at least two person-specific identifiers (e.g., name and date of birth or name and medical record number), according to employer policy.
2. Review health care provider's prescriptions for type of VAC as well as frequency of dressing change, amount of negative pressure, type of foam or gauze to use, and pressure cycle (intermittent or continuous), if applicable.
3. Review medical record for signs and symptoms related to condition of patient's wound.
4. Assess patient's level of comfort using an appropriate pain rating scale.
5. Perform hand hygiene. Apply clean gloves. Assess location, appearance, and size of wound (see Procedural Guideline 39.1). Remove and dispose of gloves. Perform hand hygiene.
6. Assess patient's and caregiver's knowledge of purpose of dressing and whether they will participate in dressing wound.

Ensures correct patient. Complies with Accreditation Canada's standards and improves patient safety (Accreditation Canada, 2019).
Determines frequency of dressing change, negative-pressure setting, and special instructions.

Provides baseline to compare findings with previous dressing change assessments and reflects wound-healing progress.
Serves as baseline to measure response to dressing therapy.

Provides information regarding status of wound healing, presence of complications, and proper type of supplies and help needed.

Identifies patient's learning needs. Prepares patient and caregiver if dressing will need to be changed at home.

NURSING DIAGNOSES

- Acute pain
- Chronic pain
- Insufficient knowledge regarding purpose of dressing
- Reduced skin integrity
- Potential for infection

Related factors/Risk factors are individualized on the basis of patient's condition or needs.

PLANNING

1. Expected outcomes following completion of procedure:
   - Patient's wound shows evidence of healing as wound decreases in size with less drainage, redness, or swelling.
   - Patient reports an acceptable level of comfort on an appropriate pain scale (e.g., 0 to 10, with of 0 being no pain and 10 being worst pain ever) during and after dressing changes.

Dressing is effective in promoting healing and preventing infection.
Analgesic and comfort measures are effective in controlling pain.

STEP	RATIONALE
PLANNING	
• Dressing remains intact with airtight seal and prescribed negative pressure.	Dressing is applied correctly and maintains negative pressure.
• If relevant, patient or caregiver demonstrates correct method of dressing changes.	Indicates that patient and caregiver learning has occurred.
2. Explain procedure to patient and caregiver.	Relieves anxiety and promotes understanding of healing process.
3. Administer prescribed analgesic as needed 30 minutes before dressing change.	A comfortable patient will be less likely to move suddenly, causing wound or supply contamination.
IMPLEMENTATION	
1. Close room door or cubicle curtains and perform hand hygiene.	Provides for patient privacy and reduces transmission of microorganisms.
2. Position patient comfortably and drape to expose only wound site. Instruct patient not to touch wound or sterile supplies.	Promotes patient's cooperation and completion of procedure smoothly. Prevents contamination of sterile supplies.
3. Cuff top of disposable waterproof biohazard bag and place within reach of work area.	Cuff prevents accidental contamination of top of outer bag.
4. Apply clean gloves. If risk for spray exists, apply a protective gown, goggles, and mask.	Reduces transmission of infectious organisms from soiled dressings to nurse's hands.
5. Follow manufacturer instructions for removal and replacement because each NPWT unit varies slightly with approach. Turn off NPWT unit by pushing therapy on/off button.	Deactivates therapy and allows for proper drainage of fluid in drainage tubing.
a. Keeping tube connectors attached to NPWT unit, raise tubing connectors; disconnect tubes from one another and drain fluids into drainage collector.	Prevents backflow of any drainage in tubing back into the wound.
b. Before lowering, tighten clamp on canister tube and disconnect canister and dressing tubing at connection points.	Prevents drainage from exiting tubing when removed.
6. Remove transparent film by gently stretching it, and slowly pull it away from the skin.	Prevents injury to wound tissue. Protects periwound skin breakdown from transparent adhesive.
7. Remove old dressing one layer at a time and discard in bag. Observe drainage on dressing. Use caution to avoid applying tension on any drains that are present.	Determines type and amount of dressings needed for replacement. Prevents accidental removal of drains.
8. Assess wound. Observe surface area and tissue type, colour, odour, and drainage within the wound. Measure length, width, and depth of the wound as prescribed.	Measurement of wound is necessary to assess wound-healing progression and justify continuation of NPWT (Netsch et al., 2016). Determines condition of wound and need for replacement of dressing.

Clinical Decision Point *This is a time when a wound-care nurse or health care provider might debride the wound. Debridement of eschar or slough, if present, should be performed for removal of devitalized tissue to prepare the wound bed (Netsch et al., 2016).*

STEP	RATIONALE
9. Remove and discard gloves in waterproof bag. Avoid having patient see old dressing because the sight of wound drainage may be upsetting. Perform hand hygiene.	Reduces transmission of microorganisms. Lessens patient anxiety during procedure.
10. Clean wound.	Irrigation removes wound debris and cleans wound bed.
a. Apply sterile or clean gloves, depending on employer policy and wound status.	Prevents transmission of microorganisms.
b. If prescribed, irrigate wound with normal saline or other solution prescribed (see Skill 39.2). Gently blot periwound with gauze to dry thoroughly.	Cleaning periwound is essential for an airtight seal.

Clinical Decision Point *If drainage appears purulent or has a foul odour or if there is a change in amount or colour, notify the health care provider about the potential for increased bioburden. A wound culture may be appropriate, and this may be an indication that NPWT should be discontinued (Hasan, Teo, & Nather, 2015).*

STEP	RATIONALE

IMPLEMENTATION

11. Apply skin protectant, barrier film, solid skin barrier sheet, or hydrocolloid dressing to periwound skin.

Maintains airtight seal needed for NPWT wound therapy and protects periwound skin from moisture-associated skin damage (Netsch et al., 2016).

12. Fill any uneven skin surfaces (e.g., creases, scars, and skinfolds) with skin-barrier product (e.g., paste, strip).

Further helps to maintain airtight seal (Netsch et al., 2016).

13. Remove and discard gloves. Perform hand hygiene.

Prevents transmission of microorganisms.

14. Depending on type of wound, apply sterile or new clean gloves (see employer policy).

Fresh sterile wounds require sterile gloves.
Chronic wounds require clean technique (WOCN, 2016).

15. Apply NPWT.

   a. Prepare NPWT filler dressing. Consult with wound-care expert for appropriate type.

Filler dressing depends on NPWT used and can include foam or gauze dressings with or without antimicrobials such as silver. The type of dressing may be adjusted based on undermining, tunneling, or sinus tracts present (Netsch et al., 2016).

     (1) Measure wound and select appropriate-size dressing.

Establishes baseline for wound size.
Black polyurethane (PU) foam has larger pores and is most effective in stimulating granulation tissue and wound contraction. White soft foam is denser, with smaller pores, and is used when growth of granulation tissue needs to be restricted (Netsch et al., 2016).

     (2) Using sterile scissors, cut filler dressing foam to wound size, making sure to fit exact size and shape of wound, including tunnels and undermined areas.

Proper size of foam dressing maintains negative pressure to entire wound (Netsch et al., 2016).

Clinical Decision Point *In some instances, an antimicrobial product such as sliver-impregnated gauze or topical antibiotic is required. These products help reduce the bioburden of the wound.*

   b. Place filler dressing in wound, following manufacturer instructions. Be sure that filler dressing is in contact with the entire wound base, margins, and tunneled and undermined areas. Count number of filler dressings and document in patient's chart. *Dressing must **not** be placed over intact periwound skin.*

Maintains negative pressure to entire wound. Edges of foam dressing must be in direct contact with the patient's skin.
Dressing count provides nurse who removes dressing with number of filler dressings that should be removed.

   c. Place suction device per manufacturer instructions.

   d. Apply NPWT transparent dressing over foam wound dressing.

     (1) Trim transparent dressing to cover wound and dressing so it will extend onto periwound skin approximately 2.5 to 5 cm (1 to 2 inches).

Prepares dressing of appropriate size for wound.

     (2) Apply transparent dressing, keeping it wrinkle-free (see illustration).

Ensures that wound is properly covered and negative-pressure seal can be achieved (Box 39.4). Dressing should be airtight with no tunnels or gaps to ensure a good seal when suction is activated.

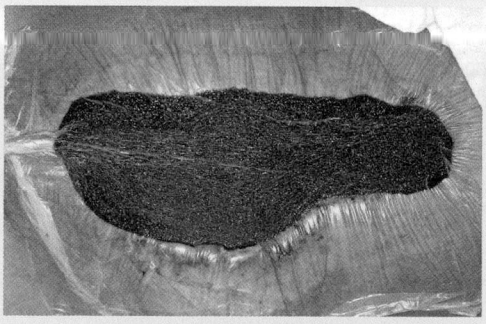

STEP 15d(2) Foam wound filler; transparent dressing over existing wound.

STEP	RATIONALE

IMPLEMENTATION

    (3) Secure tubing to transparent film, aligning drainage holes to ensure occlusive seal. Do not apply tension.

    (4) Secure tubing several centimetres away from dressing, avoiding pressure points.

16. After wound is completely covered, connect tubing from dressing to tubing from canister and NPWT unit and set at prescribed suction level.

    a. Remove canister from sterile packing and push unit until you hear click. **NOTE:** An alarm sounds if canister is not properly engaged.

    b. Connect dressing tubing to canister tubing. Make sure that both clamps are open.

    c. Place on a level surface or hang from foot of the bed. **NOTE:** Unit alarms and deactivates therapy if it is tilted beyond 45 degrees.

    d. Press power button (commonly this is a green-lit button) and set pressure as prescribed.

17. Inspect NPWT system.

    a. Verify that the system is on. This is different for each type of NPWT unit. For example, on some units the display screen shows "Therapy On." Check employer policy and procedure for specific information.

    b. Verify that all clamps are open and all tubing is patent.

    c. Examine system to be sure that seal is intact and that therapy is working.

    d. If a leak is present, use strips of transparent film to patch areas around edges of the wound.

18. Record initials, date, and time on new dressing.

19. Help patient to a comfortable position. Patients may ambulate with NPWT.

20. Discard gloves and dispose of any dressing material. Perform hand hygiene.

Rationale column:

Excessive tension may compress foam dressing and impede wound healing. It also produces shear force on periwound area (Kinetic Concepts International, 2013).

Drainage tubes over bony pressure prominences can cause medical device–related pressure injuries (Netsch et al., 2016; Pittman et al., 2015).

Intermittent or continuous negative pressure can be administered at 80 to 125 mm Hg (Netsch et al., 2016; WOCN, 2016).

Negative pressure is achieved when a tight seal is present (Netsch, 2016).

Provides reference for next dressing change.

Enhances patient comfort and relaxation.

Prevents transmission of microorganisms.

EVALUATION

1. Inspect condition of wound on an ongoing basis; note drainage (any evidence of bleeding) and odour.

2. Ask patient to rate pain using an appropriate pain rating scale.

Rationale column:

Determines status of wound healing.

Determines patient's level of comfort following procedure.

BOX 39.4

Maintaining an Airtight Seal With Negative-Pressure Wound Therapy

To avoid loss of suction (negative pressure), the wound and dressing must stay sealed after therapy is initiated. Problem seal areas include wounds around joints; near skin creases and folds; and near moisture such as diaphoresis, wound drainage, and urine or stool. The following points may help to maintain an airtight seal:

- Clip hair on skin around wound (check employer policy).
- Fill uneven skin surfaces with a skin-barrier product such as paste or strips.
- Make sure that the periwound skin surface is dry.
- Cut transparent film to extend 2.5 to 5 cm (1 to 2 inches) beyond wound perimeter.

- Frame periwound area with skin sealant, solid skin barrier, hydrocolloid, or transparent film dressing.
- Cut or mould transparent dressing to fit wound.
- Avoid wrinkles when applying transparent film.
- Identify any air leaks with a stethoscope and repair them with a sealant dressing (e.g., transparent dressing). Use only one or two additional layers for large leaks. Multiple layers reduce moisture vapor transmission and cause maceration of the wound.
- Avoid adhesive remover because it leaves a residue that hinders film adherence.

Data from Netsch, D. S. (2016). Refractory wounds. In Wound Ostomy and Continence Nurses Society, *Core curriculum: wound management.* Philadelphia: Wolters Kluwer; Netsch, D. S., Nix, D. P., & Haugen, V. (2016). Negative-pressure wound therapy. In R. A. Bryant & D. P. Nix (Eds.), *Acute and chronic wounds: Current management concepts* (5th ed.). St. Louis: Mosby.

STEP	RATIONALE

EVALUATION

3. Verify airtight dressing seal and correct negative-pressure setting.

4. Measure wound drainage output in canister on a regular basis.

5. **Use Teach-Back:** "I want to be sure I explained clearly what your wound should look like as it is healing and the signs of infection before you are discharged. Explain to me what your wound will look like as it begins to heal." Develop revised teaching plan if patient or caregiver is not able to teach back correctly.

Determines effective negative pressure being applied.

Monitors fluid balance and wound drainage.

Determines patient's and caregiver's level of understanding of instructional topic.

Unexpected Outcomes

1. Wound appears inflamed and tender, drainage has increased, and odour is present.

2. Patient reports increase in pain.

3. Negative-pressure seal has broken.
4. Wound hemorrhages.
5. Patient discharged home with NPWT.

Related Interventions

- Notify health care provider.
- Obtain wound culture.
- Increase frequency of dressing changes.
- Patient may need more analgesia.
- Instill normal saline to moisten foam and other filler dressings to allow them to loosen from granulation tissue.
- If using black foam, switch to polyvinyl alcohol (PVA) white soft foam.
- Decrease pressure setting.
- Change from intermittent to continuous cycling.
- Change type of NPWT system.
- Take preventive measures (see Box 39.4).
- Stop NPWT immediately and notify health care provider.

Ensure patient has prescriptions for NPWT products to continue treatment.

Communication and Documentation

- Document appearance of wound, characteristics of drainage, placement of NPWT (type of dressing, pressure mode and setting), and patient response to dressing change on flow sheet in nurses' notes in electronic health record (EHR) or chart.
- Document your evaluation of patient and caregiver learning.
- Report brisk, bright red bleeding, evidence of poor wound healing, evisceration or dehiscence, and possible wound infection to the health care provider immediately.

Special Considerations

Teaching

- Successful NPWT relies on the patient's and caregiver's cooperation with treatment. NPWT can be difficult to use when the patient is unable to consciously cooperate (e.g., dementia) (Netsch et al., 2016).
- If relevant, patients and caregivers need to learn how to administer analgesics appropriately. Patient tolerance of and adherence to NPWT are difficult if dressing changes are painful (Netsch et al., 2016).
- Educate patients and caregivers about the signs and symptoms that indicate development of an infection and to report this to the health care provider immediately.
- Teach patient and caregiver points to follow to maintain negative-pressure seal.
- Explain how NPWT works and why dressing is not changed daily.

Pediatric

- NPWT therapy is not appropriate for fragile neonatal skin.
- For older pediatric patients, the same approach is used as for adult patients.

Gerontological

- Older persons have fragile skin and decreased healing potential, related to numerous factors. Ensure that the patient is appropriate for NPWT (e.g., adequate nutrition, perfusion).
- Use skin-care practices to protect periwound tissue. Transparent film may be irritating to fragile skin. A skin protectant is one method to reduce the risk for tissue injury.
- Therapy may need to start with lower negative pressures (e.g., 75 mm Hg) and slowly titrate to more negative pressure.

Care in the Community

- The patient and caregiver are usually not required to change the larger NPWT treatment methods; however, small units may be managed by a patient or caregiver. Provide support and ongoing follow-up to ensure appropriate use of the NPWT product, including maintaining the seal, observing for infection, and changing the dressing (if appropriate).
- Provide information to the patient and caregiver regarding proper disposal of contaminated products.

◆ CLINICAL DEBRIEF

A patient is 6 days postoperative from a colon resection for a perforated diverticulum. She has been readmitted because of excessive drainage from her midline abdominal incision; on admission, one-half of the staples in her incision were removed by the admitting resident. The wound has been left to heal by secondary intention; moist saline gauze dressings to be applied every 12 hours. At admission, she had a computed tomography (CT) scan that showed a fluid accumulation that was drained in interventional radiology, and the drain was left and attached to a bulb syringe.

1. The abdominal wound will heal by which type of wound healing, and what principle will guide the wound toward healing?
2. Name two types of wound irrigation that may be appropriate for the twice-daily irrigation prescribed by the health care provider.
3. The patient was discharged with an open wound and instructed to use twice-daily irrigation and to apply a saline-moistened nonadherent gauze wound dressing. The patient returns to the wound clinic 1 week after discharge. She indicates increased tenderness around the wound and some light yellow drainage. The nurse takes the patient's vital signs and notes a temperature of 38.7°C (101.6°F). Wound assessment reveals yellow, foul-smelling purulent drainage and red wound edges. Use SBAR documentation to communicate these findings to the health care team.

◆ REVIEW QUESTIONS

1. A patient has recently undergone a colon resection and has an abdominal wound healing by secondary intention. For 4 days following the surgical procedure she has had a moist saline gauze dressing changed twice a day. The UCP calls the nurse to the room because of excessive drainage from under the abdominal wound dressing. Which of the following assessments will the nurse plan to do, based on this finding? *(Select all that apply.)*
   1. Ask the UCP to obtain vital signs and note the temperature.
   2. Reinforce the dressing and call the surgical team.
   3. Remove dressings and assess how many of the dressings are soaked with drainage; note the drainage colour consistency and any presence of odour.
   4. Suggest ambulation to help the wound drain additional fluid.
   5. Instruct the UCP to change the dressing as needed.
   6. Observe the wound tissue for colour and presence of abnormal drainage and the periwound area for redness or warmth.
2. A patient has an extensive abdominal wound and is to have half of the staples removed and the incision cleaned. Place the following steps in correct order for preparation of and interaction with the patient.
   1. Assess healing ridge and skin integrity of suture line.
   2. Describe to the patient how you will remove the staples.
   3. Place upper tip of the staple remover under the staple to ease removal.
   4. Assess patient for pain.
   5. Lift up on staple when depressing the extractor handles.
   6. Clean incision before removing staples, starting at sides next to incision.
3. The nurse notes approximately 60 mL of bright red drainage in the Jackson-Pratt drain 6 hours after surgery. Which two nursing interventions should be included in the care for this patient?
   1. Emptying the drain in 24 hours
   2. Shaking the bulb to thin the drainage
   3. Calling the surgeon to report the finding
   4. Securing the drain above the level of the wound
   5. Emptying the drain immediately and checking the volume again in 2 hours

Ⓔ *Visit the Evolve site for a complete list of Clinical Debrief and Review Questions answers.*

REFERENCES

Accreditation Canada. (2019). *Required organizational practices handbook—Version 14.* Ottawa, ON: Author. Retrieved from http://www.wrha.mb.ca/quality/files/2019ROPHandbook.pdf

Allard, J. P., Keller, H., Jeejeebhoy, K. N., et al. (2016). Malnutrition at hospital admission—Contributors and effect on length of stay. *Journal of Parenteral and Enteral Nutrition, 40*(4), 487–497.

Ayello, E. A., & Braden, B. (2002). How and why do pressure ulcer risk assessment. *Advances in Skin & Wound Care, 15*(3), 125.

Bååth, C., Engström, M., Gunningberg, L., & Muntlin Athlin, M. (2016). Prevention of heel pressure ulcers among older patients from ambulance care to hospital discharge: A multi-centre randomized controlled trial. *Applied Nursing Research, 30,* 170–175. doi:10.1016/j.apnr.2015.10.003

Beitz, J. M. (2014). Providing quality skin and wound care for the bariatric patient: An overview of clinical challenges. *Ostomy/Wound Management, 60*(1), 12–21.

Beitz, J. M. (2016). Wound healing. In Wound Ostomy and Continence Nurses Society (Ed.), *Core curriculum: Wound management.* Philadelphia: Wolters Kluwer.

Black, J., Clark, M., Dealey, C., et al. (2015). Dressings as an adjunct to pressure ulcer prevention: Consensus panel recommendations. *International Wound Journal, 12*(4), 484–488. doi:10.1111/iwj.12197

Black, J., & Kalowes, P. (2016). Medical device–related pressure ulcers. *Chronic Wound Care Management and Research, 3,* 91–99. doi:10.2147/CWCMR.S82370

Braden, B. J., & Bergstrom, N. (1989). Clinical utility of the Braden Scale for predicting pressure sore risk. *Decubitus, 2*(3), 44.

Braden, B. J., & Bergstrom, N. (1994). Predictive utility of the Braden scale for predicting pressure sore risk. *Research in Nursing & Health, 17*(6), 459–470.

Brienza, D., Antokal, S., Herbe, L., et al. (2015). Friction-induced skin injuries—Are they pressure ulcers? An updated NPUAP white paper. *Journal of Wound Ostomy & Continence Nursing, 42*(1), 62–64. doi:10.1097/WON

Bryant, R. A., & Nix, D. P. (2016a). Developing and maintaining a pressure ulcer prevention program. In R. A. Bryant & D. P. Nix (Eds.), *Acute and chronic wounds: Current management concepts* (5th ed.). St. Louis: Mosby.

Bryant, R. A., & Nix, D. P. (2016b). Principles for practice development. In R. A. Bryant & D. P. Nix (Eds.), *Acute and chronic wounds: Current management concepts* (5th ed.). St. Louis: Mosby.

Bryant, R. A., & Nix, D. P. (2016c). Principles of wound healing and topical management. In R. A. Bryant & D. P. Nix (Eds.), *Acute and chronic wounds: Current management concepts* (5th ed.). St. Louis: Mosby.

Byrne, J., Nichols, P., Sroczynski, M., et al. (2016). Prophylactic sacral dressing for pressure ulcer prevention in high-risk patients. *American Journal of Critical Care, 25*(3), 228–234. doi:10.4037/ajcc2016979

Canadian Patient Safety Institute (CPSI). (2016). *Pressure ulcer: Introduction.* Retrieved from http://www.patientsafetyinstitute.ca/en/toolsResources/Hospital-Harm-Measure/Improvement-Resources/HHI-Pressure-Ulcer/Pages/default.aspx

Chong, S. J., Kok, Y. O., Choke, A., Tan, E. W., Tan, K. C., & Tan, B. K. (2017). Comparison of four measures in reducing length of stay in burns: An Asian centre's evolved multimodal burns protocol. *Burns: Journal of the International Society for Burn Injuries, 43*(6), 1348–1355.

Coyer, F. M., Gardner, A., Duobrovsky, A., et al. (2015). Reducing pressure injuries in critically ill patients by using a patient skin integrity care bundle (InSpire). *American Journal of Critical Care, 24*(3), 199–209. doi:10.4037/ajcc2015930

Doughty, D. B., & McNichols, L. L. (2016). General concepts related to skin and soft tissue injury caused by mechanical factors. In *Core curriculum: Wound management.* Philadelphia: Wolters Kluwer.

Doughty, D. B., & Sparks-Defriese, B. (2016). Wound-healing physiology. In R. A. Bryant & D. P. Nix (Eds.), *Acute and chronic wounds: Current management concepts* (5th ed.). St. Louis: Mosby.

Elias, P. M. (2015). Stratum corneum acidification: How and why? *Experimental Dermatology, 24*(3), 179–180. doi:10.1111/exd.12596

European Pressure Ulcer Advisory Panel (EPUAP) and National Pressure Ulcer Advisory Panel (NPUAP). (2009). *Treatment of pressure ulcers: Quick reference guide.* Washington, DC: NPUAP.

Fearns, N., Heller-Murphy, S., Kelly, J., & Harbour, J. (2017). Placing the patient at the centre of chronic wound care: A qualitative evidence synthesis. *Journal of Tissue Viability, 26*(4), 254–259.

Hasan, M. Y., Teo, R., & Nather, A. (2015). Negative-pressure wound therapy for management of diabetic foot wounds: A review of the mechanism of action,

clinical applications, and recent developments. *Diabetic Foot & Ankle, 6,* doi:10.3402/dfa.v6.27618

Jaszarowski, K. A., & Murphree, R. W. (2016). Wound cleansing and dressing selection. In Wound Ostomy and Continence Nurses Society (Ed.), *Core curriculum: Wound management.* Philadelphia: Wolters Kluwer.

Kinetic Concepts International (KCI). (2013). *VAC therapy for wounds, product information.* San Antonio, TX: Kinetic Concepts International (KCI).

Krasner, D. L. (2016). Wound pain: Impact and assessment. In R. A. Bryant & D. P. Nix (Eds.), *Acute and chronic wounds: Current management concepts* (5th ed.). St. Louis: Mosby.

Lian, Y. (2016). Barrier products in the treatment of incontinence-associated dermatitis. *Nursing Standard, 30*(47), 59–67. doi:10.7748/ns.2016.e10298

Makic, M. B. (2015). Medical device–related pressure ulcers and intensive care. *Journal of Perianesthesia Nursing, 30*(4), 336–337. doi:10.1016/j.jopan.2015.05.004

National Pressure Ulcer Advisory Panel (NPUAP). (2016). *National Pressure Ulcer Advisory Panel announces a change in terminology from pressure ulcer to pressure injury and updates the stages of pressure injury, April 2016.* Retrieved from https://www.npuap.org/national-pressure-ulcer-advisory-panel-npuap-announces-a-change-in-terminology-from-pressure-ulcer-to-pressure-injury-and-updates-the-stages-of-pressure-injury/

National Pressure Ulcer Advisory Panel (NPUAP), European Pressure Ulcer Advisory Panel (EPUAP), Pan Pacific Pressure Injury Alliance (PPPIA), & Haesler, E. (Eds.), (2014). *Prevention and treatment of pressure ulcers: Quick reference guide.* Osborne Park, Western Australia: Cambridge Media.

Nelson, V. S., Crumbley, D. R., & Elster, E. (2016). Traumatic wounds: Bullets, blasts, and vehicle crashes. In R. A. Bryant & D. P. Nix (Eds.), *Acute and chronic wounds: Current management concepts* (5th ed.). St. Louis: Mosby.

Netsch, D. S. (2016). Refractory wounds. In Wound Ostomy and Continence Nurses Society (Ed.), *Core curriculum: Wound management.* Philadelphia: Wolters Kluwer.

Netsch, D. S., Nix, D. P., & Haugen, V. (2016). Negative pressure wound therapy. In R. A. Bryant & D. P. Nix (Eds.), *Acute and chronic wounds: Current management concepts* (5th ed.). St. Louis: Mosby.

Nix, D. P. (2016). Skin and wound assessment. In R. A. Bryant & D. P. Nix (Eds.), *Acute and chronic wounds: Current management concepts* (5th ed.). St. Louis: Mosby.

Orsted, H. L., Keast, D. H., Forest-Lalande, L., et al. (2018). *Foundations of best practice for skin and wound management.* Wounds Canada. Retrieved from https://www.woundscanada.ca/docman/public/health-care-professional/bpr-workshop/165-wc-bpr-prevention-and-management-of-wounds/file

Pieper, B. (2016). Pressure ulcers: Impact, etiology, and classification. In R. A. Bryant & D. P. Nix (Eds.), *Acute and chronic wounds: Current management concepts* (5th ed.). St. Louis: Mosby.

Pittman, J., Beeson, T., Kitterman, J., Lancaster, S., & Shelly, A. (2015). Medical device–related hospital-acquired pressure ulcers: Development of an evidence-based position statement. *Journal of Wound Ostomy & Continence Nursing, 42*(2), 151–154. doi:10.1097/WON.0000000000000113

Ramundo, J. (2016). Wound debridement. In R. A. Bryant & D. P. Nix (Eds.), *Acute and chronic wounds: Current management concepts* (5th ed.). St. Louis: Mosby.

Schallom, M., Cracchiolo, L., Falker, A., et al. (2015). Pressure ulcer incidence in patients wearing nasal-oral versus full-face noninvasive ventilation masks. *American Journal of Critical Care, 24*(4), 349–356. doi:10.4037/ajcc2015386

Stotts, N. A. (2016a). Nutritional assessment and support. In R. A. Bryant & D. P. Nix (Eds.), *Acute and chronic wounds: Current management concepts* (5th ed.). St. Louis: Mosby.

Stotts, N. A. (2016b). Wound infection: Diagnosis and management. In R. A. Bryant & D. P. Nix (Eds.), *Acute and chronic wounds: Current management concepts* (5th ed.). St. Louis: Mosby.

Tayyib, N., & Coyer, F. (2016). Effectiveness of pressure ulcer prevention strategies for adult patients in intensive care units: A systematic review. *Worldviews on Evidence-based Nursing, 13*(6), 432–444.

Thayer, D. M., Rozenboom, B., & Baranoski, S. (2016). Top down injuries: Prevention and management of moisture-associated skin damage, medical adhesive–related skin injury and skin tears. In Wound Ostomy and Continence Nurses Society (Ed.), *Core curriculum: Wound management.* Philadelphia: Wolters Kluwer.

Whitehead, F., Giampieri, S., Graham, T., & Grocott, P. (2017). Identifying, managing and preventing skin maceration: A rapid review of the clinical evidence. *Journal of Wound Care, 26*(4), 159–165.

Whitney, J. D. (2016). Surgical wounds and incisional care. In R. A. Bryant & D. P. Nix (Eds.), *Acute and chronic wounds: Current management concepts* (5th ed.). St. Louis: Mosby.

World Health Organization (WHO). (2016). *Global guidelines for the prevention of surgical site infection.* Geneva: Author. Retrieved from http://www.patientsafetyinstitute.ca/en/toolsResources/Documents/WHO%20global%20SSI%20guidelines_2016_10_22.pdf

Wound Ostomy and Continence Nurses Society (WOCN). (2016). *Guideline for prevention and management of pressure ulcers (injuries).* Mount Laurel, NJ: Author.

Wysocki, A. (2016). Anatomy and physiology of skin and soft tissue. In R. A. Bryant & D. P. Nix (Eds.), *Acute and chronic wounds: Current management concepts* (5th ed.). St. Louis: Mosby.

Yates, A. (2018). Incontinence-associated dermatitis in older people: Prevention and management. *British Journal of Community Nursing, 23*(5), 218–224.

40 | Wound Care Management and Dressings

Written by **Rosemary Kohr, RN, MScN, PhD; and Janice C. Colwell, RN, MS, CWOCN, FAAN**

SKILLS AND PROCEDURES

OBJECTIVES

Mastery of content in this chapter will enable the nurse to:
- Assess a wound correctly.
- Understand the purposes and techniques of dressings, bandages, and abdominal binders.

- Understand how to choose the correct dressing for a wound based on its characteristics.
- Apply dressings correctly.
- Apply an abdominal binder correctly.

MEDIA RESOURCES

- evolve http://evolve.elsevier.com/Canada/Perry/clinicalskills/
- Review Questions

- **NSO** Nursing Skills Online
- Clinical Debrief and Review Questions Answers

PURPOSE

Correct use of dressings, bandages, and binders support underlying tissues and promote wound healing. Knowledge and use of proper wound dressing techniques are essential nursing practices. Selection of the type of dressing is based on specific characteristics of the wound; the expected outcomes desired; and, for chronic wounds, the practicality and feasibility of caregivers performing the dressing changes in the home setting.

STANDARDS OF CARE

- Accreditation Canada, 2019—*Required Organizational Practices Handbook—Version 14* (http://www.wrha.mb.ca/quality/files/2019ROPHandbook.pdf)
- Canadian Patient Safety Institute (CPSI), 2016—*Pressure Ulcer: Resources* (http://www.patientsafetyinstitute.ca/en/toolsResources/Hospital-Harm-Measure/Improvement-Resources/HHI-Pressure-Ulcer/Pages/Resource-Library-Pressure-Ulcer-Resources.aspx)
- Harris, Kuhnke, Haley, et al., 2018—*Best Practice Recommendations for Prevention and Management of Surgical Wound Complications* (https://www.woundscanada.ca/docman/public/health-care-professional/bpr-workshop/555-bpr-prevention-and-management-of-surgical-wound-complications-v2/file)
- National Pressure Ulcer Advisory Panel (NPUAP), European Pressure Ulcer Advisory Panel (EPUAP), & Pan Pacific Pressure Injury Alliance (PPPIA), 2014—*2014 Prevention and Treatment of Pressure Ulcers: Clinical Practice Guideline* (https://www.npuap.org/resources/educational-and-clinical-resources/prevention-and-treatment-of-pressure-ulcers-clinical-practice-guideline/)
- Orsted, Keast, Forest-Lalande, et al., 2018—*Foundations of Best Practice for Skin and Wound Management* (https://www.woundscanada.ca/docman/public/health-care-professional/bpr-workshop/165-wc-bpr-prevention-and-management-of-wounds/file)

PRINCIPLES FOR PRACTICE

- Acute wounds go through a predictable, standard process as they heal. The following phases of wound healing occur: hemostasis, inflammation, proliferation (repair), and maturation (remodelling). Chronic wounds stall in this trajectory, often remaining in the inflammatory or proliferation phase (Ermer-Seltun & Rolstad, 2016).

- The T.I.M.E. framework addresses barriers to wound healing and identifies key clinical assessments and treatment options (Chamanga, Hughes, Hilston, et al., 2015; Ermer-Seltun & Rolstad, 2016; Mudge, 2015):
  - **Tissue management:** Removes nonviable, nonhealthy tissue from the wound bed. In addition, tissue management also reduces bioburden of the wound which impedes wound healing. Wound debridement reduces bioburden and in turn reduces risk for wound infection. Tissue management also controls for hypergranulation and hypertrophic scar formation, both of which affect wound healing.
  - **Inflammation and infection:** Influenced by the presence of nonviable tissue, high bacterial loads, and impaired leukocytes. The goal is to identify and treat wound infection and inflammation promptly.
  - **Moisture:** When a wound surface is too wet or too dry, the repair process is delayed. The goal is to keep a wound surface moist, not wet.
  - **Edge:** Affects the integrity of the perimeter of the wound. A closed or compromised wound edge prevents resurfacing and wound repair. The goal is to have a proliferative wound edge.
- The key principles of a physiological wound environment are adequate moisture, temperature control, pH, and control of bacterial burden.
- Effective dressings control wound moisture and drainage, debride dead tissue, protect a wound, and reduce the spread of infection.
- Primary wound healing occurs when tissue is cut cleanly and margins are reapproximated (i.e., surgical incisions).
- Secondary wound healing occurs when skin is left open, healing from granulation tissue at the base of the wound combined with epithelialization from the sides.
- Dressing material is selected on the basis of its characteristics, to promote wound healing (Box 40.1).

PERSON-CENTRED CARE

- Numerous dressings and products are available for the management of acute and chronic wounds; select dressings to achieve individual patient care outcomes (Table 40.1).
- A priority in wound care management is patient comfort:
  - Select dressings that help to reduce pain. For example, nonadherent (e.g., silicone) dressings will generally reduce wound-related pain (Hopf, Shapshak, Junkins, et al., 2016; Krasner, 2016).
  - If a patient's pain is from eroded or denuded skin around the margin of a wound, use skin sealants or barriers, or a dressing with a silicone-based border (Bryant & Best, 2016).
  - If required, provide patients with an appropriate analgesic dose 30 minutes before a dressing change to maximize comfort when the dressing and tissues will be manipulated.
- Patients may not admit to requiring pain relief related to dressing change. Discuss with the patient in advance the issue of pain relief. Culture may play a role in a patient's approach to pain. As well, individuals sometimes feel the need to experience pain "to know what's going on." However, it is important to explain the benefit of pain management for wound healing. If acceptable and appropriate, recommend pharmacological and nonpharmacological pain-relief measures before dressing changes. These measures may include altering sensory stimulus (e.g., providing a squeeze ball), letting the patient remove the dressing or perform the dressing change, and allowing for "time-outs" during painful dressing changes (Hopf et al., 2016).

BOX 40.1

Dressing Characteristics and Outcomes

Characteristics

- Nontraumatic and able to absorb exudate and allow for moisture-vapour transfer*
- Keeps wound bed moist and surrounding periwound tissues dry and intact
- Appropriate for infected wounds*
- Can be removed without trauma, pain, or leaving dressing fragments in the wound
- Conforms to body part for ease of movement
- Maintains stable physiological wound environment
- Easy to apply and remove with easy-to-follow patient and caregiver instructions
- Cost-effective

Outcomes

- Reduces volume of exudate and amount of necrotic tissue
- Resolves or prevents periwound erythema or maceration
- Reduces wound dimensions or depth of sinus tract
- Reduces pain intensity during dressing changes

Data from Bryant, R. A., & Nix, D. P. (2016). Principles of wound healing and topical management. In R. A. Bryant & D. P. Nix (Eds.), *Acute and chronic wounds: Current management concepts* (5th ed., pp. 306–324). St. Louis: Mosby; Orsted, H. L, Keast, D. H., Forest-Lalonde, L., Kuhnke, J. L., O'Sullivan-Drombolis, D., Jin, S., Haley, J., & Evans, R. (Eds.). (2018). *Best practice recommendations for the prevention and management of wounds*. Toronto, ON: Canadian Association of Wound Care. Retrieved from https://www.woundscanada.ca/docman/public/healthcare-professional/bpr-workshop/165-wc-bpr-prevention-and-management-of-wounds/file.

*Not including hydrocolloid dressings.

- Provide an opportunity for caregivers to be present during dressing changes if acceptable to the patient. Caregivers can then see the actual dressing change, thus enabling them to give the patient comfort and emotional support. Provide relevant teaching (e.g., phases of wound healing, rationale for dressing selection) and answer questions during this time.
- If a patient has a chronic wound, assess the patient's or caregiver's knowledge about proper wound care. Patients might have preferences regarding the time of day to change a dressing or before or after a certain activity.
- If it is likely that the patient will continue to have the same type of dressing while at home, educate them and the caregiver on the proper techniques for changing it and disposing of medical waste and how to assess for increased bioburden and for infection.
- Person-centred care includes recognizing how an individual's culture may attribute different meanings to wounds and trauma, blood loss, and disposal of soiled dressings and linens. In addition to ensuring privacy, the act of changing a dressing may require gender-congruent (e.g., female for female patient) caregivers. It is important to ensure that culture and religion have been assessed, to determine if there are additional steps to take in caring for the patient and family.

EVIDENCE-INFORMED PRACTICE

- Management of chronic wounds is a challenge. These wounds often have bacterial bioburden and slough. The T.I.M.E framework (see Principles for Practice, earlier) provides an organized approach to wound healing (Chamanga et al., 2015; Mudge, 2015).
- Wounds change as they move through the healing phases. Pay attention to the wound itself: the absorption requirements to

TABLE 40.1

Wound Care Dressing Categories*

Gauze Dressings

Composition: Cotton or /synthetic material; woven or non-woven. Comes in sterile or /non-sterile and in multiple sizes (square, ribbon) and sterile/ flat (Nu-gauze) for packing; not absorptive.

Use: To *protect* surgical or minimally draining wounds or wound-packing. They require a cover dressing to keep dressing intact.

Not for: Contact layer in granulating wounds or for heavily draining wounds; they do not support moisture-vapour transfer so have a limited role in absorbing drainage.

Characteristics: Gauze dressings for wounds should be nonwoven if touching the wound bed, to avoid potential of gauze fibres to irritate wound bed. Gauze can sometimes be used when first assessing a wound, to provide protection and some absorption of drainage. Gauze dressings are used mostly to clean wounds, occasionally for packing—packing should be *light* to avoid compression of wound edges.

Frequency of Dressing Change: Daily or when saturated or soiled.

Examples: Curity Gauze Sponges, KERLIX Super Sponge, KLING Gauze, NU GAUZE Packing Strips

Transparent Film

Composition: A waterproof adhesive membrane, impermeable to fluids and bacteria.

Use: Best for securing intravenous (IV) tubing, etc. Generally, a transparent film is useful to keep a dressing intact and occlusive—for example, in negative-pressure wound therapy (NPWT).

Not for: Because of the limited moisture-vapour transfer effect, these dressings are not suitable for wounds with moderate to large amounts of drainage. Not recommended for wounds with fragile periwound skin (e.g., skin tears) or drainage, since these dressings tend to hold in moisture and thus may macerate periwound skin and inhibit cell migration in the base of the wound. Should not be used on wounds where infection is suspected, or on third-degree burns.

Characteristics: *Advantage:* Can visualize wound and skin underneath dressing. Must be removed with lateral pull: Support dressing and begin to remove it at transverse edge. Pull and allow adhesive to be lifted through the mechanical pulling action. Go slowly. Avoid using adhesive remover as it will further dry patient's skin.

Frequency of Dressing Change: Every 3–4 days or when drainage or exudate remains on the wound or periwound skin (maceration of the underlying tissue).

Examples: Bioclusive Plus, OPSITE, POLYSKIN, Suresite

Hydrocolloids

Composition: Gel-forming agents which, once in contact with the wound bed, create autolysis of slough in the wound bed. They maintain a moist environment by forming a gelatinous mass as an occlusive dressing. Hydrocolloids are self-adhesive (or with transparent film borders), mould to body contours, and are considered occlusive—waterproof and, if intact, resistant to external contaminants.

Use: Autolytic debridement of noninfected wounds with slough or necrotic tissue; most commonly used for pressure injuries (stage II, III, or unstageable). Thin hydrocolloid may be used to protect area from friction or shearing.

Not for: Critically colonized or infected wounds, or on a wound with moderate to significant drainage. Not for third-degree burns. Not for arterial wounds. Not for patients with fragile skin at risk of further damage from an adhesive dressing. Avoid using on dry eschar (e.g., diabetic heel ulcers) if debridement will not be of benefit.

Characteristics: Available in different shapes and sizes; select one that provides coverage of the wound bed and allows 2–3 cm of intact hydrocolloid dressing around the wound (i.e., avoid using an over-large dressing). Protect periwound skin with barrier wipe or spray prior to application of dressing as there is potential for periwound maceration. Ensure dressing is completely sealed on application to support autolysis. Dressing will begin to wrinkle, and cream-coloured material is visible through the dressing as autolysis occurs. Odour may be noted when the dressing is removed—this is characteristic of hydrocolloids and not to be confused with infection.

Frequency of Dressing Change: Every 5–7 days or when the autolyzed material is within 1.5 cm of the border (avoid strike-through/leakage). Irrigate and cleanse wound well; apply fresh hydrocolloid if additional autolysis is required. Protect periwound skin.

Examples: Tegaderm®, Duoderm®, Granuflex, NU-DERM hydrocolloid, ULTEC

Hydrogel

Composition: Glycerin- or water-based polymers; dressings are designed to provide moisture to a dry wound bed; they support autolytic debridement by providing moisture to the wound bed.

Use: Most effective in promoting moisture in a dry wound bed, which supports wound healing. Can be used in partial- or full-thickness wounds and pressure injury; shallow to deep wounds; dry to light exudate; necrotic wounds.

Not for: Third-degree burns; wounds with existing drainage. Not generally in conjunction with hydrocolloids or other dressings where its addition may macerate the periwound or wound bed.

Characteristics: Can be in sheet or tube format. Apply sparingly to the wound bed (approximately 1.5 mm). Can be used to moisten ribbon or gauze dressing to decrease trauma to wound bed. Can also be mixed with Iodosorb® (cadexomer iodine) to help with application. Requires a cover dressing.

Frequency of Dressing Change: As per the wound bed requirement and the selected cover dressing. Generally, every 2–4 days to allow time for the hydrogel to interact with the wound bed tissue.

Examples: IntraSite Gel, Normlgel, Skintegrity Gel, Spenco 2nd Skin (most products end in *gel*)

TABLE 40.1

Wound Care Dressing Categories*—cont'd

Alginates and Hydrofibre Dressings

Composition: These two types of dressings are similar in use but different in composition. The main difference between these two types of dressings is that when wet, the hydrofibre dressing turns into a gel form that is atraumatic and easy to remove from a wound (retains shape: the needle-bonding threads).

Alginates are made of highly absorbent, nonwoven material that strengthens or forms hydrophilic gel when exposed to wound drainage; composed of fibrous product derived from seaweed (contains sodium and calcium).

Hydrofibres are soft, sterile, nonwoven pad or ribbon dressings composed of sodium carboxymethylcellulose, which is incorporated in the form of a fleece held together by a needle-bonding process.

Use: For moderately to heavily draining wounds; shallow or deep wounds; pressure injury; venous ulcers. Can be used in conjunction with other cover dressings to provide additional absorption of exudate.

Not for: Dry wounds; third-degree burns; wounds covered with dry eschar; not in combination with hydrogels (which are designed for the opposite purpose).

Characteristics: Come in sheets or ribbon so can be fluffed into a wound bed or to provide light packing in a tunnelling wound. These dressings are highly absorbent—they must be removed in one piece from the wound bed (if using ribbon, ensure amount is measured and documented on use and removal). Alginates also have hemostatic properties so are useful for postsurgical debridement, for example. Determine if nonwoven gauze or packing ribbon could be used instead, since alginate and hydrofibre dressings are more expensive, but they are more effective than gauze to absorb drainage.

Frequency of Dressing Change: As per wound requirements—generally aim for at least 2 days minimum (otherwise gauze may be used if the wound requires daily change).

Examples: ALGICELL calcium alginate, AQUACEL, Maxorb II, NU-DERM Alginate, Sorbsan

Foam Dressings

Composition: Absorbent, nonadherent polyurethane or film-coated layer used to protect wounds and maintain moist healing environment through moisture-vapour transfer from wound bed. Available in adhesive and nonadhesive forms, also "regular" or "lite" versions.

Use: Moderate-to-heavy exudate wounds; partial- and full-thickness wounds; shallow and deep wounds; stage III–IV pressure injuries.

Not for: Dry wounds; ischemic wounds with dry eschar; third-degree burns.

Characteristics: Foam dressings come in many varieties, shapes, and sizes. They may be simple pads or with a border (either adhesive or silicone). Some foam dressings are silicone based, which provides hydrophobic protection for healing tissue and protects the periwound skin (so no skin preparation is required). Foam dressings are designed to absorb drainage and permit rapid moisture-vapour transfer, which decreases maceration to the wound bed and periwound skin and supports an optimal moist wound environment. Soft and conformable, the borderless foam dressing can be used on several areas of the body (e.g., elbows, heels) and secured with gauze wrap (e.g., Kling).

Frequency of Dressing Change: Given moisture-vapour transfer and fluid handling capabilities, foam dressings should be changed when drainage appears to fill the dressing (with approximately 1–2 cm [0.4–0.8 inches] of nonsaturated foam dressing at the edges). Dressings should be changed as needed—usually every 3–5 days—but generally can be left intact for 7 days if there is no sign of infection or dressing saturation.

Examples: ALLEVYN, Biatain, Mepilex, Restore Foam, Tegaderm Foam

Modified from Bryant, R. A., & Nix, D. P. (2016). Principles of wound healing and topical management. In R. A. Bryant & D. P. Nix (Eds.), *Acute and chronic wounds: Current management concepts* (5th ed., pp. 306–324). St. Louis: Mosby.

*Please refer to manufacturers' monographs regarding specific dressings.

maintain a moist wound environment, bacterial load, and the need to remove slough or eschar and devitalized tissue (Powers, Higham, Broussard, et al., 2016).

- Wound cleaning and irrigation using noncytotoxic solutions with surfactants are used to remove loose devitalized tissue, thus reducing bioburden in chronic wounds and improving wound healing (Percival, Mayer, Malone, et al., 2017).

Comprehensive wound assessment not only helps to predict pressure injury risk but also aids in identifying hard-to-heal wounds in a timely manner (Mudge, 2015).

- Some studies have shown that various dressings may be effective in the following ways: reducing surgical site infection in postoperative wounds (Arroyo, Casanova, Soriano, et al., 2015) and preventing pressure injuries (Brindle & Wegelin, 2012; Santamaria, Gerdtz, Sage, el al., 2015).

SAFETY GUIDELINES

- Know the underlying cause of the wound and its identified type. Wounds related to vascular insufficiency, diabetes mellitus, pressure, trauma, and surgery have specific factors that need to

be considered when developing the treatment plan. Health care providers with additional skill and training, such as enterostomal therapists (ETs; also called nurses specialized in wound, ostomy, and continence), may be required to assess and participate in planning for appropriate wound care. Not knowing the cause of a wound can have serious negative effects if treatments are used that are contraindicated for certain types of wounds (Bryant & Nix, 2016).

- Identify appropriate wound-cleaning agents and appropriate concentration. Some products, used full-strength, may be cytotoxic and impede wound healing. Verify the type and frequency of wound-cleaning agents (World Health Organization [WHO], 2016).

- Be aware of the anticipated amount and type of wound exudate or drainage (Box 40.2). Select dressings that provide adequate exudate management. Heavily draining wounds may require more frequent dressing changes or benefit from use of superabsorbent polymer materials to absorb and wick away drainage from the wound or periwound. Also, increased drainage is an indicator of a wound potentially tipping into critical bacterial colonization or infection.

BOX 40.2

Types of Wound Drainage

Serous, which is a clear, watery plasma

Sanguineous, which indicates fresh bleeding, bright red

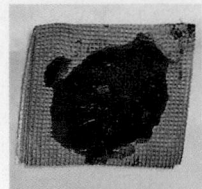

Serosanguineous, which is a pale, red, more watery drainage than sanguineous drainage

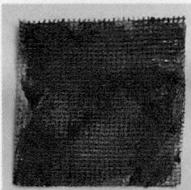

Purulent, which is a thick, yellow, green, tan, or brown drainage

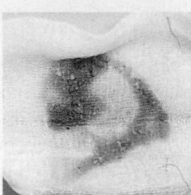

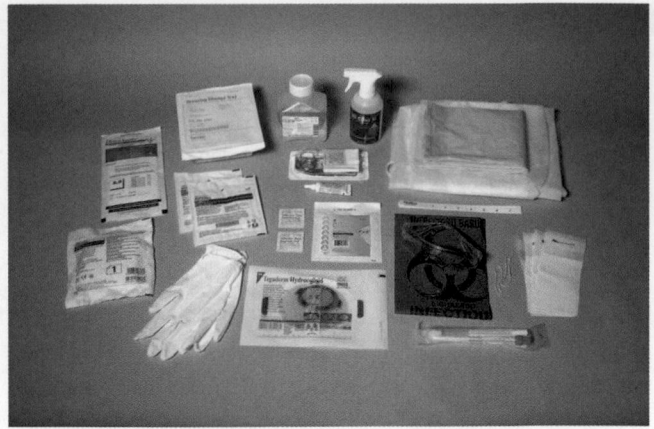

FIG 40.1 Dressing set with personal protective equipment and wound cleaners.

- Determine if wound-drainage devices are present in the wound to prevent their accidental dislocation when you remove the old dressing (see Skill 40.3).
  - Verify that any wound-drainage devices do not cause pressure on adjacent skin, which can result in medical device pressure injury (MDPI) (Pittman, Beeson, Kitterman, et al., 2015).
- A wound is a break in skin integrity that increases a patient's risk for infection. Perform hand hygiene before and after a dressing change. This aids in reducing the risk for surgical site infections in the postoperative phase (WHO, 2016).
- To protect yourself and the patient, use surgical gloves when changing a dressing.
- In the home setting, assess the patient's and caregiver's knowledge of infection control practices and provide patient education as needed.

✦ SKILL 40.1 Applying a Dry Dressing

NSO *Nursing Skills Online Wound Care Module 19 / Lesson 3*

Dry, nonwoven gauze dressings may be used for wound healing by primary intention with little drainage (Fig. 40.1). Dry dressings protect the wound from injury, reduce discomfort, and promote healing. Dry gauze dressings do not interact with wound tissues and should cause minimal wound irritation (Bryant & Nix, 2016). These dressings are commonly used for abrasions and nondraining postoperative incisions (see Table 40.1).

Dry dressings have the disadvantage of moisture evaporating quickly, which can cause a dressing to dry out. As a result, frequent dressing changes are usually needed, and there are increased infection rates when compared with those with semiocclusive dressings (Bryant & Nix, 2016). However, dry gauze may come impregnated with a variety of substances, such as zinc oxide paste, iodinated agents, petrolatum, and crystalline sodium chloride. Impregnated gauze can hydrate a wound and absorb exudate or deliver antimicrobial agents.

Dry dressings are not appropriate for actively healing wounds where the gauze adhering to wound drainage or the wound bed will disturb the healthy tissue when the gauze is removed. If gauze is adherent to the wound, moisten the dressing with normal saline or water before removing it, to minimize wound trauma and pain. Damp-to-dry dressings (also called *wet-to-dry* or *moist-to-dry*) are rarely used as mechanical debridement because this method is not selective for nonviable versus healing tissue and is painful. This practice is no longer considered an appropriate method for debridement.

The current options for debridement include autolysis (e.g., hydrocolloids), enzymatic, and surgical and maggot therapy. Hydrotherapy is considered mechanical debridement but should be used only when the bath or pool can be thoroughly decontaminated. Enzymatic debriding agents applied directly to the wound bed (or the scored eschar) work by digesting collagen in necrotic tissue (NPUAP, EPUAP, & PPPIA, 2014; Ramundo, 2016). Enzymatic debridement and maggot therapy are less commonly used, but when available, they provide effective and selective tissue debridement. Surgical debridement remains the gold standard for debridement but may not be readily available or not appropriate for the patient with underlying medical or other conditions (David & Chiu, 2018).

Some wounds require packing to promote healing. The purpose of packing a wound is to fill dead space and avoid the potential of abscess formation by a wound closing too soon (Bryant & Nix, 2016). Gauze impregnated with simple hydrogel can be used when there is *undermining* (i.e., the destruction of tissue under intact skin around the wound perimeter) or wound *tunnelling* (i.e., a channel has formed that extends from any part of the wound through

Principles for Packing a Wound

- Use the wound characteristics to decide which type of packing is appropriate.
- Make sure that the packing material can be safely used to pack a wound.
- Clean the periwound and wound; apply barrier to the periwound skin.
- Moisten the packing material with a noncytotoxic solution such as normal saline, or a scant amount of hydrogel. Never use cytotoxic solutions (e.g., povidone-iodine) to pack a wound.
- Use nonwoven gauze, if available (woven gauze may leave fibres in the wound bed). Loosen or "fluff" the gauze before packing it into the wound.
- Loosely pack the wound. Tight packing of a wound will result in pressure to the walls of the wound, slowing down the healing process.
- Do not let the packing material drag or touch the surrounding wound tissue before you put it into the wound (avoid contamination).
- Lightly fill all the wound dead space with the packing material.
- When the wound surface has been reached, make sure the packing can be affixed and readily removed; never pack the wound higher than the wound surface.
- Document and measure the amount of packing going into the wound, and being removed.

subcutaneous tissue or muscle). The hydrogel gauze will prevent the gauze from sticking to the wound edges and potentially harming granulating tissue. Ribbon gauze is used to fill the narrow areas in the channel so that the complete dressing can be removed easily during a dressing change. Alginate or hydrofibre ribbon dressings are optimal for wounds with moderate to significant exudate. Box 40.3 summarizes principles for correctly packing a wound. Keep in mind the importance of measuring and documenting the ribbon or packing dressing used in wounds to ensure no dressing is unintentionally left in the wound.

Open wounds require cleaning with each dressing change to remove surface bacteria and debris (Ramundo, 2016). Usually normal saline is the solution of choice, but commercially prepared wound cleaners are also appropriate. Municipal (treated) tap water may also be used. Use an irrigating catheter or syringe for cleaning if a wound is deep (see Chapter 39).

Delegation and Collaboration

The nurse is responsible for wound assessments, care of acute new wounds, wound care requiring sterile technique, and evaluation of wound healing; none of these actions can be delegated to an unregulated care provider (UCP). The nurse instructs the UCP about:

- Any unique modifications of the dressing change, such as the need for use of special tape or taping techniques to secure the dressing.
- Reporting pain, fever, bleeding, or wound drainage to the nurse immediately.

Equipment

- Clean gloves
- Sterile gloves (*optional*)
- Sterile dressing set (scissors, forceps) (*optional*, check employer policy)
- Sterile drape (*optional*)
- Sterile dressings: fine mesh gauze, 10 × 10–cm (4 × 4–inch) gauze, absorbent pads
- Sterile basin (*optional*)
- Antiseptic ointment (as prescribed)
- Wound cleaner (as prescribed)
- Sterile normal saline or prescribed solution
  - Debriding gel as prescribed
  - Tape, Montgomery ties, hypoallergenic tape (*optional*)
  - Skin barrier (optional if using Montgomery ties or silicone-based dressings)
- Protective waterproof underpad
- Biohazard bag
- Measurement devices: cotton-tipped applicator, measuring guide, camera
- Personal protective equipment (PPE): gown, goggles, mask as needed
- Additional lighting if needed (e.g., flashlight, treatment light)

STEP	RATIONALE

ASSESSMENT

1. Identify patient using at least two identifiers (e.g., name and date of birth or name and medical record number), according to employer policy.	Ensures correct patient. Complies with Accreditation Canada's standards and improves patient safety (Accreditation Canada, 2019).
2. Assess patient for allergies, especially antiseptics, tape, or latex, and acquire specific prescriptions for dressing change.	Reduces risk for localized or systemic allergic reactions to these supplies.
3. Ask patient to rate level of pain using a pain scale of 0 to 10, where 0 = no pain and 10 = worst pain ever—or use a visual scale, such as the FACES scale, if the patient is nonverbal or has cognitive deficits—and assess character of pain. Administer prescribed analgesic as needed 30 minutes before dressing change.	Superficial wounds with multiple exposed nerves may be intensely painful, whereas deeper wounds with destruction of dermis should be less painful (Krasner, 2016). A comfortable patient is less likely to move suddenly, which could cause wound or supply contamination. Serves as baseline to measure response to dressing therapy.
4. Assess size, location, and condition of wound. Review previous nurses' notes in electronic health record (EHR) or chart.	Helps to plan for proper dressing type and securement of supplies needed and if help is needed during dressing procedure.
5. Assess patient's and caregiver's knowledge of purpose of dressing change.	Determines level of support and explanation required.

STEP	RATIONALE

ASSESSMENT

6. Assess need for and readiness and willingness of patient or caregiver to participate in dressing wound.

Identifies areas for patient education to prepare patient or caregiver if dressing must be changed at home.

7. Review health care provider prescriptions for type of dressing.

Indicates types of dressing supplies needed.

8. Identify patients at risk for wound-healing problems, including older adults; premature infants; and those with obesity, diabetes mellitus, circulation disorders, nutritional deficit, immunosuppression, radiation therapy, high levels of stress, and use of steroids.

Physiological changes resulting from aging, chronic illness, poor nutrition, medications that affect wound healing, and cancer treatments have the potential to affect wound healing (Doughty & Sparks, 2016).

NURSING DIAGNOSES

- Acute pain
- Chronic pain
- Insufficient knowledge regarding need for specific type of dressing

- Reduced skin integrity
- Potential for infection

- Potential for caregiver role strain (e.g., taking on dressing changes between nurse visits)

Related factors/Risk factors are individualized on the basis of patient's condition or needs.

PLANNING

1. Expected outcomes following completion of procedure:
   - Patient's wound shows evidence of healing by decrease in size and reduced drainage, redness, or swelling.

   Indicates that wound is healing appropriately.

   - Patient reports less pain than that at previous assessment after dressing change.

   Indicates that patient has appropriate analgesia.

   - Dressing remains clean, dry, and intact.

   Indicates that proper application and securement are used for dressing.

   - Patient or caregiver explains purpose of dressing and method of dressing application.

   Indicates understanding and that learning has occurred.

2. Explain procedure to patient.

   Decreases patient's anxiety.

IMPLEMENTATION

1. Close room or cubicle curtains. Perform hand hygiene.

   Provides for privacy.

2. Position patient comfortably and drape to expose only the wound site. Instruct patient not to touch wound or sterile supplies.

   Draping provides access to wound while minimizing exposure. Dressing supplies become contaminated when touched by the patient's hand.

3. Place disposable biohazard bag within reach of work area. Perform hand hygiene and apply clean gloves. Apply gown, goggles, and mask if risk for splashing exists.

   Ensures easy disposal of soiled dressings.
   Use of PPE reduces transmission of microorganisms.

4. Gently remove tape, bandages, or ties: use your nondominant hand to support the dressing and, with your dominant hand, pull tape parallel to skin and toward dressing. If dressing is over a hairy area, remove it in the direction of hair growth. Get patient permission to clip or shave area (check employer policy). Remove any adhesive from skin.

   Pulling tape toward the dressing reduces stress on the suture line or wound edges, irritation, and discomfort.

5. With gloved hand or forceps remove dressing one layer at a time, observing appearance and drainage of dressing. Carefully remove outer secondary dressing first; then remove inner primary dressing that is in contact with wound bed. If drains are present, slowly and carefully remove dressings (see illustration) and avoid tension on any drainage devices. Keep soiled undersurface from patient's sight.

   Purpose of primary dressing is to remove necrotic tissue and exudate. Appearance of drainage may be upsetting to patient. Avoids accidental removal of drain.

   If dressing adheres to wound, moisten dressing and remove gently, alerting patient of potential discomfort.

   Prevents injury to wound surface and periwound during dressing removal.

STEP	RATIONALE

IMPLEMENTATION

6. Inspect wound and periwound for appearance, colour, size (length, width, and depth), drainage, edema, presence and condition of drains, approximation (wound edges are together), granulation tissue, or odour (see Chapter 39). Use measuring guide or ruler to measure size of wound (see Chapter 39). Gently palpate wound edges for bogginess or patient report of increased pain.

   Assesses condition of wound and periwound condition. Indicates status of healing.

7. Fold dressings with drainage contained inside and remove gloves inside out. With small dressings remove gloves inside out over dressing (see illustrations). Dispose of gloves and soiled dressing according to employer policy. Cover wound lightly with sterile gauze pad and perform hand hygiene.

   Contains soiled dressings, prevents contact of nurse's hands with drainage, and reduces cross-contamination.

8. Describe appearance of wound and any indicators of wound healing to patient.

   Wounds may be unsettling and frightening to patients. It helps the patient to know that wound appearance is as expected and whether healing is taking place.

9. If required, use sterile dressing tray or individually wrapped sterile supplies on over-bed table (see Chapter 6). Pour any prescribed solution into sterile basin.

   Sterile dressings remain sterile while on or within sterile surface. Preparation of all supplies before dressing change prevents break in technique during dressing change.

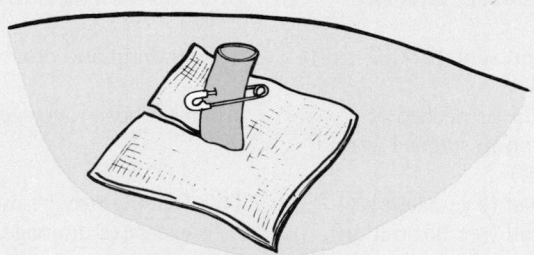

STEP 5 Penrose drain with split gauze.

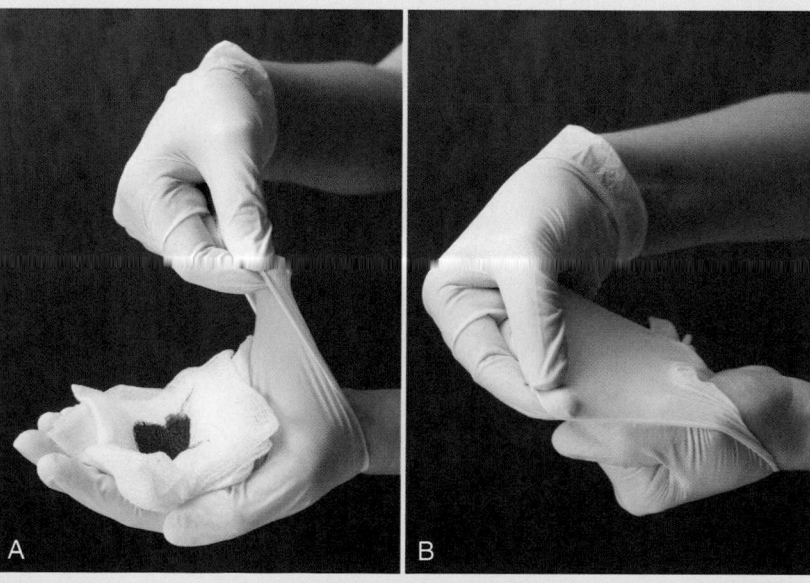

STEP 7 A and **B,** Dispose of soiled dressings by placing in gloved hand and pulling glove off over dressing and then off hand.

STEP	RATIONALE

IMPLEMENTATION

10. Clean/irrigate wound (see Chapter 39):

    a. Perform hand hygiene and apply clean gloves. Use normal saline, municipal (treated) water, sterile water, or wound cleanser set to "stream" or "spray" as needed (irrigating or cleaning the wound).

       Gauze pads may be used to gently cleanse surface of the wound and remove any soiled matter.

Removes nonadherent sloughy matter and other loose debris from the wound which interfere with the healing process. Prevents transfer of organisms from previously cleaned area.

    b. Clean from least to most contaminated area (see Chapter 39) (see illustration).

Cleaning in this direction prevents introduction of microorganisms into wound.

    c. Clean around any drain (if present), using circular strokes starting near drain and moving outward and away from insertion site (see illustration) (see Chapter 39).

Correct aseptic technique in cleaning helps prevent contamination.

11. Use sterile dry gauze to blot wound bed in same manner as in Step 10.

Drying reduces excess moisture, which could eventually harbor microorganisms.

12. Apply antiseptic ointment (if prescribed) with sterile Q-tip or gauze, using same technique to apply it as for cleaning. Dispose of gloves. Perform hand hygiene.

Helps reduce growth of microorganisms.

13. Apply dressing (see employer policy).

    a. *Dry sterile dressing:*

      (1) Apply clean gloves (see employer policy).

Some agencies or condition of wounds may require sterile gloves.

      (2) Apply loose, woven gauze as contact layer (see illustration).

Promotes absorption of drainage.

      (3) If drain is present, apply precut, split 10 × 10–cm (4 × 4–inch) gauze around drain.

Secures drain and promotes drainage absorption at site.

      (4) Apply additional layers of gauze as needed or dressing designed for absorption in surgical wound dressing (e.g., Aquacel Extra®)

Ensures proper coverage and optimal absorption.

      (5) If required, apply absorbent pad (e.g., Mesorb®) and affix with tape or gauze roll (see illustration).

This dressing may be used on postoperative wounds when there is excessive drainage.

Clinical Decision Point *Determine if there are regulations or policies in your workplace regarding who can apply packing into a wound.*

If using "packing strips," use sterile scissors to cut the amount of dressing that you will use to pack the wound. Do not let the packing strip touch the side of the bottle. Place packing strip in a container of prescribed sterile solution. Wring out excess solution.

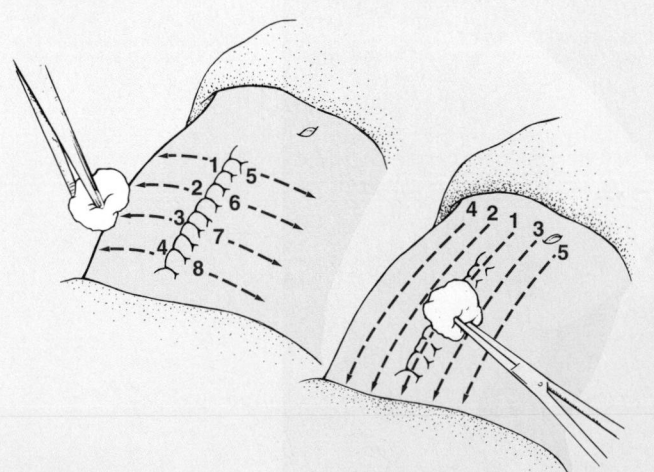

STEP 10b Methods for cleaning a wound; cleaning from least to most contaminated area.

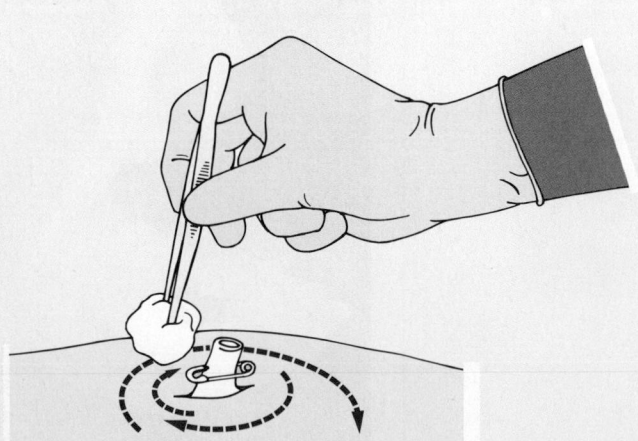

STEP 10c Cleaning around a drain site.

STEP	RATIONALE

IMPLEMENTATION

b. *Packing with gauze:*

(1) Apply damp nonwoven gauze as a single layer directly onto the wound surface. If wound is deep, gently pack gauze into wound with sterile gloved hand or forceps until all wound surfaces are in contact with moist gauze, including dead spaces from sinus tracts, tunnels, and undermining (see illustration A). Be sure that the gauze does not touch periwound skin (see illustration B).

Inner gauze should be moist, not dripping wet, to absorb drainage and adhere to debris. When packing a wound, gauze should conform to the base and side of the wound (Bryant & Nix, 2016). The wound is loosely packed to facilitate wicking of drainage into the absorbent outer layer of dressing. Moisture that escapes the dressing often macerates the periwound area.

Clinical Decision Point *Be sure to count and document how many pieces of gauze are packed in the wound, especially deep wounds. This practice ensures that all gauze from previous dressing change is removed from the wound.*

Clinical Decision Point *When packing the wound, do not overpack or underpack it (Bryant & Nix, 2016). Packing should fill the wound but should not be above the level of the skin.*

(2) Cover with absorbent pad (e.g., Mesorb®), or gauze.

Protects wound from entrance of microorganisms.

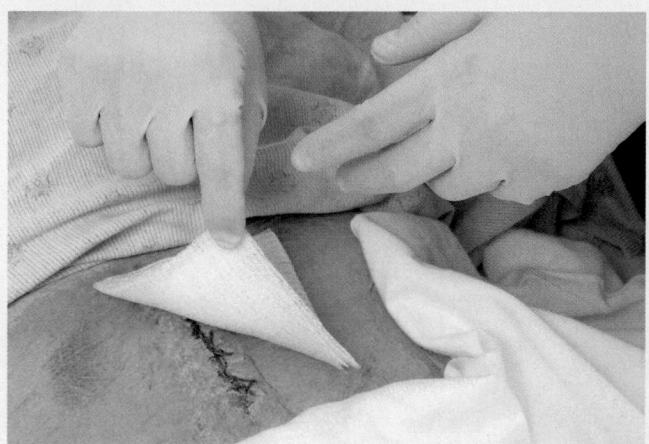

STEP 13a(2) Placing dry gauze dressing over simple wound.

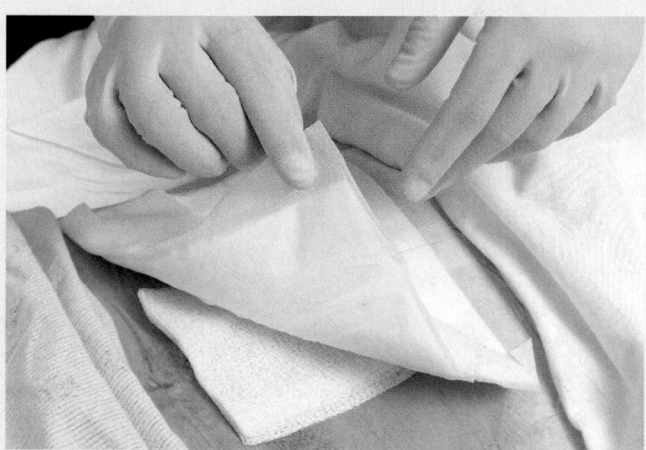

STEP 13a(5) Placing ABD pad over gauze dressing.

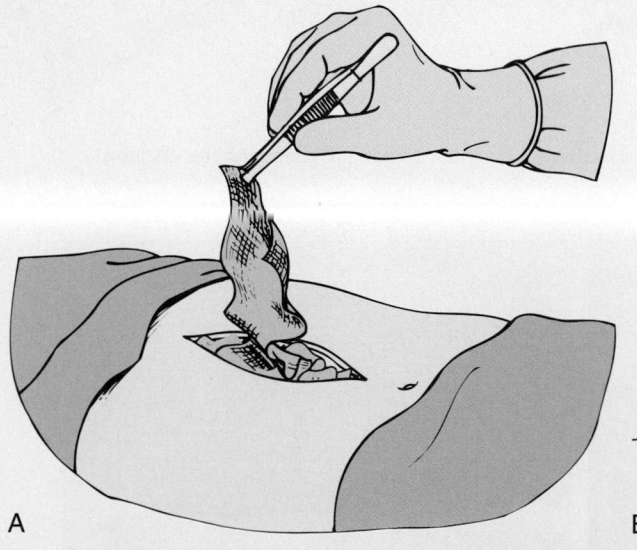

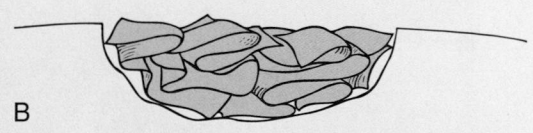

STEP 13b(1) A, Packing wound with fine-mesh gauze. **B,** Cross-section of deep wound packed loosely with gauze roll.

STEP	RATIONALE

IMPLEMENTATION

14. Secure dressing.

a. *Tape:* Apply tape 2.5 to 5 cm (1 to 2 inches) beyond dressing. Use hypoallergenic tape when necessary.

b. *Montgomery ties* (see illustrations):

   (1) Be sure that skin is clean. Application of skin barrier is recommended (see Chapter 39).

   (2) Expose adhesive surface of tape ends.

   (3) Place ties on opposite sides of dressing over skin or skin barrier.

   (4) Secure dressing by lacing ties across dressing snugly enough to hold it secure but without placing pressure on skin.

c. *For protective window:*

   (1) Cut strip of stomahesive or hydrocolloid pad into approximately 1- to 2.5-cm strips, depending on size required.

   (2) Use skin barrier to wipe areas of skin where strips will be applied.

   (3) Apply adhesive strips dressing to frame a "window" around the wound using four strips, one on each side, one on the top, and one on the bottom of the dressing material (see illustrations).

   (4) Apply dressing; secure tape ends to adhesive strips (see illustration).

Supports wound and ensures placement and stability of dressing.

Prevents skin irritation. Ties allow for repeated dressing changes without removal of tape.

Skin barrier (e.g., Cavilon® wipe) protects intact skin from stretch and tension of adhesive tape.

A protective window is an alternative to Montgomery ties for smaller wounds. There is less skin irritation by placing tape on window strips.

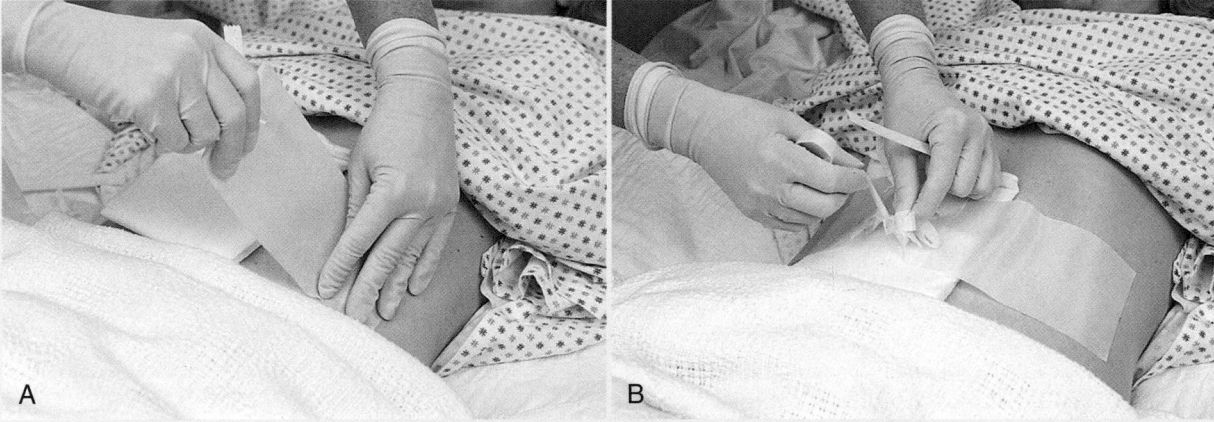

STEP 14b Montgomery ties. **A,** Each tie is placed at side of gauze dressing. **B,** Securing ties encloses dressing.

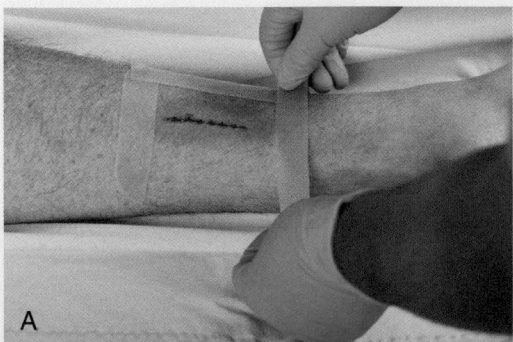
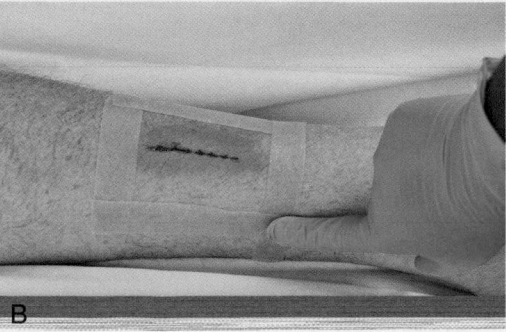

STEP 14c(3) **A** and **B,** Apply adhesive strips to frame a "window" around wound using four strips.

STEP	RATIONALE

IMPLEMENTATION

d. For dressing extremity, secure with roll gauze (see illustration) or elastic net.

15. Dispose of all dressing supplies. Remove cover gown and goggles; remove gloves inside out; dispose of them according to employer policy.

16. Label tape over dressing with your initials and date dressing is changed.

17. Help patient to a comfortable position.

18. Perform hand hygiene.

Roll gauze can conform to the contour of a foot or hand.

Reduces transmission of microorganisms. A clean environment enhances patient comfort.

Provides timeline for when next dressing change is to be scheduled.

Promotes patient's sense of well-being.

Reduces transmission of microorganisms.

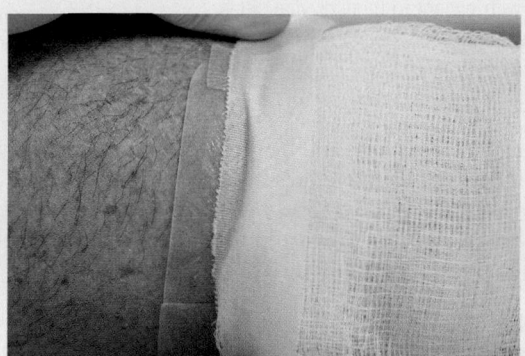

STEP 14c(4) Apply dressing; secure tape ends to adhesive strips.

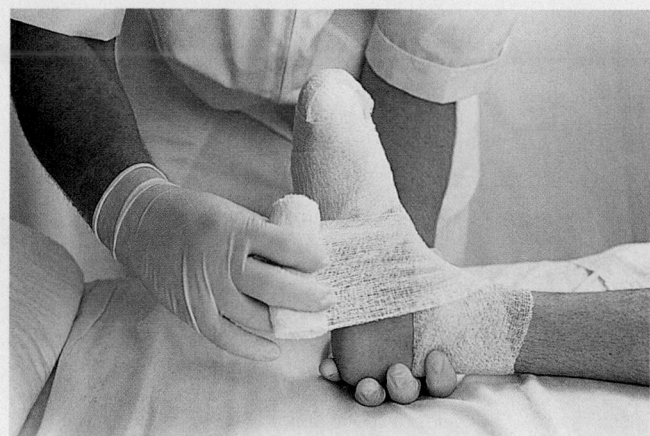

STEP 14d Wrap roller gauze around extremity to secure dressing.

EVALUATION

1. Observe appearance of wound for healing: measure size of wound; observe amount, colour, and type of drainage and periwound erythema or swelling.

2. Ask patient to rate pain level using a pain scale of 0 to 10, where 0 = no pain and 10 = worst pain ever, or using a visual scale, such as the FACES scale, if the patient is nonverbal or has cognitive deficits.

3. Inspect condition of dressing at least every shift.

4. **Use Teach-Back:** "I want to be sure I explained why and how often you need to continue these dressing changes in the hospital and at home. Tell me why it is important to change your dressing and how often you will do this." Develop a revised teaching plan if patient or caregiver is not able to teach back correctly.

Determines rate of healing.

Increased pain is often an indication of wound complications such as infection or a result of the dressing pulling on tissue.

Determines status of wound drainage.

Determines patient's and caregiver's level of understanding of instructional topic.

Unexpected Outcomes

1. Wound appears inflamed and painful, drainage is evident, and/or odour is present, periwound skin is warmer than adjacent skin.

Related Interventions

- Monitor patient for signs of infection (e.g., fever, increased white blood cell count).
- Notify health care provider.
- Obtain wound cultures as prescribed.
- If there is yellow, tan, or brown necrotic tissue, use interprofessional collaboration (e.g., wound care specialist, health care provider) to determine need for debridement (Table 40.2).

STEP	RATIONALE

Unexpected Outcomes

2. Wound bleeds during dressing change.

3. Patient reports sensation that "something has given way under the dressing."

Related Interventions

- Observe colour and amount of bloody drainage. If excessive, you may need to apply direct-pressure dressing and/or calcium alginate (e.g., Kaldostat®).
- Inspect area along the dressing and directly underneath patient to determine amount of bleeding.
- Obtain vital signs as needed.
- Notify health care provider.
- Observe wound for increased drainage or dehiscence (partial or total separation of wound layers) or evisceration (total separation of wound layers and protrusion of viscera through wound opening).
- If dehiscence or evisceration occurs, protect the wound. Cover it with a sterile moist dressing.
- Instruct patient to lie still.
- Stay with patient to monitor vital signs.
- Immediately notify health care provider.

TABLE 40.2

Problems Associated With Wound Care and Dressings

Problem	Nursing Activities
Solutions or dressings used may be irritating to periwound skin	Protect healthy skin with protective periwound barrier composed of dimethicone (e.g., Cavilon® wipes) or petrolatum or zinc oxide. If zinc oxide is used, it should be removed with mineral oil. Avoid scrubbing the skin because scrubbing can cause harm to the epithelial layer.
Wound becomes excessively dry	Wounds change over time. Consider selecting a dressing that donates moisture to the wound bed (e.g., hydrogel). This can be mixed with nonwoven gauze to lightly fluff into the wound bed. Cover with a simple gauze pad.
Wound is deep, and retention of dressing in cavity is suspected	Irrigate wound copiously with prescribed solution to loosen dressing for removal. Use continuous "ribbon" or strip of gauze to dress deep wounds and secure to the periwound skin if there is danger of the packing slipping into the deep wound.
Wound drainage is damaging healthy tissue	Always protect periwound skin with a barrier product. If drainage is significant and difficult to manage with a superabsorbent dressing, consider a drainage collection device.
Patient's skin is irritated by tape	Use silicone tape or, if there are frequent dressing changes, use Montgomery ties or straps as needed, or fabric tape that has multidirectional stretch. Secure dressing with a binder or burn-net, or wrap with roll gauze if on an extremity.

Communication and Documentation

At each dressing change, document on the flow sheet and nurses' notes in the EHR or chart.

- Document appearance and wound measurement (length × width × depth), characteristics of drainage, presence of necrotic tissue, type of dressing applied, the patient's response to dressing change, and level of comfort.

- Document patient's and caregiver's understanding through teach-back for effective dressing change.
- Report any unexpected appearance of wound drainage, accidental removal of a drain, bright red bleeding, or evidence of wound dehiscence or evisceration.

Special Considerations
Teaching

- Explain expected wound appearance and risks of improper wound care. Provide patient and caregiver with a list of signs to report to the health care provider, taking into account your assessment of the literacy level of the patient and caregiver. A written list or illustrations and images may be appropriate.
- Demonstrate wound care and, if appropriate, encourage the patient or caregiver to perform a dressing change with and without supervision. Provide supportive information for reference (e.g., steps to follow, with illustrations).

Pediatric

- Some pediatric patients are fearful of dressing changes. If appropriate, explain the procedure and allow the child to handle and see dressings (in sterile packaging or sample). Prepare to take time to engage in activities to decrease anxiety and fear. If a play therapist is available or other care provider or family member available, plan in advance for their support to assist in keeping the child cooperative during the dressing change procedure (Hockenberry & Wilson, 2015).
- Older children may need something to do during dressing changes. Listening to music or watching a video helps to relieve some of the boredom or stress during the procedure (Hockenberry & Wilson, 2015).

Gerontological

- Normal aging changes of skin and tissue and the inflammatory response may delay wound healing (Wysocki, 2016).
- Adhesive tape often irritates older persons' skin and causes skin tears. Use paper tape, nonallergenic (e.g., silicone) tape, wraps, or a burn-net to avoid skin trauma.
- Another option is to create a stomahesive window. Cut strips of stomahesive into approximately 1- to 2.5-cm strips. Use a skin barrier to wipe areas of intact skin where you will place the

strips. Apply the adhesive strips to two or four sides of the wound, framing it. Apply dressing. Apply tape to the stomahesive strips.

Care in the Community

While patients at home initially receive nursing visits for wound care and dressing changes, when possible, patients and caregivers are encouraged to become adept at managing the wound care with less frequent visits from the community health nurse.

- Consider resources within the home, the caregiver's ability, as well as time required for dressing change when selecting the dressing procedure to be done in the home setting.

- Provide education for the patient and caregiver to increase confidence and their ability to perform independent dressing changes. The nurse provides support and reassurance and monitors the wound's progress, as required.
- Select dressings that can remain intact longer, if appropriate (to decrease frequency of dressing changes and home visits).
- If the patient or caregiver will be changing the dressing, provide instruction on proper techniques for disposing of medical waste.

◆ SKILL 40.2   Applying a Pressure Bandage

A pressure bandage is a temporary treatment to control excessive, sudden, unanticipated bleeding. Hemorrhage may occur during surgical intervention (e.g., cardiac catheterization, arterial puncture, organ biopsy) or after surgery or be a life-threatening occurrence related to accidental trauma (e.g., stabbing, suicide attempt). Pressure dressings are essential to stopping the flow of blood and promoting clotting at the site until definitive action can be taken to stop the source.

Given the emergent nature of an acute bleeding episode, the aseptic techniques considered essential in most dressing applications are secondary to halting the bleeding. A pressure dressing applied in an emergency is usually temporary; the wound can be cleaned, and the dressing changed once the bleeding has been controlled.

Delegation and Collaboration

The skill of applying a pressure dressing in an emergency situation cannot be delegated to an unregulated care provider (UCP). However,

if the application requires more than one person, the UCP can assist the nurse. The nurse directs the UCP to:

- Assist the nurse as required.
- Observe the pressure dressing during care activities to make sure that it remains in place and that there is no visible bleeding from the site.
- Check underneath the patient and observe for bleeding after dressing has been applied.

Equipment

- Necessary dressings: nonadherent gauze and absorbent pads, hemostatic dressings, roller gauze
- Adhesive tape; hypoallergenic if necessary
- Adhesive remover (*optional*)
- Clean gloves
- Personal protective equipment (PPE) (e.g., gown, goggles, mask) as needed
- Equipment for vital signs

STEP	RATIONALE

ASSESSMENT

1. If the situation permits, identify patient using two person-specific identifiers (e.g., name and date of birth or name and medical record number), according to employer policy.	Ensures correct patient. Complies with Accreditation Canada's standards and improves patient safety (Accreditation Canada, 2019).
2. Anticipate patients at risk for unexpected bleeding, including those with traumatic injury, arterial puncture, a donor graft site, postoperative incision, or wounds after surgical debridement, and surgical patients with a history of bleeding disorder.	Familiarity with conditions associated with unexpected bleeding allows you to rapidly respond to the bleeding.
3. Assess location where hemorrhage occurred.	Helps identify proper type and amount of supplies needed.
4. Assess patient for allergies to antiseptics, tape, or latex. If patient is nonresponsive and no history is available, use nonlatex or nonallergenic supplies.	Prevents localized or systemic allergic reaction.
5. Quickly assess patient's anxiety level.	Determines need for education and positive reinforcement during procedure.
6. Assess patient's baseline vital signs before onset of hemorrhage.	If data are available, baseline vital signs indicate status of circulatory function.

NURSING DIAGNOSES

- Reduced skin integrity
- Potential for imbalanced fluid volume

Related factors/Risk factors are individualized on the basis of patient's condition or needs.

STEP	RATIONALE

PLANNING

1. Expected outcomes following completion of procedure:
   - Patient shows cessation of bleeding and no evidence of hematoma formation.
   - Patient maintains stable blood pressure and heart rate.
   - Distal circulation is maintained with intact pulses (distal to site of injury).

Hemostasis is achieved.
Hemodynamic stability is achieved with minimal blood loss.

IMPLEMENTATION

Phase I: Immediate Action—First Nurse

1. Identify external bleeding site. To observe underneath patients with large absorbent pads you will need to turn the patient. **NOTE:** Wounds to the groin area also can result in large amounts of blood loss, which is not always visible.
2. Apply immediate manual pressure to bleeding site.
3. Seek help.

Quick identification increases response time to stop bleeding. Maintaining asepsis and privacy is considered only if time and severity of blood loss permit.

Hemostasis is maintained as supplies are prepared.
Bandage must be secured quickly. Situation could be life-threatening.

Phase II: Applying Pressure Bandage—Second Nurse

4. Quickly identify source of bleeding.
   - *Arterial bleeding* is bright red and gushes forth in waves, related to the patient's heart rate; if the vessel is very deep, flow is steady.
   - *Venous bleeding* is dark red and flows smoothly.
   - *Capillary bleeding* is oozing of dark red blood; self-sealing controls this bleeding.
5. Elevate affected body part (e.g., extremity) if possible.
6. The first nurse continues to apply direct pressure as the second nurse unwraps a roller bandage and places it within easy reach. The second nurse quickly cuts three to five lengths of adhesive tape and places them within reach; *do not take the time to clean wound until bleeding is controlled.*
7. *In simultaneous coordinated actions:*
   a. Rapidly cover bleeding area with multiple thicknesses of gauze compresses. The first nurse slips fingers out as the other nurse exerts adequate pressure to continue controlling bleeding (see illustrations).
   b. Place adhesive strips 7 to 10 cm (3 to 4 inches) beyond width of dressing with even pressure on both sides of fingers as close as possible to central bleeding source. Secure tape on distal end, pull tape across dressing, and keep firm pressure as the proximate end of tape is secured.
   c. Remove fingers temporarily and quickly cover centre of area with third strip of tape.

Determines method of application and supplies to use.

Helps slow rate of bleeding.
Pressure dressing controls bleeding temporarily. Preparation allows for securing pressure bandage quickly.

Gauze is absorbent. Layers provide bulk against which local pressure can be applied to bleeding site.

Tape exerts downward pressure, promoting hemostasis. To ensure blood flow to distal tissues and prevent a tourniquet effect, adhesive tape must not be continued around the entire extremity.

Provides pressure to source of bleeding.

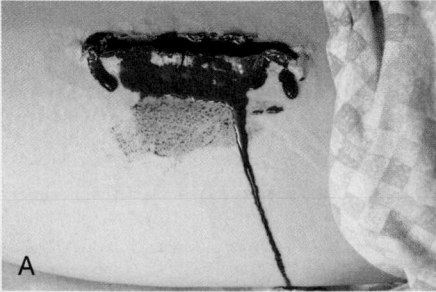 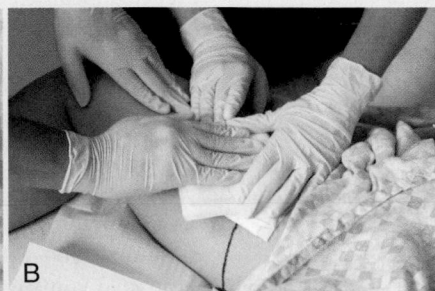 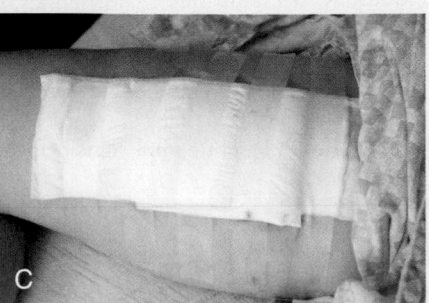

STEP 7a A, Bleeding wound. **B,** Nurses apply pressure dressing. **C,** Dressing applied.

STEP	RATIONALE

IMPLEMENTATION

d. Continue reinforcing area with tape as each successive strip is overlapped on alternating sides of centre strip. Keep applying pressure.

Prevents tape from loosening.

e. When pressure bandage is on the extremity, apply roller gauze: apply two circular turns tautly on both sides of fingers that are pressing the gauze. Compress over bleeding site. Simultaneously remove finger pressure and apply roller gauze over centre. Continue with figure-eight turns. Secure end with two circular turns and a strip of adhesive (see Procedural Guideline 40.1).

Roller gauze acts as a pressure bandage, exerting more even pressure over the extremity.

Clinical Decision Point *Start pressure bandage from distal to proximal, working toward the heart. If bleeding continues, contact the health care provider.*

EVALUATION

1. Observe dressing for control of bleeding.

An effective pressure bandage controls bleeding without blocking distal circulation.

2. Evaluate adequacy of circulation (distal pulse, skin characteristics).

Determines level of perfusion to distal body parts.

3. Estimate volume of blood loss (e.g., count number of dressings used, weigh saturated dressing).

Helps to determine blood and fluid replacement needs.

4. Monitor vital signs.

Identifies patient's response to blood loss and early stages of hypovolemic shock.

Unexpected Outcomes

1. There is continued bleeding. Fluid and electrolyte imbalance, tissue hypoxia, confusion, hypovolemic shock, and cardiac arrest develop.

2. Pressure dressing is too tight and occludes circulation.

Related Interventions

- Notify health care provider.
- Reinforce or adjust pressure dressing.
- Initiate intravenous (IV) therapy per prescription.
- Place patient in Trendelenburg's position; provide covers for warmth.
- Monitor vital signs every 5 to 15 minutes (apical pulse, distal pulses, and blood pressure) (see employer policy).
- Inspect areas distal to pressure dressing to ensure that circulation has not been occluded.
- Adjust dressing as needed.

Communication and Documentation

- Immediately report to the health care provider the current status of patient's bleeding control, time the bleeding was discovered, estimated blood loss, nursing interventions (including effectiveness of applied pressure bandage), apical and distal pulses, blood pressure, patient's mental status, signs of restlessness, and need for health care provider to assess the patient without delay.
- Document assessment, application of pressure dressing, and patient response on flow sheet in nurses' notes in electronic health record (EHR) or chart.

Special Considerations
Teaching

- Explain to patient and caregiver (if present) the need to monitor vital signs.
- Explain need for patient to remain quiet and stay in position to reduce bleeding.

Pediatric

- If family members and health care providers can remain calm, a child may calm down and be more cooperative.

Gerontological

- Because of the normal changes of aging, the older person has an increased risk for vascular and tissue changes distal to the pressure dressing. Evaluate skin and pulse distal to the pressure bandage frequently.

Care in the Community

- If the patient is at risk for hemorrhage, instruct on the following:
  - How the caregiver or patient should apply pressure with clean towels or linen
  - Immediate activation of emergency system (9-1-1)
  - How to position patient by elevating the affected body part (if extremity)
  - **CAUTION:** If a puncture wound occurs from a penetrating object (e.g., knife, toy, building materials), instruct caregivers not to remove the object. Removal will cause more rapid blood loss and may damage underlying structures.
  - How to position patient to promote elevation of the affected body part (if extremity) and relaxation

✦ SKILL 40.3 Applying a Transparent Dressing

NSO *Nursing Skills Online Wound Care Module 19 / Lesson 3*

A transparent film dressing is a clear, adherent, nonabsorptive, polyurethane sheet that is impermeable to fluids and bacteria (Bryant & Nix, 2016). Once it is applied, a moist exudate forms over the wound surface, which prevents tissue dehydration and allows for rapid, effective healing by speeding epithelial cell growth. However, transparent film dressings may contribute to maceration of the wound or periwound skin because of the occlusive nature of these dressings, which have limited moisture-vapour transfer capabilities.

The most appropriate use for transparent dressings is over an intravenous (IV) catheter insertion site to stabilize the catheter. The synthetic membrane acts as a temporary second skin, adheres to undamaged skin to contain exudate, and minimizes wound contamination from exterior environment.

Transparent film dressings should not be used on skin tears or fragile skin, since in addition to the occlusive nature, these dressings are difficult to remove without damaging periwound skin—particularly if the lateral pull technique is not used to release the adhesive in a gradual manner.

When applying dressings, including transparent film, hydrocolloid, foam, hydrogel, and other specialty dressings, follow the general principles discussed below.

Delegation and Collaboration

The assessment of the wound and care of a new acute wound cannot be delegated to an unregulated care provider (UCP). However, the nurse directs the UCP to:

- Report any signs of bleeding, drainage, infection, or poor wound healing immediately to the nurse.

Equipment

- Sterile gloves *(optional)*
- Dressing set *(optional)*
- Sterile saline or other cleansing agent (as prescribed)
- Clean gloves
- Cotton swabs
- Biohazard bag for disposal
- Transparent dressing (size as needed)
- Sterile 10 × 10–cm (4 × 4–inch) gauze pads
- Skin-preparation materials *(optional)*
- Personal protective equipment (PPE) as needed

STEP	RATIONALE

ASSESSMENT

1. Identify patient using at least two person-specific identifiers (e.g., name and date of birth or name and medical record number), according to employer policy.

Ensures correct patient. Complies with Accreditation Canada's standards and improves patient safety (Accreditation Canada, 2019).

2. Assess location, appearance, and size of wound. Determine size of dressing needed. Plan appropriate dressing based on fragility of patient's periwound skin and the amount of drainage or exudate from the wound.
Review previous nurses' notes in electronic health record (EHR) or chart.

Determines type of materials needed for dressing change. These dressings are applied over clean, debrided wounds that are not actively bleeding.

3. Review health care provider's prescriptions for frequency and type of dressing change.

Health care provider prescribes frequency of dressing changes and special instructions.

4. Assess patient for allergies, especially antiseptics, tape, or latex.

Prevents local or systemic allergic reaction.

5. Ask patient to rate level of pain using an appropriate pain rating tool. Administer prescribed analgesic as needed 30 minutes before dressing change.

A comfortable patient will be less likely to move suddenly, which can cause wound or supply contamination. Serves as baseline to measure response to dressing therapy.

6. Assess patient's knowledge of purpose of dressing.

Identifies patient's learning needs.

7. Assess patient's risks for impaired wound healing (e.g., aging, poor nutrition).

Physiological changes caused by aging, chronic illness, poor nutrition, medications, and cancer treatments have the potential to affect wound healing (Doughty & Sparks, 2016).

NURSING DIAGNOSES

- Acute pain
- Impaired skin integrity
- Risk for infection

Related factors/Risk factors are individualized on the basis of patient's condition or needs.

STEP	RATIONALE

PLANNING

1. Expected outcomes following completion of procedure:
   - Wound heals *appropriately*.

     Dressing is effective in preventing infection and promoting healing.
   - Patient experiences minimal discomfort during dressing change.

     Adequate pain control is achieved.
2. Explain procedure to patient. — Relieves anxiety and promotes understanding of healing process.
3. Position patient comfortably and to allow for access to dressing site. — Facilitates application of dressing.

IMPLEMENTATION

1. Close door or room curtains; keep sheet or gown draped over body parts not requiring exposure. — Provides privacy and decreases transfer of microorganisms.
2. Expose wound site, minimizing exposure. Instruct patient not to touch wound or sterile supplies. — Dressing supplies become contaminated when touched by the patient's hand.
3. Place biohazard bag within reach of work area. — Ensures easy disposal of soiled dressing.
4. Perform hand hygiene and apply clean gloves. Apply PPE (e.g., gown, mask, goggles) as needed. — Reduces transmission of infectious organisms from soiled dressings to nurse's hands.
5. Remove old dressing by stretching film in direction parallel to wound rather than pulling it. — Stretching action gently breaks dressing seal (Bryant & Nix, 2016). Reduces excoriation, tearing, or irritation of skin after dressing removal.
6. Dispose of soiled dressing in waterproof bag, remove gloves by pulling them inside out, dispose of them in waterproof bag, and perform hand hygiene. — Reduces transmission of microorganisms.
7. Prepare dressing supplies. Ensure dressings are sterile (package sealed) prior to use. — Reduces risk for break in sterile technique.
8. Pour saline or prescribed solution over 10 × 10–cm (4 × 4–inch) sterile gauze pads. — Maintains sterility of dressing.
9. Apply clean or sterile gloves (check employer policy). — Allows you to handle dressings.
10. Clean wound and periwound area gently with 10 × 10–cm (4 × 4–inch) sterile gauze pads moistened in sterile saline or spray with wound cleaner. Clean from least to most contaminated area (see Skill 41.1). — Reduces introduction of microorganisms into wound.
11. Pat skin around wound; dry thoroughly with dry 10 × 10–cm (4 × 4–inch) sterile gauze pads. — Transparent dressing with adhesive backing does not adhere to a damp surface (Bryant & Nix, 2016).
12. Inspect wound for tissue type, colour, odour, and drainage; measure it if indicated. — Provides baseline for monitoring wound healing.

Clinical Decision Point *If the patient has thin or fragile skin, use a skin barrier on the skin around a wound before dressing application to protect patient's skin from further injury* (Bryant & Best, 2016).

13. Remove gloves and perform hand hygiene. — Reduces transmission of microorganisms.

Clinical Decision Point *If the wound has a large amount of drainage, choose another dressing that can absorb drainage and provide effective moisture-vapour transfer.*

14. Apply clean gloves and apply transparent dressing according to manufacturer directions. *Do not stretch film during application and avoid making wrinkles.* — Wrinkles provide tunnel for exudate drainage.
    a. Remove paper backing, taking care not to allow adhesive areas to touch one another.
    b. Place film smoothly over wound without stretching (see illustrations). — Ensures coverage of wound. Prevents shearing of skin from dressing that is too tight. Stretching can also break wound seal.
    c. Use your fingers to smooth dressing and help it adhere.
    d. Label dressing with date, your initials, and time of dressing change on outer label of dressing (see illustration). — Provides record for determining when to next change dressing.

STEP	RATIONALE

IMPLEMENTATION

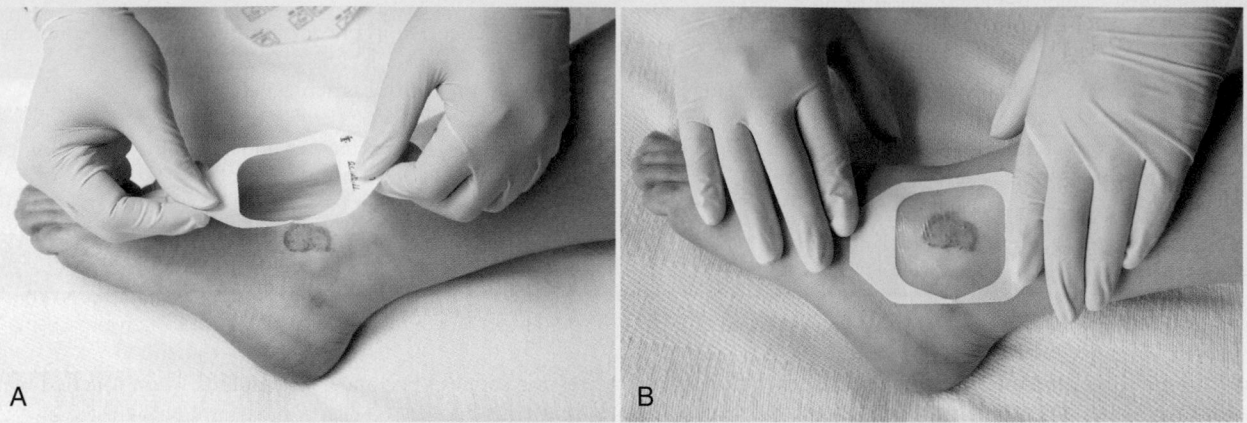

STEP 14b A, Transparent dressing placed over a small wound on ankle. **B,** Place film smoothly without stretching it.

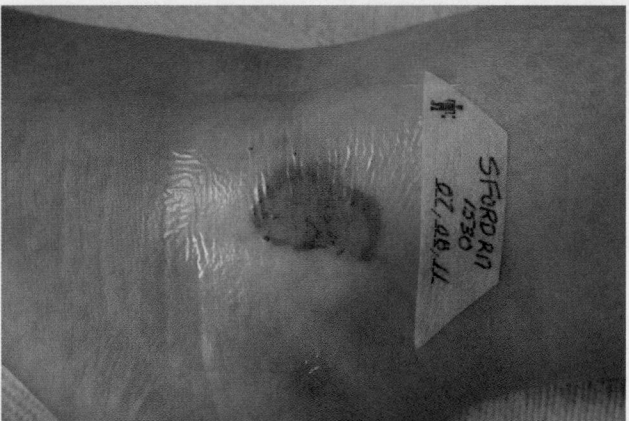

STEP 14d Transparent dressing correctly labelled.

STEP	RATIONALE
15. Discard soiled dressing materials properly. Remove gloves by pulling them inside out and discard in prepared bag. Perform hand hygiene.	Reduces transfer of microorganisms.
16. Help patient to a comfortable position.	Enhances patient comfort and relaxation.

EVALUATION

1. Inspect appearance of wound and amount of drainage and measure size.	A clear dressing allows you to observe the wound and status of wound healing.
2. Inspect periwound areas.	Identifies any injury to surrounding skin.
3. Ask patient to rate pain using an appropriate pain rating scale.	Determines any change in pain during procedure.
4. **Use Teach-Back:** "I want to be sure you understand how to apply this transparent dressing, since you will be using it at home. Show me how you will apply this dressing." Develop a revised teaching plan if patient or caregiver is not able to teach back correctly.	Determines patient's and caregiver's level of understanding of instructional topic.

STEP	RATIONALE

Unexpected Outcomes

1. Wound is inflamed and tender; accumulation of fluid with a white, opaque appearance and erythema of surrounding tissue; increased drainage or change in the colour of drainage; necrosis; and/or odour is present.

2. Dressing does not stay in place.

3. Outer layer of patient's skin tears on removal of dressing.

Related Interventions

- Remove dressing and obtain wound culture according to employer policy.
- A different type of dressing may be required.
- Notify health care provider.

- Evaluate size of dressing used for adequate wound margin (2.5 to 3.75 cm [1 to $1\frac{1}{2}$ inches]).
- Assess for increased drainage from wound.
- Dry patient's skin thoroughly before reapplication.
- Adhesive backing may be too strong for patient's skin.
- Consider other nonadhesive-backed transparent dressing, or use gauze wrap and secure wrap with tape.

Communication and Documentation

- Document appearance of wound, presence and characteristics of drainage, and presence of odour on flow sheet in nurses' notes in EHR or chart.
- Document patient's and caregiver's understanding through teach-back for effective application of dressing.
- Report any signs of infection to health care provider.

Special Considerations
Teaching

- Explain need to change dressing should edges loosen.
- Explain to patient and caregiver that collection of wound fluid under the dressing is not "pus" but normal interaction of body fluids with the dressing.

Pediatric

- Adhesive backing may cause skin tears on premature infants' immature skin (Hockenberry & Wilson, 2015).

- Children may find this procedure more tolerable if they know that the longer the dressing is left on, the easier it is to remove (Hockenberry & Wilson, 2015).

Gerontological

- Adhesive backing may be too strong for the skin of older persons. Do not use a film dressing that has an adhesive backing with a stronger bond to the epidermis than the epidermis has to the dermis.

Care in the Community

- The wound may be cleaned in the shower if approved by the health care provider.
- Many types of transparent dressings exist. Some newer options allow for moisture-vapour transfer (to some degree) and can remain in place for several weeks (e.g., absorbent acrylic dressings). Ensure that the patient understands how the dressing functions and ways to keep it intact.

◆ SKILL 40.4 | **Applying a Hydrocolloid, Hydrogel, Foam, Alginate Dressing, or Hydrofibre Dressing**

NSO *Nursing Skills Online Wound Care Module 19 / Lesson 3*

Current wound care dressings have several different characteristics and provide differing types of action for wounds, depending on the needs of a particular wound at a particular time in the wound-healing process (see Table 40.1).

Hydrocolloid dressings promote statistically significant better wound healing outcomes compared with conventional gauze (Chowdhry & Chen, 2015; Bryant & Nix, 2016). The moulding and length of time a hydrocolloid adhesive dressing can be left intact diminish pain and protect the wound and periwound skin. This type of dressing conforms well to different body contours and protects the periwound from blister formation when a dressing over a joint (e.g., knee or hip) is flexed with movement (Chowdhry & Chen, 2015). Hydrocolloid dressings are often the choice for sacral pressure injury wounds requiring autolytic debridement when there is no evidence of infection in the wound bed.

Hydrogel dressings promote moist wound healing and autolysis (Bryant & Nix, 2016). The gel dressings are nonadherent and less painful to remove. A dry wound still requires a dressing—and if

debridement or enhanced healing is of benefit, hydrogel dressings donate moisture to the wound bed.

Polyurethane foam dressings are sheets of foamed polymers that contain small, open cells capable of holding wound exudate away from a wound bed (Bryant & Nix, 2016). Foam dressings are not appropriate when there is wound tunnelling because the dressing expands, which can enlarge the tunnel. The foam dressings protect the wound surface while maintaining a moist, insulated environment. These dressings are designed to wick away moisture from the wound through moisture-vapour transfer, thus avoiding saturation of the wound bed and periwound skin.

Alginate and hydrofibre dressings create a moist environment and promote autolysis, granulation, and epithelialization (Bryant & Nix, 2016). The dressing may come as a sheet or rope that can be packed into a wound. The nurse can safely pack deep tracking wounds with either of these types of absorptive dressings, which provide easy removal with little risk for retained dressing deep in the wound cavity (Bryant & Nix, 2016).

Delegation and Collaboration

The skill of applying a hydrocolloid, hydrogel, foam, or alginate dressing cannot be delegated to an unregulated care provider (UCP). The nurse directs the UCP to:

- Help position the patient during dressing application.
- Immediately report to the nurse any pain, fever, bleeding, wound drainage, or slippage of dressing.

Equipment

- Sterile gloves (optional)
- Clean gloves

Dressing Set *(optional)*

- Sterile scissors (optional)
- Sterile drape (optional)

- Necessary primary dressings: gauze, hydrocolloid, hydrogel, foam, or alginate
- Secondary dressing of choice
- Sterile 10 × 10–cm (4 × 4–inch) gauze pads
- Sterile saline or other cleaning solution (as prescribed)
- Skin barrier wipe
- Tape (nonallergenic paper or adhesive), ties as needed
- Measuring guide (tape measure, tracing paper, camera as needed)
- Adhesive remover (if required)
- Biohazard bag
- Debriding gel (as prescribed)
- Sterile 10 × 10–cm (4 × 4–inch) gauze pads
- Irrigating solution if indicated (see Skill 40.1)
- Personal protective equipment (PPE) (e.g., gown, goggles, and mask) as needed

STEP	RATIONALE

ASSESSMENT

1. Identify patient using at least two person-specific identifiers (e.g., name and date of birth or name and medical record number), according to employer policy.	Ensures correct patient. Complies with Accreditation Canada's standards and improves patient safety (Accreditation Canada, 2019).
2. Assess for presence of allergies, especially antiseptics, tape, or latex.	Prevents localized or systemic reaction to supplies.
3. Inspect location, size, and condition of wound.	Determines supplies and help needed.
4. Ask patient to rate pain using an appropriate pain rating scale. Administer prescribed analgesic as needed 30 minutes before dressing change.	Patient may require pain medication before dressing change. Allows for peak effect of drug during procedure.
5. Review health care provider's prescriptions for frequency and type of dressing change. *Do not use alginate or absorptive dressings on nonexudative wounds.*	Prescription indicates type of dressing or application to use. Wounds change in their requirements over time. If dressing prescription is no longer appropriate, contact the health care provider to provide an up-to-date wound description for relevant prescription change.
6. Review previous nurses' notes in electronic health record (EHR) or chart. Note possible need to use customized shape or size of dressing to fit body parts that are difficult to size (e.g., sacrum, heels, or elbows).	Customized shapes aid in person-centred dressing selection and better dressing adherence.
7. Assess patient's knowledge of purpose of dressing and determine need to include caregiver in dressing wound.	Identifies patient's and caregiver's learning needs.

NURSING DIAGNOSES

- Acute pain
- Chronic pain
- Insufficient knowledge regarding application of hydrocolloid, hydrogel, foam, or alginate dressing
- Reduced skin integrity
- Potential for infection

Related factors/Risk factors are individualized on the basis of patient's condition or needs.

PLANNING

1. Expected outcomes following completion of procedure:	
• Patient's wound shows evidence of healing as it becomes smaller in size or shallower in depth with less drainage, redness, or swelling.	Dressing is effective in promoting healing.
• Patient reports pain that is less than previously assessed level, using an appropriate pain rating scale during and after dressing change.	Pain control is achieved during dressing removal and reapplication.
• Dressing remains clean, dry, and intact.	Dressing is applied correctly.
• Patient or caregiver explains procedure correctly.	Indicates that learning has occurred.

STEP	RATIONALE

PLANNING

2. Explain procedure to patient or caregiver.
3. Position patient comfortably to allow access to dressing site.

Relieves anxiety and promotes understanding of healing process.
Facilitates application of dressing.

IMPLEMENTATION

1. Close room door or room curtains.
2. Expose wound site and drape patient. Instruct patient not to touch wound or sterile supplies.

Provides for patient privacy.
Draping provides access to wound while minimizing exposure. Dressing supplies become contaminated when touched by the patient's hand.

3. Place biohazard bag within reach of work area. Fold top of bag to make a cuff.
4. Perform hand hygiene and apply clean gloves. Apply appropriate PPE as needed if there is risk for splashing.

Ensures easy disposal of soiled dressings. The nurse should not reach across a sterile field.
Reduces transmission of infectious microorganisms.

5. Using nondominant hand, gently remove tape, bandages, or ties of existing dressing. Pull tape parallel to skin and toward dressing. If dressing is over hairy areas, remove tape in the direction of hair growth and get patient's permission to clip or shave area before applying new dressing (check employer policy). Remove any adhesive from skin.

Pulling tape toward dressing reduces stress on wound edges, irritation, and discomfort.

6. With gloved hand or forceps, remove old dressing one layer at a time. Note amount and character of drainage (see illustration). Use caution to avoid placing tension on any drains.

Reduces irritation and possible injury to skin. Prevents accidental removal of drain.

Clinical Decision Point *Check removal directions for the specific brand of dressing used. Some brands need to have an old dressing soaked, irrigated, or moistened for removal. If necessary, use adhesive remover to ease off the dressing, but avoid contact of adhesive remover with the wound.*

7. Fold dressings with drainage contained inside and remove gloves inside out. With small dressings, remove gloves inside out to enclose dressing (see Skill 40.1). Dispose of gloves and soiled dressing according to employer policy. Cover wound lightly with a sterile 10 × 10–cm (4 × 4–inch) gauze pad. Perform hand hygiene.

Contains soiled dressings; prevents contact of nurse's hands with drainage; reduces cross-contamination.

Clinical Decision Point *Hydrocolloid dressings interact with wound fluids and form a soft, whitish-yellowish gel, which is sometimes hard to remove and may have a faint odour. A residual gel substance occurs in wound beds with some absorption dressings. This is a normal occurrence; do not confuse these findings with pus or purulent exudate, wound infection, or wound deterioration (Bryant & Nix, 2016). Foam dressings should have a well-marked area of saturation of wound fluid or exudate (with approximately 1.5 cm of nonsaturated foam at dressing edges).*

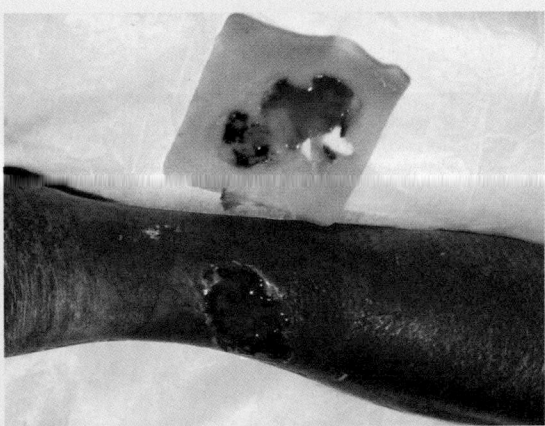

STEP 6 Hydrocolloid dressing after removal from venous injury. Purulent-appearing exudate is present on dressing and wound. This is expected with autolysis under the dressing and is not evidence of infection. *(From Bryant, R., & Nix, D. [2016]. Acute and chronic wounds: Current management concepts [5th ed.]. St. Louis: Mosby.)*

STEP	RATIONALE

IMPLEMENTATION

8. Prepare sterile field with sterile dressing kit or individually wrapped sterile supplies on over-bed table (see Chapter 6). Pour prescribed solution into sterile bowl.

Creates sterile work area.

9. Remove gauze cover over wound.

10. Clean wound:

   a. Perform hand hygiene. Apply clean gloves. Sterile gloves are optional (see employer policy). Clean wound and periwound area gently with 10 × 10–cm (4 × 4–inch) sterile gauze pads moistened in sterile saline or spray with noncytotoxic wound cleanser.

Reduces introduction of organisms into wound. Cleaning and irrigating effectively remove residual dressing gel or slough without injuring newly formed delicate granulation tissue in healing wound bed.

   b. Clean from least contaminated to most contaminated area.

Cleaning in this direction prevents introduction of microorganisms into noncontaminated areas.

   c. Clean around any drain, using circular stroke starting near drain and moving outward away from insertion site (see Skill 40.1).

11. Use sterile, dry gauze to blot dry wound bed and on skin around wound.

Dressing will not adhere to damp surface. Periwound maceration can enlarge wound and impede healing.

12. Inspect appearance and condition of wound (see Chapter 39). Measure wound length, width, and depth.

Appearance and measurement indicate state of wound healing.

13. Remove gloves and perform hand hygiene,

Reduces transmission of microorganisms.

14. Apply dressing (see manufacturer directions).

Ensures proper application of dressing. Different brands of dressings require different application techniques.

   a. Hydrocolloid dressings:

     (1) Select proper size, allowing dressing to extend onto intact periwound skin at least 2.5 cm (1 inch) (Bryant & Nix, 2016) (see illustration). Do not stretch dressing; avoid producing wrinkles and tenting.

Hydrocolloid design prevents shear and friction from loosening edges and circumvents need for tape along dressing borders (Bryant & Nix, 2016).

     (2) For a deep wound, apply hydrocolloid granules, impregnated gauze, or paste before the wafer.

Functions as filler material to ensure contact with all wound surfaces.

     (3) Remove paper backing from adhesive side and place over wound. Do not stretch, and avoid producing wrinkles or tenting. Hold dressing in place for 30 to 60 seconds after application.

Moulds dressing at body temperature (Bryant & Nix, 2016).

     (4) If cut from a larger piece, tape edges with nonallergenic tape to avoid rolling or adherence to clothing.

Clinical Decision Point *Edges may be notched to help mould around wound. Consider using custom shapes to better conform to certain parts of the body, such as heels, elbows, and sacrum.*

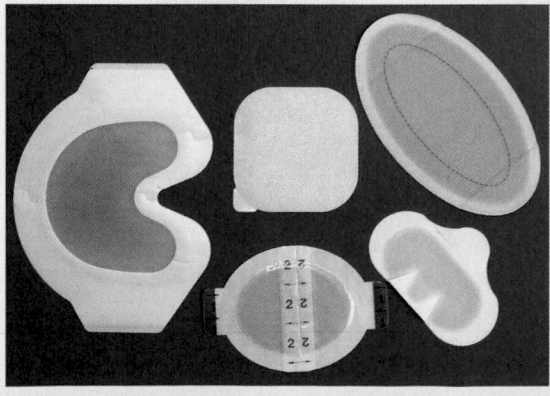

STEP 14a(1) Variety of sizes and shapes of hydrocolloid dressings. *(Courtesy Bonnie Sue Rolstad.)*

STEP	RATIONALE

IMPLEMENTATION

b. Hydrogel dressings:

(1) Apply skin barrier wipe to surrounding skin that will encounter any adhesive or gel.

Protects periwound skin. Because of the high water content of gels, care must be taken to protect periwound skin through use of a skin barrier (Bryant & Nix, 2016).

(2) Apply gel or gel-impregnated gauze directly into wound, spreading evenly over wound bed (see illustration). Apply gel to wound cavity no more than about one-third full or pack gel-impregnated gauze loosely, including any undermined or tunnelled areas. Cover with appropriate moisture-retentive dressing that will still allow for moisture-vapour transfer. *Option:* Hydrogel sheets composed of water should be cut to size of wound *only.*

Hydrogels hydrate and facilitate autolytic debridement of wounds. Filling the wound cavity partially full allows for expansion with absorption of exudate (Bryant & Nix, 2016).

(3) Apply skin barrier cream or spray to periwound skin.

Protects skin around wound from maceration.

(4) Secure dressing with nonallergenic tape if secondary dressing is not self-adhering.

c. Foam dressings:

(1) Know removal and application characteristics of the specific brand of foam dressing.

Some foam dressings have silicone in the dressing itself; some have a silicone dressing border only. With silicone dressings, no skin barrier wipe is required.

(2) If dressing is not silicone foam, a skin barrier wipe is required. Apply to the surrounding skin that will come in contact with dressing adhesive.

Protects periwound skin from maceration or irritation from adhesive.

(3) If using a foam dressing without a border, use an appropriate-sized dressing; if required, a nonborder foam dressing can be cut to extend 2.5 cm out onto intact periwound skin. Nonborder foam requires a "window-pane" border created with tape. Do not cover the entire foam dressing, just the borders.
Foam dressings with a border should extend approximately 2.5 cm (1 inch) on all sides over intact periwound skin.
Verify which side of the foam dressing should be placed toward the wound bed and which side should be facing away from it; check product instructions.

Ensures proper absorption and keeps wound exudate away from wound bed (Bryant & Nix, 2016).

(4) Cut foam to fit around drain or tube.

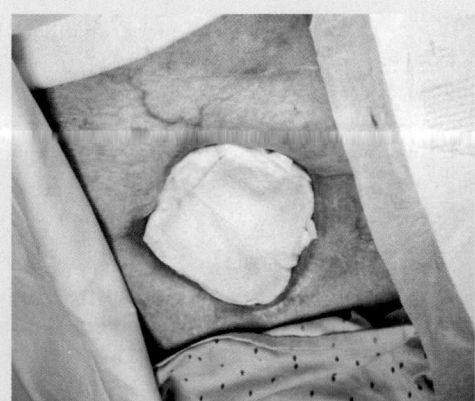

STEP 14b(2) Hydrogel-impregnated gauze used to maintain moist wound bed and fill dead space in this deep abdominal wound with undermining. *(From Bryant, R., & Nix, D. [2016]. Acute and chronic wounds: Current management concepts [5th ed.]. St. Louis: Mosby.)*

STEP	RATIONALE

IMPLEMENTATION

d. Alginate or hydrofibre dressings:

    (1) Cut sheet or rope to fit size of wound or loosely pack into wound space (see illustration), filling ½ to ⅔ full.

        Highly absorptive product expands with absorption of serous fluid or exudate (Bryant & Nix, 2016).

    (2) Apply secondary dressing: absorbent pad (e.g., Mesorb®) or foam dressing to cover. Base cover dressing selection on anticipated frequency of primary dressing change.

        Secondary dressing helps maintain appropriate moisture in the wound bed, supports moisture-vapour transfer, and prevents drainage on bed linens and clothing.

15. Label dressing with your initials and the date dressing is changed.

    Provides timeline for next dressing change.

16. Discard soiled dressing materials properly. Remove gloves by pulling them inside out and discard in prepared bag. Perform hand hygiene.

    Reduces transfer of microorganisms.

17. Help patient return to a comfortable position.

    Enhances patient comfort and relaxation.

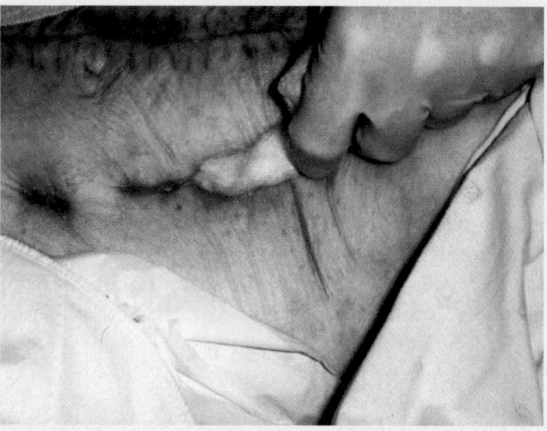

STEP 14d(1) Alginate dressing applied to fill dead space and absorb exudate in full-thickness abdominal wound. (*From Bryant, R., & Nix, D. [2016]. Acute and chronic wounds: Current management concepts [5th ed.]. St. Louis: Mosby.*)

EVALUATION

1. Inspect appearance of wound: measure length × width × depth of wound, observe amount and colour of drainage; observe presence of periwound edema or erythema. Palpate around wound for tenderness.

    Determines status of wound healing.

2. Evaluate patient's level of comfort.

    Documents patient's level of comfort after procedure.

3. Inspect condition of dressing at least every shift or as prescribed.

    Determines integrity of wound dressing.

4. Use Teach-Back: "I want to be sure I explained why I need to use this type of dressing for your wound. Tell me why this dressing material is the best option for your wound." Develop revised teaching if patient or caregiver is not able to teach back correctly.

    Determines patient's and caregiver's level of understanding of instructional topic.

Unexpected Outcomes	Related Interventions
1. Wound develops more necrotic tissue and increases in size.	• In rare instances, some wounds do not tolerate hypoxia induced by hydrocolloid dressings. In these patients, discontinue use. Notify the health care provider. • Evaluate appropriateness of wound care protocol. • Assess and treat the underlying conditions. Evaluate for other factors impairing wound healing.

STEP	RATIONALE

Unexpected Outcomes

2. Dressing does not stay in place.

3. Periwound skin is macerated.

Related Interventions

- Evaluate size of dressing used for adequate margin (2.5 to 3.5 cm [1 to 1.4 inches])
- Ensure that periwound skin is not macerated and has an appropriate skin barrier wipe to assist in keeping dressing intact.
- If patient is incontinent or diaphoretic, some dressings may be difficult to adhere. Consider alternatives (e.g., using gauze roll or burn-net/stockinet).
- Consider custom shapes for body parts that are difficult to fit.
- Dressing may be secured with roll gauze, tape, or transparent dressing (assess for fragile skin).
- Assess moisture-control property of dressing or application technique, including barrier skin protectant; incontinence or diaphoresis may also require management.

Communication and Documentation

- Document appearance, colour, and size of wound; characteristics of drainage; response to dressing change; condition of periwound skin; and patient's level of comfort on flow sheet in nurses' notes in EHR or chart.
- Graph wound surface area (L × W) or volume (L × W × D) if wound is chronic. Wound progress should demonstrate 30% wound closure at 3–4 weeks of treatment (Jørgensen, Sørensen, Jemec, et al., 2016).
- Document patient's and caregiver's understanding through teach-back for proper wound dressing.
- Report signs of infection, necrosis, or deteriorating wound status to health care provider immediately.

Special Considerations
Teaching

- Explain expected wound appearance, fluid or gel accumulation in wound bed, and possible odour with use of specific dressing.

- Because application techniques can vary with different brands, tell the patient and caregiver not to purchase a brand different from the one for which the nurse gave instructions. If a different brand must be used, the patient and caregiver should check with the nurse for any additional instructions or modifications in application and removal techniques.

Pediatric
- See Pediatric Considerations for Skills 40.1, 40.2, and 40.3.

Gerontological
- See Gerontological Considerations for Skills 40.1, 40.2, and 40.3.
- Avoid early and frequent removal of a hydrocolloid dressing to reduce injury to surrounding intact skin.

PROCEDURAL GUIDELINE 40.1 *Applying Gauze and Elastic Bandages*

NSO *Nursing Skills Online Wound Care Module 19 / Lesson 1*

Gauze and elastic bandages secure or wrap hard-to-cover areas of the body such as dressings on extremities and amputation stumps. Bandages are a secondary dressing, providing protection, pressure, immobilization, and anchoring of underlying dressings or splints. There are numerous types of and applications for bandages. They are available in rolls of various widths and materials, including gauze, elastic, webbing, elasticized knit, and muslin. Gauze bandages are lightweight and inexpensive, mould easily around body contours, and permit air circulation to prevent skin maceration. Elastic bandages apply compression to a body part. Elastic compression to a lower extremity prevents edema by promoting the return of blood from the peripheral to the central circulation.

When applying a bandage, select a type of bandage turn (Table 40.3) and width, depending on the size and shape of the body part to be bandaged. For example, 7.5-cm (3-inch)–wide bandages are commonly used for the adult leg.

Delegation and Collaboration
The skill of applying an elastic bandage for compression cannot be delegated to an unregulated care provider (UCP). A nurse assesses the condition of any wound or dressing before applying a bandage. The skill of applying bandages to secure nonsterile dressings can be delegated to a UCP (refer to employer policy). The nurse directs the UCP about:
- Modifying the bandage application such as with special taping.
- Reviewing what to observe and report back to the nurse (e.g., patient's indication of pain, numbness, or tingling after application or changes in patient's skin colour or temperature).

Continued

PROCEDURAL GUIDELINE 40.1 *Applying Gauze and Elastic Bandages—cont'd*

Equipment
- Correct width and number of gauze or elastic bandages
- Clips or adhesive tape
- Clean gloves if wound drainage is present
- *Option:* Pillow

Procedural Steps
1. Identify patient using at least two person-specific identifiers (e.g., name and date of birth or name and medical record number), according to employer policy.
2. Review patient's medical record for specific prescriptions related to application of gauze or elastic bandage. Note area to be covered, type of bandage required, frequency of change, and previous response to treatment.
3. Assess patient's level of comfort using an appropriate pain rating scale. Administer prescribed analgesic as needed before dressing change.
4. Observe adequacy of circulation by palpating temperature of skin and pulses, presence of edema, and sensation (distal to area to be bandaged). Observe skin colour and movement of body part to be wrapped. **NOTE:** Impaired circulation may result in pain, coolness to touch when compared with the opposite side of the body, cyanosis or pallor of skin, diminished or absent pulses, edema or localized pooling, and numbness and/or tingling of body part.
5. Perform hand hygiene and apply clean gloves (if drainage or a break in skin is present). Inspect skin of area to be bandaged for alterations in integrity as indicated by presence of abrasion, discoloration, or chafing. Pay close attention to areas over bony prominences.
6. Inspect the condition of any wound for appearance, size, and presence and character of drainage and be sure that it is covered with a proper dressing. If not, reapply dressing (check employer policy for type of gloves to use). Remove clean gloves and perform hand hygiene.
7. Assess for size of bandage:
   a. *Gauze or basic elastic bandage to secure a dressing:* Assess size of area to be covered. Each successive roll of gauze or elastic should overlap the previous layer. Use smaller widths for upper extremities, larger widths for lower extremities.
   b. *Elastic bandage to provide simple compression:* Assess circumference of lower extremity before or shortly after patient gets out of bed in the morning or after patient has been in bed for at least 15 minutes. Select width that will cover and overlap without bulkiness.
8. Identify patient's and caregiver's present knowledge level and their ability to manipulate the bandage if bandaging will be continued at home.
9. Close room door or curtains. Position patient comfortably in an anatomically correct supine position in bed.
10. Perform hand hygiene and apply clean gloves if drainage is present.
11. Apply gauze or elastic bandage to secure dressings:
    a. Elevate dependent extremity for 15 minutes before applying elastic bandage to promote venous return.
    b. Make sure that primary dressing over wound is securely in place.
    c. Begin elastic bandage application at the distal body part. Hold the roll of bandage in your dominant hand and use the other hand to lightly hold the beginning layer.
    d. Apply even tension during application and begin with two circular turns to anchor the bandage. Continue to maintain even tension and transfer roll to your dominant hand as you wrap the bandage (see illustration).

TABLE 40.3
Types of Bandage Turns

Type	Description	Purpose or Use
Circular turn 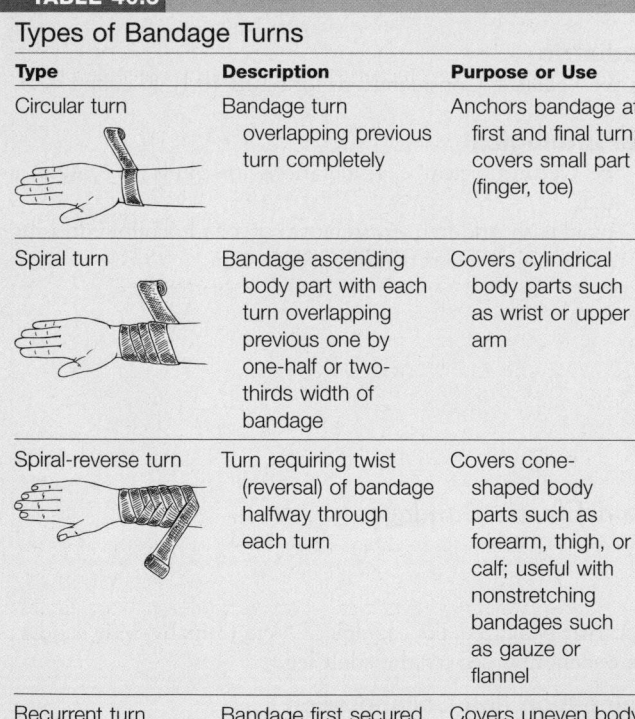	Bandage turn overlapping previous turn completely	Anchors bandage at first and final turn; covers small part (finger, toe)
Spiral turn	Bandage ascending body part with each turn overlapping previous one by one-half or two-thirds width of bandage	Covers cylindrical body parts such as wrist or upper arm
Spiral-reverse turn	Turn requiring twist (reversal) of bandage halfway through each turn	Covers cone-shaped body parts such as forearm, thigh, or calf; useful with nonstretching bandages such as gauze or flannel
Recurrent turn 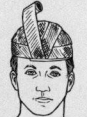 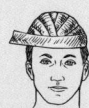	Bandage first secured with two circular turns around proximal end of body part; half turn made perpendicular up from bandage edge; body of bandage brought over distal end of body part to be covered, with each turn folded back over on itself	Covers uneven body parts such as head or stump

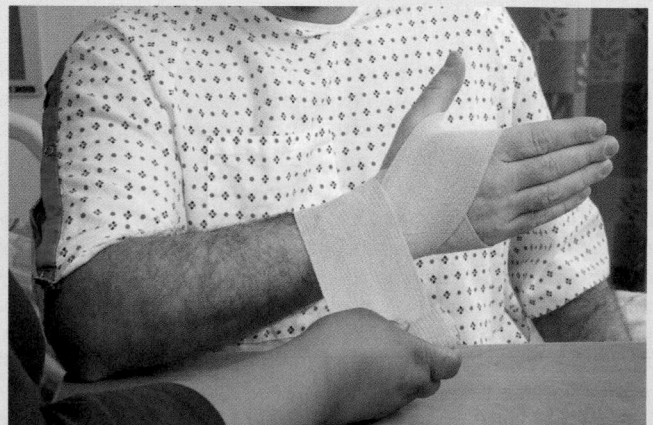

STEP 11d Hold elastic bandage in dominant hand and apply with circular turns.

PROCEDURAL GUIDELINE 40.1 *Applying Gauze and Elastic Bandages—cont'd*

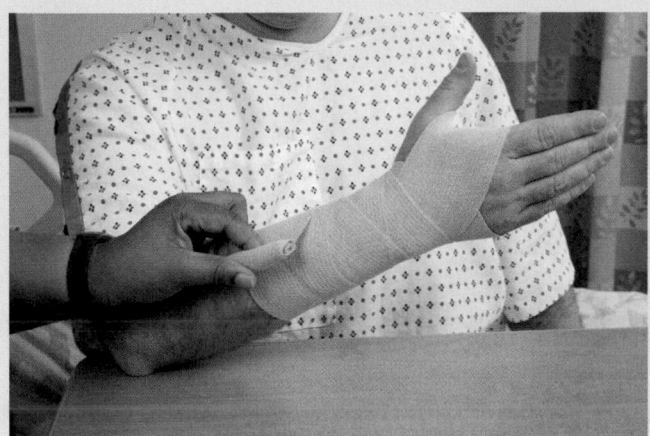

STEP 11e Apply bandage from distal to proximal area.

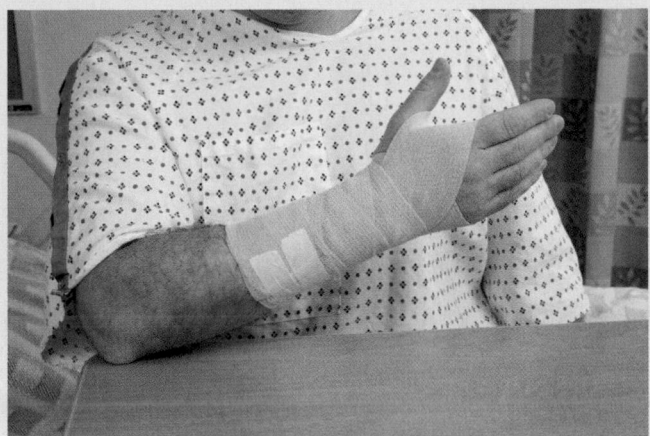

STEP 11h Secure with tape or closure device.

e. Apply bandage from distal point toward proximal boundary (see illustration), using appropriate turns to cover various shapes of body parts (see Table 40.3). Roll gauze, overlapping each layer by one-half to two-thirds the width of the bandage.

f. Double check tension and ensure that the bandage is snug but not tight and that the primary dressing or splint is positioned correctly. A tight bandage may cause numbness and tingling from impaired circulation or pressure on peripheral nerves.

g. While unrolling an elastic bandage, stretch the bandage slightly. Explain to the patient that smooth, even pressure will be applied to improve circulation, reduce swelling, immobilize the body part, and provide pressure.

h. End bandage with two circular turns; secure end of gauze or elastic bandage to outside layer of bandage, not skin, with tape or clips (see illustration).

Clinical Decision Point *Keep toes or fingertips uncovered and visible for follow-up circulatory assessment, except in cases in which toes or fingers are treated because of wounds.*

12. Apply elastic bandage over stump (see illustrations):
    a. Elevate stump with a pillow or support it with the help of another person.
    b. Secure bandage by wrapping it twice around the proximal end of the stump or person's waist (depending on size of stump).
    c. Make a half turn with bandage perpendicular to its edge.

d. Bring body of bandage over distal end of stump.
e. Continue to fold bandage over stump, wrapping from distal to proximal points.
f. Secure with metal clips, Velcro if provided, or tape.

13. Remove gloves if worn and perform hand hygiene.

14. Assess degree of tightness of bandage, wrinkles, looseness, and presence of drainage.

15. Evaluate distal circulation when bandage application is complete, at least twice during next 8 hours, and then at least every shift.
    a. Observe skin colour for pallor or cyanosis.
    b. Palpate skin for warmth.
    c. Palpate distal pulses and compare bilaterally.
    d. Ask patient to rate pain using an appropriate pain rating scale and to describe any numbness, tingling, or other discomfort, to evaluate for neurological and vascular changes.

16. Observe mobility of extremity.

17. **Use Teach-Back:** "I want to be sure I explained how to apply the elastic roll to your sprained ankle. Show me how you would apply this elastic roll to your ankle." Develop a revised teaching plan if patient or caregiver is not able to teach back correctly.

18. Record patient's level of comfort, circulation status, type of bandage applied, presence of swelling, and range of motion at baseline and after bandage application on flow sheet in nurses' notes in electronic health record (EHR) or chart.

19. Report any changes in neurological or circulatory status to health care provider.

Continued

PROCEDURAL GUIDELINE 40.1 *Applying Gauze and Elastic Bandages—cont'd*

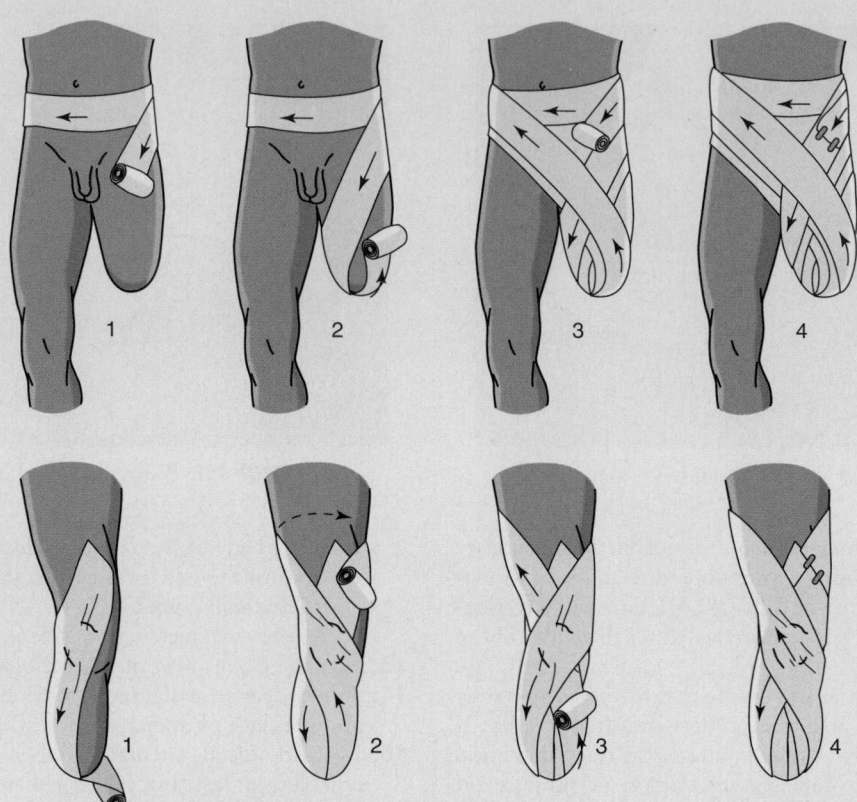

STEP 12 Top, Correct method for bandaging midthigh amputation stump. Note that bandage must be anchored around patient's waist. **Bottom,** Correct method for bandaging midcalf amputation stump. Note that bandage need not be anchored around waist. *(From Monahan, F., et al. [2006]. Phipps' medical-surgical nursing: Health and illness perspectives [8th ed.]. St. Louis: Mosby.)*

PROCEDURAL GUIDELINE 40.2 *Applying an Abdominal Binder*

Binders are bandages made of large pieces of material specially designed to fit a specific body part. Most binders are made of elastic or cotton. The most common type is the abdominal binder. Breast binders are not used as often in current practice because sports bras are preferred for breast support following certain surgeries.

An abdominal binder supports large abdominal incisions that are vulnerable to tension or stress as a patient moves or coughs (Fig. 40.2). The binder also lessens pain in postoperative patients. In addition, abdominal binders provide a noninvasive intervention for enhancing recovery of walk performance, controlling pain, and improving the patient's experience following major abdominal surgery (Gallagher, 2016). Binders support underlying muscles and large incisions, lessening muscle stress, which helps a patient move more freely without additional discomfort.

Delegation and Collaboration
The skill of applying a binder may be delegated to an unregulated care provider (UCP), depending on employer policy. A nurse is responsible for assessing the condition of any incision, the skin, and patient's ability to breathe before binder application. The nurse instructs the UCP about:

- How to modify the skill, such as using special wrapping or the

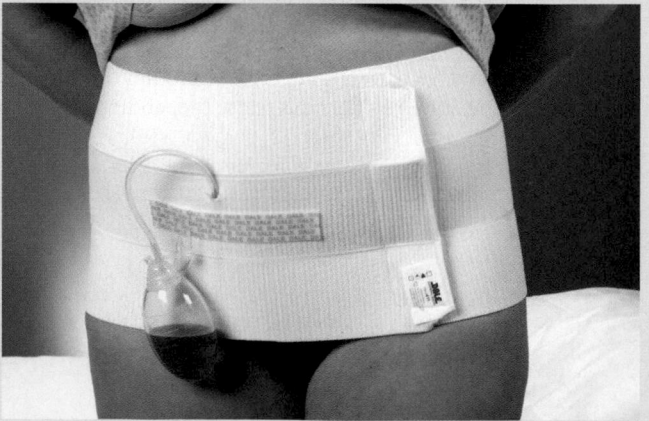

FIG 40.2 Abdominal binder with Velcro closures. *(Courtesy Dale Medical Products, Plainsville, MA.)*

PROCEDURAL GUIDELINE 40.2 *Applying an Abdominal Binder—cont'd*

manner of securing the binder.
- Reporting patient's indication of pain, numbness, tingling, or difficulty breathing after abdominal binder has been applied or any changes in patient's skin colour or temperature.

Equipment
- Clean gloves if wound drainage is present
- Gauze bandage as needed
- Correct type and size of binder
- Closures for cloth binder

Procedural Steps
1. Identify patient using at least two person-specific identifiers (e.g., name and date of birth or name and medical record number), according to employer policy.
2. Review medical record for prescription for binder (check employer policy).
3. Observe patient who needs support of thorax or abdomen; observe their ability to breathe deeply, cough effectively, and turn or move independently.
4. Inspect skin for actual or potential alterations in integrity. Observe for irritation, abrasion, and skin surfaces that rub against one another.
5. Inspect any surgical dressing for intactness, presence of drainage, and coverage of incision. Change any soiled dressing before applying binder (using clean gloves).
6. Determine patient's comfort level. Ask patient to rate pain using an appropriate pain rating scale. Administer prescribed analgesic 30 minutes before dressing change.
7. Gather necessary data regarding size of patient and appropriate binder to use (see manufacturer guidelines) to ensure proper fit.
8. Determine patient's knowledge of the purpose of the binder.
9. Close curtains or room door.
10. Perform hand hygiene and apply clean gloves (if likely to contact wound drainage).
11. Apply abdominal binder:
    a. Position patient in supine position with head slightly elevated and knees slightly flexed.
    b. Help patient roll on the side away from you toward raised side rail while patient firmly supports abdominal incision and dressing with their hands. Fanfold far side of binder toward midline of binder.
    c. Place binder flat on bed, right side up. Fanfold far side of

binder toward midline of binder so patient can roll over with minimal effort.
    d. Place fanfolded ends of binder under patient.
    e. Instruct patient or help them roll over folded binder. For overweight patients consider asking a nurse colleague to help.
    f. Unfold and stretch ends out smoothly on far side of bed. Then stretch out ends on near side of bed.
    g. Instruct patient to roll back into supine position.
    h. Adjust binder so supine patient is centred over binder, using symphysis pubis and costal margins as lower and upper landmarks.
    i. If patient is very thin, pad iliac prominences with gauze bandage.
    j. Close binder. Pull one end of binder over centre of patient's abdomen. While maintaining tension on that end of the binder, pull the opposite end of the binder over the centre and secure with Velcro closure tabs or metal fasteners. This provides continuous wound support and comfort.

Clinical Decision Point *After binder is in place, assess patient's ability to breathe deeply and cough effectively. When applied correctly, an abdominal binder over midline abdominal incisions should not have any effect on the patient's pulmonary function.*

12. Assess patient's comfort level and adjust binder as necessary.
13. Remove gloves and perform hand hygiene.
14. Ask patient to rate pain using an appropriate pain rating scale.
15. Remove binder and surgical dressing to assess skin and wound characteristics at least every 8 hours.
16. Evaluate patient's ability to ventilate properly, including deep breathing and coughing, every 4 hours to determine presence of impaired ventilation and potential pulmonary complications.
17. Document baseline and post binder condition of skin, circulation, integrity of underlying dressing, and patient's comfort level in nurses' notes in the electronic health record (EHR) or chart. Also record type of bandage applied.
18. Report any complications (e.g., pain, skin irritation, impaired ventilation) to the nurse in charge.
19. Report reduced ventilation (e.g., pulse oximetry, pulmonary function tests) to health care provider immediately.

✦ CLINICAL DEBRIEF

A 75-year-old male is postoperative day 2 after having an exploratory laparotomy with a total gastrectomy for gastric cancer. He has developed a fever of 38.5°C (101.3°F). There was purulent drainage coming from his midline incision and surrounding erythema. The patient rates his pain a 6 out of 10 and he has not received any pain medication in the past 4 hours. Temp is 38.5°C (101.3°F), BP 130/80, pulse 95, RR 20, SaO_2 96%. Approximately 5 cm (2 inch) of the incision was opened at bedside by removal of 10 staples.

1. Based on the type of wound and amount of wound drainage, which type of dressing would be appropriate?
2. On assessing the patient on postoperative day 3, the nurse notices a large amount of bright red blood coming from the base of the open wound. How should the nurse proceed, and which type of dressing should be chosen?
3. Using SBAR, show how the nurse would communicate with the health care team about this patient.

✦ REVIEW QUESTIONS

1. Of the following dressings, which are most appropriate for a shallow wound with minimal exudate? *(Select all that apply.)*
   1. Nonadherent gauze dressing
   2. Calcium alginate dressing
   3. Hydrogel dressing
   4. Transparent film dressing
   5. Hydrocolloid dressing

2. Match the following wound drainage with the appropriate definition:

Serous	1. Yellow, green, or brown drainage
Serosanguineous	2. Indicates fresh bleeding, bright red
Sanguineous	3. Pale, red, more watery drainage
Purulent	4. Clear, watery plasma

3. Which of the following are necessary to prepare the patient for changing the dressing on an open abdominal wound? *(Select all that apply.)*
   1. Assessing size, location, and condition of wound
   2. Explaining procedure to the patient
   3. Reviewing all blood results
   4. Asking the patient to rate their pain level
   5. Assessing the patient about allergies

ⓔ *Visit the Evolve site for a complete list of Clinical Debrief and Review Questions answers.*

REFERENCES

Accreditation Canada. (2019). *Required organizational practices handbook—Version 14.* Ottawa, ON: Author. Retrieved from http://www.wrha.mb.ca/quality/files/2019ROPHandbook.pdf

Arroyo, A. A., Casanova, P., Soriano, J., Torra, I., & Bou, J. E. (2015). Open-label clinical trial comparing the clinical and economic effectiveness of using a polyurethane film surgical dressing with gauze surgical dressings in the care of postoperative surgical wounds. *International Wound Journal,* 12(3), 285–292. doi:10.1111/iwj.12099

Brindle, C. T., & Wegelin, J. A. (2012). Prophylactic dressing application to reduce pressure ulcer formation in cardiac surgery patients. *Journal of Wound Ostomy & Continence Nursing,* 39(2), 133–142. doi:10.1097/WON.0b013e318247cb82

Bryant, R. A., & Best, M. (2016a). Management of draining wounds and fistulas. In R. A. Bryant & D. P. Nix (Eds.), *Acute and chronic wounds: Current management concepts* (5th ed., pp. 541–561). St. Louis: Mosby.

Bryant, R. A., & Nix, D. P. (2016b). Principles of wound healing and topical management. In R. A. Bryant & D. P. Nix (Eds.), *Acute and chronic wounds: Current management concepts* (5th ed., pp. 306–324). St. Louis: Mosby.

Canadian Patient Safety Institute (CPSI). *2016—Pressure ulcer: Resources.* Retrieved from http://www.patientsafetyinstitute.ca/en/toolsResources/Hospital-Harm-Measure/Improvement-Resources/HHI-Pressure-Ulcer/Pages/Resource-Library-Pressure-Ulcer-Resources.aspx

Chamanga, E. T., Hughes, M., Hilston, K., Sparke, A., & Jandrisits, J. M. (2015). Chronic wound bed preparation using a cleansing solution. *British Journal of Nursing,* 24(12), S30, S32–S36. doi:10.12968/bjon.2015.24

Chowdhry, M., & Chen, A. F. (2015). Wound dressings for primary and revision total joint arthroplasty. *Annals of Translational Medicine,* 3(18), 268. doi:10.3978/j.issn.2305-5839.2015.09.25

David, J. A., & Chiu, E. S. (2018). Surgical debridement. In D. Orgill (Ed.), *Interventional treatment of wounds* (pp. 3–15). Cham, Switzerland: Springer International.

Doughty, D., & Sparks, B. (2016). Wound-healing physiology and factors that affect the repair process. In R. A. Bryant & D. P. Nix (Eds.), *Acute and chronic wounds: Current management concepts* (5th ed., pp. 63–81). St. Louis: Mosby.

Ermer-Seltun, J., & Rolstad, B. S. (2016). General principles of topical therapy. In D. B. Doughty & L. L. McNichol (Eds.), *Wound Ostomy and Continence Nurses Society core curriculum: Wound management.* Philadelphia: Wolters Kluwer.

Gallagher, S. (2016). Skin care needs of obese patient. In R. A. Bryant & D. P. Nix (Eds.), *Acute and chronic wounds: Current management concepts* (5th ed., pp. 507–515). St. Louis: Mosby.

Harris, C. L., Kuhnke, J., Haley, J., et al. (2018). Best practice recommendations for prevention and management of surgical wound complications. Retrieved from https://www.woundscanada.ca/docman/public/health-care-professional/bpr-workshop/555-bpr-prevention-and-management-of-surgical-wound-complications-v2/file

Hockenberry, M. J., & Wilson, D. (2015). *Wong's nursing care of infants and children* (10th ed.). St. Louis: Mosby.

Hopf, H. W., Shapshak, D., Junkins, S., & O'Neill, D. K. (2016). Managing wound pain. In R. A. Bryant & D. P. Nix (Eds.), *Acute and chronic wounds: Current management concepts* (5th ed., pp. 399–407). St. Louis: Mosby.

Jørgensen, L. B., Sørensen, J. A., Jemec, G. B., & Yderstræde, K. B. (2016). Methods to assess area and volume of wounds—A systematic review. *International Wound Journal,* 13(4), 540–553.

Krasner, D. L. (2016). Wound pain: Impact and assessment. In R. A. Bryant & D. P. Nix (Eds.), *Acute and chronic wounds: Current management concepts* (5th ed., pp. 386–398). St. Louis: Mosby.

Mudge, E. J. (2015). Recent accomplishments in wound healing. *International Wound Journal,* 12, 4–9. doi:10.1111/iwj.12230

National Pressure Ulcer Advisory Panel (NPUAP), European Pressure Ulcer Advisory Panel (EPUAP), & Pan Pacific Pressure Injury Alliance (PPPIA). (2014). *New 2014 prevention and treatment of pressure ulcers: Clinical practice guidelines.* Retrieved from http://www.npuap.org/resources/educational-and-clinical-resources/prevention-and-treatment-of-pressure-ulcers-clinical-practice-guideline/

Orsted, H. L., Keast, D. H., Forest-Lalande, L., et al. (2018). *Foundations of best practice for skin and wound management.* Retrieved from https://www.woundscanada.ca/docman/public/health-care-professional/bpr-workshop/165-wc-bpr-prevention-and-management-of-wounds/file

Percival, S. L., Mayer, D., Malone, M., Swanson, T., Gibson, D., & Schultz, G. (2017). Surfactants and their role in wound cleansing and biofilm management. *Journal of Wound Care,* 26(11), 680–690. doi:10.12968/jowc.2017.26.11.680

Pittman, J., Beeson, T., Kitterman, J., Lancaster, S., & Shelly, A. (2015). Medical device–related hospital-acquired pressure ulcers. *Journal of Wound Ostomy & Continence Nursing,* 42(2), 151–154. doi:10.1097/WON.0000000000000113

Powers, J. G., Higham, C., Broussard, K., & Phillips, T. J. (2016). Wound healing and treating wounds: Chronic wound care and management. *Journal of the American Academy of Dermatology,* 74(4), 607–625.

Ramundo, J. M. (2016). Wound debridement. In R. A. Bryant & D. P. Nix (Eds.), *Acute and chronic wounds: Current management concepts* (5th ed., pp. 295–305). St. Louis: Mosby.

Santamaria, N., Gerdtz, M., Sage, S., et al. (2015). A randomized controlled trial of the effectiveness of soft silicone multi-layered foam dressings in the prevention of sacral and heel pressure ulcers in trauma and critically ill patients: The border trial. *International Wound Journal,* 12(3), 302–308. doi:10.1111/iwj.12101

World Health Organization (WHO). (2016). *Global guidelines for the prevention of surgical site infection.* Geneva: Author. Retrieved from http://www.patientsafetyinstitute.ca/en/toolsResources/Documents/WHO%20global%20SSI%20guidelines_2016_10_22.pdf

Wysocki, A. B. (2016). Anatomy and physiology of skin and soft tissue. In R. A. Bryant & D. P. Nix (Eds.), *Acute and chronic wounds: Current management concepts* (5th ed., pp. 40–62). St Louis: Mosby.

41 | Therapeutic Use of Heat and Cold

Written by **Anne Griffin Perry, RN, MSN, EdD, FAAN, and Nancy Logue, RN, MN, PhD**

SKILLS AND PROCEDURES

OBJECTIVES

Mastery of content in this chapter will enable the nurse to:
- Identify the physiological effects of heat and cold.
- Differentiate the types of injuries or conditions that benefit from heat and cold applications.
- Identify the potential risks related to heat and cold applications.
- Explain common guidelines used to protect patients from risks associated with heat and cold applications.
- Correctly apply heat and cold applications.

MEDIA RESOURCES

- **evolve** http://evolve.elsevier.com/Canada/Perry/clinicalskills/
- Review Questions
- Audio Glossary
- Clinical Debrief and Review Questions Answers

PURPOSE

Local application of moderate heat and cold to areas of the body provides comfort and pain relief, reduces muscle spasm, improves mobility, and promotes healing. Safe use of heat and cold therapies requires understanding of the physiological responses and potential risks associated with these therapies. The choice of heat or cold therapy depends on the local responses desired, such as reducing local inflammation, promoting wound healing, or controlling body temperature.

STANDARDS OF CARE

- Accreditation Canada, 2019—*Required Organizational Practices Handbook—Version 14* (http://www.wrha.mb.ca/quality/files/2019ROPHandbook.pdf)
- American Physical Therapy Association (APTA), 2019—*Scope of Practice* (http://www.apta.org/ScopeOfPractice/)
- Canadian Nurses Association (CNA), 2011—*Position Statement: Interprofessional Collaboration* (https://www.cna-aiic.ca/-/media/cna/page-content/pdf-en/interproffessional-collaboration_position-statement.pdf)
- Canadian Physiotherapy Association (CPA), 2012—*Position Statement. Inter-professional Collaboration and Practice* (https://physiotherapy.ca/sites/default/files/positionstatements/inter-professional-collaboration_en.pdf)
- Registered Nurses' of Ontario (RNAO), 2013—*Clinical Best Practice Guidelines: Assessment and Management of Pain* (3rd ed.) (http://rnao.ca/sites/rnao-ca/files/AssessAndManagementOfPain_15_WEB-_FINAL_DEC_2.pdf)

PRINCIPLES FOR PRACTICE

- Exposure to heat or cold causes systemic and local responses (Table 41.1). Body temperature is affected by environmental and internal factors. When the skin is exposed to warm or hot temperatures, vasodilation and perspiration occur to promote heat loss. As perspiration evaporates from the skin, cooling occurs. When the skin is exposed to cool or cold temperatures, the systemic response includes vasoconstriction and piloerection (hair erection or bristling) to conserve heat. Shivering occurs in response to cooler temperatures, producing heat through skeletal muscle contraction (Hannon & Porth, 2017).
- Cold constricts the vasculature in adjacent tissues and slows bleeding into damaged tissues. Application of cold therapy decreases the release of inflammatory mediators from the damaged tissues, which hinders protein release from the vasculature and decreases edema (da Costa Santos, dos Santos Cardoso, Figueiredo, et al., 2015).
- Sensory adaptation to local temperature extremes occurs quickly within the body. Eventually excessive heat causes a burning

TABLE 41.1

Pathophysiological Effects of Heat and Cold Applications

	Cold	Hot
Pain	↓	↓
Spasm	↓	↓
Metabolism	↓	↑
Blood flow	↓	↑
Inflammation	↓	↑
Edema	↓	↑
Joint Stiffness	↓	↓

Data from da Costa Santos, V., dos Santos Cardoso, C., Figueiredo, C. P., & de Souza Guerino Macedo, C. (2015). Effect of cryotherapy on the ankle temperature in athletes: Ice pack and cold water immersion. *Fisioterapia em Movimento, 28*, 1; Denegar, C. R., Saliba, E., & Saliba, S. (2018). *Therapeutic modalities for musculoskeletal injuries* (4th ed.). Windsor, ON: Human Kinetics; and LeBlanc, K. (2018). Skin integrity and wound care. In B. J. Kozier, G. Erb, A. T. Berman, et al. (Eds.), *Fundamentals of Canadian nursing: Concepts, process and practice* (4th Canadian ed., pp. 930–982). Don Mills, ON: Pearson Canada.

sensation and excessive cold causes a numbing sensation before pain is sensed.

- Contrast therapy, consisting of alternating applications of heat and cold, may be useful in treating athletic injuries. Sensory contrasts between heat and cold appear effective in reducing pain and muscle spasm (Denegar, Saliba, & Saliba 2018).
- Factors that determine when to use heat, cold (cryotherapy), or contrast therapy include acute or longstanding injury, severity of pain or muscle spasm, ease of application, patient preference, and contraindications for heat or cold (Denegar et al., 2018). In health care facilities (e.g., hospitals, long-term care settings) a health care provider's prescription for heat or cold applications is always necessary. The prescription should include the location and duration of treatment, and the desired temperature to be used when settings can be controlled.
- Hypothermia and hyperthermia devices are used selectively for specific clinical conditions. They are designed to raise, lower, or maintain body temperature through heat or cold transfer between the device and the patient.

PATIENT-CENTRED CARE

- The meaning and significance of heat and cold therapy may have varied interpretations, based on a patient's culture (Giger, 2017; Xu, Rich, & Connor, 2016). Therefore, as part of person-centred care, it is important to assess the culture-specific perceptions of heat and cold for each patient and caregiver:
  - Reinforce the purpose of the therapy and identify patient concerns or questions to promote understanding of the purpose and benefits of the therapy.
  - During application of heat or cold therapy, the patient, or their extremities, may be exposed; maintain comfort and privacy with additional blankets, privacy curtains, and closed room doors. Some patients may refuse exposure to reduce body temperature.
  - Include family members or professional interpreters to promote acceptance of critical therapies such as hypothermia or ice packs that may contradict a patient's or family's cultural beliefs and practices.

- Inform the patient and caregiver about the rationale for heat and cold as primary or adjuvant therapies. Lack of education about benefits of heat or cold therapies may contribute to perceptions that pain is being trivialized (RNAO, n.d.).
- Heat or cold may be used with other nonpharmacological measures such as physiotherapy, massage, or other interventions to reduce pain and improve sleep, mood, and general well-being. Nonpharmacological approaches are not intended to replace adequate pharmacological management. Interprofessional collaboration is critical in determining an appropriate treatment plan (RNAO, 2013).
- Assess the patient's and caregiver's past experiences with heat and cold therapies. Prior experiences will influence preference for heat or cold and willingness to participate in the treatment plan (Denegar et al., 2018; RNAO, 2013).

EVIDENCE-INFORMED PRACTICE

- The application of ice or cryotherapy is one of the most widely used therapeutic modalities in the management of acute musculoskeletal injuries. Patients who use a numerical rating score for pain have reported decreased pain following application of ice on their neck. Cold therapy reduces the conduction of pain impulses, which occurs when the skin temperature is lowered (da Costa Santos et al., 2015; Denegar et al., 2018).
- Ice compresses applied after scleral buckling eye surgery help to reduce swelling and pain in the operative area (Li & Wang, 2016).
- Cold therapy decreases nerve conduction velocity, formation and accumulation of edema, and blood flow to injured tissues. As a result, the physiological effects of cold therapy include reduced inflammation, pain, and edema and they help control bleeding (Bech, Moorhe, Cho, et al., 2015; Hannon & Porth, 2017; Li & Wang, 2016).
- Cold therapy is recommended for treatment of acute injury to reduce inflammation, pain, spasm, and edema. Heat is recommended for longstanding injuries due to physiological effects of increasing blood flow and tissue temperature (Arankalle, Wardle, & Nair, 2016; Denegar et al., 2018).
- Contrast therapy using alternating cold-to-heat ratios of 1 to 3 minutes or 1 to 4 minutes is effective for musculoskeletal injuries to reduce inflammation and edema and improve joint function (Denegar et al., 2018).
- There are varied recommendations about optimal length of time for heat or cold applications (Denegar et al., 2018). Treatment length is determined by the health care provider and adjusted according to individual needs and situation.

SAFETY GUIDELIINES

- Know the patient's risk for injury from heat or cold, as some individuals are more predisposed to injury than others (Table 41.2).
- Exposed layers of skin are more sensitive to temperature variations than intact skin. Therefore damaged skin should be protected when applying heat or cold therapy.
- Do not microwave towels or medical products used for heat application, as this may provide excessive heat and increase risk of tissue injury.
- Many devices such as heating pads or water-flow pads have thermostats to regulate temperature. Always check the temperature of a heating device or moist compress prior to applying it directly to the skin.

TABLE 41.2

Characteristics of Heat and Cold Application

	Examples of Conditions	Precautions	Adverse Outcomes
Cold application	Immediately after direct trauma such as sprain, strains, fractures, muscle spasms; after superficial lacerations or puncture wounds; minor burns; chronic pain from arthritis, joint trauma; delayed-onset muscle soreness; inflammation	Circulatory insufficiency Sensory impairment Radiation therapy Diabetes mellitus	Cardiovascular effects (bradycardia) Nerve and tissue damage Impaired wound healing Frostbite
Heat application	Inflamed or edematous body area; new surgical wound; infected wound; arthritis; degenerative joint disease; localized joint pain, muscle strains; low back pain; menstrual cramps; hemorrhoid, perianal, and vaginal inflammation; local abscess	Pregnancy Laminectomy sites Spinal cord injury Malignancy Vascular insufficiency Radiation therapy Acute injury Extreme caution when using heat or cold therapies with eyes, testes, heart area	Burns Infections Increased pain Increased inflammation Secondary tissue injury

- Burns and skin injuries sustained from heat or cold therapies are serious reportable events and are preventable. Prompt reporting to the appropriate health team member enables early, appropriate treatment to minimize discomfort and tissue damage.
- It is important to individualize care to meet a patient's needs and preferences. Patient teaching, safety, comfort, and privacy are important when using heat or cold therapies.
- Consider patient age, skin and circulation, vital signs, ability to sense temperature, and ability to communicate before applying heat or cold therapies. Children, older persons, or patients with sensory impairment or peripheral vascular diseases have a greater risk for injury from heat and cold applications (see Table 41.2).
- Heat or cold therapies should be used with caution in patients who have diabetes mellitus, peripheral vascular disease, or any alterations in sensation or pain perceptions. Patients with these conditions also require more frequent skin assessment during treatment. Heat or cold applications should be avoided in an area of radiation therapy for at least 5 days after treatment (RNAO, n.d.).
- Cold or contrast therapy cannot be used if patients have Raynaud's phenomenon or cold urticaria (cold allergy) (Denegar et al., 2018; LeBlanc, 2018).
- Heat should not be used for an area that is bleeding, is being treated with products that contain menthol, has decreased sensation, or within 24 hours after acute injury (LeBlanc, 2018; RNAO, n.d.).
- Dry or moist applications may be used in heat or cold therapies, depending on the expected outcome for the patient. Temperature travels from an external source such as a compress or a heating pad to the surface of the skin. A substance that conducts temperatures poorly is a good insulator and thus protects skin and tissues. However, there are distinct advantages to using both dry and moist applications (Table 41.3).
- Extremities or perineal areas have decreased fat and underlying tissue and are more sensitive than others to temperature extremes. Modify the intensity of heat and cold when treating sensitive skin areas.
- Check the patient frequently during a heat or cold application. The condition of the skin indicates whether tissue injury may be occurring. Observe for signs of excessive redness, maceration, or blistering.

TABLE 41.3

Heat Application: Moist Versus Dry

Type	Advantages	Disadvantages
Moist application	Reduces drying of skin and softens wound exudate Conforms well to body area being treated Penetrates deeply into tissue layers Lessens sweating and insensible fluid loss	Skin maceration with prolonged exposure Cools rapidly because of moisture evaporation Increases risk for burns because moisture conducts heat
Dry application	Less likely to burn skin Does not cause skin maceration Retains temperature longer because it is not influenced by evaporation	Increases insensible fluid loss through sweating Does not penetrate deep into tissue Increases drying of skin

- Inform the patient to not adjust temperature settings.
- Position the patient so it is possible for them to move away from the temperature source to decrease the risk of injury from temperature exposure. A hospitalized patient should always have a call light within reach.
- Do not leave a patient who is unable to sense temperature changes or move away from the temperature source unattended.
- Be aware of the systemic effects of heat in dilating blood vessels and increasing local blood flow. If vasodilation is significant, the patient's blood pressure may decrease, causing dizziness and increased risk for falls. While heat applications may reduce swelling and transmission of pain impulses, excessive use of heat is a noxious stimulus that may increase pain and tissue damage (Hannon & Porth, 2017).

✦ SKILL 41.1   Application of Moist Heat (Compress and Sitz Bath)

Moist heat is beneficial in increasing muscle and ligament flexibility, promoting relaxation and healing, and relieving muscle spasm. Moist heat applied as a compress may also be beneficial for treating arthritic or sprained joints, strained muscles, back pain, rheumatoid arthritis, or in any treatment where heat is applied to the skin to promote circulation. Factors to consider before application include level of temperature and duration of the heat therapy and the nature of the tissues being treated.

Compresses and commercial packs (Fig. 41.1) are examples of moist heat applications used for a variety of conditions. A warm compress is sterile or clean gauze moistened with a prescribed heated solution (i.e., normal saline or sterile water) that is applied directly to an affected area. Commercially packaged sterile, premoistened compresses, available in some facilities, require a special infrared lamp to heat them. Plain sterile or clean gauze is heated by adding the gauze to a container of warmed solution. A commercial heat pack produces its own moisture by drawing moisture from humidity in the air and retaining it in the outer flannel cover of the hot pack.

Moist heat application also includes the use of warm baths, soaks, and Sitz baths. A warm bath or soak involves immersion of a body part into a warmed solution. Warm soaks and Sitz baths promote circulation, reduce edema and inflammation, promote muscle relaxation, debride wounds, and may contain medicated solutions. In particular, a Sitz bath causes localized vasodilation that may result in decreased blood pressure. A body part that is too large to immerse may be soaked by wrapping it in a dressing saturated with the warmed solution.

Sitz baths require a special tub or chair basin that allows a patient to sit in water without immersing the legs, feet, and upper trunk (Fig. 41.2). Sitz basins are disposable and especially easy to use in the home. Portable baths fit easily on top of toilets. Patients who have undergone perineal or rectal surgery, had an episiotomy during childbirth, or have painful hemorrhoids or perineal inflammation benefit from a Sitz bath.

When preparing a soak or bath, remember that the heated solution is in direct contact with the patient's skin. Assess the patient's skin for excessive redness or blistering after 10 to 15 minutes and check water temperature frequently to prevent burns. The solution temperature should be kept constant to enhance the therapeutic effects of the moist heat. When adding heated solution to a soak basin or bath, remove the patient's body part and re-immerse it once the solution has mixed and the temperature has been checked.

Delegation and Collaboration

The skill of applying moist heat may be delegated to an unregulated care provider (UCP) (see employer policy). If there are risks or expected complications, the skill cannot be delegated. In most settings the nurse applies any sterile applications. Explanation of the purpose of the treatment, assessment of the patient's overall condition and the skin and tissues in the area being treated, and evaluation of the patient's response cannot be delegated. Where applicable, the nurse instructs a UCP about:
- Proper temperature of the application.
- Skin changes to immediately report to the nurse (e.g., burning, blistering, or excessive redness).
- Specific patient concerns and changes in vital signs to immediately report to the nurse (e.g., pain, dizziness or light-headedness, increased or decreased pulse, decreased blood pressure).
- Specific positioning and application time requirements based on employer policy and manufacturer instructions.
- Reporting when treatment is completed so the nurse can evaluate the patient's response.

Equipment
All Moist Heat Applications
- Prescribed analgesia (if prescribed)
- Dry bath towel, bath blanket
- Prescribed solution (i.e., heated normal saline) or commercially prepared compresses or commercial heat pack
- Biohazard waste bag

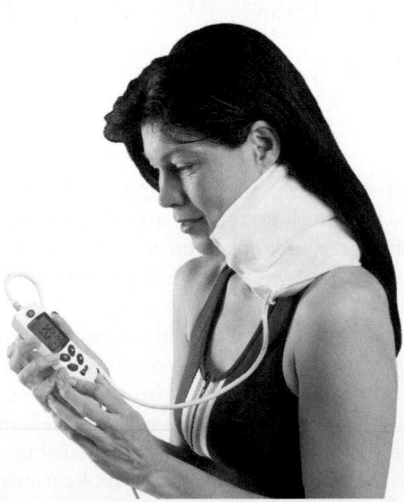

FIG 41.1 Digital moist-heat pack. (*Image used with permission from Theratherm, Chattanooga, a DJO Company. All rights reserved.*)

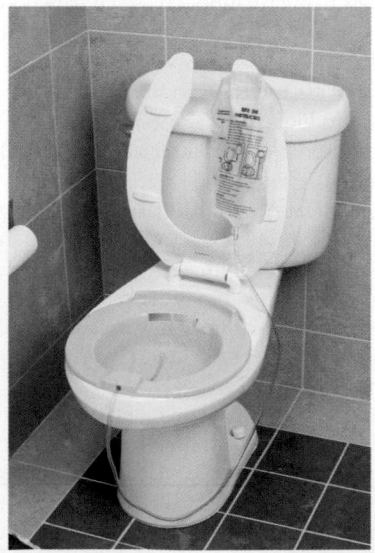

FIG 41.2 Disposable Sitz bath. (*Used with permission, Briggs Corporation.*)

- Clean gloves
- Compress
- Clean basin
- Waterproof pad
- Ties or cloth tape
- Clean gauze or towel

- Moist heat application options according to the health care provider prescription:
  - Sterile compress: sterile basin, sterile gauze, and sterile gloves
  - Aquathermia pad
  - Disposable Sitz bath: prescribed solution and any topical medication to be applied after the soak

STEP	RATIONALE

ASSESSMENT

1. Identify patient using at least two person-specific identifiers (e.g., name and date of birth or name and medical record number), according to employer policy.	Ensures correct patient. Complies with Accreditation Canada's standards and improves patient safety (Accreditation Canada, 2019).
2. Refer to health care provider's prescription for type of moist heat application, location and duration of application, desired temperature, and employer policies regarding temperature.	Ensures safe practice by verifying specific location for therapy and type and duration of heat application.
3. Perform hand hygiene and assess skin around area to be treated. Perform neurovascular assessments for sensitivity to temperature and pain by measuring light touch, pinprick, and temperature sensation (see Chapter 8).	Conditions that alter conduction of sensory impulses that transmit temperature and pain predispose patients to injury from heat applications. Patients with diminished sensation to heat or cold must be monitored closely during treatment.

Clinical Decision Point *Patients living with diabetes mellitus, vascular diseases, paralysis, rheumatoid arthritis, peripheral neuropathy, or other alterations in sensation or pain perceptions, as well as those using certain cardiovascular medications, are at greater risk for thermal injury.*

4. Refer to patient's medical record to identify any contraindications to moist heat application: unstable cardiac conditions, active bleeding, therapeutic medicinal patch, acute inflammatory reactions, recent musculoskeletal injury or radiation therapy, and skin conditions such as eczema.	Patients with certain cardiovascular conditions and who exhibit adverse effects of certain medications such as cardiac, hypertensive, and vasoactive medications may be at risk for sudden changes in blood pressure and blood flow caused by vasodilation. Heat causes vasodilation, which aggravates active bleeding, which can increase hemorrhage or bleeding into soft tissues adjacent to musculoskeletal injury (LeBlanc, 2018). Vasodilation increases the rate of medication absorption when direct heat is applied over the medication patch.
5. Assess patient's level of consciousness and responsiveness (e.g., confusion, disorientation, dementia).	Patients with altered level of consciousness are unable to sense or report reduced sensation of discomfort and will require close supervision during therapy.
6. Assess patient's mobility: ability to position self for soak application, position self in bath, and sit up from bath.	Determines level of help needed to position patient for treatment.
7. When applying moist heat, apply clean gloves and assess the wound for size, colour, drainage volume, pain (use a pain assessment method appropriate for the patient's age, culture, or cognitive state) (RNAO, 2013), and odour (this may be deferred until dressing is removed [see Step 5c in Implementation section, below] and heat is applied). Remove and discard gloves	Provides baseline to determine change in wound following heat application. Provides baseline for patient's comfort level.
8. Assess patient's blood pressure and pulse.	Establishes baseline to determine response to therapy.
9. Assess patient's range of motion (ROM) of affected area if being treated for muscle sprain.	Provides baseline to determine if ROM improves following therapy.
10. Assess patient's and caregiver's understanding of application and related safety factors.	Determines need for health teaching.

NURSING DIAGNOSES

- Acute pain
- Chronic pain
- Inadequate peripheral tissue perfusion

- Insufficient knowledge regarding heat therapy
- Reduced physical mobility

- Reduced skin integrity
- Potential for injury

Related factors/Risk factors are individualized on the basis of patient's condition or needs.

STEP	RATIONALE

PLANNING

1. Expected outcomes following completion of procedure:

- Affected area is pink and warm to touch immediately after heat application.

  Vasodilation increases blood flow to site.

- After multiple applications, wound shows signs of healing (e.g., tissue granulation; reduced edema, inflammation, drainage).

  Moist heat increases blood flow, enhances white blood cell infiltration, and removes waste products from cells (da Costa Santos et al., 2015).

- Patient denies burning sensation.

  Indicates temperature applied appropriately.

Clinical Decision Point *Heat applications may cause pain signals to be overridden by activating the spinal gating mechanism, which decreases pain perception (gate control pain theory) (Maeda, Yoshida, & Sasaki, 2017).*

- Patient reports increased mobility and decreased pain in affected region.

  Heat reduces edema and inflammation and relaxes stiff and strained muscles. Heat used in conjunction with physical therapy, exercise, or both improves function and mobility (da Costa Santo et al., 2015; Denegar et al., 2018).

- Blood pressure and pulse are within patient's normal range.

  No systemic vascular changes occur. Goal of therapy is to achieve localized vascular response.

- Patient or caregiver demonstrates how to apply therapy safely.

  Measures level of understanding necessary for home care.

2. Assemble and prepare equipment and supplies.

Organization of supplies prevents unnecessary delays in procedure.

3. Explain steps of procedure and purpose to patient. Describe expected sensations such as warmth and wetness. Explain precautions to prevent burning.

Minimizes anxiety and promotes cooperation during procedure.

IMPLEMENTATION

1. Close room door and close bedside curtains.

Decreases drafts, thus decreasing transmission of microorganisms. Provides privacy.

2. Perform hand hygiene and apply clean gloves.

Reduces transmission of microorganisms.

3. Position patient in bed, keeping affected body part in proper alignment. Expose body part to be covered with heat application and drape patient with bath blanket or towel as needed.

Limited mobility in an uncomfortable position causes muscular stress. Draping prevents cooling and maintains privacy.

4. Place waterproof pad under patient (not required with Sitz bath or commercial heat pad).

Protects bed linen from moisture and soiling.

5. **Apply moist clean or sterile compress:**

- **a.** Heat prescribed solution to desired temperature by immersing closed bottle of solution in a basin of warm water.

  Prevents burns by ensuring proper temperature of solution.

- **b.** Prepare aquathermia pad if needed. Temperature is usually preset by manufacturer or bioengineering.

  Prevents burning by using proper temperature.

- **c.** Remove any existing dressing covering the wound. Inspect the wound and surrounding skin. Dispose of gloves and dressing in a biohazard bag.

  Reduces transmission of microorganisms. Provides baseline to measure wound healing.

Clinical Decision Point *An inflamed wound appears reddened, but the surrounding skin is less red in colour. If skin surrounding the wound is inflamed or reddened or has active bleeding or drainage, moist heat application may be contraindicated. Verify with health care provider.*

- **d.** Perform hand hygiene.

  Reduces transmission of microorganisms.

- **e.** Prepare compress with appropriate aseptic or sterile technique.

  A sterile compress is needed when applied to open wound.

  - **(1)** Pour warmed solution into container. If sterile asepsis is required, use sterile technique to open sterile gauze and add it to warmed sterile solution (see Chapter 6).

    A sterile compress is needed when applied to an open wound.

  - **(2)** If using a commercially prepared compress, follow manufacturer instructions for warming.

Clinical Decision Point *To avoid injury to a patient, test the temperature of sterile solution by applying a drop to your forearm (without contaminating solution). It should feel warm to the skin without burning.*

STEP	RATIONALE

IMPLEMENTATION

f. Apply clean gloves, or if sterile asepsis is needed apply sterile gloves.

Allows manipulation of sterile dressing and touching an open wound.

g. Pick up one layer of immersed gauze, wring out excess solution, and apply it lightly to wound; avoid surrounding unaffected skin. *Option:* Apply commercial compress or heat pack over wound only; only use with clean wounds.

Excess moisture macerates skin and increases risk for burns and infection. Skin is sensitive to a sudden change in temperature.

h. After a few seconds, lift edge of gauze to assess for redness.

Increased redness indicates burn.

i. If patient tolerates compress, pack gauze snugly against wound. Ensure all wound surfaces are covered with the warm compress.

Packing the compress prevents rapid cooling from ambient air currents.

j. Cover moist compress with dry sterile dressing and towel. If necessary, pin or tie in place. Remove and dispose of gloves and perform hand hygiene.

Dry sterile dressing prevents transfer of microorganisms to wound via capillary action caused by moist compress. Towel insulates compress to prevent heat loss.

k. *Option:* When using a gauze compress, apply aquathermia, a commercial heat pack, or waterproof heating pad (see Skill 41.2) over the towel. Keep it in place for the desired duration of application.

Provides constant temperature to compress.

l. Leave compress in place for 20 minutes or per health care provider's prescription or employer policy. If aquathermia pad or commercial heat pack is *not* used, change warm compress using sterile technique every 5 to 10 minutes or as prescribed during duration of therapy.

Maintains constant temperature for best therapeutic benefit. Moist heat promotes transfer of heat to underlying subcutaneous tissues, which helps to reduce thermal injury to skin. Rebound phenomenon, in which the opposite effect begins, occurs after maximum therapeutic effect is achieved. Maximum vasodilation from heat occurs in 20–30 minutes (LeBlanc, 2018).

m. After prescribed time, perform hand hygiene and apply clean gloves. Remove pad, towel, and compress. Evaluate wound and skin and replace dry sterile dressing (using sterile gloves) as prescribed.

Continued exposure to moisture macerates skin. Prevents entrance of microorganisms into wound site.

n. Assist patient to preferred position.

Maintains patient's comfort.

o. Dispose of equipment and soiled compress. Perform hand hygiene.

Reduces transmission of microorganisms.

6. Sitz bath or warm soak to intact skin or wound:

a. Remove any existing dressing covering the wound. Inspect the wound and surrounding skin. Dispose of gloves and dressing in a biohazard bag and perform hand hygiene.

Provides baseline to determine response to warm soak. Reduces transmission of microorganisms.

b. When exudate or drainage is present, apply new clean gloves and cleanse intact skin around open area with clean cloth and soap and water. Sterile gloves and gauze may be needed to clean an open wound. Dispose of gloves and perform hand hygiene.

Cleaning removes organisms so bath or soak solution does not spread infection.

c. Fill Sitz bath or bathtub in bathroom with warmed solution. Check temperature. *Option:* If using normal saline, warm per employer policy or health care provider's prescription.

Ensures proper temperature and reduces risk for burns.

d. Assist patient to bathroom to immerse body part in Sitz bath, bathtub, or basin. Cover patient with bath blanket or towel as needed.

Prevents falls. Covering patient prevents heat loss through evaporation, maintains temperature and privacy.

e. Assess heart rate and that the patient does not feel light-headed or dizzy. Ensure the call light is within reach.

Provides baseline to determine if vascular response to vasodilation occurs during treatment.

f. After 15 to 20 minutes remove patient from soak or bath; dry body areas thoroughly. (Wear clean gloves.)

Avoids excess cooling. Enhances patient's comfort.

g. Drain solution from basin or tub. Clean the basin or tub according to employer policy. Dispose of soiled linen and gloves; perform hand hygiene.

Reduces transmission of microorganisms.

STEP	RATIONALE

EVALUATION

1. Inspect condition of body part or wound treated for evidence of healing. Assess skin colour, temperature, edema, and sensitivity to touch.

2. Assess patient's comfort level using an appropriate pain assessment method (see employer policy). Consider the patient's age, clinical condition, cognitive or developmental level, literacy, ability to communicate, culture, and ethnicity when using a pain assessment method such as verbal or face picture rating scales or nonverbal indicators of pain (RNAO, 2013).

3. Obtain blood pressure and pulse and compare with baseline.

4. Evaluate ROM of affected body part.

5. **Use Teach-Back:** "I want to be sure I demonstrated how to apply a warm, moist compress so you can do this at home. Show me how you would apply this compress at home." Develop a revised teaching plan if the patient or caregiver is unable to teach back correctly.

Rationale column:

Evaluates effectiveness of treatment and risk for potential injury.

Determines if patient was exposed to temperature extreme that may cause injury. Evaluates patient's subjective response to therapy.

Determines if systemic vascular response to vasodilation has occurred.

Determines if edema or muscle spasm is relieved.

Determines patient's and caregiver's level of understanding about applying a warm, moist compress.

Unexpected Outcomes

1. Patient's skin is reddened and sensitive to touch, either during treatment or 30 minutes after, or patient reports burning.

2. Patient describes burning and increased discomfort.

Related Interventions

- Discontinue moist application immediately.
- Verify proper temperature or check device for proper functioning.
- Notify health care provider and, if there is a burn, complete an incident or adverse event report (see employer policy).
- Reduce temperature of compress.
- Assess for skin breakdown.
- Notify health care provider.

Communication and Documentation

- Document procedure, noting type, location, and duration of application; solution and temperature; condition of body part, wound, and skin before and after treatment; and patient's response to therapy on flow sheet in nurses' notes in electronic health record (EHR) or chart.
- Document preprocedure and postprocedure vital signs.
- Document your evaluation of patient and caregiver learning.
- Report any unexpected changes in condition of skin or wound to health care provider.

Special Considerations
Teaching

- If a patient needs to continue heat applications after discharge, have the patient or caregiver give a return demonstration before discharge.
- Caregivers and patients need to learn and demonstrate the assessments that are needed for patients with reduced sensation to determine appropriate compress temperature.

Pediatric

- The skin of infants and children is thin and fragile and therefore easily damaged. Use special caution with application of heat in this population (Hockenberry & Wilson, 2015). Remain with children during the procedure for safety.
- It may be helpful to incorporate play into the time a child is required to soak. Place clean water toys in the basin or bath soak. Adult supervision is necessary.

Gerontological

- Normal aging results in thinning and increased fragility of a patient's skin, which increases risk for skin damage. If an older person is receiving long-term steroid therapy or is malnourished, the skin becomes even more fragile. Skin also becomes less elastic and more prone to tears. Chronic diseases may contribute to impaired circulation to a skin area or impaired sensation for pain or temperature (Touhy, Jett, Boscart, et al., 2019).
- Older persons who have lost subcutaneous tissue and fat have lost the insulating effect of these tissues and may experience alterations in thermoregulation and have an increased risk of injury from heat applications (Touhy et al., 2019).

Care in the Community

- When necessary, assess availability of a caregiver to help patient apply moist heat, the caregiver's understanding of the purpose of the procedure, and their willingness to comply with the procedure.
- Assess physical environment to determine adequacy of facilities for use by patient. The patient may need assistive devices to get in or out of a tub or a commode chair to set up a Sitz bath.
- Assess the patient's health state to determine whether continuous supervision is needed during therapy.

◆ SKILL 41.2 Applying Aquathermia and Dry Heat

A water-flow pad such as an aquathermia pad, electric heating pads, and commercial heat packs (Fig. 41.3) are common forms of dry heat therapy. Air-activated wearable heat wraps that maintain a temperature of 40°C (104°F) can be worn from 8 to 10 hours. The aquathermia pad (water-flow pad) consists of a waterproof rubber or plastic pad connected by two hoses to an electrical control unit that has a heating element and motor. Distilled water circulates through hollowed channels in the pad to the control unit where water is heated (or cooled).

Dry heat devices are applied directly to the surface of the skin. For this reason, extra precautions need to be taken to prevent burns and skin and tissue injury. Conventional heating pads use dry heat and are often used in the home. A cotton or flannel cloth must cover the heating pad. The pad has a temperature-regulating unit for high, medium, or low settings. Instruct patients not to turn the setting higher once they have adapted to the temperature.

Delegation and Collaboration

The skill of applying aquathermia and dry heat may be delegated to an unregulated care provider (UCP) (see employer policy). The nurse must assess and evaluate the condition of the skin and tissues in the area being treated and explain the purpose of the treatment. If there are risks or expected complications, this skill cannot be delegated. The nurse instructs the UCP about:

- Specific positioning and time requirements to keep the application in place based on the health care provider's prescription or employer policy.
- Observing and reporting immediately excessive redness or pain during application.
- Reporting to the nurse when treatment is completed so the patient's response can be evaluated.

Equipment

- Aquathermia or commercial heat pack
- Distilled water (for aquathermia pad)
- Bath towel or pillowcase
- Tape, ties, or gauze roll

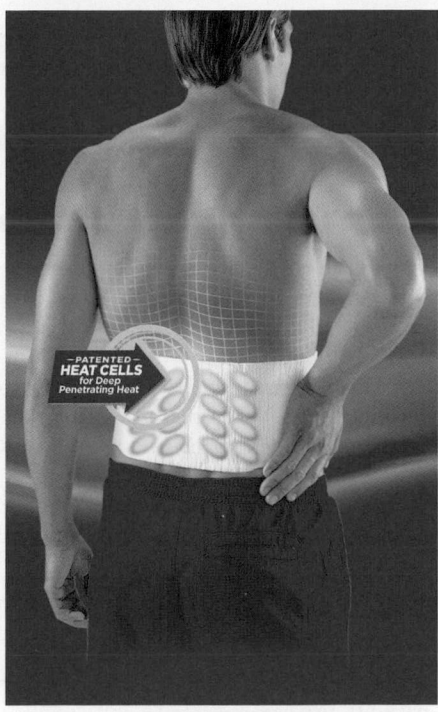

FIG 41.3 Dry heat wrap. (*Image used with permission, ThermaWrap, Pfizer Consumer Healthcare. All rights reserved.*)

STEP	RATIONALE

ASSESSMENT

1. Identify patient using at least two identifiers (e.g., name and date of birth or name and medical record number), according to employer policy.

   Ensures correct patient. Complies with Accreditation Canada's standards and improves patient safety (Accreditation Canada, 2019).

2. Refer to health care provider's prescription for location, duration of therapy, and desired temperature. Employer policy usually sets recommended temperature for aquathermia pad.

   A prescription is required to help ensure the patient's safety. Preset temperature on the device reduces risk of skin and tissue injury.

3. Perform hand hygiene and assess skin integrity around the area being treated. Assess skin colour, temperature, sensitivity to touch, blistering, and excessive dryness (see Chapter 8).

   Provides baseline to determine change in skin condition after heat application.

4. Assess patient's level of consciousness and responsiveness.

   Patients with reduced level of consciousness are unable to sense or report reduced sensation or discomfort.

5. Assess patient's comfort level using a pain assessment method that can be understood by the person or caregiver. Consider the patient's age, clinical condition, cognitive or developmental level, literacy, ability to communicate, culture, and ethnicity when using a pain assessment method such as verbal or face picture rating scales or nonverbal indicators of pain (RNAO, 2013). Assess range of motion (ROM) if patient is being treated for muscle sprain.

   Provides baseline to determine if pain relief or improved ROM is achieved.

STEP	RATIONALE

ASSESSMENT

6. Check electrical plugs and cords for obvious fraying or cracking.	Prevents injury from accidental electrical shock.
7. Determine patient's or caregiver's knowledge of procedure, including steps for application and safety precautions.	Heating pads are frequently used in the home. Assessment determines extent of health teaching required.

NURSING DIAGNOSES

- Acute pain
- Chronic pain
- Insufficient knowledge regarding heat
- application
- Reduced physical mobility
- Reduced skin integrity
- Reduced peripheral tissue perfusion
- Potential for injury

Related factors/Risk factors are individualized on the basis of patient's condition or needs.

PLANNING

1. Expected outcomes following completion of procedure:	
• Skin is pink and warm to touch after application.	Vasodilation from heat exposure increases blood flow to affected part.
• Patient reports increased ROM and a decrease in pain of inflamed tissues or strained muscles.	Thermoreceptors are activated by changes in skin temperature. Superficial heat increases joint mobility by increasing connective tissue extensibility, reducing pain, and tissue viscosity (LeBlanc, 2018).
• Patient or caregiver correctly applies pad.	Measures level of understanding necessary for safe home care.
2. Prepare equipment and supplies.	Organization of supplies prevents unnecessary delays in procedure.
3. Explain procedure, purpose, and precautions.	Improves likelihood of patient's adherence to therapy.

IMPLEMENTATION

1. Close room door and close bedside curtains.	Provides for patient's privacy.
2. Perform hand hygiene, apply clean gloves, and position patient to expose area being treated.	Reduces transfer of microorganisms. Patient must be able to assume position for several minutes during application.
3. Apply heat therapy.	
a. Aquathermia heating pad:	
(1) Cover or wrap area to be treated with single layer of bath towel or enclose pad with a pillowcase.	Prevents heated surface from touching patient's skin directly and increasing risk for injury to patient's skin.

Clinical Decision Point *Do not pin wrap to the pad because this may cause a leak in the device.*

(2) Place pad over the affected area and secure it with tape, a tie, or gauze as needed (see illustration).	Pad delivers dry, warm heat to injured tissues. Pad should not slip onto a different body part.

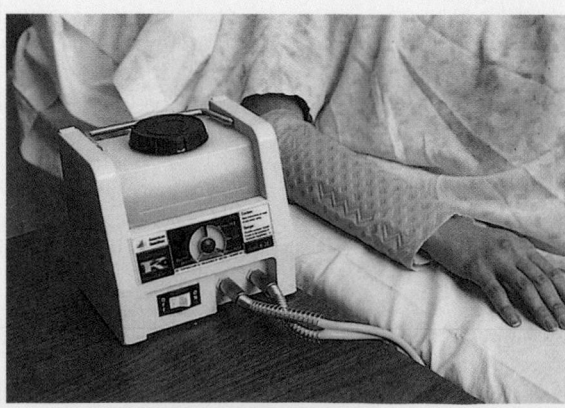

STEP 3a(2) Aquathermia pad.

STEP	RATIONALE

IMPLEMENTATION

(3) Turn on aquathermia unit and check temperature setting. Temperature of unit is usually set by employer's bioengineering department.	Prevents exposure of patient to temperature extremes.
b. Apply commercially prepared heat pack (follow manufacturer guidelines to break pouch inside the larger pack).	Activates chemicals within pack to warm outer surface.

Clinical Decision Point *Never position the patient to lie directly on the heating device. This position prevents dissipation of heat and increases risk for burns.*

4. Remove and dispose of gloves; perform hand hygiene.	Reduces transmission of microorganisms.
5. Monitor skin condition over site every 5 minutes and ask patient about sensation of burning.	Determines if heat exposure is causing any burn, blistering, or injury to underlying skin.
6. After no more than 20 minutes (or time prescribed by health care provider), perform hand hygiene, apply clean gloves, and remove pad and store it.	Rebound phenomenon, in which the opposite effect begins, occurs after maximum therapeutic effect is achieved. Maximum vasodilation from heat occurs in 20–30 minutes (LeBlanc, 2018).
7. Assist patient to preferred position, dispose of soiled linen and gloves, and perform hand hygiene.	Promotes comfort. Reduces transmission of microorganisms.

EVALUATION

1. Inspect condition of skin for integrity, colour, temperature, dryness, and blistering. Evaluate again 30 minutes following treatment.	Evaluates response of skin to heat exposure.
2. Evaluate ROM. Assess comfort level using a pain assessment method that can be understood by the patient or caregiver. Consider the patient's age, clinical condition, cognitive or developmental level, literacy, ability to communicate, culture, and ethnicity when using a pain assessment method such as verbal or face picture rating scales or nonverbal indicators of pain (RNAO, 2013).	Heat reduces edema and relieves pain from muscle stiffness and spasm (Denegar et al., 2018).

Clinical Decision Point *Instruct the patient not to actively exercise the muscle to evaluate results of therapy. Active exercise can aggravate muscle strain.*

3. Use Teach-Back: "I want to be sure I explained how to safely use a heating pad at home. Explain to me why a layer of cloth between the pad and your skin is important." Develop a revised teaching plan if patient or caregiver is unable to teach back correctly.	Determines patient's and caregiver's level of understanding of safe application of a heating pad.

Unexpected Outcomes
1. See Skill 41.1, Unexpected Outcomes.
2. Body part remains painful to move.

3. Patient or caregiver applies heat incorrectly or is unable to explain precautions.

Related Interventions

- Discontinue aquathermia pad or heat pack use.
- Observe for localized swelling.
- Notify health care provider.
- Reinstruct patient or caregiver as necessary. Consider possible home health referral.

Communication and Documentation

- Document appearance and condition of skin, degree of ROM of affected part, type of application, temperature and duration of therapy, and patient's response on flow sheet in nurses' notes in electronic health record (EHR) or chart.
- Document evaluation of patient and caregiver learning.
- Report increased pain, reduced ROM, burn, blistering, or other injury to the skin to health care provider.

Special Considerations
Teaching

- Highlight safety precautions during the procedure so these will be followed by the patient or caregiver.
- Instruct patient and caregiver not to use the highest setting and check frequently for redness or blistering on the skin exposed to the heating device.

Pediatric
- Infants and children have skin that is thin and fragile and therefore easily damaged. Use special caution in this population (Hockenberry & Wilson, 2015) when using dry heat therapy. Remain with children during the procedure for safety and effectiveness.

Gerontological
- Older persons are more at risk for burns because of loss of heat sensation and they have thin, fragile skin that is susceptible to burns.
- Check site frequently during all treatments.

Care in the Community
- Assess patient's and caregiver's understanding of and ability and motivation to adhere to procedure.
- Assess home environment for safety of facilities (e.g., condition of electrical outlets and equipment).
- Discourage use of a conventional heating pad. However, if the patient has limited resources and chooses to use this pad at home, instruct them on all safety precautions.

♦ SKILL 41.3 Application of Cold

A variety of cold (cryotherapy) modalities such as ice packs, moist cold compresses, chemical cold packs, electromechanical or compression devices, or cold-soak immersion of a body part are available. Cold therapy treats localized inflammatory responses that lead to edema, hemorrhage, muscle spasm, or pain (see Table 41.1). Improvement to joint mobility following cold therapy is related to facilitating mobility, relieving pain, inhibiting muscle spasm, and reducing muscle tension (Denegar et al., 2018).

Cold exerts a profound physiological effect on the body, reducing inflammation caused by injuries to soft tissue and the musculoskeletal system (APTA, 2019). Cold is one step in the PRICE principle (i.e., the acronym used in treating sprains and strains) (Maughan, 2018). The overall goal of the PRICE principle is to limit the amount of swelling at the injury site and promote healing:
- P—Protect from further injury
- R—Restrict/Rest activity
- I—Apply Ice
- C—Apply Compression
- E—Elevate injured area

Vasoconstriction resulting from cold application reduces blood flow to the injured part and thus reduces fluid accumulation and slows bleeding and hematoma formation associated with trauma. The lower temperature also suppresses muscle spasm and produces a local anaesthetic response (Denegar et al., 2018; Hannon & Porth, 2017). Cold applications produce maximal analgesia, control the inflammatory response, decrease nerve conduction, and improve mobility (da Costa Santos et al., 2015).

A cold compress usually consists of a commercial cold pack or a gauze dressing or washcloth that has been immersed in iced or chilled solution to achieve the desired temperature. Although a clean compress is most common, open wounds require sterile applications. The size or thickness of gauze depends on the site of injury. For example, a cold compress to the eye requires thicker gauze that fits a small area to maintain a cold temperature. Thin gauze works more effectively for larger areas such as the face.

Ice bags and cold packs come in a variety of sizes to fit different body parts (Fig. 41.4). When a commercial ice bag or cold pack is unavailable, use a plastic bag or glove filled halfway with crushed ice. Squeeze the bag or glove to expel the air, which hampers cold conduction. Wrap all of these items in a towel or cloth before application.

Electrically controlled continuous cold-flow therapy devices simultaneously provide cold and compression (e.g., Cryo/Cuff [Fig. 41.5]). Compression acts with cold to reduce the blood flow and edema formation while providing support to the soft tissues. The

cooling pad has the advantage of delivering a constant cool temperature. Elevating the extremity during treatment further augments venous return. Treatment with one of these devices provides all components of the PRICE method for managing this type of injury (APTA, 2019).

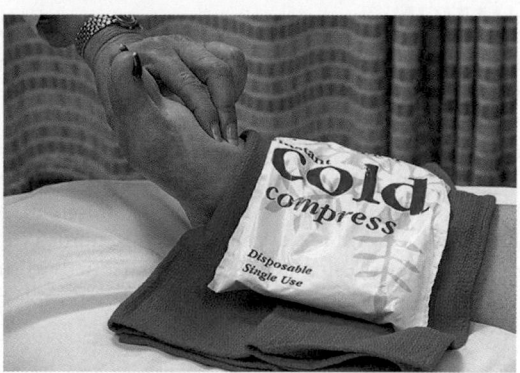

FIG 41.4 Commercial ice pack.

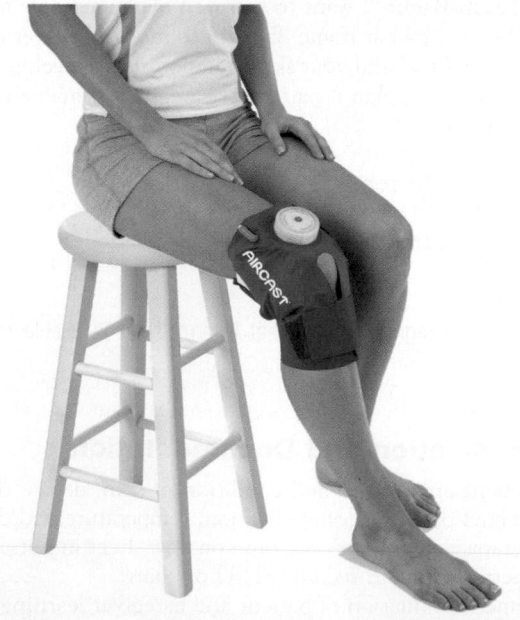

FIG 41.5 Cryo/Cuff includes integrated cooler. (*Image of AirCast Cryo/Cuff used with permission of DJO Global.*)

Delegation and Collaboration

The skill of applying cold applications may be delegated to an unregulated care provider (UCP) (see employer policy). The nurse must assess and evaluate the patient and explain the purpose of the treatment. If there are risks or possible complications, this skill cannot be delegated. The nurse instructs the UCP to:

- Keep the application in place for only the time specified in the health care provider's prescription.
- Immediately report to the nurse any excessive redness on the skin, increase in pain, or decrease in sensation.
- Report when treatment is completed so the nurse can evaluate the patient's response.

Equipment
All Compresses, Bags, and Packs
- Clean gloves (if blood or body fluids are present)
- Cloth tape or ties or elastic wrap bandage
- Soft cloth cover: towel, pillowcase, or stockinette
- Bath towel or blanket and waterproof pad

Cold Compress
- Absorbent gauze (clean or sterile) folded to desired size
- Basin
- Prescribed solution at desired temperature

Ice Bag or Gel Pack
- Ice bag
- Ice chips and water or
- Reusable or disposable commercial gel pack (cold pack)

Electrically Controlled Cooling Device
- Cool water-flow pad or cooling pad and electrical pump
- Gauze roll or elastic wrap

STEP	RATIONALE
ASSESSMENT	
1. Identify patient using at least two person-specific identifiers (e.g., name and date of birth or name and medical record number), according to employer policy.	Ensures correct patient. Complies with Accreditation Canada's standards and improves patient safety (Accreditation Canada, 2019).
2. Refer to health care provider's prescription for type, location, and duration of application. Temperature of the cooling pad will be prescribed or preset.	A health care provider's prescription is required for all cold applications in most facilities (e.g., hospitals, long-term care).
3. Perform hand hygiene and inspect condition of the injured or affected part. Gently palpate area for edema (apply clean gloves if there is risk of exposure to body fluids).	Reduces transmission of microorganisms. Provides baseline for determining change in condition of injured tissues.
Clinical Decision Point *Keep injured part in alignment and immobilized. Movement can cause further injury to strains, sprains, or fractures.*	
4. Perform neurovascular check and inspect surrounding skin for integrity, presence of pulses, colour, temperature, and sensitivity to touch (see Chapter 8).	Determines if patient is insensitive to cold extremes, which increases risk for injury.
5. Consider time elapsed since injury occurred.	Apply cold therapy as soon as possible after injury to reduce swelling, inflammation, tissue bleeding, and pain (Brooks & Hergenroeder, 2017; Maughan, 2018).
6. Assess patient's level of consciousness and responsiveness.	Patients with reduced level of consciousness are unable to sense or report reduced sensation or discomfort.
7. Assess patient's comfort level using an appropriate pain assessment method (see employer policy). Assess range of movement (ROM) of affected part if muscle sprain is involved.	Provides baseline for determining pain relief and ROM with therapy.
8. Review medical history for conditions that contraindicate cold therapy: peripheral vascular diseases (e.g., Raynaud's disease, diabetic neuropathy, rheumatoid arthritis, frostbite).	These conditions increase risk for skin and tissue injury when exposed to cold.
9. Assess patient's or caregiver's understanding and knowledge of procedure.	Cold applications are frequently used at home. Determines extent of instruction required.

NURSING DIAGNOSES

- Acute pain
- Chronic pain
- Reduced peripheral tissue perfusion
- Insufficient knowledge regarding cold application
- Reduced physical mobility
- Potential for injury

Related factors/Risk factors are individualized on the basis of patient's condition or needs.

STEP	RATIONALE

PLANNING

1. Expected outcomes following completion of procedure:

- Affected area is slightly pale and cool to touch.

Result of vasoconstriction.

- There is decreased edema, bleeding, or both in tissues at site of injury.

Cold reduces blood flow to the affected part by reducing protein extravasation from vasculature and subsequent edema formation (Brooks & Hergenroeder, 2017).

- Patient reports or shows evidence of decreased pain as determined by an appropriate pain assessment method.

Cold creates a localized analgesic effect by decreasing local swelling, reducing the inflammatory response, and decreasing nerve conduction (Brooks & Hergenroeder, 2017).

- Patient's ROM increases.

Cold reduces swelling.

- Patient or caregiver correctly states how to apply cold and provides demonstration.

Measures level of understanding necessary for safe home care.

2. Prepare equipment and supplies.

Organization prevents unnecessary delays.

3. Explain procedure and precautions.

Improves likelihood of adherence to therapy.

IMPLEMENTATION

1. Close room door and bedside curtain. Perform hand hygiene and apply clean gloves.

Provides privacy for patient. Reduces spread of microorganisms.

2. Position patient to keep body part in proper alignment and only expose area to be treated; drape patient with bath blankets.

Prevents further injury to body part. Avoids unnecessary exposure of body parts, maintaining patient's comfort and privacy.

3. Place towel or absorbent pad under area to be treated.

Prevents soiling of bed linen.

4. Apply cold compress:

  a. Place ice and water in basin and test temperature on inner aspect of arm.

Extreme temperature can cause tissue damage.

  b. Submerge gauze into basin filled with cold solution; wring out excess moisture.

Excess moisture is uncomfortable to patient.

  c. Apply compress to affected area, moulding it gently over site.

Ensures that cold is directed over site of injury.

  d. Remove, remoisten, and reapply to maintain temperature as needed.

Ensures consistency of treatment.

5. Apply ice pack or bag:

  a. Fill bag with water, secure cap, and invert.

Ensures that there are no leaks.

  b. Empty water and fill bag two-thirds full with small ice chips and water.

Partially filled bag is easier to mould over body part.

  c. Express excess air from bag, secure bag closure, and wipe bag dry.

Excess air interferes with cold conduction. Allows bag to conform to area and promotes maximum contact.

  d. Squeeze or knead commercial ice pack according to manufacturer's directions.

Releases alcohol-based solution to create cold temperature.

  e. Wrap pack or bag with single layer of towel, a pillowcase, or stockinette. Apply over injury. Secure with tape as needed.

Protects patient's tissue and absorbs condensation. Prevents direct exposure of cold against patient's skin.

6. Apply commercial gel pack:

  a. Remove from freezer.

  b. Wrap pack with a towel, pillowcase, or stockinette. Apply pack directly over injury.

Protects patient's tissue and absorbs condensation. Prevents direct exposure of cold against patient's skin.

  c. Secure with gauze, cloth tape, or ties as needed.

Clinical Decision Point *Do not reapply the ice pack to red or bluish areas; continual use of the ice pack increases ischemia.*

7. Apply electrically controlled cooling device:

  a. Prepare device following manufacturer's directions. Some devices are gravity-fed and require you to manually fill with iced water. Motorized units circulate chilled water.

Ensures safe temperature application.

STEP	RATIONALE

IMPLEMENTATION

b. Make sure that all connections are intact and the temperature, if adjustable, is set (see employer policy).

Ensures safe temperature application.

c. Wrap cooling device in a single layer of towel or pillowcase.

Prevents adverse reactions from cold such as burn or frostbite.

d. Wrap cooling device around body part.

Ensures even application of cold temperature.

e. Turn device on and check correct temperature. Temperature is usually preset in health care settings (see employer policy).

Ensures effective therapy. Preset temperature reduces risk of skin and tissue injury.

f. Secure with elastic wrap bandage, gauze roll, or ties.

Ensures cold is distributed to the correct body part.

8. Remove and dispose of gloves in a proper container. Perform hand hygiene.

Reduces transmission of microorganisms.

9. Check condition of skin every 5 minutes for duration of application.

Determines if there are adverse reactions to cold (e.g., mottling, redness, burning, blistering, numbness).

a. If area is edematous, sensation may be reduced; use extra caution during cold therapy and assess site more often.

b. Numbness and tingling are common sensations with cold applications and indicate adverse reactions only when severe and coupled with other symptoms. Stop treatment if the patient experiences a burning sensation or the skin begins to feel numb.

When applying cold, the skin will initially feel cold, followed by relief of pain. As cryotherapy continues, the patient will feel a burning sensation, pain, and finally numbness.

10. After 20 minutes (or as prescribed), perform hand hygiene, apply clean gloves, remove compress or pad, and gently dry off any moisture.

Drying prevents maceration of skin.

Clinical Decision Point *Areas with little body fat (e.g., knee, ankle, and elbow) do not tolerate cold as well as fatty areas (e.g., thigh and buttocks). For bony areas decrease time of cold application.*

11. Assist patient to a comfortable position.

Maintains comfort.

12. Remove and dispose of supplies. Dispose of soiled linen and gloves. Perform hand hygiene.

Reduces transmission of microorganisms.

EVALUATION

1. Inspect affected area for integrity, colour, temperature, and sensitivity to touch. Re-evaluate 30 minutes after the procedure.

Determines reaction to cold application.

2. Palpate affected area gently for edema, bruising, and bleeding (apply gloves if there is risk of exposure to body fluids).

Determines effectiveness of treatment and development of skin or tissue injury.

3. Assess the patient's comfort level using an appropriate pain assessment method (see employer policy).

Determines if pain has been relieved.

4. Measure ROM of affected body part.

Determines if edema or muscle spasm is decreased.

5. **Use Teach-Back:** "I want to be sure I showed you how to apply an ice pack. Show me how to apply an ice pack." Develop a revised teaching plan if patient or caregiver is unable to teach back correctly.

Determines patient's and caregiver's level of understanding of safe application of an ice pack.

Unexpected Outcomes	Related Interventions
1. Skin appears mottled, reddened, or bluish after exposure to cold.	Stop treatment. Notify health care provider.
2. Patient reports burning pain and numbness.	Stop therapy. Notify health care provider.
3. Patient or caregiver is unable to describe or demonstrate therapy.	Provide further instruction and demonstration.

Communication and Documentation

- Document appearance and condition of the skin and affected body part; procedure, including type, location, and duration of application; and patient's response on flow sheet in nurses' notes in electronic health record (EHR) or chart.
- Document evaluation of patient and caregiver learning.
- Report sensations of burning, numbness, or unrelieved skin colour changes to health care provider.

Special Considerations
Teaching

- Injuries requiring this type of therapy usually occur outside of acute care settings. Patients at risk for injury such as those active in sports should know how to minimize the extent of injury using cold.

Pediatric

- A greater metabolic rate and larger trunk in relation to the rest of the body make children more prone to hypothermia (Hockenberry & Wilson, 2015).
- Infants have an immature temperature control mechanism; thus mottling of extremities is common and does not always indicate an adverse reaction (Hockenberry & Wilson, 2015).
- Cool soaks decrease itching with some skin lesions.
- The same precautions and play techniques as with warm soaks may be useful in cold therapy with children.

Gerontological

- Older persons are more at risk for tissue damage because of altered responses to change in body temperature; therefore, they need frequent skin assessment during treatment (Touhy et al., 2019).

✦ SKILL 41.4   Caring for Patients Requiring Hypothermia or Hyperthermia Blankets

A hypothermia or hyperthermia blanket raises, lowers, or maintains body temperature through conductive heat or cold transfer between the blanket and the patient (Fig. 41.6) Adjusting body temperature using a hypothermia or hyperthermia blanket must be carefully controlled to avoid overwhelming the body's thermoregulatory center and cardiopulmonary functions. Because oral temperatures are inaccurate in circumstances of vasoconstriction and sluggish blood flow, the patient's temperature is continuously monitored with a special thermistor probe capable of measuring core temperatures as low as 25°C (Hannon & Porth, 2017).

Patients may develop high, prolonged fevers from infectious neurological diseases, as adverse effects of anaesthesia, and following severe brain injury. Induced hypothermia prevents or moderates neurological outcomes following neurosurgery, traumatic brain injury, and acute stroke (Rittenberger & Callaway, 2018). Therapeutic hypothermia decreases cerebral metabolic rate and oxygen demand and has been found to improve neurological outcomes and survival (Moeller & Webber, 2017). The Canadian Cardiovascular Critical Care Society and the Canadian Association of Interventional Cardiology recommend a temperature range of 33–36° C (96.8–104° F) for targeted temperature management (Wong, van Diepen, Ainsworth, et al., 2017).

Following severe trauma or major surgery such as cardiac surgery, thermoregulation is essential. Hypothermia causes vasoconstriction, shivering, increased oxygen demand, altered coronary blood flow, cardiac dysrhythmias, acid–base imbalances, and impaired coagulation. Rapid rewarming can be life-threatening. Interventions to progressively raise body temperature should be directed by an experienced health care provider and focused on heat retention, restoration of normal core temperature, and tissue preservation (Zieber, 2018).

Delegation and Collaboration

The skill of applying a hypothermia or hyperthermia blanket cannot be delegated to an unregulated care provider (UCP). The nurse is responsible for assessing and evaluating treatment and related patient education. The nurse instructs the UCP to:

- Maintain proper temperature of the blanket throughout the treatment and discontinue the therapy as specified in the health care provider's prescription.
- Report any unexpected patient outcomes (e.g., shivering or redness to the skin) to the nurse.
- Inform the nurse when treatment is completed to evaluate patient response to treatment.

Equipment

- Hypothermia or hyperthermia blanket with control panel and rectal probe
- Sheet or thin bath blanket
- Distilled water to fill the unit if necessary
- Clean gloves
- Rectal thermometer

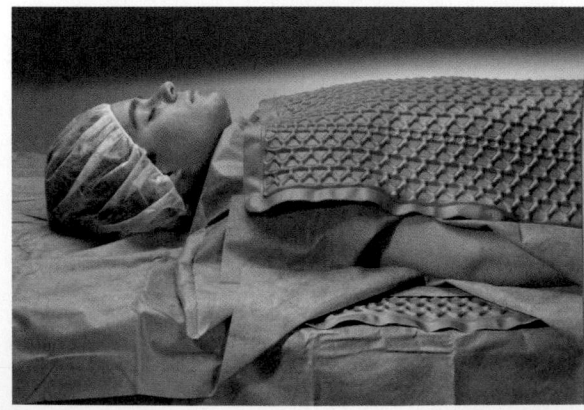

FIG 41.6 Hypothermia cooling blanket is applied over a paper sheet before additional top sheet is applied to bed. (*Courtesy Cincinnati SubZero Maxi-Therm Hyper-Hypothermia Blanket.*)

STEP	RATIONALE

ASSESSMENT

1. Identify patient using at least two person-specific identifiers (e.g., name and date of birth or name and medical record number), according to employer policy.	Ensures correct patient. Complies with Accreditation Canada's standards and improves patient safety (Accreditation Canada, 2019).
2. Refer to health care provider's prescription and check that patient's current body temperature indicates use of hypothermia or hyperthermia blanket.	Instituting therapy requires a health care provider's prescription.
3. Perform hand hygiene. Obtain vital signs and assess neurological status, mental status, and peripheral circulation.	Establishes baseline data to use for comparison during therapy.
4. Verify that other, less intensive measures are not able to restore the patient's body temperature to the desired level.	Use of a hypothermia or hyperthermia blanket is not without risk and should be instituted only when other measures are not effective.

Clinical Decision Point *Antipyretic therapy may be used in combination with a cooling blanket. Very high fevers at temperatures greater than 41°C (105.8°F) damage parenchymal cells throughout the body, particularly in the brain, which may result in irreversible neuron damage (Hannon & Porth, 2017; Zieber, 2018).*

5. Assess patient's skin on the chest and extremities, with close attention to bony prominences such as hands and feet.	Areas that are more exposed to the blanket are at greater risk for skin and tissue injury. Baseline data enable determination if skin injury or development of pressure injury is the result of therapy.

NURSING DIAGNOSES

- Hyperthermia
- Hypothermia
- Reduced peripheral tissue perfusion
- Reduced skin integrity
- Potential for skin injury

Related factors/Risk factors are individualized on the basis of patient's condition or needs.

PLANNING

1. Expected outcomes following completion of procedure:	
• Temperature is within normal range.	Indicates that therapy is effective.
• Absence of shivering with hypothermia blanket.	Shivering increases metabolic rate, heat production, and oxygen consumption. Shivering also causes vasoconstriction, which can injure skin of distal body regions (Rittenberger & Callaway, 2018).
• Skin does not show signs of injury or burns.	Indicates that treatment is not causing adverse effects.
2. Explain procedure and precautions to patient or caregiver.	Increases cooperation with treatment and reduces anxiety.
3. Prepare blanket according to employer policy, manufacturer instructions, and prescription. Manufacturer instructions are usually located on the machine.	Facilities have specific policies on maintaining and using equipment. Ensures correct and safe use of equipment.

IMPLEMENTATION

1. Perform hand hygiene and apply clean gloves. Position patient comfortably.	Reduces transmission of microorganisms.
2. Turn on blanket and observe that cool or warm light is on. Set the blanket temperature to desired level.	Verifies that blanket is set correctly for prescribed therapy to reduce or increase patient's body temperature.
3. Verify that blanket temperature limits are set at desired safety ranges.	Safety ranges prevent excessive cooling or warming. Blanket automatically shuts off when preset body temperature is achieved.
4. Cover hypothermia or hyperthermia blanket with thin paper, a cloth sheet, or bath blanket.	A thin covering prevents direct contact with the blanket, thus reducing risk for injury to skin. Covering provides insulation between the patient and appliance and protects skin from contact with the plastic blanket.
5. Position hypothermia or hyperthermia blanket following manufacturer directions.	Provides distribution of blanket against patient's skin.
a. Wrap patient's hands and feet in gauze.	Reduces risk for thermal injury to distal areas of body.
b. Wrap scrotum with towels.	Protects sensitive tissue from direct contact with cold or heat.

STEP	RATIONALE

IMPLEMENTATION

6. Continuously monitor patient's temperature using a thermistor probe according to the blanket manufacturer directions.	Accurate and continuous monitoring of the patient's core interior temperature is required during warming or cooling to prevent overwhelming thermoregulation mechanisms and cardiopulmonary functions.
7. Turn and position patient regularly to protect from pressure injury development and impaired body alignment (see Chapter 11). Keep linens free of perspiration and condensation.	Reduces risk for pressure injury development due to skin moisture created by blanket and patient's body temperature.
8. Double-check fluid thermometer on control panel of blanket before leaving room.	Verifies that blanket temperature is maintained at desired level.
9. Remove gloves and perform hand hygiene.	Reduces transmission of microorganisms.

EVALUATION

1. Monitor patient's temperature and vital signs every 15 minutes during the first hour of therapy. Evaluate automatic temperature control thereafter every 30 minutes visually and every 4 hours by assessing the patient's temperature.	Provides continuous evaluation of patient's response to therapy during initial and continual therapy. Ensures appropriate discontinuation of treatment when the patient's temperature reaches desired level. Decreases risk for subnormal body temperature. Verifies accuracy of thermistor probe and automatic temperature control device.
2. Observe skin for indications of burns, change in colour, and other injury.	Hypothermia and hyperthermia blankets have the potential to cause skin injuries.
3. Observe patient for signs of shivering.	Early signs of shivering, which may result in negative outcomes, include electrocardiographic changes, facial muscle twitching, or hyperventilation.
4. Determine patient's level of comfort.	Prompt assessment reduces risk for severe injuries.
5. **Use Teach-Back:** "I want to be sure I explained why this blanket is important for your loved one's care. Tell me why we are using the blanket." Develop revised teaching if caregiver is not able to teach back correctly.	Determines caregiver's level of understanding about the purpose of the blanket.

Unexpected Outcomes

1. Patient's core body temperature decreases or rises rapidly. This indicates that temperature is extreme and may result in injury to patient.

2. Patient's core temperature remains unchanged.

3. Patient begins to shiver. Shivering increases metabolic rate and heat production, causing patient's core body temperature to rise, and increases oxygen consumption.

Related Interventions

- Adjust blanket temperature no more than 0.6°C (1°F) every 15 minutes to avoid complications.
- Report temperature changes to health care provider.
- Patient may need hypothermic or hyperthermic treatment to axilla, groin, and neck in addition to those areas covered by blanket.
- Discuss use of antipyretic with health care provider.
- Adjust temperature range and assess if shivering decreases.
- If shivering continues, stop treatment and notify health care provider.

Communication and Documentation

- Document baseline data: vital signs, neurological and mental status, peripheral circulation, and skin integrity when therapy was initiated. Include type of hyperthermia-hypothermia unit; control settings (manual or automatic and temperature settings); temperature monitoring method, date, time, and duration; and patient's response to treatment in nurses' notes in electronic health record (EHR) or chart.
- Document repeated measurements of vital signs on temperature graphic EHR or chart to document response to therapy.
- Document evaluation of caregiver learning.
- Report any unexpected outcome to health care provider.

Special Considerations

Teaching

- Instruct patients and their families not to move the patient off the blanket.

Pediatric

- Infants have an immature temperature-control mechanism; thus mottling of extremities is common and does not always indicate an adverse reaction (Hockenberry & Wilson, 2015).

Gerontological

- Some older persons are more at risk for tissue damage because of loss of cold sensation. Check patient frequently during all treatments (Touhy et al., 2019).

◆ CLINICAL DEBRIEF

The nurse is assigned to care for a 58-year-old patient with diabetes mellitus who is postoperative day 1 following total left knee arthroplasty. The patient has type 1 diabetes mellitus that is regulated with insulin. The surgeon prescribed an electronically controlled cold compression cuff to be applied to the left knee for 2 to 3 hours, followed by a 1- to 2-hour break with compression loosened. The patient is receiving oral pain medication every 4 hours for pain.

1. Place in correct order how the nurse will begin the cold application. Explain your choice(s).
   1. Refer to the health care provider's prescription for location and duration of the application.
   2. Explain the procedure and precautions to the patient to avoid injury to the skin.
   3. Assess condition of the injured or affected body part.
   4. Assess the patient's current pain level.
2. What is the major risk associated with cold application for this patient and how should the nurse assess for this risk?
3. After 24 hours of intermittent cold therapy using a compression cuff, the patient reports a burning sensation and the nurse observes a reddened 2-cm area and a blister on his skin under the compression cuff. The left leg is warm with normal colour and pulses present distal to the compression cuff. The patient denies incisional pain and the incision is clean and intact. Show how the nurse should communicate with the health care team about this patient, using SBAR.

◆ REVIEW QUESTIONS

1. Which of the following situations would place a patient at risk for injury from heat application? *(Select all that apply.)*
   1. Acute ankle sprain
   2. A large amount of body fat
   3. Receiving treatment for anxiety
   4. Peripheral vascular disease
   5. Skin lesions
   6. Altered sensation
2. The nurse is preparing to apply an electronically cooled device to a patient's shoulder. Place the following steps in the correct sequence.
   1. Place cooling pad in a pillowcase or wrap in a towel.
   2. Assess patient's level of pain.
   3. Secure device with elastic bandage or roll.
   4. Turn device on and check correct temperature.
   5. Apply device to patient's shoulder.
3. A patient placed on a hypothermia blanket develops shivering and an increased temperature. Which of the following body responses are associated with an increase in temperature?
   1. Increases oxygen consumption
   2. Causes vasoconstriction
   3. Increases metabolic demand
   4. Increases amount of heat lost
   5. Increases body temperature

ⓔ *Visit the Evolve site for a complete list of Clinical Debrief and Review Questions answers.*

REFERENCES

Accreditation Canada. (2019). *Required organizational practices handbook—Version 14.* Ottawa, ON: Author. Retrieved from http://www.wrha.mb.ca/quality/files/2019ROPHandbook.pdf

American Physical Therapy Association (APTA). (2019). *The physical therapist scope of practice.* Retrieved from http://www.apta.org/ScopeOfPractice/

Arankalle, D., Wardle, J., & Nair, P. M. K. (2016). Alternate hot and cold application in the management of heel pain. *The Foot, 29,* 25–28. doi:10.1016/j.foot.2016.09.007

Bech, M., Moorhe, J., Cho, M., Lavergne, M. R., Stothers, K., & Hoens, A. M. (2015). Device or ice: The effect of consistent cooling using a device compared with intermittent cooling using an ice bag after total knee arthroplasty. *Physiotherapy Canada, 67*(1), 48–55. doi:10.3138/ptc.2013-78

Brooks, G., & Hergenroeder, A. (2017). Musculoskeletal injury in children and skeletally immature adolescents: Overview of treatment principles for nonoperative injuries. *UpToDate.* Retrieved from https://www.uptodate.com/contents/musculoskeletal-injury-in-children-and-skeletally-immature-adolescents-overview-of-treatment-principles-for-nonoperative-injuries

Canadian Nurses Association (CNA). (2011). *Position statement: Interprofessional collaboration.* Retrieved from https://www.cna-aiic.ca/-/media/cna/page-content/pdf-en/interproffessional-collaboration_position-statement.pdf

Canadian Physiotherapy Association (CPA). (2012). *Position statement: Inter-professional collaboration and practice.* Retrieved from https://physiotherapy.ca/sites/default/files/positionstatements/inter-professional-collaboration_en.pdf

da Costa Santos, V., dos Santos Cardoso, C., Figueiredo, C. P., & de Souza Guerino Macedo, C. (2015). Effect of cryotherapy on the ankle temperature in athletes: Ice pack and cold water immersion. *Fisioterapia em Movimento, 28*(1), 23–30. doi:10.1590/0103-5150.028.001.AO02

Denegar, C. R., Saliba, E., & Saliba, S. (2018). *Therapeutic modalities for musculoskeletal injuries* (4th ed.). Windsor, ON: Human Kinetics.

Giger, J. (2017). *Transcultural nursing: Assessment and interventions* (7th ed.). St. Louis: Mosby.

Hannon, R. A., & Porth, C. M. (2017). *Pathophysiology: Concepts of altered health states* (2nd Canadian ed.). Philadelphia: Wolters Kluwer.

Hockenberry, M. J., & Wilson, D. (2015). *Wong's nursing care of infants and children* (10th ed.). St. Louis: Elsevier.

LeBlanc, K. (2018). Skin integrity and wound care. In B. J. Kozier, G. Erb, A. T. Berman, et al. (Eds.), *Fundamentals of Canadian nursing: Concepts, process and practice* (4th Canadian ed., pp. 930–982). Don Mills, ON: Pearson Canada. Chapter 35.

Li, Z., & Wang, Q. (2016). Ice compresses aid the reduction of swelling and pain after scleral buckling surgery. *Journal of Clinical Nursing, 25*(21–22), 3261–3265. doi:10.1111/jocn.13362

Maeda, T., Yoshida, H., & Sasaki, T. (2017). Does transcutaneous electrical nerve stimulation (TENS) simultaneously combined with local heat and cold applications enhance pain relief compared with TENS alone in patients with knee arthritis? *Journal of Physical Therapy Science, 29*(10), 1860–1864. doi:10.1589/jpts.29.1860

Maughan, K. (2018). Ankle injury. *UpToDate.* Retrieved from https://www.uptodate.com/contents/ankle-sprain

Moeller, A. D., & Webber, J. C. (2017). Adverse effects of therapeutic hypothermia in a 55-year-old man with cardiac arrest. *Canadian Medical Association Journal, 189*(43), E1337–E1340. doi:10.1503/cmaj.170682

Registered Nurses' Association of Ontario (RNAO). (n.d.). *RNAO nursing best practice guidelines. Management of pain: Non-pharmacological interventions.* Retrieved from https://bpgmobile.rnao.ca/node/764

Registered Nurses' Association of Ontario (RNAO). (2013). *Clinical best practice guidelines: Assessment and management of pain* (3rd ed.). Toronto, ON: Author. Retrieved from http://rnao.ca/sites/rnao-ca/files/AssessAndManagementOf-Pain_15_WEB-_FINAL_DEC_2.pdf

Rittenberger, J., & Callaway, C. (2018). Post-cardiac arrest management in adults. *UpToDate.* Retrieved from http://www.uptodate.com/contents/post-cardiac-arrest-management-in-adults

Touhy, T. A., Jett, K. F., Boscart, V., & McCleary, L. (2019). *Ebersole and Hess' gerontological nursing & healthy aging* (2nd Canadian ed.). Toronto: Elsevier Canada.

Wong, G. C., van Diepen, S., Ainsworth, C., et al. (2017). Canadian Cardiovascular Society/Canadian Cardiovascular Critical Care Society/Canadian Association of Interventional Cardiology position statement on the optimal care of the postarrest patient. *The Canadian Journal of Cardiology, 33*(1), 1–16. doi:10.1016/j.cjca.2016.10.021

Xu, Y., Rich, E., & Connor, J. (2016). Culturally based remedies for initial home treatment of acute musculoskeletal injuries. *Medsurg Nursing, 25*(5), 360–364.

Zieber, E. M. P. (2018). Vital signs. In B. Kozier, G. Erb, A. Berman, et al. (Eds.), *Fundamentals of Canadian nursing: Concepts, process and practice* (4th Canadian ed., pp. 630–667). Don Mills, ON: Pearson Canada. Chapter 29.

42 | Safety in the Community

Written by **Nancy LaPlante, PhD, RN, AHN-BC; and Lisa MacNaughton-Doucet, RN, BTHM, MN**

SKILLS AND PROCEDURES

Skill 42.1 **Home Environment Assessment and Safety, p. 1127**

Skill 42.2 **Adapting the Home Setting for Patients With Cognitive Deficits, p. 1137**

Skill 42.3 **Medication and Medical Device Safety, p. 1143**

OBJECTIVES

Mastery of content in this chapter will enable the nurse to:
- Identify patients at risk for safety problems and possible accidents in the home.
- Promote self-care of patients in the home.
- Describe the factors within a home environment that create risks for patient injury.
- Perform a home safety risk assessment.

- Identify interventions that modify the home environment for physical safety.
- Identify interventions to reduce safety risks for persons with sensory, cognitive, and mental status alterations.
- Recommend strategies to ensure safe medication administration within the home.
- Perform a falls risk assessment.

MEDIA RESOURCES

- evolve http://evolve.elsevier.com/Canada/Perry/clinicalskills/

- Review Questions
- Clinical Debrief and Review Questions Answers

PURPOSE

Safety for patients in the community setting includes health promotion and injury prevention (Public Health Agency of Canada [PHAC], 2015a). The home has many safety hazards; the key to preventing home-related injuries is to eliminate risks before any injuries occur (Canada Safety Council, n.d.). Safety in the home begins before a patient is discharged from a health care facility. Nurses need to use interprofessional collaboration to assess the home environment for risks, with a goal of selecting appropriate interventions for preventing unintentional injuries. The patient's health condition is included in the home assessment when applicable.

STANDARDS OF CARE

- Alzheimer's Society of Canada (ASC), 2018e—*Safety in the Home* (http://alzheimer.ca/en/Home/Living-with-dementia/Day-to-day-living/Safety/Safety-in-the-home)
- Canadian Patient Safety Institute (CPSI), 2018—*Home Care Safety* (https://www.patientsafetyinstitute.ca/en/Topic/Pages/Homecare-Safety.aspx)
- Community Health Nurses of Canada (CHNC), 2019—*2019 Canadian Community Health Nursing Professional Practice Model & Standards of Practice* (https://www.chnc.ca/standards-of-practice)
- Parachute, 2019—*Home Safety* (http://www.parachutecanada.org/injury-topics/topic/C13)
- Registered Nurses' Association of Ontario (RNAO), 2017—*Preventing Falls and Reducing Injury From Falls* (3rd ed.) (http://

rnao.ca/sites/rnao-ca/files/bpg/Preventing_Falls_FINAL_WEB.pdf)

PRINCIPLES FOR PRACTICE

- Person-centred care ensures that patients are at the centre of care decisions affecting them (Fazio, Pace, Flinner, et al., 2018).
- Safety in the home involves communication among a patient, caregiver(s), and interprofessional care providers.
- The ultimate goal is to create an environment in which a patient and the caregiver can provide self-care safely and effectively.
- Insurance coverage, including Medicare, can be very limited for services offered in the community. Therefore, the time spent in the home with the patient must be well planned and used to the fullest.
- Patients living in socioeconomically disadvantaged areas may be at increased risk for injury because of violence in their community or poor living conditions.
- Falls prevention is a critical aspect of care for older persons, especially in the community.
- A patient history to assess injury prevention and risk of falls in the home and immediate environment is part of the plan of care.

PERSON-CENTRED CARE

- As a nurse conducting home safety assessments, it is important to respect a person's home, as you are a guest. Take time to listen

to the patient's health concerns and apply the knowledge you have about the person to understand which interventions within the home are likely to be accepted by the person and caregiver.

- Communication is essential and is a continuous process between you and the patient, whether they are in the community or in a facility. At the first meeting introduce yourself, explaining how you would like the patient to address you, and ask the patient how you should refer to them. If a language barrier exists, it may be necessary to request assistance from a translator.

- Collaborate with the patient in assessing their home environment. Ask them if they are willing to give you a tour of their home, and explain the purpose of a tour. Do not focus on what is wrong (e.g., barriers or features in disrepair), rather point out why safety is an issue for the person (based on health condition), and explain why a change in the immediate environment of the home may make them safer.

- Assess for culture-specific health-related beliefs that may impact a patient's willingness to use home care services. For example, an Indigenous person may have a sense of mistrust, reluctance, and suspicion based on previous experiences with residential care systems and authority figures (Gerlach, Browne, & Greenwood, 2017).

- When assessing the availability of caregivers, recognize that families, neighbours, and friends can have valuable roles in caring for the patient. Caregivers may live with the patient, live in the community, or may even live a great distance away. Regardless, all members of the patient's care circle can contribute to the health and safety of the patient living in the community. With the patient's permission, include these caregivers when performing the home safety assessment.

- Assess and provide support for any caregivers; the presence or absence of a caregiver could be the difference between a person remaining in the home or being readmitted to a facility.

EVIDENCE-INFORMED PRACTICE

Safety issues involve extrinsic factors, such as the physical environment, and intrinsic factors that can affect the person's ability to remain at home in a safe environment. In-home safety threats are common and may lead to high rates of mortality, morbidity, and incapacity. They often affect persons from lower socioeconomic groups or ethnic minorities.

Lorainne and colleagues (2017) ranked a top-10 list of safety threats for patients with dementia living at home. These included high economic burden, lack of proper training and qualifications of professional caregivers, lack of caregiver training and education, patient self-neglect, social isolation, forgetting to take medication, unsafe design of the home, patient's poor mobility and falls, caregiver inability to manage the patient, and health deterioration of the caregiver due to the burden of caring. The authors concluded that investment in both professional and caregiver education was a key factor in promoting the well-being of persons living at home with dementia.

SAFETY GUIDELINES

- Injury prevention begins with making timely and adequate home repairs (e.g., replacing loose floor tile, securing railings on stairwells). When patients do not have the resources for maintaining a safe home environment, a nurse's role is to help identify appropriate resources or services in the community.

- The nurse plays an important role in interprofessional collaboration by working within a team of health care providers, family members, and the patient to determine the best approaches for meeting a patient's safety needs.

- The ultimate goal is to create a healthy environment in which the patient can optimize self-care safely and effectively.

- When helping a patient alter their home environment, retain as much of their independence and ability to provide self-care as possible. Ask if the patient or caregiver has concerns or questions about safety and if they have suggestions to improve safety (RNAO, 2017).

- Modifications to the home environment should be made only after collaboration with the interprofessional team (e.g., occupational therapist) and should match the patient's physical strengths, remaining functional abilities, and resources.

✦ SKILL 42.1   Home Environment Assessment and Safety

The home environment should be a place where individuals feel healthy, comfortable, and safe. People want to be able to move about freely within their homes, regardless of the size of the home, and to have a sense of control over daily living routines. This requires maintaining personal space and a sense of privacy. As the nurse, you can help a patient maintain independence and reduce risk in the home environment by conducting a home safety assessment.

Patients requiring care in the community often experience physical alterations (e.g., progressive physical changes of aging) that require modifications in their home environment. For example, if a patient has poor balance but good upper-arm strength, you may need to collaborate with an occupational therapist to make modifications (e.g., install handrails on both sides of a staircase and in the bathroom) so the person can safely walk or move throughout the house, ascend and descend stairs, and enter and exit a bathtub or shower. Teaching a patient to safely use assistive devices (e.g., walker or cane) may help them increase mobility and maintain independence (Fig. 42.1).

Respect the concept of personal space. Making changes too rapidly without a patient's consent causes more problems than benefits. Appreciate the arrangement of a patient's space within the home and do not move things or suggest modifications without permission. Provide a rationale to the patient as to why changes are beneficial or needed. Knowing the rooms that a patient uses most frequently can help in making the adjustments to create a safe environment.

Delegation and Collaboration

As part of interprofessional collaboration, the unregulated care provider (UCP), under the direction of and in collaboration with a regulated health care provider, may contribute to a home safety assessment while maintaining scope-of-practice guidelines and employer regulations.

Equipment

- Home safety checklist

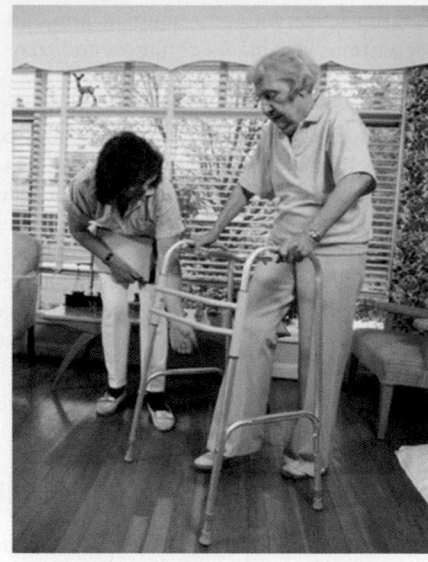

FIG 42.1 Use of a walker may help a patient remain mobile.

STEP	RATIONALE

ASSESSMENT

1. Review risk factors that predispose patients to injuries within the home:

a. Visual impairment

Reduced visual function alters a patient's balance, depth perception, or adaptation to dark or glaring light (Parsons, 2017).

b. Hearing impairment

Prevents patient from hearing normal environmental sounds (e.g., call-out by caregiver). Prevents clear perception of home-installed alarms (e.g., smoke alarm).

Interferes with communication; patient unable to hear clearly and interpret what you are saying (Parsons, 2017).

c. Neuromuscular alterations (e.g., lower-extremity weakness, unsteady gait, impaired balance, poor ankle dorsiflexion)

Age-related changes of the neurological system include slowing of reaction time (Feldman & Landry, 2017). Gait disorders make patients vulnerable to trips and falls (RNAO, 2017).

d. Reduced energy or fatigue

Predisposes patients to falls.

e. Incontinence or nocturia

Frequent trips to the bathroom may cause a patient with other deficits to accidentally trip or fall. Dementia affects the patient's ability to locate the bathroom and recognize the need to void (Saboe Rose, 2018, p. 1345).

f. History of stroke, parkinsonism, delirium, seizures, dementia, syncope

These conditions present multiple reasons for falls (Beghi, Gervasoni, Pupillo, et al., 2018), including impaired gait and coordination, visual changes, diminished cognition, pain, and muscle weakness.

g. Cardiopulmonary conditions: postural hypotension, arrhythmias, palpitations, difficulty breathing, shortness of breath

These conditions present multiple reasons for falls, including dizziness, light-headedness (Jumani & Powell, 2017), fatigue, and unsteady gait.

h. Medication usage and history, including polypharmacy and use of sedatives, antihypertensives, antidepressants, and diuretics

Polypharmacy (use of five or more medications) and medications that alter the patient's sense, balance, and judgement increase risk of falls (Pfaff, 2018, p. 357).

i. History of previous fall—obtain detailed description of previous fall

Increases risk for future fall. Helps identify circumstances that may lead to a fall (RNAO, 2017).

2. Determine if patient has had other injuries within the home, or has had near-falls, slips, and missteps.

Onset, location, and activity associated with a fall provide further details on causative factors and how to prevent future falls (RNAO, 2017).

STEP	RATIONALE

ASSESSMENT

3. Have patient who has had a near fall or actual fall maintain a fall diary (Box 42.1).

Information in a fall diary is very helpful in determining antecedents and consequences of falling (Meiner, 2015).

4. Conduct *Timed Up and Go (TUG)* test for basic mobility (see Skill 14.1).

This simple screening examination is useful in detecting difficulties with balance or gait. Collaborate with the interprofessional team, such as physiotherapist, pharmacist, dietitian, gerontologist, or neurologist, for further assessment (RNAO, 2017). *TUG* is a quick assessment to assess a patient's balance and gait (Buck, 2018, p. 776).

5. Determine if patient has a fear of falling. Indicators while ambulating are apprehension (observed in facial expressions); sweating or trembling; clutching people or objects; reluctance to change position; and wobbly, reduced mobility after fall.

Some patients may restrict mobility and participation in activities of daily living (ADLs) or instrumental activities of daily living (IADLs) because of fear of falling (RNAO, 2017).

Clinical Decision Point *In addition to the patient, include caregivers as a resource in assessments because they may witness accident trends or patterns.*

6. Partner with patient and caregivers to conduct home safety assessment:

Provides comprehensive review of all areas within home that pose hazardous situations.

a. Front and back entrances:

   (1) Are walkways to front and back door even and free from holes or cracks?

Entrances pose barriers in surfaces over which patient must walk. Uneven pavement and holes may not be seen by patient, causing tripping and falls.

   (2) Are home entrances, including walkways, well lit?

Poorly lit areas prevent individuals from seeing variations in walking surface.

   (3) Does patient have nonskid strips and safety treads or bright-coloured paint on outdoor steps? Which colours are most easily seen by patient? Are these colours used?

Nonskid surfaces can help prevent slips on stairs. Colour on steps enables individual to see edges, accommodating for any reduced depth perception.

   (4) Are doormats in good repair with nonskid backing and tapered edge?

Raised edges pose risk for tripping. Doormats without nonskid backing slide when stepped on, causing patient to lose balance.

   (5) Are doors in good repair, and do they open and close easily? Can patient open and close all doors easily?

Opening and closing a door is difficult if grasp is weak. Tripping may occur while opening door and cause a fall.

   (6) Are there sturdy handrails on both sides of stairs leading to entrance?

Handrails are recommended to be on both sides of the hallway and stairs.

   (7) Are steps in good condition with even, flat surfaces?

Uneven surfaces predispose to tripping.

   (8) Are doorways and stairs free of clutter?

Reduces risk for tripping or falling.

b. Kitchen:

The kitchen is one of most hazard-oriented rooms in the home. Poses serious hazards for fire.

   (1) Does patient wear clothing with short or close-fitting sleeves when cooking?

Short or close-fitting sleeves are less likely to accidentally catch on fire when person works at stove.

   (2) Does patient always stay in kitchen when cooking?

Lack of attention when using fire is risk.

   (3) Does patient have a loud timer to signal when food is cooked?

Prevents burning food and risk for fire.

   (4) Does patient keep stove top and oven clean and grease free?

Grease is highly flammable.

   (5) Are stove control dials easy to see and use?

Patient may accidentally use higher flame than is necessary for cooking safely.

   (6) Is charged, easy-to-use fire extinguisher close at hand?

Extinguisher should be ready for use at all times.

BOX 42.1

Fall/Near-Fall Diary

- Keep a notebook and create across the longest edge of the paper these headings: "Date," "Time of Fall," "Activity at Time of Fall," "Symptoms," and "Injury."
- As soon as possible after a fall, have patient or caregiver complete information under each heading.

- List emergency contact numbers at the bottom of the fall diary for the patient to call in case a fall results in serious injury.
- Instruct patient to bring the diary to the health care provider's office at the next scheduled visit or share information with the community care nurse on the next home visit.

Modified from Meiner, S. E. (2015). *Gerontologic nursing* (5th ed.). St. Louis: Mosby.

STEP	RATIONALE

ASSESSMENT

Clinical Decision Point *Have the patient demonstrate steps of how to use a fire extinguisher.*

(7) Are emergency numbers for police, fire, and poison control posted on or near telephone or listed in contacts on cellular phone?	Emergency phone numbers and extinguisher ensure quick response if fire occurs.
(8) Can items in kitchen cabinets and shelves be reached without climbing on a stool or chair?	Climbing on step stools or chairs creates risks for falls.
(9) Is there adequate lighting over the sink, stove, and work areas?	Good lighting makes it easier to see control knobs or dials and increases patient safety when they are using sharp knives or utensils.
(10) Are kitchen throw rugs and mats slip resistant?	Rugs or mats that are not slip resistant can easily slide on tile or wood floors.
(11) Assess food safety: Are perishable foods in the refrigerator and nonperishable foods safe to eat? Is food stored appropriately? Are expiration dates past? Is there evidence that food has spoiled? Does patient know how to prepare and store food safely?	Proper food storage and preparation can prevent foodborne illnesses. One basic of food safety is cooking food to its proper temperature. Foods are properly cooked when they are heated for long enough time and at a high enough temperature to kill harmful bacteria that cause foodborne illness (Government of Canada, 2017a). Eating foods that have spoiled or with expiration dates that have passed puts patient at risk for foodborne illness (e.g., food poisoning).

c. Bathroom:

(1) Can patient unlock the bathroom door from both sides of the door?	Functional locks prevent person from being trapped in bathroom.
(2) Is tub or shower equipped with nonskid mats, abrasive strips, or surfaces that are not slippery?	Bathrooms are hazardous. Tub or shower bottoms can be very slippery, creating risk for falls (PHAC, 2015b).
(3) Does bathroom floor have a nonslip surface or rug with nonskid backing?	Wet floors can create risk for falls.
(4) Does patient avoid using slippery bath oils when bathing?	Use of bath oils makes tub surface slippery and increases risk for falls.
(5) Do bathtub and shower have at least one grab bar or handrail placed where the patient can reach it?	Grab bars provide extra support while manoeuvring into and out of tubs or showers. Grab bars placed correctly where patient can safely reach them help to steady gait and lessen chance of falls (PHAC, 2015b).
(6) Is patient careful not to place towels on grab bars?	Some patients accidentally grab towel instead of bar when needing support. Towel can slip off bar.
(7) Does shower have stable stool or chair and handheld sprayer? Is shower easy to access (walk-in versus step-in to tub area)?	Shower stool allows patient to sit while showering.
(8) Are cold and hot water faucets clearly marked, and is temperature on water heater 48.8°C or lower?	Accidental burns can occur from exposure to hot water.

d. Bedroom:

(1) Is night-light placed in bedroom or bath?	Older persons have altered night vision.
(2) Is a working smoke detector just outside the bedroom door?	Alarm situated just outside bedroom can awaken person early enough to escape fire.
(3) Can patient turn on light without having to get out of bed in the dark? Is a flashlight available at bedside? A flashlight can be attached to a walker or cane.	Getting out of bed without proper lighting or the ability to adjust to light changes and reaching for necessary objects put patient at risk for falls.
(4) Is furniture arranged to provide clear path from bed to bathroom?	Obstructed path creates barrier that causes tripping and falls.
(5) Is phone with emergency numbers within easy reach of bed?	If patients develop physical symptoms while in bed, they need to be able to reach the phone without having to get out of bed.
(6) Are other alarm systems available? Push buttons that call for help? Nursery listening devices for cognitively impaired or nonambulatory patients?	Alarm systems placed in a readily accessible location can alert caregivers when person requires immediate help. Bedside phone, cellular phone, intercom buzzer, or lifeline can be placed in readily accessible location.

STEP	RATIONALE

ASSESSMENT

e. Living room and other rooms:

(1) Are electrical or extension cords removed from under furniture and carpeting? Kept out of the way of traffic?

Patients can easily trip or fall over electrical cords. Hidden cords are trip and fire hazards.

(2) Can patient turn on light without having to walk into a dark room?

Darkened room can disorient and prevent patient from seeing uneven surfaces.

(3) Are hallways and walkways free from objects and clutter?

Objects and clutter in common walkway can cause patient to trip, resulting in falls.

(4) Are loose area rugs securely attached to floor and not placed over carpeting? (For best safety, consider removing throw rugs.)

Loose edges of rugs are easy for persons to trip over.

(5) Is furniture arranged in each room so patient can walk around easily?

Furniture creates obstacles to walking in room.

(6) Is all furniture steady and without sharp edges?

Patients often use edges of furniture for support when standing.

f. Around the house:

(1) Are all living areas and stairways well lit?

Adequate lighting helps people see any barriers or uneven walking surfaces.

(2) Is flooring or carpeting throughout house in good repair?

Frayed carpet or irregular surfaces can cause tripping and result in fall.

(3) Are all thresholds level with floor or no more than 1.25 cm (0.5 inch) in height?

Uneven thresholds can cause tripping.

(4) Is light switch at both top and bottom of stairs?

Prevents individual from having to walk up or down part of stairs in dark.

(5) Does lighting produce glare or shadows on stairs or floor surfaces?

Older persons are sensitive to glare because their visual pathway becomes distorted.

(6) Do handrails run continuously from top to bottom of flights of stairs?

Handrails provide source of physical support when ascending and descending stairs.

(7) Are handrails securely attached to the wall?

Ensure a least one handrail is installed on the stairs. It is recommended that handrails be installed on both sides of the hallway or stairwell to reduce risk of fall (PHAC, 2015a).

(8) Are step coverings in good condition?

Loosened covering can cause tripping.

(9) Are guns kept in the house? Are trigger locks installed on all guns? Are guns stored unloaded? Is ammunition in a secure location?

Following gun safety standards decreases risk for injury and death related to gun use (Government of Canada, 2019).

g. General fire safety:

(1) Does patient have properly working smoke detectors with fresh batteries?

Smoke alarms should be properly located and have batteries checked monthly and replaced annually (Buck, 2018, p. 773).

Clinical Decision Point *Check to see when the smoke-alarm battery was last changed; the battery should be changed annually. Instruct patients to change the battery each time they change their house clocks for daylight savings.*

(2) Does patient have several emergency exit plans in case of fire?

Exit plan helps people anticipate route of escape when fire does occur. Exit should not have locks that are difficult to open or any physical barriers.

(3) Has patient determined a meeting place in event of emergency, such as at mailbox in front of home?

Use of a common emergency meeting location is an efficient method for determining that all members are safely out of the house.

(4) Does patient use portable space heaters? Are they kept at least 1 meter away from flammable items?

Heating equipment was the second most common cause of home fire fatalities from 2007 through 2011 (Statistics Canada, 2017).

(5) Is furnace area free of things that can catch on fire?

Heaters, furnaces, and chimneys pose risks for fire.

(6) Does a qualified professional check the furnace and chimney annually?

Buildup of creosote within the chimney can catch on fire. An overheated motor in the furnace can burn out and possibly cause fire.

(7) Does patient who smokes report smoking in bed?

Approximately 60% of residential fires are caused by smoking and cooking (Statistics Canada, 2017). Smoking in bed has added risk of patient falling asleep while cigarette is lit.

STEP	RATIONALE

ASSESSMENT

h. General electrical safety:

(1) Are electrical cords in good condition (i.e., not frayed, spliced, or cracked)?

Damaged cords can short circuit and lead to fire.

(2) Are electrical cords kept away from water?

Use of any appliance or device that is exposed to water creates risk for electrical shock.

(3) Does patient use extension cords or outlet extenders with a built-in circuit breaker or fuse?

Prevents overloading of circuit that can lead to fire.

(4) Do all wall outlets and switches have cover plates?

Prevents physical contact with wiring.

(5) Does patient use light bulbs of correct wattage for each fixture?

Use of excessive wattage can lead to fire.

(6) Is main electrical fuse box for home easily accessible and clearly labelled?

In event of emergency, fuse box should be easy to access so proper circuit can be cut off.

i. Carbon monoxide (CO) safety:

(1) Are furnace flues checked regularly for patency?

Obstructed flues are a common cause of CO toxicity.

(2) Is there a working CO detector in the home?

CO is a colourless and odourless toxic gas that can be emitted from a furnace and can lead to serious injury or death (Buck, 2018, p. 780).

7. Assess patient's financial resources; determine monthly income used for ongoing expenses.

Determines potential for making repairs to home. Reveals need for low-cost community service support.

8. Assess patient's and caregiver's willingness to make changes. Has patient accepted limitations that pose risk for injury? Determine how important functional independence is for patient.

Some patients perceive attempts to improve safety within home as intrusive. If you show that necessary revisions to their home environment will preserve independence, the patient will participate more willingly.

NURSING DIAGNOSES

- Reduced physical mobility
- Anxiety
- Reduced memory

- Insufficient home maintenance
- Insufficient knowledge regarding safety risks

- Potential for injury and falls
- Potential for foodborne illness

Related factors/Risk factors are individualized on the basis of patient's condition or needs.

PLANNING

1. Expected outcomes:
- Patient and caregiver describe potential environmental risks within home that predispose to accidents.

Demonstrates patient's and caregiver's recognition of safety risks that are of greatest concern.

- Patient and caregiver initiate actions to correct environmental risks, making home safer.

Patient sees value in altering living environment.

- Patient remains free of injury.

Environmental barriers are reduced or removed to minimize injuries.

2. Prioritize with patient and caregiver environmental barriers that pose greatest risk.

Patient's physical and/or cognitive deficits make certain environmental risks more hazardous. Prioritization helps patient make best choices.

3. Recommend calling in a reliable contractor if major home repairs are necessary and acceptable to patient.

Ensures that repairs are made safely and correctly.

IMPLEMENTATION

1. General home safety:

a. Provide direct light source in areas where patient reads, cooks, uses tools, or conducts hobby work. High-intensity light on the object or surface that is involved works best.

Visual impairment in older persons usually is a result of cataracts, macular degeneration, glaucoma, or diabetic retinopathy (Feldman & Landry, 2017).

Clinical Decision Point *Avoid fluorescent lighting because it creates excessive glare.*

b. Consider satin and nonglossy finishes for walls, cabinets, and countertops in kitchen. Have sheer curtains or adjustable shades in other living areas.

Reduces glare for older persons.

STEP	RATIONALE

IMPLEMENTATION

c. Apply coloured tape or paint to colour code controls of stove, oven, dryer, toaster, and other appliances.

Persons with reduced visual acuity may adjust appliance to wrong setting, creating potential risk for fire or burning.

d. Consider installing drawers with glide mechanisms in kitchen cabinets. Install C-ring handles in lower cabinets.

Makes access to food and kitchen supplies easier.

e. Install automatic door openers, level doorknob handles, and hook-and-chain locks (Touhy, Jett, Boscart, et al., 2019).

Devices may be easier to grasp and use. Remote-controlled door locks can also provide additional security.

f. Place heavier items such as pots and pans in lower cupboards

This will reduce risk of injury and falls (PHAC, 2015b).

2. **Fall prevention steps:**

a. Paint edges of concrete stairs bright yellow, orange, or white.

Person can see edge of stairs more clearly.

b. Install treads with uniform depth of 22.5 cm (9 inch) and 22.5-cm (9-inch) risers (vertical face of steps).

If stairs are of uniform size, person does not have to continually adjust vision or stride.

c. Rearrange furniture to open up space through hallways and major rooms.

Creates unobstructed pathway for ambulation.

d. Reduce clutter within living areas (e.g., footstools, flower pots, extension cords, children's toys, stacked newspapers or magazines).

Mobility hazards resulting from clutter are especially risky at night.

e. Secure all carpeting, mats, and tile; place nonskid backing under small rugs and doormats. Remove throw rugs or mats in nonessential (dry) areas.

Reduces chance of patient slipping when stepping on rug surface (PHAC, 2015b).

f. Use interprofessional collaboration when appropriate. For example, collaborate with occupational therapist for use of specialized floors that absorb the impact of falls; collaborate with physiotherapist for use of low-rise beds, if not contraindicated.

May cushion patient's fall.
Lowers distance to the floor's surface.

g. Have enough electrical outlets installed to be able to plug light or electronic device (e.g., television, video, stereo) into nearby outlet. Secure electrical cords against baseboards.

Prevents need to run extension cords across walkways.

h. Install nonskid strips on surface of bathtub and in shower stall. Be sure that floor is clean and dry, wipe up spills immediately.

Reduces chances of slipping on tub or shower stall surface.

i. Have grab bar installed in studs at tub, toilet, and shower (see illustration). Have patient select vertical or horizontal placement if choice is available. If possible, be sure that bar is a different colour than the wall and is easy to see.

Grab bars placed in the correct place where patient can safely reach them help to steady their stance and gait and lessen chance of falls (PHAC, 2015b).

j. Have handrails installed along side of any stairway (see illustration). Be sure that stairways are well lit, with switches at top and bottom of steps.

Handrails in stairwell provide greatest stability for patient. Older persons have difficulty seeing edges of stairs.

k. Install appropriate broad-beam lighting for outside walkways.

Provides full illumination.

l. Keep lighted phone easily accessible, next to patient's bed.

Prevents patient from having to get up out of bed, often in dark.

m. Install motion-sensor exterior lighting for walkways and driveway.

Reduces risk for patient falls caused by dark surroundings.

n. Use interprofessional collaboration (e.g., occupational therapist, physiotherapist) for use of padding or types of clothing that will cushion bony prominences.

Specially designed hip protectors may be available to help cushion falls.

3. **Prevent spread of infection.**

a. Wash hands before, during, and after meal preparation.

Wash hands for at least 15 seconds. Cleaning hands will help reduce the risk of food poisoning (Government of Canada, 2015).

STEP	RATIONALE

IMPLEMENTATION

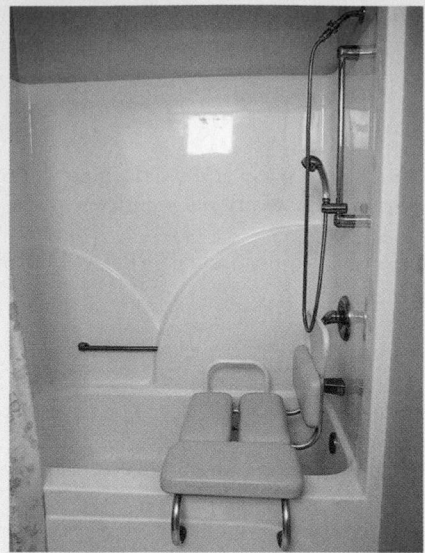

STEP 2i Grab bars and safety seat installed in shower.

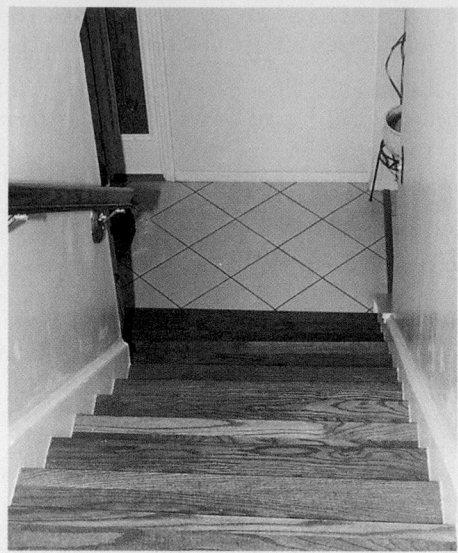

STEP 2j Handrails installed along stairways provide security for patients with visual, balance, and coordination issues.

b. Teach patient and caregiver cleaning practices to prevent spread of infection.

Cleaning kitchen surfaces and utensils will help eliminate bacteria and reduce the risk of food poisoning (Government of Canada, 2015).

c. Instruct patient not to share eating and drinking utensils.

Some infections are spread by saliva.

d. Instruct patient to clean appliances and surfaces daily.

Regular cleaning prevents risk for contamination and spread of infection (Government of Canada, 2015).

e. Instruct patient in safe food preparation and storage.

Ensures safe thawing and cooking of foods. Safe storage times for food in refrigerator and freezer help prevent foodborne illnesses (Government of Canada, 2015).

f. Set refrigerator at 4°C (39.2°F) or lower and freezer –18°C (–0.4°F) or lower.

This will keep food out of the temperature danger zone for refrigerated foods between 4°C (39.2°F) and 60°C (140°F), where bacteria can grow quickly (Government of Canada, 2014).

4. Fire safety:

a. Have smoke detectors installed near each bedroom, in kitchen, and in basement. Be sure that detector is on each floor of the home. Alarm should be close to alert patient and when sleeping.

Fires most frequently start in the basement near the furnace, dryer, or electrical wiring; in the kitchen; or in living areas where there is extensive wiring.

b. Have patient select fire extinguisher that is easy to handle and manipulate (see illustration). Ask them to read instructions and demonstrate its proper use.

Some older persons or patients with disabilities have difficulty gripping mechanisms on certain extinguishers.

c. Have area around furnace cleared of any flammable items.

Reduces risk for fire.

d. Instruct patient to be sure that any portable space heater has emergency shut-off and that equipment housing and electrical cords are intact (CSA Group, 2018).

Space heaters can be overturned by accident, which can cause fire; the safety mechanism on newer models will turn the unit off immediately (CSA Group, 2018).

e. Have patient make appointments for maintenance of furnace and chimney cleaning in appropriate season.

Furnace maintenance prevents short circuits and fires. Accumulation of creosote on chimney walls can lead to fire.

f. Have patient check light-bulb wattage in all fixtures.

Ensures proper wattage being used; wattage that exceeds recommendation can cause fire.

g. Have patient establish routine during cooking that keeps them in the kitchen. Be sure that cooking range is clean and items such as potholders and towels are away from burners.

Food cooking on stove can easily boil over or begin to burn when unattended.

STEP	RATIONALE

IMPLEMENTATION

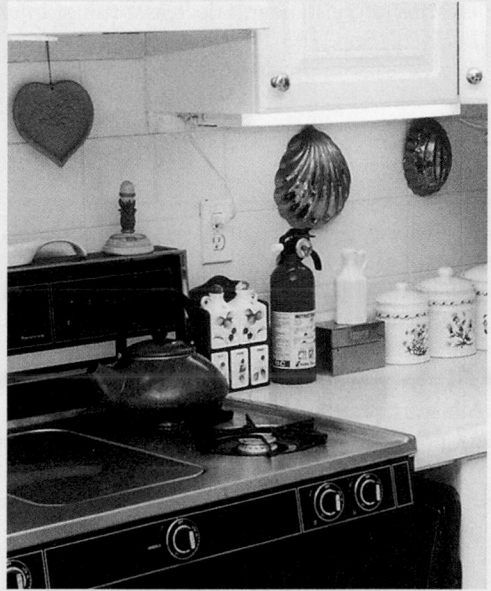

STEP 4b Fire extinguisher accessible in kitchen.

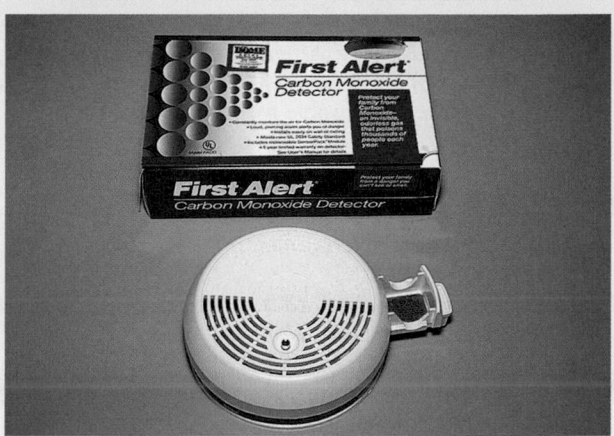

STEP 6c CO detector.

h. If patient is a smoker, review need to keep ashtrays clean and emptied. Placing a small amount of water or sand in the bottom of the ashtray is useful if patient is visually impaired.	Patients with reduced vision may be unable to tell if a cigarette, cigar, or match has extinguished.
i. Strongly discourage smoking in bed, smoking in a chair when there is possibility of falling asleep, and smoking after taking medication that diminishes alertness. Instruct patient and caregiver to put their cigarette or cigar out at first sign of feeling drowsy.	Risks factors for burns and fire. Patient's reaction time may be slower when tired.
j. Recommend that patient install power strips or surge protectors for plugging in multiple appliances and devices.	Prevents risk for electrical short, which can cause fire.

5. Burn safety:

a. Have setting on hot water heater adjusted to 49°C (120.2°F) or lower (Buck, 2018, p. 773).	Prevents scalding.
b. Instruct patient to always turn cold water on first.	Prevents direct exposure to hot water.
c. Install touch pads on lamps.	Light is easy to turn on without risk of touching hot light bulb.
d. Use colour codes of red for hot and blue for cold on water faucets. (If patient has difficulty distinguishing these colours, choose two that are easily distinguished.)	Prevents accidental burning from turning on wrong faucet.

6. CO safety:

a. Have condition of furnace venting checked annually just before turning on furnace for colder season.	Improper venting prevents escape of CO, a poisonous gas that alters hemoglobin to prevent formation of oxyhemoglobin and reduces oxygen supply to tissues.
b. Caution patients against using gas stove or barbecue grill for heating inside home.	Both are sources of CO.
c. Have battery-operated CO detector installed in home; check or replace battery when changing clocks in the fall and spring (see illustration).	Detector produces alarm when CO reaches unsafe levels. Battery operation is not affected by power outages.

7. Firearm safety:

a. Teach patient about dangers associated with keeping guns in home.	Following firearms safety standards decreases risk of injury and death (Buck, 2018, p. 782).

STEP	RATIONALE

IMPLEMENTATION

b. If guns are in the home, teach patient to store them unloaded in a locked cabinet. Teach patient to store ammunition in a secured area separate from guns. Store keys in a place inaccessible to children.

Following firearms safety standards decreases risk of injury and death (Buck, 2018, p. 782).

EVALUATION

1. Have patient and caregiver(s) identify safety risks revealed in home safety assessment.

2. During follow-up visit or call to home ask patient to discuss plans for making any modifications and observe changes patient has implemented.

3. During follow-up visits or calls ask if patient has experienced any falls or other injuries within home.

4. During subsequent home visits, reassess for progression of dementia.

5. Use Teach-Back: "I want to be sure I explained why you should make changes to your home to make it safer. Tell me why this is important." Develop a revised teaching plan if patient or caregiver is not able to teach back correctly.

Demonstrates what patient recognizes as risk and its relative importance for changing.

Evaluates extent to which patient sees risks as potentially harmful and carries out suggested changes.

Reveals if risks have been eliminated, depending on patient's previous history of injury.

Evaluates for potential new risks to patient and caregiver.

Determines patient's and caregiver's level of understanding of instructional topic.

Unexpected Outcomes	Related Interventions
1. Patient and caregiver do not acknowledge risks identified from home safety assessment.	• Determine reason or reasons patient is reluctant to make changes. Consider limited resources, disbelief concerning need to make changes, fear of loss of autonomy, or other reasons. • Review implications of risks to patient's safety and welfare.
2. Patient fails to make changes agreed on in previous plan.	• Determine reason for failure to make changes. • Help prioritize greatest risks. • Suggest making a single change and gauge patient's response.
3. Patient suffers fall or burn within home.	• Conduct assessment of contributing factors and conditions in environment at time of injury. • Make revisions based on assessment findings.

Communication and Documentation

• Retain a copy of the home safety assessment in patient's record.
• Document any instruction provided, patient's and caregiver's response, and changes made within the environment in nurses' notes in the electronic health record (EHR) or chart.

Special Considerations
Teaching

• Caregivers will benefit from learning how to safely help the patient ambulate or transfer from bed to chair or wheelchair to chair, depending on patient's mobility limitations (see Chapter 11).
• Instruct patient and caregiver about what to do in case the patient falls, including access to emergency help and how to prevent further injury.
• When appropriate, teach caregiver and patient how to use any emergency assistive devices (e.g., devices that are worn around the patient's neck and a special monitor connected to the patient's telephone). The patient summons help by pressing a button on the device if the phone is inaccessible. Refer the caregiver to local health care facilities or community support organizations for options.

• Reinforce the importance of preserving patient autonomy as much as possible with caregivers.

Pediatric

• Caution parents when working in the kitchen to never pour hot liquids when an infant or young child is near.
• Parents need to ensure that all small or sharp objects are out of the child's reach and place safety gates at stairs (McKinney, James, Murray, et al., 2018, p. 122).
• Safety measures appropriate to developmental level (e.g., cabinet locks and gates) should be installed.
• Young children should not use the sink or tub without adult help; when the child is in the tub, an adult must stay with them at all times.

Gerontological

• As a nurse assessing home safety, use "aging in place" resources and designs to practise person-centred care of older persons, considering their personal health and context, without having to completely redesign the home. Resources include community and government agencies and initiatives such as local councils on aging and the National Council on Aging (2018). Resources

also focus on helping older persons continue to live in the home of their choice, with a focus on quality of life. For example, grab bars can be installed in bathrooms, and movable cabinets under the sink so someone in a wheelchair can use the space. Light switches and electrical outlets need to be at heights that can be reached easily.

- A bedside commode (with bedpan removed) can be placed over a conventional toilet seat. Commode level is usually higher than the toilet and can also be moved near the bed for nighttime use.

✦ SKILL 42.2   Adapting the Home Setting for Patients With Cognitive Deficits

Patients with cognitive impairments and their caregivers need help to make adaptations to preserve the patient's abilities to function safely within their home. An important aspect of safety is a person's ability to perform routine activities of daily living (ADLs) and instrumental activities of daily living (IADLs). This requires a patient to make correct decisions about home-management activities. ADLs include a patient's ability to bathe, dress, go to the toilet, transfer, and feed oneself. IADLs include the ability to use a telephone, prepare meals, travel, do housework, take medication, and shop. When there are cognitive limitations, a person's independence is threatened. Caregivers often do not understand changes in a patient's cognition and thus require help to determine whether a patient is competent to stay at home safely. Three common cognitive conditions that affect patients are depression, dementia, and delirium (the "3 Ds"). Signs and symptoms of these illnesses can, at first, exhibit similarities, yet they are different. Dementia and depression are progressive illnesses. Delirium has a rapid onset within hours to days (Mayo Clinic, 2018). Depression may result from social isolation (e.g., an older person becomes homebound and has few visitors and lives alone). Depression is very common among older persons receiving care in the community and is characterized by functional impairment, lethargy, and isolation (St-Hilaire, Hudon, Préville, et al., 2017). Patients with depression are less likely to adhere to medical regimens and neglect their personal-care needs (e.g., poor diet, poor hygiene, limited activity or exercise). Compared to other patients in the community, depressed patients have been shown to have a higher risk of hospitalization and higher health care costs (Chiu, Lebenbaum, Cheng, et al., 2017).

Dementia is a progressive cognitive illness that involves memory loss and difficulties with thinking, problem-solving, language, and changes in mood or behaviour (ASC, 2018f). It leads to a decline in the ability to perform basic ADLs and IADLs. In 2016, there were an estimated 564 000 Canadians diagnosed with dementia, a number expected to increase 66% by 2031 (ASC, 2018a). Alzheimer's disease is the most common form. Some patients with dementia are at risk for wandering. Wandering in a safe environment is not harmful and can be a healthy outlet (ASC, 2018b). However, a wandering patient may try to leave their place of residence unattended, necessitating the caregiver to intervene. Caregivers also need to learn how to make the home safe.

Delirium is an acute cognitive condition. Signs and symptoms of delirium include onset of short-term confusion, excitement, disorganization, disorientation, hallucinations, illusions, being easily distracted, switching from subject to subject, rambling, irrelevant or pressured speech, and disturbance in sleep–wake cycles (Saboe Rose, 2018, p. 1319). Once the underlying issue is treated, symptoms of delirium diminish. It is important to seek immediate treatment if delirium is suspected.

Delegation and Collaboration

The skill of assessing and adapting the home environment for patients with cognitive deficits cannot be delegated to an unregulated care provider (UCP). The nurse is responsible for the assessment of cognitive function. The nurse directs the UCP to:

- Inform the nurse when there is a change in the patient's mood, memory, and ability to maintain the home or perform self-care.

Equipment

- An appropriate tool to assess cognitive and functional status (e.g., Mini-Mental State Examination [MMSE], Short Geriatric Depression Scale [SGDS], Barthel Index, or the index of ADLs)
- Calendar
- Paper for making lists
- Medication organizer (*optional*)
- Bulletin board or poster board (*optional*)
- Electronic location device (*optional*)

STEP	RATIONALE

ASSESSMENT

1. Assess patient over several short periods of time and be ready to adapt assessment if patient has sensory disabilities.

Respects dignity of patient. Improves likelihood of gathering relevant data.

2. Be sure that the room in which you meet with the patient is well lit with minimal outside noises or interruptions. Listen carefully and speak clearly and in a normal tone of voice.

Optimal environment for assessment of patient's cognitive, functional, and mental status provides a more valid assessment.

3. Ask patient to describe their own level of health and have them describe how it affects their ability to perform ADLs and IADLs. Ask caregivers (if available) to confirm description. Screen for at-risk behaviours (e.g., medication nonadherence, unsupervised use of stove)

Question requires patient to focus on one topic. Allows you to assess attention and concentration. Also determines if patient is fully perceptive of physical and cognitive capabilities.

STEP	RATIONALE

ASSESSMENT

STEP	RATIONALE
4. Ask patient and caregiver, if appropriate, how they are handling home-management responsibilities: "Tell me which bills you pay each month. Can you tell me what each one is for?" Regarding ADLs: "Can you tell me about your normal day? When do you get up, eat meals, get dressed? Tell me what you do to dress or bathe each morning."	Provides comparison of patient and caregiver perceptions. Interaction helps to measure short-term memory, judgement, and problem solving.
5. Assess patient's adherence to taking medications. Review the number and type of medications being taken, the patient's understanding of each medication's purpose as prescribed (or as chosen for over-the-counter [OTC] medications), time of day taken, and dosages. Conduct pill count over the course of a week (caregivers may need to help). Also assess where patient stores medications. Give special attention to pain medications, anticonvulsants, antihypertensives (especially beta-adrenergic blockers), diuretics, digoxin, aspirin, and anticoagulants. Have patient or caregiver keep an updated list of medications that can be brought to the emergency department if needed. Ask to see medications and the list used.	Depression, dementia, and delirium can lead to poor medication adherence. Older persons frequently suffer medication interactions from polypharmacy. Some medications or combinations of medications place the patient at risk for adverse effects that increase chances of injury as a result of physical or cognitive changes. Patient-related factors such as disease-related knowledge, health literacy, and cognitive function; medication-related factors such as adverse effects and polypharmacy; and other factors, including patient–provider relationship, can be barriers to medication adherence. Keeping a list of medications allows health care providers easy access to medication history.
6. Determine if the patient has caregivers who help with self-care or home-management responsibilities. What level of support is provided? How frequently is the caregiver available? Does the patient perceive satisfaction in caregiver's support? What level of satisfaction does the caregiver perceive? Does the caregiver have access to or take advantage of respite care?	Relationship between caregivers and the patient helps define how difficult it is to provide support. The role of the caregiver is often stressful, particularly if the individual has other responsibilities such as parenting, work, or school. Determines availability of resource to patient and quality of that support.
7. During discussion, observe patient's dress, nonverbal expressions, appearance, and cleanliness.	Conditions such as depression and dementia can result in patient's inability to attend to personal appearance.

STEP	RATIONALE
8. Observe immediate home environment.	Behavioural changes associated with cognitive dysfunction are evident in a disorderly home and inappropriate placement of objects (e.g., carton of orange juice placed inside kitchen cabinet instead of in refrigerator).
9. If you suspect cognitive or mental status change: **a.** Complete MMSE (e.g., Folstein's examination) for dementia.	Test screens orientation, attention and calculation, recall, language, and intelligence. The highest possible score is 30. A score of less than 24 is often considered impaired cognition (Folstein, Folstein, & McHugh, 1975).
b. Complete SGDS for depression. (**NOTE:** Other depression scales such as the Beck Depression Inventory [BDI] are available.)	SGDS is recommended because it takes 5 minutes to administer and has been tested, validated, and used extensively for depression in older persons (Guse, 2018, p. 667).
10. If you suspect the patient is at risk for wandering or is wandering, observe for following behaviours (caregivers might provide information as well): • Repeated shadowing or seeking whereabouts of caregiver • Revisiting one destination many times • Inability to locate landmarks or getting lost in a familiar setting • Going into unauthorized or private places • Searching for "missing" people or places	Alerts caregivers to potential safety risks. When wandering extends outside a safe environment, the patient is at increased risk for injury or death.

STEP	RATIONALE

ASSESSMENT

- Walking with no apparent destination or purpose
- Haphazard or continuous moving, walking, or pacing
- Walking that cannot easily be redirected

11. Assess which current environmental strategies caregivers are using to deal with wandering (e.g., latches and alarms on doors, visual cues such as STOP signs, constant supervision, and wearing identification band).	Helps to determine level of intervention necessary. Allows for assessment of how caregiver (who may or may not be a family member) is dealing with issues of wandering and need for additional outside support.
12. Assess caregiver for signs and symptoms of stress.	Helps to determine if caregiver is feeling burdened or overwhelmed and is in need of help.

NURSING DIAGNOSES

- Acute confusion
- Reduced self-care deficit (feeding, toileting, bathing and hygiene, dressing and grooming)

- Caregiver role strain
- Wandering
- Reduced memory
- Reduced role performance

- Insufficient health maintenance
- Insufficient home maintenance
- Potential for injury

Related factors/Risk factors are individualized on the basis of patient's condition or needs.

PLANNING

1. Expected outcomes following completion of procedure:	
• Patient can complete home-management responsibilities within existing limitations.	Modifications are made that help patient apply remaining cognitive functions.
• Patient receives appropriate combination of medications for diagnosed conditions.	Assistive devices enable patient to adhere to prescribed medication regimen.
• Patient is able to perform self-care activities or receives appropriate help.	Interventions preserve patient's autonomy and maximize their functionality.
• Caregiver describes steps to take to minimize wandering.	Instruction prepares caregiver with wandering-management strategies.
• Patient experiences fewer episodes of wandering.	Wandering-management strategies are effective.
• Caregiver identifies community resources for support.	Services available can include respite care (where an alternate [respite] caregiver provides relief to usual caregiver), adult day care programs, and support groups.
2. If patient has difficulty with self-care or fine-motor skills, use interprofessional collaboration to identify the best plan of care (e.g., collaborate with occupational therapy, home support services, respite care).	Occupational therapists can provide assistive devices and recommend self-care adaptations. Home support services provide added resources for meal preparation and home cleaning. Respite care provides caregiver a temporary rest away from continuous responsibilities.
3. Consider patient's level of cognitive impairment when making changes in their living environment. Some patients may require only minor adaptations, and others will depend more on the help of caregivers.	Retention of patient's independence and autonomy is the ultimate goal.
4. Determine best time of day for approaches that result in desired response.	Some patients are more alert and responsive in the morning than in the afternoon or vice versa.

IMPLEMENTATION

1. If patient has difficulty remembering when to perform tasks (e.g., paying bills, making appointments), help to create a list or post reminder notes in a conspicuous location (e.g., bulletin board, front of refrigerator).	Lists and organizers help the patient cope with memory loss and still safely perform activities.
2. If patient has difficulty remembering when to take medicines, help to create list or reminder note, provide medication container organized by days of week, or recommend wristwatch with alarm or schedule of text messages to signal medication administration times.	Reminder systems have benefit if the patient or caregiver is motivated and willing to adhere to them.

STEP	RATIONALE

IMPLEMENTATION

3. When patient has difficulty completing tasks such as writing checks for bills or bringing groceries into the home from the store, reduce steps it takes to complete task. Consolidate steps or simplify task.

Prevents frustration in completing task or in forgetting step that leads to task being unfinished.

4. If patient has difficulty bathing, dressing, writing, and feeding, offer assistive devices (see illustrations).

Assistive eating devices have larger handles, cup handles, or plate edges to help with meals. Assistive dressing devices use Velcro, large zippers, and elastic to facilitate independence when dressing.

5. Help patient and caregiver determine a routine schedule for ADLs such as eating, bathing, daily exercise, home cleaning, and napping. Have a large calendar posted in a conspicuous area to write in appointments or special planned events.

Consistency creates a sense of security and keeps patient oriented to daily activities. Routines are important for providing security and to decrease frustration (Ondrejka, 2018, p. 549).

6. Instruct caregiver to focus on patient's abilities rather than disabilities. Use abilities in modifying approaches to perform daily activities (e.g., if patient has limited use of right hand, try approaches that maximize use of left hand).

Retains patient's autonomy and sense of self-worth.

7. Have caregiver help set up activities so patient can complete tasks (e.g., chopping vegetables before cooking, placing wash basin on table in bedroom for sponge bath, placing clothes to wear for day on the bed, unpacking groceries on countertop for eventual storage, arranging food on plate with items in clockwise orientation [e.g., vegetables at 0900h, salad at 1500h, meat at 1800h]).

Helps patient master task even though they are unable either physically or cognitively to perform all the steps.

8. Use interprofessional collaboration, and include the patient and caregiver, to generate options for scheduling medications.

Medications sometimes cause physiological changes that create risk for injury.

   a. Have medications that are likely to cause confusion prescribed to be given at bedtime.

Reduces risk for confusion during waking hours that contribute to disorientation and risk for falling.

Clinical Decision Point *Do not recommend bedtime medication administration if patient has nocturia, because the patient will be at greater risk for falling.*

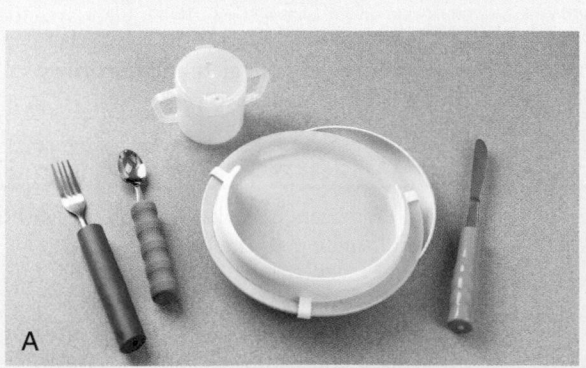
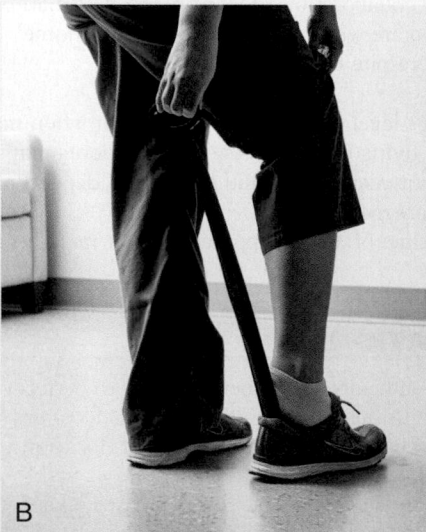

STEP 4 A, Assistive feeding devices. **B,** Assistive device to help put on shoes. (*Image used with permission ArcMate Manufacturing Corporation. All rights reserved.*)

STEP	RATIONALE

IMPLEMENTATION

b. Space antihypertensives and antiarrhythmics at different times to minimize adverse effects.

These medications cause blood pressure changes and dizziness, thus increasing risk for falls.

c. When possible, reduce the number of pain medications used.

These medications create sedative effects, increasing risk for falls.

d. Have diuretics taken early in the day and not at night.

Diuretic effect occurs during the day while patient is awake.

e. Discuss with health care provider the possibility of patient taking medications at the same time.

If safe and appropriate, taking medications at the same time will alleviate the problem of patient remembering multiple administration times.

f. Discuss use of medication organizer and dispenser (see illustration).

Organizing medications in a daily dispenser helps the patient and caregiver avoid medication errors of duplicating or missing medications.

9. Teach caregiver how to use simple and direct communication:

Relays care and support through therapeutic communication techniques.

a. Sit or stand in front of patient in full view.

Promotes reception of verbal and nonverbal messages.

b. Face patient with hearing impairment while speaking; do not cover the mouth and do not speak in a loud tone.

Patient can see a speaker's lips. Prevents voice distortion.

c. Use a calm and relaxed approach.

Helps patient feel less anxious.

d. Use eye contact and touch.

Helps to reinforce messages.

e. Speak slowly, in simple words and short sentences.

Enhances understanding of messages.

f. Use nonverbal gestures that complement verbal messages.

Provides clear messages.

10. Place clocks, calendars, and personal mementos (e.g., pictures, scrapbooks) throughout rooms within the home. Enhance environment with the addition of tactile boards or three-dimensional art.

Maintaining familiar surroundings maximizes cognitive function.

11. Have caregiver routinely orient patient to which activities they are going to complete.

This strategy is useful in patients with progressive dementia. Behavioural symptoms in later stages include delusions, agitation, and hallucinations (ASC, 2017).

12. Be sure that patient has regular naps or rest periods during the day.

Fatigue adds to any mental status changes. Provides patient energy to perform planned activities.

13. Have caregiver encourage and support frequent visits by family and friends. Teach caregiver how to use humour and reminiscing about favourite stories to promote social interaction.

Participation in social activities prevents boredom and restlessness.

14. Provide a safe place for the person to wander (e.g., large room or fenced yard).

Reduces risk for injury and leaving residence (Townsend & Morgan, 2018, p. 381).

15. Recommend installation of door locks or electronic guards if patient wanders.

Reduces chance of patient exiting home unsupervised.

16. Create a calm, safe setting that is appropriate for the patient's abilities (Townsend & Morgan, 2018, p. 381).

Prevents falls and minimizes behavioural symptoms.

17. Teach caregiver to assess for pain using an appropriate pain assessment tool (see employer policy).

Untreated pain can lead to depression, loss of appetite, social withdrawal, restlessness, aggression, and agitation (ASC, 2018d).

18. Monitor patient for personal comfort (e.g., hunger, thirst, constipation, full bladder, and comfortable temperature).

Reduces stimuli that prompt wandering (Townsend & Morgan, 2018, p. 380).

18. Keep a list of places to which patient may wander (e.g., former homes or workplaces).

Patient may seek a familiar place.

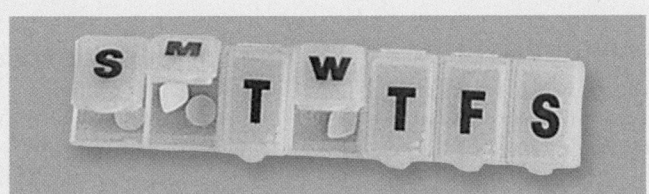

STEP 8f Weekly medication organizer.

STEP	RATIONALE

IMPLEMENTATION

STEP	RATIONALE
19. Install motion detector near exit site, with portable alarm that can accompany the caregiver.	Alerts caregiver to patient's attempt to exit residence.
20. Consider having patient wear an electronic locating device.	Alerts caregiver to patient's location (ASC, 2018b) and enhances patient safety.
21. Consider need for full-time care.	

EVALUATION

STEP	RATIONALE
1. During follow-up visits ask patient to review home-management activities completed the morning of that day and previous day.	Determines patient's ability to recall events and evaluates if patient completed planned activities.
2. Review with patient and caregiver the revised schedule for medication administration.	Evaluates understanding of regimen.
3. Check pill count you asked patient or caregiver to maintain for a week.	Tracking doses confirms if patient is adherent to regimen.
4. Ask caregiver to describe ways that will increase the patient's success in completing home-management and self-care activities.	Measures learning.
5. Have caregiver show schedules of daily routines and review specific approaches used. Observe environment for presence of reality orientation cues.	Determines caregiver's success in applying information and making environmental changes.
6. Have caregiver describe options for minimizing wandering.	Measures learning.
7. Have caregiver report number of occurrences of wandering.	Determines if reduction in wandering has occurred.
8. **Use Teach-Back:** "I want to be sure I explained how you can help reduce your partner's wandering. Tell me some ways you can do this." Develop revised teaching if caregiver is not able to teach back correctly.	Determines caregiver's level of understanding of instructional topic.

Unexpected Outcomes	Related Interventions
1. Patient is unable to complete ADLs or IADLs as planned.	• Further modifications are sometimes necessary. • Reassess what occurred when task was not completed. • Have caregiver offer suggestions.
2. Patient experiences medication interaction from multiple medications.	• Have health care provider evaluate patient's medication regimen. • Recommend feasibility of pharmacy consultation.
3. Caregiver is unable to describe or implement techniques that will improve patient's orientation and ability to complete activities.	• Reinstruction and discussion are necessary. • Support for caregiver is sometimes necessary before caregiver can learn how to support someone else. • Consider that caregiver is not able to provide necessary support; need to analyze other options.
4. Caregiver is unable to describe or implement strategies to decrease wandering.	• Reinstruction and discussion are necessary. • Caregiver may not have resources available to adapt environment. • Reconsider strategies used.
5. Patient's wandering increases.	• Reassess factors prompting wandering.
6. Patient misses medication doses or takes wrong dosage.	• Review list of medications and method for administering (e.g., medication dispenser). • Reconsider strategies to organize and schedule medications. • Assess patient for adverse effects (Hanora Lavan & Gallagher, 2016).

Communication and Documentation

- Document assessment of patient's cognitive, functional, and mental status; recommended interventions; and patient's and caregiver's response in nurses' notes in electronic health record (EHR) or chart.
- Report to health care provider any change in patient's behaviour that reflects a decline in status.

Special Considerations
Teaching

- Instruct caregiver in signs and symptoms of dementia, depression, and delirium. If delirium is suspected, contact health care provider immediately. If patient's functionality continues to decline, the caregiver may choose to learn more ADL support skills (e.g., how to help with hygiene, dressing, transfer and turning, toileting).

Pediatric

- Children with cognitive impairment often are not aware of the inherent dangers during play and other activities. Adult supervision is critical.

Gerontological

- Early diagnosis of the cause of dementia is best for the patient and caregiver so prompt treatment can begin. Ensure person-centred care by including the patient in treatment decisions as much as possible, and ensure that the caregiver has an understanding of the behaviour (Fazio, Pace, Flinner, et al., 2018).
- Elder abuse is becoming a growing concern as the population ages and more older persons are living at home longer. Older persons with cognitive decline are particularly vulnerable to abuse. *Elder abuse* is described as any form of intentional physical, emotional, mental, financial, sexual, or spiritual maltreatment by a person in a position of trust and power (Royal Canadian Mounted Police [RCMP], 2017, p. 3). Types of abuse include physical abuse (e.g., hitting, rough handling, giving too much or too little medication, use of restraints), sexual abuse (e.g., unwanted sexual activity or sexually suggestive behaviour), emotional abuse (e.g., intimidation, insults, humiliation), financial abuse (e.g., threatens or persuades another out of money or possessions), violation of rights and freedoms (e.g., withholding information, denying spiritual practices), and neglect (e.g., failing to provide food, clothing, safe shelter, medical attention, personal care, and necessary supervision) (Canadian Network for the Prevention of Elder Abuse, 2017). The nurse must monitor for signs and symptoms of elder abuse and report them immediately if suspected. These include unexplained injuries, changes in financial situation, conflicts between the patient and caregiver, the patient being nervous or afraid of the caregiver, lack of hygiene, and neglected environment.
- Caregivers may need access to respite programs, which will allow them planned time away from their caregiving role (Ondrejka, 2018, p. 579).
- Consider that patients may not have caregivers who are able or willing to care for them. Additional help of a paid caregiver may be required if available; this may also affect the patient's ability to stay in their home and not be placed in assisted or skilled care.
- If wandering is an ongoing problem, have caregiver provide current photographs of the patient to local police. Recommend enrolling the patient in the national MedicAlert Safely Home® program through the Alzheimer's Society of Canada, which provides 24-hour emergency and wandering response services and support services (ASC, 2018c). Local resources of informal caregivers (e.g., neighbors and members of the spiritual community) can also be explored to ensure safety for the patient inside and outside the home.

◆ SKILL 42.3 Medication and Medical Device Safety

The first time a nurse visits a patient's home the nurse will review and list all of a patient's medications and medication bottles. It is important to note medication name, dosage, frequency, and route and compare that list with any previous lists (e.g., known medications ordered by primary health care provider and any specific instructions). This process is known as *medication reconciliation*; the goal is to ensure that there are no errors or omissions in a patient's medication regimen, while also assessing if there is any need for change in medications (Buck & Picinbono-Larose, 2018, p. 812). Community pharmacies are a valuable resource for information on medications.

Patients in the home frequently manage the administration of medications and use of medical devices such as syringes, blood glucose monitoring equipment, dressing supplies, and even intravenous (IV) devices. This includes administration, storage, and disposal of medications and medical devices. It is critical that a patient administer medications correctly, use devices properly, clean equipment, and remove waste properly. Infection control is just one safety principle that a patient and caregiver must learn for the home setting. Nurses need to make sure that patients know regulations regarding waste disposal and follow the procedures consistent with local and provincial/territorial laws (e.g., place soiled dressings in securely fastened plastic bags before adding to regular garbage and use garbage containers with tight lids to avoid attracting animals).

One of a nurse's responsibilities within the home environment is to help a patient with sensory, mobility, or cognitive deficits.

Patients who require special consideration include those with acute sensory or neurological impairment; those with chronic illness such as diabetes mellitus or arthritis; and older persons, who frequently have physical limitations that make manipulating medical devices and dispensing medications difficult. For example, patients with arthritic hands are often unable to open medication containers because of weakness in the hands and the pain created by pressure on the joints.

Delegation and Collaboration

The skill of assessing for and monitoring medication and medical device safety cannot be delegated to an UCP. The nurse directs the UCP to:

- Make suggestions that further ensure patient safety regarding the use of basic infection-control practices.
- Make suggestions as to how to properly dispose of sharps, needles, and contaminated supplies in the home.

Equipment

- Coloured marking pens
- Labels
- Puncture-resistant sharps container or 2-L hard plastic bottle with cap
- Duct, masking, or adhesive tape
- Assistive devices (e.g., syringe magnifier)
- Medication organizers

STEP	RATIONALE

ASSESSMENT

1. Assess patient's sensory, musculoskeletal, and neurological function (see Chapter 8)—specifically hand strength, ability to read labels on containers, ability to read doses on syringe, and ability to prepare medicine in a syringe.

Reveals any deficits that will affect preparation and use of medications or medical devices. Print size on the label may be too small to read.

2. If caregiver provides routine help, ask caregiver if there are any concerns about being able to care for patient.

Assesses caregiver's health. Nurses can help educate caregivers on the need for help and provide information to avoid injury (Hughes, 2018, p. 226).

3. Assess patient's medication regimen and length of time that the patient has been receiving each medication. Ask patient to describe doses taken daily for each medication.

Determines complexity of medication regimen and how familiar patient or caregiver is with the regimen.

4. Assess patient's and caregiver's health literacy level (e.g., ask them to read a medication label out loud to you).

Helps to ensure that patient and caregiver can read and understand medication that patient is taking. Helps prevent medication errors.

Clinical Decision Point *Be sure that medication labels are not confusing for a patient. For example, the Spanish word for eleven is written as "once." A Spanish-speaking patient could confuse a medication direction that requires them to take a medication 1 time a day as 11 times a day.*

5. Ask patient to show you where medications are stored in the home. Look at each container.

Determines condition and labelling of containers.

6. Assess temperature of storage area.

Medication should not be stored in extreme heat. Insulin should not be stored near extreme heat or cold (Diabetes Canada, 2019) or near food in the refrigerator.

7. Assess patient's daily schedule for medication administration. Ask patient to describe schedule and whether there are any problems in following that schedule.

Helps to reveal patient's adherence to or misunderstanding of instructions.

8. If patient self-administers injections, ask to see where they store supplies and what they use to dispose of used syringes and needles.

Determines sterility of equipment and whether method of disposal creates risk to patient, caregiver, or nurse for needle-stick injuries.

9. If patient uses a glucose-monitoring device, ask to see where the monitor, lancets, and glucose strips are stored. Also ask how patient disposes of lancets.

Allows you to examine cleanliness of equipment, sterility of lancets, and condition of glucose strips. Sharps should be disposed of in a puncture-proof container.

NURSING DIAGNOSES

- Insufficient knowledge regarding medication safety
- Insufficient health maintenance
- Nonadherence
- Caregiver role strain
- Potential for injury
- Potential for infection

Related factors/Risk factors are individualized on the basis of patient's condition or needs.

PLANNING

1. Expected outcomes following completion of procedure:
   - Patient and caregiver discuss principles of medication safety.

   Patient education includes information and techniques for safe medication administration.

   - Patient and caregiver prepare medications independently.

   Adaptations successfully accommodate patient's and caregiver's deficits in handling and manipulating equipment.

   - Patient and caregiver identify correct conditions for storing medications, medical devices, and supplies.

   Instruction focuses on ensuring infection-control measures.

   - Patient and caregiver dispose of used medical equipment and supplies correctly.

   Appropriate receptacles and methods for disposal are made available and used.

IMPLEMENTATION

1. Teach patient and caregiver the following principles to ensure that medications are safe to use:
   a. Always use prescriptions provided by your pharmacy (Government of Canada, 2017b).

   Medications must be of full strength and used for an appropriate pharmacological reason to have therapeutic benefit.

STEP	RATIONALE

IMPLEMENTATION

b. Do not take any medicine more than 1 year old or past the expiration date on the container.

Expired medication is sometimes toxic or no longer effective.

c. Do not place different medicines in the same container.

Prevents accidental "mix-up" of medications and medication error.

d. Do not place medications in pill containers different from their original ones.

Prevents accidental "mix-up" of medications and confusion as to expiration dates.

e. Always finish prescribed medication; do not save for future illness.

Prevents underdosing or inappropriate dosing.

f. Wash hands before and after administering or taking medication.

Contaminated hands are source of infection transmission.

2. Recommend approaches for preparation of medications:

a. For patients with weakened grasp or pain in hands and fingers, have the local pharmacist place medications in a screw-top container.

Tops of childproof containers are difficult to remove, especially if hand and finger grasp is weakened.

Clinical Decision Point *If the patient has children or grandchildren who have easy access to the medication storage area or patient's purse, be sure that medications are stored in a secure place.*

b. For patients with visual alterations, have the pharmacy type larger labels on all medication containers.

Ensures that patient is able to read medication name and dosage schedule clearly.

c. For patients who are legally blind, have Braille labels placed on medication containers.

Labels embossed with medication name, strength, and prescription numbers are easy to read for a patient trained in use of Braille.

d. For patients taking multiple medications, ask if they wish to try to introduce a colour-coding system. Use the same colour for medications that patient needs to take at same time. Mark tops of bottle caps with a coloured marking pen.

Technique helps patient take correct medications and doses at correct times of day. Best used when patient is reliable in self-administration.

e. Provide specially designed syringes with large numerals or syringe magnifier for patients with visual alterations (see illustration).

Ensures that accurate dose of medication is prepared in syringe.

f. For patients who have difficulty manipulating syringes, offer spring-loaded needle insertion aid.

Delivers injection safely without manipulation of plunger.

Clinical Decision Point *Teach caregivers what to do following a needle-stick injury. Wash the affected area thoroughly with soap and water and dry. If the patient has acquired immunodeficiency syndrome (AIDS), hepatitis, or some other communicable disease, caregivers should pursue appropriate laboratory testing.*

g. Teach caregivers how to properly draw up prescribed volume of medication into syringe. When necessary, have caregiver prepare extra prefilled syringes for patient's use when the caregiver is absent.

Ensures that caregiver knows proper preparation techniques and that patient has access to injections. Watch patient and caregiver draw up and dispense medications to determine if more teaching is needed.

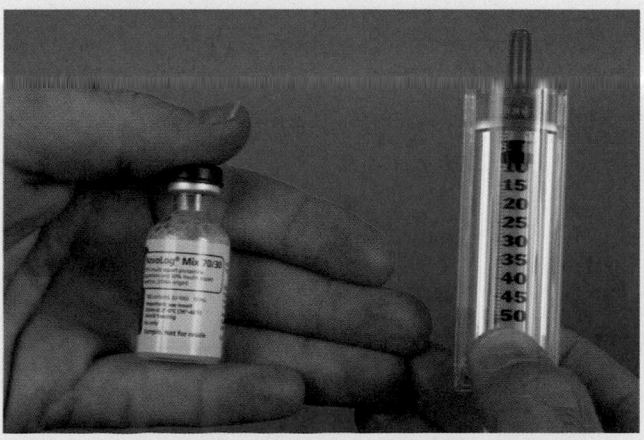

STEP 2e Syringe with magnifier.

STEP	RATIONALE

IMPLEMENTATION

3. Recommend approaches for medication and supply storage:

a. Store medications in a safe, dry place, preferably in the kitchen away from the microwave or stove.

Moisture and excessive heat may cause medications to decompose

b. Keep liquid medications and parenteral medications, especially insulin, in a cool place.

Prevents decomposition of medication.

Clinical Decision Point *Although manufacturers recommend storing insulin in the refrigerator, injecting cold insulin can sometimes make the injection more painful. To avoid this, store the bottle of insulin being used at room temperature. Insulin kept at room temperature will last approximately 1 month. However, remember to store extra bottles in the refrigerator if a patient buys more than one bottle at a time (Diabetes Canada, 2019). If insulin is stored in the refrigerator, be sure that medication is in a bin or container, away from food.*

c. Keep medical supplies such as syringes, dressing supplies, and glucose meter in an airtight container (e.g., plastic storage bin) and store in a cool place, such as a bedroom closet.

Ensures that supplies are not exposed to moisture or other contaminants.

d. Instruct patient and caregiver to use a new needle with each medication administration.

Multiple use of the same needle puts patient at risk for infection.

4. Review for patient and caregiver proper techniques for disposal of medications, "sharps," and disposable medical supplies:

Proper practices are necessary to prevent patient injury.

a. Return expired and unused prescription medications to the pharmacy for disposal (Pharmacy Association of Nova Scotia, 2019).

Medications can be harmful to the environment when disposed of improperly (Public Safety Canada, 2018).

(1) DO NOT FLUSH unused medications.

Recent environmental impact studies report that flushing medications down the toilet could be having an adverse impact on the environment (Public Safety Canada, 2018).

(2) Best practice is to return all unused medications to the community pharmacy. Patients are advised against disposing of any medications in the home setting (Public Safety Canada, 2018).

Medication return programs at local pharmacies will ensure safe and proper disposal of medications (Public Safety Canada, 2018).

b. Obtain a sharps container from a medical supply store or IV equipment supplier. (If finances are limited, have patient use a small-neck plastic bottle such as a soda bottle.) Dispose of all needles and lancets in container.

A puncture-proof container prevents exposure to contaminated needle-stick. A small-neck container makes it difficult for anyone to easily retrieve a used needle or sharp.

c. Caution against filling a sharps container to the point where needles protrude out the opening. Return it to the pharmacy when three-fourths full, securing top with duct tape or adhesive tape.

Prevents needle-sticks.

d. Store sharps container in an area inaccessible to children.

Prevents injury to child.

e. Dispose of soiled dressings, used glucose testing trips, and IV tubing in a separate, sealed, plastic garbage bag. Place in a second plastic bag (double bagged) and discard appropriately as garbage.

Prevents contamination with other items in the home. Minimizes chances of caregiver being exposed to infectious waste.

EVALUATION

1. Have patient and/or caregiver describe steps to take to ensure that medications are safe to use.

Demonstrates learning.

2. Observe patient and/or caregiver prepare and administer medication dose.

Evaluates ability to physically manipulate medications and necessary equipment.

3. Observe home setting for location of medications and supplies.

Evaluates patient's and/or caregiver's adherence to recommendations.

4. Have patient or caregiver describe how sharps or medical equipment is discarded.

Demonstrates learning.

5. Do medication counts (pills remaining in containers) at successive intervals, such as twice a week for 2 weeks.

Helps to verify that patient takes correct number of medications over a period of time.

STEP	RATIONALE

IMPLEMENTATION

6. Use Teach-Back: "I want to be sure I explained the importance of not throwing needles and sharp objects (e.g., lancets) in the garbage. Tell me how to dispose of these safely and why it is important." Develop a revised teaching plan if patient or caregiver is not able to teach back correctly.

Determines patient's and caregiver's level of understanding of instructional topic.

Unexpected Outcomes	Related Interventions
1. Patient or caregiver is unable to recall principles for safe use of medications.	• Reinstruction is necessary, or patient and caregiver need a chance to ask more questions regarding benefit of precautions. • Offer simple, plain language and written instructions.
2. Patient or caregiver has difficulty or is unable to prepare and self-administer medication.	• Offer further help to set up equipment. • Offer assistive aids. • Reinstruct in steps used to prepare medication.
3. Medications and medical devices are not stored in a secure or appropriate location.	• Assess whether patient chooses to store items conveniently rather than safely or has limited resources. • Reinstruction and discussion are necessary.
4. Sharps and disposable medical equipment are not disposed of properly.	• Provide reinstruction. • Arrange to provide appropriate containers.
5. Excess or insufficient number of pills found during pill count.	• Review with patient and caregiver daily medication prescribed. • Re-evaluate use of dosage reminders. • Notify health care provider.

Communication and Documentation

• Document instructions and recommendations to patient and caregiver and results of return demonstrations in nurses' notes in electronic health record (EHR) or chart.
• Report to health care provider any unsafe situation.

• All medicines and cleaning products should have child safety caps (McKinney et al., 2018, p. 121).
• If teaching self-management skills, include adult supervision and input. Never refer to medications as candy.

Special Considerations
Pediatric
• It is vital to keep medications and other equipment such as cleaning products out of the reach of children (McKinney et al., 2018, p. 121).

◆ CLINICAL DEBRIEF

A 79-year-old woman lives with her 84-year-old sister in a split-level four-bedroom home that she has owned for over 50 years. She has a history of metastatic bone cancer and was recently diagnosed with heart failure. In addition to taking multiple oral medications, she undergoes weekly intravenous chemotherapy for progression of her cancer. She has no other family closer than a 2-hour drive, and her older sister has advanced glaucoma and diminished hearing. Both women refuse to move from their home, even at the urging of her three children to move closer to one of them. The patient no longer drives, nor does her sister, and she is unable to climb the few steps needed to move beyond the lower living level of the home. She has begun to show signs of depression. When the nurse talks to her sister, the nurse recognizes that the sister is overwhelmed by the amount of care she needs to provide. Because of the patient's immobility, she cannot reach the upstairs bathrooms, where the shower is located, and she relies on her older sister to help care for her and maintain the house on a daily basis.

1. Give three examples of how the nurse might adapt the home setting to make it safer for the patient and her sister.
2. Which equipment might the nurse bring to the home to perform the initial home assessment?
3. The patient now lives in an assisted-living facility in a private room. The nurse visits her at the facility and plans to meet with the health care team on site to give a report. Her sister passed away the month before, and her children convinced her to move to the facility, believing she would be safer in this environment. Her apartment is on the second floor of the facility, and the dining/socialization areas are on the first floor. When the nurse visits her, she appears to be confused as to why she is in the assisted-living facility and asks when she can return "home." Using SBAR, show how the nurse would communicate with the health care team at the assisted-living facility about this patient.

✦ REVIEW QUESTIONS

1. The nurse is speaking with the caregiver who states that the patient is confused more than usual. Which of the following information will help determine the patient's physical and mental health status? (Select all that apply.)
   1. Medications the patient is taking
   2. Decrease in cognitive function within the past few months
   3. Ability to perform instrumental activities of daily living (IADLs)
   4. History of wandering
   5. Current photograph of patient available
   6. Last visit to patient's health care provider

2. The nurse is teaching a patient with diabetes mellitus how to maintain diabetic supplies. Which of the following responses by the patient indicates that the teaching was successful? (Select all that apply.)
   1. "Insulin cannot harm my grandchildren, so I don't need to keep it locked up when they visit."
   2. "I keep the insulin vials in the kitchen freezer until about 2 hours before I need to use them."
   3. "I store extra bottles of insulin that I am not using in my refrigerator in the bin with the eggs so that they will not break."
   4. "I can store my glucometer and insulin syringes in an airtight bag when I'm not using them."
   5. "When my daughter comes to visit, I'll ask her to prepare extra prefilled syringes for me."

3. The nurse is visiting an older person who is recovering from hip replacement surgery at home. Which of the following findings would indicate that the patient is at risk for falls? (Select all that apply.)
   1. Handrails are present on the staircase.
   2. The outdoor steps are all one colour, blending in with the sidewalk.
   3. There are slip-resistant mats in the kitchen and bathroom.
   4. The patient is taking morphine tablets for pain every 8 hours.
   5. The patient has a history of previous falls in the past 6 months.

ⓔ *Visit the Evolve site for a complete list of Clinical Debrief and Review Questions answers.*

REFERENCES

Alzheimer's Society of Canada (ASC). (2017). *Delusions and hallucinations.* Retrieved from http://alzheimer.ca/en/Home/Living-with-dementia/Understanding-behaviour/Delusions-and-hallucinations

Alzheimer's Society of Canada (ASC). (2018a). *Latest information and statistics.* Retrieved from http://alzheimer.ca/en/Home/Get-involved/Advocacy/Latest-info-stats

Alzheimer's Society of Canada (ASC). (2018b). *Locating devices.* Retrieved from http://alzheimer.ca/en/Home/Living-with-dementia/Day-to-day-living/Safety/Locating-devices

Alzheimer's Society of Canada (ASC). (2018c). *MedicAlert® Safely Home.* Retrieved from http://alzheimer.ca/en/Home/Living-with-dementia/Day-to-day-living/Safety/Safely-Home

Alzheimer's Society of Canada (ASC). (2018d). *Pain matters.* Retrieved from http://alzheimer.ca/en/on/We-can-help/Resources/Pain%20Matters

Alzheimer's Society of Canada (ASC). (2018e). *Safety in the home.* Retrieved from http://alzheimer.ca/en/Home/Living-with-dementia/Day-to-day-living/Safety/Safety-in-the-home

Alzheimer's Society of Canada (ASC). (2018f). *What is dementia?* Retrieved from http://alzheimer.ca/en/Home/About-dementia/What-is-dementia

Beghi, E., Gervasoni, E., Pupillo, E., et al. (2018). Prediction of falls in subjects suffering from Parkinson disease, multiple sclerosis, and stroke. *Archives of Physical Medicine and Rehabilitation*, 99(4), 641–651. doi:10.1016/j.apmr.2017.10.009

Buck, M. (2018). Safety. In B. Kozier, G. Erb, A. Berman, et al. (Eds.), *Fundamentals of Canadian nursing: Concepts, process, and practice* (4th ed., pp. 761–791). Don Mills, ON: Pearson Canada.

Buck, M., Picinbono-Larose, S., et al. (2018). Medications. In B. Kozier, G. Erb, & A. Berman (Eds.), *Fundamentals of Canadian nursing: Concepts, process, and practice* (4th ed., pp. 792–874). Don Mills, ON: Pearson Canada.

Canada Safety Council. (n.d.) *Home safety.* Retrieved from https://canadasafetycouncil.org/category/home-safety/

Canadian Network for the Prevention of Elder Abuse. (2017). *Forms of abuse.* Retrieved from https://cnpea.ca/en/what-is-elder-abuse/forms-of-abuse

Canadian Patient Safety Institute (CPSI). (2018). *Home care safety.* Retrieved from https://www.patientsafetyinstitute.ca/en/Topic/Pages/Homecare-Safety.aspx

Chiu, M., Lebenbaum, M., Cheng, J., de Oliveira, C., & Kurdyak, P. (2017). The direct healthcare costs associated with psychological distress and major depression: A population-based cohort study in Ontario, Canada. *PLoS ONE*, 12(9), e0184268. doi:10.1371/journal.pone.0184268

Community Health Nurses of Canada (CHNC). (2019). *2019 Canadian community health nursing professional practice model and standards of practice.* Retrieved from https://www.chnc.ca/standards-of-practice

CSA Group. (2018). *Safety tips from CSA International for the safe use of cord-connected, fan-forced electric space heaters.* Retrieved from http://www.csagroup.org/recall/electric-space-heaters-various-15-08/

Diabetes Canada. (2019). *Getting started with insulin.* Retrieved from https://www.diabetes.ca/diabetes-and-you/healthy-living-resources/blood-sugar-insulin/getting-started-with-insulin

Fazio, S., Pace, D., Flinner, J., & Kallmyer, B. (2018). The fundamentals of person-centered care for individuals with dementia. *The Gerontologist*, 58(1), S10–S19. doi:10.1093/geront/gnx122

Feldman, R., & Landry, O. (Eds.), (2017). *Discovering the lifespan.* Upper Saddle River, NJ: Pearson.

Folstein, M. F., Folstein, S. E., & McHugh, P. R. (1975). Mini-mental state: A practical method for grading the cognitive state of patients for the clinician. *Journal of Psychiatric Research*, 12(3), 189–198. doi:10.1016/0022-3956(75)90026-6

Gerlach, A. J., Browne, A. J., & Greenwood, M. (2017). Engaging Indigenous families in a community-based Indigenous early childhood programme in British Columbia, Canada: A cultural safety perspective. *Health & Social Care in the Community*, 25(6), 1763–1773. doi:10.1111/hsc.12450

Government of Canada. (2014). *Safe food storage.* Retrieved from https://www.canada.ca/en/health-canada/services/general-food-safety-tips/safe-food-storage.html

Government of Canada. (2015). *Safe cooking temperatures.* Retrieved from https://www.canada.ca/en/health-canada/services/general-food-safety-tips/safe-internal-cooking-temperatures.html

Government of Canada. (2017a). *Safe food handling in the home.* Retrieved from https://www.canada.ca/en/health-canada/services/general-food-safety-tips/safe-food-handling-home.html

Government of Canada. (2017b). *Using medications safely.* Retrieved from https://www.canada.ca/en/health-canada/services/drugs-medical-devices/using-medications-safely.html

Government of Canada. (2019). *Storage, display, transportation and handling of firearms by individuals: Regulations.* Retrieved from http://laws.justice.gc.ca/eng/regulations/SOR-98-209/page-1.html#h-4

Guse, L. (2018). Comprehensive assessment of the older adult. In K. Mauk (Ed.), *Gerontological nursing: Competencies for care* (4th ed., pp. 620–702). Burlington, MA: Jones & Bartlett Learning.

Hanora Lavan, A., & Gallagher, P. (2016). Predicting risk of adverse drug reactions in older adults. *Therapeutic Advances in Drug Safety*, 7(1), 11–22. doi:10.1177/2042098615615472

Hughes, J., et al. (2018). Nursing care of families. In B. Kozier, G. Erb, & A. Berman (Eds.), *Fundamentals of Canadian nursing: Concepts, process, and practice* (4th ed., pp. 223–245). Don Mills, ON: Pearson Canada.

Jumani, K., & Powell, J. (2017). Benign paroxysmal positional vertigo: Management and its impact on falls. *The Annals of Otology, Rhinology, and Laryngology*, 126(8), 602–605. doi:10.1177/0003489417718847

Lorainne, T. C., El-Khatib, M., Perneczky, R., et al. (2017). Prioritizing problems in and solutions to homecare safety of people with dementia: Supporting carers, streamlining care. *BMC Geriatrics*, 17(26), 1–8. doi:10.1186/s12877-017-0415-6

Mayo Clinic. (2018). *Delirium.* Retrieved from https://www.mayoclinic.org/diseases-conditions/delirium/symptoms-causes/syc-20371386

McKinney, E., James, S., Murray, S., Nelson, K. A., & Ashwill, J. (2018). *Health promotion during early childhood.* St. Louis, MO: Elsevier.

Meiner, S. E. (2015). Safety. In S. E. Meiner (Ed.), *Gerontologic nursing* (5th ed.). St. Louis: Mosby.

National Council on Aging. (2018). *For older adults & caregivers.* Retrieved from https://www.ncoa.org/older-adults-caregivers/

Ondrejka, D. (2018). Teaching and communication with older adults and their families. In K. Mauk (Ed.), *Gerontological nursing: Competencies for care* (4th ed., pp. 524–619). Burlington, MA: Jones & Bartlett Learning.

Parachute. (2019). *Home safety.* Retrieved from http://www.parachutecanada.org/injury-topics/topic/C13

Parsons, J. (2017). Sensory alterations. In P. A. Potter, A. G. Perry, P. A. Stockert, & A. M. Hall (Eds.), *Fundamental of nursing* (9th ed., pp. 1241–1260). St. Louis: Elsevier.

Pfaff, K., et al. (2018). Older adults. In B. Kozier, G. Erb, & A. Berman (Eds.), *Fundamentals of Canadian nursing: Concepts, process, and practice* (4th ed., pp. 344–363). Don Mills, ON: Pearson Canada.

Pharmacy Association of Nova Scotia. (2019). *Medication storage and disposal.* Retrieved from http://pans.ns.ca/medication-storage-disposal

Public Health Agency of Canada (PHAC). (2015a). *The safe living guide.* Retrieved from https://www.canada.ca/content/dam/phac-aspc/migration/phac-aspc/seniors -aines/publications/public/injury-blessure/safelive-securite/pdfs/safelive -securite-eng.pdf

Public Health Agency of Canada (PHAC). (2015b). *You CAN prevent falls!* Retrieved from https://www.canada.ca/content/dam/phac-aspc/migration/phac-aspc/ seniors-aines/alt-formats/pdf/publications/public/injury-blessure/prevent-eviter/ prevent-eviter-e.pdf

Public Safety Canada. (2018). *Prescription drug return initiatives in Canada.* Retrieved from https://www.publicsafety.gc.ca/cnt/rsrcs/pblctns/prscptn-drg-rtrn/index-en .aspx

Registered Nurses' Association of Ontario (RNAO). (2017). *Preventing falls and reducing injury from falls (3rd ed.)* Retrieved from http://rnao.ca/sites/rnao-ca/ files/bpg/Preventing_Falls_FINAL_WEB.pdf

Royal Canadian Mounted Police (RCMP). (2017). *Seniors' guidebook to safety and security.* Retrieved from http://www.rcmp-grc.gc.ca/wam/media/1971/original/ 1aad45a3f33f4b16c4f91340a803ae1a.pdf

Saboe Rose, S. (2018). Chapter 13: Delirium. In K. Mauk (Ed.), *Gerontological nursing: Competencies for care* (4th ed., pp. 1317–1361). Burlington, MA: Jones & Bartlett Learning.

Statistics Canada. (2017). *Fire statistics in Canada, selected observations from the National Fire Information Database 2005 to 2014.* Retrieved from http:// nfidcanada.ca/wp-content/uploads/2017/09/Fire-statistics-in-Canada-200 5-to-2014.pdf

St-Hilaire, A., Hudon, C., Préville, M., & Potvin, O. (2017). Utilization of healthcare services among elderly with cognitive impairment no dementia and influence of depression and anxiety: A longitudinal study. *Aging & Mental Health, 21*(8), 810–822. doi:10.1080/13607863.2016.1161006

Touhy, T. A., Jett, K. F., Boscart, V., & McCleary, L. (2019). *Ebersole and Hess' gerontological nursing & healthy aging* (2nd Canadian ed.). Toronto: Elsevier Canada.

Townsend, M., & Morgan, K. (Eds.), (2018). *Psychiatric mental health nursing concepts of care in evidence-based practice.* Philadelphia: F.A. Davis Company.

43 | Self-Care Teaching in the Community

Written by **Theresa Pietsch, PhD, RN, CRRN CNE, and Amanda Parrott, RN, CMSN(c), OHN, CCNE**

SKILLS AND PROCEDURES

OBJECTIVES

Mastery of content in this chapter will enable the nurse to:
- Identify factors that influence patients' abilities to learn and care for themselves at home.
- Discuss the collaborative nature of home care teaching with the patient and/or caregiver.
- Assess safety factors that may impair or prohibit a patient's ability to perform skills in the home setting.
- Discuss situations and conditions that require a patient

and/or caregiver to learn skills that support and achieve health maintenance.
- Choose evidence-informed teaching strategies to use in the home setting.
- Implement and evaluate evidence-informed learning strategies that support patients' ability to care for themselves in the home.

MEDIA RESOURCES

- evolve http://evolve.elsevier.com/Canada/Perry/clinicalskills/
- Review Questions
- Audio Glossary
- Clinical Debrief and Review Questions Answers

PURPOSE

Many patients recover from or are treated for illnesses at home. The need for home care services has both increased and broadened due to the increase in early hospital discharge and the incidence of chronic illness and to the acuity of patients managing their illnesses at home (Canadian Home Care Association, 2015). In these situations, patients assume greater responsibility for managing their own care and are supported by nurses providing care to them in their community. Home care nurses provide health education and resources by collaborating with a patient or caregiver to address the patient's health needs, preferences, and values and incorporating their strengths, skills, and capacity into the treatment plan (Nies & McEwen, 2015).

Home care services are not publicly insured through the *Canada Health Act* in the same way as hospital and health care provider services are (Government of Canada, 2016). Most home care and community care services are delivered by provincial, territorial, and some municipal governments. It is the nurse's responsibility to be aware of specific provincial/territorial eligibility requirements for

home care (e.g., Newfoundland and Labrador's requirements are available at https://www.health.gov.nl.ca/health/index.html).

STANDARDS OF CARE

- Accreditation Canada, 2019a—*Health and Social Services Standards* (https://accreditation.ca/standards/)
- Canadian Patient Safety Institute (CPSI), 2014—*Resource Guide for Supporting Caregivers at Home—For Home Care Service Providers* (http://www.patientsafetyinstitute.ca/en/toolsResources/HomeCareSafety/Documents/Resources%20for%20home%20care%20providers%20-%20Resource%20guide%20for%20supporting%20caregivers%20at%20home.pdf)
- Canadian Public Health Association (CPHA), 2014—*Examples of Health Literacy in Practice* (https://www.cpha.ca/sites/default/files/uploads/resources/healthlit/examples_e.pdf)
- Community Health Nurses of Canada (CHNC), *2019—2019 Canadian Community Health Nursing Professional Practice Model & Standards of Practice* (https://www.chnc.ca/standards-of-practice)

PRINCIPLES FOR PRACTICE

- Home care nurses thoroughly assess factors that affect a patient's abilities and willingness to manage self-care. Nurses need to determine what patients want to know, how they learn, and what motivates them to learn new information (CHNC, 2019).
- Patient teaching is an essential part of nursing practice. Information needs to be relevant, current, and clearly presented (Bergh, Friberg, Persson, et al., 2015).
- Home care nurses creatively adapt teaching strategies to meet each patient's unique physical, psychosocial, and cultural needs (CHNC, 2019).
- For collaboration to be successful, home care nurses identify who is involved in the patient's care and establish mutual trust and respect through open and honest communication (Nies & McEwen, 2015).
- Nurses need to consider principles of diversity when providing person-centred care for patients in their homes. Everyone's cultural background and beliefs must be respected.
- Documentation is a necessary part of home care to ensure that information regarding the patient's condition is communicated to health care provider.
- Patients and caregivers need to be familiar with the records being used and what information they need to record.

PERSON-CENTRED CARE

- Nurses need to engage the patient and caregiver(s) as participants in care (Saita, Acquati, & Molgora, 2016).
- Patients must understand how to manage their health and illnesses, take discharge medications correctly and safely, and perform related care at home. In home care, nurses help patients and caregivers make well-informed decisions about their health practices (Parker, Zimmerman, & Rodriquez, 2014).
- Patient health literacy is an important consideration for their ability to safely and successfully manage their own care. The role of the home care nurse is to assess health literacy and focus their activities and teaching to improve health literacy (Eggertson, 2011).
- Teach-back is a way to confirm that patient teaching is understood. Patient understanding is confirmed when a patient explains or demonstrates a topic back to the nurse (Almkuist, 2017).
- Respectful communication includes addressing a patient in an appropriate manner and using acceptable body language. For example, direct eye contact during an interview may not be appropriate in all cultures (Giger, 2017).
- Verbal instructions need to be reinforced with printed, patient education information in the preferred reading-level language and other audiovisual materials used when possible (Eggertson, 2011).

EVIDENCE-INFORMED PRACTICE

Patients are discharged sooner from hospitals than previously and can have more complex health care needs that must be met at home. Thus the home care nurse is challenged to teach patients and help them feel secure, along with coordinating their care among their health care providers.

- A review of outcomes in home health care identified the importance of care coordination among providers when patients transition from acute care to home care. Patients' health can be improved with efficient coordination and interprofessional collaboration.
- Nurses possess the knowledge and skills to strengthen care coordination and improve patient outcomes in home care when home care facilities create positive practice environments (Jarrin, Kang, & Aiken, 2017).
- One quality-improvement project examined postacute patients' perceptions of discharge teaching and readiness for discharge. The findings suggested that interprofessional teaching and patient engagement improve patient satisfaction scores, patients' readiness for discharge, and perceptions of the usefulness of discharge instructions (Knier, Stickler, Ferber, et al., 2015).
- Recent studies comparing different teaching modalities to improve health outcomes with chronic diseases determined that Internet education programs may improve patient engagement and management of chronic diseases, such as diabetes (Pereira, Phillips, Johnson, et al., 2015).
- A low level of therapeutic self-care ability may be a risk factor associated with the occurrence of adverse events in home care (Sun, Doran, Wodchis, et al., 2017).

The National Institutes of Health (NIH, 2018) provide best practice strategies from its health literacy research. Following are pertinent findings about literacy and providers' communication:

- Patients who are struggling to understand health information may feel judged for not understanding.
- Regardless of education level, everyone is at risk for misunderstanding health education and patient teaching material.
- Embarrassment may prevent patients from asking questions or seeking clarification from the health care provider.

SAFETY GUIDELINES

- Assess if a patient in the home setting is able to safely perform a skill. If they are unable to execute a skill independently, identify a caregiver who will provide it safely in the home setting.
- Assess and determine if the patient has home medical equipment and knows how to use it properly for safe and successful self-care management.
- Include teaching interventions for other people in the household who positively or negatively influence the patient's self-care management.
- Provide an opportunity for the patient and caregiver to demonstrate skill.
- Assess the home environment and teach appropriate disposal of patient care medical products. For example, after patients use needles and other sharps, the items should be placed in sharps disposal containers. Containers should be placed at a height that is not accessible to children and pets.
- An additional challenge facing home care nurses today is health literacy. Health literacy is the ability to get the health information one needs and understand it (Eggertson, 2011).
- It is estimated that approximately 60% of Canadians are not health literate (CPHA, 2014). Individuals with low health literacy are generally less likely to self-manage chronic conditions and use more resources.
- To improve health literacy, nurses need to use simple and plain words when speaking to patients and providing written instructions (Eggertson, 2011).

✦ SKILL 43.1   Teaching Patients to Measure Body Temperature

An elevation in body temperature may be an early warning sign of serious health problems. Patients who are susceptible to temperature alterations (e.g., immunosuppressed patients) and their caregivers need to know how to measure temperature correctly so patients can seek medical attention earlier. Parents need to know how to measure their children's temperature because children can develop high fevers very quickly; older persons and their caregivers need to know the techniques for temperature measurement because older persons have impaired temperature-control mechanisms. Nurses need to teach patients and caregivers the skills of measuring body temperature and techniques to lower temperature when a fever occurs at home.

A variety of body temperature thermometers are currently available, including disposable single-use, electronic digital, noncontact, temporal, and tympanic thermometers. The Canadian Paediatric Society (CPS, 2017) recommends the use of nonmercury thermometers. If a mercury thermometer breaks or is not disposed of properly, the mercury vapour gets into the air, posing a major health risk in the home and community (CPS, 2017). Nurses need to educate patients about the environmental hazards associated with mercury in the home and encourage them to purchase mercury-free thermometers. Patients should be encouraged to remove mercury thermometers from their homes and dispose of them at a toxic waste facility.

The nurse helps a patient choose the most appropriate thermometer to use in the home based on the patient's normal dexterity, vision, and financial resources. For example, a patient with visual impairment from glaucoma or retinopathy can read a thermometer with a large digital display more easily. The need for an oral, rectal, or axillary temperature depends on the patient's age and health status (see Chapter 7).

Delegation and Collaboration

The skill of teaching patients to measure body temperature cannot be delegated to an unregulated care provider (UCP). The nurse instructs the UCP to:

- Inform the nurse of patient or caregiver concerns about measuring body temperature.

Equipment

- Thermometer
- Disposable probe cover (if needed)
- Water-soluble lubricant (for rectal measurements)
- Paper and pencil or pen or computer if frequent measurements are to be taken
- Disposable clean gloves (for rectal temperature taken by a caregiver)

STEP	RATIONALE

ASSESSMENT

1. Identify patient using at least two person-specific identifiers during first visit. Facial recognition can be used as one of two identifiers for ongoing visits.

   Ensures correct patient. Complies with Accreditation Canada's standards and improves patient safety (Accreditation Canada, 2019b).

2. Assess patient's and caregiver's ability to manipulate and read thermometer. Have patient put on eyeglasses if necessary.

   Physical restrictions in handling or reading a thermometer can prevent a patient from being able to read the thermometer and often require teaching the caregiver as well as the patient.

3. Assess patient's knowledge of normal temperature range, symptoms of fever and hypothermia, and patient's risk for body temperature alterations.

   Identifies patient's ability to recognize alterations in body temperature and to initiate preventive health measures.

4. Assess patient's ability to determine appropriate type of thermometer to be used in varying situations (see Chapter 7).

   Determines knowledge of age-related or medical conditions that determine selection of temperature.

5. Assess patient's learning readiness and ability to concentrate; consider presence of pain, nausea, or fatigue and patient interest in instruction.

   Presence of significant illness, frailty, or confusion affects a patient's ability to attend to a teaching plan. Indicates need to rely on caregiver for learning and implementation (if available) on a short- or long-term basis.

6. Assess patient's and caregiver's previous knowledge of and experience in measuring temperature and maintaining a thermometer. Have the patient or caregiver perform a return demonstration if they indicate ability to measure temperature.

   Allows assessment of patient's and caregiver's knowledge and use of safety precautions, aseptic technique, and time period for insertion.

NURSING DIAGNOSES

- Inadequate thermoregulation
- Insufficient knowledge regarding temperature measurement skill
- Potential for imbalanced body temperature
- Potential for infection

Related factors/Risk factors are individualized on the basis of patient's condition or needs.

STEP	RATIONALE

PLANNING

1. Expected outcomes following completion of procedure:
   - Patient or caregiver is able to correctly measure body temperature.
   - Patient or caregiver demonstrates proper cleaning and storage of equipment.
   - Patient or caregiver states normal temperature range and factors that affect temperature, signs and symptoms of fever and hypothermia, and measures to take with abnormal temperatures.
2. Select setting in the home where patient or caregiver is most likely to measure temperature.
3. Select setting in the home where patient is most likely to measure temperature and is a good location for teaching session:
   a. Select a room that is well lit with comfortable seating.
   b. Be sure that the patient is close and can see the nurse clearly.
   c. Control sources of noise and distractions.

4. Discuss and demonstrate with patient and caregiver normal temperature ranges; instruct caregiver to remain with patient during measurement if age or physical status requires.

(RATIONALE column)

Indicates that skills are learned.

Prevents transfer of microorganisms and maintains integrity of thermometer.
Cognitive learning is achieved.

Considers person-centred care.

Improves likelihood of patient and caregiver being attentive to instruction.

Room environment needs to minimize existing sensory alterations. A comfortable environment free of distractions increases patient's attention.
Learning by doing; active engagement is more effective than passive models (Peter, Robinson, Jordan, et al., 2015).

IMPLEMENTATION

1. Demonstrate steps of thermometer preparation, insertion, and reading. Provide rationale for steps to patient and caregiver.
   a. Instruct patient to take oral temperature 20 to 30 minutes after smoking or ingesting hot or cold liquids or foods and to wait at least an hour after a hot bath or vigorous exercise. Explain indications for selecting temperature site other than oral.
   b. Perform hand hygiene. Instruct caregiver to wear clean, disposable gloves.
   c. Teach patient and caregiver the proper position for patient for temperature measurement (see Chapter 7).
   d. Demonstrate temperature measurement technique and have patient or caregiver perform each step with guidance. Do not rush them.
   e. Explain any special precautions in using thermometers: oral thermometer must be placed in the sublingual pocket; rectal thermometers must be lubricated with water-soluble lubricant; use rectal thermometer only for measuring rectal temperatures; never force a rectal thermometer into the rectum.
   f. Discuss typical time frame needed for each type of temperature to register (based on thermometer type) and how to take reading.
   g. Teach proper method for removing, cleaning, and storing thermometer (when applicable) and select a suitable storage location.
2. Discuss common symptoms of fever: warm, dry, flushed skin; feeling warm; chills; piloerection; malaise; and restlessness.

(RATIONALE column)

Observing and evaluation of demonstration is cornerstone of person-centred care (Almkuist, 2017).

Waiting at least 15 minutes after drinking hot or cold liquids or foods improves accuracy of temperature reading (Vorvick, 2019).

Patient and caregiver must be knowledgeable about infection prevention techniques.
Improves accuracy of readings.

Allows for correction of errors in technique as they occur and for discussion of potential consequences of errors.

Ensures accurate reading and avoidance of injury to patient.

Ensures accurate reading.

Prevents transmission of infection. Thermometer is stored properly so it does not break or become inaccurate when not in use.
Patient or caregiver needs to recognize onset of fever for early detection and intervention.

STEP	RATIONALE

IMPLEMENTATION

3. Discuss common signs and symptoms of hypothermia: cool skin, uncontrolled shivering, loss of memory, and signs of poor judgment. Explain that people with inadequate home heating, older persons, or those unaware of the potential dangers of cold conditions are at risk.

Patient or caregiver needs to recognize onset of hypothermia for early detection and intervention.

Clinical Decision Point *Teach patient and caregiver to take temperature after chills or shivering subsides, to obtain an accurate temperature.*

4. Discuss importance of notifying the health care provider when temperature elevations occur. Review common therapies for temperature reduction that are safe to perform at home, including when to use antipyretics; exposing skin to air; reducing room temperature; increasing air circulation; applying cool, moist compresses to skin (e.g., forehead); and drinking fluids (Hockenberry & Wilson, 2015). Patients receiving chemotherapy should be cautioned that any fever is a medical emergency and that they should immediately seek medical attention (Canadian Cancer Society, 2019a).

Treating fever enhances patient comfort. Lowering the temperature can reduce risk of febrile seizures in children (Hockenberry & Wilson, 2015).

5. Provide set of written guidelines for patient's reference at appropriate level of health literacy.

Patients prefer written materials that are clear and concise; bulleted lists are preferred to text blocks (NIH, 2018).

6. Give patient or caregiver a paper or digital log to time and record temperature if frequent monitoring is required. Instruct patient and caregiver to use a written record to report temperatures to the health care provider.

Keeping an organized record of temperatures helps patient validate and report temperature fluctuations to the health care provider.

EVALUATION

1. Have patient or caregiver independently demonstrate technique for temperature measurement, including body placement and ability to read thermometer, three separate times.

When psychomotor skill is performed correctly, patient confidence is increased.

2. Ask patient or caregiver to identify the normal temperature range and the influence of smoking and hot and cold liquids or foods on oral readings; discuss safety implications for temperature measurement.

Measures cognitive learning and confirms understanding of information.

3. Have patient or caregiver describe common signs and symptoms of fever and hypothermia and methods for controlling these.

Measures cognitive learning.

4. Watch patient or caregiver clean and store equipment.

Proper cleaning prevents bacterial growth, and proper storage preserves accuracy of thermometer.

5. Watch patient or caregiver record temperature values and times in log. Review patient's log periodically to ensure that temperatures are being recorded correctly.

Health care providers make changes in patient care based on information provided by the patient. To ensure that changes are made appropriately, patient or caregiver needs to record accurate information.

6. **Use Teach-Back:** "I want to be sure I explained the importance of monitoring your temperature. Explain in your own words why it is important to know how to take your own temperature." Develop a revised teaching plan if patient or caregiver is not able to teach back correctly.

Determines patient's and caregiver's level of understanding of instructional topic.

Unexpected Outcomes	Related Interventions
1. Patient or caregiver is unable to measure temperature, clean and store thermometer correctly, or verbalize knowledge about fever and temperature measurement.	• Ask patient or caregiver to describe difficulties experienced while performing temperature measurement. • Use a different teaching strategy. • Plan for patient to perform another return demonstration during the next scheduled home care visit or plan to teach the caregiver.
2. Patient reports breaking mercury glass thermometer.	• Teach patient steps to dispose of thermometer safely (Box 43.1).

Steps to Take in the Event of a Mercury Spill

- If possible, close the room off from the rest of the house and increase ventilation in the affected room by opening windows or turning on a fan.
- Put on rubber, nitrile, or latex gloves. Do not touch the mercury. Do not allow children to help clean up the spill. Remove all pets from the area.
- Pick up glass pieces, place them in a folded paper towel, and place glass and towel into a plastic zip lock bag.
- Use a squeegee or cardboard to gather mercury beads. Use an eyedropper to collect or draw up visible mercury beads. Slowly and carefully squeeze mercury onto a damp paper towel. Place the paper towel in a zip lock bag and secure. Then put shaving cream on a small brush and "dot" the area or press duct tape in the area to pick up smaller beads.
- Place mercury, material used to pick up mercury, and broken glass in a plastic zip lock bag. Triple bag the contaminated objects (place in a total of three sealed bags).
- Place gloves, mercury, and all other wastes into a trash bag. Secure and label the bag.
- Call local health department to determine where to dispose of mercury safely.
- If possible, keep windows open and room well ventilated for at least 24 hours after cleanup.
- Instruct patient not to use a vacuum cleaner, a broom, or household cleaners when cleaning up mercury spill. Also instruct patient not to put mercury down the drain or place contaminated clothing into the washing machine.

Data from Environment and Climate Change Canada. (2016). *Cleaning up small mercury spills.* Retrieved from https://www.ec.gc.ca/mercure-mercury/default.asp?lang=En&n=D2B2AD47-1.

Communication and Documentation

- Document information taught and patient's and caregiver's return demonstration in the home care record.
- Document temperature in home care record and home documentation system (e.g., log).
- Report high and low temperatures to health care provider.

Special Considerations
Teaching

- Instruct patient or caregiver to never force a thermometer into the rectum or to use a rectal thermometer after rectal surgery, when the patient has a rectal disorder such as tumour or severe hemorrhoids, when the patient has a low platelet count, or when it is difficult to position the patient for proper thermometer placement.
- Use caution in recommending aspirin or any other over-the-counter (OTC) drug or antipyretic medicine to patients whose conditions contraindicate their use (e.g., gastric ulcer, bleeding tendencies, allergic reactions, drug interactions, liver or kidney dysfunction). Encourage patient to contact the health care provider before using OTC antipyretics.
- Patients receiving chemotherapy who develop an increased temperature should seek immediate medical attention even if feeling well (Canadian Cancer Society, 2019a).
- Instruct patient to never use sponging with isopropyl alcohol to lower a fever because of its neurotoxic effects (Hockenberry & Wilson, 2015).
- Always leave a phone number and instructions on how to reach a home care nurse if needed.

Pediatric

- The stage of growth and development of a child will determine the site of measurement and type of equipment used (see Chapter 7).
- Different types of thermometers are available for use with children (e.g., temporal artery, tympanic). Reliability of these different thermometers varies; ensure that parents know how to use the equipment correctly and detect the signs and symptoms of a fever (Hockenberry & Wilson, 2015).
- Teach parents to take a child's temperature whenever the child feels warm to the touch, even if the temperature was recently normal (Hockenberry & Wilson, 2015).
- Avoid using aspirin in children under the age of 19 to prevent Reye's syndrome.

Gerontological

- Older persons' normal temperatures are often below 36.1°C (97°F); therefore, a normal temperature range for adults sometimes reflects a fever in the older person (Touhy, Jett, Boscart, et al., 2019).
- Older persons are more sensitive to temperature changes and tend to demonstrate symptoms of delirium or dementia with variations of body temperature.
- Altered internal temperature regulation or dehydration occurs frequently in frail, debilitated patients. Temperature measurement becomes very important to prevent severe states of hypothermia or hyperthermia.
- Consider common age-related sensory changes in the older person and direct teaching strategies to compensate for any alterations (e.g., a magnifying glass to read thermometer).

SKILL 43.2   Teaching Blood Pressure and Pulse Measurement

Patients with a variety of illnesses such as cardiac, kidney, or vascular diseases are susceptible to wide variations in their blood pressure (BP) and pulse. They benefit from knowing how to assess their own BP and pulse because they are able to seek medical attention early when readings vary from their acceptable ranges. In addition, healthy people who exercise learn how their body responds to exercise and are able to determine appropriate exercise plans based on knowing what their pulse and BP are before, during, and after exercise.

Research related to home monitoring of BP has illustrated the importance of regular monitoring outside of acute care settings and medical offices so that the health care provider can treat patients with hypertension appropriately (Shimbo, Abdalla, Falzon, et al., 2015). If treatment is based on single readings during an office visit, health care providers do not have an accurate picture of a patient's health. To gather this essential information about patients living at home, nurses can teach them to measure their BP and pulse regularly and to interpret readings that are outside of their individualized normal values. For example, patients should be taught about factors that affect the accuracy of BP readings, such as cuff placement, movement of the tubing, speaking during measurement, and position and movement of the extremity or body.

Aneroid sphygmomanometers are available to measure BP in the home (see Chapter 7). Aneroid manometers are safe, lightweight, compact, and portable. In the home, many patients choose to use commercial automatic electronic BP devices. These devices may measure pulse rate and produce a BP measurement without needing to use a stethoscope. The devices involve placing a cuff around the arm, the wrist, or a fingertip. A reading is displayed electronically for the patient. Electronic BP monitors are often easier to use, but their accuracy compared to manual BP monitoring is still a focus of debate. However, home monitoring of BP is still recommended because of the increased number of BP readings that can be obtained (Heart and Stroke Foundation of Canada, 2018). It is essential for patients to keep a record of all of their BP readings and compare those obtained by a health care provider with their electronic monitor to assess the accuracy of readings.

Additional factors that affect the accuracy of BP monitoring are cuff size and placement (Fallon, 2015). Patients need to learn to place a cuff directly on their skin. BP cuffs that are too small tend to overestimate BP, whereas cuffs that are too large tend to underestimate it (Fallon, 2015). Not all electronic home BP monitors come with interchangeable cuff sizes, which can complicate BP monitoring at home. Nurses need to help patients and caregivers determine cuff size, calibration, and accuracy of electronic equipment before they determine which type of BP monitor to purchase.

Delegation and Collaboration

The skill of teaching patients to measure BP and pulse cannot be delegated to an unregulated care provider (UCP). The nurse instructs the UCP to:

- Report concerns related to BP (e.g., episodes of suspected orthostatic hypotension) and measurements to the nurse.

Equipment
For Blood Pressure

- Sphygmomanometer or electronic BP reading device (Fig. 43.1) Cuff should be secure and fit snugly, encircling the arm (Box 43.2). Most often, patients have an electronic BP machine in the home setting.
- Stethoscope (two-headed teaching stethoscope is ideal) if using sphygmomanometer

For Pulse

- Wristwatch or clock with a second hand

For Both Blood Pressure and Pulse

- Paper or digital log

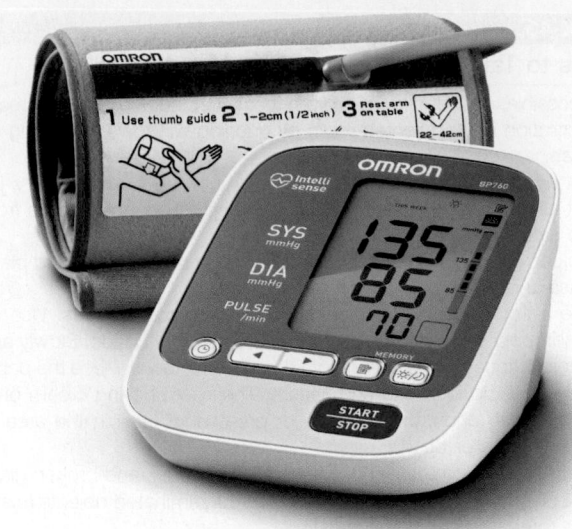

FIG 43.1 Home blood pressure monitoring device. (*Courtesy Omron Healthcare, Bannockburn, IL.*)

BOX 43.2

Guidelines for Blood Pressure Cuff Size

Adult Sizes
- For "small adult" size: 10 × 24 cm (4 × 9.5 inches)
- For "adult" size: 13 × 30 cm (5 × 11.8 inches)
- For "large adult" size: 16 × 38 cm (6.3 × 15 inches)
- For "adult thigh" size: 20 × 42 cm (7.8 × 16.5 inches)

Pediatric Sizes
- For newborn or premature infants, use "newborn" size: 4 × 8 cm (1.5 × 3 inches)
- For infants, use "infant" size: 6 × 12 cm (2.3 × 4.7 inches)
- For older children use "child" size: 9 × 18 cm (3.5 × 7 inches)
- A standard adult cuff, a large adult cuff, and a thigh cuff for use in children with very large arms may be needed.

Pediatric sizes data from Hockenberry, M. J., & Wilson, D. (2015). *Wong's nursing care of infants and children* (10th ed.). St. Louis: Mosby.

STEP	RATIONALE

ASSESSMENT

STEP	RATIONALE
1. Identify patient using at least two person-specific identifiers during the first visit. Facial recognition can be used as one of two identifiers for ongoing subsequent visits.	Ensures correct patient. Complies with Accreditation Canada's standards and improves patient safety (Accreditation Canada, 2019b).
2. Assess patient's and caregiver's psychomotor function: visual (see dial and clock) and auditory (hear Korotkoff sounds) acuity, ability to manipulate BP monitoring equipment, and ability to feel pulse.	Vision or hearing problems require use of equipment that has been adapted for these conditions (e.g., larger print). Other deficits may require the caregiver to perform skills.
3. Assess patient's and caregiver's knowledge of normal BP and pulse range for the patient and the symptoms of high or low readings. (Consult with health care provider regarding normal range desired.)	Identifies patient's and caregiver's ability to know when to initiate preventive health measures and recognize alterations in BP and pulse.

STEP	RATIONALE

ASSESSMENT

4. Assess patient's and caregiver's knowledge of what BP and pulse measure, specific medical issues that affect them, and why awareness of variations is important to the patient's health.

Identifies patient's and caregiver's understanding of potential cause-and-effect relationships between variations in BP and pulse and health status.

5. Assess patient's and caregiver's previous knowledge of and experience in measuring BP and pulse. Have patient or caregiver perform return demonstration if they indicate ability to measure BP or pulse.

Allows nurse to assess patient's and caregiver's knowledge and skill performance.

6. Assess patient's learning readiness and ability to concentrate; consider presence of pain, nausea, or fatigue and patient interest in instruction.

Presence of significant illness, frailty, or confusion affects a patient's ability to attend to a teaching plan. Indicates need to rely on caregiver for learning and implementation (if available) on a short- or long-term basis.

7. Assess home environment for a favorable place to measure BP and pulse (e.g., quiet room with comfortable place to sit) along with quality of home BP equipment.

Ensures more accurate measurement (Jung, Kim, Kim, et al., 2015).

NURSING DIAGNOSES

- Insufficient knowledge regarding pulse/BP measurement
- Inadequate health maintenance

Related factors/Risk factors are individualized on the basis of patient's condition or needs.

PLANNING

1. Expected outcomes following completion of procedure:
   - Patient or caregiver accurately measures BP and pulse.
   - BP and pulse are within range expected for patient's age and condition (see Chapter 7).
   - Patient or caregiver explains importance of measuring BP and pulse, common causes of changes, the best time for measurement, and when to communicate with the health care provider to evaluate changes in treatment regimen.

Learning has occurred.
Cardiovascular status is stable at level that is determined for patient by their health care provider.
Measures cognitive learning.

2. Encourage patient or caregiver to perform measurements on a routine schedule for long-term monitoring plan.

Daily activities and many extrinsic and intrinsic factors affect measurement fluctuations. A routine schedule allows for daily comparisons.

3. Encourage patient to avoid exercise, caffeine, and smoking for 30 minutes before assessment to avoid inaccuracy.

These factors cause elevations in BP and pulse (Heart and Stroke Foundation of Canada, 2018).

4. Have patient or caregiver perform measurement on patient in a comfortable position, with arm supported and feet flat on the floor and in a warm and quiet environment.

Maintains patient's comfort during measurement. Systolic and diastolic BP increase with crossed-leg position (Das & Sharma, 2017).

IMPLEMENTATION

1. **BP measurement:**
   a. Explain the importance of having patient sit quietly for 5 minutes with their back supported and feet on the floor before measurement. If patient cannot sit in this position, select a position that patient can maintain.

Reduces anxiety, which can falsely elevate BP readings (Fallon 2015).
It is important for patient to maintain the same position for each reading.

   b. Discuss with patient and caregiver the best sites for assessing BP. For self-measurement, the brachial artery is almost always used. If patient cannot sit in this position, select a position that patient can maintain. Instruct patient and caregiver to avoid applying cuff to an arm with:
   - Intravenous (IV) catheter with or without fluids infusing
   - Arteriovenous shunt
   - Breast or axillary surgery
   - Trauma, inflammation, or disease

The most accessible sites are easiest to measure for accuracy of assessment. Appropriate site selection promotes accuracy in reading and minimizes potential for trauma. It is important for the patient to maintain the same position for each reading. Application of pressure from an inflated bladder temporarily impairs blood flow and compromises circulation in the extremity that already has impaired circulation.

STEP	RATIONALE

IMPLEMENTATION

c. Demonstrate steps for measuring BP (see Chapter 7):	Eventual evaluation of psychomotor skill is measured through patient's performance and ability to follow instructions.
(1) *Use of sphygmomanometer and stethoscope:*	
(a) Teach palpation of artery, positioning cuff, wrapping cuff, placing stethoscope, inflating and releasing cuff, and listening for Korotkoff sounds.	Prepares patient or caregiver for measuring BP.
(b) Describe sounds of measurement and relationship to observation of gauge during BP reading. Caution patient and caregiver about level and length of time appropriate for cuff inflation.	Ensures accurate reading. Prolonged inflation of cuff impairs circulation to extremity.
(c) Teach patient and caregiver to routinely clean diaphragm and earpieces of stethoscope with rubbing alcohol or damp cloth.	Stethoscopes are frequently contaminated with microorganisms. Cleaning stethoscope routinely prevents transmission of microorganisms.

Clinical Decision Point *If the patient or caregiver needs to use a stethoscope to take BP, use a double-headed teaching stethoscope to verify accuracy of the reading or read BP 1 to 2 minutes after the patient's attempt, to verify accuracy. If the patient is having difficulty hearing Korotkoff sounds, ensure that they are applying the cuff appropriately and using the correct size cuff. Also determine correct use of equipment (e.g., cuff may have been deflated too quickly or too slowly; cuff may not have been pumped high enough for systolic readings).*

(2) *Use of electronic BP monitor:*	
(a) Teach correct placement of cuff and use of electronic equipment for proper cuff inflation.	Using electronic equipment correctly helps ensure accurate BP readings.
2. Pulse measurement:	
a. Discuss with patient and caregiver the best sites for assessing pulse: radial and carotid.	Radial and carotid sites are accessible and usually easiest to palpate.

Clinical Decision Point *If a carotid site is chosen, caution the patient against vigorously massaging their neck while attempting to locate pulse or attempting to locate both arteries at the same time. Stimulation of carotid sinus leads to reflex slowing of the heart rate from vagal stimulation. In addition, simultaneous occlusion of both carotid arteries decreases blood to the brain, resulting in fainting.*

b. Demonstrate steps for palpating pulse (see Chapter 7): position of artery on wrist or neck, how to locate artery, using fingertips for palpation, compressing artery, palpating pulse before counting, counting pulse, and calculating pulse rate (see illustration).	Eventual evaluation of psychomotor skill is measured through patient's performance and ability to follow instructions.
(1) Instruct in use of gentle pressure; reinforce not to press hard over the pulse site.	Pressing too hard may occlude the artery.

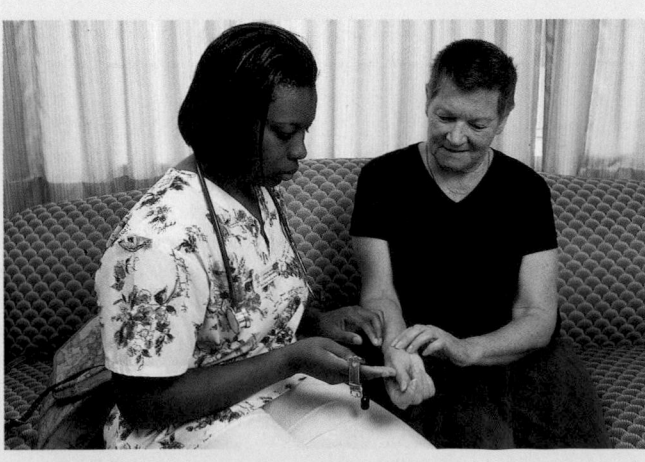

STEP 2b Nurse observes patient checking radial pulse.

STEP	RATIONALE

IMPLEMENTATION

(2) Instruct in use of watch or clock with second hand to count pulse.	Ensures correct timing of pulse.
(3) Instruct to count for a full 60 seconds, starting with the second hand at 12:00 position.	Consistent timing of procedure reduces confusion or forgetfulness about time period or starting point used for pulse measurement. A full 60-second count increases accuracy of measure.
3. Educate patient and caregiver about normal desired BP and pulse ranges, the purposes for monitoring, and when to take measurements (e.g., before and after taking cardiac or antihypertensive medications; before, during, and after exercise).	Patient or caregiver needs to be able to determine when values are not in desired ranges and when measurements need to be taken.
4. Describe symptoms that indicate the need to perform BP and/or pulse measurement.	Promotes understanding of health status alterations that need medical intervention.

Clinical Decision Point *Discuss the importance of notifying the health care provider and withholding medications when abnormal values in BP or pulse occur (e.g., hypotension or bradycardia). The patient needs to understand preventive measures to take and to follow the health care provider's directions if alterations develop.*

5. Have patient or caregiver attempt each step of skill on you or a family member.	You can correct any errors in technique as they occur.
6. Observe patient demonstrate techniques to measure pulse and BP on self. When patient is measuring BP, do not allow multiple repetitive BP attempts on any one limb.	After developing confidence in measuring values in others, the patient is ready to measure their own values. Making multiple repetitive BP attempts restricts circulation and alters measurement.
7. Teach patient and caregiver to monitor BP and pulse, even if they remain in normal range.	Continuous monitoring provides important information that evaluates the effectiveness of medications or other treatments.
8. Provide patient and caregiver with printed instructions with a written or pictorial guide or with a DVD or online demonstration of procedure if possible.	Printed and audiovisual teaching materials help stimulate patient's visual and auditory senses, which enhances learning (Shabiralyani, Hasan, Hamad, et al., 2015).
9. Give patient or caregiver a paper or digital log to record BP and pulse and the time(s) they were taken. In addition, the patient must record whether or not medications that affect BP or pulse were taken. Instruct patient and caregiver to use a written record to report readings to the health care provider.	Keeping an organized record of BP and pulse readings and medications empowers the patient and provides accurate information to health care providers.
10. Instruct patient and caregiver in proper care of equipment (e.g., storage, cleaning, and battery care).	Improper care and storage of equipment affect accuracy of measurement.

EVALUATION

1. Observe patient or caregiver demonstrate technique for BP and pulse measurement on at least three different occasions and verify that patient or caregiver adds information to log correctly.	Feedback through return demonstration of psychomotor learning is the best means to evaluate learning.
2. Ask patient and caregiver if readings are within the desired range and when to report abnormal readings to the health care provider.	Determines patient's and caregiver's ability to know when readings are within the proper range and what to do when abnormal readings are obtained.
3. Ask patient and caregiver to describe the reason for BP and pulse monitoring and any related medications (e.g., antihypertensives, antidysrhythmics) or treatment (e.g., diet and exercise).	Determines if patient understands monitoring and related therapies.
4. Have patient or caregiver demonstrate proper care of equipment.	Demonstrates learning.
5. **Use Teach-Back:** "I want to be sure I explained the importance of monitoring your BP. Explain to me how your medications can affect your BP readings." Develop a revised teaching plan if patient or caregiver is not able to teach back correctly.	Determines patient's and caregiver's level of understanding of instructional topic.

STEP	RATIONALE

Unexpected Outcomes

1. Patient or caregiver is unable to measure BP or pulse (e.g., inability to manipulate equipment, visualize numbers on equipment or clock, hear BP sounds).

2. Patient or caregiver has difficulty explaining purposes of measurement or implications of therapy.

Related Interventions

- Alter teaching plan to accommodate patient's or caregiver's problems (e.g., use other types of equipment that are easier to manipulate, see, or hear).
- Reinforce information taught and continue return demonstrations until patient or caregiver can perform skill.
- Teach skill to a different caregiver.
- Review and reinforce information that patient or caregiver does not understand.

Communication and Documentation

- Document teaching, patient and caregiver responses, and demonstration in the home care record.
- Document BP and pulse in home care record and home documentation system (e.g., logbook).
- Report BP and/or pulse findings that deviate from the patient's normal values to the health care provider.

Special Considerations
Teaching

- Educate patient and caregiver about risks for hypertension, hypotension, or change in pulse rate (see Chapter 7).
- Ensure that patient or caregiver understands health care provider's recommendations for treatment regimen, including potential adverse effects and interactions of any medication therapies (e.g., patients taking thyroid medications might need to withhold them when BP is above normal range or pulse is above 100 beats/min). Confirm specific guidelines for BP and pulse with the health care provider; document information in home care record; and provide clear, written instructions for the patient and caregiver.
- Always leave a phone number and instructions about how to reach the home care nurse if needed.

Pediatric

- Readings (BP or pulse) are often inaccurate if an infant or child is anxious and uncooperative. BP is also inaccurate when

the cuff size is inappropriate. Having others divert the child's attention or taking their BP or pulse while they are seated on the parent's lap usually helps calm the child (Hockenberry & Wilson, 2015).

- Young children will be more likely to cooperate if allowed to touch or play with equipment before the procedure. Consider performing the procedure first on the parent or another person significant to child. This allows the child to observe that the procedure is safe.
- Use the radial pulse in children over 2 years of age. Femoral or brachial pulse is the best site for palpation of pulse for children under 2 years of age (Hockenberry & Wilson, 2015). When the child is under the age of 1 year, use a stethoscope to obtain the apical heart.

Gerontological

- Musculoskeletal changes such as arthritis or other joint conditions may impair a patient's ability to position a limb comfortably or perform fine-motor skills required to measure BP and pulse (Touhy et al., 2019).
- Older persons, especially those who are frail or who have lost upper-arm mass, require a smaller BP cuff.
- Home BP monitoring among older persons is not a replacement for BP monitoring by health care providers, but it can serve to provide more information to ensure the best treatment.

◆ SKILL 43.3 | Teaching Intermittent Self-Catheterization

Most people urinate and empty their bladder four or five times a day (Society of Urologic Nurses and Associates [SUNA], 2010). However, some patients are not able to empty their bladder. Infections in the bladder or kidneys and damage to the kidneys sometimes result from incomplete emptying of the bladder. Clean intermittent self-catheterization (CISC) is a safe and effective way to empty the bladder. The patient performs self-catheterization with clean technique, eliminating the need to wear gloves. Patients who use CISC have a variety of health problems that affect the neuromuscular control of the bladder (Leach, 2018). Current practice supports CISC for use in the home to provide a means to completely empty the bladder, prevent urinary tract infections (UTIs), and prevent further bladder and kidney damage

(Lamin & Newman, 2016). Inadequate or excessive fluid intake, poor catheterization technique and catheter care, and traumatic catheterization can cause UTI. Teaching proper self-catheterization technique is crucial in preventing infections (Lamin & Newman, 2016).

Use of CISC helps patients believe that they are more in control of their daily needs, which enhances their quality of life. It helps some patients become continent, maintain a positive body image, and experience less anxiety and embarrassment. In addition, CISC allows patients to express their sexuality and sustain satisfying relationships with significant others. However, the skill requires physical and manual dexterity, and patients must adhere to a regular schedule for it to be successful (Lamin & Newman, 2016).

When the patient is unable to perform CISC independently, teach the caregiver how to perform the skill. For patients with certain medical conditions, sterile or aseptic technique is the recommended method of self-catheterization, rather than CISC (Lamin & Newman, 2016).

Delegation and Collaboration

The skill of teaching intermittent self-catheterization cannot be delegated to an unregulated care provider (UCP). The nurse instructs the UCP to:

- Document the amount of urine in the paper or digital log if the patient is unable to do so.
- Report to the nurse changes in the colour, odour, or amount of urine.

Equipment

- Soap, water, and clean washcloth
- Mirror *(optional)*
- Urethral catheter (smallest size that can pass easily into the bladder and completely drain patient's urine)
- Lubricant (e.g., water-soluble jelly) if catheter is uncoated
- Container for collection of urine (e.g., urinal)—not needed for patients emptying urine directly into toilet
- Mild soap (e.g., Ivory)
- Catheter storage item or container (e.g., brown paper bag, clean towel)
- Disposable clean gloves (for caregiver)
- Paper or digital log *(optional)*

STEP	RATIONALE

ASSESSMENT

1. Identify patient using at least two person-specific identifiers during first visit. Facial recognition can be used as one of two identifiers for ongoing subsequent visits.	Ensures correct patient. Complies with Accreditation Canada's standards and improves patient safety (Accreditation Canada, 2019b).
2. Review patient's medical record, including prescription for CISC and nurses' notes. Gather information about voiding history, existing medical and surgical history, patient's usual daily fluid intake, postvoid residual amounts, and daily voiding routine.	Determines reason for CISC, frequency of catheterization, and previous responses to patient education.
3. Assess patient's ability to perform CISC, including developmental level, level of consciousness, motor function, and psychosocial status.	Patient must be physically able to reach urethra and move equipment as needed. Patient who cannot see urethra can be taught to feel for proper location of urethral opening (Wilson, 2015).
4. Assess patient's and caregiver's knowledge about CISC and observe performance of CISC if patient has performed previously.	Effective patient and caregiver education builds on previous knowledge; observation is effective way to assess performance of psychomotor skills.

NURSING DIAGNOSES

- Reduced urinary elimination
- Reflex urinary incontinence
- Urinary retention

- Insufficient knowledge regarding self-catheterization

- Readiness for enhanced urinary elimination

Related factors/Risk factors are individualized on the basis of on patient's condition or needs.

PLANNING

1. Expected outcomes following completion of procedure:	
• Patient or caregiver states signs and symptoms that indicate need for CISC.	Indicates ability to identify appropriate times to use CISC.
• Patient or caregiver correctly demonstrates how to perform CISC and clean and store equipment.	Return demonstration of skill indicates learning (Alo, 2017).
• Patient or caregiver verbalizes signs and symptoms of complications of CISC (e.g., UTI, urethral bleeding, urethritis, stricture, creation of false passage) and when to contact health care provider (Lamin & Newman, 2016).	Urinary complications such as UTI can occur in patients who use CISC (Canadian Urological Association [CUA], 2014). Verbalization of signs and symptoms of complications helps patients and caregivers identify potential problems early and seek appropriate care.
2. Select setting in the home that patient or caregiver will most likely use when performing CISC.	Respecting patient's needs, values, and choices is key in person-centred care.
3. Help patient or caregiver select catheter that is easiest to use, causes the least amount of trauma, and is most comfortable.	A variety of single-use and reusable catheters is available.

STEP	RATIONALE

IMPLEMENTATION

1. Teach patient and caregiver how to perform appropriate hand hygiene using soap and water. If caregiver is performing skill, have them apply a pair of disposable clean gloves.

Prevents risk for UTI and trauma, which can lead to urethral strictures (Wilson, 2015). Prevents transmission of infection.

2. Perform hand hygiene. Help patient get into a comfortable position. Some men prefer to stand, whereas others prefer to sit. Female patients often need to try different positions to decide which position is most comfortable (Wilson, 2015). Position patient in a place that has adequate lighting.

Reduces transmission of infection. Patient needs adequate lighting to see meatus and equipment.

3. Teach patient or caregiver how to clean urethral meatus:

  a. *For women:* Have patient spread labia with one hand. She uses the other hand to clean urethral opening with a washcloth containing warm, soapy water, and then uses a clean, moist washcloth to rinse. Have female clean in the direction from urethral meatus toward rectum.

Retraction of labia allows for female urethral meatus to be cleaned, reducing risk for infection (Wilson, 2015). Reduces transmission of infection from rectal area to meatus.

  b. *For men:* If patient has not been circumcised, teach him to retract foreskin to expose urethral meatus. Teach him to hold the penis perpendicular to the body with one hand, use the other hand to clean urethral opening with a washcloth containing warm, soapy water, and then use a clean, moist washcloth to rinse. Have male clean in a circular motion from meatus outward.

Ensures cleaning of meatus and reduces risk for infection (Wilson, 2015).

4. Teach female patient or caregiver how to insert catheter:

  a. Catheter selection depends on patient preference and includes single-use or reusable catheter.

Single-use catheter is disposed of after one use. This decreases the risk of UTIs. Reusable catheter is cleaned and stored between uses (Lamin & Newman, 2016).

  b. Using a mirror, help patient locate meatus. Explain that it is just below the clitoris and just above the vaginal opening.

Mirror helps female patient visualize anatomy (Wilson, 2015).

Clinical Decision Point *If a female patient wants to learn how to find the meatus while in a sitting position, teach touch technique by helping her use her fingers to find her urethral opening (Wilson, 2015). Teach her to put one finger over the clitoris and another finger over the vaginal opening. Then help her use these two fingers to find the urethral opening. Another method is the tunnel technique. When women sit with their hips flexed forward, the labia create a "tunnel" that leads to the urethral opening. Teach the woman to slightly separate labia near the clitoris and angle the catheter backward into the urethral opening while placing a finger over the vaginal opening.*

  c. If an uncoated catheter is selected, have patient lubricate tip of catheter with water-soluble jelly by rotating tip to spread lubricant around bottom 2.5 to 5 cm (1 to 2 inches) of catheter. Coated catheters do not require use of separate lubrication.

Lubrication reduces urethral trauma (Lamin & Newman, 2016).
Coated catheter uses hydrophilic or other coatings that do not require use of separate lubricant (Wilson, 2015).

  d. Place outflow end of catheter into urine collection container or let hang over toilet bowl. Slowly and gently insert tip of catheter 5 to 10 cm (2 to 4 inches) into meatus until urine begins to flow.

Appearance of urine indicates that catheter tip is in bladder.

Clinical Decision Point *If the patient feels resistance at the internal sphincter, teach her to apply firm, gentle, steady pressure until muscles relax and allow the catheter to pass (SUNA, 2010).*

5. Teach male patient or caregiver how to insert catheter:

  a. Catheter selection depends on patient preference and includes single-use or reusable catheter.

Patient preference is important for adherence to CISC (Dean, 2015). Single-use catheter is disposed of after one use. Reusable catheter is cleaned and stored between use (Lamin & Newman, 2016).

STEP	RATIONALE

IMPLEMENTATION

b. Lubricate tip of uncoated catheter with water-soluble jelly by rotating tip to spread lubricant around bottom 13 to 18 cm (5 to 7 inches) of catheter. Coated catheters do not require separate lubricant (Wilson, 2015).

Lubrication reduces urethral trauma in uncoated catheters. Dry catheters may cause excoriations in the urethra, which can lead to an entry point for bacterial contamination (Lamin & Newman, 2016).

c. Place outflow end of catheter into urine collection container or let hang over toilet bowl. Slowly and gently insert tip of catheter 15 to 20 cm (6 to 8 inches) into meatus until urine begins to flow. For an uncircumcised male, retract foreskin before inserting the catheter. Tell patient that catheter often needs to be inserted all the way for urine to begin to flow.

The male urethra is longer than the female urethra. Flow of urine indicates that catheter tip is in the bladder.

Clinical Decision Point *Men may experience some resistance when the catheter reaches the prostatic urethra or the neck of the bladder. If the patient feels resistance, do not pull the catheter in and out. Teach him to apply firm, gentle, steady pressure to fatigue the external sphincter and cause muscle relaxation (Wilson, 2015).*

6. Instruct patient or caregiver to hold the catheter in place while urine flows into the container or toilet.

Release of catheter during the procedure often causes catheter to accidentally come out before the bladder is completely emptied.

7. When urine flow stops, teach patient to slowly and gently remove the catheter. For an uncircumcised male, bring foreskin back over glans penis. Then perform hand hygiene.

Removing catheter slowly allows pockets of urine that can accumulate at base of the bladder to drain (SUNA, 2010).

8. Give patient log to record amount of urine if needed.

Some patients need to keep track of their urinary output.

9. Single-use catheters are discarded after self-catheterization is complete (Lamin & Newman, 2016). Instruct patient to clean reusable catheter with mild soap (e.g., Ivory) and water immediately after use. Rinse catheter completely, allow to air dry, and store in clean, dry towel or brown paper bag.

Minimizes risk of UTIs.

10. Teach patient or caregiver to replace reusable catheters as directed by their health care provider.

Appropriate disposal and replacement of equipment prevent complications of CISC.

EVALUATION

1. Observe patient or caregiver independently demonstrate technique for CISC.

Feedback through return demonstration of psychomotor skill is the best means of evaluating learning of skill.

2. Ask patient to identify plan for timing of CISC and steps to take when problems arise.

Measures patient's cognitive learning and ability to problem solve.

3. Review patient's log and observe patient enter information about urine output if indicated.

Confirms that patient understands record keeping and the importance of tracking urine output.

4. Use Teach-Back: "I want to be sure I explained the steps clearly for how to clean and store your catheter. Explain to me how to clean and store your reusable catheter." Develop a revised teaching plan if patient or caregiver is not able to teach back correctly.

Determines patient's and caregiver's level of understanding of instructional topic.

Unexpected Outcomes	**Related Interventions**
1. Patient is unable to easily pass catheter into the bladder.	• Teach patient not to force catheter into the bladder. • Tell patient to go to the nearest urgent care centre or emergency department if the bladder is full and patient is unable to insert catheter. • Use interprofessional collaboration (e.g., urologist) when appropriate.
2. Patient states that they are having symptoms of UTI (e.g., intense urge to urinate; flank or abdominal pain, malaise, fever, chills).	• Inform patient's health care provider of symptoms and anticipate treatment with antibiotic.

Communication and Documentation

- Document teaching, patient and caregiver responses, and demonstration in the home care record.
- Document urine output in home care record and home documentation system (e.g., log).
- Report signs and symptoms of UTIs and difficulty performing CISC to health care provider.

Special Considerations
Teaching

- It is common for patients who perform CISC routinely to have an abnormal urinalysis. Patients should only be treated for UTI if they have symptoms of an infection (e.g., back pain, pelvic tenderness, malaise, confusion, foul-smelling urine, urgency) (CUA, 2014).
- Always leave a phone number and instructions on how to reach the home care nurse if needed.

Pediatric

- Children who are motivated and physiologically and developmentally ready are encouraged to learn how to catheterize themselves. Consult a pediatric urologist; children need special assessment (Dean, 2015).
- When teaching children to perform CISC, use developmentally appropriate teaching strategies. Urinary diversion requires special care (see Chapter 34).
- Concerns of children and adolescents who use CISC include leakage and being wet. They also are often concerned about what their peers know. Allow children to voice their concerns and help them problem solve what they will do in a variety of situations.

Gerontological

- CISC is very effective in older persons because it helps restore continence, decreases urinary urge and nocturia, and improves quality of life.
- Older persons may have difficulty performing CISC because of limited manual dexterity. Individualize care for a patient's needs and functional abilities. Educate the patient or caregiver (Touhy et al., 2019).

◆ SKILL 43.4   Using Home Oxygen Equipment

Medical oxygen is classified by Canada's *Food and Drug Act* as a drug; therefore, a prescription from a health care provider is required for home use (Government of Canada, 2012). The prescription includes the following components: drug/apparatus, dose, route of administration, and duration. The route of administration of oxygen in the home may include a nasal cannula, face mask, tracheal mask, or tracheal catheter. Equipment selection needs to support as much patient independence as feasible (Tiep & Carter, 2019)

Oxygen-conserving devices (OCDs) were introduced to reduce the weight of portable oxygen systems and extend operating time by not wasting oxygen through continuous flow. There are three types of OCDs:

- *Reservoir nasal cannula:* Stores oxygen in a small chamber during exhalation for subsequent delivery during early-phase inhalation.
- *Demand pulsing oxygen-delivery systems:* Deliver a burst of oxygen at the onset of inspiration; small oxygen pulses are very effective in oxygenating a patient.
- *Transtracheal oxygen catheter:* Delivers oxygen directly through a catheter placed between the second and third tracheal rings (Torres & Schwartz, 2017) (Table 43.1).

Oxygen sources in the home include liquid oxygen systems, compressed oxygen in tanks, or oxygen concentrators (Fig. 43.2, A) (Lewis, Bucher, Heitkemper, et al., 2019). Some oxygen tanks (e.g., compressed) are large and stationary. Portable tanks weighing more than 4.5 kg (10 lb) are not designed to be carried and deliver oxygen for about 5 hours at 2 L/min. Ambulatory tanks weigh less than 4.5 (10 lb), are designed to be carried (Fig. 43.2, B), and deliver oxygen for at least 4 hours at 2 L/min. Table 43.2 compares the different types of home oxygen-delivery systems.

Compressed oxygen requires a regulator and flowmeter. The patient receives delivery of several large oxygen tanks to the home. The size of the tank and flow rate determine how long compressed oxygen tanks will last (Table 43.3). Liquid systems take up less space because oxygen is stored in a liquid state. Liquid oxygen is stored at or below −183°C (−297°F) and requires the use of a small ambulatory tank that is filled from a reservoir in the home (Fig. 43.3). Table 43.4 shows how long a liquid oxygen system will last, depending on the prescribed flow rate. The oxygen concentrator method extracts oxygen from room air and supplies oxygen to the patient at prescribed flow rates. Oxygen concentrators deliver a lower percentage of oxygen to the flowmeter. Therefore, if a patient is switched to a concentrator, the flow rate usually needs to be adjusted. The patient who uses a concentrator needs to have a backup system such as a portable oxygen tank in case of power failure.

TABLE 43.1

Oxygen Flow and Appropriate Uses for Oxygen-Delivery Devices

Device	Flow (L/min)	FiO₂ Range (%)	Uses
Nasal cannula	1–6	24–44	Patients who require low concentrations of oxygen therapy
Simple face mask	6–12	35–50	Patients who require short-term oxygen therapy with moderate FiO₂ needs
Oxygen-conserving cannula	8	Up to 30–50	Patients in need of long-term home therapy
Partial and nonrebreather mask	10–15	60–90	Patients in acute respiratory failure or in emergency situations

Data from Lewis S. L., Bucher, L., Heitkemper, M., Harding, M. M., Barry, M. A, Lok, J., Tyerman, J., & Goldsworthy, S. (2019). *Medical-surgical nursing in Canada: Assessment and management of clinical problems* (4th Canadian ed.). Toronto: Elsevier Canada.

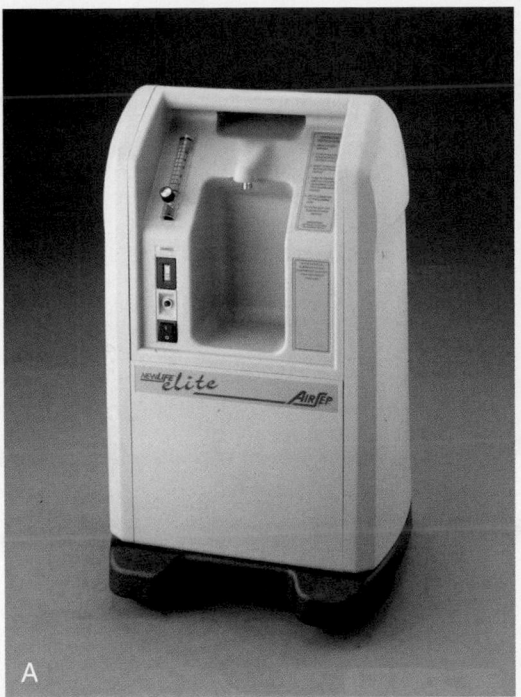
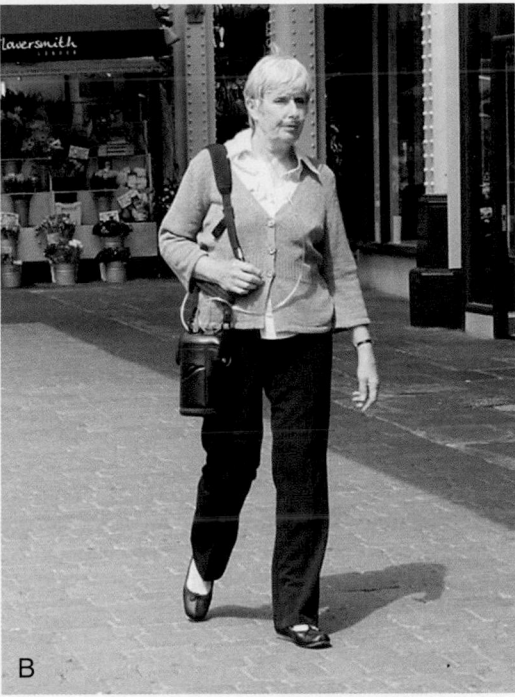

FIG 43.2 A, Portable oxygen concentrator for home use. **B,** Ambulatory tank is small enough to be carried easily. *(Courtesy AirSep Corporation.)*

TABLE 43.2		
Home Oxygen Delivery Systems		
	Advantages	**Disadvantages**
Compressed Oxygen		
Oxygen is stored under pressure in a cylinder equipped with a regulator that controls the flow rate.	An oxygen-conserving device may be attached to the system to avoid waste; the device releases gas only on inhalation and cuts it off with exhalation; it does not require an electrical source; smaller tanks are available.	Large tanks are heavy and only suitable for stationary use. Patient must know how to read the regulator and understand when to call the medical supplier for a replacement cylinder.
Liquid Oxygen System		
Oxygen is stored as a very cold liquid in a vessel very similar to a thermos. When released, the liquid converts to a gas and is breathed in just like compressed gas.	Storage method takes up less space than the compressed gas cylinder; it can transfer the liquid to a small, portable vessel at home.	It is more expensive than compressed gas, and the vessel vents when it is not in use. An oxygen-conserving device may be built into the vessel to conserve the oxygen.
Oxygen Concentrator		
It separates the oxygen out of the air, concentrates it, and stores it.	It does not have to be resupplied, and it is not as costly as liquid oxygen. Extra tubing permits the user to move around with minimal difficulty. Small, portable systems have been developed that afford even greater mobility.	It must have a cylinder of oxygen as a backup in the event of a power failure.

Provincial/territorial health coverage or private health insurance often pays for home oxygen therapy if there is a written prescription from the health care provider.

Patients and their caregivers need extensive teaching to use oxygen therapy correctly and safely. Instruct a patient to have an all-purpose fire extinguisher nearby and learn how to use it and to keep the oxygen supplier's number handy. In addition, provide patient education about the safe use of oxygen in the home (Box 43.3). When initiating and managing ongoing oxygen therapy, collaborate with the patient, health care provider, caregivers, and medical equipment provider.

Delegation and Collaboration

- The skill of teaching patients how to use home oxygen equipment cannot be delegated to an unregulated care provider (UCP).

TABLE 43.3
Oxygen Cylinder Timetable*

| | Large (H-K) Tank | | Small (E) Tank | |
L/min	998 kg (2200 lb) Full	454 kg (1 000 lb) ½ Full	625 L Full	284 L ½ Full
1	115 hr	52 hr	10 hr	5 hr
2	56 hr	26 hr	5 hr	2 hr
3	37 hr	17 hr	3 hr	1 hr
4	28 hr	13 hr	3 hr	1 hr
5	22 hr	10 hr	2 hr	54 min
6	18 hr	8 hr	<2 hr	47 min

The following formulas can also be used to determine the length of time a tank will last:

For E Cylinders

Pressure on cylinder gauge (psi): 500 psi (safety factor) × 0.3 (E cylinder factor) ÷ L/min = minutes

For H Cylinders

Pressure on cylinder gauge (psi): 500 psi (safety factor) × 3.1 (H cylinder factor) ÷ L/min = minutes

EXAMPLE: If E cylinder reads 1500 psi and liter flow rate is 4 L/min:
Time left: 1500 − 500 × 0.3 ÷ 4 = 1000 × 0.3 ÷ 4 = 300 ÷ 4 = 75 minutes (1 hr 15 min)

NOTE: Do not allow oxygen cylinder pressure to fall below 500 psi, or the patient may run out of oxygen.

*All times are approximate.

TABLE 43.4
Liquid Oxygen Timetable

| | Stationary Reservoirs | | Portable Units | |
L/min	41 L	31 L	½ L	1 L
0.25	1400 hr	1060 hr	28 hr	44 hr
0.50	1125 hr	850 hr	18 hr	27 hr
1	560 hr	425 hr	9 hr	15½ hr
1.5	375 hr	283½ hr	6 hr	11½ hr
2	281 hr	213 hr	4½ hr	8½ hr
3	187½ hr	142 hr	3 hr	6 hr

BOX 43.3
Safe Home Oxygen Therapy

Fire Safety
Although oxygen is not flammable, if it comes in contact with fire it will burn; therefore:
- Use and store oxygen in a well-ventilated area.
- Keep cylinders and vessels at least 1.5 metres (5 feet) from heat sources, open flames, or electrical devices.
- Do not use open flames (e.g., matches, fireplaces, stoves, space heaters, candles) when oxygen is in use.
- Do not allow smoking in the house. Post "No Smoking" signs inside and outside the house.
- Install smoke detectors and have a fire extinguisher available in the home. Test smoke detectors twice a month.
- Help patient or caregiver plan a fire evacuation route. Have two routes out of every room and an outside meeting place.

Oxygen Storage and Handling
- Store oxygen tanks upright in carts or stands to prevent tipping or falling, or place tanks flat on the floor when not in use.
- Do not store oxygen tanks in the trunk of a car.
- When transporting oxygen in a vehicle, ensure that tanks are secured properly in the passenger area with the windows opened 5 to 7.5 cm (2 to 3 inches) to allow adequate ventilation.

Concentrator Safety
- Plug concentrators into properly grounded outlets.
- Do not use extension cords, power strips, or multi-outlet adapters with concentrators.
- Ensure that the power supply or circuit meets or exceeds the amperage requirements of the concentrator.

Liquid Oxygen Safety
- Avoid direct contact with liquid oxygen because it can cause frostbite. The vapors are also extremely cold; they can damage delicate tissues such as eyes.
- Do not touch connectors that are frosted or icy.
- Keep ambulatory tanks upright; do not lay them down or place on their side.

Adapted from Lewis S. L., Bucher, L., Heitkemper, M., Harding, M. M., Barry, M. A., Lok, J., Tyerman, J., & Goldsworthy, S. (2019). *Medical-surgical nursing in Canada: Assessment and management of clinical problems* (4th Canadian ed.). Toronto: Elsevier Canada; National Fire Protection Association. (2015). *Public education. Safety tip sheets.* Retrieved from http://www.nfpa.org/safety-information/safety-tip-sheets.

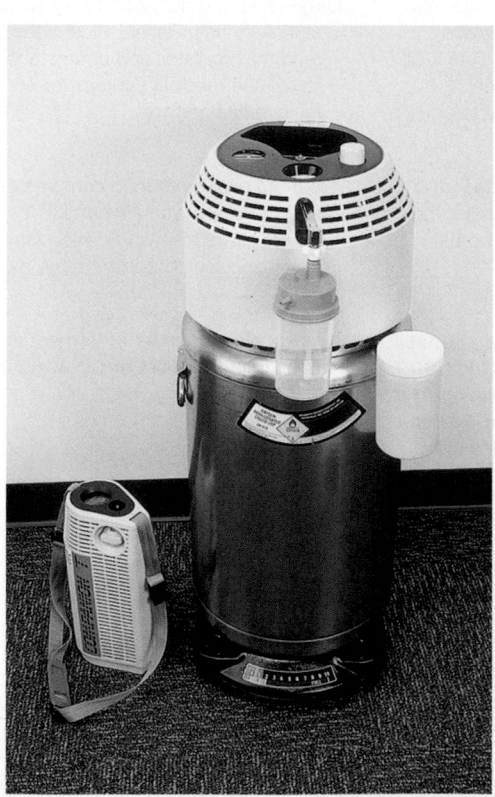

FIG 43.3 Oxygen reservoir and ambulatory tank.

Equipment

- Nasal cannula, oxygen mask (see Chapter 23), OCD, or other prescribed delivery device
- Oxygen tubing
- Home oxygen-delivery system (compressed oxygen, oxygen concentrator, or liquid oxygen) with all required equipment (varies with supplier and system used)
- "No Smoking/Oxygen in Use" sign for each entrance to the home

STEP	RATIONALE

ASSESSMENT

1. Identify patient using at least two person-specific identifiers during hospital and first home visit. Facial recognition can be used as one of two identifiers for ongoing subsequent home visits.	Ensures correct patient. Complies with Accreditation Canada's standards and improves patient safety (Accreditation Canada, 2019b).
2. While patient is still in hospital, determine patient's or caregiver's ability to apply and regulate oxygen equipment correctly. In home setting reassess for appropriate use of equipment.	Physical or cognitive impairments indicate need to teach caregiver how to operate home oxygen equipment. Determines specific components of skill that patient and caregiver are able to complete easily. Home assessment is critical for patient and community safety (Wiles, 2015).
3. Determine appropriate resources in community for equipment and assistance, including maintenance and repair services and medical equipment supplier.	Ensures readily available help for patients with home oxygen systems (Wiles, 2015). Home oxygen risk assessment is a priority with home oxygen therapy for patient and caregiver safety.
4. Determine appropriate backup systems for compressor in event of power failure (e.g., notify local emergency medical services [EMS]). Have a spare oxygen tank available for emergency use.	Many municipalities require that patients who have home oxygen equipment notify EMS before putting equipment in the home. In case of power outage, EMS will call the home, and in some cases, the home is on a priority list for having power restored.
5. Assess patient's learning readiness and ability to concentrate; consider presence of pain, nausea, or fatigue and patient interest in instruction.	Presence of significant illness, frailty, or confusion affects patient's ability to attend to teaching plan. Indicates need to rely on caregiver for learning and implementation (if available) on a short- or long-term basis.

NURSING DIAGNOSES

- Anxiety
- Insufficient knowledge regarding oxygen therapy
- Inadequate health maintenance

Related factors/Risk factors are individualized on the basis of patient's condition or needs.

PLANNING

1. Expected outcomes following completion of procedure:	
• Patient receives oxygen at prescribed rate.	Oxygen system is set up correctly.
• Patient or caregiver verbalizes purpose and correct use of home oxygen.	Provides measurable criteria to determine level of understanding.
• Patient or caregiver demonstrates how to apply, regulate, and maintain oxygen system.	Indicates learning has occurred.
• Patient or caregiver states indications for calling medical equipment provider to replenish oxygen supply and reorder oxygen-delivery supplies.	Patient needs a constant supply of oxygen at home.
• Patient or caregiver verbalizes safety guidelines for oxygen use (e.g., place "No Smoking/Oxygen in Use" signs at entrances to home; educate about safety for patient who continues to smoke) (Homecare Medical, 2017; Wiles, 2015).	Provides measure of understanding of oxygen use.
• Patient or caregiver verbalizes emergency plan of care (Wiles, 2015).	Ensures safe, continuous delivery of home oxygen.
2. Select a setting in the home where patient is most likely to use oxygen equipment and is conducive to a teaching session:	Practising in the same environment where skill is routinely performed facilitates comprehension and learning.

STEP	RATIONALE

PLANNING

- Select a room that is well lit with comfortable seating.
- Be sure that patient is close and can see the nurse clearly.
- Control sources of noise and distractions.

Room environment needs to minimize existing sensory alterations. A comfortable environment free of distractions increases patient's attention.

IMPLEMENTATION

1. Teach patient or caregiver how to perform hand hygiene before handling oxygen equipment.

    Reduces transmission of microorganisms.

2. Place oxygen-delivery system in a clutter-free environment that is well ventilated; away from walls, drapes, curtains, bedding, and combustible materials; and at least 2.4 metres (8 feet) from heat sources.

    Keeps system balanced and prevents injury.

Clinical Decision Point *Do not place oxygen-delivery system in a closet.*

3. Demonstrate steps for preparation and maintenance of oxygen therapy:

    Demonstration is a reliable technique for teaching psychomotor skill and enables the patient to ask questions.

    a. **Compressed oxygen system:**
       (1) Turn cylinder valve counterclockwise two to three turns with a wrench.

       Turns on oxygen.

       (2) Check cylinders by reading amount on pressure gauge.

       Verifies adequate oxygen supply for patient use.

       (3) Store wrench with oxygen tank or in other safe place.

       Storing wrench in a safe place ensures that it is available whenever needed.

    b. **Oxygen concentrator system:**
       (1) Plug concentrator into appropriate outlet.

       Provides power safely to concentrator.

       (2) Turn on power switch.

       Starts concentrator motor.

       (3) Alarm will sound for a few seconds.

       Alarm shuts off when desired pressure inside concentrator is reached.

    c. **Liquid oxygen system:**
       (1) Check liquid system by depressing button at lower right corner and reading dial on stationary oxygen reservoir or ambulatory tank.

       Verifies adequate oxygen supply for patient use.

       (2) Collaborate with medical equipment provider to provide instruction in refilling ambulatory tank when it becomes empty.

       Ensures that continuous oxygen therapy is not interrupted.

Clinical Decision Point *Ambulatory tanks are only filled when they are empty. Liquid oxygen is stored at or below −183°C (−297°F) inside the reservoir, and the temperature inside the ambulatory tank is warmer. If cold oxygen from the reservoir mixes with warmer oxygen left in the ambulatory tank, the ambulatory tank malfunctions. Keep the medical equipment supplier contact number in a visible location for asking questions about the equipment.*

   (3) To refill liquid oxygen tank:
       (a) Wipe both filling connectors with a clean, dry, lint-free cloth.

       Removes dust and moisture from system.

       (b) Turn off flow selector of ambulatory unit.

       (c) Attach ambulatory unit to stationary reservoir by inserting female adapter from ambulatory tank into male adapter of stationary reservoir (see illustration).

       Secures connection between oxygen reservoir and ambulatory tank.

       (d) Open fill valve on ambulatory tank (e.g., lever, button, key) and apply firm pressure to top of stationary reservoir (see illustration). Stay with unit while it is filling. You will hear a loud hissing noise. The tank should be filled in about 2 minutes.

       Prevents leakage of oxygen during filling process. If oxygen leaks during filling process, the connection between the ambulatory tank and reservoir potentially ices up, and ambulatory and reservoir tanks stick together.

STEP	RATIONALE

IMPLEMENTATION

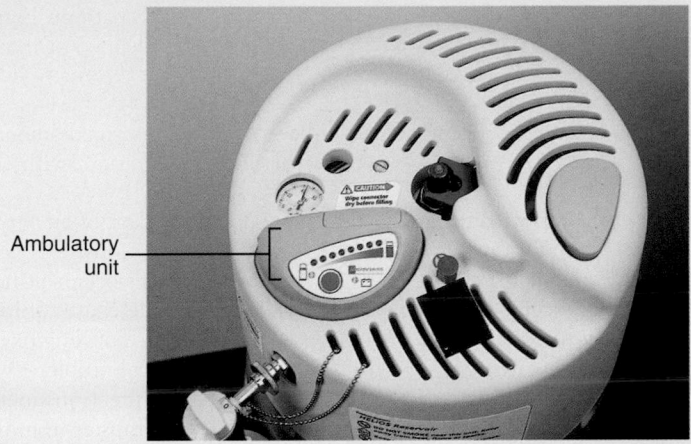

STEP 3c(3)(c) Top view of stationary reservoir.

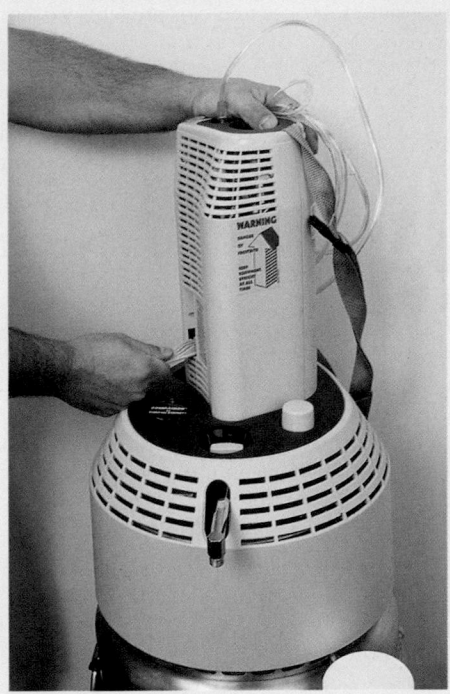

STEP 3c(3)(d) Fill valve on ambulatory tank is opened while applying firm pressure to top of ambulatory tank.

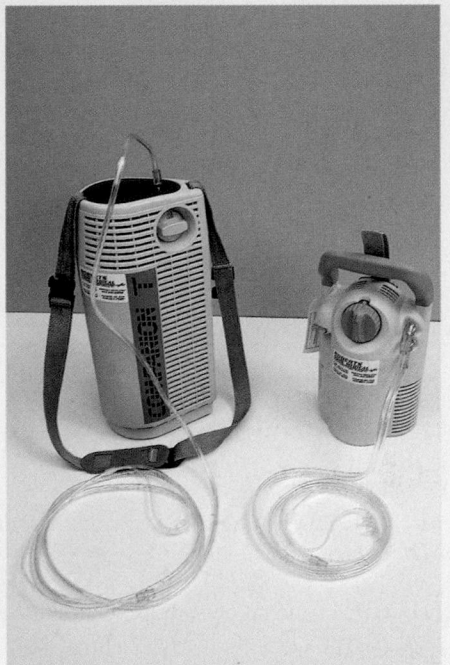

STEP 4 Oxygen-delivery device (nasal cannulas) and tubing attached to ambulatory oxygen tanks.

STEP	RATIONALE
(e) Disconnect ambulatory unit from stationary reservoir when hissing noise changes and vapor cloud begins to form from stationary unit.	Overfilling causes ambulatory unit to malfunction as a result of high pressure in the tank.

Clinical Decision Point *If the ambulatory unit does not separate easily, valves from the reservoir and ambulatory unit are frozen together. Wait until valves warm to disengage (about 5 to 10 minutes). Do not touch any frosted areas because contact with skin causes skin damage from frostbite.*

STEP	RATIONALE
(f) Wipe both filling connectors with a clean, dry, lint-free cloth.	Ice often forms during the filling process. Removes moisture from oxygen system.
4. Connect oxygen-delivery device (e.g., nasal cannula) to oxygen-delivery system (see Chapter 23) (see illustration).	Connects oxygen source to delivery method.
5. Adjust oxygen flow rate (L/min) to prescribed rate.	Ensures that prescribed oxygen dose is delivered.

STEP	RATIONALE

IMPLEMENTATION

6. Have patient or caregiver apply oxygen-delivery device (e.g., nasal cannula) correctly (see Chapter 23). Ensure that patient has two sets of oxygen-delivery devices and tubing.

Delivers oxygen to patient. Extra set of equipment is used when equipment is cleaned or in case of equipment malfunction.

7. Instruct patient and caregiver not to change oxygen flow rate.

Exceeding the prescribed amount of oxygen is sometimes harmful (e.g., patient with chronic obstructive pulmonary disease [COPD]).

8. Have patient or caregiver perform each step with guidance. Provide written material for reinforcement and review.

Allows for correction of any errors in technique and discussion of their implications.

9. Instruct patient or caregiver to notify the health care provider if signs or symptoms of hypoxia occur, including apprehension, anxiety, decreased ability to concentrate, decreased levels of consciousness, increased fatigue, dizziness, behavioural changes, increased pulse, increased respiratory rate, pallor, and cyanosis or respiratory tract infection (e.g., fever, increased sputum, change in colour of sputum, foul sputum odour).

Hypoxia sometimes occurs at home when the patient uses oxygen. Possible causes of hypoxia include poor tubing connections; use of long oxygen tubing; or worsening of patient's physical problem, with change in respiratory status.
Respiratory tract infections increase oxygen demand and often affect oxygen transfer from the lungs to blood, creating exacerbation of the patient's pulmonary disease.

10. Discuss emergency plans for power loss, natural disaster, and acute respiratory distress. Have patient or caregiver call 9-1-1 and notify the health care provider and home care employer.

Ensures appropriate response and can prevent worsening of patient's condition.

11. Instruct patient and caregiver in safe home oxygen practices, including placing "No Smoking/Oxygen in Use" signs at each entrance to the home, not allowing smoking in the house, keeping oxygen tanks 2.4 metres (8 feet) away from open flames, and storing oxygen tanks upright.

Ensures safe use of oxygen in the home and prevents injury to the patient and family (Galligan, Markkanen, Fantasia, et al., 2015).

EVALUATION

1. Monitor rate at which oxygen is being delivered during each home visit.

Determines if patient or caregiver is regulating oxygen at prescribed rate.

2. Ask patient or caregiver about ease or problems associated with home oxygen.

Determines ability of patient or caregiver to deal with stressors associated with home oxygen use. Also indicates patient's risk for inappropriate oxygen use.

3. Ask patient or caregiver to state safety guidelines, emergency precautions, and emergency plan.

Determines patient's or caregiver's knowledge of what to do if power fails, there is a failure in equipment, or patient's status worsens.

4. **Use Teach-Back:** "I want to be sure I explained the importance of oxygen. Tell me in your own words why you need oxygen and the signs and symptoms of lack of oxygen." Develop a revised teaching plan if patient or caregiver is not able to teach back correctly.

Determines patient's and caregiver's level of understanding of instructional topic.

Unexpected Outcomes

1. Patient has signs and symptoms associated with hypoxia.

Related Interventions

- Determine if oxygen-delivery device and oxygen source are delivering oxygen properly.
- Determine if prescribed oxygen flow rate is set properly.
- Assess patient for change in respiratory status, such as airway plugging, respiratory tract infection, or bronchospasm.
- Teach patient or caregiver when to notify health care provider or activate EMS because of signs of hypoxia.

2. Patient uses unsafe practices with oxygen therapy, uses oxygen around fire or cigarette smoking, or sets incorrect flow rate.

- Reinforce patient education and perform follow-up reassessment (see Box 43.3).
- Include caregiver in instruction and set up problem-solving exercises with patient.

3. Patient is unable to fill ambulatory system.

- Identify and instruct caregiver who can help patient fill tank.

Communication and Documentation

- Document teaching plan, information provided to patient, and patient's and caregiver's ability to discuss information in the home care record.
- Communicate patient's or caregiver's learning progress to other health care providers involved in the patient's care.
- Document oxygen-delivery system, related supplies, and prescribed oxygen flow rate in home care record.
- Report respiratory complications or concerns to the health care provider.

Special Considerations
Teaching

- Potential for oxygen desaturation and decreased oxygen delivery to the brain impairs the patient's ability to remember previous learning. Provide frequent teaching sessions and written or pictorial instructions to reinforce previous learning of teaching plan.
- Teach the patient or caregiver that oxygen is a medication (Hart, 2015).
- Explain to the patient and caregiver signs of hypoxia. Hypoxia sometimes occurs at home when a patient uses oxygen. Possible causes of hypoxia include poor tubing connections, use of long oxygen tubing, or worsening of the patient's physical problem, with change in respiratory status.
- Teach the patient or caregiver not to smoke within the home, for the safety of all occupants. Post "Oxygen in Use" signs on all exterior doors and on the bedroom door.

- Instruct the patient or caregiver in appropriate cleaning, disinfecting, and maintaining of all oxygen-delivery systems and supplies. Verify instructions with manufacturer guidelines and medical equipment provider's instructions.
- Instruct patient or caregiver to check the mask and tubing by placing hands or face over the mask or cannula to feel airflow and check that the mask is not too tight. A tight mask often leaves marks on the skin.
- Always leave a phone number and instructions on how to reach a home care nurse if needed.

Pediatric

- Keep equipment out of reach of any children in the home. Do not allow children to handle or operate home oxygen equipment.
- Keep children away from fire and flames always; as appropriate, educate about dangers of oxygen coming into contact with fire (Wiles, 2015).

Gerontological

- Older persons have less efficient respiratory systems and less surface area for gas exchange; thus, they are at greater risk for cerebral anoxia and confusion when they experience decreased oxygen levels. They may be unable to recognize respiratory problems or problems with their oxygen-delivery system. Therefore, they need frequent contact with a designated caregiver.

✦ SKILL 43.5   Teaching Home Tracheostomy Care and Suctioning

Performing tracheostomy care and suctioning in the home is similar to performing these skills in the hospital except for one key variable: the use of *medical asepsis* or *clean technique*. The home environment has fewer germs than hospitals; therefore, clean technique can be used. Aseptic technique is used in the hospital because the patient is more susceptible to infection and more virulent or pathogenic microorganisms are usually present. In the home setting the majority of patients use clean technique. Nurses need to use judgement in choosing the correct technique for each patient (e.g., use aseptic technique with patients who are immunocompromised; are infected [not colonized]; or have caregivers infected with viral, bacterial, or fungal microorganisms). Patients who live in unclean conditions also need to be suctioned with aseptic technique whenever possible to try to prevent infection. All caregivers need to use standard precautions when suctioning with either clean or aseptic technique.

Caring for a tracheostomy at home begins in the hospital (see Chapter 25) with teaching and return demonstration. The patient or caregiver usually learns better when instruction in less invasive techniques such as tracheal stoma care precedes more invasive techniques such as inner cannula care and suctioning. The nurse needs to continually develop, implement, and evaluate the teaching plan based on patient performance. It is imperative that patients and their caregivers have the ability to practice suctioning frequently before discharge to develop confidence with skill performance; otherwise, arrangements to provide 24-hour care are necessary before discharge.

Delegation and Collaboration

The skill of teaching home tracheostomy care and suctioning cannot be delegated to an unregulated care provider (UCP). In some community settings the skill of suctioning a patient with an established tracheostomy can be performed by a UCP (check employer policy). The nurse instructs the UCP to:

- Document changes in the patient's level of consciousness, irritability, vital signs, or decreased pulse oximetry.
- Report increased airway secretions.

Equipment

- Suction machine with connecting tube
- Clean or sterile gloves
- Three small basins
- Hydrogen peroxide
- Normal saline
- Appropriate-size sterile or clean and disinfected suction catheter (diameter no greater than half the diameter of the tracheostomy tube [e.g., if tracheostomy tube is 8 mm (0.3 inches), use 16-Fr or smaller suction catheter])
- Tracheostomy care kit or clean 10 × 10–cm (4 × 4–inch) gauze pads (nonshredding)
  - Small nylon bottle brush or pipe cleaners
  - Replacement inner cannula if patient has disposable inner cannulas

- Cotton-tipped applicators
- Tracheostomy ties (twill tape [⅛-inch preferably] or Velcro-type tie holders)
- Mirror
- Wet washcloth or paper towel (optional)

- Dry cloth, towel, or paper towel (optional)
- Protective eyewear (optional)
- Trash bag (plastic, leak proof preferred)
- Disposable apron (optional)
- Bag-valve-mask (BVM) with oxygen supply (optional)

STEP	RATIONALE

ASSESSMENT

1. Identify patient using at least two person-specific identifiers during first home visit. Facial recognition can be used as one of two identifiers for ongoing subsequent home visits.

Ensures correct patient. Complies with Accreditation Canada's standards and improves patient safety (Accreditation Canada, 2019b).

2. Assess patient's and caregiver's vision and fine-motor function for the ability to perform tracheostomy care and suctioning properly. Also assess patient's level of consciousness and ability to attend to care and problem solve.

Instructing the caregiver is essential if the patient's physical and cognitive impairment prevents ability to perform tracheostomy care and suctioning. Emergency situations usually require a caregiver to suction.

3. Assess patient's and caregiver's knowledge of indications for the need to perform:

   a. Tracheostomy care, including presence of excess peristomal secretions, excess intratracheal secretions, soiled or damp tracheostomy dressing and ties, and diminished airway through the tracheostomy tube.

   Knowledge needed for patient or caregiver to accurately assess need to provide tracheostomy care. Signs and symptoms are related to presence of secretions at the stoma site or within the tracheostomy tube.

   b. Suctioning, including patient's perceived need for suctioning, presence of gurgling, wheezes on inspiration or expiration, restlessness, ineffective coughing, tachypnea, cyanosis, acutely decreased level of consciousness, tachycardia or bradycardia, acutely shallow respirations, or acute dyspnea.

   Knowledge allows patient or caregiver to accurately determine the need to perform tracheostomy tube suctioning. Physical signs and symptoms result from lower-airway obstruction and tissue hypoxia.

4. Assess patient's or caregiver's ability to assess pulse rate and respirations.

Necessary for appropriate monitoring in the home.

5. Assess patient's learning readiness and ability to concentrate; consider presence of pain, nausea, or fatigue and patient interest in instruction.

Presence of significant illness, frailty, or confusion affects a patient's ability to attend to a teaching plan. Indicates need to rely on a caregiver for learning and implementation (if available) on a short- or long-term basis.

6. Observe patient or caregiver perform complete tracheostomy tube care and suctioning.

Determines which specific components of skill that patient or caregiver can complete easily, and which are more difficult and require reinforcement.

NURSING DIAGNOSES

- Inadequate breathing pattern
- Insufficient knowledge regarding tracheostomy care
- Inadequate health maintenance
- Potential for caregiver role strain
- Potential for infection

Related factors/Risk factors are individualized on the basis of patient's condition or needs.

PLANNING

1. Expected outcomes following completion of procedure:
   - Patient or caregiver identifies signs and symptoms, indicating need for tracheostomy care and suctioning.

   Patient or caregiver can institute preventive means to maintain airway.

   - Patient or caregiver states factors that influence tracheostomy airway functioning.

   Tracheostomy often impairs normal airway clearance, humidification, and gas exchange.

   - Patient or caregiver correctly demonstrates complete tracheostomy tube care and suctioning in a controlled setting.

   Provides validation of ability to perform procedure.

   - Patient or caregiver identifies signs of stoma inflammation or respiratory tract infection and when to notify health care provider.

   Measures cognitive learning.

STEP	RATIONALE

PLANNING

- Lower and upper airways are cleared of secretions, as evidenced by absent or diminished wheezes and gurgles in large airways, normalization of pulse and respiratory rate, increased depth of respirations, absence of cyanosis, improved colour, and decreased dyspnea. | Suctioning by patient or caregiver is successful.

- Stoma site is clean and free of an infection and transesophageal fistula. Signs of transesophageal fistula include frequent coughing when eating, aspiration, or fever. | Tracheostomy care is successful.

- Inner cannula is free of secretions. |

2. Select a setting in the home where the patient or caregiver is most likely to perform tracheostomy tube care: | Practising skill in the same setting where skill will be routinely performed facilitates comprehension and learning.

- Select a room that is well lit with comfortable seating. |
- Be sure that the patient is close and can see the nurse clearly. |
- Control sources of noise and distractions. | Room environment needs to minimize existing sensory alterations. A comfortable environment free of distractions increases patient's attention.

3. Discuss and demonstrate with patient or caregiver proper position for procedure (high-Fowler's position in front of mirror). | Promotes understanding of comfort and safety principles and facilitates visibility.

IMPLEMENTATION

1. Suctioning:

a. Verify health care provider's prescriptions for suctioning. Ensure that patient and caregiver understand suctioning prescription. | Invasive procedure requires prescription.
Prescription may be written for as-needed suctioning; ensures that patient and caregiver understand what this means.

b. Teach patient or caregiver techniques for hand hygiene and application of clean gloves. | Reduces transmission of microorganisms.

c. Explain and demonstrate step-by-step preparation and completion of tracheostomy tube suctioning using either open or closed suctioning (see Chapter 25) (see illustration). | Demonstration is a reliable technique for teaching psychomotor skill and enables the patient or caregiver to ask questions throughout the procedure. Steps used to suction patients in the hospital are also used in the home.

Clinical Decision Point *Instillation of normal saline before suctioning, once a common practice, is no longer recommended. Use of normal saline adversely affects arterial and global tissue oxygenation (Ayhan, Tastan, Iyigun, et al., 2015).*

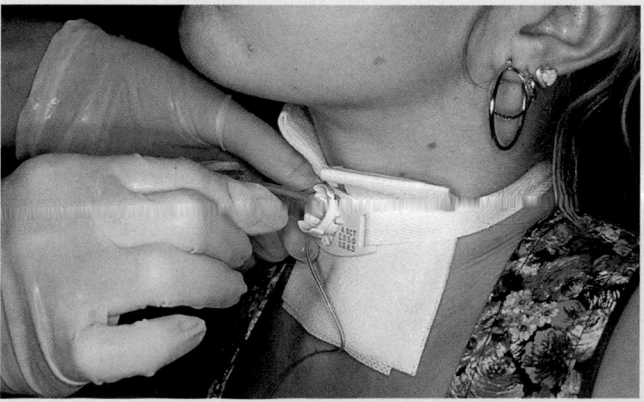

STEP 1c Insertion of suction catheter into tracheostomy tube.

STEP	RATIONALE

IMPLEMENTATION

d. After the patient or caregiver suctions tracheostomy, teach them how to suction the nasal and oral pharynx and perform mouth care. Encourage patient or caregiver to brush teeth with a small, soft toothbrush two times a day and use mouth moisturizer to moisturize the lips every 2 to 4 hours.

Suctioning removes secretions from trachea and lower airway that patients are not able to clear by coughing (Credland, 2016). Dental plaque harbours microorganisms.

e. At conclusion of the procedure, have patient take two to three deep breaths; reassess status of breathing.

Deep breathing reduces oxygen loss and prevents hypoxia. Expect patient's respiratory status to improve following suctioning.

f. Demonstrate how to disconnect suction catheter; coil and discard catheter in an appropriate receptacle. If catheter is to be cleaned and disinfected, set it aside. Have patient or caregiver remove soiled gloves and dispose of them in an appropriate container; perform hand hygiene.

Prevents transmission of microorganisms.

2. Tracheostomy care:

a. Have patient sit at a table with a mirror. Instruct patient or caregiver how to perform hand hygiene and apply clean gloves with you. Teach skills of tracheostomy care, including cleaning stoma and tracheostomy tube and changing tracheostomy ties and dressing (see illustrations and Chapter 25). *Exception:* Clean inner cannula with hydrogen peroxide and a small brush (Cleveland Clinic, 2019).

Prevents transmission of microorganisms. Steps used to provide tracheostomy care in the hospital are also used in the home.

Clinical Decision Point *During tracheostomy care a patient is at risk for the tracheostomy tube coming out. Instruct patient or caregiver to never remove the old tracheostomy tube ties until the new ties are secured properly. Keep two tracheostomy tubes, one the same size as the patient's and one a size smaller, accessible to the patient so a new tube can be inserted if the tube comes out. If the patient has a disposable inner cannula they need to have replacement cannulas available.*

b. Have patient or caregiver remove and dispose of gloves. Perform hand hygiene.

Reduces transmission of microorganisms.

c. Instruct patient or caregiver to apply clean gloves. Demonstrate technique for cleaning reusable supplies in warm, soapy water. Rinse thoroughly and dry between two layers of clean paper towels. Store supplies in a loosely closed clear plastic bag; label the bag.

Prevents transmission of microorganisms. Air must circulate, or humidity in bag can promote microorganism growth.

d. Have patient or caregiver remove and discard gloves. Perform hand hygiene.

Reduces transmission of microorganisms.

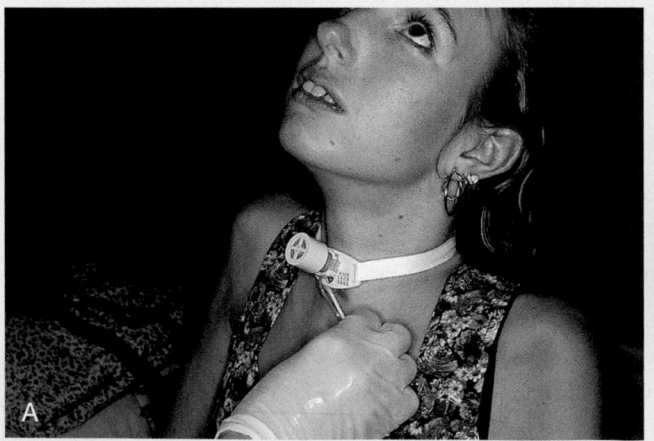
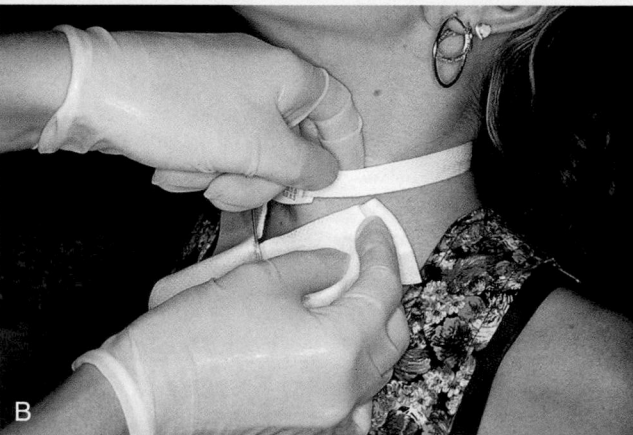

STEP 2a A, Cleaning area around tracheal stoma. **B,** Applying clean tracheostomy dressing.

STEP	RATIONALE

IMPLEMENTATION

3. Disinfecting supplies:

   a. Explain procedure for disinfecting reusable supplies. Disinfection needs to be done at least weekly. To disinfect supplies, use one of following methods:

      (1) *Method 1:* Boil reusable (boilable) supplies for 15 minutes. Allow to cool and dry.

      (2) *Method 2:* Soak reusable supplies in equal parts of vinegar and water for 30 minutes. Remove, rinse thoroughly, and dry.

      (3) *Method 3:* Soak reusable supplies in prepared solutions of quaternary ammonium chloride compounds according to manufacturer instructions. Rinse and dry.

Rationale: Removes microorganisms and reduces risk for infection.

4. Have patient or caregiver perform each step with guidance from you.

Rationale: Adults learn psychomotor skills best by active participation, and you can correct any errors in technique as they occur and discuss their implications.

5. Teach patient or caregiver signs and symptoms of the following:

   a. Stoma infection (redness, tenderness, drainage)

   b. Respiratory tract infection (fever, increased sputum, change in colour of sputum, foul sputum odour, increased cough, chills, night sweats)

   c. Transesophageal fistula (air leaking through stoma, nose, or mouth with cuff properly inflated; more air needed to inflate cuff; aspiration of food or liquid during suctioning; excessive belching; coughing when swallowing)

Rationale: Patient or caregiver must be able to recognize the onset of complications associated with long-term tracheostomy use early so that medical treatment can begin, reducing risk for more serious negative outcomes. Emphasize the importance of notifying the health care provider when signs and symptoms of complications occur.

EVALUATION

1. Observe patient or caregiver demonstrate technique for tracheostomy tube care and suctioning.

Rationale: Feedback through independent demonstration of psychomotor skill is a reliable method to evaluate learning.

2. Ask patient or caregiver to describe signs and symptoms indicating need for tracheostomy care and suctioning and the factors that influence tracheostomy airway functioning.

Rationale: Demonstrates learning and patient's and caregiver's ability to respond when airway problems develop.

3. Have patient and caregiver explain the problems that need to be reported to their health care provider.

Rationale: Demonstrates patient's and caregiver's ability to take steps for emergent care.

4. Use Teach-Back: "I want to be sure I explained how you will feel and what you may see if you develop problems or complications with your tracheostomy. Tell me the signs and symptoms for needing to suction your tracheostomy." Develop a revised teaching plan if patient or caregiver is not able to teach back correctly.

Rationale: Determines patient's and caregiver's level of understanding of instructional topic.

Unexpected Outcomes

1. Stoma site is reddened or hard, with or without drainage.

2. Copious coloured secretions are present around stoma or when patient or caregiver suctions tracheostomy.

Related Interventions

- Evaluate patient's or caregiver's technique.
- Increase frequency of tracheostomy care.
- Have patient use sterile technique for suctioning and tracheostomy care.
- Secretions may be pink, rust-coloured, or blood-tinged, depending on problem; documenting colour helps health care provider diagnose the problem.
- Evaluate for adequate humidity (use room humidifier or tracheostomy collar humidity, if needed) (see Chapter 25).
- Notify health care provider.

STEP	RATIONALE
Unexpected Outcomes 3. Bloody secretions are suctioned.	**Related Interventions** • Evaluate suctioning technique, suctioning frequency, and size of catheter used. • Usual length to insert catheter is length of tracheostomy tube plus $\frac{1}{4}$ inch. • Assess for signs of infection. • Assess patient for use of anticoagulant medications.
4. No secretions are suctioned.	• Evaluate patient's fluid status, need for increased humidity. • Determine if appropriate-size suction catheter is used. • Reassess need to suction.
5. Skin breakdown is present at stoma site.	• Assess site for pressure areas or site infection. • Remove pressure source.

Communication and Documentation

• Document patient instruction and patient's and caregiver's ability to demonstrate tracheostomy care, suctioning skills, and disinfecting skills in the home health record.
• Develop a system for patient or caregiver to document and keep track of tracheostomy care provided.

Special Considerations
Teaching

• The nose and mouth normally provide warmth, filtering, and moisture for the air we breathe. A tracheostomy tube bypasses these mechanisms. Humidification must be provided to keep secretions thin and to avoid mucous plugs.
• Caution patients and caregivers against using alcohol-based products to clean supplies because they can cause the materials to become hard and brittle. Do not place equipment or supplies in the dishwasher.
• Always leave a phone number and instructions on how to reach a home care nurse if needed.

Pediatric

• Encourage parents to give tracheostomy care as soon as the child is stable in the hospital. The more time they have to practice these skills, the more comfortable they become in caring for the child at home.
• Children with tracheostomies need to socialize and play with other children who are close to their own age. Encourage caregivers to take children out of the home. However, an additional adult needs to travel with the child to help if problems arise while in the car (Hockenberry & Wilson, 2015).
• To prevent hypoxia, teach caregivers that suctioning needs to last no more than 5 seconds. Allow the child to rest for at least 30 to 60 seconds between suctioning passes and to not suction more than three times (Hockenberry & Wilson, 2015).

• Teach caregivers pediatric cardiopulmonary resuscitation (CPR), including use of BVM or mouth-to-tracheostomy technique. They also need to notify the local EMS of the child's condition and the presence of a tracheostomy and provide EMS with a list of equipment in the home (Hockenberry & Wilson, 2015).
• Encourage caregivers to have a cool-mist humidifier in the same room as the child; humidity helps keep secretions thin and decreases the likelihood of mucous plugging (Hockenberry & Wilson, 2015).
• Caring for a child with a tracheostomy often disrupts caregivers' ability to socialize and can cause sleep deprivation. Develop a plan that includes respite care to allow caregivers time to meet their own needs (Hockenberry & Wilson, 2015).
• Teach caregivers to avoid dressing the child in clothes that could cover the tracheostomy opening, such as turtlenecks and clothes that have a tight-fitting collar. Avoid clothing, toys, and pets that shed fine hair or lint because it could get into the tracheostomy and cause breathing problems (Hockenberry & Wilson, 2015).

Gerontological

• Older persons lose some properties of elastic recoil and often have greater difficulty clearing airway secretions through cough. As a result, they require more suctioning and airway care and have increased risk for infection (Touhy et al., 2019).
• Assess for cognitive, mobility, or sensory impairments that decrease ability to manage an artificial airway at home and teach the caregiver if the patient is unable to manage the airway independently.
• Anxiety accompanies decreased ability to breathe and may cause the older person to become too nervous to perform suctioning independently.

◆ SKILL 43.6 Teaching Medication Self-Administration

A patient's medication regime can undergo various changes, either from a hospital stay or a doctor's visit (Institute for Safe Medication Practices [ISMP] Canada, 2017). The nurse can find resources and address issues that may influence patients' adherence to their medication regimen (e.g., ability to purchase medications, transportation to pharmacy, adverse effects). Teaching patients how to correctly administer medications is very important, but first the nurse needs to identify and address any issues that are of concern.

The word *compliance* was used in the past to describe whether patients' behaviours matched that of health care providers' recommendations when it came to taking prescribed medications

or adhering to prescribed treatments. Recent literature supports the term *adherence,* since this emphasizes a patient's role in decision making, considering freedom of choice (Iihara, Nishio, Okura, et al., 2014). One method that has been identified to increase adherence is to understand and then support patients' decisions in how to take their medications. Nurses need to use teaching methods that incorporate active listening so that they can adapt patients' needs and concerns into the medication regimen.

Some barriers to medication adherence include fear of adverse reactions from medications, belief that a medication does not help, inconvenience of taking medication, cost of medication, inadequate knowledge, forgetfulness, and relationship with the health care provider (Müller, Kohlmann, & Wilke, 2015). Considering these potential barriers, nurses can provide information and support to ensure that a patient or caregiver is making a well-informed decision when it comes to whether to take a medication. Once a patient has mastered the skill of administering medications, the nurse must continue to validate that the skill is being performed correctly and assess for new issues and concerns.

Delegation and Collaboration

Interprofessional collaboration (e.g., pharmacist) is required to explore methods of administration such as dosettes and blister packs that would aid in self-administration and adherence. The skill of teaching patients medication self-administration cannot be delegated to an unregulated care provider (UCP). The nurse directs the UCP to:

- Communicate to the nurse problems that the patient reports with medication self-administration.

Equipment

- Medication
- Liquid to take with medication
- Medication administration record or other up-to-date list of current medications from health care provider
- Medication log
- Container for daily or weekly preparation
- Measuring devices, as needed (e.g., medicine cup, teaspoon)
- Teaching tools (e.g., charts, written instructions, colour codes for medicine containers)

STEP	RATIONALE

ASSESSMENT

1. Identify patient using at least two person-specific identifiers during first home visit. Facial recognition can be used as one of two identifiers for ongoing subsequent home visits.

Ensures correct patient. Complies with Accreditation Canada's standards and improves patient safety (Accreditation Canada, 2019b).

2. Assess patient's cognitive, sensory, and motor function: level of consciousness, sight, hearing, touch, health literacy level, swallowing ability, mobility, activity tolerance, social support, and willingness to cooperate.

Cognitive, sensory, and motor deficits frequently influence a patient's ability to take or prepare prescribed medication correctly and participate in instruction.

3. Assess resources patient and caregiver have to obtain medications when needed (e.g., finances, social support, and transportation).

Lack of resources is major factor that negatively affects adherence to medication self-administration regimen (Müller et al., 2015).

4. Assess patient's learning readiness and ability to concentrate (consider presence of pain, nausea, or fatigue and patient interest in instruction) and learning style preference.

Presence of significant illness, frailty, or confusion affects a person's ability to attend to a teaching plan. Indicates need to rely on caregiver for learning and implementation (if available) on a short- or long-term basis. Learning style affects the choice of teaching resources.

5. Assess patient's and caregiver's knowledge of medication therapy: names of medications, how to administer them, purpose or action, daily doses and times to be taken, adverse effects to expect, and what to do if problems occur.

Patients need to be able to understand information about their medications and remember it (Ingadóttir & Zöega, 2017).

Caregiver's confidence in administering medication influences their ability to manage medication for the patient.

6. Assess patient's belief in need for medication therapy. Consider prior experiences, ethnic values, religious beliefs, personal experiences with medications, and caregiver's values about medications.

Many factors influence a patient's willingness to follow a drug regimen.

7 Assess patient's prescribed and over-the-counter (OTC) medications, including use of herbal supplements: Has more than one health care provider prescribed medications? Are labels clearly marked? Are time schedules confusing? Do different medications look alike? Does patient store medications together or out of original containers? Are expiration dates on bottles still current?

Determines sources of confusion affecting patient's adherence. Adherence to medication therapy (especially in older persons) is often complicated by polypharmacy (multiple chronic conditions are often treated with multiple medications, sometimes prescribed by more than one health care provider). Adherence is more complicated when medication regimens are complex.

8. Be sure that caregiver knows patient's drug allergies.

As new medications are prescribed, the caregiver often becomes the one to monitor for inappropriate drug prescription.

STEP	RATIONALE

ASSESSMENT

9. Consult with health care provider to review medications that patient is receiving and simplify regimen if possible.

Review of medications helps minimize risk for drug interactions from multiple medications and ensures accuracy of medication regimen. Simplification of regimen improves adherence, particularly related to daily frequency of prescribed doses.

NURSING DIAGNOSES

- Anxiety
- Insufficient knowledge regarding medication self-administration
- Inadequate health maintenance
- Readiness for enhanced knowledge

Related factors/Risk factors are individualized on the basis of patient's condition or needs.

PLANNING

1. Expected outcomes following completion of procedure:
   - Patient or caregiver is able to state the purpose of each medication and why it is beneficial. If a medication has been discontinued, patient or caregiver correctly explains why this was done.

   Demonstrates cognitive learning.

   - Patient or caregiver identifies common adverse effects and relief measures.

   Encourages adherence to medication therapy.

   - Patient or caregiver can state when to notify health care provider about medication problems.

   Empowers patient to participate in care.

   - Patient or caregiver reads each label and explains when each medication should be taken.

   Prevents medication administration errors.

   - Patient or caregiver demonstrates self-administration of medication by prescribed route.

   Demonstrates skill achieved.

2. Prepare environment for teaching session:

   Improves likelihood of patient and caregiver being attentive to instruction.

   - Select a room that is well lit and offers comfortable seating.
   - Be sure that the patient is close and can see the nurse clearly.
   - Control sources of noise and distractions.

   Room environment needs to minimize existing sensory alterations. A comfortable environment free of distractions increases patient's attention.

3. Prepare teaching materials:

   Person-centred care focuses on working in partnership with patients.

   a. Plan an approach that matches the patient's learning preference (visual, auditory, read or write, kinesthetic):

   Using an instructional approach that matches the patient's learning style in the context in which learning occurs allows for a person-centred approach that incorporates teaching modalities to maximize patient learning.

      (1) Written materials printed in large, bold letters (set in 14-point or larger type)

      Assists patients with visual limitations.

      (2) DVD or Internet instructional programs
      (3) Illustrations of medication safety guidelines
      (4) Handling equipment and supplies

4. Ensure that patient is wearing glasses or hearing aids if needed during teaching session.

   Use of glasses or hearing aids increases the patient's sensory perception and likelihood of attending to teaching session and understanding content.

5. Arrange teaching time to allow participation of caregiver (see illustration).

   Caregivers can serve as a positive resource to patients and often reinforce information provided.

STEP	RATIONALE

PLANNING

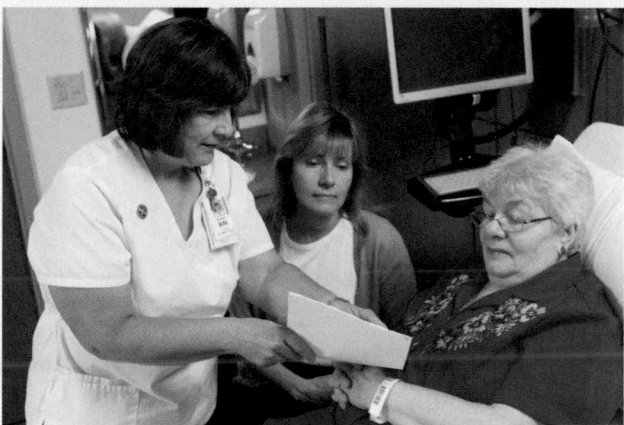

STEP 5 Patient and caregiver participate in medication self-administration teaching program.

IMPLEMENTATION

STEP	RATIONALE
1. Instruct patient or caregiver about the importance of performing hand hygiene before medication self-administration.	Reduces transmission of microorganisms.
2. Present information clearly and concisely:	Improves patient's ability to attend to and understand instruction (Ingadóttir & Zöega, 2017).
a. Face learner in a well-lit room.	Allows visualization of patient's nonverbal responses to education. A patient with hearing loss or visual impairment is able to see your expressions, read written information, and hear your voice more clearly.
b. Use short sentences and speak slowly, in a low-pitched voice.	Enhances understanding of information.
c. Provide descriptions in understandable terms.	Prevents confusion of terminology. Patients learn more quickly when you present information at the level of the learner (Ingadóttir & Zöega, 2017).
3. Provide frequent pauses so patient or caregiver can ask questions and express understanding of content.	Increases learner participation. Ongoing feedback ensures that patient is acquiring information.
4. Instruct patient or caregiver on following content: purpose of regularly scheduled and prn (as needed) medications and their desired effects, how medication works and why it helps, dosage schedules and rationale, common adverse effects, what to do to relieve adverse effects, what to do if a dose is missed, when to call the health care provider with problems, who to call with problems, medication safety guidelines, and implications when medications are not taken.	Provides patient or caregiver with sufficient information to understand medications and their effects and to take them safely at home.
5. Instruct patient or caregiver in the appropriate route of medication delivery, including oral, subcutaneous, intramuscular, inhalation, and topical.	Patients need to be proficient in all routes of medication administration. Adverse effects often occur if medications are administered incorrectly.
6. Provide frequent, short teaching sessions. Plan to have several teaching sessions, especially if patient needs to take multiple medications.	Frequent sessions improve patient's attention to and retention of information discussed.
7. Provide teaching about OTC medications and herbal supplements.	Patients may not understand the effects of OTC and herbal supplements (Government of Canada, 2017).
8. Provide patient with written schedules or individualized instruction sheets for review. Offer special charts, diagrams, learning aids, written information, weekly pill organizers, and Internet resources (see illustration).	Clearly written information, charts, and other resources such as Internet sites enhance patient learning and allow for reinforcement of information (Ingadóttir & Zoëga, 2017).

STEP	RATIONALE

IMPLEMENTATION

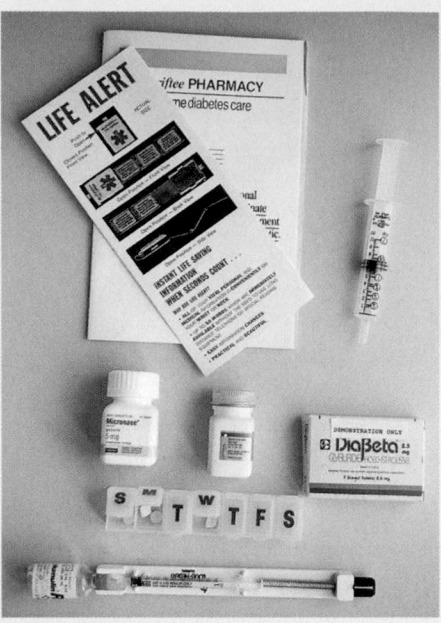

STEP 8 Examples of aids for patient self-administration of medication.

9. Offer help as the patient practices preparing medication (e.g., "Let's prepare the medications you will take with your meals or the medicines you take first in the morning").	Allows for observation of patient's ability to read labels correctly and prepare all medications for prescribed times.
10. Have pharmacy provide clear, large-print labels for medication bottles and medication teaching handouts, if appropriate.	Improves patient's ability to read and follow directions.
11. Have pharmacy provide containers that patient can open independently if manual dexterity is limited.	Most pharmacies dispense pills in "childproof" containers, which a patient with limited mobility of fingers and hands often find difficult to manipulate or open.

Clinical Decision Point *If there are pets or small children in the home or children who frequently visit the home, help the patient establish a safe place for medication storage to reduce risk of accidental ingestion by pets or children.*

12. Facilitate arrangements for pharmacy to receive written prescriptions in a timely fashion if required for dispensing. Arrange for pharmacy to deliver medications to the home if patient is unable to arrange for transportation to the pharmacy.	Availability of medications influences adherence.
13. Discuss with patient or caregiver how to dispose of discontinued or expired medications.	Ensures safe disposal.

EVALUATION

1. Ask patient or caregiver to explain information about each drug: its purpose, actions, and routes; timing of medications and maximum frequency of use of either prescribed or OTC medications; adverse effects and interactions; and foods, herbals, or OTC medications to avoid.	Patients and caregivers need to be able to understand information they are given and remember this information (Almkuist, 2017).
2. Ask patient or caregiver to describe when to call the health care provider or refer to printed information for resources.	Developing techniques to gain information and solve problems can increase patient adherence and reduces potential problems with carrying out the medication regimen.
3. Have patient or caregiver prepare and administer doses for all prescribed medications.	Indicates understanding of medication dosages and schedules.

STEP	RATIONALE

EVALUATION

4. Use Teach-Back: "I want to be sure I explained how to safely dispose of medicines you are no longer taking. Tell me in your own words the correct way to dispose of your tablets here in the home." Develop a revised teaching plan if patient or caregiver is not able to teach back correctly.

Determines patient's and caregiver's level of understanding of instructional topic.

Unexpected Outcomes

1. Patient or caregiver makes errors in preparing medications or is unable to recall or explain information discussed in teaching sessions.

Related Interventions

- Provide additional instruction and teaching materials for consultation when information is forgotten or unclear.
- Ensure that written instructions are at the patient's level of understanding. Some commercially prepared booklets contain instructions that are too complex or contain medical jargon that is difficult to understand.
- Consider use of different pictures, colour coding, diagrams, and recorded instructions for patients with visual impairment or a reading disability.
- Consider use of weekly pill organizers.
- Periodically observe patient or caregiver prepare and administer medications.

2. Medication self-administration plan is not possible because of patient's self-care deficits. This is very common when the patient develops cognitive changes.
3. Patient refuses to take medications as prescribed.

- Develop an alternative plan, which often relies on caregivers to provide safe administration of home medication regimen.

- Explore and identify reasons for nonadherence, which often include the following: cost, adverse effects, complexity of regimen, problems with swallowing or other adverse effects, and cultural preferences.
- See Box 43.4.

Communication and Documentation

- Document instruction provided and learning outcomes achieved by patient and caregiver in the home care record.
- Develop a system of recording (patient diary/log) for patient or caregiver to use to document adherence to dosage schedules and self-monitoring of any problems.
- Always leave a phone number and instructions on how to reach a home care nurse if needed.

BOX 43.4

Evidence-Informed Nursing Interventions to Enhance Adherence to Medication Therapy

- Involve patients as partners in collaboration. Encourage them to express their views and share in the decision making with you.
- Encourage patients to take medications.
- Use medication reminders and devices such as smartphone alarms and pill boxes.
- Be empathetic regarding patients' feelings.
- Encourage a sense of control for the patient by providing information about diagnosis and treatment.
- Recognize caregiver needs and provide information and support. Understand that the caregiver may have competing responsibilities (e.g., employment, other dependents).
- The patient's attitude will affect their willingness to work with health care providers and adhere to treatments.

Modified from Kinney, R. L., et al. (2015). The association between patient activation and medication adherence, hospitalization, and emergency department utilization in patients with chronic illnesses: A systematic review. *Patient Education and Counseling, 98*(5), 545; Mantri, P. (2014). Patient adherence to medication. *Practice Nursing, 25*(12), 590; Shin, J. Y., Habermann, B., & Pretzer-Aboff, I. (2015). Challenges and strategies of medication adherence in Parkinson's disease: A qualitative study. *Geriatric Nursing, 36*(3), 191.

Special Considerations
Teaching

- See Chapter 42 for guidelines for medication safety in the home.
- If it is difficult to plan a separate teaching session, teach patient while administering medications.
- Examples of learning aids include homemade calendars for each week that contain plastic bags containing medications to take at specific times, egg cartons divided into colour-coded sections with medications for the day, clock faces for patients who cannot read or see clearly, colour coding for drug types (e.g., blue for sedative, red for pain pill), and pillboxes that identify days of the week and times of day.

Pediatric

- Instruct adults to keep all medications locked and securely out of reach of children.
- Encourage caregivers not to tell children that medications are treats because this increases the risk for the child overdosing by mistaking medicine for candy.
- Successful medication teaching involves the child's parents or other caregivers and the child and siblings whenever possible. To provide effective medication teaching to children, take the child's developmental and cognitive abilities into consideration when planning teaching sessions (Hockenberry & Wilson, 2015).
- Caregivers need to supervise older children as they begin taking responsibility for their own treatment.

Gerontological

- The capacity for learning new information remains as people age (in the absence of dementia); however, older patients often need additional time to accomplish learning. Allow adequate

time and number of teaching sessions to support successful learning. Effective teaching strategies for older persons include memory aids, information written in large letters, involvement of a caregiver, follow-up teaching sessions either over the telephone or in person, and computer-assisted teaching guides (Touhy et al., 2019).

- Cognition problems coupled with complexity of medication regimens have a negative effect on older persons' ability to self-administer medication safely. Try to decrease the complexity

of medication regimens in patients with cognitive deficits whenever possible to promote safe medication self-administration practices.

- Older persons often must take medications in multiple routes (e.g., oral, inhaled, injections). Many times, problems with physical dexterity, eyesight, cognitive skills, and memory negatively affect adherence to medication schedules. Establish a therapeutic nurse–patient relationship as part of person-centred care to help patients overcome these barriers to adherence.

◆ SKILL 43.7 Managing Feeding Tubes in the Home

Patients benefit when they can see tube-feeding equipment and devices when learning how to administer home enteral nutrition. Nurses need to provide hands-on experience and patient involvement with decision making about home enteral nutrition whenever possible. Enteral nutrition therapy in the home setting is usually effective when a patient tolerates at least 70% of feeding intake without complications and is medically stable, the patient or caregiver can administer feedings, and there is sufficient time in a controlled environment to learn the skill.

This procedure in the home setting follows the guidelines and skills described in Chapter 32. Most patients who receive enteral nutrition in the home have either gastrostomy or jejunostomy tubes. This skill focuses on teaching the patient or caregiver how to administer such feedings in the home. Frequently in the home setting the nurse is responsible for reinsertion of gastrostomy feeding

tubes, and the health care provider is responsible for reinsertion of jejunostomy tubes.

Delegation and Collaboration

The skill of teaching patients and caregivers how to manage feeding tubes in the home cannot be delegated to an unregulated care provider (UCP). The nurse directs the UCP to:

- Report when the patient has difficulty with feeding, coughing, gagging, respiratory distress, discomfort, or vomiting.

Equipment

See Skills 32.1 through 32.4 and Procedural Guideline 32.1 for lists of equipment.

- Log to record daily weights, intake and output (I&O), temperature, feeding residuals

---

STEP	RATIONALE
ASSESSMENT	
1. Identify patient using at least two person-specific identifiers during first home visit. Facial recognition can be used as one of two identifiers for ongoing subsequent home visits.	Ensures correct patient. Complies with Accreditation Canada's standards and improves patient safety (Accreditation Canada, 2019b).
2. Assess patient's current health status and tolerance of enteral feedings (if already being administered).	Determines if any changes are needed in feeding schedule.
3. Assess patient's and caregiver's physical (visual, fine motor) function. Also assess emotional, financial, and community resources.	Determines patient's and caregiver's ability to manipulate equipment. Availability of resources increases ability to manage self-care at home.
4. Assess environmental conditions of home (sanitation, storage of equipment, work area, supplies, and power source).	Determines if home environment is safe for enteral feeding, with minimal risks for infection and complications.
5. Assess patient's and caregiver's understanding of the purpose of enteral feedings and positive expected outcomes.	Understanding the rationale of treatment is critical to enhancing participation and cooperation in care.
6. Assess patient's and caregiver's understanding of storage and management of equipment and supplies and where and how to obtain supplies.	Ensures safe home management and decreases risk for complications. Home care delivery companies usually deliver a month's supply at a time. If the patient stores feeding containers in the garage, they must be brought into the house a couple hours before use in colder months to warm to room temperature (Canadian Cancer Society, 2019b). The garage is not a good storage place during hot weather; the basement should be used, if possible.
7. Assess patient's learning readiness and ability to concentrate (consider presence of pain, nausea, or fatigue and patient interest in instruction) and learning style preference.	Presence of significant illness, frailty, or confusion affects a patient's ability to attend to a teaching plan. Indicates need to rely on caregiver for learning and implementation (if available) on a short- or long-term basis. Learning style affects the choice of teaching resources.

STEP	RATIONALE

ASSESSMENT

8. Observe patient or caregiver administer an enteral feeding (when already prescribed).

Determines which specific components of skill the patient or caregiver can complete easily and which ones are more difficult and require reinforcement.

NURSING DIAGNOSES

- Anxiety
- Insufficient knowledge regarding tube feeding self-administration
- Reduced ability to self-feeding
- Inadequate nutrition
- Inadequate health maintenance
- Potential for aspiration

Related factors/Risk factors are individualized on the basis of patient's condition or needs.

PLANNING

1. Expected outcomes following completion of procedure:
   - Patient or caregiver verbalizes purpose of enteral feedings and enhanced nutritional health.
   - Patient or caregiver demonstrates proper use of equipment and handling of formulas.
   - Patient or caregiver demonstrates accurate administration of enteral feedings and medications.
   - Patient or caregiver verbalizes understanding of signs, symptoms, and management of complications of feeding.
2. Prepare environment for teaching session:

   - Select a room that is well lit with comfortable seating.
   - Be sure that the patient is close and can see the nurse clearly.
   - Control sources of noise and distractions.

Provides measurable criteria to determine level of cognitive understanding.

Provides demonstration of skills needed to manage home enteral nutrition.

Provides demonstration of skills needed to administer home enteral nutrition and medications.

Confirms that patient or caregiver has knowledge needed to respond when problems with feedings develop.

Improves likelihood of patient and caregiver being attentive to instruction.

Room environment needs to minimize existing sensory alterations. A comfortable environment free of distractions increases a patient's attention.

IMPLEMENTATION

1. Have patient or caregiver perform hand hygiene with you and explain the importance of skill.
2. Discuss with patient or caregiver the purpose of enteral feeding and enhanced nutritional health.
3. Help patient or caregiver determine a feeding schedule that will maintain nutritional requirements, fit within the patient's or caregiver's schedule, and fit the health care provider's prescription.

Reduces transmission of microorganisms. Reinforces importance of infection control.

Reinforces importance of regular feedings.

Promotes adherence to enteral nutrition therapy.

A person-centred approach increases patient confidence in managing their own feedings (Kirby, Mitchell, & Hendrickson, 2017).

Clinical Decision Point *Explain that the caregiver needs to communicate to home health or the health care provider any changes in feeding schedules made to fit the daily routine.*

4. Have patient or caregiver apply clean gloves with you. If a patient has a nasoenteral tube, demonstrate how to identify placement of feeding tube: aspirating gastric fluid, checking pH of gastric fluid, and acceptable pH range (see Skill 32.2).

Reduces transmission of microorganisms.

Some nasally placed tubes are inadvertently placed in the respiratory system and migrate to the esophagus or into the respiratory tract. In these cases, check pH periodically (Taylor, McWilliam, Allan, et al., 2015). Aspirated secretions with low pH are a strong indicator of gastric placement. However, high pH cannot be used to differentiate between aspirated secretions obtained from respiratory and intestinal tube placements.

Clinical Decision Point *Instruct patient or caregiver to avoid administration of all feedings, flushes, or medications if there is any doubt as to placement of the enteral feeding tube.*

STEP	RATIONALE

IMPLEMENTATION

5. Observe patient or caregiver demonstrate placement of nasally placed tube.

Return demonstration identifies if there are areas for further teaching.

6. When the patient has a gastrostomy or jejunostomy tube, observe patient or caregiver check for gastric residual volume (GRV) by aspirating gastric contents (Fan, Tan, & Aug, 2017). Have patient return aspirated contents to the stomach unless the volume exceeds 250 mL (see employer policy).

Checking gastric residual in a small-bore nasogastric tube can easily lead to occlusion or displacement. GRV in the range of 200 to 500 mL should raise concern and lead to implementation of measures to reduce the risk of aspiration, such as changing from intermittent to continuous feedings, evaluating the possibility of decreasing opioid analgesics, and starting medication that enhances gastric motility (e.g., metoclopramide). Automatic cessation of feeding should not occur for GRV less than 500 mL in the absence of other signs of intolerance (McCarthy & Martindale, 2015).

7. Discuss use of medical asepsis in setting up and changing administration sets, mixing formulas (do not add formula to hanging bag), refrigerating unused formula, limiting amount of formula "hung" at one time to the amount that can be infused in a 4- to 6-hour period (less time in warmer weather), and maintaining and caring for the bag.

Medical aseptic technique minimizes risk for microorganism contamination. Refrigeration and limiting "hang" time reduce growth of microorganisms. Changing administration sets every 24 hours reduces microorganism growth.

8. Instruct patient or caregiver that the patient needs to sit up in a chair or have head of bed elevated at least 30 degrees, preferably 45 degrees, while receiving feedings or medications or when tube is flushed.

Decreases risk for aspiration. Aspiration is indicated by increased coughing, difficulty breathing, or increased sputum (Canadian Cancer Society, 2019b).

9. Observe the patient or caregiver mixing, administering, and storing formulas. Discuss flushing of tube after administration of feedings or medications.

Identifies competence and need for further teaching. Regular flushing of tube prevents clogging.

10. Observe the patient or caregiver change administration sets and clean bags. Have them dispose of supplies, remove gloves, and perform hand hygiene.

Reduces transmission of infection.

11. Observe patient or caregiver administering medications and flushing tube (see Skill 21.2).

Ensures that medications are given correctly.

Clinical Decision Point *Verify that medications do not include any sublingual, enteric-coated, or sustained-release medications. These medications cannot be crushed for administration.*

12. Discuss and observe use of infusion pump if patient is receiving continuous feeding (see Chapter 32).

Use of tube-feeding infusion pumps is complex and requires reinforcement.

13. Discuss measures to stabilize feeding tube in patients with abdominal tubes and to clean and protect skin insertion site (see Chapter 32).

Prevents tube from dislodging and skin breakdown.

14. Provide contact information for ordering equipment and supplies or who to call in case of equipment failure.

Ensures that caregiver can respond in an emergency.

15. Discuss emergency plan and actions to take for signs and symptoms of aspiration, such as elevating head of bed, oral suctioning, and calling the health care provider.

Ensures understanding of management of equipment, supplies, emergency plan, and collaboration.

16. Discuss who to contact and when for signs of diarrhea, constipation, or weight loss.

Provides support to patient or caregiver.

EVALUATION

1. Ask patient or caregiver to state the purpose of home enteral nutrition therapy.

Demonstrates cognitive learning.

2. Observe patient or caregiver performing medical asepsis techniques, checking tube placement, aspirating residuals, administering medications and feedings, and using and cleaning equipment.

Demonstrates psychomotor learning.

3. Ask patient or caregiver to state the measures used to prevent complications (e.g., verification of tube position before each feeding, elevation of patient's head during feeding, stabilization and flushing of tubing).

Ensures safe home management and identification of areas for teaching.

STEP	RATIONALE

EVALUATION

4. Ask patient or caregiver how to care for open formula cans.
5. **Use Teach-Back:** "I want to be sure I explained how to manage problems that can occur with your tube feedings. Tell me how to manage nausea, stomach fullness, and diarrhea." Develop a revised teaching plan if patient or caregiver is not able to teach back correctly.

Ensures safe home management for preventing foodborne illness. Determines patient's and caregiver's level of understanding of instructional topic.

Unexpected Outcomes	Related Interventions
1. Feeding tube becomes displaced.	• Instruct patient or caregiver to stop feeding and notify the home care nurse. • The nurse or health care provider will reposition feeding tube and verify placement before initiating any enteral feeding.
2. Signs and symptoms of aspiration are present.	• Stop feeding. Raise head of bed. • Verify tube position. • Notify health care provider.
3. Patient develops diarrhea.	• Notify health care provider. • Use interprofessional collaboration (e.g., dietitian, health care provider) to consider a change in strength, type, or rate of enteral feeding, soluble fibre; review medications; or use antidiarrheal medications (Englert, 2017).
4. Skin surrounding stoma breaks down, or drainage around insertion site develops.	• Clean stoma area more frequently. • Apply antibiotic ointment around stoma as prescribed. • Contact health care provider.

Communication and Documentation

- Document instructions given to patient and caregiver and their response in the home care record.
- Document specifics of enteral feeding plan, including type and size of tube in the home, formula, and amounts to be administered in specific time frames.
- Patient or caregivers need to document I&O, daily weights, amount of gastric fluid aspirated before each feeding (or every 4 hours if receiving continuous feeding), date and time of feedings, amount and type of formula, any additives, and date and time that administration sets are changed.

Special Considerations
Teaching

- Performing a skill without a nurse in attendance provokes anxiety. Always leave a phone number and instructions on how to reach a home care nurse if needed.
- Teach patient and caregiver the maximum hang time for any enteral feeding. After a can of formula has been opened, it should remain at room temperature for no longer than 8 to 12 hours.
- If the patient has a nasoenteral tube, encourage frequent mouth care to prevent dryness of oral mucous membranes.

Pediatric

- Children are at risk for aspiration and fluid and electrolyte imbalance; thus, teach parents to monitor the child carefully (Hockenberry & Wilson, 2015).
- Children who receive long-term home enteral feedings often experience developmental and growth delays. Other common problems include sleep disturbance, tube blockages, problems with delivery of equipment, and equipment malfunction. Therefore, these children require close follow-up and frequent nutritional monitoring.
- Teach the caregiver to position a child who cannot sit up during or after a tube feeding on their right side during the tube feeding and for approximately 1 hour after it (Hockenberry & Wilson, 2015).

Gerontological

- Assess for changes and limitations in sensory function, mobility, or dexterity that indicate a need to teach a caregiver how to administer feedings.
- Patients living with dementia who are receiving enteral tube feeding are at higher risk for restraint use (Bentur, Sternberg, Shuldiner, et al., 2015).

♦ SKILL 43.8 Managing Parenteral Nutrition in the Home

Parenteral nutrition (PN) in the home is indicated for patients who cannot take adequate nutrition by mouth and when enteral feedings are contraindicated (e.g., cancer, chronic respiratory or gastrointestinal disorders [Ojo, 2017]). Nurses who manage PN in the home collaborate frequently with dietitians and other health care providers to ensure that patients receive sufficient calories, protein, and fluid. PN is administered through a long-term central venous catheter (CVC) such as a tunneled CVC (e.g., Groshong or Hickman catheter), an implantable port, or a peripherally inserted central catheter (PICC) (see Chapter 29). Potential complications are

associated with PN infusion, including intravenous (IV)–related blood clots and bloodstream infection.

PN is individually formulated and includes a mixture of amino acids, dextrose, fat emulsions, vitamins, electrolytes, minerals, and trace elements. Administering PN in the home requires an inter-professional approach and a patient and caregiver who demonstrate competency in its preparation and administration (Hamilton Health Services, 2016).

Usually administration of PN in the home takes about 12 hours; thus many patients choose to receive their PN during the night. Because of the risks involved with PN and because management in the home is very complex, patients receive their first infusion in an acute care setting. After discharge, a home care nurse visits frequently. The home care nurse will need to carefully assess the reaction of the patient or caregiver to use of the technology needed to administer PN at home and provide emotional support. Although administering PN in the home increases patients' autonomy, it often interferes with their ability to maintain their normal routines. Nurses need to work with the patient or caregiver in a person-centred manner to stress the benefits and offer support in dealing with related issues.

Delegation and Collaboration

The skill of managing PN in the home cannot be delegated to an unregulated care provider (UCP). The nurse instructs the UCP to:

* Report findings of blood glucose monitoring.
* Report vital signs outside of normal range.
* Report patient statements of shortness of breath, headache, weakness, or discomfort.
* Report if the catheter dressings are wet or bleeding at the site.

Equipment

* IV solution of PN
* IV tubing with optional filter
* Electronic IV infusion pump with alarms and protection from free flow
* Home blood glucose monitoring equipment
* Alcohol swabs
* Clean gloves
* Log

STEP	RATIONALE

ASSESSMENT

1. Identify patient using at least two person-specific identifiers during first home visit. Facial recognition can be used as one of two identifiers for ongoing subsequent home visits.

   Ensures correct patient. Complies with Accreditation Canada's standards and improves patient safety (Accreditation Canada, 2019b).

2. Assess patient's ongoing nutritional status and risk for malnutrition by using a nutrition screening tool (see Chapter 31) and performing a physical examination. Identify signs and symptoms of malnutrition (e.g., weight loss or weight below ideal level; muscle atrophy, wasting, or weakness; lethargy; unable to eat for more than 6 days). Include measurement of vital signs.

   Nutritional assessment helps in identifying a patient's baseline to determine their response to PN.

3. Assess patient's fluid and electrolyte levels, serum albumin, total protein, transferrin, prealbumin, triglyceride, and glucose levels.

   Provides additional baseline assessment data (Hamilton Health Services, 2016).

4. Assess patient's venous access device for edema, drainage, tenderness, and signs of inflammation (see Chapter 29). Measure circumference of the upper arm if the patient has a PICC; mark place on the arm where measurement was taken.

   Infection is a common complication when a patient has a venous access device. Measurement of the arm helps in detecting infiltration of the PICC. The mark on the arm ensures consistent measurements over time.

5. Verify health care provider's prescription for PN, including amino acids, dextrose, fat emulsions, vitamins, minerals, trace elements, electrolytes, and flow rate.

   Ensures safe and accurate PN administration.

6. Assess patient's learning readiness, anxiety, and ability to concentrate (consider presence of pain, nausea, or fatigue and patient interest in instruction) and learning style preference.

   Presence of significant illness, frailty, or confusion affects a patient's ability to attend to a teaching plan. Indicates need to rely on caregiver for learning and implementation (if available) on a short- or long-term basis. Learning style affects the choice of teaching resources.

7. Assess patient's or caregiver's previous knowledge and experience in managing PN in the home. Have patient or caregiver perform return demonstration if they are able to perform the skill.

   Determines level of understanding before beginning teaching session.

STEP	RATIONALE

NURSING DIAGNOSES

- Inadequate nutrition: less than body requirements
- Anxiety
- Insufficient knowledge regarding total parenteral nutrition
- Fatigue
- Readiness for improved nutrition
- Caregiver role strain
- Potential for infection
- Potential for social isolation

Related factors/Risk factors are individualized on the basis of patient's condition or needs.

PLANNING

STEP	RATIONALE
1. Expected outcomes following completion of procedure:	
• Patient or caregiver can administer PN correctly.	Indicates that skills are effectively learned.
• Patient or caregiver demonstrates proper care of CVC.	Prevents infection and ensures patency of venous access device.
• Patient or caregiver explains how to properly store and maintain formulas for feeding.	Knowledge of infection control principles prevents foodborne illness.
• Patient or caregiver states signs and symptoms of alterations that need to be reported to health care provider.	Ensures safe administration of PN in home.
• Patient or caregiver demonstrates correct measurement of blood glucose.	Necessary for safe monitoring of patient's response to PN therapy.
2. Select setting in the home where patient is most likely to administer PN and that is conducive to a teaching session:	Practicing in the same environment where the skill is routinely performed facilitates comprehension and learning.
• Select a room that is well lit with comfortable seating.	
• Be sure that the patient is close and can see the nurse clearly.	
• Control sources of noise and distractions.	Room environment needs to minimize existing sensory alterations. A comfortable environment free of distractions increases patient's attention.

IMPLEMENTATION

STEP	RATIONALE
1. Provide the name and phone number of people or resources available 24 hours a day, 7 days a week in case problems arise.	Provides assurance and allows patient or caregiver to troubleshoot problems and answer questions.
2. Explain the type and name of infusion, volume and infusion rate, expected outcomes, and components of PN. Explain that PN needs to be stored in refrigerator.	Allows patient or caregiver to verify that correct PN is infused and that patient or caregiver understands expected outcomes of care. Refrigeration maintains integrity of PN.
3. Have patient or caregiver perform each of the following steps with guidance from nurse. Do not rush them.	Allows you to correct errors in technique as they occur and discuss implications.
4. Instruct patient or caregiver to inspect the IV solution bag label, ensure that patient's name is on the label, ensure that solution has not expired, and check bag for leaks.	Ensures that patient or caregiver knows how to check pharmacy-prepared solution to ensure the right patient receives right PN. Bag needs to be intact to maintain a closed system and to ensure that patient receives all prescribed nutrients.
5. Suggest taking PN solution out of the refrigerator for 30 to 60 minutes before scheduled infusion time.	Chilled solution often causes discomfort; allowing solution to warm enhances comfort during infusion.
6. Explain the need to inspect fluid in the bag for colour and precipitates.	Changes in colour or precipitates in bag indicate disruption in PN.

Clinical Decision Point *If precipitate appears, components of mixture are separated, or colour changes, explain that solution needs to be discarded.*

STEP	RATIONALE
7. Have patient or caregiver perform hand hygiene and apply clean gloves with you. Demonstrate how to attach IV tubing to bag, how to attach filter to IV tubing (*optional*), how to prime IV tubing, and how to load IV tubing into the electronic infusion pump (see Chapter 29).	Reduces transmission of infection. Prepares PN solution for IV administration.
8. Wipe CVC port with alcohol and show how to flush CVC and connect IV tubing to port (see Chapter 29). Use needleless system whenever possible.	CVC needs to be patent, and IV tubing needs to connect to CVC to allow PN to be administered. Needleless systems prevent needle-stick injuries.

STEP	RATIONALE

IMPLEMENTATION

9. Explain how to determine the appropriate rate of infusion and program the infusion pump (see Skill 29.2). Caution patient and caregiver against changing rate to "catch up."

Ensures that PN is administered at an appropriate rate.

10. Have patient and caregiver remove and dispose of gloves; perform hand hygiene.

Prevents spread of microorganisms.

11. When infusion is completed, explain and demonstrate how to disconnect IV tubing and flush CVC (see Chapter 29). Ensure that patient or caregiver performs hand hygiene before and after disconnecting line.

Flushing CVC following infusion maintains patency of vascular access device. Meticulous hand hygiene prevents infection.

12. Describe appropriate use and storage of infusion pump and supplies. Explain appropriate tubing replacement schedules (e.g., every 24 hours for total nutrition admixture [TNA], 72 hours for three-in-one solutions).

Maintains integrity of equipment; appropriate timing of tubing changes prevents infection.

13. Help to develop a plan for appropriate disposal of supplies, including needles, syringes, and unused medications or solutions, using principles of standard precautions.

Implementation of standard precautions is necessary to prevent transmission of communicable diseases and needle-stick injuries.

14. Demonstrate appropriate care of CVC site; discuss how to change dressings, frequency of dressing changes, and signs of infection (see Skill 29.6).

Prevents infection at CVC insertion site.

15. Teach patient and caregiver about signs and symptoms that indicate potential complications from PN therapy (e.g., infection and phlebitis at CVC site, refeeding syndrome, hyperglycemia, hypernatremia, hypophosphatemia, hypokalemia, hypomagnesemia) and when to call for help.

Knowledge of complications of PN therapy allows for early detection and appropriate action.

16. Demonstrate use of self–blood glucose monitor. Explain frequency of testing, normal glucose values, and what to do if values fall outside of the expected range (see Chapter 9).

PN increases blood glucose levels, which negatively affects patient outcomes. Frequent monitoring of glucose level helps in detecting problems early. Expect testing frequency to decrease as patient's condition and response to PN stabilizes.

17. Provide patient with log to record administration of PN, weights, intake and output, and blood glucose levels.

Enables health care provider and patient to evaluate outcomes and detect adverse effects of nutritional therapy.

18. Help patient develop a plan to reorder supplies, PN fluid, and prescribed additives; for emergencies (e.g., what to do if power goes out); and for home safety plan (e.g., how to get to bathroom without tripping over IV tubing).

Plans allow for continuous, safe, and effective administration of PN.

EVALUATION

1. Have patient or caregiver independently demonstrate initiation, infusion, and discontinuation of PN infusion and CVC site care.

Feedback through return demonstration of psychomotor skill is the best means of evaluating mastery of skill.

2. Watch patient or caregiver clean and store PN, equipment, and supplies.

Proper cleaning and storage help prevent bacterial growth.

3. Ask patient or caregiver to identify expected outcomes of nutritional therapy.

Measures patient's and caregiver's cognitive learning and confirms understanding of information.

4. Have patient or caregiver independently demonstrate blood glucose monitoring and recording.

Ensures mastering of skill needed for effective evaluation of patient status.

5. Watch patient or caregiver record information in log. Review patient's or caregiver's log periodically to ensure that information is being recorded correctly.

Health care providers make changes in patient care based on information provided by patient. To ensure that changes are made appropriately, the patient or caregiver needs to record accurate information.

6. **Use Teach-Back:** "I want to be sure I explained the common signs and symptoms of infection and other potential complications of PN. Tell me the signs and symptoms of infection." Develop a revised teaching plan if patient or caregiver is not able to teach back correctly.

Determines patient's and caregiver's level of understanding of instructional topic.

STEP	RATIONALE

Unexpected Outcomes

1. Patient or caregiver is unable to manage home PN therapy or verbalize information that was taught.

2. Patient or caregiver reports signs and symptoms of complications from PN or CVC.

Related Interventions

- Ask patient or caregiver to describe difficulties experienced while performing skill.
- Use a different teaching strategy.
- Teach caregiver further and evaluate need to increase frequency of home visits to ensure safe administration of PN at home.
- Inform health care provider.
- Tell patient or caregiver to call emergency medical services (EMS) if signs and symptoms are severe.

Communication and Documentation

- Document information taught, patient's and caregiver's response, and outcomes of PN therapy (e.g., weight, electrolyte and glucose levels, physical assessment findings) in the home care log.
- Document appearance of CVC site, infusions, glucose monitoring results, and patient's weight in the home care log.

Special Considerations
Teaching

- Assess patient's psychosocial status while providing information. Many patients experience a decrease in quality of life when PN feedings are started in the home, which often increases anxiety and decreases comprehension of information.
- Eating is often a social event. When patients do not eat, they tend to feel socially isolated. Teach patients and caregivers the importance of maintaining social relationships and enhancing social support during PN therapy.
- Always leave a phone number and instructions on how to reach a home care nurse if needed.

Pediatric

- The risk for displacement of the CVC increases as the child grows. Ensure that the placement of the venous access device is confirmed with radiographic film examination as the child grows.
- Teach the caregiver to socialize the child with other children to enhance development (Hockenberry & Wilson, 2015).

Gerontological

- Frail older persons are at high risk for electrolyte disturbances. Frequently assess and monitor their response to PN and their laboratory values.
- Carefully assess the patient's ability to perform skill. Management of PN at home is complex and requires manual dexterity, visual acuity, and high-level critical thinking and decision-making skills. Include the caregiver in the teaching plan to help with management of home PN.

◆ CLINICAL DEBRIEF

The nurse is scheduled to visit an 86-year-old retired engineer who lives in a private home with his 84-year-old wife. The patient is currently hospitalized for an acute episode of bronchitis and is newly diagnosed with chronic obstructive pulmonary disease. He will be sent home on oral antibiotics and oxygen therapy. When the nurse contacts his wife about an initial home assessment, the nurse learns that, in addition to his new diagnosis and oxygen therapy, his adult son, who smokes one pack of cigarettes per day, lives in the home. This is the first home visit.

1. What information would the nurse want to have about the patient's home environment before he is discharged to help him safely manage his new home oxygen therapy?
2. During the initial home visit with the patient, wife, and son, the nurse reassesses the home environment and discovers that oxygen cylinders are being stored in the bedroom closet. What should the nurse do?
3. The nurse schedules a follow-up visit to the home and discovers that the son smokes near his father. How should the nurse address the son's smoking status and the importance of maintaining a nonsmoking environment?

◆ REVIEW QUESTIONS

1. A patient is being taught self-administration of medications. Which of the following are assessments to be completed before the teaching session? *(Select all that apply.)*

1. Purpose of regularly scheduled medications and their desired effects
2. Explanation of dosage schedules and rationale
3. Knowledge regarding medication therapy
4. Learning readiness and ability to concentrate
5. Patient's belief in need for medication therapy

2. An older person is discharged from the hospital to his home after treatment for bronchitis. The person lives independently, and his closest family is 100 miles away. Which nursing intervention will enhance adherence to his medication regimen? *(Select all that apply.)*
   1. Teaching him everything he needs to know in 1 day and returning in 2 weeks
   2. Including him in deciding the system used to help him remember to take his medications
   3. Providing 12-point font instructions that are written in red ink
   4. Providing medication information when his daughter and infant grandchild are visiting him
   5. Using medication caps that the patient can open independently

3. An older person is receiving home enteral nutrition because of dysphagia (swallowing difficulty). Which action(s) should the nurse instruct the caregiver to take with enteral feeding? *(Select all that apply.)*
   1. Have the caregiver perform hand hygiene before initiating the enteral feeding.
   2. Have the patient's head of bed elevated at least 10 to 20 degrees while receiving feedings.
   3. Verify tube placement.

4. Schedule feedings to maintain nutritional requirements.
5. Use teach-back to verify the caregiver's understanding of signs and symptoms of complications such as aspiration with enteral tube feeding.

(e) *Visit the Evolve site for a complete list of Clinical Debrief and Review Questions answers.*

REFERENCES

Accreditation Canada. (2019a). *Health and social services standards.* Retrieved from https://accreditation.ca/standards/

Accreditation Canada. (2019b). *Required organizational practices handbook—Version 14.* Ottawa, ON: Author. Retrieved from http://www.wrha.mb.ca/quality/files/2019ROPHandbook.pdf

Almkuist, K. (2017). Using teach-back method to prevent 30-day readmissions in patients with heart failure: A systematic review. *Medsurg Nursing, 26*(5), 312–351.

Alo, J. (2017). Practical return demonstration: Enactment nursing students do, believed and experienced will perk their nursing care. *International Journal of Development Research, 7*(7), 13695–14697.

Ayhan, H., Tastan, S., Iyigun, E., Akamca, Y., Arikan, E., & Sevim, Z. (2015). Normal saline instillation before endotracheal suctioning: "What does the evidence say? What do the nurses think?" Multimethod study. *Journal of Critical Care, 30*(4), 762–767. doi:10.1016/j.jcrc.2015.02.019

Bentur, N., Sternberg, S., Shuldiner, J., & Dwolatzky, T. (2015). Feeding tubes for older people with advanced dementia living in the community in Israel. *American Journal of Alzheimer's Disease and Other Dementias, 30*(2), 165–172. doi:10.1177/1533317514539726

Bergh, A., Friberg, F., Persson, E., & Dahlborg-Lyckhage, E. (2015). Registered nurses' patient education in everyday primary care practice: Managers' discourses. *Global Qualitative Nursing Research,* 1–12. doi:10.1177/233339361559

Canadian Cancer Society. (2019a). *Infection.* Retrieved from http://www.cancer.ca/en/cancer-information/diagnosis-and-treatment/managing-side-effects/infection/?region=on

Canadian Cancer Society. (2019b). *Tube feeding and parental nutrition.* Retrieved from http://www.cancer.ca/en/cancer-information/diagnosis-and-treatment/managing-side-effects/tube-feeding-and-parenteral-nutrition/?region=on

Canadian Home Care Association. (2015). *Home care in Canada: Advancing quality improvement and integrated care.* Retrieved from http://www.cdnhomecare.ca/media.php?mid=4328

Canadian Paediatric Society (CPS). (2017). *Caring for kids—How to safely dispose of a mercury thermometer.* Retrieved from https://www.caringforkids.cps.ca/handouts/mercury_thermometer

Canadian Patient Safety Institute (CPSI). (2014). *Resource guide for supporting caregivers at home—For home care service providers.* Retrieved from http://www.patientsafetyinstitute.ca/en/toolsResources/HomeCareSafety/Documents/Resources%20for%20home%20care%20providers%20-%20Resource%20guide%20for%20supporting%20caregivers%20at%20home.pdf

Canadian Public Health Association (CPHA). (2014). *Examples of health literacy in practice.* Retrieved from https://www.cpha.ca/sites/default/files/uploads/resources/healthlit/examples_e.pdf

Canadian Urological Association (CUA). (2014). *Clean intermittent self-catheterization for women.* Retrieved from https://www.cua.org/themes/web/assets/files/patient_info/secured/en/2e-self-catherization_s.pdf

Cleveland Clinic. (2019). *Tracheostomy care.* Retrieved from http://my.clevelandclinic.org/services/head-neck/treatments-services/tracheostomy-care

Community Health Nurses of Canada (CHNC). (2019). *2019 Canadian community health nursing professional practice model & standards of practice.* Retrieved from https://www.chnc.ca/standards-of-practice

Credland, N. (2016). How to suction via a tracheostomy. *Nursing Standard, 30*(28), 36–38. doi:10.7748/ns.30.28.36.s46

Das, N., & Sharma, A. (2017). Effect of standing position and sitting crossed leg position on blood pressure—A literature review. *International Journal of Nursing Care, 5*(1), 23–26. doi:10.5958/2320-8651.2017.00005.9

Dean, G. (2015). Are single-use catheters worth the expense? *Journal of Urology, 194*(1), 12–13. doi:10.1016/j.juro.2015.04.071

Eggertson, L. (2011). Health literacy: More than just the three Rs. *The Canadian Nurse, 197*(1), 18–23.

Englert, M. (2017). Components of a successful home enteral teaching program. *Support Line,* (39), 1.

Fallon, N. (2015). The challenge of measuring blood pressure accurately. *British Journal of Cardiac Nursing, 10*(3), 136. doi:10.12968/bjca.2015.10.3.132

Fan, E., Tan, S., & Aug, S. (2017). Nasogastric tube placement confirmation: Where we are and where we should be heading. *Proceedings of Singapore Healthcare, 26*(3), 189–195. doi:10.1177/2010105817705141

Galligan, C. J., Markkanen, P., Fantasia, L., Gore, R., Sama, S., & Quinn, M. (2015). A growing fire hazard concern in communities: Home oxygen therapy and continued smoking habits. *New solutions : A Journal of Environmental and Occupational Health Policy : NS, 24*(4), 535–554. doi:10.2190/NS.24.4.g

Giger, J. (2017). *Transcultural nursing: Assessment and intervention* (7th ed.). St. Louis: Elsevier.

Government of Canada. (2012). *Listing of drugs currently regulated as new drugs (the new drugs list).* Retrieved from https://www.canada.ca/en/health-canada/services/drugs-health-products/drug-products/applications-submissions/guidance-documents/listing-drugs-currently-regulated-new-drugs.html

Government of Canada. (2016). *Home and community health care.* Retrieved from https://www.canada.ca/en/health-canada/services/home-continuing-care/home-community-care.html

Government of Canada. (2017). *Using medications safely.* Retrieved from https://www.canada.ca/en/health-canada/services/drugs-medical-devices/using-medications-safely.html

Hamilton Health Services. (2016). *Patient's guide to home parental nutrition.* Retrieved from http://hamiltonhealthsciences.ca/documents/Patient%20Education/HomeParenteralNutritionADULTManual-th.pdf

Hart, M. (2015). Safety considerations when transitioning the elderly from hospital to home. *AARC Times, 39*(2), 9–10.

Heart and Stroke Foundation of Canada. (2018). *High blood pressure.* Retrieved from http://www.heartandstroke.ca/heart/risk-and-prevention/condition-risk-factors/high-blood-pressure

Hockenberry, M. J., & Wilson, D. (2015). *Wong's nursing care of infants and children* (10th ed.). St. Louis: Mosby.

Homecare Medical. (2017). *Oxygen use at home: Fire safety and guidelines for storing and handling oxygen equipment.* Retrieved from https://www.homecaremedical.com/assets/Oxygen-Use-at-Home.pdf

Iihara, N., Nishio, T., Okura, M., et al. (2014). Comparing patient dissatisfaction and rational judgment in intentional medication non-adherence versus unintentional non-adherence. *Journal of Clinical Pharmacy and Therapeutics, 39*(1), 45–52.

Ingadóttir, B., & Zoëga, S. (2017). Role of patient education in postoperative pain management. *Nursing Standard, 32*(2), 50–63. doi:10.7748/ns.2017.e10939

Institute for Safe Medication Practices (ISMP) Canada. (2017). *Errors associated with hospital discharge prescriptions: A multi-incident analysis.* Retrieved from https://www.ismp-canada.org/download/safetyBulletins/2017/ISMPCSB2017-01-HospitalDischargePrescriptions.pdf

Jarrin, O., Kang, Y., & Aiken, L. (2017). Pathway to better patient care and nurse workforce outcomes in home care. *Nursing Outlook, 65*(6), 671–678. doi:10.1016/j.outlook.2017.05.009

Jung, M., Kim, G., Kim, J., et al. (2015). Reliability of home blood pressure monitoring: In the context of validation and accuracy. *Blood Pressure Monitoring, 20*(4), 215–220. doi:10.1097/MBP.0000000000000121

Kirby, D., Mitchell, R., & Hendrickson, E. (2017). Noncompliance/nonadherence with home nutrition support: An underrecognized clinical dilemma. *Nutrition in Clinical Practice, 32*(6), 777–781. doi:10.1177/0884533617730001

Knier, S., Stickler, J., Ferber, L., & Catterall, K. (2015). Patients' perceptions of the quality of discharge teaching and readiness for discharge. *Rehabilitation Nursing, 40*(1), 30–39. doi:10.1002/rnj.164

Lamin, E., & Newman, D. (2016). Clean intermittent catheterization revisited. *International Urology and Nephrology, 48*(6), 931–939. doi:10.1007/s11255-016-1236-9

Leach, D. (2018). Teaching patients a clean intermittent self-catheterization technique. *British Journal of Nursing, 27*(6), 296–298. doi:10.12968/bjon.2018.27.6.296

Lewis, S. L., Bucher, L., Heitkemper, M., et al. (Eds.), (2019). *Medical-surgical nursing in Canada: Assessment and management of clinical problems* (4th Canadian ed.). Toronto: Elsevier Canada.

McCarthy, M. S., & Martindale, R. G. (2015). What's on the menu? Delivering evidence-based nutritional therapy. *Nursing, 45*(8), 36–43. doi:10.1097/01.NURSE.0000469233.76654.2d

Müller, S., Kohlmann, T., & Wilke, T. (2015). Validation of the adherence barriers questionnaire: An instrument for identifying potential risk factors associated with medication-related nonadherence. *BMC Health Services Research, 15*(1), 153–157. doi:10.1186/s12913-015-0809-0

National Institutes of Health (NIH). (2018). *Health literacy.* Retrieved from https://www.nih.gov/institutes-nih/nih-office-director/office-communications-public-liaison/clear-communication/health-literacy

Nies, M. A., & McEwen, M. (2015). *Community public health nursing* (6th ed.). St. Louis: Elsevier.

Ojo, O. (2017). Providing optimal enteral nutrition support in the community. *British Journal of Community Nursing, 22*(5), 218–221. doi:10.12968/bjcn.2017.22.5.218

Parker, E., Zimmerman, S., & Rodriguez, S. (2014). Exploring best practices in home health care: A review of available evidence on select innovations. *Home Health Care Management & Practice*, 26(1), 17–33.

Pereira, K., Phillips, B., Johnson, C., & Vorderstrasse, A. (2015). Internet delivered diabetes self-management education: A review. *Diabetes Technology & Therapeutics*, 17(1), 55–63. doi:10.1089/dia.2014.0155

Peter, D., Robinson, P., Jordan, M., Lawrence, S., Casey, K., & Salas-Lopez, D. (2015). Reducing readmissions using teach-back: Enhancing patient and family education. *The Journal of Nursing Administration*, 45(1), 35–42. doi:10.1097/NNA.0000000000000155

Saita, E., Acquati, C., & Molgora, S. (2016). Promoting patient and caregiver engagement in care in cancer. *Frontiers in Psychology*, 7, 1660. doi:10.3389/fpsyg.2016.01660

Shabiralyani, G., Hasan, K., Hamad, N., & Iqbal, N. (2015). Impact of visual used in enhancing the learning process care research: District Dera Ghazi Khan. *Journal of Education and Practice*, 6(19). Retrieved from https://files.eric.ed.gov/fulltext/EJ1079541.pdf. ISNN 2222-1735.

Shimbo, D., Abdalla, M., Falzon, L., Townsend, R. R., & Munter, R. (2015). Role of ambulatory and home blood pressure monitoring in clinical practice: A narrative review. *Annals of Internal Medicine*, 163(9), 691–700. doi:10.7326/M15-1270

Society of Urologic Nurses and Associates (SUNA). (2010). *Adult intermittent self-catheterization: Patient fact sheet*. Retrieved from https://cdnmedia.endeavorsuite.com/images/organizations/98e43f08-16d9-4b9d-b446-4d13f0ac5512/selfCatheterization.pdf

Sun, W., Doran, D., Wodchis, W., & Peter, E. (2017). Examining the relationship between therapeutic self-care and adverse events for home care clients in Ontario, Canada: A retrospective cohort study. *BMC Health Services Research*, 17(206), 1–13. doi:10.1186/s12913-017-2103-9

Taylor, S. J., McWilliam, H., Allan, K., & Hocking, P. (2015). The efficacy of feeding tubes: Confirmation and loss. *British Journal of Nursing*, 24(7), 371–372, 374–375. doi:10.12968/bjon.2015.24.7.371

Tiep, B., & Carter, R. (2019). *Long-term supplemental oxygen therapy*. UpToDate. Retrieved from https://www.uptodate.com/contents/long-term-supplemental-oxygen-therapy .

Torres, C., & Schwartz, M. (2017). *Transtracheal oxygen therapy*. National Jewish Health. Retrieved from https://www.nationaljewish.org/treatment-programs/medications/on-the-go-with-oxygen/transtracheal-oxygen

Touhy, T., Jett, K., Boscart, V., & McCleary, L. (2019). *Ebersole and Hess' gerontological nursing and healthy aging* (2nd Canadian ed.). Toronto, ON: Elsevier.

Vorvick, L. (2019). *Temperature measurement*. MedlinePlus. Retrieved from https://medlineplus.gov/ency/article/003400.htm

Wiles, K. S. (2015). Oxygen safety in the home … a growing concern. *AARC Times*, 39(5), 5.

Wilson, M. (2015). Clean intermittent self-catheterisation: Working with patients. *British Journal of Nursing*, 24(2), 76–80. doi:10.12968/bjon.2015.24.2.76

Answer Key

CHAPTER 1
Clinical Debrief

1. Can the use of family caregivers as physical activity coaches (I) compared with standard mobility protocol (C) for orthopedic surgery patients (P) improve patients' mobility (O) over a 6-month period (T)?

2. Several different mesh terms might apply such as *activity, exercise, exercise tolerance,* or *ambulation.* The search strategy can be included and is the "S" part of PICO(TS).

3. a. The study is an example of a randomized controlled trial.
   b. It might be useful to learn how the researcher measured postoperative ambulation (e.g., did it involve a specific measurement of distance or steps)? Even though the patients underwent knee surgery, the study might offer insights into how to train and involve family caregivers.
   c. It might not be useful for the obvious reason that it involved patients undergoing knee surgery. Second, there is no indication from the physiotherapist's presentation that family caregivers were in any way involved as coaches.

4. Mobility can be measured in numerous ways. The team must come to a method of measurement that the surgeon believes represents patient progress or improvement and that the physiotherapist perceives as measurable and indicative of improvement. For example, mobility might be measured by combined distance the patient is able to walk during stay, number of times the patient ambulates, or patients' reports of exercise tolerance during each ambulation.

Review Questions

1. 7, 3, 5, 1, 4, 2, 6
2. a. The average number of analgesic doses per patient/day in the first 48 hours increased. The pain scores dropped dramatically 24 hours after surgery after the pilot began. Pain scores at 48 hours also declined, with less of a change than was noted during the 24-hour time period. The use of ATC has increased regular dosing and shown an improvement in pain scores.
   b. Yes, the changes that occurred would be expected to happen from the EIP change. The average number of analgesic doses per patient would be expected to increase with patients receiving regularly ordered analgesics ATC instead of episodically. It would also be expected that the pain scores would drop with an increase in analgesic doses.
3. 2, 3, 4 Rationale: The number of articles is not important. Instead, there needs to be a sufficient level of evidence to determine the value, feasibility, and utility of evidence for making a practice change. Evidence must show that an EIP change is relevant and appropriate to the types of patients, local setting, and clinical situation. Setting aside time for a pilot project is important to determine feasibility of a change in practice. The number of outcomes is not important. Instead there needs to be a clear identification of outcomes to be measured to determine that the EIP change is a success.

CHAPTER 2
Clinical Debrief

1. The patient has skin breakdown on her left hip. This skin breakdown is considered a community-acquired pressure injury stage 1; and, because it is present on admission, it must be documented within 24 hours of admission. Documentation indicates that the patient was admitted with the pressure injury and it did not develop in the hospital.

2. The nurse transferring the patient completes a reconciliation of medications the patient was taking on admission and those prescribed at discharge. Warfarin is a new medication; and St. John's wort, an over-the-counter (OTC) medication, was not prescribed at discharge, but OTC medications and herbal therapies do not require a prescription. St. John's wort interferes with blood thinners such as warfarin, so it is important to provide patient education related to this interference. The nurse on the rehabilitation unit needs to educate the patient before discharge about the risks of taking St. John's wort at home and the bleeding complications for which to observe when taking warfarin. The patient will not realize the possible problem if she decides to take St. John's wort again and is uninformed.

3. S: Preparing for patient discharge. Patient's sister, who will be her caregiver, is concerned about ability to assume patient's self-care.

   B: Patient is a 69-year-old widow who experienced a left-sided stroke 7 days ago and has a history of diabetes mellitus and arthritis.

   A: Patient can help with many care activities but requires help to eat. During stay in acute care she had skin breakdown over her left hip, although it has cleared. She has a sister who will be her caregiver. Her medications on admission to rehabilitation were metformin, lisinopril, and St. John's wort.

   R: Recommend community-based nurse and social worker to determine safety of sister's home environment; review for risks relative to use of walker. Patient will require physical assistance (staying active to avoid recurrent pressure injury); determine if there are other caregiver resources.

Review Questions

1. 1, 3, 4 Rationale: The nurse needs to evaluate the patient's health literacy to plan the patient's discharge teaching and ensure it is at the appropriate level. The assessment should be done as soon as possible but no later than 24 hours after admission. Obtaining a list of medications is important to ensure patients do not miss any and to prevent any medication errors. Not all patients will need an interpreter. Skin integrity should be assessed during the admission process and no later than 24 hours after admission.
2. 1, 2, 4 Rationale: Medication reconciliation is done every time there is a transition in patient care. This occurs during admission, change of unit, or discharge.
3. 1, 2, 3, 4 Rationale: The nurse should check the prescription for discharge, complete the medication reconciliation, review the patient's discharge instructions, and ensure the patient has transportation. Discharge planning should begin upon admission.

CHAPTER 3
Clinical Debrief

1. Assess the patient's orientation status. Gather information from the son to establish the patient's baseline mental status and to inquire how he communicates with his mother. Be aware of your nonverbal cues that may affect communication and that may increase her anxiety. Reduce any distractions when communicating with the patient such as external noises. Speak clearly and directly and avoid rushing the patient. Do

not interrupt if the patient speaks. Adjust communication strategies to communicate effectively, such as the use of assistive communication devices to communicate with her. Observe for understanding of message sent and received.

2. Recognize personal level of anxiety and try to remain calm because anxiety is contagious. Prepare a quiet, calm area to interact with the patient. Assess her level of anxiety and use appropriate verbal and nonverbal techniques to provide reassurance and prevent further escalation of anxiety. Be clear and direct when communicating with her. Provide appropriate comfort measures for pain related to fracture and administer antianxiety medication as needed.

3. S: Patient presents to the hospital after falling at home, wrist fracture

   B: Diagnosed with Alzheimer's disease, lives with son at his home following death of husband 3 years ago

   A: Impaired verbal communication, disoriented, anxious, unable to complete activities of daily living without assistance

   R: Assess patient's level of orientation and anxiety level and use appropriate communication techniques to communicate with patient. May use assistive devices. Involve son in care of patient. Goal is to get patient to return to baseline functioning and be free of pain from wrist fracture.

Review Questions

1. 2, 5, 6 Rationale: Examples of nontherapeutic communication. Interrupting the patient is not therapeutic and gives the patient the impression that the nurse is not listening or interested. Nurses should never give advice to patients, but rather should support the patient in exploring and understanding important problems. Minimizing the patient's concerns or feelings is not therapeutic. All these nontherapeutic communication examples hinder effective nurse–patient communication.

2. 1, 3, 5 Rationale: Providing information to patients about common reactions to health care issues encourages open communication and validation. Using open-ended questions, such as "Tell me how you are feeling," enhances communication and avoids the risk of misinterpretation. Asking the patient how long they have been feeling this way promotes patient-centred communication by focusing on the patient's perceptions and seeking clarification. False reassurance minimizes the patient's feeling. It is not therapeutic to ask "why" questions because it sets up a defensive tone. Stereotyping the patient's responses is not therapeutic and does not validate the patient's feelings.

3. 1, 3, 4, 5 Rationale: Explaining to the patient that he will benefit by acting calmer is not effective. This will only frustrate the patient further and will not solve the immediate communication issues.

CHAPTER 4
Clinical Debrief

1. Before his surgery, he was prescribed two medications: hydrochlorothiazide 12.5-mg tablet orally once per day and fluoxetine 40-mg tablet orally once daily in the morning. You expect to find the hydrochlorothiazide and fluoxetine medications listed on his discharge medication list.

2. You and another nurse reconcile his discharge medication list. You assess the omission of the pain medication from the discharge list and contact the health care provider for a nurse–provider medication reconciliation.

3. S: The patient has a discharge order 8 hours status after herniorrhaphy. Pain medication is not included on the discharge medication list

   B: The surgical procedure was finished at 0900 this morning. He received one dose of hydromorphone 1 mg IV at 0930 for a pain rating of 10 on a scale of 0–10. At 1400 the patient was medicated with oxycodone 10 mg orally for pain of 9 on a scale of 0–10. Thirty minutes later, he rated his pain at 2 on a scale of 0–10. The patient's medications on admission were hydrochlorothiazide 12.5-mg tablet orally once per day and fluoxetine 40-mg tablet orally once daily in the morning.

   A: The patient was not ordered pain medication for discharge. Since his surgical procedure, his pain has been relieved with two oxycodone 10 mg tablets. His medications on admission are included on his discharge list.

   R: Reconcile the pain medication omission. Request a prescription to manage postoperative pain at home.

Review Questions

1. 1, 3, 5 Rationale: Assess the patient following a fall to determine if immediate interventions are needed. Always identify the patient with at least two identifiers per employer policy. The patient fall and nurse's assessment are documented in the EHR. The adverse event/incident report is completed but not documented in the record. The documentation of the fall is based on a thorough investigation of the incident.

2. 2, 3, 4 Rationale: SBAR can be used as the structure for hand-off reporting. Include the situation, background, assessment, and recommendation to the next nurse. Engage the patient in hand-off reporting to minimize errors.

3. 2, 1, 3, 4 Rationale: SBAR is a framework to organize the nurse's report at care transitions.

   S: Admission date, chief concern and diagnosis

   B: Medical history, allergies, code status, isolation, significant interventions, pain management, responses to interventions, report of abnormal studies, who was notified, any interventions, IV access

   A: Review of systems: neurological, respiratory, cardiac, gastrointestinal, genitourinary, musculoskeletal, peripheral vascular, skin, hematological, endocrine, and psychosocial

   R: Patient's daily goals, consultations, planned treatments, upcoming tests or surgery, discharge planning, and patient education

CHAPTER 5
Clinical Debrief

1. The nurse should complete hand hygiene in case there was accidental contact with bodily fluids. The nurse should then apply gloves and complete the physical examination.

2. The nurse needed to remove those gloves, complete hand hygiene, and put on new gloves before assessing the urinary catheter. If this step is not completed, the patient is going to be at higher risk for urinary tract infection related to any bacteria that may have been within the wound.

3. Situation: A 78-year-old patient transferred to the acute care hospital with confusion, fever, and decreased urinary output.

   Background: A 2 × 2 cm (0.8 × 0.8 inch) sacral lesion was assessed at admission.

   Assessment: Sacral lesion increased to 3 × 3 cm (1.2 × 1.2 inch) and is red and has thick, yellow drainage.

   Recommendation: Remove pressure with frequent position changes, including the 30-degree lateral position. Increase skin care to region. Obtain a prescription for wound irrigation and consult wound specialist for most appropriate dressing for the patient.

Review Questions

1. 2, 3, 4, 5 Rationale: The percentage of health care workers using hand hygiene has been increasing because the increased use of proper hand hygiene has led to a decrease in infection rates.

2. 1, 3, 4 Rationale: You cannot discuss the patient across the hall because you cannot discuss another patient's condition or treatment without violating PIPEDA regulations. A surgical mask does not provide adequate protection while taking vital signs in this case. An N95 or P100 mask is required. A private room is needed; it is important to explain transmission-based precautions, including isolation, to the patient. Gloves meet the requirement for routine practices.

3. 2, 3 Rationale: Personal soap may not be acceptable; the nurse must use a soap and lotion approved by the facility. Handwashing for 15 to 20 seconds is needed to be effective; therefore, doing it more quickly does not provide adequate hygiene. Gloves may be worn in appropriate situations, but proper hand hygiene must be performed after removing them and before putting on new ones.

CHAPTER 6
Clinical Debrief

1. Inserting an in-dwelling urinary catheter requires the use of sterile gloves. Irrigating a nasogastric tube, suctioning the oral cavity, and measuring blood pressure do not require sterile gloves. (Suctioning into the trachea and lungs requires sterile gloves.)

2. No action is needed at this time. All material must stay within 2.5 cm (1 inch) of the border of the drape. If the item touched within 2.5 cm (1 inch), a new sterile field would need to be established.

3. Situation: The patient is scheduled for a series of procedures in which sterile gloves and sterile equipment will be used.

Background: She reported dermatitis when she used rubber gloves while doing the dishes.

Assessment: She does not have any rashes or complaints of itching at this time.

Recommendation: Document on her flow sheet, electronic health record (EHR), or chart that she has a latex allergy and that all products must be nonlatex. In addition, her food allergies should be included on the flow sheet, EHR, or chart.

Review Questions

1. 1, 2 Rationale: Opening the pack just before the procedure, allowing minimal movement, and obtaining a nonlatex catheter for the procedure are all actions that will not compromise the sterility. When an object is positioned at the edge of the table or moved below the waist, it becomes unsterile. There is a 2.5-cm (1-inch) border around any sterile drape or wrap that is considered contaminated.
2. Position Rationale: UCP may only perform tasks delegated by the nurse.
3. 1, 3, 4 Rationale: Urinary catheterization, tracheal suctioning, and lumbar puncture are all invasive procedures that require sterile technique. Insertion of a feeding tube, administering a rectal suppository, and a sitz bath do not require entry into a sterile cavity of the body and thus do not require sterile technique.

CHAPTER 7
Clinical Debrief

1. Delegate only tympanic membrane temperature to the UCP. The patient has not been determined as stable; do not delegate other vital sign measurements. Direct UCP regarding frequency of temperature measurement and review the usual temperature values and significant changes to report to the nurse.
2. The UCP may have assessed the pulse incorrectly, therefore the nurse should obtain the heart rate, preferably using the apical pulse site. Beta blockers lower BP by blocking adrenaline and noradrenaline, thereby slowing heart rate. If the heart rate has been reported accurately at 58 beats/minute, the nurse should repeat the pulse assessment within 1 hour (or according to employer policy).
3. Situation: Patient has two fractures and sustained a concussion during a motorcycle accident.

Background: Patient received 15 mg morphine sulphate IV in the emergency department for fracture pain 2 hours ago.

Assessment: Difficult to rouse, respiratory rate of 12 and shallow, oxygen saturation 90% on room air, blood pressure 112/60 mm Hg, pulse 92 beats/min.

Recommendation: 2 L oxygen via nasal cannula; consider pharmacological reversal of morphine and neurology consultation.

Review Questions

1. 2, 4 Rationale: Deflating the cuff too slowly or using a loose-fitting cuff causes falsely elevated measurements. Positioning the arm above heart level, inflating the cuff too fast, and using an adult cuff on a paediatric patient all cause false-low readings (see Box 7.6).
2. D Rationale: D is the PMI and mitral listening area.
3. 2, 4, 5 Rationale: Hypothermia reduces peripheral circulation, which decreases blood flow to extremities. Activity of the infant causes interference with probe. Area of probe should be dry (see Box 7.9).

CHAPTER 8
Clinical Debrief

1. Focused assessment would include skin (surgical wound), body temperature, and heart and lungs (circulatory system). The patient is post CABG and indicates that he has "heart pain" and shortness of breath. He may have developed a thromboembolism (blood clot). If the clot obstructs circulation to the lungs, it can be life-threatening. Check body temperature because an infection could be developing.
2. The patient is 3 days post CABG and indicates "feeling very hot"; this may indicate an infection, which is not uncommon after surgery.
3. Pericarditis (i.e., inflammation of the pericardium associated with trauma such as recent surgery). It is characterized by fever, substernal chest pain, dyspnea, a dry nonproductive cough, a rapid and forcible pulse, a pericardial friction rub, and a muffled heartbeat over the apex.
4. Situation: The patient is 3 days post CABG and is indicating "heart pain, shortness of breath, and feeling hot."

Background: Patient is 3 days post CABG. One hour ago, temperature was 37.7°C (100°F), now it is 38.3°C (101°F).

Assessment: BP 140/86, T 38.3°C (101°F), HR 90, RR 22, oxygen saturation 91% on RA; S_1, S_2, + friction rub on auscultation, negative murmurs or gallops; lungs with course rhonchi.

Recommendation: Notify health care provider immediately.

Review Questions

1. 1, 2, 5, 6 Rationale: This follows the ABCD rule of melanoma.
2. 1, 5, 7 Rationale: The general survey includes assessment of vital signs, height and weight, general behaviour, posture, and appearance.
3. 2, 1, 4, 3 Rationale: It is important to auscultate before percussing or palpating the abdomen because these manoeuvres may alter the frequency and character of bowel sounds.

CHAPTER 9
Clinical Debrief

1. On the basis of these signs and symptoms of a potential urinary tract infection, you should expect to collect a urine culture and sensitivity using the collection method for an in-dwelling urinary catheter. Blood cultures may also be obtained to rule out sepsis. In addition, a blood specimen to evaluate fluid and electrolyte status would be necessary related to her level of consciousness, low blood pressure, and increased heart rate.
2. Teach the patient how to test his urine for ketones when ill to determine if diabetic ketoacidosis (DKA) is developing and to call his health care provider if ketones are present. Discuss the need to check his blood glucose often and not to eliminate administering insulin during times of illness and stress. In addition, review and allow him to demonstrate the correct procedure for obtaining his blood glucose by using the lateral side instead of the central part of the fingertips. You may also suggest a new meter that allows for alternative testing sites such as the forearm.
3. Situation: The patient's work of breathing has dramatically increased. He has had multiple respiratory treatments over the past 3 hours, and oxygen was initiated at 2 L per nasal cannula.

Background: The patient was admitted 2 days ago with DKA related to an upper respiratory infection. He subsequently stopped taking his insulin. He was going to be discharged home today but developed shortness of breath during the night.

Assessment: Bilateral adventitious lung sounds with intercostal muscle retractions and nasal flaring. VS: temperature 40°C, pulse 112 beats/min, B/P 158/80 mm Hg, respiratory rate 32 breaths/min, SaO$_2$ 84%.

Recommendation: Immediate interprofessional consultation (e.g., health care provider, pulmonary specialist, nurse), obtain arterial blood gases, and increase oxygen.

Review Questions

1. 1, 2, 5, 6 Rationale: Two person-specific identifiers are required to ensure the correct patient. Pericare before collection of specimen reduces the number of organisms. The head of the penis is cleaned with a circular motion, not back and forth. A 90- to 120-mL amount of urine is collected. Having the patient initially void flushes microorganisms that normally accumulate in the urethra. Holding the penis above the cup prevents touching, which would contaminate the container.
2. 1, 3, 4 Rationale: The head of the bed elevated to 45 degrees and the patient leaning back against the bed allow for easy access to oral structures. Careful insertion of the swab without touching lips, teeth, tongue, or cheeks prevents contamination with organisms of the oral cavity. Swabbing the tonsillar area is correct, but not the uvula. Having her blow her nose is not indicated for a throat culture but is recommended when obtaining a nasal culture.
3. 2, 3, 1, 5, 4 Rationale: Clamping the tube for 15 minutes allows for collection of fresh sterile urine. Cleansing the port prevents entry of microorganisms into the catheter and contamination of specimen. Use of a Luer-Lok syringe prevents injury by needlestick. Collection of proper volume is needed to perform the test. Unclamping the catheter allows drainage of urine to prevent stasis of urine in the bladder.

CHAPTER 10
Clinical Debrief

1. Cardiac catheterization poses a risk for blood loss and complications that would require emergency coronary artery bypass graft surgery. Hematocrit and hemoglobin values are needed to obtain a baseline hematological status for later comparison. Prothrombin time/international normalized ratio (PT/INR) is affected by warfarin, which the patient takes for chronic atrial fibrillation. If so, the health care provider needs to instruct the patient to stop his warfarin 1 to 2 nights before this procedure. A current PT/INR is needed to determine whether the patient is at risk for uncontrolled bleeding. Values for blood urea nitrogen and creatinine evaluate his renal function and, along with urine specific gravity, determine if he is dehydrated. Patients with baseline dehydration or impaired renal function are at risk for impaired excretion of the radiographic dye used during the cardiac catheterization procedure. Baseline electrolytes (sodium and potassium) are assessed to determine possible electromechanical problems.

2. In the presence of another nurse, ask the patient the following on arrival and just before starting the procedure: name, identifying number such as birthday, purpose of visit. Also compare the person-specific identifiers with information in his medication administration record (MAR) or medical record. Document in the patient's medical record.

3. Situation: The patient has recently experienced what he describes as "mild discomfort" in his chest when he exercises.
   Background: He is a 67-year-old Métis man who lives with his sister.
   Assessment: Postprocedure femoral pulse is strong and regular. Heart rate of 88, normal sinus rhythm on ECG monitor. Resp 16, BP 150/78, SpO$_2$ 99% on 2 L O$_2$. Femoral puncture site has small dressing intact with no signs of bleeding or edema. Patient is oriented to person, place, and time and denies pain at this time.
   Recommendation: Document vital signs, SpO$_2$, and sedation level every 15 minutes for 30 minutes after the procedure. Monitor for chest pain and postprocedure adverse effects.

Review Questions

1. 4, 1, 5, 3, 6, 2 Rationale: Review Skill 10.3.

2. 1, 2, 3, 5 Rationale: The patient may be experiencing bronchospasm and requires the nurse to support his or her airway. The nurse should monitor vital signs, call the physician immediately, and prepare for possible resuscitation. Suctioning would not be appropriate since it would worsen bronchospasm. The patient requires patent IV access, and a cricothyrotomy may be needed.

3. 1, 4, 5 Rationale: Contraindications for angiography include anticoagulant therapy such as warfarin, bleeding disorders, thrombocytopenia, dehydration, uncontrolled hypertension, renal insufficiency, and pregnancy.

CHAPTER 11
Clinical Debrief

1. Additional information before transferring includes the following: patient's motivation to be moved; cognition; ability to tolerate and help with transfer (muscle strength in legs and upper arms); presence of paralysis or paresis; bone continuity (trauma); and presence of weakness, dizziness, and vital signs.

2. A nurse supervises and helps the UCP when there is a health care provider's prescription to logroll a patient. Patients with a spinal cord injury or who are recovering from neck, back, or spinal surgery often need to keep the spinal column in straight alignment to prevent further injury. Three nurses are needed to turn the patient correctly.

3. Situation: The patient is refusing to go to radiology for a CT scan to rule out injury to the neck and spine.
   Background: The patient is 6 hours post–motor vehicle accident. He is reporting a pain level of 7 (previously 9) on a scale from 0 (no pain) to 10 (worst pain ever) after receiving his pain medication. He does not have any other prescriptions for pain medication.
   Assessment: Respiratory rate has increased from 18 to 24 breaths/min; blood pressure 190/102; pulse 118 beats/min. Very anxious and yelling, "I can't take this pain anymore."
   Recommendation: Immediate consultation with the health care provider for further prescriptions for pain medication before transferring him to a stretcher for CT scan.

Review Questions

1. 1, 2, 3 Rationale: Consider individual patient problems during transfer. For example, a patient who has been immobile for several days or longer may be weak or dizzy or may develop orthostatic hypotension when transferred. If patient is unable to transfer to chair without help, apply a transfer belt, get needed help from other nurses, and use appropriate safe-handling algorithm.

2. 7, 1, 4, 3, 2, 5, 6 Rationale: Transferring a patient from a bed to a wheelchair encompasses many of the same principles discussed in Skill 11.1. Several additional steps must be taken to maintain safety of a patient and for the nurse to prevent injury when transferring a patient from or to a wheelchair. Refer to Procedural Guideline 11.1. Check wheelchair locks and footplates for proper functioning before use.

3. 3, 5, 2, 8, 7, 4, 6, 1 Rationale: Patients who are unable to bear weight require use of a mechanical/hydraulic lift. Research supports that mechanical lifts prevent musculoskeletal injuries. Before using lift, be thoroughly familiar with its operation.

CHAPTER 12
Clinical Debrief

1. The nurse should assess the patient's beliefs, values, and perceptions regarding her current health status and her confidence in being capable of exercising. This will influence her perceived self-efficacy and capability to transfer to a chair. Physically the nurse should assess the patient's ROM and strength while she performs active ROM. In addition, the nurse should assess her current pain level (using a pain scale) because an analgesic might be necessary before she gets up to sit. A set of vital signs should be collected at rest so the nurse can compare values before and after sitting. When the patient sits on the side of the bed, the nurse can determine if she becomes orthostatic or has other symptoms that would prevent helping her to the chair.

2. The patient has had a fracture and orthopaedic surgery on her hip and has participated in limited activity while being in the CCU. She is over the age of 65.

3. Situation: 68-year-old woman transferred from CCU 24 hours ago, advanced to stage 4 mobility protocol this A.M. Assisted ambulation down hallway.
   Background: Preambulation vital signs while sitting in chair: BP 138/80; R 26, P 88, oxygen saturation 96%. Patient received analgesic 30 minutes before sitting in a chair. Had been in chair for 15 minutes before initiating ambulation. Pain score was a 4.
   Assessment: Patient was steady standing, began to walk, after approximately 7 metres (20 feet) stated she had chest pain and felt dizzy. BP is now 110/60, P 130, R 32.
   Recommendation: Patient returned to chair immediately. Consider prescription for electrocardiogram. Will reassess vital signs and oxygen saturation.

Review Questions

1. 3, 1, 4, 2 Rationale: See Skill 12.2.

2. 1, 3, 5 Rationale: When sitting for long periods of time, such as when travelling for more than 4 hours, get up and walk around every 2 to 3 hours; drink plenty of water; and exercise your legs while sitting: raise and lower your heels while keeping your toes on the floor, raise and lower your toes while keeping your heels on the floor, and tighten and release your leg muscles. Also wear loose fitting clothes. Never cross your legs when sitting.

3. 3, 4, 5 Rationale: The patient should stop doing physical activity if hypotensive (drop in systolic BP of 30 or change in diastolic BP of 10 mm Hg); with development of dizziness lasting 60 seconds, fainting, or diaphoresis; or when there is a change in breathing pattern with increase in accessory muscle use, extreme fatigue, or severe dyspnea with respiratory rate greater than baseline by >20/min.

CHAPTER 13
Clinical Debrief

1. The nurse should first stop the lateral rotation to assess the patient. The nurse should talk to the patient, providing reassurance, and assess for other factors that could make him hypotensive. Some dizziness can be normal when adjusting to the movement of the bed, but the nurse

should identify any other factors for hypotension before contacting the health care provider. The nurse should also be sure that the patient is adequately hydrated because his bed can cause dryness and dehydration, which could be contributing to the dizziness.

2. This specialty bed should be preventing pressure areas; therefore, the first step is to be sure that the bed and mattress are functioning properly. The nurse should also check that the patient is being repositioned frequently and properly.

3. Situation: Patient has been on the air-suspension bed for over 24 hours.
   Background: Patient is a 48-year-old male who was involved in a motor vehicle accident that resulted in quadriplegia. He is unable to reposition himself or transfer without help. He does not speak English.
   Assessment: With the use of a qualified medical interpreter, it has been determined that he is nauseated, has vomited × 2, and feels dizzy in the bed. Despite repositioning him, the nausea continues. Vital signs: HR 100 beats/min, RR 24 breaths/min, BP 100/60 mm Hg.
   Recommendation: Administer ondansetron 4 mg IV push × 1, then 8 mg oral disintegrating tablets (ODTs) every 12 hours as needed.

Review Questions

1. 1, 2, 3, 5 Rationale: The caregiver should report all of her notes to the nurse or case manager. The caregiver should not wait to evaluate the skin because ischial wounds can occur quickly and often tunnel, causing serious pressure injuries.

2. 3, 2, 5, 1, 4 Rationale: The mattress is applied in the deflated mode and secured first. Then the connectors are attached, and the mattress is inflated and checked for proper working order. Finally, the sheet is placed before transferring the patient to the bed.

3. 2, 3, 4 Rationale: Dehydration can become a problem because the air circulating around the patient is warm. Moving a patient out of an air-fluidized bed can be difficult because of the high edges and the fact that the patient is submerged in the bed. The air-fluidized bed is large and heavy, making it difficult to transport.

CHAPTER 14
Clinical Debrief

1. The patient has numerous fall risk factors: fatigue, weakness of lower extremities, requiring help to walk a short distance, his age, and his medications. Fall prevention strategies include establishing an elimination schedule, staying with the patient during toileting, using a gait belt to help the patient transfer to a bedside commode, removing clutter from the environment, activating a bed alarm, and placing the patient into a low bed.

2. The nurse should provide airway protection and gas exchange by correctly positioning the patient's head while rolling them onto their side (if possible). This maintains a patent airway until the seizure ends. The patient is at risk for two problems: (1) hypoglycemia—history of diabetes mellitus and requires medication but has not eaten in 7 hours; and (2) NPO status causing a risk for fluid and electrolyte imbalance. In this case, the patient has an IV line with only normal saline and no dextrose. Metabolic changes can precipitate a seizure.

3. Situation: 72-year-old patient is admitted for acute pneumonia; developed seizure with tonic and clonic activity at 0945.
   Background: Patient has a history of diabetes mellitus, heart disease, and arthritis. Takes oral hypoglycemic glyburide, receiving IV D$_5$NS infusing at 80 mL/hr, has had poor appetite, and has been NPO since 12 midnight.
   Assessment: Patient awakening from seizure exhibited tonic and clonic activity lasting approximately 3 minutes, blood glucose 3.2 mmol/L, positioned on side, breathing without difficulty, confused × 2, asking what happened?
   Recommendation: Patient hypoglycemic; will repeat blood glucose measurement, recommend review of PO diet and IV fluids for glucose sources, plan to reorient patient and include spouse in explanation of seizure event.

Review Questions

1. 3, 4, 1, 2 Rationale: The nurse takes the four steps needed in responding to a fire: Rescue patient, Activate alarm, Contain the fire, and Evacuate patient.

2. 2, 3, 5 Rationale: The selected choices are appropriate in creating a restraint-free environment designed for a patient at risk for wandering. Choice 1 is an assessment activity important for the nurse to conduct. Choice 4 is not appropriate until all restraint-free interventions are tried and the patient is at risk for injury.

3. 2, 4, 5 Rationale: The nurse assesses any previous falls using the acronym SPLATT: Symptoms at time of fall, Previous fall, Location of fall, Activity at time of fall, Time of fall, and Trauma after fall. It is important to assess medications and medical conditions to determine a patient's fall risks but not as the information relates to a previous fall.

CHAPTER 15
Clinical Debrief

1. Contamination of the nurse, ED, and other patients is a concern. The nurse will don appropriate personal protective equipment (PPE) after performing hand hygiene. Only trained personnel using required PPE may decontaminate a victim. The nurse should be briefed by appropriate emergency personnel and gather knowledge as to the type of chemical agent if possible. Institution protocol should be followed for disaster response.

2. 41-year-old burn victim; 22-year-old with cyanosis; 14-year-old with rash; 56-year-old with controlled bleeding.

3. Situation: Patient states he noticed the "funny smell" in his apartment and began to feel light-headed.
   Background: Patient is an 85-year-old white male with a history of angina and prostate cancer. He lives alone in an apartment in a retirement community.
   Assessment: Pulse 96 and irregular; respirations 28 with audible wheezing, SaO$_2$ 88%. ECG reveals possible anterior wall MI. Patient is oriented to person, place, and time and complaining of heaviness in his chest.
   Recommendation: Immediate evaluation by ED health care provider for possible MI. Placement of patient in monitored area of ED, application of O$_2$. Concerns for additional effects because of age of patient.

Review Questions

1. 2, 4 Rationale: From Skill 15-1. Skill cannot be delegated to the UCP; the UCP can gather and wear PPE and be instructed by the nurse as to the proper handling of the body after death to avoid contamination to the UCP.

2. 1, 3, 4 Rationale: Psychological responses can be severe following radiation exposure. Heightened self-care practices and planning a vacation will not be possible. Self-care practices may be impaired during this time. Planning a vacation is a positive and future-oriented activity that the patient will not be able to focus on at this time.

3. 3, 1, 5, 2, 6, 4 Rationale: The goal is to prevent further contamination and prevent patient death. Before initiating any treatment, the nurse must first remove the threat of further contamination. Cutting off clothing first will prevent contamination of head and hair. It is important to next wash the patient to dilute the chemical; flushing of eyes will prevent contamination. The nurse can then focus on disposal of clothing and initiate treatment.

CHAPTER 16
Clinical Debrief

1. The patient is only a few hours postoperative. The local anaesthetic he is receiving from his epidural may be causing a motor block to his bladder or the location of surgery might affect his ability to pass urine. In addition, the adverse effects of opioids in epidural analgesia include urinary retention.

2. Nonpharmacological approaches for pain relief may be useful for the patient. His spouse can learn how to provide distraction by conversing with him, offering to play cards or engage in a shared activity, or praying. The nurses could also demonstrate how the spouse can do a relaxing hand massage. It is important that the patient and spouse understand the rationale for these approaches and their effects on pain perception.
   Situation: Patient is status postcolectomy; has not voided urine since returning from surgery.
   Background: Vital signs stable; BP 132/86 mm Hg, P 84 beats/min, regular, RR 20 breaths/min, temp 37.6 C. Epidural dressing intact

with dose on demand infusion. Surgical dressing dry and intact. Abdomen palpated; patient expressed discomfort when palpated over bladder area. Pain at a level of 5 on a 0–10 scale.

Assessment: Patient has distended bladder with urinary retention.

Recommendation: Notified health care provider; discussed potential need for insertion of straight urinary catheter or possibility of reducing opioid dosage. Straight catheterization prescribed.

3. One basic principle to follow when preparing this patient to ambulate is to have him administer a bolus of the epidural analgesic 30 to 60 minutes before standing to maximize his pain relief. This will require some planning with the patient so a dose can be given. Prior to getting the patient to stand, it is important to check the motor function and sensation in his legs. If he is having difficulty moving his legs, do not get the patient up, and call the most responsible care provider for the epidural and inform them of the findings of your assessment. If the patient has no difficulty moving his legs, you can assist him in getting up. When you help the patient stand, it will be necessary to check vital signs to be sure that he does not have orthostatic hypotension, a common adverse effect from opioids. Explain that the first attempt to ambulate may feel strange secondary to decreased sensation, but motor (leg) function should be unaffected. You should also teach the patient how to splint his incision when transferring to and from the bed and during ambulation. On return to bed you can have him practice relaxation and guided imagery to relax any tense muscles.

4. Nonpharmacological approaches for pain relief may be useful for the patient, including walking, massage, music, and distraction. Hydromorphone prn may be administered to help reduce incisional pain.

Review Questions

1. 2, 4, 5 Rationale: When providing pain relief for an older person, remember that procedures such as distraction, relaxation, or guided imagery can be effective. Cognitive-behavioural strategies are appropriate unless the patient has cognitive impairment. Analgesic dosages should be started low and titrated upward slowly until pain relief is achieved. Also, the dosages of a combination of analgesics and/or adjuvants might need to be adjusted before relief is obtained. It is important to have glasses, hearing aids, and other assistive devices in place before attempting therapies such as guided relaxation or guided imagery. Massage is a physical pain-relief strategy that promotes comfort and alters physiological responses to pain and is generally safe and effective in older persons.

2. 3, 5 Rationale: A patient at risk for sedation is one who is "opioid naïve" (i.e., one who has never taken any opioids for any reason or who has not taken opioids in the past 5 weeks). Patients with obstructive sleep apnea (brief cessation of respirations during sleep) or obese patients with short, thick necks are at risk for becoming oversedated when receiving opioids. A patient who is cognitively impaired is not a candidate for patient-controlled analgesia but is not necessarily at risk for sedation from opioids. An allergy would contraindicate use of opioids but does not increase risk for sedation.

3.

Step	Rationale
Explain how to perform hand hygiene.	Decreases transmission of microorganisms.
Have patient reposition gently lift the adhesive dressing covering the catheter insertion site and remove any remaining tape.	Exposes catheter insertion site.
Explain to patient or caregiver to grasp the catheter as close as possible to where it enters the skin and gently pull it out.	Prevents breakage of catheter.
Instruct patient or caregiver to hold pressure over the site for 2 minutes, then apply a Band-Aid.	Achieves hemostasis.
Explain to patient that any remaining numbness should go away within 24 hours after the catheter is removed.	Enables patient and caregiver to anticipate progress and recognize problems.

CHAPTER 17

Clinical Debrief

1. Acknowledge and validate the patient's feelings using empathy and compassionate presence. Determine what he knows about his diagnosis and prognosis. Offer support and listen. Provide information he requests. Revisit his desire to transfer to another facility.

2. a. Failure to have a bowel movement may be caused by the tumour, effects of opioids in pain medications, reduced level of activity, reduced peristalsis, and reduced intake of proper foods and liquids.

   b. Request prn or daily stool softener or laxative to promote normal bowel routine. Encourage ambulation. Encourage increased fluid intake if patient is not nauseated. Educate the patient about his disease process.

3. Key points to include in discussion with this patient are the following:
   - Palliative care aims to relieve suffering and improve quality of life.
   - The goals of palliative care are to support the physical, emotional, and spiritual needs of patients and their families at any time during a serious illness.
   - A specialist palliative care team is consulted and assists regular care providers when needs are complex or difficult to manage.
   - Palliative care can be provided in any setting, including the home.
   - An interprofessional team of doctors, nurses, social workers, spiritual-care providers, and others work with the patient and family to plan and provide care.

   Situation: Spouse expressing uncertainty with suggested consult to the specialty palliative care team.

   Background: Older adult male patient was hospitalized for abdominal pain, anorexia, weight loss, and weakness. Now diagnosed with metastatic prostate cancer involving abdomen and lymph nodes.

   Assessment: Spouse is patient's primary caregiver in the home. Patient's condition is declining with weight loss, anorexia, worsening abdominal pain, and depression.

   Recommendation: Suggest interprofessional patient/family conference to discuss goals of care.

Review Questions

1. 1, 2, 5, 6 Rationale: The goals of palliative care include relief of suffering and optimizing quality of life through vigilant physical symptom management, and psychosocial and spiritual support. Palliative care can be offered at any time during a serious illness and in conjunction with life-prolonging treatments. Palliative care may contribute to prolonged life, but that is not the aim; nor is cure. Palliative care neither hastens nor postpones death. Palliative care helps facilitate a peaceful death when the time comes.

2. 2, 3, 4 Rationale: End-of-life care is *a component* of palliative care. Palliative care should be initiated early in the course of a serious life-limiting illness and can be provided in conjunction with curative treatment by care teams in a variety of settings. A specialist palliative care team may be needed to support the efforts of the regular care team to manage complex symptoms and concerns.

3. 6, 7, 5, 2, 3, 1, 8, 4 Rationale: See Skill 17.2.

CHAPTER 18

Clinical Debrief

1. Check the feet every day. Make sure there are no cuts, cracks, ingrown toenails, or blisters. Wash your foot in warm water; dry them carefully, especially between the toes. Trim toenails straight across and file sharp edges; wear clean, white socks and well-fitting shoes at all times. Shoes should be supportive and should not rub or pinch. Elevate feet when sitting and wiggle your toes and ankles for a few minutes several times a day; exercise regularly to improve circulation.

2. The correct answer is 4. Patients with diabetes mellitus are prone to dryness of the mouth, gingivitis, periodontal disease, and loss of teeth. Oral surgery causes a break in mucosa and increases infection risk. Aging causes mucosa to become thin and less elastic. Chemical injury from alcohol or tobacco irritates the oral mucosa.

3. Situation: The patient has a 3-year history of type 1 diabetes mellitus and hypertension.

   Background: The patient was discharged with a right-heal ulcer requiring daily dressing changes.

Assessment: VS: Temp 37°C, pulse 86, BP 135/85, respiratory rate 30. Right-heel ulcer is 2 cm × 2 cm (0.8 × 0.8 inch); no drainage noted. 10 cm × 10 cm (4 × 4 inch) dressing applied, covered, and wrapped with gauze cling wrap.

Recommendation: Discussed maintaining adequate foot care. Patient verbalized ways to maintain good foot care. Follow up with health care provider in 2 weeks.

Review Questions

1. 2, 3 Rationale: Presence of an endotracheal tube leads to bacteria converting to Gram-negative organisms. A reduced or absent reflex is common in critically ill patients, increasing risk of aspiration, which leads to VAP. The mucus within the endotracheal tube grows resident but not Gram-negative bacteria unless an infection develops. Regular suctioning is part of the routine care for a patient with an endotracheal tube. Critical illness typically does not cause an increase in oral secretions.

2. 1, 3, 5, 7 Rationale: To be safe, the bed must be elevated to working height. Tuck in the top sheet and blanket at the foot of the bed and then make a modified mitred corner. To save steps, apply all bottom linens on one side of the bed before moving to the opposite side. Horizontal toe pleats are made on all beds. Gloves do not need to be worn except if linen is soiled with drainage. Soiled linens should be placed in a linen bag, not on the floor. Top blankets need to be fan-folded to the end of the bed when the procedure is complete.

3. 3, 6, 1, 5, 7, 4, 2 Rationale: See Skill 18.3.

CHAPTER 19
Clinical Debrief

1. a. History: Ask both of them to identify the exact changes in his hearing (e.g., when did this start, is it present all the time, does the quality of hearing acuity change with male versus female voices, adult versus children's voices?

   b. Ask both of them what their expectations are following this clinic visit.

   c. Perform an external ear examination to determine the presence of redness, visible drainage, or tenderness of external ear structures.

   d. Perform otoscopic examination to observe tympanic membrane (i.e., inflammation, drainage, or redness).

2. Batteries are toxic if swallowed, and the one should seek emergency care if this occurs. The patient and his wife need to keep batteries and aids out of their grandchildren's reach. Children are naturally curious; therefore, to take some of the mystery of the aid away, they can show the children how the aid fits in the ear and where the batteries fit.

3. Situation: Patient is a 68-year-old male who has worn hearing aids for 10 years and was satisfied with the aids. During the last week both he and his wife noticed a decrease in his hearing ability.

   Background: Three weeks ago, he had an upper respiratory infection. Since then, he has noticed that he is not hearing as well with his hearing aids. He also believes there is drainage in his left ear.

   Assessment: Excessive wax buildup in left ear with some purulent drainage; tympanic membrane is cloudy.

   Recommendation: Further examination to verify ear infection and treat with antibiotics, and an order for an ear irrigation. Patient to follow up in 2 weeks to determine if hearing is improved once the infection is resolved.

Review Questions

1. c, f, d, e, a, b

2. 1, 2, 4, 5 Rationale: When a toxic-exposure eye emergency exists, immediate irrigation is necessary to prevent further eye or vision damage. When providing routine eye irrigations, the nurse gently removes secretions to prevent them from scratching the cornea. Pupillary response provides information about how the eye is accommodating to light and should be assessed after the irrigation. During eye irrigation, the nurse prevents injury to the patient's corneas by removing dried secretions, holding the irrigation device 2.5 cm (1 inch) from the inner canthus, and slowly irrigating the eye with prescribed solution. Securing the eyelids with paper tape is not good practice; if the patient's eyes need further protection, special eye pads or a patch could be prescribed.

3. 2, 3, 4 Rationale: Talking slowly provides the patient time to process the conversation; the nurse facing the patient provides cues from facial expression. When a hearing-impaired patient doesn't understand a question or a teaching point, rephrase. Ask them which part of the conversation they understood and which part was difficult to understand. This information will help guide rephrasing. Speaking louder or using hand gestures does not promote better hearing or understanding; these may increase the patient's anxiety and frustration.

CHAPTER 20
Clinical Debrief

1. The antidepressant, hormone, cardiac drug (beta-blocker), and antihypertensive medications all have the potential to produce adverse effects in the older person. The metoprolol and the antihypertensive both have weakness and dizziness as side effects. Summation or synergism may occur with the interaction of these many different medications. Nursing interventions should include a history to determine if issues of polypharmacy are causing these adverse effects. Identify possible electrolyte alterations that the medications may cause. Take the patient's vital signs to determine if there is any hypotension. Ask the patient if he has had any recent falls and assess him for any data to support this (e.g., bruising).

2. The medication doses may be lowered by the health care provider for the older person to determine if a therapeutic effect can still be achieved. As the nurse you need to continue to monitor the patient for these adverse effects during any change in medication dose. The dose for the patient is one-half tablet to be administered orally.

3. You need to evaluate the patient's motor dexterity and visual acuity to split the tablet if it does not come from pharmacy already split.

   Situation: The patient has been on metoprolol for 1 week and is experiencing weakness and dizziness.

   Background: The health care provider has just added this new medication twice daily in addition to his other prescribed medication and the herbal supplement melatonin.

   Assessment: The patient is alert and oriented, heart rate 64 beats/min, respiratory rate 20, BP 100/70 sitting.

   Recommendation: Repeat the blood pressure measurement sitting, standing, and lying down. Consult the pharmacist about potential interactions with the medications and melatonin. Provide the assessment data especially related to blood pressure findings to the health care provider and consult the health care provider about possible revision of the metoprolol dose.

Review Questions

1. Answer: 1, 2, 3, 4 Rationale: You need to clarify all the prescriptions. Timoptic .25% solution 1 drop OD bid has a "naked" decimal point, and it is unclear if OD means right eye or right ear. Metoprolol 12.50 mg qd has a trailing zero, and it is unclear if the dosage is to be 12.5 mg or 1250 mg. Insulin glargine 6 u SC twice a day includes the letter *u*, which makes it unclear to know if this means unit or if it is a 0 or a 4; and SC could be mistaken as SL. Enalapril 2.5 mg. PO three times a day, hold for systolic blood pressure <100 has a period after mg, which could be mistaken as the number 1, and the < sign could be mistaken as "greater than." You are not sure if the identified blood pressure parameter is systolic or diastolic.

   Correctly written prescriptions:

   Timoptic 0.25% solution 1 drop right eye bid

   Metoprolol 12.5 mg daily

   Insulin glargine 6 units SUBCUT bid

   Enalapril 2.5 mg PO tid; hold if systolic blood pressure below 100 mm Hg

2. Answer: 1, 2, 5 Rationale: Larger print and a dispensing system that allows the nurse, patient, or caregiver to set up medications for a week can ensure safe medication administration in the older person. Larger-print medication pamphlets are also available. The use of teach-back ensures that the patient understands their medications and increases safety.

3. Answer: 1, 2, 3, 4, 5 Rationale: All of these are acceptable guidelines for taking verbal and telephone orders (prescriptions) in a health care facility.

CHAPTER 21
Clinical Debrief

1. The nurse should first ask the patient why she has three nitroglycerin transdermal patches in place and if she needed to take her nitroglycerin sublingual tablets more frequently. It is important to never make assumptions (e.g., in this case, that she forgot to take the patches off) before formulating a clinical decision. It would be unsafe to assume that she forgot to remove the other patches without determining if there was an increase in angina episodes during which she took her sublingual nitroglycerin tablets and thought the transdermal patch would also help. In addition, these patches could be present because she forgot to remove them, which would indicate a need for further patient teaching.

2. The nurse should wash the old medication off, explaining to the patient the reason for removing the medication. The nurse should assess the wound to determine if it has worsened or if healing occurred, and then reapply ointment and provide wound care, explaining each step to her. The patient needs further teaching on caring for this wound. Explaining why it is necessary to remove all previous ointment and why each step of wound care is important. Nursing assessment of the wound determines if wound healing is occurring and also teaches her how to observe the wound.

3. Situation: The patient has an infected bug bite treated with bacitracin topical ointment (500 units/g). During the last two visits the nurse noted that the patient was not cleaning the wound and was applying new ointment over old ointment.
   Background: The patient was hospitalized recently for dehydration following a week of gastroenteritis. She has an abscess on her right calf from an infected bug bite.
   Assessment: Wound is now 3×5 cm (1.25×2 inches) in circumference and has two new blisters. Yellow, foul-smelling drainage is present.
   Recommendation: Immediate referral to a community care wound nurse for a revised plan to promote healing of abscess on her right calf.

Review Questions

1. 3, 4, 5, 6 Rationale: An enteral tube syringe is necessary to avoid dangerous misconnections and accidently administering the medications through another tube. Flushing the tubing after medication administration clears it of any residual medication and ensures that the tube remains patent. If gastric residuals are high, the absorption of the enteral tube medication is reduced. Elevating the head of the bed helps to reduce the risk for aspiration. Verification of tube placement is essential before administering anything via a nasogastric tube. Medications are given separately to avoid any drug–drug interactions that could clog the feeding tube.

2. 2, 5 Rationale: Gloves reduce the risk of accidental exposure to medication and systemic reaction to the nitroglycerin (e.g., vasodilation and hypotension). This accidental exposure can occur during medication application or removal of used ointment wrappers. Hand hygiene is insufficient for protecting against accidental exposure because nitroglycerin is absorbed rapidly.

3. 2, 3, 6, 1, 4, 5, 8, 7 Rationale: Obtains baseline respiratory assessment before medication. Ensures optimal delivery of medication.

CHAPTER 22
Clinical Debrief

1. The nurse needs to know the drug classification, desired effect, and nursing implications related to heparin therapy and the safe medication dose, which must be compared with the order before administration. The nurse needs to calculate how many millilitres to draw from the vial and if a filter needle is required.

2. The nurse needs to know the patient's current diet and use of over-the-counter supplements, herbal supplements, and other prescribed medications to ensure that there is no increased risk for bleeding; if anything is affecting blood flow to subcutaneous tissues of the abdomen; and any related laboratory findings of the partial thromboplastin time. The patient's weight may be an indicator for a different needle length.

3. The nurse cannot delegate administration of heparin but can direct the UCP to notify the nurse of any signs of bleeding such as blood in the urine; any changes in vital signs that may indicate bleeding such as increased heart rate or decreased blood pressure; and if there is any blood oozing from any puncture or intravenous site.

4. A 1- to 3-mL syringe is sufficient to administer subcutaneous injections. If you can grasp 5 cm (2 inches) of tissue, insert the needle at a 90-degree angle; if you can grasp 2.5 cm (1 inch) of tissue, insert the needle at a 45-degree angle.

5. Situation: The patient has received a subcutaneous injection of heparin 2.5 cm (1 inch) from the left side of the umbilicus 15 minutes ago and is indicating soreness and tenderness at the injection site.
   Background: The health care provider has administered the heparin via subcutaneous route every day. This is the fourth day of administration.
   Assessment: The patient is alert and oriented; the area around the umbilicus is reddened and tender to the touch. Hardened lumps can be palpated several areas.
   Recommendation: Consult the health care provider about possible change from the subcutaneous route to an oral medication (e.g., warfarin) after the laboratory data are collected. Review the medication reference or talk with pharmacy about administering the heparin in another site.

Review Questions

1. 6, 4, 5, 3, 1, 2 Rationale: These are the steps to administer an intradermal injection (see Skill 22.2).

2. 5, 2, 1, 3, 7, 4, 6 Rationale: These are the steps to discontinue continuous subcutaneous infusion (CSQI) (see Skill 22.4).

3. 2, 5, 4, 6, 1, 3 Rationale: These are the correct steps to administer an IV push medication in an existing line with compatible fluid running (Skill 22.6).

CHAPTER 23
Clinical Debrief

1. The nurse should focus the assessment on the patient's respiratory system, including lung sounds, respiratory rate, and respiratory effort. The patient would likely have crackles or rhonchi in the right lower lobe and maybe clear sounds in all other lobes. Respiratory rate would be greater than 20 breaths/min, and the patient's effort would be dyspneic and laboured. The patient's SpO_2 level would likely be less than 90%.

2. Patients with COPD are at risk of worsening hypercapnia when high concentrations of oxygen are administered to them. Patients with acute exacerbations of COPD who are hypoxemic would benefit more from a Venturi mask. The patient is too short of breath and clinically unstable to benefit from an incentive spirometer at this time.

3. Situation: Patient has COPD and complicated pneumonia. He was admitted today for intravenous antibiotics and oxygen therapy.
   Background: Patient was treated with full course of antibiotics at home last week. His symptoms continued and eventually worsened over the past few hours.
   Assessment: Patient with crackles in right lower lobe, clear but diminished in all other lobes. Respiratory rate of 32 breaths/min, heart rate of 110 beats/min, BP 144/76, and temperature of 38.7°C (101.8°F). He indicates he is short of breath and states he "feels like he will die."
   Recommendation: Please come reassess this patient immediately. This patient's condition has acutely worsened, and the patient likely needs respiratory consultation and transfer to a critical care unit. Would recommend NIPPV and respiratory therapy.

Review Questions

1. b, d, e Rationale: UCPs cannot perform a complete respiratory assessment; they can measure respirations in stable patients. UCPs cannot educate patients and caregivers. These tasks and skills fall under the nurse's scope of practice and should be performed by the nurse. Oxygen is a medication and should not be titrated or adjusted by UCPs. Medication administration is within the nurse's scope of practice. The UCP is allowed to reposition patients, help adjust oxygen-delivery devices if they are uncomfortable or not properly placed, and record the patient's SpO_2 level in the health record.

2. b, c, e Rationale: Oxygen is administered to treat hypoxemia as evidenced by an SpO_2 less than 90% or a PaO_2 less than 60 mm Hg. Cyanosis around oral mucous membranes can indicate hypoxemia. Shortness of breath and diminished breath sounds are not indicators for patient need of oxygen unless accompanied by the other findings.

3. b, e, a, c, d, f Rationale: Organized teaching for a peak flowmeter. Refer to Procedural Guideline 23.1 for correct order of steps.

CHAPTER 24
Clinical Debrief

1. In addition to his increased respiratory rate, the nurse would expect to see laboured respirations and some use of the clavicles to increase inspiratory volume. On auscultation, crackles and other abnormal lung sounds would be present in the lower lobes. In addition, lung sounds would be absent in the right middle lobe and diminished bilaterally in the lower lobes. The nurse should focus the assessment on the patient's pulmonary system, including lung sounds, respiratory rate, and respiratory effort. The patient would have crackles or rhonchi in the right lower lobe and possibly clear sounds in all other lobes. Respiratory rate would be greater than 20 breaths/min, and the patient's effort would be dyspneic and labored. Patient SaO_2 level would likely be less than 90%.

2. The correct position to drain the lower lobes would be a Trendelenburg position, with the foot of the bed raised 45 to 50 cm (18–20 inches); for the right lower lobe, the patient is positioned on his abdomen; for the left lower lobe, the patient is on his right side.

3. Situation: Patient has CF and complicated pneumonia. He has had 24 hours of aggressive CPT with questionable improvement.

   Background: Patient has a 22-year history of CF. He is currently on the lung transplant list. He has a history of adhering to his CPT and medication regimen.

   Assessment: Bilateral crackles and other adventitious lung sounds in both lower lobes, diminished sound in right middle lobe. This morning's X-ray showed bilateral lower lobe pneumonia and expanding lobar collapse of his right middle lobe. Temperature 40°C, pulse 100, BP 130/80 mm/Hg, respiratory rate 34 breaths/min, SaO_2 85% on oxygen at 2 L/min via nasal cannula.

   Recommendation: Immediate renewed pulmonary consultation and interprofessional collaboration required.

Review Questions

1. 1, 3, 4, 5 Rationale: Coordinating therapy around meals and activities reduces the risk for aspiration, conflict with other therapies, or fatigue. In addition, adequate fluid intake may help to liquefy secretions so the patient can easily clear the secretions. As always, informing patients of any therapy helps promote cooperation and decreases anxiety. Selection of lung regions for CPT is made on the basis of patient assessment.

2. Correct order: 5, 1, 2, 3, 4, 6 Rationale: Respiratory assessment determines the lung segments requiring PD. Baseline vital signs and oximeter provide information regarding patient tolerance of the procedure. Proper positioning and drainage techniques are needed to clear selected lung segments and airways. It is important to have the patient in the correct position before initiating therapy. Providing rest periods helps the patient tolerate the complete procedure.

3. 3 Rationale: A current assessment of the patient is a priority before decisions regarding treatment can be made. There can be a number of causes for the dyspnea and bleeding. The health care provider should be notified quickly but will expect current patient information to be available. The nurse can also ask someone to notify the health care provider while assessing the patient.

CHAPTER 25
Clinical Debrief

1. The nurse should perform oropharyngeal suctioning and assess the patient for signs of aspiration. The nurse should be prepared to administer oxygen, if not already on the patient, and to notify the health care provider if there are no signs of improvement. The nurse also needs to explain what they are doing to the patient and caregiver, if present, and should be prepared for nasotracheal suctioning.

2. Situation: The patient has pulse oximetry of 82% on 10 L nonrebreather and oral secretions he cannot control.

   Background: The patient is a 65-year-old male who had a severe stroke 2 days ago. He cannot communicate verbally. Found patient in his room a few moments ago and noticed cyanotic oral mucous membranes, pulse oximeter reading of 78%, and a large amount of oral

secretions. The patient was gasping for air and was tachypneic. Performed oropharyngeal and nasotracheal suctioning.

   Assessment: Patient continued to gasp for air, and the pulse oximeter improved only to 82%, even with the addition of 10 L oxygen via nonrebreather face mask. He is having difficulty controlling his secretions and maintaining his airway and acceptable pulse oximeter levels.

   Recommendation: Come to patient bedside and insert an artificial airway such as an endotracheal tube.

3. Change tracheostomy ties, checking cuff pressures (to prevent complications such as tracheal erosion or tracheal esophageal fistula, prevent aspiration of gastrointestinal contents), change and clean inner cannulas (to prevent obstruction and infection), know what to do in case of dislodgement or obstruction (change tracheostomy tube, suction, bag-valve-mask, as indicated).

Review Questions

1. 2, 3, 5 Rationale: Exhaled tidal volume decreases when there is a need for suctioning. Peak inspiratory pressures increases with the presence of secretions. Patients who can speak or make vocal noises around the ET are demonstrating evidence of either an air leak in the cuff or displacement or incidental extubation of the ET.

2. 2, 4, 5 Rationale: TT should only be suctioned when parameters are met, such as when secretions are noted, and not on a set schedule. The holder should not be tight against the skin, or there will be an increased risk of skin breakdown. There should be space for one loose or two snug finger widths under the neck strap. The cuff pressure of the TT and its site should be assessed and cared for a minimum of every 8 hours and as needed. Nondisposable cannulas are rinsed with sterile saline to be cleaned. Refer to Skills 25.4 and 25.5 for further clarification.

3. 2, 1, 5, 4, 3 Rationale: Assess for the need for suctioning; hyperoxygenate the patient; insert catheter into endotracheal or tracheostomy tube; withdraw catheter while applying suction; perform oropharyngeal suctioning.

CHAPTER 26
Clinical Debrief

1. The primary physical concern for this patient is myocardial ischemia. Further assessments should include updated vital signs, cardiovascular assessment, respiratory assessment, and an in-depth symptoms analysis (e.g. PQRST, COLDSPA).

2. Based on the patient's signs and symptoms, as well as the current telemetry rhythm (sinus tachycardia), anticipated prescriptions include a STAT electrocardiogram (ECG) reading with immediate interpretation by the health care provider, nitroglycerin (sublingual), oxygen 2–3 L/min via nasal prongs, and cardiac enzymes by bloodwork.

3. Situation: The patient is postoperative day 2 after colectomy. She now is experiencing a new onset of chest pain, nausea, and shortness of breath.

   Background: She has a history of MI and has two stents in place.

   Assessment: Bilateral crackles in both lower lobes. BP 100/50 mm Hg; pulse 150 beats/min; respiratory rate 28 breaths/min; SpO_2 90% on room air; temp 37.5°C (99.5°F); apical pulse regular.

   Recommendation: Immediate evaluation by a health care provider, STAT 12-lead ECG, continue with telemetry monitoring, treatment of nausea and chest pain.

Review Questions

1. 3, 5, 6 Rationale: Use soap and water to clean the area and then wipe it dry. Do not use alcohol because it will dry the skin and not allow for good electrical conduction. Other recommendations are to change electrodes at least every day and as needed. Maintain correct placement of the electrodes on the chest for ECG accuracy. Inspect them to ensure that they are securely in place. Ensure the patient's cellular phone is off as that may cause artifacts on the ECG.

2. 1, 2, 3, 5, 6 Rationale: All are possible indications for a 12-lead ECG, except for shortness of breath.

3. 1d, 2f, 3e, 4a, 5c, 6b Rationale: Correct placement of the precordial leads is crucial to fully evaluate electrical cardiac activity and correctly interpret the findings.

CHAPTER 27
Clinical Debrief

1. Vital signs document the patient's cardiopulmonary status and are used to identify any early changes. Some bleeding is expected after cardiac surgery. Drainage of blood and surgical fluids from the chest tubes should decline over the first 3 hours after surgery to less than 100 mL/hr. Patient coughing and position changes can lead to temporary increases in drainage. Excessive bloody drainage (over 200 mL/hour) may indicate unresolved bleeding. This should be reported to the health care provider immediately. Sudden cessation of bleeding may suggest chest tube occlusion and with it the risk of accumulating a hemothorax. When the chest tubes are first connected to drainage, an air leak may be present in the first hour as the lungs re-expand in the chest cavity. After the first hour, an air leak can indicate a problem at the insertion site, at the connection between the tube and the drainage device, or within the drainage device itself.

2. This sudden drainage is probably related to the position change that allowed a pocket of fluid to drain. The fluid is dark red because it is probably old blood from a pocket in the chest cavity that was not close to an eyelet on the chest tube. In most cases this is a normal finding. The nurse should continue to monitor him by taking his vital signs and assessing his cardiopulmonary status. The nurse should report any sudden increase in chest tube drainage to the interprofessional team. The nurse needs to continue to monitor his chest tube drainage to be sure that the volume does not increase excessively.

3. Situation: Patient had 50 mL of dark red fluid drain from his chest tubes after he was transferred from bed to chair.

   Background: Patient had open-heart surgery 12 hours ago. He has right pleural and mediastinal chest tubes. This is his first time out of bed after surgery.

   Assessment: He had a stable 12-hour postoperative period. He is off the ventilator. He is breathing comfortably at 16 breaths/min with SpO_2 96%. His BP is 110/64 mm Hg; pulse 86 beats/min. Chest tube output is normal postoperative drainage and is related to his position change.

   Recommendation: Continue to monitor chest tube output. Use interprofessional collaboration for plans about how long he will need to keep the chest tube.

Review Questions

1. 1, 4 Rationale: Monitoring chest tube drainage and maintaining chest tube patency are the key priorities when a patient has a chest tube.

2. 1, 3, 4, 6 Rationale: These activities are directed by the nurse and can be delegated to a UCP following the nurse's assessment of patient status.

3. 3, 2, 5, 1, 4, 6 Rationale: These represent the correct steps to safely and correctly autoinfuse chest tube drainage.

CHAPTER 28
Clinical Debrief

1. Call for help. The order for basic life support in the first 2 to 3 minutes involves checking responsiveness, which had already been performed; thus, the next step is to call for help.

2. Tell your coworker to apply the AED. Defibrillation should take place as soon as a defibrillator becomes available.

3. Situation: Found her on the bathroom floor unresponsive and pulseless. Started CPR 2 minutes ago. AED shocked ×1.

   Background: 85-year-old female admitted for heart failure

   Assessment: Pulseless

   Recommendation: Interrupt chest compressions briefly to switch chest compressors (no greater than 10 seconds), perform electrocardiograph (ECG) rhythm interpretation, check pulse. Also assign bedside crash cart and recorder nurses.

Review Questions

1. 1, 4 Rationale: No more than 10 seconds of no chest compressions should be allowed for pulse checks, intubation, or any other interventions during a pulseless cardiac arrest. Ensuring that the depth and rate of compressions meet approved guidelines improves outcomes and quality of CPR. The AED does not contribute to quality of compressions.

2. 1, 5, 2, 4, 3 Rationale: The patient's responsiveness and pulse need to be checked before chest compressions begin or the AED is applied. Begin chest compressions and, once the AED is prepared, attach it to the patient. Immediately after the first shock or advised no shock, provide two ventilations and resume 30:2 CPR.

3. 5, 1, 4, 2, 6, 3, 8, 7 Rationale: This order ensures that the provider has determined that the patient is unresponsive, pulseless, and breathless; the steps of applying the external defibrillator (automatic or manual) and initiating a shock ensure proper functioning of the device and safety to all health care providers at the scene. Following delivery of the shock, it is imperative to resume compressions to ensure adequate delivery of oxygen to the organs and tissue.

CHAPTER 29
Clinical Debrief

1. Using the information from her daughter and her past history of heart failure, the nurse would assess clinical markers of vascular and interstitial volume for fluid volume excess. There may be an increase in weight, an increase in urine volume, distended neck veins, adventitious lung sounds on auscultation, and dependent edema from increased fluid volume.

2. The nurse should anticipate orders for a change of IV solutions from a hypertonic solution, because hypertonic solutions can cause increased risk of heart failure and pulmonary edema and a decrease in the infusion flow rate caused by the history of heart failure and the signs and symptoms of fluid overload. To calculate the minute flow rate or the drops per minute, the nurse would use the formula: mL/hr × drop factor/60 min = drops (gtt)/min. To ensure accurate flow rate after calculating the drops per minute, the nurse needs to check that the IV solution container is at least 1 metre (39 inches) above the IV site and regulate the flow rate by counting drops in the drip chamber for 1 minute with a watch and adjusting the roller clamp to increase or decrease rate of infusion. An electronic infusion device would deliver a more accurate rate.

3. Situation: Patient has heart failure and gastric cancer and is receiving IV solutions for dehydration after receiving chemotherapy.

   Background: Patient developed signs and symptoms of fluid overload yesterday. Her IV solutions were changed, and the infusion rate decreased. She received the first of three daily doses of IV push furosemide yesterday. Today she is no longer showing signs and symptoms of fluid overload. Her past 24-hour intake was 1 600 mL, and output 1 700 mL. Serum electrolyte levels drawn this morning were within normal limits.

   Assessment: Today she indicates tenderness at the IV site and presents with temperature 38.2°C (100.8°F), redness, swelling, and purulent drainage at the IV site.

   Recommendation: Immediate interprofessional collaboration to assess the need for continued IV solutions. Remove current IV catheter; culture the drainage at the IV site. Replace short-peripheral IV catheter and lock with normal saline to maintain access for remaining doses of IV furosemide administration.

Review Questions

1. 3, 6, 4, 2, 5, 1 Rationale: Clean technique is used to remove the old dressing from the vascular access device (VAD). A mask is used to prevent transmission or airborne organisms once the catheter insertion site is exposed. Hand hygiene is required between glove changes. The catheter site is cleaned before application of the stabilization device and TSM. The catheter hub is disinfected before applying a new injection cap. The catheter is flushed after dressing change and injection cap change to ensure patency of the catheter.

2. 1, 2, 4, 5. Rationale: Placing the thumb proximal to the insertion site would not allow for adequate stabilization of the vein and could leave the clinician vulnerable to being stuck by the needle. The vein should be stabilized by placing the thumb distal to the insertion site and stretching the skin against the direction of insertion. The tourniquet is released once blood flashback has been observed and the catheter has been advanced into the vein. Waiting to release the tourniquet until the catheter has been secured and the dressing applied would promote backflow of blood that can occlude the catheter if the blood clots.

CHAPTER 30
Clinical Debrief

1. Assessment items would include verifying the prescription from the health care provider, obtaining past transfusion history with allergies and previous transfusion reactions, verifying that a type and cross-match has been performed in the past 72 hours, assessing laboratory values such as hemoglobin (indicates the need for the transfusion) and potassium (caution is needed when infusing an older unit of blood [donated more than 29 days before use] because red blood cells are destroyed over time and release potassium into the plasma), and ensuring that the patient has signed a transfusion consent.

2. The blood should be returned to the blood bank because blood transfusions must be initiated within 30 minutes after release from the laboratory or blood bank.

3. Situation: The patient is receiving a transfusion of PRBCs and is having a transfusion reaction.

   Background: He had surgery yesterday for repair of bleeding hemorrhoids and experienced rectal bleeding after moving his bowels today. His bleeding has stopped since he returned to the unit from the OR.

   Assessment: Patient indicates he is itchy and presents with hives on his trunk and back. His respirations are regular and easy, and his lungs are clear. Vital signs: temp 37°C, pulse 112, respiration 24, BP 126/80. The transfusion has been stopped and normal saline is infusing at a rate to keep vein open (KVO).

   Recommendation: Immediate interprofessional collaboration at bedside with nursing, health care provider(s), and blood bank representative; administer antihistamine; monitor vital signs every 15 minutes for 1 hour; and resume infusion in 1 hour if no fever, dyspnea, or wheezing is present.

Review Questions

1. 2, 3, 5 Rationale: Verification ensures that the correct patient receives the correct blood component and reduces risk for administering wrong product to wrong patient. Blood components should not be infused if the integrity of the bag or component is compromised. Because many transfusion reactions occur within the first 15 minutes of the transfusion, having a baseline at its start and end provides comparison to identify reactions.

2. 2, 4, 1, 6, 5, 3 Rationale: Stopping the infusion immediately prevents any more blood from infusing into the patient. NS keeps the intravenous (IV) line patent and provides access for emergency intervention if needed. Vital signs are taken to notify the health care team and provide comparison if the patient's clinical condition deteriorates rapidly. The health care provider and the blood bank are notified of the transfusion reaction and can provide immediate medical attention. The blood bank follows procedures when notified of a transfusion reaction. Specimens are obtained so the blood can be cross-matched to ensure that the correct blood was given to the recipient and to determine the type of reaction.

3. 1, 2, 5, 6 Rationale: Strict adherence to the verification process reduces the risk for administering blood products to the wrong patient. Using two qualified clinicians enables more consistent identification of errors. Before starting a transfusion, the verification process includes making sure that the patient is the intended recipient, the blood component and blood type match the patient's, and the transfusion record number matches the patient's identification number.

CHAPTER 31
Clinical Debrief

1. The patient's BMI is 19.8 kg/m². Based on the information in Box 31.4, he is within the normal weight range. Because of his dysphagia, he could become undernourished.

2. The daughter can help him swallow more effectively in a number of ways. She can:
   a. Provide mouth care before each meal and afterward (a moist mouth makes it easier to move a bolus of food and swallow, and risk for aspiration pneumonia has been associated with poor oral hygiene).
   b. Not have her father bend his head backward because this can cause food or liquids to enter the airway more easily; instead, teach him to use chin-tuck position.

   c. Coach him during a meal.
   d. Not give him coffee because the liquid is thin and the speech-language pathologist (SLP) recommended medium-viscosity fluids. She could add a thickener to his coffee. In addition, the oatmeal cookies do not fit a mechanically altered diet unless the daughter allows the cookies to soak in milk first.

3. Nursing note: (Date, time). 73-year-old with history of difficulty swallowing and has been placed on a mechanically altered diet. Respirations at baseline 18 breaths per minute. Found coughing and gagging while sitting at dining room table after swallowing moist meat and cooked fruit. Respirations 30 breaths per minute. Unable to express if dyspneic but appears to be gasping for breath. Possible aspiration of food suspected. Feeding has been stopped. Maintained in sitting position. Contacted health care provider for prescription for chest X-ray film and consultation with SLP. K. Weaver, RN

Review Questions

1. 3, 5 Rationale: The skill of assessing a patient's risk for aspiration, determining positioning, and interpreting patient oximetry readings cannot be delegated to a UCP. The UCP may weigh patients and may feed patients after receiving instructions in aspiration precautions.

2. 1, 4 Rationale: Options 2 and 3 should also be performed; however, they are considered assessment activities rather than interventions. Interventions should be instituted on the basis of the assessment findings.

3. Signs of nutritional alteration can include rough, dry, scaly, pale, pigmented, and irritated skin; bruises, and petechiae.

CHAPTER 32
Clinical Debrief

1. 2, 6, 5, 1, 4, 3, 7. See Skill 32.1.

2. 3, 5. Cessation of tube feedings shouldn't occur automatically for gastric residual volumes less than 500 mL in the absence of other signs of intolerance. Volumes between 200 and 500 mL should lead to implementation of measures to reduce the risk of aspiration.

3. Situation: The patient may not be tolerating his tube feeding.

   Background: The patient has recently started on a continuous tube feeding of Isosource HN at 55 mL/hr. Approximately 4 hours ago the GRV was 200 mL.

   Assessment: The patient now reports feeling nauseated. Vomited 60 mL of what appears to be formula. Abdomen is tender to touch and distended, and bowel sounds are decreased. The current GRV is 300 mL. Tube feeding has been temporarily stopped.

   Recommendation: Prescription for radiographic film and confirmation of administration of antiemetic.

Review Questions

1. 4 Rationale: Obtain radiographic confirmation of the correct placement of any blindly inserted tube before its initial use for feeding or medication administration. The most common complication of blindly inserted feeding tubes is improper placement in the esophagus or pulmonary system.

2. 3 Rationale: Use an ENFit connector for all enteral nutrition sets, syringes, and feeding tubes to improve patient safety. The ENFit connector is not compatible with Luer-Lok connections or any other small-bore medical connectors and thus prevents misadministration of an enteral feeding or medication by the wrong route.

3. 1, 3, 4 Rationale: The verification of tube placement is the responsibility of the nurse and cannot be delegated to a UCP. Checking respirations or patient symptoms of shortness of breath, coughing, or choking; performing oral hygiene; and inspecting skin around the insertion site for irritation and excoriation are all things that UCPs can do.

CHAPTER 33
Clinical Debrief

1. Serum glucose levels: Serum glucose levels provide a baseline to document the patient's tolerance of high levels of glucose in the PN solution. Fluid and electrolyte balance: High osmolality of PN solution can alter a patient's fluid balance, leading to fluid overload. Baseline respiratory Assessment: The appearance of crackles is an early indication of fluid

retention. Vital signs: Changes in baseline can indicate a patient's tolerance of fluid, or a fever can indicate infection.

2. Fever can indicate a catheter-related bloodstream infection. The catheter insertion site is a common source of infection.

3. The patient's weight gain could be related to fluid retention. Appropriate assessments are vital signs, auscultation of lung sounds, and assessment for dependent edema.

4. Situation: The patient has gained 2 kg (5 lb) over 24 hours and believes that the PN via central line (CPN) is effective in increasing his weight.

   Background: Patient is a 43-year-old patient with Crohn's disease who lost 4.5 kg (10 lb) in the last 3 weeks and has recurrent abdominal pain, cramping, and loose stools.

   Assessment: Weight gain of 2 kg (5 lb) in 48 hours. Heart rate is 100 beats/min, RR 20 breaths/min with bilateral rales, BP 130/86 mm Hg. Patient does not report any shortness of breath on exertion.

   Recommendation: Reduce rate of CPN and evaluate need for other non-PN intravenous fluids and reassess volume of current PN prescription. Draw electrolyte panel, including blood glucose. Monitor intake and output every 2 hours.

Review Questions

1. 1, 3 Rationale: The fluid for the PPN is hyperosmolar. However, as a nurse you should avoid complex terms when educating patients. The patient can understand an explanation that the smaller veins cannot tolerate the concentration of the nutrients and become irritated easily.

2. 1, 2, 3, 4 Rationale: All but No. 5 can require short-term PPN to support the patient's nutritional needs during recovery.

3. 3, 1, 2 Rationale: These are the three steps for accuracy in administration of CPN.

CHAPTER 34
Clinical Debrief

1. The nurse needs to determine cultural considerations that would be appropriate in caring for this patient. The patient's understanding and knowledge of her condition and treatment plan need to be assessed. Along with reviewing the intake and output record the nurse needs to identify any trends, voiding patterns (e.g., increased incontinence, frequency, urgency), and the last time the patient voided. The patient's ability to participate in the plan of care also needs to be assessed; this includes language, sensory and cognitive issues, and mobility. The nurse should assess the lower one third of the abdomen for distention and/or tenderness, and assess for signs and symptoms of a UTI.

2. An assessment of the PVR urine is very important for this patient. An abnormal PVR urine would indicate inadequate bladder emptying. She has a history of urinary retention plus a number of other conditions that increase her risk for bladder dysfunction and urinary retention, such as stroke, history of UTIs, and type 2 diabetes. Her incontinence needs to be further evaluated, and PVR will determine if this incontinence is caused by an overflow of urine as a result of urinary retention. In addition, if the patient's bladder is emptying, a PVR would help rule out the use of catheterization.

3. The health care provider has prescribed the option to use a bladder scanner or to catheterize the patient. Whenever possible, catheterization should be avoided because of the increased risk for UTI; thus, the use of the bladder scanner would be appropriate. The initial assessment with the bladder scanner will dictate if the nurse needs to insert an in-dwelling catheter (e.g., if the bladder scanner shows a volume greater than 400 mL).

4. The rationale for the procedure should be explained in simple, easy terminology. The nurse needs to explain the procedure, including that the measurement needs to be made within 10 minutes of voiding. The nurse should instruct the patient to void in a measurement container. It is also important to explain that the bladder scanner looks inside the body and measures the volume of urine left in the bladder after voiding and that it does not hurt.

5. Situation: The patient needs an in-dwelling catheter, but the patient's spouse has refused to let anyone except a female family member do the procedure.

Background: The patient is an 80-year-old Inuit woman with a history of a stroke who needs an in-dwelling catheter placed.

Assessment: PVR of 600 mL with an order for in-dwelling catheter placement.

Recommendation: Consult with the health care provider and talk with the spouse about allowing a female congruent care provider place the in-dwelling catheter with a female family member present, if desired.

Review Questions

1. 5, 7, 2, 4, 1, 6, 3, 8, 9 Rationale: See Skill 34-1.

2. 2, 3 Rationale: By allowing the balloon to drain by gravity, the development of creases or ridges in the balloon may be avoided, thus minimizing trauma to the urethra during withdrawal. All patients who have a catheter removed should have their voiding monitored. The best way to do this is with a voiding record or bladder diary. The size syringe used to deflate the balloon is dictated by the size of the balloon. In the adult patient balloon sizes are either 10 mL or 30 mL. Catheters should be pulled out slowly and smoothly. There is no evidence to support clamping catheters before removal.

3. 1, 3, 4 Rationale: A new suprapubic catheter insertion site is a surgical incision and should be treated similarly to other incisions, which includes sterile dressing change and inspection of the site for signs of infection. To minimize trauma and increase comfort, the catheter should be anchored to the abdomen. Wiping the catheter toward the skin violates principles of asepsis. Tension to the catheter should be avoided in all circumstances to minimize discomfort and potential for damage to the bladder wall.

CHAPTER 35
Clinical Debrief

1. The patient is only allowed touch-down weight bearing, and a commode would not be appropriate at this point in his recovery. He can use a standard bedpan because he doesn't have any restrictions to hip joint mobility.

2. The UCP needs to be instructed that the patient should be able to hold the enema solution for a few minutes and to encourage the patient to retain the solution as long as possible. The patient should pass formed stool. The UCP should not flush away contents until the nurse has observed the output. The nurse is responsible for evaluating the outcome of the enema.

3. Situation: Patient had a right total knee replacement 2 days ago for severe osteoarthritis.

   Background: Patient is taking opioids and has not had a regular bowel movement since surgery. On the second postoperative day he attempted a bowel movement with a great deal of straining and expelled a small, brown, hard stool. An enema was administered 2 days ago with small amount of formed, soft stool evacuated. No bowel movements since then.

   Assessment: His abdomen is nontender, slightly distended with active bowel sounds in all four quadrants. He has liquid stool seeping from his rectum.

   Recommendation: Obtain a prescription to check for an impaction. Explain the procedure to the patient. Have UCP assist by monitoring the patient's vital signs and report if his pulse drops below 60 beats/min.

Review Questions

1. 2, 4, 5 Rationale: As comfort measures, the nurse should place a pillow or rolled towel in the curve of the patient's back, allow the patient to wipe themselves, and place the head of the bed between a 30- and 60-degree angle to replicate sitting on the toilet. Excess linens should be removed so they are out of the way but not leave the patient exposed. The patient should bend at the knees (unless contraindicated). The nurse can provide privacy by closing the door or the curtains around the bed and leaving the room (but staying close by). The nurse should give the patient the call bell so they can return when the patient is finished defecating.

2. 1, 3, 5 Rationale: A UCP can administer a tap-water enema, place a patient on the bedpan, and provide oral care. However, because of the potential for a vagus nerve response, the nurse must digitally remove

the fecal impaction. The nurse must also place an NG tube because it requires a nurse to assess the patient before and after the procedure.

3. 5, 2, 1, 4, 6, 7, 3 Rationale: For the safety of the patient, the nurse checks the prescription from the health care provider for insertion of an NG tube, then identifies inserting the tube in the correct patient. Next the nurse measures the distance of the tip of the nose to the xiphoid process. The nurse performs hand hygiene and applies clean gloves because this is not a sterile procedure. Passing the tube along the floor of the nasal passage minimizes discomfort. With the patient's head flexed forward, the nurse continues to insert the tube to the length measured. The tube is then taped to the nose to prevent dislodging.

CHAPTER 36
Clinical Debrief

1. Preoperative stoma-site marking will provide the best location for the stoma based on the patient's body habitus, clothing preferences, and activities. A well-placed stoma will facilitate adjustment to the ostomy and successful pouching after surgery. Education about emptying and changing her pouch will be helpful because these are the things she must learn before she leaves the hospital. With shortened hospital stays, the time for education after surgery is limited.

2. Situation: Patient has been admitted to the nursing unit after surgery for a laparoscopic colectomy, ileoanal anastomosis with J-pouch formation, and a temporary ileostomy. She is drowsy but alert and oriented.

   Background: She has a 10-year history of ulcerative colitis, which has become increasingly symptomatic with bleeding and diarrhea and is not responding to medical management.

   Assessment: Abdomen is distended and firm; laparoscopic port sites are dry and intact. Ostomy pouch over her stoma is intact with no drainage noted in the pouch. Her stoma is red, round, and budded.

   Recommendation: Continued assessments at intervals per surgical unit routine; consultation to ostomy nurse for teaching about ostomy care; encourage patient to observe when pouch is filling and needs to be emptied.

3. The volume in the pouch determines when it should be emptied; overfilling could cause the pouch to pull away from the skin and leak. It should be emptied when it is too full or when it is filled with gas (flatus). A pouch should be changed on a schedule that is acceptable to the patient and allows for a predictable and reliable wear time. Change frequency is usually between 3 and 7 days.

Review Questions

1. 2, 3, 4 Rationale: Little urine is stored in the conduit; therefore, it may be necessary to insert the catheter further to reach it or change the patient's position to facilitate flow through the catheter. Urine in the pouch will have bacteria in it and would be inappropriate for a culture. A larger catheter will not stimulate the flow of urine.

2. 2, 3, 5 Rationale: A visit with an ostomy care nurse may be helpful at this time to review the patient's self-care routine and assess for other possible causes of skin breakdown. It is likely that the opening in the pouch may be too big after the stoma has decreased in size and the patient has not cut a new pattern to accommodate this change. Applying alcohol to raw skin will burn, and a pouch applied over moist raw skin will not adhere and will cause more leakage and skin damage to occur. Neither of these will address the underlying problem.

3. 5, 8, 7, 2, 6, 3, 4, 1 Rationale: It is necessary to remove the pouch and assess and measure the stoma before cutting out the pouch and placing it on the patient. Closing the pouch is the essential final step in replacing the pouch.

CHAPTER 37
Clinical Debrief

1. Obesity, diabetes mellitus, and smoking place this patient at risk for surgical site infection (SSI). Good control of diabetes mellitus will decrease her risk, as will cessation of smoking. The patient will need to be reminded that she will not be allowed to smoke in the hospital and she may be more comfortable if she is prescribed a nicotine-product substitute. Given her history of smoking, she is also at risk for postoperative pulmonary complications. Careful lung assessment will be required. Her history of obesity, birth control pills, and pelvic surgery place her at risk for venous thromboembolism (VTE), deep vein thrombosis (DVT), and pulmonary embolism (PE). She needs to be encouraged to get out of bed and ambulate, do her exercises, and wear a lower-extremity sequential compression device while in bed or sitting in a chair.

2. This patient should be taught how to do postoperative exercises, turn, cough, deep breathe, and use the incentive spirometer. She should receive instruction in pain-control measures, including how to use the patient-controlled analgesia (PCA) device and how to splint her incision with a small pillow before coughing, turning, or ambulating. Early ambulation and the need to wear lower-extremity bilateral sequential compression devices while in bed or in a chair should also be part of this patient's teaching. The nurse should include in the teaching whoever will be the caregiver and reinforce that, for safety reasons, the patient should be the only person to activate the PCA device.

3. Situation: Patient is anxious and short of breath.

   Background: She is a 52-year-old female who is postoperative day 2 following an abdominal hysterectomy for fibroid tumours and a bladder neck suspension. She has a history of smoking and birth control pills.

   Assessment: The patient has diminished lung sounds on the left when compared to the right; this is a new finding. She has an SpO_2 of 82%, and her left leg is swollen and painful.

   Recommendation: Place patient on oxygen to maintain SpO_2 >95%. Call respiratory therapy if pulse oxygenation does not improve. Stat chest X-ray film, and venous ultrasound.

Review Questions

1. 1, 2, 4, 5 Rationale: Hair should be removed using clippers so that the skin remains intact, thus reducing the chance of SSI. All other statements are true.

2. 2, 5 Rationale: Sequential compression devices are applied before surgery. With the patient immobilized and not walking, there is venous pooling (venous stasis). This puts the patient at risk for deep vein thrombosis (DVT) and pulmonary embolism. The compression devices squeeze the veins in the legs, forcing the blood up through the vena cava and preventing venous pooling and stasis. Less pooling and stasis of venous blood means less clotting and thus a decreased incidence of DVT. Preoperative teaching and return demonstration of leg exercises promote postoperative compliance.

3. 3, 4 Rationale: Management of postoperative care, assessment skills, and adjusting the IV pump should be performed by the nurse and not delegated to a UCP.

CHAPTER 38
Clinical Debrief

1. See Evidence-Informed Practice section. The patient is at risk for hypothermia because she is an older person with low body weight and has a metabolic disorder. The interprofessional surgical team should communicate and document a plan for intraoperative warming to avoid complications. All should also pay close attention to her positioning, to decrease the incidence of pressure areas.

2. See Evidence-Informed Practice section. Hypothermia can put the patient at additional risk for surgical site infection, cardiac arrhythmias, changes in medication metabolism, and increased incidence of surgical bleeding.

3. Monitor intraoperative body temperature closely. Consider using warming devices. Avoid cold irrigation solutions in the body cavity and infusion of cold solutions such as intravenous fluid and blood.

4. The SBAR should be addressed to both the surgical and anaesthesiology teams.

   Situation: Patient has not received prescribed cefazolin 1 g IV antibiotic that is to be infused within 60 minutes of time of incision. In addition, antibiotic was not sent with patient on transfer to the operating room.

   Background: Patient is 82 years old and is here in the operating room for exploratory laparotomy and lysis of adhesions.

   Assessment: The antibiotic is important for prophylactic infection control and should be administered as ordered.

Recommendation: Medical-surgical unit called to see if they can locate and send antibiotic as soon as possible. If we cannot locate antibiotic quickly, I will call pharmacy to get a stat dose. We also need to be aware of the time to correlate antibiotic administration with incisional time.

Review Questions

1. 4, 1, 5, 2, 3 Rationale: See Skill 38.1, Implementation Step 2 "Perform prescrub wash at beginning of shift." A prescrub is used to remove gross debris and superficial organisms and must be completed before performing surgical antisepsis.

2. 1, 2, 4, 5 Rationale: See Box 38.3. The circulating room nurse uses the nursing process in plan of care and is responsible for maintaining patient safety and continuity of care throughout the perioperative period. This includes conducting perioperative assessment, reviewing records for accuracy and completeness, and participating in "time-out." The circulating nurse is the member of the team who is not sterile; thus, a surgical scrub and gowning and gloving are not part of the role.

3. 1, 2, 3, 4 Rationale: See Box 38.4. Torn or contaminated gloves must be removed immediately, if possible, by the nonsterile member of the team. Regloving should be done by a sterile member of the team. The gown must not be touched while removing or changing gloves and the gown cuff should remain at the wrist level. If the glove cannot be removed immediately, a sterile glove should be donned over the contaminated or damaged glove until it can be changed.

CHAPTER 39
Clinical Debrief

1. Because the patient's wound is open and will not be resutured, this wound is healing by secondary intention and will require a moist saline gauze dressing to support healing.

2. The first option is to cleanse the wound using a syringe irrigation method. Use a syringe tip of 2.5 cm (1 inch) with a 19-gauge angiocatheter held above the upper end of the wound and over the area being cleaned. Use the amount and type of irrigant ordered. The second option is to consider teaching the patient to irrigate the wound in the shower if she goes home with this wound (if she has a shower head that she can use at home). The patient sits on the shower chair holding the shower head about 30 cm (12 inches) from her wound, using warm water.

3. Situation: Patient returns to wound clinic 1 week after discharge for follow-up of open granulating wound. Patient reports increased wound tenderness and yellow discharge.

   Background: Patient was discharged with an open wound and instructed to use twice-daily irrigation and to apply a saline-moistened nonadherent gauze wound dressing.

   Assessment: Wound assessment reveals yellow, foul-smelling, purulent drainage and red wound edges. Area is tender to palpation. Patient is febrile with a temperature of 38.7°C (101.6°F).

   Recommendation: Contact health care provider if still under their care to order a wound culture. Use best practice to obtain wound culture (cleanest part of the wound). Follow prescriptions related to appropriate systemic antibiotic. For draining an infected wound, use a hypertonic sodium dressing (e.g., Mesalt) applied dry to the wound bed and covered with absorbent dressing. Irrigate with normal saline and change dressing daily. Observe for effect of antibiotic. Inform patient and caregiver to watch for signs and symptoms of persistent infection. Follow up in wound clinic in 1 week.

Review Questions

1. 1, 3, 6 Rationale: The nurse wants to know if the patient is febrile or has other signs of possible infection, such as increased heart rate or respiratory rate; therefore, the nurse should obtain a current set of vital signs. The nurse should also review previous assessments of the wound to compare with the current status. While the nurse would contact the health care provider or surgeon, the nurse would first examine the wound. The dressings should be removed and assessed for quality and quantity of wound drainage, because a sudden increase in drainage, along with odour or drainage other than serous drainage, may indicate a change in wound status. The wound bed should be examined for red, moist granulation tissue with drainage that is serous; excessive drainage with a change in color of wound tissue can also indicate a negative change in wound status. Examination of the periwound skin will provide the nurse with details about possible impending wound infection, especially if the area around the wound is warm to the touch, possibly indicating cellulitis. If the patient is allowed to ambulate with a moist, dripping wound, the wound dressing may become dislodged and fall out of the wound, allowing wound drainage outside the wound.

2. 2, 4, 1, 6, 3, 5 Rationale: Explain to the patient how you will remove the staples. Start by assessing the patient's comfort level. Then inspect the incision for a healing ridge and skin integrity. Clean the area next to the incision to decrease surface bacteria and clean over the staples. Gently slide the extractor under one staple, depress the handles of the extractor, and lift the staple. Continue until all are removed.

3. 3, 5 Rationale: An amount of 60 mL bright red blood so soon after surgery may indicate bleeding from or around the surgical site, and this finding should be reported to the surgeon. Empty the bulb to determine if the drainage continues. To prevent accumulation of excess drainage, empty the drain before it is full. There is no reason to shake the bulb; it will drain more efficiently if it is placed below the exit of the drain.

CHAPTER 40
Clinical Debrief

1. An absorptive dressing such as hydrofibre or calcium alginate would be appropriate since there is drainage. Given the patient's temperature and erythema (plus drainage at the wound site), a more appropriate dressing might be hypertonic sodium solution (e.g., Mesalt), which would be changed daily. The hydrofibre or calcium alginate would be changed when saturated (initially, likely daily). Infected wounds would benefit from dressings containing silver (Ag).

2. The nurse would apply a pressure bandage to the wound. A pressure bandage is a temporary treatment to control excessive, sudden, unanticipated bleeding. Hemorrhage may occur during surgical intervention (e.g., cardiac catheterization, arterial puncture, organ biopsy) or after surgery, or it may be a life-threatening occurrence related to accidental trauma (e.g., stabbing, suicide attempt). Pressure dressings are essential to stopping the flow of blood and promoting clotting at the site until definitive action can be taken to stop the source. Once the dressing has been applied, the surgical team is notified immediately of these findings.

3. Situation: Patient is postoperative day 3 status postexploratory laparotomy with total gastrectomy and now has a surgical site infection.

   Background: He is a 75-year-old male with a history of gastric cancer followed by surgery 3 days ago. On postoperative day 1 he had a fever that spiked at 38.5°C (101.3°F) and he had purulent drainage and erythema around his incision. The incision was partially opened and packed at bedside.

   Assessment: The superior aspect of the incision is open with purulent drainage and mild surrounding erythema on the skin. The patient rates his pain a 6 out of 10 and he has not received any pain medication in the past 4 hours. Temp is 38.5°C (101.3°F), BP 130/80, pulse 95, RR 20, SaO₂ 96%.

   Recommendation: Provide pain medication. Clean wound with normal saline (NS); irrigate (provided base of the wound is visible and irrigant will flow out of wound without pooling). Lightly pack wound with Mesalt (hypertonic sodium) or AMD gauze, or hydrofibre/calcium alginate with silver (Ag). Cover with absorbent pad (e.g., Mesorb). Reassess pain level in 30 minutes. Change dressing daily (Mesalt) or as required, based on level of saturation.

Review Questions

1. 1. Rationale: A nonadherent gauze dressing (with gentle adhesive border) will allow moisture-vapour transfer. Transparent film dressings are occlusive and if exudate is present, the wound and periwound skin can become macerated. They are also challenging to remove from fragile skin (of older persons). Hydrocolloid dressings are designed for autolytic debridement and are occlusive. Calcium alginate dressings absorb drainage but are designed for wounds with moderate to significant drainage.

Hydrogel dressings donate moisture to the wound bed, but in an uncomplicated healing wound, this is not usually required.

2. Serous (4)
   Serosanguineous (3)
   Sanguineous (2)
   Purulent (1)

3. 1, 2, 4, 5 Rationale: Assessing pain level serves as a baseline to measure the response to dressing therapy. Assessing size, location, and condition of the wound helps in planning for the proper dressing type and supplies needed. Patients with allergies may have an allergic reaction to these supplies. Explaining the procedure to the patient helps promote cooperation and decreases anxiety.

CHAPTER 41
Clinical Debrief

1. 1, 3, 4, 2. Before initiating this or any therapy, the nurse should verify the health care provider's prescription. Then the patient's current level of pain should be assessed with an acceptable pain assessment tool (see employer policy). If the patient reports increased pain, it might be necessary to administer analgesia 20 to 30 minutes before the treatment. A surgical wound is associated with knee replacement; therefore, it is important to assess the site, noting any excessive or new redness, drainage, odour, or swelling. Finally, explaining the procedure reinforces the purpose and principles of the therapy. In addition, it is also part of an educational process to teach the patient how to self-administer this cold therapy following discharge to home.

2. The patient has some decreased peripheral circulation related to diabetes. Therefore, he is at risk for decreased tissue perfusion related to the cold application and his decreased peripheral circulation. Because of these factors, the following assessments are crucial to prevent skin and tissue injury resulting from application of cold: Observe area for pallor and diminished pulses; observe distal regions of the patient's leg for warmth, colour, distal pulses; and ask the patient about any changes in sensation (e.g., increased numbing, lack of sensation, pain).

3. Situation: Patient is postoperative 24 hours for left-knee arthroscopy and is receiving cold compression therapy. Patient indicates that he had a burning sensation under the cold compression cuff.
   Background: Patient is a 58-year-old male with diabetes mellitus who is postoperative day 1 for total left knee arthroplasty. He has had diabetes mellitus type 1 since childhood that is regulated with insulin.
   Assessment: Reddened 2-cm area under cold compression cuff. Blister is present, site is tender to touch. Left leg is warm; normal colour and pulses are present distal to the cuff area. Patient does not report any increase in incisional pain or pain related to arthroscopy. Incision is clean, without redness or drainage.
   Recommendation: Initiate skin care routine to clean 2-cm area. Increase skin assessments to every 30 minutes for affected areas. Remove compression cuff when not in use.

Review Questions

1. 1, 4, 5, 6 Rationale: Heat is applied to a musculoskeletal injury 72 hours after the acute phase. People with peripheral vascular diseases have decreased circulation to a region, and that region has a greater risk of injury from heat application. When applied to skin lesions, heat irritates the lesion, causing increased itching, redness, or burning. Finally, a patient with altered sensation to a body region cannot perceive if a heat application is too hot and therefore will not move from it.

2. 2, 1, 5, 4, 3 Rationale: Cooling devices are used for analgesia to help determine the effectiveness of therapy. Assessment of a patient's level of pain before application is important. Placing the cooling device in a pillowcase or wrapping it in a towel before the procedure ensures that the cooling device will not be in direct contact with patient's skin, which could cause skin and tissue injury. Application of the device to the shoulder provides a visual assessment that the cooling will be delivered to the area of injury. Before securing the device to the patient's shoulder, the nurse must verify the correct temperature.

3. 1, 3 Rationale: *Increased temperature* will increase the patient's oxygen consumption and metabolic demand. If left untreated, increased fever can cause shivering.

CHAPTER 42
Clinical Debrief

1. Skill 42.2 is focused on adapting the home environment. Assessment of the home environment is the first priority; the nurse needs to interview the patient and observe the environment. The immediate concerns for making adaptations include the patient's impaired mobility and depression and the sister's sensory disturbances. Adaptations to prepare the lower level of the home might include the following: removing barriers to mobility (e.g., throw rugs, unnecessary furniture); being sure that there is adequate lighting where the caregiver prepares medications (the caregiver must be able to read labels on the containers); providing chairs in which the patient can sit and from which she can exit; and adapting one room for the caregiver to safely bathe the patient. The nurse will focus on making changes with the patient's input and agreement. The nurse must also consider the sister's needs and the stress this living situation is placing on both parties.

2. A home safety checklist is essential (see Skill 42.1). In addition, the nurse can use tests such as the Short Geriatric Depression Scale (SGDS) and the Mini-Mental State Examination (MMSE) (see Skill 42.2) to evaluate her for depression and mental state.

3. Situation: Patient is a new resident of the assisted-living facility. She previously lived in a single-family home for over 50 years.
   Background: She has a history of metastatic bone cancer and was recently diagnosed with heart failure. She can no longer drive and has limited mobility; she cannot climb stairs. She had begun to show signs of depression when she lived at home with her sister. Her sister recently passed away, causing her to be moved out of her home and into the assisted-living facility.
   Assessment: She is sitting in her bedroom and states she is "very sad." Her skin is pale and dry. She is oriented to person but disoriented to time and place. She continues to ask when she can return to her home. Her vital signs are within normal ranges; however, she appears to be lethargic.
   Recommendation: Immediately inform the health care team of her remark about being "very sad." She was found to be depressed before her sister's death, and there is concern that her depression has worsened. A thorough mental state evaluation is indicated to determine orientation and level of depression.

Review Questions

1. 1, 2, 3, 4, 6 Rationale: All of these topics would be covered to determine the physical and mental status of the patient and to check that the patient is not experiencing abuse or neglect. (Skill 42.2 contains a discussion of wandering and patients with cognitive impairments.)

2. 4, 5 Rationale: Insulin and other medications need to be kept secured, away from children. Insulin may be stored in the refrigerator away from food; the freezer temperature is too low. Storing supplies in an airtight container is appropriate, and the daughter (or other caregiver) can prefill syringes for the patient. (See Skill 42.3 for an extensive discussion of medication and supplies for the patient with diabetes mellitus.)

3. 2, 4, 5 Rationale: Handrails are ideally placed on both sides of the staircase; however, one side is acceptable. Outdoor steps should not blend in with walkways; there should be reflective taping to highlight the steps. Slip-resistant mats are acceptable. Taking pain medication that can alter orientation and a history of falls are risk factors for falling.

CHAPTER 43
Clinical Debrief

1. It is recommended that a home assessment be completed before initiation of oxygen therapy. Information about functioning smoke alarms, usable fire extinguishers, oxygen-in-use signs, oxygen storage plan, and a fire evacuation route should be confirmed before initiating home oxygen. Confirmation that the local emergency medical services (EMS) and fire company were notified is also crucial information.

2. The nurse should help the patient and caregiver move the oxygen cylinders to a well-ventilated area away from heat sources and review with them the potential dangers of storing oxygen cylinders in a non-ventilated closet. The nurse can use teach-back to determine their level of understanding about safe storage of oxygen.

3. The nurse needs to implement a no-smoking contract with the son. The nurse should explain to the wife and son the dangers of smoking in the home even if the oxygen is turned off. The nurse can use teach-back to determine the level of understanding about the dangers of smoking with oxygen therapy. The health care provider should be notified of the nurse's findings and implementation of a no-smoking contract.

Review Questions

1. 3, 4, 5 Rationale: Assessments occur before the teaching session. The nurse must assess the patient's knowledge of medication therapy, learning readiness and ability to concentrate, and beliefs about medication therapy. The purpose of regularly scheduled medication and explanation of dosage schedule are facts taught during the actual teaching session.

2. 2, 5 Rationale: Involving the patient in the decision-making process demonstrates person-centred care and encourages medication adherence. A patient who takes medications independently is more likely to adhere to the medication therapy. When teaching older persons, the nurse should provide frequent, short teaching sessions using 14-point font or greater for written material. Distractions such as visitors should be minimized during teaching sessions.

3. 1, 3, 4, 5 Rationale: Hand hygiene is performed before initiating enteral feedings. Tube placement is a critical step to prevent complications such as aspiration. A feeding schedule should be used to maintain nutrition requirements of the patient. Teach-back determines the patient or caregiver's level of understanding of potential enteral feeding complications. The head of the bed is elevated 30 to 45 degrees while receiving feedings.

Appendix A

TERMINOLOGY/COMBINING FORMS: PREFIXES AND SUFFIXES

Medical terminology is similar to a foreign language. Many medical terms are derived from Latin and Greek sources. They often consist of two or more simple words or word elements. A word root or *combining form* may be put together with a *prefix* and a *suffix*.

Root—the basis of a word
    Example: *nephr/o/tic* (degenerative changes in the kidney)
    Root: nephr- (kidney)

Linking vowel—a vowel that joins the combining form to the suffix or another combining form
    Example: nephr/*o*/sis (disease of the kidneys)
    Linking vowel: o

Prefix—the beginning of a word
    Example: *hyper*/active (excessively active)
    Prefix: hyper- (excessive)

Suffix—the ending of a word
    Example: nephr/*itis* (inflammation of the kidney)
    Suffix: -itis (inflammation)

Combining form—the union of a word root with a linking vowel
    Example: *hepato*/megaly (enlargement of the liver)
    Combining form: hepato- (liver)

The following table provides some of the most commonly used terminology for your reference.

COMMON PREFIXES

Prefix	Definition
a-	without
ab-	away from
abd-	abdominal
acu-	sharp
ad-	toward
adip-	fat
ad lib-	freely, as wanted
aero-	air, gas
al-	toward
ambi-	both
an-	not
ana-	up
ante-	before, in front of
anti-	against
arteri-	artery
arthro-	joint
auto-	self
bi-	two
brady-	slow
cata-	down
chole-	bile

Prefix	Definition
cili-	eyelid
circum-	around
co-	with, together
cogni-	know
colo-	colon
con-	with, together
contra-	against
crani-	skull
cut-	skin
cyt-	cell
de-	from, lack of
demi-	half
dent-	tooth
derm-	skin
dia-	through, across
diplo-	double, twofold
dis-	to free or undo
dors-	back
dur-	hard
dy-	two
dys-	bad, painful, difficult, abnormal
ec-	out, out from
ecto-	outside
em-	in
embol-	to insert
encephalo-	brain
endo-	in, within
entero-	intestine
epi-	above, on
erythro-	red
eso-	within, inward
et-	and
eu-	good, normal
ex-	out, away from
exo-	outside
extra-	outside
faci-	face
fiss-	split, cleft
fore-	before, in front of
gastro-	stomach
glosso-	relating to the tongue
glyco-	sugar
haplo-	simple, single
heme-	iron-based
hemi-	one half
hepat-	liver
hetero-	different
histo-	tissue

Prefix	Definition
homo-	same
hydro-	wet, water
hyper-	excessive, above normal
hypo-	under, below
im-	not
in-	in, not
infra-	under, below
inter-	between
intra-	in, within
isch-	deficiency
iso-	equal, alike
lapis-	stone
lapra-	loin or flank, sometimes abdomen
latero-	side
macro-	large
mal-	bad
meato-	opening
medi-	middle
melano-	black
mesa-	middle
meso-	middle
meta-	beyond, change
micro-	small
mono-	one
morpho-	form, structure
multi-	many, much
neo-	new
nephro-	kidney
oculo-	eye
onco-	tumour
oro-	mouth
osteo-	bone
pan-	all
para-	beside, beyond
per-	through, by
peri-	around
phago-	eating
poly-	many, much
post-	after, behind
pre-	before, in front of
primi-	first
pro-	before, in front of
pseudo-	false
quadri-	four
re-	again, backward
retro-	backward, behind
rhabdo-	rod-shaped, striated
rhodo-	red
scler-	hardening
semi-	one half
stetho-	chest
sub-	under, below
super-	above, excessive
supra-	above, excessive
sym-	together
syn-	union, together, joined
tachy-	rapid
tetra-	four
therm-	heat
trans-	through, across
tri-	three

Prefix	Definition
ultra-	beyond, excess
uni-	one
vas-	vessel or duct
xantho-	yellow
xero-	dry

COMMON SUFFIXES

Suffix	Definition
-ac	pertaining to
-agra	excessive pain
-al	pertaining to
-algia	painful condition, pain
-apheresis	removal
-ar	pertaining to
-ary	pertaining to
-ase	enzyme
-bi	two, double
-blast	developing cell
-cele	hernia, swelling, sac
-centesis	puncture of a cavity
-clasis	break, fracture
-clysis	irrigation, washing
-coccus	berry shaped
-crit	to separate
-cyte	cell
-desis	fusion, binding, fixation
-drome	to run
-dynia	pain
-ectasis	expansion, dilation
-ectomy	excision, removal of a body part
-emesis	vomiting
-emia	blood
-er	one who
-gen	forming, producing, origin
-genesis	forming, producing, origin
-genic	origin, formation
-grade	to go
-gram	the record made, mark
-graph	instrument for recording, machine
-graphy	the process, process of recording
-ia	condition
-iasis	morbid condition
-iatry	treatment, medicine
-ic/-ical	pertaining to
-icle	small, minute
-ism	condition
-ist	one who specializes in, specialist
-itis	inflammation
-lith	stone, calculus
-logist	specialist in the study of
-logy	process of study
-lysis	dissolution, setting free
-malacia	softening, soft
-megaly	enlargement
-meter	instrument for measuring
-metry	act of measuring
-odynia	pain
-oid	form, shape
-ole	small, minute
-ology	study or science of

Suffix	Definition	Suffix	Definition
-oma	tumour	-rrhaphy	suturing in place
-opsy	to view	-rrhea	flow, discharge
-or	one who	-rrhexis	rupture
-orrhea	flow, discharge	-scope	instrument to visually examine
-osis	condition or state	-scopy	process of examining, visual examination
-ous	pertaining to		
-para	to bear (offspring)	-sepsis	infection
-paresis	partial paralysis	-sis	state of, condition
-pathy	disease, suffering	-spasm	involuntary spasm
-penia	deficiency, lack of, decrease	-stalsis	constriction
-pexy	fixation	-stasis	control, constant level, stop
-phagia	eating, swallowing	-stenosis	narrowing, stricture
-phasia	speech	-stomy	creation of an opening
-philia	attraction for	-therapy	treatment
-phobia	fear	-tic	pertaining to
-physis	to grow	-tome	instrument for cutting
-plasia	formation, growth	-tomy	process of cutting, incision
-plasm	growth, formation	-toxic	poison
-plasty	mold, shape, repair	-tresia	opening
-plegia	paralysis	-tripsy	surgical crushing
-poiesis	formation, production	-trophy	nourishment
-ptosis	downward displacement, falling	-ula	small, minute
-ptysis	spitting	-ule	small, minute
-rrhage	bursting forth, rupture	-y	process

Index

A

Abbreviations
  in documentation, 55–56, 56b
  official "do not use", 56b
Abdomen
  concave, 185
  flat, 185
  landmarks in, 184
  quadrants of, 185f
  round, 185
Abdominal assessment, 181–188
  anatomy, 182f
  in children, 188
  communication and documentation in, 188
  delegation and collaboration in, 183
  equipment for, 183
  in older persons, 188
Abdominal binder, 1104b–1105b, 1104f
Abdominal distention, 185
Abdominal girth, 185, 185f
Abdominal pain, 181, 182t–183t
Abdominal paracentesis, 269
Abducens nerve, 198
ABO incompatibility, 833
ABO system, 832–833, 833t
Abrasion, 466t–467t, 467f
Absorption, 528–529, 530t
Abstract, of clinical article, 7
Abuse, assessment of, 152
Acapella device, 696, 696f
Acid burns, of eye, 513
Acid mantle, 1035
Acne, 466f, 466t–467t
Acoustic stethoscope, 119f
Action cycle, in knowledge-to-action
  framework, 8–9
Active motion, 196
Activities of daily living (ADLs)
  in home setting, for cognitive deficits, 1137
  range-of-motion exercises incorporated into,
    313t
Acute hypoxia, 654b
Acute pain, defined, 407
Administration sets
  for blood transfusions, 841f
  changing, 809–811, 809t
    collaboration, 809
    communication and documentation in,
      811
    in community care, 811
    delegation, 809
    equipment for, 809
    teaching about, 811
    technique for, 809–811
Admitting patients, 13–21
  Canada's health care system in, 14–15
  in children, 21

Admitting patients (*Continued*)
  communication for, 20–21
  delegation and collaboration in, 16
  documentation for, 20–21
  equipment used in, 16
  nurse's role in, 15–16
  older persons, 21
  personnel involvement in, 14
  procedures for, 14b
  process in, 14
Adolescents. *see also* Pediatric patients
  physical assessment of, 149
Advance care plan (ACP), 443–444
Advance directives, 15, 15b, 768
Adventitious sounds, 163, 164t
Adverse effects, pharmacotherapeutics, 530
Adverse event/incident, 64b
Aerobic culture, 231
Aerosol, 529t
Aerosol sprays, 565
Aging. *see* Older persons
Air embolism, 827t–828t, 900t–901t
Air mattress, 343–344, 343f
Airborne precautions, 75, 76t
Air-filled cushion for wheelchair, 343f
Air-fluidized bed, 338t–339t
Airway
  artificial. *see* Artificial airway
  management, 700–734
    closed suction catheter systems, 715b–
      717b, 716f
    evidence-informed practice for, 701
    goal of, 700
    oropharyngeal suctioning, 702–705
    person-centred care, 701
    principles for practice, 701
    purpose of, 700
    safety guidelines for, 701–702
    standards of care, 700–701
  oropharyngeal. *see* Oropharyngeal airway,
    suctioning of
  secretions in, 688
  suctioning of, 702f, 706–715, 706f,
    710f–711f, 713f
    assessment of, 707–715
    in children, 715
    communication and documentation in,
      715
    in community care, 715
    delegation and collaboration in, 707
    equipment for, 707
    in older persons, 715
    planning of, 709
    teaching, 715
Airway pressure release ventilation (APRV),
  677t–678t
Alcohol-based products, for handwashing, 71
Aldrete score
  modified, 258t
  for postanaesthesia monitoring, 1009t

Alginate dressing
  application of, 1095–1101, 1100f
    in children, 1101
    communication and documentation in,
      1101
    delegation and collaboration in, 1096
    dressing set for, 1096
    equipment for, 1096
    in older persons, 1101
  description of, 1078t–1079t
Alkaline burns, of eye, 513
Allergic reactions
  description of, 835t
  pharmacotherapeutics, 531, 531f, 531t
  to transfusions, 835t
All-hazards approach, 385b
Alzheimer's disease, 1137
Ambulation, assisting with (without assistive
  devices), 323b–326b
  delegation and collaboration in, 323
  equipment, 323
  procedural steps, 323–326, 324f–325f
Ambulatory Surgery Discharge Criteria,
  1014b
Ambulatory tank, 1169f
American Society for Pain Management
  Nursing support, 409
Amplifier, in hearing aids, 521
Ampoules
  description of, 606
  mixing medications from, 609f, 612b–615b
  tapping, 608f
  withdrawing medications from, 607,
    607f
Anaerobic culture, 232
Analgesia
  epidural, 409, 420–426
    assessment of, 422–426
    in children, 426
    communication and documentation in,
      426
    in community care, 426
    continuous infusion of, 424
    delegation and collaboration in, 421
    equipment for, 421–422, 421f–422f
    implementation of, 423–424
    in older persons, 426
    planning of, 423
    teaching, 426
  patient-controlled, 416–420
    assessment of, 417–420
    in children, 420
    communication and documentation in,
      420
    delegation and collaboration in, 416
    discontinue, 419
    equipment for, 416
    implementation of, 417, 418f
    in older persons, 420
    teaching, 420

Page numbers followed by "f" indicate figures,
"t" indicate tables, and "b" indicate boxes.

1211

Index of Skills and Procedural Guidelines